PART 7: NERVOUS SYSTEM 715

PART 8: GASTROINTESTINAL SYSTEM 891

PART 9: ENDOCRINE SYSTEM 993

PART 10: HEMATOLOGICAL AND IMMUNE SYSTEMS 1059

PART 11: INTEGUMENTARY SYSTEM 1193

PART 12: MULTISYSTEM DYSFUNCTION 1249

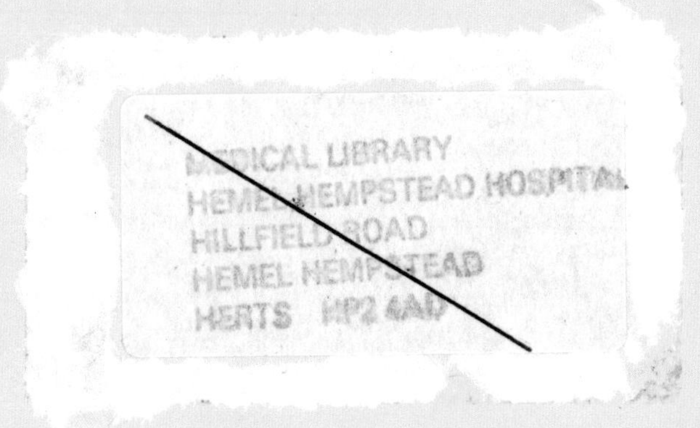

EIGHTH EDITION

Critical Care Nursing
A Holistic Approach

Patricia Gonce Morton, RN, PhD, ACNP, FAAN
Editor-in-Chief, AACN Clinical Issues: Advanced Practice in Acute and Critical Care
Professor, Assistant Dean for Master's Studies, and Coordinator of the Acute Care Nurse Practitioner and Clinical Nurse Specialist Master's Program in Trauma, Critical Care, and Emergency Nursing
University of Maryland School of Nursing
Baltimore, Maryland

Dorrie Fontaine, RN, DNSc, FAAN
Immediate Past-President, American Association of Critical-Care Nurses (AACN)
Associate Dean for Academic Programs
University of California, San Francisco School of Nursing
San Francisco, California

Carolyn M. Hudak, RN, PhD
Adult Nurse Practitioner
Denver, Colorado

Barbara M. Gallo, RN, MS, CNAA
Clinical Educator and Manager of Infusion Services
Visiting Nurse Association of Central Connecticut, Inc.
New Britain, Connecticut

Senior Acquisitions Editor: Quincy McDonald
Senior Developmental Editor: Melanie Cann
Editorial Assistant: Marie Rim
Senior Production Editor: Debra Schiff
Director of Nursing Production: Helen Ewan
Managing Editor/Production: Erika Kors
Art Director: Brett MacNaughton
Interior Design: Melissa Olson
Cover Designer: Melissa Walters
Interior Illustrations: Annelisa Ochoa/Anne Rains
Senior Manufacturing Manager: William Alberti
Compositor: Circle Graphics
Printer: RRD-Willard

8th Edition

9 8 7 6 5 4 3 2 1

Library of Congress Cataloging-in-Publication Data

Critical care nursing : a holistic approach / [edited by] Patricia Gonce Morton. [et al.]—8th ed.
p. ; cm.
Includes bibliographical references and index.
ISBN 0-7817-2759-6
1. Intensive care nursing. 2. Holistic nursing. I. Morton, Patricia Gonce, 1952–
[DNLM: 1. Critical Care. 2. Holistic Nursing. WY 154 C9328 2005]
RT120.I5C744 2005
616.02′8—dc22

2004018659

LWW.com

To my parents, Charles and Dorothy Gonce, for their many years of love and encouragement. To my husband John, for his support, help, and love throughout my career. And to Dorrie Fontaine, for always being there to help and guide me.

—Trish

To Barry and Sumner, who make all good things possible. To Eileen and Christopher Karb, for their constant love and support. And to Trish Morton, best friend for life.

—Dorrie

To the critical care nurses who have used our book throughout the many years, thanks for all you do to care for patients and their families.

—Carolyn and Bobbie

Contributors

Kara L. Adams, RN, MS, CCRN
Clinical Nurse Specialist, Critical Care
University Medical Center
Tucson, Arizona

M. Sue Apple, DNSc, RN
Adjunct Clinical Instructor
Georgetown University
School of Nursing and Health Studies
Washington, District of Columbia

Tonya Appleby, RN, MSN, CCRN, CRNP
Acute Care Nurse Practitioner, Emergency Department
Good Samaritan Hospital
Baltimore, Maryland
Clinical Instructor
University of Maryland School of Nursing
Baltimore, Maryland

Carla A. Aresco, RN, MS, CRNP
Neurotrauma Nurse Practitioner
R Adams Cowley Shock Trauma Center
University of Maryland Medical System
Baltimore, Maryland

Mona N. Bahouth, MSN, CRNP
Neurology Nurse Practitioner
University of Maryland Medical System
Baltimore, Maryland

Anne E. Belcher, PhD, RN, AOCN, FAAN
Senior Associate Dean for Academic Affairs
Johns Hopkins University School of Nursing
Baltimore, Maryland

Kathryn S. Bizek, MSN, RN, APRN, BC, CCRN
Nurse Practitioner, Cardiac Electrophysiology
Henry Ford Hospital
Detroit, Michigan

Kay Blum, PhD, CRNP
Nurse Practitioner, Heart Failure Service
University of Maryland Medical System
Baltimore, Maryland

Eileen Bohan, RN, BSN, CNRN
Senior Program Coordinator
Department of Neurosurgery
The Johns Hopkins Hospital
Baltimore, Maryland

Annushka Cesan, BSN, BS, RN
RN2
University of Washington Medical System
Seattle, Washington

Donna L. Charlebois, RN, MSN, ACNP-CS
Clinician IV, Medicine Service
University of Virginia Medical System
Charlottesville, Virginia

Dennis J. Cheek, RN, PhD, FAHA
Professor
Texas Christian University
Fort Worth, Texas

Mary C. Ciechanowski, RN, MSN, CS, CCRN
Neuroscience Clinical Nurse Specialist
Christiana Care Health Systems
Newark, Delaware

JoAnn Coleman, RN, MS, ACNP, AOCN
Acute Care Nurse Practitioner
Gastrointestinal Surgery
The Johns Hopkins Hospital
Baltimore, Maryland

Vicki J. Coombs, RN, PhD
Senior Clinical Research Associate
Midatlantic Cardiovascular Associates
Baltimore, Maryland

Therese M. Craig, MS, CRNP-A
Clinical Instructor and Adult Nurse Practitioner
University of Maryland School of Nursing
Baltimore, Maryland

Joan M. Davenport, RN, PhD
Associate Professor
York College of Pennsylvania
York, Pennsylvania

Marla J. De Jong, RN, MS, CCRN, CEN, Major
United States Air Force
Doctoral Student
University of Kentucky
Lexington, Kentucky

Jonathan L. Desamero, MSN, FNP-C
Family Nurse Practitioner, Emergency Department
Danville Regional Medical Center
Danville, Virginia

Sidenia S. Earven, RN, MSN, ACNP-CS, CCRN
Outcomes Manager, Long Term Ventilated Patients (Medicine)
University of Virginia Health System
Charlottesville, Virginia

Nancy Kern Feeley, RN, MS, CRNP, CNN
Nephrology Adult Nurse Practitioner
Johns Hopkins University School of Medicine
Baltimore, Maryland

Charles A. Fisher, RN, MSN, CCRN, ACNP-CS
Outcomes Manager, Long Term Ventilated Patients (Heart and Vascular)
University of Virginia Health System
Charlottesville, Virginia

Barbara Fitzsimmons, RN, MS, CNRN
Nurse Educator
Department of Neuroscience Nursing
The Johns Hopkins Hospital
Baltimore, Maryland

Mary Beth Flynn, RN, MS, CNS, CCRN
Clinical Nurse Specialist, Senior Instructor, and Doctoral Student
University of Colorado Health Sciences Center School of Nursing
Denver, Colorado

Dorrie Fontaine, RN, DNSc, FAAN
Immediate Past-President, American Association of Critical-Care Nurses (AACN)
Associate Dean, Academic Programs
University of California, San Francisco School of Nursing
San Francisco, California

Conrad Gordon, RN, MS, ACNP
Clinical Instructor
University of Maryland School of Nursing
Baltimore, Maryland

Christine Grady, RN, PhD
Head, Section on Human Subjects Research
Department of Clinical Bioethics
National Institutes of Health
Bethesda, Maryland

Thomasine D. Guberski, PhD, CRNP
Associate Professor and Adult Nurse Practitioner
University of Maryland School of Nursing
Baltimore, Maryland

Colonel Janet R. Harris, RN, PhD
Deputy Director, Congressionally Directed Medical Research Programs
US Army Medical Research and Material Command
Fort Detrick, Maryland

Kathy A. Hausman, RN, C, PhD
Assistant Professor
University of Maryland School of Nursing
Baltimore, Maryland

Janie Heath, RN, MS, CCRN, ANP, ACNP
Doctoral Candidate, George Mason University
Assistant Professor
Georgetown University School of Nursing and Health Studies
Washington, District of Columbia

Genell Hilton, MS, CRNP, CCNS, CCRN
Acute Care Nurse Practitioner
Surgical Intermediate Intensive Care Unit
University of Maryland Medical System
Baltimore, Maryland
Doctoral Student, Department of Physiology
University of Maryland
Baltimore, Maryland

Dorene M. Holcombe, RN, MS, ACNP, CCRN
Nephrology Acute Care Nurse Practitioner
Johns Hopkins University School of Medicine
Baltimore, Maryland

Karen L. Johnson, RN, PhD, CCRN
Assistant Professor
University of Maryland School of Nursing
Baltimore, Maryland

Dennis W. Jones, MS, RN, CFRN
Flight Nurse, STATMedevac
Johns Hopkins Hospital
Baltimore, Maryland

Kimmith M. Jones, RN, MS, CCRN
Advanced Practice Nurse
Critical Care and Emergency Department
Sinai Hospital of Baltimore
Baltimore, Maryland

Roberta Kaplow, RN, PhD, CCNS, CCRN
Clinical Professor
Nell Hodgson Woodruff School of Nursing
Emory University
Atlanta, Georgia

Jane F. Kapustin, RN, MS, CRNP
Clinical Instructor and Adult Nurse Practitioner
University of Maryland School of Nursing
Baltimore, Maryland

Kathleen Keenan, RN, MS, CCRN, ACNP
Nurse Practitioner
Massachusetts General Hospital
Boston, Massachusetts

Martha M. Kennedy, RN, PhD, CCRN, ACNP
Acute Care Nurse Practitioner
Department of Surgery
The Johns Hopkins Hospital
Baltimore, Maryland

Rose Lewis, RN, MSN, CCNS
Outcomes Manager, Long Term Ventilated Patients (Neurosciences)
University of Virginia Health System
Charlottesville, Virginia

Susan Luchka, RN, MSN, CCRN, ET
Director of Clinical Education
Memorial Hospital
York, Pennsylvania

Cathleen R. Maiolatesi, RN, MS
Case Manager GYN/OB
The Johns Hopkins Hospital
Baltimore, Maryland

Sandra W. McLeskey, RN, PhD
Professor
University of Maryland School of Nursing
Baltimore, Maryland

Alexander R. McMullen, III, RN, JD, MBA, BSN
Attorney/Principal–McMullen and Drury
Towson, Maryland

Patricia C. McMullen, DNSc, JD, CNS, CRNP
Associate Dean for Academic Affairs
The Catholic University of America School of Nursing
Washington, District of Columbia

Paul K. Merrel, RN, MSN, CCRN
Outcomes Manager, Long Term Ventilated Patients (Surgery/Trauma)
University of Virginia Health System
Charlottesville, Virginia

Sandra A. Mitchell, CRNP, MScN, AOCN
Oncology Nurse Practitioner
National Cancer Institute
Bethesda, Maryland
Doctoral Student
University of Utah, College of Nursing
Salt Lake City, Utah

Patricia A. Moloney-Harmon, RN, MS, CCNS, CCRN, FAAN
Advanced Practice Nurse/Clinical Nurse Specialist
The Children's Hospital at Sinai
Baltimore, Maryland

Patricia Gonce Morton, RN, PhD, ACNP, FAAN
Editor-in-Chief, AACN Clinical Issues: Advanced Practice in Acute and Critical Care
Professor, Assistant Dean for Master's Studies, and Coordinator of the Acute Care Nurse Practitioner and Clinical Nurse Specialist Master's Program in Trauma, Critical Care, and Emergency Nursing
University of Maryland School of Nursing
Baltimore, Maryland

Donna Mower-Wade, RN, MS, CNRN, CS
Trauma Clinical Nurse Specialist
Christiana Care Health Systems
Newark, Delaware

Nancy Munro, RN, MN, CCRN, ACNP
Acute Care Nurse Practitioner
Cardiovascular-Thoracic Services
INOVA Alexandria Hospital
Alexandria, Virginia
Clinical Instructor
University of Maryland School of Nursing
Baltimore, Maryland

Colleen K. Norton, DNSc, RN, CCRN
Assistant Professor
Georgetown University School of Nursing and Health Studies
Washington, District of Columbia

Dulce Obias-Manno, RN, BSN, MHSA
Cardiac Arrhythmia Service Nurse Coordinator
Washington Hospital Center
Washington, District of Columbia

Mary O. Palazzo, RN, MS
Director of Nursing and Operations
St. Joseph Medical Center
Towson, Maryland

Suzanne S. Prevost, RN, PhD
Professor and National Health Care Chair of Excellence
Middle Tennessee State University
School of Nursing
Murfreesboro, Tennessee

Michael V. Relf, PhD, APRN, AACRN, CCRN
Assistant Professor and Chair, Department of Professional Nursing
Georgetown University School of Nursing and Health Studies
Washington, District of Columbia

Kenneth J. Rempher, MS, RN, MBA, CCRN
Director, Professional Nursing Practice
Sinai Hospital of Baltimore
Baltimore, Maryland
Doctoral Candidate
University of Maryland School of Nursing
Baltimore, Maryland

Barbara Resnick, PhD, CRNP, FAAN
Associate Professor
University of Maryland School of Nursing
Baltimore, Maryland

Caleb A. Rogovin, CRNA, MS, CCRN, CEN
Associate Director, Nurse Anesthesia Program
University of Maryland School of Nursing
Baltimore, Maryland

Valerie K. Sabol, RN, MSN, CCNS, ACNP
Clinical Instructor and Acute Care Nurse Practitioner
University of Maryland School of Nursing
Baltimore, Maryland

Eric Schuetz, BSPharm, CSPI
Specialist
Maryland Poison Center
Baltimore, Maryland

Julie Schuetz, MS, CRNP
Acute Care Nurse Practitioner
Baltimore, Maryland

Brenda K. Shelton, RN, MS, CCRN, AOCN
Critical Care Clinical Nurse Specialist
Department of Oncology
The Johns Hopkins Hospital
Baltimore, Maryland

Jo Ann Hoffman Sikora, RN, MS, CRNP
Acute Care Nurse Practitioner, Cardiac Surgery
University of Maryland Medical System
Baltimore, Maryland

Allison G. Steele, RN, MSN, ANP
Adult Nurse Practitioner
Gastroenterology Division
University of Maryland Medical System
Baltimore, Maryland

Louis R. Stout, RN, MS
Major, United States Army Nurse Corps
Head Nurse, Burn Intensive Care Unit
Brooke Army Medical Center
Fort Sam Houston, Texas

Lieutenant Colonel Mary E. Tenhet
Chief, Medical-Surgical Nursing Section
Womack Army Medical Center
Fort Bragg, North Carolina

Paula Timmerman, RN, MSN, AOCN
Manager, Oncology Services
Advocate Good Samaritan Hospital
Downers Grove, Illinois

Terry L. Tucker, RN, MS, BA, CCRN, CEN
Critical Care Clinical Nurse Specialist
Baltimore Veterans Administration Health Center
Veterans Administration Maryland Healthcare System
Baltimore, Maryland

Mary H. van Soeren, RN, PhD, ACNP
Assistant Professor and Director
Nurse Practitioner Programs
University of Toronto
Toronto, Ontario, Canada

Kathryn Von Rueden, RN, MS, FCCM
Director, Quality and Safety
Anne Arundel Medical Center
Annapolis, Maryland

Karen Lynn Yarbrough, MS, CS, CRNP
Acute Care Nurse Practitioner
Critical Care
Upper Chesapeake Health System
Bel Air, Maryland

Elizabeth Zink, RN, MS, CCRN, CNRN
Clinical Nurse Specialist, Neuro Critical Care Unit
The Johns Hopkins Hospital
Baltimore, Maryland

Reviewers

Kara Adams, RN, MS
Clinical Nurse Specialist, Critical Care
University Medical Center
Tucson, Arizona

Kathleen C. Ashton, PhD, APRN, BC
Clinical Associate Professor
Rutgers University
Camden, New Jersey

Julia W. Aucoin, DNS, RN, BC
Assistant Professor
University of North Carolina
Greensboro, North Carolina

Denise Ayers, RN, MSN
Assistant Professor
Kent State University
Tuscarawas, Ohio

Valerie Benedix, MSN
Faculty
Clovis Community College
Clovis, New Mexico

Renea L. Breckstand, PhD, RN, CCRN
Associate Professor
Brigham Young University
Provo, Utah

Lynn Browning, MSN, RN, BC
Associate Professor
Charleston Southern University
Charleston, South Carolina

Gail M. Burns, MSN, RNC
Nursing Faculty
College of Mount St. Joseph
Cincinnati, Ohio

Nancy Burruss, MSN, RN, CS, CCRN
Assistant Professor
Bellin College of Nursing
Green Bay, Wisconsin

Terry Cicero, BSN, MN, CCRN
Instructor
Seattle University
Seattle, Washington

Ann H. Crawford, RN, PhD
Associate Professor
College of Nursing
University of Mary Hardin-Baylor
Belton, Texas

Peter E. Darwin, MD
Associate Professor of Medicine
Division of Gastroenterology
University of Maryland School of Medicine
Baltimore, Maryland

L. Angelise Davis, DSN, RN
Associate Professor, BSN Program Division Chair
University of South Carolina
Spartanburg, South Carolina

Thomas J. Doyle, MSN, RN
Coordinator, Patient Simulator Program/Instructor
Columbus State Community College
Columbus, Ohio

Barbara Draude, RN, MSN
Director, Academic and Instructional Technology Services/Assistant Professor
Middle Tennessee State University
Murfreesboro, Tennessee

George T. Fantry, MD
Director, Clinical Gastroenterology
Associate Professor of Medicine
University of Maryland School of Medicine
Baltimore, Maryland

Bruce D. Greenwald, MD
Associate Professor of Medicine
Division of Gastroenterology
University of Maryland School of Medicine
Baltimore, Maryland

Donna Gullette, DSN, RN
Associate Professor/Critical Care Chair
Mississippi University for Women
Columbus, Mississippi

Leigh Hart, RN, CCRN, PhD
Interim Dean, Nursing
Jacksonville University
Jacksonville, Florida

Frederick J. Hauf, Jr, RN, BSN
Staff Nurse
The Johns Hopkins Hospital
Department of Surgical Nursing
Baltimore, Maryland

Linda Howe, PhD, RN, CS
Assistant Professor/Critical Care Clinical Specialist
Clemson University School of Nursing
Clemson, South Carolina

Laura P. Kimble, PhD, RN
Associate Professor/Coordinator Acute Critical Care Graduate Nursing Program
Emory University
Atlanta, Georgia

Joan E. King, RNC, PhD, ACNP, ANP
Associate Professor
Vanderbilt University
Nashville, Tennessee

Louise M. LaFramboise, PhD, RN
Assistant Professor
University of Nebraska Medical Center
Omaha, Nebraska

Linda LaPointe, RN
Major, Army Nurse Corps
Deputy Director, Practical Nurse Course
Brooke Army Medical Center
Fort Sam Houston, Texas

Jacqueline Laurin, MD
Medical Director, Liver Transplantation Clinical Director, Hepatology Section
University of Maryland School of Medicine
Baltimore, Maryland

A. Renee Leasure, BSN, MS, PhD
Associate Professor
University of Oklahoma
Oklahoma City, Oklahoma

Gayle Lee, PhD, RNC, CCRN
Faculty
Brigham Young University
Rexburg, Idaho

Karen McQuillan, RN, MS, CCRN
Clinical Nurse Specialist
R Adams Cowley Shock Trauma Center
University of Maryland Medical System
Baltimore, Maryland

Sadie P. Neureuther, MSN, RN, CRNP
Faculty
University of Pennsylvania
Philadelphia, Pennsylvania

Charlotte Pooler, RN, BScN, MN
Instructor
Mount Royal College
Calgary, Alberta, Canada

Sandra L. Siedlecki, RN, MSN, CNS
Faculty
University of Akron
Akron, Ohio

Carol Smith, MSN, RN
Assistant Professor of Nursing
Lansing School of Nursing, Bellarmine University
Louisville, Kentucky

M. J. Stanley, RN, MA
Assistant Professor
University of Nebraska Medical Center
Omaha, Nebraska

Barbara Walsh, RN, CNSD
Nutrition Support Dietician
University of Maryland Medical Center
Baltimore, Maryland

Michael L. Williams, MSN, RN, CCRN
Assistant Professor
Eastern Michigan University
Ypsilanti, Michigan

Charlene A. Winters, DNSc, RN, CS
Assistant Professor
Montana State University
Missoula, Montana

Lynne Young, RN, PhD
Associate Professor
University of Victoria
Victoria, British Columbia, Canada

Karen A. Zapko, RN, MSN
RN Educator
Forum Health
Youngstown, Ohio

Preface

Through the vision and hard work of Carolyn Hudak and Barbara (Bobbie) Gallo, the first edition of *Critical Care Nursing: A Holistic Approach* was published in 1973. The discipline of critical care nursing was new at that time, and Carolyn and Bobbie pioneered a text that has become a classic in the field. When mentioning critical care books, often you hear an experienced critical care nurse say, "I grew up with the Hudak and Gallo book and I still have my original copy."

In 1998, the seventh edition of *Critical Care Nursing: A Holistic Approach* was published and that edition marked the beginning of a transition for the text. I joined the author team to help with the text and to learn from the experts so that Carolyn and Bobbie could eventually hand off the lead authorship of the book and enjoy the next phase of their careers.

This eighth edition of the text marks the final step in the author team transition. I have assumed the lead author position and have been joined by Dorrie Fontaine, a nationally known expert in critical care and the Immediate Past-President of the American Association of Critical-Care Nurses. Our goal with this edition is to continue a tradition of excellence in critical care publishing that has spanned over 30 years. We offer the next generation of critical care nurses an up-to-date, comprehensive text built on a holistic perspective.

In the 6 years that have passed since the last edition of this text, the practice of critical care nursing has witnessed many changes. Today's critical care nurse is expected to be able to care for critically ill patients in a variety of settings—no longer is critical care strictly "unit-based." And today's critically ill patient is liable to be older and even more critically ill than ever before. Advances in nursing, medicine, and technology; the rapidly changing health care climate; and the shortage of nursing staff and faculty are other factors that have come together to effect great changes on the practice of critical care nursing.

Today's critical care nurse, more than ever before, must possess a unique body of knowledge in order to provide competent and compassionate care to critically ill patients and their families. Some of this knowledge can be gained through formal education and textbooks, like the one you hold in your hand. The rest can only be gained through experience. It is our goal, with this eighth edition of *Critical Care Nursing: A Holistic Approach*, to assist readers on their journey by providing a comprehensive, up-to-date resource and reference.

As in past editions, the goal of this text is to promote excellence in critical care. Presenting theory and principles within the context of practical application helps the reader to gain competence and confidence in caring for critically ill patients and their families. As always, the patient as the center of the health care team's efforts is emphasized throughout. In the highly specialized and complicated technical environment of critical care, knowing when to merely be present with patients by sitting with them and holding their hand is just as important as knowing how to operate complex equipment and perform difficult procedures.

AN OVERVIEW OF *CRITICAL CARE NURSING: A HOLISTIC APPROACH*, 8E

Critical Care Nursing: A Holistic Approach, 8e, consists of 12 parts. The following is a brief survey of those parts and the information they contain.

Part 1: The Concept of Holism Applied to Critical Care Nursing Practice

The six chapters that make up Part 1 introduce the student to the concept of holistic care, as it applies in critical care practice. In Chapter 1, the student is introduced to critical care nursing practice. Chapters 2 and 3 review the emotional effects of critical illness on the patient and on the family, respectively. Chapter 4 describes the effect of the critical care environment on the patient, and reviews actions the nurse can take to help reduce environment-induced stress and promote healing. Chapter 5 focuses on strategies for relieving pain and promoting comfort. We conclude the part with Chapter 6, which focuses on patient and family education, a vital component of nursing care.

Part 2: Professional Practice Issues in Critical Care

This part consists of four chapters that are of concern to the nursing profession. In Chapters 7 and 8, ethical and legal issues are explored. Chapter 9, a new chapter, reviews the role genetics play in the development of disease and the determination of a treatment plan, a topic of increasing importance throughout the health care field. Part 2 concludes with a chapter about achieving professional advancement, both for the individual and the profession as a whole.

Part 3: Special Populations in Critical Care

The five chapters in this part focus on the special needs of certain groups of people who are critically ill. Chapters 11, 12, and 13 focus on the pediatric patient, the pregnant patient, and the elderly patient, respectively. Chapter 14 describes the role of the nurse in caring for a patient who is recovering from anesthesia. This part concludes with Chapter 15, which focuses on the care of the patient who is being transported between facilities.

Part 4: Cardiovascular System

This part, the first of eight organ system–based parts, focuses on the care of the patient with a cardiovascular disorder. Each organ system–based part begins with a chapter that reviews the anatomy and physiology of the organ system under discussion (Chapter 16). The part then continues with a chapter on patient assessment (Chapter 17), general patient management (Chapter 18), and common disorders (Chapter 19). In Part 4, heart failure and acute myocardial infarction are each given their own chapters (Chapters 20 and 21, respectively). The unit concludes with a discussion of the most recent developments in cardiac surgery (Chapter 22). Throughout the unit, the latest diagnostic tests, such as cardiac serum markers, the newest drugs for treating cardiovascular disorders, and updates on technologies such as the left ventricular assist device, the implantable cardioverter defibrillator, and the cardiac pacemaker are discussed.

Part 5: Respiratory System

In this part, current assessment technologies such as end tidal carbon dioxide monitoring and the newest modes of ventilation for patients in respiratory failure are discussed. Evidence-based treatment strategies for respiratory disorders such as pneumonia, pleural effusion, and chronic obstructive pulmonary disease are described. Chapter 27 is devoted to the latest developments in the assessment and management of the patient with acute respiratory distress syndrome (ARDS).

Part 6: Renal System

In this edition of the text, Part 6 includes a more in-depth discussion of the assessment and management of fluids, electrolytes, and acid-base balance. Updates on laboratory and diagnostic tests are included. The newest dialysis technologies and the latest drugs are discussed in Chapter 30. Chapter 31 focuses on common renal disorders, especially recent developments in the care of the patient with renal failure.

Part 7: Nervous System

This part offers updates on neurological diagnostic studies and the newest approaches to treating the patient with increased intracranial pressure. The latest drugs for treating neurological disorders and the most recent developments in neurosurgery are addressed. Separate chapters are devoted to care of the patient with a head injury and spinal cord injury.

Part 8: Gastrointestinal System

In Part 8, the latest diagnostic tests for evaluating patients with gastrointestinal disorders are discussed. The management of patients with gastrointestinal disorders has been updated to include the newest drugs, the latest developments in the use of enteral and parenteral nutrition, and recent trends in the treatment of common disorders such as liver failure and hepatitis.

Part 9: Endocrine System

In this edition, Part 9 includes a reorganized and expanded assessment chapter. The content is organized by the major gland, and for each gland addressed in the chapter, the reader is given information on the history, laboratory tests, and diagnostic tests. The most current information on the treatment of endocrine disorders, especially diabetic emergencies, is included in Chapter 44.

Part 10: Hematological and Immune Systems

This part continues to be a unique feature that is not included in many critical care texts. The numerous recent developments in organ and hematopoietic stem cell transplant are described in Chapter 47. Chapter 48 addresses up-to-date information on the assessment and management of patients with HIV/AIDS as well as those with oncological emergencies. The latest trends in the treatment of patients with hematological disorders such as disseminated intravascular coagulation are included in Chapter 49.

Part 11: Integumentary System

This part, which is new to this edition, includes three new chapters: the anatomy and physiology of the integumentary system, assessment of the integumentary system, and management of integumentary disorders, respectively. Evidence-based assessment and management of wounds are addressed. In addition, the chapter on burns has been moved from the multisystem dysfunction part to this part.

Part 12: Multisystem Dysfunction

In Chapter 54, hypoperfusion states such as shock, systemic inflammatory response syndrome (SIRS), and multiple organ dysfunction syndrome (MODS) are discussed. The latest understanding of the pathophysiologic process is described, as well as how this knowledge guides the selection of the most recent interventions. Chapter 55 reviews care of the trauma patient, including the latest trends in the management of these complex patients. Chapter 56 reviews care of the patient with a drug overdose or poisoning, a problem that is becoming more common in the critical care setting.

Appendices

Two appendices complete the textbook. Appendix 1 contains updated ACLS guidelines. Appendix 2 provides the reader with the correct answers to the multiple-choice questions found at the end of each chapter. In addition to the correct answer, rationales are provided.

FEATURES

Several features from past editions have been retained and revised in this edition, and several new features have been added.

Practice-Oriented Features

- **Considerations for the Older Patient boxes.** Older adults comprise the fastest growing part of our population. As a result, the number of critically ill patients who are older is also increasing. These boxes highlight the special needs of this patient population.
- **Considerations for the Pediatric Patient boxes.** Pediatric patients have special needs. These boxes give specific information about adaptations that must be made when caring for a critically ill child.
- **Red Flag boxes.** These boxes alert readers to risk factors, signs and symptoms, side effects, and complications that the critical care nurse must be vigilant for.
- **Nursing Diagnoses and Collaborative Problems boxes.** Critical care nurses work both independently and collaboratively when caring for critically ill patients. These boxes summarize common nursing diagnoses and collaborative problems for particular conditions.
- **Collaborative Care Guides.** These boxes describe how the health care team works together to manage a patient's illness and minimize complications. The information is presented in a tabular format, with outcomes in the first column and interventions in the second.
- **Nursing Intervention Guides.** These boxes present guidelines for carrying out certain key nursing interventions.
- **Patient Teaching Guides.** These boxes help the nurse to prepare patients and family members for procedures, assist patients and family members with understanding the illness they are dealing with, and explain postprocedure or postoperative activities.
- **Discharge Planning Guides.** These boxes, which were formerly called "Considerations for Home Care" boxes, outline what the nurse needs to consider when preparing a patient for discharge from the hospital.
- **Diagnostic Study Interpretation tables.** These tables summarize normal and/or abnormal findings on diagnostic tests.
- **Drug Therapy tables.** These tables summarize information about drugs used to treat selected conditions.
- **Insights Into Clinical Research boxes.** These boxes help the reader to understand the importance of research-based practice. Each research summary provides an overview of a study relevant to the chapter contents.
- **Internet Resources.** Each part begins with a list of key websites of interest that direct the reader to sources of additional information and patient education materials.

Pedagogical Features

- **Chapter Outlines** and **Learning Objectives.** Each chapter begins with an outline of the chapter and a list of learning objectives. These give the reader an overview of the chapter and help to focus his or her reading.
- **Case Studies.** Where appropriate, case studies have been included in chapters as an additional learning tool. Each case study focuses on the interventions the critical care team takes and the patient's responses to these interventions. The case studies reinforce the information in the chapter and form a basis for classroom discussion.
- **Clinical Applicability Challenges.** This feature, which appears at the end of every chapter, is divided into two sections. The first section, *Self-Challenge: Critical Thinking*, is intended to help readers develop critical thinking skills. Classroom or clinical discussion of these problems can help learners explore alternatives and apply newly learned principles to the care of the critically ill patient. The second section consists of multiple-choice *Study Questions*, which are designed to help readers test their grasp of the chapter content. Answers with rationales to the *Study Questions* are provided in Appendix 2.
- **References.** A list of current references cited in the chapter is given at the end of each chapter.
- **Other Selected Reading.** A bibliography is provided at the end of each chapter to encourage further reading of key sources relevant to the chapter.

ANCILLARY PACKAGE

- **Instructor's Resource CD-ROM.** The instructor's resource CD contains the following items:
  - A thoroughly revised and updated **Instructor's Manual,** featuring information about how to teach a critical care course in a hospital setting, teaching strategies, and student worksheets
  - A thoroughly revised and augmented **Test Generator,** featuring more than several hundred questions
  - An **Image Bank,** containing illustrations from the book in formats suitable for printing and incorporating into PowerPoint presentations and Internet sites
  - **PowerPoint lecture outlines** for each chapter

  All of these materials are also available in a course cartridge for WebCT or Blackboard.
- **Interactive Back-of-Book CD-ROM.** Packaged with the textbook at no additional charge, this CD contains a wealth of resources for the student:

- Common Drugs Used in Critical Care
- Drug Monographs
- Crisis Values of Laboratory Tests
- 20 Critical Care Nursing Procedures
- Animations
- Practice Test: Arterial Blood Gas
- Practice Test: Dosage Calculation Math Review
- Practice Test: Critical Care Comprehensive Exam
- Practice Test: Critical Care Nursing Certification Post Tests 1 & 2
- References

It is with great pleasure that we introduce these resources—the textbook and the ancillary package—to you. One of our primary goals in creating these resources has been to promote excellence in critical care nursing practice so that nurses can help patients and families cope with the consequences of critical illness. It is our intent that these resources will provide aspiring and currently practicing critical care nurses the tools to make their optimal contribution to the care of critically ill patients and their families, and to the nursing profession. We hope that we have succeeded in that goal, and we welcome feedback from our readers.

Patricia Gonce Morton, RN, PhD, ACNP, FAAN
Dorrie Fontaine, RN, DNSc, FAAN
Carolyn M. Hudak, RN, PhD
Barbara M. Gallo, RN, MS, CNAA

Acknowledgments

This project required the help and cooperation of many people. First we want to thank our many colleagues who contributed to the text, either by authoring a chapter or by sharing their expertise as a reviewer. Our publisher, Lippincott Williams & Wilkins, has gone through much change during the publishing of this edition but has remained committed to producing the best text possible. We especially want to thank Melanie Cann, Senior Developmental Editor, and Jane Velker, Director of Development—Nursing Education, for their support, humor, and words of positive encouragement as they cheered us on to the finish line with the project. Another key person in the production of this text was Debra Schiff, Senior Production Editor. Her tireless attention to detail was amazing, and she could be counted on to keep us on track with the many piles of chapters. To the numerous other members of the Lippincott Williams & Wilkins team who helped us throughout the many stages of this edition, we extend our sincere gratitude.

We also wish to express our thanks to Therese Craig for her help in editing many of the chapters and to Regina Mabrey, who compiled and checked all the websites that appear in the beginning of each part of the text. Their hours of work were an enormous help to us. And finally, we wish to express a word of thanks to our families and nursing colleagues who endured the time we took to complete this project.

Tricia, Dorrie, Carolyn, and Bobbie

Contents

26
Common Respiratory Disorders 566

27
Acute Respiratory Distress Syndrome 608

PART 6
Renal System 627

28
Anatomy and Physiology of the Renal System 629

29
Patient Assessment: Renal System 640

30
Patient Management: Renal System 658

Features Index

CONSIDERATIONS FOR THE OLDER PATIENT BOXES

CONSIDERATIONS FOR THE PEDIATRIC PATIENT BOXES

RED FLAG BOXES

NURSING DIAGNOSES AND COLLABORATIVE PROBLEMS BOXES

COLLABORATIVE CARE GUIDES

NURSING INTERVENTION GUIDES

PATIENT TEACHING GUIDES

DISCHARGE PLANNING GUIDES

INSIGHTS INTO CLINICAL RESEARCH BOXES

CASE STUDIES

PART

one

two three four five six seven eight nine ten eleven twelve

The Concept of Holism Applied to Critical Care Nursing Practice

INTERNET RESOURCES

Topic	Web Page Address
Agency for Healthcare Research and Quality (AHRQ)	www.ahrq.gov
American Association of Critical Care Nurses	www.aacn.org
American Chronic Pain Association	www.theacpa.org
American Holistic Nurses Association (AHNA)	www.ahna.org
American Pain Foundation	www.painfoundation.org
American Society of Pain Management Nurses	www.aspmn.org
Center for Medical Ethics and Mediation	www.wh.com/cmem/
Cochrane Collaboration (evidence-based practice)	www.cochrane.org
End of Life Nursing Education Center	www.aacn.nche.edu/elnec
Hospice and Palliative Nurses Association	www.hpna.org
Institute for Family Centered Care	www.familycenteredcare.org
International Center for Control of Pain in Children	www.pedspain.nursing.uiowa.edu
National Center for Complementary and Alternative Medicine	www.nccam.nih.gov
National Center for Cultural Competence	http://gucchd.georgetown.edu/nccc/cultural.html
National Guideline Clearinghouse	www.guidelines.gov
National Hospice and Palliative Care Organization	www.nhpco.org
The Patient Education Institute	www.patient-education.com
Promoting Excellence in End-of-Life Care	www.promotingexcellence.org
Transcultural Nursing Society	www.tcns.org
US Preventive Services Task Force	www.ahcpr.gov/clinic/uspstfix.htm

chapter

1

Critical Care Nursing Practice: An Integration of Caring, Competence, and Commitment to Excellence

MICHAEL RELF ■ ROBERTA KAPLOW

objectives

Based on the content in this chapter, the reader should be able to:

- Describe the value of evidence-based practice in caring for critically ill patients.
- Discuss the value of critical thinking in critical care.
- Describe the value of certification.
- Provide examples of how the Synergy Model can promote positive patient outcomes.
- Discuss the value of collaborative practice in critical care.
- List benefits of membership in the American Association of Critical-Care Nurses.
- Discuss future issues facing critical care nursing practice.

As the health care delivery system continues to evolve, so too does nursing and critical care. Today, the care of critically ill patients occurs not only in the "traditional" setting of the hospital intensive care unit (ICU), but also on the progressive care unit, the medical unit, and the surgical unit as well as in the subacute facility, the community, and the home. Since the first critical care unit (CCU) opened in the late 1960s, significant technological advances have occurred, accompanied by a knowledge explosion in critical care nursing. Consequently, critical care nurses of the 21st century are routinely caring for the complex, critically ill patient. This is accomplished by integrating sophisticated technology with the psychosocial challenges and ethical conflicts associated with critical illness, while at the same time addressing the needs and concerns of family members and other significant people in the patient's life.

In response to the ever-changing delivery system, critical care nurses are championing the needs of the patient and the family or significant others. During the last several decades, critical care nurses have experienced firsthand what nurse researchers have consistently demonstrated—however it is comprised, critical illness is not only a physiological alteration, but a psychosocial, developmental, and spiritual process. Critical illness is also a threat to the individual and his or her family constellation. As health care becomes increasingly technological, the concurrent need for humanization has become even more essential. Compatible with the need for "humanized" health care is the need to provide effective interventions that are based on evidence instead of being steeped in tradition.

EVIDENCE-BASED CRITICAL CARE NURSING PRACTICE

Today's health care system has become increasingly more costly and complex. Consequently, in this market-driven delivery system, there is a greater emphasis on outcomes, cost-effectiveness, and consumer satisfaction. These pressures operate in an environment of rapid information exchange, technological advancements, and an increasing nursing workload. Nurses are challenged to maintain clinical competence, to demonstrate how their care positively affects patient outcomes, and to participate actively in clinical decision making and practice improvements. Furthermore, nurses are now mandated to demonstrate cost-effectiveness and efficiency with the use of time and resources, while continuing to demonstrate their value-added impact on outcomes. These mandates provide a strong rationale for adopting an evidence-based model of practice.

As reported by the President's Advisory Commission on Consumer Protection and Quality in the Healthcare Industry in 1998, "improving the quality of healthcare requires a commitment to delivering healthcare based on sound scientific evidence and continuously innovating new, effective healthcare practices and preventive approaches."[1] Payers advocate the use of an evidenced-based practice model (EBP) in an effort to identify health care costs that are not beneficial.[2]

There are many instances in critical care nursing, and in nursing overall, when nurses wonder if they are providing the best possible intervention or using the best product to attain optimal patient outcomes. Too frequently, the responses may be "We've always done it that way," "That's what I learned in my undergraduate nursing program," or "I prefer to do it this way." Unfortunately, these common comments do not reflect the sophisticated knowledge base or experiential practice base that nurses use on a daily basis.

Evidence-based practice (EBP) has been defined as the use of the best clinical evidence from systemic research in making patient care decisions.[3] It is a process used by nurses to integrate the best and most timely scientific evidence with clinical expertise when making health care decisions. The methods are derived from evidence-based medicine developed as a paradigm and method in Canada.[4,5] EBP is a framework in which to determine the best means to care for patients and make informed decisions concerning nursing policies and procedures in order to influence patient outcomes. It is not intended to take the place of clinical nursing judgment and expertise. Rather, EBP combines evidence with clinical expertise and patient preferences to promote positive patient outcomes and excellence in nursing practice.

EBP is a method used by nurses as a basis for clinical decision making in an effort to optimize patient care and outcomes. It is predicated on the notion that clinical practice, guidelines, standards, and protocols should be derived from evidence from randomized clinical trials, which allows nurses to confirm or challenge the ways they provide and evaluate care.[6] Results of a meta-analysis have demonstrated that patients who receive research-based interventions and care have better outcomes than patients who receive traditional care.[7] In addition, nurses are legally responsible for the care provided in EBP. They are therefore also responsible for knowing the research foundation for practice and for determining the best interventions based on critique and application of the research.[8] Box 1-1 provides an overview of the essential steps to evidence-based critical care nursing practice.

CRITICAL THINKING IS ESSENTIAL TO CRITICAL CARE

In addition to using evidenced-based critical care nursing interventions to deliver optimal care to critically ill patients and families, critical care nurses need a strong knowledge base and critical thinking skills. Critical thinking skills

box 1-1
Steps to Evidence-Based Critical Care Nursing Practice

1. Accept the fact that health care is evolving, with the consequent need to base nursing care on evidence, rather than on tradition or previous education.
2. Identify a need for change in practice by examining less-than-favorable patient outcomes; causes of patient, family/significant other, or staff dissatisfaction; or situations in which compelling new evidence exists in an aspect of care. Targets for changing practice may include high-risk, high-volume, or high-cost procedures and interventions.
3. Frame a clinical question and search the literature for evidence regarding the topic.
4. Once current research data and evidence have been collected, evaluate the evidence for scientific merit, quality, and applicability. Inherent in this process is the need to determine if findings have been replicated and that they are relevant (applicable) to the clinical question posed, and whether the data identified constitute the best evidence.
5. Synthesize to determine the strength of the evidence to support a change in practice.
6. Conduct a comparison between current practice recommendations and current research.
7. If there is sufficient evidence to suggest a change in practice and the change in practice is practical in respect to costs, staff skill, and resources required, application of the evidence into practice can occur. Implicit in the implementation of evidence are the issues associated with change, including fear of change and the need for information, staff training, leadership, and ongoing evaluation of the change.
8. Continue to evaluate the evidence through an ongoing and systematic review to promote state-of-the-science nursing care.

allow the nurse to see the patient's "big picture" through the analysis of patient data, the evaluation of problems that emerge in the clinical setting, and the determination of appropriate interventions to solve the clinical issue. Critical thinking allows the nurse to conduct a cost–benefit analysis for any and all therapies indicated, while delving into the viability of alternative strategies to care. Although national organizations and nurses in the clinical arena identify critical thinking skills as pivotal to competent nursing practice, education often focuses on the memorization of facts regarding clinical care rather than on critical thinking as a process essential to care.[9]

Between 1995 and 1998, an international panel of expert nurses representing nine countries and the United States identified and defined 10 affective components (habits of the mind) and 7 cognitive skills of critical thinking. The affective components include confidence, contextual perspective, creativity, flexibility, inquisitiveness, intellectual ability, intuition, open-mindedness, perseverance, and reflection. The cognitive skills comprising critical thinking include analyzing, applying standards, discriminating, information seeking, logical reasoning, predicting, and transforming knowledge.[10]

All of these components are essential for providing quality care to critically ill patients. Nurses must be able to use these comprehensive skills to perform clinical decision making and problem solving as they care for patients with complex, multisystemic problems. The value of critical thinking skills has become increasingly important in the face of rapid changes in the health care environment, including procedural changes and technological advances.[11]

The development of critical thinking skills in nursing students and new critical care nurses is a major challenge confronting nurse educators in the academic and clinical settings.[12] Traditional teaching methods such as lecture, handouts, and observation do not stimulate critical thinking skills. Consequently, complementary teaching methods are essential to facilitate the application of theoretical knowledge to the bedside, particularly during the transition of the new graduate or experienced nurse into the critical care environment.

There are several strategies that may be used to enhance critical thinking skills. These include the use of case studies, simulation, videotaped vignettes, role playing, games, and clinical questioning. Clinical preceptors, managers, clinical educators, and clinical nurse specialists, along with staff nurse colleagues, need to create environments conducive to critical thinking for the new critical care nurse. By mentoring and role modeling, experienced critical care nurses can encourage creative problem solving, facilitate open dialogues, and discuss clinical issues, while at the same time facilitating the transition from novice to expert.[13] Simultaneously, new as well as experienced critical care nurses need to challenge underlying beliefs related to their practice and evaluate alternative strategies for care.[14] Critical thinking skills are required to evaluate practice and use an EBP model, which results in optimal patient outcomes.

Similar to EBP, the application of critical thinking skills has been shown to improve clinical outcomes and is associated with a decrease in errors and sentinel events.[15] Through the development and application of critical thinking, the level of competence of the critical care nurse will be increased, producing quality patient outcomes. Time, experience in the clinical arena, and the critical thinking skills themselves contribute to the development of a critical thinker. In addition, it is essential to establish a unit culture of openness, respect, and trust, which allows the novice as well as the experienced critical care nurse to ask questions, seek information, and critically analyze practice.

CERTIFICATION AND CRITICAL CARE NURSING PRACTICE

Certification is a process by which a nongovernmental agency validates, based on predetermined standards, the qualifications and knowledge of an individual nurse that are necessary for practice in a defined functional or clinical area of nursing.[16] In 1975, the American Association of Critical-Care Nurses (AACN) established the Certification Corporation. The purpose of the Certification Corporation was to develop the critical care registered nurse (CCRN) certification examination program. The purpose of the certification process, consistent with the definition of certification, is to have a means for developing, maintaining, and promoting high standards of critical care nursing practice.[17] The ultimate goal is to provide optimal care to critically ill patients and their families in a dynamic health care environment.

The CCRN credential acknowledges that the nurse has attained a knowledge base that is essential to critical care nursing practice, as well as the ability to synthesize, interpret, and apply this knowledge to the care of the patient.[18] To date, 50,000 nurses worldwide have received the CCRN credential in adult, pediatric, and neonatal critical care nursing. This credential validates to patients, peers, and hospital administrators the nurse's competence and commitment to excellence in critical care nursing. Because the standards for the examination are high, certification is well respected throughout the health care community.[18]

In May 2002, Terry Richmond[19] described the value of critical care certification in her address to the attendees of the CCRN luncheon at the National Teaching Institute. She described certified nurses as "the heroes of critical care" and noted three gifts that certified nurses give their patients. The first gift is the "gift of knowledge." The specialty of critical care requires high levels of preparation and the in-depth knowledge necessary for providing optimal care. CCRN certification is a powerful external validation of this critical knowledge and a gift that critical care nurses give themselves and their patients.

The second gift is the "gift of caring." Once a critical care nurse has attained the necessary breadth, depth, and currency of knowledge, energy can be put into other foci of care. A patient can be seen as not merely a diagnosis, but as a person with a family or significant other who likewise has needs. According to Richmond, the gift of caring is essential to being a hero. Knowledge and caring go hand in hand; one without the other does not translate into quality care.

The third gift is the "invitation into lives." A certified nurse can walk into a patient's life with knowledge and caring during the most vulnerable period in that person's life. Critical illness will never be ordinary for a patient and family. Nor should critical illness ever become ordinary for a nurse. A certified practice that uses these gifts promotes optimal patient outcomes and is nothing less than extraordinary. The process of certification enhances the profession and practice of nursing by encouraging nurses to attain the breadth and depth of knowledge required for successful completion. This is essential to the practice of giving quality nursing care to critically ill patients and their families.[19]

THE SYNERGY MODEL

In August 1999, the AACN implemented the Synergy Model to link certified practice to clinical outcomes. Synergy is an evolving phenomenon that occurs when individuals work together in mutually enhancing ways toward a common goal. The Synergy Model describes nursing practice on the basis of the needs and characteristics of patients rather than in terms of diseases and treatment modalities. The underlying premise of the Synergy Model is that the characteristics of patients and families influence and drive the characteristics and competencies of nurses. Because each patient brings a set of unique characteristics to the clinical situation, nurses must possess their own unique characteristics and competencies. When patient characteristics and nurse competencies match and synergize, optimal patient outcomes can be attained.[20]

Two major tenets of the Synergy Model are that the characteristics of the patient are of concern to nurses and that the competencies of the nurse are important to patients. Although each patient and family is unique, all patients have similar needs and experience these needs across a continuum, from low to high. The more compromised the patients are, the more complex are their needs.

Nursing practice is determined by the needs of patients and their families. Nursing care reflects an integration of the knowledge, skills, and experience necessary to meet the needs of patients and their families. The Synergy Model focuses on the unique contributions of nursing to patient care and emphasizes the role of the professional nurse. The eight patient characteristics and nurse competencies are listed and defined in Box 1-2. The eight nurse competencies also exist on a continuum, from competent to expert. Figure 1-1 provides a schematic representation of the Synergy Model and the interrelationships between the patient and family, and the patient and nurse characteristics.

There are three perspectives from which to evaluate outcomes using the Synergy Model. These are outcomes derived from the patient, the nurse, and the health care system.[20] Optimal outcomes are based on what patients define as important. These may include functional change, behavioral change, trust, satisfaction, comfort, and quality of life.

box 1-2
Patient Characteristics and Nurse Competencies as Described by the Synergy Model

Patient Characteristics

- **Resiliency:** The capacity to return to a restorative level of function using compensatory coping mechanisms; the ability to bounce back quickly after an insult
- **Vulnerability:** Susceptibility to actual or potential stressors that may adversely affect patient outcomes
- **Stability:** The ability to maintain a steady-state equilibrium
- **Complexity:** The intricate entanglement of two or more systems (e.g., body, family, therapies)
- **Resource availability:** Extent of resources (e.g., technical, fiscal, personal, psychological, social) the patient, family, and community bring to the situation
- **Participation in care:** Extent to which the patient and family engage in aspects of care
- **Participation in decision making:** Extent to which the patient and family engage in decision making
- **Predictability:** A summative characteristic that allows one to expect a certain trajectory of illness

Nurse Competencies

- **Clinical judgment:** Clinical reasoning, which includes clinical decision making, critical thinking, and a global grasp of a situation, coupled with nursing skills acquired through a process of integrating formal and experiential knowledge
- **Advocacy/moral agency:** Working on another's behalf and representing the concerns of the patient, family, and community; serving as a moral agent in identifying and helping resolve ethical and clinical concerns in the clinical setting
- **Caring practices:** The constellation of nursing activities that are responsive to the uniqueness of the patient and family and that create a compassionate and therapeutic environment, with the aim of promoting comfort and preventing suffering; these caring practices include, but are not limited to, vigilance, engagement, and responsiveness
- **Collaboration:** Working with others (e.g., patients, families, health care providers) in a way that promotes and encourages each person's contributions toward achieving optimal and realistic patient goals
- **Systems thinking:** The body of knowledge and tools that allows the nurse to appreciate the care environment from a perspective that recognizes the holistic interrelationship that exists within and across health care systems
- **Response to diversity:** The sensitivity to recognize, appreciate, and incorporate differences in the provision of care; differences may include, but are not limited to, family configuration, lifestyle, socioeconomic status, age values, and alternative medicine involving patients and their families and members of the health care team
- **Clinical inquiry or innovator/evaluator:** The ongoing process of questioning and evaluating practice, providing informed practice, and innovating through research and experiential learning; the nurse engages in clinical knowledge development to promote the best patient outcomes
- **Facilitator of learning:** The ability to facilitate learning for patients, nursing staff, physicians, and members of other health care disciplines; includes both formal and informal facilitation of learning

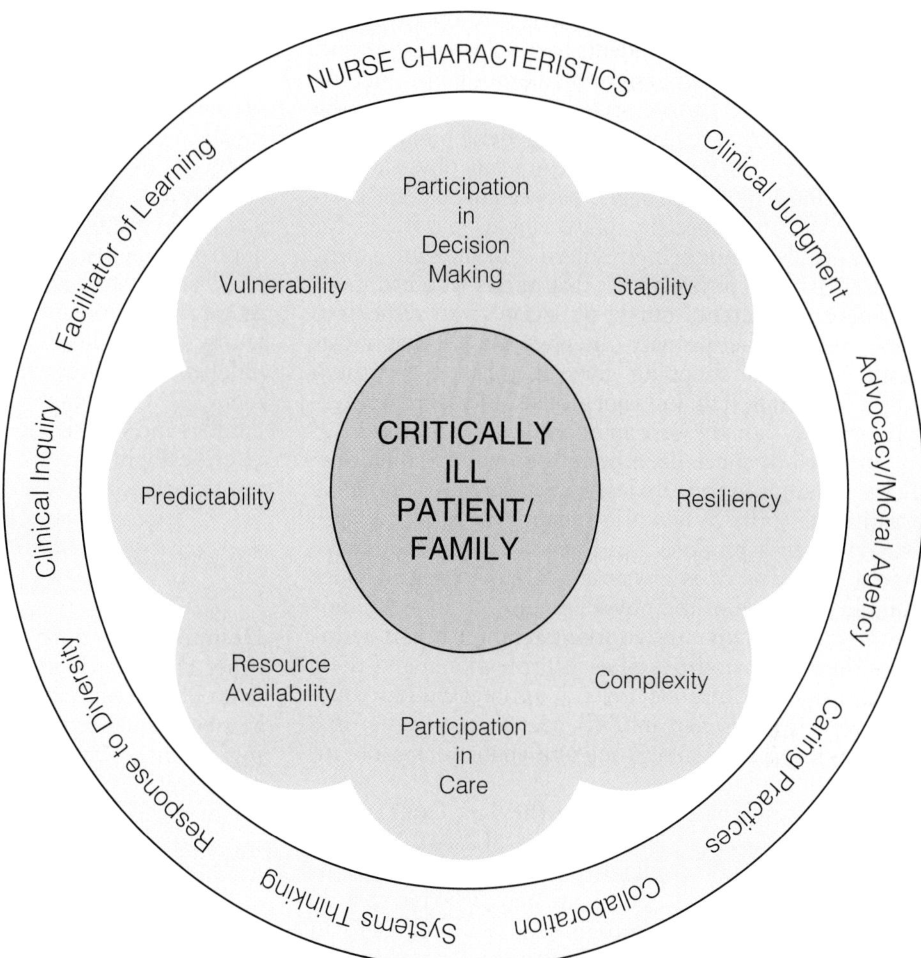

figure 1-1 The relationship between the patient/family and the nurse in the Synergy Model.

Outcomes derived from the nurse may include physiological changes, presence or absence of complications, and the extent to which treatment objectives were attained. Outcomes derived from the health care system include recidivism, costs, and resource utilization.[20]

One manner in which the Synergy Model can be used in clinical practice involves making patient care assignments. Traditionally, in an effort to enhance the continuity of care, patient assignments were made based on the person who cared for the patient the previous day. Using the Synergy Model, the nurse who demonstrates the competencies that match the patient's needs at that time would be best suited for the assignment. For example, if a patient is in a stable, unpredictable, minimally resilient, and vulnerable condition based on the model's definitions, the nurse who excelled in clinical judgment and caring practices would be ideal for this patient. If the patient was vulnerable, unable to participate in decision making, and had inadequate resource availability, the primary competencies would focus on advocacy/moral agency, collaboration, and systems thinking.

The Synergy Model is currently being evaluated to determine if nurses define their practice based on patient needs, if the patient characteristics accurately describe the full spectrum of those being cared for, and if patients experience optimal outcomes when patient–nurse synergy is achieved.

Collaboration

In the Synergy Model, the AACN defines collaboration as "working with others (e.g., physicians, families, healthcare providers) in a way that promotes/encourages each person's contributions toward achieving optimal/realistic goals. Collaboration involves intra- and interdisciplinary work with colleagues."[21] Since the publication of the Health of the Nation document in 1992, collaborative practice has been at the forefront of health service reform.[22] Effective planning of care to meet the needs of critically ill patients and their families who have complex, multisystemic problems requires a multidisciplinary approach to attain timely and optimal outcomes. In addition to meeting health care needs, collaborative practice is further encouraged so that limited federal funds may be used more efficiently.[23]

Empirical data exist that support the value of a collaborative working relationship between nurses and physicians in the intensive care setting. A collaborative relationship has been linked to higher job satisfaction and retention of nurses, a higher level of patient satisfaction, and lower-than-expected mortality rates and patient lengths of stay.[24]

Although leading organizations have put forth recommendations for multidisciplinary efforts and practitioners agree that interdisciplinary collaboration is important to attain optimal patient outcomes, there has been hesitation in adopting collaborative working practices.[24,25] One reason cited for this problem is the lack of opportunities for medical and nursing students to develop collaborative skills.[26,27] Barriers to effective collaboration also include reimbursement, territorialism, and role confusion on the part of the health care team and the general public.[28]

In one study, nurses reported "too many physicians on the case" and a "power struggle" between the patient's primary service and specialty physicians as rationales for patient problems not being resolved.[24] In the same study, one primary care physician felt that nurses who had medical opinions different from the physician's were difficult to work with. Another primary care physician felt that nurses would go "doctor shopping" for a physician to give them orders for therapy if they did not receive orders for the interventions they thought were appropriate for their patients.[24]

One area of specialized nursing in which collaboration is inherent in the job description is that of the nurse practitioner (NP). When NPs accept a position, they are usually given a practice agreement. This collaborative practice agreement is a written statement that defines the joint practice of the physician and NP in a collaborative and complementary working relationship. It delineates the responsibilities of each professional and their respective contributions toward optimal patient outcomes.[23] The physician and NP must work together in a successful, complementary, and unified manner to obtain these optimal outcomes.

In her Presidential Address at the 31st Congress of the Society of Critical Care Medicine (SCCM), Maureen Harvey described "invisible excellence." Inherent in this concept is the role of the critical care nurse who is vigilantly monitoring the patient, recognizing subtle changes in the patient's clinical status, and thwarting critical events through collaboration with the intensivist. Nurse–physician collaboration as well as collaboration with the clinical dietitian, clinical pharmacist, respiratory therapist, physical therapist, occupational therapist, and chaplain are essential for obtaining optimal patient outcomes. These outcomes should reflect the contributions made by all disciplines. Collaboration between researchers and practitioners in both disciplines is essential to provide a scientific basis for that practice.[29]

The Family, Critical Illness, and Current Evidence

Not long ago, the thought of families staying in the CCU and participating in care was almost unimaginable because of restricted and rigid visiting hours in many CCUs.[30,31] In addition, the concept that children, animals, or non–legally recognized significant others should not visit a person in the CCU was widespread and went unchallenged.[32] Today, patient, family, and significant other advocates have challenged the "status quo" and instituted a change of visitation policies based on consumer dissatisfaction and current evidence.[30] Although open visitation is not standard practice in every CCU, many CCUs have modified visiting policies to allow not only immediate family to visit, but significant others, children, friends, and, in some instances, even pets.[32–34] Expanded visitation promotes resiliency of the human spirit and allows the vulnerable critically ill patient to connect with significant people that he or she would encounter in daily life. Simultaneously, the critical care nurse must use clinical judgment to assess the impact of visitation on the physiological and psychological status of the patient and significant others, while promoting involvement in care and decision making.[32,33]

As CCUs shift from closed to open units, new clinical controversies will develop and be evaluated through clinical inquiry and research. Two of the future challenges confronting critical care nurses and the "traditions" of the CCU are the role and inclusion of families during trauma or cardiopulmonary resuscitation (CPR) and the role of family or significant other as caregivers in assisting or independently providing care in the critical care environment.[35–37] Less than a century ago in the United States, families and significant others were the primary caregivers to critically ill persons and persons at the end of life; this remains the case in much of the world today.

Spirituality and Caring During Critical Illness and at the End of Life

Despite innovations and advances in technology and other therapeutic interventions, patients still transition from life to death in the CCU. Death, whether expected as a consequence of end-stage cancer or terminal weaning, or unexpected because of trauma or postoperative complications, is viewed as the failure of caring practices for many. During critical illness and at the end of life, issues of spiritual distress, mortality, family dysfunction, grief, hopelessness, helplessness, and many other feelings and emotions may present as part of the coping mechanisms of the individual patient, his or her family or significant others, and members of the health care team.[38]

Acuity, unplanned hospitalizations, and patient–family and significant other separation are all potential sources of stress during any illness. Regardless of the acuity, the expected outcome, or the availability of interventions, a caring, competent nurse is essential.[39] During critical illness where outcomes are uncertain, the nurse competencies described in the Synergy Model are paramount. This is especially true when delivering interventions where the predictability of the outcomes is unknown, the stability of the patient is tenuous or deteriorating, and the complexity of care is ever increasing. Similarly, at the end of life, where helplessness, hopelessness, and spiritual distress may be manifested, caring nursing interventions aimed at alleviating suffering are essential. These interventions must also address patient and family involvement in care and decision making through advocacy, collaboration, and systems thinking.

PROFESSIONAL ORGANIZATIONS AND RESOURCES

American Association of Critical-Care Nurses: A Commitment to Excellence

The AACN was established in 1969 to help educate nurses working in ICUs. Currently, it is the largest specialty organization in nursing, with over 65,000 members in the

United States and abroad who care for critically ill patients across the life span. In its mission statement, AACN identifies members as the key to its success. To that end, AACN is committed to providing the highest-quality resources to maximize the nurse's contribution to caring and improving the health of critically ill patients and their families. AACN is dedicated to providing its members with the knowledge and resources necessary to help them provide optimal patient care.[18]

Holding membership in professional specialty nursing organizations has several benefits for the "card holder." It provides members with the opportunity to network with colleagues on the national, regional, and local level, while providing them with a mechanism to obtain current information in their specialty area. In addition, AACN provides members with numerous other benefits that help to enhance professional practice.[18]

AACN ONLINE

AACN Online is a comprehensive critical care Internet website. It provides members with the most recent resources in clinical practice, continuing education, and professional development. AACN Online also allows members to discuss issues and share information with other professional colleagues, obtain clinical practice information, and participate in interactive learning discussions. AACN members have 24-hour access to the website.[18]

PRACTICE RESOURCE NETWORK

The Practice Resource Network (PRN) provides members with the opportunity to network with professional colleagues. Once the PRN network is accessed from the AACN website, members begin by selecting from 1 of 32 topics about which they would like additional information. The topics include all body systems, several acute care specialties, educational content, informatics, administration/regulatory information, ethical and legal issues, and standards and guidelines for practice, to name a few. The service can be used to help problem-solve clinical dilemmas, access current practice and research information, identify public policy issues as well as resources, and connect with colleagues with similar interests.[18]

EDUCATIONAL MERCHANDISE

All members of AACN can receive educational materials at discounted prices. AACN has educational resources available in several areas, including clinical practice, research, leadership, ethics, and professional development.[18]

PUBLICATIONS

Members of AACN receive two bimonthly journals, *The American Journal of Critical Care* and *Critical Care Nurse*. The former is a scientific research journal in which critical care colleagues publish research findings, expanding the current state of the science of critical care nursing. It is an ideal journal to use as a basis for a literature review for an EBP model. *Critical Care Nurse* is a specialty journal that publishes articles related to current clinical practice topics. For example, a recent issue explored how the Synergy Model is applied in clinical practice by nurses, educators, or management. The journal also offers its readers opportunities for obtaining continuing education credits. Readers of *Critical Care Nurse* obtain information on the latest critical care trends. In addition, members receive *AACN News*, a newsletter that keeps readers apprised of current trends in health care as well as organization, chapter, and certification issues.[18]

LOCAL CHAPTER AFFILIATION

Once nurses have joined the national AACN, they can extend their membership to the local level. Local chapter affiliation provides members with the opportunity to network with peers in their immediate area, become involved with chapter activities, and attend the educational programs offered, thereby enhancing their professional development.

THE FUTURE OF CRITICAL CARE NURSING

As health care continues to evolve, so too must critical care nursing. As the past few years have demonstrated, critical care nursing will continue to be provided not only in the inpatient specialty critical care units, but on the medical, surgical, oncology, and stepdown units, as well as in the outpatient and home settings. Consequently, the demand for caring, competent, knowledgeable, and skilled critical care nurses will continue.

As the "baby boom" generation ages, and with the expansion of CCUs beyond the traditional ICU, the demand for critical care nurses will continue to rise.[40] Concurrent with an increased demand for expert critical care nurses is the need for recruiting, developing, and retaining expert clinicians in an era of nursing shortage. The ongoing and cyclical nature of the nursing shortage has had a direct impact on CCUs across the United States.[40,41] According to Needleman and colleagues,[41] the lack of trained registered nurses to provide direct nursing care has had a direct impact on the quality of patient care and consequently has also affected organizational effectiveness and outcomes. In response to an increased need for nurses, particularly critical care nurses, many organizations continue to use supplemental staffing by caring, competent, knowledgeable critical care nurses. Whether the critical care nurses are part of the organization's staff or are supplemental staff, consumers and third-party payers alike will continue to mandate competence, proven interventions derived from EBP, cost-effectiveness, and quality outcomes.

Simultaneously, the CCUs of tomorrow will be even more technologically challenging. Therefore, critical care nurses of the future must not only be technologically proficient, but competent in the psychosocial, developmental, spiritual, and caring domains to interact successfully with the patient, the family and significant others, and the other members of the health care team. With advances in technology and new interventions discovered through EBP, greater numbers of patients will be afforded interventions that sustain and improve the quality of their lives.

However, with the implementation of advances in technology, patients in the CCU will continue to require caring, competent, and knowledgeable critical care nurses. These nurses will serve as patient advocates, facilitate interdisciplinary collaboration, navigate complex delivery and reimbursement systems, and facilitate learning, while responding to diverse communities who are vulnerable owing to complex needs. These are the exciting challenges awaiting critical care nurses—challenges, it is hoped, that critical care nurses will surmount with commitment, dedication, and grace!

clinical applicability challenges

Self-Challenge: Critical Thinking

1. *Describe a patient care situation that exemplifies the use of the Synergy Model.*
2. *Identify a problem in your area of practice that needs to be changed, based on evidence in the nursing scientific literature.*
3. *Describe a situation where collaboration with other members of the health care team enhanced patient outcomes.*

Study Questions

1. *The first step to evidence-based critical care nursing practice is to*
   a. *frame a clinical question based on clinical observation.*
   b. *conduct a literature search and evaluate the evidence.*
   c. *implement a needs assessment of critical care nurses.*
   d. *accept the fact that health care is continually evolving.*
2. *According to the Synergy Model, which of the following characterizes the nurse competency of systems thinking?*
   a. *The ongoing process of questioning and evaluating practice*
   b. *The sensitivity to recognize, appreciate, and incorporate differences in the provision of care*
   c. *The ability to appreciate the care environment from a perspective that recognizes holistic interrelationships*
   d. *The ability to facilitate learning of others while fostering the work of others in a way that facilitates optimal and realistic patient goals*
3. *A domestic partner of a critically ill patient expresses an interest in learning how to provide skin care. According to the Synergy Model, this illustrates which of the following patient characteristics and nurse competencies?*
   a. *Participation in decision making and caring practices*
   b. *Participation in care and response to diversity*
   c. *Resource availability and advocacy/moral agency*
   d. *Stability and facilitator of learning*
4. *A new drug has been approved to treat coronary ischemia. Before the introduction of the drug in clinical practice, a critical care nurse conducts a series of in-services about the drug's dosing and side effects, and related nursing interventions. This is an example of*
   a. *caring practices.*
   b. *clinical inquiry.*
   c. *facilitator of learning.*
   d. *collaboration.*
5. *A certified critical care nurse uses case study analysis and reading clinical journals to maintain a personal practice of clinical excellence. These activities are essential elements of*
   a. *critical thinking.*
   b. *evidence-based practice.*
   c. *caring practices.*
   d. *advocacy/moral agency.*

REFERENCES

1. President's Advisory Commission on Consumer Protection and Quality in the Healthcare Industry: Fostering Evidence-Based Practice and Innovation, Quality First: Better Health Care for All Americans. Washington, DC, U.S. Government Printing Office, 1998
2. Goode CJ: Evidence based practice. In University of Colorado Hospital: Practice Outcomes Research Manual, 10–17. Denver, CO, University of Colorado Hospital, 2000
3. Goode C: What constitutes evidence-based practice? Appl Nurs Res 13(4):212–215, 2000
4. Schlomer G: Evidence-based nursing: A useful method for nursing practice? Pflege 13(1):47–52, 2000
5. Glanville I, Schirm V, Winemar NM: Using evidence-based practice for managing clinical outcomes in advanced practice nursing. J Nurs Care Qual 15(1):1–11, 2000
6. Jassak PF: Introduction: Evidence-based oncology nursing practice. Improving patient outcomes in the next millennium. Oncol Nurs Forum 28(2, Suppl):3–4, 2001
7. Heater BS, Becker AM, Olson RK: Nursing interventions and patient outcomes: A meta-analysis of studies. Nurs Res 37:303–307, 1988
8. Krugman M: Introduction to research. In University of Colorado Hospital: Practice Outcomes Research Manual, 5–9. Denver, CO, University of Colorado Hospital, 2000
9. Oermann M, Truesdell S, Ziolkowski L: Strategies to assess, develop and evaluate critical thinking. J Contin Educ Nurs 31(4):155–160, 2000
10. Scheffer BK, Rubenfeld MG: A consensus statement on critical thinking in nursing. J Nurs Educ 39(8):352–359, 2000
11. Thurmond VA: The holism in critical thinking: A concept analysis. J Hol Nurs 19(4):375–389, 2001
12. Youngblood N, Beitz JM: Developing critical thinking with active strategies. Nurse Educator 26(1):39–42, 2001
13. Myrick F, Yonge OJ: Creating a climate for critical thinking in the preceptor experience. Nurse Educ Today 20(6):461–467, 2001
14. May BA, Edell V, Butell S, et al: Critical thinking and clinical competence: A study of their relationship in BSN seniors. J Nurs Educ 38(3):1–10, 1999
15. Hansten RI, Washburn MJ: Facilitating critical thinking. J Nurses Staff Dev 16(1):23–30, 2000
16. American Association of Critical-Care Nurses: General information regarding certification. Available at: http://www.certcorp.org/certcorp/certcorp.nsf. Accessed April 20, 2002
17. American Association of Critical-Care Nurses: Safeguarding the patient and the profession: The value of critical care nurse certification. Am J Crit Care 12(2):154–164, 2003.
18. American Association of Critical-Care Nurses: Member services: Certification. Available at: http://www.aacn.org/AACN/MemShip.nsf. Accessed April 20, 2002
19. Anonymous: Fact sheet on the ANCC certification program. ASNA Reporter 27(2):11, 2000
20. Richmond T: Certified practice: A foundation for excellence. Keynote address at the CCRN Luncheon, National Teaching Institute, Atlanta, GA, May 2002.
21. Curley MAQ: Patient-nurse synergy: Optimizing patients' outcomes. Am J Crit Care 7(1):64–72, 1998
22. Whitehead D: Applying collaborative practice to health promotion. Nurs Standard 15(20):33–37, 2001
23. Herman J, Ziel S: Collaborative practice agreements for advanced practice nurses: What you should know. AACN Clin Issues 10(3):337–342, 1999
24. Miller A: Nurse-physician collaboration in an intensive care unit. Am J Crit Care 10(5):341–350, 2001
25. Fitzpatrick JJ, Montgomery KS: Expanding the pool of primary care clinicians: Preparation for collaborative practice. Natl Acad Pract Forum Issues Interdiscipl Care 2(3):195–201, 2000
26. Brashers VL: Medical and nursing faculty and student support for interdisciplinary skills training to promote collaborative practice. Natl Acad Pract Forum Issues Interdiscipl Care 1(3):195–201, 1999

27. Dosser DA, Handron DS, McCammon SL, et al: Challenges and strategies for teaching collaborative interdisciplinary practice in children's mental health care. Fam Syst Health 19(1):65–82, 2001
28. Neale J: Nurse practitioners and physicians: A collaborative practice. Clin Nurse Specialist 13(5):252–258, 1999
29. Harvey M: Invisible excellence. Presidential Message at the Society of Critical Care Medicine 31st Congress, San Diego, CA, Society of Critical Care Medicine, January 2002
30. Roland P, Russell J, Richards KC, et al: Visitation in critical care: Processes and outcomes of performance improvement initiative. J Nurs Care Qual 15(2):18–26, 2001
31. Clarke C, Harrison D: The needs of children visiting on adult intensive care units: A review of the literature and recommendations for practice. J Adv Nurs 34(1):61–68, 2001
32. Simon SK, Phillips K, Badalamenti S, et al: Current practices regarding visitation policies in critical care units. Am J Crit Care 6(3):210–217, 1997
33. Simpson T, Wilson D, Mucken N, et al: Implementation and evaluation of a liberalized visiting policy. Am J Crit Care 5(6):420–426, 1996
34. Carlson B, Riegel B, Thomason T: Visitation: Policy versus practice. Dimens Crit Care Nurs 17(1):40–47, 1998
35. Hupcey JE: Looking out for the patient and ourselves: The process of family integration into the ICU. J Clin Nurs 8(30):253–262, 1999
36. Morse JM, Pooler C: Patient-family-nurse interactions in the trauma-resuscitation room. Am J Crit Care 11(3):240–249, 2002
37. Williams JM: Family presence during resuscitation: To see or not to see? Nurs Clin North Am 37(1):211–220, 2002
38. Gaul AL: Care: An ethical foundation for critical care nursing. Crit Care Nurse 15(3):131–135, 1995
39. Relf MV: Illuminating meaning and transforming issues of spirituality in HIV and AIDS: An application of Parse's Theory of Human Becoming. Hol Nurs Pract 12(1):1–7, 1997
40. Steinbrook R: Nursing in the crossfire. N Engl J Med 346(22): 1757–1765, 2002
41. Needleman J, Buerhaus P, Mattkes S, et al: Nurse-staffing levels and the quality of care in hospitals. N Engl J Med 346(22):1715–1722, 2002

chapter 2

The Patient's Experience With Critical Illness

KATHRYN S. BIZEK

objectives

Based on the content in this chapter, the reader should be able to:

- Explore relationships among stress, response to illness, and anxiety.
- Construct nursing interventions to assist patients in their adaptation to critical illness.
- Compare and contrast techniques that the patient and family can learn in an effort to manage stress and anxiety.
- Discuss alternatives to the use of physical restraint in the intensive care unit.
- Describe the phases of loss and specific nursing interventions for each phase.
- Develop nursing interventions that foster the ability of patients to draw strength from their personal spirituality.
- Develop strategies to care for patients and their families at the end of life.

The patient's experience in an intensive care unit (ICU) has lasting meaning for the patient and his or her family members and significant others. Although actual painful memories are blurred by drugs and the mind's need to forget, attitudes that are highly charged with feelings about the nature of the experience survive. These attitudes shape the person's beliefs about nurses, physicians, health care, and the vulnerability of life itself.

This chapter describes specific measures that nurses use to support patients and their families through the stress of crisis and adaptation to illness, death, or a return to health. An understanding and appreciation of the intricate relationships among mind, body, spirit, and the healing process will help the critical care nurse provide emotional support to the patient and family. It is the caring and emotional support given by the nurse that will be remembered and valued.

PERCEPTION OF CRITICAL ILLNESS

Admission to a critical care unit (CCU) may signal a threat to the life and well-being of the patient who is admitted. Critical care nurses perceive the unit as a place where fragile lives are vigilantly scrutinized, cared for, and preserved. Patients and their families, however, frequently perceive admission to critical care as a sign of impending death, based on their own past experiences or the experiences of others. Understanding what critical care means to patients may help nurses care for their patients. However, effective communication with critically ill patients is often challenging and frustrating.[1,2] Barriers to communication may relate to the patients' physiological status; the existence of endotracheal tubes, which inhibit verbal communication; medications; or other conditions that alter cognitive function.

Patients' Experiences

A number of authors have sought to study and describe patients' experiences related to their ICU stay. In a review of 26 studies, Stein-Parbury and McKinley noted that between 30% to 100% of patients studied could recall all or part of their stay in the ICU.[3] Although many of the patients recalled feelings that were negative, they also recalled neutral and positive experiences. Negative experiences were related to fear, anxiety, sleep disturbance, cognitive impairment, and pain or discomfort. Positive experiences were related to feelings of being safe and secure. Often, these positive feelings were attributed to the care provided by nurses. The need to feel safe and the need for information were predominant themes in qualitative research studies conducted by Hupcey and colleagues.[4,5] Nurses' technical competence and effective interpersonal skills were cited by patients as promoting their sense of security and trust.[3–6]

STRESS

Stress has been defined as a situation that exists when an organism is faced with any stimulus that causes a disequilibrium between psychological and physiological functioning. All hormone levels can be altered by stress. Extreme levels of stress damage human tissue and may interfere with adaptive responses. If adaptive behaviors are effective, energy is freed and may be directed toward healing. If adaptive behaviors fail or are ineffective, however, the tension state is increased, as is the demand for energy. Therefore, the original stress of illness looms larger (Fig. 2-1). Hans Selye first described the stress syndrome and the general adaptation syndrome in the 1930s.[7]

Response to Stress

The characteristic problems of adapting to limitations enforced by illness can be understood by exploring the relationship between the physical and the sociopsychological response to the illness. There is an observable lag between the physical onset of illness and its emotional acknowledgment—that is, the patient experiences illness and disability physically before acknowledging them fully on an emotional level. Denial is an example of this lag. Likewise, after physical health has been stabilized, the patient still experiences concerns and fears related to acute illness. At this point, the patient is likely to resist independence

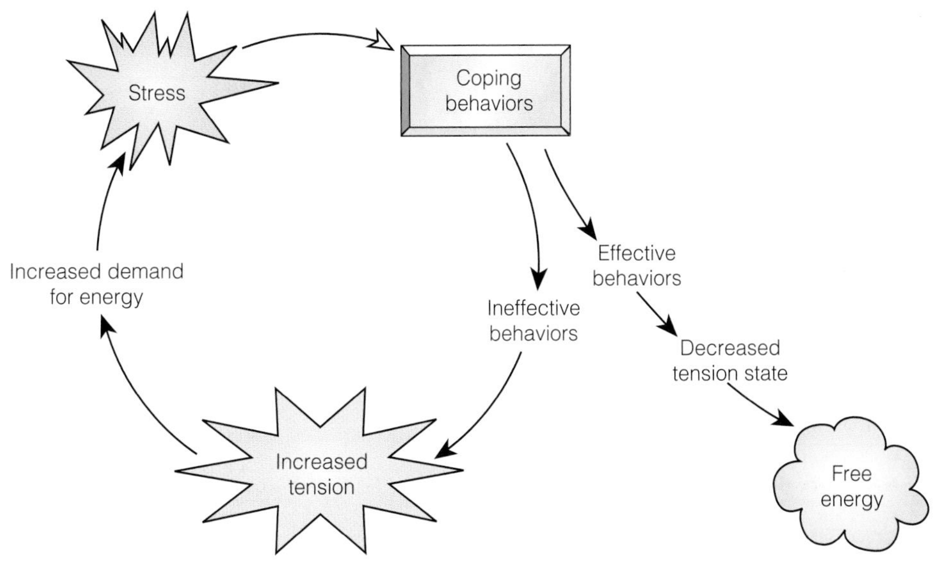

figure 2-1 Stress and coping.

and be reluctant to cooperate with increased expectations for activity and self-care. Preparation for return to health, acknowledgment of concerns about increased activity, and the reassurance of watchful eyes help alleviate anxiety as the patient progresses.

If different responses of patients to illness could be plotted on a graph, they would show both common and unique points, just as electrocardiograms (ECGs) from different people show common characteristics and individual differences. The time and congruence between physical and sociopsychological responses vary, but the stages occur predictably. Like the electrical events of the heart, response to illness, both adaptive and maladaptive, can be anticipated. The nurse has several responsibilities:

- Anticipate, assess, and monitor the response to illness.
- Recognize and support effective behaviors.
- Minimize and redirect ineffective behaviors.

ANXIETY

Causes of Anxiety

Any stress that threatens one's sense of wholeness, containment, security, and control causes anxiety. Illness is one such stress. A common cause of anxiety is a sense of isolation. Rarely is one lonelier than when in the midst of a socializing crowd of strangers. In such a situation, people attempt to include themselves, remove themselves, or emotionally distance themselves. The sick person surrounded by active and busy people is in a similar situation but with few resources available to reduce the sense of isolation. Hospital staff who ignore the presence of a patient, regardless of the patient's alertness, contribute to the patient's sense of isolation. Including the patient in conversations about treatment and providing a reassuring touch at frightening moments can reduce this sense of isolation.

Serious illness and the fear of dying also separate the patient from his or her family. The immediate development of dependent and intimate relationships with strangers is required. The reassuring cliche, "You'll be all right," often meant to comfort, only reinforces the patient's sense of distance. It shuts off the expression of fears and questions about what is to come next. The efficiency and activity that surround the patient increase the sense of separateness.

Another category of anxiety-provoking stimuli includes those that threaten the individual's security. Admission to the ICU dramatically confirms for the family and patient that their security on all levels is being severely threatened.

After the patient is admitted to the unit, the initial insecurity undoubtedly concerns life itself. Later, questions regarding such issues as length of hospitalization, return to work, financial implications, well-being of the family, and permanent limitations arise. The patient's insecurity continues and needs to be sensitively considered.

Anxiety occurs when a person experiences the following:

- Threat of helplessness
- Loss of control
- Sense of loss of function and self-esteem
- Failure of former defenses
- Sense of isolation
- Fear of dying

Responses to Anxiety

PHYSIOLOGICAL RESPONSES

The physiological responses of rapid pulse rate, increased blood pressure, increased respirations, dilated pupils, dry mouth, and peripheral vasoconstriction may go undetected in a seemingly cool, calm, self-contained patient. These autonomic responses to anxiety are frequently the most reliable index of the degree of anxiety when behavioral and verbal responses are not congruent with the circumstances.

SOCIOPSYCHOLOGICAL RESPONSES

Behavioral responses indicative of anxiety are often family-based and culturally learned. They vary from quiet composure in the face of disaster to panic in the presence of an innocuous insect. Such extremes of control and panic use valuable energy. If this energy is not directed toward eliminating or adapting to the stressor, it only perpetuates the discomfort of the tension state. The goal of nursing care is always to promote physiological and emotional equilibrium.

Patterns of Adaptation

Figure 2-2 demonstrates one pattern of adapting to various stages of illness. During stress, the patient regresses in an attempt to conserve energy. During times of acute exacerbation or heightened expectations, or during any significant change, the initial response is regression to an earlier emotional position of safety. Weaning from a respirator, removal of monitor leads, increased activity, and reduction in medication often trigger anxiety and regression. This regression may even include a retreat into increased dependency, depression, and anger. At such times, the patient may find comfort in regressing to a state that has already been mastered. Behavior at this time may seem peculiar or irrational to the nurse. The regression is usually temporary and brief and can be used to identify the cause of anxiety. Nurses may become disappointed, anxious, or angry with the patient's regression and may want to retreat. It is more helpful, however, to acknowledge that regression is inevitable and to support the patient

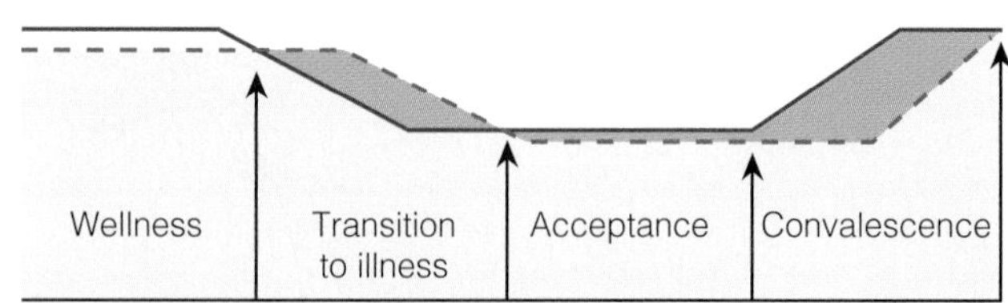

figure 2-2 One pattern of adapting to various stages of illness. The darkly shaded areas represent transition into and out of illness and show the disparity between actual health and the person's perception of his or her health. During transition to illness, there is denial. During the acceptance phase, physical and mental well-being are congruent. During the convalescence phase, an emotional lag exists between physical and emotional well-being.

with interventions appropriate to earlier stages. The nurse helps the patient understand what is happening by explaining the emotional lag phenomenon.

NURSING ASSESSMENT

Often it is not possible for the nurse simply to remove the stimuli that cause anxiety. In these circumstances, the nurse must assess the effectiveness of the patient's behaviors and either support them, help the patient modify them, or teach new behaviors. Frequently, levels of anxiety are so high that the anxious state becomes the stimulus that demands additional coping responses. After assessing coping behaviors for effectiveness, the nurse has several choices:

- Support the behaviors.
- Help the patient modify behaviors.
- Teach new behavior.

Coping behaviors may be directed either toward eliminating the stress of illness or toward eliminating the anxiety state itself. The nurse must evaluate each behavior as to whether it helps restore a steady state. Behaviors that promote movement toward a steady state can then be supported and encouraged. The nurse may also need to help the patient modify or find substitutes for behaviors that are disruptive or threatening to homeostasis. At times, the nurse must introduce new behaviors to facilitate equilibrium and promote health.

Examples of nursing diagnoses associated with critical illness and injury can be seen in Box 2-1.

NURSING INTERVENTIONS

Whenever possible, stress must be reduced or eliminated for critically ill patients. If this can be accomplished, the problem is quickly resolved, and the patient is returned to a state of equilibrium. Usually, however, the stress is not eliminated so easily because many other stressors are introduced by attempts to remedy the original problem. If adaptive behaviors are effective, anxiety is reduced, and energy is directed toward rest and healing. A number of nursing interventions may be used to reduce anxiety and promote adaptation in critically ill patients. Often a combination of interventions is used.

box 2-1 *Examples of Nursing Diagnoses and Collaborative Problems for the Patient With Critical Illness or Injury*

- Anticipatory Grieving
- Anxiety
- Body Image Disturbance
- Impaired Verbal Communication
- Ineffective Denial
- Fear
- Risk for Loneliness
- Powerlessness
- Self-Esteem Disturbance
- Spiritual Distress
- Potential for Enhanced Spiritual Well-Being

Creating a Healing Environment

Florence Nightingale is considered the founder of modern nursing. She often wrote about the nurse's role in creating an environment to allow healing to occur.[8,9] She emphasized holism in nursing—that is, caring for the whole person. In today's technological age, critical care nurses are challenged to create an environment of healing. These environments must allow critically ill patients to have their psychological needs as well as physical needs met. Manipulating the milieu may involve timing interventions to allow adequate sleep and rest, providing pain-relieving medication, playing music, or teaching deep-breathing exercises.

Fostering Trust

Almost every nurse in critical care can relate stories of special bonds that formed with individual patients and families. They can describe special situations where a trusting relationship developed and they made a difference in the patient's recovery or even dignified death. In contrast, patients have related to us, through research, that when they mistrust their caregivers, they are more anxious and more vigilant of staff behaviors, and lack the feeling of safety and security. Our goal, then, is to display a confident, caring attitude, demonstrate technical competence, and develop effective communication techniques that will foster the development of a trusting relationship.[6]

Providing Information

Besides the need to feel safe, critically ill patients identify the need for information as having a high priority. This need to know involves all aspects of the patients' care. They need to know what is happening at the moment. They also need to know what will happen to them, how they are doing, and what they can expect. Many patients also need frequent explanations of what happened to them. These explanations reorient them, sort out sequences of events, and help them distinguish real events from dreams or hallucinations.[4,5] Anxiety can be greatly relieved with simple explanations. Consider the patient, for example, who was being weaned from the ventilator who just needed reassurance that if he did not breathe, the machine would do it for him.[10] Families, too, have identified the need for information as a high priority. This is followed closely by the need to have hope. Most families identify physicians as the primary source for information. It is important for nurses to be mindful of patient confidentiality issues when speaking to family members. Nurses should have the patient's permission before giving confidential medical information to family members. If that is not possible because of the patient's condition, a family spokesperson should be identified as the person who may receive confidential information. This information should be recorded in the patient's medical record.

Allowing Control

Nursing measures that reinforce a sense of control help increase the patient's autonomy and reduce the overpowering sense of a loss of control. The nurse can help the patient to feel more control over his or her environment by:

- Providing order and predictability in routines
- Using anticipatory guidance
- Allowing the patient to make choices whenever possible
- Involving the patient in decision-making
- Providing information and explanation for procedures

Providing order and predictability allows the patient to anticipate and prepare for what is to follow. Perhaps it creates only a mirage of control, but anticipatory guidance keeps the patient from being caught off-guard and allows the mustering of coping mechanisms.

Allowing small choices when the patient is willing and ready increases the patient's feeling of control over the environment. Would the patient prefer to lie on his or her right or left side? In which arm should the intravenous (IV) line be placed? What height is preferred for the head of the bed? Does the patient want to cough now or in 20 minutes after pain medication? Any decisions that afford the patient a certain amount of control and predictability are important. These small choices may also help the patient accept lack of control during procedures that involve little choice.

Cultural Sensitivity

Interventions for individual patients must be contextually based and culturally sensitive. Transcultural nursing refers to a formal area of study and practice that focuses on providing care that is compatible with the cultural beliefs, values, and lifestyles of individuals. A cultural assessment includes the patient's usual response to illness as well as his or her cultural norms, beliefs, and world views. Because individual responses and values may vary within the same culture, the patient should be recognized as an individual within the cultural context. Exploring the meaning of the critical event with the patient, family members, and significant others may give clues to the patient's perception of what is happening. In addition, the nurse may ask if there is a particular ethnic or religious group with which the patient identifies and if there is anything the nurses may do to provide care that is sensitive to individual values or norms while the patient is hospitalized. Awareness and acceptance are the heart of cultural competence.[11]

Presencing and Reassurance

Presence, or just "being there," can in itself be a meaningful strategy for alleviating distress or anxiety in the critically ill patient. Presencing is the therapeutic use of self, adopting a caring attitude, and paying attention to an individual's needs. This presence implies more than just a physical presence, however. It means giving one's full attention to the person, focusing on the person, and practicing active listening. When a nurse uses presence, the focus is not on a task or outside thoughts. Energy and attention are directed at the patient and his or her needs or feelings. Snyder and colleagues describe a higher level of presence called transcendent presence, which conveys an energy exchange between the nurse and the patient that has a spiritual quality.[12] Quinn describes the concept of intentionality in the development of the use of self as healer. This means one makes a conscious effort to use all of one's capacity, including eyes, voice, energy, and touch, in a more intentionally healing way.[13] Reassurance can be provided to the patient in the form of presencing and caring touch. Reassurance can also be verbal. Verbal reassurance can be effective for patients if it provides realistic encouragement or clarifies misconceptions. Verbal reassurance is not valuable, however, if it prevents a patient from expressing his or her emotions or stifles the need for further dialogue. Reassurance is intended to reduce fear and anxiety and evoke a calmer, more passive response. It is best directed at patients expressing unrealistic or exaggerated fears.

Cognitive Techniques

Techniques that have evolved from cognitive theories of learning may help anxious patients and their families. They can be initiated by the patient and do not depend on complex insight or understanding of one's own psychological makeup. They can also be used to reduce anxiety in a way that avoids probing into the patient's personal life. Furthermore, the patient's friends and family members can be taught these techniques to help them and the patient reduce tension.

INTERNAL DIALOGUE

Highly anxious people are most likely giving themselves messages that increase or perpetuate their anxiety. These messages are conveyed in one's continuously running "self-talk," or internal dialogue. The patient in the ICU may be silently saying things such as, "I can't stand it in here. I've got to get out." Another unexpressed thought might be, "I can't handle this pain." By asking the patient to share aloud what is going on in this internal dialogue, the nurse can bring to awareness the messages that are distracting the patient from rest and relaxation. Substitute messages should be suggested to the patient. It is important to ask the patient to substitute rather than delete messages because the internal dialogue is continuously operating and will not turn off, even if the patient wills it to do so. Therefore, asking the patient to substitute constructive, reassuring comments is more likely to help the patient significantly reduce his or her tension level. Comments such as, "I'll handle this pain just one minute at a time" or "I've been in tough spots before, and I am capable of making it through this one!" will automatically reduce anxiety and help the patient shape coping behaviors accordingly. Any message that enhances the patient's confidence, sense of control, and hope and puts him or her in a positive, active role, rather than the passive role of victim, will increase the patient's sense of coping and well-being.

The nurse helps the patient develop self-dialogue messages that increase:

- Confidence
- Sense of control

- Ability to cope
- Optimism
- Hope

EXTERNAL DIALOGUE

A similar method can be applied to the patient's external conversation with other people. By simply requiring patients to speak accurately about themselves to others, the same goals can be accomplished. For example, patients who exclaim, "I can't do anything for myself!" should be asked to identify the things that they are able to do, such as lifting their own bodies, turning to one side, making a nurse feel good with a rewarding smile, or helping the family understand what is happening. Even the smallest movement in the weakest of patients should be acknowledged and claimed by the patient. This technique is useful in helping patients correct their own misconceptions of themselves and the way others see them. This reduces the patients' sense of helplessness and therefore their anxiety.

COGNITIVE REAPPRAISAL

This technique asks the patient to identify a particular stressor and then modify his or her response to that stressor. In other words, the patient reframes his or her perception of the stressor in a more positive light so that the stimulus is no longer viewed as threatening. The patient is given permission to take personal control of responses to the stimulus. This technique may be combined with guided imagery and relaxation training.

Guided Imagery and Relaxation Training

These are two useful techniques that can be taught to the patient to help reduce tension. The nurse can encourage the patient to imagine either being in a very pleasant place or taking part in a very pleasant experience. The patient should be instructed to focus and linger on the sensations that are experienced. For example, asking the patient, "What colors do you see?" "What sounds are present?" "How does the air smell?" "How does your skin feel?" "Is there a breeze in the air?" helps increase the intensity of the fantasy and thereby promote relaxation through mental escape.

Guided imagery also can be used to help reduce unpleasant feelings of depression, anxiety, and hostility. Patients who must relearn life-sustaining tasks, such as walking and feeding themselves, can use imagery to prepare mentally to meet the challenge successfully. In these instances, patients should be taught to visualize themselves moving through the task and successfully completing it. If this method seems trivial or silly to the patients, they can be reminded that this method demands concentration and skill and is commonly used by athletes to improve their performance and to prepare themselves mentally before an important event. Guided imagery is a way of purposefully diverting or focusing the patients' thoughts and has been shown to empower patients, improving their satisfaction and well-being.[14]

The nurse can also use techniques that induce deep muscle relaxation to help the patient decrease anxiety. Deep muscle relaxation may reduce or eliminate the use of tranquilizing and sedating drugs. In *progressive relaxation*, the patient is first directed to find as comfortable a position as possible and then to take several deep breaths and let them out slowly. Next, the patient is asked to clench a fist or curl toes as tightly as possible, to hold the position for a few seconds, then to let go while focusing on the sensations of the releasing muscles. The patient should practice this technique, beginning with the toes and moving upward through other parts of the body—the feet, calves, thighs, abdomen, chest, and so on. This procedure is done slowly while the patient gives nonverbal signals (e.g., lifting a finger) to indicate when each new muscle mass has reached a state of relaxation. Extra time and attention should be given to the back, shoulders, neck, scalp, and forehead, because many people experience physical tension in these areas.

Once a state of relaxation is achieved, the nurse can suggest that the patient fantasize or sleep as deeply as the patient chooses. The patient must be allowed to select and control the depth of relaxation and sleep, especially if the fear of death is prominent in the patient's mind. A moderately dark room and a soft voice facilitate relaxation. Asking the patient to relax is frequently nonproductive compared with directing him to release a muscle mass actively, let go of tension, or imagine tension draining through the body and sinking deeply into the mattress. Again, the patient is assisted to take an active rather than passive role by the nurse's careful use of language.

Deep Breathing

When acutely anxious, the patient's breathing patterns may change, and the patient may hold his or her breath. This could be physically and psychologically detrimental. Teaching diaphragmatic breathing, also called *abdominal breathing*, to the patient may be useful as both a distraction and a coping mechanism. Diaphragmatic breathing can be taught easily and quickly to the preoperative patient or to a patient experiencing acute fear or anxiety. The patient may be asked to place a hand on the abdomen, inhale deeply through the nose, hold briefly, and exhale through pursed lips. The goal is to have the patient push out his own hand to demonstrate the deep breath. The nurse may demonstrate the technique and perform it along with the patient, until the patient is comfortable with the technique and is in control. The mechanically ventilated patient may be able to modify this technique by concentrating on breathing and on pushing out the hand. Mechanically ventilated patients experiencing severe agitation may not be able to respond to this technique.

Music Therapy

Music therapy has been used in the critical care environment as a strategy to reduce anxiety, provide distraction, and promote relaxation, rest, and sleep.[15] The patient is provided with a choice of specially recorded audiotapes and a set of headphones. Usually, music sessions are 20 to 90 minutes long, once or twice daily. Music selections may vary by individual taste, but the most commonly used selections have a tempo of 60 to 70 beats, a simple, direct musical rhythm, and a low-pitched sound with primarily a string composition. Most patients prefer music that is familiar to them.

Humor

A good *belly laugh* produces positive physiological and psychological effects. Laughter can increase the level of endorphins, the body's natural pain relievers, which are released into the bloodstream. Laughter can relieve tension and anxiety and relax muscles. The use of humor by nurses in critical care can help reduce procedural anxiety or provide distraction. Once again, the humor must be compatible with the context in which it is offered and with the individual's cultural perspective. Many nurses report using humor cautiously after they have established a rapport with the individual. Nurses also report that they are able to take cues from the patient and visitors regarding the appropriate use of humor. Patients have reported that nurses who have a good sense of humor are more approachable and easier to talk with. In an effort to incorporate the positive effects of humor into health care settings, some institutions have developed humor resource rooms or mobile humor carts. These provide patients with a variety of lighthearted reading materials, videotapes, and audiotapes. Also included on the cart may be games, puzzles, and magic tricks. Some nurses have created their own portable therapeutic humor kits. Use of humor by patients may help them reframe their anxiety and channel their energy toward feeling better. Appropriate use of humor can relieve stress among critical care nurses who work in complex, challenging environments with significant economic pressures.[16]

Massage and Therapeutic Touch

Massage is the purposeful stroking and kneading of muscles with the goal of providing comfort and promoting relaxation.[17] Nurses have traditionally used effleurage for back rubs for patient comfort. Effleurage uses slow, rhythmic strokes from distal to proximal areas of long muscles such as the back or extremities. Consistent, firm yet flexible hand pressure is applied with all parts of the hand to conform to body contours. Lotion may be used to decrease friction and add moisture. Massage has been effective at reducing anxiety and promoting relaxation.[17] Patient selection is an important consideration when electing massage as a therapeutic intervention. Patients who are hemodynamically unstable, for example, would not be appropriate candidates. In addition, nurses require additional training in massage therapy to effectively incorporate more advanced massage techniques such as petrissage or pressure points into plans of care for critically ill patients.

Therapeutic touch is a set of techniques where the practitioner's hands move over a patient in a systematic way to rebalance the patient's energy fields.[18] An important component of therapeutic touch is compassionate intent on part of the healer. Therapeutic touch as a complementary therapy has been used successfully in acute care settings to decrease anxiety and promote a sense of well-being. It is a foundational technique of healing touch. Healing touch involves a number of full-body and localized techniques to balance energy fields and promote healing.[18] Implementation of healing touch therapy involves a formal educational program for healers, and its potential benefits are under active investigation.

Meridian Therapy

Complementary and alternative medicine (CAM) is a phrase used to describe an array of nontraditional healing approaches. Meridian therapy refers to therapies that involve an acupoint, such as acupuncture, acupressure, and the activation of specific sites with electrical stimulation and low-intensity laser.[19] Meridian therapy originates from traditional Chinese medicine. Meridians are complex energy pathways that integrate into intricate patterns.[19] These pathways contain sensitive energy points that are amenable to stimulation to relieve blockages that affect various physiological functions. Research has demonstrated the effectiveness of meridian therapy for pain relief, postoperative nausea, and other functions. Currently, research is underway to validate acupoint sites. Meridian therapy should be performed only by professionals with specialized training.

Animal-Assisted Therapy

The human–animal bond has been well documented. Pet ownership has been linked to higher levels of self-esteem and physical health. Pet therapy (or, more broadly, animal-assisted therapy) has had measurable benefits for school children and residents of nursing homes. More recently, this concept has been introduced to the acute and critical care settings with positive results. In one California hospital, a formal program exists in which volunteer owner–dog teams visit patients in the hospital on a variety of units.[20] In a small pilot study, Cole and Gawlinski described patients' delight in having fish aquariums placed in their rooms while they were awaiting heart transplantation.[20]

RESTRAINTS IN CRITICAL CARE

Physical Restraints

Historically, physical restraints have been used for patients in critical care to prevent potentially serious disruptions in patient care through accidental dislodgment of endotracheal tubes or life-saving IV lines and other invasive therapies. Other reasons that have been cited for use of restraints include the prevention of falls, behavior management, and avoidance of liability suits due to patient injury. However, research related to restraint use, especially in the elderly, has demonstrated that these reasons, although well-intentioned, often are not valid.[10,21–24] Patients who are restrained have been shown to have more serious injuries secondary to falls as they "fight" the device that limits their freedom. In addition, there are reportedly a greater number of lawsuits related to improper restraint use than to injuries sustained when restraints were not used.[25,26] Critically ill, intubated patients have been known to self-extubate despite the use of soft wrist restraints.[21, 23–24, 27]

The forced immobilization that results from restraining a patient can prolong a patient's hospitalization by contributing to skin alterations, loss of muscle tone, impaired circulation, nerve damage, and pneumonia.[25,28] Restraints have been implicated in accelerating patients' levels of agitation, resulting in injuries such as fractures or strangulation.

Physical restraints include any device that is used to restrict the patient's mobility and normal access to his or her body. These may include limb restraints, mittens with ties, vests or waist restraints, geriatric chairs, and siderails. Siderails are considered a restraint if used to limit the ability of the patient to get out of bed rather than to help him or her get up.[26]

Standards on restraint use are published and monitored by the Joint Commission on Accreditation of Healthcare Organizations (JCAHO) and the Centers for Medicare and Medicaid Services (formerly known as the Health Care Financing Administration). A summary of these standards is given in Box 2-2. These standards may be viewed on the respective agency's website. Many hospitals have revised their policies, procedures, and documentation of the use of restraints to comply with the most recent revision of these standards, effective January 2001.

box 2-2
Summary of Care Standards Regarding Physical Restraints

Initiating Restraints

- Restraints require the order of a licensed independent practitioner who must personally see and evaluate the patient within specified time periods.
- Restraints are used only as an emergency measure or after treatment alternatives have failed. (Treatment alternatives and patient responses are documented.)
- Restraints are instituted by staff who are trained and competent to use restraints safely. (A comprehensive training and monitoring program must be in place.)
- Restraint orders must be time-limited. (A patient must not be placed in a restraint for longer than 24 hours, with reassessment and documentation of continued need for restraint at more frequent intervals.)
- Patients and families are informed about the reason/rationale for the use of the restraint.

Monitoring Patients in Restraints

- The patient's rights, dignity, and well-being are to be protected.
- The patient will be assessed every 15 minutes by trained and competent staff.
- The assessment and documentation must include evaluation of adequate nutrition, hydration, hygiene, elimination, vital signs, circulation, range of motion, injury due to the restraint, physical and psychological comfort, and readiness for discontinuance of the restraint.

Chemical Restraint

Chemical restraint refers to pharmacological agents that are given to patients as discipline or to limit disruptive behavior. Medications that have been used for behavior control include, but are not limited to, psychotropic drugs such as haloperidol, sedative agents such as benzodiazepines (e.g., lorazepam, midazolam), or the anticholinergic antihistamine, diphenhydramine.[29] This definition does *not* apply to medications that are given to treat a medical condition.[29] The use of sedative, analgesic, and anxiolytic medications is an important adjunct in the care of the critically ill patient. Documentation of the use of these medications should include the indication for the drug and the patient's response.

Delirium is a common phenomenon in the ICU and may be related to sleep disturbance, the person's underlying medical condition, the unfamiliar environment, medication side effects, or a combination of these factors. Elderly patients are especially vulnerable. Delirium is a reversible cognitive disturbance associated with confusion, inappropriate behavior, decreased attention span, short-term memory impairment, and altered perceptions.[30] Dementia, however, is generally considered to be a progressive disease associated with mild to severe cognitive impairment.

Care must be taken to provide adequate comfort for patients experiencing life-threatening illnesses and a variety of noxious interventions. It is desirable to use the least amount of medication as feasible to achieve the goals of patient care because all medications have potential side effects and adverse reactions. Patients must be continually assessed for adequacy of comfort. Behaviors that seem to indicate pain may actually indicate a change in the patient's physiological status. Agitation, for example, may be a sign of hypoxemia. Caution must be exercised when using as-needed (PRN) medications to reduce pain and promote comfort. Without consistency in assessment, goal setting, and administration, PRN dosing may inadvertently lead to overmedication or undermedication in the critically ill patient. In addition, these medications can have rebound effects if abruptly withdrawn. Weaning a patient from analgesic or sedative medication may be as important as weaning a patient from a mechanical ventilator. Many CCUs incorporate assessment tools for patient comfort on their daily flow sheets.[30]

Alternatives to Restraints

What, then, is the well-meaning nurse to do when a patient is experiencing confusion or delirium and is pulling at his or her lifesaving devices and tubes? Remember that physical restraint is the last resort, to be used only when the patient is a danger to himself or others and when other methods have failed. Restraints may actually potentiate the dangerous behavior. Rather, the nurse should attempt to identify what the patient is feeling or experiencing. What is the meaning behind the behavior? Is he cold? Does she itch? Is the person in pain? Does the person know where he or she is and why he or she is there? Sometimes addressing the patient's needs or concerns and reorienting the patient is all that is needed to calm him or her. Other interventions may include modifying the patient's environment, providing diversionary activities, allowing the patient more control or choices, and promoting adequate sleep and rest[24,29,31] (Box 2-3).

LOSS AND RESPONSES TO LOSS

The threat of illness precipitates coping behaviors associated with loss. Patients must adjust to the loss of health or loss of a limb, a blow to self-concept, or a necessary change in lifestyle. Dying patients must adapt to the loss of life. All these events require a change—that is, a loss of the familiar self-image and its replacement with an altered one. All losses include at least a temporary phase of lowered self-esteem. Regardless of the nature of the loss, the dynamics of grief present themselves in some form. The response to loss can be described in the following four phases:

- Shock and disbelief
- Development of awareness
- Restitution
- Resolution

Each phase involves characteristic and predictable behaviors that fluctuate among the various phases in an unpredictable way. Through recognition and assessment of the behaviors and an understanding of their underlying dynamics, the nurse can plan interventions to support the healing process.

box 2-3
Alternatives to Physical Restraints

Modifications to Patient Environment

- Keep the bed in the lowest position.
- Minimize the use of siderails to what is needed for positioning.
- Optimize room lighting.
- Activate bed and chair exit alarms where available.
- Remove unnecessary furniture or equipment.
- Ensure that the bed wheels are locked.
- Position the call light within easy reach.

Modifications to Therapy

- Frequently assess the need for treatments and discontinue lines and catheters at earliest opportunity.
- Toilet patients frequently.
- Disguise treatments, if possible (e.g., keep intravenous [IV] solution bags behind patient's field of vision, apply loose stockinette or long-sleeved gown over IV sites).
- Meet physical and comfort needs (e.g., skin care, pain management, positioning wedges, hypoxemia management).
- When possible, guide the patient's hand through exploration of the device or tube, and explain the purpose, route, and alarms of the device or tube.
- Mobilize the patient as much as possible (e.g., consider physical therapy consult, need for cane or walker, reclining chairs, or bedside commode).

Involvement of the Patient and Family in Care

- Allow patient choices and control when possible.
- Family members or volunteers can provide company and diversionary activities.
- Consider solitary diversionary activities (e.g., music, videos or television, books on tape).
- Ensure that the patient has needed glasses and hearing aids.

Therapeutic Use of Self

- Use calm, reassuring tones.
- Introduce yourself and let the patient know he or she is safe.
- Find acceptable means of communicating with intubated or nonverbal patients.
- Reorient patients frequently by explaining treatments, devices, care plans, activities, and unfamiliar sounds, noises, or alarms.

Shock and Disbelief

In the first stage of response to loss, patients demonstrate behaviors characteristic of denial. They fail to comprehend and experience the rational meaning and emotional impact of the diagnosis. Because the diagnosis has no emotional meaning, patients often fail to cooperate with precautionary measures. For example, patients may attempt to get out of bed against the physician's advice, or they may deviate from the prescribed diet and assert, "I am here for a rest!" Denial may go so far as to allow patients to project difficulties onto what is perceived as ill-functioning equipment, mistaken laboratory reports, or, more likely, the sheer incompetence of physicians and nurses.

When such blatant denial occurs, it is apparent that the problem is so anxiety provoking to the patient that it cannot be handled by the more sophisticated mental mechanisms of rational problem solving. The stressor is temporarily obliterated. This phase of denial may be the period during which the patient's resources, briefly blocked by the shock, can be regrouped for the battle ahead. Therefore, stripping away denial may render the patient helpless. Furthermore, although denial has its obvious hazards, it has been associated with higher rates of survival after myocardial infarctions.

NURSING INTERVENTIONS

The principle of intervention consists not of stripping away the defense of denial but of supporting the patient and acknowledging the situation through nursing care.

The nurse recognizes and accepts the patient's illness by watching the monitor or changing the dressings. In these ways, the nurse communicates acceptance of the patient through tone of voice, facial expression, and touch. The nurse must reflect statements of denial back to the patient in a way that allows the patient to hear them—and eventually to examine their incongruity and apply reality. For example, the nurse may say something such as, "In some ways you believe that having a heart attack will be helpful to you?" The nurse can also acknowledge the patient's difficulty in accepting restrictions by making comments such as, "It seems hard for you to stay in bed." By verbalizing what the patient is expressing, the nurse gently confronts behavior but does not cause anxiety and anger by reprimanding and judging. In this phase, the nurse supports denial by allowing for it but does not perpetuate it. Instead, the nurse acknowledges, accepts, and reflects the patient's new circumstance.

When the patient is in denial, the nurse demonstrates acceptance in several ways:

- Tone of voice
- Congruent facial expression
- Use of touch
- Use of reflection of inaccurate statements
- Avoiding joking with patient about serious issues

Development of Awareness

In this second stage of grief, the patient's behavior is characteristically associated with anger and guilt. The anger may be expressed overtly and may be directed at the staff for oversights, tardiness, and minor insensitivities. In this phase, the ugliness of reality has made its impact. Displacement of the anger onto others helps soften the impact of reality on the patient. The expression of anger gives the patient a sense of power in a seemingly helpless state. A demanding manner and a whining tone often characterize this stage and represent the patient's primitive attempts to regain the control that appears to have been lost. However, such behavior often alienates the nurse and other personnel. The patient who does not demand or whine has probably withdrawn into depression because of anger directed toward self rather than toward others. This patient will demonstrate verbal and motor retardation, will likely have difficulty sleeping, and may prefer to be left alone.

During this phase, the nurse is likely to hear irrational expressions of guilt. Patients seek to answer the question, "Why me?" They attempt to isolate their human imperfections and attribute the cause of the malady to themselves or their past behavior. Patients and their families may look for a person or object to blame.

Guilt feelings concerning one's own illness are difficult to understand unless one examines the basic dynamic of guilt. Guilt arises when there is a decrease in the feeling of self-worth or when the self-concept has been violated. In this light, the nurse can understand that what is behind an expression of guilt is a negatively altered self-concept. Blame therefore becomes nothing more than projection of the unbearable feeling of guilt.

NURSING INTERVENTIONS

During the patient's development of awareness, nursing intervention must be directed toward supporting the patient's basic sense of self-worth and allowing and encouraging the direct expression of anger. Nursing measures that support a patient's sense of self-worth are numerous and include calling the patient by name; introducing strangers, particularly if they are to examine the patient; talking to, rather than about, the patient; and, most important, providing for and respecting the patient's need for privacy and modesty. The nurse needs to guard against verbal and nonverbal expressions of pity. It is more constructive and productive to empathize with the patient's specific and temporary feelings of anger, sadness, and guilt rather than with a condition.

The nurse can create an outlet for anger by listening and by refraining from defending the physician, the hospital, or his or her own actions. A nondefensive, accepting attitude will decrease the patient's sense of guilt, and the expression of anger will avert some of the depression. Later, when the patient apologizes for an irrational outburst, the nurse can interpret the patient's need to make this kind of verbalization as a necessary step toward rehabilitation and health.

Restitution

In this stage, the griever puts aside anger and resistance and begins to cope constructively with the loss. The patient tries new behaviors that are consistent with the new limitations. The emotional level is one of sadness, and time spent crying is useful. As the patient adapts to a new image, considerable time is spent going over significant memories relevant to the loss. Behaviors in this stage include the verbalization of fears regarding the future. Often these go unexpressed and undetected because they are unbearable for the family to hear. Furthermore, after severe trauma, which may have resulted in scarring or removal of a body part or loss of sensation, patients may question their sexual adequacy. They worry about the future response of their mates to their changed bodies. The patient probably also questions a new role in the family. Most likely, the patient has a variety of concerns that are specific to his or her lifestyle. Therefore, in the mourning process, such manifestations as reminiscing, crying, questioning, expressing fears, and trying out new behaviors help the patient modify the old self-concept and begin working with and experiencing a revised concept.

NURSING INTERVENTIONS

During restitution, nursing care should again be supportive so that adaptation can occur. Listening to the patient for lengthy periods of time is necessary. If the patient is able to verbalize fears and questions about the future, he or she will be better able to define the anxiety and solve new problems. Furthermore, hearing oneself talk about fears helps put a person into a more rational perspective. The patient may require privacy, acceptance, and encouragement to cry so that respite from sadness can be found.

During this stage, the nurse may have the patient consider meeting someone who has successfully adapted to similar trauma. This measure provides the patient with a role model as a new identity is assumed, which often occurs after the crisis period. Many support groups of recovering people with all types of illnesses and injuries will send someone to support and be a role model for patients and families.

The patient, with appropriate support from the nurse, begins to identify and acknowledge changes arising from the adaptation to illness. Relationships can and do change. Friends may respond differently to the patient who has suffered a permanent disability, causing the patient to believe that the attitudes and feelings of others have changed as a result of the injury or illness.

During this time, the family has also been going through a similar process. They too have experienced shock, disbelief, anger, and sadness. After they are ready to try to solve their problems, their energies are directed toward wondering how the changes in the patient will affect their mutual relationship and their lifestyle. They too experience the pain of turmoil and uncertainty. Nurses must also help the family. By allowing the family to ventilate their repulsion and fear and by showing acceptance of these feelings, the nurse can help the family be more useful to, and accepting of, the patient. Through intensive listening, the nurse provides a sounding board and then redirects the members of the family back to each other so that they can give and receive each other's support. Asserting the normality of untoward feelings also assists with future acceptance, while decreasing guilt and blame.

Resolution

Resolution is the stage of identity change. At first patients may *overidentify* themselves as invalids. They may discriminate against their bodies. Another method patients may use is to detach themselves emotionally from the source of trauma (e.g., a stoma, prosthesis, scar, or paralyzed limb) by naming it and referring to it in a simultaneously alienated and affectionate way. Patients are sensitive to the ways in which health care workers respond to their bodies. A patient may make negative remarks to test the acceptance of the nurse. Chiding or telling the patient that many others share the problem will be less helpful than acknowledging feelings and indicating acceptance by continuing to care for, and talk with, the patient.

As time passes and the patient adapts, the sting of the endured hurt abates, and the patient moves toward an identification as a person who has certain limitations due to illness rather than as a "cripple" or an "invalid." The patient no longer uses a defect as the basis of identity. As the resolution is reached, patients are able to depend on others, if necessary, and should not need to push beyond their endurance or to overcompensate for an inadequacy or limitation. Often, the patient reflects on the crisis as a time of growth or maturation. Such a patient achieves a sense of pride at accomplishing the difficult adaptation and is able to look back realistically on successes and disappointments without discomfort. At this time, the patient may find it useful and gratifying to help others by serving as a role model for people in the stage of restitution who are experiencing their own identity crises.

Unfortunately, the critical care nurse is rarely in a position to observe the successful outcome of resolution. However, it is useful to know the process in order to work with and communicate an attitude of hope, especially when the patient is most self-disparaging.

NURSING INTERVENTIONS

The goal of nursing care during the resolution stage is to help the patient attach a sense of self-esteem to a rectified identity. Nursing intervention centers on helping the patient find the degree of dependence that is needed and can be accepted. The nurse must accept and recognize with the patient that periods of vacillation between independence and dependence will occur. The nurse should encourage a positive emotional response to a new state of modified dependence. Certainly the nurse can support and reinforce the patient's growing sense of pride in rehabilitation. For nurses who have had the experience of successfully working through the process with one person, the challenge is to stand back and allow the patient to move away from them.

case study ■ GRIEF AND LOSS

Mr. Saunders, age 53, was admitted to the ICU conscious but unresponsive to verbal questioning. According to the accident report, a large truck had swerved out of control on an icy road, killing Mr. Saunders' fiancée and injuring him. He had been hospitalized for observation and treatment of chest wounds and blood loss. Mr. Saunders' leg was amputated above the left knee as a result of an injury incurred in Vietnam 30 years ago.

While trying to reach Mr. Saunders' family, the nurse learned that his mother had died of cancer about 1 year ago and that 3 months later his father, suffering from depression, had killed himself. He had one sister who was flying in to see him.

The primary nursing problems were maintenance of ventilation and vital signs, pain control, and immobility. Mr. Saunders remained uncommunicative, although he was tearful. When he did talk, he expressed hopelessness and said he wanted to die. He asked, "Why me, God? What have I done to deserve this?" The Collaborative Care Guide in Box 2-4 focuses on addressing Mr. Saunders' psychosocial problems. ■

SPIRITUALITY AND HEALING

Caring in nursing includes recognition and support of the spiritual nature of human beings. Spirituality refers to the realm of invisible and intangible factors that influence our thoughts and behaviors. This recognition not only includes religious beliefs, but goes beyond them. When people sense power and influence outside of time and physical existence, they are said to be experiencing the metaphysical aspects of spirituality.

Spirituality includes one's system of beliefs and values.[32–34] Intuition and knowledge from unknown sources and origins of unconditional love and belonging typically are viewed as spiritual power. A sense of universal connection, personal empowerment, and reverence for life also pertains to the existence of spirituality. These elements also may be viewed as benefits of spirituality. Spirituality includes the following:

- Religion
- Beliefs and values
- Intuition
- Knowledge from the unknown
- Unconditional love
- A sense of belonging
- A sense of connection with the universe
- Reverence for life
- Personal empowerment

Critical care patients and their families frequently pray for miraculous healing. Miracles of healing, when they are experienced by believers, can be viewed as normal healing

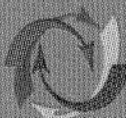

box 2-4 collaborative care guide *for the Patient Experiencing Grief and Loss*

OUTCOMES	INTERVENTIONS
Acknowledging Grief Patient will: ■ Verbally and nonverbally express his grief. ■ Describe meaning these losses have for him. ■ Share grief with another person with whom he is close.	■ Ask patient about his feelings. ■ Listen, reflect, and sit quietly with patient. ■ Acknowledge patient's reaction as a normal, expected response to multiple and severe loss. ■ Acknowledge own feelings to self regarding loss and identify separateness from patient in order not to over-identify with patient and lose objectivity. ■ Enlist other staff to act as resources for nurse and patient. ■ Assess stage of grief related to death of parents, loss of leg, and Vietnam experience. ■ Assess patient's stage of grief in relationship to ability to make sound decisions (i.e., postdischarge psychiatric follow-up). ■ Support denial, as needed to let patient move at own pace in perceiving degrees of loss. ■ Consult psychosocial liaison nurse and spiritual counselor to assist in coping and facilitating appropriate grieving. ■ Avoid the temptation to reduce pain with false reassurance. ■ Acknowledge depth and breadth of loss. ■ Offer hope by letting patient know that time will ease the degree of pain. ■ Acknowledge that the patient has already demonstrated enormous personal strength by surviving the accident and his other losses. ■ Provide hope that he will recover by talking about the future. ■ Provide positive reinforcement for crying and grieving behaviors. ("Don't apologize for your tears; it's very important that you cry as much as you need to express your grief.") ■ Reframe the catastrophic event from a tragedy to the challenge of a lifetime.
Overcoming the Sense of Powerlessness Patient will: ■ Demonstrate a sense of control over his own life by making sound decisions. ■ Experience a decrease in feelings of guilt regarding the collision.	■ Allow patient as many choices as possible. Acknowledge soundness of choices. ■ Question poor choices in a sensitive way (e.g., "You believe that giving up will somehow help you feel better about what has happened?") ■ Allow expression of irrational thoughts (e.g., "I must have done something very, very bad to deserve this."). ■ Reflect back statements emphasizing faulty logic (e.g., "You believe if you had been a better person, you could have controlled someone else's driving and the weather?"). ■ Teach patient about the stages of grieving and emphasize its necessity for health. ■ Refer patient for mental health follow-up care and support.

(continued)

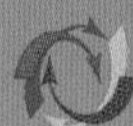

box 2-4 collaborative care guide *for the Patient Experiencing Grief and Loss (Continued)*

OUTCOMES	INTERVENTIONS
Relief of Spiritual Distress Patient will:	
■ Share spiritual belief system with nurse.	■ Ask patient to share religious or spiritual beliefs.
■ Reenlist former spiritual sources of empowerment (e.g., prayer, rosary, icons).	■ Contact appropriate religious or spiritual teacher (e.g., priest, chaplain).
■ Decrease expressions of hopelessness and the wish to die.	■ Ask patient to share other instances of spiritual distress and their outcomes. ■ Place meaningful spiritual or religious items near patient. ■ Use readings of scripture, verse, or stories with patient as he desires. Perhaps engage a friend or family member in this activity. ■ Assess patient for suicide ideation and impulse control. Observe frequently.

events occurring in collapsed time. Nursing goals related to spirituality include the recognition and promotion of patients' spiritual sources of strength. By allowing and supporting patients to share their beliefs about the universe without disagreement, nurses help patients recognize and draw on their own sources of spiritual courage. Recognition of the unique spiritual nature of each patient is thought to assist personal empowerment and healing.

Nurses who find their own spiritual values in religion must acknowledge and respect that nonreligious people may also be spiritual and experience spirituality as a life force. Regardless of personal views, the nurse is obligated to assess patients' spiritual belief systems and assist them to recognize and draw on the values and beliefs already in existence for them.

Furthermore, critical illness may deepen or challenge existing spirituality. During these times, it may be useful for the nurse or family to call on a spiritual or religious leader, hospital chaplain, or pastoral care representative to help the patient make meaningful use of the critical illness experience.

CARE AT THE END OF LIFE

Over half of the two million patients who die annually in the United States will die in the hospital.[35] Most of these patients are elderly. In CCUs, the mortality rate is high, with some estimates as high as 69%.[36] Although the goal of critical care has traditionally been to preserve and restore life, nurses working in ICU will necessarily provide care to patients at the end of life.

Experiences with patients' deaths in the CCU can be viewed on a continuum. There are times when death occurs suddenly and unexpectedly in the ICU, after aggressive resuscitative efforts have failed. Other times, death is expected, even anticipated. In such cases there may be a conscious movement that occurs over time in which treatment goals change from providing aggressive curative therapies to a comfort-focused plan of care. This comfort plan of care may involve withdrawing or withholding specific therapies.

Along this continuum of care, there is a multitude of complex issues and possible scenarios that patients and their families, physicians, and nurses must work through to optimize care of dying patients.

A Good Death

In a study of the experiences of intensive care nurses with end-of-life care, nurses described a "good" death as one where the patient was as pain free as possible and where dignity and comfort were maintained.[35] Another important component was family involvement and satisfaction with care. In caring for patients at the end of life, nurses recognized their important role in communication and continuity of care.[35] Congruence between the patient's (or family's) wishes for care and the level of care that is actually provided is also a determinant of a good death.

Barriers to Care

The landmark Study to Understand Prognoses and Preferences for Outcomes and Risks of Treatments (SUPPORT)[37] revealed several shortcomings of care provided to seriously ill hospitalized patients. Specifically, family members of half of the patients who were conscious at the end of life reported that the patients' last few days were spent in moderate to severe pain. In addition, most of the orders for "Do Not Resuscitate," indicating a transition in the plan of care, were written in the last 2 days of life. Half of the over 4,000 patients in phase I of the study spent their last days of hospitalization in undesirable states—that is, comatose or in an ICU on a mechanical ventilator. In Phase II of the study, specific interventions were undertaken to improve the quality of care at the end of life. These interventions were targeted at enhancing opportunities for more patient–physician interaction, but were not successful in improving the desired outcomes. The authors propose greater individual and societal commitment to enhancing care of the dying, hospitalized patient.

Communication about patient wishes, prognosis, goals, and treatment interventions remains a significant barrier to providing end-of-life care.[38] Only about 10% of Americans have written advance directives.[39] In patients who cannot communicate their wishes, we must rely on surrogates to help us identify patient values, beliefs, and past experiences or verbalizations that may provide clues to their wishes regarding invasive therapies or life support.

Other barriers create difficulties in providing adequate pain relief. Most nurses working in the ICU understand the principle of double effect.[36] This principle acknowledges that providing comfort or pain medications to dying patients may have a side effect of hastening the time to death, but this is preferable to having a patient in pain or distress. In establishing a pain management plan, it is important to implement the plan consistently between nurses and between shifts. Pain consultants may be asked to evaluate the patient for further recommendations and management strategies. Pain may also be a symptom of emotional or spiritual distress.[40] Interventions would therefore be directed at the etiology of the pain or distress and may be culturally based.

Nursing Interventions

COMPASSION

Most nurses recognize the importance of compassion and the development of a trusting relationship as key elements to providing quality care at the end of life. Benner describes death as a human passage[41] where nurses can help patients and families by fostering leave-taking rituals and including the family in decision making and care. Nurses use all of their skills of presencing, caring touch, cultural sensitivity, and patient advocacy to demonstrate their compassion and support in the care of the dying.

COMFORT

Caring for the patient at the end of life in the ICU may be as demanding in terms of nursing time and energy as caring for the critically ill patient who is being aggressively managed.[42] In general, attention is directed at comfort measures: positioning, skin and mouth care, pain and anxiety management, and addressing communication and spiritual needs. Campbell provides a useful manual on caring for the hospitalized patient who is near death.[43] Practical information is provided on giving bad news to patients and families, administering to patients' emotional needs, and forgoing life-sustaining therapy.

COMMUNICATION

Critical care nurses need to be involved in patient–family–physician discussions about treatment decisions and goals of care.[44] At times, physicians will discuss treatment options, including a decision to withdraw or withhold therapy, away from the patient or unit. The nurse may be in a position to understand and interpret patient wishes based on his or her intense contact with the patient. The nurse may also be able to reiterate messages about prognosis and answer patient and family questions based on his or her involvement in the discussions. Consistent, congruent messages are important for maintaining patient and family trust and optimizing satisfaction with care.

Listening well is the cornerstone of effective communication. Although we want patients and families to have realistic expectations of care, we do not want to strip them of their hope. Involving spiritual consultants in the care of dying patients may be useful for patients and families struggling to come to terms with the patient's impending death. Some patients do not want to talk about dying; to do so strips them of whatever hope they hold. Others deal with death in a symbolic way. They speak of "autumns" and "winters" and other subjects that symbolize endings. This is an effective way of terminating one's life; no interpretation is necessary, and to do so would be inappropriate.

Communication is also expressed by the nurse's attitude. Empathy and concern do not need to be expressed in a discouraging manner. Even dying people want to be cared for by a pleasant nurse. A good joke or a smile can be appreciated by a dying patient. Sensitivity to the patient's mood and a sense of timing are useful in assessing a patient's receptivity to lightheartedness.

CONFLICT RESOLUTION/DEBRIEFING

Despite our best intentions and efforts, conflicting emotions and perceptions may exist among patients, families, and caregivers regarding end-of-life care. Many institutions have established ethics committees or have ethical/palliative care experts available for consultation. These experts may be consulted proactively to help resolve a conflict or brought in to review a case for quality purposes. Debriefing after a death in the ICU rarely occurs, but may be a useful strategy for staff to support one another and identify areas for improving care.[35]

clinical applicability challenges

Self-Challenge: Critical Thinking

1. *You are the nurse caring for a patient who is scheduled for a cardiac catheterization in the morning. In report, you are told the patient has been "acting out all day—crying and very emotional." Explore the possible meaning behind the patient's behavior. Formulate an action plan, including additional data that may be needed.*
2. *You observe an elderly African-American woman clutching her Bible to her chest with her eyes tightly shut. She is moving her lips as if in animated prayer. Formulate a nursing plan to provide spiritual support for this patient.*

Study Questions

1. *Anxiety occurs when patients*
   a. *are occupied with internal dialogue.*
   b. *are overly dependent on the nurse.*
   c. *have a long-term recovery ahead.*
   d. *perceive a threat to their well-being.*
2. *The best way to help patients handle anxiety is to*
   a. *reassure them that they will receive the best possible care.*
   b. *assist them to talk about their fears and concerns.*
   c. *be direct and honest with them.*
   d. *limit visitors' time with them.*

3. *The nurse can help provide a sense of control in patients by*
   a. *providing order and predictability.*
   b. *offering as many choices as possible.*
   c. *including them in decision making.*
   d. *All of the above*
4. *Cognitive reappraisal is a technique that allows the patient to*
   a. *identify the stressor and alter the response to it.*
   b. *ignore a threatening stimulus.*
   c. *use guided imagery and progressive muscle relaxation.*
   d. *All of the above*
5. *A positive effect of laughter is*
   a. *a psychological sense of well-being.*
   b. *muscle relaxation.*
   c. *reduced tension.*
   d. *All of the above*
6. *Reassurance will not be valuable for the patient if it*
   a. *calms excessive fears.*
   b. *ceases expression of emotions.*
   c. *decreases respiratory rate.*
   d. *is combined with presencing.*
7. *Denial is a response that*
   a. *is viewed as normal in the early phase of grieving.*
   b. *helps the patient gather emotional resources to deal with problems ahead.*
   c. *is a defense that should not be stripped away by the nurse.*
   d. *All of the above*

REFERENCES

1. Happ MB: Communicating with mechanically ventilated patients: State of the science. AACN Clin Issues 12(2):247–258, 2001
2. Happ MB: Interpretation of nonvocal behavior and the meaning of voicelessness in critical care. Soc Sci Med 50:1247–1255, 2000
3. Stein-Parbury J, McKinley S: Patients' experiences of being in an intensive care unit: A select literature review. Am J Crit Care 9(1):20–27, 2000
4. Hupcey JE: Feeling safe: The psychosocial needs of ICU patients. J Nurs Scholarship 32(4):361–367, 2000
5. Hupcey JE, Zimmerman HE: The need to know: Experiences of critically ill patients. Am J Crit Care 9(3):192–199, 2000
6. Gay S: Meeting cardiac patients' expectations of caring. Dimens Crit Care Nurs 18(4):46–50, 1999
7. Chrousos GP, Elenkov IJ: Interactions of the endocrine and immune systems. In DeGroot LJ, Jameson JL (eds): Endocrinology (4th Ed), pp 571–586. Philadelphia, WB Saunders, 2001
8. Kreitzer MJ, Jensen D: Healing practices: Trends, challenges, and opportunities for nurses in acute and critical care. AACN Clin Issues 11(1):7–16, 2000
9. Tullman DF, Dracup K: Creating a healing environment for elders. AACN Clin Issues 11(1):34–50, 2000
10. Wunderlich RJ, Perry A, Lavin MA, et al: Patients' perceptions of uncertainty and stress during weaning from mechanical ventilation. Dimens Crit Care Nurs 18(1):2–8, 1999
11. Leonard BJ, Plotnikoff GA: Awareness: The heart of cultural competence. AACN Clin Issues 11(1):17–26, 2000
12. Snyder M, Brandt CL, Tseng YH: Use of presence in the critical care unit. AACN Clin Issues 11(1):27–33, 2000
13. Quinn JF: The self as healer: Reflections from a nurse's journey. AACN Clin Issues 11(1):17–26, 2000
14. Tusek DL, Cwynar RE: Strategies for implementing a guided imagery program to enhance patient experience. AACN Clin Issues 11(1):68–76, 2000
15. Chlan LL: Music therapy as a nursing intervention for patients supported by mechanical ventilation. AACN Clin Issues 11(1):128–138, 2000
16. Buxman K: Humor in critical care: No joke. AACN Clin Issues 11(1):120–127, 2000
17. Richards KC, Gibson R, Overton-McCoy AL: Effects of massage in acute and critical care. AACN Clin Issues 11(1):77–96, 2000
18. Umbreit AW: Healing touch: Applications in the acute care setting. AACN Clin Issues 11(1):105–119, 2000
19. Sutherland JA: Meridian therapy: Current research and implications for critical care. AACN Clin Issues 11(1):97–104, 2000
20. Cole KM, Gawlinski A: Animal-assisted therapy: The human-animal bond. AACN Clin Issues 11(1):139–149, 2000
21. Happ MB: Preventing treatment interference: The nurse's role in maintaining technologic devices. Heart Lung 29(1):60–69, 2000
22. Minnick A, Leipzig RM, Johnson ME: Elderly patients' reports of physical restraint experiences in intensive care units. Am J Crit Care 10(3):168–171, 2001
23. Morrison EF, Fox S, Burger S, et al: A nurse-led, unit-based program to reduce restraint use in acute care. J Nurs Care Qual 14(3):72–80, 2000
24. Wilson EB: Physical restraint of the elderly patient in critical care: Historical perspectives and new directions. Crit Car Nurs Clin North Am 8(1):61–70, 1996
25. Elk S, Ferchau L: Physical restraints: Are they necessary? Am J Nurs May Supplement:24–27, 2000
26. Rogers PD, Bocchino NL: Restraint-free care: Is it possible? Am J Nurs 99(10):26–34, 1999
27. Ellstrom K, Padilla G, Doering L, et al: Relationship of self-extubation to outcomes in medical intensive care unit (MICU) patients. Am J Crit Care 10(3):203–204, 2001
28. Johnson R, Beneda H: Reducing patient restraint use. Dimens Crit Care Nurs 18(3):34–37, 1999
29. Driscoll G: Restraints in the acute care setting. Adv Nurs 10–11, December 27, 1999
30. Bizek KS: Optimizing sedation in critically ill, mechanically ventilated patients. Crit Care Clin North Am 7(2):315–325, 1995
31. Brenner AR, Duffy-Durnin K: Toward restraint-free care. Am J Nurs 98(12):16F, 16G–H, 1998
32. Cairns AB: Spirituality and religiosity in palliative care. Home Healthcare Nurse 17(7):450–455, 1999
33. Hermann CP: Spiritual needs of dying patients: A qualitative study. Oncol Nurs Forum 28(1):67–72, 2001
34. Holt-Ashley M: Nurses pray: Use of prayer and spirituality as a complementary therapy in the intensive care setting. AACN Clin Issues 11(10):60–67, 2000
35. Kirchhoff KT, Spuhler V, Walker L, et al: Intensive care nurses' experiences with end-of-life care. Am J Crit Care 9(1):36–42, 2000
36. Puntillo KA, Benner P, Drought T, et al: End-of-life issues in intensive care units: A national random survey of nurses' knowledge and beliefs. Am J Crit Care 10(4):216–229, 2001
37. The SUPPORT Principal Investigators: A controlled trial to improve care for seriously ill hospitalized patients: The study to understand prognoses and preferences for outcomes and risks of treatments (SUPPORT). The SUPPORT principal investigators. JAMA 274:1591–1598, 1995
38. Kirchhoff KT, Beckstrand RL: Critical care nurses' perceptions of obstacles and helpful behaviors in providing end-of-life care to dying patients. Am J Crit Care 9(2):96–106, 2000
39. Levetown M: Palliative care in the intensive care unit. New Horiz 6:383–397, 1998
40. Floriani CM: The spiritual side of pain. Am J Nurs 99(5):24PP–24RR, 1999
41. Benner P: Death as a human passage: Compassionate care for persons dying in critical care units. Am J Crit Care 10(5):355–359, 2001
42. Kaplow R: Use of nursing resources and comfort of cancer patients with and without do-not-resuscitate orders in the intensive care unit. Am J Crit Care 9(2):87–95, 2000
43. Campbell M: Forgoing Life-Sustaining Therapy: How to Care for the Patient Who Is Near Death. Aliso Viejo, CA, AACN Critical Care, 1998
44. Miller PA, Forbes S, Boyle DK: End-of-life care in the intensive care unit: A challenge for nurses. Am J Crit Care 10(4):230–237, 2001

chapter 3

The Family's Experience With Critical Illness

COLLEEN NORTON

objectives

Based on the content in this chapter, the reader should be able to:

- Describe the impact of a critical illness and the critical care environment on the family.
- Describe methods to assess the needs of individual family members.
- Describe nursing behaviors that help families cope with crisis.
- Formulate a plan of care that reflects the needs of the family.
- Discuss end-of-life issues in the critical care environment that have an impact on the family.
- Identify nursing goals and behaviors associated with caring for dying patients and their families.

"There is no one practice against which I can speak more strongly from actual personal experience, wide and long, of its effects during sickness observed both upon others and upon myself. . . . I would appeal most seriously to all friends, visitors, and attendants of the sick to leave off this practice of attempting to cheer the sick by making light of their danger and by exaggerating their probabilities of recovery."

Nightingale, in her 1859 publication *Notes on Nursing*,[1] addressed the profound effect that visitors, family, and friends had on the acutely ill. To approach critical care practice from a holistic perspective, nursing must include a consideration of the patient's family. The interaction between the family/support system and the patient in the critical care environment, and the needs that result from this interaction, remain a challenge and responsibility of the contemporary critical care nurse.

The *Oxford English Dictionary* defines family as "a group of persons consisting of the parents and their children whether actually living together or not; in a wider sense, the unity formed by those who are nearly connected by blood and affinity." For the purpose of this chapter, "family" means any people who share intimate and routine day-to-day living with the critical care patient. Anyone who is a significant part of the patient's normal lifestyle is considered a family member. The term "family" describes the people whose social homeostasis and well-being are altered by the patient's entrance into the arena of critical illness or injury.

This chapter addresses the family in crisis, stressors in the critical care environment, coping mechanisms, and the family and the nursing process. Death and dying is also discussed, with emphasis given to end-of-life issues for both the patient and family.

STRESS, CRITICAL ILLNESS, AND THE IMPACT ON THE FAMILY

A critical illness is a sudden, unexpected, and often life-threatening occurrence for both the patient and the family that threatens the steady state of internal equilibrium usually maintained in the family unit. It can be an acute illness or trauma, an acute exacerbation of a chronic illness, or an acute episode of a previously unknown problem. A family member's entrance as a participant in the life–death sick role of a loved one threatens the well-being of the family and can trigger a stress response in both the patient and the family. The family enters this unplanned situation with its unexpected outcomes and often is forced into the role of decision maker. The astute critical care nurse recognizes that the fear and anxiety demonstrated by the patient and family members is an expected consequence of activation of the stress response, a somewhat protective, adaptive mechanism initiated by the neuroendocrine system in response to stressors.

Studied initially by Selye in 1956,[2] stress was defined as a specific syndrome that was nonspecifically induced. Selye also discussed the role of stressors, the stimuli that produced tension and could contribute to disequilibrium. Stressors can be physiological (trauma, biochemical, or environmental) and psychological (emotional, vocational, social, or cultural). The critical care environment is rich in both physiological and psychosocial stressors that threaten the state of well-being in the patient and family.

In response to a stressor, the "fight-or-flight" mechanism is activated, releasing through the sympathetic nervous system the catecholamines norepinephrine and epinephrine. These hormones are responsible for the increased heart rate, increased blood pressure, and vasoconstriction that comprise the physiological response to the "alarm stage," the initial stage of the general adaptation syndrome to stress described by Selye. The alarm stage is followed by the "stage of resistance," which attempts to maintain the body's resistance to stress. According to Selye's theory, all individuals move through the first two stages many times and become adapted to the stressors encountered during ordinary life. If the individual is unsuccessful at adaptation, or if the stressor is too great or prolonged, alarm and resistance are followed by the "stage of exhaustion," which can lead to death, the result of a wearing down of the human body. It is a challenge to the critical care nurse to assist both the patient and his or her family through this stress response, resulting in an adaptation to the critical care environment. Helping the patient's family resolve the crisis response and facilitate successful coping by creating a safe passage is an identified competency of the contemporary critical care nurse.[3]

After the initial fear and anxiety over the possible death of the family member, other considerations affect the family, including a shift in responsibilities and role performance, unfamiliarity with the routines of the ICU, and a lack of knowledge concerning the course and outcome of the disease. These issues can develop and persist over the duration of the patient's stay in the critical care unit (CCU).

Contributions to the family unit previously attributed to the patient are added to the responsibilities of others. Financial concerns are usually major and daily activities that were of little consequence before become important and difficult to manage. Chores such as balancing a checkbook, contributing to car pools, and shopping for groceries can become critically significant if left undone. This issue requires adding the responsibilities of the patient to the responsibilities of others.

The social role that the patient plays in the family is absent during the critical illness. Comforter, organizer, mediator, lover, friend, and disciplinarian are examples of important roles in family functioning that may be, under normal circumstances, fulfilled by the patient. When that role function is unfulfilled, havoc and grief may ensue.

The circumstances surrounding the nature of the patient's illness can also be a stressor for the family. In a sudden, unexpected event, such as a blunt trauma or an acute myocardial infarction, the life of the family can be brought to a halt in a matter of minutes. Having little or no time to prepare for such an event, the family is overwhelmed with a massive amount of unmanageable stress and can be thrown into crisis. The hospital CCU, in many instances an unknown entity, becomes the center of the life of the family. Such stress often can manifest itself as anger toward the caregiver.

In other instances, the critical event is an acute exacerbation of a chronic but life-threatening illness. Such an episode brings with it a different set of stressors, reminding the family of difficult and painful times in the past when they have faced similar circumstances. Prolonged critical illness can present emotional difficulties for the family, which may increase the likelihood of crisis.

Coping Mechanisms

Coping mechanisms can be defined as an individual's response to a change in the environment; they can be positive or negative. The critical care nurse, as caregiver to both the patient and family, should be aware of the use of coping mechanisms by the family as a means of maintaining equilibrium. A sense of fear, panic, shock, or disbelief is sometimes followed by irrational acts, demanding behavior, withdrawal, perseveration, and fainting. The family attempts to obtain some sense of control over the situation, often demonstrated by refusing to leave the bedside or, alternatively, by minimizing the severity of the illness. Reactions to crisis are difficult to categorize because they depend on the different coping styles, personalities, and stress management techniques of the family. The nurse must be able to interpret the feeling that a person in crisis is experiencing, particularly when that person cannot identify the problem or the feeling to himself or to others. The following are four generalizations about crisis:

- Whether people emerge stronger or weaker as a result of a crisis is based not so much on their character, as on the quality of help they receive during a crisis state.
- People are more open to suggestions and help during an actual crisis.
- With the onset of a crisis, old memories of past crises may be evoked. If maladaptive behavior was used to deal with previous situations, the same type of

behavior may be repeated in the face of a new crisis. If adaptive behavior was used, the impact of the crisis may be lessened.

- The primary way to survive a crisis is to be aware of it.

THE FAMILY AND THE NURSING PROCESS

Nursing Assessment

Nursing assessment by the critical care nurse involves more than an appraisal of the patient. It is also the responsibility of the nurse to include members of the family in order to provide holistic nursing care. The nursing assessment serves as a database on which care of the patient and family can be supported. It includes not only physiological responses, but psychological, social, environmental, cultural, economic, and spiritual reaction. It involves an assessment of verbal and nonverbal behavior, and requires clinical expertise. A thorough nursing assessment guides the formulation of nursing diagnoses. The standards of the American Association of Critical-Care Nurses emphasize and support the importance of an assessment of the family and the continual involvement of the family in the nursing care of the patient.[4]

An important part of the family assessment is a history of the family. Who does the patient include in the description of his family? Although all patients belong to a family, the family might not include or be restricted to blood relatives. Who are the people most upset about the patient's illness? Is there a formal or informal leader identified by the group? This becomes important when communicating with the family in decision making, as well as with legal matters, such as obtaining consent. What is the coping style of the family? Does the family have a history of dealing with a critical illness? What are the relationships between the members of the family? How close is the family? The family history can aid the nurse in interpreting how the family is coping with stress, how their coping mechanisms will affect the patient, and how they are adapting to the patient's illness.

Four intrinsic elements of an assessment of the family include:

1. Providing a human, caring presence
2. Acknowledging multiple perceptions
3. Respecting diversity
4. Valuing each person in the context of the family[5]

Numerous assessment tools are available to aid the nurse in determining the needs and problems the family faces. One of the initial assessment tools was developed by Molter in 1979.[6] This method included a 45-item needs assessment tool, which became an instrument to describe the needs of critical care family members. Leske modified the tool used by Molter by adding an open-ended item and calling it the Critical Care Family Needs Inventory (CCFNI).[7] The CCFNI continues to be used today in nursing research on the needs of critical care family members. Medonca and Warren used the CCFNI to assess the needs of family members and the importance of these needs in the first 18 to 24 hours after admission of the adult patient to the CCU.[8]

Nursing research using these tools reveals consistency in what areas should be assessed with family members. These areas include but are not limited to:

1. Family satisfaction with care given
2. Explanations that the family can understand
3. Honest information about the patient's condition
4. An understanding of why things are done
5. Staff members who are courteous and show interest in how the family is doing
6. Assurance that someone will call the family with any changes

The tools also suggest assessing how comfortable the family is in the waiting room and inquiring about what things could be made better for them. Strong communication skills on the part of the critical care nurse, as well as an atmosphere of concern and caring, help to gather the subjective and objective assessment data and formulate the appropriate nursing diagnoses for the family. Examples of nursing diagnoses appropriate to the family members of a critically ill patient are given in Box 3-1. The nursing diagnosis guides both the nurse and the family in establishing mutual goals. Addressing informational needs reflects only part of the family's adjustment to the critical illness. Nursing interventions should address cognitive, affective, and behavioral domains.[9]

Nursing Interventions

The time spent by the critical care nurse with the family is often limited because of the physiological and psychosocial needs of the patient. Therefore, it is important to make every interaction with the family as useful and

box 3-1 ***Examples of Nursing Diagnoses and Collaborative Problems for the Family With Critical Illness or Injury***

- Altered Role Performance
- Altered Family Process
- Altered Parenting
- Caregiver Role Strain
- Denial
- Spiritual Distress
- Ineffective Individual/Family Coping
- Ineffective Denial
- Decisional Conflict
- Altered Health Maintenance
- Sleep Pattern Disturbance
- Hopelessness
- Powerlessness
- Knowledge Deficit
- Impaired Memory
- Anticipatory Grieving
- Anxiety
- Fear

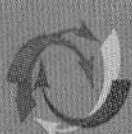

box 3-2 nursing interventions for *Care of the Family in Crisis*

- Guide the family in defining the current problem.
- Help the family identify its strengths and sources of support.
- Prepare the family for the critical care environment, especially regarding equipment and purposes of the equipment.
- Speak openly to the patient and the family about the critical illness.
- Demonstrate a concern about the current crisis and an ability to help with the initial relationship.
- Be realistic and honest about the situation, taking care not to give false reassurance.
- Convey feelings of hope and confidence in the family's ability to deal with the situation.
- Try to perceive the feelings that the crisis evokes in the family.
- Help the family identify and focus on feelings.
- Assist the family to determine the goals and steps to take in facing the crisis.
- Provide opportunities for the patient and the family to make choices and avoid powerlessness and hopelessness.
- Assist the family in finding ways to communicate with the patient.
- Encourage the family to help with the care of the patient.
- Discuss all issues as they relate to the patient's uniqueness, avoiding generalizations.
- Help the family to set short-term goals so that progress and positive changes can be seen.
- Ensure that the family receives information about all significant changes in the patient's condition.
- Advocate the adjustment of visiting hours to accommodate the needs of the family as permitted by the situation in the unit.
- Determine if there is space available in the hospital near the unit where the family can be alone and have privacy.
- Recognize the patient's and family's spirituality, and suggest the assistance of a spiritual advisor if there is a need.

therapeutic as possible. Nursing interventions should be designed to:

- Help the family learn from the crisis experience and move toward adaptation
- Regain a state of equilibrium
- Experience the normal (but painful) feelings associated with the crisis, to avoid delayed depression and allow for future emotional growth

Suggestions for nursing interventions with the family in crisis are outlined in Box 3-2. Considerations for the pediatric patient and the older patient are provided in Box 3-3 and Box 3-4, respectively.

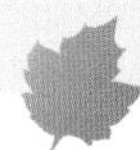

box 3-3

Providing Care for the Critically Ill Child

- Provide parents with accurate, clear, honest, up-to-date information and explanations throughout treatment.
- Consistently involve the family in care and comfort of the pediatric patient.
- Involve the family actively in preparing the plan of care.
- Allow parents open visiting time as well as private time.
- Validate the positive behaviors observed in the parents during their care of the child.
- Respect the parent's right to make as well as change decisions about treatment options for the child.
- Demonstrate the commitment of the nurse to the care and comfort of the child.
- Expose the family to all the members of the health care team, especially when making decisions.

Visitation Advocacy

The use and provision of visiting hours has long been a disputed, misunderstood topic between the nurse and the family. Visiting hours in the CCU were restricted for many years, with the rationale that rest, quiet, and an undisturbed environment were all therapeutic nursing interventions. Families often interpreted these restrictions as being denied access to their loved ones.

As early as 1978, Dracup and Breu reported that satisfying the needs of the families of patients was improved by

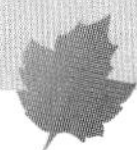

box 3-4

Providing Care for the Critically Ill Older Patient

- Respect the dignity, intelligence, privacy, and maturity of the patient at all times.
- Maintain the patient's right to make decisions as long as possible.
- Avoid the use of paternalism in patient care.
- Integrate the physiological and cognitive changes of aging with the assessment and care of the patient.
- Allow the family to share in the care of their family member.
- Provide active participation and a sense of control for the patient and family.
- Ascertain that the patient remains the focus of care, and that interventions are performed for the good of the patient.
- Assess the impact that medical and nursing interventions play on quality of life and sense of well-being.
- Determine family burden.

relaxing a policy of restricted visiting hours and initiating set communication with patients' spouses.[10] Increased visiting time was seen as a strategy to improve coping skills and strengthen the relationship between nurses and the family members of patients.[11] Over time, many units began the policy of unrestricted visiting hours. Such interventions were designed to strengthen the relationship between the family and health care provider as well as foster adaptation to the crisis on the part of the family. Through nursing research, family presence at the bedside has also been shown to decrease the patient's intracranial pressure (ICP), decrease patient and family anxiety, increase social support for the patient, and give the patient some sense of control over the situation. These findings support the need for less restrictive and individualized visiting policies for patients and families. The focus should be on what proves best for the patient, and not on what is dictated by tradition or nurse preference.

Critical care nurses must take the responsibility for revising visiting hours to meet the needs of patients and families. When choosing a less restrictive policy, the physical layout of the unit must be considered. Smaller units may not be appropriate for unrestricted visiting hours with unlimited visitors. The effectiveness of changes in visiting hours must also be evaluated. Additional nursing research is needed to determine the effect of changes in visiting hours on the needs of patients and families.

Family members should be prepared for the initial visit to the CCU because it can be an overwhelming environment. The function of monitors, intravenous drips, ventilators, and other technologies, as well as the meaning of alarms, should always be explained before and during the family visits. The names, roles, and responsibilities of all members of the health care team should also be identified to both the patient and family. The nurse, by example, can demonstrate the value of communication and touch to the family. Encouraging family members to provide direct care to the patient, if they are interested, can help to decrease anxiety and provide the family with some control. Direct care activities for the family to perform may include brushing teeth, combing hair, helping with a meal, or giving a bath.

Allowing children to visit a CCU may require special arrangements on the part of the staff. Visits should include short, simple explanations to the child concerning the patient's condition. Answering the child's questions in terms that he or she can understand helps reduce possible fears. The person who is escorting the child into the CCU should be aware that invasive monitoring and other equipment might upset a youngster. If a visit from the child is not possible, arrangements can be made for a telephone visit.

Use of the Nurse–Family Relationship

Initiating nursing interventions and establishing a meaningful relationship with the family tends to be easier during crisis than at other times. People in crisis are highly receptive to an interested, caring, and empathetic helper. When first meeting the patient's family, the nurse must demonstrate the desire and ability to help. Help that is specific to the family's needs at that time demonstrates the nurse's interest. Deciding who is to be notified of the patient's status and validating that contact person's telephone number can be an overwhelming task. Assisting the family to determine immediate priorities is essential in the early phase of crisis intervention.

With this type of timely involvement, the family will begin to trust and depend on the nurse's judgment. This process then allows family members to believe the nurse when the nurse conveys feelings of hope and confidence in the family's ability to cope with whatever is ahead of them. It is important to avoid giving false reassurance; rather, the reality of the situation should be expressed in a kind, supportive fashion.

Problem Solving With the Family

As the relationship between the nurse and the family develops from one interaction to another, the nurse is able to begin to understand the dynamics of the problem facing the family. Problem solving with the family takes into consideration items such as:

- The meaning the family has attached to the event
- Other crises with which the family may be coping
- The adaptive and maladaptive coping behaviors previously used in time of stress
- The normal support systems of the family, which might include friends, neighbors, clergy, and colleagues

Using the assessment base, the nurse is able to help the family deal with the stress. Areas to include in interventions are defining the problem, identifying support, focusing on feelings, and identifying steps.

DEFINING THE PROBLEM

A vital part of the problem-solving process is to help the family clearly state the immediate problem. Often people are overwhelmed and immobilized by the free-floating anxiety or panic caused by acute stress. Regardless of the difficulty or threat the problem implies, being able to state it as such reduces the anxiety by helping the family realize that they have achieved some sort of an understanding of what is happening. Defining the problem is a way of delimiting its parameters.

Defining and redefining problems can occur many times before the problem is solved. Stating the problem clearly helps the family assign priorities and direct needed actions. Goal-directed activity helps decrease anxiety.

IDENTIFYING SUPPORT

Under high levels of stress, some people expect themselves to react differently. Rather than turning to the resources they use daily, they become reluctant to involve them. Asking people to identify the person to whom they usually turn when they are upset, and encouraging them to seek assistance from that person now, helps to direct the family back to the normal mechanisms for handling stressful issues. Few families are truly without resources; rather, they only have failed to recognize and call on them.

Defining and redefining the problem may also help to put the problem in a different light. It is possible in time to view tragedy as a challenge and the unknown as an adventure. The process of helping the family view a problem from a different perspective is called *reframing*.

The nurse can also help the family call on its own inherent strengths. What is it as a family that they do best? How have they handled stress before? Encouraging the family members to capitalize on their strengths as a family unit is well worth the effort.

FOCUSING ON FEELINGS

A problem-solving technique emphasizing choices and alternatives helps the family achieve a sense of control over part of their lives. It also reminds them, and clarifies for them, that they are ultimately responsible for dealing with the event and that they will live with the consequences of their decisions.

Helping the family focus on feelings is extremely important to avoid delayed grief and protracted depression in the future. The reflection of feelings or active listening is necessary throughout the duration of the crisis. Valuing the expression of feelings might help the family avoid the use of unhealthy coping mechanisms, such as alcohol or excessive sleep. In difficult and sad times, the critical care nurse can promise the family, with some certainty, that things will become easier with the passage of time. Adaptation takes time.

During the difficult days of the critical illness, the family may become dependent on the judgment of professionals. The family may have some difficulty identifying the appropriate areas in which to accept the judgments of others. It is important that the nurse acknowledges the family's feelings and recognizes the complexity of the problem, while emphasizing the responsibility each member of the family has for his or her feelings, actions, and decisions.

IDENTIFYING STEPS

Once the problem has been defined and the family begins goal-directed activities, the nurse may help further by asking the family members to identify the steps that they must take. Such anticipatory guidance may help to reduce the family's anxiety. The nurse, however, must recognize moments when direction is vital to health and safety. It is often necessary to direct families, for example, to return home to rest. This can be explained by stating that by maintaining their own health, family members will, at a later date, be as helpful to the patient as possible. To make each interaction more meaningful and therapeutic, the nurse should focus on the crisis situation and avoid involvement in long-term chronic problems.

Collaborative Management

The health care providers who most often meet the needs of family members are generally thought to be nurses and physicians. Additional help comes in the form of written materials, other family members, the patient, and other hospital sources. In some cases, nurse-coached hospital volunteer programs have proven to be effective.[12] These programs consist of an inservice program taught by nurses and followed by the assignment of a nurse mentor to the volunteer. Some families benefit by a referral to a mental health clinical specialist, a social worker, a psychologist, or a chaplain. A nurse can best encourage the family to accept help from others by acknowledging the difficulty and complexity of the problem and providing several names and phone numbers. It may be appropriate for the nurse to set up the first meeting, with follow-up meetings coordinated between the family and the consultant. Many CCUs have such resources on a 24-hour on-call basis to ensure prompt interventions. An objective professional with experience in critical illness and its impact on the family can be an excellent resource.

END-OF-LIFE ISSUES IN CRITICAL CARE

The goal of CCUs has long been viewed as assisting the individual to survive a life-threatening physiological process. Integral to that survival is the critical care nurse who, with the assistance of advanced assessment modalities, multiple pharmacological agents, and sophisticated technology, directs the care of the patient and the family. Although healing is the goal, in reality the chance of being a patient in a CCU during the last 6 months of life ranges from 9% to 47%.[13] Approximately 10% of people admitted to the CCU will die there, and 20% may leave the CCU but die before discharge from the hospital.[13,14] The prevalence of debilitating chronic diseases in people older than 65 years offers a challenge to the curative model of today's CCU. This demonstrates the need for the critical care nurse, long focused on curative care, to become proficient as well in the delivery of palliative care.

Four cultural forces that are thought to influence the end-of-life care in CCUs are:

1. Biomedical knowledge as the dominant conceptual framework for understanding old age and death (that is, death has become another disease to be treated)
2. The power of the technological imperative to determine events
3. The incompatibility of lay and medical knowledge
4. An ambivalence about end-of-life goals.[15]

Family members are unprepared for what they see and the language they hear. They are confused and overwhelmed by the decision making required of them, and are unable to transfer medical terminology into lay vocabulary. Critical care nurses can bring an awareness of these issues into their units and into their individual practices.[16]

An important component of palliative care is the inclusion of the family in decision making and the provision of patient care. Families are faced with complex end-of-life decisions that must be made in the unfamiliar CCU. These decisions can be made easier with the involvement of the nurse in facilitating and guiding the decision-making process. The focus of nursing care at the end of life should be the entire family. This is often difficult in acute care units with time and space constraints. Nurses' personal issues, such as previous experiences with the death of their own family members, have the potential either to enhance or threaten assessment and intervention.

Nursing Interventions at the End of Life

Nursing care is an essential component of improving end-of-life care in today's CCUs. Miller and colleagues explored cultural issues influencing end-of-life care and factors that surround the limited involvement of critical care nurses in end-of-life decision making and care planning.[16] Their recommendations for changing nursing practice include:

insights into clinical research

Meyers T, Eichorn D, Guzzetta C, et al: Family presence during invasive procedures and resuscitation. Am J Nurs 100(2):32–42, 2000, and Meyers T, et al: Family presence during invasive procedures and resuscitation: Hearing the voice of the patient. Am J Nurs 101(5):48–55, 2001.

The purpose of this original nursing research study was to explore, both quantitatively and qualitatively, the effects of family presence at the bedside while their loved ones underwent cardiopulmonary resuscitation (CPR) or invasive procedures. Thirty-nine family members and 96 health care providers were surveyed after 43 instances of family presence.

Results of the quantitative analysis revealed that families perceived visitation as a positive experience and that they believed being with the patient was their right. Family presence helped the family members feel like active participants in the care process, and that this met their needs for knowing about, providing comfort to, and connecting with the patient. All the participating families felt that visitation was helpful to them and that they would do it again. Family members who visited with their loved ones during emergency care suffered no ill physiological effects.

The views of the health care providers differed significantly. More nurses and attending physicians supported family presence than residents. Although 88% of the health care providers thought family presence should be continued, 38% expressed concerns about possible disruptions by family members during visits, although no such instances had occurred during the study.

Results of the qualitative analysis identified seven themes. Three of these related to the positive effects that family presence had on patients—it comforted them, provided help, and served to remind providers of the patient's personhood. Two themes involved how family presence reflects the reciprocal nature of the patient–family bonds and the patient's right to have the family present. The remaining two themes characterized how patients perceived the effects of the experience on their families and the health care environment. Patients saw both positive and negative effects on those who were present but felt the benefits to families outweighed the potential problems.

Although the researchers suggest further study on this topic, it was clear that family presence appeared to deliver many benefits, with apparently few drawbacks or adverse effects to patients, their families, and their care providers. As a result of the authors' research, a hospital-wide protocol for family presence during CPR and invasive procedures was approved and implemented in their health care facility.

- Analyzing management of pain and other signs and symptoms
- Evaluating the involvement and support of the patient's family members
- Evaluating protocols for withdrawal of life support
- Developing strategies to involve family members in care planning
- Analyzing the patient's and family's preparation for death

Although end-of-life skills involve life-long learning, indicators that are important for nurses include improved listening skills, attention to the proper environment for end-of-life discussions, and a willingness to facilitate end-of-life discussions.[17]

As stated earlier, open visitation practices are beneficial in CCUs. This is especially true at the end of life. Although restricted visiting hours tend to limit noise and promote patient rest, research suggests that most nurses do not restrict visitation by family members, even where restricting visiting hours are in place.[18]

Caring for a patient's family at any point during the dying process encompasses three major areas: access, information and support, and involvement in caregiving activities. Family members of dying loved ones should be allowed more liberal access in both visiting hours and number of visitors allowed. Ensuring that a family can be with their critically ill loved one will be a source of comfort. Information has been identified as a crucial component in the family's coping, and support in the form of the nurse's caring behaviors is influential in shaping the critical care experience for both the patient and family. Honesty and truth telling are important skills in this emotionally charged time. Finally, family involvement in caregiving, in tasks as simple as being physically present to those as complex as assisting with postmortem care, may help families work through their grief. Facilitation of family involvement is a practical nursing intervention.[19]

After the Patient's Death

The manner in which a family is informed of a death has a significant impact on the grief response. The family should be escorted to a quiet, private room, near the patient's room, which is accessible to other arriving family members. Emotional support for the family at this time is critical. Specific information should also be provided to the family on an ongoing basis. When death appears to be the probable outcome, the family must be notified in a clear, concrete manner. Acceptance of death is facilitated by preparation.

The pronouncement of death requires a caring, empathetic approach. Two health care team members should be identified to approach the family, one to notify the family of the death and the other to offer support to the grieving family. It is important to use the term "death" and to avoid more abstract terms that might lead to anxiety and confusion. A warm, compassionate, honest tone should be used, and the information should be repeated.

The nurse can offer to contact a clergy member. It is important to recognize the spirituality of the patient, and contact with a spiritual advisor should be made. Requests by the family for specific people or cultural rituals after the death should be encouraged and honored.

The viewing of the body is the most difficult time for many family members, second only to the pronouncement of death. Viewing of the body has been found to be beneficial for the family because it makes the loss real, allows family members to say goodbye, and in the case of sudden death, eliminates any question or confusion. Family members should always be given the option of viewing the body and they should be allowed to make this decision on an individual basis. It is important to ask more than once, because family members may change their minds after first declining the offer.

The nurse should prepare the family for the condition of the body and describe the presence of any wounds, dressings, or tubes. The family should be allowed to stay as long as they feel is necessary and to come back and forth and stay at the bedside. Intense emotional reactions sometimes occur and may be a cultural method of grieving. Should this behavior occur, the nurse could compassionately confront the individual and escort him to a quiet place until composure is regained.

After the viewing, a health care team member should stay with the family to help complete the appropriate paperwork, to answer any questions about the patient's death, and to provide brief grief counseling. The family will benefit from a referral to a grief support group. If possible, the family should be escorted out of the hospital. A member of the staff should make a follow-up phone call 24 to 48 hours after the death.

CULTURAL ISSUES RELATED TO CRITICAL ILLNESS

Nursing interventions for the critically ill patient should also include recognition and appreciation of the cultural uniqueness of each individual. In today's diverse society, culture affects the nursing care of patients in many ways—from pain control and visitation expectations to care of the body after death. Critical care nurses must recognize the uniqueness of each individual, and the ways in which that uniqueness affects the needs of the family.

A health care provider in Western medicine often addresses a critical illness as a disease process and focuses on the physical symptoms, the pathology of organ function, or injury to a body part. The patient and family, having a different cultural perspective, may view the illness in a more psychophysiological manner, focusing on the physical, psychological, personal, and cultural ramifications of the illness. In other cultures, the patient's critical illness may be viewed as a curse or disharmony in the universe.

Although it is unrealistic to expect that the nurse should know the customs and beliefs of all critically ill patients he or she cares for, it is not unreasonable to expect some degree of cultural competence. Glass and colleagues make the following suggestions[20]:

- Be aware of one's own ethnocentrism.
- Assess the family's beliefs about illness and treatment.
- Consistently convey respect.
- Request that the family and patient act as guides for cultural preferences.
- Ask for the patient's personal preference.
- Respect cultural differences regarding personal space and touch.
- Note and allow if possible the use of appropriate complementary and alternative medical (CAM) practices.
- Incorporate the patient's cultural healing practices into the plan of care.
- Be sensitive to the need for a translator.

Cultural characteristics such as language, values, behavioral norms, diet, and attitudes toward disease prevention, death and dying, and management of illness vary from culture to culture. Critical illness may be viewed by the family from a religious or spiritual perspective. Astuteness and sensitivity on the part of the critical care nurse ensure that the beliefs of the highly technological, illness-focused health care system will not clash with cultural beliefs in folk medicine, rituals, religious healing, and medicine men.

CONCLUSION

The nature of the critical care environment exposes the nurse to repetitive achievements and losses. It is essential that the nursing staff in CCUs support each other, especially by listening in a tolerant way when a colleague is expressing what might be interpreted as an unacceptable feeling.

Critical care nursing requires concern, compassion, caring, and a quick mind. Many of these talents come with professional maturity and specific educational opportunities as well as supervision from appropriate role models. The intensity of emotion and involvement demanded by a nurse in critical care makes these nurses particularly vulnerable to the "burn-out" syndrome.

Nurses providing crisis intervention for families under stress is an important preventive mental health function. The nurse's knowledge of, and proximity to, the problem allows him or her to act as a first-line resource professional. As a patient advocate, the role of the nurse is to realize and point out that dealing with a psychological crisis in the family greatly affects the recovery and well-being of the patient and decreases the chances for further disequilibrium in the family unit.

clinical applicability challenges

Self-Challenge: Critical Thinking

1. *Mrs. Jones is a critically ill patient with multiple trauma who has been admitted to your unit. She is not expected to survive her injuries. Mrs. Jones' husband, her two children ages 6 and 10, and her parents have just arrived on your unit. Formulate a plan of care that reflects end-of-life issues that will assist the Jones family in dealing with the probable death of their loved one.*
2. *Mr. Ernest is a 73-year-old man admitted to your unit postresuscitation. He has a long-standing history of cardiac disease and collapsed at home after what has been interpreted as a life-threatening rhythm disturbance. Although he received cardiopulmonary resuscitation (CPR), he was unconscious for 10 minutes before the rescue team arrived. His older daughters are fighting over the maintenance of ventilatory support. Discuss how you would help his daughters at this difficult time.*

3. *Mr. and Mrs. Patel are the parents of a critically ill patient on your unit. They are Indian and speak very little English. Describe the criteria you would use to assess their degree of stress and anxiety. How could you be certain that the cultural needs of the Patel family will be met while their child is a patient in your unit?*

Study Questions

1. *To help the family develop a sense of control, the nurse may*
   a. *offer reassurance that the patient is receiving the best possible care.*
   b. *refer family members to a grief counselor or clergy.*
   c. *offer choices for the family whenever possible.*
   d. *all of the above*
2. *Assisting the family members to define or state a problem associated with a crisis is useful because it*
   a. *decreases their sense of understanding of the problem.*
   b. *implies parameters or limits of the problem.*
   c. *denies family members a sense of cognitive mastery.*
   d. *all of the above*
3. *The family enters a crisis under several conditions. Identify the conditions most likely to increase the probability that the family will enter a crisis.*
   a. *An event has lasting consequences for a family.*
   b. *A family's ability to problem solve is inadequate.*
   c. *The equilibrium of the family is disturbed.*
   d. *All of the above*

REFERENCES

1. Nightingale F: Notes on Nursing. London, Harrison Pall Mall, 1859
2. Selye H: The Stress of Life. New York, McGraw-Hill, 1956
3. Curley M: Critical Care Nursing of Infants and Children. New York, Elsevier, Science, 1996
4. American Association of Critical-Care Nurses: Standards of Nursing Care for the Critically Ill. Norwalk, CT, Appleton & Lange, 1989
5. Hartrick G, Lindsey AE, Hills M: Family nursing assessment: Meeting the challenge of health promotion. J Adv Nurs 20:85–91, 1994
6. Molter NC: Needs of relatives of critically ill patients. Heart Lung 8:332–339, 1979
7. Leske J: Internal psychometric properties of the Critical Care Family Needs Inventory. Heart Lung 20:236–244, 1991
8. Medonca D, Warren N: Perceived and unmet needs of critical care family members. Crit Care Nurs Q 21(1):58–67, 1998
9. Naebel B, Fothergill-Bourbonnais F, Dunning J: Family assessment tools: A review of the literature from 1978–1997. Heart Lung 29:196–209, 2000
10. Dracup KA, Breu CS: Using nursing research to meet the needs of grieving spouses. Nurs Res 27:212–216, 1978
11. Stillwell SB: Importance of visiting needs as perceived by family members of patients in the intensive care unit. Heart Lung 13:238–242, 1984
12. Appleyard M, Gavaghan S, Gonzalez C, et al: Nurse-coached interventions for the families of patients in critical care units. Crit Care Nurse 20(3):40–48, 2000
13. Levetown M: Palliative care in the intensive care unit. New Horiz 6:383–397, 1998
14. Kirchoff K, Beckstrand R: Critical care nurses' perceptions of obstacles and helpful behaviors in providing end-of-life care to dying patients. Am J Crit Care 9(2):96–105, 2000
15. Kaufman SR: Intensive care, old age, and the problem of death. Gerontologist 38:715–725, 1998
16. Miller P, Forbes S, Boyle D: End of life care in the intensive care unit: A challenge for nurses. Am J Crit Care 10(4):230–237, 2001
17. Levy MM: End of life care I: The intensive care unit: Can we do better? Crit Care Med 29:56–61, 2001
18. Simon SK, Phillips K, Badalamenti S, et al: Current practices regarding visitation policies in critical care units. Am J Crit Care 6(3):210–217, 1997
19. Davies B: Supporting families in palliative care. In Ferrell B, Coyle N (eds): Textbook of Palliative Nursing. Oxford, Oxford University Press, 2001
20. Glass E, Cluxton D, Rancour P: Principles of patient and family assessment. In Ferrell B, Coyle N (eds): Textbook of Palliative Nursing. Oxford, Oxford University Press, 2001

OTHER SELECTED READING

Azoulay E, Pochard F, Cheveret S, et al: Meeting the needs of intensive care unit patient's families: A multidisciplinary study. Am J Respir Crit Care Med 163(1):135–139, 2001

Baystate Medical Center: A quality improvement approach to meeting the needs of critically ill patients and their families. Dimens Crit Care Nurs 19(1):30–34, 2000

Benner P: Death as a human passage: Compassionate care for persons dying in critical care units. Am J Crit Care 10(5):355–359, 2001

Bijttebier P, Vanoost S, Delva D, et al: Needs of relatives of critical care patients: Perceptions of relatives, physicians, and nurses. Intens Care Med 27(1):160–165, 2001

Bisaillon S, Li-James S, Mulcahy V, et al: Family partnership in care: Integrating families into the coronary care unit. Can J Cardiovasc Nurs 8(4):43–46, 1997

Board R, Ryan-Winger N: State of the science on parental stress and family functioning in pediatric intensive care units. Am J Crit Care 9(2):106–122, 2000

Burr G: The family and critical care nursing: A brief review of the literature. Aust Crit Care 10(4):124–127, 1997

Copstead L, Banasik J: Pathophysiology: Biological and Behavioral Perspectives. Philadelphia, WB Saunders, 2000

Coyle MA: Meeting the needs of the family: The role of the specialist nurse in management of brain death. Intens Crit Care Nurse 16(1):45–51, 2000

Curtis JR, Patrick DL, Shannon S, et al: The family conference as a focus to improve communication about end of life care in the intensive care unit: Opportunities for improvement. Crit Care Med 29:N26–N33, 2001

Fox S, Jeffrey J: The role of the nurse with families of patients in ICU: The nurse's perspective. Can J Cardiovasc Nurs 8(1):17–23, 1997

Jastremski C, Harvey M: Making changes to improve the intensive care unit experience for patients and their families. New Horiz 6(1):99–109, 1998

Johnson D, Wilson M, Cavanaugh B, et al: Measuring the ability to meet family needs in an intensive care unit. Crit Care Med 26(2):266–271, 1998

Lissman I: Maintaining confidentiality and information giving in intensive care. Crit Care Nurs 5(4):187–193, 2000

Mendocona D, Warren NA: Perceived and unmet needs of critical care family members. Crit Care Nurs Q 21(1):58–67, 1998

Offord RJ: Should relatives of patients with cardiac arrest be invited to be present during cardiopulmonary resuscitation? Intens Crit Care Nurse 14(6):288–293, 1998

Quinn S, Redmond K, Begley C: The needs of relatives visiting adult critical care units as perceived by relatives and nurses: Part one. Intens Crit Care Nurs 12(3):168–172, 1996

Roland P, Russell J, Richards K, et al: Visitation in critical care: processes and outcomes of a performance improvement initiative. J Nurs Care Q 15(2):18–26, 2001

Snyder M, Brandt CL, Tseng YH: Use of presence in the critical care unit. AACN Clin Issues 11(1):27–33, 2000

Tin M, French P, Leung K: The needs of the family of critically ill neurosurgical patients: A survey of nurses' and patients' perceptions. J Neurosci Nurs 31(6):348–356, 1999

Waters CM: Professional nursing support for culturally diverse family members of critically ill adults. Res Nurs Health 22(2):107–117, 1999

Wesson JS: Meeting the informational, psychosocial and emotional needs of each ICU patient and family. Intens Crit Care Nurse 13(2):111–118, 1997

chapter 4

Impact of the Critical Care Environment on the Patient

DORRIE K. FONTAINE

objectives

Based on the content of this chapter, the reader should be able to:

- Identify current trends in health care that affect the intensive care unit (ICU) environment.
- Describe the ICU environment in terms of physical and emotional features.
- Explain the role of the nurse in controlling the environment to promote healing.
- Identify five interventions to decrease noise, lights, and frequent interruptions in the ICU.
- Explain the use of music as an intervention to reduce patient anxiety.
- Examine the evidence to support nonpharmacologic interventions to create a healing environment for the patient and family.
- Describe strategies to promote sleep for critically ill patients.
- Identify a process for allowing family presence at the bedside during the patient's end of life.

Critical care nursing practice occurs at the interface of the nurse with the patient and family in an environment that requires humanism and compassion, despite aggressive technology. The challenge to create an environment where healing can occur has historically been difficult. Intensive care units (ICUs) were established for the close monitoring of the sickest patients within the hospital walls. Often this monitoring meant that patients were cared for in close proximity to nurses and each other, with the environmental effects of noise, lights, and frequent interruptions common occurrences. The effect of this environment on the patient has been examined, with some positive and negative factors reported. This chapter reviews these factors and suggests strategies to highlight the positive effects and limit the negative. The nurse is in charge of the environment and the physical and emotional tone in the ICU. Creating an environment where patients feel secure is a major goal.

THE ENVIRONMENT OF THE HEALTH CARE SYSTEM AND THE INTENSIVE CARE UNIT

The ICU is a major component of the health care environment as hospitals are rapidly becoming occupied by older and sicker patients. An example of the expansion of critical care services due to this increased patient demand is the proliferation of progressive care units. The knowledge explosion, technology, and communication challenges all affect the way critical care is delivered. Patients and families have increased expectations for outcomes from critical care even while hospital stays become shorter. Advances in science that expand the knowledge of treatment options have an impact on all providers of health care in hospitals, as patients and families expect care based on the best evidence for proven outcomes. Communication among health care providers and patients through technology will improve treatment and bring new challenges to caring, including the "virtual ICU" or the e-ICU.

Environmental trends include not only the increase in elderly patients, but concern over the growing workforce shortage. The shortage of acute care nurses is an impetus for nurse managers to create a more rewarding work environment and retain experienced nurses at the bedside. Technology can help to limit the effects of a shortage by encouraging efficiency in scheduling, medication administration, clinical decision support, and ergonomics. New technologies should make it easier for nurses to move patients and prevent injuries. Advances in imaging, robotics, and genomics may enable the critical care nurse of the future to place an even greater emphasis on teaching and prevention. Use of personal digital assistants (PDAs) will become the norm for nurses. There will be an increase in data in the critical care environment, and the nurse must function as a critical decision maker integrating complex information. To ensure a safer health care system, strong partnerships between the patient, family, nurses, and other health care providers continue to be critical.

In the e-ICU, intensivists and critical care nurses who are located at an off-site command center use real-time audio and video to monitor patients in critical care units that are miles away. Critical care nurses at the patient's bedside are able to interact with their e-ICU colleagues by telephone and camera. In the year 2000, this scenario became a reality in the first e-ICU. Benefits include a reduction in mortality and morbidity as well as a decreased length of stay. The role of the nurse in the e-ICU environment will evolve and has the potential for keeping older and experienced nurses with strong clinical wisdom in the workforce.

Critical care occurs in an environment where the technology to keep patients alive is ever-increasing and costly. In 2002, there was an estimated $180 billion annual investment for the 6000 ICUs in the United States.[1] New mechanical ventilators, the latest cardiac monitors or intra-aortic balloon pumps, and end-tidal carbon dioxide monitors are just a few examples of technology that raises the total costs of ICU care. Technology-driven ICU care saves lives, but is expensive. Debates regarding who should receive expensive critical care and futility discussions will continue in society as a whole. The quality of ICU care must be examined, however, because expensive care does not always equate with best-quality care or efficient and effective care. Concerns over patient safety will continue to be one of several drivers of change to come in ICU care. These concerns will create improved systems of medication administration, order entry, and documentation, along with other improvements. What will remain a constant in the environment of care is the need for a steady supply of nurses, whether experienced or novice, and other health care workers to replace the aging workforce. Competent nursing leadership that inspires health care providers to incorporate the best evidence to standardize care in ICUs will be another essential component of a cost-effective health care system.

The Intensive Care Unit: Physical Features

"Thus the nurse's attempt to alter the environment through controlling the noise, light and emotional climate at the bedside is always against great environmental odds." (In Benner P, Hooper-Kyriakidis P, Stannard D: Clinical Wisdom and Interventions in Critical Care, 1999, p. 271)

Walk into any ICU and you will find the following common physical features: blinking monitors, ventilators, intravenous (IV) pumps, noise from equipment and the many disciplines talking at the bedside, bright lights, and a rushed sense of pace in a crowded space. Intra-aortic balloon pumps, extracorporeal membrane oxygenation (ECMO) machines, and other sophisticated technologies are increasingly commonplace. Critical care nursing was invented to flourish in this setting, where the most acutely ill and injured receive concentrated nursing care to enhance survival. In the early ICUs of the 1950s, nurses were confronted daily with pain, suffering, and death, while caring for patients in a confined open space.[2] Fifty years ago, ICUs were often a few beds carved out of existing wards in older hospitals that brought the sickest patients to one area. The most distinctive feature of the first ICUs was this concentration of nursing care, and the specialty of intensive care nursing was born. The design of ICUs has changed over the decades and provides a rationale for why care needs for the patient and family have also evolved. The concept of healing environments in hospitals emerged as one where the environment can make a difference in how quickly the patient recovers.[3]

Table 4-1 summarizes the key design features of ICUs from the 1950s to an envisioned future.[4] Common to all these designs is the notion of close observation and rapid intervention. Meeting patient needs through continuous monitoring is the hallmark of all critical care. However, the close monitoring has led to patient complaints of noise, lighting with no day–night distinction, and frequent interruptions of sleep and rest. Intensive care beds were often so close to each other that patients could hear everything happening to the critically ill patient in the next bed. Lack of privacy and fears related to overheard procedures and conversations in the unit created undue anxiety and the potential for physiological instability in vulnerable patients.

The evolution of ICUs has demonstrated increasing use of the precepts of family-focused care. Early units typically had no space for family to visit and visits were not encouraged. A good example of how the structure and function of ICUs has changed is the shift to family-focused care.[5] Emphasis today is on how the design of the ICU can best meet the needs of patients and families as a unit, in spite of the important life-sustaining technology. Although there is no scientific basis for restricting visitors in ICUs, restrictive policies were the norm in the past and seem to remain unnecessarily and cruelly restrictive in many hospitals.[6] Designs that create more room and furnishings at the bedside that encourage the presence of family members

table 4-1 Intensive Care Unit (ICU) Designs

	First Generation (1950s)	Second Generation (1970s)	Third Generation (1980s–Present)	Fourth Generation—Future
Characteristics	Open unit/ward. No partitions except curtains or screens. Nurses' station/desk in center or at the foot of beds. Unit lighting control often on one switch.	Individual rooms or walled cubicles. Rooms often on either side of a hall containing an open nursing station or surrounding an open nursing station on three to four sides (square configuration). Central monitoring. Some units without external patient room windows (increased incidence of delirium). Patient room lighting with separate switch(es) from nursing station. Calendars and clock in patient rooms.	Individual rooms. Folding or sliding glass doors. Rooms often arranged on a semicircle or circle with the nursing station in the center. Some units configured with decentralized nursing stations. Patient room windows with external views/lighting. Increased control of patient room lighting levels.	Individual rooms. Folding or sliding glass doors with privacy curtains/blinds. Circular/pod-shaped floor plan. Increased noise reduction designing. Patient windows with a view of outdoors (natural or contrived). Patient-controlled lighting—artificial and natural. Planned areas for family in patient rooms. Increased use of color and texture in wall, floor, and ceiling coverings.
Advantages	Increased nurses' proximity to patients	Increased patient privacy. Better control of lighting, noise, and infection.	Increased nursing access during high-intensity activities.	Nursing access and availability of high-tech care in a more homelike environment.
Disadvantages	Lack of privacy. Inability to control noise or light. Infection control issues.	Less direct patient access/observation. Less than optimal control of noise and lighting.	Glass doors reduce patient privacy.	

From Fontaine DK, Prinkey Briggs L, Pope-Smith B: Designing humanistic critical care environments. Crit Care Nurs Q 24(3):21–34, 2001, with permission.

(e.g., chairs that can be changed into beds) may serve to welcome families as key partners in healing instead of just visitors.

Signs that welcome family and visitors to the ICU often suggest the philosophy of the hospital and the culture of the unit. Is it a "Stop, Do Not Enter" sign or a "Welcome to the ICU" notice on the door? The more welcoming the ICU is to visitors, the more open the environment will be to a healing culture of care and support.

Patients experience a positive outcome in an environment that incorporates natural light, elements of nature, soothing colors, meaningful and varied stimuli, peaceful sounds, and pleasant views.[3] In fact, research demonstrates less pain medication is needed and a faster recovery may occur when careful attention is given to providing a soothing environment. Hospitals that combine creative design elements with an emphasis on family-focused care are the leaders in creating healing spaces for recovery.

NOISE

Despite third-generation unit design and architecture, the problems of noise and bright lighting have remained a challenge. Beds surrounded by noisy machines and equipment are intimidating to patients, family, and novice nurses in critical care. Noise is an environmental hazard that creates discomfort in a patient. Consequences of noisy environments include disrupted sleep, impaired wound healing, and activation of the sympathetic nervous system. Moderate noise levels may produce vasoconstriction. Hyperarousal due to noise can occur over many days to even weeks for patients with prolonged ICU stays.

Patient complaints include listening to banging noises, alarms going off at all times, water sounds (such as the bubbling of chest tubes), and doors opening and closing. Sources of noise include equipment, alarms, telephones, televisions, ventilators, and staff conversations. Health care providers are often unaware of the loudness of their conversations and the irritation they may create in the minds of patients. Individuals differ in their perceptions of noise as irritating; therefore, an objective assessment of the environment should be performed by the nurse.

Noise is measured in decibels using a logarithmic scale. An increase of 10 decibels makes a sound seem twice as loud. Sleep occurs best below 35 decibels. The Environmental Protection Agency (EPA) recommends unit noise be less than 45 decibels during the day and 35 decibels at night. Numerous studies measuring noise levels in the ICU demonstrate consistent elevations as high as 80 to 90 decibels. New technology can be an additional source of noise, although several manufacturers attempt to provide equipment that lowers the total unit volume of sound.

Decades of studies consistently point to noise as a key aspect of the ICU environment. Noise was measured in two ICUs using a sound meter placed at the head of a patient's bed.[7] Over 50% of the noise in the environment was attributed to human behavior, with a mean sound level in the medical ICU of 84 decibels. Television and talking were some of the most frequent disruptive sounds for patients. Another study investigated the perceptions of 203 patients who filled out a questionnaire on discharge from the ICU and found that noise from talking and alarms was the most disruptive to sleep.[8] Sound peaks greater than 80 decibels are common in ICUs and are directly related to arousals from sleep.[9] Noise levels in ICUs have remained fairly unchanged despite the evolution of unit design.

LIGHTS AND COLOR

Light is a powerful zeitgeber, or environmental synchronizer, that assists in entraining sleep by promoting the normal circadian cycle of sleep and wakefulness. Many critical care settings could benefit from more natural lighting and lights that are lowered during normal sleep times. In addition to natural lighting, providing a soothing view for the patient to look on instead of the ceiling or a hospital curtain may foster recovery. A classic study found that when a patient had a view of natural scenery and the outdoors, as opposed to viewing a brick wall, less pain medication was used and the hospital stay was shorter.[10] Other studies have demonstrated that impaired cognition occurs more often in windowless units than in those with windows.[11]

In the hospital setting, artificial light is provided by fluorescent bulbs and tubes. This creates a harsh type of light that leads to visual fatigue and headaches, if unshielded. Glare can occur when light is reflected off environmental surfaces such as glass, shiny metal, mirrors, and enameled or polished finishes. Any glare is especially troublesome to the elderly. Bright lights may be left on for many hours in ICUs, even when no direct patient care is being performed. Lack of control over artificial lighting is a source of frustration to critical care patients.

Interruptions in normal light–dark patterns can disrupt normal physiological processes. For example, artificial light exposure for as little as 20 minutes during a normal sleep cycle caused a drop in melatonin levels.[12] In addition, constant lighting and high-intensity light can lead to a complete disruption of the normal melatonin concentration rhythm. This has important implications in the critical care setting because melatonin facilitates sleep and modulates corticosteroid and thyroid hormone levels.[13]

In the future, the ideal ICU environment will have windows with natural views, soothing artwork, and calm colors.[14] The nurse and other health care providers will have access to work and computer stations with glass soundproof partitions that permit proximity to the patient (for easy observation) while shielding the patient from noise. Equipment will be selected for its low noise level. Stress created by unnecessary noise and light will be diminished for the good of the patients, family, and staff. This vision may already be a reality in some institutions. For example, muted colors of beige, blue, and green were used to design a holistic nursing unit in a Minnesota Hospital.[15] Art on the walls depicts many different cultures and the peacefulness of nature. This goal of a more peaceful, healing ICU environment is possible to attain.

The Intensive Care Unit: Emotional Features

The emotional features of the ICU environment are as critical as the physical elements, and may be even more important to patient outcomes. These elements include the symptoms evoked in patients by a stay in the ICU as well as the communication patterns of all who provide care in this stressful unit. Even for one-time visitors to an ICU, the overwhelming sense of the place can be fear-evoking. The ICU environment creates a sense of vulnerability because of physical and emotional dependency,[16] lack of information, and depersonalized care that fosters fear and anxiety.

PATIENT RECOLLECTIONS OF THE INTENSIVE CARE UNIT

In a review of 26 studies of patient experiences in ICUs, the positives noted were a sense of safety and security promoted by nurses, while impaired cognitive functioning and problems with sleep, pain, and anxiety were negative factors.[11] Patients reported a lack of privacy, loneliness, fear, and uncertainty. Pain is a common experience of most critically ill patients despite the ability to control pain with a combination of powerful narcotics and nonsteroidal agents. Lack of control of the environment is a major stressor for patients who often complain that they "just need to sleep." In fact, pain and anxiety promote sleep deprivation and a vicious cycle develops where sleep deprivation worsens perceived pain, with anxiety driving further sleeplessness. McKinley and colleagues state that this lack of sleep and rest contributes to fear and anxiety in patients, as noted in their analysis of the results of interviews of 14 former ICU patients.[16] "Vulnerability decreased when patients were kept informed of what was occurring while in ICU, received care that was personalized to their individual needs, and when their families were present."[16] In a study of 45 ICU patients interviewed during their hospitalization, it was noted that the overwhelming patient need was to feel safe.[17]

One of the major stressors of the environment for ICU patients is the endotracheal tube and mechanical ventilation. Rotondi and colleagues studied the stressful experiences of 150 patients who received mechanical ventilation for more than 48 hours.[18] Many did not remember the experience, but for those who did, the top stressors they recalled were trouble speaking, being thirsty, feeling tense, not being in control, difficulty swallowing, loneliness, and nightmares. Other studies report that patients receiving mechanical ventilation complain of pain during suctioning, sore throat, and feeling as if they are choking. Patients who have experienced the inability to communicate due to the endotracheal or tracheostomy tube have special fears when the basic inability to tell someone what is needed (such as, "I can't breathe") disappears. Even when a communication system is established between nurse and patient, a patient often limits the communication to essentials (e.g., "I hurt") with no discussions of fears regarding prognosis, recovery, or disability. The ability to connect with patients on this human level despite technology is a standard of excellence in critical care practice. The nurse has a special role here in what Patricia Benner refers to as "taming the technology."[19]

One classic account of a physician's recollections of his ICU stay, during which he spent 31 days on the ventilator, highlighted the importance of the nurse in the environment: "The patient lives in a very circumscribed world. Accordingly, everyone who enters his day assumes a magnified role . . . it is the nurse with whom the patient literally lives his day, who is really the most important of all."[20] He and others have noted that although technical competence is essential, the caring of the nurse at the bedside is paramount to healing.[20] Assessing and treating or preventing distressing symptoms experienced by patients in the ICU is the reason for critical care nursing.

Identifying the emotional features and responses to the ICU environment is critically important because many are amenable to nursing interventions. The first step is awareness and understanding of the paradox in the ICU environment. The hostile environment must become a healing place for patients, families, and nurses. The nurse needs to have a good understanding of the environment and the potential havoc it can play on a patient's already compromised physiological and emotional status. Turning a potentially hostile environment into one of healing is a challenge for all critical care nurses.

COLLABORATION AND COMMUNICATION

The emotional tone of the environment is often set by the degree of collegiality, collaboration, and caring for one another exhibited by the entire health care team. Patients literally live and die by the degree to which physicians and nurses communicate about the patient.[21] Attention to organizational structures that foster this collaboration and equal partnership between the physician and nurse as coleaders of the unit is essential. Creating a culture where respectful communication occurs between all members of the health care team is a standard of excellence that is an essential ingredient to all environments of healing. Novice nurses need to learn and practice patient advocacy skills during bedside clinical rounds in the ICU. The manner in which families are treated and respected as full partners in care is a key measure of the emotional tone and positive culture in an ICU.

ASSESSMENT OF THE PATIENT–ENVIRONMENT INTERFACE

Together, the ICU environment and the patient's critical illness create responses of anxiety, confusion, agitation, pain, and sleeplessness. Without appropriate anticipation and accurate assessment of these distressing patient responses, management strategies cannot be designed. The nurse must stay attuned to the environment and assess the patient. The nurse assesses for factors from the simple (e.g., is the room too cold or too hot as perceived by the patient?) to the complex (e.g., how can the patient best sleep with physical pain due to multiple fractures from a traumatic vehicle crash and simultaneously endure the emotional pain from the loss of his wife and child in the same accident?). These examples and other situations like them are critical assessments the nurse must be prepared to initiate.

Anxiety Assessment

Anxiety is the psychophysiological signal that the stress response has been initiated. Because intense anxiety can create further morbidity in vulnerable patients, the ability to assess anxiety is important. Patients experience anxiety as a result of the interface of the illness with the ICU environment. Over 70% of ICU patients experience anxiety. A survey of 2500 members of the American Association of Critical-Care Nurses (AACN) found that five of the most important clinical indicators of anxiety are agitation, increased blood pressure and heart rate, the patient's verbalization, and restlessness.[22] This is problematic because physiological and behavioral signs may underestimate the degree of anxiety. Anxiety is an uncomfortable feeling that precedes these outward signs. Efforts to develop a comprehensive anxiety assessment tool are under way. The best assessment method is asking the patient specific questions about his or her anxiety and fears. For example, the patient may be afraid of dying, although no one even asks the question or offers support. Fear of the unknown creates anxiety; therefore, communicating and establishing a strong relationship is essential. Anxiety often prevents restful sleep from occurring.

Sleep Assessment

Sleep is composed of two very distinct types of brain activity: rapid eye movement (REM) sleep and non-REM sleep. A description of these sleep stages can be found in Box 4-1. Patients progress through sleep stages in a specific order, from a light stage to a deeper stage, in 90-minute cycles. REM sleep increases later in the normal nighttime sleep patterns of most individuals.

Although sleep patterns are very individual, most patients can tell when they feel rested and have had a "good night's sleep." Unfortunately, this is a rare occurrence in the hospital. Sleep, once thought to be a quiescent state, actually involves physiological activation while the brain and body rejuvenate themselves. Sleep is often appreciated only when it has been "lost" and is typically taken for granted by health care providers, who often do not make sleep a priority for patients.

Sleep deprivation in ICU patients can have cumulative effects and lead to altered cognition, confusion, impaired wound healing, and the inability to wean from the ventilator owing to muscle fatigue and carbon dioxide retention. Promotion of sleep for patients is therefore not only a humanistic intervention but can be a life-sustaining one as well.

The complex brain biology that enables sleep to occur is not fully understood. Melatonin, synthesized from tryptophan, is secreted by the pineal gland, and this is inhibited by light and stimulated by darkness. It is easy to see how melatonin secretion could be out of normal rhythm in an ICU setting. In fact, septic patients in an ICU are likely to have disrupted melatonin secretion not linked to the normal circadian pattern.[23]

Sleep in patients with critical illness is greatly disrupted. In over three decades of research, patients in ICUs have been noted to have frequent awakenings, little to no REM sleep, shorter total sleep time than at home, and perceived poor quality of sleep.[24] This poor sleep pattern

box 4-1
Stages and Characteristics of Sleep

1. Transitional stage between wakefulness and sleep
   Relaxed state where person is somewhat aware of surroundings
   Involuntary muscle jerking that may waken the person
   Normally lasts only minutes
   Easily aroused
   Constitutes only about 5% of total sleep
2. Beginning of sleep
   Arousal occurs with relative ease
   Constitutes 50% to 55% of sleep
3. Depth of sleep increased and arousal increasingly difficult
   Constitutes about 10% of sleep
4. Greatest depth of sleep (*delta sleep*)
   Arousal from sleep difficult
   Physiological changes in the body—slow brain waves on electroencephalogram; decreased pulse and respiratory rates; decreased blood pressure; relaxed muscles; slow metabolism and low body temperature
   Constitutes about 10% of sleep
5. Sleep with vivid dreaming (REM)
   Rapid eye movement, fluctuating heart and respiratory rates, fluctuating blood pressure
   Skeletal muscle tone lost
   Most difficult to arouse
   Duration of REM sleep increased with each cycle and averages 20 minutes

Adapted from Taylor C, Lilias C, LeMone P: Fundamentals of Nursing: The Art and Science of Nursing Care (4th Ed). Philadelphia, Lippincott Williams & Wilkins, 2001.

insights into clinical research

Olson DM, Borel CO, Laskowitz DT, et al: Quiet time: A nursing intervention to promote sleep in neurocritical care units. Am J Crit Care 10(2):74–78, 2001.

Nurses at Duke University Medical Center wanted to see the effect of nursing care on improving sleep. So they turned off all the lights twice a day for quiet time and arranged care so that patients were left undisturbed in a dark, quiet environment. Here is what happened:

This study examined a protocol for a quiet time in a neurocritical care unit to see if it helped patients to achieve sleep. A total of 239 patients were observed; 118 patients were in the control group and 121 received the intervention. The intervention was the implementation of a "quiet time" where environmental sounds and lights were decreased between 2 AM and 4 AM and from 2 PM to 4 PM. Data on sleep, light, and noise levels were collected at 2:45 AM, 3:30 AM, 2:45 PM, and 3:30 PM on all patients with a Glasgow Coma Scale score greater than 10.

Results demonstrated that the percentage of patients observed asleep was significantly higher during the months of the "quiet time" intervention than during the control period.

It was concluded that a concentrated effort by staff to reduce the environmental stimuli at intervals definitely increased the likelihood of sleep in these patients.

Comment: According to the staff who worked on the study, "You really have to work and plan your work time around quiet time. You have to prioritize and plan. The culture is geared to 'I have to get my work done' but now we are focusing more on the patient and trying to provide more patient-centered care. It is odd that such a simple idea can seem so revolutionary." (Green MA: Shhhhh! It's quiet time. Inside DUMC 8[1]:1999.)

is true across all age groups, from the elderly to pediatric patients.[25] The impact of sleep disruption on the clinical outcome of ICU patients is not fully known. However, patients often report that sleep disruption is the most unpleasant aspect of their illness.

The patient's own report of sleep quality is the best measure of sleep adequacy. Similar to pain assessment, only the individual can make the assessment: "I slept well or I didn't sleep at all." Monitoring brain waves by polysomnography is the gold standard for measuring patient sleep, but is not feasible as a standard measure in the ICU. If self-report of sleep is unobtainable, systematic observation of patients by nurses has been shown to be valid and reliable.[26] In addition, a visual analog scale is recommended for select patients at high risk for sleep disruption owing to extended stay in the ICU.[27]

Delirium Assessment

Delirium is an underrecognized brain dysfunction in critical care. The syndrome can be facilitated by an ICU environment or illness that limits mobility and produces sleep deprivation and sensory overload with a lack of meaningful verbal or cognitive stimulation. Delirium is a clinical diagnosis based on the patient's behavior. Box 4-2 identifies the key differences between many psychological syndromes in critically ill patients, which can range from agitation to confusion, delirium, and dementia. Agitation is a common occurrence in patients on mechanical ventilators and, when not adequately assessed and treated, may lead to patient-initiated device removal or unplanned extubations.[28] In one study, significant agitation in patients was documented 2 hours before the patient removed tubes and devices. Ten patients removed a total of 42 devices during their hospital stays, demonstrating that agitation is a distressing symptom to patients and clinicians.[28]

A delirium assessment scale, the Confusion Assessment Method for the ICU (CAM-ICU), has shown promise as a method to accurately assess this complex syndrome in a variety of patients.[29] Appropriate sedation can be provided once assessment is accurately made.

The term "ICU psychosis" should no longer be used. Experts caution against using this term for two reasons. First, agitation or delirium, not psychosis, is what is usually meant by this term. Second, the patient, not the ICU, has the symptoms.[30]

box 4-2
Cognitive Syndromes

Anxiety: Sustained state of apprehension in response to a real or perceived threat; associated with motor tension, increased sympathetic activity, and vigilance scanning.

Delirium: Reversible organic mental syndrome of global mental impairment that can result from severe medical illness and may be manifested as random, purposeless movement, fragmented thought processes, or both; can fluctuate in severity in minutes and may be worse at night. *Think:* rapid onset, clouded consciousness, bewildered or confused, often fluctuating, and worse at night.

Agitation: Excessive, usually nonpurposeful motor activity associated with internal tension; may be accompanied by anxiety, panic, depression, delusions.

Psychosis: Persistent, bizarre, but often well-organized and consistent thought processes without organic cause. *Think:* hallucinations, delusions, impaired reality testing, inappropriate mood and impulse control, no clouding of consciousness.

Confusion: A feature of delirium resulting in an altered state of consciousness, and characterized by deficits in attention, memory, and executive functions. *Think:* disturbed orientation with respect to person, place, and time.

Dementia: Development of a state of generalized cognitive deficits in which there is a deterioration of previously acquired intellectual abilities, usually developing over weeks and months. *Think:* gradual onset, intellectual impairment, memory disturbance, personality and mood changes, with no clouding of consciousness.

Adapted from Harvey M: Managing agitation in critically ill patients. Am J Crit Care 5:7–16, 1996, p 8; and Ely EW, Siegel MD, Inouye SK: Delirium in the intensive care unit: An under-recognized syndrome of organ dysfunction. Semin Respir Crit Care Med 22:115–126, 2001, p 116.

The Vicious Cycle: Anxiety, Pain, and Sleeplessness

Patients have multiple reasons for anxiety in ICUs. Patients may be worried about a diagnosis, prognosis, treatment plan, finances, loneliness, or disturbing dreams. Pain leads to anxiety and inability to sleep. Sleep is also disrupted by environmental factors, including noise and bright lights that disrupt the natural light–dark rhythm. Sleeplessness may make the perception of pain seem that much worse. It is important to recognize this cycle because the nurse has the ability to intervene and promote resolution of the cycle and healing. Sleeplessness increases patient vulnerability.[16] Oncology patients in an ICU setting reported multiple distressing symptoms, including unrelieved, excruciating pain, anxiety, and sleep disturbance.[31]

CREATING A HEALING INTENSIVE CARE UNIT ENVIRONMENT

The nurse in the ICU is referred to as an "environmental activist"[32] and a "tamer of technology."[19] To create a positive, healing environment for family-focused care, strategies that are directed toward titrating the environmental stimuli, ensuring the comfort of the patient and family members, and fostering collaboration and communication must be pursued. The environment and the technology can be "tamed."

By controlling excessive noise and lighting, providing nonpharmacologic approaches to alleviating anxiety, and promoting sleep, the nurse demonstrates care and compassion. Actions such as turning a piece of noisy equipment away from the patient's ear, lowering a light, massaging a back, or pulling a chair up close to the bedside for a family member suggest to the patient and his or her family members, "You are the reason this unit exists; we are partners in your healing." Scientific evidence is increasingly demonstrating that many of these approaches will work to provide improved patient outcomes, indicating that they are more than just "nice to do." Two good examples include providing back massage and instituting quiet times; both of these actions increase sleep in ICU patients.

Controlling Excessive Noise and Lights

Because noise may be the most aversive effect of the ICU environment, efforts need to be directed to limiting the sounds of the ICU. Paying attention to the behavior of health care providers is the key to noise control. Behavior modification programs have had positive effects on altering the routines of staff related to noise in the ICU setting.[7,33] Using headsets for patients, making periodic assessment of noise through noise level monitors, and selecting sound-absorbent surface coverings in the ICU are recommended interventions. One of the simplest interventions is turning off unused equipment.

Natural lighting is desirable but should not be so intense that it is uncomfortable to patients. The use of slightly tinted or reflective glass can effectively reduce glare and heat production from natural sunlight.[34] Vertical blinds and other window treatments can enable the nurse to adjust light intensity as desired by the patient. Interventions to eliminate the negative effects related to disruptions in natural light include the incorporation of windows or skylights in patient rooms or their proximate vicinity.[34] The maximum intensity of light used at night should be 6.5 foot-candles for continuous lighting and 19 foot-candles for lighting used for short periods. Again, the simplest intervention may be to turn down lights that are not needed for direct observation of patients. Asking a patient about his or her lighting preference is another important strategy.

Using Nonpharmacological Therapies

Interest in complementary therapies such as relaxation, guided imagery, massage, and meditation has increased owing to the 1993 finding that over one third of all Americans use these therapies and others (such as chiropractic interventions and acupuncture) without telling their health care providers. Ten years later, this percentage has doubled, with billions of dollars spent on complementary therapies each year. Because positive results with the use of these therapies are becoming increasingly common in healthy individuals and those with illness and injury, the nurse assesses patient readiness and provides the opportunity to use alternative, nonpharmacological techniques such as relaxation, guided imagery, and music therapy.

Although sedation of patients is often indicated in the ICU, it does not have to be a first choice for all patients.[35] Complementary therapies such as relaxation and music therapy "complement" other treatment modalities (such as sedative agents) and may also negate the need for drugs or at least lower the dose required. Knowing the patient as an individual and assessing how stress was dealt with before admission can give the nurse clues as to whether this patient would be a good candidate for alternative therapy. When patients become critically ill, they should continue to use what has worked for them in the past in terms of stress reduction.

Music therapy is one example of a nonpharmacological treatment for reducing the stress and anxiety of critically ill patients. Music therapy is defined as the use of music in a therapeutic manner to promote patient well-being.[36] The use of music decreases stress and anxiety, as evidenced by cardiovascular parameters in patients with acute myocardial infarction, those who are recovering from cardiac surgery, and those on mechanical ventilators.[36–38] To begin to use music therapy, the ICU needs to have the equipment, including earphones, a variety of relaxing tapes for patients to choose, and tape or compact disk (CD) players. Music relaxes patients as body rhythms are entrained. Reductions in heart rate, blood pressure, and breathing patterns suggest the efficacy of music in achieving relaxation. Music therapy is not just turning on a patient's radio and leaving the room. It is thoughtfully working with a patient, and suggesting to him or her that listening to music on headphones in a darkened room with no interruptions can facilitate the relaxation response.

Promoting Sleep

Despite three decades of research into reasons why patients do not sleep in the ICU, little is done to facilitate what patients often rate as their number-one priority: sleep. Box 4-3 outlines strategies that are most often recommended to promote sleep. The challenging environment dictates that the nurse is first sensitive to the patient's needs and attuned to the environment, and then has the tools and resources to try both new and old ideas to aid sleep. An old idea is the 5-minute back rub. A newer idea is using music therapy, previously described.

The concept of using back massage to ease patients to sleep seems intuitive; however, it was not systematically studied until recently. In a study of 69 patients in an ICU, a 5-minute slow back massage (or *effleurage*) promoted increased sleep by 1 hour, compared with a control group.[39] If back massage was a hypnotic medication, it would be routinely ordered for ICU patients. The effective back rub was not the cold application of lotion and a quick one-handed massage while holding the patient on his side with the other hand. These powerful results came from a soothing slow-stroke massage, where the nurse first centered herself to be truly present with the patient.

One promising intervention is using a sleep protocol to institutionalize the importance of sleep,[40] block sleep times, and truly control the environment. The role of the nurse as a gatekeeper to protect patient sleep time will be harder to fulfill as patient–nurse ratios escalate, but must remain a priority.[41] According to the 2002 clinical practice guidelines for sedatives and analgesics in the critically ill adult, written by a multidisciplinary team of physicians, pharmacists, and nurses, sleep promotion should include optimization of the environment and nonpharmacologic methods to promote relaxation, with adjunctive use of hypnotics.[42]

Sleep of the health care provider is also an important aspect of the healing dyad in the ICU. Nurses who work nights are routinely sleep-deprived and may have young children to care for at home or school to attend when the next day begins. Antidotes for working at night include scheduling of shifts to phase-advance the sleep

box 4-3 nursing interventions for *Promoting Sleep*

- Provide large clocks and calendars.
- Block sleep times.
- Provide a quiet time.
- Have the patient use earplugs.
- Assess sleep time and quality of sleep by asking the patient when possible.
- Provide opportunity for music therapy.
- Provide a 5-minute backrub before sleep.
- Consider using white noise or ocean sounds.
- Eliminate pain.
- Position patient for comfort with pillows.
- Stop the practice of bathing patients in the middle of the night for the convenience of the nursing staff.
- Titrate environmental stimuli: turn down lights, turn down alarms, and decrease noise from television and talking.
- Evaluate the need for nursing care interruptions.
- At bedtime, provide information to lower anxiety. Do a review of the day and remind patient of progress made toward recovery, then add what to expect for the next day.
- Institute "PM Care" back to basics, brushing teeth, washing face before "bedtime."
- Allow family to be with the patient.
- Use relaxation techniques and guided imagery.
- Ensure patient privacy: close door or pull curtains.
- Post sign at designated times: "Patient Sleeping."

cycle (i.e., going from days to evenings to nights), eating healthy snacks, using bright lights during a shift away from patient rooms, and obtaining regular exercise.[41] Compassionate caring includes the nurse caring for self to meet better the demands of patients, families, and colleagues.

Family Visiting

Families of critically ill patients are a key influence on the environment of the ICU. Patient and family needs have remained stable over the decades since ICUs were invented, with family proximity to the patient highly valued. A scientific basis to restrict visitors simply does not exist.[43] However, nurses have varying philosophies about family visiting, and a breakdown in care can easily occur if there is an effort by nurses to distance families from the patient and the patient's bedside at those times when the patient is most critically ill.[44] Each ICU should develop a unit culture that accepts families as having a right to be with the patient and act as partners on the healing team with the nurse. A consistent visiting policy that allows nurses to coordinate visits depending on the needs of the patient and family (as opposed to establishing rigid rules) provides the best chance for patient, family, and nurse satisfaction.[5] Inflexible rules for visiting may set up a "good nurse/bad nurse" scenario and result in loss of confidence for families and job dissatisfaction in nurses. The presence of family decreases patient vulnerability and enhances feelings of security and comfort.[16] According to Kirchhoff, extending this visiting flexibility to the end of life is essential because this may be the "ultimate visit."[45]

Family Presence at the End of Life

Providing family members with the option to be present with their loved one at the end of life in an ICU setting, especially during cardiopulmonary resuscitation (CPR), is gaining increasing acceptance because of the demands of the public and professional nursing organizations like the Emergency Nurses' Association (ENA) and the AACN.[46] The ENA has published guidelines, endorsed by AACN, that clearly outline a policy and a process for bringing family members to the bedside during CPR. Less than 5% of all nurses are even aware that these guidelines exist.[47] Family members and a majority of nurses and physicians support family presence.[48] Barriers to family presence include physician and nurse resistance and lack of knowledge of the ENA guidelines.

Because family presence evokes strong feelings from staff, a decision to discuss and adopt a policy for family presence similar to the one that exists at Parkland Hospital in Dallas is recommended. Just as the delivery room was closed to fathers many decades ago and now no obstetrics area would consider excluding the father, so should families have the option to be with their loved one for what may be the final visit. In pediatric resuscitation, the movement to allow parents to be with their child during CPR is strong, with over 80% of parents desiring the option.[49] Creating a healing, humanistic environment in the ICU means building a culture where family presence is an option.

clinical applicability challenges

Self-Challenge: Critical Thinking

1. *Do an environmental ICU assessment. Consider the ICU where you practice and note carefully the sounds, noise, light, and pace. Sit in the unit and close your eyes and listen. Note what patients may hear or smell. Think of how well you would sleep in this unit if you were the patient. How many family members are visiting patients?*
2. *Think of patients who would benefit from a music therapy intervention. How would you go about initiating this therapy?*
3. *The nurse manager asks you to assist her in changing attitudes about bathing patients at night; she wants this to stop because patients are complaining. How do you go about getting other nurses to agree?*

Study Questions

1. *Patients in ICUs have many needs. One of the most overwhelming is to*
   a. *feel safe.*
   b. *achieve 2-hour sleep periods.*
   c. *visit with family members twice a day.*
   d. *receive opioids for pain.*
2. *Music therapy, a nonpharmacologic adjunct to decrease anxiety, works by*
   a. *raising sympathetic tone to decrease heart rate and blood pressure.*
   b. *entraining breathing with specific musical rhythms.*
   c. *relaxing the body and then the mind.*
   d. *distracting the patient so that no pain medication is needed.*
3. *Sleep deprivation in patients who are critically ill is most often attributed to*
   a. *bed baths during the evening shift.*
   b. *untreated pain and anxiety.*
   c. *family visiting.*
   d. *altered melatonin levels.*
4. *ICU design should consider which one of the following?*
   a. *Bright, overhead lighting*
   b. *Waiting rooms to keep family members out of the patient room*
   c. *Thick carpets to muffle sound*
   d. *Soft, calm colors*

REFERENCES

1. Pronovost PJ, Angus DC, Dorman T, et al: Physician staffing pattern and clinical outcomes in critically ill patients: A systematic review. JAMA 288(17):2151–2162, 2002
2. Fairman J, Lynaugh J: Critical Care Nursing: A History. Philadelphia, University of Pennsylvania Press, 1998
3. Stichler JF: Creating healing environments in critical care units. Crit Care Nurs Q 24(3):1–20, 2001
4. Fontaine DK, Prinkey Briggs L, et al: Designing humanistic critical care environments. Crit Care Nurs Q 24(3):21–34, 2001
5. Henneman EA, Cardin S: Family-centered care: A practical approach to making it happen. Crit Care Nurse 22(6):12–19, 2002
6. Simon SK, Phillips K, Badalamenti S, et al: Current practices regarding visitation policies in critical care units. Am J Crit Care 6:210–217, 1997

7. Kahn DM, Cook TE, Carlisle CC, et al: Identification and modification of environmental noise in an ICU setting. Chest 114:535–540, 1998
8. Freedman NS, Kotzer N, Schwab RJ: Patient perception of sleep quality and etiology of sleep disruption in the intensive care unit. Am J Respir Crit Care Med 159(4 Pt 1):1155–1162, 1999
9. Aaron JN, Carlisle CC, Carskadon MA, et al: Environmental noise as a cause of sleep disruption in an intermediate respiratory care unit. Sleep 19:707–710, 1996
10. Ulrich RS: View through a window may influence recovery from surgery. Science 224:420–421, 1984
11. Stein-Parbury J, McKinley S: Patients' experiences of being in an intensive care unit: A select literature review. Am J Crit Care 9:20–27, 2000
12. Vinall PE: Design technology: What you need to now about circadian rhythms in healthcare design. J Healthcare Design 9:141–144, 1997
13. Holtzclaw BJ: Thermal balance. In Kinney MR, Dunbar SB, Brooks-Brunn JA, et al. (eds): AACN Clinical Reference for Critical Care Nursing (4th Ed). St. Louis, Mosby, 1998
14. Jastremski CA: ICU bedside environment: A nursing perspective. Crit Care Clin 16(4):723–734, 2000
15. Horrigan B: Region's hospital opens holistic nursing unit. Alt Ther Health Med 6(4):92–93, 2000
16. McKinley S, Nagy S, Stein-Parbury J, et al: Vulnerability and security in seriously ill patients in intensive care. Intens Crit Care Nurs 18(1):27–36, 2002
17. Hupcey J: Feeling safe: The psychosocial needs of ICU patients. J Nurs Scholarsh 32(4):361–367, 2000
18. Rotondi AJ, Chelluri L, Sirio C, et al: Patients' recollections of stressful experiences while receiving prolonged mechanical ventilation in an intensive care unit. Crit Care Med 30:746–752, 2002
19. Benner P, Hooper-Kyriakidis P, Stannard D: Clinical Wisdom and Interventions in Critical Care. Philadelphia, WB Saunders, 1999
20. Viner ED: Life at the other end of the endotracheal tube: A physician's personal view of critical illness. Prog Crit Care Med 2:3–13, 1985
21. Baggs JG, Schmitt MH, Mushlin AI, et al: Association between nurse-physician collaboration and patient outcomes in three intensive care units. Crit Care Med 9:1991–1998, 1999
22. Frazier SK, Moser DK, Riegel B, et al: Critical care nurses' assessment of anxiety: Reliance on physiological and behavioral parameters. Am J Crit Care 11:57–64, 2002
23. Mundigler G, Delle-Karth G, Koreny M, et al: Impaired circadian rhythm of melatonin secretion in sedated critically ill patients with severe sepsis. Crit Care Med 30:536–540, 2002
24. Redeker NS: Sleep in acute care settings: An integrative review. J Nurs Scholarsh 32:31–38, 2000
25. Cureton-Lane RA, Fontaine DK: Sleep in the pediatric ICU: an empirical investigation. Am J Crit Care 6:56–63, 1997
26. Edwards GB, Schuring LM: Pilot study: Validating staff nurses' observations of sleep and wake states among critically ill patients using polysomnography. Am J Crit Care 2:125–131, 1993
27. Richardson SJ: A comparison of tools for the assessment of sleep pattern disturbance in critically ill adults. Dimens Crit Care Nurs 16:226–239, 1997
28. Fraser GL, Prato S, Riker RR, et al: Frequency, severity, and treatment of agitation in young versus elderly patients in the ICU. Pharmacotherapy 20(1):75–82, 2000
29. Truman B, Ely EW: Monitoring delirium in critically ill patients: Using the confusion assessment method for the intensive care unit. Crit Care Nurse 23(2):25–36, 2003
30. Harvey M: Managing agitation in critically ill patients. Am J Crit Care 5:7–16, 1996
31. Nelson JE, Meier DE, Oei EJ, et al: Self-reported symptom experience of critically ill cancer patients receiving intensive care. Crit Care Med 29:277–282, 2001
32. Topf M, Bookman M, Arand D: Effects of critical care unit noise on the subjective quality of sleep. J Adv Nurs 24:545–551, 1996
33. Moore MM, Nguyen D, Nolan SP, et al: Interventions to reduce decibel levels on patient care units. Am Surg 64:894–899, 1998
34. Guidelines/Practice Parameters Committee of the American College of Critical Care Medicine, Society of Critical Care Medicine: Guidelines for intensive care unit design. Crit Care Med 23:582–588, 1995
35. Chlan L: Integrating nonpharmacological, adjunctive interventions into critical care practice: A means to humanize care? Am J Crit Care 11:14–16, 2002
36. Chlan LL: Music therapy as a nursing intervention for patients supported by mechanical ventilation. AACN Clin Issues 11(1):128–138, 2000
37. Guzzetta CE: Effects of relaxation and music therapy on patients in a coronary care unit with presumptive acute myocardial infarction. Heart Lung 18(6):609–616, 1989
38. Byers JF, Smyth KA: Effect of a music intervention on noise annoyance, heart rate, and blood pressure in cardiac surgery patients. Am J Crit Care 6:183–191, 1997
39. Richards KC: Effect of a back massage and relaxation intervention on sleep in critically ill patients. Am J Crit Care 7(4):288–299, 1998
40. Edwards GB, Schuring LM: Sleep protocol: A research-based practice change. Crit Care Nurse 13(2):84–88, 1993
41. Dracup K, Bryan-Brown CW: To work: Perchance to sleep. Am J Crit Care 9:224–226, 2000
42. Jacobi J, Fraser GL, Coursin DB, et al: Clinical practice guidelines for the sustained use of sedatives and analgesics in the critically ill adult. Crit Care Med 30:119–141, 2002
43. Tullman DF, Dracup K: Creating a healing environment for elders. AACN Clin Issues 11(1):34–50, 2000
44. Chesla CA, Stannard D: Breakdown in the nursing care of families in the ICU. Am J Crit Care 6:64–71, 1997
45. Kirchhoff KT: Promoting a peaceful death in the ICU. Crit Care Nurs Clin North Am 14:201–206, 2002
46. Tucker TL: Family presence during resuscitation. Crit Care Nurs Clin North Am 14:177–185, 2002
47. MacLean S, Guzzetta CE, White C, et al: Family presence practices of critical care and emergency nurses in the United States. Am J Crit Care 12:246–257, 2003
48. Meyers TA, Eichorn DJ, Guzzetta CE, et al: Family presence during invasive procedures and resuscitation. Am J Nurs 100(2):32–42, 2000
49. McGahey PR: Family presence during pediatric resuscitation: A focus on staff. Crit Care Nurse 22(6):29–34, 2002

chapter 5

Relieving Pain and Providing Comfort

SUZANNE PREVOST

objectives

Based on the content in this chapter, the reader should be able to:

- Identify at least three factors that exacerbate the experience of pain in the critically ill.
- Describe at least three common sources of procedural pain in intensive care.
- Compare and contrast tolerance, physical dependence, and addiction.
- Discuss the national guidelines and standards for pain management.
- Identify five analgesics commonly used in the care of the critically ill.
- Describe four nonpharmacological interventions for alleviating pain and anxiety.

Pain is the greatest concern of patients in intensive care units (ICUs).[1,2] Most critically ill patients experience moderate to severe pain.[3] Pain management has become a national priority in recent years,[4–7] yet pain continues to be misunderstood, poorly assessed, and undertreated in ICUs and many other health care settings.[8,9] Uncontrolled pain triggers physical and emotional stress responses, inhibits healing, increases the risk of other complications, and increases the length of ICU stay. Critical care nurses need a clear understanding of concepts related to pain assessment and management to achieve effective pain control. This chapter provides an overview of key concepts related to the management of acute pain and comfort in the critically ill adult patient.

PAIN DEFINED

Pain is a complex, subjective phenomenon. It is a protective mechanism, causing one to withdraw from or avoid the source of pain and seek assistance or treatment. The International Society for the Study of Pain defined pain as "an unpleasant sensory and emotional experience associated with actual or potential tissue damage or described in terms of such damage."[10] McCaffery provides an operational definition of pain that considers the subjectivity and individuality of the pain experience and is based on the premise that the individual experiencing the pain is the true authority:

"Pain is whatever the experiencing person says it is, existing whenever he or she says it does."[11]

The pain most ICU patients experience is classified as *acute* because it has an identified cause and is expected to resolve within a given time frame. For example, the pain experienced during endotracheal suctioning or a dressing change can be expected to end when the treatment is completed. Similarly, pain at an incision or area of injury is expected to cease once healing has occurred. In contrast, *chronic* pain is caused by physiological mechanisms that are less well understood. Chronic pain differs from acute pain in terms of etiology and expected duration. It may last for an indefinite period and may be difficult, if not impossible, to treat completely.[12]

PAIN IN THE CRITICALLY ILL

Critical illness is painful. Consider the most common conditions treated in the ICU—myocardial infarction, recovery from thoracic surgery or neurosurgery, multiple trauma, and extensive burns—all are associated with severe pain. Nearly all ICU patients experience acute pain; but many, particularly those who are elderly, suffer with the combination of both acute and chronic pain. For some of these patients, the pain is considered continuous because it persists for more than half of each day.[13] Previously it was thought that critically ill patients were unable to remember their painful experiences because of the acute nature of the illness or injury. More recent research demonstrates that ICU patients do remember painful experiences and they describe their pain as being moderate to severe in intensity.[3,14]

Multiple factors inherent in the ICU environment affect the patient's pain experience. These factors include anxiety, sleep deprivation, unfamiliar and unpleasant surroundings, loss of control, and separation from family or significant others. The effects of each of these factors increase when they are experienced together. For example, pain and anxiety act in a synergistic and cyclical fashion to exacerbate each other.[9] Box 5-1 summarizes the physical, psychosocial, and environmental factors that contribute to pain and discomfort in the critically ill.

box 5-1
Factors Contributing to Pain and Discomfort in the Critically Ill

Physical

- Symptoms of critical illness (e.g., angina, ischemia, dyspnea)
- Wounds—post-trauma, postoperative, or post-procedural
- Sleep disturbance and deprivation
- Immobility, inability to move to a comfortable position because of tubes, monitors, restraints
- Temperature extremes associated with critical illness and the environment—fever, hypothermia

Psychosocial

- Anxiety and depression
- Impaired communication, inability to report and describe pain
- Fear of pain, disability, or death
- Separation from family and significant others
- Boredom or lack of pleasant distractions

Intensive Care Unit Environment or Routine

- Continuous noise from equipment and staff
- Continuous or unnatural patterns of light
- Awakening and physical manipulation every 1–2 hours for vital signs or positioning
- Continuous or frequent invasive, painful procedures
- Competing priorities in care—unstable vital signs, bleeding, dysrhythmias, poor ventilation—may take precedence over pain management

Procedural Pain

Efforts to provide pain relief and comfort measures are complicated by the fact that critical care nurses must continuously perform procedures or treatments that cause pain to the patient. Procedures like chest tube insertion and removal, endotracheal suctioning, and wound debridement are obviously painful. Recent research reveals that simple procedures, such as turning the patient, can also cause considerable pain.[15,16]

A national, multicenter research study supported by the American Association of Critical-Care Nurses (AACN), referred to as the Thunder II Project, examined procedural pain in more than 6000 critically ill patients, including 5957 adults and 176 children.[15] The investigators documented the patients' responses to six procedures that are frequently performed on critically ill patients: central venous catheter placement, femoral sheath removal, tracheal suctioning, turning, wound care, and wound drain removal. The most painful and least painful procedures for each age group are noted in Table 5-1.

The Thunder II investigators also discovered that very few of the patients (less than 20%) received opioid analgesics before their procedures. Many of the patients had even reported that they were in pain before the procedure, and still did not receive an analgesic to control their pain during the procedure.[15] The patients in the study were also asked to use words to describe the pain they were feeling before and after each procedure. The word "aching" was most frequently used to describe pain before the procedure. During and after the procedure, "sharp" was the most commonly used description.[16]

Before any procedure known to be associated with pain is performed, patients should be premedicated, and the procedure should be performed only after the medication has taken effect. National guidelines for acute pain management clearly state that "only when immediate treatment of cardiorespiratory instability is required, or if a competent patient declines treatment, should analgesia be withheld for a painful procedure."[4]

During procedures, intravenous (IV) opioids, such as morphine or fentanyl, are usually used for analgesia. The IV bolus dose of morphine is individualized and depends on the patient's age and weight, the pain intensity, and the type of procedure being performed. The patient's response must be monitored during the procedure, with additional doses

table 5-1 Procedures Causing the Most and Least Pain Intensity by Age Group

	Children (4–7 yr)	Children (8–12 yr)	Adolescents (13–17 yr)	Adults (≥18 yr)
Central line placement	*	*	*	*
Femoral sheath removal	*	*	*	Least painful
Tracheal suctioning	Least painful	Most painful	Least painful	*
Turning	Most painful	Second most painful	Second most painful	Most painful
Wound care	*	Least painful	Most painful	*
Wound drain removal	*	*	*	Second most painful

*No data were available for these procedures in these age groups.
From Puntillo KA, White C, Morris A, et al: Patients' perceptions and responses to procedural pain: Results from Thunder II Project. Am J Crit Care 10(4):238–251, 2001.

given as needed for breakthrough pain. Anxiolytic medications, such as midazolam or propofol, can be given to relieve anxiety during the procedure; however, these agents should be used as *adjuncts* because they provide only sedation, and will not relieve the pain associated with the procedure.

From the Thunder II study, nurses have learned that the pain associated with routine procedures differs across age groups. Some of the procedures that seem benign, like turning, can be the most painful. Critical care nurses must be attuned to the pain the patient is experiencing before the procedure to provide the best interventions to help the patient during the procedure. In addition to providing preprocedural analgesic medication, the nurse can educate the patient to help him or her prepare and plan for procedures, and the nurse can use interventions like imagery, distraction, and family support during procedures.[16]

CONSEQUENCES OF PAIN

Pain produces many harmful effects that inhibit healing and recovery from critical illness. The autonomic nervous system (ANS) responds to pain by causing vasoconstriction and increased heart rate and contractility. Pulse, blood pressure, and cardiac output all increase. This increases myocardial workload and oxygen use, both of which can cause or exacerbate myocardial ischemia in the already compromised critically ill person. Respiratory alterations resulting from pain include splinting, decreased respiratory effort, and reduced pulmonary volume and flow. Pulmonary complications, such as atelectasis and pneumonia, can result. In the gastrointestinal system, gastric emptying and intestinal motility decrease, which can result in impaired function and ileus. Pain also negatively affects the musculoskeletal system by causing muscle contractions, spasms, and rigidity. Because movement increases pain, the patient is hesitant to move, cough, or breathe deeply. Unrelieved pain suppresses the immune functions, predisposing the patient to pneumonia, wound infections, and sepsis.[17] Patients who have a high level of uncontrolled pain during an acute hospitalization are at risk for delayed recovery and development of chronic pain syndromes after discharge.[18]

Patients who are pain free have better outcomes than those stressed by unrelieved pain. In a classic study, patients whose pain was controlled with epidural anesthesia and epidural analgesia had shorter ICU stays, shorter hospital stays, and half as many complications as patients receiving standard anesthesia and analgesia.[19] The benefits of effective pain relief are summarized in Table 5-2.

BARRIERS TO EFFECTIVE PAIN CONTROL

Pain continues to be undertreated in many critical care settings, even though the negative consequences of uncontrolled pain and the benefits of pain relief have been well documented.[8,9,20] Pain relief is often relegated to a low priority owing to the life-threatening nature of the patient's illness and the other lifesaving interventions that are required. Critical care nurses are often concerned that analgesic administration may create problems, such as hemodynamic and respiratory compromise, oversedation, or drug addiction.

The fear of addiction is one of the greatest concerns and impediments associated with analgesia and pain control. This fear causes anxiety for patients and their families as well as health care providers. Critical care nurses must have a clear understanding of the differences between, and implications of, tolerance, physical dependence and addiction (Table 5-3). Patients who require medication for pain control should not be considered addicted, regardless of the size of their dose or the length of their medication regimen.[2]

table 5-2 Benefits of Effective Pain Relief

Cardiovascular	Decreased pulse, blood pressure, and myocardial workload
Pulmonary	Enhanced respiration and oxygenation, decreased incidence of pulmonary complications
Neurologic	Decreased anxiety and mental confusion, enhanced sleep
Gastrointestinal/nutritional	Enhanced gastric emptying, promotion of positive nitrogen balance
Musculoskeletal	Earlier ambulation, reducing complications of immobility
Economic	Decreased length of stay, decreased costs, enhanced patient satisfaction with care

RESOURCES TO PROMOTE EFFECTIVE PAIN CONTROL

During the past decade, government agencies, professional organizations, health care institutions, and pain management experts have given focused attention to improving pain management across the United States. These efforts have produced abundant resources to support nurses in their efforts to provide effective pain management. Three major events triggered this nationwide interest and movement:

- Introduction of clinical practice guidelines, specifically the guidelines for Acute Pain Management in 1992[4] and Cancer Pain Management in 1994,[5] by the Agency for Health Care Policy and Research (AHCPR), now known as the Agency for Healthcare Research and Quality (AHRQ)
- Publication of the SUPPORT (Study to Understand Prognoses and Preferences for Outcomes and Risks of Treatment) Trial in 1995[21]
- Implementation of nationwide pain management accreditation standards by the Joint Commission on Accreditation of Healthcare Organizations (JCAHO) in 2001[7]

Clinical Practice Guidelines

Early in the 1990s, the AHCPR introduced the concept of clinical practice guidelines. These guidelines were intended to serve as nationwide standards of care for specific clinical problems. This concept arose from the recognition that in the midst of a rapidly expanding body of health care research and literature, there were still wide variations in opinions and practice patterns regarding the best interventions for common clinical problems. The AHCPR convened multidisciplinary panels of national experts to review the research, provide expert opinions, summarize the current knowledge, and make recommendations for practice for each targeted clinical problem. Acute pain management was the topic of the first guideline that was published and disseminated by this agency.[4] Two years later, a practice guideline for cancer pain was published.[5]

Over the next few years, several national agencies, including the AACN, the American College of Cardiology,

table 5-3 Tolerance, Physical Dependence, and Addiction

	Definition	Implication
Tolerance	The need for increasing doses of a drug to attain the original effect	Increase dose by 50% and assess effect. Tolerance to side effects, such as respiratory depression, will increase as the dose requirement increases.
Physical dependence	A physiological phenomenon, occurring with prolonged opioid administration, manifested by the occurrence of withdrawal symptoms if the drug is abruptly reduced or discontinued	Gradually taper opioid dosage to discontinuation to avoid withdrawal symptoms.
Addiction	A pattern of compulsive drug use characterized by a continued craving for an opioid and the need to use the opioid for effects other than pain relief	Rarely seen in critical care patients, unless patient is admitted for drug overdose or other sequelae of illicit drug use.

From American Pain Society: Principles of Analgesic Use in the Treatment of Acute Pain and Cancer Pain (4th Ed). Glenview, IL, 1999; and Pasero C, McCaffery M: Multimodal balanced analgesia in the critically ill. Crit Care Nurs Clin North Am 13(2):195–206, 2001.

and the Society of Critical Care Medicine, assembled their own panels of experts to develop clinical practice guidelines for their target populations. In 1996, the AHCPR discontinued their support for producing clinical practice guideline documents and instead entered into a collaborative relationship with the American Medical Association and the American Association of Health Plans to sponsor the web-based National Guideline Clearinghouse.[22] This website currently contains more than 900 practice guidelines developed by a variety of organizations.

The AHCPR's pain guidelines have been disseminated throughout the United States and have served as a catalyst for several improvements in pain management over the past decade. These guidelines are also used as legal documents representing the national standard of care for pain management in medical liability cases.

One practice guideline that is particularly useful to critical care nurses and physicians is the guideline published jointly by the Society of Critical Care Medicine and the American Society of Health-System Pharmacists on *Sustained Use of Sedatives and Analgesics in the Critically Ill Adult.*[23] Table 5-4 contains information about this and other important guidelines and standards for pain management.

The SUPPORT Trial

The SUPPORT[21] trial was a research study involving more than 9000 seriously ill hospitalized patients. The intent of the project was to provide a supportive intervention, through specially trained nurse facilitators, to improve decision making and ease the pain and suffering associated with end-of-life care. More than a third of the patients spent over 10 days in an ICU and nearly half of them received mechanical ventilation before their death. In spite of the targeted interventions by the nurse facilitators, 50% of the conscious patients experienced moderate to severe pain during their last days of life.[21]

Results of this project were widely publicized in both professional and public media, creating national recognition of the need to provide better pain management, specifically for patients at the end of life. This movement has prompted an increase in pain management educational programs and an increase in funding for research related to pain management and end-of-life care.

Joint Commission on Accreditation of Healthcare Organizations Standards for Pain

In response to the findings of the SUPPORT trial and other pain management deficiencies, JCAHO revised their accrediting standards to include specific expectations directed toward improving the management of pain. The new standards, implemented in January, 2001, include explicit expectations related to assessment, patient and staff education, interventions, documentation, and process improvement initiatives for pain management. The standards are published in their accreditation manuals and can be found on their website.[7]

These JCAHO standards have served as a catalyst to prompt hospitals to invest more heavily in providing support for pain management. As a result, most hospitals now offer staff development and continuing education programs on pain management. Many hospitals have implemented interdisciplinary pain management consultation teams or pain management process improvement teams. Several facilities have also created new positions and hired pain management experts and consultants. This trend has created a new demand for nurse specialists in pain management, as described in the role delineation study conducted by the American Society of Pain Management Nurses.[24]

PAIN ASSESSMENT

According to the American Pain Society, the failure of staff routinely to assess pain and pain relief is the most common reason for unrelieved pain in hospitalized patients.[6] Assessment of pain is as important as any method of treatment. The patient's pain should be assessed at regular intervals to determine the effectiveness of therapy, the presence of side effects, the need for dose adjustment, or the need for supplemental doses to offset procedural pain. Pain should be reassessed at an appropriate interval after pain medications or other interventions have been administered, such as 30 minutes after an IV dose of morphine. In critical care, a number of conditions may exist making assessment of the patient's pain and subsequent treatments difficult. These conditions include the following:

- Acuity of the patient's condition
- Altered levels of consciousness
- Inability to communicate pain
- Restricted or limited movement
- Endotracheal intubation

A common misconception among health care professionals is that they are the most qualified to determine the presence and severity of the patient's pain. Absence of physical signs or behaviors is often incorrectly interpreted as the absence of pain. To perform an effective pain assessment, the critical care nurse must elicit a self-report from the patient. Behavioral observation and changes in physiological parameters should be considered along with the patient's self-report.

Patient Self-Report

Because pain is a subjective experience, the patient's self-report is the most reliable source of information about the presence and intensity of pain.[25] The patient's self-report should be obtained not only at rest, but during routine activity, such as coughing, deep breathing, and turning. Nurses working with the critically ill frequently are more attuned to objective indicators of pain than to the patient's self-report. If the patient can communicate, the critical care nurse must accept the patient's description of pain as valid. In the conscious and coherent patient, behavioral cues or physiological indicators should never take precedence over the self-report of pain. Behavioral and physiological manifestations of pain are extremely variable and may be minimal or absent, despite the presence of excruciating pain.[8]

In assessing pain quality, the nurse should elicit a specific verbal description of the patient's pain, such as "burn-

table 5-4 National Standards and Guidelines Related to Pain Management

Agency or Source	Standard or Guideline	Content Highlights
Agency for Health Care Research and Quality (AHRQ); formerly known as Agency for Health Care Policy and Research (AHCPR)	Acute Pain Management: Operative and Medical Procedures and Trauma: Clinical Practice Guideline No. 1, United States Department of Health and Human Services (1992)[4]	The AHCPR guidelines evolved from four main goals: • Reduce the incidence and severity of acute postoperative and posttraumatic pain. • Educate patients about the need to communicate unrelieved pain so that they can receive prompt evaluation and effective treatment. • Enhance patient comfort and satisfaction. • Contribute to decreased postoperative complications and, in some cases, shorter hospital stays after surgical procedures. Encourages a proactive, interdisciplinary approach to pain management with patient and family involvement. Incorporates both pharmacological and nonpharmacological interventions with specific recommendations based on research. Used widely across the United States and other countries to direct pain management efforts in critical care units, as well as in a wide variety of other acute care settings and populations.
Society of Critical Care Medicine (SCCM) and the American Society of Health-System Pharmacists (ASHP)	Clinical Practice Guidelines for the Sustained Use of Sedatives and Analgesics in the Critically Ill Adult (2002)[23]	Developed by a national panel of experts in critical care medicine, critical care nursing, and pharmacy. Includes summaries and recommendations of recent research related to analgesia and sedation specifically in the critically ill population. The summary contains 28 explicit recommendations targeted to the critically ill, including the following: • Patient report is the most reliable standard for pain assessment, and a numeric rating scale should be used when possible. • Scheduled doses or continuous infusions of opioids are preferred over an "as-needed" or prn regimen. • Fentanyl, hydromorphone, and morphine are the drugs of choice for intravenous opioid analgesia. • Fentanyl is preferred for rapid onset of analgesia in acutely distressed patients. • Sedation of agitated patients should be provided only after providing adequate analgesia. • Lorazepam is recommended for sedation of most patients by intermittent or continuous intravenous infusion. • Midazolam or diazepam should be used for rapid sedation of acutely agitated patients. • Haloperidol is the preferred agent for treatment of delirium (pp 140–141).[23]
Joint Commission on Accreditation of Healthcare Organizations (JCAHO)	JCAHO Standards on Pain Management for Accreditation of Healthcare Organizations (Implemented—January, 2001)	Affirms patients' rights to appropriate assessment and management of pain. Reinforces this right by requiring hospitals and other health care facilities to: • Make pain relief a priority. • Assess each patient on admission and then regularly reassess patients who have pain or are likely to experience pain. Pain assessment must include: pain intensity using a rating scale; location, quality, character, onset, duration and pattern of the pain; aggravating and alleviating factors; current regimen and its effectiveness; pain history; effect of pain on activities of daily living; the patient's goal or expectation for pain control; examination and observation of each painful site. • Educate staff to ensure pain management competency. • Teach patients that pain management is an important part of their care. • Teach patients and families their roles in managing pain. • Incorporate relevant cultural, spiritual, and ethnic beliefs of each patient related to their pain. • Include pain management in clinical pathways, transfer, and discharge plans. • Measure patient satisfaction and other results of process improvement activities to enhance pain management.
American Pain Society (APS)	Principles of Analgesic Use in the Treatment of Acute Pain and Cancer Pain (4th Ed) (1999)[6]	This 64-page, pocket-sized booklet, compiled by a national panel of experts from the APS, can be used as a clinical reference tool for selecting and administering nonopioid and opioid analgesics and analgesic adjuvants in a variety of patient care situations. Includes compilation of recent research on analgesics and consensus of expert opinions regarding analgesics.

insights into clinical research

Renaud KL: Cardiovascular surgery patients' respiratory responses to morphine before extubation. Pain Manage Nurs 3(2):53–60, 2002.

In this study, postoperative intensive care unit (ICU) patients who were having pain and who were ready to be weaned from their ventilators were identified. Eleven of these patients were given doses of intravenous (IV) morphine to relieve their pain. Their weaning parameters (respiratory rate, tidal volume, vital capacity, and negative inspiratory force) were measured before and after receiving the morphine. The investigator found that some of the results did not change significantly, and some of them (tidal volume and negative inspiratory force) significantly improved.

These results are important because many critical care nurses and physicians have historically withheld opioid pain medications from similar patients because they feared that the medication would decrease their respiratory force and volume, and inhibit their ability to be weaned from the ventilator.

This study should be replicated with a larger sample. If the findings are similar, it will support the theory that better pain management can enhance, rather than inhibit, effective respiration and weaning from mechanical ventilation.

ing," "crushing," "stabbing," "dull," or "sharp" whenever possible. These terms help pinpoint the cause of the pain.

The JCAHO Pain Management Standards[7] recommend the use of a pain scale in the assessment of pain. Pain scales and rating instruments based on the patient's self-report provide a simple but consistent measure of pain trends over time. Numeric rating scales and visual analog scales are used to measure pain intensity. With these scales, the patient is asked to choose a number, word, or a point on a line that best describes the amount of pain he or she is experiencing. The Society of Critical Care Medicine clinical practice guideline suggests that the numeric rating scale is the preferred type of scale for use in critical care units (CCUs).[23] With this type of scale, the patient is asked to rate the pain, with 0 being no pain and 10 being the worst possible pain imaginable (Figure 5-1).

Pictures or word boards can also facilitate communication regarding the patient's pain. The board should include open-ended questions, such as "Do you have pain?" "Where is the pain located?" "How bad is your pain?" and "What helps your pain?" Developing a simple system of eye movements ("blink once for yes and twice for no") or finger movements can be effective for the patient who cannot speak.[13]

Pain assessment and subsequent treatment are dilemmas if the patient is unable to use any of the aforementioned methods to verbalize or indicate that he or she is in pain. In this situation, it may be appropriate to observe for the behavioral cues or physiological indicators, as discussed in the next section. However, the absence of physiological indicators or behavioral cues should *never* be interpreted as absence of pain.[8] AHCPR guidelines recommend that if the procedure, surgery, or condition is believed to be associated with pain, the presence of pain should be assumed and treated appropriately.[4]

Observation

The patient in pain may exhibit specific behavioral manifestations. Protective behaviors such as guarding, withdrawal, and avoidance of movement protect the patient from painful stimuli. Attempts by the patient to seek relief, such as rubbing the area, changing positions, or requesting pain medications, are palliative behaviors. Crying, moaning, or screaming are affective behaviors and reflect an emotional response to pain. Changes in facial expressions may also indicate pain.

Patients who are unable to speak may use eye or facial expressions or movement of hands or legs to communicate their pain. Restlessness or agitation may be seen in the unresponsive patient. However, nonverbal cues are difficult to interpret as specific indicators for the presence of pain and its location. In some situations, family input may be helpful in interpreting specific behavioral manifestations of pain based on their knowledge of the patient's behavior before hospitalization.

Physiological Parameters

Critical care nurses are skilled in assessing the patient's physical status in terms of changes in blood pressure, heart rate, or respirations. Therefore, it could be reasoned that observation of the physiological effects of pain will assist in pain assessment. With critically ill patients, however, it may be difficult to attribute these physiolog-

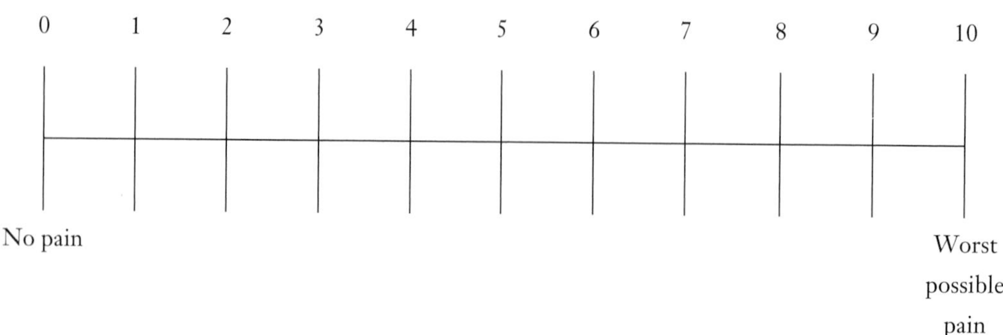

figure 5-1 Numeric rating scale for pain assessment.

ical changes specifically to pain rather than another cause. For example, an unexpected increase in the severity and intensity of the patient's pain associated with hypotension, tachycardia, or fever must be evaluated immediately. These findings may signal the development of life-threatening complications such as wound dehiscence, infection, or deep venous thrombosis (DVT).

Pain assessment is an ongoing process. In addition to the initial pain assessment, assessment after pain management interventions and before procedures is essential. After pharmacological therapy, pain reassessment should correspond to the time of onset or peak effect of the drug administered and the time the analgesic effect is expected to be dissipated. Response to therapy is best measured as a change from the patient's baseline pain level. Occasionally there may be discrepancies between the patient's self-report and behavioral and physiological manifestations. For example, one patient may report pain as a 2 out of 10, while being tachycardic, diaphoretic, and splinting with respirations. Another patient may give a self-report of 8 out of 10 while smiling. These discrepancies can be due to use of diversionary activities, coping skills, beliefs about pain, cultural background, fears of becoming addicted, or fears of being bothersome to the nursing staff. When these situations occur, they should be discussed with the patient. Any misconceptions or knowledge deficits should be addressed and the pain treated according to the patient's self-report. Box 5-2 lists common nursing diagnoses for the patient in pain.

box 5-2 *Examples of Nursing Diagnoses and Collaborative Problems for the Patient in Pain*

- Pain
- Chronic Pain
- Anxiety
- Fear
- Powerlessness
- Ineffective Individual Coping
- Impaired Physical Mobility

PAIN INTERVENTION

The nurse plays an important role in providing pain relief. Although pharmacological intervention is the most commonly used strategy, nursing management of pain also includes physical, cognitive, and behavioral measures. In addition to administering medications or providing alternative therapies, the nurse's role involves measuring the patient's response to those therapies. Because pain may diminish or the pain pattern may change, therapy adjustments may be needed before improvements are seen. General guidelines for nursing interventions for pain relief are listed in Box 5-3.

Pharmacological Interventions

In general, the ideal method of analgesia should allow adequate serum drug levels to be achieved and maintained quickly and easily. Medications should be titrated based on the patient's response, and the drug should be quickly eliminated when analgesia is no longer needed. Most clinicians agree that when using a numeric scale for assessment, pain medications should be titrated according to the following goals:

- The patient's reported pain score is less than his or her own predetermined pain management goal (e.g., 3 on a scale of 1 to 10).
- Adequate respiration is maintained.[4]

The efficacy of analgesia depends on the presence of an adequate and consistent serum drug level. Regardless of the method being used, scheduled opioid doses or a continuous infusion are preferred over as-required ("prn") administration.[23] The traditional prn analgesic order is a major barrier to effective pain control in all patient populations. The prn order allows the nurse to administer a dose of analgesic only when the patient requests it and only after a certain time has elapsed since the previous dose. Invariably, a delay occurs between the time of the request and the time the medication is actually administered. In some cases this delay can be up to an hour. The prn order poses another problem when the patient is asleep. As serum drug levels decrease, the patient is suddenly awakened by severe pain, and a

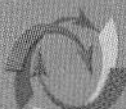

box 5-3 *nursing interventions for Pain Management*

- Perform systematic pain assessments in all critically ill patients.
- Reassess hourly the need for rescue doses of analgesic.
- If the patient is experiencing a condition or procedure that is thought to be painful, and the patient's report cannot be obtained, assume that pain is present and treat it.
- Remember that critically ill patients who are unconscious, sedated, or receiving neuromuscular blockade are at high risk for undertreatment of pain.
- Prevent pain by treating it in advance.
- If the patient has frequent or continuous pain, give analgesics by continuous intravenous (IV) infusion or around the clock, rather than on an as-required (prn) basis.

From Pasero C, McCaffery M: Pain in the critically ill. Am J Nurs 102(1):59–60, 2002; and Puntillo KA, White C, Morris A, et al: Patients' perceptions and responses to procedural pain: Results from Thunder II Project. Am J Crit Care 10(4):238–251, 2001.

greater amount of the drug is needed to achieve adequate serum levels.

NONOPIOID ANALGESICS

According to the American Pain Society Guidelines, any analgesic regimen should include a nonopioid drug, even if the pain is severe enough also to require an opioid.[6] In many patient populations, nonsteroidal anti-inflammatory drugs (NSAIDs) are the preferred choice for the nonopioid component of analgesic therapy. NSAIDs decrease pain by inhibiting the synthesis of inflammatory mediators (prostaglandin, histamine, and bradykinin) at the site of injury and effectively relieve pain without causing sedation, respiratory depression, or problems with bowel or bladder function. AHCPR guidelines recommend NSAIDs as the initial choice for managing mild to moderate postoperative pain.[4] When NSAIDs are used in combination with opioids, the opioid dose can often be reduced and still produce effective analgesia. This decreases the incidence of opioid-related side effects.

Controversy exists regarding whether NSAIDs are desirable in the critically ill population.[23] Many NSAIDs are supplied only in oral forms, which is not sufficient for critically ill patients whose oral intake is restricted. Ketorolac is available in parenteral form, but it can cause renal impairment if administration exceeds 5 days; therefore, it must be used with caution in patients with renal insufficiency or those receiving dialysis.[6] Indomethacin is available in suppository form and can be combined with opioids to provide effective pain relief, but indomethacin should not be used alone for moderate to severe pain.[4]

In addition to the concerns about route of administration, a major concern associated with NSAID use is the potential for adverse effects, including gastrointestinal bleeding, platelet inhibition, and renal insufficiency. Second-generation NSAIDs, such as celecoxib and rofecoxib, are more selective in their site of action, and therefore do not cause these harmful adverse effects, but they have not been widely used or evaluated in ICUs. Their slow onset of action may decrease their utility in critically ill patients.[23,26]

Acetaminophen is commonly used in critical care. When it is used in combination with opioids it produces a greater effect than opioids alone. In addition to providing mild analgesia, acetaminophen is an effective antipyretic; however, it does have the potential to cause hepatic damage. Dosages should be limited to a maximum of 2 g per day if patients have a history of, or high potential for, liver impairment.[23] Nonopioid analgesics that are commonly used in critical care and their recommended doses are listed in Table 5-5.

OPIOIDS

Opioids have been the pharmacological cornerstone of postoperative pain management. They provide pain relief by binding to various receptor sites in the spinal cord, central nervous system (CNS), and peripheral nervous system (PNS), thereby changing the perception of pain.

Opioids are selected based on individual patient needs and the potential for adverse effects. A comparison of commonly used opioids can be seen in Table 5-6. According to the Society of Critical Care Medicine, morphine sulfate, fentanyl, and hydromorphone are the preferred agents when IV opioids are needed.[23] Other opioids in use include codeine, oxycodone, and methadone.

Meperidine is the least potent opioid and is administered in the largest doses. For example, to produce a level of analgesia comparable to 10 mg of morphine every 4 hours, 100 to 150 mg of meperidine every 3 hours would be needed. Meperidine is commonly underdosed and given at intervals too infrequent to be effective.[4] Even though meperidine continues to be widely used in some settings, national experts and national practice guidelines do not recommend it for most patients.[4,6,23] Rationales for avoiding the use of this drug are summarized in Box 5-4.

table 5-5 Nonopioid Analgesic Drugs

Drug	Adult Dose	Usual Pediatric Dose	Comments
Acetaminophen	325–650 mg q4h	10–15 mg/kg q4h	Available in liquid form, lacks anti-inflammatory action
Aspirin	325–650 mg q4h	10–15 mg/kg q4h	Can cause gastrointestinal or postoperative bleeding
Celecoxib (Celebrex)	100–400 mg bid		Less adverse effects than other NSAIDs, considerably more expensive
Ibuprofen (Motrin)	200–400 mg q4–6h	10 mg/kg q6–8h	Available in liquid form
Indomethacin (Indocin)	25 mg q8–12h		Available in rectal and IV forms, but high incidence of side effects
Ketorolac (Toradol)	Initially, 30–60 mg IM or 15–30 mg IV Then, 15–30 mg IM or IV q6h Maintenance, 10 mg PO q4–6h		Available in parenteral form, limit use to 5 days, contraindicated with renal insufficiency
Naproxen (Naprosyn)	500 mg initially, then: 250 mg q6–8h	5 mg/kg q12h	Available in liquid form

All doses are oral, unless noted otherwise.

table 5-6 Opioid Analgesic Drugs

Drug	Equianalgesic Dose (mg) Oral	IM/IV	Comments	Precautions
Morphine	30	10	Considered the gold standard of comparison for opioids. Oral sustained-release, once-a-day, and rectal forms available.	Use caution with impaired ventilation. Not recommended with hemodynamic instability or renal insufficiency.
Fentanyl		0.1	Drug of choice for rapid onset of analgesia in acutely distressed patients. Rectal and transdermal forms available.	With transdermal form—12- to 24-hr delay to peak effect, and fever increases dose and absorption rate.
Hydromorphone (Dilaudid)	7.5	1.5	More potent and slightly shorter duration than morphine. Rectal form available.	
Meperidine (Demerol)	300	75	Not recommended (see Box 5-4). Slightly shorter-acting than morphine.	Toxic metabolite accumulates, causing CNS excitation.
Methadone (Dolophine)	20	10	Good oral potency, long half-life (24–36 h).	Accumulates with repetitive dosing, causing excessive sedation.
Oxycodone	20–30		Used for moderate pain when combined with a nonopioid agent (e.g., Percocet). As a single entity—useful for severe pain.	Dosing must be individualized due to high variability in pharmacokinetics.

Dosing Guidelines

Equianalgesia means "approximately equal analgesia." This term is used when changing a patient's regimen from one analgesic to another. Morphine, 10 mg intramuscularly, is usually considered the gold standard dose for comparison. Dosing guidelines for opioid analgesics are presented in Table 5-6.

box 5-4 *Precautions and Concerns Associated With Meperidine Use*

- Low potency—requires unusually high doses.
- Produces toxic metabolite (normeperidine).
- Can cause central nervous system (CNS) excitation, anxiety, tremors, seizures.
- Intramuscular administration produces fibrosis.
- Contraindicated in patients with compromised renal function.
- Contraindicated in elderly patients.
- Should not be used for more than 48 hours.
- Dose should not exceed 600 mg/24 hours.
- Should not be used for chronic pain treatment.
- Use in sickle cell disease creates high risk for seizures.
- Coadministration with monoamine oxidase (MAO) inhibitors can be lethal.

Adapted from Acute Pain Management: Operative or Medical Procedures and Trauma: Clinical Practice Guideline. AHCPR Publication Number 92-0032. Rockville, MD, U.S. Department of Health and Human Services, Public Health Service, 1992; and American Pain Society: Principles of Analgesic Use in the Treatment of Acute Pain and Cancer Pain (4th Ed). Glenview, IL, American Pain Society, 1999.

Opioid dosage varies depending on the individual patient, the method of administration, and the pharmacokinetics of the drug. Adequate pain relief occurs once a minimum serum level of the opioid has been achieved. Each patient's optimal serum level is different, and this level can change as pain intensity changes. Therefore, the dosing and titration of opioids must be individualized and the patient's response and any undesirable effects, such as respiratory depression or oversedation, must be closely assessed. If the patient has previously received an opioid (e.g., before surgery), doses should be adjusted above the previous required dose to achieve an optimal effect.[4] Factors such as age, individual pain tolerance, coexisting disease(s), type of surgical procedure, and the concomitant use of sedatives warrant consideration as well. Older patients are often more sensitive to the effects of opioids; therefore, decreasing the initial opioid dose and slow titration are recommended for older patients.

Methods of Administration

Oral Administration. Oral administration is simple, noninvasive, inexpensive, and provides effective analgesia. Oral is the preferred route for patients with cancer and chronic nonmalignant pain. The oral route is used infrequently in the ICU setting, however, because many patients are unable to take anything by mouth. Serum drug levels obtained after oral administration of opioids are variable and difficult to titrate. In addition, the transformation of oral opioids by the liver causes a significant decrease in serum levels.

Rectal Administration. Morphine and hydromorphone are also available in a rectal form. This provides an alternative for patients who cannot take anything by mouth. Unfortunately, this mechanism has many of the same disadvantages as oral administration, including variability in dosing requirements, delays to peak effect, and unstable serum drug levels.

Transdermal Administration. Fentanyl is available in a transdermal patch format. This form is used primarily to control chronic cancer pain because it takes 12 to 16 hours to see substantial therapeutic effects and up to 48 hours to achieve stable serum concentrations. If used for acute pain, such as postoperative pain, high serum concentrations may remain after the pain has subsided, putting the patient at risk for respiratory depression.[6]

Intramuscular Administration. Intramuscular injections should not be used to provide acute pain relief for the critically ill patient for the following reasons:

- Intramuscular injections are painful.
- Intramuscular drug absorption is extremely variable in critically ill patients because of alterations in cardiac output and tissue perfusion.[23]
- Anticipated discomfort associated with the injection increases the patient's anxiety.
- Repeated intramuscular injections can cause muscle and soft tissue fibrosis.

Intravenous Administration. Intravenous administration is usually the preferred route for opioid therapy, especially when the patient requires short-term acute pain relief—for example, during procedures such as chest tube removal, diagnostic tests, suctioning, or wound care. IV administration may be intermittent, continuous, or patient controlled. IV opioids have the most rapid onset and are easy to administer. With morphine, the time to peak effect is 15 to 30 minutes; for fentanyl, peak effect is achieved within 1 to 5 minutes.[27] However, the duration of analgesia is shorter with intermittent IV injections, and this can cause serum drug levels to fluctuate.

Continuous IV administration of opioids has many benefits for critically ill patients, especially those who have difficulty communicating their pain because of an altered level of consciousness or an endotracheal tube. Continuous IV infusions are easily initiated and maintain consistent serum drug levels. For continuous IV opioid infusions, fentanyl and morphine are commonly used because of their short elimination half-life (compared with other available opioids). Before starting a continuous IV infusion, an initial IV loading dose (or doses) is given to achieve an optimal serum level. Appropriate dosing and titration must be individualized, and this can be difficult because many critically ill patients have hepatic or renal dysfunctions that result in decreased metabolism of the opioid. A disadvantage of continuous IV infusions is that pain occurring during procedures may not be managed unless additional IV bolus injections are given.

Patient-controlled analgesia (PCA) is an effective method of pain relief for the critically ill patient who is conscious and able to participate in the pain management therapy.[23] The patient-controlled method of opioid administration produces good-quality analgesia, stable drug concentrations, less sedation, less opioid consumption, and fewer adverse effects.[23,28] Effective use of PCA is based on the assumption that the patient is the best person to evaluate and manage his or her pain. PCA individualizes pain control therapy and offers the patient greater feelings of control and well-being.

With PCA, the patient self-administers small, frequent IV analgesic doses using a programmable infusion device. Most often, morphine sulfate or fentanyl is used. The PCA device limits the opioid dose within a specific time period; thereby preventing oversedation and respiratory depression. If the patient is physically or cognitively unable to use "conventional" PCA, other adaptations can be made. For example, the PCA pump can be activated by a designated family member. This family member will need thorough education in terms of how to assess for the presence of pain, how to administer the medication, and how to assess for oversedation and respiratory depression. The PCA pump can also be activated by the patient's nurse.

Subcutaneous Administration. In some situations, venous access may be limited or impossible to obtain. When this occurs, continuous subcutaneous infusion and subcutaneous PCA may be used.

Spinal Administration. Spinal opioids can provide superior pain management for many patients. Spinal opioids selectively block opioid receptors while leaving sensation, motor, and sympathetic nervous system function intact. This results in fewer opioid-related side effects than oral, intramuscular, or IV routes of administration. Analgesia from spinal opioids has a longer duration than other routes, and significantly less opioid is needed to achieve effective pain relief.[29] Opioids such as fentanyl or morphine can be given as a single injection in the epidural or intrathecal space, as intermittent injections, as a continuous infusion through an epidural catheter, or through epidural PCA.

Epidural analgesia is noted for providing effective pain relief and improved postoperative pulmonary function. This method is especially beneficial for critically ill patients after thoracic, upper abdominal, or peripheral vascular surgery, those with rib fractures or orthopedic trauma, or in postoperative patients with a history of obesity or pulmonary disease.[29] With epidural analgesia, opioids are administered through a catheter inserted in the spinal canal between the dura mater and vertebral arch. Opioids diffuse across the dura and subarachnoid space and bind with opioid receptor sites.

Intermittent injections may be given before, during, or after surgical procedures. For more sustained pain relief, continuous epidural infusions are recommended. For patient-controlled epidural analgesia (PCEA), the same parameters are used as with IV PCA, except that smaller opioid doses are used. Contraindications to epidural analgesia include systemic infection/sepsis, bleeding disorders, and increased intracranial pressure (ICP).

Preservative-free morphine and fentanyl are most commonly used for epidural analgesia because preservatives can be neurotoxic and may cause severe spinal cord injury. Morphine is more water soluble than fentanyl and therefore is more likely to accumulate in the cerebrospinal fluid (CSF) and systemic circulation. With increased accumulation, side effects are more likely. Fentanyl diffuses more quickly to the opioid receptors and causes fewer opioid-related side effects.[6] The most serious adverse effect of epidural analgesia is respiratory depression. Although the incidence of serious respiratory depression is less than 1%

with epidural analgesia, respiratory assessments should be performed hourly during the first 24 hours of therapy and every 4 hours thereafter.[29]

Because epidural analgesia is more invasive than the other methods discussed, the patient must be closely monitored for signs of local or systemic infections. The insertion site is covered with a sterile dressing, and the catheter is taped securely. To avoid accidental injection of preservative-containing medications, the epidural catheter, infusion tubing, and pump should be clearly marked.

With intrathecal analgesia, the opioid is injected into the subarachnoid space, located between the spinal cord and dura mater. Intrathecal opioids are approximately 10 times more potent than those given epidurally; therefore, less medication is needed to provide effective analgesia.[29] The intrathecal method is usually used to deliver a one-time dose of analgesic, such as before surgery, and is infrequently used as a continuous infusion because of the risk of CNS infection.

With epidural or intrathecal analgesia, a local anesthetic, such as bupivacaine, can be added to the continuous opioid infusion. Local anesthetics block pain by preventing nerve cell depolarization. They act synergistically with the intraspinal opioid and have a dose-sparing effect. Less opioid is needed to provide effective analgesia, and the incidence of opioid-related side effects is decreased. This combination is more commonly administered by the epidural route.[29]

Side Effects

Opioids cause undesirable side effects, such as constipation, urinary retention, sedation, respiratory depression, and nausea. These side effects represent a major drawback to their use. Opioid-related side effects are best managed in the following ways:

- *Decreasing the opioid dose.* This is the most effective strategy because it is directed at the *cause* of the side effect. Side effects are usually seen with excessively high serum levels of the drug. Decreasing the opioid dose can alleviate the side effect while still providing effective pain relief.
- *Avoiding prn dosing.* When opioids are administered on an as-required basis, fluctuating serum drug levels occur, causing a greater tendency toward sedation and respiratory depression. Around-the-clock administration of analgesics, including opioids, is recommended.
- *Adding an NSAID to the pain management plan.* Using an NSAID in addition to an opioid can decrease the amount of opioid needed, still provide effective pain relief, and decrease opioid-related side effects.

Medications can be given to minimize or alleviate some side effects (e.g., stool softeners for constipation, antihistamines for pruritus, and antiemetics for nausea). However, medications commonly prescribed to treat the opioid-related adverse effects can actually cause other adverse effects. For example, promethazine, a commonly prescribed antiemetic, can cause hypotension, restlessness, tremors, and extrapyramidal effects in the older patient.[29]

Respiratory depression, a life-threatening complication of opioid administration, is often a concern for nurses and physicians. The incidence of true opioid-induced respiratory depression is low in most patients. Respiratory depression is defined as a clinically significant decrease in the rate and depth of respirations from the patient's usual pattern. In some cases, a respiratory rate as low as 10 breaths per minute may not be significant if the patient is still breathing deeply.[29] Patients most at risk for respiratory depression are infants, elderly people who have not recently used opioids, and patients with coexisting pulmonary, renal, or hepatic disease.

Opioid Antagonists

If serious respiratory depression does occur, naloxone (Narcan), a pure opioid antagonist that reverses the effects of opioids, can be administered. The dose of naloxone is titrated to effect—which means reversing the oversedation and respiratory depression, not reversing analgesia. This reversal usually occurs within 1 to 2 minutes. After giving naloxone, continue to observe the patient closely for oversedation and respiratory depression because the half-life of naloxone (1.5 to 2 hours) is shorter than most opioids.

Naloxone should be diluted (0.4 mg in 10 mL of saline) and given IV, very slowly. Giving the drug too quickly or giving too much can precipitate severe pain, withdrawal symptoms, tachycardia, dysrhythmias, and cardiac arrest. Patients who have been receiving opioids for more than 1 week are particularly at risk.[2]

SEDATION AND ANXIOLYSIS

Acute pain is frequently accompanied by anxiety, and anxiety is thought to increase the patient's perception of pain.[4] When treating acute pain, anxiolytics can be used to complement analgesia and improve the patient's overall comfort. This is an important consideration, especially before and during painful procedures.

Benzodiazepines

Benzodiazepines, such as midazolam, diazepam, and lorazepam, can control anxiety and muscle spasms and produce amnesia for uncomfortable procedures. In the ICU, benzodiazepines may be given IV as an intermittent bolus or by continuous infusion and titrated according to the patient's response. Because these medications have no analgesic effect (except for controlling pain caused by muscle spasm), an analgesic must be administered concomitantly to relieve pain. If an opioid and benzodiazepine are used together, the doses of both medications should usually be reduced because of their synergistic effects. The patient should also be closely monitored for oversedation and respiratory depression.[2]

Midazolam is recommended for conscious sedation and short-term relief of anxiety because of its rapid onset (1 to 5 minutes with IV administration) and its short half-life (1 to 12 hours). Another advantage is its retrograde amnesia effect, which is particularly beneficial during procedures. The duration of effect of midazolam can be longer in older or obese patients and those with liver disease.[2,23]

A major advantage of benzodiazepines is that they are reversible agents. If respiratory depression occurs due to benzodiazepine administration, flumazenil can be administered IV. Flumazenil is a benzodiazepine-specific reversal agent that reverses the sedative and respiratory depressant effects without reversing opioid analgesics. The dosing of flumazenil should be individualized and titrated so that only the smallest effective amount is used. After prolonged benzodiazepine therapy, flumazenil should be used with caution owing to the potential for stimulating withdrawal symptoms.[23]

Propofol

Propofol is a rapid-acting sedative/hypnotic agent that has no analgesic properties and minimal amnesic effects. With appropriate airway and ventilatory management, propofol can be an ideal agent for patients requiring sedation during painful procedures. Because of its ultrashort half-life, discontinuing the infusion reverses the effect, and patients awaken within a few minutes. Propofol can also be used as a continuous infusion for mechanically ventilated patients who require deep, prolonged sedation.[2]

Because propofol is only slightly water soluble, it is formulated in a white, oil-based emulsion containing soybean oil, egg lecithin, and glycerol. It is contraindicated, therefore, in patients who are allergic to eggs or soy products. Propofol contains no preservatives, and each ampule or vial must be used as a "single-dose" product to minimize the risk of systemic infections. Adverse effects commonly associated with propofol include respiratory depression, hypotension, elevated triglycerides, and pain and stinging at the injection site. Table 5-7 provides a comparison of sedatives commonly used in critical care.[30]

Nonpharmacological Comfort Measures

The combination of nonpharmacological and pharmacological interventions has been shown to provide better pain control, with less analgesics, decreased incidence of anxiety and depression, increased activity, and increased family involvement in care.[31] These nonpharmacological approaches, which include interventions such as distraction, relaxation, music, therapeutic touch, and massage, can be a challenge to provide in the critical setting.

ENVIRONMENTAL MODIFICATION

In critical care, the most basic and logical nonpharmacological intervention is environmental modification. The excessive noise and light in ICUs can disrupt sleep and increase anxiety and agitation, in turn contributing to pain and discomfort. Care should be preplanned to minimize noise and disruptions during normal sleeping hours and to create a pattern of light that mimics normal day–night patterns. Earphones, with music of the patient's choice, and earplugs have also been recommended for use in the ICU.[32]

DISTRACTION

Distraction helps patients direct their attention away from the source of pain or discomfort toward something more pleasant. Patients, families, and nurses often use distraction routinely without giving it much consideration. Initiating a conversation with the patient during an uncomfortable procedure, watching television, and visiting with family are all excellent sources of distraction.

RELAXATION TECHNIQUES

Relaxation exercises involve repetitive focus on a word, phrase, prayer, or muscular activity, and a conscious effort to reject other intruding thoughts. Relaxation can give the patient a sense of control over a particular body part. Most relaxation methods require a quiet environment, a comfortable position, a passive attitude, and concentration. Each of these can be challenging to achieve in an ICU.

Breathing exercises have been used with much success in childbirth. They can also be used successfully in the critically ill patient. The quieting reflex is a breathing and relaxation technique that reduces stress and can easily be taught to the conscious and coherent patient. Instructions for performing the quieting reflex can be seen in Box 5-5. The nurse encourages the patient to perform the quieting reflex frequently during the day. This relaxation technique requires only 6 seconds to do, calms the sympathetic nervous system, and gives the patient a sense of control over stress and anxiety.

TOUCH

Historically, one of the greatest contributions nurses have made is in providing the comfort and caring of presence and touch. These contributions still have an important place in today's highly technological ICUs. Nurses may

table 5-7 ■ Comparison of Sedatives Commonly Used in Critical Care

Agent	Recommended Use	Onset (IV)	Unique Adverse Effects
Diazepam	For rapid sedation of acutely agitated patients	2–5 min	Phlebitis
Lorazepam	For long-term sedation of most patients by intermittent or continuous infusion	5–20 min	Acidosis or renal failure with high doses
Midazolam	For conscious sedation and rapid sedation of acutely agitated patients; for short-term use only	2–5 min	Prolonged wakening and delayed weaning from ventilator, if used long-term
Propofol	Preferred sedative when rapid awakening is important	1–2 min	Pain on injection and elevated triglycerides

Adapted from Jacobi J, Fraser G, Coursin D, et al: Clinical practice guidelines for the sustained use of sedatives and analgesics in the critically ill adult. Crit Care Med 30(1):119–141, 2002.

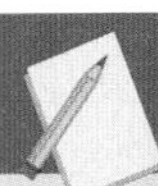

box 5-5
Instructions for the Quieting Reflex

1. Inhale an easy, natural breath.
2. Think "alert mind, calm body."
3. Smile inwardly (with your internal facial muscles).
4. As you exhale, allow your jaw, tongue, and shoulders to go loose.
5. Allow a feeling of warmth and looseness to go down through your body and out through your toes.

feel that touching is too simple to be effective. However, few medical advances can replace the benefits of warm and caring touch. The need for touch is thought to intensify during times of high stress and cannot be totally met by other forms of communication. Nurses, when using touch, are usually trying to convey understanding, support, warmth, concern, and closeness to the patient. Touching not only contributes to the patient's sense of well-being, but also promotes physical recovery from disease. It has a positive effect on perceptual and cognitive abilities and can influence physiological parameters, such as respiration and blood flow. Touch represents a positive therapeutic element of human interaction.

The effects of touch in the clinical environment are far-reaching. Touch has played a major role in promoting and maintaining reality orientation in patients prone to confusion about time, place, and personal identification. Nursing touch may be most helpful in situations in which people are experiencing fear, anxiety, depression, or isolation. It may also be beneficial for patients who have a need for encouragement or nurturing, who have difficulty verbalizing needs, or who are disoriented, unresponsive, or terminally ill. Patients often feel that the desire for touch increases with the seriousness of the illness.

MASSAGE

Superficial massage initiates the relaxation response and has been shown to increase the amount of sleep in ICU patients.[33] Although the back is the most common location used for massage, backs are often difficult to access in ICU patients. Hands, feet, and shoulders are also good sites for massage. Massage is an excellent intervention for family members to use in their attempts to provide comfort to the critically ill.

Patient Education

To educate the patient about pain and pain relief, the critical care nurse must be familiar with the patient's pain management plan and therapy being used. Communication between the nurse and patient is essential. Any information given should be reinforced periodically during the course of therapy, and the patient should be encouraged to verbalize any questions or concerns. Family members should be included whenever possible.

Plans for pain management should be discussed with patients when they are most able to understand, such as before surgery rather than during the recovery period. Emphasis is on the prevention of pain because it is easier to prevent pain than to treat it once it becomes severe.[4]

Patients need to know that most pain can be relieved and that unrelieved pain may have serious consequences for physical and psychological well-being and may interfere with recovery. The nurse helps patients and families understand that pain management is an important part of their care and that the health care team will respond quickly to reports of pain.[4]

Patients should also be given instructions about nonpharmacological interventions and traditional methods to minimize pain. Splinting the incisional area with a pillow while coughing or ambulating is a traditional pain relief measure.

The potential for drug addiction or overdosage is often a major concern for the patient and family. These issues should be addressed and clarified because they create a barrier to effective pain relief. The patient needs a clear understanding of any specialized pain management technology, such as PCA, to alleviate the fear of overdosage. The discharge planning guide in Box 5-6 summarizes points about pain management that should be covered with the patient and his or her caregiver before discharge.

PAIN MANAGEMENT IN SPECIAL POPULATIONS

Some critically ill populations create unique pain management challenges. Special considerations for pediatric and elderly patients are given in Boxes 5-7 and 5-8, respectively. A third population that is particularly challenging is patients who are known to be dying. Pain is a primary concern for patients and their families at the end of life. Since the publication of the SUPPORT trial,[21] health care providers have become much more diligent in their efforts to understand and control pain at the end of life.

Progression toward death is often marked by decreased cardiac output, decreased perfusion, and failure of major organ systems. This can create problems with excessive accumulation of analgesics and their metabolites because of limited hepatic and renal function. In such cases, hydromorphone, oxycodone, and fentanyl are preferred agents because of their short half-lives. If pain or dyspnea becomes uncontrollable despite aggressive analgesic administration, high doses of sedatives may also be used. In such cases, the

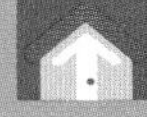

box 5-6 *Pain Management at Home*

- Teach family caregivers to assess the impact of analgesics on pain and respiratory status.
- Encourage the use of prophylactic medications, such as stool softeners, to prevent opioid-induced constipation.
- Help caregivers to understand the difference between tolerance and addiction.
- Assure that fears of addiction do not impede necessary analgesic administration.
- Reinforce the importance of preventing pain before it occurs or becomes severe.

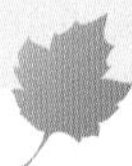

box 5-7

Considerations for the Pediatric Patient in Pain

- Pain experienced in newborns can have long-lasting effects on future pain perception and behavior.[35]
- Because of their limited ability to communicate, critically ill children should never be limited to receiving pain medication on an as-required (prn) basis only.[6]
- Intramuscular analgesics should not be used in children with a functional intravenous (IV) line.
- Analgesic dosages should be based on the child's weight, rather than age.
- Many children will deny pain because they fear shots or needles.
- Most school-aged and adolescent children have concerns about addiction because of "just-say-no" campaigns.
- Whenever possible, parents should be encouraged to provide support to their child during painful procedures.

goal of sedation is comfort and relief of suffering, and the common byproduct is end-stage unconsciousness.[34]

box 5-8

Considerations for the Older Patient in Pain

- Painful chronic diseases often compound the acute pain of critical illness in older patients.
- Arthritis, the most common cause of chronic pain in older patients, often affects the back, hips, knees, and shoulders, increasing the pain of turning in the intensive care unit (ICU).
- Some older patients can experience acutely painful conditions, such as myocardial infarction or appendicitis, without the presence of pain.
- Older patients often use words such as "aches" or "tenderness," rather than "pain."
- Family caregivers can help assess pain in older patients with cognitive or language impairments.
- Older patients are particularly sensitive to opioids, achieving higher peak concentrations and longer duration.
- Meperidine, pentazocine, propoxyphene, and methadone should not be used to treat pain in older adults.[36]
- Older patients often have an increased need for meaningful touch during episodes of crisis.

case study ■ PAIN MANAGEMENT

Ms. Breyers is 78 years old and 36 hours postoperative from a coronary artery bypass graft (CABG). She has a history of hypertension, renal insufficiency, and osteoarthritis. Her postoperative orders include 50 mg meperidine intramuscularly every 3 to 4 hours as needed for pain. She received a meperidine injection 3 hours ago, and she indicates to you that her pain is now a "9" on a scale of 0 to 10. You notice that her hands and forearms are shaking. Her heart rate is 95 beats/minute, her respiratory rate is 20 breaths/minute, and her blood pressure is 155/90 mm Hg. Ms. Breyers' surgeon plans to wean her from mechanical ventilation and discontinue her chest tubes within the next 4 hours. ■

clinical applicability challenges

Self-Challenge: Critical Thinking

1. *What concerns would you have regarding the analgesic order for Ms. Breyers?*
2. *How would you collaborate with other members of the health care team to provide interventions in response to Ms. Breyers' current symptoms?*

Study Questions

1. *Unrelieved pain may result in all of the following physiological effects except*
   a. *myocardial ischemia.*
   b. *hypotension.*
   c. *atelectasis.*
   d. *musculoskeletal contractions or spasms.*
2. *The critical care nurse should recognize that the most reliable indicator of pain in the conscious patient is*
   a. *observation of the patient's behavior.*
   b. *physiological parameters, such as heart rate and blood pressure.*
   c. *the patient's self-report of pain.*
   d. *family input regarding the presence of pain.*
3. *The best way to manage an opioid-related side effect is to*
   a. *discontinue the medication.*
   b. *administer medications to treat the side effect, such as antiemetics for nausea.*
   c. *reduce the dose of the opioid.*
   d. *only give the medication on an as-required ("prn") basis.*
4. *Although respiratory depression is rare with appropriate opioid dosing, which medication should be readily available?*
   a. *Diphenhydramine*
   b. *Nifedipine*
   c. *Naloxone*
   d. *Flumazenil*
5. *Which sedative should be used during painful procedures when rapid awakening is important?*
   a. *Diazepam*
   b. *Lorazepam*
   c. *Midazolam*
   d. *Propofol*

REFERENCES

1. Lang JD Jr: Pain: A prelude. Crit Care Clin North Am 15:1–16, 1999
2. Pasero C, McCaffery M: Multimodal balanced analgesia in the critically ill. Crit Care Nurs Clin North Am 13(2):195–206, 2001
3. Caroll, KC, Atkins, PJ, Herold GR, et al: Pain assessment and management in critically ill postoperative and trauma patients: A multisite study. Am J Crit Care 8(2):105–117, 1999

4. Agency for Health Care Policy and Research: Acute Pain Management: Operative or Medical Procedures and Trauma: Clinical Practice Guideline. AHCPR Publication Number 92-0032. Rockville, MD, U.S. Department of Health and Human Services, Public Health Service, 1992
5. Jacox A, Carr DB, Payne R, et al: Management of Cancer Pain: Clinical Practice Guideline. AHCPR Publication Number 94-0592. Rockville, MD, U.S. Department of Health and Human Services, Public Health Service, 1994
6. American Pain Society: Principles of Analgesic Use in the Treatment of Acute Pain and Cancer Pain (4th Ed). Glenview, IL, American Pain Society, 1999
7. Joint Commission on Accreditation of Healthcare Organizations: Pain Management Standards. Available at: http://www.jcaho.org/standard.html. Accessed July 1, 2002
8. McCaffery M: Pain management: Problems and progress. In McCaffery M, Pasero C (eds): Pain: Clinical Manual (2nd Ed), pp 1–14. St. Louis, Mosby, 1999
9. Cullen L, Greiner J, Titler M: Pain management in the culture of critical care. Crit Care Nurs Clin North Am 13(2):151–166, 2001
10. International Association for the Study of Pain: Pain terms: A list with definitions and notes on usage. Pain 6:249, 1979
11. McCaffery M: Nursing Practice Theories Related to Cognition, Bodily Pain and Man–Environment Interaction. Los Angeles, University of California at Los Angeles, 1968
12. Cox DS: Definitions pertaining to pain management. In St. Marie B (ed): Core Curriculum for Pain Management Nursing, pp 31–42. Philadelphia, WB Saunders, 2002
13. Pasero C, McCaffery, M: Pain in the critically ill. Am J Nurs 102(1):59–60, 2002
14. Stanik-Hutt J, Soeken K, Belcher A, et al: Pain experiences of traumatically injured patients in a critical care setting. Am J Crit Care 10(4):252–259, 2001
15. Puntillo KA, White C, Morris A, et al: Patients' perceptions and responses to procedural pain: Results from Thunder II Project. Am J Crit Care 10(4):238–251, 2001
16. Thompson CL, White C, Wild L, et al: Translating research into practice: Implications of Thunder Project II. Crit Care Nurs Clin North Am 13(4):541–546, 2001
17. Pasero C, Paice J, McCaffery M: Basic mechanisms underlying the causes and effects of pain. In McCaffery M, Pasero C (eds): Pain: Clinical Manual (2nd Ed), pp 15–34. St. Louis, Mosby, 1999
18. Swope E: Benefits of proper pain management. In St. Marie B (ed): Core Curriculum for Pain Management Nursing, pp 55–66. Philadelphia, WB Saunders, 2002
19. Yeager MP, Glass DD, Neff RK, et al: Epidural anesthesia and analgesia in high-risk surgical patients. Anesthesiology 66:729–736, 1987
20. Wild LR: Pain management: An organizational perspective. Crit Care Nurs Clin North Am 13(2):297–309, 2001
21. SUPPORT Principal Investigators: A controlled trial to improve care for seriously ill hospitalized patients. JAMA 274:1591–1598, 1995
22. National Guideline Clearinghouse. Available at: http://www.guideline.gov. Accessed July 1, 2002
23. Jacobi J, Fraser G, Coursin D, et al: Clinical practice guidelines for the sustained use of sedatives and analgesics in the critically ill adult. Crit Care Med 30(1):119–141, 2002
24. Pellino TA, Willens J, Polomano RC, et al: The American Society of Pain Management Nurses Practice Analysis: Role delineation study. Pain Manage Nurs 3(1):2–15, 2002
25. Kwekkeboom K, Herr K: Assessment of pain in the critically ill. Crit Care Nurs Clin North Am 13(2):181–194, 2001
26. Aschenbrenner D: Drugs used to control pain. In Aschenbrenner D, Cleveland L, Venable S (eds): Drug Therapy in Nursing, pp 375–419. Philadelphia, Lippincott Williams & Wilkins, 2002
27. Nickel E, Smith T: Analgesia in the intensive care unit. Crit Care Nurs Clin North Am 13(2):207–219, 2001
28. Gust R, Pester S, Gust A, et al: Effect of patient-controlled analgesia on pulmonary complications after coronary artery-bypass grafting. Crit Care Med 27:2218–2223, 1999
29. Pasero C, Portenoy R, McCaffery M: Opioid analgesics. In McCaffery M, Pasero C (eds): Pain: Clinical Manual (2nd Ed), pp 15–34. St. Louis, Mosby, 1999
30. Venable S: Drugs producing anesthesia and neuromuscular blockade. In Aschenbrenner D, Cleveland L, Venable S (eds): Drug Therapy in Nursing, pp 203–226. Philadelphia, Lippincott Williams & Wilkins, 2002
31. Titler M, Rakel B: Nonpharmacologic treatment of pain. Crit Care Nurs Clin North Am 13(2):221–232, 2001
32. Wallace C, Robins J, Alvord L, et al: The effect of earplugs on sleep measures during exposure to simulated intensive care unit noise. Am J Crit Care 8:210–219, 1999
33. Richards K: Effect of a back massage and relaxation intervention on sleep in critically ill patients. Am J Crit Care 7:288–299, 1998
34. Panke J: Difficulties in managing pain at the end of life. Am J Nurs 102(7):26–34, 2002
35. Oakes L: Assessment and management of pain in the critically ill pediatric patient. Crit Care Nurs Clin North Am 13(2):281–291, 2001
36. Luggen A: Pain. In Lueckenotte A (ed): Gerontologic Nursing (2nd Ed), pp 281–301. St. Louis, Mosby, 2000

OTHER SELECTED READING

Blakely W, Page, G: Pathophysiology of pain in critically ill patients. Crit Care Nurs Clin North Am 13(2):151–166, 2001

Blum J, Schadler A, Prush-Cooper S: Assessment and management of acute cardiac chest pain. Crit Care Nurs Clin North Am 13(2):259–270, 2001

Ferrell B, Coyle N: Textbook of Palliative Nursing. Oxford, Oxford University Press, 2001

Stanik-Hutt J: Pain management in the acutely ill. In Chulay M, Molter N (eds): Protocols for Practice. Aliso Viejo, CA, American Association of Critical-Care Nurses, 1998

Stenger K, Schooley K, Moss L: Moving to evidence-based practice for pain management in the critical care setting. Crit Care Nurs Clin North Am 13(2):319–328, 2001

Wall P, Melzack R: Textbook of Pain (4th Ed). Edinburgh, Churchill Livingstone, 1999

Wong D: Whaley & Wong's Nursing Care of Infants and Children (6th Ed). St. Louis, CV Mosby, 1999

chapter

6

Patient and Family Education in Critical Care

MARY O. PALAZZO

objectives

Based on the content in this chapter, the reader should be able to:

- Describe the barriers to learning that are unique to the critical care setting.
- Describe and differentiate between the concepts of education and learning.
- Identify the six principles of adult learning.
- Identify the three domains of learning.

Patient and family education is a vital component of nursing care. In the critical care setting, it is always a challenge to meet the educational needs of patients and families because of the life-threatening nature of critical illness. The nurse must deal with the anxiety and fear that is associated with a diagnosis of critical illness, while trying to teach difficult concepts in an environment that is poorly suited to learning. Beyond the immediate nurse–patient relationship, there are many global forces affecting health care that are reshaping every dimension of nursing care, including patient education.

Health care is no longer solely defined in terms of sound clinical decision making; now, it also encompasses prudent use of resources and financial accountability. Insurers are questioning the value-added component for every patient care interaction.[1] This change in the health care climate necessitates clear definitions and quantification of nursing care. The financial constraints of managed care have resulted in an overall decrease in hospital length of stay and the subsequent discharge of patients and families, sometimes before they are ready to learn. Today, it is not unusual for a patient to be discharged home from an intensive care unit (ICU), placing even greater responsibility on the patient and family to provide for high-intensity care at home. The critical care nurse not only manages the hemodynamic instability that often accompanies critical illness, but prepares the patient and family for the likelihood of early discharge from the hospital.

At the same time, hospitals are facing an ongoing shortage of critical care nurses. ICUs that were once reserved for the most experienced nurses are now training grounds for the newly graduated nurse. The novice nurse focuses on learning how to manage the myriad of technological devices used to support the critically ill patient, while understanding the pathophysiology of multisystemic illness. For the new nurse, however, it may be very difficult to move beyond the essential nursing tasks that are an integral part of patient care to address the educational needs of the patient and family. In addition, the expanded use of contract nurses to meet the demands of a variable patient census or to fill staff vacancies can also have a negative impact on patient and family education. A nurse working only one or two shifts a week may not develop a relationship with the patient and family or be able to follow up and validate learning. Difficulties mount when there is little or no continuity of care to assess learning needs and promote education.

These are just a few examples of the realities of health care. The fragmentation of patient care across the health care system presents many obstacles and barriers to patient education. The purpose of this chapter is to assist students and nurses in developing the skills and tools needed to meet the challenge of patient and family education in the presence of critical illness. Nurses who understand the learning barriers that are unique to the critical care setting will be better prepared to address the learning needs of patients and families.

BARRIERS TO LEARNING

Critical Illness and Stress

Typically, the patient and family enter an ICU quite unexpectedly owing to a life-threatening event. The onset of illness signals the beginning of a physical and emotional crisis for all involved. Altered metabolic responses, exposure to general anesthesia, use of cardiopulmonary bypass, episodes of hypoxia, and marked sleep deprivation are common events for the critically ill. Each of these factors can compromise mental acuity and decrease one's learning capacity and recall. In addition, combating a severe illness consumes most of the patient's energy, leaving him or her with a limited ability to learn.

The patient experiences not only the physical effects related to the disease process, but emotional and spiritual distress. Patients express feelings of helplessness, loss of control, and fear of death when facing serious illness. The vigilant critical care nurse recognizes a patient's fear and anxiety and guides him or her through the unfamiliar course of illness, treatment, and recovery. These are special opportunities for patient education despite the extreme stress of critical illness. However, in the critical care setting, it is not unusual for the focus of education to quickly shift away from the patient and be redirected to meet the learning needs of the family members.

An emotional and physical toll is exacted on the family members of critically ill patients, with stress levels peaking within 72 hours of admission to the unit.[2] The descriptive study by Halm and colleagues demonstrates changes in the sleeping and eating patterns of family members, as well as an increased use of cigarettes, over-the-counter medications, and alcohol and prescription drugs while coping with the crisis of a critically ill patient.[2] Other signs of fear and anxiety include hypervigilance, frequent visits, telephone calls, repetitive questions, and the inability to recall information.[3] Intense anxiety and the fear of death evoked by critical illness may cause families to forget much of the information that has been given to them. Often, the critical care nurse must repeat the same information and answer identical questions repeatedly. Nursing interventions that are aimed at reducing family anxiety and supporting the family throughout the course of critical illness decrease the barriers to learning. The following case study demonstrates how the interventions of the critical care nurse are used to support the educational and emotional needs of a family in crisis.

case study ■ A PATIENT AND FAMILY IN CRISIS

The electronic doors to the cardiovascular intensive care unit (CVICU) swing open and John and Margaret enter their 40-year-old daughter's room. Mary Ann has just returned to the CVICU after a mitral valve replacement and a tricuspid valve repair. Unfortunately, the valve replacement was complicated and the patient had a prolonged course on cardiopulmonary bypass. Mary Ann's heart was quite weak before the surgery and now she requires an intra-aortic balloon pump and multiple medications to support her cardiac output. She has also developed a coagulopathy related to the extended time on cardiopulmonary bypass and continues to bleed. Her vital signs are stable, but Mary Ann requires a continuous infusion of blood products to keep up with the blood loss from her chest tubes.

John and Margaret are shocked by their daughter's appearance. Mary Ann's pale, edematous face and lifeless expression are certainly not what they expected to see. There is little about their daughter that resembles the person they know and love. Equipment surrounds her bed and supports nearly every bodily function. Visibly shaken, they look at each other with tears in their eyes, wondering how a seemingly routine valve operation could turn out this way.

Suzanne, the critical care nurse caring for Mary Ann, greets John and Margaret and begins to talk about their daughter's appearance. She carefully explains the purpose of all the bedside equipment as she cares for Mary Ann. Suzanne tells the worried parents what she is doing and why she is performing each procedure. It is the nurse's calm and caring approach that engenders a sense of hope for their daughter's eventual recovery. John and Margaret begin to relax a little and start to ask questions about what to expect in the next few hours.

This brief example illustrates the unpredictability of illness and just how quickly the crisis can occur. In this scenario, the bedside nurse initiates family education through an informal discussion of the patient's status. The initial interaction with family members is extremely important because it helps to establish a foundation of trust and respect between the nurse and family.[4] In the course of talking with the parents, the nurse is continually assessing their learning needs and developing an understanding of their coping mechanisms. She is helping the family to deal with the crisis phase of this illness by providing consistent and accurate information about the condition of their loved one. Research has demonstrated that up-to-date information is the highest priority for family members who are coping with critical illness.[5] The critical care nurse teaches families about the pathophysiology of the illness, the diagnostic studies that are performed, and the treatment plan that is underway. The primary education goal for most families is to learn all that they can about their loved one. ■

Prolonged Illness and Stress

Frequently, the period of illness extends well beyond the initial crisis phase and creates additional burdens for the patient and the family. Families are forced to balance their home and work schedules with time spent at the hospital. Over time, it may become increasingly difficult for the family to obtain information and patient status reports from the health care team. Often, physician schedules are unpredictable and do not mesh with the family visits. This further underscores the vital role that the critical care nurse plays as a link to the family. With protracted critical illness, many families often struggle to keep the lines of communication open to the extended family, creating opportunities for conflict and misinformation.

As a patient and family advocate, the nurse provides accurate information and shares the plan of care with the family. Additional interventions such as a patient care or ethics conferences may be arranged by the critical care nurse to give the family an opportunity to discuss the case with the entire health care team. Patient care conferences afford open communication with the family and may be a therapeutic method for dispelling misinformation and misconceptions about the patient's progress.

Clearly, the critical care nurse plays a vital role in assisting the patient and family to cope with the crisis of critical illness by providing education from admission to discharge.

Environmental Stress

Ringing telephones, chiming call lights and pagers, overhead announcements, equipment alarms, staff conversations, banging automatic doors, and pneumatic tubes are just a few examples of the sounds that fill the air of a typical ICU. It is easy for nurses to become desensitized to these familiar noises because they are an integral part of the work environment. However, taking a moment to listen to the background sounds from a patient's bedside will quickly remind one of how stressful noise can be. Patients and families are not accustomed to the normal sounds of an ICU. Yet, as difficult as it may be, we are asking patients and families to learn in this setting.

Optimal learning environments are quiet moments spent with the patient and family using comfortable chairs that are arranged to optimize discussion along with the use of audiovisual aids, if possible. This hardly describes a typical ICU setting. However, there are common measures that can help to reduce the environmental stress and enhance the success of learning. The simple act of closing the door to the patient's room or placing a comfortable chair at the bedside can reduce the background noise sufficiently and enhance the learner's attention span. Reducing the alarm volumes on bedside equipment while the nurse is talking with the patient or family helps to minimize the number of interruptions, and may improve the learner's ability to focus on the topic of a teaching session.

Ensuring privacy while sensitive or confidential information is being exchanged can markedly reduce the anxiety of a patient or family member. Often, strangers witness the emotional outbursts and intimate interactions of families who are agonizing over the illness of a loved one. Health care providers are not always mindful of their surroundings when discussing confidential details of a patient's case. Critical care nurses can direct health care team members and families to a quiet room away from the general waiting area to afford privacy when discussing patient specifics.

This regard for the patient also applies to teaching rounds or patient care rounds that are held in the halls of an ICU. Patients should be treated with respect, and they often wish to be included in bedside presentations. Research indicates that patients prefer to be introduced to the health care team members and expect an explanation of medical terminology used in the discussion, privacy, and a seated presentation.[6] It may not always be practical for the entire team to sit down at every patient's bedside during rounds, but the patient should be given the option of participating in the discussion of his or her care whenever possible.

Cultural and Language Barriers

As the United States population transforms, the patients and families that nurses care for in hospitals and critical care settings are becoming increasingly diverse. The National Center for Health Statistics estimates that the population will be 50% ethnic minorities by the year 2050.[7] Beliefs about health and illness are deeply rooted in culture. How a patient or family member responds to the diagnosis or a proposed treatment and education may be strongly influenced by his or her values and culture.[8] Although the nursing literature readily acknowledges the importance of providing culturally sensitive patient care, in practice there is little evidence of cultural awareness in the nurse's daily assessments and interactions with patients and families. Culturally competent nursing care is defined as being sensitive to issues related to culture, race, gender, sexual orientation, social class, and economic situation.[9] In addition, culturally competent nursing also considers the family structure and gender role as it relates to the patient. For example, in the Asian culture, important health care decisions should be discussed with the family. An individual would not make an independent decision because the family is considered to be the smallest decision-making unit.[8]

Successful education of culturally diverse patients and families requires more than just basic knowledge regarding ethnic groups. Critical care nurses must recognize their own individual biases and examine their personal values and beliefs about health and nursing care. Many of our health beliefs are based on commonly held Euro-American values such as belief in individualism, belief in informed consent, orientation toward clock time, and belief in God as the most powerful being.[10] Other shared beliefs also exist, such as the belief that technology and science will improve the overall human condition.[10] The imposition of these Euro-American values on other cultures may impede communication

box 6-1
Key Pieces of Information to Obtain as Part of the Cultural Assessment

- Place of birth
- Length of time in this country
- Ethnic affiliation and ethnic identity
  - Does the patient live in an ethnic community?
  - Who are the patient's major support people?
- Primary and secondary languages (speaking and reading ability)
- Religious practices
- Health and illness beliefs and practices
- Communication practices (verbal and nonverbal)
- How decisions are made in the context of the patient and family

Adapted from Lipson JG: Culturally competent nursing care. In Lipson JG, Dibble SL, Mainarik PA (eds): Culture and Nursing Care: A Pocket Guide, pp 1–6. San Francisco, UCSF Nursing Press, 1998.

box 6-2
Guidelines for Communication Using an Interpreter

- Before the session, meet with the interpreter to give background information and explain the purpose of the session.
- If possible, have the interpreter meet with the patient or family to determine their educational level, health care beliefs, and health care attitudes to plan the depth of information needed.
- Speak in short units of speech and avoid long explanations, use of medical jargon, abbreviations, and colloquialisms.
- When communicating to the patient or family, look directly toward the person and not at the interpreter. Watch the patient's and family members' body language and nonverbal communication response.
- Be patient. Interpreted interviews take a long time to complete and may become tiresome for the patient.
- Have the patient and family members validate the information given to them through the interpreter, to make sure that they understand the instructions or message that has been given.

between the nurse and patient and hinder the education process. Although critical care nurses do not have the time to complete a thorough cultural assessment, several key pieces of information should be obtained. This information is outlined in Box 6-1.

Language barriers also pose a major obstacle to patient and family education, especially in the stressful critical care environment. Every effort should be made to provide an interpreter to translate information for the patient and family. It is convenient for health care providers to rely solely on a family member or friend to translate complex medical information and terminology that is likely to be unfamiliar to them. However, it may be difficult for a family member or friend to keep personal bias from entering the context of the conversation. In addition, the information that may be exchanged between the health care provider and the patient may be personal or embarrassing to either the patient or to the family member who is pressed into service. Box 6-2 offers some suggestions for communicating with a patient and his or her family through an interpreter. Written instructions should also be translated and reviewed in the presence of an interpreter so that any questions can be addressed immediately. Printed instructions in several languages should be readily available for use in the ICU.

EDUCATION AND LEARNING

It is important to discriminate between education and learning. Many times, these two terms are used interchangeably, but there is a difference in the concepts. Education is defined as an activity, initiated by one or more persons, that is designed to effect changes in the knowledge, skill, and attitudes of individuals, groups, or communities.[11] Education places more emphasis on the person facilitating the learning, whereas learning itself is defined as a phenomenon of internal change. The learner experiences a flash of insight that results in behavioral changes.[12] The key concept in learning is changing to a new state of mind.[13] The focus shifts from the role of the educator to that of the individual who experiences the change.

Three Domains of Learning

Three domains of human behavior or learning to consider when developing an education plan are the cognitive domain, the affective domain, and the psychomotor domain. Keeping these domains in mind while assessing and developing a teaching plan can assist the nurse in selecting suitable teaching methods.

The cognitive domain of learning involves the development of insight or understanding that provides a basis or guideline for behavior.[13] In this domain, knowledge expands and teaching–learning material is organized from simple to complex. Learning is enhanced when information builds on previous knowledge. Therefore, the basic ideas should be well introduced before attempting to teach the hard-to-remember facts. As an example, cognitive learning occurs when a family member learns to assess wound healing. The critical care nurse provides basic information about the normal healing process and the appearance of a healthy incision. Once the family member understands how a healed incision should look, the nurse can explain the signs and symptoms of infection and when to call the physician. Once prepared, the family member should then be able to apply the learned principles to provide appropriate home care for the patient.

The affective domain pervades all spheres of learning because it encompasses the patient's values, attitudes, and feelings.[13] Attempting to modify an attitude or emotional response requires a safe and trusting relationship between the patient and the nurse. When formulating a teaching plan, the nurse should take a nonthreatening approach to assessing what the patient considers important enough to learn. A helpful teaching strategy may be the interactive group learning that is typical of a smoking cessation class. In this situation the teacher demonstrates behaviors that the learner wants to imitate and provides positive feedback to the participants to encourage them to stop smoking cigarettes. If the learning experiences are satisfying and the patient associates positive feelings with the experience, it may help to influence the change in behavior.

The psychomotor domain involves motor skills that are composed of an ordered sequence of movement that must be learned.[13] To learn a particular skill, the patient must have a neuromuscular system that is able to perform the skill and the capacity to form a mental image of the act.[13] A mental image is created when the learner watches a demonstration while the teacher points out the relevant steps that are required to successfully complete the task. The nurse may use a written, step-by-step guide as a reference while demonstrating the skill and allowing the patient to ask questions. It will take practice for the patient or family member to become proficient at performing the task. Many adults are intimidated by learning a new skill; therefore, it is important for the nurse to provide praise and encouragement with each teaching session. Learning to inject insulin is an example of psychomotor learning.

Teaching methods that are based on the three domains of learning are displayed in Figure 6-1.

Adult Learning Principles

The principles of adult learning are based on multiple learning theories that originate in many different disciplines, such as developmental psychology, sociology, philosophy, and education. Adult learning is a relatively new field (approximately 40 years old), with the fundamental principles grounded in childhood learning and

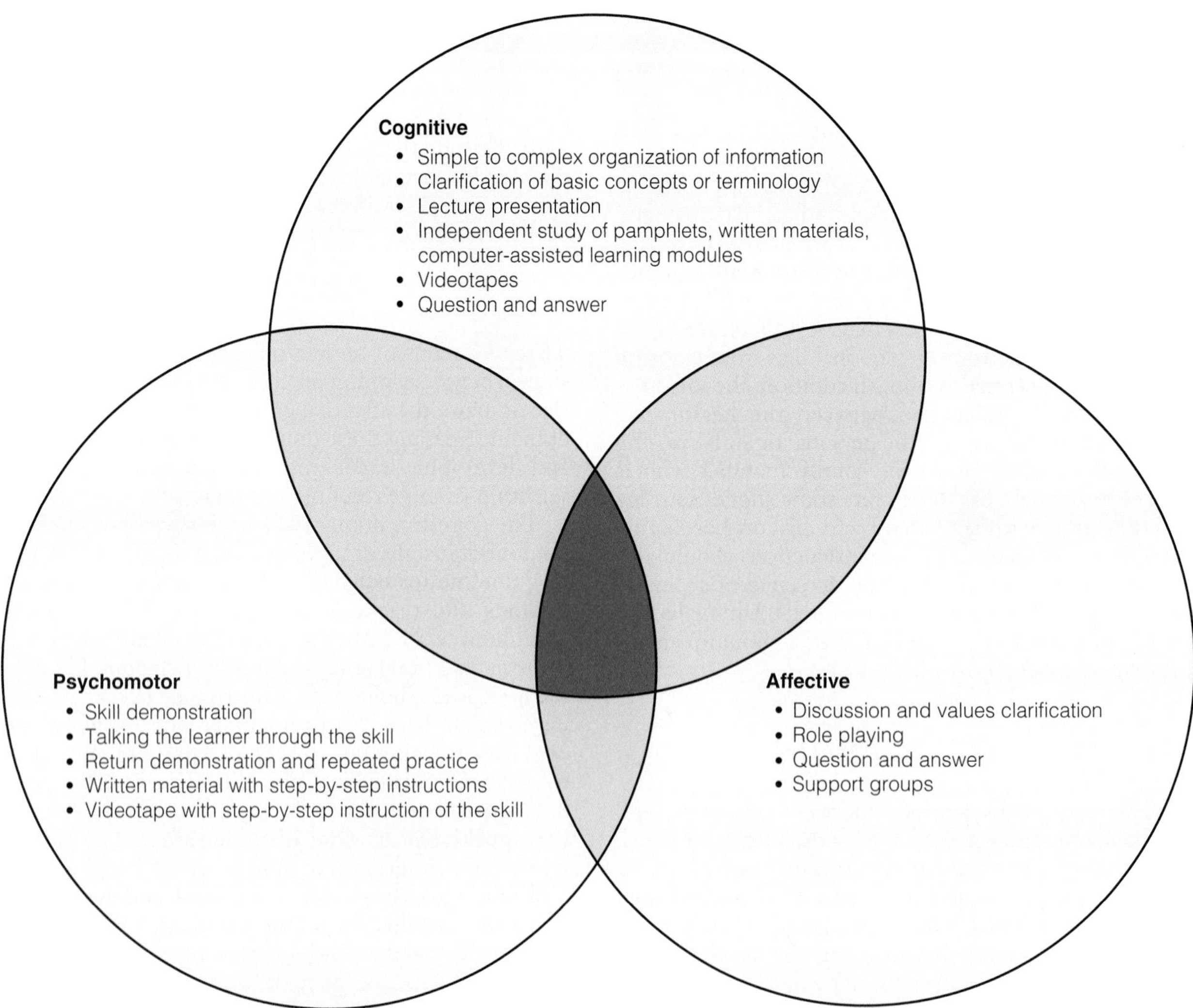
Cognitive
• Simple to complex organization of information
• Clarification of basic concepts or terminology
• Lecture presentation
• Independent study of pamphlets, written materials, computer-assisted learning modules
• Videotapes
• Question and answer
Psychomotor
• Skill demonstration
• Talking the learner through the skill
• Return demonstration and repeated practice
• Written material with step-by-step instructions
• Videotape with step-by-step instruction of the skill
Affective
• Discussion and values clarification
• Role playing
• Question and answer
• Support groups

figure 6-1 Teaching methods based on the domains of learning.

education. A new conceptual framework known as the *andragogical model* emerged from research studies that identified some of the unique characteristics of adult learners.[14] The core principles of the andragogical model of adult learning are:

1. *The need to know.* Adults need to understand why they need to learn something before they are willing to commit the energy and time to learn it. It is important for the learner to understand and be aware of the "need to know." To raise the learner's level of awareness, the facilitator may need to use real or simulated experiences to help the learner discover the lack of knowledge.
2. *The learner's self-concept.* Adults are self-directed and responsible for their own decision making. In general, adults resent the feeling that others are making choices for them. Adult educators need to create learning situations that are more self-directed and independent.
3. *The learner's life experience.* Adults have lived longer and accumulated more life experiences than children. Life experience defines and shapes adult beliefs, values, and attitudes. Adult education methods emphasize experiential techniques such as case method, simulation, and problem-solving exercises. In addition, adults learn well from their peers, making group learning an effective teaching method to use.
4. *Readiness to learn.* Adults are ready to learn the things they need to know. The information should be applicable to real-life situations.
5. *Orientation to learning.* Adults are motivated to learn if the information will help them to perform useful tasks or to deal with problems in their life.
6. *Motivation to learn.* Adults are more motivated by internal forces such as improved quality of life, increased job satisfaction, and improved self-esteem. External factors such as job promotion or increased salary are less likely to sustain learning.[14]

An example of how the critical care nurse might use adult learning principles in the practice setting is presented in the following scenario. Mr. Jones underwent a coronary artery bypass graft (CABG) procedure 2 days ago. He questions the nurse about the breakfast tray that contains scrambled eggs and ham, while explaining that the eggs contain too much cholesterol and that he has been told to avoid all high-cholesterol foods. The nurse replies that the scrambled egg is an egg substitute product that is actually part of a heart-healthy diet. At this point, Mr. Jones is demonstrating his readiness to learn and is attempting to apply the new knowledge to alter his eating habits. His learning motivation stems from an intrinsic desire to change that is now focused on his overall quality of life and improving his health. His question affords the nurse an opening to discuss other heart-healthy activities and lifestyle changes that will help the patient to achieve wellness in his recovery.

The critically ill patient and family are highly motivated to learn because a life-threatening event has triggered an intense need for information. Successful teaching plans should incorporate adult learning principles and relevant information that will readily apply to real life and assist with recovery from critical illness.

THE PROCESS OF ADULT EDUCATION

The process of patient and family education entails more than just providing an educational brochure or turning on an instructional videotape. It is an interactive process based on a therapeutic relationship, which uses the fundamental steps of assessment, diagnosis, goals, intervention, and evaluation.[13,15] Frequently, the nursing process is used informally by critical care nurses because teaching is so highly integrated into routine nursing care and family interactions. Just as the bedside nurse uses clinical judgment to recognize and treat the hemodynamic instability that often accompanies critical illness, he or she also diagnoses and intervenes to meet the learning needs of the patient and family. As nurses advance in practice, learning assessment becomes more refined and focuses on meeting the educational goals. Each learning session enhances the knowledge of the patient and family and offers the nurse a chance to evaluate the success or failure of what he or she has taught.

Although the focus of this chapter is on educating the adult patient, the principles of assessment, intervention, and evaluation remain in effect regardless of the age of the patient. Special considerations when teaching pediatric patients are listed in Box 6-3.

Assessing Learning Needs in a Time of Crisis

The critical care nurse must be very sensitive to the heightened anxiety that accompanies an admission to the ICU. Anxiety markedly reduces the ability of the patient and family to concentrate. Therefore, the nurse should avoid long explanations or tedious questions. The first step in the assessment process is to get to know the patient and family. This often begins with a simple introduction. Taking a few minutes to learn the family names and their relationship to the patient signifies respect and begins to build a therapeutic and trusting relationship. It gives the nurse a chance to orient the patient and family to the ICU, as well as to teach them about some of the equipment used in the care of the patient.

Understanding the learning needs of patients and families does not need to entail a protracted interview or use of formal assessment tools with overly generic questions about health beliefs and learning styles.[16] It is better to use an informal and open-ended dialogue between the nurse and the family to establish the "need to know." Use of open-ended questions such as "What is your understanding of your mother's condition?" or "What did the physician tell you about the surgery?" will give the nurse a starting point for teaching the family. It also validates whether the patient or family member clearly understands previous explanations given by other members of the health care team.

box 6-3

Guidelines for Teaching the Pediatric Patient

- Children learn more easily from their parents; therefore, a parent should be used as often as possible during teaching.
- If parents cannot do the actual teaching, they should be present to answer questions and give the child more confidence.
- Children learn through play (games, toys, and role playing).
- Teaching can be more effective if related to home routines.
- Teaching should be related to the child's life experiences (developmental level or personal).
- Questions should be answered immediately and in a language the child understands.
- Trust is important to teaching. If the nurse says a procedure will not hurt, and it does hurt, the child will not trust the nurse.
- Learning should be evaluated frequently to ensure that the child understands.
- The nurse should praise the child often or offer rewards.
- School-age children usually are eager to learn.
- School-age children can understand cause and effect.
- Children should be included in planning and setting goals.
- Younger children have short attention spans (about 10 minutes). School-age age children can usually tolerate teaching sessions of 30 minutes or less. Adolescents can have sessions of 45 to 50 minutes.

Informal assessment often provides the nurse with a baseline evaluation of literacy and the person's level of education. Literacy assessment can be very difficult and requires sensitivity because most adults with a reading difficulty spend a lifetime hiding it.[17] Nonthreatening questions such as, "Do you prefer to learn new information by reading or watching a program on television?" may give the nurse a clue about a patient or family member's level of literacy. With about 20% of the United States population considered to be functionally illiterate, it is very likely that the educational brochures or the operative consent that is given to patients or families will be beyond their reading level.[11] Every day, critical care nurses assume that the consent form given to a patient or family member to read is clearly understood when the form is returned signed and unquestioned. Written educational material should always be in the active voice and targeted for a fifth- to eighth-grade reading level.[18] In addition, the nurse should verbally review any written material with the patient or family, in case they are unable to read the document and are too embarrassed to admit it.

Assessment is a dynamic and ongoing process, providing the critical care nurse with many opportunities to assist patients and families to cope with the stress and anxiety associated with critical illness, while meeting their learning needs. It also entails knowing when the patient or family is unable to learn. For example, patients who are experiencing pain will not be able to focus on learning a new skill such as insulin administration without first having adequate pain control. A family member who has just learned that a loved one has suffered a cardiac arrest is not likely to be able to assimilate the intricate details of myocardial ischemia. Setting unrealistic educational goals hinders learning and frustrates both the nurse and the learner. The teaching plan must be continually evaluated and altered if it is ineffective, poorly timed, or not meeting the learner's needs.

Intervention: Effective Teaching Strategies in Critical Care

TEACHABLE MOMENTS

Teachable moments are those instances when the nurse and learner together recognize the need for education and the learner is open to hearing information.[12] Life-threatening illness often stimulates changes in unhealthy behavior patterns, only then igniting a patient's interest in learning. Much of the learning required of a patient who is recovering from critical illness involves behavior changes that will require alterations in lifestyle. Smoking cessation, dietary restrictions, and activity limitations are the types of lifestyle changes that patients frequently struggle to achieve and maintain. Teachable moments often occur in the course of routine patient care. Therefore, the nurse should be ready to incorporate teaching while providing care. For example, the nurse can review postoperative incision care in a brief teaching session, while performing skin assessment. The review can include the signs and symptoms of infection, proper wound cleansing, and a description of a healthy healing incision. Teaching pertinent information about the indications or side effects of medications, while giving them to the patient, is another way to reinforce learning. Both of these examples highlight the importance of focusing on a single concept, especially considering the limited attention span that is typical of a patient who is recovering from a critical illness. Learning is best accomplished when the message is consistent and the knowledge progresses from simple to more complex concepts.

THE FAMILY CONNECTION

Often the critical care nurse recognizes the limitations of the patient's ability to comprehend information, and then turns to the family to provide instruction. It is well known that patients retain only about 50% of the information that they receive in the hospital.[19] It is likely that retention of information by the critically ill patient is much worse. Therefore, family participation in teaching sessions helps to ensure the success of the teaching plan. In addition, providing written materials that the patient can review after discharge from the hospital helps to bridge the retention gap. Guidelines for developing printed materials that are appropriate for use with older patients are presented in Box 6-4.

Another effective teaching strategy for the adult learner is group learning. For example, postoperative cardiac surgical patients can benefit from a class on posthospital care.

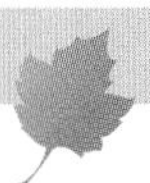

box 6-4

Guidelines for Printed Educational Materials

- Font should be 12 points or greater.
- Serif type is preferred over sans-serif type.
- Avoid script or stylized types.
- Avoid the use of all uppercase letters for body type.
- Line lengths should be no longer than 5 inches.
- Paper with a glossy finish should be avoided because the glare makes reading difficult. Use matte-finish paper instead.
- Legibility is enhanced when black ink is printed on white or off-white paper.
- Avoid printing over a designed or customized background.

A group teaching session allows patients the chance to share common experiences and concerns about recovery with each other. Including families in the group may stimulate questions and allow them to express concerns about potential complications and fears about taking care of a loved one at home. Many times families are fearful of caring for a loved one who has recovered from a life-threatening illness. They are afraid that they will miss an important symptom or that something will go wrong and their loved one will become ill again or even die. The critical care nurse should acknowledge these feelings and provide the family with emotional support while giving the tools and information to ensure safe care at home. The family interaction also provides the nurse with an assessment of potential home health care needs. It may become apparent that a home health care consultation is indicated for further teaching, and reinforcement of newly learned skills may be needed to facilitate a safe transition from the hospital to home.

Evaluating the Learning Process

Evaluation is a measurement of the critical learning elements established in the teaching plan. It provides evidence about patient accomplishments or skills that may need further development.[20] Evaluation also reinforces correct behavior on the part of learners and helps teachers determine the adequacy of their instruction.[20] Questions provide the teacher and learner with immediate feedback and validate the learner's grasp of the information presented. The nurse should avoid using leading questions to achieve a desired answer. True evaluation is based on the learner's responses, which indicate whether additional reinforcement of the key concepts is needed or not. Direct observation of newly learned skills or procedures should also be part of the evaluation. Because adults do not want to appear awkward or clumsy when performing a task, it is important to have a relaxed, positive learning environment where the teacher and student have a good rapport before asking a patient or family member to demonstrate a new task or skill. The learner should be able to successfully answer or perform 94% of all the critical elements outlined in the teaching plan.[20] Often the success or failure of patient and family education influences the discharge plans. Patients who are unable reliably to perform new tasks will need supervision and further practice to learn the new skill. Therefore, adequate evaluation of the learning process is an essential component of the health care continuum.

There are many ways to develop a patient and family teaching plan. Given a homogeneous population, standardized patient teaching plans and records can be used. Plans should include information that is essential for most patients, but can also be flexible enough to accommodate individual needs. Teaching plans include nursing diagnoses, outcome criteria, and interventions.

The nursing diagnosis assists the nurse to identify the appropriate content to teach. It also helps to formulate the outcomes that will be used to evaluate the progress of the patient and family and the effectiveness of the teaching plan. The outcomes should be stated in measurable terms, and the teaching should be outlined in a logical sequence. Each nursing intervention should include the content, method, and media used for teaching. In addition, the patient's barriers to learning should be addressed, and the nursing interventions aimed at meeting those personal needs. In critical care, families are often included in the teaching plans because of the limited learning ability of the patient.

case study ■ PATIENT EDUCATION

Mr. Chang is a 50-year-old married Asian man who was admitted to the hospital after experiencing chest pain while at work. He had mild elevation in his cardiac enzymes and was taken to the cardiac catheterization laboratory within a few hours of the onset of the chest pain. The interventional cardiologist found two arteries 50% occluded. He was able to perform an angioplasty, place a stent in the arteries, and successfully restore the blood flow to the affected myocardium. Mr. Chang spoke with the Cardiac Rehabilitation nurse the morning after his procedure and she reviewed his cardiac risk factors. He was noted to be 30 pounds overweight, his cholesterol was 250 mg/dL, and he smokes two packs of cigarettes per day. After this procedure, Mr. Chang is anxious to learn of ways to reduce his risk of myocardial infarction. The Collaborative Care Guide in Box 6-5 is a sample teaching plan for Mr. Chang. ■

THE STANDARDS OF PATIENT AND FAMILY EDUCATION

There is great emphasis on patient and family education that stems from the Joint Commission on Accreditation of Healthcare Organizations (JCAHO) patient care standards. These standards serve to promote overall patient care quality in health care organizations. Hospitals voluntarily participate in JCAHO surveys to ensure that the patient care

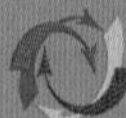

box 6-5 collaborative care guide
for Educating a Patient About Myocardial Infarction

OUTCOMES	INTERVENTIONS
Patient will be able to state content presented.	■ Plan teaching sessions for a period of time with minimal interruptions. ■ Include patient's wife and family in teaching sessions. ■ Provide written information to reinforce the verbal information. ■ Review the diagnosis of myocardial infarction and the therapies used to prevent further damage to the heart muscle. ■ Review cardiac risk factors for this patient and identify those risk factors that he can control. ■ Consult the dietitian for weight reduction and meal planning. ■ Discuss the sodium content of foods related to Asian cuisine. ■ Discuss the target cholesterol level for this patient and the medications and dietary changes needed to reduce the risk for myocardial infarction. ■ Discuss tobacco use related to myocardial oxygen demand and the vasoactive effects of nicotine. ■ Offer information about smoking cessation programs and medical options available to assist him with stopping smoking. ■ Refer the patient to a formal Cardiac Rehabilitation program after discharge from the hospital.
Patient will participate in goal setting for weight loss, decreased tobacco consumption, and cholesterol targets, and will participate in an exercise program, lose weight, reduce tobacco use, and decrease cholesterol according to his personal goals.	■ Plan and set goals with the patient for weight loss, reduction in tobacco use, and target cholesterol levels. ■ Have the patient identify appropriate menu selections and portion control to achieve weight loss. ■ Have the patient identify the triggers for tobacco use and steps that he might find useful to reduce or stop smoking. ■ Refer the patient to a weight loss and a smoking cessation support group. ■ Have the patient identify appropriate exercises post-myocardial infarction.
Patient will begin to demonstrate effective coping mechanisms.	■ Discuss the patient's feelings about multiple lifestyle changes and the diagnosis of myocardial infarction. ■ Discuss the patient's feelings about participating in both a weight loss and smoking cessation program. ■ Mobilize the patient's resources for support. ■ Help the patient to design a chart to use to map his progress with weight loss, smoking cessation, and cholesterol targets. ■ Acknowledge all questions and concerns that the patient expresses as meaningful.

provided meets or exceeds the criteria set forth in the standards. Some examples of JCAHO standards related to patient and family education include the following:

- "The hospital plans, supports, coordinates activities and resources for patient and family education."
- "The patient receives education and training specific to the patient's assessed needs, abilities, learning preferences and readiness to learn as appropriate to the care and services provided by the hospital."[21]

The goal of these educational standards is to guide hospitals to create an environment where both the patient and the health care team members are responsible for teaching and learning. The medical record should reflect an interdisciplinary approach toward patient education throughout the hospital stay. This begins on admission with the initial assessment of the patient's current health problems, based on socioeconomic status, cultural and religious practices, motivation and ability to learn, family support, and current knowledge base.[22] The JCAHO educational assessment guidelines are detailed in Box 6-6. Teaching records should illustrate documentation of the information taught, and how it relates to specific illness, medications, safe and effective use of medical equipment, restraint/seclusion, pain management, and available community resources.[22]

Finally, the teaching record should also reflect an evaluation of how well the patient and family absorbed the information. The details of teaching record documentation are outlined in Box 6-7. A sample patient education record is shown in Figure 6-2.

How do these standards affect patient education in the critical care setting? It may be difficult for critical care nurses to think in terms of teaching plans and interdisciplinary learning because critically ill patients have so much instability and require great vigilance just to maintain physiological function. However, remember that much of the patient teaching is informal and may not be clearly visible at first glance. Nurses are taught to explain each procedure, medication, intervention, or diagnostic test to the patient beforehand. This is patient education. For example, the nurse who explains that the medication she is hanging is an antibiotic that is given through the intravenous (IV) line to fight the patient's abdominal wound infection is teaching. Yet, many nurses would not recognize this action as patient education, nor would they document it in the teaching record. Nonetheless, this type of informal instruction meets the JCAHO standard for patient education. Critical care nurses teach patients and families routinely, but often the patient education record is left blank because "there isn't enough time to teach." If critical care nurses would only remember to note each informal teaching session, the patient's educational records would be filled with entries after just one day in the unit.

box 6-6
Joint Commission on Accreditation of Healthcare Organizations (JCAHO) Guidelines for Patient and Family Education Assessment

- Cultural background
- Religious beliefs and values
- Family support
- Literacy level
- Primary language
- Ability to read and comprehend information
- Barriers to learning
- Physical limitations such as visual or hearing impairment
- Emotional barriers
- Preferred learning methods
- Motivation to learn

Adapted from Iacono J, Campbell A: Patient and Family Education: The Compliance Guide to the JCAHO Standards (2nd Ed), pp 25–36. Marblehead, MA, Opus Communication, 2000.

box 6-7
Components of Teaching Documentation

- Participants (Who was taught?)
- Content (What was taught?)
- Date and time (When was it taught?)
- Patient status (What was the patient's condition at the time?)
- Evaluation of learning (How well was the information absorbed?)
- Teaching methods (How was the patient taught?)
- Follow-up and learning evaluation (If teaching was incomplete, what was the reason? What additional education needs does the patient have?)

clinical applicability challenges

Self-Challenge: Critical Thinking

1. *Discuss nursing interventions that have effectively reduced patient and family anxiety in a clinical situation that you have encountered.*
2. *Discuss when patient and family anxiety would preclude all learning.*

Study Questions

1. *What factors may reduce the critically ill patient's attention span and concentration?*
   a. *Background noise, such as bedside alarms*
   b. *Interrupted sleep patterns*
   c. *Inadequate privacy*
   d. *All of the above*
2. *Which of the following principles of adult learning should the critical care nurse assess?*
   a. *The need to know*
   b. *Readiness to learn*
   c. *Motivation to learn*
   d. *All of the above*

KEY

Barriers to Learning	**Learners**	**Tools/Method**	**Level of Learning (LOL)**
1. No barrier 2. Language/Communication/Literacy 3. Cultural/Religious Practices 4. Cognitive/Sensory Impairment 5. Severity of illness/pain 6. Motivation 7. Physical limitation	P = patient F = family/significant other O = other	C = Class/group D = Demonstration A = Audiovisual L = Literature T = Translator TV = Video/ed channel M = Model 1:1 One to one	8. Needs further reinforcement 9. Demonstrates partial skill or knowledge 10. Demonstrates skill with minimal assistance 11. Demonstrates competent skill and knowledge

EDUCATION	**Content**	**Date**	**Barrier**	**Learner**	**Tool**	**LOL**	**Initials**
Outcome Criteria **Discharge Plan of Care** • Identifies disease process • Cause • Signs and symptoms • Risk factors • Prevention							
Medications/ Food and Drug Interactions • Identifies purpose of medications • States side effects of medications • Demonstrates administration of medications • Reviews food–drug interactions							
Activity • Verbalizes activity restrictions after discharge • Identifies need for assistive apparatus as needed • Identifies safety precautions							
Equipment • States purpose • Demonstrates correct use of equipment • Identifies safety measures							
Treatments • States the purpose of the treatment • Demonstrates correct technique • Identifies findings that should be reported to health care provider							
Follow-up Care and Community Resources							

figure 6-2 Example of a patient education record. (Adapted from Georgetown University Hospital: Interdisciplinary Patient Education. Washington, DC, author, 2000.)

REFERENCES

1. Fralic MF: Nursing leadership for the new millennium: Essential knowledge and skills. Nurs Health Care Perspect 20(5):260–265, 1999
2. Halm MA, Titler MG, Kleiber C, et al: Behavioral responses of family members during critical illness. Clin Nurs Res 2:414–437, 1993
3. Oka R, Burke LE, Sivarajan Froelicher ES: Emotional responses and inpatient education. In Woods S, Sivarajan Froelicher ES, Jean H, et al. (eds): Cardiac Nursing (3rd Ed), pp 672–689. Philadelphia, JB Lippincott, 1995
4. Leske JS: treatment for family members in crisis after critical injury. AACN Clin Issues 9(1):129–139, 1998
5. Davis-Martin S: Perceived needs of families of long-term critical care patients: A brief report. Heart Lung 23:515–518, 1994
6. Lehmann LS, Brancati FL, Chen MC, et al: The effect of bedside case presentation on patient's perceptions of their medical care. N Engl J Med 336(16):1150–1155, 1997
7. National Center for Health Statistics: Changing America: Indicators of social and economic well-being by race and Hispanic origin. Council of Economic Advisors for the President's Initiative on Race. Washington, DC, United States Government Printing Office, 1999. Also available at: www.access.gpo.gov/su_docs/search/html
8. Ersek M, Kagawa-Singer M, Barnes D, et al: Multicultural considerations in the use of advance directives. Oncol Nurs Forum 25: 1683–1690, 1998
9. Meleis A, Isenberg M, Koerner J, et al: Diversity, marginalization, and culturally competent health care: Issues in knowledge development. Washington, DC, American Academy of Nursing, 2000

10. Lipson JG: Culturally competent nursing care. In Lipson JG, Dibble SL, Mainarik PA (eds): Culture and Nursing Care: A Pocket Guide, pp 1–6. San Francisco, UCSF Nursing Press, 1998
11. Hartman RA, Draegar JO, Bernstein MM: Patient literacy training: New challenge for patient education. Patient Educ Counsel 17:142–152, 1991
12. Campbell KN: Adult education: Helping adults begin the process of learning. Am Assoc Occup Health Nurse J 47:31–40, 1999
13. Redman BK: The Practice of Patient Education (9th Ed), pp 7–36. St. Louis, Mosby, 2000
14. Knowles MS, Holton EF, Swanson RA: The Adult Learner (5th Ed), pp 35–72. Houston, TX, Gulf Publishing, 1998
15. Rankin SH, Stallings KD: Patient Education: Issues, Principles, Practices (3rd Ed), pp 1–19. Philadelphia, JB Lippincott, 1996
16. Palazzo MO: Teaching in crisis: Patient and family education in critical care. Crit Care Nurs Clin North Am 13(1):83–92, 2001
17. Weinrich SP: The high risk of low literacy. Reflections 25:22–24, 1999
18. Fisher E: Low literacy levels in adults: Implications for patient education. J Contin Educ Nurs 30:56–61, 1999
19. Scalzi C, Burke L, Greenland S: Evaluation of an inpatient education program for coronary patients and families. Heart Lung J Crit Care 9:846–853, 1980
20. Redman BK: The Practice of Patient Education (9th Ed), pp 81–103. St. Louis, Mosby, 2000
21. Joint Commission on Accreditation of Healthcare Organizations: CAMH Comprehensive Accreditation Manual for Hospitals: The Official Handbook, pp 1–12. Oakbrook Terrace, IL, Joint Commission, 2000
22. Iacono J, Campbell A: Patient and Family Education: The Compliance Guide to the JCAHO Standards (2nd Ed), pp 25–36. Marblehead, MA, Opus Communication, 2000

PART
one
two
three
four
five
six
seven
eight
nine
ten
eleven
twelve

Professional Practice Issues in Critical Care

INTERNET RESOURCES

Topic	Web Page Address
The American Association of Critical-Care Nurses	www.aacn.org
The American Association of Legal Nurse Consultants	www.aalnc.org
The American Association of Nurse Attorneys	www.taana.org
The American Nurses Association	www.nursingworld.org
The Canadian Association of Critical Care Nurses	www.caccn.ca
Canadian Bioethics Society	www.bioethics.ca/english/
The Center for Ethics and Human Rights	www.nursingworld.org/ethics/
Genetics Program for Nursing Faculty at the Cincinnati Children's Hospital Medical Center	www.cincinnatichildrens.org/education/gpnf
Genomics and Disease Prevention at Centers for Disease Control and Prevention	www.cdc.gov/genomics/activities/ogdp.htm
Human Genome Project of the U.S. Department of Energy	www.ornl.gov/hgmis
The ICN Code of Ethics for Nursing	www.icn.ch/icncode.pdf
Introduction to Genetics: GlaxoSmithKline	www.genetics.gsk.com/overview.htm
National Coalition for Health Professional Education in Genetics (NCHPEG)	www.nchpeg.org
National Human Genome Research Institute	www.genome.gov/glossary.cfm
The National League for Nursing	www.nln.org
Nursing Ethics	www.nursingethics.ca/
Online Mendelian Inheritance in Man (OMIM)	www.ncbi.nlm.nih.gov/omim
Sigma Theta Tau International Honor Society of Nursing	www.nursingsociety.org
The Society of Critical Care Medicine	www.sccm.org

chapter 7

Ethical Issues in Critical Care Nursing

CHRISTINE GRADY

objectives

Based on the content in this chapter, the reader should be able to:

- Explain the way ethics assists clinicians in resolving moral problems.
- Name and describe the ethical principles most frequently appealed to in clinical ethics.
- Describe steps in the process of ethical decision making.
- Identify resources available to nurses to resolve ethical dilemmas.
- Discuss an ethical issue confronted by critical care nurses in practice and how applying ethical principles may assist in its resolution.
- Recognize the applicability of the American Nurses Association's (ANA) *Code of Ethics for Nurses* to everyday practice

Mechanical replacement of kidney function was once science fiction. Now we routinely replace the mechanical function of the kidneys through dialysis, replace the kidney itself through transplantation, and soon may be able to predict genetically who is at risk for kidney failure. The incorporation of sophisticated technology into the clinical arena has made the once simpler questions of life and death increasingly more complex. Progress in health care technology and information is a double-edged sword. Although there are indisputable benefits from the availability and use of technology and access to information, there are also profound ethical, legal, economic, and social challenges and dilemmas.

Questions regarding the appropriate use of technology and information in patient care are fundamental, and nowhere is this more true than in critical care. The intensive care unit (ICU) is dense with complicated technology and is a place where crucial decisions about life and health are made with striking frequency and urgency. Also, patients in the ICU tend to be older and more acutely ill than in the past. Although nurses and other health care providers make moral choices constantly in everyday practice, sometimes the choices are difficult and create feelings of uncertainty, conflict, or distress. The function of ethics is to help clarify and illuminate moral issues and obligations and to provide systematic methods for reaching resolutions.

How does ethics illuminate moral issues? Identifying a problem as a source of moral uncertainty, distress, or dilemma begins the process of reasoning through the complexity. According to Jameton,[1] *moral uncertainty* exists if one is unable to identify clearly a moral conflict within a situation but experiences the troublesome feeling that "something is not quite right." *Moral dilemmas* occur if two or more conflicting principles or alternatives exist, and to choose one would be to violate or compromise another. *Moral distress* is caused if one can clearly identify a moral conflict and the right action to resolve it, but institutional protocol, disagreement between members of the health care team, or professional rules or lines of authority prevent morally appropriate action.

Ethics education, interdisciplinary dialogue, collaboration, communication, consultation with institutional ethics committees, and the use of institutional ethics policies and professional codes of ethics can help nurses reason through moral conflicts in the clinical environment. The major purposes of ethical analysis in the clinical area are to clarify the moral issues and principles involved in a situation, to examine one's responsibilities and obligations, and to provide an ethically adequate rationale for any decision or action taken. This chapter presents an overview of ethics, some principles and guidelines for nursing ethics, and a process by which to apply them clinically.

ETHICS AND THE NURSE

The *Code of Ethics for Nurses* begins with the statement "Ethics is an integral part of the foundation of nursing."[2] But, what exactly is ethics? And how does it form part of the foundation of nursing? Are morals and ethics the same? Does the nursing profession have its own realm of ethics different from that of the medical profession? On what are the tenets of nursing ethics based?

Morals are personal or codified standards of conduct derived from societal expectations of behavior. They are the standards of behavior and values to which we are committed as members of society. *Ethics*, a more formal term, refers to the systematic study of those standards and values. Ethical inquiry, a form of philosophical or theological inquiry, allows us to think reasonably about, to question, to critique, and ultimately to understand the dimensions of moral conduct. Specifically, ethics is a method of inquiry that helps us answer questions about what is right or good, what ought to be done in specific situations, and what kind of people—and what kind of nurses—we ought to be, and why.

Sometimes the term *ethics* is used to refer to the formal beliefs or practices of a particular group of people, such as "Jewish ethics," "business ethics," or "medical ethics." Most professional groups have formal codes of ethics for their members; the nursing profession is guided by the American Nurses Association's (ANA) *Code of Ethics for Nurses with Interpretive Statements* (Box 7-1). Other professional associations, such as the American Association of Critical-Care Nurses (AACN), support the ANA code.

box 7-1
The American Nurses Association's (ANA) Code of Ethics for Nurses

1. The nurse, in all professional relationships, practices with compassion and respect for the inherent dignity, worth, and uniqueness of every individual, unrestricted by considerations of social or economic status, personal attributes or the nature of health problems.
2. The nurse's primary commitment is to the patient, whether an individual, family, group, or community.
3. The nurse promotes, advocates for, and strives to protect the health, safety, and rights of the patient.
4. The nurse is responsible and accountable for individual nursing practice and determines the appropriate delegation of tasks consistent with the nurse's obligation to provide optimum patient care.
5. The nurse owes the same duty to self as to others, including the responsibility to preserve integrity and safety, to maintain competence, and to continue personal and professional growth.
6. The nurse participates in establishing, maintaining, and improving health care environments and conditions of employment conducive to the provision of quality healthcare and consistent with the values of the profession through individual and collective action.
7. The nurse participates in the advancement of the profession through contributions to practice, education, administration, and knowledge development.
8. The nurse collaborates with other health professionals and the public in promoting community, national, and international efforts to meet health needs.
9. The profession of nursing, as represented by associations and their members, is responsible for articulating nursing values, for maintaining the integrity of the profession and its practice, and for shaping social policy.

Bioethics, a form of normative applied ethics, is the study of ethical issues and ethical judgments made within the biomedical sciences, including care of patients, the delivery of health care, and biomedical research. Bioethics takes into account the difficult and practical realities found in the clinical care of people with everyday or unusual health problems and illnesses. Some have argued that nursing ethics is just a subset of bioethics, that there is little that is morally unique to nursing. According to this schema, nursing ethics is the ethical analysis of judgments made by nurses, and the same moral issues emerge whether one is the nurse, physician, or patient.[3] Others have contended that nursing ethics is a separate and unique field of inquiry built on an understanding of the nature and philosophy of nursing and the nurse–patient relationship.[4] In either case, nursing ethics is best understood as being built on the specific professional roles and responsibilities of the nurse and on the relationships the nurse has with patients, other health care providers, the institutions with which he or she is affiliated, and society. In fact, a nurse never practices in isolation. Decision making, conflict resolution about ethical issues, and ethical practice are accomplished through communication and collaboration with patients, peers, and colleagues on the health care team.

Specific concerns of nursing ethics include what our obligations and responsibilities as nurses are, what makes a good nurse, and what ends nursing ought to seek. The answers to these questions guide our everyday practice. Codes of professional ethics, bioethical principles, and ethical theories all provide nurses with guidance for addressing these questions. They are general guidelines for professional conduct that should be applied to specific clinical situations and when making judgments about individual cases.

The ANA *Code of Ethics for Nurses* was recently revised to reflect the expanded and increasingly complex role of nurses in our current health care environment. The *Code* describes desired normative behaviors for nurses and reflects the actual work of nurses; it also makes explicit to society the commitments and obligations of professional nurses.

THE TOOLS OF ETHICS

Resolution may sometimes seem very difficult when we are involved in moral conflict. Systematically applying the tools of ethics, basic moral principles, and the professional guidelines of nursing, however, helps us identify our ethical obligations and decide which "right" actions can help us meet them. A systematic decision-making process is a tool that can help us identify the issues and carefully and justifiably resolve them. Multidisciplinary collaboration and dialogue and sometimes consultation with ethics committees or experts can also be critical to achieving the satisfactory resolution of problems.

Ethical decision making does not promise absolute answers, however. Ethical dilemmas are dilemmas precisely because compelling reasons exist for taking each of two or more opposing actions. Decisions about which action to take should be analyzed and justified using guidelines such as the bioethical principles discussed later. Careful ethical reflection and analysis do not preclude the possibility that reasonable people may disagree. However, the value of thoughtful debate and reflection in making ethical judgments cannot be overestimated.

Approaches to Ethics

Within normative ethics, there are several general approaches or orientations used in the process of determining what is right or wrong. One approach, *consequentialism*, includes theories that determine an action to be right or wrong on the basis of its consequences. *Utilitarianism*, a popular form of consequentialism, asserts that the right action is that which offers the greatest possible benefit with the least amount of burden for all affected by the decision. A second approach, the *deontologic* or *nonconsequentialist* approach, includes theories that judge an action right or wrong on the basis of features other than consequences, usually on the basis of the conformity of the action to a moral rule. Both utilitarian and deontologic theories use principles and rules, although for different reasons. *Principlism*, an approach that depends on a specific set of principles used to identify, discuss, and analyze the ethics of a situation, is widely used in bioethics. *Virtue ethics*, another approach, emphasizes what agents do and how their actions reflect their virtues. Faced with an ethical problem, virtue ethics looks to persons of good character and judgment for direction in determining what is best rather than applying rules or calculating consequences. An *ethics of care* approach emphasizes the salience and characteristics of caring relationships between people as essential in determining right actions. Sympathy, compassion, trust, fidelity, and discernment are emphasized over rules and principles.

In addition to ethical theories, general moral principles, and professional guidelines, personal values, emotions, and judgment help guide actions and decisions that the nurse takes in a particular situation. How we feel about an issue is a manifestation of our moral convictions that should not be ignored. We should strive, though, to reach ethical decisions by allowing reason to temper emotions and emotions to tutor reason. Although nursing is a moral endeavor based on the idea of service, the nurse must be allowed to practice in a manner that maintains the practitioner's sense of self-respect while also maintaining the dignity of the patient.

When applying basic moral principles to specific situations, we should also remain aware of professional values and obligations that color our ethical reasoning. Awareness of differences in professional and personal obligations can provide insight into sources of interprofessional or interpersonal ethical conflict. Nursing practice takes place within a team of health care professionals, reflecting a multiplicity of values that can be in conflict. Differing personal, professional, and institutional values can compound moral conflict; all must be considered. In the end, competing values must be weighed and assigned priority in light of the ethical norms that guide us.

Principles of Bioethics and the Ethics of Care

Four widely accepted bioethical principles are often applied to ethical problems in health care.[5] These principles, useful in analyzing moral choices and conflicts faced by practicing nurses, include nonmaleficence, beneficence, respect for autonomy, and justice (Box 7-2). Two other principles often cited as relevant to nursing practice are fidelity and veracity.[5] *Fidelity* is the duty to be faithful to one's patients, to keep promises, and to fulfill contracts and commitments. It is the moral covenant between individuals in a relationship. *Veracity* is the duty to tell the truth and not to lie or deceive others. All of these principles stipulate *prima facie* obligations. A *prima facie* obligation is binding unless it is in conflict with another obligation of equal or stronger claim.

Because the principle-based approach to ethical problem solving is sometimes seen as too abstract to reflect the complex, human dimensions of real cases, a "care ethic" adds an important dimension, especially for nursing. The

box 7-2
Principles of Bioethics

Nonmaleficence: An obligation to never deliberately harm another

Beneficence: An obligation to promote the welfare of others, to maximize benefits and minimize harms

Respect for autonomy: An obligation to respect, and not to interfere with, the choices and actions of autonomous individuals (i.e., those capable of self-determination)

Justice: An obligation to be fair in the distribution of burdens and benefits and in the distribution of social goods, such as health care or nursing care

Veracity: An obligation to tell the truth

Fidelity: An obligation to keep promises and fulfill commitments

care ethic is built on the understanding that individuals are unique, that relationships and their value are crucial in moral deliberations, and that emotions and character traits have a role in moral judgment. Caring is considered essential to the nursing role and has been long valued in the nurse–patient relationship. Nurse caring is directed toward the protection of the health and welfare of patients and indicates a commitment to the protection of human dignity and the preservation of human health. Caring has been called a central art and moral virtue of nursing practice.[5] The AACN describes its "mission, vision and values as framed within an ethic of care and ethical principles."[6]

NONMALEFICENCE AND BENEFICENCE

The principle of nonmaleficence says that we have an ethical duty not to inflict harm or evil. It is a duty foundational to our society. In other words, the duty not to harm others bears more weight than the duty to benefit others. Citing statements from the Hippocratic oath and the words of Florence Nightingale, Jameton (p. 93) argues that "it is more important to avoid doing harm than it is to do good."[1]

Beneficence involves taking deliberate steps to benefit another person. Beauchamp and Childress state that this duty compels us to provide benefits by preventing and removing harm and to balance benefits and harms by performing a risk–benefit analysis, such as weighing the side effects of a drug against its therapeutic actions.[5]

Nonmaleficence or the noninfliction of harm is a strong *prima facie* principle (which means that it is usually given greater weight than other principles). The following case study illustrates a situation in which appeal to the principles of nonmaleficence and beneficence may facilitate decision making:

case study ■ BALANCING RISKS AND BENEFITS

George Edwards, a 59-year-old man, came into the emergency department complaining of dizziness and chest pain for the past week. A cardiac monitor showed ventricular tachycardia, and he was successfully cardioverted and placed on Tridil. After admittance to the coronary care unit, Mr. Edwards required multiple cardioversions for recurrent ventricular tachycardia. At one point, he required cardiopulmonary resuscitation (CPR) for sustained symptomatic ventricular tachycardia. Laboratory work indicated a massive myocardial infarction, and an echocardiogram showed an ejection fraction of 25%. Mr. Edwards' cardiologist planned electrophysiology studies, with a possible implantable defibrillator when the patient became stable.

On day 14 of his hospital stay, Mr. Edwards went into congestive heart failure and sustained ventricular tachycardia, requiring CPR and multiple defibrillations. The cardiologist continued to show optimism that the electrophysiology studies and the automatic implantable cardiac defibrillator (AICD) would provide good results. Mr. Edwards was tired, confused at times, and began to seek frequent reassurance from the nurses that he would live long enough for the AICD insertion. He expressed fear about the frequent cardioversions and the discomfort they caused him. The nurses began to question what kind of long-term benefit such treatment would offer this severely compromised patient. ■

This patient care study shows the dilemma of providing treatment that might offer the benefit of defibrillation for recurrent ventricular tachycardia to a patient who already has sustained severe cardiac damage. An analysis of the risks and benefits leads to the following questions: Are we helping or harming the patient with recurrent cardioversions? What are the long-term benefits of AICD implantation? How do the benefits of recurrent cardioversions in someone with already severe cardiac damage compare with the discomforts and suffering caused by the same procedures? Without the therapy, the patient is likely to die, but how do we determine if the benefits of avoiding sudden cardiac death outweigh the risks of physical and emotional harm caused by repeated cardioversions and defibrillations while he awaits implantation of the AICD?

Clinicians who work in the ICU frequently use aggressive treatment to try to stabilize a patient and keep him or her alive. Stepping back to ascertain the complex factors that contribute to suffering and comfort for an individual patient often is not easy. Sometimes clinicians forget that relief of suffering is a fundamental goal in health care. In addition to careful pain management, we must be attentive to other components of individual suffering. The desire to prevent harm by postponing death is shaped by beneficence. In some situations, however, perhaps a greater harm than death is the physical and psychological suffering that can be caused by aggressive treatment, especially if it is of uncertain or slight benefit. In some cases, less aggressive treatment and more comfort may be a more beneficent course. It is crucial to involve the patient or surrogate in discussions and decisions about goals and risks and benefits of treatment and care. Respect for the considered opinions, preferences, and decisions of the patient based on and guided by the principle of respect for autonomy can be very helpful in deciding appropriate action in a case like the one involving Mr. Edwards.

RESPECT FOR AUTONOMY

Respect for autonomy involves respecting the capacity of an individual to be self-determining; that is, the capacity to deliberate about actions and life choices, and to act on those deliberations without interference from others. Informed consent is an application of the principle of respect for autonomy in the health care setting. The nurse's duty regarding informed consent is to see that the patient is adequately informed, has the capacity to understand available options, and can deliberate and make a health care decision. Promoting respect for autonomy includes being honest with the patient and family, protecting the patient's privacy and confidentiality, and helping the patient make important decisions.

If a patient is incapable of making an informed decision about a treatment or intervention, a surrogate is asked to give consent for the patient. A surrogate decides for the patient in a way that is consistent with what the patient would want, if known, or that is consistent with the patient's best medical interests. The surrogate is usually a spouse, parent, adult child, or someone previously designated by the patient as possessing durable power of attorney for health care. Most important, if possible, the surrogate is someone who knows and can represent the preferences and interests of the patient regarding the treatment options.

To be fully informed, the patient or surrogate needs all the information a "reasonable person" would need to make a particular decision. Sometimes, because of age, physical condition, educational level, position, language, culture, emotional stress, or other factors, the health care team may need to spend additional time and care providing information and ensuring that the patient or surrogate understands. Providers are always responsible for presenting information in an understandable and sensitive manner and for assessing the patient's or surrogate's understanding.

Consistent with respect for autonomy, consent given as part of informed consent is voluntary. The patient is not to be subject to coercion, fraud, or deceit. A fully informed, freely consenting patient has a right to make an autonomous decision, regardless of whether it corresponds with what others think he or she should do, as long it does not harm others.

It is not uncommon for patients in the ICU to have compromised autonomy and decision-making capacity owing to critical illness and its management. Although important in every health care interaction, assessment of an individual's ability to understand treatment options and make decisions in the ICU should be frequent and careful. Respect for the autonomy of the patient may be manifested through a surrogate decision maker or an advance directive. Respect for persons is the overriding principle under which respect for autonomy falls.

Making Treatment and Care Decisions

Historically, health care professionals and hospitals have occasionally sought to override the autonomy of the patient by giving the patient treatment or continued treatment unwanted by the patient, but deemed necessary for the patient's benefit by the health care team. However, in most cases, according to both ethical and legal standards, the wishes of the patient or surrogate take priority. The right to refuse treatment is a corollary of the right to informed consent and is grounded in the principle of respect for autonomy. The famous words of former Supreme Court Justice Cardozo articulate this respect for a patient's decision to refuse treatment: "Every human being of adult years and sound mind has a right to determine what shall be done with his body. . . ."[7] The *Code of Ethics for Nurses* (section 1.4) states "patients have the moral and legal right to determine what will be done with their own person, to be given adequate, complete, and understandable information in a manner that facilitates an informed judgment, to be assisted in weighing the benefits, burdens, and available options in their treatment, including the option of no treatment; to accept, refuse, or terminate treatment without deceit, undue influence, duress, coercion, or penalty; and to be given necessary support throughout the decision making and treatment process."[2]

A major concern of the public is over the possibility of being forced to endure an existence supported by machines without hope of a meaningful life and without the ability to have a say in the decision. The Patient Self-Determination Act of 1990 requires all health care facilities that receive federal funds to provide written information to patients about their rights to make decisions about medical care, including the right to accept or refuse care. Included should be information about the right of the patient to formulate a health care advance directive.

All states in the United States and the District of Columbia have statutes regarding advance directives for health care. There are two main kinds of advance directives, instructional and designation of proxy, and it is not uncommon for an individual to have both. A living will or instructional advance directive allows a person to specify in advance specific wishes regarding treatment and care for such time that he or she may lose the capacity to make decisions. A durable power of attorney for health care designates a proxy, familiar with the patient's treatment preferences, to make decisions in the event of the patient's incapacity. Advance care planning is the process that offers the patient an opportunity to deliberate about and express his or her preferences and values for treatment and care in advance of such time when the patient can no longer deliberate or decide for himself. Encouraging patients to reflect on preferences, talk to their loved ones and health care providers, and implement a durable power of attorney or living will in case of future need is a demonstration of respect for the autonomy of the patient. The *Code of Ethics for Nurses* (section 1.4) reminds us, though, that "support of autonomy in the broadest sense also includes recognition that people of some cultures place less weight on individualism and choose to defer to family or community values in decision making. Respect not just for the specific decisions but also for the patient's method of decision making is consistent with the principle of autonomy."[2] In addition to respecting the process and decisions, honoring the patient's expressed preferences and wishes, including those found in a patient's advance directive, is also a demonstration of respect. Despite efforts to encourage advance care planning, a remarkably small number (less than 25%) of even seriously ill patients have written advance directives. And unfortunately, even when an advance directive exists, the patient does not always have a copy available, or the language of the written instructions is vague and can be difficult to apply to a particular, often unforeseen, situation.

Withholding and Withdrawing Treatment, Especially at the End of Life

How should nurses understand a patient's or surrogate's decision to "withhold" or "withdraw" treatment, especially at the end of life? "Withholding" refers to never initiating a treatment, whereas "withdrawing" refers to stopping a treatment once started. The distinction between not starting a treatment and stopping it is not itself of ethical significance; what matters is whether the decision is consistent with the patient's interests and preferences. Ending treatment for sound moral reasons does not violate professional obligations. Health care professionals may find it emotionally more difficult to withdraw a treatment than to withhold it in the first place. On the other hand, it is often important to start a treatment to evaluate whether it works in the situation, until a diagnosis is confirmed, or a patient or family has the time to deliberate about the situation and make often-difficult decisions. The Hastings Center's *Guidelines on the Termination of Life-Sustaining Treatment and Care of the Dying* states that "there is strong reason to prefer stopping treatment over not starting it in some cases. . . . There is often uncertainty about the efficacy of a proposed treatment, or the burdens and benefits it will impose on the patient. It is better to start the treatment and later stop if it is ineffective than not to start treatment for fear that stopping will be impossible."[8]

When the patient or surrogate decides in good faith that a proposed treatment will impose undue burdens and refuses such treatment, it is morally correct for the health care professional to respect that decision. If the patient or surrogate decides that a treatment in progress and the life it provides have become too burdensome for the patient, then the treatment may permissibly be stopped. Imposing harmful or futile treatment against the patient's wishes violates the autonomous patient's right to self-determination, and even when the patient's wishes cannot be known, can sometimes violate the nonautonomous patient's best interests. Stopping treatment acknowledges that a patient has an autonomous right to refuse treatment and to determine what constitutes "benefit" for him or her. It also acknowledges the principle of nonmaleficence, or not harming the patient's dignity and quality of life by forcing unwanted, painful, or futile treatment on him or her. Because withdrawing an intervention can be a difficult and emotional activity for the nurse, the physician, and other members of the health care team, communication and mutual support are critically important.

One familiar example of a decision to withhold treatment is the decision not to attempt cardiopulmonary resuscitation (CPR) in the event of an arrest, recorded as a "do not resuscitate" (DNR) order. The original intent of CPR was to resuscitate or revive patients suffering specific types of sudden cardiac or pulmonary arrest: victims of drowning, electric shock, untoward effects of drugs, anesthetic accidents, heart block, and acute myocardial infarction. Now, CPR is a routine medical intervention extended to almost all patients suffering cardiac or pulmonary arrest, no matter what the underlying disease process. Although CPR has proven dramatically effective for some groups of patients, it is of little, if any, benefit for many others.

The immediate, reflexive intervention to preserve life without the express consent of the patient is supported by the principle of beneficence. Health care personnel assume that a "reasonable person" would wish to be resuscitated and act on the assumption that death is undesirable to the patient. However, some patients can express or have expressed their wishes not to be resuscitated. In such cases, to presume to understand the needs of a patient and act against the patient's expressed wishes (or to avoid ascertaining what those wishes might be) is paternalistic. Paternalism is the act of overriding another's autonomous actions or requests to bring about what is believed to be the best outcome for that person. Paternalism violates respect for the patient's autonomy. To ensure respect for patient self-determination and the opportunity to refuse treatment, discussion about CPR preferences should ideally occur when the patient is alert and has a reasonably clear sensorium. Before making a voluntary and informed decision to accept or to refuse CPR, the patient or surrogate must understand what CPR is and how it will most likely affect the disease process and future quality of life. This process applies to consideration of all treatments, including life-sustaining treatments.

The ANA *Code of Ethics for Nurses* (section 1.3) acknowledges that "Nurses are leaders and vigilant advocates for the delivery of dignified and humane care. Nurses actively participate in assessing and assuring responsible and appropriate use of interventions in order to minimize unwarranted or unwanted treatment and patient suffering. The acceptability and importance of carefully considered decisions regarding resuscitation status, withholding or withdrawing life-sustaining treatment, forgoing medically provided nutrition and hydration, aggressive pain and symptom management and advance directives are increasingly evident."[2] Wright and colleagues state, "All critical care nurses are expected to master the skills necessary for assisting patients and families through the harrowing experience of life-threatening illness . . . [and] must assume responsibility . . . [for] working through the ethical issues which often include end-of-life decisions and organ donation."[9] Decisions about treatment at the end of life are often difficult[10] and best made after careful discussions between the health care professional and the patient (or patient surrogate). The health care team supplies the necessary information about realistic outcomes and possible interventions. The nurse ensures that the patient or surrogate understands the information by clarifying technical terms and helping the patient weigh treatment options. By providing the patient an opportunity to discuss personal choices about end-of-life care, the nurse assists the patient. The patient then considers his or her own values and wishes in the context of prognoses and realistic options. The final decision reflecting the patient's wishes should be supported by the nurse and other members of the health care team.

Intensive care nurses may have a limited role in some decisions about end-of-life care.[11] In some cases, the nurse may have a personal moral conviction contrary to a certain decision or may believe that the certain decision is against the patient's best interests or wishes. The nurse is morally permitted to refuse to participate in withholding or withdrawing treatment from the patient. As stated in section 5.4 of the *Code of Ethics*, "Where a particular treatment, intervention, activity, or practice is morally objectionable to the nurse, whether intrinsically so or because it is inappropriate for the specific patient, or where it may jeopardize both patients and nursing practice, the nurse is justified in refusing to participate on moral grounds. . . . The nurse . . . must communicate the decision in appropriate ways. . . . The nurse is obliged to provide for the patient's safety, to avoid patient abandonment and to withdraw only when assured that alternative sources of nursing care are available to the patient."[2]

Limits to Treatment

In contrast to cases in which health care workers want to treat patients against their wishes, cases also arise in which the patient or surrogate wants treatment that physicians or other members of the health care team feel is inappropriate.

A landmark case of this type involved 86-year-old Helga Wanglie, who had been in a persistent vegetative state and on a ventilator in the ICU for more than 1 year. The health care team treating her felt continued treatment was futile, but her husband disagreed. The court upheld the right of Mr. Wanglie to act as surrogate decision maker for his wife. Another case of this type involved a hospital's request to withhold ventilator treatment from Baby K, an anencephalic baby. The court upheld the wishes of the baby's mother for continued ventilation and treatment. These and other cases stimulated a great deal of discussion among ethicists, health care professionals, and patients' rights groups about under what conditions, if any, a patient's request for treatment can be denied because the physician or health care team believes it is futile. In addition to lack of consensus on a definition of or criteria for futility, there is concern about whether health care providers can be objective enough to make these determinations. In fact, in the best-publicized court cases involving issues of futility, the courts' decisions focused only on who had the right to make decisions about treatment, and have upheld the autonomy rights of family members. Ethicists have argued that no one is better able to judge what is beneficial to patients than patients themselves,[12] and noted that physicians have "no particular expertise in making decisions about subjective matters such as futility."[13] As efforts to formulate criteria for futility were stymied by disagreement, some institutions developed a process-based approach to decisions about stopping or not offering treatments. The Council on Ethical and Judicial Affairs of the American Medical Association recommends that institutions adopt a policy that follows a "fair process approach" to determining futility of interventions.[14] Most such policies require deliberation by multidisciplinary committees, such as ethics committees, rather than unilateral decisions by a physician, and require genuine attempts to transfer the patient's care.[15]

The issue of futility arises in relation to the use of CPR.[16] As previously mentioned, CPR is usually initiated unless there is a DNR order. In some cases, however, CPR could be more harmful than beneficial. Patients can request that resuscitation not be attempted for them or that other aggressive, possibly futile or harmful efforts be foregone, especially when death is imminent and inevitable. Most DNR orders are written at the request of, or with the consent of, the patient or surrogate. However, when a patient or family member wants resuscitation, but the physician or health care team believes CPR is inappropriate, some institutions have a process that may make it possible for the physician, after consultation with others, to write a DNR order without the consent of the patient or family.

Nurses and other health care professionals promise to act in their patients' best interests, respect their autonomy, and advocate for them. Communicating honestly with patients and their significant others, discussing and respecting their wishes regarding treatment and care, convening patient care conferences for all involved parties when indicated, and facilitating advance care planning discussions and the use of advance directives are all important methods of fulfilling these obligations, as the following case study illustrates.

case study ■ RESPECTING AND ADVOCATING FOR THE PATIENT

Jane Crawford was a 44-year-old woman with severe and persistent pain from metastatic cancer. After a stay in the ICU marked by slow deterioration, Mrs. Crawford, who was weak, short of breath, anasarcic, and in considerable pain, confided to her primary care nurse, Ms. B., that she was ready to die and did not want any life-sustaining treatments. Ms. B. knew that Mr. Crawford had not accepted his wife's prognosis, was hoping for a miracle, and insisted on aggressive treatment to extend his wife's life. Ms. B. dreaded the impending conflict between the unit's aggressive oncologist, the patient with no hope of a life without pain, and the husband who was not ready to let his wife die.

As the primary nurse, Ms. B. had worked to develop a trusting relationship with Mrs. Crawford and her husband and felt it was her responsibility to act as her patient's advocate. She felt that Mrs. Crawford trusted her to facilitate communication about her wishes to the physician and the rest of the health care team and to help ensure that they were followed.

Ms. B contacted the physician and set up a family conference to discuss the plan of care with the Crawfords, the physician, the nursing staff, and the social worker. She also spoke to the physician and to Mrs. Crawford about the potential usefulness of a written advance directive, and offered some examples. She hoped that the Crawfords and the health care team could discuss Mrs. Crawford's prognosis and desires and come to an agreement on current goals of care and what types of treatment would be of benefit to her and consistent with her wishes. ■

JUSTICE

Justice is a principle of fairness. In the context of health care, the most frequent appeal is to distributive justice, which requires a fair or equitable distribution of burdens and benefits. A principle of justice is appealed to when determining how health care should be distributed in society; whether people are entitled to receive health care, regardless of their ability to pay; and whether they should receive a similar amount (e.g., type, quality) of health care. Fairness means that decisions about the distribution of health care should be based on morally significant characteristics. Therefore, for example, health care distribution should not be based on factors such as race, ethnicity, gender, social standing, or religious beliefs. Several substantive criteria have been proposed as useful for making distribution decisions for social goods, such as health care. These include that everyone should have equal access to health care, or that health care should be distributed according to need, contribution, or free market exchange.[5]

Criteria such as these are useful in deliberation and decisions not only about how health care resources are distributed in society but for decisions about allocation of limited resources, treatments, and even time and attention between and among patients. Every time a decision is made to transplant a kidney into one person and not another, to answer one patient's bell before another's, or to put one patient instead of others in an ICU bed, criteria such as those listed previously are used. Some egalitarians argue that because absolute equality is not possible in the distribution of health care goods, the only fair methods of deciding include random selection or first-come, first-served, thereby avoiding the use of any criteria that make distinctions between people. Allocation decisions are ordinarily made independent of the wishes of the patient or family and usually require balancing potential harms and benefits between people. Allocation decisions can be very difficult, and not everyone will be happy with decisions made; hence the need for well-thought-out and carefully applied criteria. Two important examples of difficult allocation decisions are organs for transplantation and beds in the ICU, both resources for which the demand exceeds the supply.

Allocation of Organs for Transplantation

Despite great technological successes in the transplantation of organs such as kidneys, hearts, and pancreas, there is a greater need for organs than there are available organs. In great part, this is because people do not donate organs even when they could. Critical care nurses may be at the bedside of a brain-dead patient when discussions with the family about procuring organs are initiated. Usually, a procurement coordinator from the nearest Organ Procurement Organization (OPO) works with hospital staff to discuss the option of donating organs with the patient's family. Because of the scarce supply of organs, difficult decisions must also be made about who gets the organs that are available. The Task Force on Organ Transplantation in the United States proposed that donated organs be considered a national, public resource that should be distributed according to the needs of the patients and the probability of success of the transplantation. There are many factors that influence the likelihood of an individual patient receiving a transplanted organ. All patients put onto a transplant center's waiting list are registered with the United Network for Organ Sharing (UNOS) Center. When an organ becomes available, information is entered into the computerized organ matching system. The computer program generates a list of potential recipients according to objective criteria agreed on by UNOS. Each organ has its own specific criteria, including such factors as blood type, human leukocyte antigen (HLA) type, size of the organ, time on the waiting list, medical urgency, and distance between donor and recipient, but not ethnicity, gender, or financial status.[17] However, the criteria used for deciding whether someone who needs an organ is put on a transplant center waiting list in the first place are less transparent.

Allocation of Intensive Care Unit Beds

Sometimes a patient requires care in the ICU and all the beds are already filled with critically ill patients, or admitting another patient would endanger the care of patients already in the ICU because of the level of staffing available. Decisions about admitting or discharging patients from the ICU often involve some sort of triage to maximize the effective and efficient use of resources. Triage decisions are usually based on considerations of medical utility; that is, a comparative judgment about the probability of success of ICU care for the individual patients involved. Beauchamp and Childress argue that "principles and rules of justice mandate attention to medical utility followed by the use of chance or queuing for scarce resources when medical utility is roughly equal for eligible patients."[5] Lanken and colleagues point out that "studies of how ICU resources have been allocated during times of scarcity indicate that, in general, when beds are scarce, the average severity of illness of those admitted to ICU increases. However, in some hospitals, political or economic factors appear to play important roles in determining who has access to scarce ICU beds."[18]

Zoloth-Dorfman and Carney[19] discuss the case of James Ramsey, a young patient with acquired immunodeficiency syndrome (AIDS) who was admitted through the emergency department (ED) in acute respiratory distress and diagnosed with *Pneumocystis carinii* pneumonia. Unable to obtain a bed in the ICU, the ED physician transferred Mr. Ramsey to an AIDS ward. Despite the valiant efforts of the evening nurses and the house staff, his condition continued to worsen. The resident was informed that there were "no available beds" in the ICU but later found out that one bed was being reserved for a "code." The patient continued to deteriorate throughout the night, with development of acute respiratory distress and hypotensive shock; eventually a code was called, but the patient died in transit to the ICU.

ICU staff felt intensive care in this case was futile, and bed space was limited. AIDS unit staff felt their patient had been discriminated against because he had AIDS and worried about the appeal to "futility" as an excuse. This case raises many interesting questions about the way patient selection and resource allocation decisions are made. Perhaps institutional clarification of ICU admitting criteria, including when the bed saved for codes could be used, would have helped in this case.

Increasingly, decisions about allocation of health care services and resources, such as ICU care, are influenced by the number of qualified nurses available to take care of patients. Given the current nursing shortage and the personnel cutbacks that have been made by many hospitals, this is a growing problem. Studies have demonstrated that higher patient-to-nurse ratios are associated with higher mortality rates and more complications among surgical patients, as well as higher burnout and job dissatisfaction among nurses.[20]

To comply with Joint Commission on Accreditation of Healthcare Organizations (JCAHO) requirements, hospitals and other health care institutions must have policies and procedures that ensure fair and equitable standards for admissions, care, discharge, and billing.[21] Ethical principles applied to some of the business practices of the organization are important in helping a health care organization meet its obligations as a business while maintaining its commitment to the ethical care of patients. Nurses, as members of the multidisciplinary team and as an essential but scarce resource, have a valuable and critical perspective to bring to the development of these organizational and societal policies.

Health Care in the United States

Justice also applies to the distribution of health care services in the country. Health care in the United States has been described as fragmented, inefficient, and unjust.

The United States spends approximately 14% of its gross national product on health care, and costs have continued to escalate in recent years. Nonetheless, an estimated 40,000,000 or more people in the United States, most of them poor, have no health insurance.[22] In addition, eligibility, coverage, and reimbursement provided by different health plans, including Medicaid, vary dramatically. A large percentage of health care in the United States is managed care, in which health insurance companies, industrial health care plans, or groups of patients contract with health care providers to provide a specified level of health care services at a predetermined cost. The goal of managed care is to reduce waste and control costs. A major concern expressed by some health care providers is that in striving to "manage" patients efficiently, we may be ignoring significant individualized needs for "care," even subverting the interests of the patient to those of the plan.[23] The ANA published their *Agenda for Health Care Reform* in 1991, and it remains a solid and ethical proposal for equitable and appropriate care according to the needs of patients and consumers. Continued changes in the structure and payment of health care delivery in the United States are likely to occur.

ETHICAL DECISION MAKING WITHIN A NURSING PROCESS MODEL

Ethical decisions made in the health care context should take into consideration the interests of the patient, the professional and personal values of health care professionals, institutional values, personal feelings, moral principles, and legal issues. At first glance, it might seem impossible to integrate these into anything other than an incoherent mass of conflicting possible actions, but with careful reflection and deliberation, acceptable resolutions can usually be achieved. The ANA *Code of Ethics for Nurses* (section 5.2) states that "nurses are required to have knowledge relevant to the current scope and standards of nursing practice, changing issues, concerns, controversies, and ethics."[2]

Ethical decision-making models provide a process for systematically and thoughtfully examining a conflict, ensuring that participants consider all important aspects of a situation before taking action. The steps of ethical analysis and evaluation are much like the steps of the nursing process and, as such, are a skill that can be learned. Both provide an orderly approach to problems. There are usually five steps to resolution of an ethical problem in the clinical setting (Box 7-3).

box 7-3
Model for Ethical Decision Making

Analysis of an ethical problem in the clinical setting usually involves the following five steps:

1. Gather the relevant facts and identify the decision maker(s) and the stakeholders.
2. Identify the ethical problem(s). Involve others in the process and use consultation resources as appropriate.
3. Analyze the problem using ethical guidance and resources.
4. Deliberate about the action alternatives in light of guidance; choose one and justify the choice.
5. Evaluate and reflect.

Gather the Relevant Facts

The first step is to identify information needed to understand the situation fully. What are the medical facts (i.e., diagnoses, prognoses, treatment alternatives)? Who are the principal agents involved? Who are the decision makers and the stakeholders? Are the values and goals for treatment and care of the patient clear? How do the values, interests, and relationships of others involved affect the problem? Are cultural, religious, or other aspects relevant to the case? It is important to understand the various contexts of the situation, including the physiological, psychosocial, and legal dimensions. Are there legal ramifications, institutional policies, or economic factors to consider?

Identify the Problem

The next step is to identify the ethical problem or problems. Is this truly a problem involving a question about or conflict between ethical principles or values, or is the problem primarily a legal or organizational issue or a communication problem? Communication problems and legal restrictions are often part of an ethical problem; however, some problems can be resolved simply through better communication or legal counsel without ethical analysis.

Analyze the Problem Using Ethical Principles and Rules

It is essential to identify the person or people who have the responsibility and authority to make a decision. Is the patient competent, fully informed, and free to make a choice (consistent with application of the principle of respect for autonomy)? Is there a family member able to speak to the best interests of a comatose patient (beneficence) or a designated durable power of attorney for health care who knows the patient's wishes (respect for autonomy)? How is the family involved? Are there vested interests to consider?

Consider ethical principles. Is harm being avoided or minimized? What are the benefits, and who will benefit? What are the harms, and who will be harmed? Are rights being protected? Have the patient's wishes and interests been articulated? Have promises been made? Has fairness been considered? Which principles are most applicable to the case? How can the principles be specified to provide guidance in the particular situation? Consider the role of care and compassion. There may be competing claims, all of which are reasonable and justifiable, and a conflict of principles. There may also be conflicts between principles and legal or institutional requirements. These should be clearly articulated.

Analyze Alternatives and Act

Identify all the possible and reasonable alternatives, and evaluate each of them on their conformity to principles and rules and their compatibility with care and compassion for the patient. Which option most promotes respect for the autonomy of the patient? How will each proposed action and its outcome benefit or harm those involved? Which of the possible alternatives seems fairest in terms of process, outcome, or both? Will the action strengthen or jeopardize patient–professional bonds and reaffirm society's expectations of health care professionals? After reflection and careful reasoning, nurses and other health care professionals should choose and act on the option that is most consistent with sound ethical analysis and personal moral convictions.

When considering alternatives, nurses must evaluate their position and involvement in the case. The nurse may not be the primary decision maker. However, because the nurse is an integral member of the health care team, it is important that she or he contribute to the dialogue, facilitate communication, articulate relevant personal views and values, and cooperate in implementation of the course of action. The nurse's role may also include planning a multidisciplinary conference or arranging for an ethics consultation.

Evaluate and Reflect

After the action has been taken, the ethical problem, the process of resolution, and the outcome must be further analyzed. The outcome should be compared with what was hoped for or intended. How can a similar situation be handled with greater sensitivity or wisdom in the future? Evaluation is especially helpful if it is undertaken in a nonjudgmental and nonthreatening atmosphere conducive to reflection and constructive change.

BIOETHICS RESOURCES AND SERVICES

Informed clinicians and clear organizational policies and support help in preventing and resolving ethical dilemmas in health care organizations. In addition, most health care organizations have some ethics services, which may consist of an ethics committee or an ethics consultation service or program. Services provided usually include education, policy development, and consultation at the bedside for ethical problems that arise in patient care.

Ethics Committees and Consultant Services

Institutional ethics committees are multidisciplinary and usually include representatives of the professions and disciplines involved in patient care (e.g., nursing, medicine, social work, spiritual care). In addition, many committees have one or more member of the lay community, as well as a lawyer, an ethicist, or clergy, as members of the committee or as *ad hoc* consultants.

Ethics committee members are involved in self-education as well as education of the professional staff and community on issues related to clinical ethics. Ethics committees may serve as an institutional resource for policy studies and the drafting of institutional policies concerning ethical issues. JCAHO requires policy statements and guidelines on a number of clinical issues, including the process of addressing ethical issues, informed consent, use of surrogate decision makers, decisions about care and treatment at the end of life, and confidentiality of information. Well-thought-out and articulated policies about these types of issues offer useful guidance to clinicians in often-difficult situations. Ethics consultation is offered in one or both of two modes: an initial bedside consultation by a consultant or small group of consultants, or a consultation by the committee. A bedside consultation by one or more trained consultants may be sufficient to provide the education, clarification, or dialogue necessary to assist decision makers in resolving an ethical problem. In some more complicated cases or when there is conflict among decision makers, consultation by the whole ethics committee may be appropriate. After deliberation, some committees aim to make a single recommendation for the resolution of the ethical problem, whereas for others the goal is to frame the morally acceptable options and assist key decision makers in choosing an acceptable course of action. In seeking consultation, it is useful to clarify the structure, process, and approach of available bioethics services in each institution. Limited data show that physicians and nurses find ethics consultation helpful in difficult situations.[24]

In addition to services provided by an ethics committee or bioethics consultant service, other resources are available to nurses. Some institutions have nursing ethics committees, which, although possibly coordinated with an existing institutional ethics committee, often function independently. These committees are designed to meet the needs of nurses in the institution by providing education and addressing issues unique to nursing, such as refusal of assignment, staffing patterns, or allocation of beds. Some institutions sponsor periodic ethics rounds, which may be general, unit based, or specific to nursing, and serve primarily an educational function. Pastoral care, quality assurance, and peer support activities are other examples of institutional resources that may facilitate the resolution of ethical problems.

Professional Nursing Organizations

Professional nursing organizations also address ethical issues of concern to nursing practice. The ANA addresses professional issues and moral dilemmas common to all nurses in the United States. In addition to the aforementioned ANA *Code of Ethics for Nurses*, the ANA's Center for Ethics and Human Rights publishes position statements and guidelines on many issues for which nurses seek ethical guidance. The AACN also has an active ethics committee, which develops policy statements and position papers that set standards for ethical behavior and decision making for critical care nurses. The AACN's ethics committee works closely with other professional nursing organizations and interfaces with other professional organizations, such as the

insights into clinical research

Schneiderman L, Gillmer T, Teetzel H: Impact of ethics consultation in the intensive care setting: A randomized, controlled trial. Crit Care Med 28(12):3920–3924, 2000.

The purpose of this study was to determine if ethics consultations in the intensive care setting reduced non-beneficial treatments to patients and whether physicians, nurses, social workers, and families thought ethics consultation was beneficial. In recent years, ethics consultation has been offered in many health care institutions as a way to help health care providers resolve conflicts and make difficult decisions about medical treatment. Empirical research evaluating ethics consultation, however, is very limited. One of the largest empirical studies, the SUPPORT study, demonstrated no improvement in end-of-life decision making or reduction in the use of life-prolonging care after intervention by a nurse specially trained to facilitate advance care planning. The need for further empirical research is great.

This study was conducted in both medical and pediatric intensive care units (ICUs) in a university medical center. Seventy-four patients for whom value-based treatment conflicts arose were randomized to receive or not to receive an ethics consultation. Medical data and ICU hospital days were compared between the intervention and control groups. Interviews of responsible physicians, nurses, social workers, and families were conducted within 1 month of the patient's death or hospital discharge. Interviewees were asked whether ethics consultation helped to identify, analyze, and resolve ethical issues; educate about ethical issues; and present personal views.

Patients were entered into the study because of disagreements about whether to pursue aggressive life-sustaining treatment or comfort care; because physicians or nurses expressed concerns about futile treatment; or because of conflicts or questions about the appropriate decision maker for the patient. Results showed that although there were no differences in mortality between the control patients and those receiving ethics consultation, for patients who received an ethics consultation, there was a reduction in ICU hospital days and life-sustaining treatments in those who died before discharge. The majority of health care providers and family members interviewed found ethics consultation to be helpful and would seek ethics consultation again in similar circumstances.

Society of Critical Care Medicine (SCCM), to examine issues shared by both professions.

Adequate information, multiple perspectives, deliberate thought, ethical principles and guidance, and organizational support are extremely important in enabling clinicians to exercise professional judgment and make sound decisions. Seeking advisory and consultative services from an appropriate resource often assists in this process.

clinical applicability challenges

Self-Challenge: Critical Thinking

1. *You believe that CPR is inappropriate for your patient, who is terminally ill with metastatic cancer. Construct plans for proceeding. Identify the people with whom you would talk and in what order you would speak to them. Structure arguments you would make to support your position.*
2. *A patient in your unit has severe and intractable pain, which you believe is being inadequately managed. Consider whether this is an ethical issue, and state why or why not. Explain what you would do to resolve the problem. Defend your position by using the American Nurses Association's (ANA)* Code of Ethics for Nurses.
3. *You receive a call from the emergency department regarding a septic patient who needs to be admitted to your unit. At the time of the call, however, your unit is full. Explain the criteria you would use to determine if there is a patient who could be moved to another unit to accommodate the patient from the emergency department. Determine who would make this decision, and construct how the decision would be made. Describe the ethical principle relevant to this situation.*

Study Questions

1. *An ethic of care is primarily based on*
   a. *acknowledgment of the history of nurses providing care to patients.*
   b. *recognition of the uniqueness of individuals, the value of relationships, and the importance of emotions in moral judgments.*
   c. *expectations of the American Nurses Association (ANA).*
   d. *None of the above*
2. *Ethics helps people reach answers to moral dilemmas by*
   a. *clarifying the moral issues and principles involved in a situation.*
   b. *helping the person to examine his or her responsibilities and obligations.*
   c. *providing an ethically adequate rationale for a decision.*
   d. *All of the above*
3. *A nurse believes that the medical treatment being given a particular patient is ethically inappropriate and refuses to give the patient care, leaving the workplace that day to avoid being involved in the situation. This is an example of*
   a. *a nurse standing up for his or her right not to participate in morally objectionable care.*
   b. *violation of the principles of beneficence and fidelity through patient abandonment.*
   c. *a nurse's support for the principle of nonmaleficence (noninfliction of harm).*
   d. *the exercise of professional nursing judgment.*
4. *Which of the following is not true?*
   a. *Withholding life-sustaining treatment is ethically acceptable, but withdrawing such treatment is not.*
   b. *To be truly autonomous, a patient must be fully informed and freely consenting.*
   c. *"Do Not Resuscitate" (DNR) is a medical order to withhold cardiopulmonary resuscitation (CPR).*
   d. *A nurse's duty always to act in the best interests of his or her patient is based on the principle of beneficence.*

REFERENCES

1. Jameton A: Nursing Practice: The Ethical Issues. Englewood Cliffs, NJ, Prentice-Hall, 1984
2. American Nurses Association: Code of Ethics for Nurses With Interpretive Statements. Washington, DC, American Nurses Publishing, 2001
3. Veatch R, Fry S: Case Studies in Nursing Ethics (2nd Ed). Sudbury, MA, Jones and Bartlett, 2000
4. Fry S: Toward a theory of nursing ethics. Adv Nurs Sci 11(4):9–22, 1989
5. Beauchamp T, Childress J: Principles of Biomedical Ethics (5th Ed). New York, Oxford University Press, 2001
6. American Association of Critical-Care Nurses: Our mission: An ethic of care. Available at: www.aacn.org
7. *Schloendorff v. Society of N.Y. Hospital*, 211 N.Y. 125, 105 N.E. 92, 93 (1914)
8. The Hastings Center: Guidelines on the Termination of Life-Sustaining Treatment and Care of the Dying. Briarcliff Manor, NY, The Hastings Center, 1987
9. Wright F, Cohen S, Caroselli C: How culture affects ethical decision making. Crit Care Nurs Clin North Am 9(1):63–73, 1997
10. Stroud R: The withdrawal of life support in adult intensive care: An evaluative review of the literature. Nurs Crit Care 7(4):176–184, 2002
11. Miller P, Forbes S, Boyle D: End-of-life care in the intensive care unit: A challenge for nurses. Am J Crit Care Nurs 10(5):369, 2001
12. Lantos J, Singer P, Walker R, et al: The illusion of futility in clinical practice. Am J Med 87:81–84, 1989
13. Veatch R. Why physicians cannot determine if care is futile. J Am Geriatr Soc 42:871–874, 1994
14. Council on Ethical and Judicial Affairs, American Medical Association: Medical futility in end-of-life care. JAMA 281:937–941, 1999
15. Helft P, Siegler M, Lantos J: The rise and fall of the futility movement. N Engl J Med 343:293–296, 2000
16. Kite S, Wilkinson S: Beyond futility: To what extent is the concept of futility useful in clinical decision making about CPR? Lancet Oncol 3:638–642, 2002
17. The Organ Procurement and Transplantation Network: About transplantation. Available at: http://www.optn.org/about/transplantation. Accessed on November 26, 2002
18. Lanken P, Terry P, Osborne M: Ethics of allocating intensive care resources. New Horiz 5(1):38–50, 1997
19. Zoloth-Dorfman L, Carney B: The AIDS patient and the last ICU bed: Scarcity, medical futility, and ethics. QRB 17(6):175–181, 1991
20. Aiken L, Clarke S, Sloane D, et al: Hospital nurse staffing and patient mortality, nurse burnout, and job dissatisfaction. JAMA 288(16):1987–1993, 2002
21. Marsee V: Ethical perspectives of reimbursement under economic pressures. Crit Care Nurs Clin North Am 12(3):365–372, 2000
22. Committee on the Consequences of Uninsurance: Care Without Coverage: Too Little, Too Late. Washington, DC, National Academy of Sciences, 2002
23. Darragh M, McCarrick P: Managed health care: New ethical issues for all. Kennedy Inst Ethics J 6(2):189–297, 1996
24. Schneiderman L, Gilmer T, Teetzel H: Impact of ethics consultation in the intensive care setting: A randomized, controlled trial. Crit Care Med 28(12):3920–3924, 2000

chapter 8

Legal Issues in Critical Care Nursing

PATRICIA C. MCMULLEN ■ ALEXANDER R. MCMULLEN

objectives

Based on the content in this chapter, the reader should be able to:

- Describe major areas of the law that affect critical care nursing practice.
- Define the four elements of malpractice (professional negligence).
- Delineate allegations commonly made against nurses.
- Explain types of vicarious liability.
- Apply knowledge of advance directives to patient care situations.

Because society seems to be more litigious than ever, legal issues involving critical care are of increasing concern. The number of malpractice suits that name or involve nurses is increasing. Issues such as refusal and termination of treatment have been widely discussed and addressed in the literature. Even legislators have become involved by enacting so-called "living will statutes" in their jurisdictions.

This chapter begins with a discussion of the major areas of law that may have an impact on the practice of nursing. After this discussion, the legal principle of negligence is reviewed and pertinent critical care case examples are provided. The chapter then proceeds to identify and address certain current legal issues most applicable to the critical care nurse.

AN OVERVIEW OF MAJOR AREAS OF THE LAW

There are three areas of the law that affect the practice of the critical care nurse: administrative law, civil law, and criminal law.

Administrative Law

Administrative law exists as a consequence of state and federal laws and regulations related to the practice of nursing. In all states, the legislatures have enacted nurse practice acts. Within each of these acts, the practice of nursing is defined, and powers are delegated to a state agency, usually the State Board of Nursing. These agencies develop regulations that dictate how the nurse practice act is to be interpreted and implemented.

Nurses practicing in a state are expected to know the provisions of their nurse practice act and any regulations dealing with the practice of nursing. Therefore, if a nurse is unfamiliar with the nurse practice act, it is important that he or she contact the State Board of Nursing to request and review a copy of this act. Copies of the nurse practice act are also available in state statutes. Law libraries in every state maintain copies of their state statutes and many public libraries have state statutes as well. A number of state boards of nursing also place their nurse practice act and regulations on a website.

State government is charged with protecting the health, safety, and well-being of the citizens in each state. If a citizen feels that he or she did not receive reasonable nursing care, that person may contact the State Board of Nursing and file a complaint against the nurse or nurses involved in the care. The state is then responsible for conducting an investigation to determine whether the patient's claim has merit.

Under the Fifth Amendment of the United States Constitution, all citizens are afforded the right to due process before any property can be taken by a state or federal government. Case law indicates that a nurse's license is a form of property because it helps an individual to earn a living. Because due process rights are attached to a nursing license, certain due process requirements must be met before a State Board of Nursing can revoke, discipline, or place conditions on a nursing license. First, the nurse is entitled to a notice that someone has filed a claim on his or her license. Next, the nurse must be given an opportunity to answer any charges that are alleged. This opportunity usually takes the form of a hearing before the State Board of Nursing. Usually, the nurse will want to attend the hearing with an attorney to make sure all rights are respected.

At the hearing, the investigators for the State Board of Nursing present the complaint that was filed and any investigation that was performed. The nurse may call witnesses who have knowledge of facts surrounding the complaint. These witnesses may include the person who filed the complaint, any witnesses to the incident, and individuals who supervised the nurse. At this hearing, the nurse, either directly or through legal counsel, can question witnesses and introduce evidence or testimony to refute the allegations in the complaint. Based on these presentations, the State Board of Nursing makes a determination as to whether reasonable nursing care was given and what, if any, discipline is warranted. Typically, the decision of the State Board of Nursing is final, and unless there were violations of the nurse's due process rights, a court will uphold the State Board's findings.

Although the nurse's right of due process cannot be abridged, state boards of nursing have the right temporarily to suspend a nurse's license immediately for acts the Board deems dangerous to the welfare of the general public. When the state immediately suspends a nursing license, it must afford the nurse a right to a hearing within a prescribed short time from the date of suspension.

Civil Law

Civil law is the second area of the law that affects the practice of nursing. One specific area of civil law, tort law, forms the foundation of most civil cases involving nurses. Torts are civil wrongs. The torts of negligence, malpractice, assault, and battery are addressed later in this chapter. The civil concepts of vicarious liability and product liability also are discussed.

Criminal Law

The third area of the law relevant to nursing practice is *criminal law*. Unlike civil law, where private parties sue one another, criminal law encompasses cases where the local, state, or federal government has filed a lawsuit against a nurse. Criminal cases include criminal assault and battery, negligent homicide, and murder. Criminal cases are extremely rare in nursing situations. An example of a criminal case is presented with the case studies given later in this chapter.

NURSING NEGLIGENCE IN CRITICAL CARE

The legal responsibility of the registered nurse in critical care settings does not differ from that of the registered nurse in any work setting. The registered nurse adheres to five principles for the protection of the patient and the practitioner (Box 8-1). The most common lawsuits against nurses and their employers are based on the legal concept of malpractice, known as negligence by a professional. The following discussion emphasizes the major elements of malpractice and provides some case examples for clarification.

Duty and Breach of Duty

A duty is a legal relationship between two or more parties. Several different kinds of situations can create this type of duty. In most nursing cases, duty arises out of a contractual

box 8-1
Five Legal Responsibilities of the Registered Nurse

- Performs only those functions for which he or she has been prepared by education and experience
- Performs those functions competently
- Delegates responsibility only to personnel whose competence has been evaluated and found acceptable
- Takes appropriate measures as indicated by observations of the patient
- Is familiar with policies of the employing agency

relationship between the patient and the health care facility. That is, when a patient receives health care, an implied contract arises. The patient, his insurer, or both agree to pay for any health care services the patient receives; in return, the health care facility agrees to supply "reasonable care." A nurse who cares for a patient is legally responsible for providing reasonable care under the circumstances present at the time of the incident. The critical care nurse who fails to provide reasonable care under the circumstances has breached (violated) his or her duty toward the patient.

Many different methods are used to determine whether the nurse complied with reasonable standards of care that existed at the time of the incident. The following factors can be used to determine if the care of the critical care nurse was reasonable:

- Testimony from experts in critical care
- Agency procedure and protocol manuals
- Nursing job descriptions
- Nursing texts, professional journals, medication books
- Professional organization standards (Advanced Cardiac Life Support [ACLS] and Certified Critical Care Registered Nurse [CCRN] standards)
- Equipment manufacturers' instructions

Once duty is established, a breach of that duty is required; that is, the nurse must have been negligent. Negligence is found or refuted by a comparison of the nurse's conduct with the standard of care. In general, negligence is either ordinary or gross. Ordinary negligence implies professional carelessness, whereas gross negligence suggests that the nurse willfully and consciously ignored a known risk of harm to the patient. Most cases involve ordinary negligence, but gross negligence can be present if the nurse ignored sound nursing advice or harmed a patient while under the influence of drugs or alcohol.

Causation

Malpractice law also requires that there be a causal relationship between the conduct of the critical care nurse and the injury to the patient, and that the injury that the patient suffers must be reasonably anticipated. For example, if a critical care nurse administered digoxin to a cardiac patient who had a pulse of 30 beats/minute and the patient suffered a cardiac arrest, it is likely that the critical care nurse would be found to have caused the patient's arrest; that is, the wrongful administration of the digoxin will be deemed to be the "proximate cause" of the arrest. However, if the patient had a pulse of 70 beats/minute when the digoxin was administered, and the patient suffered a totally unanticipated seizure, it is probable that the nurse would not be found to have caused the seizure. In this case, the seizure was not caused by the digoxin, and the nurse would be exonerated because seizures are not an expected complication of digoxin administration.

Injury

The intent of the law is to make "the injured patient whole." That is, the law attempts to return the plaintiff to a position he or she would have been in had an injury not been suffered. Unfortunately, injuries sustained usually cannot be "undone." As such, most court awards attempt to give monetary damages to compensate for the injuries sustained by a plaintiff.

In a malpractice suit, the plaintiff has to show that some type of injury or harm occurred as a result of the nurse's actions or inaction. The law allows several different types of monetary damages. These are grouped under the broad headings of economic and noneconomic damages.

Economic damages relate to those damages that can be calculated within a degree of certainty. Things such as medical costs and lost wages are the two major types of economic damages. Attorneys have a special type of accountant, called an actuary, to estimate how much an injured patient was likely to earn over the course of a normal life expectancy and how the injury has affected this earning capacity. This monetary amount comprises the "lost wages" part of the award. Similarly, the actuary is able to use past figures and inflation factors to estimate how much present and future medical expenses will cost the plaintiff.

Noneconomic damages are somewhat more difficult to calculate. These damages include pain and suffering and loss of consortium (services) that occurred as a result of the malpractice. Many state and federal governments place monetary limits on the amount a patient can recover for pain and suffering, regardless of the amount that may be awarded by a jury. Loss of consortium damages deal with such things as the patient's inability to perform household tasks or loss of marital relations.

In a number of cases, the spouse and minor children of a patient may also be able to recover both economic and noneconomic damages that they suffer as a consequence of injuries to the patient. When a minor child is the plaintiff, it is not unusual for the parents to file for noneconomic losses due to the loss of society and affection of their child. On the economic side, a parent can sue for his or her own lost wages due to a need to care for the child.

Many types of malpractice complaints are lodged against critical care nurses. The following cases illustrate reasons nurses are often named in malpractice suits.

case 1 ■ FAILURE TO COMPLY WITH REASONABLE STANDARDS OF CARE

Mr. Scott, a 46-year-old man with a history of ventricular tachycardia, was prescribed Tambocor for his heart condition. One evening he reported his heart "started feeling funny" and had a friend take him to the emergency room. An ECG on admission to the emergency room revealed he was experiencing ventricular tachycardia.

Mr. Scott told those in the ER that he did not want to be cardioverted. The ER physician, in telephone consultation with a cardiologist, ordered 5 mg of verapamil. Within 2 minutes, Mr. Scott's blood pressure crashed, and he seized and went into cardiac arrest. Due to the arrest, Mr. Scott suffered brain damage and was forced to reside in a nursing home due to lack of any independent motor function and inability to speak.

The ER nurse, physician, and hospital were sued for several reasons, including malpractice. During deposition, the nurse testified that she was ACLS certified and admitted to knowing that verapamil was contraindicated in patients with ventricular tachycardia. Additionally, she related that she had serious questions about administering the verapamil but acceded to the physician's orders.

The court found that the standard of reasonable nursing care required her to intervene to prevent complications and that failure to intervene was a violation of the nursing standard of care. Further, the court determined that the standard of nursing care requires nurses to exercise independent nursing judgment if they feel an order may have adverse consequences to the patient. ■

case 2 ■ IMPROPER MEDICATION ADMINISTRATION

Kelsey Martin, a 26–28 week premature infant, was brought to Stephens County Hospital when she was unexpectedly delivered at home. Stephens County Hospital arranged to have Kelsey transported to Crawford Long Hospital, which had a neonatal ICU (NICU). A registered nurse and respiratory therapist were sent for the transport. During the course of the transport, Kelsey received an overdose of heparin, which caused a cerebral hemorrhage, resulting in brain damage and physical and mental impairments.

Kelsey's parents sued the transport nurse, the respiratory therapist, and the transport system for malpractice. The defendants in the case claimed the transport was for emergency services and that they should be absolved from liability under Georgia's "Good Samaritan" statute, which provides immunity from suit for responding to certain types of emergencies. The court found that Kelsey's medical assistance coverage had paid for the transport services, so that the "Good Samaritan" statute was not applicable. A trial was ordered on the malpractice suit.[2]

In this case, an overdose of heparin was the alleged cause of malpractice. Such medication errors often form the basis of malpractice suits against critical care nurses. ■

case 3 ■ CRIMINAL LIABILITY IN CRITICAL CARE

Virgil Dykes was an 86-year-old man who was admitted to the hospital with abdominal pain. He was diagnosed with a perforation in the proximal duodenum, causing diffuse peritonitis. The day after his surgery, he was found to have a serum potassium level of 3.2 mEq/L, below the normal levels of 3.3 to 5.5 mEq/L. The ICU nurse administered an ordered dose of potassium chloride elixir through his nasogastric tube. However, subsequent laboratory tests showed this had not been well absorbed.

Mr. Dykes' physician, Dr. Wood, ordered the ICU nurse to run in an intravenous (IV) bag with 40 mEq of potassium chloride in 100 mL of saline. When the nurse informed Dr. Wood that the potassium chloride would need to be infused over the course of 1 hour, he ordered her to draw up a syringe of 40 mEq of potassium chloride in 30 to 50 mL of saline. The nurse drew up the syringe, but refused to administer it, knowing that this was dangerous.

Another ICU nurse was also present and informed Dr. Wood that it was contrary to hospital policy to administer a maximum dosage of 40 mEq of potassium chloride over 1 hour. Dr. Wood then took the syringe from the nurse and administered the potassium chloride himself. During the injection, Mr. Dykes stopped breathing and efforts at cardiopulmonary resuscitation (CPR) were unsuccessful.

Dr. Wood was convicted of involuntary manslaughter, "the unlawful killing of a human being without malice in the commission, without due caution and circumspection, of a lawful act which might produce death." He was sentenced to 5 months' imprisonment, 36 months' supervised parole, a $100 assessment, and a $25,000 fine.[3]

Dr. Wood's failure to use reasonable standards of medical care and his total disregard of the cautions given by the ICU nursing staff resulted in criminal liability. His criminal conviction was upheld by the United Sates Court of Appeals for the 10th Circuit. ■

Vicarious Liability

In some cases, a person or institution can be held liable for the conduct of another. This is called *vicarious liability*. There are various types of vicarious liability, including respondeat superior, corporate liability, negligent supervision, and rule of personal liability.

RESPONDEAT SUPERIOR

The doctrine of *respondeat superior* is translated as "let the master answer for the sins of the servant." This is the major legal theory under which hospitals are held liable for the negligence of their employees. Respondeat superior is a public policy type of legal doctrine. The philosophy behind respondeat superior is based on the idea that because a hospital typically generates profits from the patients seeking care, if negligence occurs, the hospital should pay for some of the damages caused by hospital personnel. This doctrine applies only when hospital employees act within the scope of their employment.

In some situations, respondeat superior is not applicable. For instance, hospitals are not usually responsible for temporary agency personnel because they are usually employees of the agency, not the hospital. Physicians, unless they are employed by the hospital, do not typically come within the sphere of this doctrine. Actions by hospital nurses who cause malpractice outside of their employment rarely fall into the respondeat superior category.

Because the hospital may be held liable for nursing activities conducted by their employees, they carry professional liability insurance for the activities of their employees. Usually, a hospital will defend a nurse named in a malpractice case. However, many nurses also carry their own malpractice insurance for off-the-job nursing activities, and in order to retain independent counsel in the event they are sued.

CORPORATE LIABILITY

Another type of vicarious liability is called *corporate liability*. Corporate liability occurs when a hospital is found liable for its own unreasonable conduct. For example, if it is found that a unit is chronically understaffed and a patient suffers an injury as a result of short staffing, the hospital can be held accountable. It is reasonable to expect any hospital that has an ICU or an emergency department (ED) to take precautionary measures to ensure that it is adequately staffed or that beds or admissions are reduced. Failure to ensure adequate staffing can lead to payment of monetary damages under the theory of corporate liability.

Corporate liability may also occur within "floating" situations. A nurse working in a critical care setting must be competent to make immediate nursing judgments and to act on those decisions. If the nurse does not possess the knowledge and skills required of a critical care nurse, he or she should not be rendering critical care. A nurse who is not well versed in critical care should notify the charge nurse or nursing supervisor of this fact. The nurse needs to clearly state which nursing care activities he or she can and cannot implement. The supervisor and charge nurse must then delegate the remaining nursing duties to staff members with adequate education, training, and experience. Box 8-2 addresses issues of concern to the floating nurse.

NEGLIGENT SUPERVISION

A third type of vicarious liability is *negligent supervision*. Negligent supervision is claimed when a supervisor fails to reasonably supervise people under his or her direction. For example, if a nurse is rotated to an unfamiliar unit and informs the charge nurse that she has never worked in critical care, it would be unreasonable for the charge nurse to ask her to perform invasive monitoring. If the charge nurse did assign such responsibilities to the floater and a patient injury resulted, the charge nurse could be held accountable to the patient for negligent supervision.

CAPTAIN OF THE SHIP DOCTRINE

Finally, a fourth type of vicarious liability is known as the *captain of the ship doctrine*. At one time, the physician was viewed as the captain of the ship. Therefore, any order by the doctor was expected to be implemented by the nurse. This doctrine has largely been replaced by a legal concept known as *the rule of personal liability*. That is, by virtue of specialized education, training, and experience, nurses are expected to make sound decisions. If they are unsure about the propriety of a physician's order, they need to seek clarification from the physician or, if needed, from their supervisor.

Establishment of Protocols

If the critical care nurse is required to perform medical acts and is not under the direct and immediate supervision of a delegating physician, the activities must be based on established protocols. These protocols should be created by the medical and nursing departments and should be reviewed for compliance with state nurse practice acts. They must be reviewed frequently so that health care professionals can determine whether they reflect current medical and nursing standards of care. In the event of a malpractice suit, the critical care protocols and procedures can be introduced as evidence to help establish the applicable standard of care. Although it is important that protocols provide direction, excessive detail restricts the critical care nurse's flexibility when selecting a proper course of action.

box 8-2
Commonly Asked Questions When Rotating to an Unfamiliar Unit

1. **If I am asked to go to another unit, must I go?**
   Usually, you will be required to go to the other unit. If you refuse, you can be disciplined under the theory that you are breaching your employment contract or that you are failing to abide by the policies and procedures of the hospital. Some nursing units negotiate with hospitals to ensure that only specially trained nurses rotate to specialty units.
2. **If I rotate to an unfamiliar unit, what types of nursing responsibilities must I assume?**
   You will be expected to carry out only those nursing activities that you are competent to perform. In some instances, this will be the performance of basic nursing care activities, such as blood pressures, and uncomplicated treatments. If you are unfamiliar with the types of medications used on the unit, you should *not* be administering them until you are thoroughly familiar with them. Consider the medication cards the student completes in nursing school. They were assigned because a reasonable, prudent nurse does not give medications without knowledge of their pharmacology, dosage, method of administration, side effects, and interactions with other medications. The same reasoning applies for any other type of critical care monitoring.
3. **What should I do if I feel unprepared when I get to the unit?**
   Suggest that you assist the unit with basic nursing care requirements and that specialized activities (e.g., invasive monitoring, cardiac monitoring, or the administration of unfamiliar drugs) be performed by staff who are adequately prepared. Do not feel incompetent because you are not familiar with all aspects of nursing care. After all, when is the last time you saw the neurologist go to labor and delivery and perform a cesarean section?
4. **What if the charge nurse orders me to do something I am not able to do safely?**
   You are obligated to say you are unqualified and request that another nurse carry out the task. The charge nurse also needs to remember that she could be held liable for negligent supervision if she orders you to do an unsafe activity and a patient injury results.

The Questionable Medical Order

In addition to protocols, a policy statement should exist (in procedures or by directive) that indicates the manner of resolving the issue of the "questionable" medical order. This is important for all medical orders, but particularly for those given for critically ill patients because of the unusual doses of medication that are frequently ordered. The nurse who questions a particular order should express his or her specific reasons for concern to the physician who wrote the order. This initial approach frequently results in an explanation of the order and a medical justification for the order in the patient's medical record. If this approach is unsuccessful, many hospitals require that the attending physician or the nursing supervisor be notified; others have a policy that the chief of the service must be consulted about questionable orders. If these options are unavailable or are unsuccessful, a critical care nurse or any other nurse can refuse to give a medication.

As was demonstrated in the Bush case, an order that is patently wrong can harm the patient if it is followed. A secondary consequence can be liability for the physician, the nurse, and the hospital (as the employer) if the patient suffers harm as a direct result of the order.

Liability for Defective Medical Equipment

A medical device, defined as virtually anything used in patient care that is not a drug, includes intricate pieces of equipment (e.g., intra-aortic balloon pumps, endotracheal tubes, pacemakers, defibrillators), along with less complicated ones, such as bedpans, suture materials, patient restraints, and tampons. Before 1976, medical devices were unregulated; since 1976, medical devices have been regulated by the U.S. Food and Drug Administration (FDA). Before November 1991, hospitals, their employees, and staffs were permitted, but not required, to report device malfunctions to the device manufacturer or to the FDA.

On November 28, 1991, the Safe Medical Devices Act of 1990 (Fl 10 1-629) became effective just after proposed regulations (called the Tentative Final Rule) were published for comment. This act requires user facilities (which include hospitals and ambulatory surgery facilities, but not physician offices) to report to the manufacturer medical device malfunctions that result in serious illness, injury, or death to a patient. They are also required to report to the FDA those that result in a patient's death. A serious illness or injury includes not only a life-threatening injury or illness, but an injury that requires "immediate medical or surgical intervention to preclude permanent impairment of a body function or permanent damage to a body structure."[4] Therefore, the rupture of an intra-aortic balloon pump that requires that the balloon-dependent patient immediately be transported to the operating room for removal and replacement of the device is a reportable event.

Nursing and other staff must now participate in reporting device malfunctions, including those associated with user error, to a designated hospital department. Personnel in that area are usually responsible for determining which malfunctions engender an obligation to report and to whom they should be reported.

More recently, the FDA has implemented a new tracking system in which hospitals must participate. As of March 1, 1993, facilities that implant certain devices (e.g., pacemakers, heart valves, or silicone breast implants) must notify the manufacturer when the devices are implanted. They must also maintain files that the hospital can use to determine the identities and certain other information about patients in whom the devices have been implanted.[5]

There is a duty not to use equipment that is patently defective. If the equipment suddenly ceases to do what it was intended to do, makes unusual noises, or has a history of malfunction and has not been repaired, the hospital could be liable for damage caused by it. Likewise, the nurses could be liable if they know or should know of these problems and use the equipment anyway. The following cases involved liability for defective equipment.

case 4 ■ MEDICAL EQUIPMENT AND PATIENT INJURIES

Mr. Carter was admitted to the hospital for hemorrhaging and underwent a partial gastrectomy. After surgery, x-rays were ordered to assess his status. Two nursing students tried to assist transfer of a portable x-ray machine into his room for the x-ray studies. The wheels of the machine became tangled in the cord and the portable x-ray machine fell onto Mr. Carter's abdomen and pinned his left arm and hand. Mr. Carter suffered excruciating pain and had to undergo a second operation for gastric hemorrhaging. Mr. Carter recovered $17,500 actual damages for his injuries.[6] ■

case 5 ■ DEFECTIVE EQUIPMENT AND NEGLIGENCE

An infant suffered a cardiac arrest during surgery and was treated after surgery with a hypothermia machine. Although the nurse knew that the continuous-readout thermometer often malfunctioned, she did not check it with a glass thermometer. After the infant's temperature did not decrease, the nurse did not use other methods to lower body temperature, nor did she call the physician. The infant had a seizure and required mechanical ventilation. The nurse noticed poor air exchange but did not correct a kink in the ventilator tubing. The infant suffered permanent neurological damage. The court held that the injury was proximately caused by the negligence of the hospital's employees and by the defective equipment used in the ICU.[7] ■

The Need for Consent

In most instances, the law requires that the patient be given enough information before a treatment to make an informed, intelligent decision. However, in some situations, such consent is not required. For example, an emergency situation does not require informed consent, and a patient can waive informed consent by stating that he or she does not want information about a proposed treatment or procedure. In addition, some courts allow a physician to avoid full disclosure if the information disclosed might lead to further patient harm. This exception is known as *therapeutic privilege*.

Usually, obtaining informed consent from the patient or the family is the responsibility of the physician, but the nurse is frequently asked to witness the consent form. In these cases, the nurse is attesting that the signature on the consent form is the patient's or the family member's. When the nurse actually witnesses the physician's explanation concerning the nature of the proposed treatment, the risks and benefits of the treatment, alternative treatments, and potential consequences if the patient decides to do nothing, the nurse may want to place a note on the consent form or in the nurse's notes stating "consent procedure witnessed." This information may be vital in the rare case in which the patient or family sues the physician for lack of informed consent.

ISSUES THAT INVOLVE LIFE-SUPPORT MEASURES

Several basic issues regarding refusal and termination of treatment can involve the critical care nurse. Do not resuscitate (DNR) orders, refusal of treatment for religious reasons, advance directives, and withdrawal of life support are all complex topics that fall into this category.

Do Not Resuscitate (DNR) Orders

CPR success rates for those receiving in-hospital care are quite variable and are affected by patient environment and resuscitative factors.[8] However, CPR is not appropriate for all patients who experience a cardiac arrest because it is highly invasive and may constitute a "positive violation of an individual's right to die with dignity." Furthermore, CPR may not be indicated when the illness is terminal and irreversible and when the patient can gain no benefit.

Prestigious authorities (e.g., the President's Commission for the Study of Ethical Problems in Medicine and Biomedical and Behavioral Research; hereafter "the President's Commission") have recommended that hospitals have an explicit policy on the practice of writing and implementing DNR orders.[9] Most hospitals and medical societies, and some states, have published DNR policies.[10]

Whether to resuscitate any patient is a decision that is made by the attending physician, the patient, and the family, although critical care nurses and other nurses often have substantial input into the decision. In general, however, the consent of a competent patient should be required when a DNR order is written. If the patient is incompetent, the physician and family members make the decision. The situation can be more complex, and the physician and the family or patient can disagree.

Once the DNR decision has been made, the order should be written, signed, and dated by the responsible physician. It should be reviewed periodically; hospital policies may require review every 24 to 72 hours. The more informal methods of designating patients with whom CPR is not to be undertaken can lead to errors if an arrest occurs. For example, the wrong patient can be allowed to die.

If an arrest occurs in an ED or in another situation in which a formal DNR decision has not been made and written, the presumption of the medical and nursing staffs should be in favor of life, and a code should be called. A "slow code" (in which the nurse takes excessive time to call or the health care team takes its time responding) is never permissible. Either CPR is indicated, or it is not.

Courts may be involved in DNR decisions. In 1978, a Massachusetts appellate court ruled that an attending physician may lawfully write a DNR order for an incompetent patient for whom there is no lifesaving or life-prolonging treatment.[11] In a 1984 case, a New York grand jury investigated a hospital that indicated DNR decisions by using purple dots stuck to nursing cards that were discarded after the death of the patient. Nurses from the hospital complained that the decals could be stuck to the wrong patient's card; in one case, a card had two dots affixed to it. The grand jury found that the dot system "virtually eliminated professional accountability, invited clerical error and discouraged physicians from obtaining informed consent from the patient or his family."[12]

case 6 ■ DECISIONS CONCERNING VENTILATOR DISCONTINUATION

Mrs. Law, a 64-year-old woman with diabetes, was admitted to Greenwich Hospital with complaints of weakness, a low-grade fever, a nonproductive cough, frequent urination, anorexia, and malaise. On admission, her blood glucose was low and she was indeed febrile. Her attending physician placed her on Unasyn, a broad-spectrum antibiotic, and adjusted her insulin dosage. The day after her admission, Mrs. Law suffered a respiratory arrest, was resuscitated, and had her cardiac function restored. She was intubated and placed on mechanical ventilation. During the arrest she sustained severe neurologic damage.

Two days after her arrest, Mrs. Law remained unresponsive and had fixed, dilated pupils and no purposeful movements, and did not respond to external stimuli. The chief of neurology consulted with the family, suggesting that no significant recovery was possible. The neurologist proposed that Mrs. Law be removed from mechanical ventilation and placed on patient-assisted ventilation. If Mrs. Law had no brain function, she would not breathe and would die. Her family was aware that if she could not assist with ventilation she would die.

Mrs. Law was removed from the mechanical ventilator and died shortly after being placed on patient-assisted ventilation. Mrs. Law did not have a living will, health care proxy, or notation concerning her wishes regarding life support. Further, she had never made her wishes known to her family. Mrs. Law's family subsequently sued the physicians and the hospital, alleging medical malpractice on the grounds that the physicians did not act according to Connecticut's statute pertaining to continuation or removal of life support systems, nor did they follow the hospital's protocol.

After review of applicable state law and the hospital's policies, the trial court concluded that brain death was not necessary in order to place Mrs. Law on assisted ventilation. The lawsuits against the physicians and hospital were dismissed. This dismissal was upheld on appeal.[13] ■

Unfortunately, it is estimated that as few as 4% to 24% of Americans have an advance directive.[14–16] An advance directive can help with troublesome decisions such as those that were faced by both the family and the health care team in this case. The case was unclear as to whether Mrs. Law received advance directive information at the time of her admission, but this certainly would have been helpful in her case. It is also important for patients to speak with their families and their attending physician concerning end-of-life decisions. Relevant references on the ethical issues surrounding advance directives are found in the works cited previously.

Refusal of Treatment for Religious Reasons

case 7 ■ LIFESAVING TRANSFUSION FOR JEHOVAH'S WITNESS

Gregory Novack, a 16-year-old boy, was seriously injured in an automobile accident. On admission to Kennestone Hospital, he informed the staff not to give him blood because it was against his religious beliefs as a Jehovah's Witness. During orthopedic surgery, Gregory lost a considerable amount of blood. The hospital staff became convinced he would die without a transfusion. The hospital petitioned the court for a guardian ad litem to determine whether a blood transfusion would be in Gregory's best interests. A trial judge conducted an emergency hearing, and a transfusion was ordered against Gregory's and his parents' wishes. Gregory received the transfusion, and subsequently he and his parents claimed his rights of freedom of religion had been violated. The trial and appeals courts found no violation of constitutional rights on the part of the hospital and staff.[17]

The courts are split as to whether blood transfusions violate the religious rights of the patient or family. For example, in *Vega*, the Connecticut Supreme Court found that the hospital cannot "thrust unwanted medical care on a patient who . . . competently and clearly denied that care." Consequently, ICU nurses need to consult the hospital's risk management department in such situations to ensure proper handling of these types of legal issues.[18] ■

Advance Directives: Living Wills and Powers of Attorney

A living will is a written directive from a competent patient to family and health care team members concerning the patient's wishes in the event the patient is unable to express these wishes. One difficulty associated with a living will is its limited applicability. In most states, a living will becomes effective only if the patient is terminally ill or permanently comatose. Consequently, when the patient is critically ill or temporarily unable to make health care decisions, the living will is not operative.

To provide broader coverage, many patients opt for a durable power of attorney for health care. A durable power of attorney allows the patient to appoint a surrogate decision maker, known as a health care agent or proxy, who has authority to make treatment and health care decisions in the event that the patient is not able to do so. This type of document allows a trusted friend or relative to "stand in the shoes of the patient" when the patient is not able to make health care decisions.

Many savvy patients elect to combine the living will and the durable power of attorney for health care into one document, commonly called an *advance directive.* An advance directive allows the patient to communicate his or her wishes in the event of terminal illness or a permanently comatose state. It also names an agent who assists in decision making. Many advance directives give the health care agent specific instructions concerning health matters. For example, the advance directive may provide instructions concerning artificial nutrition and hydration, or it may outline specific treatments, such as a "no code" status under specified circumstances.

In response to federal law, all 50 states have statutes that allow patients to execute living wills, durable powers of attorney for health care, and advance directives. Each state, however, may place unique requirements on the drafting of these documents. Some states require that the directive be notarized. Other states mandate that the patient be counseled by a state-appointed ombudsman who outlines the pros and cons associated with the advance directive. Witness requirements also vary from state to state. Consequently, it is important to know the laws concerning advance directives that apply in your state. An excellent starting point is the living wills/advance directive web page of the American Association of Retired Persons (AARP). This group provides lay people and health care providers with up-to-date information on laws applicable in their state.

In most states, it is likely that a recent living will would be taken as evidence of what the patient would have wanted had he or she been competent when the decision was presented. Although there have not been any cases concerning a written living will, there have been several involving patients who had expressed wishes orally about life-sustaining measures.

Patient Self-Determination Act

On December 1, 1991, the Patient Self-Determination Act went into effect.[19] This federal statute is applicable to facilities that receive Medicare reimbursement for patient care. As a condition of reimbursement, the law requires that hospitals, nursing facilities, home health care services, hospice programs, and certain health maintenance organizations (HMOs) provide information to adults about their rights concerning decision making in that state. For hospitals, this information must be provided to every adult on admission regardless of diagnosis and regardless of whether the individual is eligible for Medicare coverage. The material distributed must include information about the types of advance directives that are legal in that state. Documentation that the patient has received this information must be placed in the medical record. If the patient is incapacitated on admission, the information must be provided to a family member, if available. This action, however, does not relieve the hospital of its duty to provide information to the patient once he or she is no longer incapacitated.

Withdrawal of Life-Support Measures

What constitutes life support, when these measures must be used, and when they may be terminated have been issues raised in many court cases. However, the law in these areas is still developing and will continue to do so as each state creates its own guidelines.

Given the regularity with which life-support decisions must be made in health care facilities, it is remarkable that it was not until 1976 that the first case, *In re Quinlan*, focused national attention on the "right to die" controversy. The cases concern competent minors and adults who have a disease or condition that would eventually be terminal. States have not been consistent in their decisions, even when the situations are arguably similar. For example, the New Jersey court in the case of Karen Ann Quinlan, a 21-year-old woman in a persistent vegetative state, held that the decision about treatment is in the hands of the patient's guardian in consultation with the hospital ethics committee.[20] Massachusetts, however, rejected the New Jersey approach in favor of judicial review of decisions made by physicians and family members.[21] The President's Commission stated (p. 6) that judicial review of these decisions should be reserved for occasions when "adjudication is clearly required by state law or when concerned parties have disagreements that they cannot resolve over matters of substantial import."[9]

case 8 ■ RIGHT TO REFUSE TREATMENT

Elizabeth Bouvia was a 28-year-old woman who suffered from severe cerebral palsy and was a quadriplegic. She was a patient at a public hospital and was totally dependent on the care of others. She was mentally competent. Eventually, her physical condition deteriorated to the point that she required nasogastric tube feedings. Ms. Bouvia requested that the hospital remove the nasogastric tube and resort only to those feedings that she could tolerate orally. The trial court concluded that physically Ms. Bouvia tolerated the nasogastric tube and that it was not a great physical discomfort. The California Court of Appeals, Second District reversed the trial court and ordered that the hospital remove Ms. Bouvia's nasogastric tube and that they not replace it or aid in replacing it without Ms. Bouvia's express consent.[22] ■

case 9 ■ RIGHT TO RESTRICT FOOD AND FLUIDS

Nancy Cruzan was a young woman who suffered anoxic brain damage in an automobile accident. She remained in a persistent vegetative state in Missouri and was fed by gastrostomy. After rehabilitation was unsuccessful, Ms. Cruzan's parents (as co-guardians) requested withdrawal of the feeding tube. After the employees of the residential rehabilitation center where Ms. Cruzan was receiving care refused to withdraw the feedings, the Cruzans sought judicial review of their request. After testimony, the trial court approved the parents' request.

On appeal, the Missouri Supreme Court reversed the lower court. First, it held that Missouri law does not permit surrogate decision making in decisions of this importance. For a person to exercise the right to terminate artificial feeding in Missouri, that person must have previously expressed his or her wishes, either orally or in writing. Evidence of those wishes had to meet a relatively high evidentiary standard, a standard that the court held had been met in the lower court proceeding.

This case was appealed to the United States Supreme Court, and in 1990, it was affirmed on constitutional grounds.[23] After the decision was issued, the Cruzans returned to the Missouri lower court and presented further evidence (through additional witnesses) about what their daughter had expressed while competent. The lower court found that they had presented clear and convincing evidence and affirmed the rights of the co-guardians to authorize withdrawal of the feeding tube. After withdrawal of the tube, Nancy Cruzan died on December 26, 1990.[23] ■

It is important to note that although *Cruzan* is still applicable law, the way in which this landmark case has been interpreted and implemented has been extremely variable at state court levels. Although this case received much publicity, it did not change the law in any state but Missouri. Most states continue to permit surrogate decision making by relatives and require a lower evidentiary standard than that required in Missouri.

case 10 ■ RIGHT TO TERMINATE TREATMENT

In the case *In re the Conservatorship of Wanglie*, a patient who was ventilator dependent and competent had a cardiopulmonary arrest. After this event, she remained in a persistent vegetative state. Pursuant to the wishes of the family, she was nourished by feeding tube and treated aggressively for recurrent pneumonia. Hospital staff disagreed with the family in this case; intervention by the hospital ethics committee did not resolve the conflict. Therefore, the hospital filed an application for a non-family member guardian to decide for the patient. The Minnesota court instead appointed the husband as guardian, finding that he was in the best position to know his wife's wishes. The court found that the hospital had requested the appointment of a non–family member not because Mr. Wanglie was incompetent to be guardian, but because he disagreed with hospital staff.[24] ■

In recent years, as health care providers have become more comfortable recommending termination of treatment in selected cases, they have met resistance from some families who wish to continue treatment no matter what its chance of success. Although no law or legal principle requires that extraordinary, but clearly futile, treatment be provided, it is probably also true that health care providers have no legal recourse against families who refuse to withdraw life support. (That is, unless the patient has left written indications of his or her wishes before incompetence.)

In most states, problems of terminating treatment need not be resolved in court. Decisions regarding treatment or nontreatment that meet accepted medical standards and with which the patient concurs are made virtually every day in health care settings. If the patient is not competent to decide, usually family members may do so, although they may not refuse therapy that would benefit the patient. Finally, a distinction should be made between termination of treatment and termination of care. Even patients who are not being treated for their terminal condition require competent and sensitive nursing and medical care so that their final days are as comfortable as possible. The families of these patients may also require information along with sensitive emotional support. The need for good nursing care does not end with the decision not to treat.

For an excellent review of all of the issues concerning advance directives, right to refuse treatment, and restriction of patient treatments, refer to Beauchamp and Walter's book, *Contemporary Issues in Bioethics.*[10]

Brain Death

In 1968, the Harvard criteria established standards for determining brain death. The criteria have been found quite reliable. Some states adopted the Harvard criteria by statute, whereas other states enacted legislation defining brain death in broader, less restrictive terms.

The President's Commission published *Defining Death* in July 1981. The Commission recommended a uniform statute defining death; it recommended that the statute address "general physiological standards rather than medical criteria and tests, which will change with advances in biomedical knowledge and refinements in technique."[25] All states have laws addressing the definition of "death" in the state. Some states use brain death as the sole criterion; other states rely on a number of factors, such as response to pain and cessation of cardiac function. It is important for the nurse to know the legal definition of death in any state where he or she is practicing, although such a determination typically rests with the patient's attending physician, and may also require the concurrence of other consulting physicians.

A patient who is brain dead is legally dead, and there is no legal duty to continue to treat him or her. It is not necessary to obtain court approval to discontinue life support on a patient who is brain dead. Furthermore, although it can be desirable to obtain family permission to discontinue treatment of a brain-dead patient, there is no legal requirement. However, before terminating life support, physicians and nurses should be sure that organs are not intended for transplant purposes.

Organ Donation

Every state in the United States has a law based on the Uniform Anatomical Gift Act. The statutes establish the legality of organ donation by individuals and their families and set procedures for making and accepting the gift of an organ. Every state also has some provision to enable people to consent to organ donation using a designated place on a driver's license. More recently, many states have enacted "required request" laws. These laws attempt to increase the supply of organs for transplant by requiring hospital personnel to ask patients' families about an organ gift at the time of the patient's death.

clinical applicability challenges

Self-Challenge: Critical Thinking

1. *You are the charge nurse in the ICU on night shift. One of the nurses on your shift reports to work smelling of alcohol. What should you do? What legal principles may be applicable if you allow this nurse to care for patients and a patient is subsequently injured?*
2. *Mr. Michaels is a patient on your unit. He has chronic obstructive pulmonary disease (COPD) and suffers a respiratory arrest. He has not drafted any type of advance directive, but you are aware that he has spoken to his family about his wishes in the event he is no longer to make his desires known concerning extraordinary care. As a nurse caring for Mr. Michaels, what legal issues do you feel are of relevance? Whom can you turn to concerning this dilemma?*

Study Questions

1. *The doctrine of respondeat superior is the legal theory under which*
   a. *a hospital is directly liable for its corporate hiring decisions.*
   b. *a health care provider is personally liable for acts of negligence.*
   c. *an employer is vicariously liable for the negligent acts of its employees as long as they act within the scope of employment.*
   d. *a hospital is liable for injuries to its employees.*
2. *The Patient Self-Determination Act went into effect in 1991. This federal law requires that hospitals, nursing homes, and certain other providers*
   a. *provide patients with information about advance directives and require them to execute at least one type of advance directive.*
   b. *provide patients with information about living wills only.*
   c. *provide patients with information about all types of advance directives applicable in that state.*

d. *provide patients with information about all types of advance directives, regardless of whether the information is applicable in that state.*

3. *A living will is applicable under which of the following circumstances?*
   a. *The patient is incapacitated and is terminally ill.*
   b. *The patient is incapacitated and has a life-threatening but curable illness.*
   c. *The patient is competent to express his or her wishes, has a desire to be treated, and has subsequently become incapacitated.*
   d. *The patient is competent but wants his or her grown children to make the health care decisions.*

REFERENCES

1. *Las Collinas Medical et al v. Bush*, 122 SW3d 835 (2003) (TX App 2nd Dist)
2. *Martin v. The Fulton-DeKalb Hospital Authority d/b/a Grady Memorial Hospital d/b/a Grady Health System et al*, 2001 Ga.App. LEXIS 762, 1 Fulton County DR 2168 (2001)
3. *US v. Wood*, 207 F.3d 1222; 2000 U.S. App. LEXIS 5475, 2000 Colo J. C.A.R. 1645 (2000)
4. U.S. Department of Health and Human Services, Food and Drug Administration: Medical devices: Medical device, user facility, distributor, and manufacturer reporting, certification and registration. Federal Register 56:64004–64182 (December 6), 1991
5. U.S. Department of Health and Human Services, Food and Drug Administration: Medical devices: Device tracking. Federal Register 57:22971–22981 (May 29), 1992
6. *Carter v. Anderson Memorial Hospital*, 325 S.E.2d 78 (S.C.App. 1985)
7. *Rose v. Hakim*, 335 F. Supp. 1221 (DDC 1971, affirmed in part, reversed in part, 501 F.2d 806 (DC Cir 1974)
8. Dumot JA, Burval DJ, Sprung J et al: Outcome of adult cardiopulmonary resuscitations at a tertiary referral center including results of "limited" resuscitations. Arch Intern Med 161(14), 1751–1758, 2001
9. President's Commission for the Study of Ethical Problems in Medicine and Biomedical and Behavioral Research: Deciding to Forego Life-Sustaining Treatment. Washington, DC, Government Printing Office, March, 1983
10. Beauchamp TL, Walters L. Contemporary Issues in Bioethics (5th Ed). Belmont, CA, Wadsworth, 1999
11. Matter of Dinnerstein; 380 NE2d 134, Massachusetts, 1978
12. Panel accuses hospital of hiding denial of care. New York Times, March 21, 1984
13. *Law v. Camp et al*, 116 F.Supp.2d 295 (CT 2000)
14. Center for Bioethics: Advanced directives. Available at: http://www.bioethics.umn.edu/resources/topics/advance_directives.shtml. Accessed March 2004
15. Huffman GB: Benefits of discussing advance directives with patients. Available at http://www.aafp.org/afp/20010715/tips/4.html. Accessed March 2004
16. Ackermann RJ: Withholding and withdrawing life-sustaining treatment. Available at http://www.aafp.org/afp/20001001/1555.html. Accessed March 2004
17. *Novak v. Cobb County Kennestone Hospital Authority*, No 94-8403 (11th Cir., Feb. 14, 1996)
18. *Stamford Hosp. v. Vega*, 646 (CT 1996)
19. Omnibus Budget Reconciliation Act of 1990. Pub.L.No. 101-508 §§4206, 4751 (codified in scattered sections of 42 U.S.C., particularly §§1395cc, 1396a) (West Supp. 1991)
20. *In re Quinlan*, 70 NJ 10, 355 A2d 647, New Jersey, 1976
21. *Superintendent of Belchertown State School v. Saikewicz*, 373 Mass. 728, 370 NE2d 417, Massachusetts, 1977
22. *Bouvia v. Superior Court*, 225 Cal.Rptr. 297 (Cal.App. 2 Dist)
23. *Cruzan v. Director*, Missouri Department of Health et al, III L Ed2d 224, 110 SCt 2841 (1990)
24. *In re the Conservatorship of Wanglie*, No. PX-91-283 (Minn Dist Ct. Probate Ct Division, July 1991)
25. President's Commission for the Study of Ethical Problems in Medicine and Biomedical and Behavioral Research: Defining Death, p 1. Washington, DC, Government Printing Office, July, 1981

chapter 9

Genetic Issues in Critical Care Nursing

DENNIS J. CHEEK ■ JONATHAN L. DESAMERO ■ ANNUSHKA CESAN

objectives

Based on the content in this chapter, the reader should be able to:

- Explain basic genetics terminology and concepts.
- Name and describe the main categories of genetic disease.
- Describe the interplay between the environment and genetics in disease.
- Identify the potential roles of the nurse in the critical care setting.
- Discuss the emerging applications of pharmacogenetics in nursing practice.

HUMAN GENOME PROJECT

Overview

An extraordinary challenge called the *Human Genome Project* was proposed in the mid-1980s to identify the entire human genetic code. It required sifting through and deciphering a tremendous amount of biological information, with the goal of mapping out the sequences of every human gene, letter by letter. It was expected that the elaboration of the fundamental building blocks that made up the human genome would lead to a greater understanding of many diseases and bring about the development of new treatment modalities.

Such a massive project required the collaboration of groups from several countries, including the United States, the United Kingdom, Japan, France, Germany, and China. They generated a draft sequence of the human genome. Both the February 15, 2001 issue of *Nature* and the February 16, 2001 issue of *Science* published the sequence of the human genome, and recently the Human Genome Project has been completed.

Several discoveries will be made through analysis of the published code. For instance, it was realized that humans have far fewer genes than once believed. The old paradigm of "one gene makes only one protein" is no longer valid, because humans make approximately 100,000 proteins from far fewer genes. We now know that the total human

box 9-1
Core Competencies in Genetics Essential for All Health Care Professionals (Continued)

3.5 Seek coordination and collaboration with interdisciplinary team of health professionals
3.6 Speak out on issues that undermine client's rights to informed decision making and voluntary action
3.7 Recognize the limitations of their own genetics expertise
3.8 Demonstrate willingness to update genetics knowledge at frequent intervals
3.9 Recognize when personal values and biases with regard to ethical, social, cultural, religious, and ethnic issues may impact or interfere with care provided to clients
3.10 Support client-focused policies

From National Coalition for Health Professional Education in Genetics (NCHPEG) website: http://www.nchpeg.org.

Another emerging tool that nurses will need to learn is gene therapy, or the therapeutic transfer of human genes into the patient to temporarily correct a genetic defect. Human gene transfer still faces several barriers in its application, but very soon nurses will need to learn specifics about its route of administration, mechanism of action, potential for cure, risk of side effects, and ratio of success. In the field of nursing, the learning never stops.

CONCEPTS IN GENETICS

To understand the types of genetically influenced diseases that present in adult critical care, it is essential that nurses understand relevant terminology.

Cells Contain DNA

The human body is composed of billions of cells. There is usually one nucleus for each cell, and each nucleus contains *deoxyribonucleic acid*, or DNA, arranged on chromosomes. Specific segments of DNA are called *genes*, and genes code for proteins. Proteins perform the necessary cellular functions. Virtually all the body's cells contain exactly the same full set of genes.[6,11]

Because there is a diversity of cell types and functions, some cells may have certain genes turned "on," whereas others have the same genes turned "off." Although virtually all of the cells have the same genes, certain genes are expressed in certain cells only at certain times. Not all genes are or should be "on," or expressed, in every tissue. A given cell type may need to express some genes sometimes and other sets of genes at other times.

Cells exhibit diverse patterns of protein production because certain genes are expressed at specific times. This diversity in gene expression leads to the different functions performed by cell or tissue types. Altering gene expression also allows for the changing pattern of protein production during development, creating different tissue types in the body. During normal human development, different cells express different sets of genes in a precisely regulated fashion. This ensures that an embryo can develop into a normally formed human being. Problems with development are sometimes caused by errors in the gene expression.

Most cells are *somatic*, or body cells, although a small fraction consists of *germline* cells, from which the gametes (egg and sperm) are derived. Each somatic cell has 46 chromosomes, made up of 22 identical pairs called *autosomes* and 1 pair of *sex chromosomes* (XX or XY). A *karyotype* is a photographic representation of the chromosomes of a single somatic cell. Somatic cells are termed *diploid* because they have a total of 23 pairs of chromosomes. The germline cells are called *haploid*, because they have only one set of the same 23 types of chromosomes.[1,6,11]

The two types of cell division are *mitosis* (somatic cells) and *meiosis* (generates gametes). Nuclear division is called *mitosis*, and it is a carefully programmed process in the cell cycle. Sperm and eggs have a different form of division from somatic cells because they have only 23 chromosomes, and they must maintain this haploid number in their daughter cells. Each type of cell division makes new cells of the same type and number as their parent cells. Although in mitosis the daughter cells are genetically identical to their parent cells, there is a recombination of genes in meiosis, thereby introducing an extra source of genetic variation for germline cells.

Chromosomes Contain DNA

The basis of all genetic disease ultimately originates from changes in the DNA and the chromosomes into which it is arranged. Each chromosome is composed of proteins and DNA. Each chromosome is composed of only *one* long DNA molecule that is double-stranded and highly coiled. The DNA coil is tightly wound around proteins called *histones*, and together the unit is referred to as a *nucleosome* (some of the regions of DNA are free of histones).

Segments of DNA Are Called Genes

Each DNA strand contains thousands of genes arranged in linear fashion. A gene is a small region or segment of the long DNA molecule, and humans have about 30,000 to 35,000 genes. Genes hold the cellular information that encodes for a function, or directs the assembly of large molecules called proteins. Genes are also the basic unit of heredity because they are transferred on the sperm or egg DNA during conception. Therefore, they are inherited by the new developing embryo.

DNA is a long, linear molecule composed of repeating subunits called *nucleotides*. A nucleotide consists of a sugar (deoxyribose), phosphate group, and an attached base. One end of a single DNA strand is called the 3' (three prime) end, whereas the other end is labeled 5' (five prime). In each chromosome, DNA consists of two individual nucleotide chains wrapped around each other to form a *double helix*. The backbone of each DNA strand of the double helix consists of a sugar-phosphate-sugar-phosphate polymer. The phosphates are attached by ester bonds to their 3'- and 5'-hydroxyl groups. There are four types of *bases:* adenine (A), thymine (T), cytosine (C), and guanine (G). The bases, all nitrogen-containing, are attached to the 1' (one prime) position of the sugar ring. The bases cytosine and thymine are called *pyrimidines*, and the bases adenine and guanine are called *purines*. These subunits are repeated down the length of the strand in a varying linear arrangement[1,6,11] (Fig. 9-1).

Each DNA molecule contains many genes, or specific segments of DNA that have been found to code for a protein. Because genes are sections of the DNA strand, genes are made up of base sequences. This is the actual "code." The two strands are weakly connected through the hydrogen bonding of base pairing, where an A from one strand always binds with a T from the other, or a C from one strand always binds with a G from the other. This is called *complementary base pairing*. Because the two strands are made to be perfect matches for one another, the strands themselves are called *complementary* (for example, if one is 5'-ATGCCAG-3', the other must be 3'-TACGGTC-5'). They are also antiparallel, or facing in opposite directions, so that the 3' end of one strand is next to the 5' end of the other.

Genes Code for Proteins

The DNA structure provides a means of storing and coding massive amounts of information. This information is based on the *sequence* of the bases present. Before cellular division occurs, the DNA replicates its own information so that all cells generated will have the same code. This enzyme-directed process is called *DNA replication* (or *synthesis*): The double-stranded DNA "denatures," or separates into two strands; the strands are replicated into a total of four strands of DNA; and each pair "anneals," or binds into a set of double-stranded DNA.

Each strand contains the full informational content of the DNA molecule and can serve as a template for synthesis of a new complementary strand as the complex

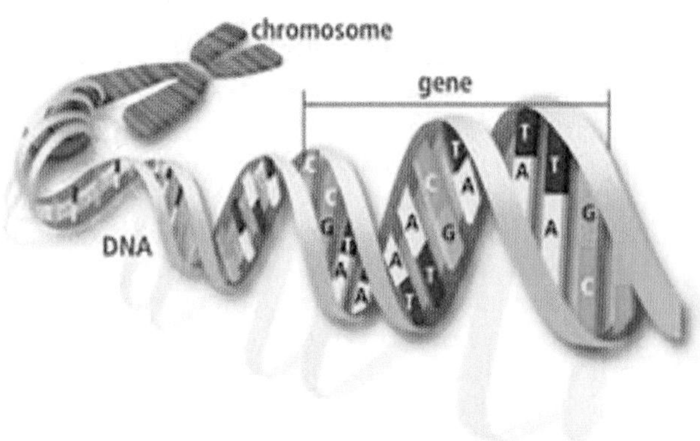

figure 9-1 The DNA sequence is the particular side-by-side arrangement of bases along the DNA strand (e.g., ATTCCGGA). This order spells out the exact instructions required to create a particular organism with its own unique traits. (Courtesy of U.S. Department of Energy Human Genome Program, http://www.ornl.gov/hgmis.)

unwinds and replicates. The complementary strand also provides a defense against information loss through DNA damage because a base on one strand that is damaged or lost can be replaced using the complementary strand to direct its repair. This is an example of only one way a cell attempts to repair its own damage and thus prevent the perpetuation of an erroneous code and its resulting potential for disease.

Genes code for proteins. The gene's information is transcribed into messenger ribonucleic acid (mRNA), and then this mRNA is translated into proteins. The sequence of the base pairs in a gene determines its protein product. RNA is similar to DNA, except that it is single-stranded, has a different sugar, and the pyrimidine base uracil (U) replaces thymine (T). Both mRNA and proteins are gene expression products.[1,6,11]

Transcription is the generation of a single-stranded RNA molecule from a gene, or section of the double-stranded DNA template. It is directed by enzymes. Transcription begins in the nucleus as genes are first coded for mRNA. This process is described generally: Enzyme binds to the DNA strands, the two strands separate into "sense" and "antisense" strands, the mRNA is synthesized in the 5' to 3' direction and has the same sequence as the 5' to 3' DNA strand (the "sense" strand), the DNA reanneals, and the formed mRNA leaves the nucleus and goes into the cytoplasm.

In the cytoplasm, the mRNA serves as the template for the creation of a protein strand. This process is called *translation*, and it occurs with the assistance of ribosomal RNA (rRNA), transfer RNA (tRNA), assembled amino acids, and enzymes. The *genetic code* defines rules by which the base sequence of mRNA is translated into an amino acid sequence (Fig. 9-2). During translation, a *codon* (set of three nucleotides) specifies a single amino acid. As the mRNA strand is "read," a corresponding amino acid sequence is constructed. Three bases specify for an amino acid. There is "degeneracy" in the code, so that several codons may result in the same amino acid (for example, UUA, UUG, CUU, CUC, CUA, and CUG all code for the amino acid leucine). This process continues until a "stop codon" is reached. "Stop codons" (UUA, UAG, and UGA) do not code for an amino acid, but instead cause translation to terminate. After translation is completed, the short-lived mRNA is quickly destroyed.

Only the genes on the DNA strand code for proteins. For genes to bring about their effects, they must create a protein. Proteins are made in the cell cytoplasm. They are linear arrays of amino acid subunits that are joined by chemical bonds, and they are composed of varying combinations of only 20 amino acids. Therefore, only 20 amino acids make up every protein in the body. It was once believed that one gene coded for only one protein, but as a result of the Human Genome Project, it is now understood that the 30,000 to 35,000 genes can make more than 100,000 proteins. Because there are 64 possible codons (each of three bases can be A, U, G, or C) and only 20 amino acids, it becomes clear how more than one codon can code for the same amino acid.

Proteins cause processes to happen in the body, and there are several types and functions of proteins. Some examples include structural proteins, such as tubulin, keratin, and col-

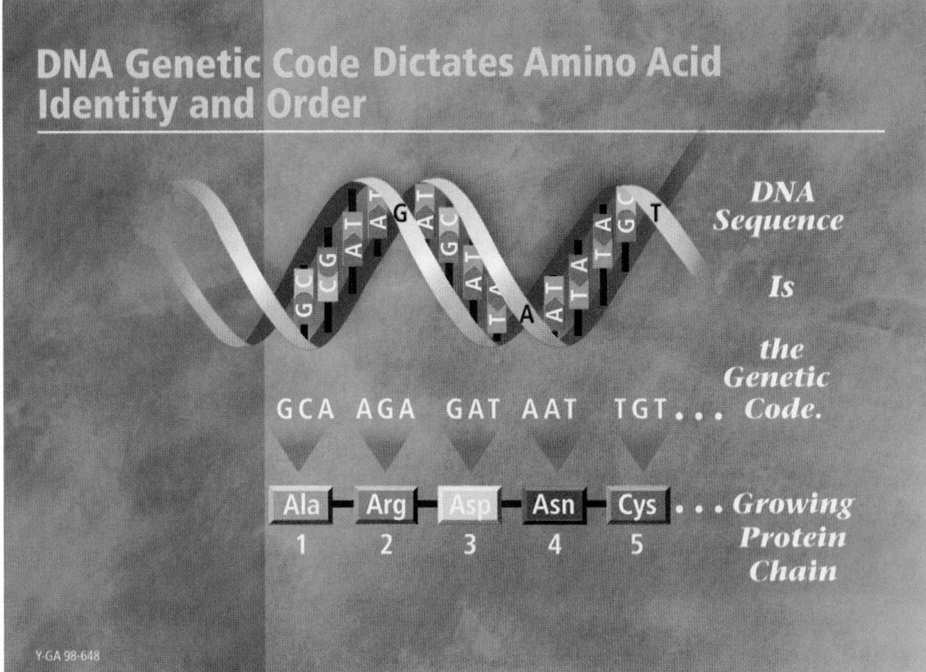

figure 9-2 Within the gene, each sequence of three DNA bases (codons) directs the cell's protein-synthesizing machinery to add specific amino acids to the growing protein chain. (Courtesy of U.S. Department of Energy Human Genome Program, http://www.ornl.gov/hgmis.)

lagen; enzymes, which catalyze countless biochemical reactions; hormones, the chemical messengers of the body; and immunoglobulins, which make up the antibodies of the immune system. Each amino acid has a certain set of biochemical properties that helps determine the final structure and function of the protein. The function of a protein is determined by its amino acid sequence and three-dimensional structure.

Mutations Can Cause Disease

Each somatic cell carries two copies of each gene, one on each *homologous chromosome* (the two paired chromosomes). These can be identical or different, but they are called *alleles* if they are alternate forms of the same gene. Therefore, alleles are alternate forms of a gene (or DNA sequence) at a given *locus*, or position on the chromosome. The variant allele is a *mutation*, or any sequence alteration in a gene from its natural (or "wild-type") state. A mutation can be benign, a normal variant, protective, or pathological. Most mutations are "silent," and their presence is not detected because the balancing gene on the homologous chromosome is normal. New mutations can take various forms at the molecular level. Germline mutations may not always be present in all tissues of the body, but these mutations can be passed to the individual's offspring.

A *genotype* is the genetic composition of an individual, and it also refers to alleles at a specific genetic locus. A *phenotype* is the observed interaction of the genotype with environmental factors. It is the observable expression of a gene or genes, and it includes factors like eye color or biochemical makeup. If both alleles at a locus are identical, a person is described as being *homozygous* at that locus; if the alleles are different, the individual is *heterozygous*.[1,6,11]

Dominance and recessivity refer to traits, or phenotypes, and not to genes. Conditions are *dominant* if they are expressed in heterozygotes, or individuals who have one copy of a mutant allele and one copy of a normal, "wild-type" allele. Conditions are *recessive* if a person is homozygous for the allele, or has a double dose of the abnormal gene. The term *autosomal* can be applied to "dominant" or "recessive" to designate a gene on one of the 22 non-sex chromosomes. Transmission is described as *X-linked* if a faulty gene is transmitted from parent to child on the X chromosome, either by the mother or father. X-linked traits can also be either dominant or recessive, or even lethal in some cases. These concepts are important in single-gene defects, also known as *mendelian disorders*.

The relationship between a mutation and its phenotype is complex. Sometimes mutations at different genes can produce identical phenotypes, resulting in separate genetic disorders with symptoms so similar that they are labeled the same disease (an example is osteoporosis, which can present as autosomal dominant in one family and recessive in another). Mutations permanently alter the structure of a gene, and thus its informational content and expression. In other words, DNA damage causes a permanent sequence alteration in all future progeny for that given cell.

An altered gene can produce new proteins or it can stop producing proteins altogether. A mutated gene that fails to code for protein production is often a cause of genetic disease. It is a permanent and often heritable change in the ability of a gene to encode a protein. The damaged gene in itself does not cause the disease—rather, its protein product is the problem. There are several built-in mechanisms for the detection or repair of errors during DNA synthesis, transcription, and translation, but mutations do not always get recognized. Essentially, diseases can result from problems at any step of the process, or from errors at the gene to the protein levels. Genes can be erroneously turned "off" or "on." Protein production can be absent, faulty, or excessive. In addition, mutations have been identified in more than 1,000 genes, and it is probable that nearly all human genes are capable of causing disease if they are substantially altered.

Mitochondrial DNA

Most of the cellular DNA is on chromosomes in the nucleus, but mitochondria carry separate genetic information. Mitochondria have chromosomes, DNA, and genes required for their own organelle functioning. Mitochondria are the energy-producing organelles in a cell. Ova are rich with mitochondria, but sperm are not. Consequently, mitochondrial DNA is usually inherited from the mother. Its genes, and the diseases due to variants in them, are transmitted in a matrilinear pattern, which is a distinctly different pattern of inheritance than that demonstrated by nuclear genes. Almost all mutations in this DNA are inherited from the mother. Little is known about the range of mitochondrial disorders, but they include several multisystem disorders involving sight, hearing, muscle function, and the brain.[12]

GENETICALLY DETERMINED DISEASES

Chromosomal Disorders

Cytogenetic disorders, or those pertaining to chromosomes, are rarely diagnosed in the adult population. These diseases result from the addition or deletion of entire chromosomes or parts of a chromosome. Because each chromosome contains tens of thousands of genes, these types of alterations can have a significant impact on the individual. Most of these disorders are characterized by growth or mental retardation, or a variety of somatic abnormalities, and most are diseases of childhood onset, rather than adult onset. A well-known example of a cytogenetic disorder is Down syndrome.

Monogenic Conditions

Also called mendelian diseases, monogenic conditions are the result of a single mutant gene. If the mutation exists in only a single nucleotide in a gene, then it is called a *single-nucleotide polymorphism* (SNP, pronounced "snip").[13] One example of a heritable clinical disease caused by a SNP is sickle cell anemia, in which the diseased phenotype arises from a mutation in a single nucleotide. Monogenic conditions can arise from either a SNP or from changes in several nucleotides in a single gene, or section of DNA.

Single-gene disorders have a large impact on phenotype, and are usually inherited in simple patterns as described by Mendel's laws of inheritance. There are thousands of these types of disorders, some rare and others more common. Some mutations can inactivate genes, leading to a loss of function, whereas others stimulate gene functioning to cause disease. Although the major impact of single-gene disorders occurs between the newborn period and early childhood, their significance in diseases of adult life is also becoming more apparent.

Familiar examples include adult-onset cystic fibrosis, muscular dystrophy, autosomal dominant polycystic disease, alpha$_1$-antitrypsin deficiency in chronic obstructive pulmonary disease (COPD), familial breast and prostate cancers, hereditary colon cancer, early-onset Alzheimer's disease, and Huntington's disease. Mutations in the genes BRCA1 (on chromosome 17) and BRCA2 (on chromosome 13) cause well-known examples of autosomal dominant forms of breast cancer, resulting in 5% of cases of breast cancer in the United States.[14] Single-gene disorders can also arise from mutations on mitochondrial chromosomes, resulting in mitochondrial diseases (Table 9-1). These and thousands of other monogenetic disorders are catalogued in the on-line compendium called OMIM (On-line Mendelian Inheritance in Man; Fig. 9-3).

The patterns of inheritance of several monogenic traits are now understood by observing the transmission of these traits in families. This is done by constructing and analyzing pedigrees, or diagrams that describe genetic relationships of family members. A pedigree uses standardized nomenclature and displays modes of inheritance. The primary ways that single-gene disorders are expressed include in an autosomal dominant, autosomal recessive, or X-linked fashion.[1,6,11]

Autosomal diseases are encoded by genes on any one of the 22 pairs of autosomes, or non-sex chromosomes. A large proportion of disorders of adult onset are autosomal dominant because this requires a mutation in only one of a gene pair. Individuals with autosomal disease and unaffected parents are apparently demonstrating a new mutation for that family line, unless there is no access to the patient's family history for pedigree analysis or it is a disease of delayed onset. Examples of autosomal dominant disorders that manifest later in life are Huntington's disease and a type of polycystic kidney disease. Autosomal dominant polycystic kidney disease usually does not show symptoms until the fourth decade of life, and it is characterized by bilateral enlargement of the kidneys with multiple cysts, hematuria, hypertension, abdominal pain, and progressive renal failure. Huntington's disease typically manifests by age 35 years, and it is a degenerative neurological disorder characterized by chorea and dementia. Late-onset disorders demonstrate that genetic diseases are not always congenital, or present at birth.

As with multifactorial disorders, single-gene disorders do not always express a mutation when it is present. A phenomenon called *penetrance* describes the percentage of individuals in a population that exhibit clinical symptoms of a mutant gene. A disorder has complete penetrance if it is expressed by all individuals with the mutation, or incomplete penetrance if only some carriers evidence expression.

The old paradigm of "one gene, one protein, and one disease" is no longer a valid concept for many disorders because different types of mutations in one gene can sometimes result in clinically different disorders. One example is with chromosome X, where different mutations to the

table 9-1 Common Genetic Disorders

Disorder	Pathophysiology	Signs and Symptoms
Autosomal Recessive Disorders		
Cystic Fibrosis (CF) Inborn error in a cell membrane transport protein. Dysfunction of the exocrine glands affects multiple organ systems. The disease affects men and women. It is the most common fatal genetic disease in white children.	Most cases arise from the mutation that affects the genetic coding for a single amino acid, resulting in a protein (cystic fibrosis transmembrane regulator [CFTR]) that does not function properly. The CFTR resembles other transmembrane transport proteins, but it lacks the phenylalanine in the protein produced by normal genes. This regulator interferes with cystic adenosine monophosphate (cAMP)-regulated chloride channels and transport of other ions by preventing adenosine triphosphate from binding to the protein or by interfering with activation by protein kinase. The mutation affects volume-absorbing epithelia in the airways and intestines, salt-absorbing epithelia in sweat ducts, and volume-secretory epithelia in the pancreas. Lack of phenylalanine leads to dehydration, which increases the viscosity of mucus gland secretions and consequently obstructs glandular ducts. CF has varying effects on electrolyte and water transport.	• Chronic airway infections leading to bronchiectasis • Bronchiolectasis • Exocrine pancreatic insufficiency • Intestinal dysfunction • Abnormal sweat gland function • Reproductive dysfunction
Phenylketonuria (PKU) Inborn error in metabolism of the amino acid phenylalanine. PKU has a low incidence among blacks and Ashkenazic Jews and a high incidence among people of Irish and Scottish descent.	Patients with classic PKU have almost no activity of phenylalanine hydroxylase, an enzyme that helps convert phenylalanine to tyrosine. As a result, phenylalanine accumulates in the blood and urine, and tyrosine levels are low.	• By age 4 months, signs of arrested brain development, including mental retardation • Personality disturbances • Seizures • Decreased IQ • Macrocephaly • Eczematous skin lesions or dry, rough skin • Hyperactivity • Irritability • Purposeless, repetitive motions • Awkward gait • Musty odor from skin and urine excretion of phenylacetic acid
Sickle Cell Anemia Congenital hemolytic anemia resulting from defective hemoglobin molecules. In the United States, sickle cell anemia occurs primarily in persons of African and Mediterranean descent. It also affects populations in Puerto Rico, Turkey, India, the Middle East, and the Mediterranean.	Abnormal hemoglobin S in red blood cells becomes insoluble during hypoxia. As a result, these cells become rigid, rough, and elongated, forming a crescent or sickle shape. The sickling produces hemolysis. The altered cells also pile up in the capillaries and smaller blood vessels, making the blood more viscous. Normal circulation is impaired, causing pain, tissue infarctions, and swelling. Each patient with sickle cell anemia has a different hypoxic threshold and different factors that trigger a sickle cell crisis. Illness, exposure to cold, stress, acidotic states, or a pathophysiological process that pulls water out of the sickle cells precipitates a crisis in most patients. The blockages then cause anoxic changes that lead to further sickling and obstruction.	• Symptoms of sickle cell anemia do not develop until after the age of 6 months because fetal hemoglobin protects infants for the first few months after birth. • Chronic fatigue • Unexplained dyspnea on exertion • Joint swelling • Aching bones • Severe localized and generalized pain • Leg ulcers • Frequent infections • Priapism in men *In sickle cell crisis:* • Severe pain • Hematuria • Lethargy

(continued)

table 9-1 Common Genetic Disorders (Continued)

Disorder	Pathophysiology	Signs and Symptoms
Tay-Sachs Disease Also known as GM_2 gangliosidosis, the most common lipid storage disease. Tay-Sachs affects Ashkenazic Jews about 100 times more often than the general population.	The enzyme hexosaminidase A is absent or deficient. This enzyme is necessary to metabolize gangliosides, water-soluble glycolipids found primarily in the central nervous system (CNS). Without hexosaminidase A, lipid molecules accumulate, progressively destroying and demyelinating CNS cells.	• Exaggerated Moro (startle) reflex at birth and apathy (response only to loud sounds) by age 3 to 6 months • Inability to sit up, lift head, or grasp objects; difficulty turning over; progressive vision loss • Deafness, blindness, seizures, paralysis, spasticity, and continued neurological deterioration (by 18 months of age) • Recurrent bronchopneumonia
Autosomal Dominant Disorders *Marfan's Syndrome* Rare degenerative, generalized disease of the connective tissue that results from elastin and collagen defects. The syndrome occurs in 1 of 20,000 individuals, affecting men and women equally.	The syndrome is caused by mutation in a single gene on chromosome 15, the gene that codes for fibrillin, a glycoprotein component of connective tissue. These small fibers are abundant in large blood vessels and the suspensory ligaments of the ocular lenses. The effect on connective tissue is variable and includes excessive bone growth, ocular disorders, and cardiac defects.	• Increased height, long extremities, and arachnodactyly (long, spider-like fingers) • Defects of sternum (funnel chest or pigeon breast, for example), chest asymmetry, scoliosis, or kyphosis • Hypermobile joints • Myopia • Lens displacement • Valvular abnormalities (redundancy of leaflets, stretching of chordae tendineae, or dilation of valvulae annulus) • Mitral valve prolapse • Aortic regurgitation
X-Linked Recessive Disorders *Hemophilia* Bleeding disorder; severity and prognosis vary with the degree of deficiency, or nonfunction, and the site of bleeding. Hemophilia occurs in 20 of 100,000 male births. Hemophilia A, or classic hemophilia, is a deficiency of clotting factor VIII; it is more common than type B, affecting more than 80% of all hemophiliacs. Hemophilia B, or Christmas disease, affects 15% of all hemophiliacs and results from a deficiency of factor IX. There is no relationship between factor VIII and factor IX inherited defects.	Abnormal bleeding occurs because of specific clotting factor malfunction. Factors VIII and IX are components of the intrinsic clotting pathway; factor IX is an essential factor and factor VIII is a critical cofactor. Factor VIII accelerates the activation of factor X by several thousandfold. Excessive bleeding occurs when these clotting factors are reduced by more than 75%. Hemophilia may be severe, moderate, or mild, depending on the degree of activation of clotting factors. A person with hemophilia forms a platelet plug at a bleeding site, but clotting factor deficiency impairs the ability to form a stable fibrin clot. Delayed bleeding is more common than immediate hemorrhage.	• Spontaneous bleeding in severe hemophilia • Excessive or continued bleeding or bruising • Large subcutaneous and deep intramuscular hematomas • Prolonged bleeding in mild hemophilia after major trauma or surgery, but no spontaneous bleeding after minor trauma • Pain, swelling, and tenderness in joints • Internal bleeding, often manifested as abdominal, chest, or flank pain • Hematuria • Hematemesis or tarry stools
Polygenic (Multifactorial) Disorders *Cleft Lip and Cleft Palate* May occur separately or together. Cleft lip with or without cleft palate occurs twice as often in boys as in girls. Cleft palate without cleft lip is more common in girls. Cleft lip deformities can occur unilaterally, bilaterally, or, rarely, in the midline. Only the lip may be involved, or the defect may extend into the upper jaw or nasal cavity. Incidence is highest in children with a family history of cleft defects.	During the second month of pregnancy, the front and sides of the face and the palatine shelves develop. Because of a chromosomal abnormality, exposure to teratogens, genetic abnormality, or environmental factors, the lip or palate fuses imperfectly. The deformity may range from a simple notch to a complete cleft.	• Obvious cleft lip or cleft palate • Feeding difficulties due to incomplete fusion of the palate

(continued)

table 9-1 Common Genetic Disorders (Continued)

Disorder	Pathophysiology	Signs and Symptoms
	A cleft palate may be partial or complete. A complete cleft includes the soft palate, the bones of the maxilla, and the alveolus on one or both sides of the premaxilla. A double cleft is the most severe of the deformities. The cleft runs from the soft palate forward to either side of the nose. A double cleft separates the maxilla and premaxilla into freely moving segments. The tongue and other muscles can displace the segments, enlarging the cleft.	
Spina Bifida Incomplete fusion of one or more vertebrae, resulting in dimpling of the area (spina bifida occulta) or protrusion of the spinal tissue (spina bifida cystica). Spina bifida occulta occurs in as many as 25% of births, and spina bifida cystica occurs in 1 in 1,000 births in the United States. Incidence varies greatly with countries and regions.	Neural tube closure normally occurs at 24 days' gestation in the cranial region and continues distally, with closure of the lumbar regions by 26 days. As the nervous system develops and differentiates, it is vulnerable to teratogenic effects. The specific cause of spina bifida, incomplete fusion of the vertebrae in the developing nervous system of the embryo, is unknown, but neural tube defects have been associated with such noninfectious maternal disorders as folic acid deficiency. Spina bifida occulta rarely affects the structure or function of the cord and peripheral nerve roots. Spina bifida cystica can occur as a meningocele, in which the meninges protrude in a cerebrospinal fluid–filled sac, or as a myelomeningocele, in which peripheral nerves, root segments, or the spinal cord also protrude. Varying degrees of sensory and motor dysfunction below the level of the lesion are present.	• Weak feet • Bowel and bladder disturbances • Dimple, tuft of hair, soft fatty deposits, port wine nevi, or combination over spine (spina bifida occulta) • Saclike protrusion over the spine due to meningocele or myelomeningocele (spina bifida cystica) • Possible permanent neurological dysfunction due to meningocele or myelomeningocele (spina bifida cystica)
Disorders of Chromosome Number *Down Syndrome (Trisomy 21)* Spontaneous chromosome abnormality that causes characteristic facial features, other distinctive physical abnormalities (cardiac defects in 60% of affected persons), and mental retardation. It occurs in 1 of 650 to 700 live births.	Nearly all cases of Down syndrome result from trisomy 21 (3 copies of chromosome 21). The result is a karyotype of 47 chromosomes instead of the usual 46. In 4% of patients, Down syndrome results from an unbalanced translocation or chromosomal rearrangement in which the long arm of chromosome 21 breaks and attaches to another chromosome. Some affected persons and some asymptomatic parents may have chromosomal mosaicism, a mixture of two cell types, some with the normal 46 and some with an extra chromosome 21.	• Distinctive facial features (low nasal bridge, epicanthic folds, protruding tongue, and low-set ears); small, open mouth and disproportionately large tongue • Single transverse crease on the palm (simian crease) • Small white spots on the iris (Brushfield's spots) • Mental retardation (estimated IQ of 20 to 50) • Developmental delay • Congenital heart disease, mainly septal defects and especially of the endocardial cushion • Impaired reflexes

Reprinted with permission from Anatomical Chart Company: Atlas of Pathophysiology. Springhouse, PA, Springhouse, 2002.

dystrophin gene can produce either Duchenne's or Becker's muscular dystrophy. Some mutations exhibit *variable expressivity*, where expression varies based on environmental influences or interaction with other significant genes. Individuals with these types of mutations differ in the age of onset and severity of clinical symptoms, and sometimes even affected members in the same family have different presentations. Some genes are capable of both dominant and recessive expression, depending on the presence or absence of other factors.

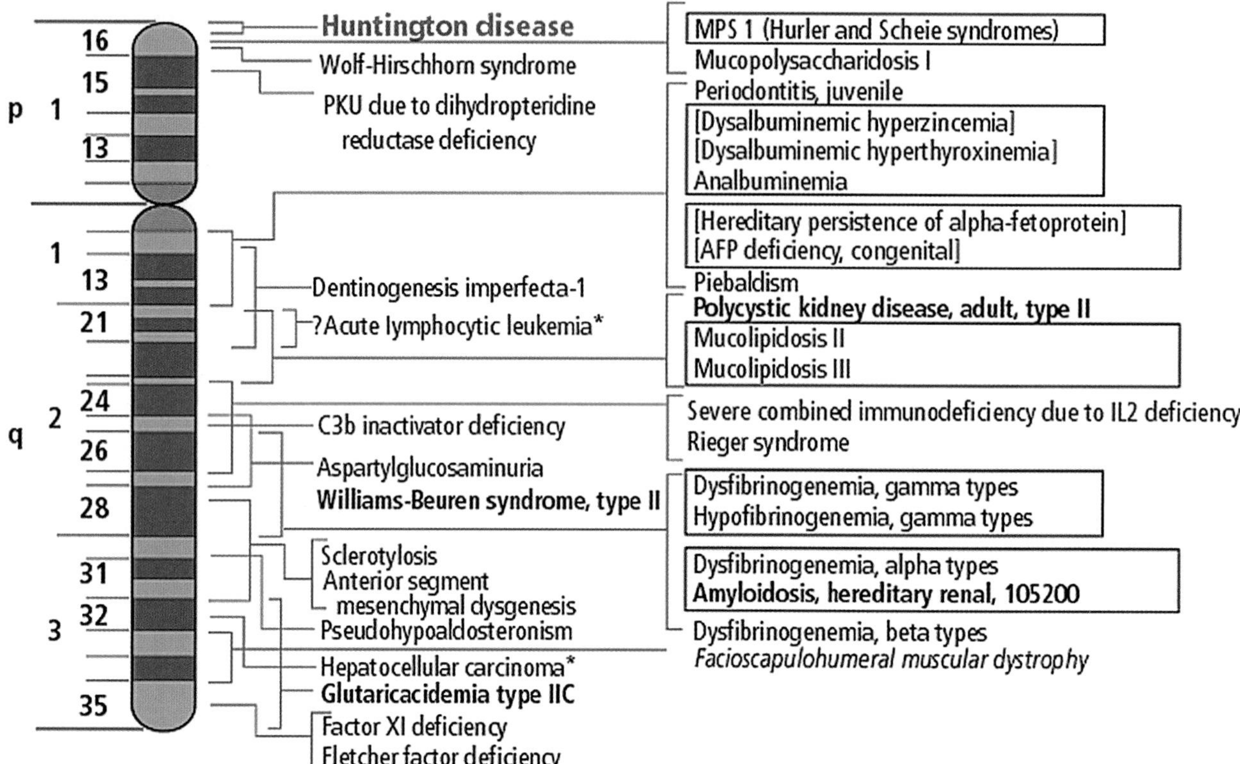

figure 9-3 Sequencing and analysis of human chromosomes has allowed researchers to characterize in detail a number of genes associated with diseases. (Courtesy of U.S. Department of Energy Human Genome Program, http://www.ornl.gov/hgmis.)

Multifactorial Disorders

These disorders are often described as *polygenic*, or resulting from the interaction of more than one gene with multiple environmental factors. There is not a direct cause-and-effect relationship between a given set of genes and their associated disease because environmental factors throughout the lifetime of an individual contribute to an unknown and significant degree in their expression. These describe cases where an individual may have a *genetic predisposition* to a disease, or enhanced susceptibility, based on the presence of one or multiple known suspect genes. Nurses can make a significant impact on these patients by emphasizing lifestyle changes to modify the environment and decrease the probability of disease manifestation.

These are the most common genetic diseases, yet the least understood. The nurse may see patients whose syndrome was not diagnosed early, or they may present with new signs and symptoms of a multifactorial disorder at any stage in adulthood. Several disorders of adult onset require years to be symptomatic, so a patient could present in early, middle, or late adulthood. Many of these disorders are potentially preventable, especially if a patient presents with risk factors or is in the early stages of symptom presentation. These disorders present a significant challenge in understanding ways in which multiple genes interact to produce disease in the presence of specific environmental triggers. Although many traits reflect the interaction of an individual's genotype with the environment, some require a threshold number of deleterious alleles before a given phenotype, such as disease, is exhibited.

Multifactorial inheritance underlies clinically important human traits, such as disease susceptibility or predisposition. An example of a gene–environment interaction involves the gene for alpha$_1$-antitrypsin, where a mutation causes an enzyme deficiency that leads to a much earlier diagnosis of emphysema in smokers than nonsmokers. Other multifactorial disorders that commonly present in adults are hypertension, atherosclerosis, COPD, coronary heart disease, diabetes, stroke, osteoporosis, some types of breast and colon cancer, human immunodeficiency virus (HIV) disease, tuberculosis, Parkinson's disease, types of Alzheimer's disease, schizophrenia, major affective disorders, alcoholism, and obesity. Childhood disorders include cleft lip, cleft palate, neural tube defects, and congenital heart diseases. A diagnosis of a genetic disease of multifactorial origin is often suspected if there is a positive family history, multisystem involvement, or multifocal presentation. An example of multifocal presentation is familial adenomatous polyposis, where multiple polyps are found throughout the colon.[9]

Multifactorial inheritance is defined by four general rules. First, the trait tends to run in families. These traits, including those that express disease, exhibit no distinctive pattern of inheritance within a single family, such as autosomal dominance or recessivity. However, an individual with an affected family member is at a much greater risk for developing the disease than a member of the general population. First-degree relatives to the affected person, such as parents, siblings, or offspring, are at a greater risk for developing the disorder than second-degree relatives. In turn, more distant relatives have an even smaller risk.

The second rule states that an individual has a much higher risk for developing the disease when more than one family member is affected. Because the expression of multifactorial traits could be influenced by the number of deleterious alleles present, a family that accumulates these alleles could confer greater risk to its members. This risk increases even more when a child in the family is the product of a consanguineous union, or mating of genetically related individuals.

The third rule states that a trait is more likely to occur in relatives of the affected individual if the expression of the given disease is particularly severe. This is because the severity of the phenotype is directly proportional to the number of deleterious alleles carried.

The final rule of this mode of inheritance reflects genetic information gained from studies of identical twins. Because identical twins theoretically have identical genetic information and thus carry the same inherited mutations, it seems probable that they will exhibit the same genetically determined diseases. However, this is not always the case for multifactorial disorders. Studies with identical twins show that they are not always concordant with respect to a given trait, which means that there are unknown, nongenetic factors involved in its expression. Environmental exposure begins in the womb and exerts its pressures on an individual throughout the life span.

Somatic Cell Disorders

The categories of genetic disorders described so far (cytogenetic, monogenic, and multifactorial disorders) all describe situations where the genetic abnormality can be found in the DNA of all the cells in the body, including the germ cells. Mutations contained in the sperm and egg are transmitted at human conception. Somatic cell disorders arise only in specific somatic cells, or non-sex cells, during the lifetime of an individual. The primary example of a somatic disorder of adult onset is cancer, although many types of cancer do follow mendelian patterns of inheritance or exhibit familial predisposition.

Cancer is a disease that results from just a single somatic cell overriding the normal controls of cell division. It is promoted by mutations in normal genes called *proto-oncogenes.* These genes normally code for protein products that stimulate cellular proliferation. The mutations activate genes in tissues that should stay suppressed and nonfunctional. Malignancy is the consequence of mutations in genes that control cellular growth. Sources of mutations include radiation, chemical exposure, viruses, and other unknown environmental factors.[1,6,11]

Mitochondrial Disease

Abnormal mitochondrial functioning may cause many common adult diseases. Mitochondrial dysfunction can be devastating to an individual's entire level of functioning because these organelles are responsible for energy production. Mitochondrial diseases can affect almost every organ system, and they can manifest at any point throughout the life span.

Mitochondrial DNA significantly differs from nuclear DNA, and it has a much larger probability of gaining mutations. Mitochondrial functioning depends on proteins coded by nuclear *and* mitochondrial DNA. These organelles also rely on nuclear genes for repair mechanisms in DNA replication, transcription, and translation. Mitochondrial DNA is more vulnerable to oxidative stress, so it can mutate at much faster rates than nuclear DNA. In addition, mitochondrial DNA contains no introns, so mutations are more likely to occur in coding regions.[12]

Mitochondrial dysfunction may play a role in exercise intolerance, aging, and metabolism. Diseases can affect several body systems, including the cardiovascular, central nervous, endocrine, gastrointestinal, renal, and pulmonary systems. Several pulmonary manifestations may present in a critical care setting, such as lactic acidosis in the absence of hypoxia or sepsis, respiratory failure, neurological or cardiac abnormalities, unexplained dyspnea, muscles weakness, or sleep apnea. Pathological changes in mitochondria deprive cells of the adenosine triphosphate (ATP) necessary for cellular functioning. Cells that function at high metabolic rates are particularly vulnerable, such as the heart, brain, or skeletal muscles. Deprivation of ATP facilitates an alternative metabolic pathway, and this can lead to the accumulation of harmful lactate.

Mitochondria are usually inherited in a matrilinear pattern. Their associated diseases can be expressed in an autosomal dominant or autosomal recessive way, or they can occur spontaneously. They may be acquired as a result of environmental or drug exposure. The mutations may be transient, or they can accumulate throughout the lifetime of an individual. Female offspring from the same mother can demonstrate wide variation in the expression of mitochondrial disease because eggs have multiple copies and random concentrations of mitochondrial DNA. This variation can make these diseases very difficult to recognize, diagnose, or treat.

PHARMACOGENETICS

The terms *pharmacogenetics* and *pharmacogenomics* are frequently used interchangeably because they are closely related. However, there is a slight difference in the two fields of research. The study of pharmacogenomics is relatively new, having emerged only within the past decade. The field of pharmacogenomics studies how the variations between chemicals affect gene expression in tissues. It covers a broader spectrum than pharmacogenetics, and applies advancing genetic technology to drug development with the goal of attaining more desirable results and fewer negative side effects. Advancing technology in molecular genetics enables researchers to determine genotypes of individuals and monitor differences in drug response.[15–17]

There are three main areas of pharmacogenomics. One aspect is drug response profiling by studying SNPs as genetic markers. SNPs are one frequently occurring form of genetic variation, and some are more common in a population than others. Identifying SNPs, especially those positioned in a coding or regulatory gene region, shows correlations between sequence variations and drug metabolism. Not only do differing genotypes result in drug kinetic variations, but SNPs affect gene response. Several SNPs among a group of genes can collectively affect drug interactions when they lead to changes in protein expression or binding site modifications. The second aspect of pharmacogenomics studies the role drugs play in altering gene expression, and measures their overall effects. The third aspect is drug development. The discovery of specific DNA sequences and proteins in a cell that increase the risk of disease will enable the creation of drugs that target those sites. In addition, because SNPs occur so frequently, pharmacogenomics attempts to design drugs that are still effective regardless of small mutations.[13,15–17]

People can have different reactions to the same medications. Pharmacogenetics aims to choose the medication and dosage that will best interact with each individual patient. It concentrates on a small, select group of genes that influence the resulting variation of responses between individuals for the specific drug of interest. The differences in drug effectiveness and adverse reactions are partially due to individual genetic makeup. When creating a new drug, researchers consider the drug and binding site interaction, and the method by which the compound assimilates, circulates, and is eliminated from the body.[10,13] Gene mutations can inactivate the therapeutic effect of the drug, which can then build up to toxic levels and lead to adverse reactions. Mutations can also lead to a premature elimination of the chemicals, rendering them ineffective. Because each person is unique in his or her genetic profile and environment, the same drug that helps one person can be ineffective or harmful to another. In fact, the identical dosage can produce ideal results in one yet be toxic in another individual.

Drug metabolism is determined by enzymes, proteins that control the activation and transformation of the chemical compounds. Because enzymes are genetically determined, there is variation in drug metabolism within the human population. The levels of metabolism for the same drug can vary among people. The population is generalized into three groups of metabolizers. Individuals who are considered the norm are those who readily metabolize many compounds, and hence are called *extensive metabolizers* (EM). People with little to no ability to metabolize drugs are classified as *poor metabolizers* (PM). The third subset is those who have higher-than-normal drug metabolism, and are referred to as *ultraextensive metabolizers* (UEM). Screening patients to determine metabolizing ability before prescribing a medication helps prescribers choose a correct dose the first time and eliminate the trial-and-error method of determining dosage.

A particular group of enzymes known as cytochrome P450 have come under intense study because of their extensive participation in drug metabolism. Drugs are usually metabolized by oxidative processes, and cytochrome P450 catalyzes most drug oxidation reactions in the liver. Some individuals cannot effectively metabolize drugs through the cytochrome P450 system, whereas others have a poorer response or even accumulate toxic byproducts. Appropriate drug selection, partially based on the patient's genetically coded enzymes, decreases unwanted side effects and enhances drug efficacy.[16]

Genetic testing will soon allow health care professionals to determine the most effective and safest drug for a patient based on his or her genetic makeup. In the near future, it is probable that nurses will be responsible for genetic testing to predict individual responses to drugs, and will also be expected to educate patients on their specific gene-based drug therapy. Currently, the information gained from genotype testing is limited for many reasons. First, most of the time drug metabolism does not depend on one enzyme. It is usually regulated by several enzymes. Another restraint is that analysis of gene expression entails obtaining sample tissues, which are not readily available. Also, the regulatory sequences that control the amount of gene expression may also vary between individuals. Even if a gene is identified as a good target for a drug, it may be more effective in those patients who produce a higher level of transcription for that gene.[16]

Genetic screening has positive future applications. An example is the apolipoprotein E (ApoE) gene, one of the genes correlated to inherited and sporadic Alzheimer's disease. All people have two copies of the gene. One form of the gene, ApoE isoform 4 (ApoE-4), is believed to increase the risk of early-onset sporadic Alzheimer's disease if both faulty copies are present. Pharmacogenetics can be useful in a situation with a patient who has the disease because ApoE-4 individuals do not have positive responses to the drug tacrine, whereas non–ApoE-4 patients respond well.[10]

Pharmacogenetics has the potential of individualizing drug therapy for patients with cancer. One person may have more adverse reactions to some forms of chemotherapy than others. The compounds that would be undesirable for a specific individual can be removed from his or her therapy without eliminating the elements that destroy the cancerous cells. One such example occurs with dihydropyrimidine dehydrogenase–deficient (DPD) patients. The frequently used chemotherapy, 5-fluorouracil, causes neurotoxicity in individuals with DPD. Therefore, chemotherapy treatment that does not include 5-fluorouracil will still benefit such patients and not produce adverse reactions. Another example is HER2, a gene correlated with breast cancer. Some patients with breast cancer overexpress HER2. Herceptin is a monoclonal antibody that can inhibit HER2 expression. A patient with breast cancer who does not overexpress the gene would not benefit from this drug. Genetic screening will soon be able to identify which patients are good candidates for the drug.[12]

clinical applicability challenges

Study Questions

1. *Which item is* not *listed in the* Core Competencies in Genetics for All Healthcare Professionals *defined by the National Coalition for Health Professional Education in Genetics (NCHPEG)?*
   a. *Knowledge of basic genetic terminology and science*
   b. *Understanding of the role that genetic factors have in maintaining health and preventing disease*
   c. *Ability to diagnose a genetic disorder*

d. *Appreciation for the sensitivity of genetic information and the need for privacy and confidentiality*

2. *What is the final product of translation?*
   a. *DNA segments called genes*
   b. *Amino acids assembled into proteins*
   c. *Cells*
   d. *Messenger RNA (mRNA)*
3. *Which statement is true regarding mutations?*
   a. *All mutations cause disease.*
   b. *Most mutations are "silent" and cause no disease.*
   c. *All mutations are inherited.*
   d. *Mutations are never inherited.*
4. *What is the most common type of genetically influenced disorders in the adult population?*
   a. *Multifactorial*
   b. *Cytogenic (chromosomal)*
   c. *Monogenic*
   d. *Mitochondrial*

REFERENCES

1. Guttmacher AE, Collins FS: Genomic medicine: A primer. N Engl J Med 347(19):1512–1527, 2002
2. Hawley RS, Mori CA: The Human Genome: A User's Guide. San Diego, Academic Press, 1999
3. Tinkle MB, Cheek DJ: Human genomics: Challenges and opportunities. J Obstet Gynecol Neonatal Nurs 31(2):30–38, 2001
4. Persing BF, Cheek DJ: Pharmacogenomics. Nurs Clin North Am 35(4):975–980, 2000
5. National Coalition for Health Professional Education in Genetics (NCHPEG): Core Competencies in Genetics Essential for All Health-Care Professionals. Available at: http://www.nchpeg.org. Accessed January 3, 2004
6. Sommers MS, Beery T: Foundations of genetics: Genetic structure, function, and therapeutics. AACN Clin Issues 9(4):467–482, 1998
7. Prows DR: Optimizing drug therapy based on genetic difference: Implications for the clinical setting. AACN Clin Issues 9(4):499–512, 1998
8. Gilchrist DM: Medical genetics: 3. An approach to the adult with a genetic disorder. CMAJ 167(9):1021–1029, 2002
9. Jorde LB: Genes, environment, and common diseases. In McCance KL, Huether SE (eds): Pathophysiology: The Biological Basis for Disease in Adults and Children, pp 153–173. St. Louis, Mosby, 1998
10. McCarthy A: Pharmacogenetics. BMJ 322:1007–1008, 2001
11. Gelehrter TD, Collins FS, Ginsburg D: Principles of Medical Genetics (2nd Ed). Baltimore, Williams & Wilkins, 1998
12. Clay AS, Behnia M, Brown KK: Mitochondrial disease: A pulmonary and critical-care medicine perspective. Chest 120(2):634–648, 2001
13. McCarthy JJ: Turning SNPs into useful markers of drug response. In Licinio J, Wong M (eds): Pharmacogenomics: The Search for Individualized Therapies, pp 24–32. Weinheim, Germany, Wiley-Vch, 2002
14. Amlung S, Huelsman K, Skinn B: Genetic predisposition to breast and ovarian cancer: A case study. AACN Clin Issues 9(4):555–562, 1998
15. American Pharmacists Association, Rostogi M: An Overview of Pharmacogenomics. Committee report background paper. Available at: http://www.aphanet.org/govt/policycomm2000/pharmacobackground.html. Accessed May 13, 2003
16. Dean P, Gane P, Zanders E: Pharmacogenomics and drug design. In Licinio J, Wong M (eds): Pharmacogenomics: The Search for Individualized Therapies, pp 56–64. Weinheim, Germany, Wiley-Vch, 2002
17. Meyer UA: Introduction of pharmacogenomics: Promises, opportunities, and limitations. In Licinio J, Wong M (eds): Pharmacogenomics: The Search for Individualized Therapies, pp 1–8. Weinheim, Germany, Wiley-Vch, 2002

OTHER SELECTED READING

Gelehrter TD, Collins FS, Ginsburg D: Principles of Medical Genetics (2nd Ed). Baltimore, Williams & Wilkins, 1998

International Human Genome Sequencing Consortium: Initial sequencing and analysis of the human genome. Nature 409(6822):860–921, 2001

Jenkins J: Genetics competency: New directions for nursing. AACN Clin Issues 13(4):486–491, 2002

Licinio J, Wong M: Pharmacogenomics: The Search for Individualized Therapies. Weinheim, Germany, Wiley-Vch, 2002

Porth C: Genetic and congenital disorders. In Pathophysiology: Concepts of Altered Health States (6th Ed), pp 131–148. Philadelphia, Lippincott Williams & Wilkins, 2002

Venter JC, Adams MD, Meyers EW, et al: The sequence of the human genome. Science 291(5507):1304–1351, 2001

Williams J: Education for genetics and nursing practice. AACN Clin Issues 13(4):492–500, 2002

Zawacki K: Hereditary cancer syndromes of the gastrointestinal system. AACN Clin Issues 13(4):523–539, 2002

chapter 10

Building a Professional Practice Model for Excellence in Critical Care Nursing

JANIE HEATH

objectives

Based on the content of this chapter, the reader should be able to:

- Discuss nursing professionalism and nursing excellence.
- Recognize characteristics of professional development.
- Explore personal and professional attributes to build a professional practice model of critical care nursing excellence.

In today's fast-paced critical care environment, nurses respond to the needs of patients and families who have entered a chaotic and frightening world of illness, trauma, and pain. Often, finding the time for professional growth can be challenging. Building a professional practice of excellence requires a "passion" to profoundly affect the lives of patients and families. At the same time, it requires advancing the critical care nursing profession through evidence-based practice (EBP), best practice models of care, or both. This chapter discusses how a professional practice for excellence in critical care nursing can be built with the attributes of values, vision, mastery, passion, action, and balance as the framework.

DEFINING THE CRITICAL CARE NURSE

Like their patients and patients' families, critical care nurses are an exceptional and diverse group of individuals. Knowledgeable, highly skilled, and caring are a few of the professional attributes that can be applied to critical care nurses. However, the term *nursing professionalism* may bring to mind different images, especially to health care consumers. To some, nursing professionalism means wearing a crisp, clean, white uniform, whereas to others it means demonstrating a high level of intellectual, interpersonal, ethical, and technical skills. Kalisch and Kalisch first reported on the image of nursing in the early 1980s. They found that "90% of the public thought nurses were nice ladies who help doctors."[1]

Critical care nurses know all too well that responding to lethal dysrhythmias, administering blood products, and weaning patients from ventilators requires education and clinical experience in holistic nursing, not just "niceness." For both the novice and the experienced critical care nurse, the journey of nursing professionalism and nursing excellence goes beyond the bedside skills required to take care of the sickest and most vulnerable patients and families. Critical care nursing has been recognized as a specialty for over 30 years, yet Buresh and Gordon (2000) have found increasing evidence of a large communication gap between the profession and the greater public.[2] If critical care nursing is to be recognized as a respected and valued profession, nurses must speak up to define who they are and what they do.

The characteristics of today's registered nurse (RN) in critical care are illustrated in a demographic survey conducted in 2000 by the American Association of Critical-Care Nurses (AACN), the world's largest specialty nursing organization.[3] Approximately half of AACN's 65,000 RN members participated in this study about critical care nursing attributes (n = 32,500). It was reported that the typical critical care nurse is 45 years old and has an average income of $47,000 per year.[3] Although the profession continues to be predominantly female (92%), the

AACN study reported that the number of men in critical care is increasing (8%).[3] In addition, the AACN study reported that the largest ethnic background for critical care nurses was white (84%) followed by Asian (9%), African American (4%), Hispanic (2%), and Native American (1%) populations.[3] Of interest, these AACN data are consistent with the average findings of today's 2.7 million RNs reported by the 2000 National Sample Survey.[4]

It is important to look at numbers as reported in the AACN study to determine trends, issues, implications for policy, and advocacy for the profession and the patients and their families. Currently, 79% of critical care nurses work full time. Of this 79%, 18% work in combined intensive care unit (ICU)/critical care unit (CCU) settings, 13% work in ICU settings, 9% work in cardiovascular/surgical ICU settings, 8% work in CCU settings, 5% work in telemetry stepdown units, 5% work in surgical ICU settings, 5% work in emergency department (ED) settings, 4% work in medical ICU settings, 4% work in recovery room settings, 3% work in pediatric ICU settings, and 3% work in catheterization laboratories.[3] Most of the critical care nurses in the AACN survey (66%) are staff nurses working in cardiovascular, cardiology, medical–surgical, or pulmonary units (Fig. 10-1). Almost half of the critical care nurses surveyed work in nonprofit community hospitals (49%), followed by 13% employed by university medical centers and 13% employed by for-profit community hospitals. Furthermore, the size of hospitals in which critical care nurses work varies; however, most (38%) have an average of 300 beds and 6% have 900 or more beds.[3]

DEFINING NURSING PROFESSIONALISM

The struggle to define nursing professionalism expands beyond critical care environments. For many years there has been an ongoing dialogue about whether nursing is a true profession. Kelly (1981) emphasizes that the status of nursing as a profession is important because it reflects the value society places on the work of nurses.[5] However, some think that nursing is, at best, an emerging profession because entry into the nursing profession does not require a baccalaureate degree.[5] Still others believe that the nursing profession has made adequate progress to meet full-fledged professional status.[5]

One of the first definitions of professionalism came from Abraham Flexner, who wrote the classic "Flexner report" in the early 1900s to reform medical education.[6] He defines professionalism as a process by which an occupation achieves professional status. Although other professions have developed their own criteria, Flexner's work remains the benchmark and foundation for many. Kelly (1981) was the first to expand his work for the nursing profession.[5,7] Kelly's criteria give a theoretical framework from which professional nursing characteristics are defined today[5,7] (Box 10-1).

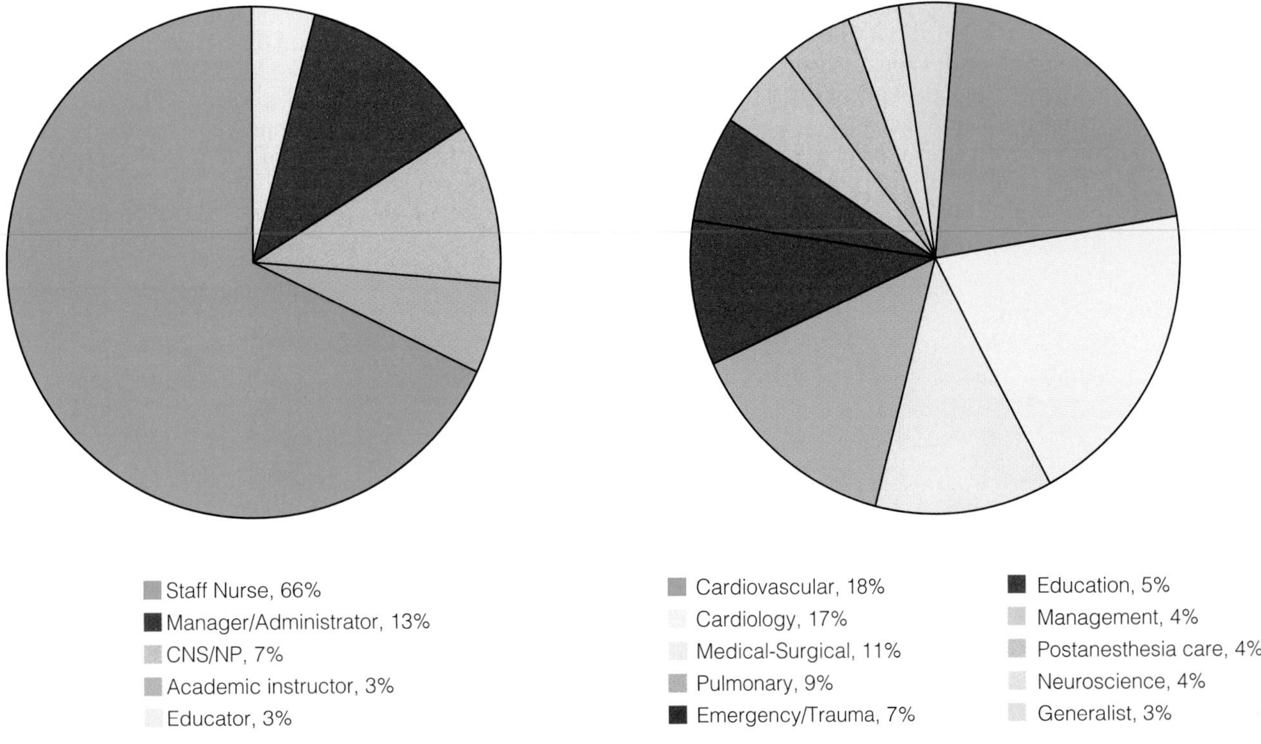

figure 10-1 Who are critical care nurses? (**A**) The positions held by critical care nurses. (**B**) Break-out of the profession by clinical specialty. *CNS,* clinical nurse specialist; *NP,* nurse practitioner. (Redrawn with permission from American Association of Critical-Care Nurses: Who are critical care nurses? Critical Care Nurse. AACN Critical Care Careers Supplement, 9–12, 2001.)

box 10-1
Kelly's Characteristics of a Profession

- The services provided are vital to humanity and the welfare of society.
- There is a special body of knowledge that is continually enlarged through research.
- The services provided involve intellectual activities where accountability is a strong feature.
- Practitioners are educated in institutions of higher learning.
- Practitioners are motivated by service, and work is an important component of their lives.
- There is a code of ethics to guide the decisions and conduct of practitioners.
- There is an association that encourages and supports standards of practice.

From Kelly L: Dimensions of Professional Nursing. New York, Macmillan, 1981; and Kelly L, Joel L: Dimensions of Professional Nursing (8th Ed). New York, McGraw-Hill, 1999.

To a great extent, the criteria addressed by Flexner and Kelly are only as good as the person who takes personal responsibility and accountability for committing to a professional role. Many of Kelly's criteria have been used to evaluate professionalism in critical care nursing. In 1994, Holl investigated such characteristics as professional beliefs, decision making, level of education, membership of professional nursing organization, and certification.[8] Holl found that nurses (n = 133 RNs) who continue their education and belong to professional organizations are more likely than others to be independent thinkers and to participate in creative problem solving.[8]

In a similar study, Heath and colleagues (2001) found that there was a high level of "passion about nursing and promoting the profession" and that self-motivation was the leading influential factor for fostering individual professional development in critical care nurses (n = 100).[9] Other professional development characteristics evaluated included participation in employing agency committees, community service, and recognition of peers.[9] Of note, the professional characteristics initially identified by Kelly and studied by others[8,9] are identified as the "cornerstone for nursing excellence" and contribute to the professional practice model described in this chapter.

DEFINING NURSING EXCELLENCE

The term "excellence" can be a misnomer similar to the expression "best practice." There is no single definition that captures the essence of "excellence" for everyone. For some it is something that is "seen," "heard," or "felt" that describes excellence in nursing. For example, the way a critical care nurse "sees" a patient "going bad" before laboratory values or hemodynamic numbers are known may be evidence of excellence. Other descriptions of excellence may be the way a critical care nurse "hears" an S_3 or S_4 heart sound before a patient becomes symptomatic, or the way a critical care nurse "feels" the pain of a postoperative patient on neuromuscular blockade without analgesics.

Weston and colleagues (1998) define nursing excellence as a dynamic process that is continually redefined and reinforced.[10] They further describe excellence as an ongoing comparison with a standard that one continuously tries to improve.[10] Six attributes for advanced-practice nursing excellence have been identified by Weston and colleagues as values, vision, mastery, passion, action, and balance.[10] These attributes have been adopted and modified for this chapter to propose a professional practice model for critical care nursing (Fig. 10-2). The foundation for this model consists of strong values and a vision. The supporting structures of the model are composed of mastery, passion, action, and balance. The top of the model captures the essence of the structure: critical care nursing excellence. Each structure of the professional practice model has

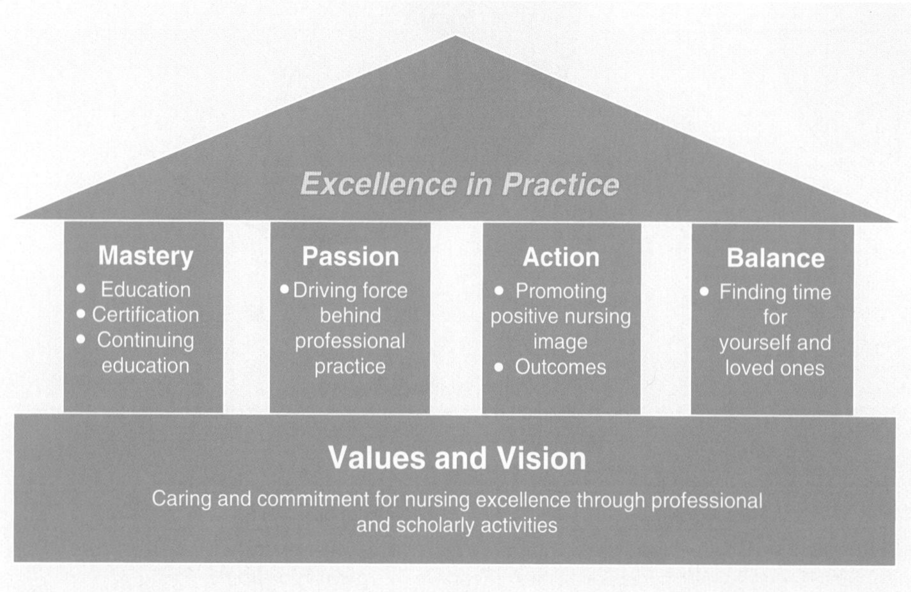

figure 10-2 A professional practice model for critical care nursing.

defining characteristics that are instrumental for ongoing self-reflection, which is necessary to develop and commit to excellence in critical care nursing.

Values

"*Only a lived life for others is worth living.*" (Albert Einstein)[11]

> ***Real Moments of "Values" in Critical Care Nursing Excellence***
>
> *Carolyn was a 52-year-old admitted to the ICU after a cardiac arrest in the ED. She was successfully resuscitated, but engaged in a life-and-death roller coaster ride for 6 long weeks. Her family placed trust in me to care for her. Carolyn's last great hurdle was severe depression and psychosis. Her family did not have a clue how the system worked but they knew she needed something. They trusted that I would get the appropriate help for her. I would not and could not let them down. I am the patient's advocate. After the appropriate referral and treatment, Carolyn was discharged to a rehabilitation facility 1 week later. Unfortunately, Carolyn died 3 days after she returned home from the rehabilitation facility. Her family called to tell me that Carolyn died and invited me to her funeral. When I look back on just this one opportunity to make a difference in someone's life, I feel richer. Just think how many opportunities we have, as critical care nurses, to make that kind of an impact. Each day renews the power, the passion, and the promise that I must uphold to fulfill my commitment to clinical excellence.*
>
> ***AACN Circle of Excellence Awards 2000***
> ***Judy N. Nichols, RN, CCRN***
> *3M Health Care: Excellence in Clinical Practice Award Recipient*
> *Palmetto Richland Memorial Hospital*
> *Columbia, South Carolina*

True excellence is seen when professionals reflect their core values. The values of one's profession, the values of one's employing organization, and one's own personal values are the behaviors that guide professional practice for excellence. The unique contributions that critical care nurses bring to the bedside are often a reflection of an inner core value of caring. It is this deep and personal connection to caring that brings many into the nursing profession. The word *nursing* is derived from the Latin word *nutrire*, which means "to nourish." Nurturing implies an ability to care for, sustain, and provide for another. Critical care nurses are privileged to care for individuals who face life-threatening conditions during the most vulnerable and private time of their lives. It is through this value of altruism (the desire to help others) that critical care nurses have the ability to creatively bridge "high-tech" and "high-touch" with everyday practice.

The everyday "busyness" of critical care nursing is labor intensive, but the "real moments" of taking the time to share joyful, painful, and tearful experiences with complex patients and families is the core of critical care nursing's existence. The "art" of nursing is probably what dominates the image of nursing for the public. Gallup polls continue to report that the public rates nursing as the most honest and ethical profession.[12,13] Seventy-three percent of the participants rated the nursing profession in 2000 as high or very high in honesty and ethical standards, significantly above the next-highest-rated groups, pharmacy (69%), veterinary medicine (63%), and physicians (58%).[12] In 2001, firefighters were the frontrunners in the Gallup poll, and now nurses are once again the most highly rated profession.[13]

In their book, *From Silence to Voice*, Buresh and Gordon (2000) report that these Gallup poll results reflect a paradox.[2] As non-nurse authors, they discuss how the public holds nurses in the highest regard, yet they have limited information about what nurses really do.[2] There is power in the nursing profession when nurses articulate not only the core values of "caring," but of advocacy, accountability, autonomy, and collaboration. Buresh and Gordon believe nurses have been silent for too long and that the days of "It is just my job" or " I am just a nurse" need to come to an end.[2] Campaigns such as AACN's "Making Waves" and "Bold Voices: Fearless and Essential" help to ensure that critical care nurses make their voices heard for their patients, families, and profession.[14,15] Strong personal and professional core values, such as those promoted by AACN,[16] guide the dedication and vision for critical care nursing excellence. Box 10-2 outlines core values for nurses.

Vision

"*To see our future, we must embrace our past.*" (Patricia Donahue RN, PhD, FAAN)[17]

box 10-2
Core Values: American Association of Critical-Care Nurses (AACN)

- **Be accountable** to uphold and consistently act in concert with ethical values and principles.
- **Advocate** for organizational decisions that are driven by the needs of patients and families.
- **Act with integrity** by communicating openly and honestly, keeping promises, honoring commitments, and promoting loyalty in all relationships.
- **Collaborate** with all essential stakeholders by creating synergistic relationships to promote common interest and shared values.
- **Provide leadership** to transform thinking, structures and processes to address opportunities and challenges.
- **Demonstrate stewardship** through fair and responsible management of resources.
- **Embrace life-long learning,** inquiry, and critical thinking to enable each to make optimal contributions.
- **Commit to quality and excellence** at all levels of the organization, meeting and exceeding standards and expectations.
- **Promote innovation** through creativity and calculated risk taking.
- **Generate commitment and passion** to the organization's causes and work.

From American Association of Critical-Care Nurses: Core values. Available at www.aacn.org. Accessed June 2001; and American Association of Critical-Care Nurses: Who are critical care nurses? Crit Care Nurse. AACN Critical Care Careers Supplement, February: 9–12:2001.

Real Moments of "Vision" in Critical Care Nursing Excellence

Just as the ocean waves continually shape the landscape by moving the sand one grain at a time, critical care nurses can make a difference in healthcare, one life at a time. My message is to "make waves" by having the courage to influence practice. The word courage is derived from the French word coeur, which means "heart." Thus, practicing courage means exercising acts of the heart. Courage can guide us and strengthen our pursuits. More than a single heroic act, courage comes from the day-to-day actions that spring from our hearts and our core values. Courage means taking risks, letting go of the status quo, and facing hardship and possible failure, as well as confronting our own self-doubts. Often, "taking heart" inspires and motivates others, who then follow us and become aware of our vision and integrity as we engage in daily acts of courage.

Denise Thornby, RN, MS, CCRN
AACN President 2000–2001
Closing Session Address, National Teaching Institute and Critical Care Exposition 2000
Orlando, Florida

A clear vision, based on core values, is essential to building a professional practice model of critical care nursing excellence. It requires envisioning the future's possibilities and then taking the challenge of making the vision a reality. In *Nursing the Finest Art: An Illustrated History*, Donahue gives numerous examples of the vision the founding leaders had for nursing.[17] Stories are told about men and women who withstood public ridicule and hindered reputations all because they had a "vision" that change was necessary. As risk takers and agents for change, today's critical care nurses are making history by taking control of establishing nursing practice and educational standards. From the boardroom to the classroom to the bedside, critical care nurses have been agents of change in providing patients and families a safe passage in the increasingly complex health care system. Buresh and Gordon (2000) encourage today's nurses to tell their "bold and courageous" stories.[2] Advancing the nursing profession through scholarly activities is one way to be heard. It can start simply as writing a letter to the editor of a local newspaper, to giving a regional or national presentation, to publishing about the unique contribution that critical care nurses make in the lives of their patients and families.

Winston Churchill once said, "The pessimist sees difficulty in every opportunity and the optimist sees the opportunity in every difficulty."[18] It is challenging to have a positive "21st century nursing vision" in today's health care environment. Concerns about nurse-to-patient ratios, mandatory overtime, unionization, nursing recruitment, and retention are on the minds of all. It is increasingly difficult to provide critical care nurses with the tools, resources, and support needed to effectively meet patient and family needs, and at the same time enhance their growth, learning, and satisfaction. Nursing has a long tradition of taking "bumpy" roads to make a vision reality, and we are still on the road. No matter how many times we fall down and get bruised on the way to reaching our vision, we maintain our resilience by having the courage to believe in ourselves and in our profession.

Mastery

"*Education is our passport to the future for tomorrow belongs to the person who prepares for today.*" (Malcolm X)[11]

Real Moments of "Mastery" in Critical Care Nursing Excellence

It is 3:00 A.M. and Jane is working her first night shift after finishing orientation. She is caring for a fresh cardiac surgery patient who arrived from the operating room a few hours ago. Jane came on at 7:00 P.M. and has done a good job keeping up with frequent assessments and hemodynamic monitoring, and with following laboratory data and chest tube drainage on this patient. At 3:05 A.M., her patient goes into ventricular tachycardia (VT). Jane stares at the monitor, and a million thoughts rush through her head in a split second. Until tonight she could turn to her preceptor, educator, or clinical nurse specialist and they would problem-solve with her. Now she is alone with the patient, and the critical electrocardiography alarm is sounding. How will she organize her thoughts, what her preceptor taught her, and the information she learned over the last 4 months in the critical care course? At such times, theory from the electrocardiography course, patient assessment parameters, advanced cardiac life support (ACLS) principles, pharmacology, and acute postoperative management of patients all must be integrated and applied to deliver appropriate care. Jane must think critically and function appropriately to help her patient. Seconds count in situations such as this, and sound critical thinking is essential.

Carol Rauen, MS, RN, CCRN
Using simulation to teach critical thinking skills: You can't just throw the book at them. Critical Care Nursing Clinics of North America 13(1):93–103, 2001

Senge, author of *The 5th Discipline: The Art and Practice of the Learning Organization*, believes that "people with high levels of personal mastery are continually expanding their ability to create the results in life they truly seek" (1990, p. 80).[19] To value lifelong learning and to have a vision for personal mastery is essential to building a professional practice model for critical care nursing excellence (see Fig. 10-2). There are many pathways for personal mastery. Weston and colleagues (1998) believe seeking feedback and peer review for self-improvement is one of the most effective pathways for building mastery.[10] Other pathways for personal mastery include seeking a degree in higher education, making a commitment to ongoing continuing education, and demonstrating competence through certification. The rewards of mastery often go beyond these pathways. Mastery combines expert professional skills with leadership, interpersonal, and organizational proficiency and often leads to the most coveted role of all, the role of mentoring.

Evidence of mastery can also be seen in Benner's model of "novice to expert," where nursing experience evolves through five steps to reach expertise.[20] Wojner (2000) believes true expertise is gained only through years of study and practice that include support by expert mentors; a commitment to lifelong learning; a humility that allows one to recognize his or her boundaries and limitations; and an approachability and willingness to change.[21] Regardless of the chosen pathway, personal mastery is well demonstrated throughout critical care nursing practice.

The AACN reports that 48% of critical care nurses participating (n = 32,500) in a recent study held a baccalaureate degree, followed by 30% with an associate or diploma degree, 19% with a master's degree, and 2% with a doctorate[3] (Fig. 10-3A). The number of years of experience in critical care nursing varied in the AACN study; however, a significant majority of critical care nurses (81%) had more than 5 years of experience, including 8% with between 26 and 35 years of critical care experience[3] (see Fig. 10-3B). Sixty-nine percent of the participants are certified critical care nurses (CCRN; see Fig. 10-3C), and

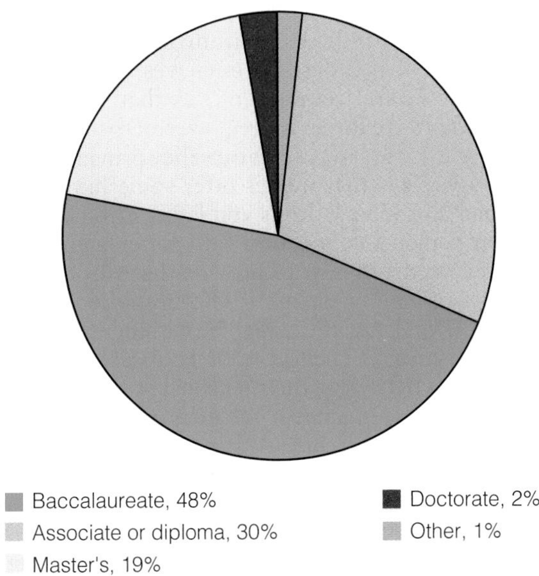

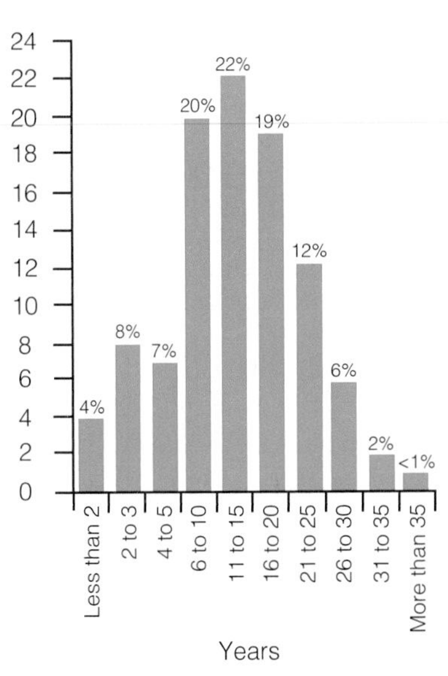

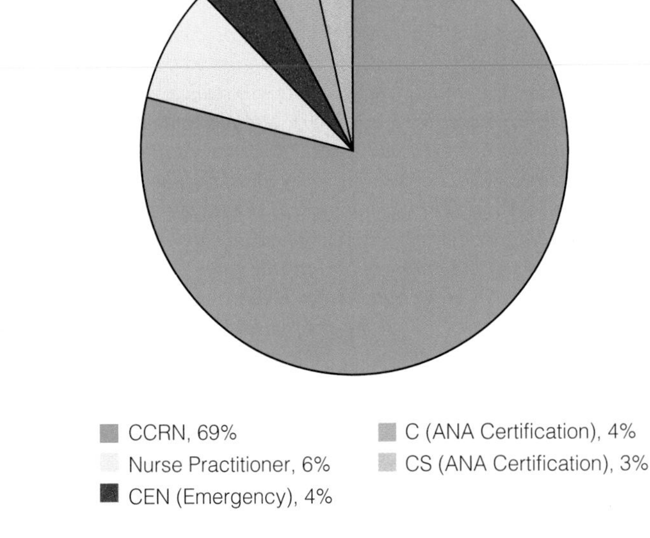

figure 10-3 Mastery of the profession. (**A**) The nursing degrees earned by critical care nurses. (**B**) Years of experience in critical care nursing. (**C**) Professional certifications held by critical care nurses. *ANA,* American Nurses Association; *C,* certified; *CCRN,* certified critical care nurse; *CEN,* certified emergency nurse; *CS,* clinical specialist. (Redrawn with permission from American Association of Critical-Care Nurses: Who are critical care nurses? Critical Care Nurse. AACN Critical Care Careers Supplement, 9–12, 2001.)

a separate study by the AACN Certification Corporation indicated that more than 70% of the CCRN participants (n = 2,000) received some form of compensation or recognition for certification from their employers.[3]

Cary (2001) reported that there are four avenues through which certification status can be recognized: public acknowledgment, financial compensation, career advancement, and retention.[22] In addition, Cary's study revealed that there is a perception, especially among newly certified nurses, that certification gives autonomy, enhances collaboration with other health care providers, allows control over practice, and results in higher patient satisfaction ratings.[22] Of interest, these findings are similar to those reported by critical care nurses who responded to the AACN Certification Corporation study.[3]

The AACN recently released a white paper on the value of certification. The AACN believes that certification validates competency of knowledge, skills, and experience for quality patient care.[23] Consumers of nursing services must be able to recognize the contributions critical care nurses make to ensure high-quality care to patients and families. Barden (2003) believes that there are two types of critical care nurses at the bedside: (1) those who are certified, and (2) those who are not.[24] Certification is a process of achieving the highest recognition of excellence. It is more than "another initial"[25]; it is a mark of excellence that can be referred to as "the Good Housekeeping Seal of Approval." Credentials on name badges, such as CCRN or (critical care clinical nurse specialist), make personal mastery visible to the consumer and ensure public protection.

Passion

"*Perpetual optimism is a force multiplier.*" (General Colin Powell)[11]

Real Moments of "Passion" in Critical Care Nursing Excellence

On December 6, 1996, I sustained a dirty needlestick from a high-risk patient for human immunodeficiency virus (HIV). The patient was unconscious and no family could ever be located. Consequently under the law, an HIV test could not be administered, and for 6 weeks I had to take two protease inhibitors and zidovudine (AZT) as a precautionary measure. The drugs made me very ill. The hospital took the matter to the probate court to have a conservator appointed who could authorize the test. Based on the wording of the law, the judge denied this request. I contacted my state senator and assemblyman regarding what was happening to me and showed them this portion of the state health and safety code. SB-1385 was introduced in January, 1998, by my state senator on my behalf. I testified four times before committees in the Senate and the Assembly and gathered hundreds of signatures in support of the bill.

In June, 1998, SB-1385 was passed by the legislature and on September 13, 1998, Governor Pete Wilson signed this bill into law. Due to SB-1385, the law now states that with documentation by an attending physician of a significant exposure, and following a documented good faith effort to locate family or an authorized representative, that the HIV test can be completed. The source patient in my case died and an HIV test was completed. The test was completely negative and I have tested negative. Because I had such limited rights and protections as a healthcare worker, I undertook to change the law. I am proud that I was able to make a difference and that this new law has already helped so many healthcare workers in my state.

AACN Circle of Excellence Awards 2000
Diana B. Mertrude, RN
Ross Products Pioneering Spirit Award Recipient
UCSD Medical Center
San Diego, California

Just as a link is seen between values, vision, and mastery, passion is the essential thread to link together all the professional practice attributes for critical care nursing excellence (see Fig. 10-2). Passion involves enthusiastically striving for what is best for ourselves and those we serve. Thornby (2000) reminds nurses that sometimes they feel as if there are forces more powerful than they are determining the quality of patient care they provide.[14] Yet, Thornby emphasizes that nurses offer something more powerful than all the new drugs and latest medical technology: their personal connection with patients in knowing what they need and how to provide that all-powerful healing effect of simply caring.[14] Thornby often quotes Staub's book, *The 7 Acts of Courage*,[26] to influence critical care nursing practice. She believes that if critical care nurses would encompass these acts, their personal power, efficacy, and ability would be enhanced.[14] Staub's acts include the courage to dream; the courage to see reality; the courage to confront; the courage to be confronted; the courage to learn and grow; the courage to be vulnerable and to love; and the courage to act.[26]

Whether encompassing Staub's seven acts of courage or developing your own, a sense of purpose and devotion is essential for the attribute of passion. Weston and colleagues state that "passion involves ardently striving for the best, even when repeated efforts seem tedious or appear exceedingly strenuous" (1998, p. 310).[10] The truly passionate critical care nurse will not be satisfied with providing less than the highest-quality care possible to patients and families. Achieving this goal often requires going beyond an 8- or 12-hour shift.

Acts of passion for critical care nursing excellence can be seen in bringing the latest research findings to the bedside, revising unit policy and procedure books with the most up-to-date procedures, and teaching coworkers the most effective therapies to produce the best outcomes for patients and families.

There is an energy of "passion" that can be felt in critical care nursing not only at the bedside but throughout the profession. Nursing leaders in critical care are partnering with multidisciplinary groups and talking to legislators to improve workplace issues such as the nursing shortage, mandatory overtime, workplace injuries, recruitment, and retention. Being passionate about something requires time, energy, and commitment. Peters and Austin state "the adventure of excellence is not for the faint of heart" (1985, p. 414).[27] Passion is a contagious gift that requires self-discipline to prevent inflexibility and loss of perspective. Carlson reminds us in his book, *Don't Sweat the Small Stuff*, that we must not get lost and overwhelmed in the chaos, responsibilities, and goals of life, and that it is best to keep asking the question, "What is really important?" (1997, p. 22).[28]

Action

"*We are what we repeatedly do. Excellence then is not an act but a habit.*" (Aristotle)[11]

Real Moments of "Action" in Critical Care Nursing Excellence

The morning news sent chills up my spine. A 34-year-old man with burns over 65% of his body was now at the trauma center where I worked as the critical care clinical nurse specialist. I pulled together the burn-care team and developed the plan of care, which included sending a skin biopsy to grow cultured epidermal autographs (CEAs). In 4 weeks, delicate epidermal skin (costing $60,000) would return for final skin grafting. Jim's course was highly complicated with septic shock, renal failure, gastrointestinal bleeding, and acute respiratory distress syndrome (ARDS). The skin healed with a 99% take while the narcotics and sedation were tapered off. Jim did not awaken. A neurologist painted a grim prognosis. I searched the literature and engaged my medical director in a thorough case review coupled with exotic tests to find a cause of the encephalopathy. Jim's wife, Anne, sought my advice. The neurologist was recommending withdrawal of life support, but Anne shared with me that she wanted Jim back, even if he was a little goofy. I suggested giving it more time. Two weeks later, Jim woke up! He gradually developed motor movement and is now home joyfully watching his daughter grow. He can walk and enjoys life. The neurologist related a visit with Jim, telling him, "You owe your wife your life. She insisted we keep you going. Thank her every day that you are alive!" I just smiled.

AACN Circle of Excellence Awards 2000
Jane Cunneen, RN, MSN, CCRN
Outstanding Advanced Practice Nurse Award Recipient
Clarian Health Partners, Methodist Hospital
Indianapolis, Indiana

Florence Nightingale once said "one's feelings waste themselves in words, they ought all to be distilled into action which brings results" (1859, p. 44).[29] In other words, part of professionalism in critical care nursing is "to walk the talk." As values, vision, mastery, and passion for critical care nursing excellence build, the attribute of "action" (see Fig. 10-2) becomes another pathway for our voice to make itself heard. The leading charge of action today for the nursing profession is to promote a professional and exciting image. One way this can be done is by demonstrating the impact nurses have on patient and family outcomes. Increasingly, critical care nurses are influencing changes in practice through reported research studies.[30] Informal structures, such as raising questions about practice, often start the process for quality improvement and best practice models of care.

Critical care nurses have been using their innate gift of inquiry for decades. However, Nightingale is perhaps our most famous leader who first used research to change practice.[29] Even though she lacked the theoretical bases that we have today, she had a core set of values, a vision, the mastery, and a passion to improve England's hospital care in the mid-19th century. Today critical care nurses are seeing "sacred cows" that were once revered being thrown out of practice. Nursing research has shown us that we do not need to use saline to suction endotracheal tubes, we do not need to bathe all postoperative coronary artery bypass graft (CABG) patients at 4:30 AM, and we do not need to restrict visitation in ICUs.

It does not take a doctorate-prepared critical care nurse to raise questions and put a plan in place for collecting, analyzing, and reporting patient and family outcomes. Kleinpell (2001) states that the purpose of outcomes includes the following: (1) describe the impact of care on patients and their families, (2) establish a basis for clinical decision making, (3) evaluate the effectiveness of care, and (4) identify areas for improvement. Once nursing integrates outcome management into daily nursing practice, there will be a greater sense of accountability and advancement of the science of nursing.[30]

Outcome-based practice is the responsibility of all nurses, whether one is actually doing the research, disseminating the research to the bedside, or reporting the research findings. In addition, it is important for all nurses to celebrate and showcase high-quality nursing outcomes, no matter what nursing specialty provided the body of knowledge. The recent and often-cited study by Mundinger and colleagues (2000)[31] may not at first glance seem relevant to every critical care nurse. However, its implications for the nursing profession as a whole are significant. This study was completed by a team led by an advanced-practice nurse and was reported in a prestigious medical journal. Mundinger and colleagues' study revealed that the patient outcomes in a nurse practitioner–managed practice were the same as those in a physician-managed practice in a number of areas, including health status, asthma peak flow, glycosylated hemoglobin (HbA_{1c}) testing, and hypertension management.[31]

This is the voice that needs to be heard. Outcomes must be reported to increase awareness of what nurses do. Buresh and Gordon (2000) remind nurses that the public cannot protect a social resource that it does not know and understand; only nurses can give the public the knowledge and understanding necessary to protect human caregiving.[2] Critical care nurses have a great opportunity to promote that powerful image of "high-tech to high-touch" through positive nursing outcomes.

Balance

"*Balance isn't either/or, it's AND.*" (Steven Covey)[11]

Real Moments of "Balance" in Critical Care Nursing Excellence

Charlie was 21 years old when she entered nursing. She had wanted to be a nurse for as long as she could remember. For more than 20 years, Charlie exemplified the beauty of critical care nursing as she blended the art and science of nursing into masterful human caring. However, Charlie recently died after a difficult battle with breast cancer. She asked me to give you this message:

"Life is the most wonderful gift, and to be a nurse, touching the lives of so many others, is by far the most significant of roles. You have but a precious small amount of time here on this Earth, and it is not by chance that each one of you became

a nurse. Don't waste your time here in frustration and anger. Pull together, support one another through difficult times and, most of all, stay focused on caring for our patients. You should be so proud of what you do everyday."

Anne Wojner, RN, PhDc, CCRN
AACN President 1999–2000
Opening Session Address, National Teaching Institute and Critical Care Exposition 2000
Orlando, Florida

Balance is the final component of the professional practice model for critical care nursing excellence (see Fig. 10-2). Balance brings renewal to our spirit, which often breaks down in our hectic lives. DeAngelis (1994) reminds us in *Real Moments: Discover the Secrets for True Happiness* that "yesterday is history, tomorrow is a mystery, today is a gift; that's why we call it 'the present' " (p. 22).[32] Taking the time to take care of ourselves is essential to keeping our bodies and mind in balance. Otherwise, we have difficulty keeping our perspectives clear. Today, nurses are increasingly blurring the lines between home and work and work and leisure. The lines of communication are continuously open owing to the proliferation of pagers, cell phones, facsimile machines, e-mail, and voicemail. It is time to say "no" to being "super nurse" and "super mom or dad" and find the time to take care of ourselves. We do not do our patients, our families, or ourselves any good if we consistently place the needs of others above our own. Critical care nurses listen to patients and families 24 hours a day, 7 days a week. They must also have time to listen to their minds and hearts and those who love them most.

In *Thinking in the Future Tense: Leadership Skills for a New Age*, James describes how tension shuts down the mind and heart. When one is stressed from an unexpected or unwelcome event, the capacity for altruism (caring for others) is drained.[33] We cannot stop the beeps, alarms, and phone calls at work, but when our shift is over, it is time to "shut down." We can turn the television off and read to our children, take a leisurely walk with our pet, or sit quietly listening to the sounds of life. Our minds and hearts need time to renew and be recharged for the next day of taking care of critically ill patients and their families. When we are balanced it is easier not to give in to the cynicism and frustration that abounds in the workplace or home. To be truly engaged and energized requires nurturing ourselves first and then empowering others to do the same. Look around your unit today and ask yourself some questions. Who are the critical care nurses who reach out to others the most? Who are the critical care nurses who smile the most? Who are the critical care nurses who say "thank you" and give compliments the most? You may find that your answer is those nurses who have been on an inner journey to discover the joy of creating "real moments of balance" in life.

CONCLUSION

Excellence comes from an inner core deep inside each of us. The desire and commitment for critical care nursing excellence requires self-reflection about the values, vision, mastery, passion, action, and balance in one's professional practice (see Fig. 10-2). It also requires raising the public's awareness of our "inner core" and articulating the essence of this "thing we do" called critical care nursing excellence. Nurses must move "from silence to voice"[2] in their everyday practice to make a difference in the quality of care received by critically ill patients and their families.

Buresh and Gordon define voice of agency as "the capacity for acting or the condition of exerting power" (2000, p. 35).[2] As the largest health care profession, nursing collectively is large and powerful enough to be a "voice of agency." Critical care nurses are a powerful vehicle for a voice of agency. Building a professional practice model of excellence can give critical care nurses the confidence needed to articulate their thoughts and tell their stories about the value of their role. Once this collective voice of agency is created and maintained, we will realize Buresh and Gordon's goal for nurses to have the long overdue "3 Rs": recognition, respect, and rewards.[2]

Critical care nurses can use their voice and presence to make significant contributions for improving the delivery of care to the patients and families who have entered a chaotic and frightening world of illness, trauma, and pain. Even in the fastest-paced critical care environments of today, finding the time for professional growth is challenging but essential. For the profession of critical care nursing to advance, each of us must look at how we are acquiring the skills necessary to provide best practice models of care to our critically ill patients and their families. Whether it is participating on a hospital committee or recruiting youth to critical care nursing, endless opportunities exist for building a professional practice of excellence. The days of landmark studies reporting that nursing is a silent and unknown profession[34,35] will soon come to an end as more voices are heard about how critical care nurses achieve excellence in their practice every day.

Closing Thoughts on Real Moments in Critical Care Nursing Excellence

Most of us have no idea how often we profoundly affect others with our nursing care. That is why we need to stop periodically and take account. Sometimes someone we touched tells us how we affected them. It is important that we accept that we are responsible for this significant event. Never say, "It was nothing," because it is not so. Allow yourself to bask in the sunshine of knowing that you have made a difference.

Linda Carpenito, RN, MSN, CRNP
Another opportunity to change the odds.
Nursing Forum 34(1):3, 4, 1999

clinical applicability challenges

Self-Challenge: Critical Thinking

1. *If more critical care nurses were prepared at the baccalaureate of nursing degree level or higher, how would that influence the profession (or would it)?*
2. *How would requiring "mandatory" certification for critical care nursing influence the profession (or would it)?*

3. *As a critical care nurse, what is one nursing or public health issue that you could use your "voice" for to make a difference? How would you do that?*

Study Questions

1. *Identify two current non-nursing authors who specifically address how to help nurses "find their voice" and bring awareness to the public about the value of nursing.*
   a. *Connie Barden and Denise Thornby*
   b. *Abraham Flexner and Lucie Young Kelly*
   c. *Bernice Buresh and Suzanne Gordon*
   d. *Barbara DeAngelis and Ann Wojner*
2. *According to a 2000 survey by the American Association of Critical-Care Nurses (AACN), approximately how many nurses are members of AACN?*
   a. *25,000*
   b. *45,000*
   c. *65,000*
   d. *85,000*
3. *Which of the following attributes (as discussed in this chapter) can help build a professional practice model for critical care nursing excellence?*
   a. *Values and vision*
   b. *Mastery and passion*
   c. *Action and balance*
   d. *All of the above*
4. *How can the critical care nursing profession be advanced?*
   a. *Letting "our voices" be heard about the art (high-touch) and science (high-tech) of nursing that is delivered every day through evidenced-based practice (EBP), best practice models of care, or both.*
   b. *Nothing needs to be done; the profession is just fine.*
   c. *Nothing needs to be changed; continue to be silent partners in health care delivery.*
   d. *None of the above.*
5. *Which of the following best demonstrates a critical care nurse who follows a professional practice model of excellence?*
   a. *One who is certified*
   b. *One who is educated at the baccalaureate of nursing level or higher*
   c. *One who is published with research in nursing*
   d. *One who is continually self-assessing his or her inner core values about how to bring the best critical care nursing performance to patients, families, and the profession*

REFERENCES

1. Kalisch P, Kalisch B: Working together for nursing. Focus Crit Care 10:12–14, 1983
2. Buresh B, Gordon S: From Silence to Voice: What Nurses Know and Must Communicate to the Public. Ottawa, Canada, Canadian Nurses Association, 2000
3. American Association of Critical-Care Nurses: Who are critical care nurses? Crit Care Nurse. AACN Critical Care Careers Supplement, February: 9–12, 2001
4. Division of Nursing, Bureau of Health Professionals in the Health Resources and Services Administration, U.S. Department of Health and Human Services: 2000 National Sample Survey of Registered Nurses. Available at: www.hrsa.gov. Accessed March 2003
5. Kelly L: Dimensions of Professional Nursing. New York, Macmillan, 1981
6. Flexner A: A Medical Education in the United States and Canada: A Report to the Carnegie Foundation for the Advancement of Teaching. Bethesda, MD, Science & Health Publications, 1910
7. Kelly L, Joel L: Dimensions of Professional Nursing. New York, McGraw-Hill, 1999
8. Holl R: Characteristics of the registered nurse and professional beliefs and decision making. Crit Care Nurs Q 17:60–66, 1994
9. Heath J, Andrews J, Graham-Garcia J: Assessment of professional development of critical care nurses: A descriptive study. Am J Crit Care 10(1):17–22, 2001
10. Weston M, Buchda V, Bergstrom D: Creating excellence in practice. In Sheehy CM, McCarthy MC (eds): Advanced Practice Nursing: Emphasizing Common Roles, pp 304–318. Philadelphia, FA Davis, 1998
11. Famous Quotations Network. Available at www.famous-quotations.com. Accessed March 2003
12. Carlson D: Nurses remain at top of honesty and ethics poll. The Gallup Organization, November 27, 2000. Available at www.gallup.com. Accessed May 2001
13. The Gallup Organization: Effects of year's scandals evident in honesty and ethics ratings. Available at www.gallup.com. Accessed March 2003
14. Thornby D: Make waves: Find courage to influence practice. AACN News 17(7):2–3, 2000
15. Barden C: Bold voices make sure our story is heard. AACN News 19(7):2, 2002
16. American Association of Critical Care Nurses: Core values. Available at www.aacn.org. Accessed March 2003
17. Donahue MP: Nursing the Finest Art: An Illustrated History. St. Louis, CV Mosby, 1985
18. A day by day account of the life of Winston Churchill. Available at www.winstonchurchill.org. Accessed March 2003
19. Senge PM: The Fifth Discipline: The Art and Practice of the Learning Organization. New York, Doubleday, 1990
20. Benner P: From Novice to Expert: Excellence and Power in Clinical Nursing. Boston, Addison-Wesley, 1984
21. Wojner A: Pioneering in a world of innovation. AACN News 17(6):2, 10, 2000
22. Cary AH: Certified registered nurses: Results of the study of the certified workforce. Am J Nurs 101(1):44–52, 2001
23. American Association of Critical-Care Nurses and AACN Certification Corporation: Safeguarding the patient and the profession: The value of critical care nurse certification. Am J Crit Care 12(2):154–164, 2003
24. Barden C: Certification: Good for whom? AACN News 20(2):2, 2003
25. Mason D: What's in a letter. Am J Nurs 101(1):7, 2001
26. Staub RE II: The 7 Acts of Courage: Bold Leadership for a Wholehearted Life. Provo, UT, Executive Excellence Publishing, 1999
27. Peters T, Austin N: A Passion for Excellence: The Leadership Difference. New York, Random House, 1985
28. Carlson R: Don't Sweat the Small Stuff. New York, Hyperion, 1997
29. Nightingale F: Notes on Nursing: What It Is, and What It Is Not. London, Harrison and Sons, 1859
30. Kleinpell R: Outcome Assessment in Advanced Practice Nursing. New York, Springer, 2001
31. Mundinger MO, Kane RL, Lenz ER, et al: Primary care outcomes in patients treated by nurse practitioners or physicians. JAMA 283:59–68, 2000
32. DeAngelis B: Real Moments: Discover the Secret for True Happiness. New York, Delacorte Press, 1994
33. James J: Thinking in the Future Tense: Leadership Skills for a New Age. New York, Simon & Schuster, 1996
34. Buresh B, Gordon S, Bell N: Who counts in news coverage of health care. Nursing Outlook 39(5):204–208, 1991
35. Sigma Theta Tau International: The Woodhull Study on Nursing and the Media: Health Care's Invisible Partner. Indianapolis, IN, author, 1998

PART

one two **three** four five six seven eight nine ten eleven twelve

Special Populations in Critical Care

INTERNET RESOURCES

Topic	Web Page Address
Chapter 11: The Critically Ill Pediatric Patient	
Congenital Heart Information Network	www.tchin.org/index.htm
Manitoba Pediatric Nursing Resource Centre	http://www.cche.net/nurses/default.html
National Association of Pediatric Nurse Practitioners, Inc	www.napnap.org
Pediatric Critical Care Medicine	www.pedsccm.org
Chapter 12: The Critically Ill Pregnant Woman	
Association of Women's Health, Obstetric and Neonatal Nurses	www.awhonn.org
The American College of Obstetricians and Gynecologists	www.acog.org
The Universe of Women's Health	www.obgyn.net
Chapter 13: The Critically Ill Older Patient	
American Geriatrics Society	www.americangeriatrics.org
Gerontological Society of America	www.geron.org
National Family Caregivers Association Association	www.nfcacares.org
National Gerontological Nurses Association	www.ngna.org
Chapter 14: The Postanesthesia Patient	
American Association of Nurse Anesthetists	www.aana.com
American Association of PeriAnesthesia Nurses	www.aspan.org
Association of periOperative Registered Nurses	www.aorn.org
Malignant Hyperthermia Association of the United States	www.mhaus.org
Chapter 15: Interfacility Transport of the Critically Ill Patient	
Air and Surface Transport Nurses Association	www.astna.org
American College of Emergency Physicians	www.acep.org
Association of Air Medical Services	www.aams.org
Emergency Nurses Association	www.ena.org
Society of Critical Care Medicine	www.sccm.org

chapter

11

The Critically Ill Pediatric Patient

PATRICIA A. MOLONEY-HARMON

objectives

Based on the content in this chapter, the reader should be able to:

- Analyze anatomical and physiological differences in the infant and child that necessitate the modification of physical assessment parameters and intervention techniques.
- Describe special considerations in ventilatory management and medication administration for the critically ill child.
- Evaluate pain assessment tools that can be used for the critically ill child.
- Examine important aspects of interaction with the critically ill child and family that will enhance interventions.

Most adult critical care clinicians feel ill-equipped to manage the percentage of children seen in adult intensive care units (ICUs), emergency departments (EDs), procedural suites, and recovery rooms. To facilitate smooth and optimal care of the critically ill child, it is wise to adopt a framework for the modification of the adult critical care practice to include the pediatric patient. A comprehensive framework is beyond the scope of this chapter, but readers are referred to the "PEDS" framework discussed in more detail elsewhere.[1,2] This chapter highlights prominent anatomical and physiological differences and related implications, equipment selection, recognition of the decompensating child, and unique challenges in caring for the pediatric patient in a critical care environment.

PROMINENT ANATOMICAL AND PHYSIOLOGICAL DIFFERENCES AND IMPLICATIONS

Vital Signs

Infants and young children have an age-appropriate, but higher, heart rate and respiratory rate than adults. The higher heart and respiratory rates assist in meeting the need for a higher cardiac output, despite a smaller stroke volume and a higher basal metabolic rate. Blood pressure in children is lower than that of adults. Vital signs (Table 11-1), although important parameters, should not be evaluated in isolation, but rather in a trending fashion.

Tachycardia is a nonspecific response to a variety of entities, such as anxiety, fever, shock, and hypoxemia. Although the child is predisposed to bradycardia, tolerance is poor. Persistent bradycardia produces significant changes in perfusion because cardiac output is heart rate–dependent. Bradycardia is most often caused by hypoxemia, but any vagal stimuli, such as suctioning, nasogastric tube insertion, and defecation, may precipitate an event.

As for respiratory rate, an infant or child increases his or her respiratory rate to compensate for an increased oxygen demand. Tachypnea is often the first sign of respiratory distress. A slow respiratory rate in a sick child often indicates impending respiratory arrest. Associated conditions, such as fever and seizure activity, which further increase the metabolic rate, also increase oxygen requirements. These conditions can cause rapid deterioration in an already-compromised child.

Unlike the adult, the child's blood pressure is the last parameter to fall in the face of shock. Children can

table 11-1 Pediatric Vital Signs

Age	Heart Rate (beats/min)	Respirations (breaths/min)	Systolic Blood Pressure (mm Hg)
Newborn	100–160	30–60	50–70
1–6 wk	100–160	30–60	70–95
6 mo	90–120	25–40	80–100
1 y	90–120	20–30	80–100
3 y	80–120	20–30	80–110
6 y	70–110	18–25	80–110
10 y	60–90	15–20	90–120
14 y	60–90	15–20	90–130

compensate for up to a 25% blood loss before the systolic blood pressure falls. A normal blood pressure should never discourage interventions for the child showing signs of circulatory failure. The pulse pressure is often a more reliable indicator for assessing the adequacy of perfusion. Hypertension is uncommon unless the child has renal disease.

Neurological System

Brain growth occurs at a rapid rate during the first few years of life. Because brain growth is rapid during this time, measurement of head circumference is important in the child until 2 years of age. The circumference of the child's head is related to intracranial volume and estimates the rate of brain growth.

The child's cranial sutures are not completely fused until 18 to 24 months of age. The posterior fontanel closes by 3 months of age, and the anterior fontanel closes by 9 to 18 months of age. The fontanels provide a useful assessment tool in the infant. The characteristics of the fontanels can be used to assess hydration status or the presence of increased intracranial pressure (ICP). Bulging fontanels may indicate increased ICP or fluid overload. Sunken fontanels may be seen with fluid deficit.

Like adults, infants and children have protective reflexes (e.g., the cough and gag reflexes). There are also several newborn reflexes (i.e., the Moro, rooting, grasp, and Babinski reflexes), which differ from adult reflexes. For example, the Babinski reflex is present until 9 to 12 months of age or until the child starts walking. A positive Babinski reflex response (fanning of the toes and dorsiflexion of the big toe when the lateral aspect of the sole of the foot is stroked) is expected in an infant, yet is considered an abnormal finding in an older child or adult. In-depth discussion of these reflexes is beyond the scope of this chapter; the reader is referred to a developmental anatomy text for further information.

An infant's or child's mental status is assessed the same way as an adult's, by noting the level of consciousness, interaction with the environment, and appropriateness of behavior for age. Level of consciousness is assessed by noting whether the child is arousable and oriented. This can be done by observing for spontaneous arousability or by providing verbal, tactile, or noxious stimuli. Even though the assessment is the same, the assessment techniques must be age-appropriate. Specific techniques are provided in the section in this chapter on interaction. An important difference when interacting with the child is paradoxical irritability. This is present with meningeal irritability, nuchal rigidity, and positive Brudzinski's and Kernig's signs.

Infants and young children are at high risk for ineffective thermoregulation, resulting in physiological instability, owing to a variety of maturational and environmental factors.[3] Close monitoring of body temperature and providing a temperature-controlled environment help manage temperature regulation. The temperature is measured at regular intervals, and external factors affecting body temperature should be controlled.

Cardiovascular System

Decreased perfusion to the skin is an early and reliable sign of shock. Because a child's skin is thinner than an adult's, skin characteristics change easily and rapidly with changes in perfusion. Skin color, texture, and temperature and capillary refill are of great significance during assessment of the child. Before assessing the skin, it is important to note the room temperature because some findings may be a normal response to the environment (such as mottling in a drafty operating room). Mottling in a bundled infant or warm environment is reason for further investigation. The nurse assesses skin temperature and the line of demarcation between extremity coolness and body warmth. Coolness or the progression of coolness toward the trunk may be a sign of diminishing perfusion.

Peripheral cyanosis is normal in newborns but abnormal in young children and adults. Central cyanosis (circumoral) is always an abnormal finding. Capillary refill time is normally recorded in seconds rather than as "brisk, normal, or slow" and normally is no longer than 2 seconds. Estimated blood volume varies with age; despite a higher volume per kilogram of body weight in children, the overall total circulating volume is small. A small amount of blood loss can be significant in the child.

Respiratory System

The infant's or child's large head (in proportion to body size), weak, underdeveloped neck muscles, and lack of cartilaginous support to the airway lead to an easily compressible or obstructed airway. The nurse must avoid overextending or overflexing the neck because the airways are easily collapsible. Head and neck position alone can facilitate a patent airway. Ideal positioning for the decompensating child is in a neutral ("sniffing") position and can be accomplished by placing a small roll horizontally behind the shoulders (Fig. 11-1). Infants, until 6 months of age, are obligate nose breathers, so any obstruction of nasal passages can produce significant airway compromise and respiratory distress. Secretions, edema, inflammation, poorly taped nasogastric tubes, or occluded nasal cannulas can cause obstructed nasal passages in an infant. The infant's and young child's airways are smaller in diameter and in length, thus requiring smaller artificial airways. Airway compromise can be caused by the slightest amount of inflammation or edema of the natural airway or from a mucus plug in either the natural or artificial airway. The narrowest part of the child's airway (until approximately 8 years of age) is at the level of the cricoid ring, as opposed to the glottic opening in the adult.

The young child's thin, compliant chest wall allows for easy assessment of air entry. Air entry is assessed by observing the rise and fall of the child's chest with adequate ventilatory efforts. Unequal chest movement may indicate the development of a pneumothorax or atelectasis but also may indicate endotracheal tube obstruction or displacement into the right mainstem bronchus. The child's flexible rib cage and poorly developed intercostal muscles offer little stability to the chest wall; therefore, suprasternal, sternal, intercostal, and subcostal retractions may be seen during respiratory distress. The presence and location of retractions should be noted. Accessory muscles also are poorly developed, so an infant or child may use the abdominal muscles to assist with breathing. This gives the appearance of "seesaw" breathing, a paradoxical movement of the chest and abdomen. Seesaw breathing becomes more exaggerated with respiratory distress. Like in the adult, the major muscle of respiration is the diaphragm. However, the child is more diaphragm dependent.

Because of the thin chest wall, breath sounds are more audible than in the adult. In addition, obstructed airways often produce sounds that are easily heard during assessment. The nurse listens for expiratory grunting, inspiratory and expiratory stridor, and wheezing. Expiratory grunting is a sound produced in an attempt to increase physiological positive end-expiratory pressure (PEEP) to prevent small airways and alveoli from collapsing. The infant's and child's thin chest wall may allow breath sounds to be heard over an area of pathology when sounds are actually being referred from another area of the lung. The nurse listens for changes in the breath sounds as well as for their presence or absence.

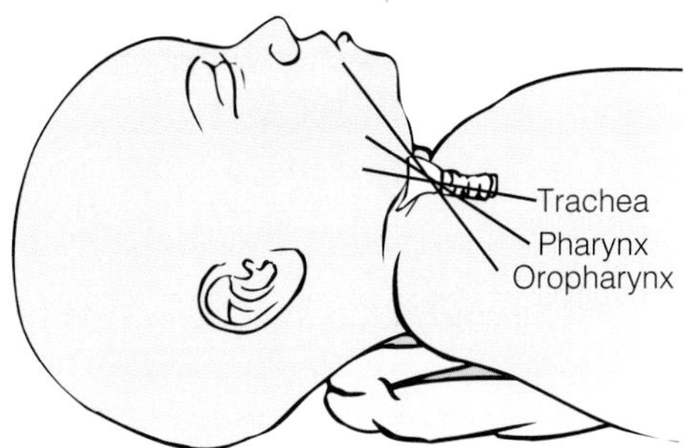

figure 11-1 The neutral ("sniffing") position can improve airflow in a decompensating child by aligning the oropharynx, pharynx, and trachea with the mouth.

Gastrointestinal System

Children normally have protuberant abdomens; however, there are numerous causes of abnormal abdominal distension. A nasogastric or orogastric tube should be inserted early rather than later to minimize the risk of distension. Abdominal distension can interfere with respiratory excursion and may even cause respiratory arrest. Active removal of air with a syringe may be necessary if distension is not relieved by putting the tube to straight drainage. In addition, the abdominal girth is measured every shift or more often if there is a concern about abdominal distension.

Stomach capacity varies with the age of the child. A newborn's stomach capacity is 90 mL, a 1-month-old's is 150 mL, a 12-month-old's is 360 mL, and an adult's is 2,000 to 3,000 mL. Because stomach capacity is smaller, care is taken when formula and other fluids are instilled into the abdomen. Bolus feedings are of an appropriate amount, consistent with the child's stomach capacity.

The infant and young child have a gastric emptying time of 2½ to 3 hours, which increases to 3 to 6 hours in the older child. An appropriate amount of time to allow for absorption of formula is taken into account when measuring residuals. If the child is receiving chest physiotherapy, the amount of time between therapy and feeding is considered or the gastric contents are checked to avoid problems with reflux and aspiration.

Renal System

Infants have less ability to concentrate urine and therefore have a normal urine output of 2 mL/kg/h. For children and adolescents, normal urine output is 1 mL/kg/h and 0.5 mL/kg/h, respectively. Because of the infant's limited ability to concentrate urine, a low specific gravity does not necessarily mean that the infant is adequately hydrated. The immaturity of the child's kidney means that the child may not process fluid as efficiently as the adult and will be less able to handle sudden large amounts of fluid, leading to fluid overload.

Infants and young children have a larger body surface area in relation to body weight. Maintenance fluid requirements are determined based on body weight (Table 11-2). Children have a higher percentage of total body water, most of which is composed of extracellular fluid (ECF), compared with adults. The ECF comprises 50% of the body weight in infants but 20% in adults. In addition, children have a higher insensible water loss because of a

table 11-2 Calculation of Maintenance Fluid

Body Weight (kg)	Fluid Requirements per Day	Fluid Requirements per Hour
<10	100 mL/kg	4 mL/kg
10–20	1,000 mL/kg + 50 mL/kg for each kg above 10	2 mL/kg for each kg above 10
>20	1,500 mL/kg + 20 mL/kg for each kg above 20	1 mL/kg for each kg above 20

From Roberts KE: Fluid and electrolyte regulation. In Curley MAQ, Moloney-Harmon PA (eds): Critical Care Nursing of Infants and Children, pp 369–392, 2001, with permission of Elsevier Science.

higher basal metabolic rate, higher respiratory rate, and larger body surface area. The child's higher percentage of total body water and higher insensible water loss increase the risk for dehydration. Sudden weight loss or gain may indicate fluid imbalance. Children should be weighed daily at the same time using the same scale.

Signs of dehydration include dry mucous membranes, decreased urine output, increased urine concentration, sunken fontanels and eyes, and poor skin turgor (Table 11-3). The severity of dehydration varies with the degree of dehydration and the child's fluid and electrolyte status. Circulatory compromise accompanies severe dehydration. Treating a child's dehydration in an adult ICU requires pediatric consultation.

Fluid overload is manifested by bulging fontanels, taut skin, edema (usually periorbital and sacral), hepatomegaly, and other signs of congestive heart failure.

Endocrine System

Infants and young children have smaller glycogen stores and increased glucose demand because of their larger brain to body size ratio. The smaller stores and increased demand predispose infants and young children to the development of hypoglycemia. Blood glucose levels are closely monitored, especially when the infant or child is not permitted to have anything by mouth and numerous adjustments are being made to nutritional support.

table 11-3 Clinical Assessment of Severity of Dehydration

	Mild Dehydration	Moderate Dehydration	Severe Dehydration
Physical appearance			
Infants and young children	Thirsty, alert, restless	Thirsty, restless, or lethargic but irritable to touch or drowsy	Drowsy, limp, cold, sweaty, cyanotic extremities, may be comatose
Older children and adults	Thirsty, alert, restless	Thirsty, alert, postural hypotension	Usually conscious, apprehensive, cold, sweaty, cyanotic extremities, wrinkled skin of fingers and toes, muscle cramps
Radial pulse	Normal rate and strength	Rapid and weak	Rapid, feeble, sometimes impalpable
Respiration	Normal	Deep, may be rapid	Deep and rapid
Anterior fontanel	Normal	Sunken	Very sunken
Systolic blood pressure	Normal	Normal or low	Low, may be unrecordable
Skin elasticity	Pinch retracts immediately	Pinch retracts slowly	Pinch retracts very slowly (>2 sec)
Eyes	Normal	Sunken (detectable)	Grossly sunken
Tears	Present	Absent	Absent
Mucous membranes	Moist	Dry	Very dry
Urine output	Normal	Reduced amount and dark	None passed for several hours, empty bladder
Body weight loss (%)	3–5	6–9	≥10
Estimated fluid deficit (mL/kg)	30–50	60–90	≥100

Data from Adelman RD, Solhaug MJ: Pathophysiology of body fluids and fluid therapy. In Behrman RE (ed): Nelson Textbook of Pediatrics (15th Ed), pp 185–222, 1996, with permission from Elsevier Science.

SELECTED PEDIATRIC CHALLENGES

Ventilatory Issues

The most common cause of cardiopulmonary arrest in children is respiratory in nature. This mandates that respiratory distress and failure be recognized early and that airway management interventions be immediate (Table 11-4). Signs of respiratory decompensation include diminished level of consciousness, tachypnea, minimal or no chest movement with respiratory effort, evidence of labored respirations with retractions, seesaw breathing, minimal or no air exchange noted on auscultation, and the presence of nasal flaring, grunting, stridor, or wheezing.

table 11-4 Quick Examination of a Healthy Versus Decompensating Child

Assessment	Healthy Child	Decompensating Child
Airway		
Patency	Child requires no interventions; child verbalizes and is able to swallow, cough, gag.	Child self-positions and requires interventions, such as head positioning, suctioning, adjunct airways. Unmaintainable airway requires intubation.
Breathing		
Respiratory rate	Breathing is within age-appropriate limits.	Breathing is tachypneic or bradypneic compared with age-appropriate limits and conditions.* **Note:** Warning parameter: > 60 breaths/min
Chest movement (presence)	Chest rises and falls equally and simultaneously with abdomen with each breath.	Child has minimal or no chest movement with respiratory effort.
Chest movement (quality)	Child has silent and effortless respirations.	Child shows evidence of labored respirations with retractions. Asynchronous movement (seesaw) is observed between chest and abdomen with respiratory efforts.
Air movement (presence)	Air exchange is heard bilaterally in all lobes.	Despite movement of the chest, minimal or no air exchange is noted on auscultation.
Air movement (quality)	Breath sounds are of normal intensity and duration.	Nasal flaring, grunting, stridor, wheezing are noted.
Circulation		
Heart rate (presence)	Apical beat is present and within age-appropriate limit.*	Heart rate is absent; bradycardia or tachycardia occurs as compared with age-appropriate limits.* **Note:** Warning parameters: Infant: <80 beats/min; Child <5 y: >180 beats/min; Child >5 y: >150 beats/min
Heart rate (quality)	Heart rate is regular with normal sinus rhythm.	Heart rate is irregular, slow, or very rapid; common dysrhythmias include supraventricular tachycardia, bradyarrhythmias, and asystole.
Skin	Extremities are warm, pink with capillary refill ≤ 2 seconds; peripheral pulses are present bilaterally with normal intensity.	Child has pallor, cyanotic, or mottled skin color and cool-to-cold extremities. Capillary refill time is ≥ 2 seconds; peripheral pulses are weak or absent; central pulses are weak.
Cerebral perfusion	Child is alert to surroundings, recognizes parents or significant others, is responsive to fear and pain, and has normal muscle tone.	Child is irritable, lethargic, obtunded, or comatose; has minimal or no reaction to pain; has loose muscle tone (floppy).
Blood pressure	Blood pressure is within age-appropriate limits.	Blood pressure falls from age-appropriate limits,* a late sign of decompensation. **Note:** A fall of 10 mm Hg systolic pressure is significant. Lower systolic blood pressure limit: Infant ≤1 mo, 60 mm Hg; Infant ≤1 y, 70 mm Hg; Child, 70 + (2 × age in years)

*All vital signs are interpreted within the context of age, clinical condition, and other external factors, such as the presence of fever.

Adapted from Moloney-Harmon PA, Rosenthal CH: Nursing care modifications for the child in the adult ICU. In Stillwell S (ed): Mosby's Critical Care Nursing Reference, pp 588–670, 1992, with permission from Elsevier Science.

The initial intervention for respiratory decompensation is positioning the child to open the airway. If the child does not respond to position alone, manual ventilation with 100% oxygen using a bag-mask device is initiated. There are several sizes of pediatric manual resuscitation bags; the correct size is determined by noting the child's tidal volume and deciding if the bag is capable of delivering one and one-half times the child's tidal volume. Even though a pressure manometer may assist in minimizing pressure, the true indicator of delivery of an adequate tidal volume is a clinical one. The adequate amount of tidal volume delivered during a manual resuscitation breath is the amount that causes rise and fall of the child's chest.

If bag-mask ventilation is not successful in restoring the child's ventilatory status, endotracheal intubation is required. Numerous sizes of endotracheal tubes are available for infants and children. To estimate the correct size endotracheal tube, the size of the child's little finger or the following formula can be used:

$$\text{Internal diameter} = (16 + \text{age in years}) \div 4$$

Because these are both estimations of endotracheal tube size, tubes one-half size smaller and larger should be available for immediate use. Table 11-5 provides information regarding endotracheal tube sizes and other equipment issues. In general, uncuffed endotracheal tubes are used in children younger than 8 years of age because the narrow cricoid cartilage provides an anatomical cuff in the presence of anatomically normal lungs. Pediatric endotracheal tubes with cuffs are available for use with stiff lungs that are difficult to ventilate.

Monitoring the patient during intubation is critical to assess for desaturation or bradycardia. Once the child

table 11-5 Recommended Resuscitation Equipment for Infants and Children

	Child's weight						
	4–8 kg (8.8–17.6 pounds)	*8–11 kg (17.6–24.2 pounds)*	*11–14 kg (24.2–30.8 pounds)*	*14–18 kg (30.8–39.6 pounds)*	*18–24 kg (39.6–52.8 pounds)*	*24–32 kg (52.8–70.4 pounds)*	*32+ kg (70.4+ pounds)*
Oxygen mask	Newborn	Pediatric	Pediatric	Pediatric	Pediatric	Adult	Adult
Oral airway	Infant	Small child	Child	Child	Child	Small adult	Small adult
Resuscitation bag	Infant	Child	Child	Child	Child	Adult	Adult
Laryngoscope blade	0–1 straight	1 straight	2 straight or curved	2 straight or curved	2 straight or curved	2–3 straight or curved	3 straight or curved
Endotracheal tube (mm)	2.5 preterm; 3.0–3.5 term infant	4.0 uncuffed	4.5 uncuffed	5.0 uncuffed	5.5 uncuffed	6.0 cuffed	6.5 cuffed
Endotracheal tube (cm at the tip)	10–10.5	11–12	12.5–13.5	14–15	15.5–16.5	17–18	18.5–19.5
Stylet	Small	Small	Small	Small	Large	Large	Large
Suction catheter	6–8	8	8–10	10	10	10–12	12–14
Nasogastric tube (F)	5–8	8–10	10	10–12	12–14	14–18	18
Urinary catheter	5–8	8–10	10	10–12	10–12	12	12
Chest tube (F)	10–12	16–20	20–24	20–24	24–32	28–32	32–40
Blood pressure cuff	Newborn or infant	Infant or child	Child	Child	Child	Child or adult	Adult
IV catheter (G)	22–24	22–24	20–22	18–22	18–20	18–20	16–20
Butterfly catheter	23–25	23–25	21–23	21–23	21–23	20–22	18–21
Vascular catheter	3.0 F 5–12 cm	3.0–4.09 F 5–12 cm	3.0–4.0 F 5–12 cm	4.0–5.0 F 5–25 cm	4.0–5.0 F 5–25 cm	4.0–5.0 F 5–25 cm	5.0–8.0 F 5–30 cm
Guide wire (mm)	0.46	0.46–0.53	0.53–0.89	0.53–0.89	0.53–0.89	0.53–0.89	0.89

References: Chameides L, Hazinski M. Textbook of Pediatric Advanced Life Support, Dallas, Tex., American Heart Association, 1997; Hazinski M (ed). Nursing Care of the Critically Ill Child, 2nd edition, St. Louis, Mo., Mosby-Year Book, Inc. 1992; Slota M. AACN Core Curriculum for Pediatric Critical Care Nursing, Philadelphia, Pa., W. B. Saunders Co., 1998.

From the AACN Pediatric Critical Care Pocket Reference Card. © 1998 American Association of Critical-Care Nurses (AACN). Adapted with permission of the publisher. The card (product #400825) costs $4 for nonmembers and $2 for AACN members. To order, or to request a catalog of the AACN's other pocket reference cards, books, audiotapes, and more, call the AACN at 1-800-899-AACN or visit the on-line bookstore at http://www.aacn.org.

Reprinted from Dimens Crit Care Nurs 20(1): 23, 2001, with permission.

is intubated, observation of chest movement and auscultation of the lungs help determine correct placement. An x-ray is used to confirm proper placement. Once placement is confirmed, the tube is securely taped to avoid accidental displacement. In addition, soft restraints should be used to prevent the child from removing the tube. Adequate sedation and analgesia are provided to increase the child's comfort and manage anxiety while intubated.

Medication Administration

Because a child may differ in weight significantly from the average child in the associated age group, medications are prescribed on a microgram, milligram, or milliequivalent per kilogram of body weight basis rather than on a standard dose according to age. Confirming the weight (in kilograms) that is being used to determine drug dosages is important. This same weight should be used during the child's entire hospitalization unless there is a significant change in the child's weight. Because pediatric dosages may be unfamiliar to the adult clinician, precalculated emergency drug sheets are helpful. The emergency drug sheet should include the recommended resuscitation medication dosages, medication concentration, and the final medication dose and volume the individual child is to receive. The recommended dosages should reflect the American Heart Association's Pediatric Advanced Life Support (PALS) standards.

An important recommendation for medication administration in the pediatric patient is the single-dose system. The single-dose system involves preparing one syringe to contain only the prescribed medication dose. The syringe should be properly labeled with the drug name and dose. The nurse administers the entire volume of the syringe to ensure that the prescribed dose has been given. The single-dose system prevents overmedication or undermedication of the child.

Pain Management

Because of the nature of the environment and associated procedures, the critically ill child is at high risk for pain. The first step in assessing pain in children is to understand the child's response to, and communication of, pain. This is based on a variety of factors, including the child's developmental level, past and present experience with pain, cultural aspects, personality, parental presence, age, and the nature of the illness or injury.[4] For instance, critically ill children may be in severe pain but may be unable to communicate because of sedation, paralytic agents, mechanical ventilation, or coma.

Pain assessment is multidimensional. There are a variety of parameters that, when synthesized, provide information that can be used to make a decision about the level of the child's pain and the most appropriate intervention. Assessment of pain by nurses is influenced by factors such as educational level, skills, experience, personal beliefs, and different strategies adopted for assessment.[5,6] A recent study demonstrated that nurses use mainly physiological parameters, followed by behavioral indicators to determine pain in critically ill children.[7] Another study reported that the indicators of pain and agitation used most frequently by nurses caring for critically ill infants were nurses' and parents' judgment and documentation; environment; and infant's cues (e.g., cry, sleep patterns, physiological responses, and body movements). Medical diagnosis was used most frequently to determine pain.[5]

Physiological parameters used in pain assessment include heart rate, respiratory rate, blood pressure, and oxygen saturation. Other parameters described by Anand and Carr[8] include sweating, increased muscle tone, and skin color changes. These parameters return to normal as physiological adaptation occurs. This adaptation can actually occur within minutes, and the nurse must realize that the child may still be in pain. The physical signs are not necessarily specific for pain but may be the only parameter available to the nurse caring for the critically ill child.

Behavioral responses may be helpful for pain assessment, especially in the child who cannot communicate. The next section on interaction with children and families discusses the continuum of responses related to pain and comfort. Another dimension of pain assessment is self-report. Many tools are available; however, these often require children to interact or use their hands. Because of this, these tools are not usually helpful in the critical care setting. Examples of self-report tools include the numeric rating scale (see Chapter 5, Fig. 5-1), the faces scale (Fig. 11-2), and the color scale. If the child is unable or unwilling to give a report, the parent's report of pain is often helpful. Multidimensional scales, such as the COMFORT, Modified Motor Activity Assessment, and the FLACC (Face, Legs, Activity, Cry, Consolability) scales (see Fig. 11-2), are helpful because they combine dimensions of behavioral and physiological distress and do not require interaction or use of the hands.

Pain management interventions are multidimensional whenever possible, including nonpharmacological and pharmacological approaches. However, pharmacological intervention is never withheld when it is appropriate. Opioids are usually the first-line drugs for pain management in the critically ill child. A variety of pharmacological agents are available, and the choice of drug depends on the child's response and the practitioner's preference. Nursing responsibilities include assessing the child's need for the drug, administering the appropriate dose, and monitoring the child's response.

Other methods of pain control include intravenous patient-controlled analgesia (PCA) and epidural analgesia. PCA helps the child maintain a steady state of pain relief and also gives the child some control over pain. Epidural analgesia is also helpful for a variety of children. Epidural narcotics provide selective analgesia but do have associated side effects, including respiratory depression, nausea and vomiting, pruritus, and urinary retention.[9]

Nurses may consider the use of nonpharmacological methods, such as distraction, relaxation, massage, and hypnosis, in conjunction with pharmacological agents. The method must be age-appropriate, and parental presence is considered. Whatever methods are used, a critical determinant of their effectiveness is the child's response.

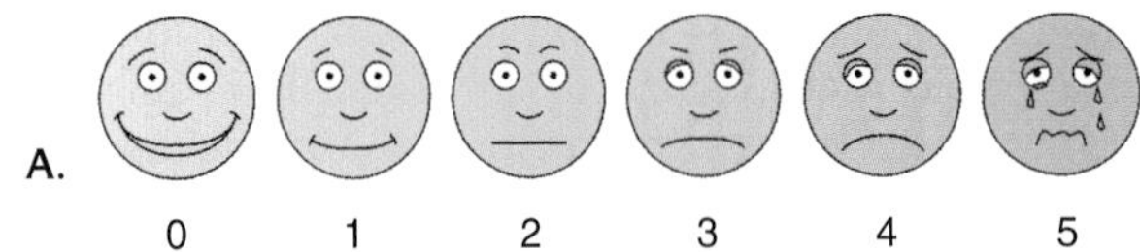

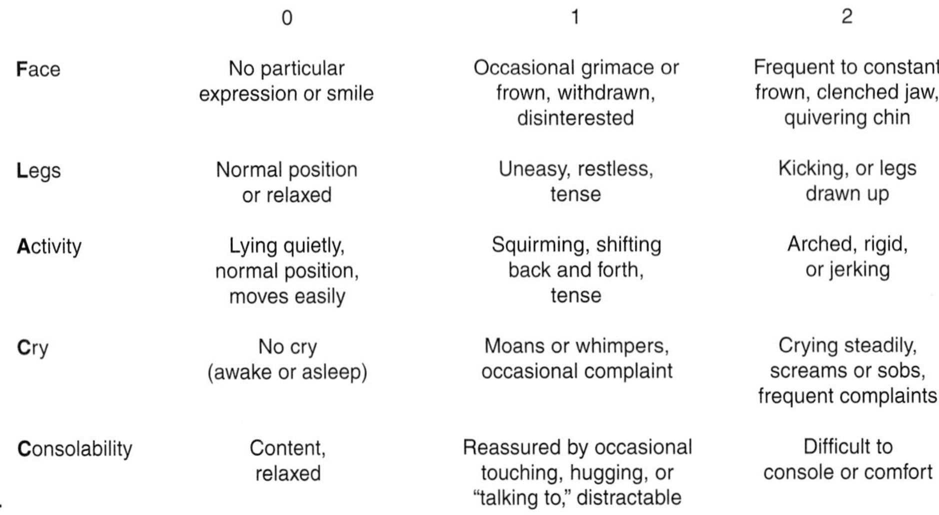

	0	1	2
Face	No particular expression or smile	Occasional grimace or frown, withdrawn, disinterested	Frequent to constant frown, clenched jaw, quivering chin
Legs	Normal position or relaxed	Uneasy, restless, tense	Kicking, or legs drawn up
Activity	Lying quietly, normal position, moves easily	Squirming, shifting back and forth, tense	Arched, rigid, or jerking
Cry	No cry (awake or asleep)	Moans or whimpers, occasional complaint	Crying steadily, screams or sobs, frequent complaints
Consolability	Content, relaxed	Reassured by occasional touching, hugging, or "talking to," distractable	Difficult to console or comfort

B.

figure 11-2 Tools for assessing pain in children. (**A**) The faces scale. This scale may be used in children 3 years and older. Explain that FACE 0 is a very happy face because there is no pain. FACE 1 hurts just a little bit. FACE 2 hurts a little bit more. FACE 3 hurts even more. FACE 4 hurts a whole lot. FACE 5 hurts very much; the pain can make you cry. Ask the child to choose the face that best describes the pain he or she is feeling. (From Wong DL, Hockenberry-Eaton M, Wilson D, Winkelstein ML, Schwartz P: Wong's Essentials of Pediatric Nursing, [6th Ed], p 1301. St Louis, Mosby, 2001. Copyrighted by Mosby, Inc. Reprinted by permission.) (**B**) The FLACC (**F**ace, **L**egs, **A**ctivity, **C**ry, **C**onsolability) scale. This scale can be used with children younger than 3 years. To use the FLACC scale, assess the child in each category, assigning a score between 0 and 2. Total the score, and then evaluate the total using the 0–10 pain scale parameters. (Reprinted with permission from Merkel SI, Voepel-Lewis T: The FLACC: A behavioral scale for scoring post-operative pain in young children. Pediatr Nurs 23(3):293–297, 1997.)

INTERACTION WITH CHILDREN AND FAMILIES

Interacting with children demands familiarity with their developmental capabilities and psychosocial needs. Categorization of children into groups according to physical and cognitive age can assist the nurse in predicting the child's expected social, cognitive, and physical capabilities. Developmental and psychosocial assessment is beyond the scope of this chapter; therefore, the reader should consult an appropriate growth and development reference. Although each age group of children has common developmental capabilities, tasks, and fears, it is helpful to recognize the common fears of all children despite their age. These fears include loss of control, threat of separation, painful procedures, and communicated anxiety.[10]

Unlike the adult patient, the young child does not consciously screen most behavior and spoken words. The young child subconsciously communicates behaviorally through verbal, nonverbal (body language, behaviors), and abstract (play, drawing, story telling) cues. Although the child's behavior is more natural in a familiar environment, the cues available to the clinician can suggest how a child is feeling or perceiving an event or the presence of an individual. In general, the child's behavior is more activity oriented and more emotional than that of adults.[10] These qualities of a child's behavior should be expected as the norm of average, healthy children and may be used as parameters against which to contrast the behavior of the critically ill child (Table 11-6).

Behavioral responses are particularly helpful during the assessment of pain or comfort. The infant or child may display body movement that spans the entire activity continuum from minimal movement, such as rigidity and guarding, to high activity, such as thrashing and kicking. Assessing various behavioral responses (e.g., gestures, posture, movement, and facial expression) and examining the congruency between these responses are particularly helpful.

Interaction with pediatric patients and their families is also facilitated by the appreciation of the child's significant others. The philosophy of family-centered care is essential to the optimal care of the pediatric patient.[11] Gone are the days when parents dropped their children for care at the entrance of the hospital. Although there are several components of family-centered care, the salient concept is to

table 11-6 Contrasting Nonverbal Behavioral Cues of the Healthy and the Critically Ill Child

Healthy	Critically Ill
Posture	
Moves, flexes	May be loose, flaccid May prefer fetal position or position of comfort
Gestures	
Turns to familiar voices	Responds slowly to familiar voices
Movement	
Moves purposefully	Exhibits minimal movement, lethargy
Moves toward new, pleasurable items	Shows increased movement, irritability (possibly indicating cardiopulmonary or neurological compromise, pain, or sleep deprivation)
Moves away from threatening items, people	
Reactions/Coping Style	
Responds to parent(s) coming, leaving	Exhibits minimal response to parent presence, absence
Responds to environment and equipment	Exhibits minimal response to presence or absence of transitional objects
Cries and fights invasive procedures	Displays minimal defensive responses
Facial Expressions	
Looks at faces and makes eye contact	May not track faces, objects
Changes facial expressions in response to interactions	Avoids eye contact or has minimal response to interactions
Responds negatively to face wash	Minimally changes facial expression during face wash
Blinks in response to stimuli	Exhibits increased or decreased blinking
Widens eyes with fear	Avoids eye contact
Is fascinated with own mouth	Avoids or dislikes mouth stimulation
Holds mouth "ready for action"	Drools or displays loose mouth musculature
	Sucks intermittently or weakly

Taken from Moloney-Harmon P, Rosenthal CH: Nursing care modifications for the child in the adult ICU. In Stillwell S (ed): Critical Care Nursing Reference Book, p 590, 1992, with permission from Elsevier Science.

value, recognize, and support the family in the care of their child. The family is the constant in the child's life and is ultimately responsible for responding to the child's emotional, social, developmental, physical, and health care needs.[12] Appropriate support and incorporation of parents may buffer the threats of the ICU environment on the child.[12] Parents may assist or influence the child's cognitive appraisal of the environment, personnel, and events.[13] The child often uses the reactions of the parent as a barometer in interpreting events in ways ranging from threatening to beneficial.

The tone and manner in which the clinician approaches the bedside of a pediatric patient and his or her family are important. Communicated anxiety refers to the anxious feelings conveyed to the child by the parents, the health care team members, or both. Interventions to relieve the anxiety of parents and fellow health care team members will have a direct impact on the child's well-being. Interventions may include assisting parents and staff in anticipating the child's responses to therapy and illness and guiding parents and staff in therapeutic communication techniques.[14]

Examples of nursing diagnoses and collaborative problems for the pediatric patient in the ICU are given in Box 11-1.

case study ■ RESPIRATORY DISTRESS IN A PEDIATRIC PATIENT

Donald is a 3-year-old, 15-kg boy who is admitted for status asthmaticus. On admission, his vital signs are a heart

box 11-1 ***Examples of Nursing Diagnoses and Collaborative Problems for the Critically Ill Pediatric Patient***

- Airway Clearance, Ineffective related to obstructed airway
- Anxiety related to environment
- Risk for Imbalanced Body Temperature
- Interrupted Family Processes related to shift in health status of a family member
- Deficient Fluid Volume related to active fluid volume loss, failure of regulatory mechanisms
- Delayed Growth and Development related to separation from significant others

insights into clinical research

Crain N, Dilton H, Slanim A: End of life care for children: Bridging the gap. Crit Care Med 29(3):695–697, 2001.

Although issues for dying children and their families are similar in many ways to the issues that affect adult patients, the roles of family members in the decision-making process contribute to a set of circumstances that are unique to the care of children. In this study, the authors used a survey questionnaire design to query the attitudes and perceived practices of pediatric intensive care physicians and nurses caring for children at the end of life. The results showed that the majority of practitioners agreed with consensus statements offered concerning end of life. The only significant characteristic of the practitioners who disagreed was fewer years of experience. Other differences noted by the authors as a result of the survey were the attitudes of nurses toward end of life and the difference in priorities and factors influencing decision making between nurses and physicians. Nurses were less likely than physicians to agree that ethical issues were less discussed among members of the health care team and between the team and the family.

End-of-life care is an important component of pediatric critical care. However, this study and others demonstrate a gap between theory and practice for many practitioners, gaps between practitioners of different disciplines, and gaps between practitioners with different levels of experience. The challenge is to enhance and standardize the approach to dealing with end-of-life issues for children and their families.

rate of 150 beats/min, a respiratory rate of 48 breaths/min, a blood pressure of 100/60 mm Hg, an axillary temperature of 100.4° F (38° C), and an oxygen saturation of 94%.

Physical examination reveals an agitated, irritable, and crying young boy with intercostal and substernal retractions and nasal flaring. His expiratory wheezing can be heard across the room. The child's respiratory rate is slightly high for his age, although tachypnea is to be expected for his clinical condition. He has a low-grade fever and is anxious, which may also account for the tachypnea. The anxiety, agitation, and increased work of breathing increase his oxygen demand, while at the same time lower airway obstruction is decreasing oxygen transport. The warning parameters of mild tachypnea, nasal flaring, retractions, and wheezing indicate a child with respiratory distress who is at risk for the development of respiratory failure.

Initial management priorities include having the child assume a position of comfort and administering oxygen while assessing his response. Albuterol, an inhaled β_2-agonist, is administered. After these interventions, the child's vital signs are a heart rate of 150 beats/min, a respiratory rate of 42 breaths/min, a blood pressure of 105/62 mm Hg, and an oxygen saturation of 98% on 40% oxygen by face mask.

One hour later, the child is noted to have a heart rate of 100 beats/min, a respiratory rate of 20 breaths/min, a blood pressure of 98/58 mm Hg, and an oxygen saturation of 90%. His retractions are more pronounced and wheezing is not audible by auscultation. He is extremely lethargic. Arterial blood gases (ABGs) reveal the following: pH 7.25; $PaCO_2$ 56 mm Hg; PaO_2 80 mm Hg; and HCO_3^- 27 mEq/L on a fraction of inspired oxygen (FIO_2) of 0.5. The child is demonstrating signs of fatigue and respiratory failure. Warning parameters include an unmaintainable airway, bradypnea, worsening retractions, lethargy, and no air movement (indicated by lack of wheezing). Management priorities at this time include bag-mask ventilation and intubation.

Treatment is directed toward ensuring oxygenation and ventilation while reversing bronchospasm. Medications include inhaled bronchodilators, anticholinergics, corticosteroids, and intravenous magnesium sulfate. Mechanical ventilation is also provided until the child shows improvement, as demonstrated by his ABGs, vital signs, and clinical condition. ■

clinical applicability challenges

Self-Challenge: Critical Thinking

1. *What were the signs of impending respiratory failure in Donald, the young boy who was the subject of the case study?*
2. *Determine management priorities for the child with signs of impending respiratory failure.*

Study Questions

1. *An early sign of shock in a child is*
   a. *increased capillary refill time*
   b. *bradycardia*
   c. *hypotension*
   d. *decreased pulse pressure*
2. *You are caring for an 8-year-old child who requires intubation. The child weighs 25 kg. What size endotracheal tube would you select?*
   a. *5.0 mm*
   b. *5.5 mm*
   c. *6.0 mm*
   d. *6.5 mm*
3. *You are caring for a 3-year-old, 15-kg child who presents with grunting, nasal flaring, and retractions. You note that he has both inspiratory and expiratory wheezing. His oxygen saturation is 91% on room air. Your initial intervention is to*
   a. *administer oxygen*
   b. *begin an inhalation bronchodilator*
   c. *intubate*
   d. *begin a terbutaline infusion.*

REFERENCES

1. Rosenthal CH: Pediatric Critical Care Nursing in the Adult ICU: Essentials of Practice. National Conference on Pediatric Critical Care Nursing. New York, Contemporary Forums, 1990
2. Moloney-Harmon P, Rosenthal CH: Nursing care modifications for the child in the adult ICU. In Stillwell S (ed): Critical Care Nursing Reference Book, pp 588–670. St. Louis, Mosby-Year Book, 1992

3. Pate MFD: Thermal regulation. In Curley MAQ, Moloney-Harmon PA (eds): Critical Care Nursing of Infants and Children, pp 443–460. Philadelphia, WB Saunders, 2001
4. Oakes LL: Caring practices: Providing comfort. In Curley MAQ, Moloney-Harmon PA (eds): Critical Care Nursing of Infants and Children, pp 547–576. Philadelphia, WB Saunders, 2001
5. Ramelet AS: Assessment of pain and agitation in critically ill infants. Aust Crit Care 12(3):92–96, 1999
6. Fuller BF, Connor DA: Distribution of cues across assessed levels of infant pain. Clin Nurs Res 5(2): 167–184, 1996
7. Coffman S, Alvarez Y, Pyngolil M, et al: Nursing assessment and management of pain in critically ill children. Heart Lung 26(3): 221–228, 1997
8. Anand KJS, Carr DB: The neuroanatomy, neurophysiology, and neurochemistry of pain, stress, and analgesia in newborns and children. Pediatr Clin North Am 36(4):795–821, 1989
9. Macfayden AJ, Buckmaster MA: Pain management in the pediatric intensive care unit. Crit Care Clin 15(1):185–199, 1999
10. Smith J, Martin SA: Caring practices: Providing developmentally supportive care. In Curley MAQ, Moloney-Harmon PA (eds): Critical Care Nursing of Infants and Children, pp 17–46. Philadelphia, WB Saunders, 2001
11. Shelton TL: Family-centered care in pediatric practice: when and how? J Dev Behav Pediatr 20:117–118, 1999
12. Rushton CH: Family-centered care in the critical care setting: Myth or reality. Child Health Care 19(2):68–78, 1990
13. Curley MAQ: Effects of the nursing mutual participation model of care and parental stress in the pediatric intensive care unit. Heart Lung 17:682–688, 1988
14. Curley MAQ, Meyer EC: Caring practices: The impact of the critical care experience on the family. In Curley MAQ, Moloney-Harmon PA (eds): Critical Care Nursing of Infants and Children, pp 47–67. Philadelphia, WB Saunders, 2001

OTHER SELECTED READING

Beckstrand R: Understanding chest radiographs of infants and children: The AIR systematic approach. Crit Care Nurse 21(3):54–65, 2001

Bettler J, Roberts K: Nutritional assessment in the critically ill child. AACN Clin Issues 11(4):498–506, 2000

Champi C, Gaffney-Yocum P: Managing febrile seizures in children. Dimens Crit Care Nurs 20(5):2–7, 2001

Irving S, Simone S, Hicks F, Verger J: Nutrition for the critically ill child: Enteral and parenteral support. AACN Clin Issues 11(4):541–558, 2000

Jenkins T: Sickle cell anemia in the pediatric intensive care unit: Novel approaches for managing life-threatening complications. AACN Clin Issues 13(2):154–168, 2002

Kimberly A: Caring for adolescents in the adult intensive care unit. Crit Care Nurse 22(2):80–99, 2002

LeRoy S: Clinical dysrhythmias after surgical repair of congenital heart disease. AACN Clin Issues 12(1):87–99, 2001

Oakes L: Assessment and management of pain in the critically ill pediatric patient. Crit Care Nurs Clin North Am 13(2):281–296, 2001

Velsor-Friedrich B, Foley M: School-based management of the child with an acute asthma episode. AACN Clin Issues 12(2):282–292, 2001

Ware L: Inhaled nitric oxide in infants and children. Crit Care Nurs Clin North Am 14(1):1–6, 2002

Wedekind C, Fidler B: Compatibility of commonly used intravenous infusions in a pediatric intensive care unit. Crit Care Nurse 21(4):45–51, 2001

chapter

12

The Critically Ill Pregnant Woman

CATHLEEN R. MAIOLATESI

objectives

Based on the content in this chapter, the reader should be able to:

- Summarize normal physiological changes that occur in the cardiovascular, respiratory, renal, and hematological systems during pregnancy.
- Differentiate the signs and symptoms of preeclampsia and severe preeclampsia.
- Explain the pathophysiology of severe preeclampsia.
- Describe parameters of nursing assessment of a severely preeclamptic patient on intravenous magnesium sulfate.
- Name three obstetrical conditions that predispose a woman to development of disseminated intravascular coagulation.
- Summarize the psychosocial support needed for an obstetrical patient in the intensive care unit (ICU).
- Compare and contrast the care of an obstetrical trauma patient to a nonobstetrical trauma patient.

Most women experience a normal pregnancy. A small percentage of women, however, experience life-threatening complications that may result from the pregnancy itself or may be part of a preexisting condition. Such critically ill pregnant women provide a unique challenge to nurses.

The general principles of diagnosis and management are similar to those used for other intensive care unit (ICU) patients. However, physiological changes inherent in pregnancy must be considered to decrease morbidity and mortality.[1] Critical care nurses caring for these patients must understand the physiological changes that occur in pregnancy to distinguish normal from abnormal responses. Table 12-1 outlines these changes.

PHYSIOLOGICAL CHANGES IN PREGNANCY

Cardiovascular Changes

Normal cardiovascular changes that occur during pregnancy affect pulse, blood pressure, cardiac output, and blood volume (see Table 12-1). Maternal blood volume increases 40% to 50% above baseline. This increase, which is mostly plasma, begins in the first trimester and continues throughout pregnancy. The increase is necessary to provide adequate blood flow to the uterus, fetus, and changing maternal tissues and to accommodate blood loss at birth. Red blood cell volume increases by 20% and

table 12-1 Physiological Changes in Pregnancy

	Change	Pregnancy Levels
Cardiovascular Changes		
Blood volume	>40%–50%	1,260–1,625 mL
Red blood cells	>20%	250–450 mL
Blood pressure		
Systolic	<5–12 mm Hg	
Diastolic	<10–20 mm Hg	
Cardiac output	>30%–50%	6–7 L/min
Heart rate	>10%–30%	Increased by 15–20 beats/min
Systemic vascular resistance	<20%–30%	1,210 ± 266 dynes/sec/cm^{-5}
Pulmonary vascular resistance	<34%	78 ± 22 dynes/sec/cm^{-5}
Colloid osmotic pressure	<10%–14%	<22.4 ± 0.5
Respiratory Changes		
Functional residual capacity	<10%–21%	1343–1530
Tidal volume	>30%–35%	600 mL
Renal Changes		
Renal blood flow	>25%–50%	1,500–1,750 mL/min
Glomerular filtration rate	>50%	140–170 mL/min
Creatine clearance	>50%	100–150 mL/min

is disproportionate to the plasma increase, resulting in maternal physiological anemia. Heart rate increases 10 to 15 beats/minute as early as 7 weeks' gestation and returns to the prepregnancy level by 6 weeks postpartum.[2] Changes in blood volume and heart rate lead to an increase in cardiac output of 30% to 50% (6 to 7 L/minute) during pregnancy.[2] Cardiac output increases slightly more intrapartum as a result of the shunting of blood from the placental–fetal unit. Immediately after birth, a larger increase in cardiac output (59% to 80%) occurs when the empty uterus contracts and shunts approximately 1,000 mL of blood back into the systemic circulation[3] (Table 12-2). A woman loses approximately 500 mL of blood during a vaginal birth and approximately 1,000 mL of blood during a cesarean birth.

Development of the uteroplacental unit provides a low-resistance network for the expanded blood volume, which reduces cardiac afterload.[4] The pulmonary vascular resistance, or right afterload, also decreases in response to increased blood volume and vasodilation. Under hormonal influence, smooth muscles and vascular beds relax, lowering systemic vascular resistance. Blood pressure decreases during the first and second trimesters and returns to prepregnancy levels by the third trimester. Blood pressure during pregnancy is affected by maternal position more so than in the nonpregnant state. Supine hypotension occurs when the mother remains in a flat position. The side-lying position is recommended, but if the patient must be supine, the uterus should be tilted away from the inferior vena cava by using a wedge under the hip.

table 12-2 Cardiac Output Changes in Pregnancy and Labor and Delivery

Stage of Pregnancy, Labor, or Delivery	Cardiac Output
By 8 weeks' gestation	22%–30% increase
By 20 weeks' gestation	50% increase
Repositioned from supine to left lateral decubitus	21% increase
Early first stage of labor (dilated <3 cm)	13%–17% increase
Late first stage of labor (dilated 4–7cm)	23% increase
Second stage labor (dilated >8 cm)	34% increase
During each contraction	11%–15% increase
Immediately after delivery (10 min)	59%–80% increase (dependent on type of anesthesia)
Within 1 hr of delivery	49% increase

Respiratory Changes

Respiratory changes as seen in Table 12-1 occur to accommodate the enlarged uterus and the increased oxygen demands of the mother and fetus. Structural changes include the upward shift of the diaphragm, which decreases functional residual capacity, and rib cage volume displacement, which increases tidal volume by 30% to 35%.[4] Airway mucosal changes include hyperemia, hypersecretion, increased friability, and edema. These changes are significant when inserting nasogastric tubes or nasotracheal tubes because of the risk of epistaxis. Respiratory rate remains unchanged, although some women experience tachypnea or shortness of breath at some time during their pregnancy. The exact cause of dyspnea is unknown, but it may be related to hyperventilation, increased oxygen consumption, or decreased partial pressure of arterial carbon dioxide ($Paco_2$).

Oxygen consumption increases by 15% to 20% during pregnancy and may increase by 300% during labor.[5] This results in an increased partial pressure of arterial oxygen (Pao_2) to 104 to 108 mm Hg. $Paco_2$ decreases to 27 to 32 mm Hg and allows for the increased diffusion of carbon dioxide from the fetus to the mother.[5] Renal excretion of bicarbonate causes a slight increase in maternal pH, which is usually insignificant.

Renal Changes

Changes in renal function, also outlined in Table 12-1, accommodate the increase in metabolic and circulatory requirements of pregnancy.[4] Renal blood flow increases by 30% and glomerular filtration rate (GFR) by 50%.[4] These increases allow elevations in the clearance of many substances, such as creatinine and urea, and are reflected in lower serum levels.

Gastrointestinal and Metabolic Changes

Gastrointestinal changes in pregnancy occur as a result of the growing uterus. Displacement of the esophageal sphincter into the thoracic cavity allows stomach contents to enter the esophagus passively. The pregnant woman is prone to passive regurgitation and aspiration, especially when under general anesthesia or any time she may be unconscious.[4] Hormonal influences cause delayed gastric emptying and increased gastric acid secretion in the third trimester. Smooth muscle relaxation contributes to nausea, heartburn, and constipation. Pregnancy creates a diabetogenic state because the body becomes increasingly resistant to insulin and hyperinsulinemia occurs. Hepatic and maternal fasting blood glucose levels decrease owing to the constant transfer of glucose to the fetus. Whenever a pregnant woman fasts for more than 12 hours, the fetus is at risk for ketonemia.[4]

Hematological Changes

Hematocrit laboratory values decrease because of the hemodilution effect of increased plasma volume. Normal hematocrit values are 32% to 40% during pregnancy.[1] The white blood cell count (WBC) is elevated from the normal range of 5,000 to 10,000/mm^3 to 6,000 to 16,000/mm^3.[4] There is an increase in clotting factors VII through X and a decrease in factors XI and XIII, which inhibit coagulation. Fibrinogen increases to 300 to 600 mg/dL. Bleeding and clotting times and platelet counts remain the same in pregnancy.

Fetal and Placental Development Considerations

Clinicians must carefully balance the effects and risks of all treatment decisions on the pregnant woman and her fetus. Maternal circulation and nutrition and exposure to teratogens influence embryonic and fetal development.

There are three stages in fetal development: preembryonic (first 14 days), embryonic (day 15 through 8 weeks), and fetal (8 weeks through 40 weeks/delivery). During the embryonic stage, vital organs such as the heart and brain are in development. It is during this stage that the fetus is most vulnerable to teratogens (Fig. 12-1).

Certain medications used in treating the critically ill pregnant woman may cross the placenta and have teratogenic effects on the fetus. For this reason, the clinician must consider the risks and benefits of medication therapy. In 1998, the U.S. Food and Drug Administration (FDA) revised the five risk categories for labeling drug use in pregnancy (Table 12-3).

The placenta is the organ responsible for the metabolic exchange of oxygen, nutrition, and waste removal between the pregnant woman and the fetus. In early pregnancy, the placenta produces four hormones necessary to maintain the pregnancy. The hormone human chorionic gonadotropin (hCG) is the basis for pregnancy tests and preserves the function of the corpus luteum. Another hormone, human placental lactogen (hPL), stimulates maternal metabolism to supply needed nutrients for fetal growth. This hormone is responsible for the increase in insulin resistance associated with pregnancy. The hormones progesterone and estrogen are eventually produced by the placenta and are responsible for uterine growth and uteroplacental blood flow.

Placental function depends on maternal blood flow. Diseases and conditions that cause vasoconstriction, such as hypertension, cocaine use, or smoking, can diminish blood flow to the placenta and fetus. Even excessive maternal exercise can shunt blood away from the placenta and fetus.

CRITICAL CARE CONDITIONS IN PREGNANCY

During pregnancy, normal physiological changes occur to provide for growth of the fetus and prepare the mother for birth. Medical or obstetrical complications may alter this adaptation and shift an uncomplicated pregnancy into a critical situation. ICU admissions become necessary in 1% to 3% of pregnancies, with the majority of indications being hemodynamic instability and respiratory failure.[6,7] The most common complications requiring ICU admission are severe preeclampsia, disseminated intravascular coagulation (DIC), amniotic fluid embolus, acute respira-

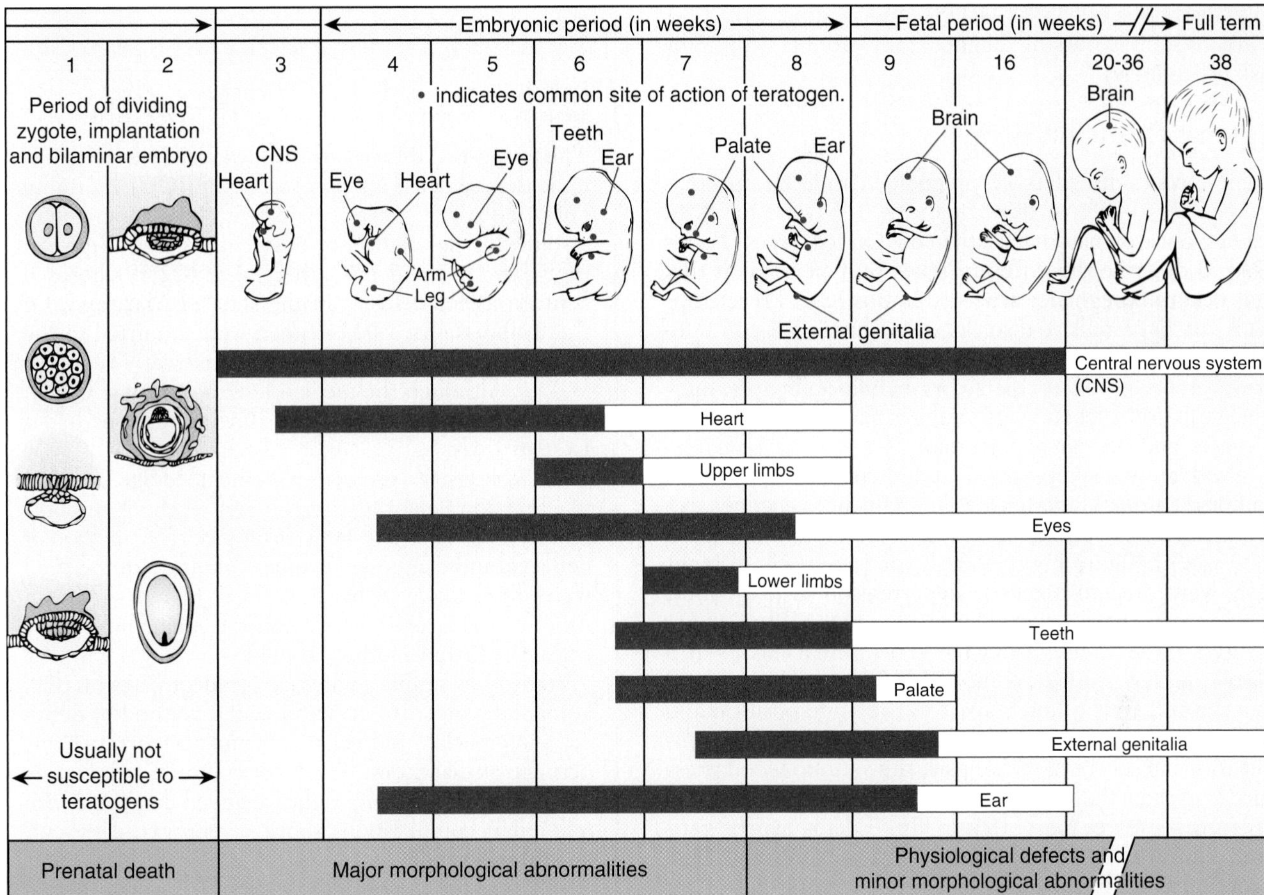

figure 12-1 Critical periods of development. *Red* denotes highly sensitive periods. (Reprinted with permission from Moore K: The Developing Human [6th Ed]. Philadelphia, WB Saunders, 1998.)

table 12-3 **Teratogenic Medication Risk Categories**

Category	Description
A	Adequate studies in pregnant women have not demonstrated a risk to the fetus in the first trimester of pregnancy and there is no evidence of risk in later trimesters.
B	Animal studies have not demonstrated a risk to the fetus, but there are no adequate studies in pregnant women; or animal studies have shown an adverse effect, but adequate studies in pregnant women have not demonstrated a risk to the fetus in the first trimester of pregnancy, and there is no evidence of risk in later trimesters.
C	Animal studies have shown an adverse effect on the fetus, but there are no adequate studies in humans; the benefits from the use of the drug in pregnant women may be acceptable despite its potential risks; or there are no animal reproduction studies and no adequate studies in humans.
D	There is evidence of human fetal risk, but the potential benefits from the use of the drug in pregnant women may be acceptable despite its potential risks.
X	Studies in animals or humans demonstrate fetal abnormalities, or adverse reaction reports indicate evidence of fetal risk. The risk of use in a pregnant woman clearly outweighs any possible benefit.

tory distress syndrome (ARDS), and trauma. Box 12-1 contains sample nursing diagnoses for patients with high-risk pregnancies.

Severe Preeclampsia

Hypertensive disorders of pregnancy occur in approximately 3% to 10% of all pregnancies.[8] They are the third leading cause of maternal death in the United States. Terms used to describe the different types of hypertension that may occur in pregnancy are listed in Box 12-2. Preeclampsia is one hypertensive disorder occurring in 5% to 7% of pregnancies.[9] The etiology of preeclampsia is unknown; however, predisposing risk factors include nulliparity, multiple gestation, diabetes, age younger than 18 or older than 35 years, and chronic hypertension.

Preeclamptic symptoms include hypertension, edema, and proteinuria. Hypertension in pregnancy is defined as a blood pressure of greater than 140/90 mm Hg.[8] In the past, increases of 30 mm Hg systolically or 15 mm Hg diastolically were used to diagnose hypertension in pregnancy. These criteria have become unreliable and should no longer be used. If the prepregnancy blood pressure is unknown, a blood pressure measurement of 140/90 mm Hg obtained twice at intervals 6 hours apart in the same position and using the same arm is appropriate to diagnose this complication. In severe preeclampsia, the systolic blood pressure is greater than 160 mm Hg, and the diastolic blood pressure is greater than 110 mm Hg.[9] Edema may be generalized but is more pronounced in the hands and face. Proteinuria is diagnosed by protein concentrations of 5 g or greater in a 24-hour urine specimen. Oliguria may occur and is defined as a urine output less than 30 mL/hour or less than 500 mL/24 hours. Other symptoms of severe preeclampsia include visual and cerebral disturbances, such as blurred vision and headaches, epigastric pain, impaired liver function, thrombocytopenia, and pulmonary edema.

PHYSIOLOGICAL PRINCIPLES

Severe preeclampsia is associated with vascular endothelial damage caused by arteriolar vasospasms and vasoconstriction.[9] Arterial circulation is disrupted by alternating

insights into clinical research

Panchal S, Arria A, Harris A: Intensive care utilization during hospital admission for delivery. Anesthesiology 92(6):1537–1544, 2000

The purpose of this case-controlled study was to determine the use of the intensive care unit (ICU), mortality rates, and risk factors associated with ICU admission in a statewide population of obstetric women. Between the years 1984 and 1997, there were 822,591 hospital admissions for delivery in the state of Maryland. Of these admissions, 1,023 women were admitted to the ICU (0.12%), and 34 ICU deaths were reported (3.3%). Although the median length of stay (LOS) in the ICU was 2 days, 45% of ICU admissions had a LOS of 1 day.

Variables that were examined included age, hospital of admission (major teaching, minor teaching, or community), race, marital status, insurance type, method of delivery, and diagnoses. Women admitted to the ICU were more likely to be older than 35 years, African American, and cared for in a minor teaching hospital or transferred from another hospital.

Statistically significant risk factors identified with ICU admissions included cesarean as the method of delivery and preeclampsia, eclampsia, and postpartum hemorrhage as diagnoses. The most common risk factors associated with ICU mortality included diagnoses with pulmonary complications, shock, cerebrovascular event, and drug dependence.

ICU use for the obstetric patient is low and developing a dedicated obstetric ICU may not be cost effective. This information may be useful for health care institutions and providers who are involved in planning care for critically ill obstetric patients and planning facilities/resources for them.

box 12-1 *Examples of Nursing Diagnoses and Collaborative Problems for Critically Ill Pregnant Patients*

- Anxiety, Stress related to poor/uncertain pregnancy outcomes
- Anticipatory Grieving related to threat to self
- Fear related to fetal well-being
- Potential Injury related to infection
- Alterations in Family Coping related to hospitalization
- Decreased Cardiac Output related to increased intrathoracic pressures (patient receiving mechanical ventilation)
- Impaired Fetal Oxygen Transport related to maternal position, blood loss, or placental trauma

box 12-2 *Clinical Terminology: Hypertensive Disorders of Pregnancy*

Pregnancy-induced hypertension: Onset of hypertension after the 20th week of pregnancy

Preeclampsia: Development of hypertension after the 20th week of pregnancy complicated by renal involvement leading to proteinuria

Eclampsia: Preeclampsia complicated by central nervous system involvement leading to seizures

HELLP syndrome: Development of hypertension after the 20th week of pregnancy complicated by hepatic and hematological manifestations

Chronic hypertension: Hypertension developing before the 20th week of pregnancy

From American College of Obstetricians and Gynecologists: Technical Bulletin, Hypertension in Pregnancy. Washington, DC, American College of Obstetricians and Gynecologists, 1996.

areas of constriction and dilation. Damage to the endothelium results in leakage of plasma into the extravascular space and allows platelet aggregation to occur. Colloidal osmotic pressure decreases as protein enters the extravascular space, and the woman is at risk for hypovolemia and alteration in tissue perfusion and oxygenation.[8] Pulmonary edema may develop and can be noncardiogenic or cardiogenic. Noncardiogenic pulmonary edema develops because pulmonary capillaries become more permeable and are susceptible to fluid leakage. Cardiogenic pulmonary edema occurs because of an increase in hydrostatic pressure in the pulmonary capillaries; this increase occurs because of fluid buildup in the pulmonary bed.[10] Symptoms of pulmonary edema include coughing, dyspnea, chest pain, tachycardia, cyanosis, and pink, frothy sputum.[10]

Arterial vasospasm and endothelial damage also decrease perfusion to the kidneys. The decreased kidney perfusion results in a decreased GFR and leads to oliguria. Oliguria may not be an indication of hypovolemia and should not be treated with diuretics. Glomerular capillary endothelial damage permits protein to leak across the capillary membrane and into the urine, resulting in proteinuria, increased blood urea nitrogen (BUN), and increased serum creatinine. If vasospasm and hypercoagulability are long lasting, ischemia occurs in the glomeruli. Complete recovery of renal function usually occurs after delivery.[9]

The liver is also affected by multisystem vasospasm and endothelial damage. Decreased perfusion to the liver can cause ischemia and necrosis. The liver may become edematous as a result of inflammatory infiltrates and obstructed blood flow.[11] Liver damage is reflected in elevated liver function study results, such as serum aspartate aminotransferase (AST), lactate dehydrogenase (LDH), and serum alanine aminotransferase (ALT).[1]

Neurological sequelae may include seizures, cerebral edema, and cerebral hemorrhage.[10] Symptoms associated with neurological progression are headaches, blurred vision, hyperreflexia and clonus, and changes in level of consciousness. Increased intracranial pressure (ICP) and decreased perfusion can lead to hypoxia, coma, and death.[9]

MEDICAL MANAGEMENT

The only cure for severe preeclampsia is delivery of the fetus. The decision to deliver the fetus versus continuing expectant management (i.e., to maintain the pregnancy and monitor changes) is individualized.[8]

Usually these patients require invasive hemodynamic monitoring, frequent blood pressure measurements, strict intake and output monitoring, laboratory report monitoring, aggressive anticonvulsant and antihypertensive drug therapy, and, if undelivered, fetal surveillance. Management is focused on preventing seizures and respiratory complications, monitoring cardiovascular status, and maintaining fluid status. If the woman does not deliver, fetal monitoring is necessary. Critical care and obstetrical staff must collaborate to provide close fetal observation.

Hemodynamic monitoring permits accurate assessments of cardiac output and fluid volume status. Normal hemodynamic values during pregnancy are listed in Table 12-4.[12] Elevated pulmonary artery wedge pressure (PAWP) and pulmonary artery pressure (PAP) values may indicate hypervolemia, thereby placing the woman at risk for cardiogenic pulmonary edema. (See Chapter 17 for a more detailed discussion of hemodynamic monitoring.) Interventions to reduce preload include restricting intravenous fluids, repositioning the patient on her side, and administering diuretics when fluid overload or pulmonary edema is present. Decreased central venous pressure (CVP), PAP, and PAWP values indicate hypovolemia, and the patient may need a fluid challenge.

Drug therapy is directed at preventing seizures and hypertensive crises. Intravenous magnesium sulfate is the drug of choice for severe preeclampsia to prevent maternal seizures (Box 12-3). Magnesium sulfate blocks the reuptake of acetylcholine at the nerve end synapses and relaxes smooth muscles. Side effects include drowsiness, flushing, diaphoresis, hyporeflexia, hypocalcemia, and respiratory paralysis.[9] A therapeutic serum level of 4 to 7 mg/dL is maintained through a continuous infusion of 1 to 3 g/hour. Serum levels higher than 15 mg/dL may result in respiratory arrest.

Hydralazine hydrochloride is the antihypertensive agent most commonly used during pregnancy. It causes arterial vasodilation and decreases mean arterial pressure and systemic vascular resistance. Hydralazine increases cardiac output, heart rate, and renal blood flow. Doses are commonly given in 5- to 10-mg boluses intravenously every 20 minutes until a satisfactory reduction in blood pressure is achieved. Other antihypertensive agents used include nitroprusside, nifedipine, and labetalol hydrochloride. These drugs may be used when hydralazine therapy fails.

table 12-4 Hemodynamic Values in Nonpregnant and Pregnant Women

	Nonpregnant	Pregnant
Central venous pressure	5–10 mm Hg	1.1–6.1 mm Hg
Pulmonary artery pressure		
Systolic	20–30 mm Hg	18–30 mm Hg
Diastolic	8–15 mm Hg	6–10 mm Hg
Mean	10–20 mm Hg	11–15 mm Hg
Pulmonary artery wedge pressure	6–12 mm Hg	5.7–9.3 mm Hg
Cardiac output	4.3–6.0 L/min	5.2–7.2 L/min

box 12-3
Magnesium Sulfate Administration

Dose concentration: 20 g in 500 mL normal saline or D_5W = 2 g/50 mL
Loading dose: 4–6 g intravenous bolus over 10–20 min
Maintenance dose: 2–3 g/hr by intravenous infusion

NURSING INTERVENTIONS

The nurse must assess the patient for increased risk of seizures by evaluating neurological symptoms. To reduce the risk of seizures, the nurse can decrease light and sound stimulation to the patient. Treatments and interventions are coordinated to optimize rest periods. If seizures occur, the nurse protects the patient from injury, ensures a patent airway, provides adequate oxygenation, and evaluates possible aspiration.[9] After stabilizing the patient, uterine and fetal activity are quickly assessed. In most instances, immediate delivery of the fetus is indicated.

If the patient is receiving magnesium sulfate therapy, the nurse continuously assesses for symptoms of magnesium toxicity, such as respiratory depression and hyporeflexia. Magnesium is excreted in the urine, and prolonged oliguria allows blood levels to accumulate to toxic levels.[9]

If the patient has delivered, magnesium sulfate therapy should be continued for 24 hours. The nurse must assess uterine bleeding. The uterus should be firm after delivery, and if not, uterine massage and oxytocin therapy are needed. Box 12-4 summarizes some of the key nursing interventions for patients with severe preeclampsia.

case study ■ PREECLAMPSIA

Ms. Vile is a 31-year-old, para 1001 (one previous full-term pregnancy, child is living) at 30 6/7 weeks by dates who has been admitted to Labor and Delivery to rule out preeclampsia. Her blood pressure has ranged from 144 to 167/77 to 98 mm Hg, and she has 4+ proteinuria (by dipstick). She denies headache, visual changes, right upper quadrant pain, nausea, or vomiting. She reports good fetal movement. Initial laboratory results are 24-hour urine 21.7 g of protein and a creatinine clearance of 129 mL/minute, WBC 6.4/mm^3, hemoglobin 10.8 g/dL, hematocrit 32.3%, platelets 180,000/mm^3, ALT 28 U/L, AST 23 U/L, LDH 183 IU/mL, and uric acid 6.2 mg/dL.

Physical examination reveals the following: lungs clear to auscultation; respiratory rate 20 breaths/minute; head, eyes, ears, nose, and throat (HEENT) normal; pulse rate 84 beats/minute and regular; abdomen soft, nontender; extremities slightly edematous; 2 to 3+ reflexes; and weight 138 pounds. The patient was not contracting and the fetal heart rate was 140 beats/minute. An intravenous line was initiated, the patient was placed on strict bed rest in left lateral tilt, and an external fetal monitor was applied.

After several hours of observation, the patient began to complain of a severe headache, blurred vision, and black and green spots in her vision. She was given a 6-g intravenous drip bolus of magnesium sulfate and maintained on 2 g/hour.

Repeat laboratory tests revealed the following: hemoglobin 11.8 g/dL, hematocrit 35.0%, platelets 207,000/mm^3, BUN 14 mg/100 mL, creatinine 0.5 mg/dL, ALT 22 U/L, AST 29 U/L, and LDH 280 IU/mL. The patient's blood pressure range was 100 to 150/50 to 80 mm Hg, and her urine output was 20 to 100 mL/hour. A repeat 24-hour urine was also obtained and the results were 5,643 g of protein and a creatinine clearance of 101.9 mL/minute. The fetal heart rate tracing was reassuring. Observation continued in Labor and Delivery.

On hospital day 4, the patient's blood pressure was 170/102 mm Hg, and her urine output was 50 mL in 5 hours. The patient vomited, and complained of epigastric pain. A central line was placed for better intravenous access. Laboratory tests revealed the following: hemoglobin 11.7g/dL, hematocrit 35.7%, platelets 151,000/mm^3, BUN 20 mg/100 mL, creatinine 0.6 mg/dL, ALT 81 U/L, AST 116 U/L, LDH 280 IU/mL, and uric acid 6.9 mg/dL. On ultrasound, the baby was found to be breech, and the patient was taken to the operating room for a cesarean section. A 2-lb, 8-oz boy was delivered and transferred to the neonatal ICU (NICU).

The estimated blood loss was 1,000 mL, the urine output was 0 mL, and the intravenous intake was 3,700 mL. During surgery, the patient's blood pressure range was

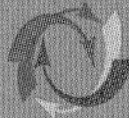

box 12-4 nursing interventions for *Severe Preeclampsia*

Strict Bed Rest in Left Lateral Tilt

- Explain rationale and expected benefits.
- Encourage family and friends to visit and provide activities that may prevent boredom.
- Explain seizure precautions.

Medications

- Explain the action of drugs such as magnesium sulfate and hydralazine.
- Explain the frequency of laboratory tests, vital sign assessment, and urinary output measurement.

Fetal Surveillance

- Explain external fetal monitoring and tests used to monitor fetal well-being, such as the nonstress test, the biophysical profile, Doppler flow studies, and fetal pulse oximetry.
- Explain the rationale used to determine adequate uteroplacental function.

Delivery

- Prepare the patient for the possibility of cesarean delivery.
- Explain the rationale for the need to deliver.
- Explain how neonatal intensive care unit (NICU) works if unable to physically take the patient on a tour.
- Arrange for a discussion with a neonatologist, if the infant is premature or expected to be admitted to NICU.

150 to 160/100 to 115 mm Hg. Laboratory results after surgery were hemoglobin 6.4g/dL, hematocrit 19.3%, platelets 69,000/mm^3, BUN 24 mg/100 mL, creatinine 1.4 g/dL, ALT 140 U/L, AST 23 U/L, LDH 1,143 IU/mL, and uric acid 6.7 mg/dL. Magnesium sulfate administration was continued and two units of packed red blood cells (PRBC) were transfused. No urine output was noted. Intravenous hydralazine was begun for the patient's blood pressure. A Swan-Ganz catheter was inserted. The patient's hemodynamic values were: CVP 6 mm Hg, PAWP 12 mm Hg, mean arterial pressure (MAP) 110 mm Hg, and cardiac output 12 L/minute. Laboratory results were hemoglobin 8.5 g/dL, hematocrit 25.4%, platelets 19,000/mm^3, BUN 36 mg/100 mL, creatinine 3.0 mg/dL, ALT 516 U/L, AST 942 U/L, LDH 6,190 IU/mL, and uric acid 7.9 mg/dL. The patient was transferred to the ICU for continued invasive monitoring and assessment.

Subsequent hemodynamic monitoring revealed the following: blood pressure 138 to 165/81 to 92 mm Hg, CVP 4 to 8 mm Hg, PAWP 11 to 15 mm Hg, cardiac output 12 L/minute, and a systemic vascular resistance (SVR) of 700 dynes/cm/second. The patient's profound oliguria continued. A total of 10 units of platelets were transfused and a Shiley catheter was placed for hemodialysis. On postoperative day 11, the patient's blood pressure was 120/60 mm Hg, her urine output was 50 mL/hour, her CVP was 3 to 6 mm Hg, her PAWP was 7 to 9 mm Hg, her cardiac output was 9 L/minute, and her SVR was 900 dynes/cm/second. Laboratory results were as follows: hemoglobin 8.1 g/dL, hematocrit 24.0%, platelets 121,000/mm^3, BUN 22 mg/100 mL, creatinine 2.1 mg/dL, ALT 15 U/L, AST 34 U/L, LDH 923 IU/mL, and uric acid 6.6 mg/dL.

The patient was transferred back to the postpartum floor. On day 14, hemodialysis was discontinued. The patient continued to improve and was discharged home. ■

HELLP Syndrome

HELLP syndrome (*h*emolysis, *e*levated *l*iver enzymes, and *l*ow *p*latelets) may accompany severe preeclampsia/eclampsia in approximately 10% to 20% of diagnosed cases.[8,9] Maternal mortality rates may be as high as 30%.[13] It is often considered a variation of severe preeclampsia. Women in whom HELLP syndrome develops are usually older than 27 years, white, and multiparous.[8] Patients with HELLP syndrome are at an increased risk for development of complications such as renal failure, pulmonary edema, DIC, placental abruption, acute respiratory distress syndrome, and liver hematoma/rupture.

Signs and symptoms of HELLP syndrome may be similar to those of severe preeclampsia and include epigastric pain, nausea, malaise, and right upper quadrant tenderness. Laboratory results reveal decreased platelets (<100,000/mm^3), and elevated liver enzymes.

PHYSIOLOGICAL PRINCIPLES

Hemolysis occurs when red blood cells pass through vasospastic vessels, producing burr cells or schistocytes.[9] Liver enzymes become elevated as liver damage occurs as a result of ischemia secondary to vasospasm.[1] Prolonged vasospasm can lead to hepatic necrosis. Platelets are consumed because of the aggregation at endothelial damage sites.

MANAGEMENT

As with severe preeclampsia, delivery is the treatment of choice for HELLP syndrome; however, the timing of delivery remains controversial. If the woman remains undelivered, management includes bed rest, frequent blood pressure assessments, frequent laboratory evaluation of liver function, coagulation status, and intensive fetal surveillance.[9] The patient is managed in the same manner as severe preeclampsia, and magnesium sulfate and antihypertensive agents are given as needed. Blood products may be given to correct coagulation abnormalities.[14]

HELLP syndrome may mimic other disease entities and differential diagnosis must be made to rule out autoimmune thrombocytopenic purpura, chronic renal disease, pyelonephritis, cholecystitis, gastroenteritis, hepatitis, pancreatitis, thrombotic thrombocytopenic purpura (TTP), hemolytic–uremic syndrome (HUS), or acute fatty liver disease of pregnancy.[1]

Monitoring changes in vital signs, bleeding, pain, and laboratory values is necessary when caring for patients with HELLP syndrome. Fetal surveillance is important and should include assessments for fetal heart rate and signs and symptoms of placental abruption. Nurses must be aware of the complications that can occur in patients with HELLP syndrome. Signs of worsening pain, vascular collapse, or shock may indicate liver hematoma/rupture. Accurate monitoring of intake and output must be maintained to assess renal status.

Disseminated Intravascular Coagulation

Several conditions predispose a pregnant woman to DIC because of changes in the coagulation and fibrinolytic systems. These conditions include preeclampsia, abruptio placentae, amniotic fluid embolus, fetal death, and sepsis.[15] Although the incidence of sepsis has decreased because of antibiotic therapy, it is responsible for 3% to 8% of the maternal deaths in the United States.[16] Sepsis during pregnancy is a result of bacterial invasion of the uterine cavity. Immunosuppression is a normal consequence of pregnancy and thought to occur so that the fetus is not rejected by the maternal immune system. This alteration increases the susceptibility to infection and decreases the body's ability to fight infection. Septic shock may develop in a few days or several hours. Manifestations of septic shock include tachycardia, tachypnea, temperature instability, increased cardiac output, and decreased peripheral resistance.

Abruptio placentae is the premature separation of the placenta from the uterine wall and is one of the most common causes of DIC. Blood collects between the uterus and placenta, causing consumption of clotting factors. The placental unit contains high concentrations of thromboplastin. When the placenta prematurely separates, thromboplastin continues to be released systemically, activating the clotting and fibrinolytic systems throughout the body. Parallel to the activation of the fibrinolytic system, the hemostatic system initiates clot formation at the site of the separation.[17] Clinical signs of abruption include acute abdominal pain, uterine tenderness, premature contractions, and vaginal bleeding. Abruptions may be subtle, and blood may not be visible.

Intrauterine fetal death can also lead to DIC. Tissue thromboplastin is released from the dead fetus into the maternal circulation activating the procoagulant system. Coagulopathy is gradual and consistent with chronic, low-grade DIC.[15]

MANAGEMENT

Management of patients with DIC includes identifying the underlying condition and initiating appropriate therapy, evaluating and monitoring the coagulation system to restore hemostasis, and preventing further hemorrhage and thrombosis. Management of DIC due to sepsis includes prompt delivery of the fetus and intravenous administration of broad-spectrum antibiotics. For abruptio placentae, prompt delivery of the fetus is necessary to control further bleeding.

Nursing care is aimed at preventing further bleeding, monitoring coagulation studies, and assessing the patient for multisystem involvement, altered tissue perfusion, and fluid volume deficits.[17] Nursing care includes monitoring respiratory status, administering intravenous fluids to prevent hypovolemia, assessing hemodynamic values, and administering and evaluating antibiotics, blood replacement products, and antipyretics.[17] (See Chapter 49 for a more detailed discussion of DIC.)

Amniotic Fluid Embolism

Amniotic fluid embolism (AFE) is responsible for approximately 10% of maternal deaths in the United States.[15] AFE occurs when amniotic fluid gains entry into the maternal circulation. This entry may occur during cesarean section or uterine rupture, or through small tears in the endocervical veins during a vaginal delivery. Once amniotic fluid enters the maternal circulation, it is rapidly transported to the pulmonary vasculature, resulting in pulmonary emboli. The pulmonary response to AFE is vasospasm, which produces transient pulmonary hypertension and profound hypoxia. The maternal system becomes hemodynamically compromised, similar to anaphylactic shock, with elevated PAP and left ventricular failure.[15] Predisposing factors that may lead to AFE include preeclampsia, multiple gestation, polyhydramnios (excess amniotic fluid), low insertion of placenta, post-term pregnancy, hypertonic contractions during labor, abruptio placentae, uterine rupture, maternal seizures, and umbilical cord prolapse. Clinical manifestations of AFE include sudden onset of dyspnea, cyanosis, and hypotension, followed by cardiopulmonary arrest.

MANAGEMENT

Management of AFE is directed at maintaining left ventricular output and an adequate airway.[15] Interventions include intubation and ventilation with 100% oxygen, intravenous administration of vasopressors and crystalloid fluids, cardiopulmonary resuscitation (CPR), administration of blood products, and pulmonary artery catheterization. In extreme cases, extracorporal membrane oxygenation (ECMO) may be used to provide adequate oxygenation and ventilatory support during treatment of the AFE. Potential sequelae include acute pulmonary edema, respiratory distress, DIC, hemorrhage, and multisystem failure.

The nurse must react quickly when AFE is suspected. Following the basic ABCs (airway, breathing, and circulation), the nurse can prioritize interventions needed in this stressful situation. If the patient is not intubated, oxygen must be administered using a face mask and oxygen saturation assessed using a pulse oximeter. The nurse can anticipate that after intubation, a resuscitation bag or mechanical ventilation will be needed. To maximize venous return, the woman should be positioned on her side or a wedge placed under her hip. A large-bore intravenous line is needed to administer intravenous fluids and blood products and to correct hypotension. Assessment is focused on the cardiovascular, pulmonary, hematological, and neurological systems.

Acute Respiratory Distress Syndrome

Acute respiratory distress syndrome (ARDS) is characterized by progressive respiratory distress, severe hypoxemia, low lung compliance, noncardiogenic pulmonary edema, and diffuse infiltrates on chest radiography.[5] Precipitating factors of ARDS associated with pregnancy include abruptio placentae, severe preeclampsia, pyelonephritis, DIC, sepsis, AFE, aspiration, systemic infections, and fetal death in utero.[5] Maternal hypoxemia can lead to spontaneous labor and fetal hypoxia, acidosis, and death; therefore, it should be aggressively managed. Perfusion to vital organs, including the fetus, must be maintained to reduce morbidity and mortality.

MANAGEMENT

Pregnant women with ARDS require cardiovascular support and mechanical ventilation using positive end-expiratory pressure (PEEP).[5] Hemodynamic monitoring is essential for evaluating changes associated with ARDS, such as central hypovolemia and noncardiogenic pulmonary edema. Ventilator settings include a rate of 12 breaths/minute, a tidal volume of 12 to 15 mL/kg body weight, 100% oxygen, and a PEEP of 5 cm H_2O.

Nursing care of pregnant women with ARDS is primarily supportive. Interventions are directed at optimizing oxygen transport to tissues and restoring pulmonary capillary integrity.[15] A complete respiratory assessment is made, including evaluation of arterial oxygen saturation using pulse oximetry; observation of respiratory rate, character, and effort; and auscultation of lungs. While the symptoms of noncardiogenic pulmonary edema are similar to cardiogenic pulmonary edema (i.e., tachypnea, tachycardia, rales, shortness of breath), the nurse should be aware that a decrease in PAWP and PAP (from the obstetrical normal; see Table 12–4) may indicate noncardiogenic pulmonary edema. Noncardiogenic pulmonary edema in obstetrical patients can be caused by aspiration of gastric contents, sepsis, blood transfusion reactions, DIC, and amniotic fluid embolism. Nursing interventions to improve uteroplacental blood flow include positioning the patient on her side and maintaining adequate fluid volumes.[15]

Nursing care for women who are mechanically ventilated includes psychosocial support to help relieve anxiety, fear, and separation from family. Nurses can facilitate communication between the patient and family and keep them informed about maternal and fetal conditions.

In extreme cases of ARDS in the postpartum period, ECMO may be used to provide adequate oxygenation and ventilatory support.

Trauma

Accidental injuries occur in 6% to 7% of all pregnancies and are associated with spontaneous abortion, preterm labor, abruptio placentae, and fetal death. Trauma is the leading cause of nonobstetrical maternal death.[18] Common types of trauma include blunt trauma from motor vehicle accidents (67%), falls, and domestic violence (10% to 31%), and penetrating trauma from stab wounds or gunshots (13% to 22%).[18] Fetal survival depends on maternal survival, so immediate care and stabilization of the pregnant woman are essential.

Hemodynamic instability may not be initially apparent because of the normal physiological cardiovascular changes during pregnancy. A pregnant woman can lose up to 2,000 mL of blood before becoming hemodynamically unstable.[18]

MANAGEMENT

Management consists of immediate stabilization and care. Immediate stabilization of all trauma patients consists of applying the ABCs of resuscitation: establishment of airway, breathing, and circulation. First an airway is established, and oxygen is provided at a rate of 10 to 12 L/minute to produce a Pa_{O_2} level of 60 mm Hg or higher. This Pa_{O_2} level is necessary for optimal fetal oxygenation. A nasogastric tube should be inserted to avoid aspiration.

If CPR is necessary, the anatomical and physiological changes in pregnancy must be considered to maximize efforts.[19] The uterus compresses major abdominal vessels and displaces abdominal contents, which decreases chest compliance. Placing a wedge under the woman's right hip displaces the uterus and decompresses the vessels. Standard Advanced Cardiac Life Support (ACLS) procedures are used, including defibrillation and most drugs. The administration of vasopressors should be avoided because the vasoconstrictive action can impair uteroplacental perfusion.[18] Medical antishock trousers (MAST) or pneumatic antishock garment (PASG) equipment may be used, but the abdominal compartment should not be inflated.[19]

Intravenous access using large-bore catheters is needed, and aggressive intravenous infusions are used to increase stroke volume and maintain cardiac output. If hemorrhage occurs, bleeding must be controlled. A decrease in arterial blood pressure may not be an indication of hypovolemia because of low resistance in the uteroplacental system. A 30% to 35% loss can occur with severe consequence to the fetus before hypotension is noted. Fluid replacement therapy must be administered at a higher rate.[19]

Once the pregnant woman has been stabilized, her neurological status is assessed. After this assessment, a fetal assessment, including determination of life, is made. The fetal heart rate can be auscultated using a fetoscope, stethoscope, fetal Doppler, or ultrasound. Additional assessments can be made on arrival at the hospital or trauma center. These assessments include electrocardiography, a complete physical examination, and laboratory tests, such as arterial blood gases (ABGs; Table 12-5), complete blood count (CBC), platelet count, electrolytes, blood type and cross-match, and the Kleihauer-Betke test. The Kleihauer-Betke test identifies red blood cells from the fetus that have entered the maternal circulatory system and quantifies fetomaternal hemorrhage.[19] Assessments should include parameters such as the onset of regular contractions (indicating labor may have begun), vaginal bleeding, and leakage of fluid from the vagina (indicating ruptured membranes).

table 12-5 Arterial Blood Gas Values in Nonpregnant and Pregnant Women

	Nonpregnant	Pregnant
Pa_{O_2}	80–100 mm Hg	87–106 mm Hg
Pa_{CO_2}	36–44 mm Hg	27–32 mm Hg
pH	7.35–7.45	7.40–7.47
HCO_3^-	24–30 mEq/L	18–21 mEq/L

PROVIDING EMOTIONAL SUPPORT

Emotional support is very important to all critically ill pregnant women and their families. If the woman labors in the ICU, her coach or significant other should be allowed to remain at the bedside. When she gives birth, breast-feeding and bonding can be encouraged when feasible. The mother needs access to her newborn and family during this time. If the newborn is not able to be at the bedside, frequent updates about the newborn are important and can be provided by the staff. Providing a flexible and individualized atmosphere to a new family is a challenge in the ICU. The importance of coordinating obstetrical and critical care cannot be overemphasized. Box 12-5 outlines strategies for promoting emotional well-being in high-risk pregnancies.

If the fetus dies as a result of maternal complications, grief support may be needed. The nurse may collaborate with Labor and Delivery staff (who may have additional grief training), psychiatric liaison nurses, social workers, psychologists, psychiatrists, or clergy to offer emotional support to a grieving mother and family.

box 12-5
Strategies for Promoting Emotional Well-Being in High-Risk Pregnancies

- Shift orientation from the health care team to family-centered care.
- Incorporate cultural beliefs into the environment. Maintain family rituals when possible.
- Understand the role of the pregnant woman and her family members and assist them with their tasks to optimize family function.
- Provide names of family support groups.
- Provide information and education to family members.
- Encourage the family when they are coping well.
- Validate the family's emotions.

CONCLUSION

When pregnant women become critically ill and require intensive care, it is essential for ICU nurses to understand the physiological changes that occur during pregnancy. This knowledge can help staff recognize subtle changes, thereby reducing morbidity and mortality. Collaboration between the obstetrical team and the critical care team facilitates appropriate management for both the mother and her fetus. Childbirth is an emotional experience, and nursing care must address the psychosocial needs of these patients. Providing a supportive, family-centered environment is essential in the care of critically ill pregnant women.

clinical applicability challenges

Self-Challenge: Critical Thinking

1. *Compare the parameters that need to be assessed in a patient with severe preeclampsia and determine when the diagnosis of HELLP syndrome becomes evident.*
2. *Compare the cardiac output values of Ms. Vile (in the case study presented in this chapter) with those of a pregnant woman with an uncomplicated pregnancy and a nonpregnant woman.*
3. *Develop a nursing care plan for Ms. Vile that includes the promotion of infant bonding.*
4. *List pertinent nursing priorities for Ms. Vile for days 1 to 4, days 4 to 14, and days 14 to discharge.*

Study Questions

1. *Indications for hemodynamic monitoring during pregnancy include*
   a. *oliguria responsive to a fluid challenge.*
   b. *severe preeclampsia with oliguria and pulmonary edema.*
   c. *preterm labor.*
   d. *diagnosis of HELLP syndrome.*
2. *Initial resuscitation to the fetus when maternal trauma has occurred includes*
   a. *immediate cesarean section delivery.*
   b. *fetal monitoring, oxygen, and amniocentesis.*
   c. *maternal airway management, oxygenation, and fluid resuscitation.*
   d. *all of the above.*
3. *Which of the following complications are associated with amniotic fluid embolism (AFE)?*
   a. *Hemorrhage, pulmonary edema, cardiac arrest*
   b. *Hemorrhage, hypertension, oliguria*
   c. *Increased cardiac output and right-sided heart failure*
   d. *Loss of consciousness, decreased platelets, and increased liver enzymes*
4. *A severely preeclamptic patient is being treated with intravenous magnesium sulfate. Her laboratory results indicate a magnesium level of 9.3 mg/dL. The nurse has also assessed for which signs and symptoms of magnesium toxicity?*
   a. *Heart rate greater than 140 beats/minute, hypotension, and muscle twitching*
   b. *Loss of deep tendon reflexes, respiratory rate less than 10 breaths/minute, drowsiness*
   c. *Increased urine output, epigastric pain, elevated liver enzymes*
   d. *Hyperreflexia, hypertension, and bradycardia*

REFERENCES

1. Clark S, Cotton D, Hankins G, et al (eds): Critical Care Obstetrics. Boston, Blackwell Science, 1997
2. Comport K, Seng J: Aortic stenosis in pregnancy: A case report. J Obstet Gynecol Neonatal Nurs 26(1):67–77, 1997
3. Ridley D, Smiley R: The parturient with cardiac disease. Anesthesiol Clin North Am 16(2):419–440, 1998
4. Harvey M: Physiologic changes in pregnancy. In Mandeville LK, Troiano N (eds): High-Risk and Critical Care Intrapartum Nursing, pp 2–33. Philadelphia, Lippincott Williams & Wilkins, 1999
5. Catanzarite V, Cousins L: Asthma and allergy during pregnancy. Immunol Allergy Clin North Am 20(4):775–806, 2000
6. Mahutte N, Murphy-Kaulbeck L, Le Q, et al: Obstetric admissions to the intensive care unit. Obstet Gynecol 94(2):263–266, 1999
7. Mabie WC: Critical care obstetrics. In Gabbe S, Niebyl J, Simpson J (eds): Obstetrics: Normal and Problem Pregnancies. New York, Churchill Livingstone, 1996
8. Kelley M: Triage and management of the pregnant hypertensive patient. J Nurse Midwife 44(6):558–571, 1999
9. Leicht T, Harvey C: Hypertensive disorders in pregnancy. In Mandeville LK, Troiano N (eds): High-Risk and Critical Care Intrapartum Nursing, pp 159–173. Philadelphia, Lippincott Williams & Wilkins, 1999
10. Dorman K: Pulmonary disorders in pregnancy. In Mandeville LK, Troiano N (eds): High-Risk and Critical Care Intrapartum Nursing, pp 185–200. Philadelphia, Lippincott Williams & Wilkins, 1999
11. Walker J: Pre-eclampsia. Lancet 356:1260–1265, 2000
12. Drummond S, Troiano N: Cardiac disorders during pregnancy. In Mandeville LK, Troiano N (eds): High-Risk and Critical Care Intrapartum Nursing, pp 173–185. Philadelphia, Lippincott Williams & Wilkins, 1999
13. Isler C, Rinehart B, Terrone D, et al: Maternal mortality associated with HELLP (hemolysis, elevated liver enzymes, and low platelets) syndrome. Am J Obstet Gynecol 181(4):924–928, 1999
14. Vigil-De Gracia P: Pregnancy complicated by preeclampsia-eclampsia with HELLP syndrome. Int J Gynecol Obstet 72(1):17–23, 2001
15. Bick R: Syndromes of disseminated intravascular coagulation in obstetrics, pregnancy, and gynecology. Hematol Oncol Clin North Am 12(5):999–1044, 2000
16. Arafeh J: Sepsis and systemic inflammatory response syndrome: Critical complications during pregnancy. In Mandeville LK, Troiano N (eds): High-Risk and Critical Care Intrapartum Nursing, pp 200–214. Philadelphia, Lippincott Williams & Wilkins, 1999
17. Sisson M, Ruth D: Disseminated intravascular coagulation. In Mandeville LK, Troiano N (eds): High-Risk and Critical Care Intrapartum Nursing, pp 214–224. Philadelphia, Lippincott Williams & Wilkins, 1999
18. Stone K: Trauma in the obstetric patient. Obstet Gynecol Clin 26(3):459–467, 1999
19. Henderson S, Mallon W: Trauma in pregnancy. Emerg Med Clin North Am 16(1):209–228, 1998

OTHER SELECTED READING

Brewer JM, Williams PA: Epilepsy and pregnancy: Maternal and fetal effects of phenytoin. Crit Care Nurse 23(2):93–98, 2003

Bridges EJ, Womble S, Wallace M, McCartney J: Hemodynamic monitoring in high-risk obstetrics patients, I. Crit Care Nurse 23(4): 53–62, 2003

Bridges EJ, Womble S, Wallace M, McCartney J: Hemodynamic monitoring in high-risk obstetrics patients, II. Crit Care Nurse 23(5): 52–57, 2003

Deitcher S, Gardner J: Physiologic changes in coagulation and fibrinolysis during normal pregnancy. Clin Liver Dis 3(1):83–96, 1999

DeJong MJ, Fausett MB: Anaphylactoid syndrome of pregnancy: A devastating complication requiring intensive care. Crit Care Nurse 23(6):42–48, 2003

Dekkar G, Sibai B: Primary, secondary, and tertiary prevention of preeclampsia. Lancet 357:209–215, 2001

Finkel M, Nadel E, Brown D: Respiratory distress and hypertension in pregnancy. J Emerg Med 17(6):1039–1043, 1999

Garland M: Pharmacology of drug transfer across the placenta. Obstet Gynecol 25(1):21–42, 1998

Jayasinghe C, Blass N: Pain management in the critically ill obstetric patient. Crit Care Clin 15(1):201–228, 1999

Mackay A, Berg C, Atrash H: Pregnancy-related mortality from preeclampsia and eclampsia. Obstet Gynecol 97(4):533–538, 2001

Mandeville L, Troiano N (eds): High-Risk and Critical Care Intrapartum Nursing. Philadelphia, Lippincott Williams & Wilkins, 1999

Martin-Arafeh J, Wilson C, Baird S: Promoting family-centered care in high risk pregnancy. J Perinat Neonatal Nurs 13(1):27–42, 1999

Minotti D: Pregnancy and atopic diseases. Immunol Allergy Clin North Am 19(1):191–211, 1999

Naylor LL, Toal K, Goodwin SA: Two lives on the line: A case study in obstetric critical care. Crit Care Nurse 22(6):20–26, 2002

Pak L, Reece E, Chan L: Is adverse pregnancy outcome predictable after blunt abdominal trauma? Am J Obstet Gynecol 179(5):1140–1144, 1998

chapter 13

The Critically Ill Older Patient

BARBARA RESNICK

objectives

Based on the content in this chapter, the reader should be able to:

- Explain physical changes occurring as a result of the normal aging process.
- Describe the developmental tasks of the older person.
- Discuss prevalent conditions that affect the major body systems of the older person.
- Explain cognitive changes that may occur in the older patient.
- Compare and contrast delirium and dementia in the older patient.
- Describe assessment indicators of potential abuse or neglect of the older person.
- Describe why the principle *start low, go slow* is important for the older patient in regard to the absorption, distribution, metabolism, and excretion of medications.

Data from the United States Bureau of the Census indicate a threefold increase since 1900 in the percentage of Americans 65 years of age and older (Fig. 13-1). Since 1990, the number of older Americans has increased by 2.6 million, or 8%, compared with an increase of 6% for the population younger than 65 years of age. Although older Americans enjoy good health, many older adults have physical disabilities. Chronic disease is the leading cause of disability among older adults. When older adults have acute exacerbations of their diseases, they often require hospitalization in an intensive care unit (ICU).

As a result, critical care nurses need to understand age-related physiological changes that occur normally with aging. Many physiological processes alter as a person ages. These alterations are progressive and usually are not apparent or pathological. These age-related changes, however, put the critically ill older adult at increased risk for complications. Aggressive nursing care should be implemented, focusing on the prevention of potential problems.

The leading causes of death among older patients are heart disease, malignant neoplasms, cerebrovascular accidents (CVAs), influenza, and chronic obstructive pulmonary disease (COPD). Chronic conditions are prevalent among older people (e.g., arthritis, hearing and visual deficits). With advancing age, these conditions become more common and result in increased hospitalizations. A longer life span has been the single most important cause of the increased numbers of older patients with multiple chronic and acute illnesses.

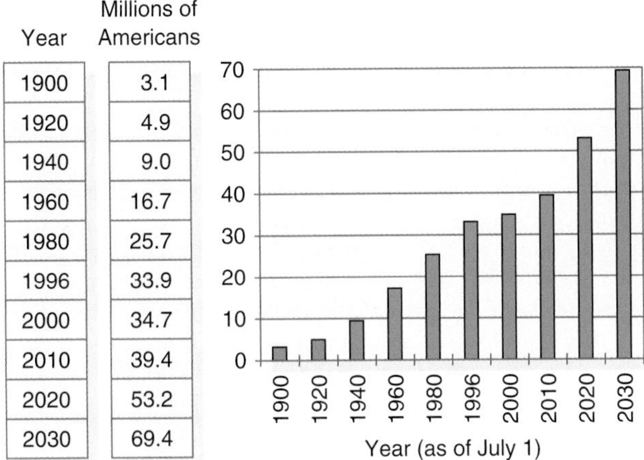

Year	Millions of Americans
1900	3.1
1920	4.9
1940	9.0
1960	16.7
1980	25.7
1996	33.9
2000	34.7
2010	39.4
2020	53.2
2030	69.4

figure 13-1 Profile of Americans age 65 years and older (based on data from the United States Bureau of the Census). Data from the year 1900 to present were used to predict the number of Americans age 65 years and older in the year 2030. (Source: Smeltzer SC, Bare BG: Brunner & Suddarth's Textbook of Medical-Surgical Nursing [9th Ed], p 149. Philadelphia, Lippincott Williams & Wilkins, 2000.)

NORMAL PSYCHOBIOLOGICAL CHARACTERISTICS OF AGING

Biological Issues

Intrinsic aging refers to characteristics and processes that occur universally with all older adults. Changes resulting from the aging process must be distinguished from those resulting from a particular disease process, disuse, or environmental factors, such as ultraviolet radiation. Extrinsic aging is composed of factors that influence aging to varying degrees in different individuals. Extrinsic factors include such things as lifestyle or exposure to environmental influences. Normal aging is defined as the sum of intrinsic aging, extrinsic aging, and idiosyncratic or individual genetic factors specific to each individual.[1]

In most physiological systems, the normal aging processes do not result in significant impairment or dysfunction in the absence of disease and under resting conditions. It is only in response to stress that an age-related reduction in physiological reserves causes a loss of homeostatic balance. The following are some examples of intrinsic age changes:

- Reduced resistance to stress
- Poor tolerance to extremes of heat and cold because of hypothalamic and skin changes
- Reduced sensory perceptions
- Greater fluctuation in blood pH

Aging, in one organ or the entire body, may be premature or delayed in relation to actual chronological age. The effect of aging on cellular tissues is asymmetrical. For example, the changes resulting from aging in relation to the brain, bone, cardiovascular, and lung tissues may be fairly obvious, whereas changes affecting the liver, pancreas, gastrointestinal tract, and muscle tissues are less obvious. Several organic changes that result from aging are listed in Box 13-1.

box 13-1

Organic Changes With Aging

- The amount of connective and collagen tissue is increased.
- Cellular elements in the nervous system, muscles, and other vital organs disappear.
- The number of normally functioning cells is reduced.
- The amount of fat is increased.
- Oxygen use is decreased.
- During rest, the amount of blood pumped is decreased.
- Less air is expired by the lungs.
- Excretion of hormones is decreased.
- Sensory and perceptual activity is decreased.
- Absorption of lipids, proteins, and carbohydrates is decreased.
- Presbyesophagus occurs.
- The arterial lumen thickens.

Psychosocial Issues

In addition to physical signs of aging, nurses caring for acutely ill older patients must be aware of the older person's normal developmental tasks and the specific dreams or wishes of a particular senior. Developmental tasks of older people are listed in Box 13-2.

The need for support and meaningful relationships continues throughout life. Support can be described as a feeling of belonging or a belief that one is an active participant in the surrounding world. The feeling of mutuality with others in the environment lends strength and

box 13-2

Developmental Tasks of the Older Person

- Deciding where and how to live for his or her remaining years
- Preserving supportive, intimate, and satisfying relationships with spouse, family, and friends
- Maintaining an adequate and satisfying home environment relative to health and economic status
- Providing sufficient income
- Maintaining a maximum level of health
- Attaining comprehensive health and dental care
- Maintaining personal hygiene
- Maintaining communication and adequate contact with family and friends
- Maintaining social, civic, and political involvement
- Initiating new interests (in addition to former activities) that increase status
- Recognizing and feeling that he or she is needed
- Discovering the meaning in life after retirement and when confronted with illness of self or spouse and death of spouse and other loved ones; adjusting to death of loved ones
- Developing a significant philosophy of life and discovering comfort in a philosophy or religion

helps decrease the sense of isolation. Support by family, friends, and the community can provide an older patient with a greater sense of stability and security.

Self-worth and perceived well-being are feelings that usually coincide in older adults. The perception of well-being arises from the satisfaction of meeting an acceptable proportion of one's life goals. It can be described as an inner contentment one has in life as a whole. Related to this, a feeling of self-worth is derived not only from a sense of well-being, but from satisfaction with one's image or acceptance by others. Self-worth also reflects the quality of interactions with family and friends.

Family environment for the older adult includes, among others, dimensions of interpersonal relationships, personal growth, integrity of the family unit, and adaptation to stress. As family members age, all of these areas of concern intensify because of changes in roles of family members, alterations in the family power structure, and changes in financial and decision-making dynamics. Acute illness increases the urgency for effective cooperation among all family members as the traditional family structure is suddenly challenged.

When older patients are admitted to intensive care, issues of family cohesion and adaptability often surface. Frequently, families face immediate changes in roles, with adult children and grandchildren assuming the roles of caretakers and nurturers for the older family members. The family must suddenly adjust to dramatically different demands. Frequent visits to the hospital; dialogues with nurses, physicians, and social workers; and efforts to support and communicate with the patient become primary tasks. Amid these activities, family members (particularly those who have been given power of attorney) find themselves being pressed for decisions about immediate and long-term care. At this time, the issue of the individual's end-of-life care preferences, competency, and ability to be involved in treatment decisions may arise. Effective communication and a willingness to listen to and respect the wishes of the older patient become foremost. If this is achieved, the stress on families is reduced because of increased acceptance of the plan of care by all family members.

PHYSICAL CHALLENGES

Chronic changes in one organ system may be associated with changes in other systems. Moreover, there is individual variation in age-related changes. Therefore, each person must be evaluated based on the age-related changes actually present rather than on those that are "normal" for a particular age.

It is equally important to distinguish age-related changes from those associated with a chronic disease or acute illness and to avoid prematurely attributing some findings to age if they are caused by illness. A discussion of the effects of aging on various body systems follows; age-related changes and the clinical implications of these changes are summarized in Table 13-1.

Auditory Changes

With age there is a change in the shape of the ear such that the auricle becomes elongated and broader, the cartilage is less elastic and less flexible, and tophi may appear on the pinna. The hairs on the external ear canal become longer and more coarse, the tympanic membrane is thicker and more fixed, and there are fewer cerumen glands (leading to thicker, drier cerumen). In the cochlea, hair cells, neuron-supporting cells, ganglion cells, and fibers are decreased, causing decreased hearing and balance. It is estimated that 7 million people older than 65 years have significant hearing loss, and continuation of current trends indicates that by 2000, more than 11 million people will have this problem.[2] Specifically, the aging process affects hearing in two critical ways: reduction in threshold sensitivity and reduction in the ability to understand speech. Threshold elevations that occur between 8,000 and 20,000 Hz are not detectable with a routine hearing test. Therefore, hearing loss because of aging or other factors is not documented clinically until frequencies are at or below 8,000 Hz.

Presbycusis is defined as a sensorineural hearing loss and is the most common form of hearing loss in older adults. Presbycusis is characterized by a gradual, progressive, bilateral, symmetrical, high-frequency sensorineural (perceptive) hearing loss with poor speech discrimination. Sensorineural hearing loss is due to degeneration or changes in the neural receptors in the cochlea, cranial nerve VIII (the acoustic nerve), and the central nervous system (CNS). Treatment may vary dramatically from simple removal of impacted earwax to surgical removal of an auditory nerve tumor. Thirteen percent of people 65 years of age and older, if tested, would show signs of presbycusis.[3] Conductive hearing loss is due to the blockage of sound transmission from the external ear through the tympanic membrane and small bones in the middle ear. Like presbycusis, conductive hearing loss is commonly found in older adults, and it is not unusual for older people to have both sensorineural and conductive hearing loss.

FINDINGS ON PHYSICAL EXAMINATION AND MANAGEMENT

The ear canal of the older adult should be evaluated at regular intervals (every few months) because of the tendency to have thicker, drier cerumen, which can occlude the canal and affect hearing. The older patient may retain the ability to hear pure tones, but if these pure tones are grouped to form words, the ability to understand and perceive these sounds as intelligible speech may be lost. This loss is known as *impairment of discrimination ability*. The patient has increased difficulty hearing high-frequency, stimuli-sibilant sounds (*-f-*, *-s-*, *-th-*, *-ch-*, and *-sh-*). Noisy environments further hamper the ability to hear certain sounds. Therefore, the individual may respond inappropriately to questions, withdraw, or frequently ask for the speaker to repeat what is said. Eliminating background noise, speaking lower and louder, and using multiple means of getting information across (e.g., verbal as well as written formats) can facilitate communication. These individuals may also have problems with balance during transfers and ambulation, and experience frequent falls. Activity and exercise interventions should be implemented as soon as possible to strengthen muscles and bones and improve balance.

Visual Changes

Like all other body systems, the eye is affected by aging. Structural and functional changes occur slowly and gradually. Visual perception depends on the integration of

table 13-1 Summary of Age-Related Changes, Clinical Implications, and Key Nursing Interventions

System	Clinical Implications	Key Nursing Interventions
Cardiovascular		
• Atrophy of muscle fibers that line the endocardium • Atherosclerosis of vessels • Increased systolic blood pressure • Decreased compliance of the left ventricle • Decreased number of pacemaker cells • Decreased sensitivity of baroreceptors	• Increased blood pressure • Increased emphasis on atrial contraction with an S_4 heard • Increased arrhythmias • Increased risk of hypotension with position change • Valsalva maneuver may cause a drop in blood pressure • Decreased exercise tolerance	• To prevent falls related to positional hypotension, make sure the person changes position slowly and waits before ambulating.
Neurologic		
• Decreased number of neurons and increase in size and number of neuroglial cells • Decline in nerves and nerve fibers • Atrophy of the brain and increase in cranial dead space • Thickened leptomeninges in spinal cord	• Increased risk for neurological problems: cerebrovascular accident (CVA), parkinsonism • Slower conduction of fibers across the synapses • Modest decline in short-term memory • Alterations in gait pattern: wide based, shorter stepped, and flexed forward • Increased risk of hemorrhage before symptoms are apparent	• To compensate for the decline in short-term memory, provide more time to complete memory-associated tasks.
Respiratory		
• Decreased lung tissue elasticity • Thoracic wall calcification • Cilia atrophy • Decreased respiratory muscle strength • Decreased partial pressure of arterial oxygen (Pao_2)	• Decreased efficiency of ventilatory exchange • Increased susceptibility to infection and atelectasis • Increased risk of aspiration • Decreased ventilatory response to hypoxia and hypercapnia • Increased sensitivity to narcotics	• To prevent infection and atelectasis, encourage deep breathing and coughing.
Integumentary		
• Loss of dermal and epidermal thickness • Flattening of papillae • Atrophy of sweat glands • Decreased vascularity • Collagen cross-linking • Elastin regression • Loss of subcutaneous fat • Decreased melanocytes • Decline in fibroblast proliferation	• Thinning of skin and increased susceptibility to tearing • Dryness and pruritus • Decreased sweating and ability to regulate body heat • Increased wrinkling and laxity of the skin • Loss of fatty pads protecting bone and resulting in pain • Increased need for protection from the sun • Increased time for healing of wounds	• To prevent damage to fragile skin, avoid shearing forces. • To counteract dryness, immerse skin in water daily and apply emollients. • To minimize pain, pad thinned areas with additional layers (e.g., extra socks for feet). • Encourage sunscreen use.
Gastrointestinal		
• Decreased liver size • Less efficient cholesterol stabilization *and* absorption • Fibrosis and atrophy of salivary glands • Decreased muscle tone in bowel • Atrophy of and decrease in number of taste buds • Slowing in esophageal emptying • Decreased hydrochloric acid secretion • Decreased gastric acid secretion • Atrophy of the mucosal lining • Decreased absorption of calcium	• Change in intake due to decreased appetite • Discomfort after eating related to slowed passage of food • Decreased absorption of calcium and iron • Alteration of drug effectiveness • Increased risk of constipation, esophageal spasm, and diverticular disease	• Encourage small, frequent meals to avoid discomfort and improve intake. • Encourage fluids and fiber to improve bowel function.

(continued)

table 13-1 Summary of Age-Related Changes, Clinical Implications, and Key Nursing Interventions (Continued)

System	Clinical Implications	Key Nursing Interventions
Urinary		
• Reduced renal mass • Loss of glomeruli • Decline in number of functioning nephrons • Changes in small vessel walls • Decreased bladder muscle tone	• Decreased glomerular filtration rate (GFR) • Decreased sodium-conserving ability • Decreased creatinine clearance • Increased blood urea nitrogen (BUN) • Decreased renal blood flow • Altered drug clearance • Decreased ability to dilute urine • Decreased bladder capacity and increased residual urine • Increased urgency	• To prevent complications from medical therapy, monitor drug clearance and alter dosing as necessary. • Monitor for urinary tract infections.
Reproductive		
• Atrophy and fibrosis of cervical and uterine walls • Decreased vaginal elasticity and lubrication • Decreased hormones and reduced oocytes • Decreased seminiferous tubules • Proliferation of stromal and glandular tissue • Involution of mammary gland tissue	• Vaginal dryness and burning and pain with intercourse • Decreased seminal fluid volume and force of ejaculation • Reduced elevation of the testes • Prostatic hypertrophy • Connective breast tissue is replaced by adipose tissue, making breast examinations easier	• To compensate for vaginal dryness or pain, encourage the use of lubricating creams, estrogen cream, or both. • Monitor for urinary retention in men.
Musculoskeletal		
• Decreased muscle mass • Decreased myosin adenosine triphosphatase activity • Deterioration and drying of joint cartilage • Decreased bone mass and osteoblastic activity	• Decreased muscle strength • Decreased bone density • Loss of height • Joint pain and stiffness • Increased risk of fracture • Alterations in gait and posture	• Encourage resistive exercises to reverse a decline in muscle strength. • Encourage exercise and intake of calcium and vitamin D. • Encourage activity and exercise.
Sensory		
Vision		
• Decreased rod and cone function • Pigment accumulation • Decreased speed of eye movements • Increased intraocular pressure • Ciliary muscle atrophy • Increased lens size and yellowing of the lens • Decreased tear secretion	• Decreased visual acuity, visual fields, and light/dark adaptation • Increased sensitivity to glare • Increased incidence of glaucoma • Distorted depth perception with increased falls • Less able to differentiate blues, greens, and violets • Increased eye dryness and irritation	• Provide materials with large print. • Make sure there is adequate lighting without glare. • Use contrasting colors for print material.
Hearing		
• Loss of auditory neurons • Loss of hearing from high to low frequency • Increased cerumen • Angiosclerosis of ear	• Decreased hearing acuity and isolation (specifically, decreased ability to hear consonants) • Difficulty hearing, especially when there is background noise, or when speech is rapid • Cerumen impaction may cause hearing loss	• Make sure to face the person; use touch and visual cues to facilitate communication. • Evaluate for cerumen impaction, and remove cerumen as necessary.
Smell		
• Decreased number of olfactory nerve fibers	• Inability to smell noxious odors • Decreased food intake	
Taste		
• Altered ability to taste sweet and salty foods, bitter and sour tastes remain		• Use alternative seasonings.

(continued)

table 13-1 Summary of Age-Related Changes, Clinical Implications, and Key Nursing Interventions (Continued)

System	Clinical Implications	Key Nursing Interventions
Touch		
• Decreased sensation	• Safety risk with regard to recognizing dangers in the environment: hot water, fire alarms, or small objects that result in tripping	• Avoid a cluttered environment.
Endocrine		
• Decreased testosterone, growth hormone (GH), insulin, adrenal androgens, aldosterone, and thyroid hormone • Decreased thermoregulation • Decreased febrile response • Increased nodularity and fibrosis of thyroid • Decreased basal metabolic rate	• Decreased ability to tolerate stressors such as surgery • Decreased sweating and shivering and temperature regulation • Lower baseline temperature; infection may not cause an elevation in temperature • Decreased insulin response, glucose tolerance • Decreased sensitivity of renal tubules to antidiuretic hormone (ADH) • Weight gain • Increased incidence of thyroid disease	• Monitor the temperature of the room. • Provide adequate clothing and blankets to keep the patient warm. • Closely monitor blood glucose levels of patients with diabetes.

various neurosensory systems and structures that age at different rates.

Normal changes associated with aging may include a loss of elasticity in the eyelids and subsequent wrinkling, ptosis (upper eyelid drooping), and "pouches" resulting from changes in the tissues beneath the eyelid skin and the subsequent formation and accumulation of fatty tissue. The conjunctiva may develop a yellowish or discolored membrane or become thickened as a result of environmental hazards, such as dust and exposure to drying and irritating pollutants. Arcus senilis, which is a white or gray ring around the limbus (junction of the cornea and sclera), may be related to a high blood level of fatty substances accumulated with advancing age. Although there is a decrease in the

insights into clinical research

Epstein C, Mokadem N, Peerless J: Weaning older patients from long-term mechanical ventilation. Am J Crit Care 11(4):369–377, 2002

As the number of older persons in the United States increases, the number of older adults who experience traumatic injuries and undergo surgical procedures will also increase. In the United States, the percentage of older adults in the intensive care unit (ICU) ranges from 42% to 48%. With greater numbers of older adults requiring intensive care, the use of long-term mechanical ventilation has increased. This study group defined long-term mechanical ventilation as lasting 3 days or more. This pilot study looked at 10 trauma/surgical patients older than 60 years of age who required 3 or more days of mechanical ventilation. The purpose of this study was to describe the clinical course of weaning in critically ill older adults who were receiving long-term ventilation to determine whether differences exist between patients who can be weaned and those who cannot, and whether systemic factors (age) play a role in these differences.

Participants were monitored daily until they were successfully weaned for 24 hours. Available clinical data were collected every day and weaning decisions were made using these data and the Burns Weaning Assessment Program (BWAP). The BWAP is a 26-item checklist of general and respiratory factors to assess readiness for weaning. Results of this pilot study showed that the six patients who could be weaned from ventilatory support were significantly younger (mean age = 70 years, median age = 71.5 years, with a range of 60 to 80 years) than the four patients who could not be weaned (mean age = 76 years, median age = 80 years, with a range of 63 to 82 years). Patients who could be weaned, however, were ready by day 11 of their stay in the ICU, and those who could not be weaned were not ready until day 17.

Results of this study are not surprising and support the findings of other gerontological studies. Older critically ill patients must generate enormous adaptive responses to the stressors of injury to regain hemostasis. Older adults have many of the risk factors that prolong mechanical ventilation, including respiratory muscle weakness, a blunted ventilatory response to hypoxemia, increased atelectasis due to diminished production of surfactant, and a greater susceptibility to infection. The multidimensional and interactive effects of these factors on weaning from mechanical ventilation most likely are more problematic for older patients than for younger patients.

amount of lacrimation with age, overflow of tears may occur because of impaired drainage of the ductal system.

The iris loses its ability to accommodate rapidly to light and dark and develops an increased need for light. With age, the pupil becomes smaller and fixed. The lens becomes inflexible with less complete accommodation for near and far vision, and is the site of cataract formation. The vitreous humor behind the lens may pull on the retina, producing holes or tears and predisposing the older person to retinal detachment. The ciliary muscle becomes stiff, which contributes to the problems of accommodating to distances. By the age of 60 years, presbyopia may develop. Presbyopia is the inability to shift focus from far to near. A possible rationale for this loss is that the older, aging lens is less flexible and cannot easily change shape from the action of the focusing muscle to which it is attached. Dark–light adaptation slows as the pupillary response slows and rods degenerate. As the lens yellows with increasing age, color discrimination becomes less acute, especially in the blue-green tones. Peripheral vision may decline because of decreased extraocular muscle strength, and depth perception may decline because of a thickening lens. Therefore, time must be provided for the person to adapt when moving between dark and light environments and when getting out of bed.

In addition to normal changes in vision, there is an increased incidence of cataracts, glaucoma, senile macular degeneration, and diabetic retinopathy. These diseases must be studied in relation to normal aging of the eye structure.

A cataract is a clouding of the normally clear and transparent lens of the eye. When a cataract interferes with the transmission of light to the retina, some loss in visual acuity may result. The older patient may complain of increased sensitivity to glare, a blurring of vision, halo images, cloudiness, decreased visual acuity, and decreased contrast sensitivity. Risk factors for cataract formation include diabetes mellitus, heredity, ultraviolet-B radiation exposure, smoking, corticosteroid drugs, alcohol use, and insufficient ingestion of antioxidant vitamins. The visual changes can progress to complete loss of vision. Cataracts account for one sixth of all cases of visual impairment in the United States and mostly occur in individuals older than 50 years.

Glaucoma is one of the major causes of blindness and is especially prevalent in the older adult. Glaucoma is due to increased intraocular pressure. This pressure may result in compression of the optic disk of the eye and damage to cranial nerve II (the optic nerve). This results in loss of peripheral vision and visual acuity. Risk factors for glaucoma include African-American race, a family history of glaucoma, ocular hypertension, advanced age, myopia, retinal vascular disturbance, corticosteroid drug use, diabetes mellitus, and vascular crisis (elevation in blood pressure). Age-related changes in the canal of Schlemm, infection, injury, swollen cataracts, and tumors are also etiological factors for glaucoma. Glaucoma is classified based on whether the angle of the anterior chamber is open or narrow and whether the glaucoma is primary or secondary. Primary, open-angle glaucoma is the most common type found in older adults. This type progresses slowly. Narrow-angle closure primary glaucoma is less common and is characterized by a sudden and marked increase in intraocular pressure with accompanying redness and pain in the eye, headache, nausea or vomiting, corneal edema, and decreased vision. Secondary glaucoma is characterized by an anatomical or functional blockage of the outflow channels. These glaucomas can be open-angle (such as those that occur from corticosteroid-induced pressure increases) or closed-angle (such as those caused by a swollen cataract). Early diagnosis is important because the earlier treatment is started, the easier it is to control the disease.

Retinal degeneration, or macular degeneration, is the third major source of visual disability in the older adult. Macular degeneration is a pigmentary change of the macular area of the retina caused by small hemorrhages. Individuals see a gray shadow in the center of the visual area but can see well at the outer border. This condition rarely results in total blindness; however, visual loss can progress to legal blindness. Early symptoms include a slight blurring of vision, followed by a blind spot. Compensation techniques include wearing sunglasses or visors, looking to the side, and use of magnifiers.

Diabetic retinopathy is the leading cause of blindness in the United States. It is caused by the deterioration of the blood vessels nourishing the retina at the back of the eye. Microaneurysms and small hemorrhages in the eye may leak fluid or blood and cause swelling of the retina. If this leaking blood or fluid damages or scars the retina, the image sent to the brain becomes blurred, and the condition eventually can progress to blindness.

FINDINGS ON PHYSICAL EXAMINATION AND MANAGEMENT

The older adult is likely to have smaller pupils, decreased visual acuity, difficulty with depth perception, decreased peripheral vision, and dry eyes. Ectropion and entropion are commonly noted with age. Ectropion is eversion of the eyelid (usually the lower lid) resulting in exposure of the lid, thickening and keratinization, and chronic irritation. Entropion is inversion of the eyelid and results in the eyelashes rubbing against and scratching the cornea. Entropion can result in corneal trauma and scarring and ultimately may result in decreased vision. When cataracts are present, there is opacity of the lens, and the red reflex may be absent during funduscopic examination. The older adult with cataracts presents with dimming of his or her vision, and complains that everything appears clouded. Individuals who have glaucoma present with complaints of blurred vision, halos around lights, or decreased peripheral vision. Funduscopic examination in these individuals shows cupping of the optic disc and atrophy of the optic nerve. Last, older adults with macular degeneration present with a gradual decline in vision, particularly central vision, without a change in peripheral vision. Good lighting, avoiding glare, and using contrasting colors (e.g., black letters on white paper) and large print can facilitate vision. As with interventions for hearing changes, providing information in various ways is effective for facilitating vision and compensating for losses. Selected nursing interventions for people with impaired vision are listed in the Box 13-3.

Other Sensory Changes

Although hearing and vision changes are the most researched sensory changes occurring in older people, there also may be declines in other senses.

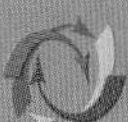

box 13-3 **nursing interventions for *Visually Impaired Patients***

- Identify yourself on approach.
- Approach blind patients from the front.
- Assess impact of failing vision and patient's ability to adapt during hospitalization and after discharge.
- Assess stress level because increased stress can necessitate higher dosages of eye medication for patients with glaucoma.
- Be alert to side effects that other medications may have on the eyes (i.e., medications containing antihistamines, caffeine, and atropine-like substances).
- Provide eye lubrications when eyes are dry.
- Instill all prescribed medications.

The number of taste buds is reported to decrease with age, in conjunction with a decline in the ability to taste substances. Sweet and salty substances are less detectable as one ages; therefore, many older adults complain that food tastes bitter or sour. There is very little information on smell sensation, but it is thought that a decrease in the sense of smell can result from atrophy of the olfactory organ and increased hair in the nostrils.[4] The loss of taste and smell affects the older person's ability to identify food and make odor discriminations.

The threshold of touch varies with the part of the body stimulated. There is a loss of tactile sensation as one ages, although this varies individually. Older adults may not feel the effects of lying too long in one position. A key nursing intervention is to vary the positions of the immobile older patient. The older adult also has decreased kinesthetic sense, which is the person's awareness of his or her body in space. Decreased kinesthetic sense results in postural instability and difficulty reacting to bodily changes in space.

FINDINGS ON PHYSICAL EXAMINATION AND MANAGEMENT

With age, the lips tend to become thin and pale and the tissue of the oral mucosa is thinner, paler, and less elastic. Small yellow sebaceous glands may be seen in the buccal mucosa. The dorsum and margins of the tongue may have decreased number and size of papillae and may be coated with a thin white film. There may also be increased fissures on the dorsal aspect of the tongue, whereas the undersurface is smooth with a bluish-purple hue from increased varicosities. Taste buds and the submaxillary, pituitary, and salivary glands atrophy. The gums are thinner and receded, and there is decreased tooth enamel, dry and less translucent dentin, decreased dental pulp, and diminished perfusion and sensitivity of the gums. Decreased taste sensitivity (especially for sweets and salt) and increased difficulty swallowing food (due to less saliva production) may cause the older adult to present with weight loss. To facilitate taste and improve oral intake, the nurse provides frequent mouth care (before meals), offers foods in a pleasant setting using liberal seasonings to stimulate taste, and encourages the use of interventions, such as sugar-free candies, to stimulate salivation.

Older adults with decreased sensation may present with complaints of increased difficulty performing fine motor activities such as buttoning clothes or picking up objects. They may also have pressure sores and decreased balance. Frequent position changes of older patients are essential and should be instituted every 30 minutes.

Sleep Changes

It is estimated that sleep disturbances occur in more than one half of those older than 65 years.[5] An important aspect of the critical care nurse's assessment is to determine whether sleep problems are the result of normal aging, sleep disorders, or sleep disturbances due to the acute care environment.

Although some age-related changes in sleep patterns are the normal consequences of aging, the prevalence and potential for severe sleep disorders calls for increased clinical awareness and evaluation. Such complaints as habitual snoring, frequent awakening, nocturnal sweating, and awakening with anxiety may be signs of a genuine sleep disorder.

The loss of neurons in the brain may be responsible for the normal age changes in the sleep cycle. These include:

- A longer time to fall asleep
- Increased time spent in the lighter stages of sleep (stages 1 and 2)
- Decreased time spent in the deeper stages of sleep (stages 3 and 4) and in rapid eye movement (REM) sleep
- Increased and shorter repetitions of the sleep cycle

The amount of sleep needed for each individual does not change with age. There is, however, an increased tendency for older adults to sleep less at night, to be somnolent late in the day or early evening, and to awaken early in the morning. This has been referred to as the *advanced sleep phase syndrome*.[6] Older adults also have shortened sleep latency, resulting in daytime napping. Daytime napping further compounds the problem as it reduces the need for nighttime sleep. Common complaints (e.g., anxiety, waking up due to choking, headaches, sweating at night, nocturia, and snoring) are not normal age-related changes and should be assessed more thoroughly.

The most prevalent and most serious age-related sleep disorder is sleep apnea. There is evidence of an association between sleep apnea and circulatory disorders, including hypertension, stroke, and angina pectoris. There also may be a link between sleep apnea and reduced life expectancy. The prevalence of disordered breathing in the older patient is high. Moreover, there may be an association among habitual snoring, stroke, and angina pectoris in older men.[6]

FINDINGS ON PHYSICAL EXAMINATION AND MANAGEMENT

Older adults with sleep disorders present with an inability to fall asleep, an inability to stay asleep, or both. They may exhibit daytime napping, and fall asleep during activities. Conversely, there may be evidence of sleep deprivation with altered mental status being the major presenting sign. Loud snoring with multiple apnea–hypopnea events is indicative of sleep apnea. These individuals may have daytime hypersomnolence, fatigue, irritability, and decreased cognitive function because of impaired nighttime sleep patterns.

Normal aging, chronic illness, and drug therapy increase the older person's susceptibility to insomnia. Treatment depends on the problem. Before drug therapy is considered, poor sleep hygiene habits should be addressed. Good sleep hygiene includes:

- Avoiding daytime naps that are longer than 30 minutes
- Maintaining regular bedtimes and rising times
- Avoiding heavy evening meals, excessive fluids, alcohol, and caffeine
- Increasing daytime activity, even if this is as simple as sitting up out of bed for extended periods of time
- Keeping the sleep environment quiet, sufficiently dark, at a comfortable temperature, and safe

Behavior modification has been used successfully for many sleep problems. The conservative use of medications may be indicated in more problematic sleep disorders, periodic movements of sleep, and dementing illness.[7] Drug treatment is best when accompanied by improved sleep hygiene and patient education about age-related changes in sleep.

Care should be taken in dispensing sedative–hypnotics for people with risk factors for sleep apnea. Nursing interventions include encouraging older patients with disordered breathing to sleep on their sides and to lose weight if obese. Other interventions include giving supplemental oxygen if hypoxemia, caused by chronic lung disease or hypoventilation, is present.

Skin Changes

Although a variety of cutaneous changes have been associated with age, some of these changes are due to normal or intrinsic age factors, whereas others are due to chronic solar exposure.[8] Photoaging is the combined effect of repeated sun exposure and intrinsic aging on the skin, and it is the cause of what is generally associated with the clinical (and histological) changes that are consistent with "aging." With age, there is a thinning of the skin and a decrease in skin flexibility. This puts the older adult at risk for epidermal tearing from shearing forces. Likewise, there is a loss of elasticity resulting in fine wrinkling, looseness, and sagging. Over time, there is a decrease in the number of dermal blood vessels, and these blood vessels become thinner and more fragile. These changes result in the hemorrhaging (known as senile purpura) commonly seen in older adults, in impaired body temperature management and healing of wounds, and decreased absorption of topical treatments. With age, there is decreased density and activity of the eccrine and apocrine glands and decreased sebum production. Overall, due to a combination of skin changes in older adults, there tends to be a quicker breakdown in the skin barrier and a slower recovery of skin integrity. Common interventions to maintain skin integrity are shown in Box 13-4.

FINDINGS ON PHYSICAL EXAMINATION AND MANAGEMENT

The skin of older adults tends to sag, especially on the hands and forearms, and causes underlying tissue injury. The individual may appear pale, and may not be able to correctly perceive surface temperature (e.g., how hot water is). The hair becomes gray and is coarser and the nails may break and become more brittle. Additional hairs develop on the eyebrows, nose, and ears. Wound healing is prolonged and there is increased risk of contact dermatitis due to increased skin sensitivity. Xerosis, or dry skin, is a common problem for the older adult and is the most common cause of pruritus in this group. The treatment for dry skin focuses primarily on the replacement of water, which is the major cause of dryness. Older adults should be encouraged to do the following:

- Maintain a sufficient oral intake of fluid, approximately 2,000 mL of liquids daily.
- Increase bathing time so there is total body water immersion 10 minutes daily, with water temperature ranging from 90°F to 105°F (32.2°C to 40.5°C).
- Avoid the use of soaps.
- Use an emollient after bathing.

Skin lesions are more common in the older adult, and certainly any change in a skin growth or any lesion that does not heal in a reasonable time should be suspect for malignancy. Malignant lesions tend to occur in sun-exposed areas, but may also be present in other areas.

box 13-4 nursing interventions for ***Maintaining Skin Integrity in the Older Adult***

- Avoid shearing forces when turning the patient.
- Turn the patient frequently.
- Keep the patient appropriately covered for warmth.
- Bathe the patient daily, preferably with total immersion in water 32.2°C to 40.5°C (90°F to 105°F).
- Apply oil-based emollient to the patient's skin after bathing.
- Monitor responses from transdermal medications.
- Monitor wounds closely for healing and signs and symptoms of infection.

Cardiovascular Changes

A number of cardiovascular changes occur with aging (see Table 13-1). These age-related changes, overt and occult cardiovascular disease, and reduced physical activity all affect cardiovascular function in elderly persons. With age there is a loss of myocytes in both the left and right ventricles, with a progressive increase in myocyte cell volume per nucleus in both ventricles.[9] With age there is also a progressive reduction in the number of pacemaker cells in the sinus node, with only 10% of the number of cells at 20 years of age still remaining at 75 years. Aging changes in the heart have an impact on afterload, preload, contractility, diastolic function, and the cardiovascular response to exercise.

Afterload is the resistance to the ejection of blood by the left ventricle and is composed of (1) peripheral vascular resistance and (2) characteristic aortic impedance. With age, the large elastic arteries become dilated, with a reduction in compliance. Progressive thickening of the aortic media and intima is associated with aortic enlargement. There is an age-associated increase in arterial stiffness resulting from changes in the arterial media (e.g., thickening of the smooth muscle layers, increased fragmentation of elastin, an increase in the amount and characteristics of collagen, and increased calcification). These structural changes are associated with a reduction in aortic distensibility due to increased aortic stiffness with an increase in pulse wave velocity. The reduction in arterial compliance contributes more to the age-related increase in afterload than does the loss of peripheral vascular beds.

The decrease in vessel compliance affects large and small arteries. As a result, even a small increase in intravascular volume can be accompanied by a substantial rise in aortic pressure (and, in turn, systolic blood pressure), which may lead to pressure-produced ventricular hypertrophy.[10]

Circulating levels of catecholamines increase with age, especially related to stress. Specifically, β-adrenergic vasodilation of vascular smooth muscle decreases with aging, and α-adrenergic vasoconstriction of vascular smooth muscle does not change with aging. The impaired vasodilator response to β-adrenergic stimulation with age is particularly important during exercise.

With aging there is an increase in systolic blood pressure and a widened pulse pressure. A slight reduction in diastolic blood pressure occurs after the sixth decade.[11] The increase in systolic blood pressure is due to an interaction of many factors, with age being only one of them.

Posterior left ventricular wall thickness increases (i.e., left ventricular hypertrophy develops) with age and this is mediated by an increase in systolic blood pressure.[11] This hypertrophy is due to volume, not the number of cardiac myocytes. Fibroblasts undergo hyperplasia and collagen is deposited in the myocardial interstitium. Increased afterload causes an increase in left ventricular systolic stress and the addition of sarcomeres. These changes result in an increased left ventricular wall thickness with a normal or decreased left ventricular chamber size, and an increased relative wall thickness.

Preload is the filling volume of the left ventricle, and is determined by numerous factors that influence blood return to the heart. Resting preload does not change with age,[12] although left ventricular early diastolic filling is reduced with age. With age, left ventricular stiffness is increased, left ventricular compliance is decreased, left ventricular wall thickness is increased, left ventricular relaxation is impaired, and left ventricular diastolic filling is decreased. An age-related increase in systolic blood pressure also impairs left ventricular early diastolic filling, leading to hypotension if preload is reduced. Despite this age-related reduction, preload is maintained because left atrial contraction becomes more vigorous and thereby increases late diastolic filling of the left ventricle.[12]

An age-related increase in left atrial size from increased wall stress counteracts the effects of decreased left ventricular compliance with aging. Left atrial contraction can contribute up to 50% of left ventricular filling in a poorly compliant left ventricle. Consequently, in older adults, development of atrial fibrillation may cause a marked reduction in cardiac output because of the loss of left atrial contribution to left ventricular late diastolic filling.

The intrinsic ability of the heart to generate force does not change with age, although the duration of contraction and relaxation is prolonged in older adults. There is no reduction of resting left ventricular ejection fraction or circumferential fiber shortening in healthy older adults.

Aging is associated with prolongation of isovolumic relaxation time, a reduction in early diastolic filling of the left ventricle, and augmentation of the late diastolic filling of the left ventricle.[12] Also with aging, there is a slowing of the rate at which calcium enters the sarcoplasmic reticulum after myocardial excitation, and a subsequent decrease in relaxation of the left ventricle.[13] Reduced oxidative phosphorylation and cumulative mitochondrial peroxidation occurring with aging may also impair left ventricular diastolic function.

The maximum amount of oxygen uptake ($\text{V}O_2$ max) decreases with age, although the degree to which oxygen uptake decreases is affected by physical conditioning, subclinical coronary artery disease (CAD), smoking, and body weight. With exercise, older adults have a decrease in heart rate, cardiac index, and left ventricular ejection fraction, and increases in the left ventricular end-diastolic and end-systolic volume indices.[14]

FINDINGS ON PHYSICAL EXAMINATION AND MANAGEMENT

In the absence of vascular disease, these changes should not interfere with normal tissue perfusion. In the older patient, however, the likelihood of atherosclerosis is increased. The narrowing of vessels, coupled with their decrease in compliance, may produce tissue ischemia. These changes, along with bed rest, contribute to tissue injury and decubitus ulcer formation.

The increased vascular stiffness of aging causes the upstroke of the arterial pulse to appear more brisk than usual, potentially masking the slowly rising carotid pulse of aortic stenosis. Older adults commonly present with an early-peaking basal systolic murmur of aortic stenosis, typically accompanied by an S_4 sound at the cardiac apex as evidence of reduced ventricular compliance. These individuals report and demonstrate a limited ability to tolerate physical activity. The older patient may also have a greater amount of pooling in the lower extremities because of decreased muscle mass and poor venous return. If the patient is placed on bed rest, this fluid pool is redistributed and may cause an overload in the cardiovascular system. The nurse must be alert for vascular overload and congestive heart failure.

Another factor to consider is the shifting of fluids when a patient arises after having been on bed rest. The sudden shift in fluid to the lower extremities and the lowered fluid volume that results from bed rest can produce extreme lightheadedness. This is further complicated by a decrease in baroreceptor sensitivity with age. A slow progression of head elevation and dangling before moving the patient to sitting or standing is necessary to prevent syncope and possible injury from falling.

Although chest pressure is the classic symptom of angina in older adults, there is an increased incidence of silent ischemia in these individuals. If angina or a myocardial infarction is suspected, a comprehensive history, vital signs, and electrocardiogram (ECG) should be obtained, and a laboratory workup (including cardiac enzymes) should be sent. If at all possible, it is important to obtain a prior ECG for comparison.

About 50% of all older adults have abnormalities on the resting ECG, most commonly PR and QT interval prolongation, intraventricular conduction abnormalities, reduction in QRS voltage, and a leftward shift of the frontal plane QRS axis. Common age-related changes to the ECG are shown in Table 13-2. Elderly men more frequently have major ECG abnormalities than do elderly women, and these abnormalities increase with age.[15]

Respiratory Changes

It is particularly difficult to distinguish age-related changes in the structure and function of the lungs from those changes caused by disease because the lungs are continually exposed to environmental stressors. However, there are some commonly identified lung changes with physiological aging, including dilatation of alveoli, enlargement of airspaces, a decrease in exchange surface area, and loss of supporting tissue for peripheral airways. These changes result in decreased static elastic recoil of the lung and increased residual volume (RV) and functional residual capacity (FRC). Chest wall compliance decreases and thereby increases the work of breathing for the older adult. The most important age-related change in the large airways is a reduction in the number of glandular epithelial cells. This results in reduced production of protective mucus and thus impaired defense against respiratory infection. There are few changes in the bronchi, but the area of the alveoli decreases and the alveoli and alveolar ducts enlarge. The FRC and RV increase, and compliance decreases. There is deposition of amyloid in lung vasculature and alveolar septa, although the significance of this is unclear. Small airways change such that there is dilatation of the alveolar ducts and air spaces, and an increased tendency for the small airways to collapse during expiration. There is as much as a 20% reduction in alveolar surface area with consequent reduction in respiratory reserve. The major age-related change in the respiratory muscles is a reduction in the proportion of type II A fibers with consequent impairment of strength and endurance.

Lung volumes fall gradually with age. Specifically, the forced expiratory volume in 1 second/forced vital capacity (FEV_1/FVC) ratio falls by approximately 0.2% per year.[16] The FEV_1/FVC ratio declines less rapidly in older men than in older women, and maximal expiratory flow and maximum voluntary ventilation (MVV) decline less rapidly in women. The ventilation–perfusion ratio heterogeneity increases and carbon monoxide transfer also decreases with age.

The most clinically important functional changes in the aging respiratory system are:

- The increased tendency for small airways to collapse sooner during expiration
- Reduction in respiratory muscle strength and endurance
- Changes in the monitoring and control of breathing

There is a tendency for older adults to have relative inefficiency in control and monitoring of ventilation. This is especially true with regard to responses to both hypoxia and hypercapnia at rest. The elderly tend to have increased ventilatory response to exercise-induced carbon dioxide production.[14]

table 13-2 Common Age-Related Changes in the Electrocardiogram (ECG)

	Age			
ECG Variable	*<30 yr*	*30–39 yr*	*40–49 yr*	*>49 yr*
R-wave amplitude (mm)	10.4	10.5	9.0	9.3
S-wave amplitude (mm)	15.2	14.2	12.2	12.4
Frontal plane axis (degrees)	48.9	48.1	36.5	38.8
PR duration (msec)	15.9	16.2	16.0	16.2
QRS duration (msec)	7.6	7.5	7.4	8.0
QT duration (msec)	37.8	37.5	37.9	39.6
T-wave amplitude (msec)	5.2	4.6	4.3	4.4

Data from Bachman S, Sparrow D, Smith LK: Age-related changes in electrocardiographic variables. Am J Cardiol 48:513, 1981.

The $\dot{V}O_2$ max declines with age due to a decrease in the diffusing capacity and alveolar capillary volume along with ventilation–perfusion mismatch. Mucociliary clearance is reduced with age, although there is some evidence to suggest that the cough reflex is unaffected by aging.[17] Older adults, however, tend to get more frequent and severe bacterial, viral, and fungal infections, but this is due to pathological processes commonly seen in these individuals, changes in other body systems, as well as some of the functional and structural changes identified.

Pulmonary function studies in healthy older adults have shown an increase in the RV and a decline in the total lung capacity (TLC). The actual declines in FVC and maximum expiratory flow rates are attributed more to changes in body weight and strength rather than to changes in the pulmonary tissue. There tends to be an increase in the partial pressure of arterial carbon dioxide ($PaCO_2$) and a decrease in the partial pressure of arterial oxygen (PaO_2) with age. The gradual decline in PaO_2 is caused by a loss of elastic recoil and a subsequent reduction in airway caliber, early airway closure, and a maldistribution of ventilation.

In spite of all these changes, however, the respiratory system remains capable of maintaining adequate gas exchange at rest and during exertion throughout the life span. Aging does tend to result in diminished reserve of the respiratory system in cases of acute disease. Specifically, decreased sensitivity of respiratory centers to hypoxia or hypercapnia results in a diminished ventilatory response in cases of heart failure, infection, or aggravated airway obstruction. Moreover, decreased perception of bronchoconstriction and diminished physical activity may result in lesser awareness of the disease and delayed diagnosis.[18]

FINDINGS ON PHYSICAL EXAMINATION AND MANAGEMENT

Older adults commonly present with barrel chest (an increased anterior–posterior diameter), which has a significant impact on appearance as well as chest wall compliance (particularly in patients who are supine), and may result in lung sounds being more distant and less discernible. It may be helpful to use a pediatric diaphragm to listen for breath sounds in older adults with predominant ribs. This allows for a more firm application of the stethoscope between the interspaces.

Dyspnea is a very common complaint and the causes may be cardiac, pulmonary, metabolic, mechanical, or hematologic, or due to deconditioning. Increased lung sounds are also common with age and may be due to deconditioning and age-related fibrotic changes rather than acute disease such as congestive heart failure. When evaluating the older adult, it is particularly important to match clinical signs and symptoms of disease with objective diagnostic findings such as chest radiography and laboratory testing.

Pulmonary infections are more common with age because of the changes described previously. Expectorated specimens in older adults, however, are often unreliable because of pharyngeal colonization. To prevent infection, careful attention to nutrition, especially to sufficient calories, protein, and fluid intake, is needed. Moreover, frequent position changes also assist in the clearance of secretions and aid ventilation and perfusion of the lungs.

Renal Changes

Age-associated kidney changes can be categorized as anatomical or functional. Anatomical changes include the loss of renal glomeruli, decreased kidney size, renal tubular changes, and renal vascular changes. There are also functional kidney changes, as described in Box 13-5. The total number of glomeruli decreases by 30% to 40% by the eighth decade. The loss of glomeruli, in conjunction with decreased kidney perfusion, results in a decreased glomerular filtration rate (GFR). A longitudinal study, however, revealed that not all people exhibit a decline in GFR.[19] Changes are likely due to a combination of lifestyle factors and associated chronic illness. The decrease in filtration may result in decreased clearance of substances normally excreted. An increase in blood urea nitrogen (BUN) or creatinine may indicate the extent to which the GFR is diminished. However, creatinine levels from muscle breakdown may be less than in younger patients and could mask an elevated creatinine. Creatinine clearance is a more accurate measure of renal function for the older patient. Evaluation of renal function is extremely important if the patient is receiving drugs normally excreted by the kidney. Table 13-3 provides an overview of normal laboratory values, including renal function, and how these change with age.

With age there is also a decrease in renal blood flow, decreased tubular function, and decreased ability to concentrate urine. Basal renin is diminished by 30% to 50% in older adults. Renin alterations and other renal changes diminish the capability of the older adult to maintain sodium and water balance, especially in the presence of stress. There may also be a lessened response to antidiuretic hormone (ADH), which can result in a decreased ability to concentrate urine. This decreased ability may lead to problems of fluid–electrolyte balance as sodium, potassium, and water are lost. Loss of hydrogen ions may also make the acid–base balance more difficult to maintain.

FINDINGS ON PHYSICAL EXAMINATION AND MANAGEMENT

Older adults tend to have decreased sensations of thirst and consequently drink less fluid. This change leaves them vulnerable to dehydration, especially when medications with

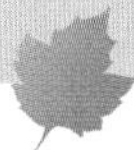

box 13-5

Age-Associated Functional Kidney Changes

- Decreased glomerular filtration rate (GFR)
- Decreased mean creatinine clearance rate
- Increased mean creatinine concentrations
- Decreased blood flow through the kidneys
- Decreased tubular transport capacity
- Decreased functional nephrons
- Decreased concentrating ability
- Decreased diluting ability
- Decreased plasma renin activity
- Impaired sodium conservation

table 13-3 Normal Laboratory Values and Age-Related Changes

Laboratory Test	Normal Values	Age-Related Changes
Urinalysis		
Protein	0–5 mg/100 mL	Rises slightly
Glucose	0–15 mg/100 mL	Glycosuria appears after high plasma levels and is very unreliable
Specific gravity	1.005–1.020	Lower maximum of 1.016–1.022
Sedimentation rate	Men 0–20 mm/hr Women 0–30 mm/hr	Increases with age; no clinical significance
Iron	50–60 μg/dL	Slight decrease
Iron binding	230–410 μg/dL	Decrease
Hemoglobin	Men 13–18 g/100 mL Women 12–16 g/100 mL	No normal decline with age
Hematocrit	Men 45%–52% Women 37%–48%	No normal decline with age
Leukocytes	4,300–10,800/mm^3	No normal decline with age
Lymphocytes	500–2,400 T cells/mm^3 50–200 B cells/mm^3	Both T- and B-cell levels decrease
Platelets	150,000–350,000/mm^3	No change with age
Albumin	3.5–5.0 g/100 mL	Declines because of a decrease in liver size and enzymes
Globulin	2.3–3.5 g/100 mL	Slight increase
Serum protein	6.0–8.4 g/100 mL	No change with age
Blood urea nitrogen (BUN)	Men 10–25 mg/100 mL Women 8–20 mg/100 mL	Can increase with age
Creatinine	0.6–1.5 mg/100 mL	Increases, although this is related to lean body mass
Creatinine clearance	104–124 mL/min	Decreases by 10% per decade after age 40 yr
Glucose	<200 mg/dL fasting	Slight increase in glucose tolerance of 10 mg/dL per decade after age 30 yr
Triglycerides	40–150 mg/100 mL	20–200 mg/100 mL
Cholesterol	120–220 mg/100 mL	Increases with age, more so in women than in men
Thyroxine (T_4)	4.5–13.5 μg/100 mL	No change
Triiodothyronine (T_3)	90–220 ng/100 mL	Decreases 25%
Thyroid-stimulating hormone (TSH)	0.5–5.0 μg/mL	No significant change with age
Alkaline phosphatase (AP)	13–39 IU/L	Increases by 8–10 IU/L, although elevations greater than 20% are likely due to disease
Prostate-specific antigen (PSA)	4 ng/mL	No change with age, although elevated levels may be seen in nonmalignant disease
Uric acid	Men 44–76 mg/L Women 23–66 mg/L	Slight increase with age

diuretic actions are administered. To prevent renal damage, care must be taken to ensure that the hospitalized older patient has adequate fluid intake by oral, enteral, or parenteral routes. Fluid balance may also be precarious because disease states such as diabetes can produce diuresis. Further, potassium and sodium levels may already be low when the patient arrives in the unit. Care must be taken to ensure that electrolyte balance remains stable or is restored. Confusion, dysrhythmias, coma, and death can occur quickly in the older patient with altered electrolyte balance.

As bladder muscle tone is lost, incomplete emptying with retention can foster the development of urinary tract infections that can ascend and become renal infections. Hypertrophy of the prostate gland also places older men at risk for urinary tract infection because the enlarged gland interrupts urine flow. Loss of muscle tone, retention with overdistension, and loss of sphincter control lead to incontinence in the older man or woman. For older patients, this loss of control is embarrassing and disconcerting.

If any type of incontinence or retention develops in an older patient during the stay in the ICU, the nurse should do a comprehensive evaluation to determine the underlying cause of the urinary problem. Specifically, consideration should be given to drugs, metabolic and neurological problems, and bladder inflammation as potential causes (Table 13-4). If an indwelling (Foley) catheter is necessary during acute illness, it should be removed as soon as the primary reason for inserting it (e.g., hourly urine measurements) has passed. Early removal may prevent deterioration of bladder function and urinary tract infection.

Gastrointestinal Changes

The gastrointestinal system undergoes many age-related changes (see Table 13-1). The mechanical and chemical processes of digestion that begin in the mouth may be impaired because of loss of teeth, poor hygiene, and a decrease in salivary secretions. Many older adults experience diminished senses of taste and smell, which may lead to decreased food intake.[20]

Flattening of the gastric mucosae and secretory changes have been noted in normal older adults. This influences active transport mechanisms for calcium, iron, and vitamin B_{12} absorption. The gastrointestinal fluid pH, gastric emptying time, intestinal transit rates, and gastrointestinal blood flow and surface area are all altered in the older adult.

Slowing of peristalsis may interfere with swallowing, gastric emptying, and passage through the bowel. The decrease in hydrochloric acid, digestive enzymes, and bile may contribute to incomplete digestion of nutrients. In some older adults, diminished intrinsic factor and decreased vitamin B_{12} synthesis may produce pernicious anemia.

Data are insufficient to make assumptions regarding changes in absorption in the large and small bowel. Some evidence indicates that absorption is somewhat impaired. Given that the eating patterns of older adults may not include all food groups, deficiencies may arise from lack of intake rather than malabsorption.

The decreased motility of the large bowel is probably not sufficient to produce constipation in the active adult. However, older adults who are on bed rest, have decreased intake of food and fluids, and are exposed to multiple medications may experience constipation and fecal impaction. Dependence on or misuse of laxatives must be assessed when the history is taken because this may further exacerbate the constipation and management of bowel function.

FINDINGS ON PHYSICAL EXAMINATION AND MANAGEMENT

Examination of the mouth in an older adult commonly reveals a wearing of dental enamel and gum recession, thereby exposing more of the teeth and increasing the likelihood of decay. The oral mucous membranes also tend to be very dry, making eating difficult. Swallowing disorders are common and can be due to functional abnormality of the oral, pharyngeal, or esophageal stage of swallowing.

Older adults commonly report constipation, and stool may be palpable in the large bowel. In addition to an abdominal examination, a rectal examination must be done to determine the consistency of stool and the anal tone, and establish an appropriate treatment plan. Heartburn (which may present as chest pain) is also a common complaint and is often associated with epigastric tenderness. Aortic aneurysms are more common in older adults and present as a pulsatile mass in the abdomen.

Acute abdominal pain in this population is a particularly challenging complaint, and causes range from diverticulitis to bowel obstruction, appendicitis, pancreatic disease,

table 13-4 Causes of Incontinence

Cause	Explanation
Drug side effects	
Diuretics	Urgency
Caffeine and alcohol	Diuretic effect and irritation
Sedatives	Inhibition of micturition, functional changes
Anticholinergics	Constipation causing obstruction
Calcium channel blockers	Constipation causing obstruction, smooth muscle relaxation
Nonsteroidal anti-inflammatory agents (NSAIDs)	Blockage of prostaglandin receptors causing decreased force of contraction
Physiological changes	
Hypoxemia	Depressed function of brain
Delirium	Depressed function of brain
Hyperglycemia	Diuretic effect of glycosuria
Hypercalcemia	Diuretic effect of hypercalciuria
Functional impairment	Inability to get to the toilet in time
Bladder inflammation	
Infection	Uninhibited bladder contractions
Atrophic vaginitis	Uninhibited bladder contractions

infarction, or cancer. Even more challenging, however, is identifying older adults with acute abdominal problems because these individuals often present without pain or any other significant signs and symptoms of an acute problem (e.g., fever, anorexia). Careful evaluation of the abdomen in older adults is essential to monitor for acute changes.

Nursing interventions for gastrointestinal changes begin with a careful history. Eating habits, including time and frequency of food intake, food preferences, usual intake, food intolerances, and taste and smell changes must be assessed. Use of laxatives, enemas, and vitamin supplementation also should be explored. Evaluation of the teeth and gums helps to establish how well food can be handled mechanically.

When planning care, the nurse must consider that bed rest slows peristalsis and aggravates any preexisting condition related to motility. Adequate fluid intake, bulk in the diet, use of natural laxatives (e.g., prune juice, warm liquids), and as much active or passive exercise as the condition of the patient allows may help maintain a normal pattern of bowel movements. Stool softeners and mild laxatives may need to be included in the regimen.

Hospitalized patients of any age can become rapidly malnourished secondary to the stress of acute illness, an increased demand for energy, and lack of nourishment. Therefore, it is important to look for indicators of nutritional risk. Indicators include a history of recent weight loss, a diet lacking in protein and calories, an albumin level <3.5 g/dL, and a lymphocyte count $<1500/\text{mm}^3$. The older patient who enters the hospital already mildly to moderately malnourished and who has a poor intake of protein and calories may quickly become severely malnourished. This malnourished state can markedly compromise the immune response and increase the incidence and severity of infection. Therefore, it is crucial to see that critically ill older patients maintain adequate nutritional intake.

Musculoskeletal Changes

Mobility limitations of the older patient may be related to loss of muscle strength. Muscle mass may be lost because of a reduction in the number and size of muscle fibers or an increase in connective tissues. These changes result in less muscle tension and decreased strength of the contraction. The decrease of lean muscle mass and the loss of elasticity contribute to lost flexibility and increased stiffness.

Skeletal calcium losses are a universal concomitant of aging and reflect an imbalance of bone remodeling, with osteoclastic bony resorption exceeding osteoblastic new bone formation. After approximately 30 years of age, when peak skeletal bone mass has been achieved, resorption begins to exceed formation with subsequent skeletal calcium losses and a decline in bone density. The rate of bone loss is approximately 0.5% to 1% yearly from age 60 years onward. The bone changes that occur are likely due to a multitude of factors in addition to normal age-related changes: lack of exercise, poor nutrition, and calcium malabsorption. Known age-related changes in factors influencing bone homeostasis occur in calcium, vitamin D, and gonadal hormone status. Dietary intake of calcium, gastrointestinal absorption of calcium, and vitamin D synthesis are all decreased with age. Decreased intake of vitamin D_2 and decreased skin absorption of 7-dehydrocholesterol as a result of inadequate sunlight exposure also may contribute to vitamin D deficiency with age. The patient on bed rest may rapidly lose bone mineral concentration. The calcaneus (heel) and spine are most susceptible, with a loss of approximately 1% per week. This loss is related to lack of weight bearing.

Musculoskeletal function is dictated largely by the size of the muscle mass that is contracting, and to a lesser extent by changes in surrounding connective tissue in the joint and neural recruitment, conduction velocities, and fatigue. Sedentary individuals lose large amounts of muscle mass over time. Unfortunately, muscle mass cannot be maintained into old age even with habitual aerobic activities in either normal or athletic adults.[21] Only loading of muscle with weight-lifting exercise has been shown to reverse muscle mass loss and strength in older adults.[22,23] There is also a decrease in oxidative and glycolytic enzyme capacity with age, a decrease in total number of muscle fibers, selective atrophy of type 2 (fast-twitch) fibers, and shortening of tendons and ligaments with decreased tissue elasticity. Bone changes, as evidenced by osteoporosis, present with decreased height, kyphosis, and scoliosis.

FINDINGS ON PHYSICAL EXAMINATION AND MANAGEMENT

Older adults with osteoporosis may have spontaneous fractures, occurring simply from moving in bed. In general, older adults have a decrease in overall muscle strength and an increased tendency to have muscle cramping. Crepitus and pain with range of motion of the joints is common, particularly in the weight-bearing joints (e.g., the knee). Gait and posture changes are frequently present and older adults tend to have a stooped posture with a slow, shuffling gait.

Forced fasting of the critically ill hospitalized patient may further accelerate muscle loss through catabolism and gluconeogenesis. The added burden of bed rest leads to a rapid loss of mobility, strength, and energy in the older patient. Maintaining nutrition, changing position frequently, active and passive exercise, and getting out of bed as much as permitted by condition are essential to preserving strength, energy, and bone mass. If the patient is comatose or has suffered loss of function, proper positioning and splinting can help prevent permanent deformity.

Endocrine Changes

The equilibrium concentrations of the principal hormones are not necessarily altered with age; however, for older adults, there may be a change in how hormonal equilibrium is achieved. With advancing age, therefore, some alterations in hormone production, metabolism, and action are found. There are subtle changes noted in pituitary dynamics, adrenal gland physiology, and thyroid function; however the changes in glucose homeostasis, reproductive function, and calcium metabolism are more apparent.[24]

Most of the principal neuroendocrine nuclei in the hypothalamus are structurally intact in old age, although there is some loss of morphologic integrity of the suprachiasmatic nucleus. Morphometric variables associated with increased cellular functional activity have been measured in several hypothalamic nuclei. Certain neurons in the human paraventricular nuclei seem activated, and the neurons that produce arginine vasopressin (AVP) increase in size and the number of neurons that express both AVP and corticotropin-releasing hormone (CRH) increase with age.

The anterior pituitary shows unchanged output of stimulating hormones, although the peripheral levels of target hormones decrease. For example, circulating levels of daytime and nighttime thyroid-stimulating hormone (TSH) and growth hormone (GH) were greatly diminished in old age.[25] In contrast, prolactin and melatonin were decreased only at night. Age-related decreases in hormonal levels were associated with a decrease in the amplitude, but not the frequency of secretory pulses.

The decline in GH with age is believed to be associated with the decrease in lean body mass, increase in body fat (especially in the visceral/abdominal compartment), adverse changes in lipoproteins, and reduction in aerobic capacity commonly noted in older adults. Research is ongoing to determine if replacement of GH in healthy older adults can reverse these changes.[25]

Normal aging is associated with insulin resistance and reduced beta-cell function, but it is not known whether changes in proinsulin and the proinsulin/immunoreactive insulin ratio are also related to reduced beta-cell function.[26] Glucose tolerance decreases with age. An increase in blood glucose to 200 mg/dL occurs in about 50% of people older than 70 years.[26] Interpretation of this glucose intolerance requires the use of age-adjusted parameters to avoid the inappropriate diagnosis and treatment of diabetes mellitus. Evaluating glycosylated hemoglobin (HbA_{1c}) or glycosylated albumin may help establish the presence or absence of diabetes mellitus in the older patient with elevated blood glucose levels. Because the renal threshold for reabsorption of glucose increases with age, higher degrees of hyperglycemia must be present before glucose spills into the urine. Therefore, monitoring for hyperglycemia with urine testing should be avoided.

Throughout life, the adrenal cortex shows significant morphogenic and steroidogenic changes. There is a subtle decline in aldosterone with age and a subtle increase in cortisol; however the adrenal androgens dehydroepiandrosterone (DHEA) and dehydroepiandrosterone sulfate (DHEAS) decline with age in a process similar to menopause. This decline is believed to aggravate some age-related diseases.[27]

The thyroid gland undergoes a progressive decrease in size with aging, although enlargement due to the presence of nodules is not uncommon. The concentration of thyroid hormones found in the blood of older adults is variable and influenced by disease. There may, however, be an alteration in the responsiveness of target tissues. Specifically, there may be an age-related reduction in the ability of aged tissues to increase receptor numbers in response to a reduction in hormone levels.[28]

FINDINGS ON PHYSICAL EXAMINATION AND MANAGEMENT

The reduction in thyroid hormone levels with increasing age is correlated with many physiological and pathological sequelae: changes in cholesterol metabolism, heart rate, cardiac output, and strength of cardiac contraction and alterations in basal metabolic rate and thermoregulation. The symptoms of thyroid disease, such as apathy, weakness, and weight loss, may not be as pronounced in the older adult as they are in younger people. Moreover, these symptoms are often attributed to old age rather than to hyperthyroidism or hypothyroidism. The older patient with hyperthyroidism is likely to present with atrial tachycardia and is more likely to be anorexic than hyperphagic; this person usually does not experience heat intolerance. The hypothyroid older adult may present with increased susceptibility to hypothermia if exposed to cold, a change in cognitive status, fatigue, dizziness, and a tendency to fall.

Being aware of the atypical presentation of thyroid disease in older adults leads the critical care nurse to recognize endocrine imbalance. Once identified, the imbalance can easily be corrected by replacing thyroid hormone or changing the dosage of thyroid replacement.

Diabetes mellitus is frequently seen in conjunction with acute illness, trauma, or surgery. The end-organ damage of diabetes mellitus is a factor in stroke, myocardial infarction, decreased renal function, and peripheral vascular disease. Long-standing non–insulin-dependent diabetes may be diagnosed only when the patient presents with a stroke or acute myocardial infarction. Therefore, it is important to distinguish among the impaired glucose tolerance of aging, a transient rise in glucose related to acute illness, and the disease process of diabetes.

Recognition of the underlying diabetes and possible end-organ damage may alter the course of the acute illness. For example, knowing that the incidence of congestive heart failure after myocardial infarction is higher in diabetic than in nondiabetic patients, the nurse can be alert for early signs of fluid retention.

Older people with diabetes are, for the most part, not insulin dependent. Therefore, even if they have extremely high blood sugars, they are rarely ketoacidotic. In fact, the coma of this age group is usually hyperglycemic, hyperosmolar, and nonketotic (HHNK). Managing this state requires a delicate balance of hydration and rapid reduction of blood sugar without massive brain edema and death. The critical care nurse must be aware that HHNK coma can be triggered by acute illness or surgery. Common problems found in older adults with diabetes, and nursing interventions to prevent these problems, are shown in Box 13-6.

Immunological Changes

With age there is a decline in immune function. Specifically, there is a decline in both T-cell and B-cell function, with a dramatic effect on cell-mediated immunity. The decline in B-cell function may be indirectly related to a decline in T-cell function. The decreased numbers of B cells secreting immunoglobulin G result in a generally poor humoral immune response. With aging, the thymus gland involutes and there is a decrease in thymic hormone levels, and the number of autoantibodies increases.[29]

FINDINGS ON PHYSICAL EXAMINATION AND MANAGEMENT

The usual symptoms of infection such as chills, fever, leukocytosis, or tachycardia may be absent or blunted in the older adult. Instead, these individuals may present with an acute change in cognition, function, or behavior. Delirium, for

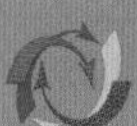

box 13-6 nursing interventions for *Prevention of Problems in the Older Adult With Diabetes*

Skin Alterations
- Monitor for decreased circulation and skin breakdown.
- Provide foot care to maintain skin integrity. Bathe the feet daily and apply emollient.

Hyperglycemia
- Maintain a controlled diet.
- Monitor blood glucose levels.

Hydration Status
- Monitor hydration.
- Encourage the intake of 2,000 mL of fluid daily.

End-organ Disease
- Monitor kidney function.
- Monitor for visual changes (e.g., blurred or decreased vision).

example, may be the only sign or symptom of a urinary tract infection in an older adult. The most common sites of infection in older adults are respiratory, urinary, and skin, and when subtle changes are noted in an older patient, consideration should be given to each of these areas.

PSYCHOLOGICAL CHALLENGES

Cognitive Changes

Cognition refers to the process of obtaining, storing, retrieving, and using information. The neuroanatomical and neurophysiological underpinnings of cognitive change are unclear. Studies[30] have shown that younger individuals have larger ventricular volumes and smaller gray and white matter volumes compared with older individuals. There is also greater prefrontal cortex activity in younger compared with older adults in the dorsolateral area during memory retrieval. These changes are believed to account for the changes in working memory with normal aging,[31] as well as executive abilities.[32] With age there is some decline in perceptual motor skills, concept formation, complex memory tasks, and quick-decision tasks. However, age itself is not the criterion for making decisions about a patient's cognitive functions. Each person's abilities must be judged individually rather than against a norm.

Cognitive function should be assessed and described on admission and monitored routinely over time and whenever the patient's condition changes. While assessing cognitive functions during the patient's stay in intensive care, it is important to remember that physiological deficits, some medications, and internal and external stress, such as environmental stressors, affect cognitive skills. In older adults, acute physical changes frequently initially present as changes in cognitive status. For example, an older adult with pneumonia may not have symptoms such as fever or cough. Rather, this individual may present with changes in cognitive status.

A mental status questionnaire, such as the Folstein Mini-Mental State Examination (MMSE), can be used to assess cognitive function systematically. (For more information regarding the MMSE, contact the publisher: Psychological Assessment Resources, Inc., 16204 North Florida Avenue, Lutz, Florida 33549.) The MMSE has 11 questions that provide information about orientation, attention, memory, perception, and thought process. It takes 5 to 10 minutes to complete, and the patient must be able to give oral and written responses.[33] Use of a consistent assessment tool helps the nurse compare responses and monitor results over time. The main drawback to the use of a questionnaire is that some critically ill patients may not be able to hear, see, talk, or write well enough to respond to the questions. Longer, more sensitive tools may also be more fatiguing for the critically ill older patient.

Several common syndromes cause cognitive impairment, including dementia, delirium, and depression (discussed later). Dementia is based on impairment of memory plus at least one of the following: a personality change or impairment in either abstract thinking, judgment, or higher cortical functions. Delirium is the abrupt onset of clouding of consciousness and is a medical emergency. Table 13-5 identifies factors to differentiate dementia from delirium. Reversible causes of dementia and delirium are listed in Box 13-7.

LEARNING

Older adults may take longer to respond to and assimilate new material. They may also be hesitant to take on new tasks. Motivation continues to be an important aspect of learning new material. If the material is irrelevant or meaningless, motivation is decreased, which is often interpreted as an inability to learn. Sensory abilities and cognition are used to teach older patients. It may be necessary to present information using small segments and varied stimuli, including touching, seeing, hearing, and (if vision permits) writing. If movements are slowed, allow time for the completion of motor tasks, such as manipulating equipment or carrying out exercises.

MEMORY

The older person's memory decline involves short-term memory rather than long-term and remote memory. Recall of memory from the past is least impaired by age. Remote memory recall (items learned many years ago) can be a positive therapeutic strategy for older patients. Reminiscence is an adaptive mechanism that helps the nurse learn about the patient and contributes to feelings of increased self-worth and competence for the patient.

DEPRESSION

Depression disorders are among the most common complaints of older adults and the leading cause of suicide in later life. Symptoms of depression are listed in Box 13-8. Based on the diagnostic criteria for major depression, at least five of these symptoms should occur almost daily for at least

table 13-5 Summary of Differences Between Dementia and Delirium

	Dementia		Delirium
	ALZHEIMER'S DISEASE (AD)	MULTI-INFARCT DEMENTIA	
Etiology	Familial (genetic [chromosomes 14, 19, 21]) Sporadic	Cardiovascular (CV) disease Cerebrovascular disease Hypertension	Drug toxicity and interactions; acute disease; trauma; chronic disease exacerbation Fluid and electrolyte disorder
Risk factors	Advanced age; genetic factor	Preexisting CV disease	Preexisting cognitive impairment
Occurrence	50%–60% of dementias	20% of dementias	20% of hospitalized older people
Onset	Slow	Often abrupt Follows a stroke or transient ischemic attack (TIA)	Rapid, acute onset A harbinger of acute medical illness
Age of onset (years)	Early-onset AD: 30s–65 Late-onset AD: 65+ Most commonly: 85+	Most commonly 50–70	Any age, but predominantly in older persons
Gender	Males and females equally	Predominantly males	Males and females equally
Course	Chronic, irreversible; progressive, regular, downhill	Chronic, irreversible Fluctuating, stepwise progression	Acute
Duration	2–20 years	Variable; years	Lasts 1 day to 1 month
Symptom progress	Onset insidious. *Early*—mild and subtle *Middle and late*—intensified Progression to death (infection or malnutrition)	Depends on location of infarct and success of treatment; death due to underlying CV disease	Symptoms are fully reversible with adequate treatment; can progress to chronicity or death if underlying condition is ignored
Mood	Early depression (30%)	Labile; mood swings	Variable
Speech/language	Speech remains intact until late in disease *Early*—mild anomia (cannot name objects); deficits progress until speech lacks meaning; echoes and repeats words and sounds; mutism	May have speech deficit/aphasia depending on location of lesion	Fluctuating; often cannot concentrate long enough to speak
Physical signs	*Early*—no motor deficits *Middle*—apraxia [70%] (cannot perform purposeful movement) *Late*—Dysarthria (impaired articulation) *End stage*—loss of all voluntary activity; positive neurologic signs	According to location of lesion: focal neurologic signs, seizures Commonly exhibits motor deficits	Signs and symptoms of underlying disease
Orientation	Becomes lost in familiar places (topographic disorientation) Has difficulty drawing three-dimensional objects (visual and spatial disorientation) Disorientation to time, place, and person—with disease progression		May fluctuate between lucidity and complete disorientation to time, place, and person
Memory	Loss is an early sign of dementia; loss of recent memory is soon followed by progressive decline in recent and remote memory		Impaired recent and remote memory; may fluctuate between lucidity and confusion
Personality	Apathy, indifference, irritability *Early disease*—social behavior intact; hides cognitive deficits *Advanced disease*—disengages from activity and relationships; suspicious; paranoid delusions caused by memory loss; aggressive; catastrophic reactions		Fluctuating; cannot focus attention to converse; alarmed by symptoms (when lucid); hallucinations; paranoid
Functional status, activities of daily living	Poor judgment in everyday activities; has progressive decline in ability to handle money, use telephone, function in home and workplace		Impaired

(continued)

table 13-5 Summary of Differences Between Dementia and Delirium (Continued)

	Dementia	Delirium
Attention span	Distractable; short attention span	Highly impaired; cannot maintain or shift attention
Psychomotor activity	Wandering, hyperactivity, pacing, restlessness, agitation	Variable; alternates between high agitation, hyperactivity, restlessness, and lethargy
Sleep-wake cycle	Often impaired; wandering and agitation at nighttime	Takes brief naps throughout day and night

From Smeltzer SC, Bare BG: Brunner and Suddarth's Textbook of Medical-Surgical Nursing (9th Ed), p 158. Philadelphia, Lippincott Williams & Wilkins, 2000.

2 weeks. These symptoms of depression in the older adult can be masked by normal age-related changes or disease states. For example, difficulty sleeping, early morning awakening, and lethargy are common physical complaints of the normal aging person. Alternatively, depression in the older adult may more commonly present with pseudohypochondriasis, preoccupation with past life events, and changes in cognitive ability. In some patients, the dominant emotional mood may not be sadness but anger, anxiety, or irritability.

Causes of depression are multifaceted and include multiple losses associated with aging, underlying illness, or drugs. Box 13-9 lists drug groups that may cause depression. Screening tools, such as the Geriatric Depression Scale,[34] shown in Box 13-10, are useful to identify individuals who are depressed. Once identified, appropriate interventions, including drug therapy, behavioral modification, and counseling, can be initiated.

The nurse must also be aware of cardiovascular side effects of tricyclic antidepressive drugs. On the ECG, ST segment and T-wave changes may become evident but are not necessarily indicative of myocardial damage. Ventricular dysrhythmias and disturbances in cardiac conduction are considered serious side effects of some antidepressant drugs, and may result in the drug being reduced or discontinued. The older person may also experience changes related to sleep, appetite, and blood pressure with antidepressant drugs. Anticholinergic effects, especially in patients with Alzheimer's disease, benign prostatic hypertrophy, or CAD, may also be seen.

Untreated depression may result in suicide, which is a serious problem among older adults. Of all suicides committed in this country annually, 25% are by people older than 65 years. White men older than 85 years are at particular risk.[35] Because of their many losses and changes, older adults may view suicide as a means of fulfilling a fantasy of "reunion" with a dead spouse or significant other. The nurse must monitor signs and symptoms of depression, explore the causes of depression, facilitate treatment, and be watchful for suicide attempts or warnings.

Abuse of the Older Person

Mistreatment of older people is a problem that affects more than 4% of the older adults in the United States.[36] Abuse of older adults occurs in homes and institutions and takes many forms. Abuse may be blatant or subtle; it may be physical, psychological, or material (e.g., financial). Abuse may involve neglect (by others or by self), exploitation, or abandonment. The abused older person is often physically or mentally frail and unable to report the abusive situation. Abuse can also happen to emotionally and intellectually stable older people who are unable to stop the abuse or report it because of their financial or emotional dependence on the abuser. They may also be afraid of being abandoned.

The abuse can be by people who may or may not live with the older person. Abuse can occur because of lack of knowledge about the older person's basic needs, lack of resources to help, and desire to protect an inheritance. The abuse can be by caretakers who are extremely stressed, or the abused older adult may be the caretaker.

box 13-7
Reversible Causes of Dementia and Delirium

Drugs
Emotional illness (including depression)
Metabolic/endocrine disorders
Eye/ear/environment
Nutritional/neurological disorders
Tumors/trauma
Infection
Alcoholism/anemia/atherosclerosis

box 13-8 ***Symptoms of Depression***

- Depressed mood
- Decreased interest in activities
- Weight changes
- Sleep changes
- Psychomotor changes
- Fatigue
- Feelings of worthlessness or guilt
- Decreased concentration
- Suicidal ideation

box 13-9
Drug Groups That May Cause Depression in the Older Person

Analgesics/anti-inflammatory agents
Anticonvulsants
Antihistamines
Antihypertensives
Antimicrobials
Antiparkinsonian agents
Hormones
Immunosuppressive agents
Tranquilizers

The nurse should be alert to the signs and symptoms of elder abuse as outlined in Box 13-11. Any suggestion by the patient or family that things are not well at home should be pursued. A statement such as, "My son hasn't been here yet. He sometimes forgets his commitments," should open the door for further conversation. It might uncover a mother who is worried about her son's drinking and perhaps about the way he treats her when he has been drinking. Attempts should be made to compare the history given by the patient with that given by the family. Inconsistencies need to be explored further. Likewise, it is helpful to ask caretakers if they were able to give the care they felt was needed. Indications that the patient was "getting to be a handful" may be a clue to mismanaged care or a caretaker

box 13-10
Geriatric Depression Scale

Patient ____________________ Examiner ____________________ Date ____________

Directions to Patient: Please choose the best answer for how you have felt over the past week.
Directions to Examiner: Present questions VERBALLY. Circle answer given by patient. Do not show to patient.

1.	Are you basically satisfied with your life?	yes	**no** (1)
2.	Have you dropped many of your activities and interests?	**yes** (1)	no
3.	Do you feel that your life is empty?	**yes** (1)	no
4.	Do you often get bored?	**yes** (1)	no
5.	Are you hopeful about the future?	yes	**no** (1)
6.	Are you bothered by thoughts you can't get out of your head?	**yes** (1)	no
7.	Are you in good spirits most of the time?	yes	**no** (1)
8.	Are you afraid that something bad is going to happen to you?	**yes** (1)	no
9.	Do you feel happy most of the time?	yes	**no** (1)
10.	Do you often feel helpless?	**yes** (1)	no
11.	Do you often get restless and fidgety?	**yes** (1)	no
12.	Do you prefer to stay at home rather than go out and do things?	**yes** (1)	no
13.	Do you frequently worry about the future?	**yes** (1)	no
14.	Do you feel you have more problems with memory than most?	**yes** (1)	no
15.	Do you think it is wonderful to be alive now?	yes	**no** (1)
16.	Do you feel downhearted and blue?	**yes** (1)	no
17.	Do you feel pretty worthless the way you are now?	**yes** (1)	no
18.	Do you worry a lot about the past?	**yes** (1)	no
19.	Do you find life very exciting?	yes	**no** (1)
20.	Is it hard for you to get started on new projects?	**yes** (1)	no
21.	Do you feel full of energy?	yes	**no** (1)
22.	Do you feel that your situation is hopeless?	**yes** (1)	no
23.	Do you think that most people are better off than you are?	**yes** (1)	no
24.	Do you frequently get upset over little things?	**yes** (1)	no
25.	Do you frequently feel like crying?	**yes** (1)	no
26.	Do you have trouble concentrating?	**yes** (1)	no
27.	Do you enjoy getting up in the morning?	yes	**no** (1)
28.	Do you prefer to avoid social occasions?	**yes** (1)	no
29.	Is it easy for you to make decisions?	yes	**no** (1)
30.	Is your mind as clear as it used to be?	yes	**no** (1)

TOTAL: Please sum all bolded answers (worth one point) for a total score. ____________

Scores: 0–10 Normal **11–20 Moderate Depression** **21–30 Severe Depression**

From Yesavage JA, Brink TL: Development and validation of a geriatric depression screening scale: A preliminary report. J Psychiatr Res 17:37–49, 1983.

box 13-11 ***Signs and Symptoms of Elder Abuse***

- Lack of compliance with management of health problems
- Unexplained injuries, such as fractures, bruises, lacerations
- Burns
- Poor personal hygiene
- Sexually transmitted disease
- Altered mood
- Depression
- Failure to thrive (underhydration/impaired nutritional status)
- Impaired skin integrity/fungal rashes

in need of support and assistance. In either situation, the nurse can provide information and support and refer the patient and caregiver to a social worker or mental health nurse for further assistance. In addition, health care workers, including nurses, should know their responsibility under state law for reporting abuse of the older patient.

Alcohol Abuse

Alcohol abuse occurs in the aging population, although there is little documentation about its prevalence.[37] Problem drinking in older adults occurs for similar reasons as during the early to middle adult years. However, smaller amounts of alcohol create larger problems for the older person, and they may be more susceptible to alcohol-induced disease. Differences in metabolism of alcohol in the older person, the smaller volume of body water, and the decrease in lean body tissue may increase the propensity to alcoholism or alcohol problems. In addition, older adults are high consumers of psychotropic drugs and are at risk for drug–alcohol interactions.

Nursing interventions include screening the older adult for alcohol use. The HEAT screening method,[38] shown in Box 13-12, is useful for screening purposes. A positive response on any item is a reason to obtain a more detailed history of alcohol use. When alcohol abuse is suspected, the immediate goal is to stabilize physiological and psychological responses to alcohol withdrawal and determine the impact of alcohol abuse on whatever other diagnoses have resulted in the need for critical care. As soon as possible, the nurse should refer the patient to a social worker, psychiatric liaison nurse, or alcohol counselor.

box 13-12
The HEAT Screening Method for Indications of Alcohol Abuse

How do you use alcohol?
Have you ever thought you used alcohol to **E**xcess?
Has **A**nyone else ever thought you used too much?
Have you ever had any **T**rouble resulting from your use of alcohol?

CHALLENGES IN MEDICATION USE

The rule for giving therapeutic medications to the older patient is *start low, go slow*. In other words, be patient. Changes related to aging can have a great impact on drug response. Changes in renal function, gastrointestinal secretions and motility, and cell receptor sites and concurrent disease states can alter the absorption, distribution, and excretion of drugs. These changes are summarized in Table 13-6.

Before admission to the ICU, older patients may have been taking many different medications, including over-the-counter (OTC) medications such as vitamins, tonics, laxatives, antacids, and pain relievers. They may also have a history of heavy alcohol intake. Any of these drugs can cause problems if combined with medications administered in the hospital.

The nurse needs to elicit a careful history of drug use from the patient and family. The family can be asked to bring in all medications the patient has been using; these include OTC medications and herbal remedies. Although alcohol use may be a sensitive topic, establishing the pattern of use can be essential in preventing untoward drug interactions and anticipating problems with liver damage or withdrawal.

Special considerations concerning administration of drugs to the older patient include knowing the drugs the patient has been taking; assessing renal, hepatic, endocrine, and digestive systems; and evaluating lean body mass. Impaired body systems may affect the absorption, metabolism, and excretion of drugs. Additional considerations are listed in Box 13-13. A decrease in lean body mass and an increase in total body fat may alter the distribution of the drug in the body.

Drug Absorption

Drug absorption is affected by the following age-related changes: decreased gastric acid, decreased gastrointestinal motility, decreased gastric blood flow, changes in gastrointestinal villi, and decreased blood flow and body temperature in the rectum. The increased pH of gastric secretions and delayed stomach emptying time can alter the degradation, and thus the absorption, of drugs. Drugs that are not stable in an acid medium can be severely reduced in bioavailability if they remain in the stomach for long periods. Drugs that are designed to be acted on in the small intestine may be affected by the higher pH of the aging stomach. A coated, pH-sensitive medication, such as erythromycin, may lose its coating in the stomach and be degraded before reaching the absorption sites in the small intestine. Coated gastric irritants may lose their coatings and cause bleeding or nausea and vomiting.

Some drugs are eliminated from the body before they enter the systemic circulation by a process called *first-pass metabolism*. In general, the enzymes responsible for this

table 13-6 Altered Drug Responses in Older People

Age-Related Changes	Impact of Age-Related Change	Applicable Drugs
Absorption		
Reduced gastric acid; increased pH (less acid)	Rate of drug absorption—possibly delayed	
Reduced GI motility; prolonged gastric emptying	Extent of drug absorption—not affected	
Distribution		
Decreased albumin sites	Serious alterations in drug binding to plasma proteins (the unbound drug gives the pharmacologic response); highly protein-bound drugs have fewer binding sites, leading to increased effects and accelerated metabolism and excretion	*Selected highly protein-binding drugs:* Oral anticoagulants (warfarin) Oral hypoglycemic agents (sulfonylureas) Barbiturates Calcium channel blockers furosemide (Lasix) Nonsteroidal anti-inflammatory drugs (NSAIDs) Sulfonamides quinidine phenytoin (Dilantin)
Reduced cardiac output	Decreased perfusion of many bodily organs	
Impaired peripheral blood flow	Decreased perfusion	
Increased percentage of body fat	Proportion of body fat increases with age and thus gives the body an increased ability to store fat-soluble drugs; this causes drug accumulation, prolonged storage, and delayed excretion	*Selected fat-soluble drugs:* Barbiturates diazepam (Valium) lidocaine Phenothiazines (antipsychotics) Ethanol morphine
Decreased lean body mass	Decreased body volume allows higher peak levels of drugs	
Metabolism		
Decreased cardiac output and decreased perfusion of the liver	Decreased metabolism and delay of breakdown of drugs, resulting in prolonged duration of action, accumulation, and drug toxicity	All drugs metabolized by the liver
Excretion		
Decreased renal blood flow; loss of functioning nephrons; decreased renal efficiency	Decreased rates of elimination and increased duration of action Danger of accumulation and drug toxicity	*Selected drugs with prolonged action:* Aminoglycoside antibiotics cimetidine (Tagamet) chlorpropamide (Diabinase) digoxin lithium procainamide

From Smeltzer SC, Bare BG: Brunner and Suddarth's Textbook of Medical–Surgical Nursing (9th Ed), p 165. Philadelphia, Lippincott Williams & Wilkins, 2000.

first-pass effect are decreased in the elderly so bioavailability of the high–hepatic-extraction drugs may be increased with age. These drugs require dosage reduction for older adults.

Drug Distribution

Distribution of drugs in the body can be affected by a decrease in lean body mass, an increase in total body fat, or a decrease in total body fluid, all of which may accompany aging. Drugs that bind to muscle (e.g., digoxin) become more bioavailable as lean body mass diminishes, increasing the risk of toxicity. Fat-soluble drugs (e.g., flurazepam [Dalmane], chlorpromazine [Thorazine], phenobarbital) can be deposited in fat and result in cumulative effects of oversedation. In the presence of a volume deficit, drugs that are water soluble (e.g., gentamicin [Garamycin]) may have a higher concentration and may reach toxic levels rapidly.

Drug Metabolism

The liver is the major organ for biotransformation and detoxification of medications. Drug-metabolizing reactions are classified as phase I reactions, which involve adding or unmasking a polar chemical group to increase water solubility, and phase II or conjugation reactions, which involve linking the drug to another molecule such as glucose, acetate, or sulfate. In older adults, phase I metabolism is often impaired, whereas phase II metabolism is usually unaffected. In the older patient, there may be some decrease in the metabolism of drugs requiring hepatic enzymes for transformation. This results in an increased plasma level and prolonged half-life of the drug. The

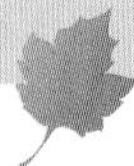

box 13-13

Considerations for Medication Use in Older People

- Drug dosage guidelines are usually based on studies in younger people, and recommended adult dosage guidelines may not be appropriate for older patients.
- Older people may be taking numerous prescription drugs and may self-medicate with borrowed, old, and over-the-counter drugs.
- The effects of alcohol use must be considered.
- The potential for drug interactions and adverse reactions is increased because of the effects of aging on drug absorption, distribution, metabolism, and excretion.
- Drug toxicities are different from those in younger people. Fewer symptoms may be identified, and they may develop more slowly but be more pronounced once they occur.
- Behavioral side effects are more common in older people because the blood–brain barrier becomes less effective. When there is an acute change in mental status, medication should always be considered as the cause.

benzodiazepines (e.g., diazepam [Valium], flurazepam), for example, have a half-life increase from 20 to 90 hours in the older patient. Hepatic oxidation of these drugs can further be affected by alcohol-induced changes in the liver. There may be a decrease in drug metabolism with occasional alcohol use. In chronic alcohol use, however, drug metabolism is increased, and excretion is accelerated.

Drug Excretion

The kidney is the primary excretory organ for clearing drugs. Drugs that are excreted unchanged (e.g., digoxin, cimetidine, antibiotics) or have renally excreted active metabolites require dosage reduction in the older adult to avoid accumulation and toxicity. Serum creatinine alone is not a good determinant of renal function in older people. A creatinine clearance study reflects a more accurate estimation for drug clearance.

case study ■ POSTOPERATIVE DELIRIUM

Mrs. Hannum, a 90-year-old white woman, is in surgical intensive care recovering from a hip fracture and open reduction internal fixation done with local anesthesia. She received one unit of autologous blood after surgery and is on enoxaparin (Lovenox; 30 units subcutaneously) for venous thrombolic embolism prevention. Thirty-six hours after her surgery, the family visited her and noted that she did not seem to recognize them, could not recall recent events or the date, and had no idea where she was or why she was there. Her normal baseline Mini-Mental Status Examination (MMSE) score was known to be 29/30.

The patient complained of vague nausea but denied chest pain, shortness of breath, and dizziness. She had easily passed some urine after surgery with no urinary symptoms. She was receiving some fluids intravenously for hydration (D_5W and half-normal saline) at 70 mL/hour and had started taking oral fluids with no difficulty. Her vital signs were stable with a blood pressure of 152/70 mm Hg and a regular heart rate of 78 beats/minute. She was afebrile. Physical examination was unremarkable, revealing a soft abdomen, normal bowel sounds, and no masses or tenderness. Lung sounds were likewise normal vesicular breath sounds without rales, rhonchi, or wheezes. Extremities were without edema on the left, unaffected side. She had 1+ edema on the right lower extremity up to the groin, but her calf was soft and nontender. The incision was draining serosanguineous drainage and staples were intact with no erythema noted. She did have a small blister secondary to tape around the incision line.

The patient's past medical history includes hypertension, skin cancer of the nose and face with multiple surgeries, and gastroesophageal reflux disease (GERD). The patient takes hydrochlorothiazide (25 mg daily); amlodipine (Norvasc; 5 mg daily); Metamucil; and ranitidine (Zantac; 150 mg every night). She has a daily alcohol intake of 2 to 3 ounces of whiskey daily before dinner and drinks a glass of wine (approximately 6 ounces) with dinner.

After the family voiced concern about Mrs. Hannum's confusion, Mrs. Hannum was reevaluated. At this time, her vital signs were as follows: supine blood pressure, 155/72 mm Hg; oral temperature, 97.2°F (36.2°C); and a regular heart rate of 72 beats/minute without an S_3, an S_4, or a murmur. Normal vesicular breath sounds without rales, rhonchi, or wheeze are heard on auscultation of the lungs. The patient's abdomen is soft with normal bowel sounds and no masses, tenderness, or organomegaly. She has full range of motion and strength 5/5 throughout (her right lower extremity was not tested). She scores 21/30 on the MMSE.

The complete blood count (CBC) is within normal limits. Electrolytes are as follows: sodium 135 mEq/L; potassium 3.5 mEq/L; chloride 84 mEq/L. The hematocrit was 36.2% after the autologous blood was given. The white blood cell count was within a normal range at 7,300 cells/mm^3. ■

clinical applicability challenges

Self-Challenge: Critical Thinking

1. *What is your immediate concern related to Mrs. Hannum's behavior?*
2. *In light of the delirium, what measures would you take to prevent iatrogenic complications and keep her safe?*
3. *What options are available for management of the delirium?*
4. *How would you support and help the family in this situation?*
5. *What care interventions are essential to help maintain and restore functional ability?*

6. *What care interventions are appropriate related to current cognitive state?*
7. *What care interventions would you implement specifically related to falls prevention?*
8. *How would you decrease Mrs. Hannum's risk of postoperative complications?*

Study Questions

1. *Physical changes that are not part of the normal aging process include which of the following?*
   a. *Reduced sensory and perceptual activity*
   b. *Reduced glomerular filtration rate (GFR)*
   c. *Decreased amounts of connective and collagen tissue*
   d. *A decline in hemoglobin and hematocrit*
2. *Drug absorption in older adults is influenced by all of the following factors except*
   a. *Increased gastrointestinal pH.*
   b. *Changes in albumin levels.*
   c. *Changes in gastrointestinal villi.*
   d. *Altered gastrointestinal motility.*
3. *Bone loss in hospitalized older adults may be further exacerbated by which one of the following?*
   a. *Dehydration*
   b. *Bed rest*
   c. *Infection*
   d. *Delirium*
4. *What is a typical sign of depression in an older person?*
   a. *Sadness and melancholy*
   b. *Acute physical problems*
   c. *An acute change in cognition*
   d. *Pseudohypochondriasis*
5. *Older adults with cataracts typically describe which one of the following symptoms?*
   a. *Acute pain radiating to the forehead*
   b. *Drainage from the eye*
   c. *Decreased peripheral vision*
   d. *Blurring and blunting of vision and visual acuity*
6. *How does infection in the older adult most commonly present?*
   a. *As a change in cognition, function, or behavior*
   b. *With fever and chills*
   c. *As leukocytosis*
   d. *As altered sleep patterns*

REFERENCES

1. Schmidt K: Physiology and pathophysiology of senescence. Int J Vitam Nutr Res 69(3):150–153, 1999
2. Maggi S, Minicuci N, Marini A: Prevalence rates of hearing impairment and comorbid conditions in older people: The Veneto Study. J Am Geriatr Soc 46:1069–1073, 1998
3. Maguire G: The changing realm of the senses. In Lewis CB (ed): Aging: The Health Care Challenge, pp 137–142. Philadelphia, FA Davis, 1996
4. Larsson M, Finkel D, Pederson N: Odor identification and influences of age. J Gerontol Psychosoc Behav 55:P304–P310, 2000
5. Ancoli-Israel S: Insomnia in the elderly: A review for the primary care practitioner. Sleep 23(Suppl 1):S23–S30, 2000
6. Agency for Health Care Policy and Research: Systemic Review of the Literature Regarding the Diagnosis of Sleep Apnea: Summary. Evidence Report/Technology Assessment No. 1 Rockville, MD, U.S. Department of Health and Human Services, Public Health Service, Agency for Health Care Policy and Research, 1998. Available at http://ahcpr.gov/clinic/apnea.htm. Accessed October 2004
7. McDowell JA, Mion LC, Lydon TJ, et al: A nonpharmacologic sleep protocol for hospitalized older patients. J Am Geriatr Soc 46:700–706, 1998
8. Adelman A: Common dermatologic problems. In Adelman A, Daly M (eds): Geriatrics: 20 Common Problems, pp 367–389. New York, McGraw-Hill, 2000
9. Chung JH, Kang S, Varani J, et al: Decreased extracellular-signal-regulated kinase and increased stress-activated MAP kinase activities in aged human skin in vivo. J Invest Dermatol 115(2):177–182, 2000
10. Florea VG, Henein MY, Anker SD, et al: Relation of changes over time in ventricular size and function to those in exercise capacity in patients with chronic heart failure. Am Heart J 139(5):913–917, 2000
11. Gryglewska B, Grodzicki T, Czarnecka D, et al: QT dispersion and hypertensive heart disease in the elderly. J Hypertens 18(4):461–464, 2000
12. Lakatta EG: Cardiovascular aging in health. Clin Geriatr Med 16(3):419–444, 2000
13. Kane RL, Ouslander JG, Abrass IB: Essentials of Clinical Geriatrics (3rd Ed), pp 256–279. New York, McGraw-Hill, 1994
14. Fiatarone-Singh MA: Exercise, Nutrition, and the Older Woman. New York, CRC Press, 2000
15. Miyajima H, Nomura M, Nada T, et al: Age-related changes in the magnitude of ventricular depolarization vector: Analyses by magnetocardiogram. J Electrocardiol 33(1):31–35, 2000
16. Janssens J, Pache J, Nicod L: Physiological changes in respiratory function associated with ageing. Eur Respir J 13(1):197–205, 1999
17. Perez-Guzman C, Vargas MH, Torres-Cruz A, et al: Does aging modify pulmonary tuberculosis? A meta-analytical review. Chest 116(4):961–967, 1999
18. Zaugg M, Lucchinetti E: Respiratory function in the elderly. Anesthesiol Clin North Am 18(1):47–58, 2000
19. Fliser D, Franek E, Joest M, et al: Renal function in the elderly: Impact of hypertension and cardiac function. Kidney Int 51(4): 1196–1204, 1997
20. Hoffman H, Ishii E, MacTurk R: Age related changes in the prevalence of smell/taste problems among the United States adult population. Ann NY Acad Sci 855:716–722, 1998
21. Nair K: Age related changes in muscle. Mayo Clin Proc 75(Suppl): S14–S18, 2000
22. Hikida R, Staron R, Hagerman F, et al: Effects of high intensity resistance training on untrained older men: II. J Gerontol A Biol Sci Med Sci 55(7):B347–B356, 2000
23. Hagerman F, Walsh S, Staron R, et al: Effects of high intensity resistance training on untrained older men: I. J Gerontol A Biol Sci Med Sci 55(7):B336–B346, 2000
24. Haden ST, Brown EM, Hurwitz S, et al: The effects of age and gender on parathyroid hormone dynamics. Clin Endocrinol (Oxf) 52(3):329–338, 2000
25. Cummings D, Merriam G: Age related changes in growth hormone secretion: Should the somatopause be treated? Semin Reprod Endocrinol 17(4):311–325, 1999
26. Roder M, Schwartz R, Prigeon R, et al: Reduced pancreatic B cell compensation to the insulin resistance of aging: Impact on proinsulin and insulin levels. J Clin Endocrinol Metab 85(6):2275–2280, 2000
27. Harper A, Buster J, Casson P: Changes in adrenocortical function with aging and therapeutic implications. Semin Reprod Endocrinol 17(4):327–328, 1999
28. Timiras P, Quay W, Vernadakis A: Hormones and Aging. Boca Raton, FL, CRC Press, 1995
29. Douek DC, Koup RA: Evidence for thymic function in the elderly. Vaccine 18(16):1638–1641, 2000
30. Resnick S, Goldszal A, Davatzikos C, et al: One year age changes in MRI brain volumes in older adults. Cereb Cortex 10(5):464–472, 2000
31. Rypma B, D'Esposito M: Isolating the neural mechanisms of age related changes in human working memory. Nat Neurosci 3(5): 509–515, 2000
32. Keys R, White D: Exploring the relationship between age, executive abilities, and psychomotor speed. J Int Neuropsychol Soc 6(1):76–82, 2000
34. Folstein M, Folstein S, McHugh P: Mini-Mental State: A practical method for grading the cognitive state of patients for the clinician. J Psychiatr Res 12:189–198, 1975

35. Yesavage JA, Brink TL, Rose TL, et al: Development and validation of a Geriatric Screening Scale: A preliminary report. J Psychiatr Res 17(1):37–49, 1983
36. Conwell Y, Lyness J, Duberstein P, et al: Completed suicide among older patients in primary care practices: A controlled study. J Am Geriatr Soc 48(1):23–30, 2000
37. Anetzberger G, Palmisano B, Sanders M, et al: A model intervention for elder abuse and dementia. Gerontologist 40(4):492–498, 2000
38. Alcohol and older people. A hidden epidemic. Mayo Clin Health Lett 18(2):6, 2000
39. Rathbone-McCuan E: Promoting help-seeking behavior among elders with chemical dependencies. Generations 12(4):37, 1988

OTHER SELECTED READING

Adelman A: Hearing and visual impairment. In Adelman A, Daly M (eds): Geriatrics: 20 Common Problems. New York, McGraw-Hill, 2001

Coll P: Sleep disorder. In Adelman A, Daly M (eds): Geriatrics: 20 Common Problems. New York, McGraw-Hill, 2001

Dobbin KR, Strollo PJ: Obstructive sleep apnea: Recognition and management considerations for the aged patient. AACN Clin Issues 13(1):103–113, 2002

Hall C: Special considerations for the geriatric patient. Crit Care Nursing Clinics of North America 14(4):427–434, 2002

Hart BD, Birkas J, Lachmann M, et al: Promoting positive outcomes for elderly persons in the hospital: Prevention and risk factor modification. AACN Clin Issues 13(1):22–22, 2002

Horner A, VanDemark M, Jensen GA: The challenge of assessing a patient with dementia and head injury. AACN Clin Issues 13(1):73–83, 2002

Michocki R: Polypharmacy and principles of drug therapy. In Adelman A, Daly M (eds): Geriatrics: 20 Common Problems. New York, McGraw-Hill, 2001

Mick D, Ackerman M: New perspectives on advanced practice nursing case management for aging patients. Crit Care Nursing Clinics of North America 14(3):281–291, 2002

Miller SK: Acute care of the elderly units: A positive outcomes case study. AACN Clin Issues 13(1):34–42, 2002

Nusbaum N: Aging and sensory senescence. South Med J 92(3):267–275, 1999

Ognibene A, Petruzzi E, Troiano L, et al: Age related changes of thyroid function in both sexes. J Endocrinol Invest 22(Suppl 10):38–39, 1999

Schretlen D, Pearlson G, Anthony J, et al: Elucidating the contributions of processing speed, executive ability, and frontal lobe volume to normal age-related differences in fluid intelligence. J Int Neuropsychol Soc 6(1):52–61, 2000

chapter **14**

The Postanesthesia Patient

CALEB ROGOVIN

objectives

Based on the content in this chapter, the reader should be able to:

- Compare and contrast anesthetic options used for surgery.
- Differentiate between anesthetic agents appropriate for the conscious patient and those appropriate for the unconscious patient.
- Summarize five potential problems encountered during the immediate postanesthetic period.
- Describe nursing interventions for the patient recovering from anesthesia.

The time immediately after surgery, when the patient is taken to the postanesthesia care unit (PACU) or the intensive care unit (ICU), is the most crucial period in the patient's recovery from anesthesia. Most patients are taken to the PACU for close observation and care by a qualified PACU nurse. Others are taken directly to the ICU, where nurses must be competent in postanesthesia nursing care. Alterations in the patient's physiological condition that occur in the immediate postoperative period are the focus of this chapter.

The critical care nurse must have a basic understanding of anesthetic options available for use during the intraoperative phase. To help with this understanding, common clinical terminology related to the use of anesthesia is listed in Box 14-1.

COLLABORATION BETWEEN THE ANESTHESIA PROVIDER AND NURSE

The anesthesia provider examines the patient before surgery. From this examination, the anesthesia provider decides which options and techniques to use. Decisions are based on the patient's condition, age, surgical and anesthetic history, and ongoing disease processes; the operation to be performed; and the position required for the surgical procedure. The anesthesia provider's options range from maintaining a conscious state with the use of minimal, regional, or intravenous (IV) agents to inducing an unconscious state with the use of IV or inhalation agents. These options are illustrated in Figures 14-1 and 14-2.

What happens in the operating room may affect the patient's immediate postoperative care and the overall recovery. To convey what has occurred in the operating suite, the anesthesia provider gives a detailed report to the nurse who is assuming postoperative care of the patient. Information given in the report is listed in Box 14-2.

While receiving the report from the anesthesia provider, the nurse must simultaneously assess the patient's condition and individualize the nursing plan of care. Initial assessment parameters reported by the anesthesia provider are the patient's vital signs (blood pressure, pulse, respiration, and temperature), pulse oximetry, and level of consciousness. Cardiac monitoring, hemodynamic parameters, and urine output monitoring also may be indicated. Vital signs are monitored every 15 minutes or more often if the patient's condition warrants. Box 14-3 provides the collaborative care guidelines for the postanesthesia patient. The American Society of PeriAnesthesia Nurses, as endorsed by the American Society of Anesthesiologists and the American

box 14-1
Clinical Terminology

Sedation: An induced state of quiet, calm, or sleep by means of a medication. The degree of sedation ranges from anxiolysis to anesthesia.

Minimal sedation: A state in which the patient responds normally to verbal stimuli. Impairment to cognition and coordination may exist.

Moderate sedation: A drug-induced depression of consciousness during which the patient responds purposefully to verbal commands either alone or in conjunction with tactile stimulation. There is some alteration of mood, drowsiness, and sometimes analgesia. The patient's protective reflexes remain intact.

Deep sedation: A drug-induced depression of consciousness during which the patient cannot be easily aroused but responds purposefully after repeated or painful stimulation. Spontaneous ventilation and the ability to maintain a patent airway may be impaired. The patient may require assistance in maintaining a patent airway.

General anesthesia: A drug-induced loss of consciousness during which a patient cannot be aroused, even by painful stimulation. The ability to independently maintain ventilatory function is often impaired. The patient may require assistance in maintaining a patent airway, and positive-pressure ventilation may be required. Cardiovascular function may be impaired.

Monitored anesthesia care (MAC): Describes a specific anesthesia service in which an anesthesia provider has been requested to participate in the care of a patient undergoing a therapeutic or diagnostic procedure. It does not describe a continuum of depth of sedation.

Regional anesthesia: This state of anesthesia produces analgesia in a specific body part. Regional anesthesia is achieved by placing local anesthetics close to appropriate nerves to achieve a conduction block.

Spinal anesthesia: In this type of anesthesia, local anesthetic is injected into the lumbar intrathecal space. The anesthetic blocks conduction in spinal nerve roots and dorsal ganglia. Analgesia occurs below the level of injection.

Epidural anesthesia: A local anesthetic is injected via a catheter into the epidural space. The effects are similar to spinal analgesia.

Peripheral nerve block: A local anesthetic is injected at a specific site to achieve a defined area of anesthesia.

Association of Nurse Anesthetists, recommends all assessment data be collected and documented on the patient's postoperative record.[1]

MODERATE SEDATION

Moderate sedation is an anesthetic technique that provides a drug-induced depression of consciousness during which the patient responds purposefully to verbal commands, either alone or associated with light tactile stimulation. No interventions are required to maintain airway patency or spontaneous ventilation. In addition, cardiovascular function is maintained. A patient under moderate sedation adheres to three major criteria: He or she will be able independently to maintain a patent airway, retain protective airway reflexes, and respond to verbal and physical stimulation. If these three conditions are not met, then the patient is not receiving moderate sedation, and perhaps this is not the correct anesthetic choice for the patient or the procedure. The advantage of moderate sedation is that it allows the patient to respond to the verbal directives of the practitioner and to physical stimulation. Moderate sedation is used for certain ambulatory surgical, therapeutic, and diagnostic procedures. The regimen usually consists of an opiate, an amnestic, a sedative, and a local anesthetic.[2]

Initial objectives for moderate sedation were developed by Scammon and colleagues in 1985.[2] The main goal of moderate sedation is to decrease patient anxiety associated with the proposed procedure. The least amount of medication to achieve sedation and comfort is the goal. In addition, moderate sedation alters the patient's mood and enhances cooperation, maintains stable vital signs, elevates the pain threshold, provides amnesia, and allows for rapid recovery.[2]

Standards for administration of moderate sedation are regulated by multiple entities. Individual State Boards of Nursing, the Joint Commission on Accreditation of Healthcare Organizations (JCAHO), and individual hospital and unit policies are available. Standards for planning and providing moderate sedation are available to practitioners and should be followed.[3]

A group of 14 nursing societies developed standards for the role of the registered nurse in managing patients receiving IV moderate sedation. These standards are published in Standards of Perianesthesia Nursing Practice[1] and include management and monitoring before, during, and after the procedure. Among the standards are the following skills required of the registered nurse who is managing the care of patients receiving IV moderate sedation:

- Demonstrate the required knowledge of anatomy, physiology, pharmacology, cardiac dysrhythmia recognition, and complications related to IV moderate sedation and medications.
- Assess total patient care requirements during moderate sedation and recovery. Physiological measurements should include, but are not limited to, respiratory rate, oxygen saturation, blood pressure, cardiac rate and rhythm, and patient's level of consciousness.
- Understand the principles of oxygen delivery, respiratory physiology, transport, and uptake, and demonstrate the ability to use oxygen delivery devices.
- Anticipate and recognize potential complications of IV moderate sedation in relation to the type of medication being administered.
- Possess the requisite knowledge and skills to assess, diagnose, and intervene in the event of complications or undesired outcomes and to institute nursing interventions in compliance with orders (including standard orders) or institutional protocols or guidelines.
- Demonstrate skills in airway management resuscitation.

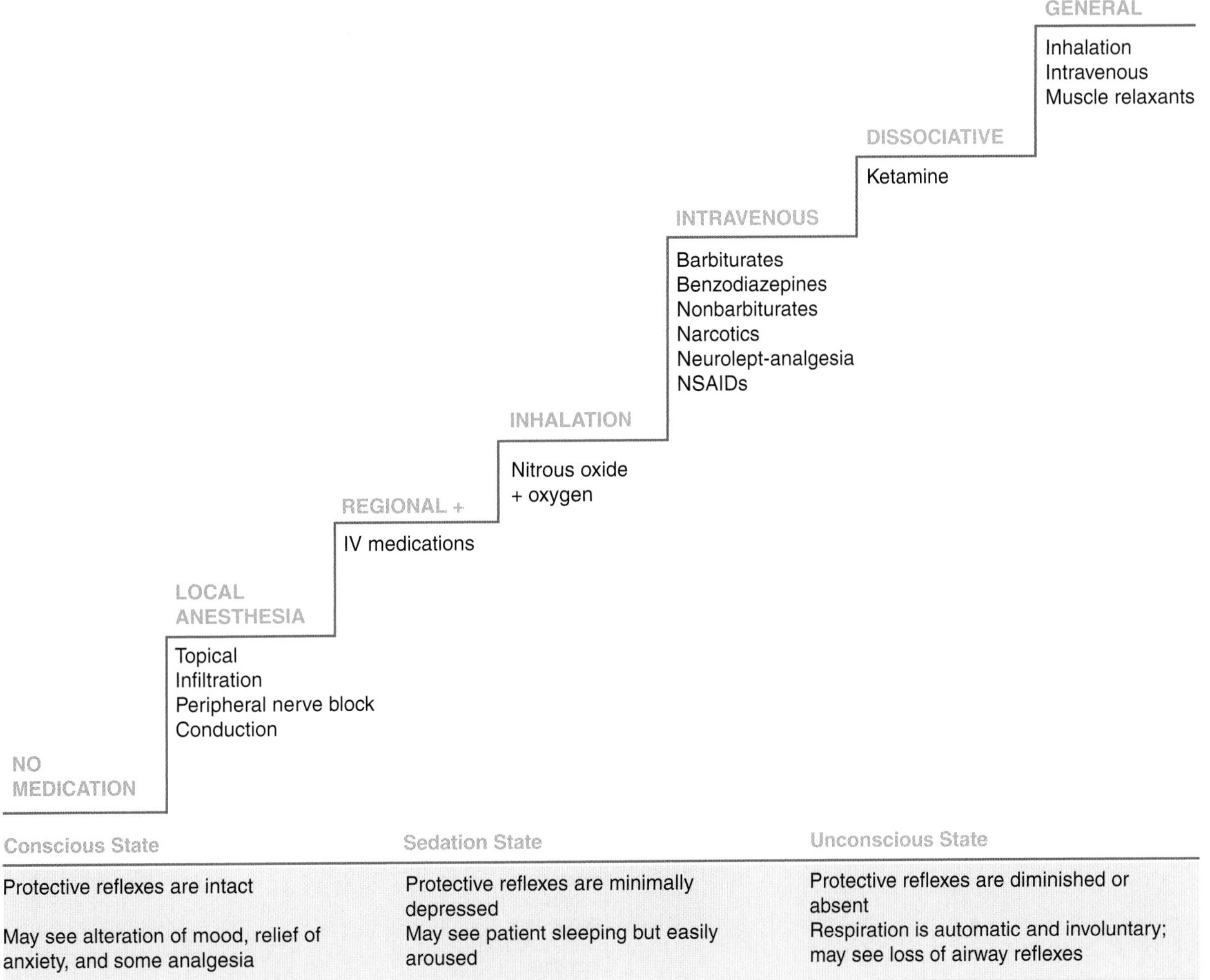

NSAIDs, nonsteroidal anti-inflammatory drugs; IV, intravenous.

figure 14-1 Anesthetic options for surgery.

- Demonstrate knowledge of the legal ramifications of administering IV moderate sedation or monitoring patients receiving IV moderate sedation, including the registered nurse's responsibility and liability in the event of an untoward reaction or life-threatening complication.

Monitored anesthesia care (MAC) describes a specific anesthesia service in which the anesthesia provider has been requested to participate in the care of a patient undergoing a therapeutic or diagnostic procedure. The main difference between moderate sedation and MAC is that the anesthesia provider deviates from the major goal of having the patient maintain his or her own airway and follow commands. To facilitate the surgical/diagnostic procedure and experience, the patient may be rendered unconscious or apneic for a period of time. IV agents are used in conjunction with local anesthetics that are injected by the surgeon. Postoperative or postprocedural care of the patient who has received moderate sedation or MAC is similar, although the patient who has received MAC may require more intervention in the postanesthesia phase. Table 14-1 provides a comparison of moderate sedation and MAC.

POTENTIAL PROBLEMS IN THE POSTANESTHESIA PATIENT

There are common potential problems in the postanesthesia patient for which the nurse must assess. They are discussed in the following sections.

Hypoxemia

Hypoxemia is a common occurrence in the immediate postoperative period. Severe hypoxemia is characterized by a partial pressure of arterial oxygen (PaO_2) of less than 50 mm Hg and is life-threatening. Hypoventilation leads to hypoxia, which is difficult to diagnose because of its multiple presentations. Clinical manifestations of hypoxia may include hypotension or hypertension, tachycardia or bradycardia, cardiac dysrhythmias, dyspnea, tachypnea,

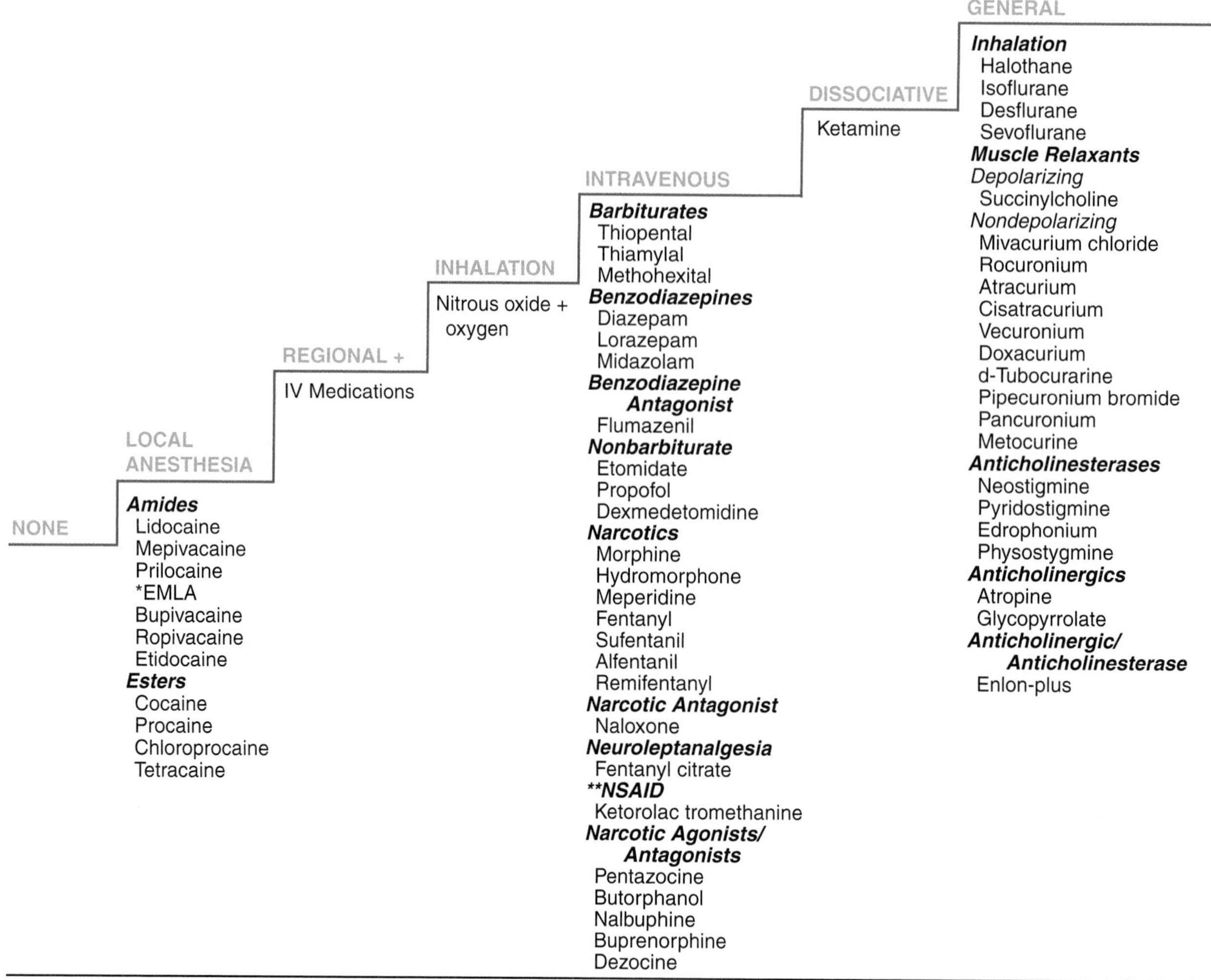

figure 14-2 Medication choices for anesthetic options.

> **box 14-2**
> ***Anesthesia Provider-to-Nurse Report: Information to Convey***
>
> Name of patient
> Surgical procedure
> Anesthetic options (agents and reversal agents used)
> Estimated blood loss/fluid loss
> Fluid/blood replacement
> Vital signs—significant problems
> Complications encountered (anesthetic or surgical)
> Preoperative condition (e.g., diabetes, hypertension, allergies)
> Considerations for immediate postoperative period (pain management, reversals, ventilator settings)
> Language barrier
>
> Ideally, the anesthesia provider should not leave the patient until the nurse is satisfied with the patient's airway and immediate condition.

hypoventilation, disorientation, agitation, decreased partial pressure of arterial carbon dioxide ($Paco_2$), and cyanosis.

When investigating the etiology of hypoxemia related to anesthetic agents, the nurse considers the effects of a spinal or epidural block that has traveled too high, narcotic use, deep sedation, use of inhalation agents, and the use of neuromuscular blocking agents, particularly if they have not been adequately reversed. Diffusion hypoxia may occur when nitrous oxide is used, but because administering 100% oxygen for 3 to 4 minutes after the nitrous oxide is discontinued may prevent this complication, diffusion hypoxemia usually is not seen in the PACU patient.

All patients who receive a general anesthetic or sedation should receive supplemental oxygen in the immediate postoperative period. The oxygen may be weaned subsequently using pulse oximetry. Because pulse oximetry offers a noninvasive method of continuously monitoring oxygen saturation, increasing numbers of patients are receiving supplemental oxygen for 24 hours after surgery.

In addition to being aware of hypoxia, the nurse uses a "stir-up" regimen for patients in the postoperative period.

table 14-1 Comparison of Moderate Sedation and Monitored Anesthesia Care

	Moderate Sedation	Monitored Anesthesia Care (MAC)
Responsiveness	Purposeful response to repeated or painful verbal or tactile stimulation	Purposeful response after stimulation
Airway	No intervention required	Intervention may be required
Spontaneous ventilation	Adequate	May be inadequate
Cardiovascular function	Usually maintained	Usually maintained

This regimen involves encouraging the patient to deep breathe, cough, and move in bed, as allowed by the procedure or intervention. An integral part of recovery from anesthesia, this routine should be included every time vital signs are checked. It also allows the nurse to identify subtle changes in the patient's condition and to make appropriate interventions.

Reversal agents may be required while the patient is still under the effects of muscle relaxants, benzodiazepines, and opioids. Close monitoring is always indicated when reversal agents are administered. The effects of muscle relaxants, benzodiazepines, and opioids may last longer than the reversal medication, resulting in hypoventilation and hypoxia at some point after the reversal medication is administered. It is important for the nurse to be knowledgeable about the onset and duration of action of reversal agents, and the drugs they are being used to reverse. This knowledge allows for appropriate intervention in the event of a change in the patient's condition.[4]

Hypoventilation

Hypoventilation leading to hypercarbia may result from the following:

- Inadequate respiratory drive secondary to the effects of residual anesthesia (i.e., opioids, sedatives, and inhalation agents)
- Inadequate functioning of the respiratory muscles (the lungs may be unable to move an adequate tidal volume because of pain or inadequate reversal of neuromuscular blockade)

box 14-3 collaborative care guide *for the Postanesthesia Patient*

OUTCOMES	INTERVENTIONS
Oxygenation/Ventilation	
Depth and rate of respiration after extubation will be normal.	■ Monitor respiratory rate and breathing pattern every 15 min and PRN.
Arterial blood gases are within preoperative normal values.	■ Assess weaning parameters before extubation. ■ Monitor end-tidal CO_2 and pulse oximetry of mechanically ventilated patients.
Airway will be maintained with intact protective reflexes.	■ Encourage patient to cough and deep breathe. ■ Elevate head of bed if not contraindicated. ■ Use jaw thrust, head tilt, or oral oropharyngeal or nasopharyngeal airway to maintain airway. ■ Stimulate patient every few minutes (e.g., call name, touch).
There will be no evidence of aspiration.	■ Administer antiemetic as indicated. ■ Position patient on side; suction and maintain airway if patient is vomiting.
Circulation/Perfusion	
Heart rate and blood pressure will return to preoperative values within 1–2 h after anesthesia.	■ Monitor vital signs every 15 min and PRN. ■ Assess pulse quality and regularity. ■ Monitor for dysrhythmias. ■ Monitor for hypotension related to bleeding. ■ Monitor for hypotension related to warming and vasodilation. ■ Administer IV solution and blood products as ordered.

(continued)

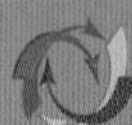

box 14-3 collaborative care guide *for the Postanesthesia Patient (Continued)*

OUTCOMES	INTERVENTIONS
Body temperature will be within normal limits.	■ Anticipate hypothermia; have warming devices readily available. ■ Measure temperature on admission and PRN until normal. ■ Warm patient at 1° to 2°C/h.
There will be no evidence of malignant hyperthermia.	■ Monitor for malignant hyperthermia, and immediately notify anesthesia provider of temperature increase of 0.5°C. ■ Administer dantrolene, and initiate cooling measures. ■ Assist with malignant hyperthermia protocol.
Fluids/Electrolytes	
Patient will have stable blood pressure and heart rate.	■ Maintain patient IV. ■ Monitor intake and output. ■ Assess skin, mucous membranes for signs of hypovolemia.
Urine output will be 0.5–2 mL/kg/h.	■ Measure specific gravity if indicated.
There will be no evidence of hypervolemia or hypovolemia.	■ Assess for signs of hypervolemia (e.g., pulmonary crackles, neck vein distension). ■ Measure serum electrolytes if indicated.
Mobility/Safety	
Patient will arouse easily and respond appropriately to commands. Patient will move all extremities purposefully and with normal strength.	■ Assess level of consciousness every 15 min and PRN. ■ Monitor motor and sensory function to assess reversal of neuromuscular blockade. ■ Assess level of regional block, epidural, or spinal anesthesia.
Skin Integrity	
Skin will remain intact.	■ Assess skin immediately postoperatively for pressure areas and burns.
Nutrition	
Nutritional intake will be reestablished without nausea or vomiting.	■ Resume enteral feeding with return of bowel sounds. ■ Begin oral fluids with return of protective airway reflexes.
Comfort/Pain Control	
Pain will be less than 4 on pain scale or visual analog.	■ Assess location, type, and severity of pain. ■ Administer opioids as indicated. ■ Monitor response to analgesics. ■ Institute nonpharmacological pain relief strategies and comfort measures. ■ Evaluate patient-controlled analgesia IV or epidural as postoperative pain management option.
Psychosocial	
Personal support systems will be used to reduce anxiety.	■ Encourage significant other visits in early postoperative phase. ■ Validate patient's significant other's understanding of surgery and illness. ■ Initiate referrals to social services, clergy, and so forth.
Teaching/Discharge Planning	
Discharge from postanesthesia care phase will occur within 1–2 h. Exercises to prevent postoperative pulmonary complications will be demonstrated.	■ Orient patient frequently. ■ Explain procedures and pain management treatment plan. ■ Teach coughing, deep breathing, incentive spirometer use. ■ Teach early mobilization. ■ Teach pain control strategies.
Patient or significant other will state understanding of surgical procedure and outcome of surgery.	■ Provide information regarding the procedure, and discuss probable outcomes.

- Intrinsic lung disease, which often requires postoperative ventilatory support of the patient (e.g., chronic obstructive pulmonary disease)
- Laryngospasm and obstruction of the airway, which must be identified and treated promptly (Box 14-4)

The nurse institutes the stir-up regimen in the immediate postoperative phase to stimulate the patient, especially if opioids and sedatives were used during surgery. Also, the nurse considers the length of time since reversal agents were administered to antagonize neuromuscular blockade. The patient may not be fully reversed and exhibit signs of residual neuromuscular blockade. Inadequate respiratory effort, inability to maintain a head lift for 5 seconds, inappropriate use of chest and abdominal wall muscles, air hunger, anxiety, and tachycardia are signs that may indicate residual paralysis.[4] Neuromuscular blocking agents are summarized in Box 14-5. Information about various muscle relaxants, their onset and duration, and other comparisons are given in Table 14-2.

Hypothermia may prolong neuromuscular blockade associated with nondepolarizing muscle relaxants; therefore, the patient's temperature must be monitored. Other conditions that increase the effects of neuromuscular blocking agents are listed in Box 14-6.

box 14-4
Managing Laryngospasm and Airway Obstruction

Laryngospasm

Laryngospasm is a spasm of the laryngeal musculature. The spasm is often caused by blood, mucus, or other oral secretions that irritate the vocal cords. Careful suctioning of the oropharynx before extubation helps to prevent spasm. In most cases, laryngospasm will break with the application of positive pressure with 100% fraction of inspired oxygen (FIO_2) via a bag-valve mask with a tight seal. If this does not break the spasm, a dose of depolarizing muscle relaxant (succinylcholine) may be given.

Upper Airway Obstruction

Upper airway obstruction must be identified and treated promptly and effectively. Airway obstruction may range from minimal to complete. Signs of obstruction include:

- Paradoxical breathing
- Stridor
- Lack of, or change in, breath sounds
- Alteration in vital signs
- Change in level of consciousness

Treatment to relieve obstruction must be provided in a systematic fashion.

1. Tilt head/lift chin.
2. Thrust jaw.
3. Call for assistance.
4. Insert an oropharyngeal or nasopharyngeal airway. (Bear in mind that an oropharyngeal airway may not be tolerated by the partially obtunded patient.)
5. Apply positive-pressure ventilation.
6. Administer succinylcholine.

box 14-5
Neuromuscular Blocking Agents

Muscle Relaxants

- Neuromuscular blockers pharmacologically paralyze patients and provide no sedation or analgesia.
- Neuromuscular blocking agents are used to facilitate endotracheal intubation, relax muscles for surgical procedures, terminate laryngospasm, eliminate chest wall rigidity, and provide for ease of mechanical ventilation if indicated.
- There are two groups of muscle relaxants, depolarizing and nondepolarizing, that work at the myoneural junction, affecting the chemical transmitter acetylcholine.

Depolarizing Agent (succinylcholine)

- This drug combines with acetylcholine receptors at the myoneural junction and mimics the action of acetylcholine.
- Onset of action is 1–2 minutes and duration of action is 4–6 minutes.
- The enzyme pseudocholinesterase removes succinylcholine from plasma, so in conditions involving a decrease in pseudocholinesterase, the length of action of succinylcholine increases, keeping patients paralyzed for longer periods.
- Increased pseudocholinesterase enzyme may be seen in pregnancy, liver disease, malnutrition states, severe anemia, cancer, and with other pharmacological agents, such as quinidine, phospholine eye drops, and propranolol.

Nondepolarizing Agents

- Nondepolarizing agents (atacurium, cisatracurium, mivacurium chloride, pipecuronium bromide, vecuronium, *d*-tubocurarine, pancuronium, doxacurium, rocuronium) compete with acetylcholine at the myoneural junction for muscle membrane receptors.
- Onset of action is within 2–3 minutes.
- Duration of action ranges from 20 minutes to 2 hours, depending on the medication and dosage.
- May be reversed pharmacologically with anticholinesterase drugs (neostigmine, pyridostigmine, edrophonium). Duration of action of anticholinesterase is brief, so there is a chance the patient may have continued muscle weakness or respiratory depression. Anticholinesterases may induce muscarinic side effects, including bradycardia, lacrimation, defecation, and increased salivary and bronchial secretions. These side effects are counteracted with the routine administration of anticholinergic drugs (atropine, glycopyrrolate) in conjunction with the anticholinesterase.

Hypotension

Probably the most common cardiovascular complication seen in the postoperative period is hypotension. It is most often caused by a decreased circulating blood volume. Hypotension is defined as a 25% to 30% decrease in systolic blood pressure from the resting baseline value.

table 14-2 Muscle Relaxant Comparisons

Drug	Onset	Duration	Dose	Metabolism Elimination	Histamine	Side Effects	Advantages
Depolarizing							
Succinylcholine	1–2 min	4–6 min	1.5–2 mg/kg	Plasmacholinesterase Renal, biliary	Possible	↓ Pulse Fasciculations Cardiac dysrhythmia Hyperkalemia ↑ ICP ↑ IOP	Short acting
Nondepolarizing							
Mivacurium chloride (Mivacron)	2–2.5 min	10–15 min	0.1–0.25 mg/kg	Plasmacholinesterase Renal, biliary	Yes	Flushing Hypotension Dysrhythmia Rash, muscle spasm Bronchospasm	Short acting Minimal CV side effects
Atracurium (Tracrium)	Within 2 min	30–45 min	0.4–0.5 mg/kg	Hoffman elimination Ester hydrolysis	Mild		Intermediate acting No CV effect Easily reversed Block not prolonged
Vecuronium (Norcuron)	Within 3 min	30–45 min	0.06–0.1 mg/kg	Hepatic, renal to none	Very mild		Intermediate acting Little or no CV effect Easily reversed
Rocuronium (Zemuron)	1–1.5 min	20–40 min	0.45–1.2 mg/kg	Renal, biliary	Low	↑ PVR	Intermediate acting Minimal CV effects
Cisatracurium (Nimbex)	2–3 min	40–60 min	0.15–0.2 mg/kg	Hoffman elimination Renal and hepatic	None		Intermediate acting Hemodynamic stability
d-Tubocurarine (Curare)	Within 3 min	45–60 min	Up to 0.6 mg/kg	Renal, hepatic	Yes	Hypotension Histamine-like reaction	Long acting
Pancuronium (Pavulon)	Within 4 min	1–1 1/2h	0.04–0.1 mg/kg	Renal, hepatic, biliary	Isolated cases	Avoid with: Myasthenia gravis Renal disease Hypersensitivity to bromide Coronary artery disease	Long acting
Doxacurium (Nuromax)	4–6 min	100–160 min	0.05–0.08 mg/kg	Renal	None	Potentiated by inhalation agents, particularly halothane Prolonged recovery in elderly	Long acting
Pipecuronium (Arduan)	3–5 min	60–120 min	0.14 mg/kg	Renal, biliary	None	Hypoglycemia Hyperkalemia CNS depressant Respiratory depressant	Long acting No CV effects

ICP, intracranial pressure; IOP, intraocular pressure; CV, cardiovascular; PVR, peripheral vascular resistance; CNS, central nervous system.

box 14-6
Conditions and Medications That Increase the Effects of Nondepolarizing Muscle Relaxants

Local anesthetics
General anesthetics
Antibiotics: aminoglycosides, polypeptides, polymyxin
Antiarrhythmics: quinidine, procainamide
Furosemide
Acid–base status: respiratory acidosis, metabolic alkalosis
Electrolyte imbalance: hypokalemia, hypocalcemia, dehydration, magnesium administration
Hypothermia

Intervention is indicated if the pressure decreases by more than 30% of the baseline value.[5] Risk factors for postanesthesia hypotension are listed in Box 14-7.

Anesthetic agents may affect the blood pressure in various ways. Regional anesthetics, such as bupivacaine and tetracaine, may decrease blood pressure by sympathetic blockade and vasodilation. IV agents, including opioids, cause vasodilation and histamine release, resulting in lowered blood pressure. Tranquilizers, especially droperidol and chlorpromazine hydrochloride, produce sympathetic blockade and subsequent decreased blood pressure. Barbiturates cause myocardial depression, as do inhalation agents such as isoflurane, enflurane, halothane, sevoflurane, and desflurane. Muscle relaxants may cause hypotension by ganglionic blockade and histamine release.

Because decreased venous return is seen with hypovolemia and myocardial depression, the nurse considers the adequacy of volume replacement, blood loss, third spacing, and excessive diuresis. The nurse evaluates the patient for orthostatic hypotension by taking vital signs with the patient supine and after raising the head of the bed 60 degrees (if not contraindicated by the surgical procedure or patient status). Cardiac dysrhythmias may cause hypotension, especially when cardiac output is decreased, as it is with supraventricular tachycardia and marked bradycardias. Other causes of early postoperative hypotension include sepsis, pulmonary embolism, transfusion reaction, and pain.

Deliberate, controlled hypotensive techniques are often used during specific procedures, such as neurosurgical procedures of the head and neck, shoulder arthroscopy, and some oncologic operations. The advantages of this technique are that it minimizes blood loss and the need for transfusion, and decreases oozing and possible hematoma formation.

Treatment of hypotension is directed to the underlying cause. A complete report from the anesthesia provider, including the techniques used during surgery and any untoward events that occurred, helps the nurse identify the underlying cause.

Various interventions may be used to treat hypotension. A priority is to ensure adequate oxygenation and ventilation of the patient while the blood pressure is being addressed. Anesthetic drugs may require reversal, including muscle relaxant reversal with anticholinesterase and anticholinergic agents, narcotic reversal with naloxone, and benzodiazepine reversal with flumazenil. Vasopressor drugs can be administered to increase blood pressure. IV fluids, including blood products, plasma expanders, and crystalloids, may be administered. Dressings, drains, and surgical sites should be inspected frequently for signs of hemorrhage.

An important consideration when assessing and treating the patient with hypotension is the possibility of technical rather than physiological problems. Is the blood pressure cuff the correct size and is it positioned correctly? Is the stethoscope positioned correctly? Is the patient's position a factor? If an arterial line is present, is the patient peripherally constricted, or does peripheral vascular disease exist? Is the transducer balanced and correctly calibrated? Troubleshooting should occur simultaneously with assessment.

box 14-7 ***Risk Factors for Hypotension Postanesthesia***

Anesthetic Agents
- Regional agents
- Opioids
- Tranquilizers
- Barbiturates
- Muscle relaxants
- Inhalation agents

Decreased Venous Return
- Hypovolemia (inadequate replacement, continued blood loss)
- Hypothermia
- Myocardial depression
- Third spacing
- Sepsis
- Transfusion reaction
- Tight abdominal dressing
- Increased intrathoracic pressure

Cardiac
- Dysrhythmias (supraventricular tachycardia)
- Myocardial infarction
- Congestive heart failure

Pulmonary
- Hypoxia
- Acidosis
- Pulmonary embolism
- Pneumothorax

Vasovagal Reactions
- Bradycardia
- Pain
- Bladder/abdominal distension

Technical Problems
- Blood pressure cuff size and position
- Transducer balance and calibration
- Stethoscope position

Hypertension

Hypertension is classified according to its degree of severity. It ranges from mild with a diastolic pressure between 90 and 104 mm Hg, to severe with a diastolic pressure between 105 and 120 mm Hg, to malignant with a diastolic pressure greater than 120 mm Hg.

The two most common causes of postoperative hypertension are a history of hypertension, and pain. Hypertension may be associated with peripheral vasoconstriction and shivering. Inhalation and IV anesthetic agents may produce hypoxia and hypercarbia with a resultant increase in catecholamine release and blood pressure elevation. Ketamine, a dissociative drug used in anesthesia, stimulates the sympathetic nervous system and may cause tachycardia and hypertension. Also, if given too rapidly, naloxone may precipitate hypertension, which in turn may precipitate pulmonary edema or cerebral hemorrhage. Other causes of hypertension include hyperthermia, anxiety, urinary bladder distention, fluid overload, pain, a too-narrow blood pressure cuff, and withholding of antihypertensive therapy before surgery.

Transient hypertension may occur during induction, intubation, or positioning, when the surgical incision is made, or during postanesthesia. Transient hypertension can be avoided by a vigilant anesthesia practitioner.

The hypertensive patient requires reassurance, close observation, and aggressive postoperative treatment. The treatment is first directed to the cause of the hypertension, if known. Unless instructed otherwise, patients should take their antihypertensive medication up to the time of the surgical procedure. Antihypertensive medications may be ordered if indicated by the severity of hypertension. Short-acting peripheral vasodilators, such as hydralazine and nifedipine, may be used. Labetalol, a beta-adrenergic blocker, may also be prescribed. Continuous vasodilator drips of sodium nitroprusside or nitroglycerin are used to bring the blood pressure within safe limits and maintain it. When hypertension accompanies emergence delirium, opioids or physostigmine, an anticholinesterase, may be required. If the patient is hypertensive due to anxiety and verbal reassurance is ineffective, tranquilizers, such as diazepam, midazolam, and lorazepam, may be indicated. Urinary catheterization and aggressive treatment with diuretics such as furosemide may be used if the hypertension is a result of fluid overload during surgery.

Cardiac Dysrhythmias

The dysrhythmias covered in this chapter are those induced by anesthetic agents and complications frequently seen in the immediate postoperative period (Table 14-3). Refer to Chapter 17 for detailed information on identifying specific cardiac dysrhythmias. There are many causes of cardiac dysrhythmias in the immediate postoperative period. Some of the most common are residual anesthetic agents, anticholinesterase drugs, hypoxemia, hypoventilation, hypovolemia, fluid overload, hyperthermia, hypothermia, and pain (Box 14-8).

Hypothermia

Hypothermia is present when the body temperature is less than 35°C (95°F). Heat loss during surgery occurs secondary to reduced basal metabolism when patients given muscle relaxants fail to shiver. Also, vasodilation caused by inhalation anesthetic agents, related to sympathetic blockade with inhibition of motor and sensory nerve fibers, and resulting when regional techniques are used, is a factor in hypothermia. Other intraoperative causes include heat loss through radiation, exposure, convection, and conduction because of prolonged exposure of body surface; lying under saturated drapes (especially in long procedures); use of antiseptic prepping solutions; and use of cold irrigation or IV solutions. Older, debilitated patients and newborns are more intolerant of temperature changes and thus more prone to hypothermia. Hats and other warming devices, such as fluid warmers and warming blankets, may prevent hypothermia.

Hypothermia, with its associated vasoconstriction and initial increase in blood pressure, requires special attention in the postoperative phase. Care must be taken in rewarming because too rapid rewarming of the patient may result in an acute drop in blood pressure and other significant problems.

Hyperthermia

Hyperthermia is a body temperature greater than 39°C (102.2°F). Elevated temperature may occur in the anesthetized patient secondary to thermal insulation from the surgical drapes and the administration of inhalation anesthetics. Anticholinergic drugs may also induce a pharmacological loss of thermoregulatory capacity. Most patients with an elevated temperature either arrive in the surgical suite with a fever or have a pyrogenic response from septicemia. Other possible causes of postoperative hyperthermia are allergic reactions to blood or drugs, central nervous system disorders, and infection.

Malignant Hyperthermia

One of the most catastrophic events that can occur in the immediate postoperative period is malignant hyperthermia. Although most cases of malignant hyperthermia occur in the operating room during the administration of a general anesthetic, the immediate 12-hour period after general anesthesia is also a critical time. Malignant hyperthermia is a hypermetabolic syndrome that may be triggered in susceptible individuals by commonly used anesthetic agents, including succinylcholine and the halogenated inhalation agents. Other anesthetic agents are safe to use, including nitrous oxide, local anesthetics, opioids, propofol, sodium thiopental, and the nondepolarizing muscle relaxants.

The exact mechanism of malignant hyperthermia is not well understood. Research points to a derangement in muscle contraction. The known triggering agents cause a release of calcium from muscle storage sites, leading to an elevated concentration of calcium. This high calcium level increases metabolism and causes muscle to contract and become rigid (masseter muscle rigidity). This process results in hyperthermia, acid–base imbalance, and muscle cell breakdown.

Malignant hyperthermia is a rare, inherited autosomal dominant disorder of skeletal muscle and is more prevalent in those with muscular abnormalities. Malignant hyperthermia has been linked to several other muscle disorders, including some forms of muscular dystrophy, but whether this is true malignant hyperthermia is not clear. Most experts on malignant hyperthermia do not believe that caffeine or stress will precipitate malignant hyperthermia. The

table 14-3 **Cardiac Dysrhythmias Associated With Anesthetic Options**

Anesthetic Option	Dysrhythmia
Local anesthesia with epinephrine	Tachycardia
Spinal and epidural	Bradycardia second-degree vagal response; PACs, PVCs, supraventricular tachycardia, atrial fibrillation second-degree sympathetic stimulation; wandering pacemaker and heart block second-degree increased vagal tone
Barbiturates	
Pentothal	Bradycardia, AV dissociation, occasional PVC
Nonbarbiturate etomidate	Sinus tachycardia
Opioids	
Morphine sulfate	Transient brachycardia
Meperidine hydrochloride	Transient tachycardia
Fentanyl	Bradycardia
Opioid antagonist	PVCs, ventricular tachycardia, occasional ventricular fibrillation
Neuroleptanalgesia (droperidol component)	Tachycardia
Dissociative agent	Myocardial depression, ventricular ectopy, tachycardia
Inhalation agents	
Halothane	AV dissociation, ventricular dysrhythmias if hypercarbia occurs
Halothane plus aminophylline, cocaine, lidocaine	Bradycardia
Halothane plus pancuronium	PACs and PVCs
Isoflurane	Tachycardia
Enflurane	AV dissociation
Muscle relaxants	
Succinylcholine	Sinus bradycardia, junctional rhythms, PVCs Patients with burns, trauma, paraplegia or quadriplegia prone to ST segment depression, peaked T waves, widening QRS complex leading to ventricular tachycardia, ventricular fibrillation, or asystole
Pipecuronium bromide	Atrial fibrillation, ventricular extrasystole
Pancuronium	Tachycardia and nodal rhythms
d-Tubocurarine	Tachycardia
Anticholinesterases	Bradycardia, slowed AV conduction, PVC
Anticholinergics	Tachycardia

PAC, premature atrial contraction; PVC, premature ventricular contraction; AV, atrioventricular.

exact incidence of malignant hyperthermia is not known. The rate of occurrence has been estimated at between 1 in 5000 and as rare as 1 in 65,000. The states with the highest incidence are Michigan, West Virginia, and Wisconsin.[6]

Clinical manifestations include an increase in temperature of 0.5°C or more every 15 minutes from the time of induction of anesthesia to as high as 46°C, muscle rigidity, hypercarbia, unexplained tachycardia, sweating, and unstable blood pressure. Masseter muscle rigidity after the administration of succinylcholine is the earliest warning sign of malignant hyperthermia. Temperature elevation is quite dramatic but is not the first sign of malignant hyperthermia. If the patient's temperature increases rapidly and the anesthetic is not discontinued and treatment rapidly instituted, death may occur.

Malignant hyperthermia is treated vigorously with dantrolene sodium (Dantrium), 100% oxygen administration, correction of acid–base imbalances, and removal of triggering agents. Cooling measures, such as icing down the patient and cold fluids, are used. Dantrolene sodium 2.5 mg/kg IV is given and may be repeated up to 10 mg/kg as necessary to control signs and symptoms. Dantrolene sodium is reconstituted with preservative-free sterile water. The administration of dantrolene is labor intensive, thus requiring assistance. Most institutions that administer anesthesia have a malignant hyperthermia kit in the operating suite. Box 14-9 lists the common contents of a malignant hyperthermia kit.

After the acute phase of the malignant hyperthermia crisis, care includes observation in a critical care unit for at least 24 hours and administration of dantrolene sodium 1 mg/kg every 6 hours for 24 to 48 hours. Oral dantrolene may then be used with monitoring of arterial blood gases, creatinine kinase, potassium, calcium, urine, serum myoglobin, and clotting studies every 6 hours. Patients should be referred to the Malignant Hyperthermia Association of the United States (MHAUS) for support and continued education about this disorder.[7]

box 14-8 ***Risk Factors That Precipitate Dysrhythmias***

- Hypoxemia (sinus bradycardia, sinus tachycardia, PVCs, supraventricular tachycardia)
- Hypoventilation/Hypercarbia (sinus tachycardia, PVCs, sinus bradycardia)
- Hypovolemia (sinus tachycardia)
- Fluid overload (PVCs, supraventricular tachycardia, PACs, atrial fibrillation/flutter)
- Hyperthermia (sinus tachycardia, PVCs)
- Hypothermia (sinus bradycardia, atrial fibrillation, atrioventricular nodal blocks)
- Pain (sinus tachycardia, PVCs)

PVCs, premature ventricular contractions; PACs, premature atrial contractions.

Nausea and Vomiting

Nausea and vomiting occur frequently in the immediate postoperative period and may result from any of the anesthetic options. Nausea is a subjective, unpleasant experience usually leading to vomiting. Although not usually life-threatening, postoperative nausea and vomiting (PONV) leaves the patient with a lasting unpleasant memory and may have an impact on future surgical and anesthetic decisions. PONV is a major complication associated with the need for admission after outpatient surgery. Frequent causes include use of preoperative and intraoperative opioids; increased gastric secretions; certain anesthetic techniques, particularly spinal anesthesia; and surgical procedures involving manipulation of eye muscles, abdominal muscles, and genitourinary muscles. Laparoscopic techniques and procedures involving the breast are also associated with an increase in postoperative nausea and vomiting.

Vomiting is controlled by the vomiting center located in the medulla. Once stimulated, efferent impulses are sent by the 5th, 7th, 9th, 10th, and 12th cranial nerves, spinal nerves, and phrenic nerves to the diaphragm, esophagus, and stomach. The vomiting center receives input directly from the gastrointestinal tract, the chemoreceptor trigger zone, the labyrinthine apparatus (motion sickness), and various cortical and visual stimuli.

The critical care nurse must be cognizant of the potential for regurgitation and aspiration in all patients who have been anesthetized. Vomiting is an active process, whereas regurgitation is passive. Adequate positioning of the unconscious patient is essential. The ideal position is on the side with the head and neck extended. If the surgical procedure precludes turning the patient on the side or the patient is unable to comply, then the patient must not be left unattended until consciousness is regained.

Antiemetics frequently are ordered in the immediate postoperative period. The critical care nurse should recognize that many antiemetics potentiate the effects of other medications, particularly opioids. Therefore, decreased doses of opioids for pain relief may be indicated.

Often, nausea and vomiting can be relieved by identifying the causative factor (e.g., gastric distension, hypotension, administration of opioids) and making the appropriate intervention.

box 14-9
Contents of Malignant Hyperthermia Kit

- Methylprednisolone
- Furosemide
- Sodium bicarbonate
- Dextrose (50%)
- Sterile water
- Insulin
- Mannitol
- Refrigerated intravenous fluids
- Dantrolene sodium
- New oxygen tubing and delivery devices
- Foley catheter tray
- Nasogastric tubes
- Blood specimen tubes
- Arterial blood gas kits

Postoperative Pain

Patients normally expect to feel pain when their surgical procedure is over. The incidence of pain and its severity depend on the individual. All pain assessment in the immediate postoperative period must be individualized. A number of factors affect the severity of pain, including the site of the operation, the psychological state of the patient, and the anesthetic technique used.

If the anesthetic option chosen was use of inhalation agents without the use of opioids or local anesthetics, then the patient may have more pain than one who received some form of analgesia during surgery. Patients who have been given analgesic medication during the procedure and who then receive naloxone at the end may also experience severe pain because naloxone reverses the analgesic effects of any prior medication. Because these patients may renarcotize, the nurse must wait 15 to 45 minutes after the administration of naloxone before medicating the patient with an analgesic. Box 14-10 outlines some factors that may influence the patient's response to pain.

INTRAVENOUS MEDICATIONS

IV titration of opioids in the immediate postoperative period offers the quickest and most effective method of pain relief. Because the patient's basal metabolic rate is decreased during surgery, the uptake of intramuscular medication is difficult to predict.

INTRAMUSCULAR MEDICATIONS

One intramuscular medication, ketorolac tromethamine (Toradol), administered during surgery, has proved effective in the management of postoperative pain. Ketorolac tromethamine is a nonsteroidal anti-inflammatory drug (NSAID) that exhibits analgesic, anti-inflammatory, and antipyretic activity. Peak analgesia occurs in 45 to 60 minutes after intramuscular or IV injection, and the analgesic effect lasts 6 to 8 hours. The medication should not be used for more than 5 days, and no more than a 30-mg dose should be used. The medication is contraindicated in

box 14-10
Factors Influencing Pain

Surgical procedure: Site and nature of the operation
Anxiety level: Fear of surgery, disfigurement, death, loss of control
Patient expectations: Effectiveness of preoperative teaching, adequately prepared for outcome
Pain tolerance: Prior use of medications, including analgesics, individual differences
Anesthesia technique: Analgesics used during the intraoperative period, use of naloxone

patients with active peptic ulcers, recent gastrointestinal bleeds, or renal insufficiency.[4]

PATIENT-CONTROLLED ANALGESIA AND EPIDURAL MEDICATIONS

Trends in pain control management include use of patient-controlled analgesia (PCA) devices and epidural analgesia. The use of PCA pumps has increased significantly during recent years, and it is believed that patients report less pain when they maintain autonomy by controlling the administration of opioids for their pain relief.

Epidural analgesia has proved successful in treating acute pain after surgery. Patients who receive epidural opioids are less sedated and therefore ambulate sooner and have improved respiratory function. Epidural medications may be administered as a bolus injection or by a continuous infusion. When administering continuous infusions, an infusion pump should be used. Safeguards to be taken include using preservative-free medications in the epidural infusion; using infusion sets that have no injection ports; and labeling the infusing pump, infusion bag, and infusion tubing with the word *epidural.* The reason for such safeguards is that accidental infusion of vasodilators, chemotherapy medications, antibiotics, and medications with any type of preservative could permanently destroy nerve tissue and paralyze or even kill the patient.

Frequently used preservative-free epidural medications include morphine, hydromorphone, meperidine, and fentanyl. The duration of sensory analgesia varies with the opioid administered. The more lipid-soluble agents penetrate the dura mater more rapidly, resulting in a more rapid diffusion away from the spinal cord and subarachnoid space and hence a shorter duration of action. The most frequently used opioids for epidural administration for which average duration times have been identified are morphine, with a duration that varies from 2 to 24 hours; hydromorphone, with an average duration of 10 to 14 hours; meperidine, with an average duration of 6 to 8 hours; and fentanyl, with an average duration of 4 to 6 hours.

Dilute local anesthetic solutions are used either in conjunction with the previously mentioned opioids or used alone. Local anesthetics used alone and in conjunction with narcotics are lidocaine, mepivacaine, prilocaine, bupivacaine, and etidocaine. The most common local anesthesia used for epidural infusions is bupivacaine. The combination of local anesthetics and opioids has been used to obtain a rapid onset and prolonged duration of analgesia. The local agents work more rapidly, and the opioids have a more prolonged action. Side effects may occur with the use of opioids and anesthetic solutions in the epidural space. Nurses have the primary responsibility for recognizing and preventing side effects when caring for patients receiving epidural analgesia, as listed in Box 14-11. Adequate pain relief during the postoperative period allows the patient to cough, deep breathe, and ambulate sooner, thus preventing complications.

OTHER MEDICATION METHODS

Other techniques investigated as alternatives in pain management include intrathecal and interpleural methods, transdermal patches, and transmucosal–nasal aerosol delivery systems. Intrathecal analgesia is injected, usually as a one-time dose, directly into the cerebrospinal fluid of the subarachnoid space.[7] Interpleural techniques involve administration of local anesthetics into the interpleural space. A series of injections are given or a catheter is placed during the perioperative period, but occasionally after surgery. Continuous infusions and bolus injections may be given.

Transdermal patches of fentanyl are being studied, as are transmucosal–nasal aerosol delivery systems.[1–3] Transdermal fentanyl is an excellent alternative to sustained-release morphine preparations, especially when oral medication is not possible or is contraindicated. Patches are constructed as a drug reservoir separated from the skin by a microporous rate-limiting membrane and adhesive polymer. The major disadvantages, to the transdermal patches are the

box 14-11
Side Effects From Epidural Analgesia

Specific protocols for epidural management are essential for each individual hospital.

Urinary retention
- Catheterize as needed.

Postural hypotension
- Give fluid (volume) replacement.
- Administer ephedrine 5 mg IV as ordered.

Pruritus (itching of face, head, and neck)
- Treat with Benadryl 25 mg PO, IM, IV.
- Treat with naloxone 0.1 mg IV.
- Treat with propofol 10 mg IV.

Nausea and vomiting
- Administer metoclopramide 10 mg IV.
- Administer scopolamine patch.
- Administer ondansetron (Zofram) 4 mg IV.
- Administer dolasetron 12.5 mg IV.

Respiratory depression (risk increases with age)
- Assess for first signs which may include change in level of consciousness.
- Assess for occurrence up to 24 hours after opioid injection with naloxone 0.1 mg up to a maximum of 0.4 mg IV.
- Observe continuously because naloxone's duration is 30 minutes.
- Have naloxone and ephedrine readily available at the bedside of patients who have received epidural opioids or anesthetics.

slow onset and the inability to change dosages rapidly in response to changing opioid requirements. Oral transmucosal fentanyl citrate has been evaluated and approved for pediatric premedication and sedation. The onset of sedation is within 5 to 10 minutes, and full recovery is within 60 minutes after administration of the "fentanyl oralet." Plasma levels rise as the patient sucks on the lozenge on a stick. These oralets should be used only in the hospital setting where 1:1 observation of respiratory function may be measured. Side effects of oral transmucosal fentanyl citrate include nausea and vomiting and facial pruritus.

clinical applicability challenges

Self-Challenges: Critical Thinking

1. *Compare and contrast the actions of the depolarizing muscle relaxants with the nondepolarizing muscle relaxants and identify medications that may be used to reverse these agents pharmacologically.*
2. *Develop a plan of care for the patient who has a known family history of malignant hyperthermia.*
3. *Relate any dysrhythmias demonstrated by the anesthetized patient to his or her clinical condition.*
4. *Discuss the admission of a postoperative patient to your unit and detail priorities of care on arrival.*
5. *Compare and contrast postoperative pain modalities for the patient who has received general anesthesia with parenteral opioids versus general anesthesia and has an epidural catheter in place.*
6. *Develop a plan of care for the patient who presents to the postanesthesia care unit (PACU) with postoperative shivering.*

Study Questions

1. *Which of the following medications should be available for a patient with suspected malignant hyperthermia?*
   a. *Dantrolene sodium*
   b. *Calcium chloride*
   c. *Succinylcholine*
   d. *Dextrose 70%*
2. *Which of the following agents is associated with the lowest incidence of postoperative nausea and vomiting?*
   a. *Thiopental*
   b. *Etomidate*
   c. *Ketamine*
   d. *Propofol*
3. *Which of the following is a major cause of postoperative hypoxemia?*
   a. *A high inspired oxygen concentration*
   b. *Hyperventilation*
   c. *Hypothermia*
   d. *Atelectasis*
4. *Which of the following should be the first monitor attached to the patient on arrival in the postanesthesia care area (PACU)?*
   a. *Pulse oximeter*
   b. *Cardiac monitor*
   c. *Noninvasive blood pressure*
   d. *Temperature monitoring device*
5. *Your postoperative patient is ready for extubation in the PACU. What objective criteria do you use?*
   a. *A negative inspiratory force greater than -20 cm H_2O*
   b. *A vital capacity greater than 5 mL/kg*
   c. *Patient is awake*
   d. *Heart rate greater than 110 beats per minute*
6. *Which of the following oxygen administration devices would you expect to use to provide supplemental oxygen to a patient in the PACU after repair of a fractured tibia?*
   a. *Simple face mask*
   b. *Bag-valve mask*
   c. *Venturi mask*
   d. *Nasal cannula*

REFERENCES

1. American Society of PeriAnesthesia Nurses: Standards of PeriAnesthesia Nursing Practice. Thorofare, NJ, American Society of PeriAnesthesia Nurses, 2002
2. Kost M: Manual of Conscious Sedation. Philadelphia, WB Saunders, 1998
3. Patterson C: New rules impact sedation and anesthesia care. Nurs Management 31:22, 2000
4. Nagelhout J, Zaglaniczny K: Nurse Anesthesia (2nd Ed). Philadelphia, WB Saunders, 2001
5. Vender JS, Spiess BD: Post Anesthesia Care. Philadelphia, WB Saunders, 1992
6. Malignant Hyperthermia Association of the United States: A concern for OR and PACU nurses. Sherburne, NY, Malignant Hyperthermia Association of the United States, 2001
7. Martin SN, Vane EA: Malignant hyperthermia: A case study. Semin Periop Nurs 9:27–36, 2000

OTHER SELECTED READING

Beyea SC: The ideal state of perioperative nursing. AORN J 73:817, 2001

Buggy DJ, Crossley AW: Thermoregulation, mild hypothermia and postanesthetic shivering. Br J Anaesth 84:615–628, 2000

Carkner H: Some good news and some truly useful nursing research. Nurs Econ 18:308, 2000

Chang AM, Ip WY, Cheung TH: Patient-controlled analgesia versus conventional intramuscular injection: A cost effectiveness analysis. J Adv Nurs 46(5):531–544, 2004

Cornish PB, Barton J, Deacon A: The impact of regional anesthesia on outcome: A patient's perspective. Anaesthesia 59(6):613–615, 2004

Duncan PG, Shandro J, Bachand R, Ainsworth L: A pilot study of recovery room bypass ("fast-track protocol") in a community hospital. Can J Anaesth 48(7):630–636, 2001

Kovac AL: Update on prophylaxis and treatment of postoperative nausea and vomiting. Anesth Analg 26:131–143, 2003

Mace L: An audit of post-operative nausea and vomiting, following cardiac surgery: Scope of the problem. Nurs Crit Care:8(5):187–196, 2003

McCarthy EJ: Malignant hyperthermia pathophysiology, clinical presentation, and treatment. AACN Clin Issues 15(2):231–237, 2004

Ng A, Smith G: Gastroesophageal reflux and aspiration of gastric contents in anesthetic practice. Anesth Analg 93:494–513, 2001

Saar LM: Use of a modified postanesthesia recovery score in phase II perianesthesia period of ambulatory surgery patients. J Perianesth Nurs 16(2):82–89, 2001

Schechter LN: Advances in postoperative pain management: The pharmacy perspective. Am J Health Syst Pharm 61:S15–S21, 2004

Sessler DJ: Perioperative heat balance. Anesthesiology 92:578–596, 2000

Troung L, Moran JL, Blum P: Post-anesthesia care unit discharge: A clinical scoring system versus traditional time-based criteria. Anaesth Intensive Care 32(1):33–42, 2004

Watcho MF: The cost-effective management of postoperative nausea and vomiting. J Adv Nurs 29:1130–1136, 2000

Wong K, Chong WK, Sia AT: Patient controlled epidural anesthesia. Anesthesia 56:1090–1115, 2001

chapter

15

Interfacility Transport of the Critically Ill Patient

KATHLEEN KEENAN ■ DENNIS W. JONES

objectives

Based on the content in this chapter, the reader should be able to:

- Describe the indications for interfacility transport of the critically ill patient.
- Compare and contrast the advantages and disadvantages of air versus ground transport.
- Discuss the specific considerations and implications for care for air transport.
- Explain the Emergency Medical Transfer Active Labor Act (EMTALA) requirements for an appropriate interhospital transfer.
- Describe key factors necessary for an effective interfacility transfer plan.
- Analyze the role of the registered nurse in the five phases of the interfacility transport of the critically ill.

Critically ill patients are transported between facilities daily. These transfers are linked to a number of factors. Typically, transport is indicated when the patient's need for complex diagnostic procedures or sophisticated medical and nursing expertise exceeds what can be provided at a facility. Family requests may also affect the decision to transport. For example, a family may want their family member transferred to a hospital closer to home.

Outcomes of evolving health care reform also have increased the demands for interfacility transport of critically ill patients. Third-party payors may require patients to be transported to a facility that is a member of their network. In addition, many hospitals vie for fewer patients and have developed their own transport teams to provide a flow of patients to their particular facility.

Whatever the reason for transporting a patient, a risk/benefit analysis of the transport should always be performed. Risks for the patient range from physical safety to physiological compromise to emotional distress.[1] Benefits from interfacility transport include access to lifesaving assessment techniques and specialized interventions that can improve the patient's outcome. When the benefits for the patient exceed the risks, an interfacility transport is warranted.

The American College of Emergency Physicians (ACEP) has outlined physician responsibilities at this point. These responsibilities are as follows:

- The sending physician performs the patient assessment and determines the appropriate level of care during transfer.
- The receiving physician ensures that his or her facility is capable of caring for the patient.
- The medical director of the transferring agency provides medical direction during transport.[2]

MODES OF TRANSPORT

Once the decision has been made to transport, the method of transport must be determined. The two primary methods of interfacility transport are ground and air. Ground transport includes ambulances and mobile intensive care units (ICUs). Air transport can occur by either a rotary-wing vehicle (helicopter) or a fixed-wing vehicle (airplane). When selecting the mode of transport, the following factors must be considered:

- Distance
- The safety of the transport environment
- Patient "out of hospital" time
- The patient's condition and the potential for complications
- The patient's need for critical or time-sensitive intervention (e.g., rescue angioplasty)
- Traffic conditions
- Weather conditions[3]

In addition, the advantages and disadvantages of ground versus air transport must be considered when selecting the mode of transport. Table 15-1 summarizes the advantages and disadvantages of ground versus air transport.

AIR TRANSPORT OF THE CRITICALLY ILL PATIENT

Table 15-2 summarizes the special considerations for air transport. It is important for the nurse who may be caring for a patient to have a basic understanding of these considerations. A more thorough understanding aids in preparing the patient before the arrival of the flight team and allows for a smoother transition at the bedside on arrival.

The environment in which the patient will be transported differs greatly from the in-hospital setting. Because the patient will be transported at a higher altitude, where the barometric pressure is reduced, the possibility of hypoxia increases. Therefore, almost all patients transported by air receive supplemental oxygen. The flight team administers the appropriate amount of oxygen to the patient based on clinical condition and altitude. If applicable, advising the patient and family members of the need for oxygen during flight may help to allay any anxiety before departure.

Any air-filled cavity in the patient's body, such as the stomach, lungs, or containers (air splint, glass intravenous bottle), can be affected physiologically by changes in barometric pressure. The primary change that occurs is an expansion of the gas as the barometric pressure decreases. Depending on the amount of gas, the location of the gas, and the degree of barometric pressure change, the patient could suffer deleterious effects if not properly screened and managed. The flight team screens the patient carefully and takes preventive measures to ensure a safe and uneventful transport. However, it is important for the sending nurse to be aware of these potential problems to assist in their prevention.

Other environmental factors affecting the patient during the transport include changes in temperature and humidity as well as the presence of noise and vibration. The degree to which each of these factors occur depends very much on both the mode of transport—that is, whether the vehicle is a fixed-wing or rotary-wing aircraft—and the type of aircraft. The flight crew will take the necessary steps in either preventing or decreasing the effects of each of these factors on the patient.

If the critically ill patient is awake and aware of the need for air transport, the sending nurse screens the patient for the presence of fear or anxiety related to flying and a history of motion sickness while in a moving vehicle. Consultation with the sending physician would be indicated if any of these factors exist because treatment with an anxiolytic or antiemetic medication could aid in preventing clinical problems during the flight. The flight crew screens the patient for the presence of these factors during the preflight assessment.

TRANSFER GUIDELINES AND LEGAL IMPLICATIONS

To facilitate the appropriate transfer of patients, ACEP has developed guidelines. These principles of appropriate patient transfer are listed in Box 15-1.

table 15-1 Advantages and Disadvantages of Ground Versus Air Transport

Mode of Transport	Advantages	Disadvantages
Ground	Adequate work space for personnel and equipment Sensitive monitoring equipment may work better No weight restrictions Adequate lighting Able to travel in most types of weather	Longer transport time Unfavorable road conditions may make transport uncomfortable for patient Interventions difficult to perform in a moving vehicle Ambulance unavailable for other calls in the community
Air	May shorten "out of hospital" time Crew generally composed of advanced level care providers Improved communication capability Ground emergency medical services remain available in the community	Weather conditions restrict availability of the vehicle Potentially more costly Limited space (helicopters) Weight limitations Physiological impact on patient and crew Psychological impact on patient (e.g., fear of flying)

Holleran R: Prehospital Nursing: A Collaborative Approach. St. Louis, CV Mosby, 1994.

table 15-2 Special Considerations for Air Transport

Stressors	Effect	Nursing Interventions
Altitude change	Hypoxia is due to the following: Decrease in the partial pressure of O_2 Decrease in the diffusion gradient for oxygen molecules to cross the alveolar membrane Decrease in oxygen availability	Provide supplemental O_2. Use pulse oximeter and end tidal CO_2 monitor.
Barometric pressure (atmospheric pressure) change	With increasing altitude, the barometric pressure decreases and gases expand. Expansion of gases affects eardrums, sinuses, gastrointestinal tract, pleural spaces, and hollow organs. Expansion of gases affects air splints, pressure bags or cuffs, balloon cuffs on endotracheal tubes, intravenous fluid bags and bottles, pneumatic antishock garments.	Insert a nasogastric tube to decompress the stomach. If possible, fill cuffs with water or saline rather than air. Monitor equipment and decompress with higher altitudes. Vent glass bottles and wrap to protect against breakage. Apply pressure cuffs to IV solution bags.
Thermal change	As altitude increases, temperature decreases. Oxygen demand increases as the body tries to maintain warmth.	Use blankets to keep the patient warm.
Humidity change	As air is cooled, it loses moisture. Mucous membranes dry.	Humidify supplemental O_2. Provide adequate fluid intake.
Gravitational change	Gravitational change affects acceleration and deceleration forces. Transient increase in venous return occurs for patients positioned with head at the back of the aircraft. Potential exists for motion sickness.	Use a head-forward position for patients with fluid overload or increased intracranial pressure. To minimize motion sickness, provide O_2, cool cloth to face, cool air to face. Administer medications, such as transdermal scopolamine patches and promethazine.
Noise	It is difficult to monitor blood pressure, breath sounds, endotracheal tube air leak.	Explain sounds to patient. Monitor blood pressure by Doppler device. Provide continuous airway assessment. Wear head sets or ear plugs.
Vibration	Vibration may distort readings on equipment. Equipment may loosen or move.	Secure all equipment. Check equipment function frequently.

Harrahill M: Interfacility transfer. In Kitt S, Selfridge-Thomas J, Proehl J, et al (eds): Emergency Nursing: A Physiologic and Clinical Perspective (2nd Ed), pp 12–18. Philadelphia, WB Saunders, 1995.

Legislation also exists that provides guidelines, regulations, and penalties for patient transfer. One such law, the Consolidated Omnibus Reconciliation Act (COBRA) of 1985, contains provisions addressing the transfer of patients from hospital to hospital. The purpose of the legislation is to prevent inappropriate transfers of patients who seek emergency department care. As a result, this legislation has become known as the "antidumping" law.

The following provisions of the COBRA legislation prevent any patient from being denied an initial screening in an emergency department or from being transferred to another hospital or discharged without receiving care:

1. Hospitals must provide screening examinations for every individual who comes to the emergency department and requests care.
2. If the patient has an emergency medical condition, the hospital must provide stabilizing treatment or transfer the patient to another medical facility. The physician must document that the medical benefits outweigh the risks of the transfer.
3. The receiving medical facility agrees to accept the patient and provide appropriate medical treatment. The receiving medical facility must have adequate space and qualified personnel to care for the patient.
4. The transfer is conducted by qualified personnel and appropriate equipment needed to provide care during the transfer is available.[4]

There may be situations when a patient is not stabilized, yet is appropriate for transfer. This would occur when:

1. The risks of remaining at the initial facility outweigh the benefits of transfer.
2. The patient or family requests the transfer.
3. A physician is not present at the initial facility but a qualified medical person certifies that the benefits outweigh the risks.
4. The transfer occurs with appropriate equipment and qualified personnel.[4]

Figure 15-1 presents the requirements for evaluating a patient's suitability for transfer, as outlined by the Emergency Medical Transfer Active Labor Act (EMTALA). In addition, the Air and Surface Transport Nurses Association (ASTNA, formerly known as the National Flight Nurses Association, or NFNA) developed nursing stan-

box 15-1
Principles of Appropriate Patient Transfer

- The health and well-being of the patient must be the overriding concern when any patient transfer is considered.
- Emergency physicians and hospital personnel should comply with state and federal regulations regarding patient transfer. A medical screening exam should be performed by a physician or by properly trained ancillary personnel according to written policies and procedures.
- The patient should be transferred to another facility only after medical evaluation and, when possible, stabilization.
- The physician should inform the patient or responsible party of the reasons for and the risks and likely benefits of transfer, and document this in the medical record.
- The hospital and medical staff should identify individuals responsible for transfer decisions and clearly delineate their duties regarding the patient transfer process.
- The patient should be transferred to a facility appropriate to the medical needs of the patient, with adequate space and personnel available.
- A physician or other responsible person at the receiving hospital must agree to accept the patient prior to transfer.
- The patient transfer should not be refused by the receiving hospital when the transfer is medically indicated and the receiving hospital has the capability and/or responsibility to provide care for the patient.
- Communication to exchange clinical information between responsible persons at the transferring and receiving hospitals must occur prior to transfer.
- An appropriate medical summary and other pertinent records should accompany the patient to the receiving institution.
- The patient should be transferred in a vehicle that is staffed by qualified personnel and contains appropriate equipment.
- When transfer of patients is part of a regional plan to provide optimal care of patients at specified medical facilities, written transfer protocols and interfacility agreements should be in place.

Adapted from: American College of Emergency Physicians: Principles of appropriate patient transfer. Ann Emerg Med 19(3):337–338, 1990.

dards for transport of the critically ill patient by rotary-wing transport.

PHASES OF TRANSPORT

Five phases of transport have been identified: (1) notification and acceptance by the receiving facility, (2) preparation of the patient by the transport team, (3) the actual transport, (4) turnover of the patient to the receiving hospital, and (5) continuous quality improvement monitoring after transport. The keys to the success of transport are a comprehensive assessment, determination of the appropriateness of the transfer, collaboration, communication, evaluation, and education of personnel (Box 15-2).

Phase One: Notification and Acceptance by the Receiving Facility

The first phase of transport requires notifying the receiving facility to determine their willingness to accept the patient, and to determine the mode of transport. Communication is an essential element in this phase of the process. The sending, transporting, and receiving personnel must have the necessary information to make the transport decision. Standards of care and protocols should be in place ahead of time so that the decision to transport and the transport process are carried out in an organized way. A transfer checklist can be used to make sure no steps in the transfer process are missed. In addition, an awareness of the policies and procedures of the transporting agencies used in an area is needed for a smooth transport process.[1]

Once it has been determined that a patient requires transport to another facility, an accepting physician must be identified and an available bed confirmed. The identification of a responsible physician is essential so that a contact person is available for consultation while en route and on arrival. ACEP has described medical direction for interfacility transfers as a shared responsibility. The transferring physician ensures that the transport team is composed of professionals appropriate to the needs of the patient, and that an appropriate vehicle and equipment are used for transport.[2] If the local emergency medical system (EMS) is not providing medical direction en route, then the responsible physician must be identified as being part of the hospital-based or private ambulance program. The Emergency Nurses Association (ENA) believes that any patient transferred to another facility should be transferred at the same level of care that he or she needed in the emergency department.[3] Transport teams should have standard orders and protocols if they are unable to maintain contact with a medical center physician en route.

Current regulations require the patient or a legally authorized representative to give informed consent for the transport. If consent cannot be obtained, documentation of the indications for the transport and the reason consent was not obtained must appear in the medical record.[1]

After the transport decision is made, the receiving facility agrees to accept the patient, and the mode of transport is selected. A qualified transport team is then notified. Initial information given to the transporting agency includes the patient's name, diagnosis, reason for transfer, vital signs, intravenous and special monitoring lines, continuous infusion medications, and airway and oxygenation or ventilation status. This information assists in determining the composition of the transport team and the equipment and medications needed. The American Association of Critical-Care Nurses (AACN), the Amer-

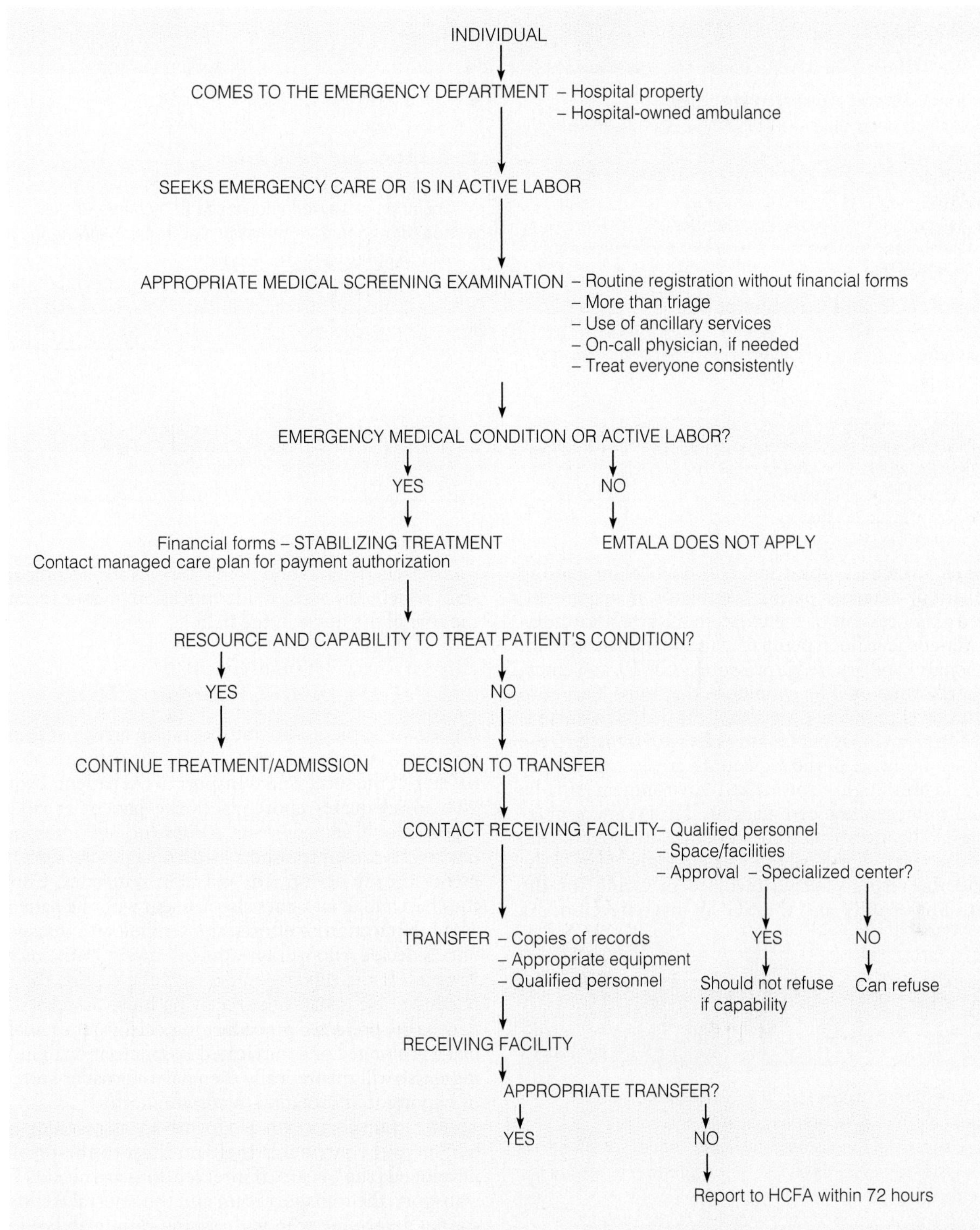

figure 15-1 Emergency Medical Transfer Active Labor Act (EMTALA) flow chart. HCFA (formerly Health Care Finance Administration) is now Center for Medicare and Medicaid Services. (Reprinted with permission from Lee NG: Legal Concepts and Issues in Emergency Care, p 140. Philadelphia, WB Saunders, 2001.)

ican College of Critical Care Medicine, and the Society of Critical Care Medicine (SCCM) offer guidelines for accompanying personnel for interfacility transfers[1] (Box 15-3). It is important to recognize, however, that these are simply guidelines and may not be followed in all cases. Therefore, it is important for the sending nurse to ascertain the credentials of the accompanying team members to ensure there is a smooth transition of care to a qualified transport team.

Individual states define the role of the nurse who may be involved in interfacility transport.[4] Some states have outlined an expanded set of specialized acts for the nurse while practicing in the prehospital setting, the interagency transport arena, or both. Examples of these specialized acts

box 15-2
Key Factors Vital to an Effective Transfer Plan

Assessment and Appropriateness

- Assess and determine available resources (quality and suitability of local technology).
- Appraise level of medical, nursing, and ancillary staff expertise.
- Assess patient benefits versus the risks of transfer.
- Determine appropriateness of transfer and appropriate receiving center.

Collaboration and Communication

- Establish a multidisciplinary team committed to quality patient care and appropriate transfer of critically ill patients.
- Promote interfacility communication that enhances transfer outcomes.

Evaluation and Education

- Approach transfer of critically ill patients as a process requiring specialized knowledge and competencies.
- Monitor and update the essential transfer knowledge and skills of appropriate personnel.
- Develop a comprehensive quality improvement program to evaluate and document problem resolution and patient transfer outcomes.

Guidelines for the Transfer of Critically Ill Patients. Prepared by the American Association of Critical-Care Nurses Transfer Guidelines Task Force and the Guidelines Committee, American College of Critical Care Medicine, Society of Critical Care Medicine, p 6. American Association of Critical-Care Nurses, Aliso Viejo, CA, 1998. Used with permission.

include endotracheal intubation, nasotracheal intubation, defibrillation, external pacing, ventilator management, needle decompression of the chest, jugular vein cannulation, intra-aortic balloon pump management, management of pulmonary capillary wedge pressure (PCWP), and emergency cardioversion. The conditions that must be met to allow this level of practice are also identified.[5] If a nurse is assigned from an inpatient unit to assist with transport, the nurse must be aware of the regulations governing nursing practice in this highly specialized environment and be qualified to meet these expectations. These state regulations should be investigated ahead of time to avoid having a nurse accompanying a patient without knowledge of the role and the responsibilities involved in caring for the patient. The AACN and the SCCM have developed a transfer curriculum and competencies for accompanying staff, which may assist in identification of issues related to the role of the nurse in the field.[1]

box 15-3
Guidelines for Accompanying Personnel for Interfacility Transfer

- A minimum of two people in addition to the vehicle operator should accompany the patient.
- At least one of the accompanying personnel should be a registered nurse, physician, or advanced emergency medical technician.
- When a physician does not accompany the patient, there should be a mechanism available to communicate with the physician any changes in the patient status and obtain additional orders. If an accompanying physician is not possible, advanced authorization by standing orders to perform acute life-saving interventions must be established.

Guidelines for the Transfer of Critically Ill Patients. Prepared by the American Association of Critical-Care Nurses Transfer Guidelines Task Force and the Guidelines Committee, American College of Critical Care Medicine, Society of Critical Care Medicine, p 11. American Association of Critical-Care Nurses, Aliso Viejo, CA, 1998. Used with permission.

Phase Two: Preparation of the Patient by the Transport Team

Phase two begins as the transport team arrives at the referral facility. A thorough report about the patient is an essential step in the successful transport of the patient. Failure to give an adequate report places the patient at risk. The report should include chief complaint, allergies, medical history, reason for transport, patient's age, vital signs, treatments already performed, and their outcomes. Copies of the chart and of all x-rays also are sent with the patient. To avoid duplication of efforts, the sending and transporting nurses decide who will give the full report to the receiving hospital. If the sending nurse calls the report, the transporting nurse updates the receiving nurse as needed. This may be the preferred procedure, especially if the patient has had a prolonged or complicated hospitalization. The sending nurse will theoretically then have a broader knowledge of important information to communicate.

The transport team performs an assessment of the patient and contributes their findings to the previously developed plan of care. If interventions are needed before transport, the transport team and the referral facility personnel determine who will assume responsibility for the interventions. Although resuscitation and stabilization are initiated at the referral hospital, full stabilization may not be achieved until the patient arrives at the receiving hospital.[4]

The psychosocial preparation of the patient and family for transport is an important step before transport begins. The sending nurse ensures that the patient and family understand the reason for transport, the transport mode, the time of transport, and the transport destination. Information about the family is also communicated at this time and includes identification of a family spokesperson and the family's plan for getting to the receiving hospital. If the transport team is unable to meet with the family, the sending nurse supplies information about how to contact the family.

Physical preparation of the patient is the next important step to ensure a safe transport. The ABCs of care (airway, breathing, and circulation) are the top priority. Adequate oxygenation and ventilation are ensured before transport begins. The need for an artificial airway is determined before leaving the sending facility so that endotracheal intubation can be performed in a more predictable environment and the endotracheal tube can be well secured. Most intubated patients are sedated to prevent them from dislodging the endotracheal tube and to decrease fear and discomfort during transport. In addition to the endotracheal tube, a nasogastric tube may be inserted to prevent aspiration of stomach contents into the airway. Because auscultation of breath sounds is difficult en route, end-tidal carbon dioxide levels and oxygen saturation are used to monitor respiratory status. If an endotracheal tube is not indicated, supplemental oxygen may still be used to maintain adequate oxygenation.

The patient's circulatory and hemodynamic status also are stabilized before transport. Any bleeding is controlled and adequate intravenous access established and well secured. For a patient with an unstable volume status, several 14-gauge intravenous lines are indicated. If the patient is already on intravenous drips, the transport team may change over to their own equipment and intravenous mixtures. The patient's circulatory status is also continuously assessed through cardiac monitoring during the entire transport process. Cardiac arrest medications and a defibrillator should be easily accessible.

Patients with actual or potential spinal injuries should have spinal and neck immobilization devices in place before transport. Patients with any skeletal fractures must have the fracture immobilized before transport to prevent pain and further complications.

Pain control during transport is also addressed. The best agents for a transport patient are those with a rapid onset, short duration, and ease of administration and storage.

Phase Three: The Transport Process

Phase three is the actual transport of the patient. The time spent in careful planning of the transport and stabilization of the patient will ease the transport process. The transport vehicle must contain the essential equipment needed for transporting a critically ill patient. Box 15-4 lists the minimal necessary equipment.[1]

The ABCs of care continue to be the primary focus of the transport team. Each member of the transport team must have a clear understanding of his or her role in the continuous assessment, planning, and intervention that takes place when caring for the patient. Throughout the transport, the team also provides explanations and reassures the patient because transport can be very stressful. The transport team is responsible for documenting the physical and psychosocial care provided during transport and the patient's response to the care.

Before arriving at the receiving facility, the transport nurse calls either a full or updated report. This report includes an estimated time of arrival at the receiving facility. The nurse also communicates any special needs, changes in patient status, and unchanged but pertinent findings.

box 15-4
Minimally Essential Equipment Necessary for Transport

- Airway and ventilary management
  - Resuscitation bag and mask of proper size and fit for the patient.
  - Oral airways, laryngoscopes, and endotracheal tubes of proper size for the patient.
  - Oxygen source with a quantity sufficient to meet the patient's anticipated consumption with at least 1-hour reserve in addition
  - Suction apparatus and catheters
- Cardiac monitor/defibrillator/transcutaneous pacemaker
- Blood pressure cuff and stethoscope
- Materials for intravenous therapy and devices for regulation of infusion
- Drugs
  - For advanced cardiac resuscitation
  - For the management of acute physiological derangements
  - For special needs of the patient
- Spinal immobilization devices
- Communication equipment

Guidelines for the Transfer of Critically Ill Patients. Prepared by the American Association of Critical-Care Nurses Transfer Guidelines Task Force and the Guidelines Committee, American College of Critical Care Medicine, Society of Critical Care Medicine, pp 11,13. American Association of Critical-Care Nurses, Aliso Viejo, CA, 1998. Used with permission.

Phase Four: Turnover of the Patient to the Receiving Facility

Phase four of transport involves handing over the patient to the receiving unit staff at the receiving facility. Backup plans on how to handle an acutely deteriorating patient in transit between the transport vehicle and the ICU should also be identified. This plan may include stopping at the emergency department to stabilize the patient; it is essential for the emergency department staff to be aware of this possibility. Once the patient arrives safely in the receiving unit, the transport team and the receiving staff determine when the receiving staff will take over the responsibility for the patient's care. A final verbal update and all medical documents are given to the receiving staff. The written report of the transport is also completed.

Phase Five: Post-transport Continuous Quality Improvement Monitoring

The final phase of transport is very important and involves continuous quality improvement monitoring. Ideally, the referring facility, the transport team, and the receiving facility are involved in the review process. The first phase of the quality improvement monitoring involves evaluation of the current transport, including any quality indicators developed by the transporting agency. These indicators may include appropriateness of the transfer, appropriateness of the accompanying personnel, timeliness of the transfer, patient outcome, management of complications, and transfer outcome. The second phase of continuous quality improvement monitoring entails the ongoing review of the transport system. Such reviews focus on system functioning, and indicators may include complications, deaths in transport, and deaths after transport.[1]

The multidisciplinary team responsible for continuous quality improvement monitoring scrutinizes the collected data for patterns and trends, identifies solutions to patient care problems, initiates corrective action, and communicates such action to all involved in the transport process. Through a quality improvement plan, the transport process is improved and results in optimal care of the critically ill patient during the transport process.[1]

clinical applicability challenges

Self-Challenge: Critical Thinking

1. *Analyze the policies and procedures for interfacility transport at an acute care facility. Identify the strengths and weaknesses of the policies and procedures, and develop recommendations for change.*
2. *Evaluate the Emergency Medical Transfer Active Labor Act (EMTALA) requirements for interhospital transfer, and identify potential areas of risk for the patient, the transferring facility, and the receiving facility.*
3. *Analyze specific clinical conditions and their implications for preparation for air transport.*

Study Questions

1. *While still at the sending facility, a patient requires additional stabilization and treatment, which the facility is capable of providing. It is best to stabilize*
   a. *at the sending facility, before arrival of the transport team and departure of the receiving facility.*
   b. *at the receiving facility, because that facility is better qualified to do it.*
   c. *en route to the receiving facility by the specialized transport team.*
   d. *none of the above.*

REFERENCES

1. American Association of Critical-Care Nurses Transfer Guidelines Task Force and the Guidelines Committee, American College of Critical Care Medicine, Society of Critical Care Medicine: Guidelines for the transfer of critically ill patients. Aliso Viejo, CA, American Association of Critical-Care Nurses, 1998
2. American College of Emergency Physicians: Position Paper: Interfacility Transportation of the Critical Care Patient and Its Medical Direction (1999). Available at: http://acep.org
3. Holleran R: Prehospital Nursing: A Collaborative Approach. St. Louis, CV Mosby, 1994
4. Lee GN: Emergency Medical Treatment and Active Labor Act. In Lee GN (ed): Legal Concepts and Issues in Emergency Care, pp 137–150. Philadelphia, WB Saunders, 2001
5. Maryland Board of Nursing: Declaratory Ruling 2003-1, Re: The Standards of Practice for the Registered Nurse When Managing and Caring for the Critically Ill Client in the Specialty Care Transport Arena (Interhospital). Baltimore, Maryland Board of Nursing, 2003

OTHER SELECTED READING

Arndt K (Ed): Standards for Critical Care and Specialty Rotor-Wing Transport. Air and Surface Transport Nurses' Association. Lexington, Kentucky, Myers Printing, 2003

Bitterman RA: Providing Emergency Care Under Federal Law: EMTALA. Dallas, Texas, American College of Emergency Physicians, 2001; Supplement, 2004

Gebremichael M, Borg U, Habashi N, et al: Interhospital transport of the extremely ill patient: The mobile intensive care unit. Crit Care Med 28:79–85, 2000

Lee GN: Aeromedical transport. In Lee GN (ed): Legal Concepts and Issues in Emergency Care, pp 137–150. Philadelphia, WB Saunders, 2001

McGrow KM, Roys R, Maloney RC, Xiao Y: Using wireless technologies to improve information flow for interhospital transfers of critically ill patients. Crit Care Nurse 24(2): 66–72, 114, 2004

Pierce PF, Evers KG: Global presence: USAF Aeromedical evacuation and critical care air transport. Crit Care Nurs Clin North Am 15(2): 221–232, 2003

Selevan J, Fields W, Chen W, et al: Critical care transport: Outcome evaluation after interfacility transfer and hospitalization. Ann Emerg Med 33:33–43, 94–96, 1999

Trauma Nursing Coalition: Resource Document for Nursing Care of the Trauma Patient. Parkridge, IL, Emergency Nurses Association, 1999

PART

one
two
three
four
five
six
seven
eight
nine
ten
eleven
twelve

Cardiovascular System

INTERNET RESOURCES

Topic	Web Page Address
American College of Cardiology	www.acc.org
American College of Chest Physicians	www.chestnet.org
American Heart Association	www.americanheart.org
Angioplasty Website	www.ptca.org
Cardiology Resource	www.theheart.org
Cleveland Clinic	www.clevelandclinic.org
Guidant Corporation (Medical Technology)	www.guidant.com/products
Guidelines Resource	www.guidelines.gov
Heart Failure Society of America	www.hfsa.org
Heart Rhythm Society	www.naspe.org
Mayo Health Clinic	www.mayohealth.org
Medtronic Corporation (Medical Technology)	www.medtronic.com
National Heart, Lung and Blood Institute	www.nhlbi.nih.gov
Patient Education	www.heartcenteronline.com
PharmWeb	www.pharmweb.net
Physician Reference on Diagnosis and Treatment	www.arrhythmiaonline.com/intro.asp
RxList: The Internet Drug Index	www.rxlist.com
Society for Vascular Nursing	www.svnnet.org
Society of Thoracic Surgeons	www.sts.org
St. Jude Medical (Medical Technology)	www.sjm.com
Transcatheter Cardiovascular Therapeutics	www.tctmd.com
United Network for Organ Sharing	www.patients.unos.org
United States Food and Drug Administration	www.fda.gov
Virtual Library Pharmacy	www.pharmacy.org
Women's Heart Foundation	www.womensheart.org

chapter

16

Anatomy and Physiology of the Cardiovascular System

PATRICIA GONCE MORTON ■ THERESE M. CRAIG

objectives

Based on the content in this chapter, the reader should be able to:

- Briefly describe the characteristics of cardiac muscle cells.
- Differentiate the electrical events from the mechanical events in the heart.
- Explain depolarization and repolarization.
- Describe the normal conduction system of the heart.
- State the formula for calculating cardiac output.
- Compare and contrast the role of the parasympathetic and sympathetic nervous systems in the regulation of heart rate.
- Explain the three factors involved in the regulation of stroke volume.
- Describe the coronary artery blood source for the cardiac chambers and conduction system.
- Explain the influence of blood volume and blood pressure on peripheral circulation.

During the 70 years in the life of the average person, the heart will pump approximately 5 quarts of blood a minute, 75 gallons an hour, 57 barrels a day, and 1.5 million barrels in a lifetime. Although the work accomplished by this organ is out of proportion to its size, for most people, the heart functions normally throughout the life span. The pumping action of the heart moves blood, a vital substance, throughout the body, supplying oxygen and nutrients to cells and removing waste. Without this action, cells die. For people in whom cardiac problems develop, the results may be dramatic and the outcome drastic. This chapter reviews the principles of cardiovascular anatomy and physiology.

CARDIAC MICROSTRUCTURE

Microscopically, cardiac muscle contains visible stripes, or striations, similar to those found in skeletal muscle (Fig. 16-1). The ultrastructural pattern also resembles that of striated muscle. The cells branch and connect freely and form a three-dimensional, complex network. The elongated nuclei, like those of smooth muscle, are found deep in the interior of the cells and not next to the cell membrane as they are in striated muscle.

Cardiac muscle (myocardial) cells are endowed with extraordinary characteristics, most of which belong to the cell membrane or sarcolemma. To pump effectively, the heart muscle must begin contraction as a single unit. To contract myocardial cells simultaneously, cell membranes must depolarize at the same time. The heart does this, without using much neural tissue, by rapidly conducting impulses from cell to cell through intercalated disks. At each end of every myocardial cell, adjacent cell membranes are folded elaborately and attached strongly. These areas comprise the intercalated disks, where depolarization is conducted extremely rapidly from one cell to the next[1] (see Fig. 16-1).

Another extraordinary characteristic of myocardial cells, seen mainly in cell membranes, is automaticity. Selected

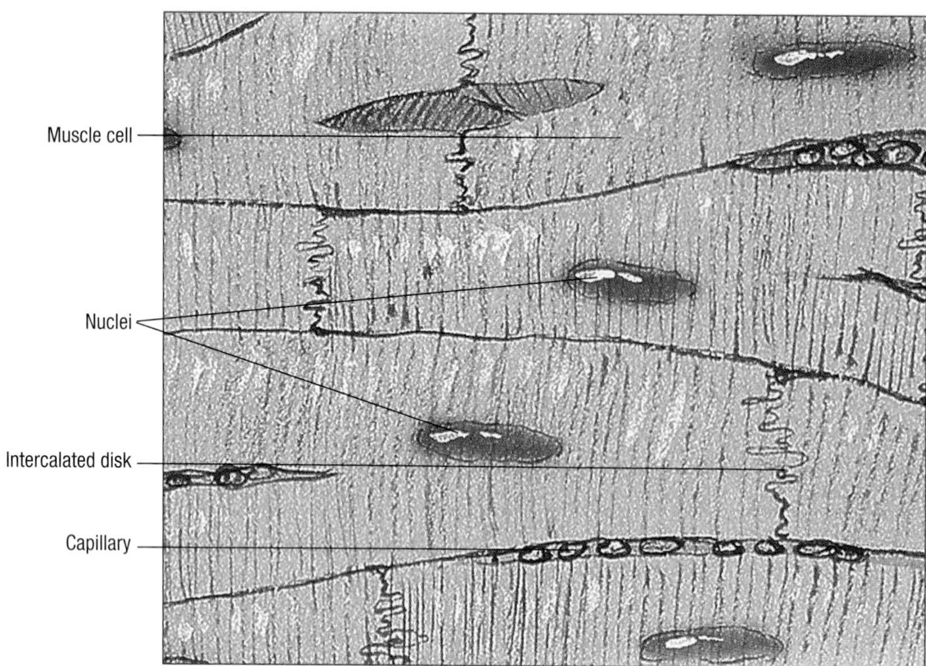

figure 16-1 Cardiac muscle fibers, showing the branching structure and intercalated disks. (From Anatomical Chart Company: Atlas of Human Anatomy, p 167. Springhouse, PA, Springhouse, 2001.)

groups of cardiac cells are capable of initiating rhythmic action potentials, and thus waves of contraction, without any outside humoral or nervous intervention.

Within each cardiac cell lie thousands of contractile elements, the overlapping actin and myosin filaments. Figure 16-2 illustrates these elements and the changes seen during diastole and systole. Not shown are the many cross-bridges that extend like rows of oars from the surface of the thicker myosin filaments. During diastole, these bridges are unattached to other filaments. The arrangement of actin and myosin filaments gives cardiac muscle its banded or striated appearance. One grouping of actin and myosin filaments is called a *sarcomere.*

MECHANICAL EVENTS OF CONTRACTION

Before mechanical contraction, an action potential travels quickly over each cell membrane and down into each cell's sarcoplasmic reticulum. When an action potential causes depolarization of the sarcoplasmic reticulum, calcium ions move from the sarcoplasmic reticulum into the myocardial cell cytoplasm and bind to troponin molecules on actin filaments. Calcium-bound troponin moves slightly to uncover binding sites on the actin, to which myosin filaments then attach. With a release of energy stored in adenosine triphosphate (ATP), these binding sites move so that actin and myosin slide past each other and new couplings between actin and myosin occur. Rapid, successive uncoupling of cross-bridges and their reattachment to new actin-binding sites lead to rapid and dramatic shortening of the sarcomere (see Fig. 16-2). This shortening is the essence of myocardial contraction (systole). Contraction ceases when the calcium ions return to their storage sites on the sarcoplasmic reticulum, thereby causing the binding sites on the actin filaments to be covered again. The separated actin and myosin filaments then slip past each other in the reverse direction, lengthening the sarcomere to its relaxed state.

Contraction requires calcium and energy. The presence of adequate ATP stores and the movement of calcium provide the essential link between the electrical events of depolarization and the mechanical events of contraction in the heart.

ELECTRICAL EVENTS OF DEPOLARIZATION

Membranes of all the cells in the human body are charged; that is, they are polarized and therefore have electrical potentials. The charges are separated at the membrane. In humans, all cell membranes, regardless of type, are positively charged at rest, with more positively charged parti-

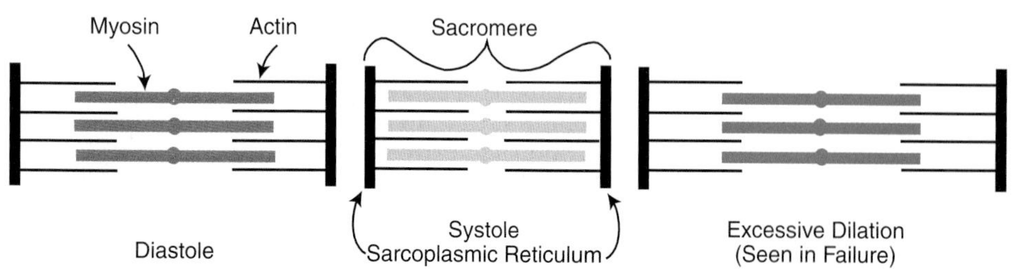

figure 16-2 Contractile elements lying inside a single sarcomere of a myocardial cell.

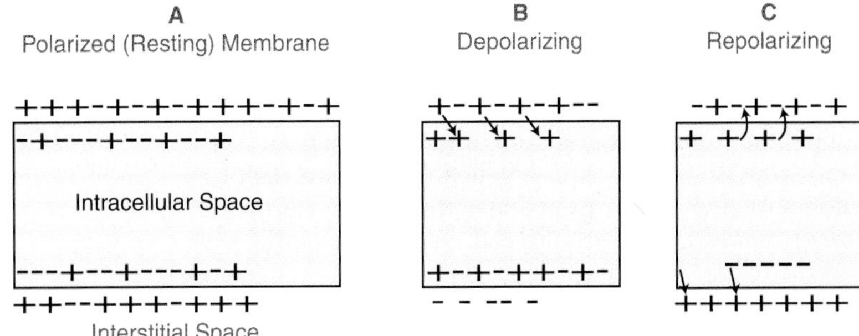

figure 16-3 Electrical events at rest (diastolic) and preceding contraction (systolic).

cles at the outer surface of the cell membrane than at the inner surface. Figure 16-3A illustrates this "resting stage."

In the depolarized state, the cell membrane is negatively charged, with more negatively charged particles at the outer surface of the cell membrane than at the inner surface. Figure 16-3B illustrates this "depolarized stage."

Cardiac muscle membranes are polarized, and the electrical potential can be measured, as it can in any of the cells in the human body. The potential results from the difference between intracellular and extracellular concentrations of electrolytes. When salt compounds of various elements are dissolved in aqueous solutions, they dissociate into their charged particles, called *ions*.

In the resting myocardial cell, there are more potassium ions inside than outside the cell and more sodium and unbound calcium ions outside than inside the cell. All three of these positively charged ions (cations) may diffuse through pores, or channels, in the cell membrane. If each ion freely obeyed the law of diffusion, however, potassium would diffuse out of the cell, whereas sodium and calcium would diffuse into it. Very soon there would be equal concentrations of each ion between the intracellular and extracellular fluids, and no resting potential would exist. It is through selective regulation of the concentrations of these ions on either side of the membrane that the resting membrane potential is maintained. Several factors contribute to this regulation. The first factor is the presence of sodium–potassium "pumps" in the cell membrane. These pumps move sodium out of the cell and potassium into the cell, with both movements occurring against the concentration gradients for each of these ions. The second factor is the active movement of calcium out of the cell against the concentration gradient in response to the passive diffusion of sodium into the cell. The third factor is the regulation of membrane channels, whereby calcium ions can enter the resting myocardial cell. The fourth factor is the presence of intracellular anions (negatively charged particles) that are too large to exit from the cell.

PHYSIOLOGICAL BASIS OF THE RESTING POTENTIAL

The cardiac cell contains large anions that cannot exit the cell. These anions attract sodium and potassium cations, which diffuse through membrane channels into the cell. The anions would attract the calcium cation also, except that the membrane channels for the entry of this ion are closed when the cell is at rest. The potassium ions remain within the cell, but the sodium ions are pumped out of the cell almost as fast as they can enter by the sodium–potassium pumps located in the cell membrane. While forcing sodium out of the cell, these pumps actively transport potassium ions into the cell against their concentration gradients. This increase in intracellular potassium still is insufficient to offset all the intracellular anions. Thus, the inside of the myocardial cell remains negative with respect to the outside—as long as the pumps are operative. As a result, the resting potential is approximately −80 mV. For each molecule of an ion pumped from the cell, one molecule of ATP is required to provide the energy necessary to effect the chemical bond between ion and carrier. Maintaining a resting potential thus requires energy. Factors that maintain resting membrane potential of myocardial cells are listed in Box 16-1.

PHYSIOLOGICAL BASIS OF THE ACTION POTENTIAL

When a stimulus is applied to the polarized cell membrane, the membrane that ordinarily is only slightly permeable to sodium permits sodium ions to diffuse rapidly into the cell. This rapid diffusion occurs because of inactivation of the sodium active transport enzymes (pumps). The result is a reversal of net charges. The outer surface is now more negative than positive, and the membrane is said to be depolarized (see Fig. 16-3B).

When the sodium influx changes the polarity from −80 mV to approximately −35 mV, the electrical change opens the previously closed "calcium channels" in the myocardial cell membrane. Once opened, these channels permit the influx of calcium. The entry of this cation, together

box 16-1
Factors That Maintain Resting Membrane Potential of Myocardial Cell

- Sodium–potassium pumps within the cell membrane
- Active movement of Ca^{2+} out of cell against its concentration gradient in response to passive diffusion of Na^{+} into cell
- Regulation of membrane channels so that Ca^{2+} ions can enter resting myocardial cell
- Presence of intracellular anions too large to exit from cell

with the continued entry of sodium, is responsible for the remainder of the depolarization, which continues until the polarity of the extracellular side equals approximately +30 mV. Such a maximal depolarization inactivates sodium–potassium pumps in nearby membranes. This can cause depolarization in these areas. When the original depolarization becomes self-propagating in this way, it is termed an *action potential.* In a myocardial cell, an action potential triggers the release of intracellular calcium from its storage sites on the sarcoplasmic reticulum. This release plus the calcium influx across the sarcolemma elevates intracellular calcium levels, thereby initiating muscular contraction, as previously described.[2]

If the depolarization remains below a certain critical (threshold) point, it dies out without having opened any calcium channel or inactivated any adjacent sodium–potassium pumps. Because it does not become self-propagating and remains localized, such a depolarization is termed a *local depolarization.*

During depolarization, the elevated intracellular sodium concentration frees potassium ions to diffuse out of the cell in accordance with their concentration gradient. Just as this potassium efflux gains some momentum, however, the sodium–potassium pumps automatically reactivate (they can be inactivated only temporarily). Once reactivated, the pumps begin to restore the original resting potential, a process termed *repolarization* (see Fig. 16-3C). During the initial phase of repolarization, the efflux of potassium and sodium ions exceeds their influx; but as the intracellular sodium ions are removed from the cell, potassium ions remain as the major cation to be electrostatically held within the cell by the intracellular anions. This halts the potassium efflux. The remainder of repolarization consists of pump activity that increases intracellular potassium and decreases intracellular sodium; thus, the resting potential is reestablished. The electrical events at the start of repolarization also reclose the calcium entry channels, thereby halting calcium influx. Intracellular calcium levels are reduced when the diffusion of sodium into the cell causes a movement of calcium out of the cell against the latter's concentration gradient.[2] The phases of the action potential are shown in Figure 16-4.

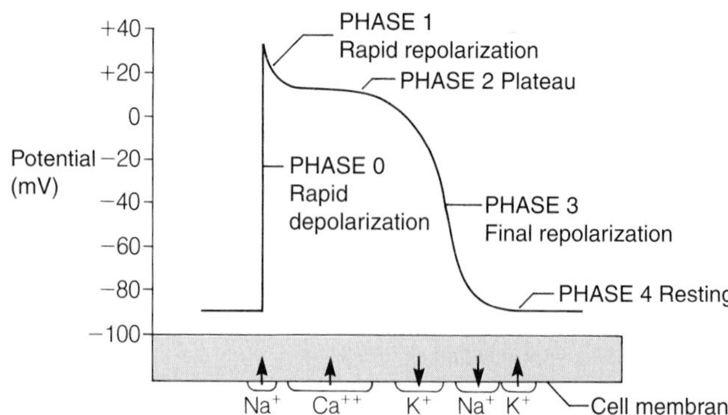

figure 16-4 Cardiac action potential. Phase 0 is the rapid depolarization phase. During this phase, the fast sodium channels in the cell membranes are stimulated to open, resulting in the rapid influx of sodium. Contraction of the myocardium follows depolarization. Phase 1 is the rapid repolarization phase and occurs at the peak of the action potential. This phase indicates the inactivation of the fast sodium channels with an abrupt decrease in sodium permeability. Phase 2 represents the plateau of the action potential. During this phase, potassium permeability is low, allowing the membrane to remain depolarized throughout phase 2. The influx of calcium that occurs during the plateau phase is much slower than that of sodium and lasts for a longer time. Phase 3 is the final repolarization phase and begins with the downslope of the action potential curve. During this phase, the influx of calcium and sodium ends and there is a rapid outward movement of potassium. By the end of phase 3, sodium and potassium return to their normal resting state. Phase 4 is the resting membrane potential and corresponds to diastole. During this phase, the sodium–potassium pump is activated resulting in the active transport of sodium out of the cell and potassium is moved back into the cell. The arrows below the diagram indicate the approximate time and direction of movement of each ion influencing membrane potential. The phase of calcium moving out of the cell is not well defined but is thought to occur during phase 4.

CARDIAC MACROSTRUCTURE

The heart is about the size of a clenched fist and comprises four layers: the endocardium, the myocardium, the epicardium, and the pericardium. The inner layer is known as the *endocardium* and consists of endothelial tissue that lines the inner surface of the heart and the cardiac valves. The *myocardium* is the middle layer and is composed of muscle fibers that enable the heart to pump. The outer layer, known as the *epicardium*, is tightly adherent to the heart and the base of the great vessels. A thin, fibrous, double-layered sac known as the *pericardium* surrounds the heart. The outer layer is known as the *parietal pericardium* and the inner layer is called the *visceral pericardium*. Between these two layers is a small amount of pericardial fluid (30 to 50 mL) that serves as a lubricant between the two layers.[1]

The heart consists of four chambers: right and left atria, and right and left ventricles. The atria are smaller, thinner-walled, low-pressure chambers. Approximately 30% of blood flow to the ventricles is the result of atrial contraction, also known as *atrial kick.* The remaining 70% of blood that reaches the ventricles is the result of pressure differences between the atria and the ventricles. The ventricles are larger, higher-pressure chambers with thicker walls than the atria. The walls of the left ventricle are thicker than the right ventricle because the left ventricle must generate a large amount of force to eject blood into the aorta. Deoxygenated blood enters the right atrium from the superior and inferior venae cavae. The blood passes through the tricuspid valve into the right ventricle, which then pumps the blood through the pulmonic valve into the pulmonary circulation. After gas exchange in the lungs, oxygenated blood returns to the left atrium, passes through the mitral valve, enters the left ventricle, passes through the aortic valve, and finally enters the aorta (Fig. 16-5).

The cardiac valves are composed of fibrous tissue and allow blood to flow in one direction. The valves open and close as a result of blood flow and pressure differences. The tricuspid and mitral valves are known as the *atrioventricular (AV) valves* because they are located between the atria and the ventricles. The chordae tendineae and the papillary muscles attach to the AV valves and help maintain closure and prevent eversion of the valve leaflets during ventricular contraction so that blood does not move into the atria. The

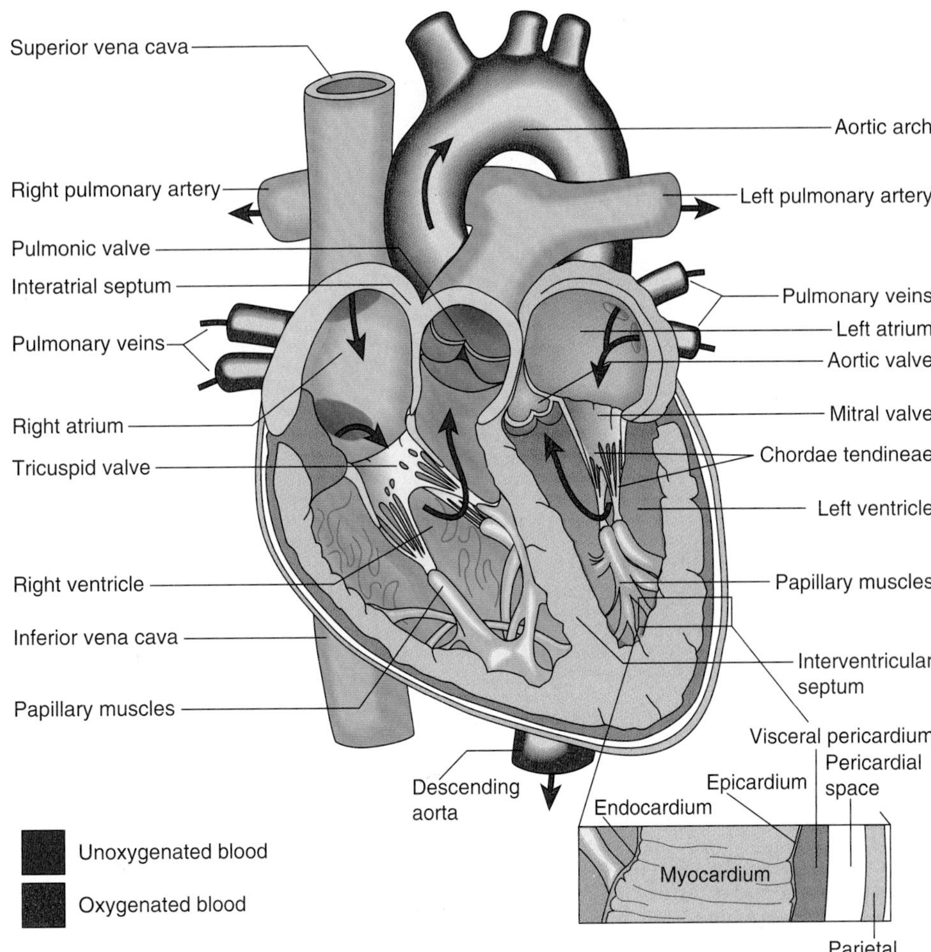

figure 16-5 Structure of the heart. Arrows show course of blood flow through the heart chambers. (From Smeltzer SC, Bare BG: Textbook of Medical-Surgical Nursing [10th Ed], p 648. Philadelphia, Lippincott Williams & Wilkins, 2004.)

pulmonic and aortic valves are known as the *semilunar valves* because each has three leaflets shaped like half-moons.

CARDIAC CONDUCTION

To pump effectively, large portions of cardiac muscle must receive an action potential nearly simultaneously. Special cells that conduct action potentials extremely rapidly are arranged in pathways through the heart. All these cells have automaticity.

The heart chambers and specialized tissues are diagrammed in Figure 16-6. The sinoatrial (SA) node is located between the opening of the inferior and superior venae cavae in the right atrial wall. The cells of the SA node have the property of automaticity. Because the SA node normally discharges faster than any other heart cell with automaticity (60 to 100 beats per minute), this specialized tissue acts as a normal cardiac pacemaker. Atrial action potentials travel through atrial cells by intercalated disks, although some specialized conductive tissue in the atria has been discovered.

In the lower right portion of the interatrial septum is the AV node, also known as the AV junction. This tissue conducts, yet delays, the atrial action potential before it travels to the ventricles. Action potentials reach the AV node at different times. The AV node slows conduction of these action potentials until all potentials have exited the atria and entered the AV node. After this slight delay, the AV node passes the action potential all at once to the ventricular conduction tissue, allowing for nearly simultaneous contraction of all ventricular cells. This AV node delay also allows time for the atria to eject fully their load of blood into the ventricles in preparation for ventricular systole.

From the AV node, the impulse travels down the bundle of His in the interventricular septum into either a right or left bundle branch and then through one of many Purkinje fibers to the ventricular myocardial tissue itself. An action potential can traverse this conducting tissue three to seven times more rapidly than it can travel through the ventricular myocardium. Thus, the bundle branches and Purkinje fibers enable a near-simultaneous contraction of all portions of the ventricle, thereby allowing a maximal unified pump action to occur.[2]

Electrocardiograms

Conduction of an action potential through the heart can be shown by an electrocardiogram (ECG; Fig. 16-7). Because ECGs are extensively covered in a later chapter, discussion here is brief. An ECG does not show mechanical events of the heart, but in the normal heart, coupling

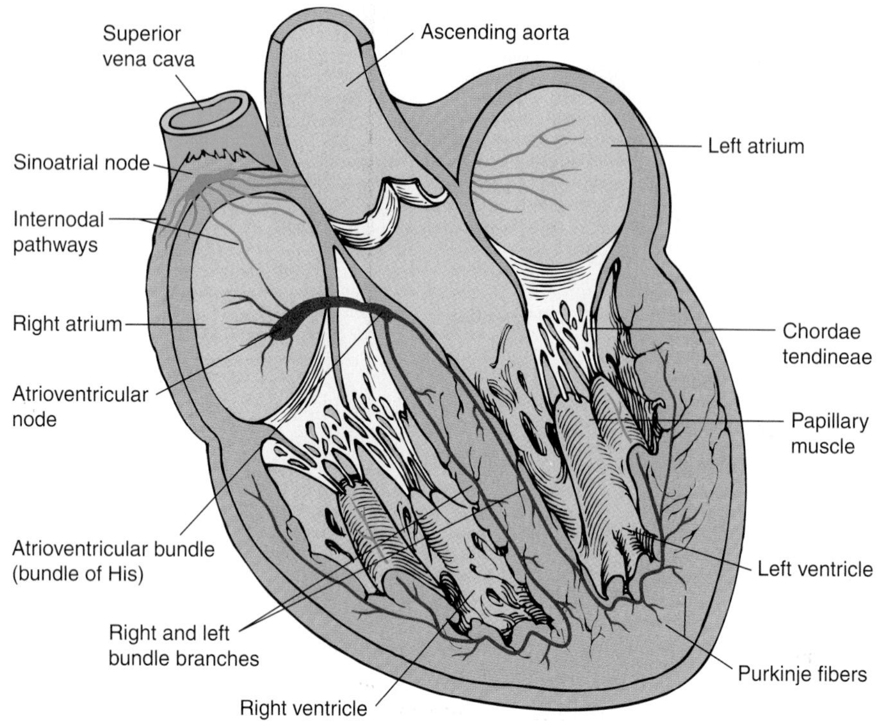

figure 16-6 The electrical conduction system of the heart begins with impulses generated by the sinoatrial node (*green*) and circuited continuously over the heart. (From Weber J, Kelley K: Health Assessment in Nursing [2nd Ed], p 305. Philadelphia, Lippincott Williams & Wilkins, 2004.)

of electrical and mechanical events can be assumed (see Chapter 17).

In Figure 16-7, point 1 shows early ventricular diastole, when the atria and ventricles are at rest. Blood from the large veins is passively filling both atria. As the atria fill, the pressure in the atria exceeds the pressure in the ventricles and the AV valves open in response to the pressure gradient. The blood from the atria now passively fills the ventricles.

At point 2, the beginning of late ventricular diastole, both ventricles remain relaxed and are about three-fourths full. The SA node fires spontaneously (due to automaticity) and both atria depolarize, generating a P wave. The atria contract and blood is actively moved from the atria into the ventricles: this "atrial kick" supplies approximately 20% to 30% of the ventricular blood volume.

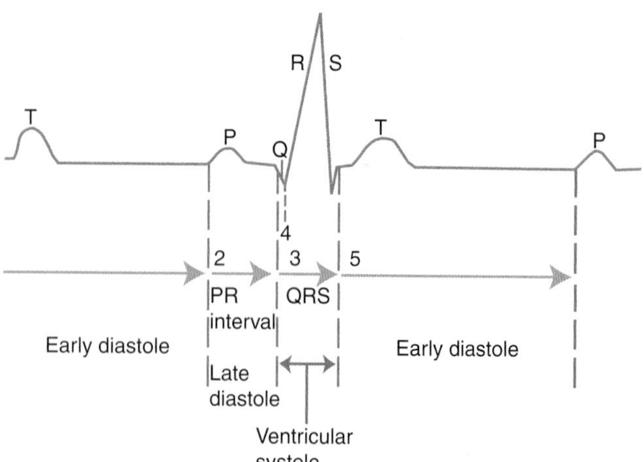

figure 16-7 Comparison of electrical and mechanical events during one cardiac cycle, using a normal electrocardiogram tracing.

At point 3, late in the PR interval, the action potential begun in the SA node is being delayed and "collected" in the AV node and travels to the bundle of His. The atria and ventricles are at rest.

At point 4, the action potential moves to the septum, which depolarizes and leads to the Q wave. Septal depolarization is rapidly followed by action potential movement down the right and left bundles into the Purkinje fibers to all cardiac muscle cells. These electrical events are seen as the RS wave on the ECG and are followed rapidly by mechanical contraction of both ventricles. The AV valves close, and the aortic and pulmonic valves open.

At point 5, the heart returns to early ventricular diastole, and the ventricles repolarize. This repolarization shows as a large, wide T wave. The aortic and pulmonic valves close about midway through repolarization.[1]

Rhythmicity and Pacing

Automaticity is an inherent property of myocardial conduction cells and occurs as a result of a spontaneous and rhythmic inactivation of the sodium pumps. Under abnormal conditions, cardiac muscle cells also gain automaticity and can produce their own rhythmic series of action potentials and thus their own stimulus for contraction. Coordination of automaticity is important for rhythmic cardiac contraction and is achieved through the varying rates of automaticity found in different cardiac tissues.

The SA node discharges normally in an adult at a resting rate of 60 to 100 times per minute. The remainder of the conduction system and ventricles have progressively slower rates of firing. The AV node discharges at a rate of 40 to 60 times per minute. The conduction tissues in the ventricles fire about 20 to 40 times per minute. The group of cells with the fastest rate of automaticity paces the heart. Normally, this is the SA node.

If conduction from the SA node to the AV node is disrupted, the fastest pacemaker tissue on both sides of this interruption will govern their respective areas, and the ECG may show independent atrial and ventricular rhythms. Atrial systole is not needed for the ventricle to fill with blood because most ventricular filling is passive and occurs in early diastole. The clinically important rhythm is that of the ventricles; they are the chambers that supply the lungs and the rest of the body with blood. Their systolic rate helps determine true perfusion. The slower the rate, the less able are the ventricles to meet the perfusion needs of the body during exercise or activities of daily living. A very rapid ventricular rhythm also compromises perfusion needs because the shorter the diastole, the less time for filling of the chambers. Decreased ventricular filling reduces cardiac output.

CARDIAC OUTPUT

A traditional measure of cardiac function, cardiac output is the amount of blood, in liters, ejected from the left ventricle each minute. Cardiac output (CO) is the product of heart rate (HR) and stroke volume (SV), which is the volume of blood ejected per ventricular contraction:

$$CO = HR\ (\text{beats/min}) \times SV\ (\text{liters/beat})$$

Normal cardiac output for an adult ranges from 4 to 8 L/minute. The output can be altered to meet changing bodily demands for tissue perfusion, but the cardiac output equation does not account for differences in body size. An output of 5 L/minute may be adequate for a 50-kg man but insufficient for a 120-kg man. Because perfusion is a function of body size, a more accurate measure of cardiac function is cardiac index, which represents the amount of blood, in liters, ejected each minute from the left ventricle (or cardiac output) per square meter of body surface area. Cardiac index (CI) typically averages 3.0 ± 0.2 L/minute and ranges from 2.8 to 4.2 L/minute/m^2:

$$CI = \frac{CO\ (\text{liters/min})}{\text{body surface area } (m^2)}$$

Regulation of Heart Rate

Although the heart has the ability to beat independently of any extrinsic influence, cardiac rate is under autonomic and adrenal catecholamine influence. Parasympathetic and sympathetic fibers innervate the SA and AV nodes. In addition, some sympathetic fibers terminate in myocardial tissues.

Parasympathetic stimulation releases acetylcholine near the nodal cells and decreases the rate of depolarization, thereby slowing cardiac rate. Stimulation of sympathetic fibers causes the release of norepinephrine. This chemical increases the rate of nodal depolarization and has inotropic effects on myocardial fibers, which are discussed later. Thus, sympathetic stimulation increases heart rate (Table 16-1). The adrenal medulla also releases norepinephrine and epinephrine into the bloodstream. These circulating catecholamines act on the heart in the same way as sympathetic stimulation.

Two reflexes adjust heart rate to blood pressure: the aortic reflex and the Bainbridge reflex. In the aortic reflex (Fig. 16-8A), a rise in arterial blood pressure stimulates aortic and

table 16-1 α and β Effects of Autonomic Nervous System on the Heart and Vascularity

Effector Organ	Cholinergic Impulses Response	Noradrenergic Impulses: *Receptor Type*	Noradrenergic Impulses: *Response*
Heart			
Sinoatrial node	Decrease in heart rate; vagal arrest	β_1	Increase in heart rate
Atria	Decrease in contractility and (usually) increase in conduction velocity	β_1	Increase in contractility and conduction velocity
Atrioventricular (AV) node and conduction system	Decrease in conduction velocity; AV block	β_1	Increase in conduction velocity
Ventricles	—	β_1	Increase in contractility and conduction velocity
Arterioles			
Coronary, skeletal muscle, pulmonary, abdominal viscera, renal	Dilation	α β_2	Constriction Dilation
Skin and mucosa, cerebral, salivary glands	—	α	Constriction
Systemic Veins	—	α β_2	Constriction Dilation

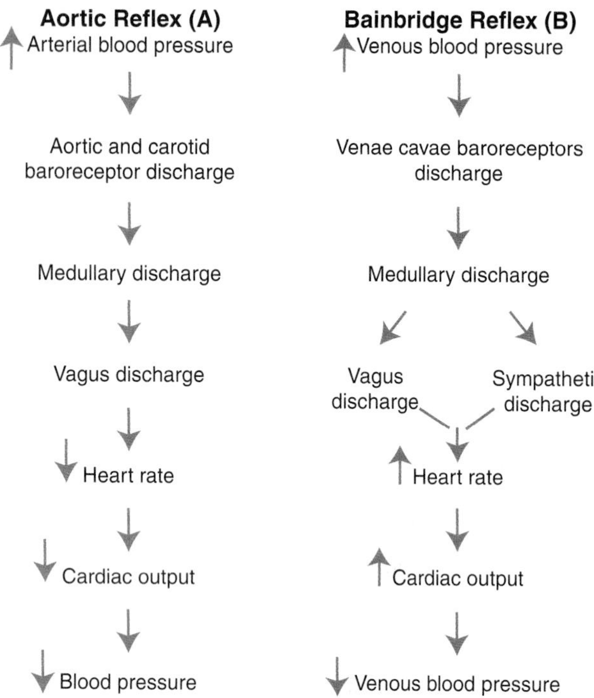

figure 16-8 Effects of (**A**) aortic reflex and (**B**) Bainbridge reflex on heart rate.

carotid sinus baroreceptors to fire sensory impulses to the cardioregulatory center in the medulla. The result is an increase in parasympathetic stimulation or a decrease in sympathetic stimulation to the heart. Thus, a rise in arterial blood pressure reflexively causes a slowing of cardiac rate. The decrease in heart rate results in a decrease in output, which can decrease arterial blood pressure. Conversely, a fall in arterial blood pressure, such as in shock, reflexively increases heart rate. This aortic reflex is an ongoing regulatory mechanism for homeostasis of arterial blood pressure.

The Bainbridge reflex (see Fig. 16-8B) uses receptors in the venae cavae. An increase in venous return stimulates these receptors, which then fire sensory impulses that travel to the cardioregulatory center. These reflexively cause a decrease in parasympathetic cardiac stimulation and an increase in sympathetic cardiac stimulation, thereby increasing cardiac rate. A fall in venous return causes a decrease in heart rate. Thus, the Bainbridge reflex adjusts cardiac rate to handle venous return.

Regulation of Stroke Volume

Stroke volume is the amount of blood ejected by the left ventricle during systole. Normal values range from 60 to 100 mL/beat. Three factors are involved: preload, afterload (or wall tension), and inherent inotropic myocardial contractility.

PRELOAD

Preload is the amount of stretch placed on a cardiac muscle fiber just before systole. Usually, the amount of stretch in any chamber is proportional to the volume of blood the chamber contains at the end of diastole, before systole. However, in some situations, the chamber can hold a large amount of volume with little change in pressure.

The concept of preload is related to Starling's law of the heart, which states that the force of myocardial contraction is determined by the length of the muscle cell fibers. Within a certain range increasing myofibril stretch increases the force of systole. Beyond optimal fibril length it is hypothesized that too few actin–myosin binding sites overlap to provide an adequate contraction. Below optimal shortening there is little room for filaments to slide, and cell walls limit further sliding. Also, actin filaments may have begun to overlap, decreasing the number of binding sites available to myosin fibers.

When the force of systole decreases, the chamber pumps poorly and does not empty properly. Excessive blood is left in the chamber at the end of systole. During diastole, when the chamber fills, this extra blood causes overfilling of the chamber and increases stretch. The next systole will be even weaker, as preload increases during every diastole.

Because preload is affected by the volume at the end of diastole, it often is equated with end-diastolic volume or pressure. Thus, left ventricular preload is represented by left ventricular end-diastolic pressure.

An example of rapid and normal adjustments to changes in preload occurs during the Valsalva maneuver. The first part of the Valsalva occurs when one holds one's breath and bears down, such as during defecation or heavy lifting. Bearing down increases intra-abdominal and intrathoracic pressures, decreasing venous return to the right atrium and ventricle. Right heart preload decreases. Bearing down also stimulates the vagus nerve, and the heart rate slows.

On exhalation, during the second part of the Valsalva maneuver, intrathoracic pressures decrease rapidly, allowing a sudden increase in venous return. Right atrial and ventricular preloads increase dramatically, stretch increases, and the right ventricular stroke volume increases. Atrial stretch receptors also signal the medulla and lead to sympathetic nervous discharge. Heart rate increases.

AFTERLOAD

Afterload is the force or pressure against which a cardiac chamber must eject blood during systole. The most critical factor determining afterload is vascular resistance, in the systemic or pulmonic vessels. Afterload often is equated with systemic vascular resistance or pulmonary vascular resistance.

Afterload affects stroke volume by increasing or decreasing the ease of emptying a ventricle during systole. A decrease in systemic vascular resistance, through vasodilation, presents the left ventricle with relatively large, open, relaxed arteries into which it can pump. Because it is easier to pump, the left ventricles empty easily, which increases stroke volume.

If systemic vascular resistance increases, for example through catecholamine-induced constriction of arteries, it takes a great deal more force for the left ventricle to pump into such a tightened vasculature. Stroke volume decreases.

CONTRACTILITY

Inotropic capabilities and cardiac workload refer to contractile forces. Cardiac muscle forces change in response to neural stimuli and circulating levels of catecholamines.

It is thought that through cyclic adenosine monophosphate (cAMP) mechanisms, cardiac cells change intracellular levels of calcium and ATP. These changes lead to increased inotropic actions, although the mechanisms remain unknown.

However, increased inotropic action increases the oxygen consumption of heart cells. This increased consumption also is called *increased workload* and *increased oxygen demand.*

Cardiac output depends on heart rate and stroke volume. Regardless of the initial cause of increased stroke volume (increased preload, increased afterload, or increased inotropic force), an increase in stroke volume increases workload. Similarly, an increased heart rate, no matter what the cause, increases oxygen demand.

CORONARY CIRCULATION

Blood supply to the myocardium is derived from the two main coronary arteries, the left and the right (Fig. 16-9). These arteries originate from the aorta, immediately above the aortic valve. The left main coronary artery has two major branches known as the left anterior descending (LAD) and the left circumflex artery (LCA). The LAD passes down the anterior wall of the left ventricle toward the apex of the myocardium. The LAD supplies blood flow to the anterior two thirds of the ventricular septum, the anterior left ventricle, the apex, and most of the bundle branches (Table 16-2).

The LCA, the other branch of the left main coronary artery, sits in the groove between the left atrium and the left ventricle and wraps around to the posterior wall of the heart. The LCA supplies blood flow to the left atrium, the lateral wall of the left ventricle, and the posterior wall of the left ventricle. In about 10% of the population, the LCA is the source of blood flow to the posterior descending coronary artery; when this pattern of flow occurs, the patient is referred to as left dominant. Branches of the LCA provide blood flow to the SA node in about 45% of people and to the AV node in about 10% of people.

The right coronary artery (RCA) also comes off the aorta and branches toward the right atrium; the anterior, lateral, and posterior regions of the right ventricle; and the posterior ventricular septum. The RCA provides blood flow to the right atrium, the right ventricle, and the inferior wall of the left ventricle. In about 90% of the population, the RCA is the source of blood flow to the posterior descending coronary artery, a pattern of flow known as right dominant. The RCA supplies oxygenated blood to the SA node in about 55% of people and to the AV node in about 90% of people.

The coronary arteries initially supply the epicardial layer of the heart and then pass deeper into the heart muscle to provide blood flow to the endocardium. As a result of this flow pattern, poor coronary blood flow initially deprives the subendocardial area of oxygenated blood. If the interruption to flow continues, the effects of decreased oxygenation expand throughout the thickness of the wall of the heart to the subepicardial surface.

Because the coronary arteries derive from the aorta (above the aortic valve) and lie between myocardial fibers, blood flow through the coronary arteries occurs when the aortic valve is closed during ventricular diastole, not systole. Therefore, anything that decreases the diastolic time (e.g., tachycardia) decreases coronary perfusion.

PERIPHERAL CIRCULATION

The biological significance of the cardiovascular system is tissue perfusion. Such perfusion supplies the body's cells with oxygen and nutrients while carrying away metabolic

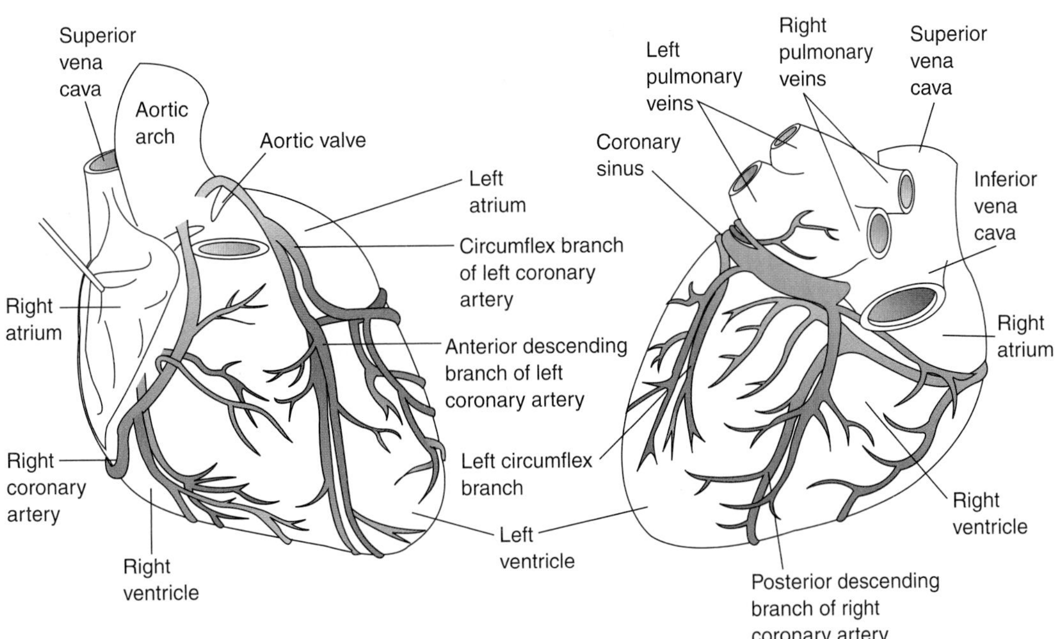

figure 16-9 Coronary arteries and some of the coronary sinus veins. (From Porth CM. Pathophysiology: Concepts of Altered Health States [6th Ed], p 492. Philadelphia, Lippincott Williams & Wilkins, 2002.)

table 16-2 Coronary Artery Blood Supply for Cardiac Muscle and Conducting System

Coronary Artery	Cardiac Muscle Supplied	Conducting Tissue Supplied
Left Main Coronary Artery		
Left anterior descending	Anterior ventricular septum Anterior left ventricle The apex	Bundle branches
Left circumflex	Left atrium Left ventricular lateral wall Left ventricular posterior wall	Sinoatrial node in 45% of hearts Atrioventricular node in 10% of hearts
Right Coronary Artery	Right atrium Right ventricle Posterior ventricular septum Inferior wall of left ventricle	Sinoatrial node in 55% of hearts Atrioventricular node in 90% of hearts

wastes, including carbon dioxide. Tissue perfusion is directly proportional to the rate of blood flow, which depends on several factors. One factor is the difference between the mean arterial blood pressure and right atrial pressure (usually represented by the central venous pressure [CVP]). The greater this difference, the faster the flow rate (all else being unchanged). Conversely, if arterial pressure falls or venous pressure rises, flow rate, and thus tissue perfusion, will be decreased.

Another factor affecting flow rate is vascular resistance. The relationship between vascular resistance and blood flow has two general applications. One is to describe the flow rate through vessels of differing diameters (e.g., arteries, capillaries). The other application concerns the ongoing regulation of blood flow by means of adjustments in arteriole diameters (i.e., constriction, dilation). Arteriole constriction reduces the radius, thereby increasing resistance and decreasing the flow rate. Conversely, arteriole dilation increases the flow rate.

The other two factors that can affect the flow rate normally are held constant. They are the sum of all vessel lengths and blood viscosity. Because these factors do not normally change significantly, they usually are omitted from flow rate considerations. Their relationships are obvious, however. The greater the length of a vessel, the more resistance and thus the slower the flow rate. Also, the more viscous the blood, the slower the rate of its flow. Blood viscosity is determined by the proportion of solvent (water) to solute and other particles, including blood cells and platelets. The less water and more particles that exist, the more viscous is the blood. The complete equation that describes all four factors is as follows:

$$\text{flow rate} = \frac{\text{mean arterial pressure} - \text{central venous pressure}}{\text{resistance} \times \text{viscosity} \times \text{vessel length}}$$

Because blood volume and pressure have such an important influence on tissue perfusion, the factors that alter and regulate them are examined.

Blood Volume

Urinary output and fluid input are the major normal mechanisms for regulating volume. If output is greater or fluid input is less, the volume is less—if all else is held constant. Factors that alter the volume of urine excreted every 24 hours include those that alter the glomerular filtration rate and the tubular reabsorption of water, with or without electrolytes. (For a more detailed explanation of these factors, see Chapter 42, specifically the discussion of normal endocrine physiology that considers the antidiuretic hormone.) Pathological conditions that promote any type of fluid loss (e.g., burns, severe diarrhea, osmotic diuresis) or a shift of water from the vascular to the interstitial compartment have the potential for reducing blood volume.

Blood Pressure

Because the difference between arterial and venous pressures is the driving force for blood circulation and tissue perfusion, factors that influence CVP are examined first, followed by the factors that regulate arterial blood pressure. CVP is, strictly speaking, the pressure of blood in the venae cavae just before its entry into the right atrium. CVP can be increased by an increase in blood volume (e.g., intravenous fluid overload) or a decrease in the pumping ability of the heart (e.g., cardiac failure). Because the pulsatile effects of the cardiac cycle are removed by capillary networks, venous pressure is recorded as an average, or mean, and reported in millimeters of mercury (mm Hg).

Arterial blood pressure is the pressure of blood in the arteries and arterioles. It is a pulsatile pressure due to the cardiac cycle, and systolic (peak) and diastolic (trough) numbers are reported in millimeters of mercury. Average or mean arterial blood pressure can be clinically useful as an indicator of average perfusion pressures.

Arterial blood pressure is regulated by the vasomotor tone of the arteries and arterioles, the amount of blood entering the arteries per systole (i.e., cardiac output), and blood volume itself. The greater the volume or output, the greater the blood pressure, and vice versa, if vasomotor tone were held constant. The normal regulation of vasomotor tone involves neural and hormonal mechanisms.

Neural regulation is mediated by the vasomotor center of the medulla oblongata. This center consists of vasopressor and depressor subdivisions. The vasomotor center receives neural input from baroreceptors in the carotid sinuses and aorta, atrial diastolic stretch receptors, the limbic system and hypothalamus, the midbrain, and pulmonary stretch receptors. In addition, the center is directly responsive to local hypoxia or hypercapnia. Neural outputs from the vasopressor center result in increased sympathetic stimulation to arterial smooth muscle cells. This increase in sympathetic stimulation results in arterial constriction and an increase in arterial blood pressure. Stimulation of the depressor area decreases such sympathetic stimulation.

Rapid adjustments in arterial blood pressure are affected primarily by the baroreceptor reflexes. An increase in the pressure on these receptors (directly by elevated blood pressure or manual compression and indirectly by increased blood volume) reflexively stimulates the depressor area. This stimulation of the depressor area results in decreased sympathetic stimulation to major arteries and the aorta, which causes a decrease in arterial blood pressure. The decreased baroreceptor stimulation caused by a fall in arterial blood pressure reflexively stimulates the pressor area and results in increased sympathetic stimulation to arterial muscles, causing a rise in arterial blood pressure. Thus, homeostasis of arterial pressure is maintained.

In orthostatic hypotension, the baroreceptor reflex is sluggish. Because arterial pressure is not elevated rapidly enough, the postural change results in a temporary decrease in brain perfusion that leads, in extreme cases, to syncope.

Other factors may alter arterial blood pressure reflexively by their influences on the vasomotor center. Nerve fibers from the limbic system and hypothalamus are believed to mediate emotionally produced alterations in blood pressure. An example of this is fainting, caused by neurally mediated vasodilation in response to the sight of blood or very bad (or good) news. Neural inputs from the midbrain and possibly from ascending spinothalamic fibers in the medulla result in the elevation in arterial pressure that initially accompanies severe pain and in the later decrease in arterial pressure that occurs when severe pain is prolonged. Lung inflation stimulates pulmonary stretch receptors. Their input to the vasomotor center reflexively decreases arterial pressure. Hypercapnia and, to a lesser extent, hypoxia of vasomotor neurons stimulate the pressor area, reflexively causing an increase in arterial pressure. Such stimuli obviously are not part of a normal daily regulatory mechanism but can operate as a normal compensatory mechanism in certain pathological situations. Elevated intracranial pressure can promote medullary hypercapnia and hypoxia. The increase in arterial pressure reflexively produced by these stimuli (Cushing's reflex) increases medullary perfusion, which can ameliorate the medullary hypoxia or hypercapnia, or both. Hormonal regulation of arterial blood pressure is affected by adrenal medullary catecholamines and the renin–angiotensin system. In the former, adrenal medullary catecholamines mimic the action of sympathetic fibers innervating the muscle layer or arteries (tunica media), causing arterial constriction and elevating arterial pressure. The renin–angiotensin system is discussed in Chapter 28. Briefly, a decreased glomerular filtration rate, which can result, for example, from a decrease in blood volume or renal perfusion, stimulates the secretion of renin from the juxtaglomerular apparatus. This stimulation of renin leads to the production of angiotensin II, which acts directly on the tunica media to promote vasoconstriction. Thus, renin elevates arterial pressure, which increases renal perfusion and glomerular filtration.

Finally, arterial blood pressure can be influenced by alterations in the level of unbound calcium in tunica media cells. Such levels are influenced by factors that open or close calcium channels in the membranes of these muscle cells. Drugs that block calcium channels ("calcium blockers") inhibit the entry of calcium into cells. Such decreased calcium influx can lower intracellular calcium levels sufficiently to decrease muscle contractility, including contractility of the heart, thereby promoting a degree of vasodilation and lowering the arterial pressure.

clinical applicability challenges

Self-Challenges: Critical Thinking

1. *Mrs. Lopez has been diagnosed with a 90% occlusion of her left anterior descending coronary artery. Describe which anatomical walls of the heart are affected. Explain which parts of her cardiac conducting system may be affected by the occlusion.*
2. *Mr. O'Keefe is a patient in the intensive care unit. His cardiac output has dropped from 8 L/minute to 4 L/minute. His heart rate has remained unchanged. Discuss possible physiological causes of his decreased cardiac output.*

Study Questions

1. *As blood leaves the left atrium and is pumped to the left ventricle, it passes through the*
   a. *mitral valve.*
   b. *aortic valve.*
   c. *tricuspid valve.*
   d. *pulmonic valve.*
2. *The normal pacemaker of the heart is the*
   a. *Purkinje fibers.*
   b. *atrioventricular (AV) node.*
   c. *sinoatrial (SA) node.*
   d. *bundle of His.*
3. *The coronary arteries fill during which phase of the ventricular cycle?*
   a. *Atrial contraction*
   b. *Ventricular contraction*
   c. *Ventricular diastole*
   d. *Ventricular systole*
4. *The left coronary artery supplies blood to the*
   a. *left ventricle and the septum.*
   b. *right ventricle and the septum.*
   c. *right posterior wall.*
   d. *left and right atria.*
5. *The best measure of the heart's effectiveness as a pump is the*
   a. *heart rate.*
   b. *systolic blood pressure.*
   c. *diastolic blood pressure.*
   d. *cardiac output.*
6. *The right ventricular wall is thinner than the left because*
   a. *the valves on the right are smaller.*

b. *the systolic pressure is higher on the right.*
c. *the workload is not as great on the right.*
d. *the workload is increased on the right.*

7. *The atrioventricular valves*
   a. *prevent backflow from atria to venae cavae during systole.*
   b. *assist forward flow to pulmonary veins during diastole.*
   c. *assist forward flow to the aorta during diastole.*
   d. *prevent backflow from ventricle to atria during systole.*

8. *The smooth layer lining the chambers of the heart and valves is called*
   a. *pericardium.*
   b. *endocardium.*
   c. *epicardium.*
   d. *myocardium.*

9. *As pressure rises in the right atria, the valve forced open is the*
   a. *pulmonic.*
   b. *aortic.*
   c. *tricuspid.*
   d. *mitral.*

REFERENCES

1. Johnson LR: Essential Medical Physiology (2nd Ed). Philadelphia, Lippincott-Raven, 1998
2. Porth CM: Pathophysiology: Concepts of Altered Health States (6th Ed). Philadelphia, Lippincott Williams & Wilkins, 2002

OTHER SELECTED READING

Berne RM, Levy MN: Principles of Physiology (3rd Ed). St. Louis, CV Mosby, 2000

Cohen BJ, Wood DL: Memmler's The Structure and Function of the Human Body (7th Ed). Philadelphia, Lippincott Williams & Wilkins, 2000

Ganong WF: Review of Medical Physiology (19th Ed). Norwalk, CT, Appleton & Lange, 2003

Guyton AC, Hall JE: Textbook of Medical Physiology (10th Ed). Philadelphia, WB Saunders, 2000

Marieb EN: Human Anatomy and Physiology (5th Ed). San Francisco, Benjamin Cummings, 2001

Scanlon V, Sanders T: Essentials of Anatomy and Physiology (4th Ed). Philadelphia, FA Davis, 2003

Thibodeau GA, Patton KT: Anatomy and Physiology (4th Ed). St Louis, Mosby, 1999

Tortora G: Principles of Human Anatomy. New York, Wiley, 2001

chapter

17

Patient Assessment: Cardiovascular System

PATRICIA GONCE MORTON ■ TERRY TUCKER ■
KATHRYN VAN RUEDEN

objectives

Based on the content in this chapter, the reader should be able to:

- Explain the components of the cardiovascular history.
- Describe the steps of the cardiovascular physical examination.
- Discuss the mechanisms responsible for the production of the first, second, third, and fourth heart sounds and their timing in the cardiac cycle.
- Explain each type of murmur, its timing in the cardiac cycle, and the area on the chest wall where it is most easily auscultated.
- Compare and contrast the usefulness of serum enzymes and myocardial proteins in diagnosing an acute myocardial infarction.
- Explain possible causes of serum creatine kinase elevations other than acute myocardial infarction and ischemia.
- Describe current techniques used for diagnostic purposes in cardiology.
- Discuss the nursing care before and after cardiac diagnostic studies.
- Outline the patient and family teaching appropriate to prepare the patient for cardiac diagnostic studies.
- Describe potential complications of cardiac diagnostic procedures.
- Explain the major features of an electrocardiogram (ECG) monitoring system.
- Compare and contrast a hard-wire monitoring system with a telemetry monitoring system.

- Explain correct electrode placement when monitoring the standard leads or the chest leads with a three-electrode and a five-electrode system.
- Discuss steps for troubleshooting ECG monitor problems.
- Describe the components of the ECG tracing and their meaning.
- Explain the steps used to interpret a rhythm strip.
- Describe the causes, clinical significance, and management for each of the arrhythmias discussed.
- Describe the parameters of a normal 12-lead ECG.
- Define electrical axis, and determine the direction of the axis for a 12-lead ECG.
- Explain the causes, clinical significance, and treatment for bundle branch blocks, atrial enlargement, and ventricular enlargement.
- Describe the ECG changes associated with serum potassium and calcium abnormalities.
- Analyze the characteristics of normal systemic arterial, right atrial, right ventricular, pulmonary artery, and pulmonary artery wedge pressure waveforms.
- Describe the system components required to monitor hemodynamic pressures.
- State nursing interventions that ensure accuracy of pressure readings.
- Discuss the major complications that can occur with an indwelling arterial line and pulmonary artery catheter.
- Describe the thermodilution method of measuring cardiac output.
- Identify the determinants of cardiac output.
- Evaluate the factors influencing oxygen delivery and consumption.
- Use $S\bar{v}O_2$ monitoring to assess oxygen delivery and consumption.

The application of complex technology to the assessment and management of cardiovascular and cardiopulmonary conditions has increased greatly in the past several decades. Use of advanced and complex technologies is an integral part of the care of critically ill patients. Nevertheless, the value of a comprehensive cardiovascular history and physical examination should never be underestimated. The chapter begins with a discussion of the cardiac history and physical examination and then discusses technological assessment techniques.

CARDIAC HISTORY AND PHYSICAL EXAMINATION

The cardiovascular history provides physiological and psychosocial information that guides the physical assessment, the selection of diagnostic tests, and the choice of treatment options. During the history, the nurse asks about the presenting symptoms, past health history, current health status, risk factors, family history, and social and personal history. The nurse also inquires about behaviors that promote or jeopardize cardiovascular health and uses this information in guiding health teaching. During the process of taking a thorough history and performing a physical examination, the nurse has an opportunity to establish rapport with the patient and to evaluate the patient's general emotional status.

History

CHIEF COMPLAINT AND HISTORY OF PRESENT ILLNESS

The nurse begins the history by investigating the patient's chief complaint. The patient is asked to describe in his or her own words the problem or reason for seeking care. The nurse then asks for more information about the present illness, using the questions in Box 17-1. Answers to these questions are essential to understanding the patient's perception of the problem. The nurse also asks the patient about any associated symptoms, including chest pain, dyspnea, edema of feet/ankles, palpitations and syncope, cough and hemoptysis, nocturia, cyanosis, and intermittent claudication.

Chest Pain

Chest pain is one of the most common symptoms of patients with cardiovascular disease. Therefore, it is an essential component of the assessment interview. Chest pain is often a disturbing or even frightening experience for a patient, so the patient may be hesitant to initiate a discussion of chest pain. The questions listed in Box 17-1 are particularly useful when assessing chest pain.

Because cardiac pain (angina pectoris) is the result of an imbalance between oxygen supply and oxygen demand, it usually develops over time. Typically, anginal pain does not start at maximal intensity. Not all chest pain is cardiac in origin, and careful reporting of the characteristics of the pain and the behaviors (or lack thereof) that precede the onset of pain is required. The nurse asks the patient about his or her *normal* baseline status before the symptoms developed. It is also important to ask about the *onset* of the symptoms to determine the date and time that the symptoms started and whether the onset was sudden or gradual.

Chest pain caused by coronary artery disease is often *precipitated* by physical or emotional exertion, a meal, or being out in the cold. *Palliative* measures to relieve anginal pain may include rest or sublingual nitrates; these measures usually do not relieve the pain of a myocardial infarction (MI). The *quality* of cardiac chest pain is often described as a heaviness, tightness, squeezing, or choking sensation. If

box 17-1
Assessment Parameters: Questions to Ask in a Symptom Assessment

N Normal: Describe your normal baseline. What was it like before this symptom developed?
O Onset: When did the symptom start? What day? What time? Did it start suddenly or gradually?
P Precipitating and palliative factors: What brought on the symptom? What seems to trigger it—factors such as stress, position change, or exertion? What were you doing when you first noticed the symptom? What makes the symptom worse? What measures have helped relieve the symptom? What have you tried so far? What measures did not relieve the symptom?
Q Quality and quantity: How does it feel? How would you describe it? How much are you experiencing now? Is it more or less than you experienced at any other time?
R Region and radiation: Where does the symptom occur? Can you show me? In the case of pain, does it travel anywhere such as down your arm or in your back?
S Severity: On a scale of 1 to 10, with 10 being the worst ever experienced, rate your symptom. How bad is the symptom at its worst? Does it force you to stop your activity and sit down, lie down, or slow down? Is the symptom getting better or worse, or staying about the same?
T Time: How long does the symptom last? How often do you get the symptom? Does it occur in association with anything, such as before, during, or after meals?

the pain is reported as superficial, knifelike, or throbbing, it is not likely to be anginal. Cardiac chest pain is usually located in the substernal *region* and often *radiates* to the neck, left arm, the back, or jaw. Although the pain is often referred to other areas, anginal pain is visceral in origin, and most complaints include a reference to a "deep, inside" pain. When the patient is asked to point to the painful area, the painful area is about the size of a hand or clenched fist. It is unusual for true anginal pain to be localized to an area smaller than a fingertip. Using a scale of 1 to 10, with 10 being the worst pain the patient has ever experienced, the patient is asked to rate the *severity* of the pain. When asked about *time*, the patient with cardiac chest pain reports the pain lasting anywhere from 30 seconds to hours.

Pain may be secondary to cardiovascular problems that are unrelated to a primary coronary insufficiency. Therefore, when obtaining the patient's history, the nurse must consider other causes. For example, if the patient reports the pain is made worse by lying down, moving, or deep breathing, it may be caused by pericarditis. If the pain is retrosternal and accompanied by sudden shortness of breath and peripheral cyanosis, it may be caused by a pulmonary embolism.

Dyspnea

Dyspnea occurs in patients with both pulmonary and cardiac abnormalities. In patients with cardiac disease, it is the result of inefficient pumping of the left ventricle, which causes a congestion of blood flow in the lungs. During history taking, dyspnea is differentiated from the usual breathlessness that follows a sudden burst of physical activity (e.g., running up four flights of stairs, sprinting across a parking lot). Dyspnea is a subjective complaint of true *difficulty* in breathing, not just shortness of breath. The nurse determines whether the breathing difficulty occurs only with exertion or also at rest. If dyspnea is present when the patient lies flat but is relieved by sitting or standing, it is *orthopnea.* If it is characterized by breathing difficulties starting after approximately 1 to 2 hours of sleep and relieved by sitting upright or getting out of bed, it is *paroxysmal nocturnal dyspnea.*

Edema of the Feet and Ankles

Although many other problems can leave a patient with swollen feet or ankles, heart failure may also be responsible because the heart is unable to mobilize fluid appropriately. Because gravity promotes the movement of fluids from intravascular to extravascular spaces, the edema becomes worse as the day progresses and usually improves at night after lying down to sleep. Patients or families may report that shoes do not fit anymore, socks that used to be loose are now too tight, and the indentations from sock bands take more time than usual to disappear. The nurse should inquire about the timing of edema development (e.g., immediately after lowering the extremities, only at the end of the day, only after a significant salt intake) and duration (e.g., relieved with temporary elevation of the legs or with constant elevation).

Palpitations and Syncope

Palpitations refer to the awareness of irregular or rapid heart beats. Patients may report the "skipping" of beats, a rushing of the heart, or a loud "thudding." The nurse asks about onset and duration of the palpitations, associated symptoms, and any precipitating events that the patient or family can remember. Because a cardiac arrhythmia may compromise blood flow to the brain, the nurse asks about symptoms of dizziness, fainting, or syncope that accompany the palpitations.

Cough and Hemoptysis

Abnormalities such as heart failure, pulmonary embolus, or mitral stenosis may cause a cough or hemoptysis. The nurse asks the patient about the presence of a cough and inquires about the quality (wet or dry) and frequency of the cough (chronic or occasional, only when lying down or after exercise). If the cough produces expectorant, the nurse records its color, consistency, and amount perceived by the patient. If the patient reports spitting up blood (hemoptysis), the nurse asks if the substance spit up was streaked with blood, frothy bloody sputum, or frank blood (bright or dark).

Nocturia

Kidneys that are inadequately perfused by an unhealthy heart during the day may finally receive sufficient flow during rest at night to increase their output. The nurse asks about the number of times the patient urinates during the night. If the patient takes a diuretic, the nurse also evaluates frequency of urination in relation to the time of day the diuretic is taken.

Cyanosis

Cyanosis reflects the oxygenation and circulatory status of the patient. *Central* cyanosis is generally distributed and best found by examining the mucous membranes for discoloration and duskiness, and reflects reduced oxygen concentration. *Peripheral* cyanosis is localized in the extremities and protrusions (hands, feet, nose, ears, lips) and reflects impaired circulation.

Intermittent Claudication

Claudication results when the blood supply to exercising muscles is inadequate. Usually the cause of claudication is significant atherosclerotic obstruction to the lower extremities. The limb is asymptomatic at rest unless the obstruction is severe. Blood supply to the legs is inadequate to meet metabolic demands during exercise, and ischemic pain results. The patient describes a cramping, "charley horse," ache, or weakness in the foot, calf, thigh, or buttocks that improves with rest. The patient should be asked to describe the severity of the pain and how much exertion is required to produce the pain.

PAST HEALTH HISTORY

When assessing the patient's past health history, the nurse inquires about childhood illnesses such as rheumatic fever as well as previous illnesses such as pneumonia, tuberculosis, thrombophlebitis, pulmonary embolism, MI, diabetes mellitus, thyroid disease, or chest injury. The nurse also asks about occupational exposures to cardiotoxic materials. Finally, the nurse seeks information about previous cardiac or vascular surgeries and any previous cardiac studies or interventions (Box 17-2).

CURRENT HEALTH STATUS AND RISK FACTORS

As part of the health history, the nurse queries the patient about use of prescription and over-the-counter medications, vitamins, and herbs. It is essential to ask the patient about drug allergies, food allergies, or any previous allergic reactions to contrast agents. The nurse inquires about use of tobacco, drugs, and alcohol. The nurse also asks about dietary habits, including usual daily food intake, dietary restrictions or supplements, and intake of caffeine-containing foods or beverages. The patient's sleep pattern and exercise and leisure activities also are noted (see Box 17-2).

Assessment of risk factors for cardiovascular disease is an important component of the history. Risk factors are categorized as major uncontrollable risk factors; major risk factors that can be modified, treated, or controlled; and contributing risk factors. Box 17-3 summarizes these risk factors.[1,2]

FAMILY HISTORY

The nurse asks about the age and health, or age and cause of death, of immediate family members, including parents, grandparents, siblings, children, and grandchildren.

box 17-2
Cardiovascular Health History

Chief Complaint
- Patient's description of the problem

History of the Present Illness
- Complete analysis of the symptoms (using the NOPQRST format; see Box 17-1)

Past Health History
- Childhood illnesses: rheumatic fever, murmurs, congenital anomalies
- Past medical problems: heart failure, hypertension, coronary artery disease, myocardial infarction, hyperlipidemia, valve disease, cardiac arrhythmias, peripheral vascular disease, diabetes
- Past surgeries: cardiovascular surgeries such as coronary artery bypass grafting, valve replacement, peripheral vascular procedures; surgeries for other health problems
- Past diagnostic tests and interventions: electrocardiogram, echocardiogram, cardiac catheterization, stress test, electrophysiological studies, percutaneous transluminal coronary angioplasty, stent placement, atherectomy, pacemaker implantation, implantable cardioverter–defibrillator placement, valvuloplasty

Current Health Status and Risk Factors
- Medications: prescription drugs, over-the-counter drugs, vitamins, herbs, and supplements
- Allergies and reactions: medications, food, contrast agents
- Tobacco, alcohol, and substance use
- Diet
- Sleep patterns
- Exercise
- Leisure activities
- Risk factors: major risk factors that cannot be altered, major risk factors that can be altered, contributing risk factors (see Box 17-3)

Family History
- Hypertension, elevated cholesterol, coronary artery disease, myocardial infarction, stroke, peripheral vascular disease, cardiac arrhythmias

Social and Personal History
- Family composition
- Living environment
- Daily routine
- Sexual activity
- Occupation
- Coping patterns
- Cultural beliefs
- Spiritual/religious beliefs

box 17-3
Risk Factors for Cardiovascular Disease

Major Uncontrollable Risk Factors

- Age: There is an increased incidence of all types of atherosclerotic disease with aging. About 85% of people who die from coronary artery disease are age 65 years or older. Women at older ages who have a myocardial infarction are twice as likely as men to die from it within a few weeks.
- Heredity: The tendency for development of atherosclerosis seems to run in families. The risk is thought to be a combination of environmental and genetic influences. Even when other risk factors are controlled, the chance for development of coronary artery disease increases when there is a familial tendency.
- Gender: Men have a greater risk for development of coronary artery disease than women at earlier ages. After menopause, women's death rate from myocardial infarction increases but is not as great as men's.
- Race: Rates of cardiovascular disease are higher for African Americans, Mexican Americans, Native Americans, Native Hawaiians, and some Asian Americans.

Major Risk Factors That Can Be Modified, Treated, or Controlled

- Tobacco smoking: A smoker's risk of a myocardial infarction is more than twice that of nonsmokers. Smokers who have a myocardial infarction are more likely to die and die within an hour than are nonsmokers. Cigarette smoking is the greatest risk factor for sudden death. Smokers have two to four times the risk of sudden death compared with nonsmokers. Chronic exposure to environmental tobacco smoke may increase the risk of heart disease.
- High blood cholesterol: The risk of coronary heart disease increases as the blood cholesterol level rises. When other risk factors are present, this risk increases even more.
- Hypertension: Known as the "silent killer," hypertension is a risk factor with no specific symptoms and no early warning signs. Men have a greater risk for hypertension than women until the age of 55 years. The risk for development of hypertension is about the same for men and women between the ages of 55 and 75 years. After the age of 75 years, hypertension is more likely to develop in women than in men. African Americans are more likely to have hypertension than whites. Hypertension increases the risk of stroke, myocardial infarction, kidney failure, and heart failure.
- Physical inactivity: A lack of physical exercise is a risk factor for coronary artery disease. Moderate to vigorous regular exercise plays a significant role in preventing heart disease and blood vessel disease. Even moderate-intensity exercise is beneficial if performed regularly and long-term. Physical activity also plays a role in controlling cholesterol, diabetes, obesity, and hypertension.
- Obesity: There is an association between obesity and an increased mortality rate from coronary artery disease and stroke. Excess weight is also linked with an increased incidence of hypertension, insulin resistance, diabetes, and dyslipidemia.
- Diabetes mellitus: Diabetes significantly increases the risk for development of cardiovascular disease. The associated risk is greater for women than for men. Three fourths of individuals with diabetes die of some form of heart or blood vessel disease.

Other Contributing Factors

- Stress: A person's response to stress may be a contributing factor to heart disease. Stress in a person's life, his or her health behaviors, and socioeconomic status may all contribute to established risk factors. For example, individuals under stress may overeat, smoke, and not exercise.
- Sex hormones: Men are at higher risk of myocardial infarction than premenopausal women. After menopause, the risk for women increases because it is believed that the loss of natural estrogen as the woman ages may be a contributing factor.
- Birth control pills: Newer low-dose oral contraceptives carry a much lower risk of cardiovascular disease than the early forms of birth control pills. If a woman using oral contraceptives has other risk factors such as smoking or hypertension, her risk for development of blood clots and having a myocardial infarction increases.
- Excessive alcohol intake: Drinking too much alcohol can raise blood pressure, cause heart failure, lead to stroke, contribute to high triglycerides and obesity, and produce arrhythmias. The risk of heart disease in individuals who drink moderate amounts of alcohol (an average of one drink for women and two drinks for men per day) is lower than in those who do not drink alcohol.
- Homocysteine levels: An association has been shown between elevated levels of homocysteine and cardiovascular disease. Homocysteine causes increased platelet adhesiveness, enhances low-density lipoprotein deposition in the arterial wall, and activates the coagulation cascade.

The nurse inquires about cardiovascular problems such as hypertension, elevated cholesterol, coronary artery disease, MI, stroke, and peripheral vascular disease (see Box 17-2).

SOCIAL AND PERSONAL HISTORY

Although the physical symptoms provide many clues regarding the origin and extent of cardiac disease, social and personal history also contribute to the patient's health status. The nurse inquires about the patient's family, spouse or significant other, and children. Information about the patient's living environment, daily routine, sexual activity, occupation, coping patterns, and cultural and spiritual beliefs contributes to the nurse's understanding of the patient as a person and guides interaction with the patient and family (see Box 17-2).

Physical Examination

Cardiac assessment requires examination of all aspects of the individual, using the standard steps of inspection, palpation, percussion, and auscultation. A thorough and careful examination helps the nurse detect subtle abnormalities as well as obvious ones.

INSPECTION

General Appearance

Inspection begins as soon as the patient and nurse interact. General appearance and presentation of the patient are key elements of the initial inspection. Critical examination reveals a first impression of age, nutritional status, self-care ability, alertness, and overall physical health.

It is necessary to note the ability of the patient to move and speak with or without distress. Consider the patient's posture, gait, and musculoskeletal coordination.

Jugular Venous Distension

Pressure in the jugular veins reflects right atrial pressure and provides the nurse with an indication of heart hemodynamics and cardiac function. The height of the level of blood in the right internal jugular vein is an indication of right atrial pressure because there are no valves or obstructions between the vein and the right atrium.

The internal jugular veins are not directly visible, because they lie deep to the sternomastoid muscles in the neck (Fig. 17-1). The goals of the examination are to determine the highest point of visible pulsation in the internal jugular veins, to note the level of head elevation, and to measure this point of visible pulsation as the vertical distance above the sternal angle. The patient is placed in the bed supine with the head of the bed elevated 30, 45, 60, and 90 degrees. The patient is examined at each elevation with the head slightly turned away from the examiner. The nurse uses tangential light to observe for the highest point of visible pulsation.[3,4]

Next, the angle of Louis is located by palpating where the clavicle joins the sternum (suprasternal notch). The examining finger is slid down the sternum until a bony prominence is felt. This prominence is known as the *angle of Louis*. A vertical ruler is placed on the angle of Louis. Another ruler is placed horizontally at the level of the pulsation. The intersection of the horizontal ruler with the vertical ruler is noted, and the intersection point on the vertical ruler is read.

Normal jugular venous pulsation should not exceed 3 cm above the angle of Louis. See Figure 17-2 for an illustration of the procedure for assessment of jugular venous pressure. A level more than 3 cm above the angle of Louis indicates an abnormally high volume in the venous system. Possible causes include right-sided heart failure, obstruction of the superior vena cava, pericardial effusion, and other cardiac or thoracic diseases. An increase in the jugular venous pressure of more than 1 cm while pressure is applied to the abdomen for 60 seconds (hepatojugular or abdominojugular test) indicates the inability of the heart to accommodate the increased venous return.

Chest

The chest is inspected for signs of trauma or injury, symmetry, chest contour, and any visible pulsations. Thrusts (abnormally strong precordial pulsations) are noted. Any depression (sternum excavatum) or bulging of the precordium is recorded.

Extremities

A close inspection of the patient's extremities can also provide clues about cardiovascular health. The extremities are examined for lesions, ulcerations, unhealed sores, and varicose veins. Distribution of hair on the extremities also is noted. A lack of normal hair distribution on the extremities may indicate diminished arterial blood flow to the area.

Skin

Skin is evaluated for moistness or dryness, color, elasticity, edema, thickness, lesions, ulcerations, and vascular changes. Nail beds are examined for cyanosis and clubbing, which may indicate chronic cardiac or pulmonary abnormalities. General differences in color and temperature between body parts may provide perfusion clues.

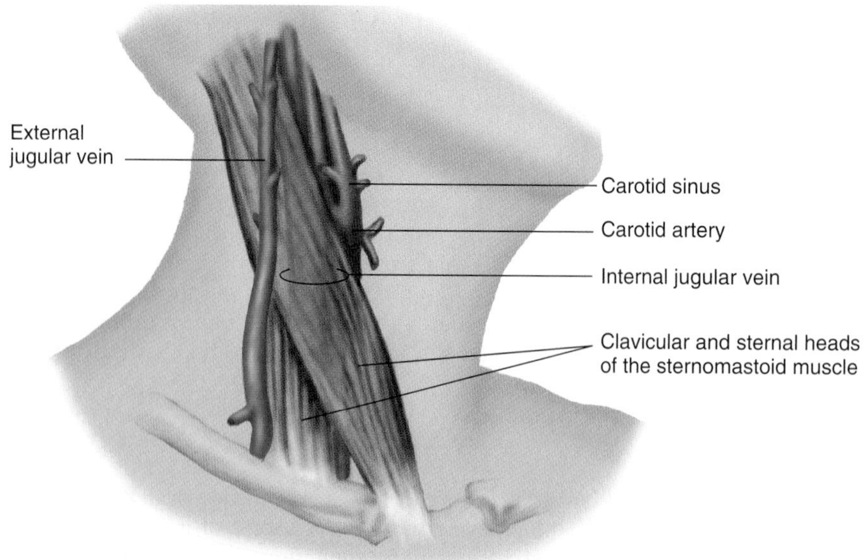

figure 17-1 Internal jugular veins. (From Bickley L: Bates' Guide to Physical Examination and Health History [8th Ed], p 32. Philadelphia, Lippincott Williams & Wilkins, 2003.)

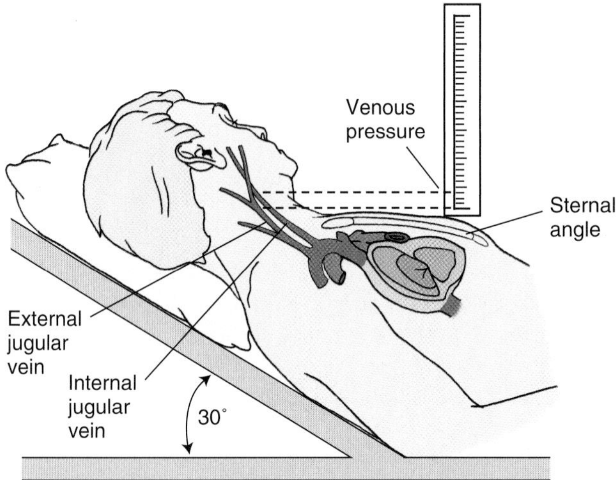

figure 17-2 Assessment of jugular venous pressure. Place the patient supine in bed and gradually raise the head of the bed to 30, 45, 60, and 90 degrees. Using tangential lighting, note the highest level of venous pulsation. Measure the vertical distance between this point and the sternal angle. Record this distance in centimeters and the angle of the head of the bed.

PALPATION

Pulses

Cardiovascular assessment continues with palpation and involves the use of the pads of the finger and balls of the hand. Using the pads of the fingers, the carotid, brachial, radial, femoral, popliteal, posterior tibial, and dorsalis pedis pulses are palpated. The peripheral pulses are compared bilaterally to determine rate, rhythm, strength, and symmetry. The 0-to-3 scale described in Box 17-4 is used to rate the strength of the pulse. The carotid pulses should never be assessed simultaneously because this can obstruct flow to the brain.

Pulses can also be described according to their characteristics. For example, pulsus alternans is a pulse that alternates in strength with every other beat; it is often found in patients with left ventricular failure. Pulsus paradoxus is a pulse that disappears during inspiration but returns during expiration. To determine if the condition is pathological, the sphygmomanometer is deflated until the pulse is heard only during expiration and the corresponding pressure noted. As the cuff continues to deflate, the point at which the pressure is heard *throughout* the inspiratory and expiratory cycle is noted. The second systolic pressure reading is subtracted from the first; if the difference is greater than 10 mm Hg during normal respirations, it is considered pathological. During the assessment of pulses, the nurse compares the warmth and size of the palpated areas to monitor perfusion.

box 17-4
Rating Scale Used for Assessing Strength of Pulses

0	Absent
1	Palpable but thready, weak, easily obliterated
2	Normal, not easily obliterated
3	Full, bounding, easily palpable, cannot obliterate

Precordium

The chest wall is palpated to assess for the point of maximal impulse (PMI), thrills, and abnormal pulsations. The nurse first uses the pads of the fingers and then places a hand flat against the patient's chest, using light pressure.

A systematic palpation sequence is used with the patient in a supine position and includes the precordial areas shown in Figure 17-3. Palpation starts with locating the PMI. In most patients, the PMI represents the point where the apical pulse is most readily felt. The PMI is palpated, noting its location, diameter, amplitude, and duration. Usually, the PMI is located in the midclavicular line at about the fourth or fifth intercostal space. If the pulse is difficult to palpate, it may be necessary to ask the patient to turn on the left side (left lateral decubitus position).

Next, the nurse palpates the lower left sternal border area, the upper left sternal border area, the sternoclavicular area, the right upper sternal border area, the lower right sternal border area, and finally the epigastric area. During palpation of these areas, the nurse feels for a thrill, which is a palpable vibration. A thrill usually represents a disruption in blood flow related to a defect in one of the semilunar valves.

PERCUSSION

With the advent of radiological means of evaluating cardiac size, percussion is not a significant contributor to cardiac assessment. However, a gross determination of heart size can be made by percussing for the dullness that reflects the cardiac borders.

AUSCULTATION

Data obtained by careful and thorough auscultation of the heart are essential in planning and evaluating care of the critically ill patient. In this section, the basic principles underlying cardiac auscultation; the factors responsible for the production of normal heart sounds; and the pathophysiological conditions responsible for the production of extra sounds, murmurs, and friction rubs are discussed.

To facilitate accurate auscultation, the patient should be relaxed and comfortable in a quiet, warm environment with adequate lighting. The patient should be in a recumbent position with the trunk elevated 30 to 45 degrees. To help hear abnormal sounds, the patient may be asked to roll partly onto the left side (left lateral decubitus position). This position helps bring the left ventricle closer to the chest wall.

A good-quality stethoscope is essential. The earpieces should fit the ears snugly and comfortably and follow the natural angle of the ear canals. Sound waves that travel a shorter distance are more intense and less distorted; therefore, the tubing of the stethoscope should be approximately 12 inches in length and somewhat rigid. It is best to have two tubes leading from the head of the stethoscope, one to each ear. The head of the stethoscope should be equipped

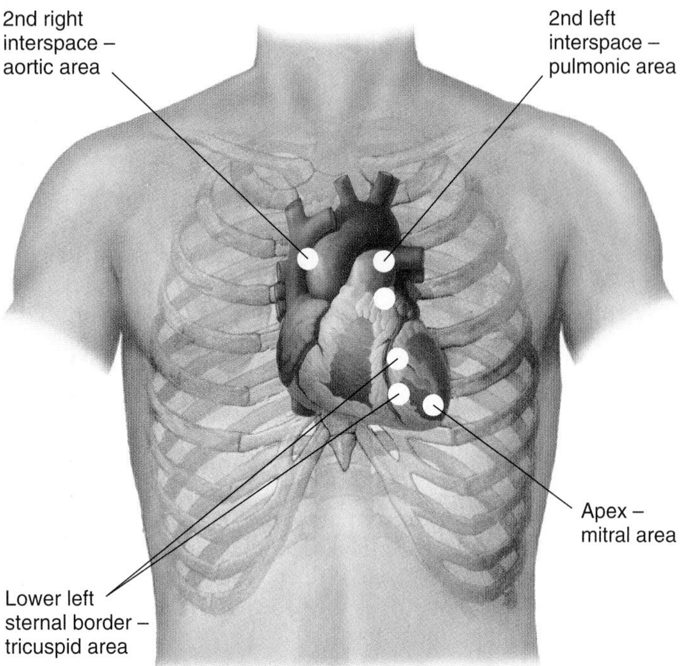

figure 17-3 Areas of auscultation. I. Aortic area (second intercostal space to the right of the sternum). II. Pulmonic area (second intercostal space to the left of the sternum). III. Tricuspid area (fifth intercostal space to the left of the sternum). IV. Mitral or apical area (fifth intercostal space midclavicular line). (From Bickley L: Bates' Guide to Physical Examination and Health History [8th Ed], p 278. Philadelphia, Lippincott Williams & Wilkins, 2003.)

with both a diaphragm and a bell on a valve system that allows the clinician to switch easily between the two components. The diaphragm is used to hear high-frequency sounds, such as the first and second heart sounds (S_1, S_2), friction rubs, systolic murmurs, and diastolic insufficiency murmurs. The diaphragm should be placed firmly on the chest wall to create a tight seal. Low-frequency sounds, such as the third and fourth heart sounds (S_3, S_4) and the diastolic murmurs of mitral and tricuspid stenosis, are best heard with the stethoscope bell, which should be placed lightly on the chest wall only to seal the edges.

The precordium should be auscultated systematically (see Fig. 17-3). Some authorities suggest the use of anatomical names for the auscultation areas (e.g., aortic and pulmonic), whereas others discourage the use of such labels because murmurs of more than one origin can be heard in a given area.[3] The nurse begins the examination by listening with the stethoscope diaphragm in the right second intercostal space along the sternum. This area is sometimes called the aortic area and is the place where S_2 is loudest. Next, the nurse places the stethoscope in the left second intercostal space along the sternum, which is known as the pulmonic listening area, and from there moves the stethoscope down the left sternal border between the second and fifth spaces, one intercostal space at a time. The lower left sternal border area is sometimes referred to as the tricuspid area. Finally, the nurse moves the stethoscope to the mitral area or apex of the heart, where S_1 is the loudest. This pattern is then repeated with the stethoscope bell.

In each area auscultated, the nurse should identify S_1, noting the intensity of the sound, respiratory variation, and splitting. S_2 should then be identified and the same characteristics assessed. After S_1 and S_2 are identified, the presence of extra sounds is noted—first in systole, then in diastole. Finally, each area is auscultated for the presence of murmurs and friction rubs.

First Heart Sound

S_1 is timed with the closure of the mitral and tricuspid valves at the beginning of ventricular systole (Fig. 17-4). Because mitral valve closure is responsible for most of the sound produced, S_1 is heard best in the mitral or apical area. The upstroke of the carotid pulse correlates with S_1 and can be used to help distinguish S_1 from S_2.

The intensity (loudness) of S_1 varies with the position of the atrioventricular (AV) valve leaflets at the beginning of ventricular systole and the structure of the leaflets (thickened or normal). A loud S_1 is produced when the valve leaflets are wide open at the onset of ventricular systole and corresponds to a short PR interval on the surface electrocardiogram (ECG) tracing. A lengthening of the PR interval produces a soft S_1 because the leaflets have had time to float partially closed before ventricular systole. Mitral stenosis also increases the intensity of S_1 due to a thickening of the valvular structures.

In general, S_1 is heard as a single sound. If right ventricular systole is delayed, however, S_1 may be split into its two component sounds. The most common cause of this splitting is delay in the conduction of impulses through the right bundle branch; the splitting correlates with a right bundle branch block (RBBB) pattern on the ECG. Splitting of S_1 is heard best over the tricuspid area.

Second Heart Sound

S_2 is produced by the vibrations initiated by the closure of the aortic and pulmonic semilunar valves and is heard best at the base of the heart (Fig. 17-5). This sound represents the beginning of ventricular diastole.

Like S_1, S_2 consists of two separate components. The first component of S_2 is aortic valve closure; the second component is pulmonic valve closure. With inspiration, systole of the right ventricle is slightly prolonged because of increased filling of the right ventricle. This causes the pulmonic valve to close later than the aortic valve and S_2 to

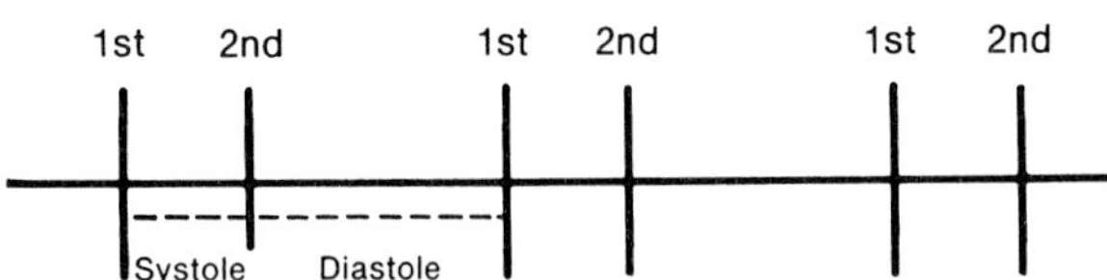

Normal: S_1 is produced by the closure of the AV valves and correlates with the beginning of ventricular systole. It is heard best in the apical or mitral area.

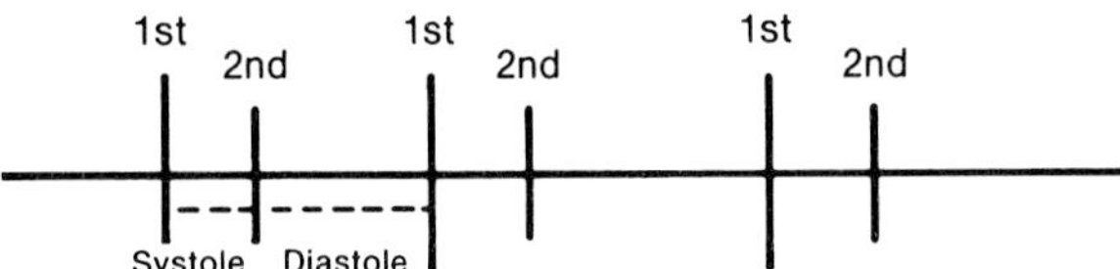

Loud First Sound: The intensity of the first heart sound may be increased when the PR interval is shortened, as in tachycardia, or when the valve leaflets are thickened, as in mitral stenosis.

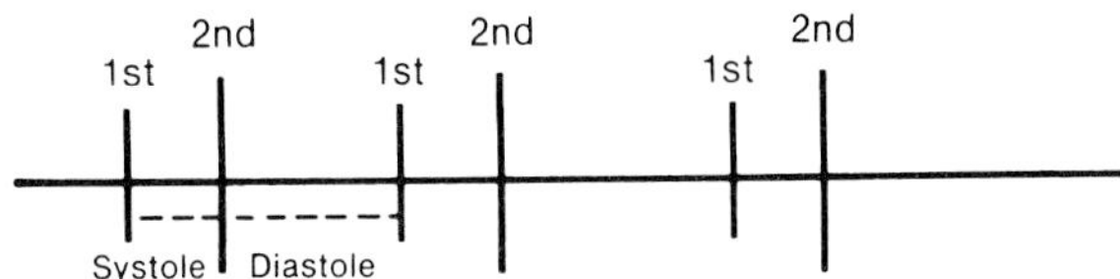

Soft First Sound: A soft S_1 is heard when the PR interval is prolonged.

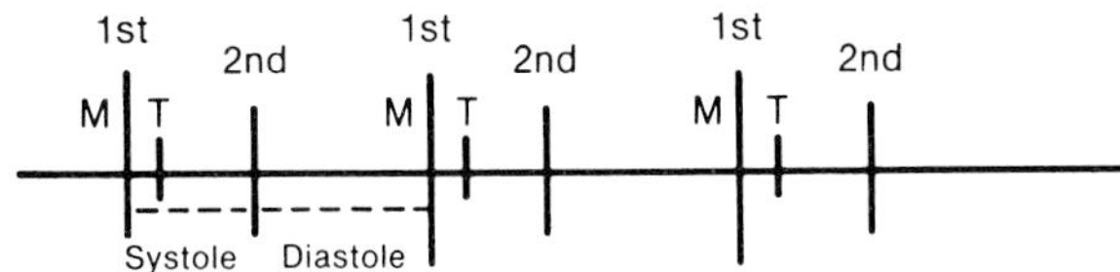

Split First Sound: A split S_1 is heard when right ventricular emptying is delayed. The mitral valve closes before the tricuspid valve and "splits" the sound into its two components.

figure 17-4 First heart sound.

become "split" into its two components. This normal finding is termed *physiological splitting* and is heard best on inspiration with the stethoscope placed in the second intercostal space to the left of the sternum.

The intensity of S_2 may be increased in the presence of aortic or pulmonic valvular stenosis or with an increase in the diastolic pressure forcing the semilunar valves to close, as occurs in pulmonary or systemic hypertension.

Third Heart Sound

An S_3 may be physiological or pathological (Fig. 17-6). A physiological S_3 is a normal finding in children and healthy young adults; it usually disappears after 25 to 35 years of age. An S_3 in an older adult with heart disease signifies ventricular failure.

An S_3 is a low-frequency sound that occurs during the early, rapid-filling phase of ventricular diastole. A noncompliant or failing ventricle cannot distend to accept this rapid inflow of blood. This causes turbulent flow, resulting in the vibration of the AV valvular structures or the ventricles themselves, producing a low-frequency sound. An S_3 associated with left ventricular failure is heard best at the apex with the stethoscope bell. The sound may be accentuated by turning the patient slightly to the left side. A right ventricular S_3 is heard best at the xiphoid or lower left sternal border and varies in intensity with respiration, becoming louder on inspiration.

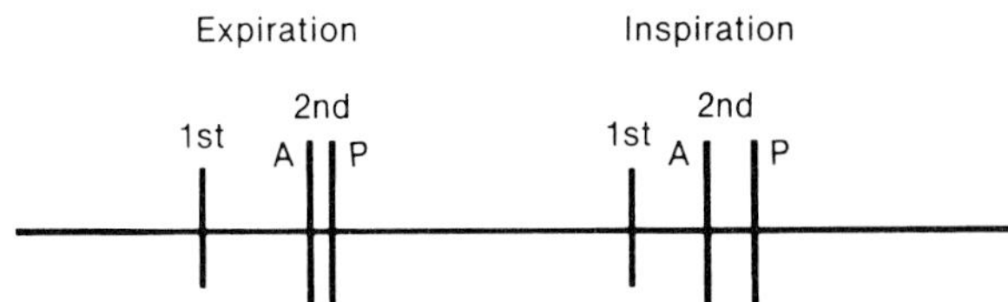

figure 17-5 Second heart sound. The second heart sound is produced by the closure of the semilunar valves (aortic and pulmonary). During inspiration, there is an increase in venous return to the right side of the heart, which causes a delay in the emptying of the right ventricle and the closure of the pulmonic valve. This allows the two components of the second heart sound to separate or split during inspiration.

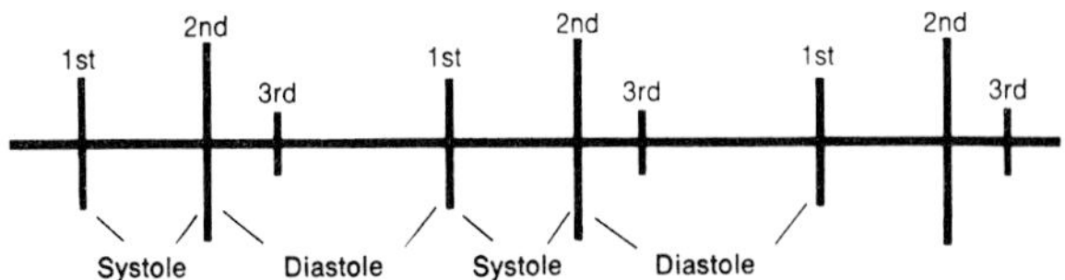

figure 17-6 Third heart sound. An S_3 or ventricular gallop is heard in early diastole, shortly after the second heart sound. The presence of a pathological S_3 may be indicative of heart failure.

Fourth Heart Sound

An S_4 or atrial gallop is a low-frequency sound heard late in diastole just before S_1. It is rarely heard in healthy patients (Fig. 17-7). The sound is produced by atrial contraction forcing blood into a noncompliant ventricle that, by virtue of its noncompliance, has an increased resistance to filling. Systemic hypertension, MI, angina, cardiomyopathy, and aortic stenosis all may produce a decrease in left ventricular compliance and an S_4. A left ventricular S_4 is auscultated at the apex with the bell of the stethoscope. Conditions affecting right ventricular compliance, such as pulmonary hypertension or pulmonic stenosis, may produce a right ventricular S_4 heard best at the lower left sternal border; it increases in intensity during inspiration.

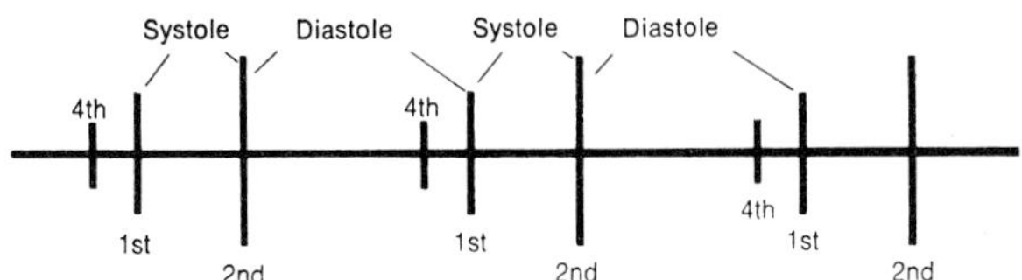

figure 17-7 Fourth heart sound. An S_4 is a late diastolic sound that occurs just prior to S_1. It is a low-frequency sound heard best with the bell of the stethoscope.

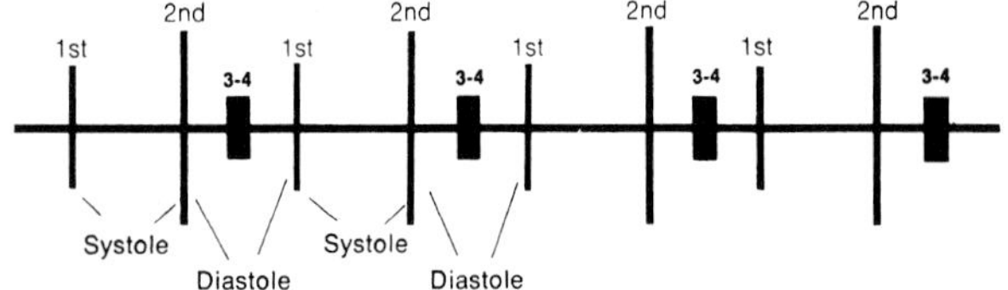

figure 17-8 Summation gallop. With rapid heart rates, S_3 and S_4 may become audible as a single, very loud sound that occurs in mid-diastole. This sound is a summation gallop.

Summation Gallop

With rapid heart rates, as ventricular diastole shortens, if S_3 and S_4 are both present, they may fuse together and become audible as a single diastolic sound. This is called a *summation gallop* (Fig. 17-8). This sound is loudest at the apex and is heard best with the stethoscope bell while the patient lies turned slightly to the left side.

Heart Murmurs

Murmurs are sounds produced either by the forward flow of blood through a narrowed or constricted valve into a dilated vessel or chamber or by the backward flow of blood through an incompetent valve or septal defect. Murmur classification is based on timing in the cardiac cycle. Systolic murmurs occur between S_1 and S_2. Diastolic murmurs occur after S_2 and before the onset of the following S_1. Murmurs are described further according to the anatomical location on the anterior chest where the sound is heard the loudest. Any radiation of the sound also should be noted. The quality of the sound produced is described as blowing, harsh, rumbling, or musical (Box 17-5). The intensity or loudness of a murmur is described using a grading system. Grade I is faint and barely audible; grade II is soft; grade III is audible but not palpable; grade IV and V murmurs are associated with a palpable thrill; and a grade VI murmur is audible without a stethoscope (Box 17-6).

box 17-5
Attributes of Heart Murmurs

- **Timing:** A systolic murmur is heard between S_1 and S_2. A diastolic murmur is heard between S_2 and S_1.
- **Location of maximal intensity:** The nurse describes the anatomical location where the murmur is heard best. The location is identified based on intercostal space and its relation to the sternum, the apex, the mid-clavicular line, or one of the axillary lines.
- **Radiation or transmission from the point of maximal intensity:** The nurse notes the site farthest from the location of greatest intensity at which the sound is still heard. The farthest site is identified using anatomical landmarks as described above.
- **Pitch:** The terms *high, medium,* or *low* are used to describe the pitch of the murmur.
- **Quality:** Terms such as *harsh, raspy, vibratory, blowing,* or *musical* are used to describe the quality of the sound.
- **Intensity:** A grading system is used to describe the intensity of the murmur. See Box 17-6 for a summary of the grading system.

box 17-6
Gradation of Heart Murmurs

Grade 1	Barely audible in a quiet room; very faint; may not be heard in all positions
Grade 2	Quiet, but clearly audible
Grade 3	Moderately loud
Grade 4	Loud with a palpable thrill
Grade 5	Very loud with an easily palpable thrill
Grade 6	Very loud; may be heard with stethoscope entirely off of the chest; thrill palpable and visible

Systolic Murmurs. As previously described, S_1 is produced by mitral and tricuspid valve closure and signifies the onset of ventricular systole. Murmurs occurring after S_1 and before S_2 are therefore classified as systolic murmurs.

During ventricular systole, the aortic and pulmonic valves are open. If either of these valves is stenotic or narrowed, a sound classified as a mid-systolic ejection murmur is heard. Because the AV valves close before blood is ejected through the aortic and pulmonic valves, there is a delay between S_1 and the beginning of the murmur. The murmurs associated with aortic stenosis and pulmonic stenosis are described as crescendo–decrescendo or diamond shaped (Fig. 17-9), meaning that the sound increases and then decreases in intensity. The quality of these murmurs is harsh, and they are of medium pitch. The murmur caused by aortic stenosis is heard best in the aortic area and may radiate into the neck. The murmur of pulmonic stenosis is heard best over the pulmonic area.

Systolic regurgitant murmurs are caused by the backward flow of blood from an area of higher pressure to an area of lower pressure. Mitral or tricuspid valvular insufficiency or a defect in the ventricular septum produces systolic regurgitant murmurs, which are harsh and blowing in quality. The sound is described as holosystolic, meaning that the murmur begins immediately after S_1 and continues throughout systole up to S_2 (Fig. 17-10).

Mitral insufficiency produces this type of murmur, heard most easily in the apical area with radiation to the left axilla. This type of murmur associated with tricuspid insufficiency is heard loudest at the left sternal border and increases in intensity during inspiration. This murmur may radiate to the cardiac apex.

A ventricular septal defect also produces a harsh, blowing holosystolic sound caused by blood flowing from the

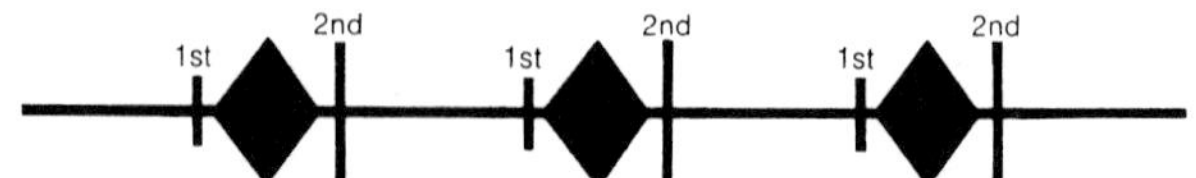

figure 17-9 Murmur associated with aortic or pulmonic stenosis. Blood flow through a stenotic aortic or pulmonic valve produces a crescendo–decrescendo midsystolic ejection murmur.

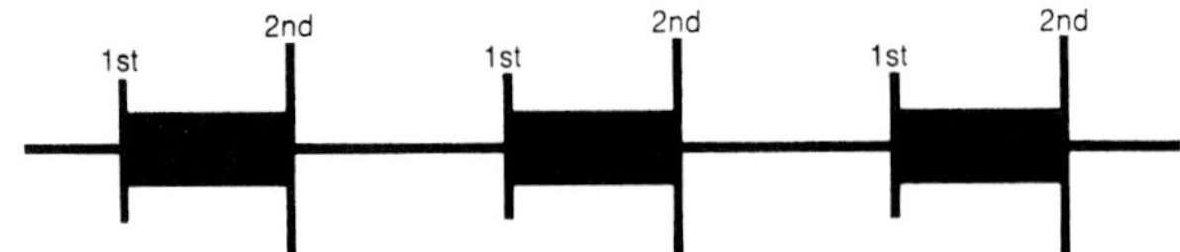

figure 17-10 Murmur associated with tricuspid or mitral regurgitation. A holosystolic murmur is caused by the regurgitant flow of blood through an incompetent mitral or tricuspid valve. Flow of blood from the left ventricle to the right ventricle through a ventricular septal defect also produces this type of murmur.

left to the right ventricle through a defect in the septal wall during systole. The associated murmur is heard best from the fourth to sixth intercostal spaces on both sides of the sternum and is accompanied by a palpable thrill.

Diastolic Murmurs. Diastolic murmurs occur after S_2 and before the next S_1. During diastole, the aortic and pulmonic valves are closed while the mitral and tricuspid valves are open to allow filling of the ventricles.

Aortic or pulmonic valvular insufficiency produces a blowing diastolic murmur that begins immediately after S_2 and decreases in intensity as regurgitant flow decreases through diastole. These murmurs are described as early diastolic decrescendo murmurs (Fig. 17-11).

The murmur associated with aortic insufficiency is heard best in the aortic area and may radiate along the right sternal border to the apex. Pulmonic valve insufficiency produces a murmur that is loudest in the pulmonic area.

Stenosis or narrowing of the mitral or tricuspid valve also produces a diastolic murmur. The AV valves open in mid-diastole shortly after the aortic and pulmonic valves close, causing a delay between S_2 and the start of the murmur of mitral and tricuspid stenosis. This murmur decreases in intensity from its onset and then increases again as ventricular filling increases because of atrial contraction; this is termed *decrescendo–crescendo* (Fig. 17-12).

The murmur associated with mitral stenosis is heard best at the apex with the patient turned slightly to the left side. Tricuspid stenosis produces a murmur that increases

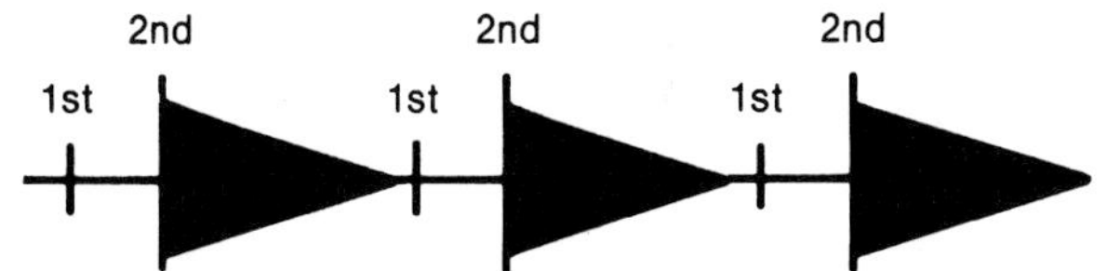

figure 17-11 Murmur associated with aortic or pulmonic insufficiency. Regurgitant flow through an incompetent aortic or pulmonic valve produces a diastolic decrescendo murmur.

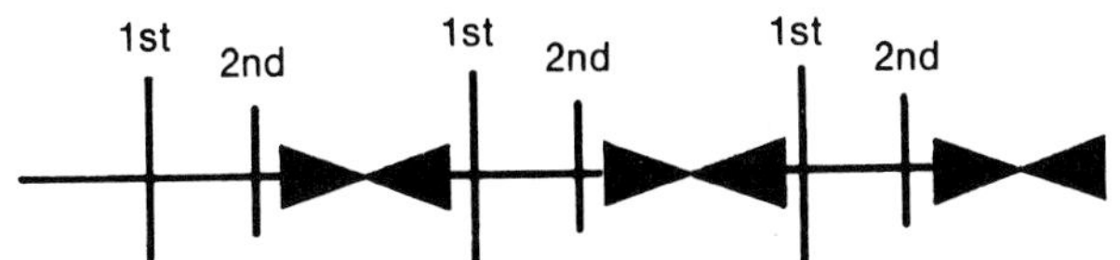

figure 17-12 Murmur associated with tricuspid or mitral stenosis. This low-frequency murmur is heard best with the bell of the stethoscope. It occurs after S_1 and has a decrescendo–crescendo configuration.

in intensity with inspiration and is loudest in the fifth intercostal space along the left sternal border.

Friction Rubs

A pericardial friction rub can be heard when the pericardial surfaces are inflamed. This high-pitched, scratchy sound is produced by these inflamed layers rubbing together. A rub may be heard anywhere over the pericardium with the diaphragm of the stethoscope. The rub may be accentuated by having the patient lean forward and exhale. A pericardial friction rub, unlike a pleural friction rub, does not vary in intensity with respiration.

CARDIAC LABORATORY STUDIES

Knowledge of the purpose and significance of laboratory values in relation to the diagnosis and prognosis of acute MI can enhance the quality of nursing care available to patients. Laboratory studies include both routine serum analysis and special studies, such as serum and cardiac enzymes. Nurses who have a basic understanding of laboratory studies can exercise judgment in interpreting results relative to other information about the patient. The ability to use this kind of judgment may well affect the patient's clinical course or prognosis.

Routine Laboratory Studies

Appropriate assessment of normal and compromised cardiac function is essential to ensure accurate evaluation and correct diagnosis of the patient experiencing symptoms consistent with a cardiovascular disorder or coronary artery disease. Nurses can more appropriately plan the care of the patient and initiate interventions if they have an understanding of these laboratory tests and recognize their implications. Valuable information may be obtained by assessing levels of hematological components, coagulation factors, electrolytes, and phospholipids. Determination of these laboratory studies may vary with institutional techniques and equipment used. Normal and abnormal assay ranges have been universally established, and a brief listing of frequently ordered laboratory studies with their normal values can be found in Table 17-1. A more extensive explanation of the effects of abnormal laboratory determinations is provided in other parts of this text and is not addressed here.

HEMATOLOGICAL STUDIES

Accurate assessment of the patient with a possible cardiac disruption merits review of hematological function. It is important for the critical care nurse to understand the role of blood cells in cardiac function and their contribution to the maintenance of healthy tissue. Blood is the transport medium for nutrients, such as oxygen and glucose, as well as electrolytes, plasma proteins, hormones, and medications. It is also the vehicle for removal of the products of metabolism. Changes in blood cell integrity and total cell count may reflect specific disorders of the cardiac system and should be considered an integral part of the laboratory assessment.

table 17-1 Normal Reference Ranges for Laboratory Blood Tests

Blood Test	Reference Range	Blood Test	Reference Range
Hematological Studies		***Blood Chemistries–(cont.)***	
Red blood cell count		Bilirubin	
Men	4.6–6.2 × 10^6	Total	0.2–1.3 mg/dL
Women	4.2–5.4 × 10^6	Direct	0–20 mg/dL
Hematocrit		Calcium	
Men	40%–50%	Total	8.9–10.3 mg/dL
Women	38%–47%	Free (ionized)	4.6–5.1 mg/dL
Hemoglobin		Creatinine	
Men	13.5–18.0 g/100 mL	Men	0.9–1.4 mg/dL
Women	12.0–16.0 g/100 mL	Women	0.8–1.3 mg/dL
Corpuscle indices		Glucose (fasting)	65–110 mg/dL
Mean corpuscular volume	82–98 FL	Magnesium	1.3–2.2 mEq/L
Mean corpuscular hemoglobin	27–31 pg	Phosphorus	2.5–4.5 mg/dL
Mean corpuscular hemoglobin concentration	32%–36%	Phosphatase, alkaline	35–148 U
		Protein (total)	6.5–8.5 g/dL
White blood cell count		Urea nitrogen	8–26 mg/dL
Total	4,500–11,000/mm³	Uric acid	65–110 mg/dL
Differential (in number of cells/mm³ blood)		Men	4.0–8.5 mg/dL
		Women	2.8–7.5 mg/dL
Total leukocytes	5,000–10,000 (100%)	***Serum Enzymes****	
Total neutrophils	3,000–7,000 (60%–70%)	CK-MM	95%–100%
Lymphocytes	1,500–3,000 (20%–30%)	CK-MB	0%–5%
Monocytes	375–500 (2%–6%)	CK-BB	0%
Eosinophils	50–400 (1%–4%)	LDH-1	Dependent on assay technique ratio
Basophils	0–50 (0.1%)		
Sedimentation rate	0–30 mm/h		
Coagulation Studies*		LDH-1:LDH-2 ratio	<1.0
Platelet count	250,000–500,000/mm³	Aspartate aminotransferase	<50 U/L
Prothrombin time	12–15 s		
Partial thromboplastin time	60–70 s	***Myocardial Proteins***	
Activated partial thromboplastin time	35–45 s	Troponin-I	0–2 ng/mL
Activated clotting time	75–105 s	Troponin-T	0–3.1 ng/mL
Fibrinogen level	160–300 mg/dL	Myoglobin	
Thrombin time	11.3–18.5 s	Men	20–90 ng/mL
		Women	10–75 ng/mL
Blood Chemistries		***Cholesterol***	
Serum electrolytes		Total blood cholesterol	
Sodium	135–145 mEq/L	Desirable	<200 mg/dL
Potassium	3.3–4.9 mEq/L	Borderline high	200–239 mg/dL
Chloride	97–110 mEq/L	High	≥240 mg/dL
Carbon dioxide	22–31 mEq/L	LDL cholesterol	
Blood gases		Desirable	<130 mg/dL
pH	7.35–7.45	Borderline high	130–159 mg/dL
Pao_2	80–105 mm Hg	High	≥160 mg/dL
$Paco_2$	35–45 mm Hg	HDL cholesterol	>35 mg/dL
Bicarbonate	22–29 mEq/L	Apolipoprotein A	120 mg/dL
Base excess, deficit	0±2.3 mEq/L	Apolipoprotein B	134 mg/dL
Sao_2	98%		
$S\bar{v}co_2$	75%		

*Examples: regional laboratory techniques and methods may result in variations.

Knowledge of normal blood values is vital to understand deviations from normal that can be seen with various cardiac disruptions. It is necessary to review both the red blood cell count, which assesses cellular nutrition, and the white cell count, which assesses defensive capability against infections, when diagnosing specific insults. Table 17-1 lists the components of these helpful hematological studies.

COAGULATION STUDIES

Coagulation studies are also warranted in the laboratory assessment of patients with cardiac disease (see Table 17-1). Establishment of a baseline for coagulation function provides important information about the patient's ability to form, maintain, and dissolve blood clots. Such information may prove instrumental in patient care decisions. This is especially true in relation to the administration of anticoagulation agents, whether for long-term management, such as warfarin for the management of atrial fibrillation, or for emergency interventions, such as the use of fibrinolytic therapy during an acute MI.

BLOOD CHEMISTRIES

Mechanisms that ensure homeostatic function at the cellular and tissue level depend on the appropriate production and modulation of intracellular and extracellular electrolytes. It is important that the nurse understand normal electrolyte functions and the unique, perhaps life-threatening, situations that may occur when they are significantly abnormal. A thorough analysis of basic electrolyte chemistries is always appropriate in screening of the patient with cardiac disease, whether in the inpatient or outpatient setting. These studies are almost universally obtained during the initial clinical examination. The blood chemistries most commonly assessed are sodium, potassium, chloride, carbon dioxide, calcium, glucose, magnesium, and phosphorus. Table 17-1 provides the normal assay values for common electrolytes.

Common Electrolytes

Sodium is the most abundant cation in the body. It is essential in the maintenance of acid–base balance and osmolality of extracellular fluids as well as in the transmission of nerve impulses. It plays a pivotal role in fluid balance, and its concentration is primarily regulated by the kidneys. Significant alterations of cellular function are evident when sodium levels are lower than normal (hyponatremia) or greater than normal (hypernatremia).

Potassium is the major intracellular cation. Its role in the evaluation of cardiac patients is important because it is released when cells are damaged. It is essential for maintenance of oncotic pressure, intracellular osmolality, and acid–base balance, as well as for its role in cellular reactions. In addition, potassium is vital to the normal functioning of skeletal, smooth, and cardiac muscle. It is particularly important in the regulation of cardiac rate and force of contraction.

Chloride is another major extracellular cation. Like sodium and potassium, it plays a role in acid–base balance and is an important component in the evaluation of acid–base balance.

The carbon dioxide electrolyte is a reflection of carbon dioxide *content* (mainly bicarbonate), not carbon dioxide *gas*. In some settings, carbon dioxide is reported as bicarbonate (HCO_3^-).

Other Blood Chemistries

Calcium, like potassium, is important for cardiac function. It plays a significant role in the initiation and propagation of electrical impulses and in myocardial contractility. It is also important for blood clotting, teeth and bone formation, and intracellular energy production. Ionized calcium (free calcium) is responsible for cardiac and neuromuscular excitability. Calcium is reported as total and free (ionized) values.

Glucose levels are important to monitor with baseline laboratory studies because they reflect the nutritive status of the cell. Alterations in glucose, such as in diabetes mellitus, can provide the clinician with both diagnostic as well as prognostic information.

Magnesium is the second major intracellular cation after potassium. It is important in many metabolic processes and is necessary for the normal functioning of the neuromuscular system. It facilitates enzyme activities, which help maintain protein synthesis and metabolism, carbohydrate and lipid metabolism, and nucleic acid synthesis. Alterations in normal magnesium levels are reflected in disruptions in neuromuscular activity, such as in the patient with arrhythmia.

Phosphorus reflects levels of serum phosphate. It is controlled by the parathyroid gland and regulated in the kidneys. Phosphate is important for normal cellular function and for oxygen delivery. It is reciprocal to calcium. Abnormalities can be seen with alterations in heart rate, alterations in neuromuscular function, and reciprocal changes in serum calcium.

SERUM LIPID STUDIES

A review of serum lipid levels can provide the nurse with a perspective on cardiovascular risk for the patient presenting with a cardiac event. Measurement of cholesterol, low-density and high-density lipoprotein, and triglycerides can aid in the evaluation for the presence of atherosclerosis and coronary artery disease. (See Table 17-1 for a list of normal lipid values.) Cholesterol, a precursor of bile acids and steroid hormones, can accumulate in arterial walls, where it can be atherogenic. Cholesterol levels vary with age, diet, level of activity, and stress. Low-density lipoproteins (LDLs), which represent 60% to 70% of the total serum cholesterol found in the serum, carry plasma cholesterol. Higher levels of LDL are associated with a higher risk for the development of cardiovascular disease. High-density lipoproteins (HDLs) are responsible for carrying 20% to 30% of the total serum cholesterol. HDL has been implicated in a protective role against atherogenesis and appears to have an inverse relationship with the development of coronary artery disease. Higher levels of HDL are associated with decreased risk of coronary heart disease. Factors that influence the serum levels of LDL and HDL can be found in Table 17-2. Triglycerides represent stored fat in tissues. The normal range for triglycerides is 40 to 200 mg/dL. Levels greater than 200 mg/dL can contribute to the development of atherosclerosis and coronary artery disease.

Enzyme Studies

Enzymes are found in all living cells and act as catalysts in biochemical reactions. They are present in low amounts in the serum of healthy individuals. However, when cells are injured, enzymes leak from damaged cells, resulting in serum enzyme concentrations greater than the usual low levels. No single enzyme is specific to the cells of a single organ. Each organ contains a variety of enzymes, and there is considerable overlap among organs in the enzymes they contain. However, the distribution of enzymes in the cells of organs is relatively organ specific. When organ damage occurs, the presence of abnormally high levels of enzymes in the serum, their distribution, and the timing of their appearance and disappearance make the clinical use of serum enzyme studies relevant.

table 17-2 Factors That Influence Low-Density Lipoprotein (LDL) and High-Density Lipoprotein (HDL) Levels

LDL Levels	HDL Levels
Increased with	Increased with
Diets high in cholesterol	Not smoking
Diets high in saturated fat	Lean body mass
Alcohol	Estrogen
Strict vegetarian diet	Vigorous exercise
Hypothyroidism	Diet low in sucrose and starch
Obesity	Increased clearance of very–low-density lipoprotein (triglyceride)
Obstructive liver disease	Alcohol
Nephrosis	Decreased with
Thiazide diuretics	Cigarette smoking
Beta-adrenergic blocking agents	Obesity
Progestin and anabolic steroids	Progesterone
Decreased with	Male sex
Low-cholesterol diet	Sedentary lifestyle
Low-fat diet	Hypertriglyceridemia
Alcohol restriction	Type 2 diabetes mellitus
Regular strenuous exercise	Strict vegetarian diet
	Hypertriglyceridemia
	Anabolic steroids
	Starvation
	Beta-adrenergic blocking agents
	Infectious illness

From Baker M: Laboratory tests using blood. In Woods S, Froelicker E, Motzer S (eds): Cardiac Nursing (4th Ed). Philadelphia, Lippincott Williams & Wilkins, 2000.

Cardiac enzymes are enzymes found in cardiac tissue. When cardiac injury occurs, as in acute MI, these enzymes are released into the serum, and their concentrations can be measured (Fig. 17-13). Cardiac tissue enzymes are present in other organs as well, so elevation of one or more of these enzymes is not a specific indicator of cardiac injury. Because cardiac damage does result in above-normal serum concentrations of these enzymes, however, the quantification of cardiac enzyme levels, along with other diagnostic tests and the clinical presentation of the patient, is routinely used for diagnosing cardiac disease, particularly acute MI.

Only three of the many enzymes present in cardiac tissue have widespread use in the diagnosis of acute MI: creatine kinase (CK), lactate dehydrogenase (LDH), and aspartate aminotransferase (AST; previously termed serum glutamic oxaloacetic transaminase [SGOT]). LDH and

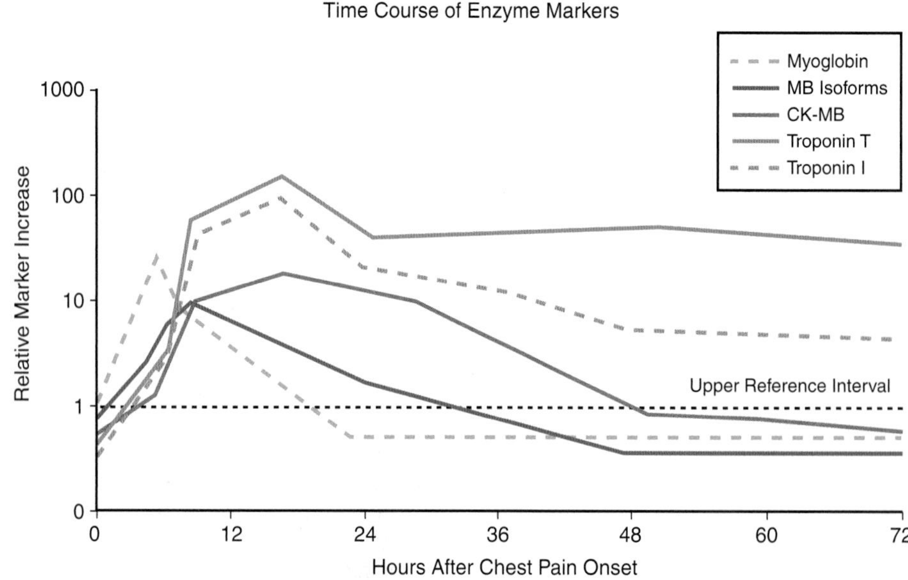

figure 17-13 Peak elevation and duration of serum enzymes after acute myocardial infarction. (Data from Antman EM: Acute myocardial infarction. In Braunweld E [ed]: Heart Disease: A Textbook in Cardiovascular Medicine [5th Ed], pp 1184–1228. Philadelphia: W. B. Saunders, 1997. Used with permission.)

AST were first used in the 1950s. Since the mid-1960s, CK has become the most important addition to the enzyme diagnosis of acute MI. None of the three enzymes is specific to cardiac tissue. However, CK and LDH can be divided further into components called *isoenzymes*. In each case, at least one of the isoenzymes is more specific for cardiac disease. The increase in these more specific components of LDH or CK relative to their other isoenzymes has resulted in their common use in diagnosis of acute MI. Because of the nonspecificity of AST and the widespread availability of CK and LDH isoenzymes, the routine sampling of serum for AST for the diagnosis of acute MI is no longer recommended. The value of drawing blood samples for measuring CK, LDH, and their associated isoenzymes for the diagnosis of acute MI is discussed in the following text.

CREATINE KINASE

The level of total CK in plasma usually becomes abnormal 6 to 8 hours after onset of MI and peaks in 24 and 28 hours. When patients appear at the hospital soon after the onset of symptoms, the initial CK frequently is within normal limits, and at the time of hospital admission, it is not possible to discriminate on the basis of CK those who are having an acute MI from those who are not. For this reason, CK is sampled every 4 to 6 hours for the first 24 hours after the onset of symptoms. Within 2 to 4 days after MI, the serum concentration of total CK usually has returned to normal. Therefore, abnormal total CK levels may be missed in patients who present more than 24 hours after the onset of infarction. The normal level of total CK typically is higher in men than in women and in African Americans than in whites. The upper limit of normal may vary among laboratories, and nurses must be aware of the normal value used in their laboratory. In general, the amount of total CK correlates with the amount of myocardial damage and is of prognostic importance. With a small infarction, total CK may increase to two to three times the initial level, but never reach the upper limit of normal, and CK isoenzymes may be valuable.

Skeletal muscle contains more CK than the heart, whereas the cerebral cortex has slightly less CK. Conditions that result in damage or injury to the brain or skeletal muscle also may result in abnormal levels of CK in plasma. Skeletal muscle diseases, such as polymyositis and muscular dystrophy, and the effects of alcohol, strenuous exercise, convulsions, trauma, surgery, and intramuscular injections in skeletal muscle may give rise to abnormal CK levels. Cerebrovascular disease also may result in abnormal CK levels. In cerebrovascular disease, the increase occurs later, lasts longer, and is not as high as the abnormal CK levels caused by acute MI. Although the clinical presentation of the patient, the ECG, and the amount and time course of abnormal CK levels are useful in determining whether the diagnosis of acute MI is appropriate, it is not always possible to distinguish MI from other clinical conditions. For this reason, CK isoenzymes, in addition to total CK, usually are obtained serially.

Creatine Kinase Isoenzymes

Electrophoresis, glass bead, and radioimmunoassay are techniques used to measure CK isoenzymes. The three CK isoenzymes routinely reported are CK-MM, CK-BB, and CK-MB, which are found to the greatest extent in skeletal muscle, brain, and heart muscle, respectively. Total CK usually consists entirely of CK-MM, and neither CK-BB nor CK-MB is present. In other words, skeletal muscle accounts for the normal levels of CK found in healthy individuals. Normal skeletal muscle may contain up to 2% CK-MB, and values of CK-MB of as much as 5% are not necessarily considered diagnostic. The amount of CK-MB in cardiac muscle is 15% to 22%, with the remainder being CK-MM. When cardiac damage occurs, as in acute MI, total CK increases, and the percentage of CK-MB is greater than 5%. Although other organs, such as the tongue, small intestine, uterus, and prostate, contain CK-MB, the presence of CK-MB in amounts greater than 5% generally is considered diagnostic for myocardial damage in the presence of chest pain or other symptoms believed to represent myocardial ischemia.

Within 6 to 12 hours after the onset of infarction, CK-MB usually begins to appear in serum, and it peaks at approximately 24 hours. However, the appearance and peak may be significantly earlier in patients who have a non–Q-wave infarction or who have undergone successful recannulation of the infarct-related coronary vessel by angioplasty or thrombolytic therapy. Patients who present more than 24 hours after the onset of symptoms may not benefit from measurement of CK isoenzymes because the levels already may have returned to normal. As with total CK, serial sampling should be performed every 4 to 6 hours for the first 24 hours after the onset of symptoms. Patients who continue to have signs or symptoms of myocardial ischemia after hospital admission should continue to undergo serial CK isoenzyme sampling.

Most laboratories report the absolute amount of each CK isoenzyme present in the serum, although some also report the percentage. Normal values for absolute amounts of each of the CK isoenzymes vary by laboratory and by the measuring technique used. The amount of CK-MB released into the serum after an acute MI offers a better correlation with infarction size than total CK because of its specificity to cardiac muscle.

Because total CK and CK isoenzymes are the cardiac enzymes whose levels become abnormal earliest after the onset of infarction, routine serial sampling for other cardiac enzymes is unnecessary. Serial analysis of CK isoenzymes is the most specific, sensitive, and cost-effective means of diagnosing acute MI. Perhaps more important, CK isoenzymes also have made it possible to "rule out" an acute MI more quickly and reliably. It no longer requires 2 to 3 days of intensive care unit (ICU) hospitalization to determine that AST or LDH enzyme levels remain normal; rather, an acute MI can be ruled out in less than 24 hours if a patient's CK isoenzyme levels do not become abnormal. Nurses and physicians not only are able to provide earlier reassurance to patients who are found not to have acute infarction, but patients can be discharged sooner to a less costly environment than the ICU.

Clinical presentation of the patient and the ECG usually are helpful in distinguishing patients with acute MI. Cardiac disorders other than acute MI, including pericarditis, myocarditis, and trauma, also may be associated with abnormal total CK and CK-MB levels. In addition, CK-MB levels have been reported to be abnormal after cardiac surgery and cardioversion.

Creatine Kinase Isoforms

The isoenzymes CK-MB and CK-MM may be divided further into isoform or subform components using electrophoretic or immunoassay techniques. Laboratory performance of these tests is time-consuming and labor intensive. However, they are used clinically in some hospitals because isoforms may offer confirmation or exclusion of MI earlier than CK isoenzymes. Efforts are underway to develop faster and less labor-intensive CK isoform measurements that will result in their widespread clinical use.

Two subforms of CK-MB and three subforms of CK-MM have been identified. Because CK-MB is more specific to cardiac muscle than CK-MM, CK-MB isoforms are appropriate for patients with suspected MI. CK-MB_2 (tissue CK-MB) is released into the serum and converted to CK-MB_1 (plasma CK-MB) by carboxypeptidase N, another enzyme present in serum. In patients without MI, the amounts of CK-MB_2 and CK-MB_1 present in serum are small, and the ratio of CK-MB_2 to CK-MB_1 is approximately one. In patients with acute MI, CK-MB_2 is released into the serum in larger quantities than normal and the amount of CK-MB_2 and the ratio of CK-MB_2 to CK-MB_1 in the serum of these patients becomes elevated.

Abnormal elevations of CK-MB_2 have been reported as early as 2 hours after onset of symptoms of MI.[1] In this study, in patients with acute MI, 59% had diagnostic CK-MB isoforms on serum samples obtained within 2 to 4 hours of onset of symptoms, whereas only 23% were diagnosed by the conventional CK isoenzyme assay. In addition, in patients in whom blood samples were obtained within 8 hours of onset of symptoms, CK-MB isoforms were positive in 100% of cases, compared with 71% for CK isoenzymes.

Because the ratio of CK-MB_2 to CK-MB_1 may remain elevated only for up to 12 hours after onset of infarction, CK-MB isoforms likely will not be as useful as CK isoenzymes in patients presenting to the hospital more than 12 hours after the onset of symptoms. Nevertheless, the importance of a reliable early laboratory marker of infarction cannot be underestimated. The period of early sensitivity of CK-MB isoforms is similar to the therapeutic window for the administration of thrombolytic therapy and may be useful in identifying additional patients who could benefit. Also, acute MI can be excluded as a diagnosis within 8 hours of symptom onset using CK-MB isoform assay, compared with the 18 to 24 hours required for the conventional CK isoenzyme assay (Table 17-3).

LACTATE DEHYDROGENASE

LDH can be found in many organs besides the heart, including the liver, skeletal muscle, kidney, lung, fat, and red blood cells. Because LDH is found in several other tissues in addition to the heart, it is no longer considered a specific test for MI and is not ordered as frequently today. However, LDH is used to help diagnose myocarditis, liver and renal dysfunction, and skeletal muscle disorders or trauma. It may be abnormally elevated in various conditions, including hemolytic anemia; pulmonary infarction; renal infarction; hepatic disorders, such as hepatitis and hepatic congestion; and skeletal muscle disorders.

Lactate Dehydrogenase in Cardiac Disease

Total LDH is less specific than CK for cardiac disease. It usually begins to appear in the serum within 24 hours after the onset of acute MI and does not peak until 2 to 3 days; it may remain elevated for 7 to 10 days before returning to normal levels. The use of LDH in the diagnosis of acute MI is unnecessary if the diagnosis can be confirmed by CK and CK-MB. Patients who present more than 24 hours after the onset of symptoms (CK and CK-MB levels already may have returned to normal) or those who have been having symptoms of myocardial ischemia for several days may be appropriate for sampling for total LDH and LDH isoenzymes. LDH may help confirm an MI that occurred several days earlier. Although LDH increases more slowly and remains elevated longer than CK, the time course of abnormal levels for both enzymes overlaps. A single sample for LDH may be obtained in patients who present more than 24 hours after symptom onset. If the LDH value is abnormally elevated, the sample may be further analyzed for LDH isoenzymes. Routine serial sampling of LDH or LDH isoenzymes in these patients is not recommended because in the face of nondiagnostic CK isoenzymes, there is no evidence that serial LDH or LDH isoenzyme sampling improves the diagnostic yield.[2]

Care must be taken when obtaining blood samples for LDH because hemolysis may result in LDH being released from red blood cells, causing falsely elevated levels. The upper limit of normal for LDH, like CK, is higher in men than women and varies by laboratory. Nurses must know the normal values for their laboratory.

Lactate Dehydrogenase Isoenzymes

Although LDH isoenzymes are not as specific as CK isoenzymes in the diagnosis of acute MI, they nevertheless are helpful in patients whose CK isoenzyme levels may have returned to normal. Electrophoretic techniques are used to measure LDH (see Table 17-3). The isoenzyme that moves most quickly toward the positive pole of the electrical field, LDH_1, is found most abundantly in heart muscle. Somewhat lower amounts of LDH_1 are present in kidney, brain, and red blood cells. LDH_5, the LDH isoenzyme that moves most slowly toward the positive electrode, is found most abundantly in liver and skeletal muscle. LDH_2, LDH_3, and LDH_4 are present in intermediate amounts in these organs between the extremes of LDH_1 and LDH_5. In healthy individuals, LDH_1 makes up between 17% and 27% of total LDH, whereas LDH_2 comprises 28% to 38%; LDH_1 is always present in a lesser percentage than LDH_2. Because the heart contains relatively more LDH_1 than LDH_2, the ratio of the percentage of LDH_1 to LDH_2 usually becomes one or more whenever cardiac injury occurs. This "flip" in the ratio of the percentage of LDH_1 to LDH_2 occurs 1 to 3 days after the onset of MI.

DIAGNOSTIC LIMITATIONS TO ENZYME STUDIES

Enzyme determinations can serve only as adjuncts to ECG and clinical diagnosis. To be of most value, they should be used with discretion. Consideration must be given to the length of time since onset of symptoms occurred because each enzyme rises and returns to normal at different intervals.

table 17-3 Biochemical Markers for Diagnosing Acute Myocardial Infarction

Test and Description	Time to Run Test	First Detectable in Serum (After Onset of Symptoms)	Peak Levels and Normal Values	Time Required for Reliable Diagnosis*
CK-MB	Electrophoresis: 1–2 h	Electrophoresis: 4–8 h	Electrophoresis: 10–24 h nl = 24–195 IU/L	8–12 h
MB isoform of CK (more abundant in myocardial tissue)	Monoclonal antibody test: 10–40 min	Monoclonal antibody test: 2–3 h	Monoclonal antibody test: 10–18 h nl = 0–9 ng/mL	2–3 h
MB2/MB1 ratio Ratio of subforms of CK-MB isoforms: MB2 in the tissue and MB1 in the plasma	25 min	1–6 h; may be detected as early as <1 h	4–8 h nl = 1:1	1 h
LDH	Varies†	Within 24 h	2–4 days; varies	2–3 days
Isoforms of LDH			normal values†	
LDH_1			nl = 17–27%	
LDH_2			nl = 28–28%	
LDH_3			nl = 16–20%	
LDH_4			nl = 2–3%	
LDH_5			nl = 0.5–1.5%	
Myoglobin Heme protein (found in myocardial and skeletal muscle)	10 min	2–3 h; may be detected as early as <1 h	2–4 h (cyclic rise and fall) nl = 30–90 ng/mL	2h
Troponin I, troponin T Contractile protein (found in myofibrils)	30 min	4–6 h	10–24 h; elevated 5–14 days Troponin I elevated for 5–7 days; troponin T elevated for 10–14 days nl = 0–0.4 ng/mL	2–3 h

* Refers to the minimal time after onset of symptoms.
† Values vary according to laboratory performing the test
From Apple S: Advanced strategies for diagnosing acute myocardial infarction. Heartbeat 6:1–12, 1995; adapted and updated from various resources.

Enzyme determinations have been of greatest value to patients whose ECG and clinical picture are equivocal for diagnosis of MI. Enzyme elevation may well confirm a suspected diagnosis. Sometimes it is difficult or impossible to interpret infarction on ECG because of previous infarction changes; effects of certain drugs or electrolyte imbalances; conduction defects, such as bundle branch block or Wolff-Parkinson-White syndrome; arrhythmias; or a functioning pacemaker. Enzyme determination may be a distinct advantage in such a setting. If a definite diagnosis can be made by ECG, enzyme tests may not be needed, except for academic and prognostic interest.

Because serum enzyme elevations are nonspecific in the diagnosis of MI, they must be considered in view of the total clinical picture. We are in a highly technical age of nursing and must not forget to look at and listen to the patient before making judgments and decisions.

Biochemical Markers: Myocardial Proteins

Two newer diagnostic markers are being used in the laboratory for evaluating myocardial damage. Myoglobin and troponin levels have shown high specificity for detecting myocardial damage. Both proteins are evaluated using the same monoclonal antibody technique used for CK-MB subform quantification. Table 17-1 presents the normal values for these proteins.

Myoglobin detection can be helpful in the determination of ischemic muscle damage. Found in skeletal and cardiac muscle, it appears in the serum earlier than CK and may be detectable in the serum less than 1 hour after the onset of symptoms. Myoglobin usually peaks in 2 to 4 hours. It is detected for *any* muscle damage and is not specific for cardiac muscle damage alone. This characteristic facilitates its value in the *exclusion* of an MI. Myoglobin levels may be very sensitive to reperfusion events after thrombolytic therapy and thereby prove to be of significant clinical value in this intervention.

Troponin is highly specific for cardiac muscle damage and is detectable in two subforms, cardiac troponin I (cTnI) and troponin T (cTnT). An advantage of troponin assays is that, unlike myoglobin, troponin is unaffected by skeletal injury. Troponin I can be detected within 4 hours after an acute MI and can remain elevated for 7 to 10 days. In a healthy person, this contractile protein is not detectable, and its high sensitivity and specificity can provide rapid diagnostic information in the patient with a suspected acute MI. Troponin values may be greater than 10 ng/mL in the presence of an acute MI. Lower levels (0.4 ng/mL) are often seen with lesser insults, such as angina pectoris. Troponin I may play a role in predicting an increase in mortality in non–Q-wave infarctions and unstable angina. Troponin T has been shown to be highly sensitive in detecting minor myocardial injury and may provide valuable prognostic information in patients experiencing angina pectoris. It has been reported that troponin T may detect smaller amounts of myocardial damage than even high-quality serial echocardiograms and may remain elevated in the plasma for 10 to 14 days after myocardial insult.

Neurohumoral Hormones: Brain-type Natriuretic Peptide

When the cardiac muscle decompensates, hormones are released from extracardiac and cardiac origins. Norepinephrine and endothelin are hormones released as a peripheral response to cardiac impairment. Natriuretic peptides are neurohumoral hormones released by the heart. Atrial natriuretic peptides are secreted as a result of atrial myocardial distension, but only minute amounts are released in response to ventricular distension. Another neurohumoral hormone, brain-type natriuretic peptide (BNP), was first isolated in the porcine brain—hence the "B." Although the human brain does secrete BNP, the primary site of release is in the cardiac ventricles, with only very small amounts released in the atria. BNP is released in response to ventricular dilation and increased intraventricular pressures.[3]

BNP levels are helpful in the diagnosis of ventricular dysfunction caused by heart failure. Results of the blood test that measures endogenous levels of BNP may be available in about 30 minutes, making this test especially useful for diagnosing heart failure in the emergency department. Endogenous BNP levels diagnose decompensated heart failure with 95% accuracy.[4] For patients with an acute MI, BNP levels increase rapidly during the first 24 hours and then plateau.[5] Elevated levels of BNP provide important prognostic information for the patient with acute coronary syndromes. In acute MI and unstable angina, elevated BNP levels are predictive of a greater risk of death, postinfarction heart failure, or reinfarction.[6]

Newer Diagnostic Markers

C-reactive protein and P-selectin are newer markers of inflammation and necrosis that have been implicated as factors that can cause disruption of fibrous cap lesions underlying acute coronary events. C-reactive protein, an acute-phase protein and marker of systemic inflammation, has been shown to be elevated in patients with acute coronary syndromes.[7,8] Normal values are 0 to 2 mg/dL. Serum values greater than 3 mg/dL in patients with acute coronary syndrome or greater than 5 mg/dL in patients who are post–coronary interventional procedure may indicate a higher risk and merit closer monitoring or more thorough evaluation.[7]

D dimer is another newer physiological marker that may be useful in predicting the risk of cardiac events. D dimer represents the end product of thrombus formation and dissolution that occurs at the site of active plaques in acute coronary syndromes; this process precedes myocardial cell damage and release of protein contents.[9,10] It is thought that D dimer, which is detected early and remains elevated for days, can identify unstable plaque in high-risk patients when troponin and CK-MB have not yet been released.[9] Universal normal serum values for D dimer are not yet established, although a threshold of 500 μg/L indicates increased sensitivity for acute MI.[10] Studies are underway to determine the effectiveness of D dimer in identifying patients who may benefit from the use of anticoagulant or antiplatelet therapy.

case study ■ ACUTE ANTEROSEPTAL MYOCARDIAL INFARCTION

Mrs. James, a 74-year-old widow, is being admitted to the coronary care unit from the emergency department with a diagnosis of acute anteroseptal MI. Her history is significant for the onset of chest pain more than 4 hours before she arrived in the emergency department.

Symptom assessment in the emergency department, using the "NOPQRST" parameters described in Box 17-1, reveals the following:

- **N**ormal: No history of chest pain
- **O**nset: 1 PM.
- **P**recipitating and palliative factors: No pain relief with rest
- **Q**uality and quantity: Pain described as heaviness in the chest
- **R**egion and radiation: Mid-sternal pain that radiates to the back
- **S**everity: Pain described as 7/10
- **T**ime: Patient in pain for 4 hours before she called an ambulance

The patient has a history of hypertension and hypercholesterolemia. She currently tales atenolol and atorvastatin (Lipitor). Previous surgeries include a hysterectomy and a right hip replacement. Mrs. James lives alone and has two daughters who live nearby.

Important findings on physical examination are:

- Vital signs: temperature 99°F (37.2°C); respirations 24 breaths/minute; pulse rate 98 beats/minute and regular; blood pressure 164/92 mm Hg
- Neck: jugular venous distension

- Cardiac: S_1, S_2, regular rhythm, and an audible S_3
- Respiratory: fine crackles in the bases
- Extremities: +1 pedal edema

Laboratory studies reveal an elevated CK with positive MB, elevated myoglobin (100 ng/mL), and elevated troponin (0.8 ng/mL).

The nurse in the emergency department tells you to expect to receive Mrs. James in about 30 minutes. She has O_2 at 2-L nasal cannula with an intravenous (IV) line of 5% dextrose in water (D_5W) at 90 mL/hour. ■

CARDIAC DIAGNOSTIC STUDIES

Cardiovascular diagnostic techniques have expanded dramatically in the past few years, especially in the area of noninvasive testing. This permits a more careful screening of the population for high-risk procedures and low-risk methods for monitoring disease progression and response to treatment. In addition, many technologies are combined for a functional assessment of the patient's cardiac status so the best treatment option can be chosen.

The critical care nurse often cares for patients who undergo one or more of these procedures. Understanding the principles on which the procedures are based enables the nurse to answer questions, incorporate diagnostic findings into the patient's plan of care, and provide high-level nursing care. The critical care nurse also can decrease the anxiety of patients and their families by providing an explanation of the procedure.

Noninvasive Techniques

STANDARD 12-LEAD ELECTROCARDIOGRAM

Purpose

The standard ECG records electrical impulses as they travel through the heart. In patients with normal conduction, the first electrical impulse for each cardiac cycle originates in the sinus node and is spread to the rest of the heart through the specialized conduction system—the intra-atrial tracts, AV node, bundle of His, and right and left bundles. As the impulse traverses the conduction system, it penetrates the surrounding myocardium and provides the electrical stimuli for atrial and ventricular contraction. The change in electrical potential in cells of the specialized conduction system as the impulse proceeds is very small and cannot be measured from electrodes outside the body. However, the change in electrical potential of myocardial cells produces an electrical signal that can be recorded from the surface of the body, as is done with an ECG.

Impulses that originate in sites other than the sinus node or impulses that are prevented from traversing the conduction system because of disease or drugs interrupt the normal order of electrical sequences in the myocardium. An ECG may be used to record these abnormal patterns of impulse formation or conduction. A clinician then has a visual record of the abnormal pattern from which to identify the arrhythmia.

In addition, an abnormal ECG tracing may result from diseased myocardial cells. For example, in patients with left ventricular hypertrophy (LVH), impulses traversing the enlarged muscle mass of the left ventricle produce a larger electrical signal than normal. In contrast, impulses are unable to traverse myocardial cells that are irreversibly damaged, such as in MI, and no electrical signal is present in the infarcted cells of the left ventricle.

Procedure

The standard 12-lead ECG is so named because the usual electrode placement and recording device permit the electrical signal to be registered from 12 different views. The four limb and six precordial leads are attached to the patient as shown in Figure 17-14. For the limb leads, the recording device alternates the combination of electrodes that are active during recording of electrical signals from the heart (Fig. 17-15). This results in six standard views or leads (I, II, III, augmented voltage of the right arm [aVR], augmented voltage of the left arm [aVL], and augmented voltage of the left foot [aVF]) that are recorded in the heart's frontal plane. The six precordial leads (V_1, V_2, V_3, V_4, V_5, and V_6) are arranged across the chest to record electrical activity in the heart's horizontal plane (see Fig. 17-14). Abnormal localized areas of myocardial conduction, such as occur with ischemia or infarction, may be identified in the leads that are nearest to that part of the heart. For example, an inferior MI produces changes in the leads that view the inferior aspect of the heart, or leads II, III, and aVF.

Used routinely in ICU patients, ECGs assess arrhythmias and myocardial ischemia or MI. An ECG is performed easily at the bedside with the patient ideally placed in the supine position and the electrodes arranged as previously described. In some patients, chest bandages may preclude placement of the precordial leads. It is important that the patient remain still during the ECG recording so that skeletal muscle movement does not result in extraneous noise or artifact in the electrical signal. Additional horizontal plane leads may be recorded by placing electrodes on the right side of the chest to view right ventricular activity or the back of the chest to view left ventricular posterior wall activity (see Fig. 17-14).

Nursing Assessment and Management

Critical care nurses often record an ECG in the event of a change in patient status. This change in status includes the development of arrhythmias. Evaluation of a rhythm strip in relationship to arrhythmias is discussed later in this chapter. Often, an ECG is obtained during episodes of chest pain before the administration of sublingual nitroglycerin. The ECG provides documentation of ST segment changes associated with the pain.

Some patients fear being shocked by the ECG recorder. Preparatory instruction for patients should include an explanation of the manner in which the electrical impulses of the heart are recorded.

HOLTER MONITORING

Purpose

Ambulatory monitoring of coronary care or telemetry patients provides a noninvasive method of assessing for arrhythmias, response to arrhythmia treatment, pacemaker failure, and ECG signs of myocardial ischemia. Patients who present to the hospital with syncope, near syncope, or palpitations may not have recurrence of symptoms while at rest. Holter monitoring permits these patients to ambulate

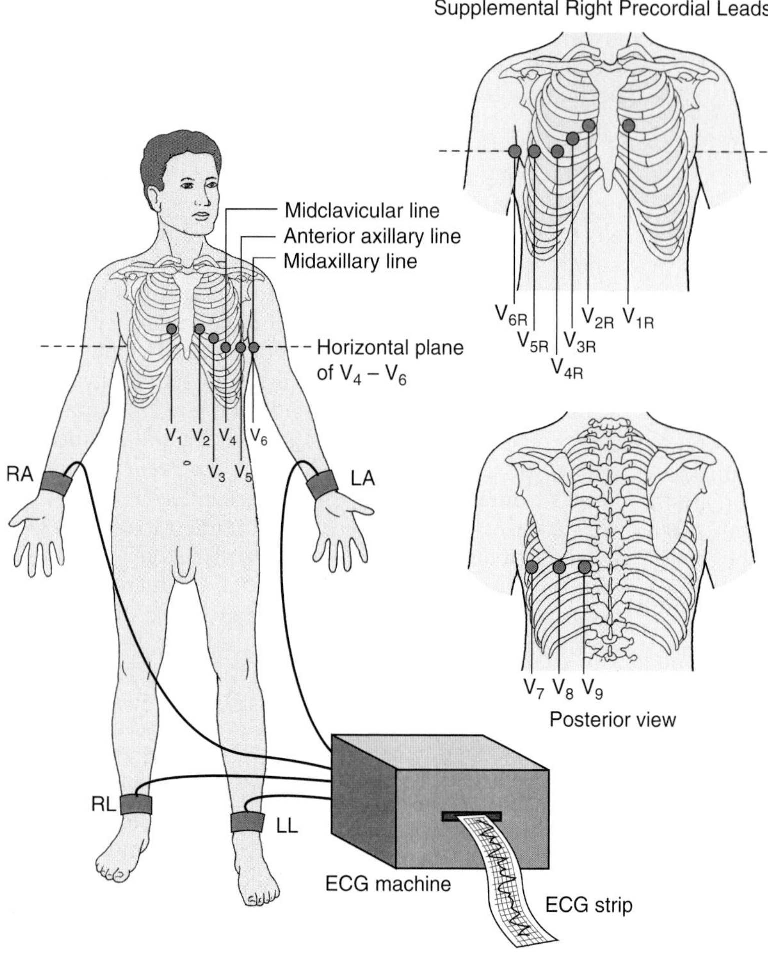

figure 17-14 Electrocardiogram electrode placement. The standard left precordial leads are V_1, fourth intercostal space, right sternal border; V_2, fourth intercostal space, left sternal border; V_3, diagonally between V_2 and V_4; V_4, fifth intercostal space, left midclavicular line; V_5, same horizontal line as V_4, anterior axillary line; V_6, same horizontal line as V_4 and V_5, midaxillary line. The right precordial leads, placed across the right side of the chest, are the mirror opposite of the left leads. For the posterior leads, V_7 is placed at the left posterior axillary line, V_8 is placed at the left midscapular line, and V_9 is placed at the left border of the spine. All are placed on the same horizontal line as V_6.

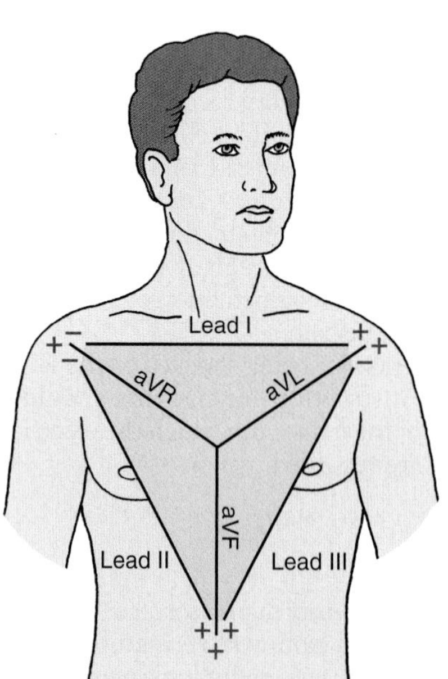

figure 17-15 Frontal plane leads = standard limb leads, I, II, III, plus augmented leads aVR, aVL, and aVF. This allows an examination of electrical conduction across a variety of planes (e.g., left arm to leg, right arm to left arm).

while their heart rhythm is recorded continuously to ascertain whether the etiology of the symptoms is caused by arrhythmia. Many patients with unstable angina have transient episodes of ST segment depression or elevation without associated angina pectoris; Holter monitoring enables the documentation and quantification of these episodes of "silent ischemia."

Procedure

The Holter monitor is a battery-powered tape-recording device that may be worn on a belt around the patient's waist or carried on a shoulder strap. Commonly, two leads are recorded continuously on tape through four or five electrodes placed on the patient's anterior chest; the electrodes are arranged so that one lead reflects the inferior wall of the heart, and the other lead reflects the anterior wall. Continuous recording of ECG leads usually is performed for 24 to 48 hours. The Holter monitor contains a clock so that time also is recorded on the tape. After completion of the test, the tape is removed and played back for identification and quantification of ST segment changes or arrhythmias.

Nursing Assessment and Management

Patients who are scheduled to undergo Holter monitoring should be instructed to bathe before the test because the electrodes cannot be removed during the 24- to 48-hour recording. Skin preparation and electrode placement are crucial to obtaining high-quality ECG recordings. It may be necessary to wrap material or fishnet over the electrodes and cables on the patient's torso to reduce movement artifact. Often, the skin under and around the electrodes becomes irritated, and the patient must be cautioned to avoid pulling at the electrodes because loss of electrical contact can mimic sinus pauses or heart block, making the diagnostic interpretation of the test difficult.

Most Holter monitors have an "event" button that can be pushed whenever symptoms occur; this button sends a signal to mark the tape. Patients are asked to maintain a diary of symptoms and activities and the time they occurred and should be instructed to record the time from the Holter monitor clock. Patients should be encouraged to maintain normal activities while wearing the monitor and told that it is desirable to record an entry in the diary at least every 2 hours. Hospitalized patients may need the assistance of nursing staff in maintaining their diaries.

IMPLANTABLE LOOP MONITOR

The insertable loop recorder (ILR) is a newer, implantable device designed to capture and record the patient's ECG during a syncopal episode. The evaluation of syncope has long been problematic; isolated measurements such as Holter monitoring and random 12-lead ECG tracings seldom provide clinicians with an accurate confirmation of the causes leading to syncopy.[1] The ILR is now used to provide longer and more inclusive surveillance for up to 1 year or longer. The device may be programmed so that a correlation can be established between the patient's intrinsic cardiac rhythm and syncopal events, and it continually monitors the patient's cardiac electrical activity, recording it in a memory loop. The patient or family member is instructed to activate the loop recorder, using a hand-held activator that works in concert with a computer programmer with a telemetry head that communicates with the device. When the activator is triggered, the ILR stores the ECG before, during, and after the syncopal event. When the ECG is retrieved by the clinician, a determination regarding the cause of the patient's syncope can be made and appropriate treatment can then be initiated, thereby reducing the risk of morbidity and mortality.[1]

SIGNAL-AVERAGED ELECTROCARDIOGRAPHY

Purpose

Signal-averaged ECG is a noninvasive method for assessing patients who are at high risk for sudden cardiac death due to ventricular arrhythmias. In recent years, it has been used primarily in patients who are recovering from or have a history of MI to define the risk of ventricular tachycardia. In addition, patients who are admitted with unexplained syncope may benefit from signal-averaged ECG after other noncardiac causes have been excluded.

The major mechanism of ventricular tachycardia in patients with a history of MI relates to an area of slow conduction in the left ventricle. This area of slow conduction depolarizes late after most of the ventricle has depolarized, producing small-amplitude and late electrical potentials not visible on the normal 12-lead ECG. The signal-averaged ECG allows these late potentials to be identified by repetitively mapping the patient's QRS complexes onto each other; filtering out noise, such as movement or electrical interference; averaging the repetitively mapped QRS complexes; and amplifying the averaged signal. There is some variation between laboratories in the definition of a positive signal-averaged ECG; however, in general, late potentials are considered to be present if the QRS complex duration is prolonged, the terminal low-amplitude portion of the QRS complex is prolonged, or the root mean square voltage of the terminal portion of the QRS complex is less than 20 mV.

Procedure

In addition to a ground electrode, six other electrodes are placed on the patient's chest during the 20 minutes required for performing the signal-averaged ECG. The six electrodes constitute three paired leads that are at right angles to each other; one set of leads is placed horizontally on the mid-right and left anterior chest, a second set is placed vertically at the top and bottom of the sternum, and the third set is placed anteroposteriorly just to the left of the sternum and on the posterior thorax. The patient must rest quietly in a supine position for the duration of the study. Extraneous noise, such as muscle movement, interferes with interpretation of the test, and patients who are restless or agitated or have difficulty lying supine are not good subjects for signal-averaged ECG.

Nursing Assessment and Management

The critical care nurse may be responsible for explaining the general format of the test and for emphasizing the need to remain as motionless as possible during the study to achieve accurate data.

CHEST RADIOGRAPHY

Purpose

Chest radiography is a routine diagnostic test used to assess critically ill patients with cardiac disease. The test can be performed easily at the bedside in patients too ill to be transported to the radiology department. The image obtained on a radiograph that allows visualization of vascular and cardiac shapes is based on the premise that thoracic structures vary in density and permit different amounts of radiation to reach the film.

Chest radiography may be used for the evaluation of cardiac size, pulmonary congestion, pleural or pericardial effusions, and position of intracardiac lines, such as transvenous pacemaker electrodes or pulmonary artery (PA) catheters.

Procedure

Cardiac size is evaluated best in the radiology department, where the procedure can be standardized with the patient standing and the radiograph taken from a posterior view at a distance of 6 feet. Portable bedside chest radiographs usually are taken from an anterior view with the patient lying supine or sitting erect and are not standardized.

Patients undergoing radiography of the chest should be instructed not to move while the radiograph is being taken. Proper positioning of the radiographic plate behind the patient is important to ensure that thoracic structures are aligned on the film. Care should be taken to remove all metal objects, including fasteners on clothing, from the field of view because metal blocks the x-ray beam. Patients usually are asked to take a deep breath and hold it when the radiograph is taken to displace the diaphragm downward; this may be uncomfortable for patients who have undergone recent thoracic surgery.

Nursing Assessment and Management

The critical care nurse's role in obtaining diagnostic thoracic radiographic films often is limited to the ICU, where portable radiographs are made. With unstable patients, the nurse must decide when the film can be taken. It is important that IV lines not become tangled or loosened while one is trying to place the radiographic plate in the proper position.

Female patients of childbearing potential should have a lead drape placed over the abdomen to protect the ovaries from any radiation scatter. For the same reason, caregivers and family members should leave the patient's room when the radiograph is taken. When caregivers cannot leave the patient's bedside, a lead apron should be worn.

ECHOCARDIOGRAPHY

Purpose

The use of echocardiography in diagnosing and monitoring heart disease has increased dramatically since its introduction in the 1960s. For many patients, echocardiography has been an invaluable substitute for more invasive procedures in the management of heart disease. Echocardiography now refers to a group of tests that use ultrasound either alone or in combination with other technologies. Its growth as a clinical tool is likely to continue. Because of miniaturization of the equipment, research concerning intravascular ultrasound (IVUS) devices that would permit the identification of intraluminal defects is being conducted.

Echocardiography is used clinically in many cardiac conditions. The type of echocardiogram performed depends on the condition being evaluated. In critical care patients, echocardiography is used most often to assess ejection fraction, segmental wall motion, systolic and diastolic ventricular volumes, and mitral valve regurgitation due to papillary muscle dysfunction, and to detect the presence of mural thrombi, valve vegetations, or pericardial fluid. Echocardiography is a helpful diagnostic tool in the presence of sudden clinical deterioration in acute MI, in which significant complications may be observed or suspected. It also may be used in the evaluation of function of all four cardiac valves, including calculation of gradients and orifice size, intracardiac tumors, and aortic dissection. In some centers, echocardiography has made it possible for young patients unlikely to have coronary artery disease to undergo valve replacement without requiring a preoperative cardiac catheterization. M-mode and two-dimensional echocardiography can be performed easily at the bedside, but the reduced noise and light levels of the laboratory usually result in better recordings.

Procedure

M-mode echocardiography is the first and simplest use of ultrasonography in patients with cardiac disease. This technique provides a rapid assessment of valvular motion and chamber wall thickness. It requires a transducer that acts both as a sound transmitter and a sound receiver. The transducer is placed on the anterior chest in an intercostal space or subcostal position to avoid bony structures. A single ultrasound beam is sent from the transducer and directed toward the heart. As the sound waves reach various structures in the path of the beam, some pass through and around the structures, and some are reflected back to the transducer by the interface between two structures of differing densities. The more distant the interface, the longer it takes for the reflected sound waves to reach the transducer. A recording device is connected to the transducer so that as the reflected sound waves are received, they are converted to an electrical signal. If only one ultrasound wave beam is emitted from the transducer, the recording contains echoes from structures in the beam's path. For example, if transducer position #1 in Figure 17-16 is used, the recording would contain sound waves reflected from the chest wall, the free right ventricular wall, a space representing the right ventricular cavity, the intraventricular septum, a space representing the left ventricular cavity, and the posterior wall of the left ventricle.

In M-mode echocardiography, ultrasound waves are transmitted intermittently; the remainder of the time, the transducer is receiving the reflected sound waves. Typically, an M-mode recording is made with the reflected sound waves on the vertical axis and time on the horizontal axis. As the heart moves during the cardiac cycle, the recording displays this movement. Because M-mode echocardiography is based on a single beam, the so-called "ice-pick" view, only a small region of the heart can be visualized at any

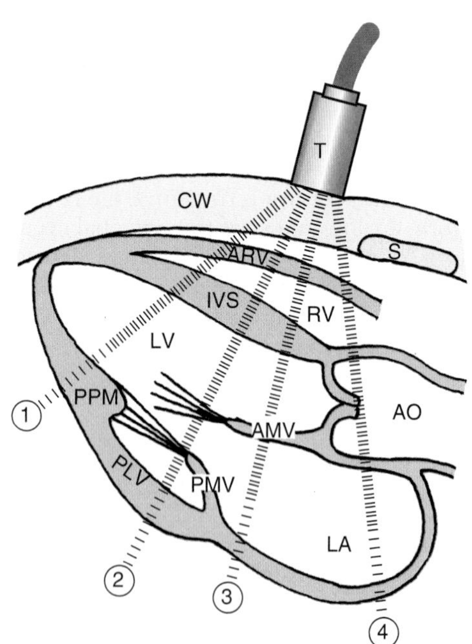

figure 17-16 Echocardiographic views of the heart. A cross-section of the heart shows the structures through which the ultrasonic beam passes as it is directed from the apex (1) toward the base (4) of the heart. *CW*, chest wall; *T*, transducer; *S*, sternum; *ARV*, anterior right ventricular wall; *RV*, right ventricular cavity; *IVS*, interventricular septum; *LV*, left ventricle; *PPM*, posterior papillary muscle; *PLV*, posterior left ventricular wall; *AMV*, anterior mitral valve; *PMV*, posterior mitral valve; *AO*, aorta; *LA*, left atrium.

one time. The four positions of the transducer depicted in Figure 17-16 are the typical views used during an M-mode echocardiogram.

Two-dimensional (2D) echocardiography is performed in a similar manner except for two major differences: The ultrasound waves are transmitted in a pie-shaped beam, resulting in a "plane" of reflected echoes, and the recording device is a video camera so that the two dimensions of the plane and movement over time are recorded. In addition to parasternal and subcostal transducer positions, apical, and suprasternal positions also may be used in 2D echocardiography.

Recently, exercise or pharmacological stress testing has been used in conjunction with 2D echocardiography. A combination of physical exercise and 2D echocardiography has long been recognized as a valuable method to confirm or evaluate the presence of coronary artery disease and the extent of its involvement. An image taken at rest is compared with an image taken immediately after exercise. In patients with significant coronary artery disease, ventricular wall motion abnormalities develop after exercise in the segments supplied by diseased arteries. In patients who are unwilling or unable to exercise because of physical or psychological constraints, pharmacological agents have been used appropriately and effectively to stress the heart physiologically. Vasodilators, such as adenosine and dipyridamole, have been used in the past to induce myocardial ischemia in several imaging modalities (e.g., thallium scan testing) and echocardiography. Observation of areas of reduced blood flow can unmask coronary artery disease and quantify myocardium at risk.

In recent years, dobutamine hydrochloride has been proven effective in pharmacological stress testing in combination with echocardiography. Dobutamine is a synthetic catecholamine with beta$_1$-receptor and alpha-receptor properties, which give the drug both inotropic and chronotropic effects that mimic physical exercise. With dobutamine stress echocardiography (DSE), global or regional wall motion abnormalities in compromised myocardial muscle may be observed before, during, and after titrated dobutamine infusion. If motion abnormalities are noted, the test is deemed positive and the patient can then be considered for surgical revascularization to improve cardiac performance. Distinct advantages of DSE include the fact that the test is noninvasive, can be safely performed a few weeks after an acute MI, and can illuminate wall motion abnormalities that cannot be assessed with electrographic monitoring.

Doppler echocardiography superimposes Doppler techniques on either M-mode or 2D images. The direction of blood flow can be assessed by measuring echoes reflected from red blood cells as they move away or toward the transducer. This type of study is particularly useful in patients with valvular stenosis or regurgitation; blood flow is quite turbulent through a stenotic valve, and in the opposite direction with regurgitation. When the direction of flow is color encoded, the study is known as a color Doppler echocardiogram. Audio signals usually are recorded during Doppler studies. Contrast material also may be used in conjunction with M-mode or 2D echocardiography. Although many agents have been used as contrast material, almost any liquid injected intravenously contains microbubbles. As the microbubbles travel through the heart, they produce multiple echoes. This technique is especially useful in identifying right-to-left intracardiac shunts because of the early appearance of the microbubble echoes in the left atrium or ventricle.

A newer use of Doppler ultrasound technology makes use of an esophageal Doppler monitor. This device can provide valuable information on heart function, patient fluid status, and the impact of therapeutic interventions.[2,3] This noninvasive, harmless technology uses a thin silicone probe that is inserted into the esophagus of an intubated, sedated patient. The probe is positioned close to the descending aorta. Data collected can provide the clinician with hemodynamic information, such as heart rate, stroke volume, preload, afterload, cardiac output, systemic vascular resistance, and cardiac index, that has been demonstrated to be as accurate as information obtained from an invasive PA catheter.[4,5] Because this technique is safe and more readily available for a wider range of patients, it has been implicated in reducing postoperative complications and lengths of hospital stays for critically ill patients.[6]

Transesophageal echocardiography (TEE) is another method of ultrasonographic study that is made possible by placing a 2D transducer on the end of a flexible endoscope and positioning it at various locations in the esophagus (Fig. 17-17). Doppler and color Doppler also can be added. Because the transducer is closer to cardiac structures, the images are usually superior to those obtained with transthoracic techniques. TEE is useful in situations where it is technically impossible to image structures of interest from the usual transthoracic position—in particular, the aorta, atria, and valves. Newer techniques such as transgastric and transthoracic echocardiography are beginning to appear and may demonstrate value in the detection of structural anomalies.

Nursing Assessment and Management

There are no specific prestudy restrictions for patients undergoing transthoracic echocardiography. During the study, the patient usually is placed in the supine position or turned slightly to the left side. Noise and light should be kept to a minimum. There is no discomfort associated with transthoracic echocardiography; however, the patient may experience chest wall discomfort due to the positioning of the transducer after the study. Suboptimal imaging may occur in patients who are obese or have obstructive lung disease.

Patients who are scheduled to undergo transesophageal echocardiography should take nothing by mouth (NPO) for 6 or more hours before the study. Mild to moderate sedation may be administered intravenously both before and during the test. Emergency equipment should be readily available in case of oversedation. A local anesthetic spray usually is applied to the posterior oropharynx to block the gag reflex before the endoscope is inserted orally. After the procedure, the patient should remain NPO until the gag reflex has returned. Table 17-4 summarizes nursing considerations for caring for the patient undergoing TEE.

PHONOCARDIOGRAPHY

Purpose

In phonocardiography, heart sounds are recorded by a microphone and converted to electrical activity that is

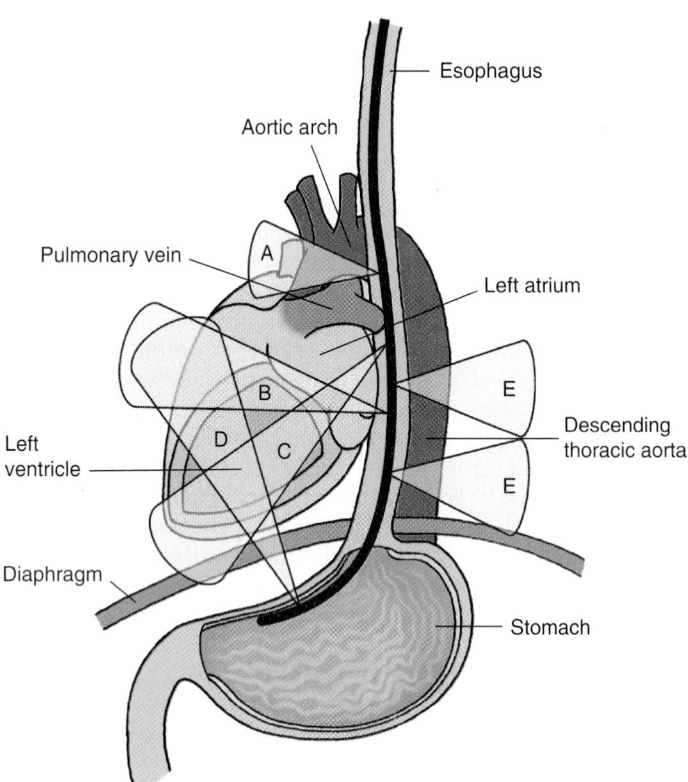

figure 17-17 Views of the heart from a transesophageal echocardiogram. (**A**) Horizontal scan plane of aortic arch and distal portion of aorta. (**B**) Basal short-axis (transverse), long-axis (sagittal) views, and short-axis views of both atria. (**C**) Four-chamber and left atrioventricular long-axis views. Sagittal scan plane can image a cross-section of the left ventricle. (**D**) Transgastric short-axis view of left and right ventricles. (**E**) Transverse and sagittal scan sections of descending aorta.

recorded. This procedure may be used to obtain precise measurements of the timing of cardiac cycle events, to determine the characteristics and timing of murmurs and abnormal heart sounds, to measure systolic time intervals, and to teach cardiac auscultation. There are no contraindications or risks associated with this procedure.

Procedure

For a phonocardiogram, the patient is brought to a quiet room and asked to lie on a comfortable table or bed. Microphones are applied to the chest wall over areas where the heart sounds and murmurs are auscultated best. The microphones pick up the sound of the heart beat and convert it to an electrical impulse that is then amplified, filtered, and recorded. Some of the microphones are allowed to lie free on the chest; others are attached by straps or Ace bandages. A recording of sound waves is obtained, usually in conjunction with an ECG and a carotid pulse wave recording. These accessory recordings provide a reference point for the timing of cardiac events.

Special maneuvers or the use of pharmacological agents may accentuate certain heart sounds and murmurs. These include the inhalation of amyl nitrate, injection of IV isoproterenol or vasopressors, changes in position (sitting or squatting), variations in breathing (deep inspiration and expiration), and the performance of a Valsalva maneuver.

Nursing Assessment and Management

Phonocardiography usually takes 1 to 2 hours. Patients should be told beforehand that they may be asked to perform certain maneuvers or may be given certain agents to facilitate the diagnostic value of the test.

EXERCISE ELECTROCARDIOGRAPHY

Purpose

Exercise ECG is used primarily as an outpatient procedure to assess patients at risk for the presence of coronary artery disease. However, its use in coronary care and telemetry units is becoming more widespread. Patients who have presented to the hospital with chest pain but without associated ECG changes, have had the diagnosis of infarction excluded, and have remained symptom free may undergo exercise ECG to evaluate the etiology of their presenting symptoms and whether continued hospitalization is warranted. In addition, exercise ECG may be used to evaluate patients with arrhythmias whose symptoms are exacerbated by exercise. Low-level exercise ECG, a modification of the standard exercise test, is commonly performed before discharge in patients hospitalized with acute MI.

Patients with significant coronary artery disease may have normal ECGs at rest when myocardial oxygen supply is sufficient to meet oxygen demands. However, with increased oxygen demands during exercise, coronary blood flow cannot increase adequately because of coronary artery stenoses, and ECG changes may occur.

Exercise ECG should not be performed in patients who have left bundle branch block (LBBB) or pre-excitation at rest because the baseline QRS complex abnormalities preclude interpreting the ST segment response to exercise. The test also is less specific in women, especially those who are young or middle-aged, than in men. It is common practice to perform a low-level exercise test before hospital discharge after acute MI to identify patients at risk for ischemic events and to determine exercise prescription.

table 17-4 Nursing Considerations for the Patient Undergoing Transesophageal Echocardiography (TEE)

Nursing Action	Rationale
Preprocedure	
1. Evaluate patient for contraindications.	Patients with history of dysphagia or esophageal disease are not candidates for TEE.
2. Instruct patient and family about procedure.	Some discomfort may occur; patient will receive moderate sedation but will be closely monitored.
3. Ensure that documented patient history is adequate and informed consent has been signed.	Medication allergies should be noted; procedure requires consent signature.
4. Ensure that patient has been NPO for 6 hours before procedure.	Aspiration precaution is vital.
5. Prepare patient for procedure.	Remove oral prosthetics, as indicated; have patient void.
6. Insert peripheral IV catheter.	IV access is required for routine medication administration; emergency vascular access line should be available.
7. Place patient on cardiac monitor with blood pressure and pulse oximetry.	Patient must be continually monitored during procedure.
8. Ensure that emergency resuscitation equipment is nearby, including medications, defibrillator, and suction apparatus.	Cardiac arrest precaution.
During Procedure	
1. Monitor cardiac rhythm, blood pressure, pulse oximetry, and airway patency per institutional policy.	Continuous observation is required after moderate sedation.
2. Assist physician with patient positioning and endoscope placement.	Allaying fears enhances patient cooperation.
3. Monitor for complications.	Vagal stimulation may occur with a resultant vasovagal reaction; transient tachycardia/bradycardia and blood pressure alterations may appear; patient may experience hypoxia or laryngospasm.
4. Reassure patient throughout procedure.	Allaying fears enhances patient cooperation.
5. Document patient response to procedures.	Per institutional protocol.
Postprocedure	
1. Assess vital signs at conclusion of procedure; document per institutional policy.	Comparison with baseline is necessary to monitor sedation recovery.
2. Assist patient to position of comfort or on one side.	Position provides comfort and patent airway support.
3. Keep patient NPO until gag reflex is assessed.	Prudent aspiration risk.
4. If gag reflex is present, encourage patient to cough; offer lozenges or ice to soothe sore throat; keep NPO per physician order.	Interventions provide patient opportunity to clear residual secretions and obtain comfort.
5. If outpatient, instruct patient not to drive for at least 12 h.	If patient was sedated during procedure, it is best if family member or another drives patient home.
6. Instruct patient to seek care or contact physician in event of dyspnea, hemoptysis, or severe pain.	If symptoms of complications occur, patient should be reevaluated.

The low-level test exercise target is approximately 70% to 80% of the predicted age-adjusted maximum. In patients with uncomplicated MI, the low-level exercise test has been performed safely as early as 3 days after infarction.

Procedure

Although there are various exercise protocols, most are based on either walking on a treadmill or riding a stationary bicycle. The test usually begins at a low level of exercise and increases every 2 to 3 minutes until the patient reaches a target level of oxygen consumption, manifests signs or symptoms of coronary artery disease, or reaches a predicted heart rate level calculation. Oxygen consumption, the amount of oxygen used in milliliters per minute per kilogram, usually is expressed in metabolic equivalents that take into account the age of the patient. If a treadmill is used to perform exercise, the speed or the uphill slope of the treadmill is increased at the beginning of each 2- to 3-minute stage; in cycling, the resistance of the pedals or braking mechanism is increased at the beginning of each stage.

Patients who have not previously undergone exercise testing should be allowed briefly to practice walking on the treadmill or riding the bicycle. Before starting the test, a resting ECG and blood pressure are obtained with the patient in sitting and standing positions. During the test, an ECG and blood pressure are obtained at the end of each stage of the protocol and immediately before termination. The test usually is terminated when signs or symptoms of myocardial ischemia develop or when the patient manifests other symptoms, such as fatigue or dyspnea, and cannot continue. In the absence of myocardial ischemia or serious arrhythmias, every effort should be made to reach the patient's predicted level of exercise to avoid a nondiagnostic test. During the recovery period, monitoring of the ECG and blood pressure continues until the patient has reached baseline values. It is mandatory that emergency resuscitation equipment and trained personnel be available in areas where exercise testing is performed.

Indications of myocardial ischemia during exercise testing are the development of (1) ST segment depression of 1 mm or more, (2) angina pectoris, or (3) failure to increase systolic blood pressure to 120 mm Hg or more or a sustained decrease of 10 mm Hg or more with progressive stages of exercise. The ECG leads in which ST segment depression occurs during exercise are not specific to the coronary artery involved. The greater the number of leads with ST segment depression, however, the more likely it is that the patient has multivessel coronary artery disease. The development of ST segment elevation or T-wave changes during exercise testing is not specific for myocardial ischemia, and its significance requires further assessment. Often, exercise ECG is performed in conjunction with echocardiography, radionuclide perfusion imaging, or radionuclide ventriculography to assess better the extent of coronary artery disease and its effect on ventricular function.

Nursing Assessment and Management

Patients who are scheduled to undergo exercise ECG should abstain from eating or drinking caffeine-containing beverages several hours before testing to prevent abdominal cramps or nausea from developing at maximal exercise and to minimize blood diversion to the gastrointestinal tract, which decreases available coronary blood supply. They also should wear comfortable shoes for walking on a treadmill or riding a bicycle. The lead system is the same as used for the standard 12-lead ECG. However, the limb leads are moved to the torso so that arm or leg movement during exercise does not interfere with ECG recording. Careful attention is paid to skin preparation and electrode attachment to permit interpretable recordings during maximal exercise. It may be necessary to wrap material or fishnet over the electrodes and cables on the patient's torso to reduce movement artifact.

The critical care nurse may be responsible for explaining the general format of an exercise test to the patient and family. It is important that patients understand why the test is indicated and what will be expected of them. Patients should be reassured that someone will observe them closely throughout the test and encouraged to express any concerns before, during, and after the procedure. Patients also should understand that they may have to continue exercising after the development of angina but will not be expected to exercise more than is safe.

RADIONUCLIDE IMAGING

The noninvasive assessment of cardiac structure and function using radiotracers has increased dramatically in the past few years. In particular, radionuclide perfusion studies are playing a larger role in the diagnosis and treatment of patients with coronary artery disease. The ability of perfusion studies to separate ischemic, viable myocardium from infarcted, nonviable myocardium is used by clinicians to select noninvasive versus invasive strategies, such as angioplasty or coronary bypass grafting, for treating the underlying coronary artery disease in patients with more severe disease.

Radionuclide perfusion studies provide information not only about the presence of coronary artery disease but about the location and quantity of ischemic and infarcted myocardium. In addition, they offer advantages over exercise ECG when ischemic changes cannot be assessed easily on the ECG, such as in patients with LBBB, with paced rhythm, or those receiving digitalis.

New on the horizon and not discussed in detail here is positron emission tomography (PET). This modality is highly sensitive and specific for diagnosing coronary artery disease. However, it is not superior to single-photon emission computed tomography (SPECT) in diagnostic accuracy. The equipment required for PET is expensive and is available in only a few centers. Because it offers the ability to image and quantify myocardial metabolism and blood flow, it is useful in distinguishing viable myocardium and evaluating the response of the myocardium to treatment with pharmacological agents.

Perfusion Imaging

Procedure. Cardiac radionuclide perfusion imaging is based on the fact that a radioactive tracer is taken up in abnormal myocardial cells in either increased or decreased amounts compared with normal myocardium. After injection of the tracer, a gamma camera is used to record an image of radioactive counts from the entire myocardium. An abnormal area with decreased uptake, or "cold spot" imaging, is the type of study used to assess myocardial perfusion. An abnormal area with increased myocardial uptake, or "hot spot" imaging, is the type of study used to assess myocardial necrosis.

Perfusion studies are performed most commonly in conjunction with exercise testing so that radionuclide scans obtained at rest and with exercise can be compared. Typically, at rest, the radiotracer is spread uniformly throughout the myocardium, and the camera reads counts equally from throughout the myocardium. A similar scan is obtained during exercise in patients without significant coronary artery stenosis as blood flow increases uniformly to meet myocardial oxygen demands.

However, in patients with significant coronary artery disease, the image obtained during exercise is altered. The amount of coronary blood flow is limited in stenotic arteries, and the quantity of tracer in myocardial segments supplied by stenotic arteries is diminished or absent compared with segments supplied by nonstenotic arteries. The presence of an area of decreased tracer uptake during exercise compared with rest is known as a *reversible perfusion defect.* In patients with previous infarction, decreased uptake may be present on both the rest and exercise scans in the infarcted segments; this pattern is known as a *fixed perfusion defect* and usually signifies nonviable myocardium. It is possible for patients to have fixed perfusion defects in some myocardial segments, reversible defects in others, and normal perfusion in the remaining segments.

Because of the many patients who are physically unable to exercise, pharmacological agents may be used to mimic the heart's response to exercise. Vasodilating agents, such as dipyridamole, adenosine, and dobutamine, administered intravenously mimic exercise conditions in the heart by dilating nonstenotic coronary arteries. Coronary blood flow is increased preferentially through normal, nonstenosed arteries; this results in relative hypoperfusion in myocardial segments supplied by stenosed coronary arteries. A radiotracer injected during the peak action of the pharmacological agent produces images similar to those seen with exercise. As of this writing, only dipyridamole is approved by the U.S. Food and Drug Administration (FDA) for use in perfusion imaging.

Two methods are used to record radioactive images—planar and tomographic. With the planar technique, images of the heart are obtained by the gamma camera from three views: anterior, left anterior oblique (45 degrees to the left of the anterior view), and left lateral (Fig. 17-18). Tomographic or SPECT images are obtained by rotating the head of the camera over a 180-degree arc from the left lateral to the anterior position while stopping to make 32 to 64 recordings of 20 to 40 seconds each. A computer uses the recorded images to reconstruct multiple slices of the heart along its short axis and both horizontal and vertical long axes.

Three radioactive tracers, thallium-201, technetium (Tc)-99m sestamibi, and Tc-99m teboroxime, are approved for perfusion imaging. Most experience in radionuclide perfusion studies has occurred with thallium because this agent has been available since 1974. Characteristics of the three agents differ and are responsible for the varying imaging protocols used.

Thallium Protocol. The cardiac half-life of thallium is approximately 7.5 hours, meaning that 50% of the tracer still is present in myocardial cells 7.5 hours after it is administered. It also redistributes readily, so thallium in normally perfused areas moves to previously underperfused areas after the myocardial blood flow demands in that territory have decreased. The standard protocol for thallium perfusion studies begins first with the exercise portion; thallium is injected at the peak of exercise, and imaging starts within 5 minutes of injection. The rest portion is obtained 2 to 4 hours later. Because of redistribution, no additional thallium is required. However, in some patients with perfusion defects on both the rest and exercise scans, significant redistribution may not occur, and it is recommended that an additional dose of thallium be administered.

Sestamibi Protocol. Perfusion imaging with sestamibi typically begins with the rest scan first. Because significant uptake also occurs in the liver, imaging is delayed for approximately 60 minutes. This delay allows sestamibi to be cleared from the liver but not the heart. In addition, a glass of milk or small fatty meal is taken shortly after radiotracer injection to enhance hepatic clearance. A second dose of sestamibi is administered during peak exercise, and the exercise scan is obtained 60 minutes after injection, again allowing time for hepatic clearance. Because sestamibi redistributes very slowly, the image obtained 60 minutes after peak exercise reflects the perfusion conditions at the time of injection. Initially, perfusion studies with sestamibi were performed on 2 different days, but it now is customary to complete both portions of the study in 1 day. It has been shown that exercise sestamibi myocardial perfusion SPECT can provide incremental prognostic information in patients who have not suffered a previous MI or undergone cardiac catheterization and who are determined to be at low risk.

Teboroxime Protocol. Because of the very short cardiac half-life of teboroxime, two injections of the tracer are required. As with sestamibi, hepatic uptake also occurs. Redistribution is not an issue because of the short half-life. Imaging must begin within 2 to 5 minutes of injection and be completed within 15 minutes. The sequence of imaging, exercise versus rest, is not of concern, and typically the two scans are obtained 60 to 90 minutes apart.

Planar imaging usually is performed with the patient in the supine position, although some laboratories place

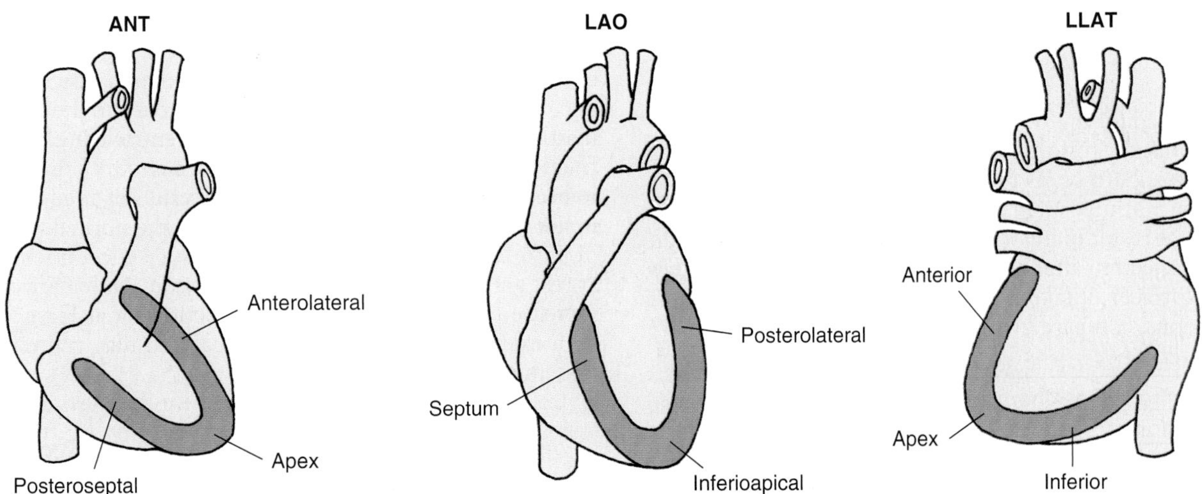

figure 17-18 Ventricular segments of the heart projected on radionuclide planar views. *ANT,* anterior; *LAO,* left anterior oblique; *LLAT,* left lateral.

patients on their right side to obtain the left lateral image. When teboroxime is used as the radiotracer, scans may be obtained with the patient in a sitting or standing position to avoid hepatic interference. With tomographic studies, it is extremely important that the patient not move during image acquisition because computer reconstruction of the images requires the same reference points. If significant movement occurs, the entire tomographic scan may have to be repeated.

Nursing Assessment and Management. All the directions and precautions that pertain to exercise ECG also apply to exercise radionuclide imaging. When pharmacological agents are used in place of exercise, minor side effects, such as flushing, headache, and nausea, may occur. Serious side effects due to the radiotracer are extremely rare. Medications to counteract serious side effects should be readily available. Some patients who receive sestamibi report a metallic taste several minutes after injection. Patients often are anxious about the radiation involved and the appearance of the equipment. It is important for the nurse to allay these anxieties.

Infarct Imaging

Procedure. Infarct or "hot-spot" imaging may be useful in patients who present to the hospital several days after MI when serum cardiac enzymes have returned to normal. Accumulation of the radiotracer in the area of myocardial necrosis compared with the surrounding normal myocardium is responsible for the hot-spot image obtained.

Tc-99m Sn-pyrophosphate, the only radiotracer currently approved by the FDA for infarct imaging, is sensitive for 1 to 5 days after onset of symptoms. Because aneurysm formation in the area of a previous infarction may result in a false-positive study, a second pyrophosphate scan may be performed 7 to 10 days after symptom onset. In patients with recent infarction, little or no radiotracer uptake is seen on the repeat scan. The diagnostic sensitivity of pyrophosphate imaging in patients with a small or non-transmural infarction is poor.

Indium-111 antimyosin is a monoclonal antibody that binds to damaged myocytes and is under investigation as an imaging agent for myocardial necrosis. Planar or tomographic images are obtained 24 to 48 hours after injection of the indium-labeled antibody. Although the study usually is performed within 1 week of an MI, a positive scan may be obtained for up to 1 year after myocardial necrosis. Initial results suggest that antimyosin is more sensitive than pyrophosphate scans for the detection of infarction. In addition, antimyosin may be useful in other clinical conditions that result in myocardial necrosis, such as myocarditis and rejection after cardiac transplantation. The pattern of radiotracer uptake is more diffuse and global in these conditions, compared with the localized pattern of uptake in infarction.

Nursing Assessment and Management. No special preparation is required for patients undergoing infarct imaging other than an explanation of the procedure. Views usually are obtained with the patient in the supine position. If an antimyosin tomographic study is to be performed, the importance of not moving during image acquisition should be reinforced. No serious side effects have been reported with either pyrophosphate or antimyosin administration.

Table 17-5 outlines some of the tests that are used to detect the presence of myocardial ischemia.

ANGIOCARDIOGRAPHY

Purpose

Radionuclide angiocardiography for the assessment of cardiac performance has been in clinical use since the 1970s. Such studies may include information about right and left ventricular ejection fractions, left ventricle regional wall motion abnormalities, ventricular volumes, and cardiac shunts. The measurement of left ventricular ejection fraction, the percentage of blood ejected with each contraction of the left ventricle, has been a key prognostic index for patients with MI or cardiac arrest.

Two approaches are used for the evaluation of cardiac performance. The technique used most commonly is known as equilibrium angiocardiography. It is performed easily at the bedside in patients too critically ill to be transported to the laboratory. The other technique, first-pass angiocardiography, likely will enjoy wider use in the future because it can use technetium radiotracers, such as teboroxime or sestamibi, and can be performed at the same time as perfusion imaging.

Procedure

With *equilibrium radionuclide studies*, an aliquot of the patient's blood is drawn, and the erythrocytes are tagged with Tc-99m radiotracer. The blood sample is then returned intravenously to the patient. Imaging can begin within a few minutes after administration and is performed serially over a period of 4 to 6 hours because the radiotracer-tagged erythrocytes remain within the vascular system. An ECG signal from the patient is used to separate radioactive counts acquired during systole from those during diastole; imaging continues over several hundred cardiac cycles, and images are averaged for both systole and diastole to obtain a representative cardiac cycle.

At the end of diastole, when the left ventricle is maximally filled with blood containing tagged erythrocytes, the amount of radioactivity is greatest. As the ventricle contracts during systole, blood is ejected into the aorta. The amount of blood and therefore radioactivity in the left ventricle is lowest at the end of systole. Because radioactive counts are proportional to the blood volume, the difference in counts obtained at the end of systole and the end of diastole permits the calculation of left ventricular ejection fraction. Left ventricular impairment caused by a previous infarction or cardiomyopathy usually results in a reduction in left ventricular ejection fraction from the normal values of 55% to 70%. Comparisons between ejection fractions at rest and with exercise also can be made. An inability to increase left ventricular ejection fraction by at least 5% with exercise is considered abnormal and may represent ischemic myocardium.

Left ventricular volumes and wall motion also can be assessed with equilibrium angiocardiography. By tracing the images obtained during the end of diastole and the end of systole, abnormalities in systolic or diastolic volumes can be ascertained. In addition, global versus regional impairment of ventricular function can be differentiated, including

table 17-5 Diagnostic Tests Used to Detect Myocardial Ischemia

Procedure	Abnormal Findings	Special Considerations
Standard 12-lead ECG	Transient ST segment and T-wave changes in patients with chest pain at rest or of prolonged duration	
Holter monitoring	Transient ST segment and T-wave changes occurring at rest or with activity	Only two ECG leads monitored
Stress echocardiogram	Segmental wall motion abnormality associated with echocardiogram obtained during exercise	May be used in patients with ventricular conduction defects Pharmacological agents may be used in patients who cannot exercise.
Exercise ECG	Transient ST segment and T-wave changes occurring with exercise	Cannot be used in patients who are unable to exercise or who have left bundle branch block or paced rhythm Does not provide good information on the location of the coronary artery disease
Radionuclide perfusion stress study	"Cold spot" image or perfusion defect associated with scan obtained during exercise	May be used in patients with ventricular conduction defects Pharmacological agents may be used in patients who cannot exercise.
Online ischemia analysis	Myocardial ischemia dynamic analysis (MIDA)* analyzing eight leads to detect ST segment levels indicating ischemia and QRS complex changes corresponding to infarct evolution	Noninvasive Hastens clinical decision making Graphic trends monitored online Reocclusion readily identified Helps differentiate chest pain related to ischemia from nonischemic symptoms

*MIDA CoroNet, Hewlett-Packard, Andover, MA, Product Literature

the identification of aneurysm formation after infarction. Baseline data may provide information about the etiology of the ventricular impairment, and serial measurements often are used to assess response to treatment.

First-pass radioangiocardiography also uses Tc-99m tracers; however, they are not tagged to any blood components. An image is obtained immediately after IV injection of the radiotracer as it enters the central circulation. The appearance time of the tracer in the various cardiac chambers and right and left ventricular systolic and diastolic counts provide diagnostic information. Because the time required for the tracer to traverse the central circulation is only a few cardiac cycles, the image acquisition time is very short.

Intracardiac shunts may be diagnosed by first-pass techniques. For example, in a patient with a ventricular septal defect and right-to-left shunt, the tracer appears in the left ventricle at the same time or before its appearance in the left atrium. In addition, this technique allows the amount of shunting to be quantified.

Right ventricular ejection fraction and volumes are measured best by first-pass angiocardiography. Because the tracer is present in the right ventricle before it appears in the left ventricle, there is no contamination of counts from the overlapping left ventricle. The methods for measuring right ventricular volumes and ejection fraction are similar to those used for the left ventricle.

Nursing Assessment and Management

Three planar views similar to those used in perfusion imaging are obtained during equilibrium angiocardiography. If exercise angiocardiography is to be performed, the patient should be instructed to wear comfortable shoes for treadmill walking or bicycle riding. As with exercise testing, emergency equipment should be readily available. Although imaging usually is performed with the patient in the supine position, semierect or erect positioning may be used. It is important that the patient not move during image acquisition for either equilibrium or first-pass studies because of the effect on systolic and diastolic images.

Nurses caring for patients who have undergone radionuclide imaging should be aware of precautions; this information is available through the radiation safety department of their institution. The length of time that any precautions may be necessary is related to the half-life of the radiotracer used. In general, nurses who are pregnant should avoid caring for patients for 24 to 48 hours after the study, and all nurses should wear gloves when handling body fluids during the 24- to 48-hour period.

COMPUTED TOMOGRAPHY

Computed tomography (CT) uses x-rays to provide a planar image of tissue structures. An x-ray source and detector rotate mechanically around the patient, and multiple cross-sectional images, or slices, are taken along a designated plane. Imaging is slow, which has proven to be a significant factor in the clear acquisition of structures in motion, such as the ventricles. The resultant blurring of images limits CT's effectiveness in viewing certain cardiac structures. However, CT is effective in illuminating nonmoving structures, such as the aorta, pericardium, and great vessels. CT can be used with or without a contrast agent.

Ultrafast Computed Tomography

Ultrafast CT is a noninvasive technique that is rapidly showing promise in the assessment of myocardial blood flow. It is similar to conventional CT but differs in the speed at which images can be relayed. Ultrafast CT has a distinct advantage: its ability to provide high-quality image acquisition that is not contaminated by the artifactual movement that occurs with cardiac contractions. Images are obtained when an electronic beam passes across four tungsten targets, creating a fan-shaped x-ray view that is transmitted, digitalized, and reconstructed as with traditional CT scanning. Segmental slices of the heart can then be obtained, which are used to evaluate myocardial perfusion. This is especially useful when clear spatial resolution is required. This technique can be used with or without contrast media.

Ultrafast CT has demonstrated an increased sensitivity in the detection of coronary calcium, which has been implicated in the development of coronary atherosclerosis. Studies have shown that the greater the amount of intimal calcium present, the greater the likelihood of obstructive coronary disease. When ultrafast CT is used to identify and quantify coronary calcium, no contrast media are required, radiation exposure is minimal, and the physician need not be present. When ultrafast CT is used with contrast media, it has shown a high degree of accuracy in the assessment of myocardial blood flow when flow is normal or reduced. However, it is less accurate when blood flow is increased.

MAGNETIC RESONANCE IMAGING

Magnetic resonance imaging (MRI) is a noninvasive imaging technique that uses a magnetic field and radiofrequency pulses to produce cross-sectional, three-dimensional images of tissues without the use of x-rays. MRI uses powerful magnetic fields that cause protons to become aligned or parallel to the magnetic field. MRI scans are used to view structural cardiovascular abnormalities when other diagnostic techniques (e.g., echocardiogram) are inconclusive or ambiguous. Because they do not visualize bone, they are superior to other techniques, such as a routine radiographic studies. Wall motion abnormalities, wall thickening, congenital defects, cardiac ejection fraction, coronary arteries, and valvular disease can be visualized on MRI. In addition, MRI scans help assess thrombus formation, major vessel malformations, and diseases of the aortic arch. Regions of MI as well as cardiac masses are best illuminated using the MRI technique.[7,8]

MRI does have limitations. The procedure is expensive, and the technology is not readily available in many treatment centers. In addition, patients must often be transported to a special MRI laboratory, thereby making the examination difficult for critically ill patients who require transport. The patient is placed in a small tube for 60 to 90 minutes; thus, the nurse should explain the procedure to the patient to allay any fears concerning close confinement. The patient should be NPO for at least 4 hours before the procedure, and premedication may be required. MRI is not a hazard to living cells, but there are significant absolute and relative contraindications to its use (Box 17-7).

Invasive Techniques

CARDIAC CATHETERIZATION

Cardiac catheterization is a generic term that refers to a variety of procedures performed in the catheterization laboratory. Such procedures include selective coronary artery, saphenous vein bypass graft, or internal mammary artery angiography, ventriculography, and right or left heart catheterization. All of the procedures are performed using invasive techniques and require a sterile environment.

Procedure

Coronary angiography is used to evaluate the presence and location of coronary artery disease. A catheter is introduced into the arterial system retrograde to the ascending aorta under fluoroscopy. The right or left main coronary artery is then selectively cannulated, and a radiopaque dye is injected directly into the artery through the catheter. As dye flows through the artery, the lumen of the artery can be visualized and the image recorded on film. Disease in the coronary artery or one of its branches delays or obstructs the flow of dye and may be visualized on the film as a site of lumen narrowing and slow filling of the artery with dye. In patients who have undergone previous coronary bypass surgery, selective injections of saphenous vein bypass grafts or internal mammary arteries can be performed in a similar manner.

box 17-7
Contraindications to Magnetic Resonance Imaging (MRI)

ABSOLUTE	RELATIVE (INDIVIDUAL ASSESSMENT REQUIRED)
Cardiac pacemaker	Prosthetic joints
Aneurysm clips	Certain foreign objects in body (e.g., dental braces)
Epicardial pacing wires	Nonmetallic prosthetic heart valves
Metal prosthetic heart valves	Surgical staples
Implanted cardioverter–defibrillator (ICD)	Coronary stents (if recently deployed)
Implanted infusion pumps	
Cochlear implants	
Metal intrauterine devices	
Metal debris (e.g., bullets, shrapnel)	

Radionuclide ventriculography is an excellent tool to assess regional decreases in contractility in areas of stenosed vessels and is useful in the evaluation of left ventricular ejection fraction at peak exercise. Ventriculography, which commonly is performed in conjunction with selective coronary angiography, is accomplished by injecting dye directly into the left ventricle. A catheter is directed retrograde into the left ventricle through the arterial system under fluoroscopy. Dye is injected rapidly, and an image of the left ventricle cavity is recorded on film as the ventricle contracts. Left ventricular ejection fraction, the percentage of blood present in the left ventricle during diastole that is ejected during systole, can be calculated from the film images. Outlines of the ventricle during diastole and systole are traced, and the areas inside each outline are proportional to the amount of blood present. In addition, regional ventricular wall motion abnormalities caused by MI or severe ischemia can be visualized. The competence of the mitral valve also may be evaluated during ventriculography. In patients with mitral regurgitation, dye is observed being ejected not only into the aorta during systole, but into the left atrium through an incompetent mitral valve. In patients with suspected aortic regurgitation, dye may be injected into the aorta; if regurgitation is present, the dye flows retrograde into the left ventricle during diastole.

Left heart catheterization is performed to measure intracardiac or intravascular pressures in the structures of the left side of the heart. The chambers are accessed with a catheter introduced retrograde through the arterial system under fluoroscopy. If either the mitral or aortic valve is stenosed, the pressures required to eject blood forward are higher than normal because of the small valve orifice. For example, with normal mitral valve function, the left atrial pressure and left ventricular pressure are nearly equal during ventricular diastole, because blood flows easily from the left atrium through the mitral valve into the left ventricle. In contrast, mitral stenosis results in a left atrial pressure that is significantly higher than the pressure in the left ventricle during ventricular diastole because the left atrium has to generate more pressure to force blood forward through the stenosed valve. This difference in pressure is known as a *gradient* and is related to the degree of stenosis. Similar pressure comparisons are made in the left ventricle and aorta during systole to evaluate aortic stenosis. If a cardiac output measurement is available, the area of either the mitral or aortic valve opening may be calculated.

Mitral or aortic valve regurgitation also may be assessed by pressure measurements and with ventriculography, as previously described. The abnormal retrograde flow of blood into the left atrium during ventricular systole that occurs with mitral regurgitation produces higher-than-normal left atrial pressures. In patients with severe mitral regurgitation, the pressure in the left atrium may nearly equal the peak systolic pressure in the left ventricle. Similar pressure measurements are made in the left ventricle and aorta to evaluate aortic regurgitation.

Right heart catheterization is performed to measure intracardiac and intravascular pressures in structures of the right side of the heart. A catheter is inserted antegrade through the venous system under fluoroscopy; the procedure is similar to the insertion of a PA catheter. Pressures are recorded from the vena cava, right atrium, right ventricle, PA, and pulmonary capillary wedge position. In addition, blood samples may be drawn from each chamber as the catheter is advanced, and the amount of oxygen present in each blood sample is measured. Because the right side of the heart normally contains venous blood, a significant increase in the amount of oxygen present in a blood sample may indicate a left-to-right intracardiac shunt.

Cardiac output, the amount of blood pumped by the heart in a minute, may be measured during a right heart catheterization using the thermodilution technique. Because cardiac output can be expected to vary with body size, the term *cardiac index*, which takes height and weight into consideration, is used more often.

Arterial and venous accesses usually are achieved with percutaneous techniques from femoral sites. Typically, a needle is inserted into the artery or vein. A guide wire is then inserted through the needle and advanced to the appropriate position in or near the heart. After removing the needle, a catheter may be placed over the guide wire and advanced to the desired position. Changing catheters over guide wires allows specific preformed catheters to be used during the procedure. In some patients, percutaneous access cannot be accomplished from a femoral site, and a cutdown at a brachial site may be required. A bolus of IV or intra-arterial heparin is administered to patients requiring arterial access to prevent clot formation on the guide wire or catheter.

Nursing Assessment and Management

Patients undergoing elective cardiac catheterization are NPO for at least 6 hours before the procedure. Because the dye may be nephrotoxic, hydration with IV fluids may be started before the procedure and continued afterward. Patients with low cardiac output or renal impairment are especially susceptible to dye nephrotoxicity, and their renal function should be monitored closely after the procedure. Patients may be prescribed a mild sedative before the procedure. When percutaneous access is used, pressure usually is applied over the site until bleeding has ceased. A pressure dressing, and in some laboratories, a sandbag, is left in place for several hours after the procedure.

Patients typically are placed on bed rest for 6 hours after the procedure and instructed not to flex the affected extremity. After the procedure, the access site should be checked frequently for signs of bleeding, swelling, or hematoma formation. If a femoral arterial access site was used, peripheral pulses in the affected extremity should be monitored. In addition, bleeding may occur in the retroperitoneal space in patients who have undergone femoral arterial access. Close monitoring of blood pressure and heart rate and an awareness that retroperitoneal bleeding frequently presents as low back pain are useful in preventing a significant bleed. Nursing considerations for patients undergoing cardiac catheterization can be found in Box 17-8.

Before catheterization, patients should be informed about the procedures that will be performed and questioned about any possible dye allergies. They should be instructed that they will be placed on a table with rounded sides and that their body will be strapped down so that they will not move as the table rotates from side to side. If they are to undergo ventriculography, they should be instructed that they may experience a temporary hot flash or flushing

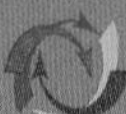

box 17-8 nursing interventions for *The Patient Undergoing Cardiac Catheterization*

Preprocedure

- Explain procedure to patient and family.
- Verify that the patient has taken nothing by mouth for at least 6 hours before the procedure *except* prescribed medications as advised by the physician.
- Ensure ordered preoperative laboratory studies have been completed and results are available.
- Verify patient allergy information; alert physician if patient is allergic to radiographic dye, medications, or specific foods.
- Ensure that informed consent has been obtained.
- Establish intravenous access per institutional protocol or physician order.
- Place patient on cardiac monitoring system with blood pressure and pulse oximetry monitoring.
- Provide supplemental oxygen as ordered/indicated.
- Premedicate patient per physician order.
- Obtain vital signs before transfer to catheterization laboratory.

During Procedure

- Continually assess patient vital signs, oxygenation, level of consciousness, and cardiac rhythm per institutional protocol.
- Alert attending physician to significant changes in vital signs, oxygenation, and presence of malignant cardiac arrhythmias (e.g., premature ventricular contractions, ventricular tachycardia, ventricular fibrillation).
- Be prepared to initiate cardiac resuscitation with emergency equipment and medications.

Postprocedure

- Ensure patient vital signs are stable before transfer.
- Check catheterization site dressing for bleeding and integrity.
- Check distal pulses below catheterization site; if femoral site was used, check distal pulse, extremity color, capillary refill, and neurosensory status.
- Keep extremity straight and instruct patient not to bend leg or arm.
- Maintain intravenous infusion per physician order or institutional protocol.
- Maintain supplemental oxygenation support as ordered or indicated.
- Encourage oral fluids as ordered.
- Check patient's coagulation status per institutional protocol before sheath removal.
- When catheter is removed:

  Apply direct pressure over invasive site for 20 to 30 minutes to prevent bleeding or apply commercial hemostatic compression device per institutional protocol.

  Check distal extremity for pulse, color, capillary refill, and sensorium.

  Remind patient to lie flat for 4 to 6 hours per institutional protocol.

  Check site dressing every 4 to 6 hours for bleeding and integrity.

when dye is injected into the left ventricle. Postcatheterization procedures also should be explained to the patient, including bed rest and monitoring of the access site and vital signs. If the patient is to be discharged after the procedure and a cutdown was used for access, the patient should be instructed to make a follow-up appointment with the physician for suture removal. A summary of patient teaching for patients undergoing cardiac catheterization can be found in Box 17-9.

INTRAVASCULAR ULTRASONOGRAPHY

IVUS is a newer approach to the assessment of coronary anatomy. Using catheters of various frequencies, miniaturized ultrasound crystals are interfaced to ultrasound imaging consoles. Generally, the higher the frequency, the greater the image resolution. IVUS differs from angiography in that IVUS provides a circumferential assessment of the vessel with a 360-degree view, whereas angiography provides a rapid means of assessing the diameter of the vessel lumen in silhouette. IVUS is capable of providing cross-sectional images of coronary arteries that can illuminate arterial wall layers as well as injured media and adventitia. Vessel diameter and the cross-sectional dimensions can be determined. This evaluation permits identification of plaque composition on the vessel wall and its morphology.

In addition to better assessment of coronary and peripheral arterial atherosclerotic lesions, IVUS has proved useful in the assessment of arterial dissections and clots as well as aortic and pulmonary arterial disorders, and it can provide guidance during various catheter-based therapeutic procedures. Studies have shown that IVUS has been useful in the identification of atheromatous disease in vessels that appear normal with angiography and in the recognition of whether such lesions are soft, fibrous, or calcified. Another common use of IVUS has been for the evaluation of coronary artery stents. Data suggest that IVUS is superior to routine angiography in the determination of expansion and underexpansion of the intracoronary stent postimplantation. IVUS catheters are also used for intracardiac echocardiographic studies. Using 10-MHz ultrasound transducers, atrial and ventricular chambers can be visualized to a greater extent, and views of the structures of the left side of the heart can be obtained through the right atrium and right ventricle.

IVUS techniques have proven to be superior for intravascular diagnostic assessment over angiographic procedures alone. Their ability to characterize plaque composition, arterial wall characteristics, areas at risk, and intracoronary stent expansion has made IVUS a powerful tool in the armamentarium of cardiac diagnostic testing.

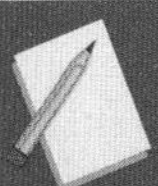

box 17-9
Patient Teaching for the Patient Undergoing Cardiac Catheterization

Preprocedure

- Instruct the patient not to take anything by mouth for at least 6 hours before the procedure *except* prescription medications as advised by the physician to reduce the chance of nausea and vomiting during the procedure.
- Tell the patient that an intravenous line will be placed to allow fluid and medication administration before, during, and after the procedure.
- Tell the patient that preoperative medication will be given before transport.
- Inform the patient that only a patient gown will be worn during the procedure.
- Advise the patient that the catheterization laboratory is usually cool, and the procedure table is firm and may be uncomfortable after a prolonged time.
- Tell the patient that he may be asked to turn his head, hold his breath, or cough during the procedure.
- Advise the patient that he may experience some discomfort during the procedure but that local anesthesia will be administered to minimize pain.
- Inform the patient that he will be placed on a cardiac monitor for the duration of the procedure and for a few hours after the procedure.
- Tell the patient that he will have to lie flat for several hours after the procedure to minimize the chance of bleeding from the catheter site.
- Inform the patient that he will be encouraged to take oral fluids as tolerated after the procedure to assist in elimination of the radiographic dye.
- Encourage the patient and family to ask questions.

During Procedure

- Instruct the patient to inform the physician and team if he is experiencing chest pain.
- Remind the patient to lie still.
- Reassure the patient and allay anxiety.
- Encourage and answer the patient's questions.

Postprocedure

- Remind the patient to lie still and keep the extremity straight.
- Instruct the patient to verbalize any chest pain or shortness of breath if present.
- Tell the patient when the catheter sheath is due for removal.
- Encourage the patient to take oral fluids as ordered.
- Advise the patient that the physician will review the catheterization findings with him.

ELECTROPHYSIOLOGY STUDIES

Purpose

Electrophysiology studies are used both for diagnosing and evaluating interventions in the treatment of arrhythmias. The testing protocol may include the measurement of conduction and recovery times in the specialized conduction system of the heart, identification of abnormal or accessory conduction pathways, and stimulation of atrial or ventricular tissues to induce arrhythmias. All of the procedures are performed using invasive techniques and require a sterile environment.

Patients presenting with symptoms suggestive of supraventricular tachycardia, ventricular tachycardia (VT), or syncope frequently are studied with electrophysiological testing. The intracardiac electrodes are used to stimulate atrial or ventricular tissue at various pacing rates and numbers of extra stimuli. The induction and subsequent recording of a supraventricular tachycardia provides information about the mechanism of the arrhythmia. If an accessory pathway is identified as the mechanism, radiofrequency or surgical ablation of the pathway may be successful in eliminating future episodes of the tachycardia.

The successful induction of VT with electrophysiological testing is of both diagnostic and prognostic value for the risk of sudden cardiac death. Treatment with pharmacological agents can be evaluated with subsequent studies. Antiarrhythmics that prevent induction or slow the rate of a VT in a patient who was inducible in the control state may be used in the long-term management of the arrhythmia. Ventricular arrhythmias usually are not treated with ablation methods because the areas of ventricular tissue responsible for the tachycardia are not easily identified and are widespread.

Procedure

To measure electrical activity from the specialized conduction system of the heart, it is necessary to place electrodes at various intracardiac sites. Special catheters with multiple electrodes are inserted through arterial or venous access and advanced to locations in the heart; a separate access site is required for each electrode. In most studies, venous access is adequate for proper positioning of the electrodes; however, arterial access may be required for blood pressure monitoring. The high right atrium, bundle of His, and right ventricular apex sites typically are used for recording and stimulation. In addition, several body surface leads are recorded simultaneously.[9]

Venous and arterial accesses usually are achieved with percutaneous techniques from femoral sites in a manner similar to that used during cardiac catheterization. A sheath may be left in place during the procedure, however, so that electrode catheters may be repositioned as necessary. In some patients, access cannot be accomplished from a femoral site, and percutaneous access through the jugular vein or a cutdown at a brachial site may be required. A bolus of IV or intra-arterial heparin is administered to patients requiring arterial access to prevent clot formation on the electrode catheter.

Conduction times from the atria to the bundle of His and bundle of His to ventricles are measured. Sites of block—supra-His or infra-His—can be identified and provide information that is used to direct treatment. In addition, the atrium can be paced over a range of rates to identify the rate at which heart block develops. Sinus node function is evaluated by pacing the atrium at various rates, suddenly stopping pacing, and measuring the amount of time it takes for the sinus node to initiate an impulse. The development of heart block at slow heart rates or prolonged sinus node recovery times may indicate a causal factor in patients presenting with syncope or presyncope.

Nursing Assessment and Management

Patients undergoing electrophysiological testing are NPO for at least 6 hours before the procedure, although a sedative administered orally may be prescribed. When percutaneous access is used, pressure is applied over the site until bleeding has ceased. A pressure dressing usually is left in place for several hours after the procedure.

Patients typically are placed on bed rest for 6 hours after the procedure and instructed not to flex the affected extremity. The access site should be checked frequently for signs of bleeding, swelling, or hematoma formation. If a femoral arterial access site was used, peripheral pulses in the affected extremity should be monitored.

Before electrophysiological testing, patients should be instructed that they will be placed on a table with straps over their torso. They should be informed that they may experience palpitations or syncope if rapid tachyarrhythmias are induced. Poststudy procedures also should be explained to the patient, including bed rest and monitoring of the access site and vital signs. If the patient is to be discharged after the procedure and a cutdown was used for access, the patient should be instructed to make a follow-up appointment with the physician for suture removal.

Patients with VT who are being initiated on antiarrhythmic therapy are at risk for sudden cardiac death because some medications may have adverse proarrhythmic effects. These patients often are kept in a monitored setting for most of their hospital stay until appropriate therapies have been identified. Because most of these patients are otherwise healthy and physically active, it becomes a challenge for the nursing staff to care for these patients as well as the more severely ill patient population.

ELECTROCARDIOGRAPHIC MONITORING

Cardiac monitoring is used in a variety of settings. Traditionally used in ICUs and operating rooms, cardiac monitors are now found in other inpatient units where it is necessary to monitor continuously a patient's heart rate and rhythm or the effects of a therapy. In addition, cardiac monitors are used outside the hospital in settings such as paramedic ambulances, surgical centers, outpatient rehabilitation programs, and transtelephonic monitoring clinics.

Although the type of monitor may differ in each of these settings, all monitoring systems have three basic components: a display system, a monitoring cable, and electrodes. Electrodes are placed on the patient's chest to receive the electrical current from the cardiac muscle tissue. The electrical signal is then carried by the monitoring cable to a screen, where it is magnified and displayed. The display can be obtained both at the patient's bedside and at a central station, along with displays from other patients' monitors.

Equipment Features

Two types of cardiac monitoring equipment are in use: continuous hard-wire monitoring systems and telemetry monitoring systems.

HARD-WIRE MONITORING SYSTEMS

Hard-wire monitors, which are commonly used in ICU settings, require the patient to be linked directly to the cardiac monitor through the ECG cable. Information is displayed and recorded at the bedside along with simultaneous display and recording at a central station. Because this type of cardiac monitoring limits patient mobility, patients using this system usually are confined to bed rest or are allowed to be up at the bedside only. Hard-wire monitors operate on electricity but are well isolated so that water, blood, and other fluids do not pose an electrical hazard as long as the machine is maintained properly.

TELEMETRY MONITORING SYSTEMS

In telemetry monitoring, no direct wire connection is needed between the patient and the ECG display device. Electrodes are connected by a short monitoring cable to a small battery-operated transmitter that the patient carries in a disposable pouch tied to his or her body. The ECG is then sent by radiofrequency signals to a receiver that picks up and displays the signal on an oscilloscope, either at the bedside or at a distant central recording station. Antennas are built into the receiver and may be mounted in the vicinity of the receiver to widen the range of signal pickup. Batteries are the power source for the transmitter, thus making it possible to avoid electrical hazards by isolating the monitoring system from potential current leakage and accidental shock. Telemetry systems are used primarily for arrhythmia monitoring in areas where the patient is fairly mobile, such as an arrhythmia surveillance or progressive care unit. Because the patient is mobile, stable ECG tracings often are more difficult to obtain. Some hard-wire systems have built-in telemetry capability so that patients may be switched easily from one system to another as monitoring needs change.

DISPLAY SYSTEMS

Modern electronic technology continues to make sophisticated advances in monitoring equipment, and current display systems incorporate features such as the following:

- Improved freeze/hold modes, which allow the ECG pattern to be held for more detailed examination
- Storage capability that permits retrieval of arrhythmias
- Automatic chart documentation, in which the ECG recorder is activated by alarms or at preset intervals
- Alarm systems for a variety of parameters
- Multilead or 12-lead ECG display, which facilitates complex arrhythmia interpretation
- ST segment analysis for monitoring ischemic events
- Multiparameter displays, which offer display of hemodynamic pressures, temperature, intracranial pressure, and respirations
- Computer systems that store, analyze, and trend monitored data, allowing the information to be retrieved

at any time to aid in diagnosis and to note trends in the patient's status

- Wireless communication devices carried by the nurse that provide data and alarms

MONITORING LEAD SYSTEMS

All cardiac monitors use lead systems to record the electrical activity generated by cardiac tissue. Each lead system is composed of a positive or recording electrode, a negative electrode, and a third electrode used as a ground. As the heart depolarizes, the waves of electrical activity move inferiorly, because the normal route of depolarization moves from the sinoatrial (SA) node and atria, downward through the AV node, His–Purkinje system, and ventricles, and to the left because the muscle mass in the left side of the heart is greater than the muscle mass of the right side of the heart. Each lead system views these waves of depolarization from a different location on the chest wall and thus produces P waves and QRS complexes of varying configuration.

The terminology used to describe lead systems can be confusing. The wires attached to the patient's chest are called leads, and the pictures produced by these wires are also called leads. A standard ECG uses 10 lead wires with electrodes at the ends (4 placed on the limbs and 6 placed on the chest) and produces 12 electrical views of the heart, known as 12 leads.

Cardiac monitoring systems currently on the market vary from two- and three-electrode telemetry devices to three-, four-, and five-electrode hard-wire systems. The two- or three-electrode systems produce limited selections of leads I, II, or III with only a single lead viewed on the screen at one time (single-channel recording). Five-electrode systems allow the possibility of viewing any of the 12 ECG leads and permit the nurse to view two or more leads on the monitor screen simultaneously (multichannel recording).

Three-Electrode Systems

Monitors that require three electrodes use positive, negative, and ground electrodes that are placed in the right arm (RA), left arm (LA), and left leg (LL) positions on the chest as designated by markings on the monitor cable. When the electrodes are placed appropriately, the standard leads (leads I, II, III) may be obtained by moving the lead selector on the bedside monitor to the lead I, II, or III position (Fig. 17-19). The lead selector automatically adjusts which electrode is positive, which electrode is negative, and which electrode is ground to obtain an appropriate tracing. When lead I is selected, the LA is positive, the RA is negative, and the LL is ground. For a lead II configuration, the LL is positive, the RA is negative, and the LA is ground. To obtain a lead III, the LL is positive, the LA is negative, and the RA is ground. The configuration of leads I, II, and III, known as *Einthoven's triangle*, is illustrated in Figure 17-20.

To obtain a chest lead on the monitor that replicates the chest lead from the 12-lead ECG, a five-wire system is needed. (See Fig. 17-14 for a review of chest lead placement.) When only three wires are available, a modified version of any of the six chest leads may be obtained. To configure a modified chest lead (MCL), the goal is to position the positive electrode in the designated chest position. For example, an MCL_1 would require the positive electrode to be placed in a V_1 position (fourth intercostal space, right sternal border). The negative electrode is always positioned under the left clavicle. The ground electrode can be positioned anywhere.

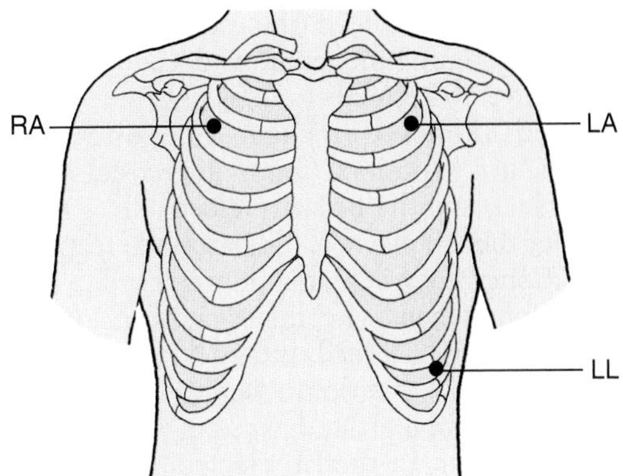

figure 17-19 Three-electrode monitoring system. Leads placed in this position allow the nurse to monitor leads I, II, or III. The left leg electrode must be placed below the level of the heart. *LA*, left arm; *LL*, left leg; *RA*, right arm.

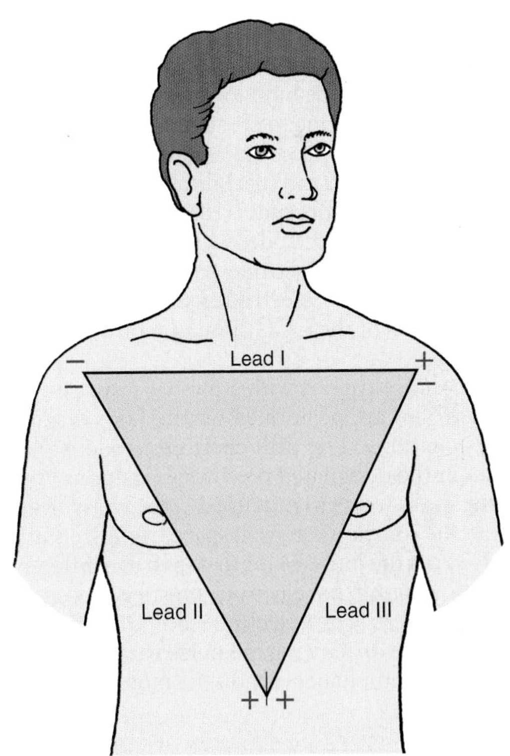

figure 17-20 Einthoven's triangle. Leads I, II, and III are known as the standard leads. When placed together over the chest, they form what is known as Einthoven's triangle.
Lead I: Left arm is positive, and right arm is negative.
Lead II: Left leg is positive, and right arm is negative.
Lead III: Left leg is positive, and left arm is negative.

To obtain an MCL_1 lead, the monitor is set to lead I (Box 17-10). By setting the monitor to lead I, the LA electrode is positive, the RA electrode is negative, and the leg wire is ground (Einthoven's triangle). The positive electrode (LA) is placed in a V_1 position (fourth intercostal space, right sternal border), and the negative electrode (RA) is positioned under the left clavicle. The ground electrode (LL) can be positioned anywhere, but if it is placed in a V_6 position, it is helpful when switching to an MCL_6 lead.

To obtain an MCL_6 lead, the goal is to place a positive electrode in a V_6 position, a negative electrode under the left clavicle, and a ground wire anywhere. By setting the monitor to lead II, the LL electrode is positive, the RA electrode is negative, and the LA electrode is ground (Einthoven's triangle). The positive electrode (LL) is placed in the V_6 position (midaxillary line, same horizontal level as V_4), and the negative electrode (RA) is placed under the left clavicle. The ground wire can be placed anywhere, but if it is placed in a V_1 position, it will be helpful when switching to an MCL_1 lead.

By arranging the electrodes as described, the nurse can monitor both MCL_1 and MCL_6 merely by switching the monitor from a lead I to a lead II without changing the electrode placement on the patient's chest. MCL_1 and MCL_6 are ideal leads for detecting bundle branch block rhythms and for differentiating supraventricular wide-QRS tachycardias from VT.

Five-Electrode Systems

The five-electrode system increases the monitor's capability beyond the three-electrode system. (The four-electrode monitor requires a right leg electrode that is the ground for all leads described in the three-electrode system.) The five-electrode monitor adds an exploring "chest" electrode that allows one to obtain any one of the six chest leads and the six limb leads. In essence, a five-wire monitor system provides all the capabilities of the 12-lead ECG machine. The only difference is that the five-wire monitor has only one chest electrode, whereas the 12-lead ECG machine has six chest electrodes. Newer cardiac monitors now have all six chest electrodes and allow the nurse to view all 12 leads of the ECG simultaneously on the monitor screen.

To monitor a patient with a five-wire system, the four limb electrodes are positioned on the body according to their designations. The fifth chest electrode is placed on the chest in the designated precordial position. For example, if the nurse wants to monitor V_1, the chest electrode is placed in the fourth intercostal space, right sternal border (Fig. 17-21). If the nurse wants to switch to a different chest lead for monitoring, the electrode must be repositioned on the patient's chest. A five-electrode monitor offers the additional advantage of allowing the nurse to view two or more different leads simultaneously on the monitor screen.[1]

Lead Selection

No single monitoring lead is ideal for every patient. Table 17-6 summarizes the use of various leads and the reasons for their use. Lead II is used commonly because it records clear upright P waves and QRS complexes that are helpful in determining the underlying rhythm. In addition to lead II, leads III, aVF, and V_1 or MCL_1 show

box 17-10
Three-Electrode System

To monitor MCL_1 using a three-electrode monitor:

1. Select lead I on the monitor.
2. Refer to Einthoven's triangle to remember that LA is positive, RA is negative, and LL is ground for lead I.
3. Place the positive electrode (LA) in a V_1 position (fourth intercostal space, right sternal border).
4. Place the negative electrode (RA) under the left clavicle.
5. Place the ground wire (LL) in the V_6 position (fifth intercostal space, left midaxillary line).

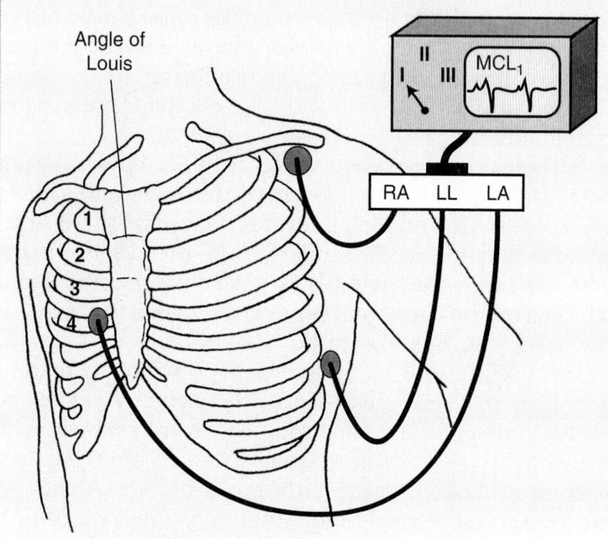

To monitor MCL_6 using a three-electrode monitor:

1. Select lead II on the monitor.
2. Refer to Einthoven's triangle to remember that LL is positive, RA is negative, and LA is ground for lead II.
3. Place the positive electrode (LL) in the V_6 position (fifth intercostal space, left midaxillary line).
4. Place the negative electrode (RA) under the left clavicle.
5. Place the ground wire (LA) in a V_1 position (fourth intercostal space, right sternal border).

Note: The electrodes are in the same position on the chest for the MCL_1 lead and the MCL_6 lead. To view the two leads, the nurse merely switches the monitor from lead I to lead II.

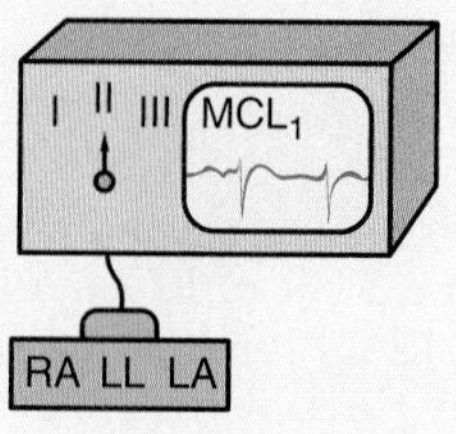

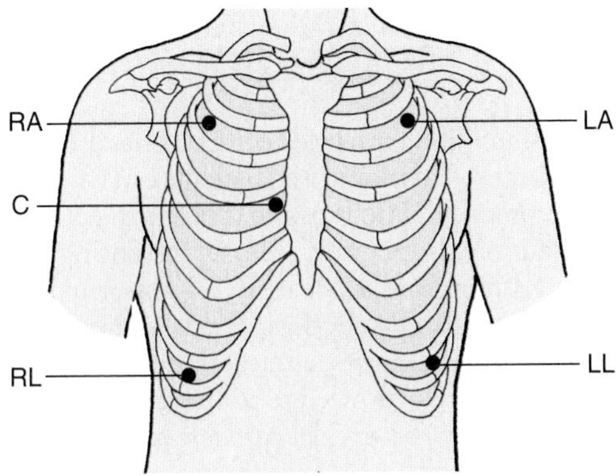

figure 17-21 Five-electrode monitoring system. Using a five-electrode system allows the nurse to monitor any of the 12 leads of the electrocardiogram. The chest electrode must be moved to the appropriate chest location when monitoring the precordial leads.

well-formed P waves and therefore are helpful in identifying atrial arrhythmias. V_1 or MCL_1 is useful in recognizing RBBB and in differentiating ventricular ectopy from supraventricular rhythms with aberrancy. V_6 or MCL_6 is helpful in identifying LBBB and also is useful in differentiating ventricular ectopy from supraventricular rhythms with aberrancy. Lead I may be tried with the patient with respiratory disease who has much artifact on the tracing because there is less movement of the positive electrode in this lead than in a lead II or a V_1.

As mentioned, there is no one ideal monitoring lead for every patient, and in several situations, multilead recording is desirable. Multilead ECG systems offer multiple views of the heart because they reflect a tracing from each of the major heart surfaces. One of the major uses of multilead monitoring is in the interpretation of complex cardiac arrhythmias, especially when differentiating aberrancy from ventricular ectopy and in identifying complex atrial arrhythmias, uncharacteristic-looking ventricular premature beats, and fascicular blocks. Another use of multilead monitoring is in assessment of myocardial ischemia, injury, and infarction. By continuously viewing one lead from each area of the heart, episodes of anginal pain or silent ischemia can be documented. As soon as possible, these changes should be confirmed by a full 12-lead ECG.

Procedure

ELECTRODE APPLICATION

Proper skin preparation and application of electrodes are imperative for good ECG monitoring. An adequate tracing should reflect (1) a narrow, stable baseline; (2) absence of distortion or "noise"; (3) sufficient amplitude of the QRS complex to activate the rate meters and alarm systems properly; and (4) identification of P waves.

The type of electrode currently used for ECG monitoring is a disposable silver- or nickel-plated electrode centered in a circle of adhesive paper or foam rubber. Most electrodes are pregelled by the manufacturer. They may have disposable wires attached to the electrodes or nondisposable wires that snap onto the electrodes. Electrodes should be comfortable for the patient. If not properly applied, undue artifact and false alarms may result.

When applying electrodes, the following procedure should be followed:

1. Select a stable site. Avoid bony protuberances, joints, and folds in the skin. Areas in which muscle attaches to bone have the least motion artifact.
2. Shave excessive body hair from the site.
3. Rub the site briskly with a dry gauze pad to remove oils and cellular debris. Skin preparation with alcohol may be necessary if the skin is greasy; allow the alcohol to dry completely before applying the electrode. Follow the electrode

table 17-6 Suggested Monitoring Lead Selection

Lead	Rationale for Use
II	Produces large, upright visible P waves and QRS complexes for determining underlying rhythm
V_1 or MCL_1	Helpful for detecting right bundle branch block and to differentiate ventricular ectopy from supraventricular rhythm aberrantly conducted in the ventricles
V_6 or MCL_6	Helpful lead for detecting left bundle branch block and to differentiate ventricular ectopy from supraventricular rhythm aberrantly conducted in the ventricles
III, aVF, V_1	Produce visible P waves; useful in detecting atrial arrhythmias
I	Useful in patients with respiratory distress Left arm and right arm electrodes involved and placements less affected by chest motion compared with other leads
II, III, aVF	Helpful in detecting ischemia, injury, and infarction in the inferior wall
I, aVL, V_5, V_6	Helpful in detecting ischemia, injury, and infarction in the lateral wall
V_1 through V_4	Helpful in detecting ischemia, injury, and infarction in the anterior wall

manufacturer's directions because the chemical reaction between alcohol or other skin-preparation materials and the adhesives used in some electrodes may cause skin irritation or nonadhesion to the skin.
4. Remove the paper backing and apply each electrode firmly to the skin by smoothing with the finger in a circular motion. Attach each electrode to its corresponding ECG cable wire. Sometimes it is necessary to tape over the cable wire connection or make a stress loop with the cable wire for extra stability.
5. Change electrodes every 2 to 3 days, and monitor for skin irritation.

While applying the electrodes, explain the purpose of the procedure to the patient. Reassure the patient that monitor alarm sounds do not necessarily indicate a problem with the patient's heart beat; alarms often occur when an electrode becomes loose or disconnected.

MONITOR OBSERVATION

Cardiac monitors are useful only if the information they provide is "observed," either by computers with alarms for programmed parameters or by the human eye, and appropriately acted on by competent, responsible individuals. Some critical care units use monitor technicians whose main responsibilities are to observe monitors, obtain chart samples, and give appropriate information to the nurse about each patient's ECG status. Those observing the monitor should know the acceptable arrhythmia parameters for each patient and should be notified of any interruptions in monitoring, such as those caused by changing electrodes or by changing the patient to a portable monitor. The observer also should be aware of the presence of artifact from chest physical therapy or hiccups so that it may be considered in arrhythmia diagnosis.

Regardless of the system used for monitor observation, certain practices always should be followed. If the monitor alarm sounds, the nurse evaluates the clinical status of the patient *before doing anything else* to see if the problem is an actual arrhythmia or a malfunction of the monitoring system. Asystole should not be mistaken for an unattached ECG wire, nor should a patient inadvertently tapping on an electrode be misread as VT. In addition, monitor alarms always should be in the functioning mode. Only when direct physical care is being given to the patient can the alarm system safely be put on "standby." This ensures that no life-threatening arrhythmia goes unnoticed. If the change on the monitor is not caused by an artifact or a disconnected wire, a full 12-lead ECG should be recorded to evaluate the rhythm change further.

Troubleshooting Electrocardiogram Monitor Problems

Several problems may occur in monitoring the ECG, including baseline but no ECG trace, intermittent traces, wandering or irregular baseline, low-amplitude complexes, 60-cycle interference, excessive triggering of heart rate alarms, and skin irritation.[2] Box 17-11 outlines the steps to follow when such problems occur.

ARRHYTHMIAS AND THE 12-LEAD ELECTROCARDIOGRAM

Arrhythmias and abnormalities of the 12-lead ECG commonly encountered in monitored patients can be recognized with a little practice. The types that occur most frequently are discussed in this chapter. Before presenting the individual arrhythmias and 12-lead ECG abnormalities, the method for evaluating a rhythm strip is addressed.

To understand the causes, clinical significance, and treatment of arrhythmias, knowledge of the conduction system is essential. Chapter 16 provides a review of the essential elements of the cardiac conducting system.

Evaluation of a Rhythm Strip

ELECTROCARDIOGRAM PAPER

An ECG tracing is a graphic recording of the heart's electrical activity. The paper consists of horizontal and vertical lines, each 1 mm apart. The horizontal lines denote time measurements. When the paper is run at a sweep speed of 25 mm/second, each small square measured horizontally is equal to 0.04 second, and a large square (five small squares) equals 0.2 second. Height or voltage is measured by counting the lines vertically. Each small square measured vertically is 1 mm, and the large square is 5 mm (Fig. 17-22). Most ECG paper also is marked by vertical slash marks across the top or bottom. The distance between two vertical markings represents 3 seconds. The distance between 6 seconds is used for rate calculation.

WAVEFORMS AND INTERVALS

During the cardiac cycle, the following waveforms and intervals are produced on the ECG surface tracing (see Fig. 17-22):

- *P wave:* The P wave is a small, usually upright and rounded deflection representing depolarization of the atria. It normally is seen before the QRS complex at a consistent interval.
- *PR interval:* The PR interval represents the time from the onset of atrial depolarization until the onset of ventricular depolarization. Included in the interval is the brief delay of the electrical signal at the AV node that allows time for the blood to move from the atria to the ventricles before the ventricles are depolarized. The interval is measured from the beginning of the P wave to the beginning of the QRS complex. A normal PR interval is 0.12 to 0.2 second.
- *QRS complex:* The QRS complex is a large waveform representing ventricular depolarization. Each component of the waveform has a specific connotation. The initial negative deflection is a Q wave, the initial positive deflection is an R wave, and the negative deflection after the R wave is an S wave. Not all QRS complexes have all three components, even though the complex is commonly called the QRS complex. A normal QRS complex is 0.06 to 0.11 second in width. Figure 17-23 illustrates different kinds of QRS complexes.

box 17-11
Troubleshooting: Electrocardiogram Monitor Problem Solving

Excessive Triggering of Heart Rate Alarms

- Is the high–low alarm set too close to the patient's heart rate?
- Is the monitor sensitivity level set too high or too low?
- Is the patient cable securely inserted into the monitor receptacle?
- Are the lead wires or connections damaged?
- Has the monitoring lead been properly selected?
- Were the electrodes applied properly?
- Are the R and T waves the same height, causing both waveforms to be sensed?
- Is the baseline unstable, or is there excessive cable or lead wire movement?

Baseline But No Electrocardiogram (ECG) Trace

- Is the size (gain or sensitivity) control properly adjusted?
- Is an appropriate lead selector being used on the monitor?
- Is the patient cable fully inserted into the ECG receptacle?
- Are the electrode wires fully inserted into the patient cable?
- Are the electrode wires firmly attached to the electrodes?
- Are the electrode wires damaged?
- Is the patient cable damaged?
- Call for service if the trace is still absent.
- Is the battery dead (for telemetry system)?

Intermittent Trace

- Is the patient cable fully inserted into the monitor receptacle?
- Are the electrode wires fully inserted into the patient cable?
- Are the electrode wires firmly attached to the electrodes?
- Are the electrode wire connectors loose or worn?
- Have the electrodes been applied properly?
- Are the electrodes properly located and in firm skin contact?
- Is the patient cable damaged?

Wandering or Irregular Baseline

- Is there excessive cable movement? This can be reduced by clipping to the patient's clothing.
- Is the power cord on or near the monitor cable?
- Is there excessive movement by the patient? Are there muscle tremors from anxiety or shivering?
- Is site selection correct?
- Were proper skin preparation and application procedures followed?
- Are the electrodes still moist?

Low-Amplitude Complexes

- Is size control adjusted properly?
- Were the electrodes applied properly?
- Is there dried gel on the electrodes?
- Change electrode sites. Check 12-lead ECG for lead with highest amplitude, and attempt to simulate that lead.
- If none of the preceding steps remedies the problem, the weak signal may be the patient's normal complex.

Sixty-Cycle Interference

- Is the monitor size control set too high?
- Are there nearby electrical devices in use, especially poorly grounded ones?
- Were the electrodes applied properly?
- Is there dried gel on the electrodes?
- Are lead wires or connections damaged?

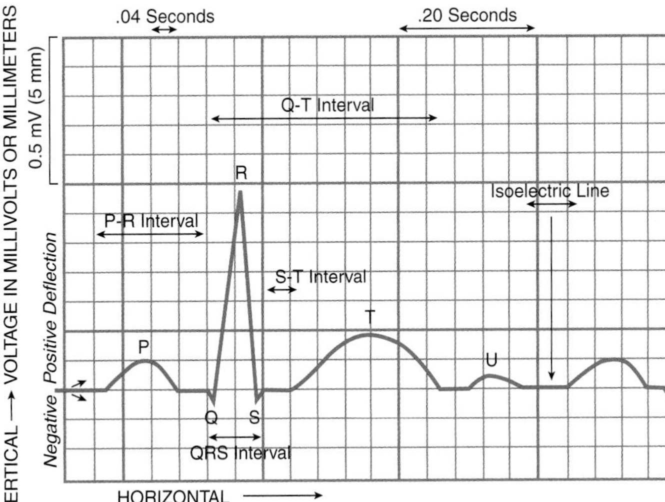

figure 17-22 Waveforms of the electrocardiogram. Schematic representation of the electrical impulse as it traverses the conduction system, resulting in depolarization and repolarization of the myocardium.

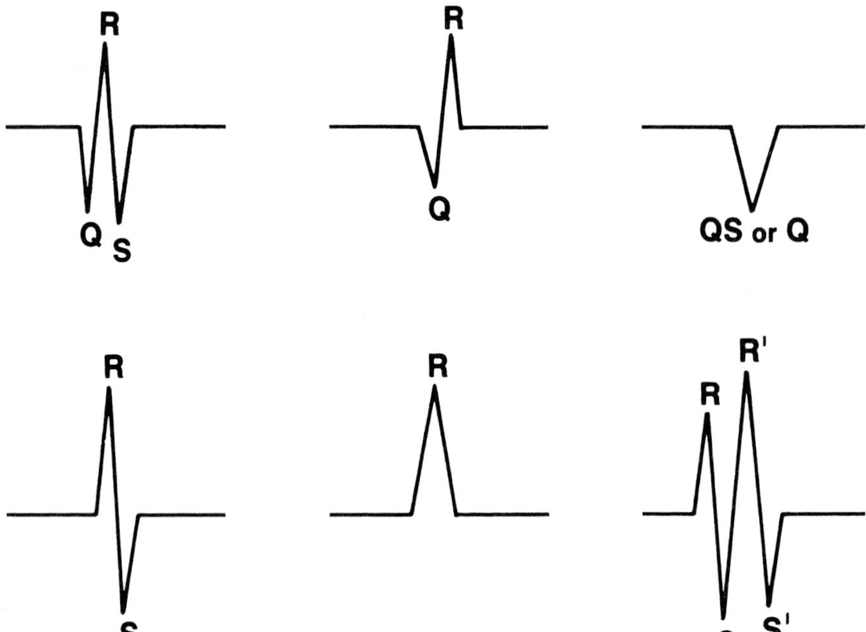

figure 17-23 Configurations of the QRS complex. A Q wave is a negative deflection before an R wave, an R wave is a positive deflection, and an S wave is a negative deflection after an R wave.

- *ST segment:* The ST segment is the portion of the tracing from the end of the QRS complex to the beginning of the T wave. It represents the time from the end of ventricular depolarization to the beginning of ventricular repolarization. Normally, it is isoelectric. An isoelectric ST segment means the ST segment joins the QRS complex at the baseline. ST segments may be elevated or depressed in a variety of conditions. Elevated ST segments could indicate acute myocardial injury. Depressed ST segments may signify acute myocardial injury or myocardial ischemia. For a more detailed discussion of ST segment abnormalities, see Chapter 21.
- *T wave:* The T wave is the deflection representing ventricular repolarization or recovery. The T wave appears after the QRS complex. The atria also have a repolarization phase. However, there is no visible wave on the ECG to represent atrial repolarization because it occurs at the same time as the QRS complex.
- *U wave:* A U wave is a rarely seen, small, usually positive deflection after the T wave. Its significance is uncertain, but it typically is seen with hypokalemia.
- *QT interval:* The QT interval is the period from the beginning of ventricular depolarization to the end of ventricular repolarization. The QT interval is measured from the beginning of the QRS complex to the end of the T wave. Because the QT interval varies with heart rate, it is necessary to use a table in which QT intervals for various heart rates are listed. Tables are available for this purpose in most texts about arrhythmias (Table 17-7). If such a table is not available, a corrected QT interval (QT_C) can be calculated for comparison with normal values. Normal QT_C usually does not exceed 0.42 second for men and 0.43 second for women. A quick method for obtaining a QT_C is to use half of the preceding RR interval (described later).

CALCULATION OF HEART RATE

Although cardiac monitors and ECG strips can be used to calculate heart rate, the calculated rate is merely an estimate of the number of times per minute the heart has been electrically excited. In the normal heart, each excitation should be followed by cardiac contraction. However, in some situations, electrical activity can occur without contraction, resulting in a lack of perfusion. Therefore, the heart rate obtained from the cardiac monitor or ECG strip should never be substituted for the determination of heart rate by palpating the pulse.

table 17-7 **Approximate Normal Limits for QT Intervals in Seconds**

Heart Rate per Minute	Men and Children	Women
40	0.45–0.49	0.46–0.50
46	0.43–0.47	0.44–0.48
50	0.41–0.45	0.43–0.46
55	0.40–0.44	0.41–0.45
60	0.39–0.42	0.40–0.43
67	0.37–0.40	0.38–0.41
71	0.36–0.40	0.37–0.41
75	0.35–0.38	0.36–0.39
80	0.34–0.37	0.35–0.38
86	0.33–0.36	0.34–0.37
93	0.32–0.35	0.33–0.36
100	0.31–0.34	0.32–0.35
109	0.30–0.33	0.31–0.33
120	0.28–0.31	0.29–0.32
133	0.27–0.29	0.28–0.30
150	0.25–0.28	0.26–0.28
172	0.23–0.26	0.24–0.26

Both the atrial and the ventricular rates can be estimated by examining the ECG. To determine the ventricular rate, count the number of QRS complexes in a 6-second strip, and multiply by 10. To estimate the atrial rate, count the number of P waves in a 6-second strip and multiply by 10. In the normal patient, the atrial and the ventricular rates should be the same. This method of rate calculation provides an estimate of heart rate for regular and irregular rhythms.

Another method of rate calculation can be used if the rhythm is regular. The ventricular heart rate is estimated by dividing 300 by the number of large boxes on the ECG paper between two R waves (the RR interval). The atrial rate is calculated by dividing 300 by the number of large boxes on ECG paper between two P waves (the PP interval).

Another quick method for estimating rate involves the use of a series of numbers. To use this method for estimating ventricular rate, the nurse first finds a QRS complex that falls directly on a dark line of the ECG paper. This dark line is the reference point. The next six dark lines of the paper are labeled 300, 150, 100, 75, 60, and 50 (Fig. 17-24). Then, the nurse finds the next QRS complex immediately after the reference point and estimates the ventricular rate using the sequence of numbers. The same method can be used for estimating atrial rate by using the P waves.

STEPS IN ASSESSING A RHYTHM STRIP

The following analysis represents a systematic approach to assessment of a cardiac rhythm strip. Whether or not this method is used, it is important to take the time to complete each step because many arrhythmias are not as they first appear.

1. Determine the atrial and ventricular heart rates.
   - Are they within normal limits?
   - If not, is there a relationship between the two (i.e., one a multiple of the other)?
2. Examine the rhythm to see if it is regular.
   - Is there an equal amount of time between each QRS complex (RR interval)?
   - Is there an equal amount of time between each P wave (PP interval)?
   - Are the PP and RR intervals the same?
3. Look for the P waves.
   - Are they present?
   - Is there one or more P waves for each QRS complex?
   - Do all P waves have the same configuration?
4. Measure the PR interval.
   - Is it normal?
   - Is it the same throughout the strip, or does it vary?
   - If it varies, is there a pattern to the variation?

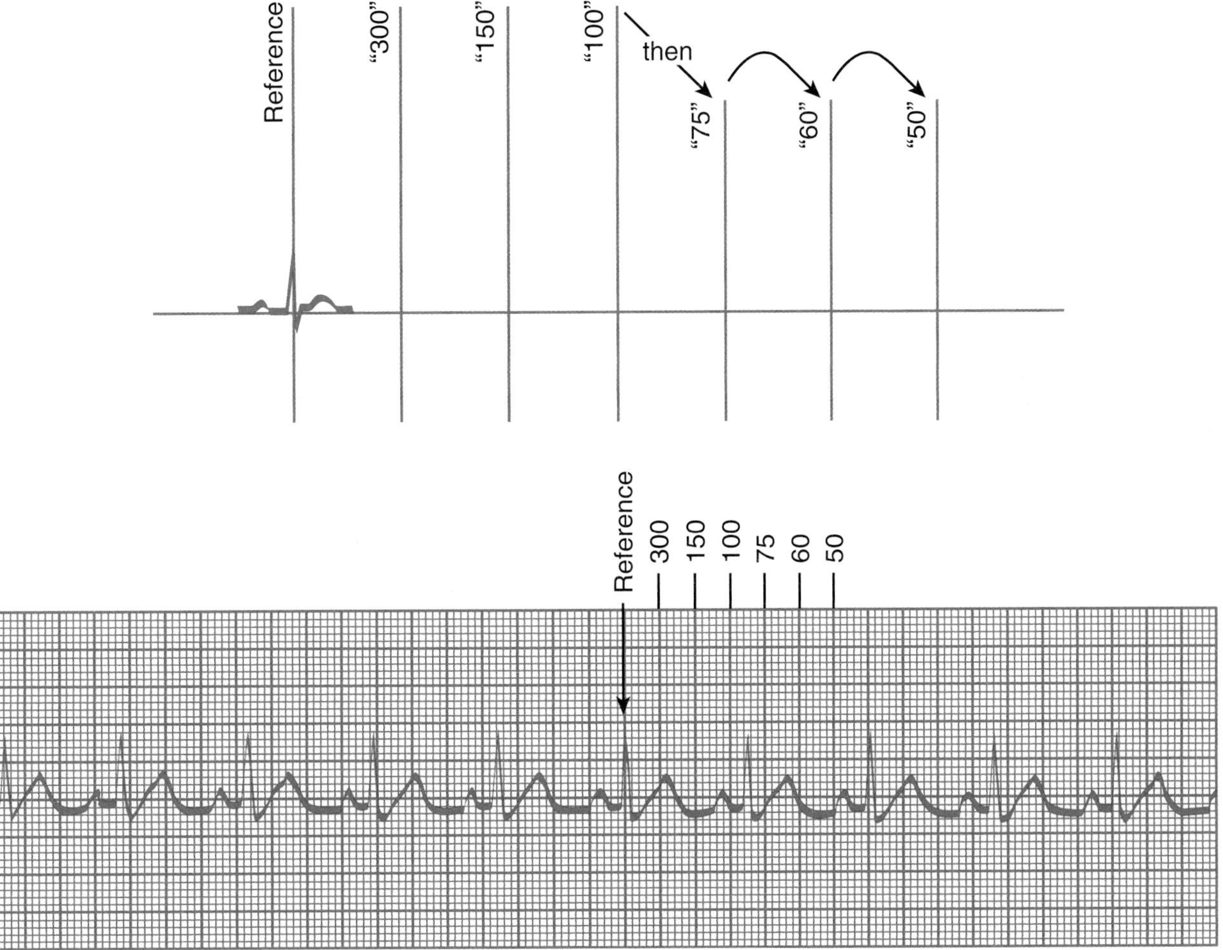

figure 17-24 Method for estimating heart rate. Using this method, the heart rate is approximately 85 beats/min.

5. Evaluate the QRS complex.
   - Is it normal in width, or is it wide?
   - Are all complexes of the same configuration?
6. Examine the ST segment.
   - Is it isoelectric, elevated, or depressed?
7. Identify the rhythm and determine its clinical significance.
   - Is the patient symptomatic? (Check skin, neurological status, renal function, coronary circulation, and hemodynamic status/blood pressure.)
   - Is the arrhythmia life-threatening?
   - What is the clinical context?
   - Is the arrhythmia new or chronic?

Normal Sinus Rhythm

Normal sinus rhythm (Fig. 17-25A) is the normal rhythm of the heart. The impulse is initiated at the sinus node in a regular rhythm at a rate of 60 to 100 beats/minute. A P wave appears before each QRS complex. The PR interval is within normal limits and of equal duration (0.12 to 0.2 second), and the QRS is narrow (<0.12 second) unless an intraventricular conduction defect is present.

Arrhythmias Originating at the Sinus Node

Table 17-8 summarizes and compares ECG characteristics of sinus rhythms.

SINUS TACHYCARDIA

In sinus tachycardia, the sinus node accelerates and initiates an impulse at a rate of 100 times/minute or more (see Fig. 17-25B). The upper limits of sinus tachycardia extend to 160 to 180 beats/minute. All other ECG characteristics, except for heart rate, are the same as in normal sinus rhythm.

Sinus tachycardia usually is caused by factors relating to an increase in sympathetic tone. Stress, exercise, and stimulants such as caffeine and nicotine can produce this arrhythmia. Sinus tachycardia also is associated with such clinical problems as fever, anemia, hyperthyroidism, hypoxemia, heart failure, and shock. Drugs such as atropine, which blocks vagal tone, and the catecholamines (e.g., epinephrine, dopamine) also can produce this rhythm.

The cause of the sinus tachycardia and the underlying state of the myocardium determine the prognosis. Sinus tachycardia alone is not a lethal arrhythmia but often signals an underlying problem that should be pursued. In addition, the rapid rate of sinus tachycardia increases oxygen demands on the myocardium and decreases the filling time of the ventricles. In individuals who already have depleted cardiac reserve, ischemia, or heart failure, the persistence of a fast rate may worsen the underlying condition.

Treatment for sinus tachycardia usually is directed at eliminating the underlying cause. Specific measures may include sedation, oxygen administration, digitalis, and diuretics if heart failure is present, or propranolol if the tachycardia is caused by thyrotoxicosis.

SINUS BRADYCARDIA

Sinus bradycardia is defined as a rhythm with impulses originating at the sinus node at a rate of less than 60 beats/minute (see Fig. 17-25C). The rhythm (RR interval) is regular and all other parameters are normal.

Sinus bradycardia is common among individuals of all ages and may be normal in highly trained athletes. It is present in both healthy and diseased hearts. It may be associated with sleep, severe pain, inferior wall MI, acute spinal cord injury, and certain drugs (e.g., digitalis, beta-blockers, verapamil, diltiazem).

Slow heart rates are tolerated well in individuals with healthy hearts. In those with severe heart disease, however, the heart may not be able to compensate for a slow rate by increasing the volume of blood ejected per beat. In this situation, sinus bradycardia leads to a low cardiac output.

No treatment is indicated unless symptoms are present. If the pulse is very slow and the patient is symptomatic,

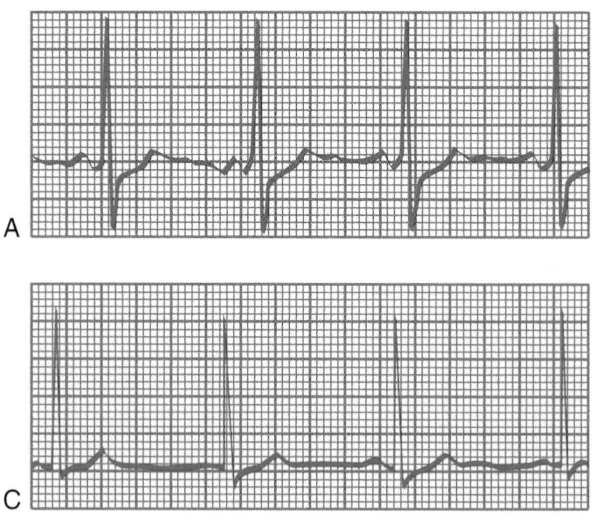

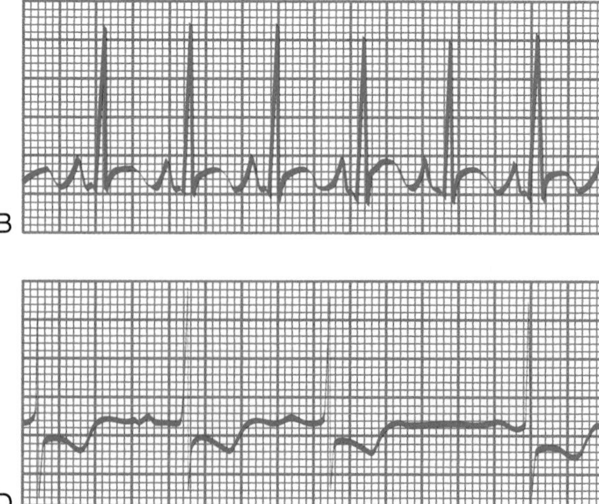

figure 17-25 Sinus rhythms. (**A**) Normal sinus rhythm. (Heart rate = 60–100 beats/min.) (**B**) Sinus tachycardia. (Heart rate = 100–180 beats/min.) (**C**) Sinus bradycardia. (Heart rate < 60 beats/min.) (**D**) Sinus arrhythmia. (Difference between shortest and longest R-R interval.)

table 17-8 A Comparison of the Electrocardiographic Characteristics of Sinus Rhythms

	Normal Sinus Rhythm	Sinus Tachycardia	Sinus Bradycardia	Sinus Arrhythmia
Rate	60–100 beats/min	>100 beats/min	<60 beats/min	60–100 beats/min
Rhythm	Regular	Regular	Regular	Irregular
P waves	Present, one per QRS	Present, one per QRS	Present, one per QRS	Present, one per QRS
PR interval	<0.20 s, equal	<0.20 s, equal	<0.20 s, equal	<0.20 s, equal
QRS complex	<0.12 s	<0.12 s	<0.12 s	<0.12 s

appropriate measures include atropine (to block the vagal effect) or cardiac pacing.

SINUS ARRHYTHMIA

Sinus arrhythmia is a disorder of rhythm (see Fig. 17-25D) that is said to be present if the RR intervals on the ECG, from the shortest RR interval to the longest, vary by more than 0.12 second. This arrhythmia is caused by an irregularity in sinus node discharge, often in association with phases of the respiratory cycle. The sinus node rate gradually increases with inspiration and gradually decreases with expiration.

Sinus arrhythmia is a normal phenomenon, seen especially in young individuals in the setting of lower heart rates. It also occurs after enhancement of vagal tone (e.g., with digitalis or morphine). Because it is a normal finding, sinus arrhythmia does not imply the presence of underlying disease. Symptoms are uncommon unless there are excessively long pauses between heart beats, and usually no treatment is required.

SINUS ARREST AND SINOATRIAL BLOCK

Sinus arrest is a disorder of impulse formation. The sinus node fails to form a discharge, producing pauses of varying lengths because of the absence of atrial depolarization. The P wave is absent, and the resulting PP interval is not a multiple of the basic PP interval. The pause ends either when an escape pacemaker from the junction or ventricles takes over or sinus node function returns.

An SA block often is difficult to differentiate from sinus arrest on a surface ECG tracing. In SA block, the sinus node fires, but the impulse is delayed or blocked from exiting the sinus node. If the block is complete, the duration of the pause is a multiple of the basic PP interval (Fig. 17-26).

Both arrhythmias may result from disruption of the sinus node by infarction, degenerative fibrotic changes, drugs (digitalis, beta-blockers, calcium channel blockers), or excessive vagal stimulation. These rhythms usually are transient and insignificant unless a lower pacemaker fails to take over to pace the ventricles. Treatment is indicated if the patient is symptomatic. The goal is to increase the ventricular rate, which may require the use of atropine or, in the presence of serious hemodynamic compromise, a pacemaker.

SICK SINUS SYNDROME

Sick sinus syndrome refers to a chronic form of sinus node disease (Fig. 17-27). Patients exhibit severe degrees of sinus node depression, including marked sinus bradycardia, SA block, or sinus arrest. Often, rapid atrial arrhythmias, such as atrial flutter or fibrillation ("tachycardia–bradycardia syndrome"), coexist and alternate with periods of sinus node depression.

Management of sick sinus syndrome requires control of the rapid atrial arrhythmias with drug therapy and, in selected cases, control of very slow heart rates, often requiring implantation of a permanent pacemaker.

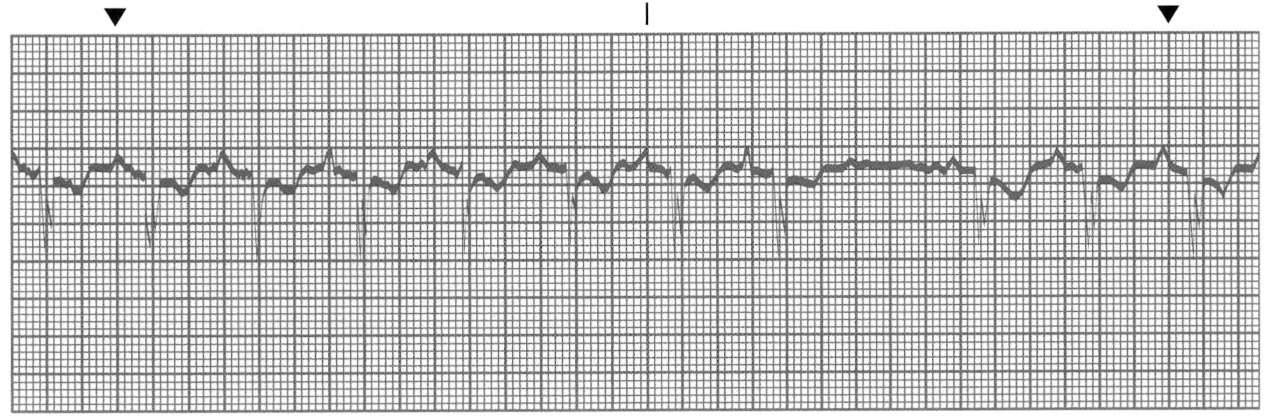

figure 17-26 Sinoatrial block. The pause is a multiple of the basic PP interval.

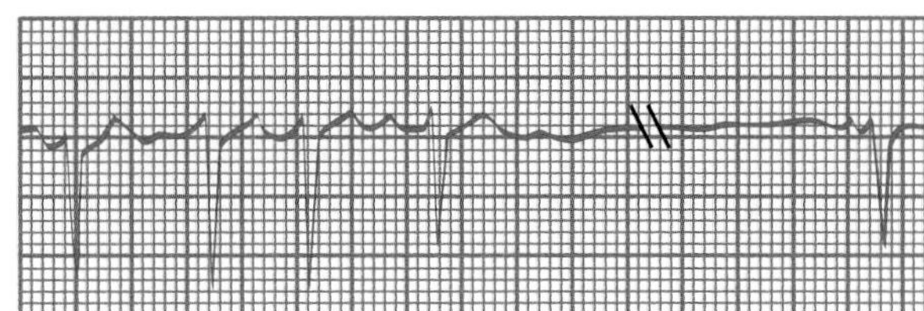

figure 17-27 Sick sinus syndrome. Atrial fibrillation is followed by atrial standstill. A sinus escape beat is seen at the end of the strip.

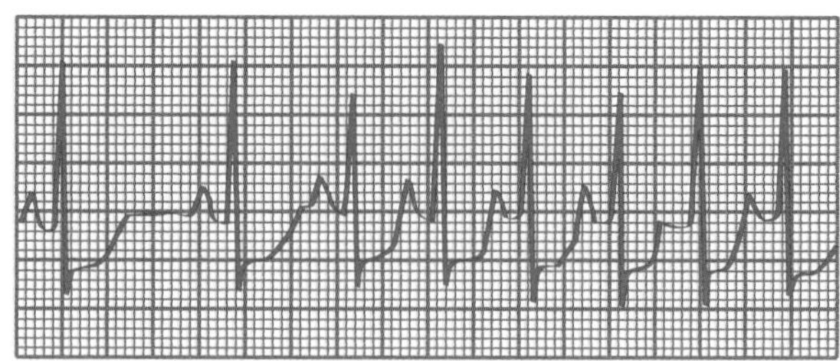

figure 17-29 Paroxysmal supraventricular tachycardia, which begins with a premature atrial contraction.

Atrial Arrhythmias

PREMATURE ATRIAL CONTRACTION

A premature atrial contraction (PAC) occurs when an ectopic atrial impulse discharges prematurely and, in most cases, is conducted in a normal fashion through the AV conducting system to the ventricles (Fig. 17-28). On the ECG tracing, the P wave is premature and may even be buried in the preceding T wave; it often differs in configuration from the sinus P wave. The QRS complex usually is of normal configuration. However, because of timing, the QRS complex may appear wide and bizarre if conducted with some degree of delay (aberrant PAC) or may not appear at all if the atrial impulse is blocked from being conducted to the ventricles (blocked PAC). A short pause, usually less than "compensatory," is present (see later definition of premature ventricular contraction).

Individuals of all ages experience PACs. PACs may occur in healthy individuals as a result of various stimuli, such as emotions, tobacco, alcohol, and caffeine. PACs also may be associated with rheumatic heart disease, ischemic heart disease, mitral stenosis, heart failure, hypokalemia, hypomagnesemia, medications, and hyperthyroidism.

Alternatively, PACs may be a precursor to an atrial tachycardia, atrial fibrillation, or atrial flutter, indicating an increasing atrial irritability. They also may indicate an underlying condition (e.g., heart failure). Patients may have the sensation of a "pause" or "skip" in rhythm when PACs are present.

No treatment is necessary in many cases. The patient should be monitored and frequency of premature beats documented. In addition, the patient should be assessed for underlying conditions and treated.

PAROXYSMAL SUPRAVENTRICULAR TACHYCARDIA

Paroxysmal supraventricular tachycardia (PSVT) describes a rapid atrial rhythm occurring at a rate of 150 to 250 beats/minute (Fig. 17-29). The tachycardia begins abruptly, in most instances with a PAC, and it ends abruptly. P waves may precede the QRS complex, but also may be hidden in the QRS complex or precede the T wave at faster rates. (If some of the P waves are not followed by a QRS complex, this is referred to as *PSVT with block* and usually is caused by digitalis toxicity.) The P waves may be negative in leads II, III, and aVF because of retrograde conduction from the AV node to the atria. The QRS complex usually is normal unless there is an underlying intraventricular conduction problem. The rhythm is regular and the paroxysms may last from a few seconds to several hours or even days.

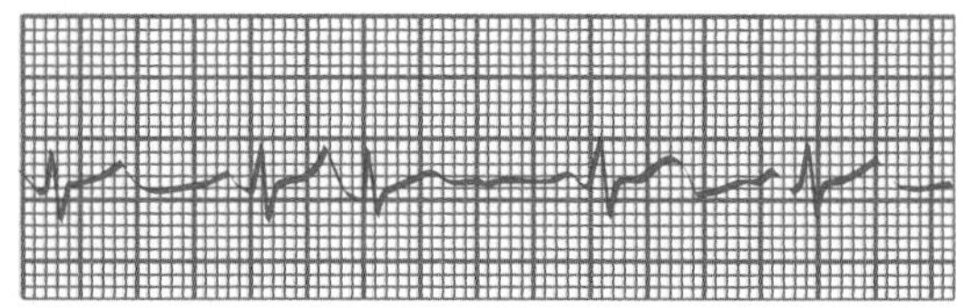

figure 17-28 Premature atrial contraction.

The term *PSVT* is used to identify rhythms previously called paroxysmal atrial tachycardia and paroxysmal nodal or junctional tachycardia, rhythms similar in all respects except in their sites of origin. PSVT also is known as *AV nodal reentrant tachycardia* because the mechanism most commonly responsible for this arrhythmia is a reentrant circuit or chaotic movement at the level of the AV node.

PSVT must be differentiated from other narrow QRS complex (supraventricular) tachycardias. Table 17-9 is a guide to the differential diagnosis. The following points favor the diagnosis of PSVT versus a sinus tachycardia:

- An atrial premature beat often initiates the rhythm.
- The tachycardia begins and terminates abruptly.
- The rate often is faster than a sinus tachycardia and tends to be more regular from minute to minute.
- In response to a vagal maneuver, such as carotid sinus massage, the ectopic tachycardia either is unaffected or reverts to a normal sinus rhythm; sinus tachycardia, however, slows slightly in response to increased vagal tone.

Like PACs, PSVTs often occur in adults with normal hearts for the same reasons (e.g., emotions, tobacco, alcohol, caffeine). When heart disease is present, such abnormalities as rheumatic heart disease, acute MI, and digitalis intoxication may serve as the background for a PSVT.

Often the patient has no underlying heart disease and may experience only palpitations and some lightheadedness, depending on the rate and duration of the PSVT. If the patient has underlying heart disease, dyspnea, angina pectoris, and heart failure may occur as ventricular filling time, and thus cardiac output, is decreased.

Vagal stimulation often terminates the PSVT, either through carotid massage or the Valsalva maneuver. If vagal stimulation is unsuccessful, IV adenosine is given. If adenosine is not effective in treating the arrhythmia, IV procainamide may be used. Cardioversion or overdrive pacing may be required if drug therapy is unsuccessful. Long-term prophylactic therapy may be indicated.

table 17-9 Differential Diagnosis of Narrow QRS Tachycardia

Type of SVT	Onset	Atrial Rate	Ventricular Rate	RR Interval	Response to Carotid Massage
Sinus tachycardia	Gradual	100–180 beats/min	Same as sinus rate	Regular	Gradual slowing
PSVT	Abrupt	150–250 beats/min	Usually same as atrial; block seen with digitalis toxicity and AV node disease	Regular, except at onset and termination	May convert to normal sinus rhythm
Atrial flutter	Abrupt	250–350 beats/min	Occurs with 2:1, 3:1, 4:1, or varied ventricular response	Regular or regularly irregular	Abrupt slowing of ventricular response; flutter waves remain
Atrial fibrillation	Abrupt	400–650 beats/min	Depends on ability of AV node to conduct atrial impulse; decreased with drug therapy	Irregularly irregular	Abrupt slowing of ventricular response; fibrillation waves remain

ATRIAL FLUTTER

Atrial flutter is a rapid atrial ectopic rhythm in which the atria fire at rates of 250 to 350 beats/minute (Fig. 17-30). The AV node functions as a "gatekeeper," preventing too many impulses from reaching the ventricle. If the ventricles are stimulated 250 to 350 times per minute, they are unable to respond with effective contractions, and cardiac output is insufficient to sustain life. The AV node may allow only every second, third, or fourth atrial stimulus to proceed to the ventricles, resulting in what is known as a 2:1, 3:1, or 4:1 flutter block.

The rapid and regular atrial rate produces "sawtooth" or "picket-fence" P waves on the ECG. It is usual for a flutter wave to be partially concealed in the QRS complex or T wave. The QRS complex exhibits a normal configuration except when aberrant conduction is present.

When the ventricular rate is rapid, the diagnosis of atrial flutter may be difficult. Vagal maneuvers, such as carotid sinus massage or the administration of adenosine, increase the degree of AV block and allow recognition of flutter waves. Atrial flutter often is seen in the presence of underlying cardiac disease, including coronary artery disease, cor pulmonale, and rheumatic heart disease. If atrial flutter occurs in conjunction with a rapid ventricular rate, the ventricular chambers cannot fill adequately, resulting in varying degrees of hemodynamic compromise. Likewise, if atrial flutter is accompanied by a very slow ventricular rate, cardiac output is diminished. The loss of "atrial kick," because atrial contraction is not occurring, is also a concern. The lack of atrial kick can compromise cardiac output. Finally, without atrial contractions, thrombi can form on the walls of the atria. If these thrombi break loose, the result could be pulmonary embolus, cerebral embolus, or MI.

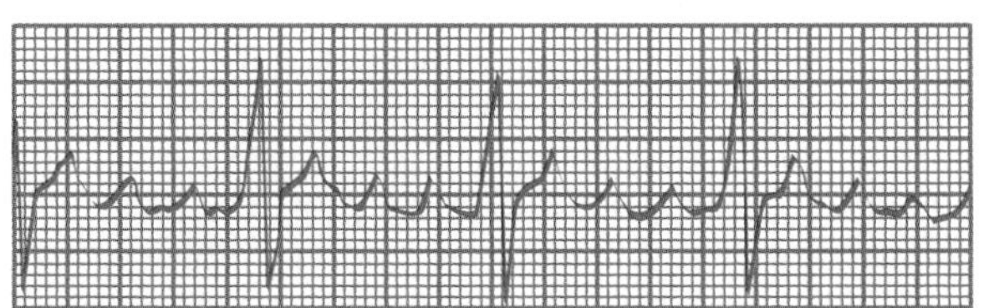

figure 17-30 Atrial flutter. (Atrial rate = 250–350 beats/min. P wave shows characteristic sawtoothed pattern.)

Treatment goals for atrial flutter are to reestablish sinus rhythm or to achieve ventricular rate control. When the ventricular rate is rapid, prompt treatment to control the rate or revert the rhythm to a sinus mechanism is indicated. Drugs may be selected to slow the conduction of the impulses through the AV node, including ibutilide, calcium channel blockers, digoxin, amiodarone, or beta-adrenergic blockers. Ibutilide also may be used to achieve pharmacological conversion of the rhythm. If pharmacological conversion is not successful, electrical cardioversion can be used. Synchronized cardioversion is especially useful in the prompt treatment of atrial flutter. The patient should be NPO before the procedure and receive sedation. (For a more detailed discussion of cardioversion, see Chapter 18.) If the patient has been experiencing atrial flutter for more than about 72 hours, anticoagulation may be needed before pharmacological or electrical conversion of the rhythm is attempted. Other modes of therapy may be indicated for the long-term management of atrial flutter, such as ablation, pacing, and implantable devices.

ATRIAL FIBRILLATION

Atrial fibrillation is defined as a rapid atrial ectopic rhythm, occurring with atrial rates of 350 to 500 beats/minute (Fig. 17-31). It is characterized by chaotic atrial activity with the absence of definable P waves. Instead, the P waves appear as small, quivering fibrillatory waves. Like atrial flutter, the ventricular rate and rhythm depend on the ability of the AV junction to function as a gatekeeper. If too many atrial stimuli pass through the AV junction, the ventricular response is rapid. If too few atrial stimuli pass through the AV junction, the ventricular response is slow. The ventricular rhythm is characteristically irregular.

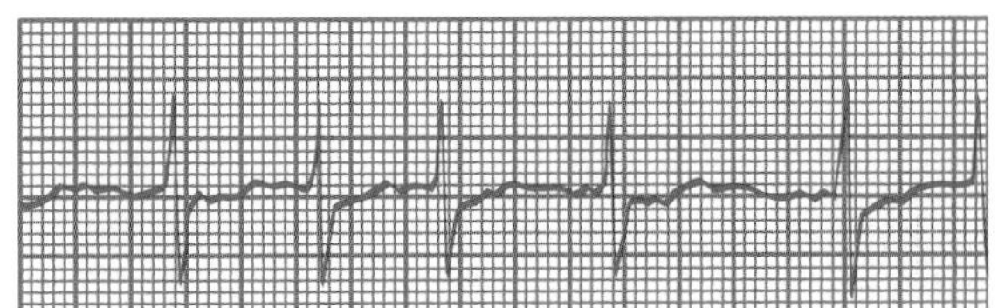

figure 17-31 Atrial fibrillation. (Atrial rate = 400–600 beats/min with a variable ventricular response. Characteristic atrial fibrillatory waves seen.)

Although atrial fibrillation may occur as a transient arrhythmia in healthy young individuals, the presence of chronic atrial fibrillation is usually associated with underlying heart disease. One or both of the following are present in patients with chronic atrial fibrillation: atrial muscle disease or atrial distension together with disease of the sinus node. This rhythm commonly occurs in the setting of heart failure, ischemic or rheumatic heart disease, pulmonary disease, and after open heart surgery. Atrial fibrillation also is seen in congenital heart disease.

The immediate clinical concern in patients with atrial fibrillation is the rate of the ventricular response. If the ventricular rate is too fast, end-diastolic filling time is decreased and cardiac output is compromised. If the ventricular rate is too slow, cardiac output may again be decreased. As in atrial flutter, patients with atrial fibrillation have lost AV synchrony and atrial kick, resulting in a compromised cardiac output. Patients also are at risk for the formation of mural thrombi and embolic events, such as stroke, MI, and pulmonary embolus.

The treatment principles for atrial fibrillation are the same as those for atrial flutter. The goal of therapy is to achieve rate control or to convert the rhythm to sinus. Drug therapy as described for atrial flutter may be used. If a patient has chronic atrial fibrillation, anticoagulant therapy is added to the drug regimen to prevent an embolic event. Cardioversion is indicated for rhythm control when drug therapy fails or in the setting of hemodynamic compromise. Ablation, pacing, and implantable devices are among the therapy options.[1,2]

MULTIFOCAL ATRIAL TACHYCARDIA

Multifocal atrial tachycardia is a rapid atrial rhythm with varying P-wave morphology, resulting from the firing of three or more atrial foci (Fig. 17-32). The atrial rate exceeds 100 beats/minute, and the rhythm usually is irregular. The P waves vary in shape because of the multiple foci. The PR intervals may vary also, depending on the proximity of the focus to the AV node. The QRS complexes are normal unless an impulse is conducted with aberrancy.

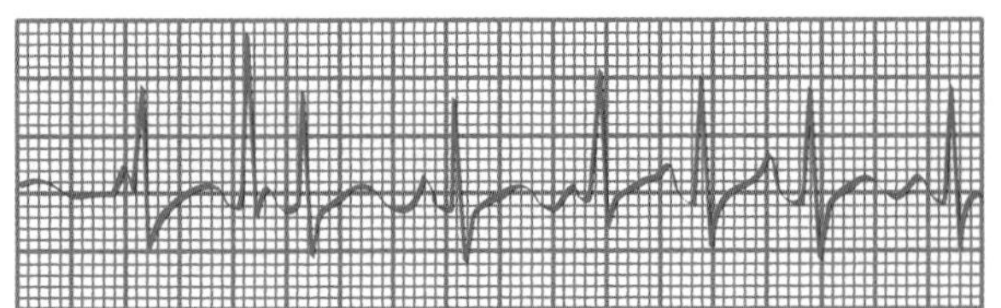

figure 17-32 Multifocal atrial tachycardia. (The atrial rate exceeds 100 beats/min with three or more different P-wave morphologies.)

This rhythm characteristically occurs in patients with severe pulmonary disease. Such patients often exhibit hypoxemia, hypokalemia, alterations in serum pH, or pulmonary hypertension. They usually manifest symptoms associated with the underlying disease rather than with the arrhythmia itself. Treatment is directed at controlling the underlying pulmonary disease and slowing the ventricular rate if necessary.

Junctional Arrhythmias

JUNCTIONAL RHYTHM

A junctional rhythm, also known as a *nodal rhythm*, is a rhythm originating in the AV node. When the SA node fails to fire, the AV node usually takes control, but the rate is slower. The rate of a junctional rhythm ranges between 50 and 70 beats/minute. The P wave in the arrhythmia can have one of three possible configurations.

1. The AV node fires and the wave of depolarization travels backward (retrograde conduction) into the atria. The impulse from the AV node then moves forward into the ventricle. When this sequence occurs, the P wave appears as an inverted wave before a normal QRS complex (Fig. 17-33A).
2. The retrograde conduction into the atria occurs at the same time as the forward conduction into the ventricles. The resulting rhythm strip shows an absent P wave with a normal QRS complex. In reality, the P wave is not absent. Instead, it is buried inside the QRS complex (see Fig. 17-33B).
3. Forward conduction of the ventricles precedes retrograde conduction of the atria. When this sequence occurs, a normal QRS complex is followed by an inverted P wave (see Fig. 17-33C).

A junctional rhythm may be the result of hypoxia, hyperkalemia, MI, heart failure, valvular disease, drugs (digoxin, beta-blockers, calcium channel blockers), or any cause of SA node dysfunction. Patients with a junctional rhythm may become symptomatic as a result of the slower rate. Hypotension, decreased cardiac output, and decreased perfusion may occur. The benefit of AV synchrony and atrial kick may be lost when the atria are stimulated with or after ventricular depolarization.

Treatment should be directed at the underlying cause. Symptomatic patients may require immediate treatment. The heart rate can be increased through the use of atropine or cardiac pacing. Interventions are also directed toward improving cardiac output.

PREMATURE JUNCTIONAL CONTRACTIONS

A premature junctional contraction (PJC) is an ectopic impulse from a focus in the AV junction, occurring prematurely, before the next sinus impulse (Fig. 17-34). As in all rhythms originating in the AV junction, the QRS complex is narrow (<0.12 second), reflecting normal AV conduction. On rare occasions, the QRS complex may be wide if the impulse is conducted aberrantly. The atria are depolarized in a retrograde fashion before, during, or after ventricular excitation, producing inverted P waves that may occur before, during, or after the QRS complex. As with PACs,

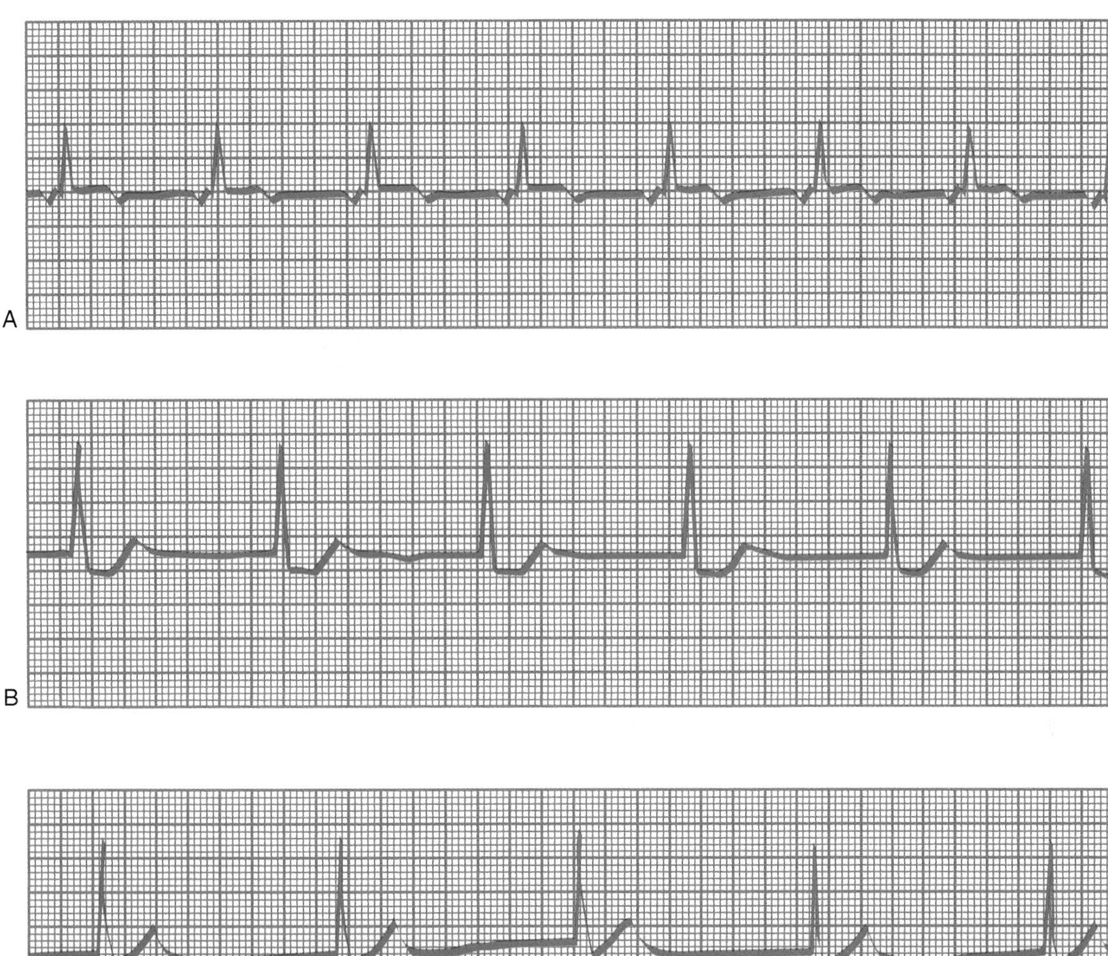

figure 17-33 Junctional rhythm. (**A**) A junctional rhythm in which the inverted P wave appears before a normal QRS complex. (**B**) A junctional rhythm in which the inverted P wave is buried inside the QRS complex. (**C**) A junctional rhythm in which the inverted P wave follows the QRS complex.

PJCs may occur in healthy individuals or in those with underlying heart disease. Ischemia or infarction may activate an ectopic focus in the AV junction, as may stimulants, such as nicotine or caffeine, or pharmacological agents (e.g., digitalis).

Frequent PJCs may indicate increasing irritability and may be a precursor of a junctional rhythm. Although usually asymptomatic, patients may experience a "skipped beat." Treatment for PJCs is not necessary.

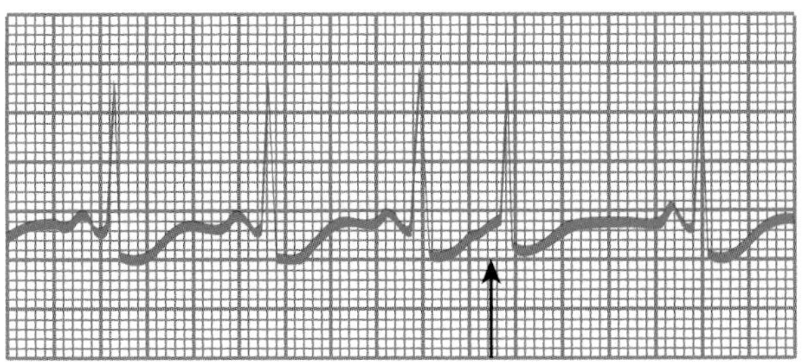

figure 17-34 Premature junctional contraction.

Ventricular Arrhythmias

PREMATURE VENTRICULAR CONTRACTIONS

A premature ventricular contraction (PVC) is an ectopic beat originating prematurely at the level of the ventricles (Fig. 17-35A). The beat is ventricular in origin and results in no electrical activity in the atria. As a result, no P waves appear. The ventricular depolarization does not travel through the normal rapid ventricular conduction system. Instead, ventricular conduction spreads more slowly through the Purkinje system, resulting in a wide QRS complex with a T wave that is opposite in direction to the QRS complex. A compensatory pause often follows the premature beat as the heart awaits the next stimulus from the sinus node. The pause is considered fully compensatory if the cycles of the normal and premature beats equal the time of two normal heart cycles.

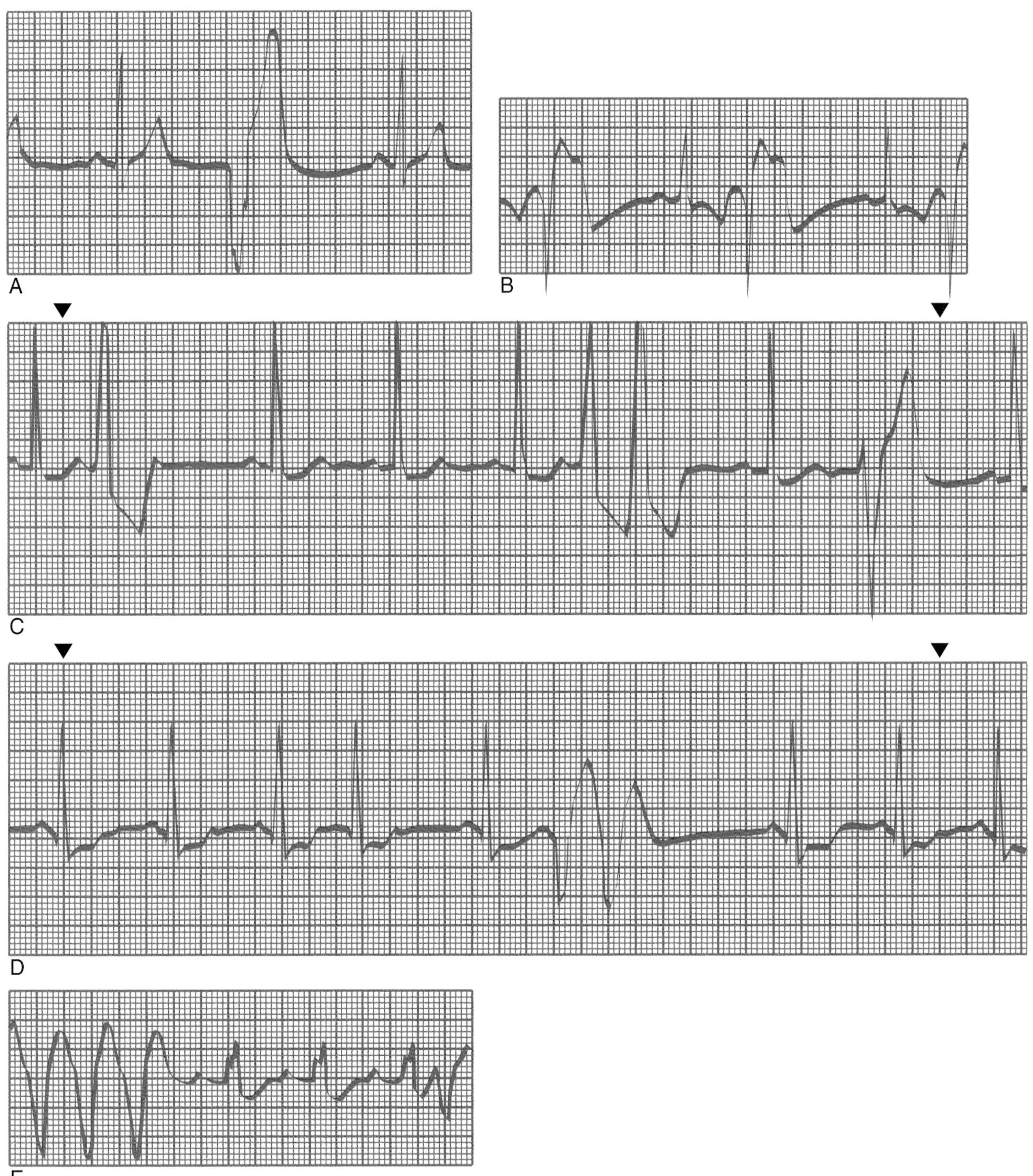

figure 17-35 Ventricular arrhythmias. (**A**) Premature ventricular contractions (PVCs). (**B**) Ventricular bigeminy. (Every other beat is a PVC.) (**C**) Multiformed PVCs. (**D**) Couplet (two PVCs in a row). (**E**) Triplet. (Short run of ventricular tachycardia [VT]; the first three beats are VT with the rhythm converting to sinus rhythm with first-degree heart block.)

Ventricular premature beats can be described by their frequency and pattern. They can be *rare*, *occasional*, or *frequent;* optimally, they are described as number of PVCs per minute. If PVCs occur after each sinus beat, *ventricular bigeminy* is present (see Fig. 17-35B). *Ventricular trigeminy* is a PVC occurring after two consecutive sinus beats. When PVCs appear in only one form (from one ventricular site), they are referred to as *uniformed*, as opposed to *multiformed*, when two or more forms (from more than one ventricular site) of the QRS complex are apparent (see Fig. 17-35C). Two PVCs in a row are a *couplet* (see Fig. 17-35D), whereas three in a row are a *triplet*, which is a short run of VT (see Fig. 17-35E).

The most common of all ectopic beats, PVCs can occur with or without heart disease in any age group. They are especially common in individuals with myocardial dis-

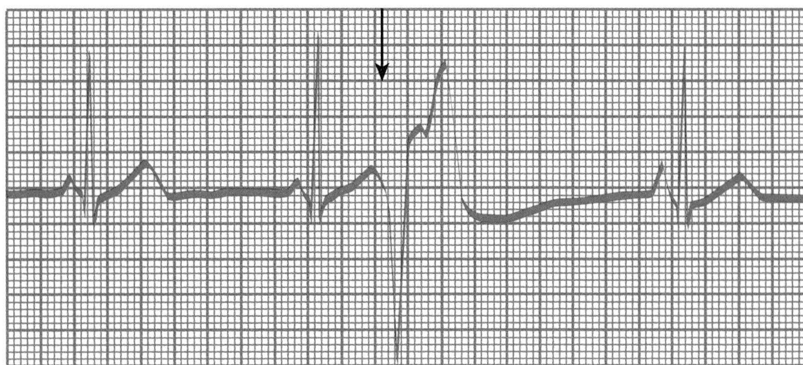

figure 17-36 R-on-T premature ventricular contraction. (From Huff J: ECG Workout [4th Ed], p 195. Philadelphia, Lippincott Williams & Wilkins, 2002.)

ease (ischemia or infarction) or with myocardial irritability (hypokalemia, increased levels of catecholamines, or mechanical irritation with a wire or catheter). The presence of PVCs is a sign of ventricular myocardial irritability and, in some patients, may lead to VT or ventricular fibrillation (VF). The nature of the patient's underlying heart disease rather than presence of PVCs as such determines the treatment and prognosis. Numerous and multiformed PVCs in the presence of serious heart disease worsen the prognosis. PVCs approaching the apex of the preceding T wave (R-on-T phenomenon) are of clinical concern. The T wave represents ventricular repolarization, when the heart should not be stimulated. If stimulation occurs during this vulnerable period, VF and sudden death may result (Fig. 17-36).

Infrequent, isolated PVCs require no treatment. Multiple or consecutive PVCs may be managed with antiarrhythmic agents. In the emergency setting, amiodarone and lidocaine are the drugs of choice. Many antiarrhythmic agents are available for chronic therapy. If serum potassium is low, potassium replacement may correct the arrhythmia. If the arrhythmia is caused by digitalis toxicity, withdrawal of the digitalis may correct it.

VENTRICULAR TACHYCARDIA

In the previous section, VT was defined as three or more PVCs in a row. VT is recognized by wide, bizarre QRS complexes occurring in a fairly regular rhythm at a rate greater than 100 beats/minute (Fig. 17-37). P waves usually are not seen and, if seen, are not related to the QRS complex. VT may be a short, nonsustained rhythm or longer and sustained.

In adults with normal hearts, VT is rare but is a common complication of MI. Other causes are the same as those described for PVCs. VT is a precursor of VF, and signs and symptoms of hemodynamic compromise (e.g., ischemic chest pain, hypotension, pulmonary edema, and unconsciousness) may be seen if the rate is fast and the tachycardia is sustained. Serious arrhythmia progression depends on the underlying heart disease.

If the patient is hemodynamically stable with the arrhythmia, lidocaine may be administered intravenously. If the patient becomes unstable, synchronized cardioversion (or in emergency situations, unsynchronized defibrillation) is indicated. Long-term treatment for this arrhythmia may involve the use of an implantable cardioverter–defibrillator (ICD). See Chapter 18 for a more detailed discussion of ICDs.

TORSADES DE POINTES

Torsades de pointes ("twisting of the points") is a specific type of VT (Fig. 17-38). The term refers to the polarity of the QRS complex, which swings from positive to negative and vice versa. The QRS complex morphology is characterized by large, bizarre, polymorphous, or multiformed QRS complexes of varying amplitude and direction, frequently varying from beat to beat and resembling torsion around an isoelectric line. The rate of the tachycardia is 100 to 180 beats/minute but can be as fast as 200 to 300 beats/minute. The rhythm is highly unstable; it may terminate in VF or revert to sinus rhythm. This form

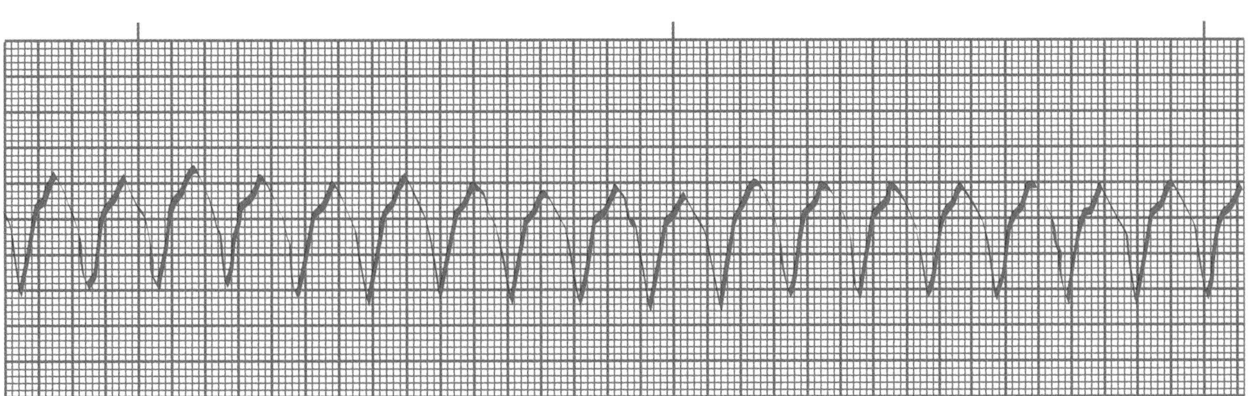

figure 17-37 Ventricular tachycardia. (From Huff J: ECG Workout [4th Ed], p 197. Philadelphia, Lippincott Williams & Wilkins, 2002.)

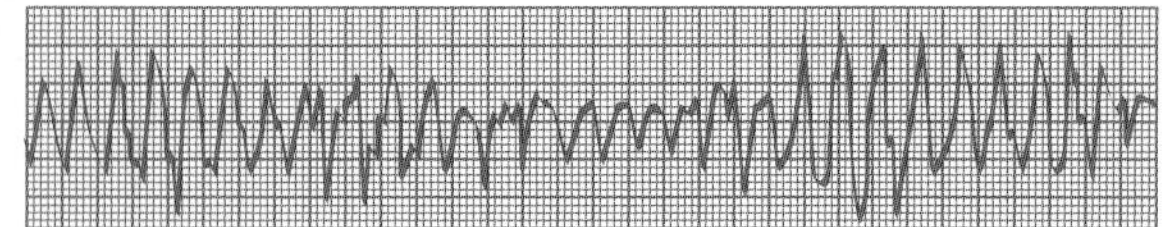

figure 17-38 Torsades de pointes.

of VT is most likely to develop in myocardial disease when the underlying QT interval has been prolonged.

Torsades de pointes is favored by conditions that prolong the QT interval. Examples include severe bradycardia; drug therapy, especially with type IA antiarrhythmic agents; and electrolyte disturbances, such as hypokalemia and hypocalcemia. Other factors that can precipitate this arrhythmia include intrinsic cardiac disease, familial QT interval prolongation, central nervous system disorders, and hypothermia. Torsades de pointes may terminate spontaneously and may repeat itself after several seconds or minutes, or it may transform into VF.

Treatment for torsades de pointes consists of shortening the refractory period (and thus the QT interval) of the underlying rhythm. IV magnesium sulfate, magnesium chloride, or isoproterenol is effective in suppression of the arrhythmia. Overdrive pacing also can be used. Treatment is directed at correcting the underlying problem and may necessitate stopping the offending pharmacological agent or correcting the electrolyte imbalance. Emergency cardioversion or defibrillation is indicated if the torsades does not revert spontaneously to sinus rhythm.

VENTRICULAR FIBRILLATION

VF is defined as rapid, irregular, and ineffectual depolarizations of the ventricle (Fig. 17-39). No distinct QRS complexes are seen. Only irregular oscillations of the baseline are apparent; these may be either coarse or fine in appearance.

VF may occur in the following circumstances: myocardial ischemia and infarction, catheter manipulation in the ventricles, electrocution, prolonged QT interval, or as a terminal rhythm in patients with circulatory failure. As in asystole, loss of consciousness occurs within seconds in VF. There is no pulse and no cardiac output. VF is the most common cause of sudden cardiac death and is fatal if resuscitation is not instituted immediately.

If VF occurs, rapid defibrillation is the management of choice (see the discussion of cardiopulmonary resuscitation in Chapter 18). The patient should be supported with cardiopulmonary resuscitation and drugs if there is no response to defibrillation. An ICD may be indicated for long-term management of VF (see Chapter 18 for a discussion of ICDs).

ACCELERATED IDIOVENTRICULAR RHYTHM

Accelerated idioventricular rhythm (AIVR) is produced by a "speeding up" of ventricular pacemaker cells, which normally have an intrinsic rate of 20 to 40 beats/minute (Fig. 17-40). When the idioventricular rate accelerates above the sinus rate, the ventricular pacemaker becomes the primary pacemaker for the heart. AIVR is characterized by wide QRS complexes occurring regularly at a rate of 50 to 100 beats/minute. AIVR may last for a few beats or may be sustained.

Typically, AIVR is seen with acute MI, often in the setting of coronary artery reperfusion after thrombolytic therapy. It may occur less commonly as a result of ischemia or digitalis intoxication. Patients usually are not symptomatic. Adequate cardiac output can be maintained, and degeneration into a rapid VT is rare.

In most cases, treatment is not necessary. If a patient is hemodynamically compromised, the sinus rate is increased with atropine or atrial pacing to suppress the AIVR.

Atrioventricular Blocks

A disturbance in some portion of the AV conduction system causes an AV block. The sinus-initiated beat is delayed or completely blocked from activating the ventricles. The block may occur at the level of the AV node, bundle of His, or the bundle branches because the AV conduction system contains all of these structures. In first- and second-degree AV block, the block is incomplete; some or all of the impulses eventually are conducted to the ventricles. In third-degree or complete heart block, none of the sinus-initiated impulses are conducted. Table 17-10 summarizes and compares heart block rhythms.

FIRST-DEGREE ATRIOVENTRICULAR BLOCK

In first-degree block, AV conduction is prolonged and equal in time. All impulses eventually are conducted to the ventricles (Fig. 17-41A). P waves are present and precede each QRS complex in a 1:1 relationship. The PR interval is constant but exceeds the upper limit of 0.2 second in duration.

First-degree heart block occurs in individuals of all ages and in healthy and diseased hearts. PR prolongation may be caused by drugs, such as digitalis, beta-blockers, or calcium channel blockers; coronary artery disease; a variety of infectious diseases; and congenital lesions. First-degree block is of no hemodynamic consequence but should be seen as an

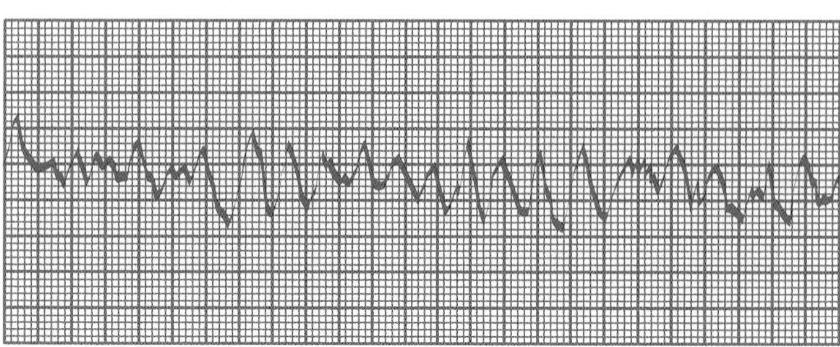

figure 17-39 Ventricular fibrillation.

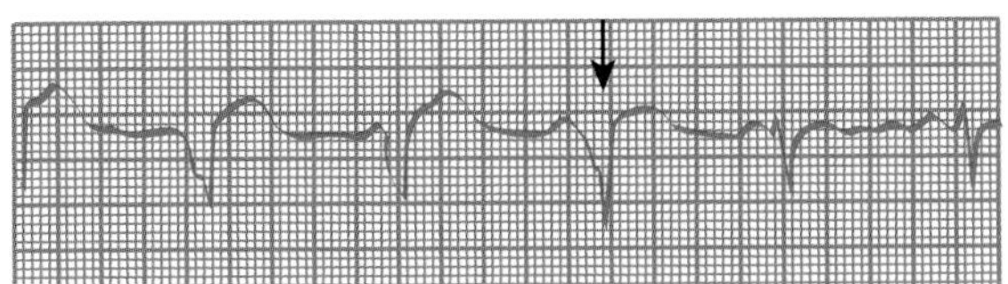

figure 17-40 Accelerated idioventricular rhythm. The first three beats are of ventricular origin. The fourth beat (*arrow*) represents a fusion beat. The subsequent two beats are of sinus origin.

indicator of a potential AV conduction system disturbance. First-degree block may progress to second- or third-degree AV block.

No treatment is indicated for first-degree heart block. The PR interval should be monitored closely, watching for further block. The possibility of a drug effect also should be evaluated.

SECOND-DEGREE ATRIOVENTRICULAR BLOCK—MOBITZ I (WENCKEBACH)

Mobitz type I (Wenckebach) block occurs when AV conduction is delayed progressively with each sinus impulse until eventually the impulse is completely blocked from reaching the ventricles. The cycle then repeats itself (see Fig. 17-41B). Of the two types of second-degree block, Mobitz I (Wenckebach) and Mobitz II, Mobitz I occurs more commonly.

On the ECG tracing, P waves are present and related to the QRS complex in a cyclical pattern. The PR interval progressively lengthens with each beat until a QRS complex is not conducted. The QRS complex has the same configuration throughout the underlying rhythm.

A Mobitz type I block usually is associated with block above the bundle of His. Therefore, any drug or disease process that affects the AV node, such as digitalis, myocarditis, or an inferior wall MI may produce this type of second-degree block.

Patients with Mobitz type I second-degree AV block rarely are symptomatic because the ventricular rate usually is adequate. Wenckebach block often is temporary, and if it progresses to third-degree block, a junctional pacemaker at a rate of 40 to 60 beats/minute usually takes over to pace the ventricles. No treatment is required for this rhythm except to discontinue a drug if it is the offending agent. The patient should be monitored for further progression of block.

SECOND-DEGREE ATRIOVENTRICULAR BLOCK—MOBITZ II

Mobitz type II block is described as an intermittent block in the AV conduction, usually in or below the bundle of His. Mobitz type II block is characterized by a fixed PR interval when AV conduction is present and a nonconducted P wave when the block occurs (see Fig. 17-41C). This block in conduction can occur occasionally or be repetitive with a 2:1, 3:1, or even 4:1 conduction pattern. Because there is no disturbance in the sinus node, the PP interval is regular. Often there is accompanying bundle branch block, so the QRS complex may be wide.

A Mobitz type II pattern is seen in the setting of an anterior wall MI and various diseases of the conducting tissue, such as fibrotic disease. A Mobitz type II block is potentially more dangerous than a Mobitz type I block. Mobitz type II block often is permanent, and it may deteriorate rapidly to third-degree heart block with a slow ventricular response of 20 to 40 beats/minute.

Constant monitoring and observation for progression to third-degree heart block are required. Medications, such as atropine or isoproterenol, or cardiac pacing may be required if a patient becomes symptomatic or if the block occurs in the setting of an acute anterior wall MI. Permanent pacing often is indicated for long-term management.

THIRD-DEGREE (COMPLETE) ATRIOVENTRICULAR BLOCK

In third-degree or complete heart block, the sinus node continues to fire normally, but the impulses do not reach the

table 17-10 **A Comparison of the Electrocardiographic Characteristics of Heart Block Rhythms**

	First-Degree Heart Block	Second-Degree Heart Block—Mobitz Type I (Wenckebach)	Second-Degree Heart Block—Mobitz Type II	Third-Degree Heart Block
Rate	Usually 60–100 beats/min	Usually 60–100 beats/min	May be slow depending on number of blocked P waves	Rate determined by ventricular focus, usually very slow
Rhythm	Regular	Irregular due to dropped QRS	Often regular but depends on pattern of block	May be regular or irregular ventricular focus
P waves	Present, one per QRS	Present, one per QRS until QRS is missed	Present, more than one P wave per QRS	Present, more than one P wave per QRS; P waves no relationship to QRS complexes
PR interval	>0.20 s, equal throughout	Progressively gets longer until QRS is missed; pattern repeats	May be normal or prolonged, equal throughout	May be normal or prolonged, unequal throughout
QRS complex	<0.12 s	<0.12 s	Usually >0.12 s	>0.12 s

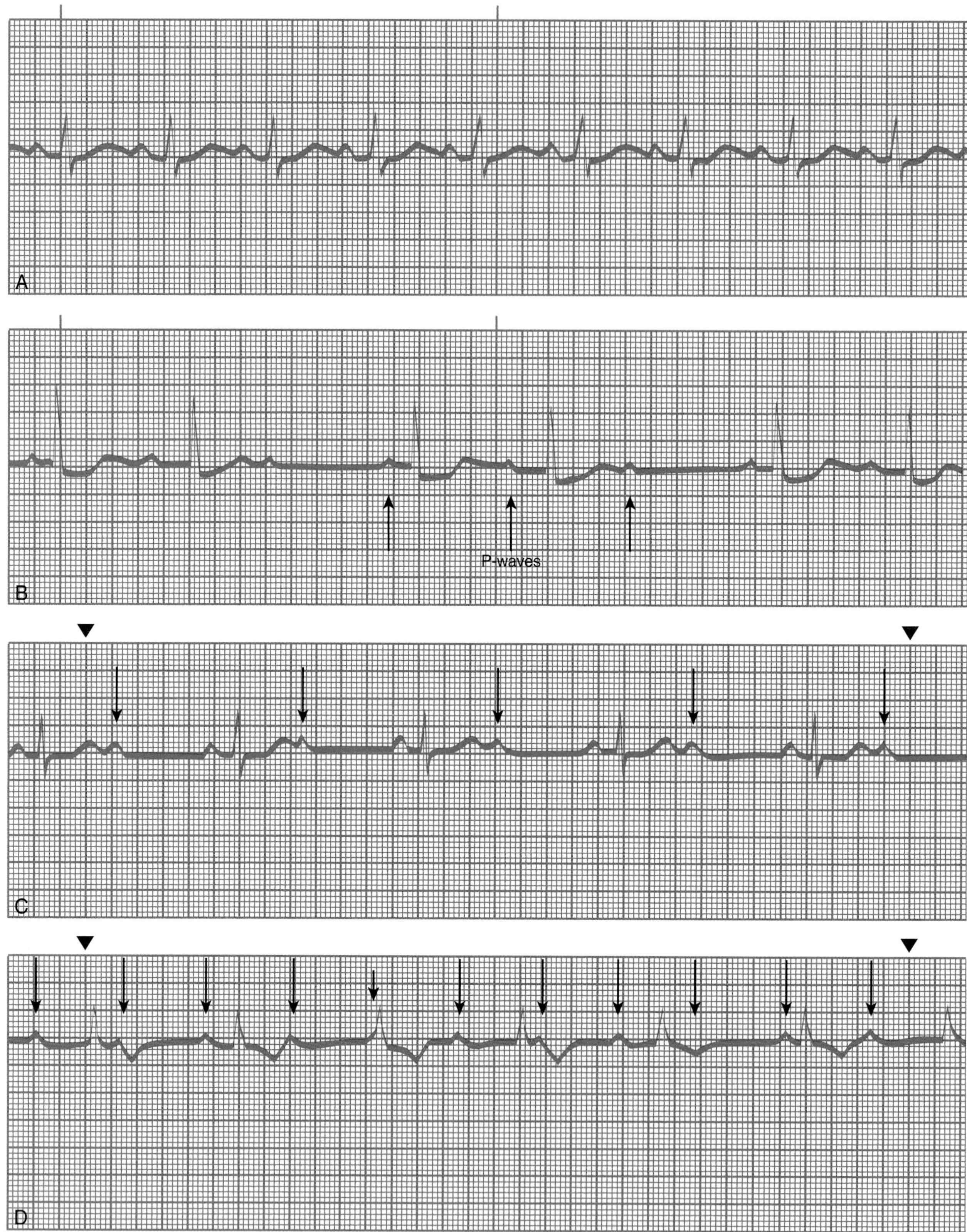

figure 17-41 Heart block rhythms. (**A**) First-degree heart block. (From Huff J: ECG Workout [4th Ed], p 156. Philadelphia, Lippincott Williams & Wilkins, 2002.) (**B**) Second-degree heart block: Mobitz type I. (From Huff J: ECG Workout [4th Ed], p 150. Philadelphia, Lippincott Williams & Wilkins, 2002.) (**C**) Second-degree heart block: Mobitz type II. Arrows denote blocked P wave (2:1 block). (**D**) Third-degree heart block (complete atrioventricular block). Arrows denote P waves. Note the lack of relationship between the atria (P wave) and ventricles (QRS).

ventricles (see Fig. 17-41D). The ventricles are stimulated from escape pacemaker cells either in the junction (at a rate of 40 to 60 beats/minute) or in the ventricles (at a rate of 20 to 40 beats/minute), depending on the level of the AV block.

On the ECG tracing, P waves and QRS complexes are both present, but there is no relationship between the two. Therefore, complete heart block is considered one form of AV dissociation. The PP and RR intervals are each regular, but the PR interval is variable. If a junctional pacemaker paces the ventricles, the QRS complex is narrow. A pacemaker site lower in the ventricles produces a wide QRS complex.

The causes of complete heart block are the same as for lesser degrees of AV block. Complete heart block is often poorly tolerated. The rate and dependability of the ventricular pacemaker depend on its location. If the escape rhythm is ventricular in origin, the rate is slow, and the pacemaker site is unreliable. The patient may be symptomatic because of a low cardiac output. A pacemaker site high in the bundle of His may provide an adequate rate and is more dependable. The patient may remain asymptomatic if the escape rhythm supports a normal cardiac output.

A temporary pacing wire is usually inserted immediately, and when the patient is stabilized, a permanent pacemaker is implanted.

The 12-Lead Electrocardiogram

THE NORMAL 12-LEAD ELECTROCARDIOGRAM

As previously described, the ECG provides 12 electrical views of the heart. The first three electrical views are provided by the standard leads I, II, and III. The next three electrical views are provided by the augmented leads, aVR, aVL, and aVF. The standard and augmented leads are referred to as the *limb leads* and provide a view from a vertical plane. The remaining six electrical views of the heart, the precordial leads, chest leads, or V leads, V_1 through V_6, provide a horizontal plane view of the heart (Fig. 17-42).

In the normal 12-lead ECG, the P wave representing atrial depolarization is usually upright and rounded. Each component of the QRS complex (ventricular depolarization) is analyzed separately. The Q wave, the initial downward deflection of the QRS complex, should be absent or small. The R component is the tallest upright portion of the QRS complex in the limb leads except aVR. In the precordial leads, the R wave begins as a small wave in V_1 and gradually progresses to a tall wave by V_6. The S wave, the downward stroke after the R wave, is small or absent in the limb leads. The S wave begins as a deep wave in V_1 and gradually disappears by V_6 in the precordial leads. The ST segment is isoelectric but may be slightly elevated in V_1 through V_3. The T wave, representing ventricular repolarization, is usually upright, although a variety of configurations can be normal. Table 17-11 summarizes the normal 12-lead ECG.

The 12-lead ECG may be useful in determining the electrical axis of the heart and detecting abnormalities that require more than one electrical view. These abnormalities include bundle branch block; atrial or ventricular enlargement; and patterns of ischemia, injury, or infarction.

ELECTRICAL AXIS

Electrical axis refers to the general direction of the wave of excitation as it moves through the heart. In the normal heart, the flow of electrical forces originates in the SA node, spreads throughout atrial tissue, passes through the AV node, and moves throughout the ventricles. This

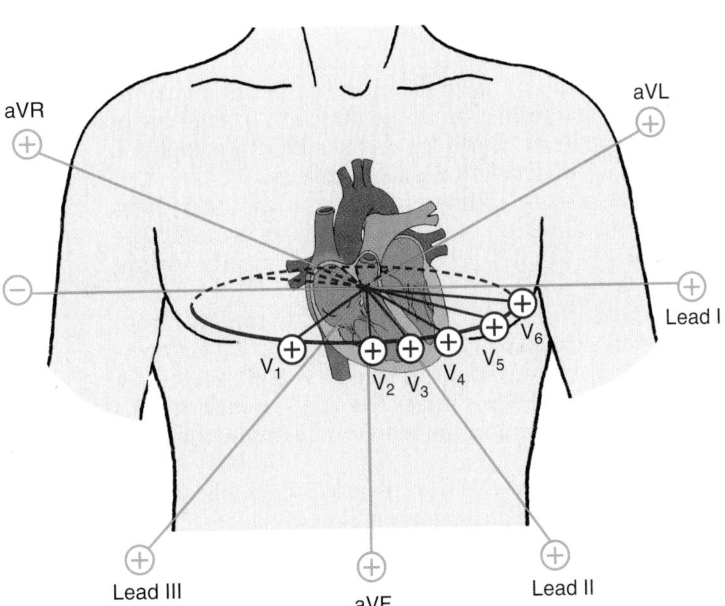

figure 17-42 Electrocardiographic views of the heart.

table 17-11 The Normal 12-Lead Electrocardiogram

Lead	P	Q	R	S	S-T	T
I	Upright	Small, 0.04 sec, or none	Dominant	<R or none	Isoelectric +1 to −0.5 mm	Upright
II	Upright	Small or none	Dominant	<R or none	+1 to −0.5 mm	Upright
III	Upright Flat Diphasic Inverted	Small or none	None to dominant	None to dominant	+1 to −0.5 mm	Upright Flat Diphasic Inverted
aVR	Inverted	Small, none, or large	Small or none	Dominant	+1 to −0.5 mm	Inverted
aVL	Upright Flat Diphasic Inverted	Small, none, or large	Small, none, or dominant	Small, none, or dominant	+1 to −0.5 mm	Upright Flat Diphasic Inverted
aVF	Upright Flat Diphasic Inverted	Small or none	Small, none, or dominant	None to dominant	+1 to −0.5 mm	Upright
V_1	Upright Flat Diphasic	None May be QS	Small	Deep	0 to +3 mm	Inverted Flat Upright Diphasic
V_2	Upright	None			0 to +3 mm	Upright Diphasic Inverted
V_3	Upright	Small or none			0 to +3 mm	Upright
V_4	Upright	Small or none			+1 to −0.5 mm	Upright
V_5	Upright	Small			+1 to −0.5 mm	Upright
V_6	Upright	Small	Tall	Small or none	+1 to −0.5 mm	Upright

flow of forces is normally downward and to the left, a pattern known as normal axis.

The ventricles make up the largest muscle mass of the heart and therefore make the most significant contribution to the determination of the direction of the flow of forces in the heart. For this reason, the QRS complex is examined when deciding the electrical axis.

A quick way to estimate the axis of the heart is to examine the direction of the QRS complex in leads I and aVF (Fig. 17-43). A QRS complex that is mainly upright in both leads represents a normal axis. A QRS complex that is upright in lead I and downward in lead aVF represents left axis deviation. A QRS complex that is downward in lead I and upright in lead aVF represents right axis deviation. A QRS complex that is downward in leads I and aVF is uncommon and represents extreme right axis deviation.

The direction of the flow of forces in the heart can change as a result of an anatomical shift of the heart in the chest wall. An anatomical shift may occur in very obese patients or in patients with large abdominal tumors or abdominal ascites. Left axis deviation can be caused by LBBB, left ventricular enlargement, or inferior wall MI.

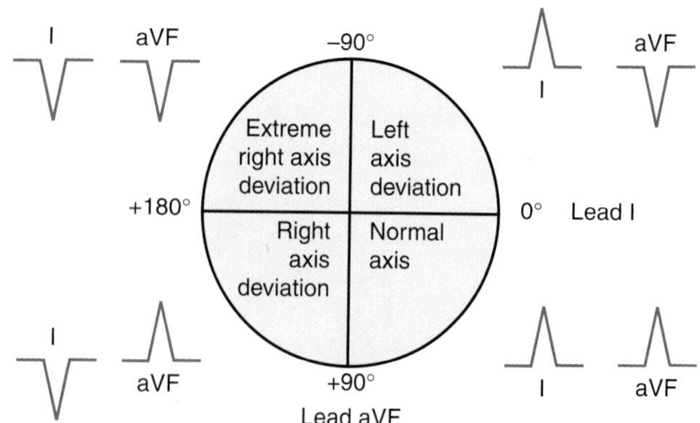

figure 17-43 Determining electrical axis. To determine the axis of the heart, examine the direction of the QRS complex in leads I and aVF.

Lead I	*Lead aVF*	*Axis*
Negative	Negative	Extreme right axis deviation
Negative	Positive	Right axis deviation
Positive	Negative	Left axis deviation
Positive	Positive	Normal axis

Right axis deviation can be caused by RBBB, right ventricular enlargement, or an anterior wall MI.[3]

Patients with an axis shift are asymptomatic. The only way an axis shift can be detected is through a 12-lead ECG. The axis shift usually represents some underlying abnormality, and treatment is directed at the underlying cause.

BUNDLE BRANCH BLOCK

A bundle branch block develops when there is either a functional or pathological block in one of the major branches of the intraventricular conduction system. As conduction through one bundle is blocked, the impulse travels along the unaffected bundle and activates one ventricle normally. The impulse is delayed in reaching the other ventricle because it travels outside of the normal conducting fibers. The right and left ventricles are thus depolarized sequentially instead of simultaneously. The abnormal activation produces a wide QRS complex, representing the increased time it takes for ventricular depolarization (Fig. 17-44). The broad QRS complex has two peaks (RSR′), indicating that depolarization of the two ventricles was not simultaneous.

An RBBB and LBBB are diagnosed on the 12-lead ECG but also can be identified on the bedside monitor using a V_1 or MCL_1 tracing and a V_6 or MCL_6 tracing (see section on Electrocardiographic Monitoring for description of lead selection). To identify the presence of a bundle branch block, the QRS complex duration must be prolonged to 0.12 second or longer, representing the delay in conduction through the ventricles. An RBBB alters the configuration of the QRS complex in the right-sided chest leads, V_1 and V_2. Normally, these leads have a small, single-peaked R-wave and deep S-wave configuration. With an RBBB, depolarization of the right ventricle is delayed, and the ECG pattern changes. An RBBB is evidenced by an RSR′ configuration in V_1. If the initial peak of the QRS complex is smaller than the second peak, the pattern would be described as rSR′. An "r" is used to describe the first, smaller peak, and an "R" is used to describe the second, taller peak. Likewise, if the initial peak of the QRS complex is taller than the second peak, the pattern is described as an Rsr′. Whenever ventricular depolarization is abnormal, so is ventricular repolarization. As a result, ST segment and T-wave

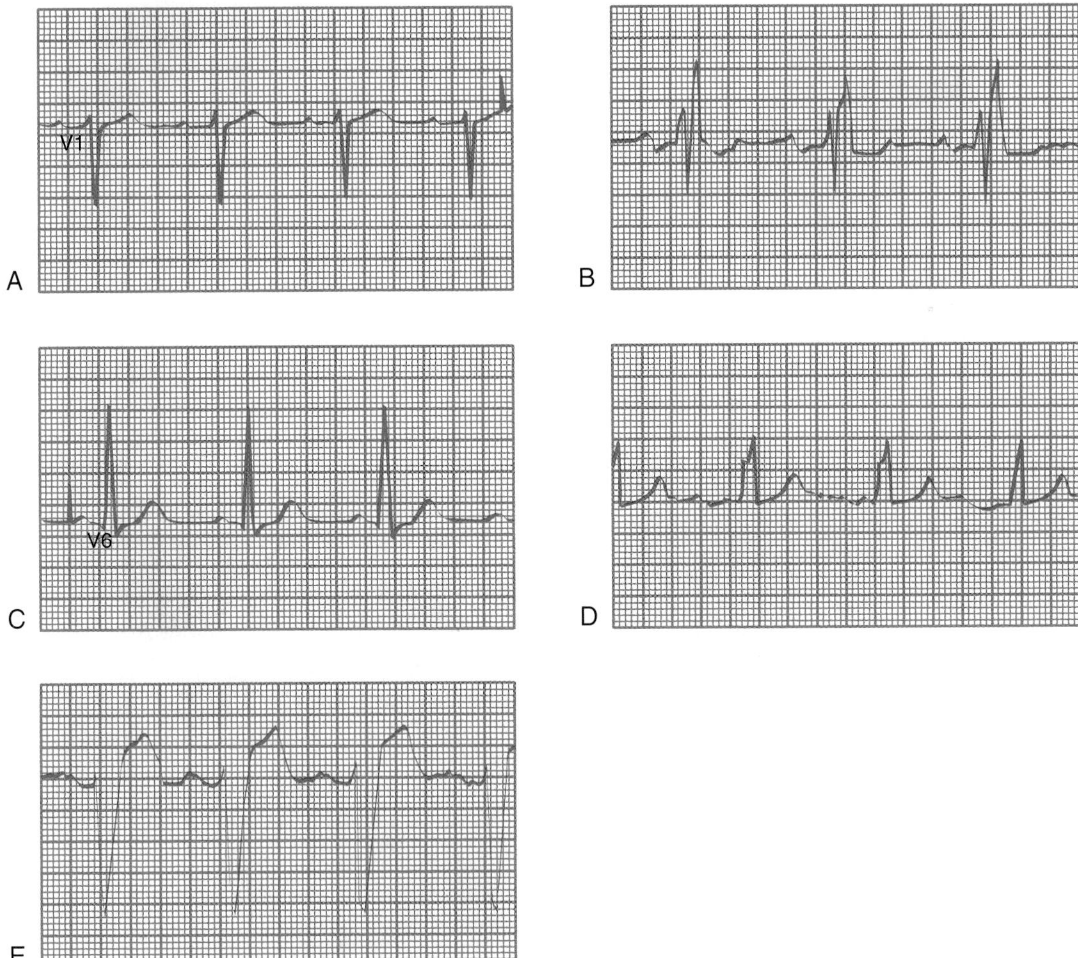

figure 17-44 Comparison of right versus left bundle branch block. (**A**) A normal V_1 tracing. Note the small narrow R and deep narrow S wave. (**B**) V_1 tracing showing the wide QRS complex and double-peaked R wave, indicating a right bundle branch block. (**C**) A normal V_6 tracing. Note the tall narrow R wave and absent S wave. (**D**) A V_6 tracing showing the side QRS complex and double-peaked R wave, indicating a left bundle branch block. (**E**) A V_1 tracing. Note the small narrow R and deep wide S wave, indicating a left bundle branch block.

abnormalities may be seen in leads V_1 and V_2 for patients with an RBBB.[4]

An LBBB changes the QRS complex pattern in the left-sided chest leads, V_5 and V_6. Normally, these leads have a tall, single-peaked R wave and a small or absent S wave. Instead, the double-peaked RSR′ pattern is noted. In addition, V_1 shows a small R wave with a widened S wave, indicating delayed conduction through the ventricles. Like RBBB, the ST segments and T waves may be abnormal in the left-sided chest leads V_5 and V_6 when the patient has an LBBB[4] (see Fig. 17-44).

The most common causes of bundle branch block are MI, hypertension, heart failure, and cardiomyopathy. RBBB may be found in healthy individuals with no clinical evidence of heart disease. Congenital lesions involving the septum and right ventricular hypertrophy are other causes of RBBB. LBBB is usually associated with some type of underlying heart disease. Long-term cardiovascular disease in the older patient is a common cause of LBBB.

Bundle branch block signifies underlying disease of the intraventricular conduction system. Patients should be monitored for involvement of the other bundles or fascicles or for progression to complete heart block. Progression of block may be very slow or rapid, depending on the clinical setting. A new-onset LBBB in conjunction with an acute MI is associated with a higher mortality rate.

The underlying heart disease determines treatment and prognosis. Patients with an MI and new-onset bundle branch block are closely monitored for progression to a type of complete heart block. A temporary pacemaker may be inserted.

ENLARGEMENT PATTERNS

Enlargement of a cardiac chamber may involve hypertrophy of the muscle or dilation of the chamber. The most common causes include pumping for a prolonged period against high pressures or pumping for a prolonged period to move blood through narrowed valves. Electrocardiography is not an ideal diagnostic tool for determining the cause of the enlargement. Echocardiography is more helpful in determining if the enlargement is the result of hypertrophy or dilation. The terminology used to describe enlargement patterns on the ECG can be confusing. The term *ventricular hypertrophy* is commonly used because hypertrophy is the most frequent cause of the enlargement pattern in the ventricles. The general terms *atrial abnormality* and *atrial enlargement* are often used rather than the specific terms *atrial hypertrophy* or *atrial dilation* because atrial changes on the ECG may result from a variety of causes, including atrial dilation, hypertrophy, or other conditions.

Right Atrial Enlargement

When the atria enlarge, changes are seen in the P wave because the P wave represents atrial depolarization. Right atrial enlargement is noted on the ECG by the presence of tall, pointed P waves in leads II, III, and aVF. The P wave in V_1 may show a diphasic wave with an initial upstroke that is larger than the downstroke (Fig. 17-45B).

The right atrium is more likely to enlarge as a result of pressures created by pulmonary causes, such as pulmonary hypertension and chronic obstructive pulmonary disease.

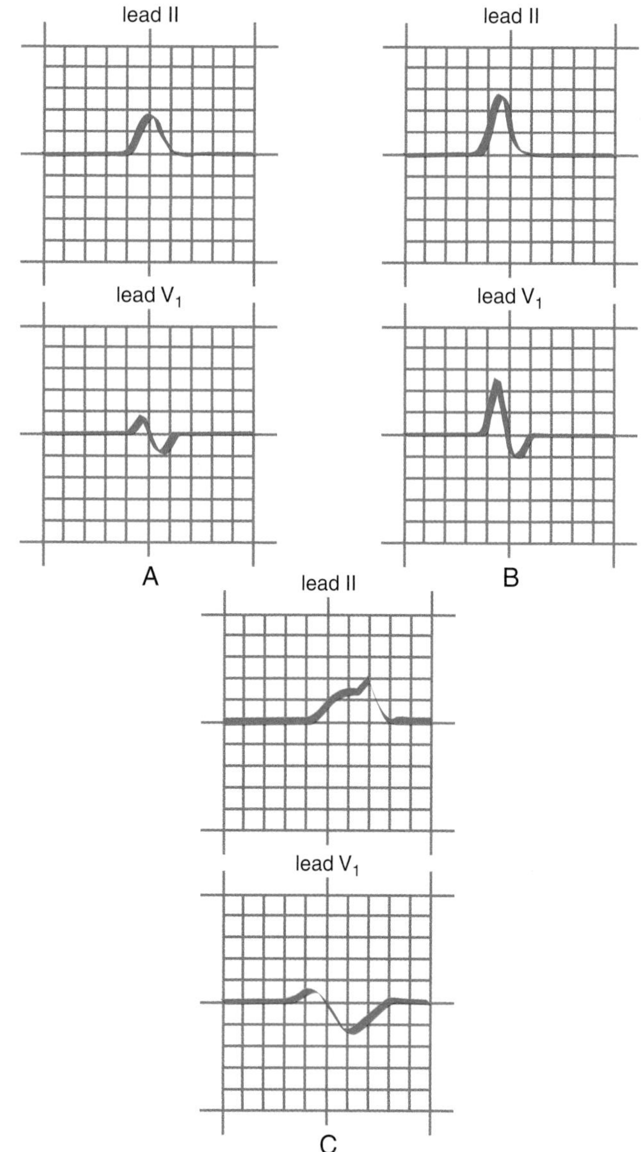

figure 17-45 Right versus left atrial enlargement. (**A**) The normal P wave in leads II and V_1. (**B**) Right atrial enlargement. Note the increased amplitude of the early, right atrial component of the P wave in V_1 and the tall, pointed P wave in lead II. (**C**) Left atrial enlargement. Note the increased amplitude and duration of the P wave in V_1 and the broad, notched P wave in lead II.

For this reason, right atrial enlargement is often referred to as P pulmonale. Right atrial enlargement is often associated with right ventricular hypertrophy.

Treatment is directed at the underlying cause. Often, however, the underlying cause may be a chronic condition that cannot be cured.

Left Atrial Enlargement

Left atrial enlargement is noted on the ECG by the presence of broad, notched P waves in leads I, II, and aVL. The P wave in V_1 may show a diphasic wave with a terminal downstroke that is larger than the initial upstroke (see Fig. 17-45C).

The left atrium is more likely to enlarge because of increased pressures created by trying to pump blood through a stenotic mitral valve. For this reason, left atrial enlargement is often referred to as P mitrale. When a left atrial enlargement pattern is noted on the ECG, the patient should be evaluated for the presence of mitral stenosis. An echocardiogram is a helpful diagnostic tool in addition to cardiac auscultation. Treatment is directed at the underlying cause. A valve replacement may be necessary.

Right Ventricular Hypertrophy

Right ventricular hypertrophy (RVH) may exist without clear evidence on the ECG because the left ventricle normally is larger than the right and can mask changes in the size of the right ventricle. ECG evidence suggestive of RVH includes right atrial enlargement and right axis deviation. In addition, the normal QRS complex pattern across the precordial leads is reversed. Normally, R waves are small in V_1 and gradually grow tall by V_6. With RVH, the R wave is tall in V_1 and progresses to small by V_6. Precordial S waves persist rather than gradually disappear.

The presence of RVH is most likely an indicator of a chronic pulmonary condition, most likely chronic obstructive pulmonary disease, pulmonary hypertension, or pulmonic stenosis. Right atrial enlargement is usually seen with an accompanying RVH. Treatment is directed at the underlying pulmonary disease.

Left Ventricular Hypertrophy

Numerous criteria exist for the detection of LVH on the ECG. The simplest criterion involves remembering the number "35." LVH is determined by adding the deepest S wave in either V_1 or V_2 to the tallest R wave in either V_5 or V_6. If the sum is 35 mm or more and the patient is older than 35 years, LVH is suspected.[4] In addition, the T waves in V_5 and V_6 may be asymmetrically inverted, and the a left axis shift is likely.

Most likely, LVH is the result of chronic systemic hypertension, a chronic cardiovascular problem, or aortic stenosis. LVH may result in a displacement of the PMI when palpating the apical pulse. Treatment of LVH is directed at the underlying condition.

ISCHEMIA, INJURY, AND INFARCTION PATTERNS

The 12-lead ECG can be very useful in detecting evidence of myocardial ischemia, injury, or infarction. Ischemia is seen on the ECG by ST segment depressions and T-wave inversions. Acute patterns of injury are noted by ST segment elevations. The presence of significant Q waves indicates an MI. For a more detailed discussion of patterns of ischemia, injury, and infarction, see Chapter 21.

EFFECTS OF SERUM ELECTROLYTE ABNORMALITIES ON THE ELECTROCARDIOGRAM

Maintenance of adequate fluid and electrolyte balance assumes high priority in the care of patients in any medical, surgical, or coronary ICU. Patients being treated for renal or cardiovascular diseases are especially vulnerable to electrolyte imbalances. The cure may well be worse than the disease if electrolyte abnormalities go undetected or ignored because they frequently are caused by the treatment rather than by the disease itself.

Diuresis can very quickly cause major shifts in electrolytes. Certainly, the often insidious drop of serum potassium levels in the patient with cardiac disease who has been taking digitalis and then starts diuretics is well known. Diuretics also are used frequently as part of the medical regimen for the control of hypertension. Any addition, deletion, or change in diuretic therapy warrants close monitoring of serum electrolytes. A history of any of these problems should alert the nurse to check the patient's serum electrolytes on an ongoing basis.

Potassium and calcium are probably the two most important electrolytes involved in the proper function of the heart. Because of their effects on the electrical impulse in the heart, an excess or insufficiency of either electrolyte frequently causes changes in the ECG (Table 17-12). The nurse who is aware of and able to recognize these changes may well suspect electrolyte abnormalities before laboratory findings or clinical symptoms appear and hazardous arrhythmias occur.

However, it is necessary to remember that just as a patient who sustains MI may not have chest pain, the patient with electrolyte abnormalities may not exhibit any of the ECG changes described in the following sections. The ECG manifestations are valuable primarily in arousing suspicion of electrolyte abnormalities. Not one of them even approaches being diagnostic.

table 17-12 **Electrocardiographic Changes Associated With Electrolyte Imbalances**

Hyperkalemia	Tall, narrow, peaked T waves; flat, wide P waves; widening QRS complex	Sinus bradycardia; sinoatrial block; junctional rhythm; idioventricular rhythm; ventricular tachycardia; ventricular fibrillation
Hypokalemia	Prominent U waves; ST segment depression; T-wave flattening or inversion	Premature ventricular beats; supraventricular tachycardia; ventricular tachycardia; ventricular fibrillation
Hypercalcemia	Shortened QT interval	Premature ventricular contractions
Hypocalcemia	Lengthened QT interval; T-wave flattening or inversion	Ventricular tachycardia

Potassium

Potassium is the primary intracellular cation found in the body. Inside the cardiac cell, potassium is important for repolarization and for maintaining a stable, polarized state.

HYPERKALEMIA

The earliest sign of hyperkalemia on the ECG is a change in the T wave. It usually is described as tall, narrow, and "peaked" or "tented" in appearance (Fig. 17-46). As the serum potassium level increases, the P-wave amplitude decreases and the PR interval is prolonged. Atrial asystole occurs, along with a widening of the QRS complex. At high, near-lethal potassium levels, the widened QRS complex merges with the T wave and starts to resemble a sine wave. Various arrhythmias may occur during this time, with progression to VF and asystole. Clinically, the described changes in T waves begin to appear at serum levels of 6 to 7 mEq/L, and QRS complex widening is seen at serum levels of 8 to 9 mEq/L. Vigorous treatment must be instituted to reverse the condition at this point because sudden death may occur at any time after these levels are reached.

The ECG changes in hyperkalemia also may be associated with other conditions. Tall, peaked T waves may be a normal finding or may occur in the early stages of MI. QRS complex widening may be seen with quinidine and procainamide toxicity.

HYPOKALEMIA

Hypokalemia is associated with the appearance of U waves. Although the presence of U waves may be normal in many individuals, these waves also may be an early sign of hypokalemia (Fig. 17-47). Usually easily recognized (best seen in lead V_3), a U wave may encroach on the preceding T wave and go unnoticed. The T wave may look notched or prolonged when it is hiding the U wave, giving the appearance of a prolonged QT interval. With increased potassium depletion, the U wave may become more prominent as the T wave becomes less so. The T wave becomes flattened and may even invert. The ST segment tends to become depressed, somewhat resembling the effects of digitalis on the ECG. Only at very low serum levels is there reasonable correlation between ECG changes and serum potassium concentrations.

The changes seen in hypokalemia also are observed in other conditions. The U wave may be accentuated in association with digitalis, LVH, and bradycardia.

Untreated hypokalemia enhances instability in the myocardial cell. Ventricular premature beats are the most common manifestation of this imbalance, but supraventricular arrhythmias, conduction problems, and eventually VT and VF may occur. Hypokalemia also increases the sensitivity of the heart to digitalis and its accompanying arrhythmias, even at normal serum levels. The severity of the arrhythmias associated with hypokalemia requires early recognition of this problem.

Calcium

Like potassium, calcium is important in normal cardiac function. It is essential for the initiation and propagation of electrical impulses and for myocardial contractility. Abnor-

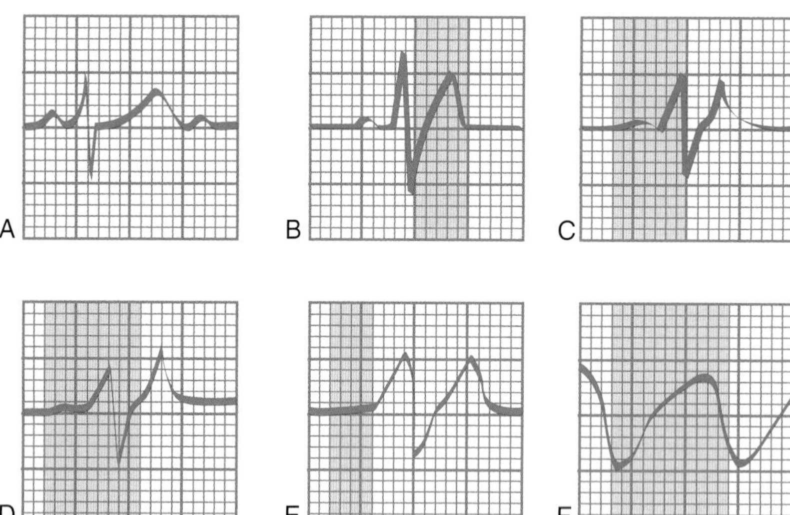

figure 17-46 The effect of hyperkalemia on an ECG. (**A**) This waveform is produced when the serum potassium level falls within the normal range—usually considered to be 3.5 to 5 mEq/L. (**B**) When the serum potassium level rises above 5.5 mEq/L, the T wave begins to peak (see highlighted area). The P wave and QRS complex are normal. (**C**) When the potassium level exceeds 6.5 mEq/L, the P wave grows wider and its amplitude falls. The QRS complex also widens (see highlighted area) as intraventricular conduction velocity diminishes. (**D**) When the potassium level reaches 10 mEq/L, the P wave becomes almost indiscernible; the QRS complex is slurred and widened (see highlighted area). (**E**) When the potassium level ranges from 10 to 12 mEq/L, the P wave is undetectable (see highlighted area), because the atria are no longer excitable. (**F**) When the potassium level exceeds 12 mEq/L, the QRS complex is no longer identifiable. The waves are known as sine waves (see highlighted area). Ventricular fibrillation and cardiac arrest follow. (From Springhouse: ECG Interpretation: Clinical Skillbuilders, p 113. Springhouse, PA, author, 1990.)

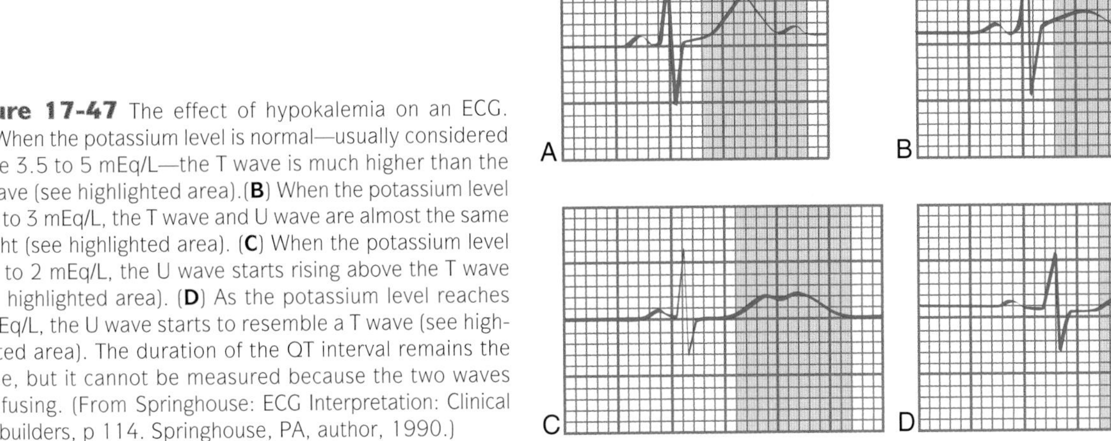

figure 17-47 The effect of hypokalemia on an ECG. (**A**) When the potassium level is normal—usually considered to be 3.5 to 5 mEq/L—the T wave is much higher than the U wave (see highlighted area).(**B**) When the potassium level falls to 3 mEq/L, the T wave and U wave are almost the same height (see highlighted area). (**C**) When the potassium level falls to 2 mEq/L, the U wave starts rising above the T wave (see highlighted area). (**D**) As the potassium level reaches 1 mEq/L, the U wave starts to resemble a T wave (see highlighted area). The duration of the QT interval remains the same, but it cannot be measured because the two waves are fusing. (From Springhouse: ECG Interpretation: Clinical Skillbuilders, p 114. Springhouse, PA, author, 1990.)

mal calcium levels are not commonly seen unless they are associated with an underlying disease, and therefore they are not as common as serum potassium abnormalities.

HYPERCALCEMIA

On an ECG, the major finding associated with hypercalcemia is shortening of the QT interval (Fig. 17-48A). Because the QRS complex and T wave usually are unaffected by changes in serum calcium levels, the shortened QT interval is a result of shortening of the ST segment. QT interval shortening also is seen in patients taking digitalis. In addition, ST segment depression occasionally occurs, and T-wave inversion may be seen.

HYPOCALCEMIA

On an ECG, low serum calcium levels prolong the QT interval because of a lengthening of the ST segment (see Fig. 17-48B). The T wave itself is not prolonged but may be inverted in some cases. The prolongation of the QT interval in hypocalcemia should not be mistaken for a prolonged QTU interval seen in hypokalemia. In patients with chronic renal failure, hypocalcemia may be associated with decreased potassium levels.

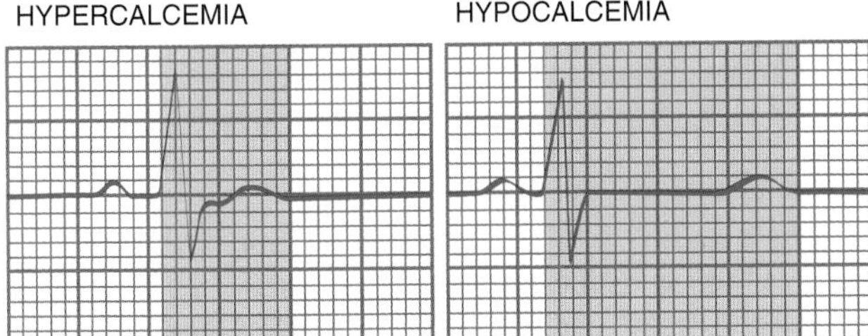

figure 17-48 The effects of hypercalcemia and hypocalcemia on an ECG. Changes in serum calcium levels are reflected in phase 2 of the action potential. Hypercalcemia shortens the QT interval, whereas hypocalcemia lengthens it (see highlighted areas). (From Springhouse: ECG Interpretation: Clinical Skillbuilders, p 115. Springhouse, PA, author, 1990.)

QT interval prolongation also may be seen in cerebral vascular disease and after cardiac arrest. Several antiarrhythmic agents produce prolonged QT intervals and always should be considered when evaluating an ECG for hypocalcemic changes.

HEMODYNAMIC MONITORING

The purposes of hemodynamic monitoring are to aid the diagnosis of various cardiovascular disorders, guide therapies to minimize cardiovascular dysfunction or treat disorders, and evaluate response to therapy. To incorporate hemodynamic data into the care of the critically ill, the nurse must understand the following:

- Cardiopulmonary anatomy and physiology
- Monitoring system components to measure pressures and cardiac output
- Rationales for interventions directed toward enhancing cardiac output, oxygen delivery, and oxygen consumption
- Potential complications
- Distinguishing between physiological changes and mechanical or monitoring system problems

Pressure Monitoring System

Basic equipment necessary to measure hemodynamic pressures includes noncompliant pressure tubing, a transducer, an amplifier, and a means of recording or displaying the information collected (Fig. 17-49). Hemodynamic pressures are transmitted from the intravascular space or cardiac chamber through the catheter and the fluid in the noncompliant pressure tubing to the pressure transducer. A transducer is a device that converts one form of energy into another. A pressure transducer senses changes in the fluid column generated by the pressures in the cardiac chambers or vessels being monitored. When pressure is applied to the diaphragm of the transducer, sensors are compressed, changing electrical flow to the amplifier or monitor. The monitor then converts the electrical signal generated by the

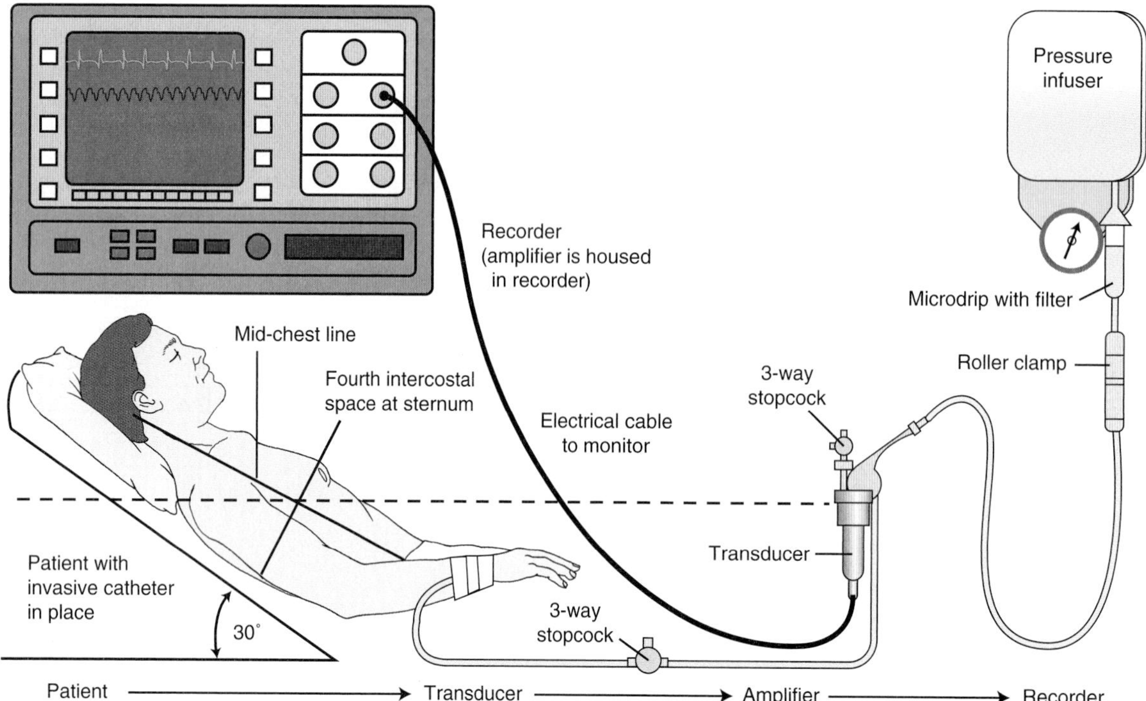

figure 17-49 Indwelling arterial catheter. The catheter is attached by pressure tubing to a transducer. The transducer is connected to an amplifier/monitor that visually displays a waveform and systolic, diastolic, and mean pressure values. The system is composed of a flush solution under pressure, a continuous flush device, and a series of stopcocks. The stopcock closest to the insertion site is used to draw blood samples from the artery, and the stopcock located near the transducer is used for zeroing.

transducer to a pressure tracing and digital value. In general, bedside monitoring systems have the capability to display several digital readings, whereas the oscilloscope displays the pressure waveforms simultaneously. The monitors also include mechanisms to set or adjust alarms and waveform size and zero the system.

Pressure transmission from the catheter in the patient to the transducer occurs through fluid-filled, noncompliant pressure tubing. The patency of the hemodynamic monitoring system is maintained by a continuous infusion of flush solution. The flush solution may be normal saline or D_5W and is usually heparinized. The solution is placed in a pressure bag that is inflated to 300 mm Hg to maintain a constant pressure through the transducer and flush device. A continuous flow of approximately 3 mL/hour prevents backflow of blood through the catheter and tubing, thereby maintaining system patency and accurate transmission of pressures. The system can be flushed manually by activation of a fast flush device.

OPTIMAL USE OF THE MONITORING SYSTEM

Several technical or mechanical factors may cause inaccuracies of the hemodynamic waveforms and values. For instance, air bubbles or blood in the tubing or transducer system distorts pressure readings. Also, as mentioned previously, the system requires continuous pressure of 300 mm Hg on the flush solution bag and noncompliant pressure tubing connecting the transducer to the indwelling catheter. The use of soft, distensible tubing distorts and reduces the amplitude of the pressure waveforms. To decrease the distance over which pressures are transmitted to the transducer, the length of the pressure tubing is kept to a minimum. Stopcocks are included in most prepackaged systems for sampling of blood and zeroing of the transducer. The number of these stopcocks and any other connections should be as low as possible, and Luer-Loks should be used to preserve the integrity of the system.

Square-Wave Test

A square-wave test helps identify whether the hemodynamic system is optimized. By activating the fast flush device for 1 or 2 seconds, the pressure waveform on the oscilloscope is replaced by a square wave. In an optimized system, the square wave has a straight vertical upstroke from the baseline, a straight horizontal component, and, most important, a straight vertical downstroke back to the baseline with two of three sharp oscillations.[1,2] Figure 17-50 depicts a normal square wave and examples of square waves from nonoptimized hemodynamic monitoring systems. Causes of nonoptimized systems include air bubbles, blood, loose connections, cracks, leaks, or soft IV tubing in the system.

Zeroing and Leveling

The position of the transducer in relation to the patient's atria and the system calibration also affects the accuracy of the hemodynamic values. Before obtaining hemodynamic parameters, the transducer is leveled and zeroed. A transducer placed above the reference point produces falsely low readings; conversely, a transducer below the reference point produces falsely high readings. Every inch the transducer is above or below the reference point produces a 2 mm Hg change in pressure reading.

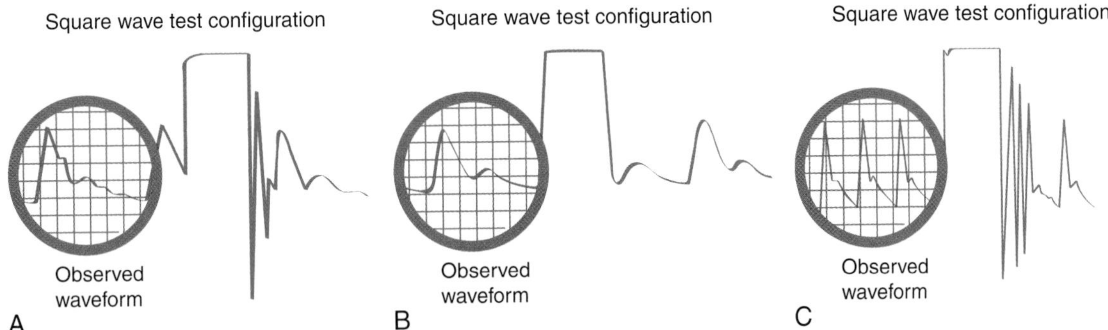

figure 17-50 Square wave test. (**A**) Optimally damped system: Activation of the fast flush device generates a sharp vertical upstroke, horizontal line, and straight vertical downstroke ending with one or two oscillations (minimal ringing) and quick return to the baseline. (**B**) Overdamped system: Activation of the fast flush device generates a slurred upstroke and downstroke with no oscillations above or below the baseline. Causes of an overdamped system include system leaks, blood clots, or air bubbles in the tubing or transducer. (**C**) Underdamped system: Activation of the fast flush device (more than three) above and below the baseline. Usually caused by a small air bubble in the system. (From Darovic GO: Hemodynamic Monitoring: Invasive and Noninvasive Clinical Application, p 161. Philadelphia, W. B. Saunders, 1995.)

The zero reference point is established at the intersection of the mid–anterior-posterior line and the fourth intercostal space (see Fig. 17-49). This point is known as the *phlebostatic axis.* Once the zero reference point has been established, the patient's chest must be marked to ensure consistent transducer placement when subsequent pressure readings are obtained by other practitioners.

The patient is placed on his or her back, and the head of the bed may be elevated. With a carpenter-type level, the transducer is placed even with the preestablished zero reference point. Further hemodynamic pressure measurements are taken with the patient in the supine position. Measurements should not be obtained in the side-lying position because of variability in the readings and inconsistent leveling of the transducer. The head of the bed may be elevated as much as 40 degrees, providing the transducer is releveled after any changes in patient position.

Zeroing the system negates any effect of atmospheric pressure on the pressure readings, ensuring measurements reflect only pressure values in the vessel or heart chamber being monitored. After leveling the transducer, the system is zeroed by turning the stopcock on the transducer off to the patient and open to air. Typically, the bedside monitor has a function key that is used to zero the system. When it is activated, the monitor adjusts the digital reading to zero and indicates that the zeroing procedure was successful. The transducer should be zeroed with any change in the bed or patient's position, elevation of the head of the bed, and patient transport. It also should be zeroed every 8 hours.

Arterial Pressure Monitoring

Arterial pressure monitoring is achieved through an intra-arterial catheter connected to the pressure monitoring system. This allows continuous monitoring of the systemic arterial blood pressure and provides vascular access for obtaining blood samples by withdrawing blood from a stopcock in the system. Arterial blood pressure monitoring is indicated for patients receiving vasoactive IV infusions or those with fluctuating, unstable blood pressures.

ARTERIAL LINE INSERTION

The most common sites for arterial catheter insertions are the radial and femoral arteries. Alternative and less frequent sites include the brachial, axillary, and dorsalis pedis arteries in adults as well as the temporal and umbilical arteries in neonates. Artery selection is made after the following factors are considered:

- Size of the artery in relation to the size of the catheter; the artery should be large enough to accommodate the catheter without occluding or significantly impeding flow.
- Accessibility of the site; the chosen site should be easily accessible and free from contamination by body secretions.
- Blood flow to the limb distal to the insertion site; there should be adequate collateral flow in the event that the cannulated artery becomes occluded.

The radial artery, which satisfies these criteria, is the most frequent site for an arterial catheter. It is superficially located and therefore easy to palpate. Cannulation of this artery also usually poses the least limitation on the patient's mobility.

Before a catheter is inserted into the radial artery, the presence of adequate collateral circulation to the hand by the ulnar artery is assessed by performing Allen's test (Fig. 17-51). Both the ulnar and radial arteries are occluded. The patient then clenches and unclenches the fist until the hand is blanched. Pressure on the ulnar artery is released, and the hand is observed for return of color. If color returns in 5 to 7 seconds, the ulnar circulation to the hand is adequate. If color returns in 7 to 15 seconds, ulnar filling is impaired. If the hand remains blanched for longer than 15 seconds, ulnar circulation is considered inadequate, in which case the radial artery should not be cannulated.

Regardless of the site chosen for arterial catheter placement, the insertion is performed under sterile technique.

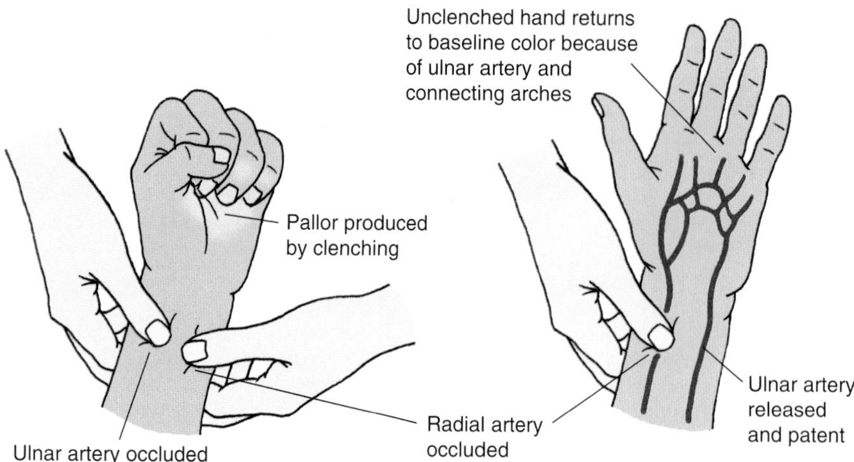

figure 17-51 Modified Allen's test.

The connecting tubing is assembled and flushed, and the transducer is leveled, zeroed, and calibrated before the catheter is inserted. Once the catheter is in place, it should be secured and the site dressed according to institutional policy.

ARTERIAL PRESSURE WAVEFORM

The normal arterial waveform should have a rapid upstroke, a clear dicrotic notch, and a definite end-diastole, as shown in Figure 17-52. The initial sharp upstroke of the waveform represents the rapid ejection of blood from the ventricle into the aorta. Note that the QRS complex precedes the rapid rise in arterial pressure. Ventricular depolarization causes ventricular contraction and the sharp increase in pressure. This increase in pressure therefore follows the QRS complex. The dicrotic notch reflects a slight backflow of blood in the aorta, reflecting closure of the aortic valve when the aortic pressure is higher than the left ventricular pressure. The dicrotic notch corresponds with the end of ventricular repolarization and the T wave on the ECG.[3]

The value measured at the peak of the waveform is the systolic pressure. A normal systolic pressure is typically 90 to 140 mm Hg. The dicrotic notch then indicates the end of ventricular systole and the beginning of diastole. As blood flows to the periphery, the pressure in the arterial system decreases. The lowest point of the waveform is the diastolic pressure, normally between 60 and 90 mm Hg.

Mean arterial pressure (MAP) is used to evaluate perfusion of vital body organs. Normal MAP is 70 to 105 mm Hg. Most bedside monitors automatically calculate and continuously display the MAP.

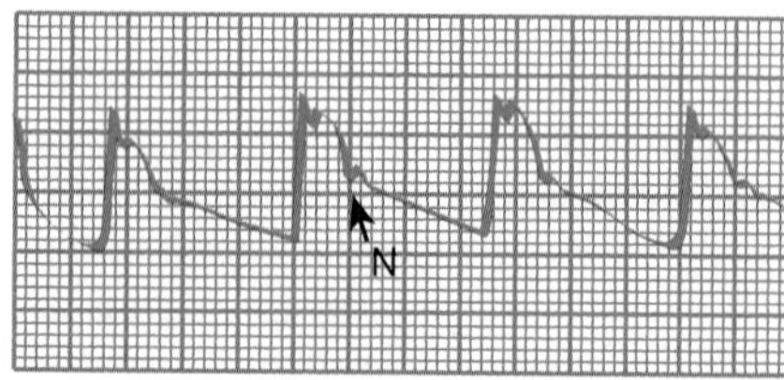

figure 17-52 Normal features of an arterial pressure wave. These include a prominent pulse pressure (50 mm Hg in this patient) and a dicrotic notch (*N*) signifying closure of the aortic valve. The crisp dicrotic notch indicates a properly responsive catheter system.

COMPLICATIONS

Infection

Proper attention to sterile technique during catheter insertion, care of the insertion site, blood sampling, and maintenance of a sterile, closed monitoring system reduce the risk of infection. The insertion site is assessed frequently for signs of infection. Sterile dressing changes, tubing changes, and flush solution changes are performed according to institutional policy, while the integrity of the system is maintained. Aspiration removes blood or air in the system through the stopcocks. The stopcocks are flushed and cleaned of any blood residue each time a blood sample is withdrawn. Sterile caps must be used to cover the stopcock ports between use.

Accidental Blood Loss

Accidental blood loss from an arterial catheter usually can be prevented. All connections in the system should use Luer-Loks. The extremity in which the catheter is placed may be immobilized (e.g., placing the wrist on an arm board). If some type of patient self-protective device is used, it should not be placed over the insertion site. Easy access to the insertion site and connections is imperative.

Impaired Circulation to Extremity

Circulation to the extremity in which the arterial line is placed must be monitored frequently. Initial assessment of color, sensation, temperature, and movement of the extremity is made after insertion of the arterial catheter and at least every 8 hours for as long as the catheter is in place. Any indication of impaired circulation may be an indication for catheter removal and is reported immediately to the physician.

NURSING CONSIDERATIONS

Blood pressures obtained using an arterial catheter are compared with auscultated pressures occasionally and whenever the accuracy of the monitored pressure is questioned. Although the two methods of blood pressure measurement reflect different physiological events and are therefore not truly comparable, they are somewhat correlated. Blood pressures obtained using an arterial catheter are usually 5 to 20 mm Hg higher than those obtained using a cuff.

Bedside monitor alarms provide warning that a change has occurred either in the system or in the patient's physiological status. The high and low alarms are set for systolic, diastolic, and mean pressures within 10 to 20 mm Hg of the patient's typical blood pressure. Nursing assessment of the patient after hearing an alarm includes evaluating the cuff blood pressure, performing the square-wave test, examining the monitoring system for disconnections, checking for bleeding at the catheter insertion site, and observing for kinking of the catheter because of extremity involvement.

If catheter patency is in question, blood and fluid are aspirated from the blood-drawing port or stopcock in an attempt to remove a blood clot, and then the system is flushed using the fast flush device. The system should not be flushed with a syringe. No IV solution or medication should be administered through the arterial pressure monitoring system at any time.

Central Venous Pressure Monitoring

Central venous pressure (CVP) reflects the pressure of blood in the right atrium or vena cava. It provides information about intravascular blood volume, right ventricular end-diastolic pressure, and right ventricular function. To a very limited degree, the CVP indirectly reflects left ventricular end-diastolic volume and function, because the left and right sides of the heart are linked by the pulmonary vascular bed. Alterations in volume status or ventricular function usually are associated with abnormally high or low CVP measurements. Although isolated CVP measurements using a water manometer generally have been replaced by hemodynamic monitoring techniques, an understanding of both methods of CVP measurements is valuable.

CATHETER INSERTION

The CVP catheter is long and flexible. It is inserted under sterile conditions with a povidone–iodine (Betadine) site preparation. The physician uses a sterile field, gloves and gown, and a mask and cap. Those assisting the physician also should wear a cap and mask and sterile gloves if near the catheter or insertion site. The CVP IV catheter is inserted into an antecubital, jugular, femoral, or subclavian vein and is threaded into position in the vena cava close to the right atrium. Occasionally, the catheter may advance into the right atrium. If a water manometer is used to measure the CVP, rhythmic fluctuations appear in the manometer corresponding to the patient's heart rate. If a pressure transducer system is used, the hemodynamic waveform tracing on the bedside monitor becomes more pronounced. In this situation, the catheter is withdrawn several centimeters until either the fluctuations cease or the pressure tracing reflects the CVP.

CENTRAL VENOUS PRESSURE MEASUREMENT

Water Manometer

Figure 17-53 illustrates a typical setup for measuring the CVP using a water manometer. A manometer with a three-way stopcock is introduced between the IV solution and the patient's IV catheter. The stopcock is manipulated to open the IV solution flow to the patient, bypassing the manometer, or it is turned off to the IV solution, allowing open communication between the CVP catheter and the manometer. Before the CVP is measured, the manometer is partially filled with solution from the IV bag by turning the stopcock off to the patient and open to the IV solution tubing and the manometer.

To measure the CVP with the water manometer, the stopcock is opened to the manometer and the patient.

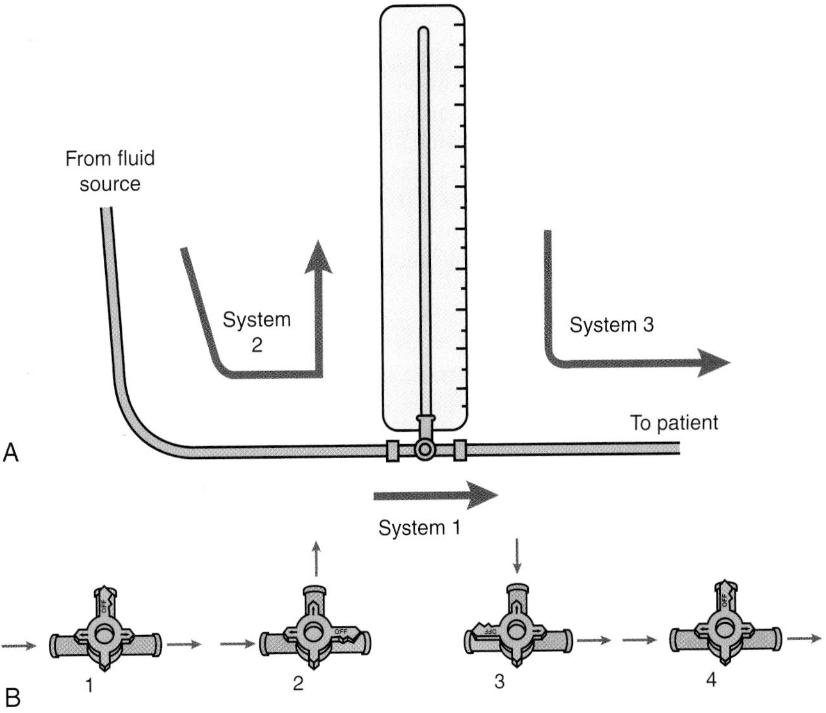

figure 17-53 Measuring central venous pressure (CVP) using a water manometer. (**A**) System 1 allows for fluid administration. System 2 fills the manometer with fluid. System 3 allows the flow of fluid from the manometer to the patient and determines the CVP reading. (**B**) Steps in measuring CVP. (1) Stopcock turned so that IV fluid flows to patient. (2) Stopcock in position to fill manometer with fluid. (3) Stopcock turned so that it is open from manometer to patient to obtain reading. (4) Stopcock returned to first position so that IV fluid flows to patient.

Pressure in the vena cava equilibrates with the pressure exerted by the column of fluid in the manometer. The point at which the fluid level settles is the CVP. A slight fluctuation in the manometer may occur; this corresponds with the patient's respiratory rate. A patent system is ensured when the fluid column falls freely and the slight fluctuation of the fluid column is apparent. The fluid level in the manometer falls on inspiration and rises on expiration because of changes in intrapulmonary pressure.

Pressure Transducer

The hemodynamic monitoring system components and preparation for CVP monitoring are identical to those described for arterial pressure monitoring. After insertion of the catheter, the pressure tubing is connected to the catheter hub. The CVP waveform and value appear on the bedside monitor.

COMPLICATIONS

Infection

Infection may occur within the catheter or around the insertion site. Systemic infection when the source is the central venous catheter is diagnosed and verified by blood cultures. Signs and symptoms of infection such as fever or elevated white blood cell count may appear as with any pyrogenic source. Routine catheter and tubing changes, as outlined by the Centers for Disease Control and Prevention and hospital policy, and adherence to sterile technique are primary measures to prevent infection.

Thrombosis

Thromboses may vary in size from a thin fibrin sheath over the catheter tip to a large thrombus. A small thrombus may be flushed away without causing harm, but a larger thrombus occluding the catheter and vein should not be flushed into the venous circulation. A large thrombus may be detected by loss of hemodynamic waveform and inability to infuse fluid or withdraw blood from the catheter. The patient may have edema of the arm closest to the catheter site, varying degrees of neck pain (which may radiate), and jugular vein distension. A large thrombus is classified as an emergency because it may impair circulation to a limb. A nurse may attempt to aspirate this clot if hospital policy permits. Frequently, hospitals also have protocols to administer small doses of thrombolytic agents to dissolve the clot. At the very least, the nurse is responsible for reporting suspected catheter occlusion to a physician.

Air Embolism

Air embolism occurs as a result of air entering the system and traveling to the right ventricle through the vena cava. Usually air entry into the catheter is associated with disconnection of the catheter from the IV tubing. Changes in intrathoracic pressure with inspiration and expiration draw air into the catheter and vena cava. Sudden hypotension from decreased cardiac output may be the first indicator of this sometimes lethal problem.

Approximately 10 to 20 mL of air must enter the system before the patient becomes symptomatic. Signs of such an emergency may include confusion, lightheadedness, anxiety, and unresponsiveness. The physiological event is the creation of foam in the ventricle with each heart contraction and loss of stroke volume due to air instead of blood in the ventricle, causing a sudden decrease in cardiac output. Cardiac arrest may occur.

If this problem is suspected, turning the patient on the left side in the Trendelenburg position may allow the air to rise to the wall of the right ventricle and improve blood flow. Oxygen should be started on the patient unless contraindicated.

Strategies to prevent disconnections include having Luer-Lok connections on all central line catheters and tubings, careful manipulation of catheter and tubing during dressing changes, and routine monitoring of the connections. There is no substitute for close observation by skilled and educated nursing staff.

NURSING CONSIDERATIONS

If a patient is changed from a water CVP monitoring system to a pressure transducer system, the nurse must remember that the normal values are different. CVP measured by a water manometer normally is approximately 5 to 8 cm H_2O, and CVP measured by a pressure transducer normally is 0 to 6 mm Hg. The values are different because mercury is heavier than water. To convert a value in cm H_2O to a value in mm Hg, the value in cm H_2O is divided by 1.36. To convert a value in mm Hg to a value in cm H_2O, the value in mm Hg is multiplied by 1.36. The trend in values is most significant as it relates to the patient's cardiovascular dysfunction and the response to interventions.[1,2]

Decreased CVP values indicate a hypovolemic state often requiring administration of fluids. The anticipated response to fluid therapy is an increase in the CVP. Similarly, diuretic therapy reduces intravascular volume and is associated with a decrease in the CVP. A low or decreasing CVP also may be related to vasodilation from sepsis or vasodilating drugs; both create a relative hypovolemia because blood volume has not changed. Rather, the intravascular space has become greater relative to the patient's blood volume.

Increased CVP values may be caused by a number of complex and interrelated factors, each of which requires scrutiny. Right ventricular failure and mechanical ventilation are two of the more common causes of increased CVP. Rarely is intravascular volume overload and hypervolemia alone a cause of increased CVP.

Mechanical ventilation increases intrathoracic pressure, which is transmitted to the pulmonary vasculature, heart, and great vessels. CVP values may be directly affected by this pressure. CVP may be increased as well because intrathoracic pressure compresses the pulmonary vessels, creating resistance to blood flow from the right side to the left side of the heart and causing blood to back up in the right ventricle, right atrium, and vena cava. In extreme cases, the increased intrathoracic pressure associated with mechanical ventilation causes significant right ventricular dysfunction, and the CVP is elevated because of reduced forward blood flow and the backup of blood and pressure in the right atrium and vena cava.

Right ventricular failure due to coronary artery disease or left ventricular failure is associated with increased CVP values. The inability of the right ventricle to pump blood through the pulmonary vasculature because of injured or infarcted myocardium results in increased volume and pressure in the right atrium and vena cava. Left ventricular failure may increase CVP as the pressure of blood volume congests the pulmonary vasculature and impairs flow from the right ventricle, causing right ventricular dilation and subsequent failure. Again, the increased pressure is reflected backward to the right atrium and vena cava. In these instances, interventions are directed toward facilitating forward blood flow by improving ventricular contractility and reducing the intravascular blood volume. A decrease in the CVP is an indication of the effectiveness of therapy.

CVP is always interpreted in conjunction with other clinical observations, such as auscultation of breath sounds, heart and respiratory rate, ECG, neck vein distension, and urine output. For example, increased CVP associated with pulmonary basilar crackles and decreased urine output is often indicative of left ventricular failure. Distended neck veins but clear breath sounds and a high CVP might be caused by increased intrathoracic pressure from mechanical ventilator effects. Patients who are septic may have a low CVP that is associated with fever, elevated white blood cell count, tachycardia, and tachypnea, whereas patients who are taking vasodilating agents may have a low CVP that is associated with an increased heart rate but none of the other aforementioned clinical signs. A CVP value alone is meaningless, but when used in conjunction with other clinical data, it is a valuable aid in managing and predicting the patient's clinical course.

Pulmonary Artery Pressure Monitoring

The PA catheter has made possible the assessment of right ventricular function, pulmonary vascular status, and, indirectly, left ventricular function. Cardiac output, right atrial, right ventricular, and PA pressures, as well as pulmonary artery wedge pressure (PAWP) are measured using a PA catheter. The pressures and cardiac output obtained using this catheter allow the clinician to calculate derived parameters and facilitate diagnosis of cardiovascular and cardiopulmonary dysfunction, determine the therapy needed, and evaluate the effectiveness of the interventions.

PULMONARY ARTERY CATHETERS

Several types of flow-directed, balloon-tipped PA catheters are available in different sizes. The type of catheter used is determined by the parameters to be monitored and additional requirements governed by the patient's condition. The 7.5-French (F; a measure of catheter size) thermodilution catheter is the size most commonly used (Fig. 17-54).

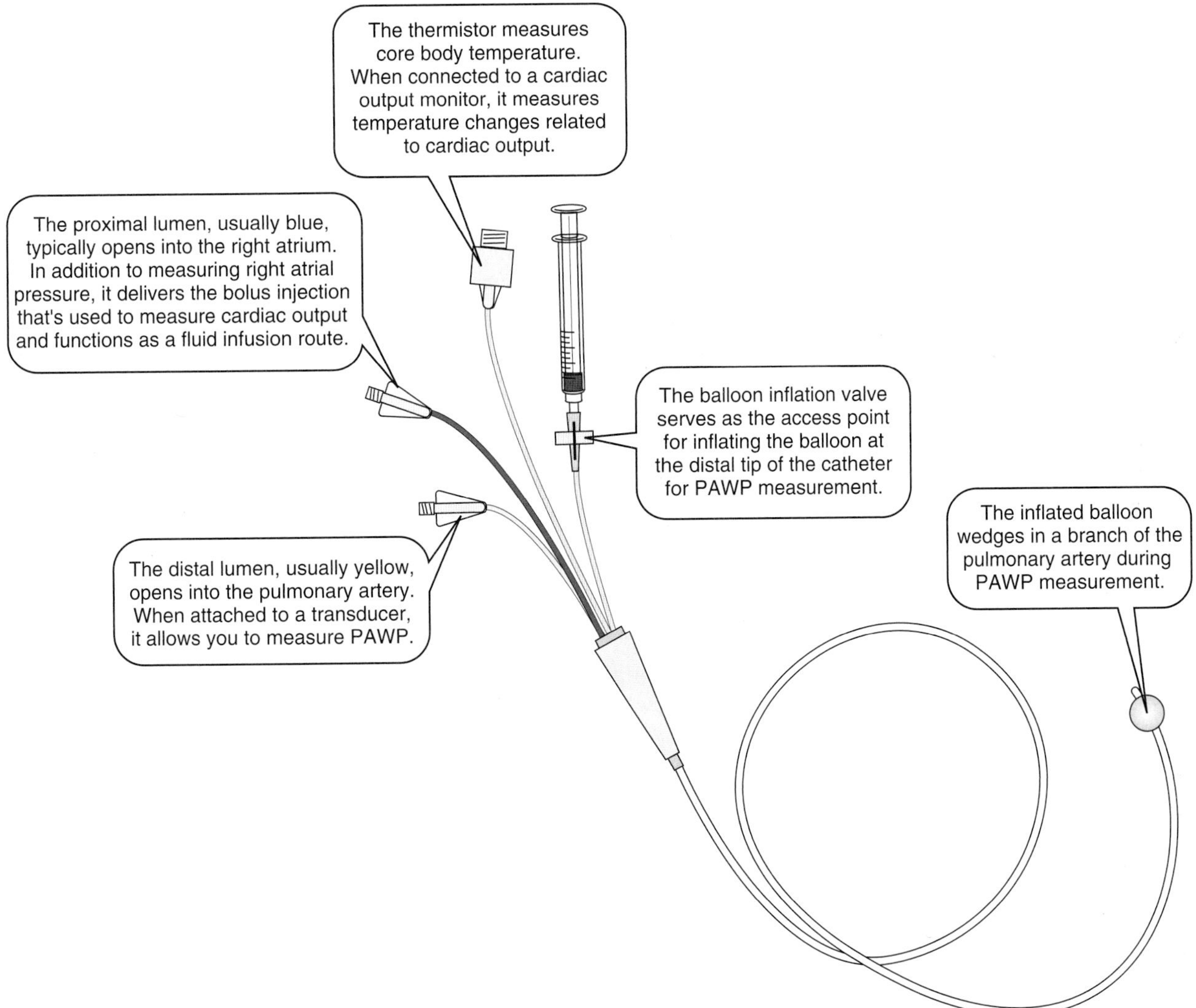

figure 17-54 Pulmonary artery catheter. *PAWP,* pulmonary artery wedge pressure. (From Springhouse: Critical Care Made Incredibly Easy, p C1. Springhouse, PA, author, 2004.)

All PA catheters have several external ports or lumen hubs corresponding to internal lumens and lumen openings into the right side of the heart and PA. There are four lumens with external hubs or ports: the proximal hub and lumen, distal hub and lumen, balloon inflation valve and lumen, and thermistor connector and lumen.

The proximal or right atrial lumen, which opens into the right atrium, may be used for infusion of fluids or medications and is connected to a transducer allowing right atrial pressure measurements and display of the right atrial pressure waveform. The right atrial lumen port also is used as the injectate port for measuring cardiac outputs.

The distal or PA lumen hub is always attached to a transducer and a continuous flush system. The PA waveform is displayed continuously, as are the PA systolic, diastolic, and mean pressures. The PA port is used for the withdrawal of mixed venous blood gases, which are necessary for oxygen extraction, oxygen consumption, and intrapulmonary shunt measurements. The PA port usually is not used for fluid or medication administration, although sometimes it may be necessary to use this port for infusions.

The balloon inflation port and lumen enable the clinician to inflate the balloon at the catheter tip with a small volume of air to measure the PA occlusion pressure, known as the PAWP. The balloon capacity of most PA catheters is 1.5 mL, and the balloon should not be inflated with more than this amount of air. Fluid is never infused through the balloon inflation port.

The tip of the PA catheter also contains a thermistor. The external thermistor port is connected to the bedside monitor or to a cardiac output computer. The thermistor permits measurement of the patient's temperature in the PA (core temperature), and it detects the blood temperature change when solution is injected through the right atrial port to obtain a cardiac output measurement.

Specialty PA catheters include the previously described components and additional features and lumens. Some of the specialty features include a second proximal lumen that serves as an additional infusion port; a right ventricular lumen that may be used for infusions or insertion of a cardiac pacemaker probe (designated for that particular type of PA catheter) if temporary ventricular pacing is required; a lumen containing fiberoptic filaments allowing continuous measurement of mixed venous oxygen saturation ($S\bar{v}O_2$); continuous measurement and display of cardiac output; and right ventricular ejection fraction determinations. Several models of PA catheters have combined specialty features, such as the continuous cardiac output and $S\bar{v}O_2$ monitoring catheter or the right ventricular ejection fraction and $S\bar{v}O_2$ monitoring catheter. Figure 17-55 shows various types of PA catheters.

PULMONARY ARTERY CATHETER INSERTION

Before the PA catheter is inserted, all necessary equipment should be assembled. The exact setup and equipment used vary depending on the institution. The flush system is connected to the transducer, which is then placed at the zero reference point, leveled, and zeroed. Each lumen of the PA catheter is flushed with sterile solution from the flush system. (Note that fiberoptic $S\bar{v}O_2$ monitoring catheters are calibrated before flushing lumens of the PA catheter.) The PAWP balloon is inflated with air and then deflated to ensure proper inflation and to check for leaks before the catheter is inserted. The PA port is then connected to the prepared transducer with pressure tubing, and the other lumens are connected to either a pressure monitoring system or to IV solution.

Strict sterile technique is required for the PA catheter insertion procedure. The physician performing the procedure wears a cap, mask, gown, and gloves. The nurse assisting wears a cap and mask and, if manipulating the catheter, gloves. The field should be sterile. The PA catheter is inserted into a large vein through an introducer catheter, which is usually placed by a percutaneous approach. The most common insertion sites are the left or right subclavian veins. Other sites that may be used are the internal or external jugular veins or femoral veins. Occasionally, the antecubital vein is used. Antecubital access requires a venous cutdown.

Once the introducer is in place, the PA catheter is inserted by the physician and threaded into place. Determination of the catheter tip location is established by monitoring the waveform and pressures on the bedside monitor as the catheter passes through the vena cava into the right atrium. When the catheter tip is in the right atrium, the PA balloon is inflated with 1.5 mL of air to help "float" the catheter through the tricuspid valve into the right ventricle, across the pulmonic valve into the PA, and eventually into the wedged position (Fig. 17-56). The balloon is allowed to deflate passively after the PA wedge waveform is noted on the monitor and return of the PA waveform is confirmed. The PA catheter is then secured, and a sterile dressing is placed over the insertion site. Catheter position is also verified with a chest radiograph after the insertion.

Nursing responsibilities during the insertion procedure include monitoring sterile technique, monitoring the changes in hemodynamic waveforms, recording the pressures in each chamber of the heart as the catheter is passed through, and monitoring the patient for complications. Ventricular arrhythmias are the most common complication during PA catheter insertion (see section on Complications). Therefore, it is advisable to have a lidocaine bolus and defibrillator available for the insertion procedure.

WAVEFORM INTERPRETATION

All hemodynamic pressures and waveforms are generated by pressure changes in the heart caused by the myocardial contraction (systole) and relaxation/filling (diastole) phases of the cardiac cycle. This mechanical activity of the heart is generated in response to the electrical activity (i.e., the depolarization and repolarization of myocardial cells). Therefore, interpretation of the hemodynamic waveforms depends on the correlation of mechanical to electrical activities using the ECG. There are three categories of hemodynamic waveforms: atrial, which includes right atrial, left atrial, and PA wedge; ventricular, which includes left and right ventricular; and arterial, which includes PA and systemic aortic. The waveforms in each category are similar because they result from the same cardiac events. The pressure measurements are different because of the different amount of pressure that is generated in the right ventricle and atrium compared with the left side of the heart.

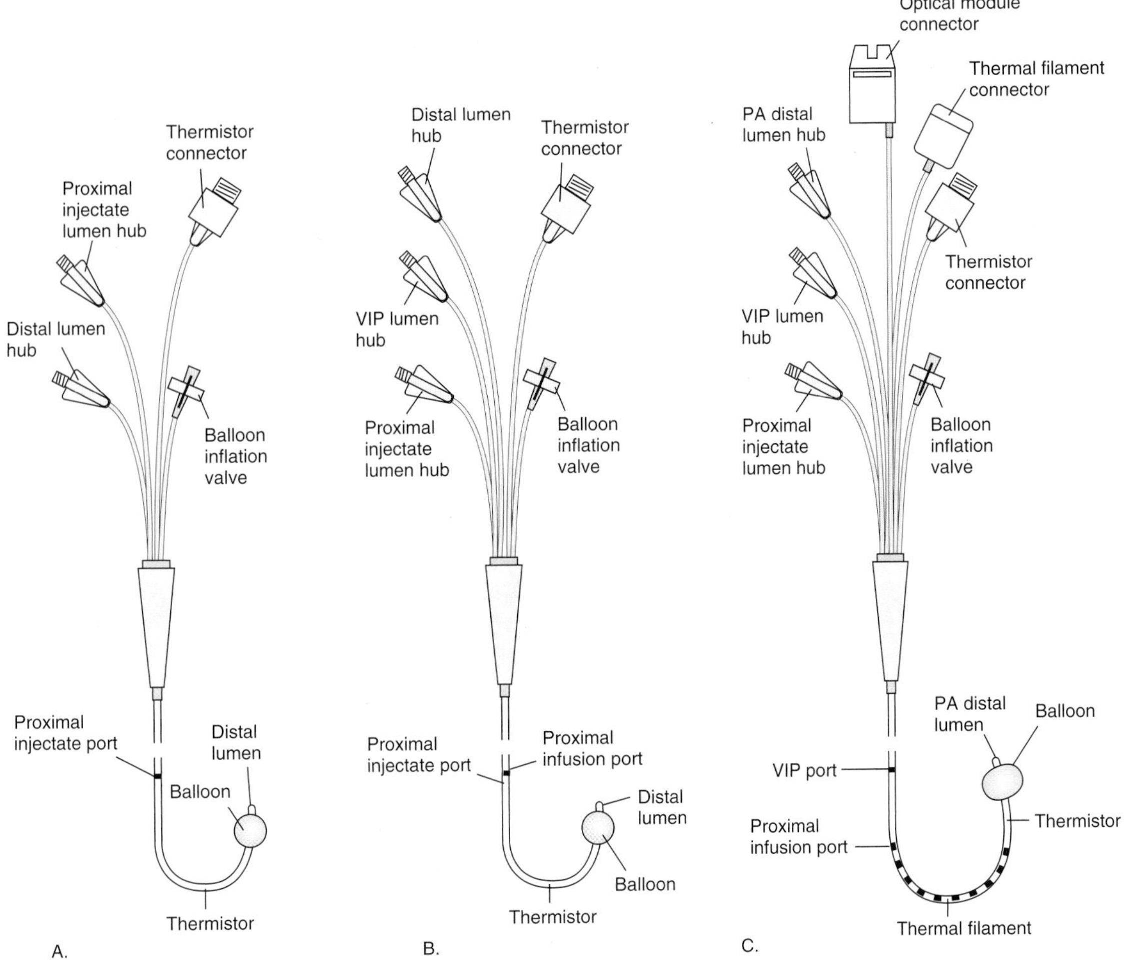

figure 17-55 Types of pulmonary artery (PA) catheters. (**A**) Four-lumen catheter. (**B**) Five-lumen catheter that includes an additional venous infusion port (VIP) into the right atrium. (**C**) Seven-lumen catheter that includes a VIP port and two additional lumens for continuous cardiac output (CCO) and thermal filament, and continuous mixed venous oxygen saturation ($S\bar{v}O_2$) monitoring (optical module connector). An additional option is to combine use of the CCO filament and the thermistor response time to calculate end-diastolic volume monitoring.

Right Atrial Pressure

The right atrium is a low-pressure chamber, receiving blood volume passively from the vena cava. The normal pressure is less than 8 mm Hg, which reflects the mean right atrial pressure.

Atrial waveforms have three positive waves: a, c, and v. The a wave reflects the increase in atrial pressure during atrial contraction with systole. The c wave, a minor wave, reflects the small increase in right atrial pressure associated with closure of the tricuspid valve and early atrial diastole. The c wave may be a distinct wave, a notch on the a wave, or completely absent. The v wave represents atrial diastole and reflects the increase in pressure caused by filling of the atrium with blood. The v wave of right atrial diastole is also affected by ventricular contraction and the bulging of the tricuspid valve up into the right atrium after right atrial systole. Figure 17-57 shows the right atrial waveform.

Accurate identification of the a, c, and v waves requires correlation of the waveform with the ECG. On the ECG, the P wave represents discharge of the SA node and atrial depolarization, which causes left atrial and right atrial contraction. Therefore, the a wave occurs after the P wave and usually in the PR interval. The QRS complex represents ventricular depolarization and causes ventricular contraction. Simultaneously the right atrium relaxes and fills with blood. The v wave generated by these events thus falls after the QRS complex and in the T-to-P interval. The c wave is not always visible because of the small increase in pressure caused in early diastole and with tricuspid valve closure. If it is visible, the c wave occurs between the a and v waves.

Atrial pressure tracings also have two primary negative waves or descents: x and y. The x descent follows the a wave and represents a decrease in pressure caused by atrial relaxation at the beginning of atrial diastole. The y descent follows the v wave and represents the initial, passive atrial emptying into the ventricle as the tricuspid valve opens.[1,2]

Right Ventricular Pressure

The right ventricle is a low-pressure chamber. Right ventricular end-diastolic pressure is usually 0 to 8 mm Hg and is equal to the right atrial pressure because the tricuspid valve is open. Right ventricular systolic pressure is normally 20 to 30 mm Hg because the right ventricle must generate only enough pressure to open the pulmonic

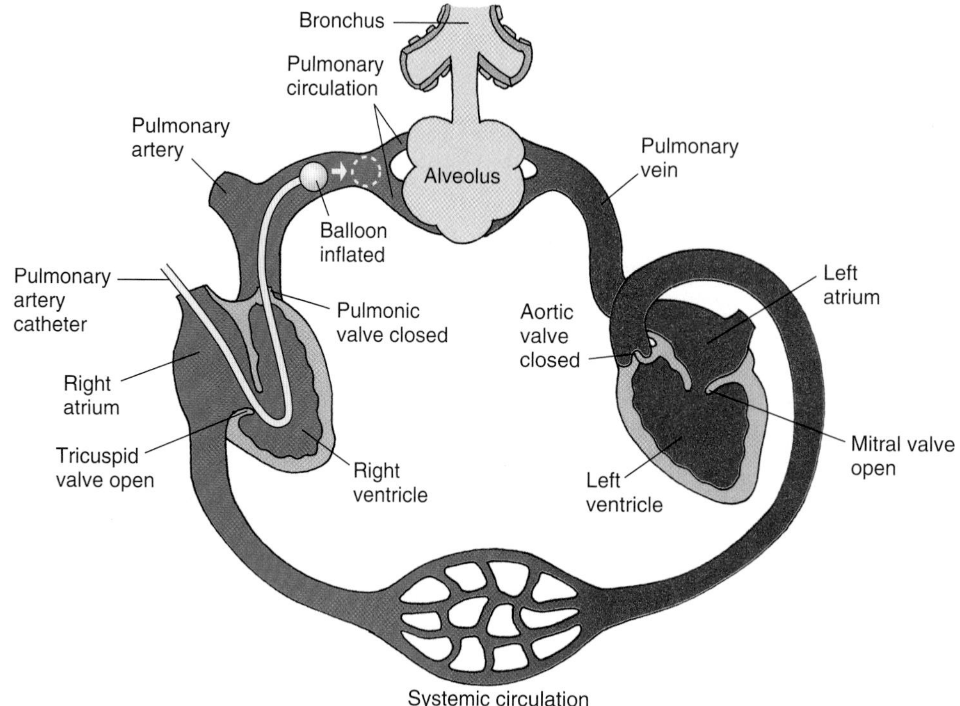

figure 17-56 Position of the pulmonary artery catheter in the right atrium, right ventricle, and the pulmonary artery. When the balloon is inflated and the catheter is in the wedge position, there is an unrestricted vascular channel between the tip of the catheter and the left ventricle in diastole. Pulmonary artery wedge pressure thus reflects left ventricular end-diastolic pressure, an important indicator of left ventricular function. (Courtesy of Hewlett Packard.)

valve and move blood through the low-pressure pulmonary vasculature.

As the PA catheter is advanced from the right atrium into the right ventricle, or if the right ventricular lumen of the PA catheter is transduced, the waveform has a distinctive "square root" configuration. Figure 17-57 shows the right ventricular waveform. The initial rapid increase in right ventricular pressure represents isovolumetric contraction, which follows the QRS complex of the ECG. The right ventricular pressure continues to increase as the tricuspid and pulmonary valves are closed until the force generated exceeds the PA pressure. Rapid ejection occurs when the pulmonic valve opens. After ventricular systole, the pulmonic valve closes, and the right ventricular pressure rapidly decreases, creating a diastolic dip. Next in the cardiac cycle, the tricuspid valve opens and the right ventricle passively fills with blood from the PA. Right ventricular diastole falls within the period from the T wave to the next Q wave on the ECG. The point on the waveform just before the rapid increase in pressure represents right ventricular end-diastole.[1,2]

Pulmonary Artery Pressure

The pulmonary vasculature is a relatively low-resistance, low-pressure system in healthy individuals. Normal systolic PA pressure is 20 to 30 mm Hg. Normal diastolic PA pressure is 8 to 15 mm Hg, with a mean of 10 to 20 mm Hg. Systolic PA pressure and the peak of the PA waveform are generated by right ventricular systolic ejection; therefore, the PA pressure and the right ventricular systolic pressure are the same. The PA waveform characteristics are similar to the systemic arterial waveform previously described (see Fig. 17-57). The dicrotic notch in the downward slope of the PA waveform corresponds with pulmonary valve closure at the beginning of right ventricular diastole and is the beginning of the PA diastolic phase. PA diastolic pressure reflects the resistance of the pulmonary vascular bed and, to a limited degree, left ventricular end-diastolic pressure. In absolutely normal conditions, PA diastolic pressure theoretically is an indirect measure of left ventricular pressure because the pulmonary vasculature, left atrium, and open mitral valve allow equalization of pressure from the left ventricle back to the tip of the PA catheter.[1,2]

Pulmonary Artery Wedge Pressure

When the PA catheter is properly positioned, the PAWP is obtained by inflating the balloon at the catheter tip. The balloon occludes forward flow in the branch of the PA, creating a static column of blood from that portion of the PA through the left atrium, an open mitral valve during diastole, and the left ventricle. In this way, the PAWP reflects left ventricular end-diastolic pressure. Normal PAWP is 8 to 12 mm Hg. The PAWP more closely measures left atrial and ventricular end-diastolic pressure than the PA diastolic pressure because balloon inflation halts blood flow past the catheter tip, thereby decreasing the influence of pulmonary vascular resistance on the pressure reading.

Inflation of the PA balloon causes the PA waveform on the monitor to become a PAWP tracing. No more than 1.5 mL of air is used to inflate the balloon. If less than 1 mL

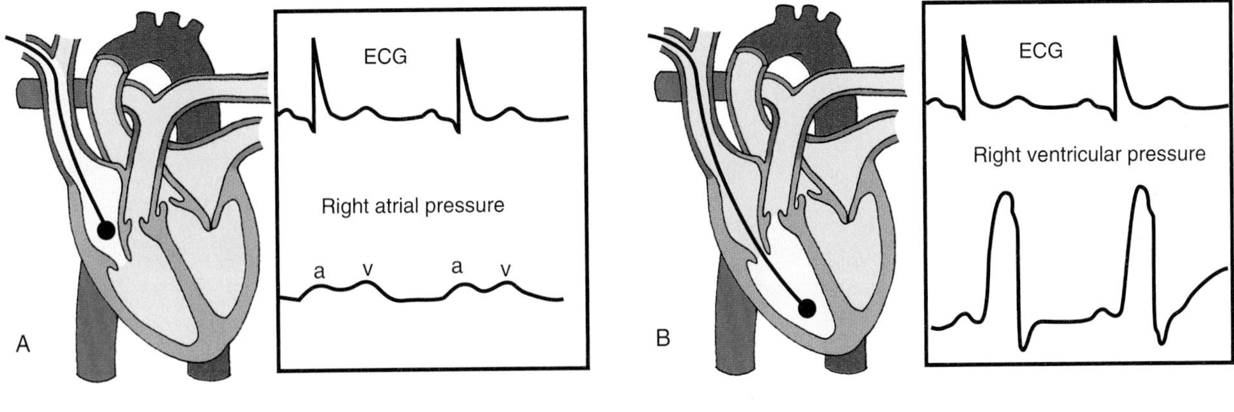

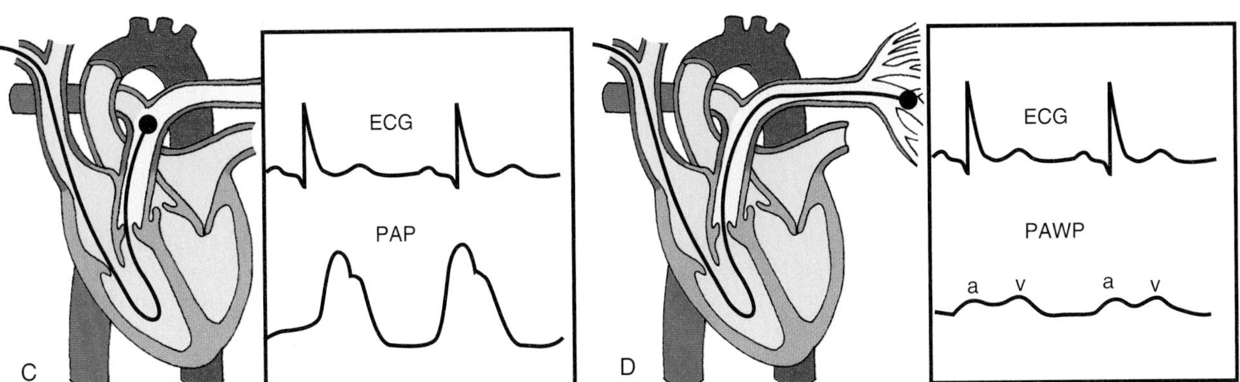

figure 17-57 Normal pulmonary artery (PA) waveforms. During PA insertion, the waveforms change as the catheter advances through the heart. (**A**) When the catheter enters the right atrium, a waveform with two small upright waves appears. The a waves represent the right ventricular end-diastolic pressure; the v waves, right atrial filling. (**B**) When the catheter reaches the right ventricle, a waveform with sharp systolic upstrokes and lower diastolic dips appears. (**C**) When the catheter "floats" into the PA, a PA pressure (PAP) waveform appears. Note that the upstroke is smoother than on the right ventricle waveform. The dicrotic notch indicates pulmonic valve closure. (**D**) When the catheter "floats" into a distal branch of the pulmonary artery, the balloon wedges where the vessel becomes too narrow for it to pass, and a pulmonary artery wedge pressure (PAWP) waveform, with two small upright waves, appears. The a wave represents left ventricular end-diastolic pressure; the v wave, ventricular filling. *ECG*, electrocardiogram. (From Springhouse: Critical Care Made Incredibly Easy, p 173. Springhouse, PA, author, 2002.)

of air generates a PAWP tracing, the PA catheter has migrated distally and needs to be withdrawn slightly, usually by a physician, for proper placement.

The PAWP tracing has a, c, and v waves and x and y descents. The electrical and mechanical events of the heart generating these waves are identical to those of the right atrial waveform, except that the PAWP waveform reflects activity from the left side of the heart. The a wave corresponds to left atrial contraction, and the v wave corresponds to left ventricular contraction and left atrial filling. The c wave is rarely visible on the PAWP tracing (see Fig. 17-57).

The ECG may be correlated with the PAWP waveform just as with the right atrial waveform. The primary difference between the PAWP and the right atrial waveforms is the slight delay of a and v waves in PAWP relative to the ECG because of the distance from the left side of the heart over which these pressures are transmitted. The a wave now falls more closely in line with the QRS complex, although it may be within the PR interval. The v wave correlates with the T-to-P interval.[1,2]

Figure 17-58 shows the PAWP tracing as the PA catheter is inserted. Note that normally, the right atrial pressure is equivalent to the right ventricular diastolic pressure, the right ventricular systolic pressure is equivalent to the PA systolic pressure, and the PA diastolic pressure is equivalent to the PAWP.

COMPLICATIONS

Pneumothorax

Pneumothorax is a complication of insertion of the PA catheter introducer through the subclavian vein. Anatomical factors can make placement of a PA catheter difficult, particularly if the patient is obese or has torturous subclavian veins. The needle or introducer sheath may puncture the lung during insertion and cause an apical pneumothorax.

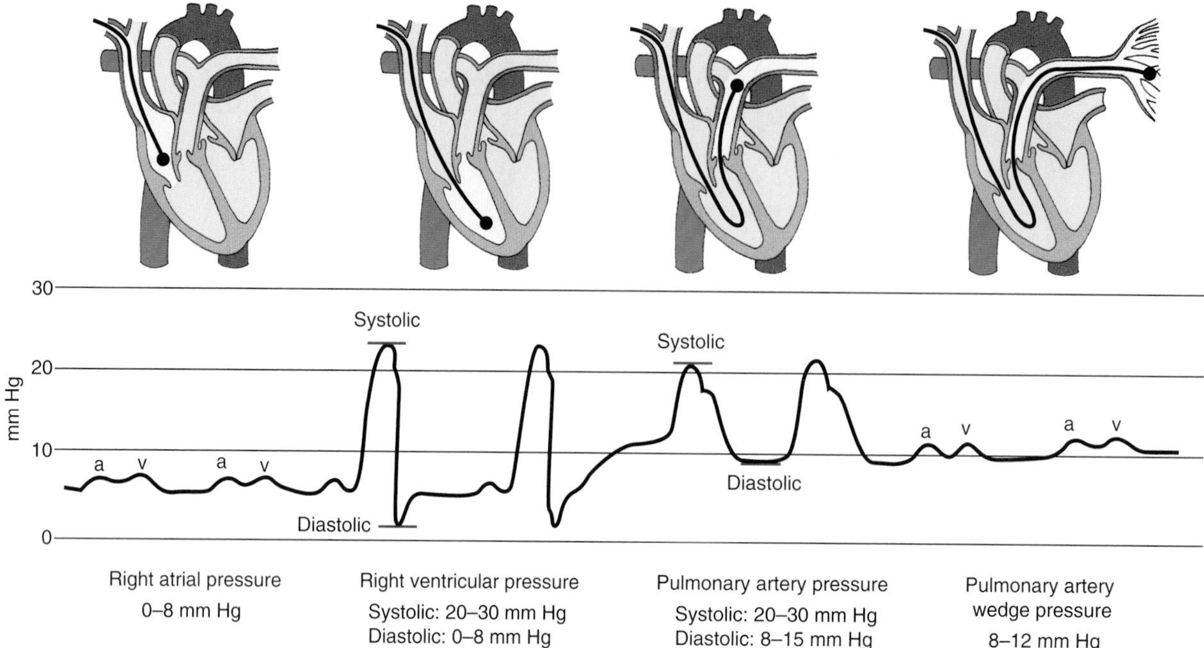

figure 17-58 Normal values and wave configurations produced by the pulmonary artery catheter.

Signs and symptoms of a pneumothorax and routine post-insertion chest radiograph are the techniques used to diagnose this complication.

Infection

Systemic infection and sepsis are caused by contamination of the PA catheter, insertion site, or pressure monitoring system. Careful attention to sterile technique during pressure tubing assembly, insertion, and dressing changes helps prevent infection. Protocols for changing the PA catheter and monitoring system should be followed carefully. Diagnosis of PA catheter–related sepsis is based on blood cultures, white blood cell count, and fever in the absence of other sources of infection.

Ventricular Arrhythmias

Ventricular arrhythmias are common during the insertion of a PA catheter. As the catheter passes through the right ventricle, it may irritate the endocardium and cause PVCs and occasionally VT. The arrhythmias typically resolve when the catheter is advanced into the PA. After the PA catheter is in proper position, it may become dislodged if it is not well secured, and the tip may "fall back" into the right ventricle. The patient may experience arrhythmias, and the hemodynamic pressures and waveform reflect those of the right ventricle. Usually in this situation, because of potential contamination at the insertion site, the physician withdraws the catheter or occasionally inflates the balloon and advances the catheter into the PA. It is essential to have ready access to emergency drugs and equipment in case the ventricular arrhythmias persist.

Pulmonary Artery Rupture or Perforation

A rare but very serious and potentially fatal complication is rupture or perforation of the PA. Perforation of the PA may occur during insertion or manipulation of the PA catheter. Patients with friable PAs may be at some risk. However, proper advancement of the catheter with the balloon fully inflated with 1.5 mL of air and avoidance of advancing the catheter too far into a small artery minimize the chance of PA perforation. Rupture of the PA is associated with overinflation of the balloon, particularly if the catheter has migrated distally into a small PA. Close observation of the PA waveform as the balloon is inflated and filling the balloon only with the amount of air necessary to obtain a PAWP tracing prevent overdistending a small PA. As previously stated, the catheter should become wedged when inflated with 1 to 1.5 mL of air. If less air is required to obtain the PAWP waveform, the catheter has migrated out of proper position.

NURSING CONSIDERATIONS

Nursing care of the patient undergoing PA pressure monitoring is complex. Critical care nurses must be able to interpret waveforms and pressure data and be alert to potential complications. It is necessary to ensure accurate readings and minimize operator error. Consistency of leveling and measurement techniques are especially important because small variations in the zero reference point elicit large and erroneous changes in the right atrial pressure and PAWP. Table 17-13 outlines problems and troubleshooting strategies associated with hemodynamic pressure monitoring.

Measurement of all hemodynamic pressures is most accurate when obtained at the end of expiration in the respiratory cycle. In the healthy individual, intrathoracic pressure at end-expiration is about equal to atmospheric pressure. During the end-expiration period, there is minimal airflow and little variation in pleural pressures that would influence cardiac structures. Thus, end-expiration provides a standard reference point for measurement that is not influenced by extravascular pressures. Mechanical ventilation causes increased intrathoracic pressure during

table 17-13 Troubleshooting: Inaccurate Pressure Measurements

Problem	Cause	Prevention	Treatment
Damped waveforms and inaccurate pressures	Partial clotting at catheter tip	Use continuous drip with 1 U heparin/1 mL IV fluid. Hand flush occasionally. Flush with large volume after blood sampling. Use heparin-coated catheters.	Aspirate, then flush catheter with heparinized fluid (*not* in PAW position).
	Tip moving against wall	Obtain more stable catheter position.	Reposition catheter.
	Kinking of catheter	Restrict catheter movement at insertion site.	Reposition to straighten catheter. Replace catheter.
Abnormally low or negative pressures	Incorrect air-reference level (above midchest level)	Maintain transducer air-reference port at midchest level; re-zero after patient position changes.	Remeasure level of transducer air-reference and reposition at midchest level; re-zero.
	Incorrect zeroing and calibration of monitor	Zero and calibrate monitor properly.	Recheck zero and calibration of monitor.
	Loose connection	Use Luer-Lok stopcocks.	Check all connections.
Abnormally high pressure reading	Pressure trapped by improper sequence of stopcock operation	Turn stopcocks in proper sequence when two pressures are measured on one transducer.	Thoroughly flush transducers with IV solution; re-zero and turn stopcocks in proper sequence.
	Incorrect air-reference level (below midchest level)	Maintain transducer air-reference port at midchest level; recheck and re-zero after patient position changes.	Check air-reference level; reset at midchest and re-zero.
Inappropriate pressure waveform	Migration of catheter tip (e.g., in RV or PAW instead of in PA)	Establish optimal position carefully when introducing catheter initially. Suture catheter at insertion site and tape catheter to patient's skin.	Review waveform; if RV, inflate balloon; if PAW, deflate balloon and withdraw catheter slightly. Check position under fluoroscope or x-ray after reposition.
No pressure available	Transducer not open to catheter Amplifiers still on *cal, zero,* or *off*	Follow routine, systematic steps for pressure measurement.	Check system, stopcocks.
Noise or fling in pressure waveform	Excessive catheter movement, particularly in PA	Avoid excessive catheter length in ventricle.	Try different catheter tip position.
	Excessive tubing length	Use shortest tubing possible (<3–4 ft).	Eliminate excess tubing.
	Excessive stopcocks	Minimize number of stopcocks.	Eliminate excess stopcocks.

PAW, pulmonary artery wedge; RV, right ventricle; PA, pulmonary artery.

inspiration; therefore, end-expiration is the lowest point of the hemodynamic waveform (Fig. 17-59). Spontaneous breathing causes negative intrathoracic pressure; therefore, end-expiration is the highest point of the waveform in these patients.

Alarm parameters are closely set to alert nurses to potential physiological or technical complications. For example, one of the first indications of a pulmonary embolus is an acute increase in PA pressures. Distal migration of the PA catheter may cause the catheter to wedge spontaneously without balloon inflation, and PA pressures decrease to that of a PAWP. Both situations are detected early if alarms are properly set.

Abnormalities of the right atrial waveform usually are large, elevated a or v waves. Increased size of the a wave is caused by impaired atrial emptying during atrial contraction and the subsequent increase in atrial pressure. Examples of pathological processes causing large a waves in the right atrial waveform are tricuspid stenosis and right ventricular failure. Elevated v waves are related to incompetence of the tricuspid valve, allowing blood to flow from the ventricle back into the atrium during ventricular contraction. These abnormalities also cause the mean right atrial pressure to be higher.

Increased PA pressures are associated with left ventricular failure, mechanical ventilation, and pulmonary vascular vasoconstriction. This vasoconstriction may result from acute respiratory distress syndrome, primary pulmonary hypertension, or pulmonary embolus.

Abnormal PAWP waveforms are more common than abnormal right atrial waveforms because left ventricular dysfunction and mitral valve disease tend to occur more frequently than right ventricular or tricuspid valve disorders. Pressure changes caused by left-sided heart disorders

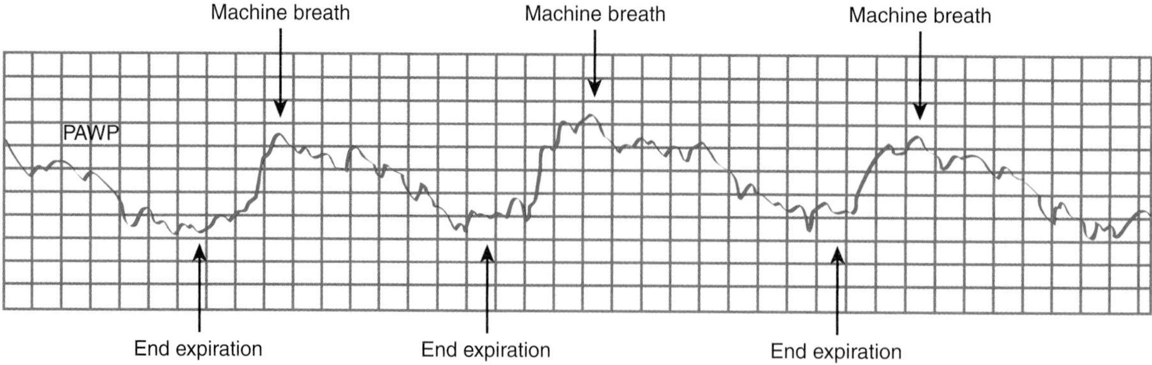

figure 17-59 Pulmonary artery wedge pressure (PAWP) tracing showing respiratory variation from positive pressure mechanical ventilation. Measurement of PAWP is made at the mean point of end expiration.

are transmitted back through the pulmonary veins to the tip of the catheter in the PA and reflected as changes in the PAWP and waveform. Mitral stenosis creates large a waves as the left atrium contracts against the semiclosed valve, increasing pressure in the left atrium. Mitral regurgitation or insufficiency allows the backflow of blood into the left atrium during ventricular contraction and generates large v waves on the PAWP tracing. However, in both these valvular diseases, the PAWP does not accurately reflect left ventricular end-diastolic pressure. Left ventricular failure usually causes elevation of both the a and v waves and significantly increases the PAWP because of reduced contractility and forward blood flow. Except for the high pressure reading, the PAWP waveform configuration is usually normal.

Elevated PAWP frequently is due to left ventricular dysfunction or hypervolemia. In some cases, such as acute respiratory distress syndrome or mechanical ventilator settings that generate extremely high intrathoracic pressure, PAWP is elevated because of noncardiogenic causes. In these cases, however, the PA diastolic pressure is greater than the PAWP. Causes of changes in hemodynamic pressures are summarized in Table 17-14.

Determination of Cardiac Output

Cardiac output is the volume of blood ejected from the heart per minute, expressed in liters per minute. Normally, it is 4 to 8 L/minute at rest. Cardiac output is a function of heart rate and stroke volume. Cardiac output and flow through the aorta are determined by the volume of blood in the ventricle at the end of diastole, impedance to flow from the heart, and the contractile ability of the myocardium. The left ventricle must generate enough pressure in systole to overcome aortic pressure and systemic vascular resistance (SVR) and eject sufficient blood volume to perfuse the organs of the body. The measurement of cardiac output and assessment of its determinants are important adjuncts to the care of critically ill patients. Routine evaluation of cardiac output is essential when technology such as a PA catheter is used. Details concerning the calculation of cardiac output and other cardiac values are presented in Table 17-15.

Cardiac output may be calculated to reflect body size; in this case, it is termed the *cardiac index*. Cardiac index is the preferred value to use clinically because it takes into account body size. The cardiac index is obtained by dividing cardiac output by the patient's body surface area (BSA). The BSA can be determined by using the Dubois body surface area chart (Fig. 17-60). Often bedside monitors and computers automatically calculate cardiac index when the patient's height and weight are entered. Normally, the cardiac index is 2.5 to 4 L/minute/m^2.

FACTORS THAT DETERMINE CARDIAC OUTPUT

Cardiac output is always evaluated based on analysis of its determinants, heart rate and stroke volume. Tachycardia may decrease cardiac output as a result of shortened diastole and decreased filling time of the ventricles. A patient with bradycardia may be symptomatic because of low cardiac output and blood pressure.

Stroke volume, the volume of blood ejected by each ventricular contraction, is influenced by preload, afterload, and contractility (see Chapter 16 for detailed discussion). Preload is the amount of stretch on the myocardial muscle fibers at end-diastole and is determined by ventricular filling (end-diastolic) volume. Within physiological limits, increases in end-diastolic volume cause stretch of the myofibrils and increases the force of ventricular contraction (Frank-Starling law of the heart). Preload is primarily influenced by total blood volume. Because the PA catheter measures pressure, not volume, assumptions are made that volume and pressure can be equated. Although many factors alter the pressure–volume relationship, pressures are used to evaluate the adequacy of end-diastolic volume. Right ventricular preload is assessed using the right atrial pressure. Left ventricular preload is assessed using the PAWP measurement.

Afterload, which is impedance to ejection of blood from the ventricles, is influenced primarily by the status of pulmonary vascular resistance or SVR and the function of the pulmonic and aortic valves. Pulmonary vascular resistance is used to assess right ventricular afterload. Left ventricular afterload is evaluated by calculating SVR (see Table 17-15). Indexed values (pulmonary vascular resistance index and SVR index) are used to account for BSA.

table 17-14 Putting Hemodynamic Monitoring to Use

Hemodynamic monitoring provides information on intracardiac pressures, arterial pressure, and cardiac output. To understand intracardiac pressures, picture the heart and vascular system as a continuous loop with constantly changing pressure gradients that keep the blood moving. Hemodynamic monitoring records the gradients within the vessels and heart chambers.

Pressure and Description	Normal Values	Causes of Increased Pressure	Causes of Decreased Pressure
Central Venous Pressure or Right Atrial Pressure			
The central venous pressure or right atrial pressure (RAP) shows right ventricular function and end-diastolic pressure.	Mean pressure: 0 to 8 mm Hg	• Right-sided heart failure • Volume overload • Tricuspid valve stenosis or insufficiency • Constrictive pericarditis • Pulmonary hypertension • Cardiac tamponade • Right ventricular infarction	Reduced circulating blood volume
Right Ventricular Pressure			
Typically, the physician measures right ventricular pressure only when initially inserting a pulmonary artery catheter. Right ventricular systolic pressure normally equals pulmonary artery systolic pressure; right ventricular end-diastolic pressure, which reflects right ventricular function, equals RAP.	Systolic pressure: 20 to 30 mm Hg Diastolic pressure: 0 to 8 mm Hg	• Mitral stenosis or insufficiency • Pulmonary disease • Hypoxemia • Constrictive pericarditis • Chronic heart failure • Atrial and ventricular septal defects • Patent ductus arteriosus	Reduced circulating blood volume
Pulmonary Artery Pressure			
Pulmonary artery systolic pressure shows right ventricular function and pulmonary circulation pressures. Pulmonary artery diastolic pressure reflects left ventricular pressures, specifically left ventricular end-diastolic pressure, in a patient without significant pulmonary disease.	Systolic pressure: 20 to 30 mm Hg Mean pressure (usually): 8 to 15 mm Hg	• Left-sided heart failure • Increased pulmonary blood flow (left or right shunting, as in atrial or ventricular septal defects) • Any condition causing increased pulmonary arteriolar resistance (such as pulmonary hypertension, volume overload, mitral stenosis, or hypoxia)	Reduced circulating blood volume
Pulmonary Artery Wedge Pressure			
Pulmonary artery wedge pressure (PAWP) reflects left atrial and left ventricular pressures, unless the patient has mitral stenosis. Changes in PAWP reflect changes in left ventricular filling pressure.	Mean pressure: 8 to 12 mm Hg	• Left-sided heart failure • Mitral stenosis or insufficiency • Pericardial tamponade	Reduced circulating blood volume

From Springhouse: Critical Care Made Incredibly Easy, p. 170. Springhouse, PA, author, 2004.

Contractility is an inherent property of the heart. It is not affected by end-diastolic volume and cannot be directly measured. Sometimes stroke work index for both the left and right ventricles are used to assess contractility. Myocardial contractility is influenced by cardiac oxygen supply and demand balance, electrolytes, and minerals (e.g., calcium).

MEASUREMENT OF CARDIAC OUTPUT

Several methods are used to measure cardiac output. The Fick method, originally developed in the 1800s by Adolf Fick, is the historic gold standard. The Fick method uses the difference between arterial and venous oxygenation, oxygen consumption, and carbon dioxide production measured by spirometry to determine the cardiac output. Dye dilution is another method. A dye indicator is injected into the venous system, and a time–concentration curve is generated from a blood sample obtained from the arterial system. Analysis of the curve allows cardiac output calculation.[1,2] Thermodilution is the most common method used to measure cardiac output. Cold or room-temperature solution is the indicator and is injected into the right atrial port of the PA catheter. A thermistor near the end of the catheter continuously measures the temperature of blood flowing past it, and a temperature curve is generated by the rate of change in blood temperature after indicator

table 17-15 Calculation of Cardiac Values

Parameter	Formula	Normal Values
CO	Heart rate × stroke volume	4–8 L/min
CI	$\frac{\text{CO}}{\text{Body surface area}}$	2.5–4 L/min/m^2
SVI	$\frac{\text{CI}}{\text{Heart rate}}$	33–47 mL/beat/m^2
MAP	$\frac{\text{Systolic BP} + (\text{diastolic BP} \times 2)}{3}$	70–105 mm Hg
RAP	Direct measurement	0–8 mm Hg
PAWP	Direct measurement	8–12 mm Hg
RVEDVI	$\frac{\text{Stoke volume index}}{\text{RV ejection fraction}}$	60–100 mL/m^2
SVRI	$\frac{(\text{MAP} - \text{RAP}) \times 80}{\text{CI}}$	1,360–2,200 dyne/s/cm^{-5}
PVRI	$\frac{(\text{MPAP} - \text{PAWP}) \times 80}{\text{CI}}$	<425 dyne/s/cm^{-5}
LVSWI	SVI(MAP – PAWP) × 0.0136	40–70 g-m^2/beat
RVSWI	SVI(MPAP – RAP) × 0.0136	5–10 g-m^2/beat

CO, cardiac output; CI, cardiac index; SVI, stroke volume index; RAP, right atrial pressure; RVEDVI, right ventricular end diastolic volume index; SVRI, systemic vascular resistance index; PVRI, pulmonary vascular resistance index; MAP, mean arterial pressure; MPAP, mean pulmonary artery pressure; LVSWI, left ventricular stroke work index; RVSWI, right ventricular stroke work index.

injection. Based on this curve, cardiac output is calculated by the computer.

Procedure for Thermodilution Cardiac Output Measurement

A computation constant, based on the catheter size and volume of injectate, is set on the computer. The injectate solution used for the procedure is sterile normal saline or D_5W. Five or 10 mL of solution is drawn into the syringe, which is attached to the atrial port. Use of 10 mL enhances accuracy. The syringe is usually part of a closed system that remains intact and attached to the right atrial port by a stopcock (Fig. 17-61). Iced (0°C to 4°C) or room-temperature solution may be used. Room-temperature injectate has little effect on accuracy compared with iced injectate. The decision to use iced solution is based on the need to have at least a 10°C difference between the patient's blood temperature and the injectate. Iced solution may be necessary in hypothermic patients and may improve accuracy in very low cardiac output states.

When the injectate syringe is filled, the computer is activated, and it signals the time for injection. The injectate must be given quickly, in less than 4 seconds, and injected smoothly. When injected, the solution passes a temperature probe in the system and flows through the right atrium and right ventricle, past the thermistor at the tip of the PA catheter. The change in temperature sensed by the thermistor generates a cardiac output curve and measurement by the computer.

The average of several cardiac output determinations is required to obtain a final measurement. Serial measurements and averaging are necessary because of the number of physiological variables and the performance of the technical procedure. Three or more consecutive measurements are usually necessary. Measurements included in the average should be within 10% to 15% of each other, and each one should be associated with a normal cardiac output curve. Cardiac output measurements associated with abnormal curves are eliminated from the averaging process.

INTERPRETATION OF CARDIAC OUTPUT CURVES

Many bedside monitors and cardiac output computers are equipped with a strip recorder or modality for visualizing the cardiac output curves. Normal cardiac output curves have a smooth upstroke followed by a gradual decline (Fig. 17-62). Curves associated with high cardiac outputs are smaller and have a steeper upstroke and decline than curves associated with low cardiac outputs.

NURSING CONSIDERATIONS

Alterations in cardiac output are caused by changes in heart rate, preload, afterload, and contractility. Therefore, analysis of these parameters is essential in directing interventions to address the underlying pathophysiological process.

Decreased cardiac output may be related to a decrease in preload (right atrial pressure and PAWP) caused by hypovolemia or decreased venous return associated with mechanical ventilation and elevated intrathoracic pressures. Vasoconstriction causes elevated afterload and has several causes. Increased SVR may be a compensatory response to hypovolemia caused by vasoconstriction to maintain cardiac

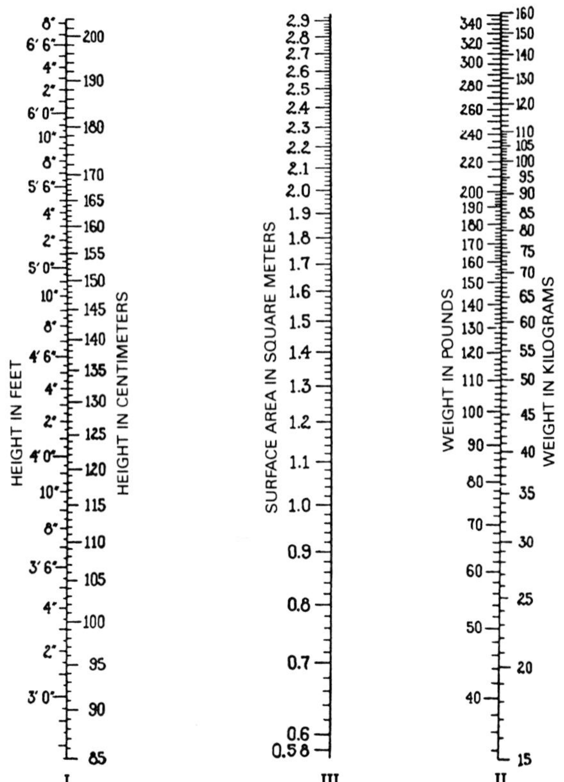

figure 17-60 Dubois body surface chart (as prepared by Boothby and Sandiford of the Mayo Clinic). To find the body surface area of a patient, locate the height in inches (or centimeters) on scale I and the weight in pounds (or kilograms) on scale II, and place a straightedge (ruler) between these two points, which intersect scale III at the patient's surface area.

output in this state. Some medications, hypothermia, and the compensatory vascular response to cardiogenic shock also increase afterload but decrease cardiac output and increase oxygen demand and the work of the heart. Reduction in contractility decreases cardiac output. Examples include insufficient oxygen delivery to the myocardium, causing myocardial ischemia and infarction; medications, such as beta-blocking agents; or metabolic imbalances, such as low serum levels of calcium, phosphorus, or magnesium.

Cardiac output increases with intravascular volume resuscitation, which increases preload. Decreased afterload due to vasodilation reduces resistance to ejection of blood, thus increasing cardiac output. Vasodilating medications, septic states, or allergic and anaphylactic reactions are all causes of vasodilation and result in elevated cardiac output. Positive inotropic agents or correction of impaired myocardial oxygenation or metabolic derangements may cause enhanced contractility, most often resulting in increased cardiac output.

Evaluation of Oxygen Delivery and Demand Balance

One of the primary objectives of hemodynamic monitoring is to apply the data obtained from the PA catheter to the evaluation of oxygen delivery or transport and the consumption of oxygen by the tissues and organs. Adequate oxygen delivery to the body's organs is essential for maintenance of cellular, tissue, and ultimately organ function. Insufficient oxygen delivery and consumption to meet the cellular requirements for oxygen, or oxygen demand, result in hypoxia and the accumulation of an oxygen deficit. Persistent oxygen deficit causes cell and organ dysfunction and eventually leads to cell death and organ failure. Table 17-16 lists the parameters that are used to evaluate oxygen delivery and demand balance, the formulas, and normal values.

DETERMINANTS OF OXYGEN DELIVERY

Arterial oxygen delivery (DaO_2) is the amount of oxygen transported to the tissues. DaO_2 depends on arterial oxygen content and cardiac output.

Oxygen Content

Oxygen content is the total amount of oxygen in the blood that is available to the cells. Most of the available oxygen (fuel) in arterial blood (more than 95%) is reversibly bound to hemoglobin in the form of oxyhemoglobin and is measured by arterial oxygen saturation (SaO_2). A very small amount of oxygen (less than 5%) is dissolved in plasma and measured as PaO_2. A sufficient amount of hemoglobin is required to ensure adequate oxygen-carrying capacity. The two primary determinants of oxygen content are hemoglobin and oxygen saturation.

Cardiac Output

Cardiac output is required to deliver oxygenated blood to the cells of the body. DaO_2 is assessed by evaluating the adequacy of cardiac output and arterial oxygen content. In nonstressed states, normal DaO_2 is 1,000 mL O_2/minute, or indexed to BSA, 600 mL O_2/minute/m^2. Increases in the body's oxygen demand associated with injury or illness are initially and primarily met by a compensatory increased cardiac output. Deficiencies of hemoglobin, arterial saturation, or cardiac output decrease DaO_2 to cells and threaten the adequacy of cellular oxygenation.[4]

DETERMINANTS OF OXYGEN CONSUMPTION

Oxygen consumption ($\dot{V}O_2$) is the amount of oxygen used by the tissues of the body. The primary determinants of $\dot{V}O_2$ are the cellular demand for oxygen, the delivery of adequate amounts of oxygen, and the extraction of oxygen from the blood for use by the cells.

Oxygen Demand

Oxygen demand is the requirement of cells for oxygen and is not directly measurable. Any stress increases the oxygen demand (e.g., surgery, infection, mobilization, pain, anxiety). Reduced oxygen demands are associated with lower metabolic rates (e.g., hypothermia, sedation, pharmacological paralysis). Oxygen demands are met through adequate delivery of oxygen and cellular extraction of oxygen.

Oxygen Delivery

Cellular use of oxygen depends on an adequate supply of oxygen. This is termed *delivery-dependent oxygen consumption* (Fig. 17-63). As oxygen delivery increases, oxygen consumption also increases to meet the oxygen demand. When the requirement for oxygen is met, further increases in oxygen delivery do not increase consumption. The level

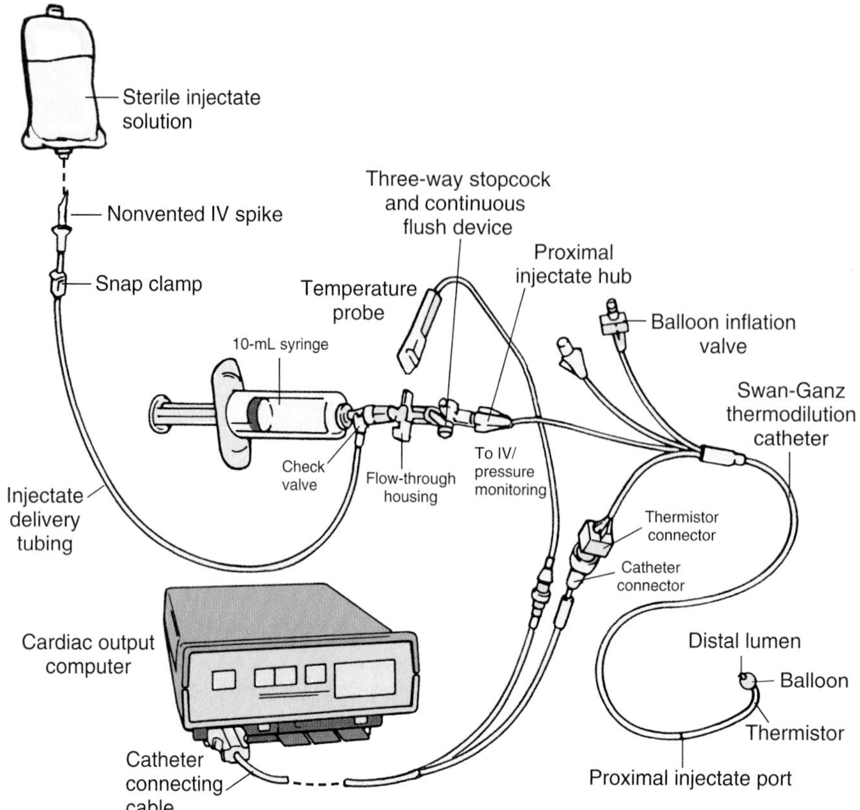

figure 17-61 A closed injectate system for measurement of cardiac output.

of critical oxygen delivery is the point at which a decrease in oxygen delivery results in decreased $\dot{V}O_2$ because of an insufficient oxygen supply.

Oxygen Extraction

Oxygen extraction ($CaO_2 - CvO_2$) is the amount of oxygen removed from the blood for use by the cells. It is measured by comparing the arterial oxygen content to venous oxygen content. Like arterial oxygen content, venous oxygen content (CvO_2) is primarily determined by the amount of hemoglobin that is saturated with oxygen. Venous saturation is obtained by withdrawing a mixed venous blood gas sample from the distal port of the PA catheter.

In normal circumstances, provided that oxygen is supplied in adequate amounts, the cells extract the oxygen they need to support tissue and organ function. Increased demand for oxygen results in a compensatory increase in oxygen extraction as more oxygen is "unloaded" from the hemoglobin for cellular use. The decreased amount of oxygen in venous blood means that the $CaO_2 - CvO_2$ difference is larger. Conversely, as oxygen demands decrease, less oxygen is required and extracted from the blood, and the $CaO_2 - CvO_2$ difference becomes smaller.[4]

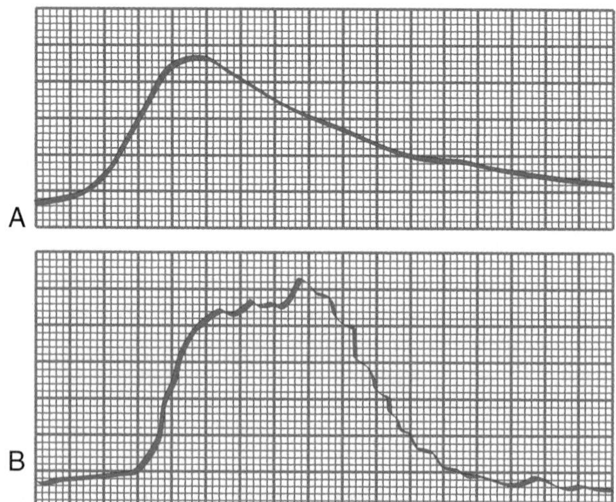

figure 17-62 Thermodilution curves produced on a strip chart recorder. (**A**) Smooth recording is accurate. (**B**) Irregular recording is distorted, probably because of irregular or uneven emptying of the injectate syringe.

OXYGEN SUPPLY AND DEMAND IMBALANCE

An imbalance of oxygen supply and demand occurs whenever oxygen delivery is inadequate to meet cellular demand or the cells are unable to extract sufficient quantities of oxygen. Specific threats to the balance of oxygen supply and demand are decreased cardiac output, hemoglobin, or arterial saturation; impaired cellular extraction of oxygen; or oxygen demands that are so great that they cannot be met by increased oxygen delivery or extraction.

Metabolic Indicators of Oxygen Debt

Inadequate oxygen consumption causes an anaerobic state and cellular hypoxia. Cells deprived of oxygen begin to acquire an oxygen debt. Over time, oxygen debt accumulation becomes irreversible, cell damage is irreparable, and cell death results. Oxygen debt is a major cause of mul-

table 17-16 Oxygen Use Variables

Parameter	Formula	Normal Values
Cao_2	$(Hb \times 1.37 \times Sao_2) + (0.003 \times Pao_2)$	20 mL O_2/dL
Cvo_2	$(Hb \times 1.37 \times S\bar{v}o_2) + (0.003 \times Pvo_2)$	15 mL O_2/dL
Dao_2I	$CI \times Cao_2 \times 10$	500–600 mL O_2/min/m^2
Dvo_2I	$CI \times Cvo_2 \times 10$	375–450 mL O_2/min/m^2
$S\bar{v}o_2$	Direct measurement	60%–80%
Pvo_2	Direct measurement	35–45 mm Hg
O_2 extraction	$Cao_2 - Cvo_2$	3–5 mL O_2/dL
OER	$\frac{Cao_2 - Cvo_2}{Cao_2}$	22%–30%
Vo_2I	$(Cao_2 - Cvo_2) \times CI \times 10$	120–170 mL/min/m^2
pHa	Direct measurement	7.35–7.45
BE/BD	Direct measurement	−2 to +2
Lactate	Direct measurement	0.5–2.2 mmol/L

OER, oxygen extraction ratio; Vo_2I, oxygen consumption index; pHa, arterial pH; BE/BD, base excess/base deficit; Cao_2, arterial oxygen content; Hb, hemoglobin; Cvo_2,venous oxygen content; Dao_2I, arterial oxygen delivery index; Dvo_2I, venous oxygen delivery index.

tisystem organ dysfunction and failure. If oxygen debt accumulation is identified before irreversible cell injury has occurred, the oxygen deficit may be reversed by increasing oxygen availability.

Several metabolic parameters can be measured to evaluate oxygen debt. When these indicators of oxygen debt are used in conjunction with hemodynamic monitoring of oxygen delivery and consumption, therapies may be more specifically directed to achieve a balanced oxygen supply and demand.

Because hypoxia and oxygen debt are associated with anaerobic metabolism, the byproducts of anaerobic metabolism can be used to assess the presence of an oxygen deficit. Lactic acid accumulation causes a metabolic acidosis in an oxygen debt state. Therefore, laboratory measurement of lactate levels, serum pH, and base deficit/excess are means to evaluate oxygen debt. Serum pH and base deficit/excess are routinely measured and reported with blood gas analysis. Elevated lactate levels (>2.2 mm/L) or metabolic acidosis ($pH < 7.35$ with normal $Paco_2$) correlate with oxygen debt, particularly when the patient has a low or even normal level of Dao_2 and $\dot{V}o_2$. As with all assessment parameters, lactate levels, pH, and base deficit should not be viewed in isolation; they should be evaluated in conjunction with other assessment parameters.[4]

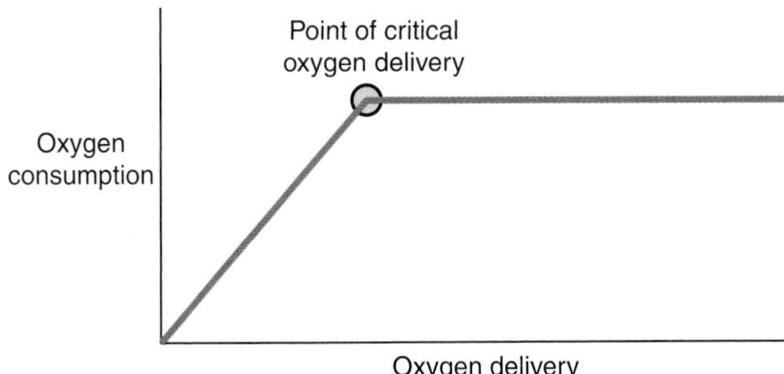

figure 17-63 Delivery-dependent oxygen consumption curve reflecting the change in oxygen consumption related to oxygen delivery. At the point of critical oxygen delivery, oxygen delivery is sufficient to meet oxygen demand, and oxygen consumption does not increase further. However, any decrease in oxygen delivery from this point results in a decrease of oxygen consumption due to an inadequate supply of oxygen.

Monitoring of Continuous Mixed Venous Oxygen Saturation

Mixed venous oxygen saturation ($S\bar{v}o_2$) may be used to reflect the balance of oxygen supply, oxygen use, and oxygen demand. $S\bar{v}o_2$ is the measurement of oxyhemoglobin in desaturated blood returning to the right ventricle and PA. The $S\bar{v}o_2$ is significantly less than arterial saturation because of the extraction of oxygen by the cells and the unloading of oxygen from hemoglobin. $S\bar{v}o_2$ is influenced by the degree of arterial saturation, the quantity of hemoglobin, the cardiac output, the determinants of oxygen delivery, and the amount of oxygen extracted and consumed by the cells. Under normal conditions of oxygen delivery, oxygen consumption, and oxygen demand, approximately 25% of the available oxygen is extracted and used to meet demand. In this situation, the $S\bar{v}o_2$ is 60% to 80%. If oxygen delivery is reduced by a decrease in arterial saturation, hemoglobin, or cardiac output, then more oxygen is extracted from the blood to meet cellular demand. The blood returning to the right side of the heart and PA has had a greater quantity of oxygen removed and is more desaturated, which is reflected by a decrease in $S\bar{v}o_2$. Similarly, if oxygen demand increases but oxygen delivery does not increase to meet this requirement, additional oxygen is extracted from the blood and consumed by the cells. Therefore, oxyhemoglobin is reduced in the venous blood, decreasing $S\bar{v}O_2$. Persistently low $S\bar{v}O_2$ is a warning that an oxygen debt may be accruing because of inadequate oxygen delivery or a high oxygen demand not met by the oxygen supply.

Three general conditions result in increasing $S\bar{v}O_2$:

- When the oxygen delivery is much greater than the oxygen demand, only a small percentage of the delivered oxygen is extracted, causing $S\bar{v}O_2$ to increase.
- When the metabolic rate and oxygen demand are low, the need for oxygen is reduced, and less oxygen is extracted and consumed. $S\bar{v}O_2$ reflects the decrease in extraction as greater amounts of oxyhemoglobin are returned to the right side of the heart.
- In pathological states in which the cells cannot extract oxygen from the blood or in which tissue beds are not well perfused with oxygenated blood, oxygen is not extracted from the blood despite the cellular oxygen demand. The $S\bar{v}O_2$, returning to the right side of the heart and PA is therefore higher because of the decreased oxygen consumption.

Although the $S\bar{v}O_2$ may be in the normal range, cells in the body may not use or receive the oxygen they require, and they may begin to accumulate an oxygen debt because of the reduced cellular oxygen extraction or the shunting of oxygenated blood past tissue beds. In such a situation, a normal $S\bar{v}O_2$ may be misleading when viewed in isolation.

$S\bar{v}O_2$ can be continuously measured at the bedside by a PA catheter containing fiberoptic filaments in one of the lumens ending at the tip of the catheter in the PA. The blood in the PA is venous blood, most of which is desaturated. An infrared light is emitted that reflects off the red blood cells that are saturated with oxygen. The percentage of saturated hemoglobin compared with the total hemoglobin is calculated by the $S\bar{v}O_2$ monitoring computer to yield the venous saturation value. The information is updated every few seconds; thus, a continuous $S\bar{v}O_2$ reading is obtained.

NURSING CONSIDERATIONS

When patients are critically ill, careful evaluation of the adequacy of oxygen delivery, oxygen extraction, and consumption with respect to oxygen demand is paramount. Scrutiny of each determinant of cardiac output (heart rate, preload, afterload, and contractility parameters), oxygen content (arterial saturation and hemoglobin), oxygen consumption (DaO_2 and $CaO_2 - CvO_2$), and oxygen debt (lactate, pH, base deficit/excess, $S\bar{v}O_2$) is important to critical care nursing.

Numerous interventions are used to enhance oxygen delivery. Measures to increase cardiac output include the addition of intravascular volume to increase preload as well as the administration of positive inotropic agents to improve contractility and vasodilating agents to reduce afterload. Interventions that may increase oxygen content include changes in mechanical ventilator settings; chest physiotherapy; positioning and mobilization; and, in nonmechanically ventilated patients, coughing and deep-breathing exercises. All of these techniques improve arterial oxygenation. Administration of packed red blood cells increases hemoglobin and oxygen-carrying capacity. In all cases, it is necessary to manage both the treatment modalities and patient response to therapy.

Many of the interventions used to decrease oxygen demand and increase oxygen consumption are important tenets of nursing care. For example, appropriate management of the environment, pain, and anxiety reduces stress, thus decreasing the demand for oxygen. Maintaining normothermia by control of the patient's temperature may decrease oxygen requirements associated with fevers and facilitate impaired perfusion and oxygen consumption associated with hypothermia.

$S\bar{v}O_2$ monitoring may be a helpful guide in nursing interventions. For example, endotracheal suctioning may cause a temporary decrease in arterial oxygenation and increase discomfort and anxiety. Monitoring $S\bar{v}O_2$ allows the nurse to judge the impact of this activity on the patient's oxygen supply and demand. A decreasing $S\bar{v}O_2$ during suctioning is usually caused by increased oxygen demand and decreased arterial oxygenation. Hyperoxygenating and hyperventilating before, during, and after suctioning helps lessen the negative effects on oxygen demand and arterial oxygenation. Before preceding to another activity such as repositioning, the nurse should monitor the $S\bar{v}O_2$ and wait until the value normalizes, thereby avoiding an additional stressor and further increase on oxygen demand.

clinical applicability challenges

Self-Challenge: Critical Thinking

The following five questions are based on the Case Study that appeared earlier in this chapter.

1. *What are the nursing priorities when a patient such as Mrs. James enters the coronary care unit?*
2. *Mrs. James' daughters accompany their mother when she arrives in the coronary care unit, and they want to know why so many blood samples have been taken from their mother. As a nurse in the unit, what do you tell them?*
3. *About 8 hours after Mrs. James' admission to the coronary care unit, you note that her heart rhythm has changed to atrial fibrillation with a ventricular response of 110 beats/minute. What are your clinical concerns about this rhythm?*
4. *Stressors of any type increase the body's oxygen demand. Develop specific interventions to reduce or minimize Mrs. James' oxygen demand and decrease the work of her heart, and outline anticipated interventions to improve oxygen delivery.*
5. *Mrs. James is scheduled for a cardiac catheterization on hospital day 3. As a coronary care nurse, how do you explain this test to her and her family?*

Study Questions

Cardiac History and Physical Examination

1. *In the case concerning Mrs. James, which of the following risk factors may have contributed to her acute myocardial infarction?*
   a. *Age*
   b. *History of hypertension*

c. *History of hyperlipidemia*
d. *All of the above*

2. *During a physical examination, the nurse palpates the precordium. Where is the apical pulse normally located?*
   a. *Left sternal border at the fifth intercostal space*
   b. *Left midclavicular line at the fourth or fifth intercostal space*
   c. *Left anterior axillary line at the fifth intercostal space*
   d. *Left sternal border at the second intercostal space*

3. S_2 *is an important heart sound that is timed with the*
   a. *beginning of diastole.*
   b. *closure of the mitral and tricuspid valves.*
   c. *closure of the pulmonic and aortic valves.*
   d. *early, rapid-filling phase of ventricular diastole.*

Cardiac Laboratory Studies

1. *The myocardial protein that is most sensitive to myocardial injury and is not influenced by other muscle damage is*
   a. *LDH.*
   b. *troponin I.*
   c. *CK-MB.*
   d. *myoglobin.*

2. *With myocardial damage, the subforms of CK-MB, CK-*MB_1 *and CK-*MB_2
   a. *normally are not affected.*
   b. *should be in a 1:1 CK-*MB_1*:CK-*MB_2 *ratio.*
   c. *usually demonstrate CK-*MB_2 > *CK-*MB_1.
   d. *usually demonstrate CK-*MB_1 > *CK-*MB_2.

3. *Troponin has a distinct advantage over other serum markers for monitoring because troponin*
   a. *peaks first before other serum markers are released.*
   b. *falls rapidly compared with CK.*
   c. *may remain elevated several days, thereby confirming myocardial damage or necrosis.*
   d. *is only moderately affected by noncardiac muscle damage.*

Cardiac Diagnostic Studies

1. *Evaluation of syncope in cardiac patients is best accomplished using*
   a. *a signal-averaged electrocardiogram.*
   b. *an implantable loop monitor.*
   c. *a Holter monitor.*
   d. *a standard 12-lead electrocardiogram.*

2. *Cardiac and vascular structural integrity is best evaluated with*
   a. *transesophageal echocardiography.*
   b. *M-mode echocardiography.*
   c. *phonocardiography.*
   d. *Doppler echocardiography.*

3. *Absolute contraindications to the use of MRI include*
   a. *history of biological (tissue) cardiac valve replacement.*
   b. *permanent cardiac pacemaker.*
   c. *use of an artificial limb.*
   d. *presence of surgical staples.*

4. *Postprocedure care for the cardiac catheterization patient includes all of the following except*
   a. *permitting leg flexion only to 30 degrees.*
   b. *continually monitoring heart rate, blood pressure, and oxygenation by pulse oximetry.*
   c. *monitoring hemostasis over the catheterization site.*
   d. *monitoring coagulation status.*

Electrocardiographic Monitoring

1. *You have decided to monitor your patient using a modified version of chest lead 6 (*MCL_6*). To achieve this electrical view of the heart, you would turn the monitor to lead II and place the lead wires in which of the following positions?*
   a. *Negative below the left clavicle and positive in the left midaxillary line, fifth intercostal space*
   b. *Negative below the right clavicle and positive left midclavicular line below lowest rib*
   c. *Negative below the right clavicle and positive below the left clavicle*
   d. *Negative below the left clavicle and positive in the fourth intercostal space right sternal border*

2. *You have decided to monitor your patient using lead II. To achieve this electrical view of the heart, you would place the lead wires in which of the following positions?*
   a. *The positive under the left clavicle and the negative under the right clavicle*
   b. *The positive on the left side of the body below the heart and the negative below the right clavicle*
   c. *The positive on the left side of the body below the heart and the negative below the left clavicle*
   d. *The positive below the right clavicle and the negative on the left side of the body below the heart*

3. *The best leads to distinguish ventricular ectopy from supraventricular rhythms with aberrancy are*
   a. *leads II, III, aVF.*
   b. *leads I, aVL,* V_5, V_6.
   c. *leads* V_1 *and* V_6.
   d. *leads* V_1, V_2, V_3.

Arrhythmias and the 12-Lead Electrocardiogram

1. *The QRS complex represents*
   a. *contraction of the ventricles.*
   b. *repolarization of the atria.*
   c. *depolarization of the ventricles.*
   d. *repolarization of the ventricles.*

2. *Sam, a healthy 20-year-old student, has normal sinus rhythm with a heart rate of 62 beats/minute at rest. During sleep, his heart rate is as low as 50 beats/minute, and during exercise, it is as high as 110 beats/minute. Which of the following statements best describes these heart rate variations?*
   a. *The heart rate varies from sinus bradycardia to sinus tachycardia, and the rate ranges would be considered extreme; this is likely due to pathological sinus node disease.*
   b. *The heart rate varies from sinus bradycardia to sinus tachycardia; although the variations in rate may not be pathological, it is doubtful they are normal.*
   c. *The heart rate variations of 50 to 110 beats/minute are well within the range of normal sinus rhythm.*
   d. *The heart rate range from sinus tachycardia to sinus bradycardia is physiological—a normal response to exercise and rest.*

3. *Patients in atrial fibrillation are at increased risk for thromboembolism. The reason for this is*
   a. *in atrial fibrillation, the contents of the atria are not sufficiently expelled, allowing thrombi to form.*
   b. *atrial fibrillation is often accompanied by platelet aggregation.*

c. *atrial fibrillation so diminishes cardiac output that patient's inactivity results in thrombus formation in the lower legs and pelvic regions.*
d. *atrial fibrillation is nearly always a symptom of underlying valvular heart disease, a common site for thrombus formation.*

4. *In atrial flutter*
   a. *the atrial and ventricular rates are both equal and rapid.*
   b. *the QRS complex is widened.*
   c. *the ventricles respond only to every second, third, or fourth atrial stimuli.*
   d. *always requires cardioversion to convert.*
5. *The ECG shows extra beats that appear early in the rhythm, have no P wave, and a wide QRS complex. These beats are*
   a. *sinus in origin.*
   b. *atrial in origin.*
   c. *nodal in origin.*
   d. *ventricular in origin.*
6. *The P wave in junctional rhythm*
   a. *is absent because the impulse starts at the AV junction.*
   b. *is normal in configuration and precedes each QRS complex.*
   c. *may be inverted before, during, or after the QRS complex.*
   d. *occurs twice as frequently as the QRS complex because the AV node blocks every other beat.*
7. *In third-degree heart block, the greatest clinical concern is*
   a. *the sluggish conduction through the AV node.*
   b. *the instability of the ventricular focus.*
   c. *the risk of SA node failure.*
   d. *the rapid ventricular response due to AV nodal problems.*
8. *Hyperkalemia may cause which of the following changes on the ECG?*
   a. *Tall, peaked T waves*
   b. *U wave*
   c. *Prolonged QT interval*
   d. *Shortened QT interval*
9. *Hypocalcemia produces which of the following changes on the ECG?*
   a. *Prolonged QT interval*
   b. *Shortened QT interval*
   c. *Prominent U waves*
   d. *Tall, peaked T waves*

Hemodynamic Monitoring

1. *What is the normal pulmonary artery pressure?*
   a. *15 to 25/0 to 8 mm Hg*
   b. *20 to 30/8 to 15 mm Hg*
   c. *110 to 160/60 to 90 mm Hg*
   d. *35 to 50/15 to 30 mm Hg*
2. *What is the most common complication encountered during a PA catheter insertion?*
   a. *Arrhythmias*
   b. *Catheter contamination*
   c. *PA perforation*
   d. *Balloon rupture*

Questions 3 through 5 are based on a man who is in the intensive care unit with a diagnosis of acute inferior wall MI. Today he seems restless and apprehensive, but he has no specific complaints of pain. The table presents the assessment data recorded:

Time	Apical Pulse (beats/min)	Arterial Blood Pressure (mm Hg)	CVP (mm Hg)
8 AM	84	100/70	3–4
10 AM	102	98/72	3–4
11 AM	120	95/75	3–4
PAP (mm Hg)	**PAWP (mm Hg)**		**Cardiac Output**
26/10	12		6 L/min
28/12	13		4 L/min
30/14	14		3 L/min

3. *The increasing pulmonary artery pressure (PAP) and PAWP probably indicate*
   a. *blood volume depletion.*
   b. *left ventricular failure.*
   c. *cardiac arrhythmias.*
   d. *right ventricular failure.*
4. *The increasing pulse rate probably indicates*
   a. *nothing, because it is only slightly above normal.*
   b. *the body's response to cardiac structural damage.*
   c. *anxiety.*
   d. *the heart's attempt to compensate for inadequate cardiac output.*
5. *The steady CVP readings show that*
   a. *cardiac function is stable.*
   b. *peripheral resistance is low.*
   c. *the right heart is still adequately handling venous return.*
   d. *the patient is dehydrated.*

REFERENCES

Cardiac History and Physical Examination

1. American Heart Association: Risk Factors and Coronary Heart Disease. Available at www.AHA.org. Accessed March 27, 2004
2. American Heart Association: Heart and Stroke Facts. Dallas, American Heart Association, 2003
3. Bickley L: Bates' Guide to Physical Examination and Health History (8th Ed). Philadelphia, Lippincott Williams & Wilkins, 2003
4. Weber J, Kelley J: Health Assessment in Nursing (2nd Ed). Philadelphia, Lippincott Williams & Wilkins, 2003

Cardiac Laboratory Studies

1. Adams J, Sicard G, Allen B, et al: Diagnosis of perioperative myocardial infarction with measurement of cardiac troponin I. N Engl J Med 330:670–674, 1994
2. Apple S: Advanced strategies for diagnosing acute myocardial infarction. Heartbeat 6:1, 12, 1995
3. Gordon C, Rempher K: Brain (B-type) natriuretic peptide: Implications for heart failure management. AACN Clin Issues 14(4):522–542, 2003
4. Dao Q, Krishnaswamy P, Kazanegra R, et al: Utility of B-type natriuretic peptide in the diagnosis of congestive heart failure in an urgent-care setting. J Am Coll Cardiol 37:379–385, 2001
5. Futterman L, Lemberg L: Novel markers in the acute coronary syndrome: BNP, IL-6, PAPP-A. Am J Crit Care 11(2):168–172, 2002
6. de Lemos JA, Morrow DA, Bentley JH, et al: The prognostic value of B-type natriuretic peptide in patients with acute coronary syndrome. N Engl J Med 345:1014–1021, 2001
7. McErlean E: New advances in the management of acute coronary syndromes: Evolving strategies for nursing practice. Presented at the AACN National Teaching Institute, Orlando, FL, May 23, 2000
8. Roettig M, Tanabe P: Emergency management of acute coronary syndromes. J Emerg Nurs 26(6 Suppl):S1–S42, 2000

9. Bays-Genis A, Mateo J, Santalo M, et al: D-Dimer is an early diagnostic marker of coronary ischemia in patients with chest pain. Am Heart J 140(3):379–384, 2000
10. Newby L: Cardiac marker testing: Where should we focus? Am Heart J 140(3):351–353, 2000

Cardiac Diagnostic Studies

1. Cerino-Toth L: Implantable loop monitor for detection of syncopy. Crit Care Nurs Clin North Am 11(3):297–302, 1999
2. Gan TJ: The esophageal Doppler as an alternative to the pulmonary artery catheter. Curr Opin Crit Care 6:214–221, 2000
3. Payen D: Oesophageal Doppler monitoring: History, physical principles and clinical applications. Int J Intensive Care 4(3):88–93, 1997
4. Marik PE: Pulmonary artery catheterization and esophageal Doppler monitoring in the ICU. Chest 116(4):1085–1090, 1999
5. Shaw AD, Weavind LM, Parnley L: Comparison of thermodilution, esophageal Doppler and transesophageal echocardiography data in the hemodynamic assessment of critically ill cancer patients. Crit Care Med 28(12 Suppl):159/M65, 2000
6. Saberi D, Caudwell L, McGloin H, et al: Proactive circulatory management in the 1st 4 hours post-cardiac surgery: Interim analysis of a nurse-led, oesophageal Doppler-guided protocol. Intensive Care Med 26(3 Suppl):S220, 2000
7. Darty S, Thomas M, Neagle C, et al: Cardiovascular magnetic resonance imaging. Am J Nurs 102(12):34–38, 2002
8. Carr M, Greg M: Magnetic resonance imaging. Am J Nurs 102(12): 26–33, 2002
9. Bosen D, Flemming M: Electrophysiologic testing. Dimens Crit Care Nurs 22(1):10–19, 2003

Electrocardiographic Monitoring

1. Huff J: EKG Workout: Exercises in Arrhythmia Interpretation (4th Ed). Philadelphia, Lippincott Williams & Wilkins, 2001
2. Springhouse: EKG Interpretation Made Incredibly Easy (2nd Ed). Springhouse, PA, Springhouse, 2002

Arrhythmias and the 12-Lead Electrocardiogram

1. American College of Cardiology/American Heart Association/ European Society of Cardiology: Guidelines for the management of patients with atrial fibrillation: Executive summary. J Am Coll Cardiol 38:1231–1265, 2002
2. Snow V, Weiss K, LeFevre M, et al: Management of newly detected atrial fibrillation: A clinical practice guideline from the American Academy of Family Physicians and the American College of Physicians. Ann Intern Med 139:1009–1017, 2003
3. Tilley P, Petersen D: Pulling axis together. Dimens Crit Care Nurs 22(5):210–215, 2003
4. Grauer K: A Practical Guide to EKG Interpretation (2nd Ed). St. Louis, Mosby, 1998

Hemodynamic Monitoring

1. Darovic G: Hemodynamic Monitoring: Invasive and Noninvasive Clinical Application (3rd Ed). Philadelphia, WB Saunders, 2002
2. Daily E: Hemodynamic waveform analysis. J Cardiovasc Nurs 15(2): 6–22, 2001
3. McGhee B, Bridges E: Monitoring arterial blood pressure: What you may not know. Crit Care Nurse 22(2):60–79, 2002
4. Von Rueden KT, Dunham CM: Evaluation and management of oxygen delivery and consumption in multiple organ dysfunction syndrome. In Secor VH (ed): Multiple Organ Dysfunction and Failure: Pathophysiology and Clinical Implications (2nd Ed), pp 384–401. St. Louis, CV Mosby, 1996

OTHER SELECTED READING

Cardiac Assessment

Martinez EA, Kim LJ, Faraday N, et al: Sensitivity of routine intensive care unit surveillance for detecting myocardial ischemia. Crit Care Med 31(9):2302–2308, 2003

Sweeney J, Cody M, O'Sullivan P, et al: Women's early warning symptoms of acute myocardial infarction. Circulation 108(21): 2619–2623, 2003

Cardiac Laboratory and Diagnostic Studies

Futterman LG, Lemberg L: High-sensitivity C-reactive protein is the most effective prognostic measurement of acute coronary events. Am J Crit Care 11(5): 482–486, 2002

Jones-Reeder S, Hoffman RL, Magdic KS, et al: Homocysteine: The latest risk factor for heart disease. Dimens Crit Care Nurs 19(1):22–28, 2000

Malinow MR, Bostom AG, Krauss RM: Homocysteine, diet and cardiovascular diseases. Circulation 99(1):178–182, 1999

MacKenzie JR: Predicting CAD events: C-reactive protein: A marker for atherosclerotic risk. The Nurse Practitioner 29(6):14–27, 2004

Reiff PA, Gutierez JD: Use of the insertable loop recorder to detect cardiac arrhythmias during syncopal episodes. Medsurg Nurs 13(2):105–109, 2004

Taylor-Chinn M: Homocysteine and atherosclerotic heart disease. Clinician Rev 10(10): 45–57, 2000

Electrocardiographic Monitoring

Adams-Hamoda MG, Caldwell MA, Stotts NA, et al: Factors to consider when analyzing 12-lead electrocardiograms for evidence of acute myocardial ischemia. Am J Crit Care 12(1): 9–16, 2003

Bosen DM: Atrio-ventricular nodal re-entry tachycardia. Dimens Crit Care Nurs 21(4):134–139, 2002

Bosen DM: Identifying inappropriate sinus tachycardia. Nursing2001, 31(7): 1–5, 2001

Brady WJ, Hwang V, Sullivan R, et al: A comparison of 12 and 15-lead ECG's on ED chest pain patients: Impact on diagnosis, therapy and disposition. Am J Emerg Med 18(3): 239–243, 2000

Hampton CT: Long QT syndrome: More common than you thought. Clin Rev 13(1): 40–45, 2003

Zimetbaum PJ, Josephson ME: Use of the electrocardiogram in acute myocardial infarction. N Engl J Med 348(10):933–940, 2003

Hemodynamic Monitoring

Bernard GR, Sopko G, Cerra F, et al: Pulmonary artery catheterization and clinical outcomes: National Heart, Lung and Blood Institute and Food and Drug Administration Workshop Report. JAMA 283(19):2568–2572, 2000

Druding MC: Integrating hemodynamic monitoring and physical assessment. Dimens Crit Care Nurs 19(4):25–30, 2000

Dulak SB: What the waveforms reveal [Online]. RN Web 66(9):56–63, 2003. Available: www.rnweb.com

Leeper B: Monitoring right ventricular volumes: A paradigm shift. AACN Clin Issues 14(2) 208–219, 2003

Moore K: Critical care hemodynamic parameters and pharmacologic interventions. Crit Care Nurs Clinics North Am 14(1):71–76, 2002

Ott K, Johnson K, Ahrens T: New technologies in the assessment of hemodynamic parameters. J Cardiovasc Nurs 15(2):41–55, 2001

Prentice D, Ahrens T: Controversies in the use of the pulmonary artery catheter. J Cardiovasc Nurs 15(2):1–5, 2001

Turner MA: Doppler-based hemodynamic monitoring: A minimally invasive alternative. AACN Clin Issues 14(2):220–231, 2003

chapter **18**

Patient Management: Cardiovascular System

MARLA DE JONG ■ VICKI COOMBS ■ KENNETH REMPHER ■
DULCE OBIAS-MANN ■ CONRAD GORDON

objectives

Based on the content in this chapter, the reader should be able to:

- Compare and contrast commonly used fibrinolytics, anticoagulants, and platelet inhibitors used to affect the thrombotic process.
- Describe the four classes of antidysrhythmic drugs.
- Explain how inotropic drugs improve myocardial function.
- Discuss the rationale for using angiotensin-converting enzyme inhibitor drugs for patients with cardiovascular disease.
- Compare and contrast the four major classes of antihyperlipidemic drugs.
- Compare and contrast the indications and contraindications for percutaneous coronary interventions (PCI), including percutaneous transluminal coronary angioplasty (PTCA), intracoronary stenting, directional coronary atherectomy (DCA), laser, brachytherapy, and percutaneous balloon valvuloplasty (PBV).
- Summarize interventions for complications associated with PCI procedures.
- List potential nursing diagnoses and the interventions for each diagnosis in the patient undergoing an interventional cardiology procedure.
- Describe the physiological effect of intra-aortic balloon pump (IABP) counterpulsation therapy.
- Explain indications for and contraindications to IABP therapy.
- Describe a ventricular assist device and its indications and mechanism of action.
- Discuss nursing interventions for the patient receiving IABP therapy or ventricular circulatory assistance.
- Describe the indications, procedure, and nursing management for cardioversion and radiofrequency catheter ablation.
- Describe the components of the pacing system and pacemaker functioning.
- Use the pacemaker code to describe modes of pacing.
- Explain complications of pacing and appropriate interventions.
- Discuss the nursing management of the patient with a pacemaker.
- Describe the indications for an implantable cardioverter–defibrillator (ICD).
- Describe the ICD system and its functioning.
- Explain the nursing management of a patient with an ICD.
- Describe causes of cardiopulmonary arrest.
- Explain steps of cardiopulmonary resuscitation.
- Discuss roles of members of the resuscitation team.
- Explain indications, procedure, and nursing management for defibrillation.
- Discuss the rationale for using hypothermia as part of cardiopulmonary arrest management.
- Describe pros and cons of having family members present in a cardiopulmonary arrest situation.

Pharmacological Therapy

Cardiovascular disease continues to be the leading cause of death in the United States. However, recent and remarkable pharmacological advances have reduced morbidity and mortality related to cardiovascular disease.

Critical care nurses are responsible for preparing and administering potent drugs that affect the patient's cardiovascular function. Furthermore, nurses continuously evaluate the effects of these drugs and use detailed patient assessment data to guide the titration of these drugs.

This section summarizes drugs that are commonly used in critical care settings to treat cardiovascular disease. Recent research data are included to provide a scientific basis for drug therapy. Pharmacotherapy advances continually occur; therefore, changes in drug therapy are common. Critical care nurses frequently use current drug books or guides because before administering drugs, nurses must know the drug's effects, contraindications, dosage and method of administration, and adverse effects. Finally, many patients require treatment with numerous cardiovascular drugs; therefore, it is important to consider how drugs interact with other drugs.

FIBRINOLYTICS, ANTICOAGULANTS, AND PLATELET INHIBITORS

Atherosclerotic plaque rupture or vascular endothelium damage initiates a complex platelet reaction, consisting of adhesion, activation, and aggregation. The platelet aggregate accelerates thrombin production through the coagulation cascade. When thrombin, a potent agonist for further platelet activation and coagulation cascade activity, converts fibrinogen to fibrin, a nonsoluble fibrin thrombus forms. For further information about the coagulation process, see Chapter 45. An arterial thrombus may transiently or persistently occlude coronary artery blood flow, causing acute coronary syndrome (ACS). Fibrinolytic, anticoagulant, and platelet inhibitor drugs affect different phases of the thrombotic process.

Fibrinolytics

Fibrinolytic agents are indicated for patients with acute ST segment elevation myocardial infarction. Fibrinolytic drugs are not effective for patients with ACS without ST segment elevation, a posterior wall acute myocardial infarction (AMI), or a new left bundle branch block. Fibrinolytic agents either directly or indirectly convert plasminogen to plasmin, which in turn lyses the thrombus. The goal of fibrinolytic therapy is to dissolve the thrombus, reestablish coronary blood flow, minimize infarct size, preserve left ventricular function, and reduce morbidity and mortality.[1] Table 18-1 summarizes commonly used fibrinolytic agents.

Many researchers continue to evaluate fibrinolytic agents, and numerous multicenter, randomized fibrinolytic trials have shown that fibrinolytic therapy significantly reduces mortality from AMI.[2] The Thrombolysis in Myocardial Infarction (TIMI) 10B trial found that a 40-mg dose

table 18-1 Fibrinolytic Drugs

	Alteplase	Reteplase	Tenecteplase	Streptokinase
Action	Binds to fibrin in a thrombus and converts plasminogen to plasmin	Catalyzes the cleavage of plasminogen to generate plasmin	Binds to fibrin and converts plasminogen to plasmin	Binds with plasminogen to produce a complex that converts plasminogen to plasmin
Indications	AMI Acute ischemic stroke Acute, massive PE Unlabeled use: to clear thrombi in central venous catheters (2 mg into blocked catheter)	AMI	AMI	AMI Acute PE Acute, extensive deep venous thrombosis Acute arterial thrombosis or embolism Occlusion of arteriovenous cannulae
Dose	100 mg IV over 90 min (15 mg IV bolus; 50 mg IV over 30 min; 35 mg IV over 60 min)	10 U + 10 U IV bolus (each 10 U given over 2 min; second bolus given 30 min after first bolus)	Weight-based dose IV over 5 sec: >60 kg = 30 mg ≥60 to <70 kg = 35 mg ≥70 to <80 kg = 40 mg ≥80 to <90 kg = 45 mg ≥90 kg = 50 mg	1,500,000 IU IV within 60 min
Half-life	<5 min	13–16 min	20–24 min	23 min

PE, pulmonary embolism.

of tenecteplase, a recently released fibrinolytic, achieved coronary artery patency and flow similar to that obtained with tissue-type plasminogen activator (tPA).[3] The Assessment of the Safety and Efficacy of a New Thrombolytic (ASSENT)-2 trial reported nearly identical mortality rates when comparing tPA and tenecteplase.[4] Although the Global Utilization of Streptokinase and tPA for Occluded Coronary Arteries (GUSTO) V trial found that half-dose reteplase plus abciximab did not reduce mortality significantly more than standard-dose reteplase, ongoing research is focused on whether mortality can be reduced by combining fibrinolytics with glycoprotein (GP) IIb/IIIa receptor antagonists or low–molecular-weight heparins (LMWHs).[5]

The decision to administer fibrinolytic therapy is based on the patient's cardiovascular physical assessment data and electrocardiogram (ECG). Unless contraindicated (Box 18-1), fibrinolytics should be given to patients with ST segment elevation greater than 0.1 mV in two or more contiguous leads, or a new-onset left bundle branch block. Fibrinolytic therapy produces the greatest mortality reduction when initiated within the first 0 to 4 hours of symptom onset; however, fibrinolytics are now administered up to 12 hours after symptom onset.[1] The goal is to administer a fibrinolytic drug within 30 minutes of presentation. Patients are at risk for recurrent thromboembolism; therefore, aspirin and heparin are given to most patients who receive fibrinolytic therapy.[6]

Reperfusion may be manifested by decreased or resolved ST segment elevation, abrupt cessation of chest pain, early peak of serum cardiac markers, and reperfusion dysrhythmias such as premature ventricular contractions (PVCs), ventricular tachycardia (VT), accelerated idioventricular rhythm (AIVR), and atrioventricular blocks. In contrast, reocclusion may be evidenced by recurrent chest pain and ST segment elevation, further myocardial ischemia or infarction, lethal dysrhythmias, cardiogenic shock, or death. The most common adverse effects of fibrinolytic therapy are bleeding, stroke, and reperfusion dysrhythmias. For more details about the use of fibrinolytic therapy for AMI, see Chapter 21.

Anticoagulants

Anticoagulants such as unfractionated heparin, LMWHs, direct thrombin inhibitors, and warfarin limit further fibrin formation and help prevent thromboembolism.[2]

box 18-1 ***Contraindications to Fibrinolytic Therapy***

- Active internal bleeding
- Prior hemorrhagic stroke
- Nonhemorrhagic stroke within the past year
- Intracranial neoplasm, arteriovenous malformation, or aneurysm
- Recent intracranial or intraspinal surgery
- Recent trauma
- Suspected aortic dissection
- Severe uncontrolled hypertension

Unfractionated heparin, the most commonly used anticoagulant drug for acute conditions, is indicated for ACS, venous thromboembolism, percutaneous coronary interventions (PCI), and surgical revascularization; and for patients receiving alteplase, reteplase, or tenecteplase. Heparin prevents clot formation by combining with antithrombin III and inhibiting circulating thrombin. However, unfractionated heparin does not lyse thrombi and is not an optimal anticoagulant due to its narrow therapeutic range, low bioavailability, varied anticoagulant response, requirement for parenteral administration and activated partial thromboplastin time (APTT) monitoring, and risk for bleeding, heparin-induced thrombocytopenia, and hypersensitivity reactions.

The dosage for unfractionated heparin varies according to its indication and route of administration. When used in conjunction with alteplase, the recommended heparin dosage is 60 U/kg intravenously (IV; maximum 4,000 U) bolus given when the alteplase infusion is started, followed by an infusion of 12 U/kg/hour (maximum 1,000 U/hour).[6] The heparin infusion rate is adjusted to maintain an APTT of 50 to 70 seconds for 48 hours. Protamine sulfate reverses the effects of heparin; however, protamine may cause a life-threatening anaphylactic reaction.

LMWHs, such as enoxaparin and dalteparin, are small fragments derived from unfractionated heparin and are appealing alternatives to heparin for patients with unstable angina, non–ST segment elevation AMI, or deep venous thrombosis (DVT). Table 18-2 summarizes these drugs, which inhibit clot formation by blocking factor Xa and thrombin. Patients with unstable angina or non–Q-wave myocardial infarction (NQWMI) who received enoxaparin had lower rates of recurrent angina, AMI, and death at 48 hours, 14 days, 30 days, and 1 year than patients who received unfractionated heparin.[7,8] Results from the TIMI 11B trial and a meta-analysis study indicated that enoxaparin and aspirin reduced death, myocardial infarction, and

table 18-2 **Low–Molecular-Weight Heparins**

	Enoxaparin	Dalteparin
Indications	USA (with aspirin) Non–ST segment elevation AMI (with aspirin) Prophylaxis of DVT	USA (with aspirin) Non–ST segment elevation AMI (with aspirin) Prophylaxis and treatment of DVT
Absolute bioavailability	87%	92%
Dose for patients with USA or non–ST segment elevation AMI	120 IU/kg (maximum 10,000 IU) SC q12h	1 mg/kg SC q12h
Peak effect	4 h	3–5 h
Half-life	3–5 h	4.5 h

USA, unstable angina.

the need for urgent revascularization more effectively than heparin and aspirin for patients with unstable angina or non–ST segment elevation myocardial infarction.[9,10]

The advantages of LMWHs are their longer half-life, more predictable anticoagulation effect, greater bioavailability, and cost-effectiveness. In addition, LMWHs are administered subcutaneously twice daily and do not require APTT monitoring.

The most common adverse effects of LMWHs include bleeding, thrombocytopenia, elevated aminotransferase levels, and pain, erythema, ecchymosis, or hematoma at the injection site. Because LMWHs have different molecular weight distribution profiles, activities, and plasma clearance rates, they must not be used interchangeably with each other or unfractionated heparin.

Lepirudin is a direct thrombin inhibitor used to prevent thromboembolic complications for patients with heparin-induced thrombocytopenia (HIT) and thromboembolic disease. After a bolus dose of 0.4 mg/kg (maximum 44 mg), an infusion is initiated at 0.15 mg/kg/hour (maximum 16.5 mg/hour). The infusion rate is adjusted to maintain an APTT ratio of 1.5 to 2.5. As with other anticoagulants, the major adverse effects of lepirudin are bleeding complications.

Warfarin, an oral drug used for chronic anticoagulation therapy, interferes with the synthesis of vitamin K–dependent clotting factors such as factors II, VII, IX, and X. The most common cardiovascular indications for warfarin include post-AMI anticoagulation for high-risk patients, dilated cardiomyopathy, atrial fibrillation (AF), congestive heart failure (CHF), venous thromboembolism, and presence of a prosthetic heart valve. The Coumadin Aspirin Reinfarction Study (CARS) investigators reported that warfarin did not provide more benefits than aspirin for patients after AMI; therefore, only high-risk patients routinely receive warfarin after AMI.[11]

Contraindications for warfarin include uncontrolled hypertension, severe hepatic or renal disease, bleeding diathesis, gastrointestinal (GI) or genitourinary (GU) bleeding, cerebral or dissecting aortic aneurysm; recent central nervous system, eye, or other major surgery; recent trauma, pregnancy (first and third trimesters), pericarditis, pericardial effusion, spinal puncture, and recent diagnostic procedures with the potential for uncontrolled bleeding. Patients on warfarin must be able and willing to comply with this somewhat complicated therapy.

Warfarin is usually started at 5 to 10 mg daily but should be decreased for the elderly and patients with liver or renal impairment and heart failure. The dose is titrated according to the patient's international normalized ratio (INR). Because warfarin does not peak for 3 to 4 days, acute anticoagulant therapy is continued until the INR is at the desired level for the patient's condition, usually 2 to 3.5. The INR is evaluated daily until it is therapeutic. Once the INR is therapeutic on a stable warfarin dose, less frequent INR monitoring is appropriate. Elevated INR levels predispose the patient to bleeding, warfarin's most common adverse effect.

Patient education is an important part of warfarin therapy. Warfarin interacts with numerous drugs and foods; safe treatment depends on the patient's knowledge of therapy and compliance.

Platelet Inhibitors

Aspirin, the most widely used platelet inhibitor, inhibits thromboxane A_2, a platelet agonist, and prevents thrombus formation and arterial vasoconstriction. Aspirin is used to decrease mortality for patients with AMI; to reduce incidence of nonfatal AMI and mortality for patients with stable angina, unstable angina, or previous myocardial infarction; and to prevent graft closure after coronary artery bypass graft surgery (CABG) and coronary artery thrombus after angioplasty. Aspirin is also indicated to reduce the risk of nonfatal stroke and death in patients with a history of ischemic stroke or transient ischemia due to platelet emboli. Patients with a history of aspirin intolerance, GI or GU bleeding, peptic ulcer, severe renal or hepatic insufficiency, or bleeding disorders should not receive aspirin.

Common aspirin dosages range from 75 to 325 mg daily. Depending on the indication, patients may take aspirin for a few weeks or indefinitely. Unless contraindicated, patients with symptoms of ACS should immediately chew 160 to 325 mg of aspirin. A 325-mg aspirin suppository is recommended for patients unable to take oral drugs or for patients with severe nausea, vomiting, or upper GI disorders. Aspirin may cause stomach pain, nausea, vomiting, GI bleeding, subdural or intracranial hemorrhage, thrombocytopenia, coagulopathy, and a prolonged prothrombin time.

The adenosine diphosphate receptor antagonists ticlopidine and clopidogrel prevent adenosine diphosphate–induced platelet activation and platelet aggregation, resulting in an irreversible and noncompetitive inhibition of platelet function. Ticlopidine is primarily used for patients who cannot tolerate aspirin. The dosage is 250 mg administered twice daily with food to increase absorption and minimize GI irritation. A loading dose of 500 mg can be given to achieve platelet inhibition more quickly. Maximum platelet aggregation inhibition occurs after 8 to 11 days of therapy. Once ticlopidine is discontinued, bleeding times and platelet function normalize within 2 weeks. Ticlopidine's major adverse effects include bleeding, neutropenia, agranulocytosis, thrombotic thrombocytopenic purpura, elevated liver aminotransferases, and GI irritation.

Clopidogrel is indicated to reduce new atherosclerotic events in patients with atherosclerosis as documented by recent stroke or AMI or by peripheral arterial disease. It is commonly used for 4 weeks after coronary artery stenting and is an alternative to aspirin. In the Clopidogrel versus Aspirin in Patients at Risk of Ischemic Events (CAPRIE) trial, patients with atherosclerotic disease were randomly assigned to receive either clopidogrel or aspirin. Clopidogrel-treated patients had an 8.7% reduction in episodes of ischemic stroke, AMI, or vascular death, plus significantly less GI upset and GI hemorrhage.[12] The dosage for clopidogrel is 75 mg daily with or without food. A loading dose of 300 to 600 mg is often used to achieve a rapid onset of action. Clopidogrel achieves steady-state platelet inhibition after 3 to 7 days of therapy. Once clopidogrel is discontinued, bleeding times and platelet function normalize within 3 to 7 days. Clopidogrel's major adverse effects include bleeding disorders, GI upset, thrombotic thrombocytopenic purpura, and neutropenia. Patients receiving clopidogrel have less GI upset, hemorrhage, and abnormal liver function than patients receiving aspirin.

Three GP IIb/IIIa receptor antagonists are currently available and include abciximab, tirofiban, and eptifibatide (Table 18-3). These drugs inhibit the GP IIb/IIIa receptor, the final common pathway for platelet aggregation, inhibit thrombus formation, and prevent platelet aggregation. Box 18-2 lists the contraindications to GP IIb/IIIa inhibitors. Adverse effects for this class of drugs include bleeding, thrombocytopenia, stroke, and allergic reactions.

Many clinical trials have been performed to evaluate GP IIb/IIIa receptor antagonists. Researchers reported that eptifibatide[13,14] and abciximab[15] significantly decreased composite end points of death, AMI, and target vessel revascularization 30 days and 6 months after stenting. The combined use of coronary artery stenting plus abciximab was more effective than alteplase in salvaging myocardium and reducing death, reinfarction, and stroke at 6 months.[16] For patients with AMI, abciximab and half-dose alteplase produced better coronary reperfusion than full-dose alteplase alone.[17] In the Platelet Receptor Inhibition in Ischemic Syndrome Management (PRISM) trial, patients with unstable angina or NQWMI who received tirofiban had significantly lower mortality rates than patients who received heparin.[18] The Platelet Receptor Inhibition in Ischemic Syndrome Management in Patients Limited by Unstable Signs and Symptoms (PRISM-PLUS) researchers studied patients with higher-risk unstable angina and NQWMI and reported that patients treated with tirofiban and heparin had a significantly lower incidence of death, AMI, and refractory ischemia at 7 days, 30 days, and

box 18-2 *Contraindications to Glycoprotein IIb/IIIa Inhibitors*

- Internal bleeding
- Bleeding diathesis within 30 days
- Intracranial neoplasm, arteriovenous malformation, or aneurysm
- Recent stroke
- Any hemorrhagic stroke
- Thrombocytopenia
- Aortic dissection
- Recent surgery or trauma
- Severe hypertension
- Pericarditis
- Concurrent use of another GP IIb/IIIa inhibitor
- Dependence on dialysis or serum creatinine ≥4.0 mg/dL (eptifibatide)

table 18-3 Glycoprotein IIb/IIIa Inhibitors

	Abciximab	Eptifibatide	Tirofiban
Indications	PCI USA that does not respond to conventional therapy and when PCI is planned within 24 h	Non–ST segment elevation ACS, including patients who are managed medically or with PCI PCI	Non–ST segment elevation ACS, including patients who are managed medically or with PCI
Dose	PCI: 0.25 mg/kg IV 10–60 min before PCI, then 0.125 μg/kg/min (maximum 10 μg/min) for 12 h USA with planned PCI: 0.25 mg/kg IV, then 10 μg/min IV for 18–24 h, concluding 1 h after PCI	ACS: 180 μg/kg bolus IV, then 2 μg/kg/min infusion up to 72 h, discharge, or CABG; if PCI performed, continue infusion 18–24 h post-PCI, allowing up to 96 h of therapy; for patients with a creatinine between 2–4 mg/dL, reduce infusion to 1 μg/kg/min PCI: 180 μg/kg IV bolus immediately before PCI, then begin a 2 μg/kg/min IV infusion, then repeat bolus 10 min after first bolus while continuing infusion until discharge or for up to 18–24 h; for patients with a creatinine between 2–4 mg/dL, reduce infusion to 1 μg/kg/min	0.4 μg/kg/min IV for 30 min, then 0.1 μg/kg/min IV infusion through angiography or for 12–24 h after angioplasty or atherectomy; for patients with severe renal insufficiency, give half the usual rate of infusion
Concurrent aspirin and heparin therapy	Yes	Yes	Yes
Half-life	First phase, 10 min; second phase 30 min; remains in circulation up to 15 days in platelet-bound state	2.5 h; platelet function returns to normal approximately 4 h after stopping the infusion	2 h; platelet function returns to near baseline 4–8 h after stopping the infusion

USA, unstable angina.

6 months than patients treated with heparin.[19] Based on these favorable findings, the Guidelines for the Management of Patients With Acute Myocardial Infarction recommend GP IIb/IIIa inhibitors for patients with non–ST segment elevation AMI who have high-risk features or refractory ischemia, provided that they do not have a contraindication due to risk of bleeding.[6]

ANTIDYSRHYTHMICS

Antidysrhythmic drugs are used to restore a normal cardiac rhythm and to prevent the life-threatening sequelae of dysrhythmias. Unfortunately, these drugs are not always effective and sometimes even worsen mortality.[20] Antidysrhythmics are classified by their effect on the cardiac action potential; however, many have more than one action (Table 18-4). Table 18-5 summarizes antidysrhythmic drugs that are commonly used in the intensive care unit (ICU). Refer to Chapter 16 for more specific information regarding the cardiac action potential.

Class I Antidysrhythmic Drugs

Quinidine, procainamide, and disopyramide are class IA antidysrhythmics. These drugs do not improve mortality, may cause life-threatening dysrhythmias, and interact with other drugs commonly used for patients with cardiovascular disease.

The class IB antidysrhythmics include lidocaine, mexiletine, and tocainide. Although lidocaine continues to be widely used, it is less efficacious than procainamide.[21] Lidocaine is no longer use prophylactically for patients with AMI or asymptomatic ventricular dysrhythmias.

Flecainide, moricizine, and propafenone are class IC antidysrhythmics. Because these drugs are prodysrhythmic and may increase mortality, they are not commonly prescribed.

In general, research data do not support the effectiveness of class I antidysrhythmics. The current trend is to use class II and class III antidysrhythmics, cardioversion, and implantable cardioverter–defibrillators rather than class I drugs.[21]

Class II Antidysrhythmic Drugs

Beta blockers are class II drugs that are also used for patients with tachydysrhythmias, ST segment elevation AMI, non–ST segment elevation AMI, continuing or recurrent ischemic pain, hypertension, and CHF. This class of drugs has a broad spectrum of activity, an established safety record, and is currently the best class of antidysrhythmics for *general* use.[21] Beta blockers interfere with sympathetic nervous system stimulation, contributing to decreased heart rate, depressed atrioventricular (AV) node conduction, decreased contractility, and decreased myocardial oxygen demand. Esmolol, propranolol, sotalol, and acebutolol are the only approved beta blockers used to treat dysrhythmias. All beta blockers, except esmolol and sotalol, are indicated for hypertension.

Beta blockers are categorized as cardioselective (inhibition of $beta_1$ receptors) or nonselective (inhibition of $beta_1$ and $beta_2$ receptors). Inhibition of $beta_1$ receptors causes a decreased heart rate, slowed conduction through the AV node, and depressed cardiac function. Inhibition of $beta_2$

table 18-4 Classification of Antidysrhythmic Medications

Class	Action	Medication Examples
IA	Inhibits fast sodium channel, decreases automaticity, depresses phase 0, and prolongs the action potential duration	Quinidine Procainamide Disopyramide
IB	Inhibits fast sodium channel, depresses phase 0 slightly, and shortens action potential duration	Lidocaine Mexiletine Tocainide
IC	Inhibits fast sodium channel, depresses phase 0 markedly, slows His-Purkinje conduction profoundly, leading to a prolonged QRS complex duration	Flecainide Moricizine (plus IA and IB effects) Propafenone
II	Depresses phase 4 depolarization, blocks sympathetic stimulation of the conduction system	Esmolol Propranolol Sotalol (plus class III effects) Acebutolol
III	Blocks potassium channel, prolongs phase 3 repolarization, prolongs action potential duration	Amiodarone Sotalol Ibutilide Dofetilide
IV	Inhibits inward calcium channel, depresses phase 4 depolarization, lengthens repolarization in phases 1 and 2	Verapamil Diltiazem

table 18-5 ■ Selected Antidysrhythmic Medications

Drug	Antidysrhythmic Indications	Antidysrhythmic Dose	Route	Effect on Electro-cardiogram	Major Adverse Effects
Procainamide	VT; SVTs including WPW syndrome, AF, atrial flutter	IV: 17 mg/kg at 20 mg/min, then infusion of 1–4 mg/min to maintain therapeutic drug level PO: Up to 50 mg/kg/day given in divided doses q3h to maintain therapeutic drug level	IV, PO	→ QRS → QTI	Hypotension with IV use, lupus syndrome, rash, fever, heart block, torsades de pointes, headache, agranulocytosis
Lidocaine	VT, VF	1.0–1.5 mg/kg IV bolus; may repeat 0.5–0.75 mg/kg IV every 5–10 min for total of 3 mg/kg Then infusion of 1–4 mg/min	IV; ETT if no patent IV (2–4 mg/kg)	None	Bradycardia, blurred vision, hypotension, tremors, dizziness, tinnitus, convulsions, mental status changes
Flecainide	PSVT including WPW syndrome and paroxysmal AF and atrial flutter; life-threatening sustained VT	100–200 mg PO q12h	PO	→ PRI → QRS 0/→ QTI	Ventricular dysrhythmias, dizziness, dyspnea, headache, fatigue, nausea, palpitations
Esmolol	SVT including AF, and atrial flutter; ST	500 μg/kg/min IV loading dose for 1 min, then 50 μg/kg/min infusion for 4 min Repeat loading dose every 5 min and increase infusion by 50 μg/kg/min increments until desired therapeutic effect or maximum of 200 μg/kg/min	IV	↓ HR 0/→ PRI 0/← QTI	Hypotension, nausea, diaphoresis, dizziness, headache, weakness, somnolence, heart block, bronchospasm, thrombophlebitis from extravasation
Propranolol	SVT, ST, VT, digitalis-induced tachydysrhythmias; ventricular rate control with AF, atrial flutter	IV: 1–3 mg not exceeding 1 mg/min PO: 10–30 mg tid–qid	IV PO	↓ HR 0/→ PRI 0/← QTI	Hypotension, heart block, bradycardia, CHF, bronchospasm, fatigue, nausea, vomiting, gastric pain, constipation, diarrhea
Sotalol	AF, atrial flutter, VT, VF	80 mg PO bid; may be increased to 240–640 mg/day given in two or three divided doses	PO	↓ HR → PRI 0/→ QTI	Bradycardia, AV block, dizziness, CHF, bronchospasm, gastric pain
Ibutilide	AF, atrial flutter	1 mg IV infusion over 10 min (<60 kg, 0.01 mg/kg); may repeat either dosage in 10 min	IV	→ QTI	Hypotension, torsades de pointes, VT, BBB, bradycardia, nausea
Dofetilide	AF, atrial flutter	125–500 μg bid depending on creatinine clearance	PO	→ QTI	Torsades de pointes, bradycardia

(continued)

table 18-5 ■ Selected Antidysrhythmic Medications (Continued)

Drug	Antidysrhythmic Indications	Antidysrhythmic Dose	Route	Effect on Electro-cardiogram	Major Adverse Effects
Amiodarone	Recurrent VF or hemodynamically unstable VT in patients refractory to other drugs; unlabeled uses: AF, atrial flutter, SVTs including WPW syndrome	IV: Loading infusion of 150 mg over 10 min; 360 mg over next 6 h; 540 mg over next 18 h; may follow with maintenance infusion of 0.5 mg/min For breakthrough dysrhythmias, 150 mg supplemental infusions PO: Loading dose of 800–1600 mg qd for 1–3 wk; then 600–800 mg qd for 1 mo Maintenance dose 100–400 mg/day	IV PO	→ PRI → QTI	Heart block, cardiac arrest, bradycardia, hypotension, VT, pneumonitis, liver disease, hypothyroidism or hyperthyroidism, photosensitivity, solar dermatitis, blue discoloration of skin, malaise, paresthesias, nausea, vomiting, constipation, visual disturbances, anorexia
Verapamil	Ventricular rate control in AF, atrial flutter; SVT	IV: 5–10 mg over 2 min; may give 10 mg 30 min after first dose PO: 240–480 mg/day in three or four divided doses	IV PO	↓ HR → PRI	Hypotension, heart block, CHF, bradycardia, headache, dizziness, edema, nausea, constipation
Diltiazem	Ventricular rate control in AF, atrial flutter; PSVT	IV: 0.25 mg/kg over 2 min; may give 0.35 mg/kg after 15 min May follow with an infusion of 5–15 mg/h for up to 24 h	IV for antidysrhythmic indications	↓/0 HR → PRI	Bradycardia, heart block, edema, hypotension, nausea, dizziness, flushing, headache, fatigue
Adenosine	Narrow-complex PSVT including WPW syndrome, idiopathic VT; used diagnostically to evaluate VT, SVT, latent preexcitation	6 mg IV over 1–3 sec followed by rapid saline flush; after 1–2 min, may give 12 mg A second 12 mg dose may be given in 1–2 min if needed	IV	→ PRI	Facial flushing, lightheadedness, headache, bradycardia, dyspnea, heart block, asystole, chest pain, nausea
Atropine	Symptomatic sinus bradycardia, AV block, asystole, bradycardic PEA	Asystole or PEA: 1 mg IV push; repeat every 3–5 min to maximum of 0.04 mg/kg Bradycardia: 0.5–1.0 mg IV every 3–5 min to maximum of 0.04 mg/kg	IV; ETT if no patent IV (1–2 mg)	↑ HR	Palpitations, tachycardia, blurred vision, dry mouth, altered taste, nausea, urinary retention
Digoxin	Ventricular rate control in AF	IV: Loading dose of 0.4–0.6 mg with additional doses of 0.1–0.3 mg q4–8h; maintenance dose of 0.125–0.5 mg qd PO: Loading dose of 0.5–0.7 mg with additional doses of 0.125–0.375 mg q6–8h Maintenance dose of 0.125–0.5 mg qd	IV PO	↓ HR → PRI ← QTI	Heart block, bradycardia, weakness; toxicity: dysrhythmias, anorexia, nausea, vomiting, headache, fatigue, depression, confusion, hallucination

VF, ventricular fibrillation; ST, sinus tachycardia; AF, atrial fibrillation; BBB, bundle branch block; PEA, pulseless electrical activity; HR, heart rate; ETT, endotracheal tube; ↑, increased; ↓, decreased; →, prolonged; ←, shortened; 0, little or no effect

receptors causes bronchoconstriction, vasoconstriction, and decreased glycogenolysis. Table 18-6 indicates the beta activity for selected beta blockers.

Numerous recent research trials have demonstrated the effectiveness of beta blockers for dysrhythmias and other cardiovascular disorders such as unstable angina and heart failure. The Carvedilol Post-Infarct Survival Control in Left Ventricular Dysfunction (CAPRICORN) investigators reported that, compared with placebo, carvedilol reduced mortality and recurrent, nonfatal AMIs for patients with AMI and left ventricular dysfunction who were being treated with angiotensin-converting enzyme inhibitors (ACEIs).[22] Three studies involving patients with heart failure were stopped early because beta blockers reduced mortality significantly more than the placebo. The Carvedilol Prospective Randomized Cumulative Survival Trial (COPERNICUS) researchers found that carvedilol significantly reduced hospitalization and mortality rates for patients with severe, chronic heart failure.[23] Patients with chronic heart failure who received controlled-release/extended-release metoprolol had a significantly lower mortality rate from all causes, sudden death, and heart failure.[24] Finally, bisoprolol reduced mortality rates for patients with symptomatic heart failure.[25]

Unless contraindicated, beta blockers should be a part of early treatment for patients with AMI or unstable angina.[6,26] Metoprolol, propranolol, atenolol, and nadolol are approved for angina, whereas metoprolol and atenolol are indicated as first-line drugs for AMI. The first dose is given IV; successive doses are usually given orally. The goal is to reduce the patient's resting heart rate to 55 to 60 beats/minute.[27]

Beta blockers are contraindicated in patients with severe asthma or bronchospasm, severe chronic obstruction pulmonary disease, cardiogenic shock, overt left ventricular failure, severe bradycardia, or greater than first-degree heart block. Cardioselective beta blockers are sometimes used with caution for patients with pulmonary disease. It is important to remember that cardioselective drugs lose their selectivity at higher doses.

Adverse effects for beta blockers include bradycardia, heart block, hypotension, heart failure, bronchospasm, cold extremities, insomnia, fatigue, and depression. Some patients who experience these adverse effects may respond better to a different beta blocker.

table 18-6 Selected Beta-Blockers

Medication	Cardioselective	Nonselective
Acebutolol	X	
Atenolol	X	
Esmolol	X	
Labetalol		X
Metoprolol	X	
Nadolol		X
Pindolol		X
Propranolol		X
Sotalol		X
Timolol		X

Class III Antidysrhythmic Drugs

Class III antidysrhythmic drugs include amiodarone, sotalol, ibutilide, and dofetilide. It is important to know each drug's unique properties because individual agents contain unique properties not shared by other class III drugs.

Amiodarone is the treatment of choice for patients with marked ventricular dysfunction and AF.[28] Amiodarone has been shown to decrease ventricular fibrillation and death due to dysrhythmias for patients after AMI.[29] In a recent study, patients who received amiodarone experienced less recurrent AF than patients who received sotalol or propafenone.[30] A small study showed that when compared with placebo, prophylactic, short-term oral amiodarone decreased postoperative AF, VT, and cerebral vascular accident (CVA) after open heart surgery for patients 60 years or older who were already receiving beta blockers.[31]

The Advanced Cardiac Life Support algorithms now include amiodarone as a first-line option for treating ventricular fibrillation/pulseless ventricular tachycardia, wide-complex tachycardia, narrow-complex tachycardia, AF, and atrial flutter.[32] Limitations of amiodarone include its variable onset of action, intolerable adverse effects, dangerous drug interactions, and life-threatening complications associated with chronic therapy.[20]

Ibutilide and dofetilide are newer class III drugs that are indicated for AF and atrial flutter. Dofetilide blocks the rapid potassium current channel, which prolongs the action potential duration and refractory period. The exact mechanism of action for ibutilide is unclear. Although these drugs may cause a prolonged QTc interval and torsades de pointes, they have fewer systemic adverse effects than amiodarone and sotalol.

Class IV Antidysrhythmic Drugs

The class IV calcium channel blocker antidysrhythmics, verapamil and diltiazem, decrease automaticity of the sinoatrial (SA) and AV nodes, slow conduction, and prolong the AV nodal refractory period. These agents have negative inotropic and peripheral vasodilation effects. In addition, calcium channel blockers have antiplatelet and anti-ischemic effects.[33] Verapamil and diltiazem are contraindicated for usual forms of ventricular tachycardia, severe sinus bradycardia, sick sinus syndrome, Wolff-Parkinson-White (WPW) syndrome with AF, digoxin toxicity, hypotension, heart failure, AV conduction defects, and severe aortic stenosis, and are not standard therapies for AMI. Adverse effects include hypotension, AV block, bradycardia, headache, dizziness, peripheral edema, nausea, constipation, and flushing.

Calcium antagonists are also used for patients with unstable angina when beta blockers or nitrates do not relieve symptoms, when there is evidence of vasospasm, or when patients cannot tolerate adequate doses of nitrates or beta blockers.[26,34] However, the use of calcium channel blockers is controversial because they have not consistently decreased morbidity or mortality for most cardiovascular disorders.

Unclassified Antidysrhythmic Drugs

Adenosine is a first-line antidysrhythmic that effectively converts narrow-complex paroxysmal supraventricular tachycardia to normal sinus rhythm by slowing conduction through the AV node. Adenosine is effective in terminating dysrhythmias due to reentry involving the SA and AV nodes; however, it does not convert AF or atrial flutter to sinus rhythm. It is also used to differentiate between VT and supraventricular tachycardia (SVT), treat rare forms of idiopathic VT, and reveal latent preexcitation in patients suspected of having WPW syndrome.[21] Adenosine's half-life is less than 10 seconds; therefore, adverse effects are short-lived.

Magnesium sulfate is the drug of choice for treating torsades de pointes. Magnesium is also used for refractory VT and ventricular fibrillation, and for life-threatening dysrhythmias due to digitalis toxicity. Its mechanism of action is unclear; however, it has calcium channel blocking properties and inhibits sodium and potassium channels. The dose for patients in cardiac arrest is 1 to 2 g diluted in 10 mL of D_5W given by IV push. Adverse effects include hypotension, nausea, depressed reflexes, and flushing.

Atropine, a parasympatholytic agent, is a first-line drug used to treat symptomatic bradycardia and slowed conduction at the AV node. It is also indicated for asystole or bradycardic pulseless electrical activity. Atropine reduces the effects of vagal stimulation, thus increasing heart rate and improving cardiac function. It is important not to increase the heart rate excessively in patients with ischemic heart disease because this may increase myocardial oxygen consumption and worsen ischemia.

Digoxin is a mild positive inotrope with antidysrhythmic and bradycardic actions. Digoxin inhibits the sodium–potassium pump, causing a rise in intracellular sodium. This rise promotes calcium influx and ultimately enhances myocardial contractility. Digoxin also activates the parasympathetic system, causing a decreased heart rate and increased atrioventricular nodal inhibition.

Although commonly prescribed for dysrhythmias, digoxin is most beneficial for patients with acute AF with a rapid ventricular rate or chronic CHF with chronic AF.[21,35] Researchers compared digoxin with a placebo for patients with chronic heart failure and reported that digoxin did not reduce overall mortality.[36] Digoxin is no longer indicated for paroxysmal AF, SVT, mitral stenosis with normal sinus rhythm, or acute left ventricular failure, and is not effective in converting AF to sinus rhythm.[28,35]

The doses and therapeutic blood levels for digoxin are controversial. Loading doses are often not required except for acute SVT that is unresponsive to other drugs.[37] Loading doses of digoxin must be given slowly and take up to 2 hours to be effective. The current trend is to administer lower doses that lessen the risk of toxicity.[35] Routine doses are individualized based on the patient's diagnosis, symptoms, underlying disease processes, age, response to therapy, and blood levels. A recently proposed therapeutic digoxin level is 0.5 to 1.5 ng/mL.[37]

Signs and symptoms of digitalis toxicity include palpitations, syncope, dysrhythmias, elevated digoxin level, anorexia, vomiting, diarrhea, nausea, fatigue, confusion, insomnia, headache, depression, vertigo, facial pain, and colored or blurred vision. Digitalis levels may be increased by the concurrent use of quinidine, verapamil, amiodarone, captopril, diltiazem, esmolol, indomethacin, quinine, or ibuprofen. Finally, hypokalemia, hypomagnesemia, and hypothyroidism may predispose the patient to digitalis toxicity.

INOTROPES

Cardiovascular function is regulated by two divisions of the autonomic nervous system, the sympathetic and parasympathetic systems. Refer to Chapter 32 to review this information. Adrenoreceptor stimulation leads to a variety of effects; therefore, it is important to understand which receptor(s) each drug stimulates (Table 18-7).

Inotropic drugs are used to increase the force of myocardial contraction and cardiac output. Inotropic drugs include sympathomimetics, such as dopamine, dobutamine, epinephrine, isoproterenol, and norepinephrine; and the phosphodiesterase inhibitors amrinone and milrinone. These drugs are commonly given to patients with ventricular dysfunction or cardiogenic shock. Enhanced ventricular contraction increases stroke volume, cardiac output, blood pressure, and coronary artery perfusion. As the ventricles empty more completely, ventricular filling pressures, preload, and pulmonary congestion are decreased. However, as contractility and heart rate increase, myocardial oxygen demand also increases. Myocardial ischemia can occur if a myocardial oxygen supply–demand mismatch develops. The nurse must closely monitor the patient for evidence of ischemia, angina, and dysrhythmias.

Dopamine

Dopamine, the most widely used inotropic drug, is administered to patients with conditions that cause hypotension, decreased cardiac output, and oliguria. Dopamine directly stimulates dopaminergic, beta-adrenergic, and alpha-adrenergic receptors and promotes release of norepinephrine from sympathetic nerve terminals. Dopamine

table 18-7 Adrenergic Receptors Affecting Cardiovascular Function

Receptor	Location	Effects of Stimulation
$Beta_1$	Heart	Positive inotropic and chronotropic actions
$Beta_2$	Bronchial smooth muscle	Bronchodilation
	Vascular smooth muscle	Vasodilation
	AV node	Positive dromotropic action
$Alpha_1$	Vascular smooth muscle	Vasoconstriction
	Heart	Weak positive inotropic and chronotropic actions
$Alpha_2$	Presynaptic sympathetic nerve endings	Inhibition of norepinephrine release
Dopaminergic	Kidney and splanchnic vessels	Renal and splanchnic vessel vasodilation

is given by continuous IV infusion and its dose is titrated to achieve the desired effect. Doses of 3 µg/kg/minute or less stimulate vasodilation of the renal arterioles and may improve renal function. Increased myocardial contractility results from dosages of 3 to 10 µg/kg/minute. Higher dosages predominantly cause vasoconstriction and increased blood pressure. Dopamine is usually given through a central line to enhance its distribution and to avoid extravasation, which may cause local vasoconstriction and tissue necrosis. Adverse effects include tachycardia, palpitations, dysrhythmias, angina, headache, nausea, vomiting, and hypertension.

Dobutamine

Dobutamine acts on $beta_1$ receptors and increases myocardial contractility. Dobutamine is used after cardiac surgery, during some cardiac diagnostic stress procedures, and for patients with heart failure, shock, or other conditions that cause poor cardiac contractility or a low cardiac output. The dosage for dobutamine is 2 to 20 µg/kg/minute by continuous IV infusion. Adverse effects include tachycardia, dysrhythmias, blood pressure fluctuations, headache, and nausea.

Epinephrine

Epinephrine stimulates $alpha_1$, $beta_1$, and $beta_2$ receptors and is given for a variety of indications, including cardiac arrest, symptomatic bradycardia, severe hypotension, anaphylaxis, and shock. In the ICU, epinephrine is given by continuous IV infusion through a central line, as an IV bolus, or through the endotracheal tube. Continuous IV dosages of 1 to 2 µg/minute stimulate $beta_1$ receptors to increase cardiac output by increasing heart rate and myocardial contractility. At higher dosages, epinephrine stimulates alpha receptors, causing profound vasoconstriction, increased blood pressure and systemic vascular resistance, and decreased renal and splanchnic perfusion. Epinephrine may cause dysrhythmias, tachycardia, cerebral hemorrhage, pulmonary edema, headache, dizziness, nervousness, myocardial ischemia, and angina. Vasopressin is now used as an alternative to epinephrine for patients with refractory ventricular fibrillation or shock associated with vasodilation.[32] This potent vasoconstrictor promotes smooth muscle contraction and increases peripheral vascular resistance. The dosage for patients with cardiac arrest is 40 U given by IV push. The drug may also be given as an infusion. Adverse effects include dysrhythmias, myocardial ischemia, angina, myocardial infarction, tremors, vertigo, sweating, and water intoxication.

Isoproterenol

Isoproterenol stimulates $beta_1$ and $beta_2$ receptors to increase myocardial contractility, cardiac output, heart rate, and blood pressure. Currently, isoproterenol is used mainly to increase heart rate after cardiac transplantation. Other indications include refractory torsades de pointes, beta blocker overdose, and symptomatic bradycardia when an external pacemaker is not available. The IV dosage is 0.5 to 10 µg/minute by continuous infusion. Isoproterenol causes a variety of adverse effects, including dysrhythmias, tachycardia, palpitations, myocardial ischemia, hypotension, pulmonary edema, bronchospasm, headache, nausea, vomiting, and sweating.

Norepinephrine

Norepinephrine primarily affects alpha receptors, causing peripheral vasoconstriction, increased blood pressure, and increased systemic vascular resistance (SVR). The increased SVR may actually increase myocardial oxygen demand and work, thus decreasing cardiac output. Norepinephrine is used for patients with cardiogenic shock and significant hypotension accompanied by a low SVR. The dosage is 2 to 12 µg/minute by continuous IV infusion. Adverse effects include tachycardia, bradycardia, dysrhythmias, headache, hypertension, and tissue necrosis from extravasation.

Amrinone

The phosphodiesterase III inhibitors, amrinone and milrinone, increase contractility, venous vasodilation, and arterial vasodilation by inhibiting an enzyme that breaks down cyclic adenosine monophosphate. Both drugs reduce ventricular filling pressures and tend to decrease arterial pressure; however, they minimally affect heart rate.

Amrinone is used for severe CHF that is refractory to other drugs. An IV bolus dose of 0.75 mg/kg is given over 2 to 3 minutes. A maintenance IV infusion of 5 to 15 µg/kg/minute is titrated to the desired effect. Adverse effects include hypotension, tachycardia, dysrhythmias, and thrombocytopenia.

Milrinone

Milrinone is used for the short-term treatment of CHF. The IV bolus dose of 50 µg/kg is given over 10 minutes and is followed by a maintenance IV infusion of 0.375 to 0.75 µg/kg/minute. Patients who receive milrinone may experience ventricular dysrhythmias, hypotension, headache, bronchospasm, and thrombocytopenia.

VASODILATORS

Vasodilator drugs decrease preload and afterload. Preload is the distending force that stretches the ventricular muscle at the end of filling. The greater the stretch, the better the contraction. However, if the cells are overstretched, contractile force decreases. Afterload is the force against which the heart has to work to eject its contents. If afterload is too low, blood pressure and tissue perfusion may be low. If afterload is too high, the heart has to work harder.

Nitrates

Patients with myocardial ischemia or infarction may have an increased preload and afterload, which further strains their hearts. Nitrates cause peripheral vasodilation, which in turn decreases venous return to the heart and reduces preload. These drugs promote coronary artery vasodilation, improve collateral blood flow, reduce platelet aggregation, enhance perfusion to ischemic myocardium, and decrease myocardial oxygen demand, thus reducing ischemia, chest pain, and infarct size. At high doses, nitrates reduce afterload by arterial vasodilator effects. Nitrates reduce blood pressure and previously elevated pulmonary vascular resistance, SVR, and central venous and pulmonary capillary wedge pressures.

Nitrates are indicated for acute angina; large anterior AMI; AMI associated with CHF, persistent ischemia, or hypertension; angina unresponsive to other therapies; and prophylaxis of angina. Contraindications to IV nitrates include, but are not limited to, hypotension, uncorrected hypovolemia, hypertrophic obstructive cardiomyopathy, and pericardial tamponade. When a right ventricular AMI is suspected, nitrates are used with extreme caution because these patients require an adequate venous return to maintain cardiac output and blood pressure. Patients should not receive nitrates for 24 hours after sildenafil (Viagra) use because this drug interaction predisposes patients to life-threatening hypotension.[38]

Nitrates are available in a variety of dosage forms. In the ICU, nitrates are often given by the IV, sublingual, or topical routes. An IV nitroglycerin drip is initiated at 5 to 20 µg/minute and increased every 5 to 15 minutes, up to 200 µg/minute, to achieve the desired effects. When used to treat or prevent angina, a 0.3- to 0.6-mg tablet is placed under the patient's tongue and may be repeated twice at 5-minute intervals. The usual dose for nitroglycerin ointment is 1 to 2 inches every 8 hours; however, treatment is often initiated with 0.5 inch and increased gradually to achieve the desired effects.

The adverse effects of nitrates include headache, hypotension, syncope, and tachycardia. Tolerance may develop to the antianginal, hemodynamic, and antiplatelet effects of nitrates, especially with continuous or high-dose therapy; however, dosing regimens that allow for nitrate-free intervals may prevent this occurrence.[27]

Nitroprusside Sodium

Nitroprusside is a potent arterial and venous vasodilator that is used to treat severe left ventricular heart failure, hypertension after coronary artery bypass grafting, hypertensive crisis, and dissecting aneurysm. Nitroprusside decreases SVR and increases cardiac output. The usual IV infusion dosage is 0.5 to 10 µg/kg/minute; however, to prevent cyanide toxicity, the maximum dose should not be given for longer than 10 minutes. The dose is titrated to effect; if blood pressure does not respond after 10 minutes, the drug is discontinued. Because nitroprusside is sensitive to light, the infusion bag is covered with an opaque material to prevent the drug's degradation. Adverse effects include hypotension, myocardial ischemia, nausea, vomiting, abdominal pain, and cyanide toxicity.

ANGIOTENSIN-CONVERTING ENZYME INHIBITORS

ACEIs are indicated to treat CHF, hypertension, AMI with or without left ventricular dysfunction or failure, and asymptomatic left ventricular dysfunction. They are also used to decrease morbidity and mortality for patients at high risk for AMI, stroke, or cardiovascular death. Unless contraindicated, patients with an anterior AMI with ST segment elevation or heart failure should receive an ACEI within 24 hours.[6]

The ACEIs block the conversion of angiotensin I to the potent vasoconstrictor angiotensin II, reduce aldosterone synthesis, and may promote fibrinolysis.[39] As a result, ACEIs increase cardiac output and decrease sodium retention, blood pressure, central venous pressure, SVR, pulmonary vascular resistance, and pulmonary capillary wedge pressure.

Numerous research trials conducted in the late 1980s and early 1990s showed that ACEIs are outstanding drugs for cardiovascular disease.[40] More recently, two large meta-analysis studies found that the early use of ACEIs after AMI significantly reduced mortality.[41,42] The Heart Outcomes Prevention Evaluation (HOPE) trial investigators reported that ramipril reduced death, myocardial infarction, stroke, revascularization procedures, cardiac arrest, heart failure, and diabetic complications for patients at high risk for cardiovascular events.[43]

Table 18-8 summarizes selected ACEIs. All ACEIs are contraindicated in pregnancy, angioedema, bilateral renal artery stenosis, and preexisting hypotension, and should be used with caution for patients with renal failure or hyperkalemia. Patients with impaired renal function, hypotension, or concurrent diuretic use should receive a lower ACEI dosage. Adverse effects of ACEIs include hypotension, dizziness, angioedema, cough, headache, fatigue, nausea, vomiting, diarrhea, hyperkalemia, and renal function impairment.

ANTIHYPERLIPIDEMICS

Cholesterol reduction is an important part of therapy for patients with cardiovascular disease. The pharmacological management of hyperlipidemia decreases morbidity and mortality from coronary heart disease.[44] According to the Adult Treatment Panel III, a low-density lipoprotein (LDL) level of less than 100 mg/dL is optimal, a total cholesterol level of less than 200 mg/dL is desirable, and a normal triglyceride level is less than 150 mg/dL.[45] Recently released practice guidelines emphasize primary prevention of coronary heart disease (CHD) for patients with multiple risk factors.[45] Primary prevention includes LDL-lowering drugs for patients with no or one risk factor and an LDL level of 160 mg/dL or greater, or two or more risk factors and an LDL level greater than 130 to 160 mg/dL.[45] Secondary prevention for patients with documented CHD or CHD risk equivalents may begin when the LDL is 130 mg/dL or greater.[45] Drug therapy is also appropriate when triglycerides are 200 mg/dL or greater.[45] Finally, patients with borderline-high triglycerides (150 to 199 mg/dL) and CHD or CHD risk equivalents may receive drugs to raise the high-density lipoprotein (HDL).[45]

There are four major classes of antihyperlipidemic drugs:

- Hydroxymethylglutaryl coenzyme-A (HMG-CoA) reductase inhibitors decrease total and LDL cholesterol, decrease triglycerides, and increase HDL cho-

table 18-8 ■ Selected Angiotensin-Converting Enzyme Inhibitors

Drug	Indications	Usual Initial Dose	Usual Maintenance Dose
Benazepril	HTN	10 mg PO qd	20–40 mg/d PO in one or two doses
Captopril	HTN	25 mg PO bid–tid	25–150 mg PO bid–tid
	CHF	6.25–12.5 mg PO tid	50–100 mg PO tid
	LVD post-AMI	6.25–12.5 mg PO tid	50 mg PO tid
Enalapril	HTN	1.25 mg IV q6h	1.25–5 mg IV q6h
		5 mg PO qd	10–40 mg/d PO in one or two doses
	CHF	2.5 mg PO bid	20 mg PO bid
	Asymptomatic LVD	2.5 mg PO bid	20 mg PO bid
Lisinopril	HTN	10 mg PO qd	20–40 mg PO qd
	CHF	2.5–5 mg PO qd	5–20 mg PO qd
	AMI	2.5–5 mg PO qd	10 mg PO qd
Ramipril	HTN	2.5 mg PO qd	2.5–20 mg/d PO in one or two doses
	CHF post-AMI	2.5 mg PO bid	5 mg PO bid
Quinapril	HTN	10–20 mg PO qd	20–80 mg/d PO in one or two doses
	CHF	5 mg PO qd	20–40 mg/d PO in two doses

HTN, hypertension; LVD, left ventricular dysfunction.

lesterol by inhibiting the rate-limiting enzyme that promotes cholesterol biosynthesis.

- Nicotinic acid inhibits lipolysis in adipose tissue and inhibits hepatic production of very–low-density lipoprotein (VLDL) thus decreasing cholesterol, triglycerides, VLDL, and LDL, and increasing HDL.
- The bile acid sequestrants bind bile acids in the intestine and form an insoluble complex that is excreted in the feces. Because bile acids are not absorbed, there is ultimately an increased hepatic synthesis of bile acids from cholesterol that may be evident by a slightly increased triglyceride level. However, plasma total and LDL cholesterol actually decrease due to an increased clearance rate.
- The fibrates inhibit peripheral lipolysis and decrease the hepatic extraction of free fatty acids, which reduces triglyceride production. These agents decrease total cholesterol, triglycerides, and VLDL, and increase HDL.

Table 18-9 summarizes selected drugs used to treat hyperlipidemia.

table 18-9 ■ Selected Lipid-Lowering Drugs

Drug	Usual Initial Dose	Major Adverse Effects
Simvastatin	20 mg PO qd in the evening	Headache, abdominal pain, constipation, cramps, liver damage, myopathy
Pravastatin	10–20 mg PO qd at bedtime	Headache, nausea, vomiting, diarrhea, abdominal pain, flatulence, constipation, dizziness, musculoskeletal pain, liver damage, myopathy
Lovastatin	20 mg PO qd with the evening meal	Headache, diarrhea, nausea, vomiting, constipation, flatulence, liver damage, myopathy
Cholestyramine	4 g PO qd–bid	Constipation, impaction, abdominal pain, flatulence, gastrointestinal bleeding, bleeding tendencies
Colestipol	5 g PO qd–bid	Constipation, impaction, abdominal pain, flatulence, gastrointestinal bleeding, bleeding tendencies
Nicotinic acid	100 mg PO tid	Flushing, sensation of warmth, itching, tingling, headache, gastrointestinal upset, dizziness, hepatotoxicity
Gemfibrozil	600 mg PO bid given 30 min before the morning and evening meals	Fatigue, dyspepsia, abdominal pain, diarrhea, nausea, vomiting, cholelithiasis, myopathy, dizziness, blurred vision, impaired hepatic and renal function

Percutaneous Coronary Interventions and Percutaneous Balloon Valvuloplasty

PERCUTANEOUS CORONARY INTERVENTIONS

Historical Background

Cardiovascular disease is the number one cause of death in the United States. The American Heart Association estimates that 1,500,000 Americans will have a myocardial infarction, and about 500,000 of them will die each year.[1]

The first major advance in the palliative treatment of coronary artery disease (CAD) was the implantation of an aortocoronary saphenous vein bypass graft in 1967. Since that time, CABG has been refined and has been the treatment of choice for many patients with CAD. The first percutaneous transluminal coronary angioplasty (PTCA), however, performed by Gruentzig in 1977, marked another major innovation in the treatment of CAD.

Since the late 1970s, techniques to treat CAD have expanded beyond PTCA. Today, the term *percutaneous coronary intervention* (PCI) is used to describe invasive procedures to treat CAD, which include PTCA, laser angioplasty, atherectomy, stents, brachytherapy, percutaneous myocardial vascularization, and gene therapy for myocardial angiogenesis. These interventions are described in this chapter.

The path to PTCA began in 1964, when Dotter and Judkins introduced the concept of mechanically dilating a stenosis in a blood vessel with a technique of inserting a series of progressively larger catheters to treat peripheral vascular disease. After experimenting with this technique, Gruentzig modified the procedure by placing on the tip of a catheter a polyvinyl balloon, which was passed into a narrowed vessel and then inflated. Because it produced a smoother luminal surface with less trauma than the Dotter-Judkins approach, this new method reduced the risk of complications such as vessel rupture, subintimal tearing, and embolism. At first, Gruentzig continued to apply his technique only to peripheral vascular lesions. Then, after successful dilation of more than 500 peripheral lesions, he designed a smaller version of the dilation catheter for use within the coronary arterial tree. This new design was tested initially on dogs with experimentally induced coronary artery stenoses. After extensive canine experimentation, Gruentzig performed the first human PTCA in 1977.[2] Since then, considerable improvements in technique and equipment have made PTCA the treatment of choice for appropriate cases of CAD.

PTCA may be used to treat patients with myocardial infarction or unstable angina, or those with lesions that occlude more than 70% of the internal lumen of a coronary artery. PTCA is the hallmark procedure and basis of almost all other intracoronary interventions. During PTCA, a coaxial catheter system is introduced into the coronary arterial tree and advanced into an area of coronary artery stenosis. A balloon attached to the catheter is then inflated, increasing the luminal diameter and improving blood flow through the dilated segment. Several inflations ranging from 30 to 300 seconds are performed. PTCA is a nonsurgical technique applied as an alternative to CABG in the treatment of obstructive CAD. When indicated and if successful, PTCA can alleviate myocardial ischemia, relieve angina pectoris, and prevent myocardial necrosis.

Physiological Principles

The process that leads to successful dilation is complex and not clearly defined. Angiographic evaluation and animal and human histological studies indicate that PTCA stretches the vessel wall, leading to fracture of the inelastic atherosclerotic plaque and to tearing or cracking within the intima and media of the vessel. This cracking or slight dissection of the inner lumen of the vessel may be necessary for successful dilation.[3]

Comparisons Between PTCA and CABG

As an alternative treatment in appropriate cases of CAD, PTCA compares favorably with CABG in terms of risk, success rate, the patient's physical capacity after the procedure, length of hospital stay, and cost.

Mortality rates associated with first-time angioplasty and CABG are similar. The in-hospital death rate for patients undergoing angioplasty ranges from 0% to 2%; the CABG mortality rate ranges from 1.5% to 4%.[3] If a second surgical procedure becomes necessary to alleviate the symptoms of progressive CAD, the mortality and complication rates for the bypass procedure are significantly greater than for second angioplasty. Current 7-year survival data in the Bypass Angioplasty Revascularization Investigation (BARI) trial reveal that CABG offers a survival benefit to diabetic patients compared with PTCA (76.4% versus 55.7%). There is no difference in the survival rates of nondiabetic patients with CABG versus PTCA (86.4% versus 86.8%).[4]

Successful PTCA, which is defined as a significant reduction of the luminal diameter stenosis without in-hospital death, myocardial infarction, or CABG, ranges from 80% to 95%, depending on the severity of the patient's angiographic and clinical presentation. In a study by Bentivoglio and colleagues, the cumulative 2-year survival rates were 96% and 95% among patients with stable and unstable angina, respectively, with event-free survival (i.e., no death, myocardial infarction, or CABG) in 79% and 76%, respectively.[5] Among patients with multivessel PTCA, the actuarial survival rates were 97% at 1 year and 88% at 5 years in a study by O'Keefe and colleagues.[6] At 7 years after PTCA, Dorros and associates reported a survival rate of 90% in patients with simple single-vessel angioplasty and 95% in patients with simple multivessel angioplasty.[7] Long-term survival data in the era of stenting should be forthcoming in the near future.

In the Coronary Artery Surgery Study, graft patency after CABG was 90% at 2 months, 82% at 18 months, and 82% at 5 years. The 10-year survival rate was 82%.[8]

Restenosis or patency data differ greatly between CABG and PTCA. Within 6 months after angioplasty, 20% to 30% of lesions recur or restenose. Intracoronary stenting reduces the incidence of restenosis by an additional 5% to 10%. The mean occlusion rate for bypass grafts is approximately 18% during the first 5 years and 4% to 5% between 5 and 10 years.[8]

Psychological advantages of PTCA over surgery may argue favorably for the less invasive procedure. The emotional stress of awaiting dilation is less than that of awaiting surgery. This reduction in anxiety, however, is partly offset by the risk of psychological crisis if the angioplasty fails and surgery—especially immediate surgery—is needed. The psychological impact of this discouraging situation is significant, but it occurs in a relatively low percentage of cases.

Barring complications with either procedure, PTCA requires a hospital stay of 12 to 24 hours, whereas CABG requires a stay of 3 to 7 days. Because the average hospital stay is shorter with PTCA and because PTCA is performed in the cardiac catheterization laboratory under local anesthesia, the average cost of PTCA may be substantially lower than that of CABG. The following factors, however, can increase the cost of PTCA:

- Complications occurring during the procedure, requiring emergency surgery
- Lesions that recur, requiring repeat dilation, or bypass surgery
- Surgical standby, which is provided in different levels to correspond to the risk associated with each PTCA
- Lesions that require multiple devices to ablate the lesion
- Complications associated with the anticoagulation regimen or arterial and venous access

A factor in favor of PTCA is the lower morbidity after the procedure compared with CABG. Patients who have undergone PTCA often return to work within 7 to 10 days after the procedure, whereas patients undergoing CABG return to work within 6 weeks.

In conclusion, the major advantages of angioplasty over bypass surgery may include reduced mortality and morbidity, shorter convalescence, and lower cost to the patient and third-party payers.

Diagnostic Tests for PTCA and CABG Patient Selection

Before deciding between PTCA and CABG, all objective evidence of coronary insufficiency must be documented. Noninvasive methods of evaluation that may be used before and after PTCA include standard treadmill stress testing and thallium stress and redistribution myocardial imaging. These tests allow the physician to discover the areas of ischemia in the myocardium when the patient is subjected to stress (i.e., exercise; see Chapter 17 for a discussion of these tests). The nurse should be familiar with the results of the thallium stress test indicated on the examination report because an understanding of the patient's diagnosis and related symptoms, and thus of the reasons for interventional angioplasty therapy, promotes more informed patient care.

Coronary arteriography with cardiac catheterization, another method of documenting coronary insufficiency, is done if the previous tests indicate coronary disease. Although this procedure is more invasive than treadmill testing and thallium imaging, it is required to pinpoint the location of any stenoses and the degree of involvement of the artery or arteries (see Chapter 17 for a discussion of this test). This procedure yields a 35-mm, VHS tape cineangiogram, or digital image of the coronary artery anatomy. The physician can then analyze closely areas of narrowing, gaining precise information to decide the mode of treatment (Figs. 18-1 and 18-2).

Equipment Features

Since the introduction of PTCA, the equipment has been continually refined, resulting in fewer contraindications and lower rates of mortality and emergency bypass surgery.

The guiding catheters used to direct and support the advancement of the dilation catheter into the appropriate coronary artery ostium have an outer diameter of 6 to 10 Fr. Like the Judkins and Amplatz coronary angiography catheters, the tips of the guiding catheters have curves that are preshaped for selective access to either the right or left coronary artery.

Balloon dilation systems have evolved since Gruentzig's original design, in which the guidewire tip and catheter shaft were integral. In the early days of angioplasty, physicians were limited by catheter performance and could address lesions only in the proximal anatomy. In 1982, Simpson introduced a coaxial "over-the-wire" system, an

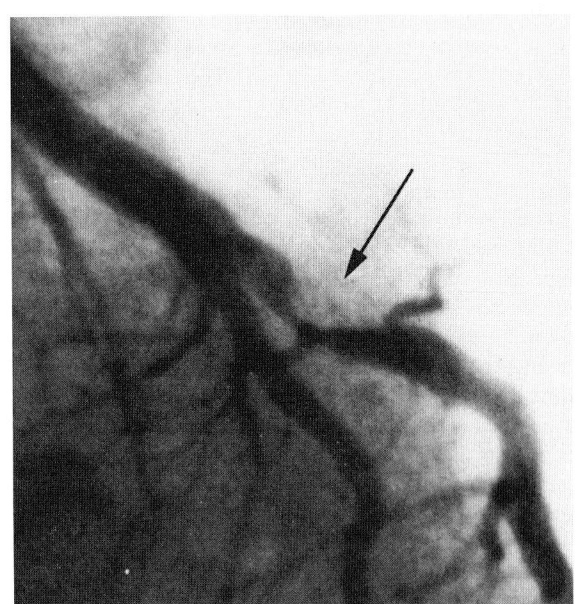

figure 18-1 An eccentric stenosis in the left anterior descending artery. The term *eccentric* defines a plaque involving only one side of the intraluminal wall. (Courtesy of John B. Simpson, MD, Palo Alto, CA.)

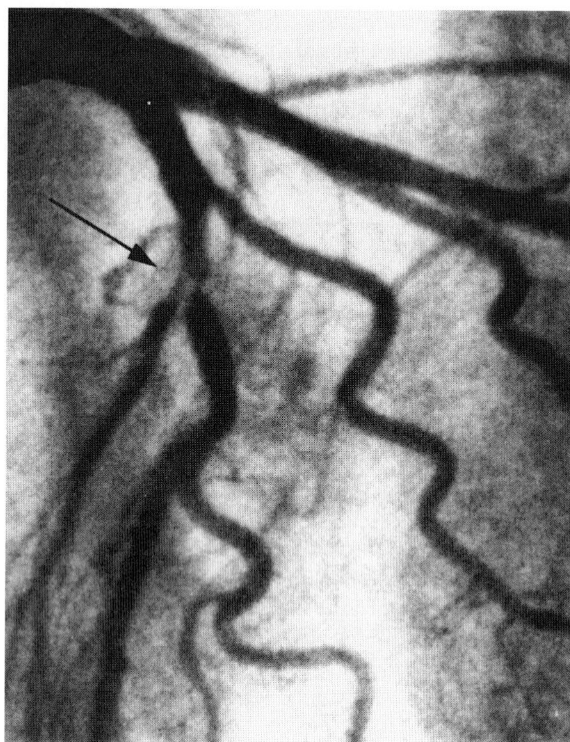

figure 18-2 A coronary arteriogram of the circumflex artery illustrating a concentric stenosis. The term *concentric* defines a plaque involving the intraluminal wall circumferentially, giving a dumbbell appearance. (Courtesy of John B. Simpson, MD, Palo Alto, CA.)

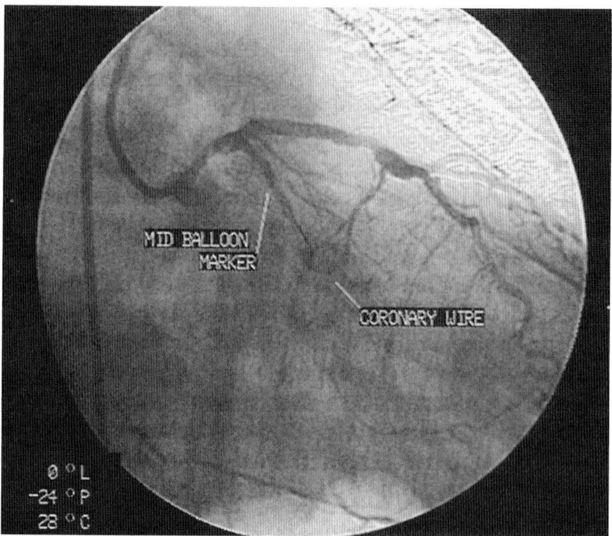

figure 18-3 Contrast injection through the guiding catheter to verify position. The coronary guidewire tip is located at the occlusion of the circumflex artery, and the coronary balloon is positioned in the proximal vessel. (Reprinted with permission of Advanced Cardiovascular Systems [ACS] Inc., Santa Clara, CA.)

improvement that has become predominant in current catheter designs. The main innovation is an independently movable guidewire within the balloon dilation catheter. This guidewire can be manipulated to select the correct vessel despite side branches and permits safe advancement of the dilation catheter across the lesion. Currently, the available guidewires measure between 0.010 and 0.018 inch in diameter and thus usually pose little threat of interference with the blood flow through a stenosis.

Coronary balloon dilation catheter shafts range in size from 1.9 to 4.2 Fr, small enough for easy passage through the guiding catheter and for visualization around the catheter during contrast injection (Fig. 18-3). The balloon dilation catheter has one or more radiopaque markers that can be imaged by fluoroscopy (Fig. 18-4). Thus, the physician can position the balloon accurately across the lesion. The inflated balloon size ranges from 1.5 to 5 mm in diameter and from 10 to 40 mm in length. The size (inflated diameter) of the balloon to be used for a particular PTCA is usually the same as the smallest-diameter segment of the coronary artery proximal or distal to the stenosis (i.e., 3-mm vessel, 3-mm balloon). Lesion and balloon length also are approximated.

The physician manually inflates the balloon with a contrast-filled, disposable inflation device that connects to the side arm or balloon lumen of the coronary dilation catheter (Fig. 18-5). The device incorporates a pressure gauge that indicates the amount of pressure exerted against the balloon wall during inflation. Balloon pressure is measured in pounds per square inch (psi) or atmospheres (atm). The average initial inflation is between 60 and 150 psi or 4 to 10 atm and lasts from 1 to 3 minutes. Longer inflations may promote a smoother, more regular vessel wall as assessed by angiography and are used primarily for the treatment of major dissections and abrupt closure. Extended inflations are performed safely with perfusion catheters that simultaneously dilate and perfuse.

Many factors must be considered when selecting the most appropriate equipment for performing PTCA. Technological advances in angioplasty equipment have made

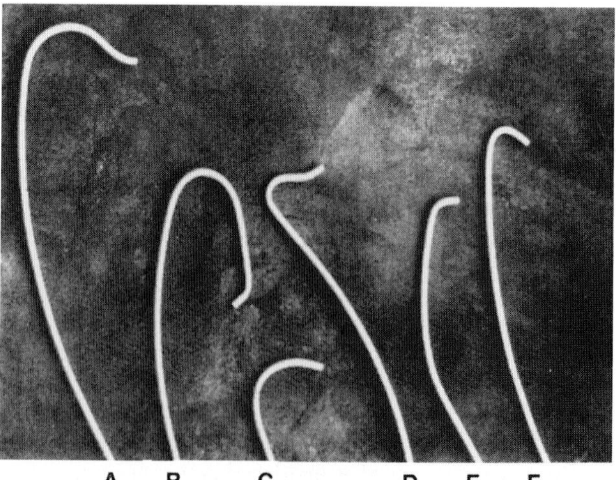

figure 18-4 A variety of guiding catheters with preshaped tips suitable for selectively engaging the appropriate coronary ostia, from left to right: (**A**) left Amplatz guiding catheter; (**B**) left Judkins guiding catheter; (**C**) hockey stick guiding catheter; (**D**) right Amplatz guiding catheter; (**E**) right Judkins guiding catheter; (**F**) left internal mammary guiding catheter. (Reprinted with permission of Advanced Cardiovascular Systems [ACS] Inc., Santa Clara, CA.)

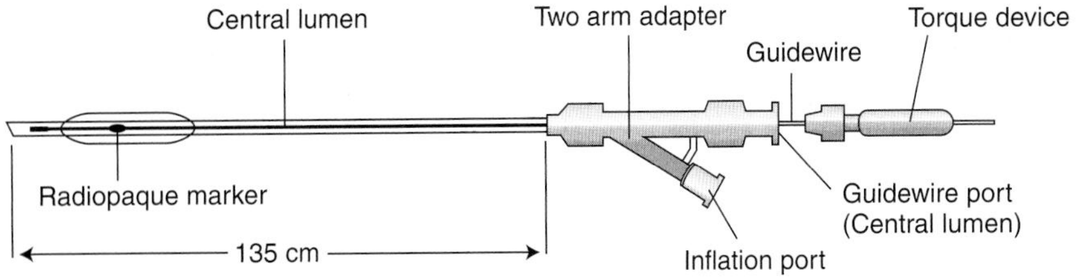

figure 18-5 PTCA balloon dilation catheter illustrating the key components of the system. (Reprinted with permission of Advanced Cardiovascular Systems [ACS] Inc., Santa Clara, CA.)

available several balloon dilation catheter systems that have been developed to improve the success and safety associated with any PTCA.

Many physicians consider the coaxial "over-the-wire" system a workhorse catheter because it can approach any anatomy well. A physician also might select a "rapid-exchange" system to accomplish more easily the dilation of a bifurcation lesion. This type of device incorporates a "rail" system that facilitates the exchange process. A "fixed-wire" catheter is used to reach and dilate lesions in distal, tortuous anatomy, and its small shaft also makes it an option for the use of two coronary dilation catheters in one guiding catheter when the strategy calls for side-by-side balloons.

Each intervention also encompasses an inflation strategy. The main elements of an inflation strategy are the duration and pressure of balloon inflation required to open a lesion. Today, balloons are available that can withstand greater pressure for the treatment of calcific lesions.

The outcome of any PTCA is greatly affected by (1) the selection of a guiding catheter that provides a platform for the advancement of the dilation system while preserving flow to the coronary artery, and (2) the selection of a balloon dilation system that best addresses the vessel's anatomy, the lesion's location, and lesion characteristics.

Indications for and Contraindications to Percutaneous Transluminal Coronary Angioplasty

INDICATIONS

When choosing to treat with PTCA (as with CABG), the physician's purpose is to alleviate angina pectoris unrelieved by maximal medical treatment and to reduce the risk of myocardial infarction in symptomatic patients and asymptomatic patients with severe stenosis. Indications for PTCA have expanded as equipment, technique, and operator experience have improved.

PTCA is indicated in patients with coronary arteries that have at least a 70% narrowing. Lesions with less narrowing are not considered appropriate for PTCA because they are equally at risk for abrupt closure, which can have serious consequences. Patients with surgical risk factors, such as severe underlying noncardiac diseases, advanced age, and poor left ventricular function, are particularly suited for PTCA because successful dilation obviates the need for an operation that would be poorly tolerated.

An example of the wide spectrum of candidacy for PTCA is the accepted practice of treating patients with multivessel disease. The common technique for dilating multiple lesions is to dilate the most critical stenosis first. With successful dilation of this "culprit" lesion, remaining lesions are dilated in stages (i.e., at different intervals during the procedure or over several days). Dilation of multiple vessels, however, is technically more demanding and carries a higher risk of complications.

Another expanded indication is the approach to treating the patient with a totally occluded vessel. Early in PTCA practice, total occlusion disqualified a patient for the procedure because the stenosis could not be crossed with the guidewire and balloon dilation catheter without causing severe trauma to the artery. Currently, due to refinement of equipment, technical advances, and greater physician experience, dilation of total occlusions may be attempted in appropriate candidates. Total occlusions of short duration (i.e., 3 months or less) are easier to cross and dilate successfully than total occlusions of longer duration.

Additional candidates for PTCA are those who have undergone CABG in whom symptoms have recurred due to stenosis and graft closure or progression of coronary disease in the native vessels. For these candidates, successful angioplasty makes second surgery, with its increased potential for complications, unnecessary. It is thought that the proliferative disease in the graft wall generates fibrous stenosis that is much less dense than most fibrotic tissue in the native vessels, so certain vein graft stenoses respond favorably to dilation.

In the past, if a patient had an AMI documented by significant ST segment elevation, increased cardiac enzyme levels, and pain unrelieved by medication, surgery or pharmacological treatment with complete bed rest in a coronary care unit were the only treatment alternatives. Now, if thrombosis and underlying stenosis are causing the infarction, thrombolytic therapy, PTCA, or both offer alternatives. When a blood clot has impeded flow to the distal myocardium and thus caused an ischemic episode, a thrombolytic agent (i.e., streptokinase, urokinase, tPA) can be administered IV or directly into the coronary artery. On successful lysis of the thrombus, dilation of the underlying stenosis often further enhances blood flow to the reperfused myocardium, reducing the risk of rethrombosis or critical narrowing caused by normal or spastic vasomotion superimposed on an organic stenosis.

Primary coronary angioplasty is a dilation of an infarct-related coronary artery during the acute phase of a myocardial infarction without prior administration of a thrombolytic agent. Meyer and associates first used PTCA in the AMI setting in 1982.[9] They reported an 81% success rate in PTCA of the infarct-related artery after intracoronary thrombolytic therapy. In 1999, Grines and associates reported a stand-alone PTCA success rate of 97% with a patency rate of 53% 2 years after PTCA.[10] Parameters routinely assessed in patients selected to receive primary angioplasty are depicted in Box 18-3.

box 18-3
Parameters Evaluated in Patients Selected to Receive Primary Angioplasty

- Age
- Hemodynamic status
- Angiographic anatomy:
  - Single-, double-, or triple-vessel disease
  - Vessel involvement: LAD, RCA, LCX
  - Lesion location: proximal, mid, or distal disease
  - Percent grade stenosis
  - Thrombolytics in Myocardial Infarction (TIMI) flow: 0, I, II, III
  - Left ventricular ejection fraction
- Presence of chest pain consistent with acute myocardial infarction
- ECG evidence of acute myocardial infarction:
  - 1 mm ST elevation in two contiguous leads
  - or
  - 1 mm ST depression believed to represent reciprocal changes to an area of infarction

LAD, left anterior descending artery; RCA, right coronary artery; LCX, left circumflex artery.

box 18-4
Indications and Contraindications for PTCA

Indications	Contraindications
Clinical	
Symptomatic (angina unrelieved by medical therapy)	
Asymptomatic but with severe underlying stenosis	
Stable/unstable angina	
Acute myocardial infarction	
High-risk surgical candidates	
Anatomical	
Severe stenosis (≥50%)	Mild stenosis (<50%)
Proximal and distal lesions	"Unprotected" left main coronary artery
Single and multivessel disease	
Bifurcation lesions	
Ostial lesions	
Totally occluded vessels	
Bypass graft lesions	
"Protected" left main coronary artery (previous LAD or LCX CABG)	

LAD, left anterior descending artery; LCX, left circumflex artery.

In the setting of AMI, PTCA may benefit patients deemed ineligible for traditional medical therapy. Such patients include those in cardiogenic shock, those believed to be at high risk for bleeding complications (CVA, prolonged cardiopulmonary resuscitation [CPR], bleeding diathesis, severe hypertension, or recent surgery), and those of advanced age (older than 75 years). Primary angioplasty does not preclude the use of thrombolytics if residual thrombus is observed. Primary angioplasty may offer distinct advantages in reducing the length of hospital stay and eliminating the need for additional intervention in many cases.[10,11] Indications for PTCA are summarized in Box 18-4.

Complications of primary angioplasty include retroperitoneal or vascular hemorrhage, other bleeding requiring transfusion, late restenosis, and early acute reocclusion. These complications occur at the same rate as those experienced in routine elective coronary angioplasty.

CONTRAINDICATIONS

There are very few contraindications to PTCA. Patients with left main CAD usually are not considered candidates for angioplasty. The obvious drawback of PTCA in left main artery disease is the possibility of acute occlusion or spasm of the left main artery during the procedure, which would result in severe left ventricular dysfunction. The only exception to this rule is the patient who has a "protected" left main artery (i.e., has had previous bypass surgery to the left anterior descending or circumflex arteries with patent grafts present). Only then might a physician consider dilating a left main artery stenosis. Most of these patients are still considered surgical candidates.

For high-risk patients (i.e., patients with left main vessel disease, severe left ventricular dysfunction, or dilation of the last remaining patent artery), percutaneous support devices may improve the safety of PTCA. Among the devices and techniques being investigated are perfusion balloons, intra-aortic balloon counterpulsation, coronary sinus retroperfusion, cardiopulmonary support, and partial left heart bypass (see Box 18-4).

Procedure

The PTCA procedure is carried out in a sterile fashion, with the use of local anesthesia and either the Judkins (percutaneous femoral) approach or, less often, the Sones (brachial cut-down) approach (Fig. 18-6).

With the Judkins approach, the physician cannulates the femoral vein and artery percutaneously by inserting a needle (usually 18-gauge) containing a removable obturator. The obturator then can be removed to confirm by the presence of blood flow that the outer needle is within the lumen of the vessel. Once proper placement is established, a guidewire is introduced through the outer cannula into the artery to the level of the diaphragm. The cannula then is removed and replaced by a valved introducer sheath. The sheath provides hemostasis and support at the puncture site in the groin and reduces potential arterial trauma if multiple catheter exchanges are necessary. The guiding catheter is preloaded with a 0.038-inch J wire and introduced into the sheath. The 0.038-inch J wire is advanced over the arch and the guiding catheter is advanced over the wire. The 0.038-inch J wire is removed, and the guiding catheter is rotated precisely to the appropriate coronary ostium. The procedure also may be accomplished by the Sones approach, in which a brachial cut-down is used to isolate the brachial

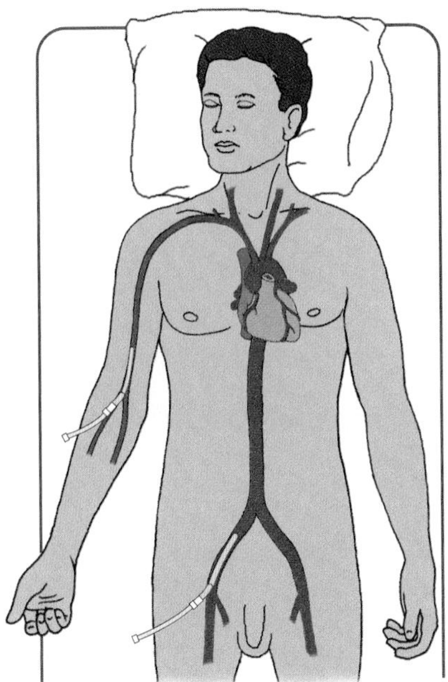

figure 18-6 Two approaches to left heart catheterization. The Sones technique uses the brachial artery, and the Judkins technique uses the femoral artery. With either method, the catheter is passed retrograde through the ascending aorta to the left ventricle. (Reprinted with permission of Advanced Cardiovascular Systems [ACS] Inc., Santa Clara, CA.)

vein and artery. A small arteriotomy is made, and the catheter is passed to the level of the aortic arch.

Regardless of the mode of access, coronary arteriography is then carried out in both the left anterior oblique (30 degrees) and right anterior oblique (60 degrees) views. These views allow for visualization of the heart along its transverse and longitudinal planes. Opposing views provide a thorough assessment of both the lesion and the anatomical approach. A "freeze frame" of each view is obtained as a road map or guide throughout the procedure. A final lesion assessment is made, confirming lesion severity and vessel diameter for appropriate balloon sizing.

If PTCA is indicated, the patient is anticoagulated with 5,000 to 10,000 units of heparin to prevent clots from forming on or in the catheter system during the procedure. Intracoronary nitroglycerin is kept on the sterile field throughout the procedure and given intermittently as needed for vasospasm and for dilation to facilitate visualization of the culprit coronary artery.

The balloon dilation catheter is introduced into the guiding catheter through a bifurcated adapter that provides access and is a port for contrast injections and aortic pressure measurement. The balloon dilation catheter and guidewire are advanced to the tip of the guiding catheter while their position is checked by fluoroscopy (Fig. 18-7). The guidewire then is advanced and manipulated to negotiate the branches of the coronary artery. Proper advancement can be confirmed by injecting contrast through the guiding catheter and fluoroscopically visualizing the coronary tree.

Once the guidewire is positioned safely beyond the stenosis, the balloon dilation catheter can be advanced slowly over the guidewire into the narrowing without risk of injury to the intima (Fig. 18-8).

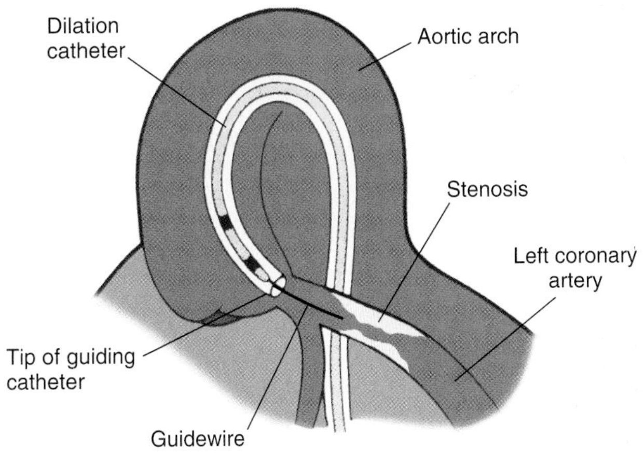

figure 18-7 The advancement of the coronary dilation catheter to the tip of the guiding catheter, which is positioned in the left coronary artery, is facilitated by fluoroscopy. (Reprinted with permission of Advanced Cardiovascular Systems [ACS] Inc., Santa Clara, CA.)

Exact placement of the dilation balloon in the stenosis is facilitated under fluoroscopy by the radiopaque marker on the balloon and by contrast injections for visualization. Initially, the balloon is inflated at 1 to 2 atm of pressure to confirm its position. Many PTCA balloon catheters expand at both ends and not in the center, where they are pinched by the stenosis (Figs. 18-9 and 18-10). The central indentation usually disappears as the stenosis is dilated. After each inflation, the physician injects a small bolus of contrast medium to assess any changes in coronary blood flow through the stenosis and to assess any increase in luminal diameter. At this time, the need for additional inflations is determined and a waiting period of 10 to 15 minutes is observed. Complications such as vessel recoil and abrupt

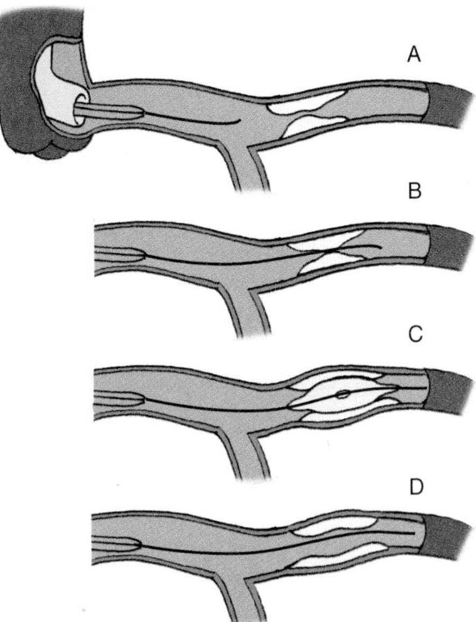

figure 18-8 (**A**) PTCA dilation catheter and guidewire exiting the guiding catheter. (**B**) Guidewire advanced across the stenosis. (**C**) Dilation catheter advanced across the stenosis and inflated. (**D**) Dilation catheter pulled back to assess luminal diameter. (Reprinted with permission of Advanced Cardiovascular Systems [ACS], Inc., Santa Clara, CA.)

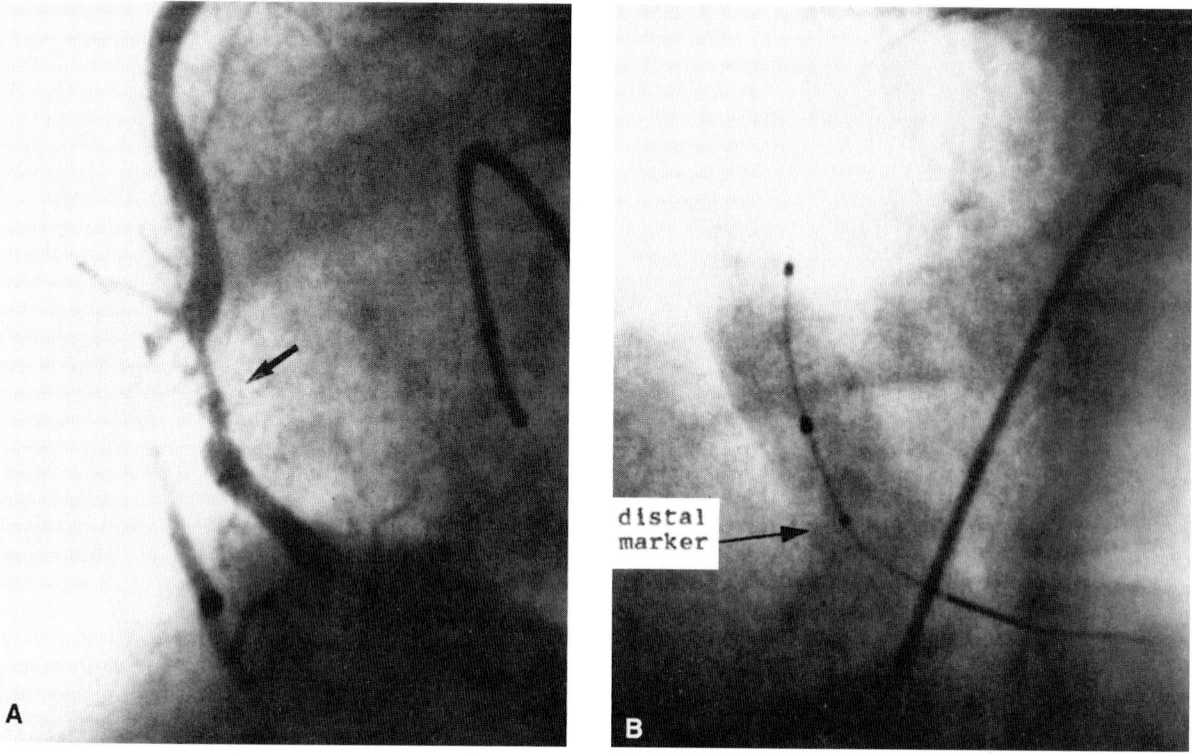

figure 18-9 Thirty-five-spot frames showing (**A**) stenosis involving the midright coronary artery and (**B**) the first and second radiopaque markers revealing the position of the dilation balloon across the stenosis, with the distal marker referring to the tip of the catheter beyond the narrowing. (Courtesy of John B. Simpson, MD, Palo Alto, CA.)

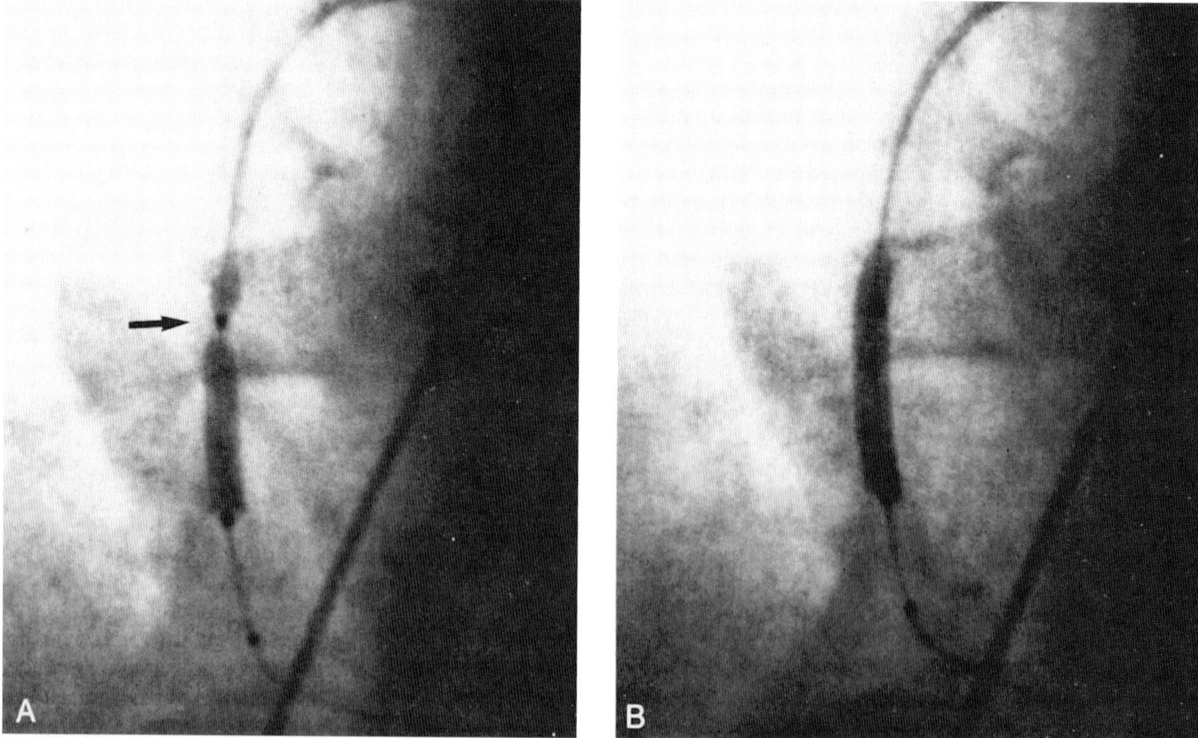

figure 18-10 Thirty-five-spot frames showing (**A**) inflation of the balloon, revealing the position of the stenosis by the "dumbbell" effect, and (**B**) absence of stenosis after dilation. (Courtesy of John B. Simpson, MD, Palo Alto, CA.)

closure occur most often during this early phase; however, their incidence is low, and redilation can be done readily at this time. After dilation is complete, the guiding catheter and the balloon dilation catheter are removed. Postdilation angiography is performed to define more clearly the results of the PTCA.

Reasons for failure to complete a PTCA procedure include inability to cross the target lesion with a guidewire or dilation catheter due primarily to chronic total occlusions; inability to dilate the lesion due to rigid lesions or severe dissection; and embolization of friable vein graft material or of thrombus.

Successful dilation of a lesion commonly is defined as a reduction of the luminal diameter stenosis by about 40% or 50%. Clinical success commonly is defined as angiographic success with clinical improvement and without significant in-hospital complications, such as death, myocardial infarction, or CABG or repeat PTCA for abrupt closure.

Angiography after successful PTCA demonstrates an immediate increase in the intraluminal diameter of the involved vessel (Fig. 18-11). Clinical improvement of the patient is demonstrated by improved or normalized myocardial perfusion deficits, as shown by comparison of a post-PTCA thallium stress image to the pre-PTCA stress image. Postangioplasty treadmill test results compared with the preprocedure test results reveal increased exercise endurance and a decrease in exercise-induced angina or angina equivalent.

Results

Excellent short- and long-term results have been achieved in patients undergoing coronary angioplasty. The results vary depending on the patient's clinical presentation (i.e., stable or unstable angina) and angiographic characteristics (i.e., subtotal or total occlusion). Among patients undergoing either single-vessel dilation or multivessel dilation, in-hospital clinical success ranges from 85% to 95%.[12] In-hospital complications are low, with a reported mortality rate of 1% to 2% in both these patient groups.[13] Long-term survival rates are high, although repeat PTCA may be necessary for recurrent or progressive disease.

Patients with high-risk clinical or angiographic presentations have lower success rates. PTCA, however, is often preferable to surgical revascularization because of the latter's increased risk of mortality in patients such as older adults or those with depressed left ventricular function.

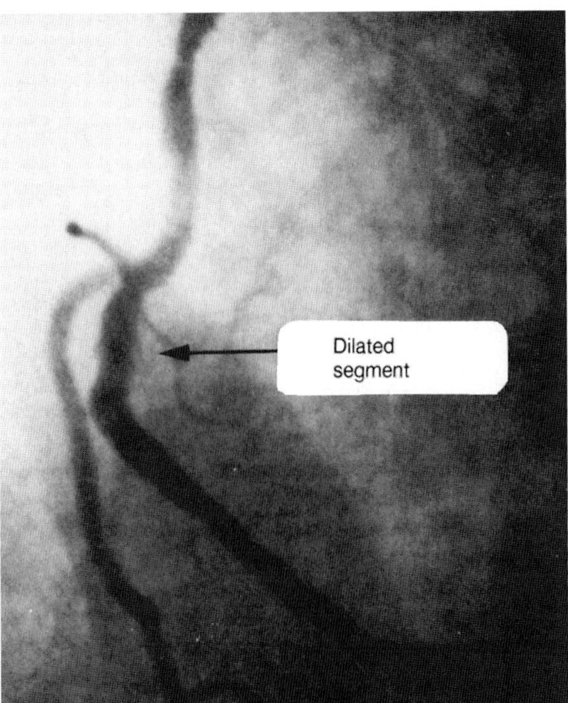

figure 18-11 Repeat angiography after PTCA of a right coronary artery stenosis showing increased flow and increased diameter of the dilated segment. (Courtesy of John B. Simpson, MD, Palo Alto, CA.)

Assessment and Management

PATIENT PREPARATION

Laboratory Tests

When the decision has been made to proceed with any PCI procedure, the patient usually is admitted to the hospital the day of the procedure. The nurse should monitor all preliminary laboratory tests, including cardiac enzymes, serum electrolytes, and coagulation studies (prothrombin time and partial thromboplastin time). Serum potassium, creatinine, and blood urea nitrogen (BUN) are particularly important.

Potassium levels must be within normal limits because low levels result in increased sensitivity and excitability of the myocardium. The cardiac muscle also is sensitive and becomes irritable when the flow of oxygen-rich blood decreases, as happens for a controlled period of time during placement and inflation of the dilation balloon across the lesion. The irritability arising from hypokalemia or ischemia or both can give rise to life-threatening ventricular dysrhythmias.

Elevation in the levels of serum creatinine, BUN, or both may indicate problems in kidney function. Good kidney function is important because during angioplasty, radiopaque contrast material (which allows fluoroscopic visualization of the coronary anatomy and of catheter placement) is introduced into the bloodstream. This contrast material is a hyperosmotic solution that the kidneys must filter from the blood and excrete. High levels of creatinine and BUN may reflect decreased renal filtration capability and vulnerability of the kidney in processing the extra load of radiopaque solution. Instances of acute renal failure have resulted from high doses of radiopaque contrast. The nurse should ensure that the patient is adequately hydrated, either orally or with IV solutions, to avoid falsely high electrolyte levels. Kidney function can be monitored by trends in creatinine and BUN levels, in conjunction with measurement of urine output.

Informed Consent

The informed consent for the PCI procedure is obtained from the patient before the procedure after a detailed discussion of the potential complications, anticipated benefit, and alternative therapies. This discussion should be conducted before any preoperative sedation. The nurse plays an important role in answering any questions that the patient and his or her family may have regarding the procedure and follow-up care.

Preoperative Medications

Twenty-four hours before the procedure, the patient's medications should include aspirin 325 mg once a day for its antiplatelet effect. Medications may be prescribed to reduce vasospastic events, including nitroglycerin and calcium channel blocking agents, such as nifedipine 10 mg three times a day, and diltiazem 30 mg three times a day. Diabetic patients taking metformin should be advised to discontinue this medication before their procedure because it is contraindicated with intravascular contrast agents. Anticoagulants such as warfarin are often held for a number of days before the PCI procedure.

Surgical Standby

Surgical standby for PTCA is arranged before the procedure. Surgical availability is required, but the degree to which the operating room is held for availability varies according to the patient's risk factors, hospital policies, or both. Many smaller community hospitals across the United States are performing PCI procedures without in-house surgical standby. These patients are typically low risk and reside near larger academic centers that can accept the patient by immediate transfer if complications arise during the PCI. A comparison of patients treated with PCI at hospitals without on-site cardiac surgery with those treated only with thrombolytic therapy reveals that the former group has better clinical outcomes at 1, 3, and 6 months.[13]

NURSING MANAGEMENT DURING PERCUTANEOUS TRANSLUMINAL CORONARY ANGIOPLASTY

During the preparation for PTCA and throughout the procedure, nurses in the cardiac catheterization laboratory are responsible for understanding all aspects of equipment use and patient care. They should be experienced in advanced cardiac life support and be knowledgeable about the proper administration of emergency medications and the correct application of emergency equipment, including the defibrillator, the ventilator, and the pacemaker. They should observe and communicate with the patient intermittently and report any changes in patient status to the physician. The nurse should monitor the ECG and arterial pressure, noting significant changes that may accompany the administration of drugs, symptoms of ischemia, or chest pain. The nurse must recognize signs and symptoms of contrast sensitivity, such as urticaria, blushing, anxiety, nausea, and laryngospasm. The nurse should understand the proper assembly and use of all angioplasty equipment and should be able to troubleshoot any situation that might arise.

The patient's anticoagulation status during the PTCA procedure is of utmost importance. Subtherapeutic levels may result in serious complications, including acute closure or thrombotic events. An activated clotting time (ACT) should be measured in the catheterization laboratory at baseline (before the PTCA), 5 minutes after the heparin bolus (usually 5,000 to 10,000 U), and every 30 minutes thereafter for the duration of the procedure. ACT levels of 250 to 300 seconds are desirable after the initial heparin bolus. Subsequent boluses of 2,000 to 5,000 units of heparin may be required to achieve and maintain these ACT levels during the PTCA procedure.

box 18-5 ***Instructions Regarding Precautions Post-PTCA***

- Remain on bed rest for 4 to 6 hours.
- Maintain the involved leg in a straight position (for Judkins technique).
- Avoid an upright position.
- Avoid vigorous use of the abdominal muscles, as in coughing, sneezing, or moving the bowels.

Patients at high risk for abrupt closure or with unstable lesions maybe administered a platelet GP IIb/IIIa antagonist in addition to aspirin and heparin. These agents are typically initiated just before or during PCI. Eptifibatide or tirofiban should be administered, in addition to aspirin and either unfractionated heparin or LMWH, to patients with continuing ischemia, an elevated troponin, or other high-risk features in whom an invasive management strategy is not planned.[14]

After the PTCA is complete, the nurse instructs the patient in the precautions necessary to prevent bleeding from the puncture site. Box 18-5 presents patient teaching.

After the procedure, the patient is transferred to a telemetry unit for observation. Common nursing diagnoses and collaborative problems for patients undergoing PTCA are listed in Box 18-6.

box 18-6 ***Examples of Nursing Diagnoses and Collaborative Problems for the Patient Having PCI or PBV***

Risk for Decreased Cardiac Output related to mechanical factors that affect preload, afterload, and left ventricular function
Risk for Decreased Cardiac Output related to electrical factors affecting rate, rhythm, or conduction
Risk for Decreased Cardiac Output related to structural changes (dissection, thrombus, or arterial spasm at PCI site), resulting in myocardial ischemia or infarction
Risk for Decreased Cardiac Output related to increased preload and pulmonary congestion related to temporary mechanical factors (eg, balloon inflation during PBV)
Risk for Decreased Cardiac Output related to left-to-right shunt with mitral PBV or late cardiac tamponade
Risk for Impaired Peripheral Perfusion related to hematoma, thrombus formation, or infection associated with cannulation site
Risk for Impaired Cerebral Perfusion related to embolism from procedure site, left ventricle, or left atrium
Risk for Pain related to angina or stretching of the valve during dilation
Risk for Fluid Volume Deficit related to renal sensitivity to contrast material or diuretic therapy
Deficient Knowledge related to illness and impact on patient's future
Anxiety/Fear related to lack of knowledge of PCI/PBV, acute care environment, and potential for surgery

NURSING MANAGEMENT AFTER PERCUTANEOUS CORONARY INTERVENTIONS

The nurse in the coronary care or telemetry unit plays an important role in observing and assessing the patient's recovery. Post-PCI care is designed to monitor the patient closely for signs and symptoms of myocardial ischemia. The most overt symptom of a possible complication, early recurrence of angina pectoris, requires prompt nursing action.

As soon as possible on receiving the patient from the cardiac catheterization laboratory, the nurse attaches the ECG monitor, which allows a quick initial cardiac assessment and establishes a baseline if the patient's condition should change suddenly. The nurse assesses the patient's status from head to toe, noting the overall skin color and temperature and carefully observing the level of consciousness. After the patient is transferred to the bed and attached to the monitor, the nurse listens closely to heart and breath sounds. The nurse evaluates the peripheral circulation by noting peripheral skin color and temperature and the presence and quality of dorsalis pedis and posterior tibial pulses.

Because the Judkins technique is used most often in PTCA to access the vasculature, most patients have an entry port in either the right or the left groin through which sheaths will have been placed percutaneously in a vein and artery. If the Sones technique was used, there is an arterial catheter in the brachial area (see Fig. 18-6). Due to elevated levels of anticoagulation required during the procedure, the sheaths are not removed immediately after the PCI procedure to avoid complications of clot formation; consequently, the effects of the heparin are not reversed but allowed to dissipate naturally, over 3 to 4 hours. Indwelling arterial and venous sheaths should not be removed until ACT levels fall below the 160-second level. A variety of mechanical devices and clamps may be used to facilitate hemostasis after sheath removal. The insertion of collagen plugs or the application of a surgical suture around the opening of the blood vessel is also routinely performed to obtain hemostasis. After sheath removal, the nurse pays careful attention to the area distal to the puncture site, checking pulses frequently and reporting immediately to the physician any changes that may indicate bleeding. Bleeding at the sheath site may result in a major hematoma that can require surgical evacuation or compromise distal blood flow to the lower extremity. To prevent excessive bleeding and to aid hemostasis, the physician may order a 5-lb sandbag placed over the puncture site after sheath removal.

The nurse instructs the patient on the importance of keeping the involved leg straight and the head of the bed angled up no more than 45 degrees. To prevent clotting in the lumens of the introducing sheaths, an IV infusion is attached to the venous sheath, and a pressurized arterial flush is attached to the arterial line. This arrangement also ensures patency should an immediate return to the cardiac catheterization laboratory be necessary because of a complication. The physician chooses both the type of solution to be infused through the venous sheath and the rate of infusion. His or her decision depends on the patient's fluid volume status.

Initial post-PCI laboratory blood tests should include coagulation studies, cardiac enzymes, and serum electrolytes. Elevation of the cardiac enzymes can indicate that a silent myocardial infarction has occurred (i.e., infarction unannounced by chest pain). If an abnormal cardiac enzyme laboratory value appears, the nurse notifies the physician immediately because the patient's postoperative care might need to be modified to prevent further injury.

The nurse plays a significant role in observing and assessing angina that recurs soon after a PCI procedure. Any chest pain demands immediate and careful attention because it may indicate either the start of vasospasm or impending occlusion. The patient may describe angina as a burning, squeezing heaviness or as sharp mid-sternal pain. Other signs and symptoms of myocardial ischemia include ischemic ECG changes (elevation of the ST segments or T-wave inversion), dysrhythmias, hypotension, and nausea. The nurse notifies the physician immediately of any such change in the patient's condition because it is impossible to tell merely by observation whether the change indicates a transient vasospastic episode, which can be resolved with vasodilation therapy, or an acute occlusion requiring emergency surgery.

If vasodilation therapy is indicated, it may be administered as described subsequently unless the patient is severely hypotensive; in that case, vasodilation is contraindicated. At the first sign of vasospasm, the nurse gives oxygen by mask or nasal cannula. For fast, temporary (and possibly permanent) relief, 0.4 mg of nitroglycerin, 5 mg of isosorbide, or 10 mg of nifedipine is administered sublingually. In addition, the IV drip of nitroglycerin should be titrated to maintain a blood pressure adequate to ensure coronary artery perfusion and to alleviate chest pain.

In conjunction with the onset of the chest pain, a 12-lead ECG reading is recorded to document any acute changes. If the angina resolves and any acute ECG changes caused by medical therapy disappear, it is safe to assume that a transient vasospastic episode occurred; however, if the angina continues and the ECG changes persist, redilation or emergency bypass surgery should be considered.

If the post-PCI course is uncomplicated, the sheaths are removed after 3 to 4 hours, and a pressure dressing is applied to the site. A variety of mechanical clamps or hemostasis devices may be used to facilitate hemostasis after sheath removal. The patient must continue complete bed rest for 4 to 6 hours after the sheaths are removed. A normal, low-sodium, or low-cholesterol diet may be resumed, depending on the preference of the physician and the needs of the patient.

During the recovery period, the nurse can introduce the patient to the rehabilitation process, emphasizing ways to combat the advance of CAD. Efforts should be made during this instruction to reinforce the importance of aerobic conditioning with regular, moderate exercise and reasonably paced increases. Also, the nurse explains that such abuses as frequent stress, excessive weight, and smoking promote CAD and that the patient has the power and responsibility to avoid these abuses by behavior modification. See Box 18-5 for instructions for the patient post-PCI. Box 18-7 describes implications for the older patient.

After PCI, the patient is asked to take medications that help prevent thrombus formation and maintain maximal

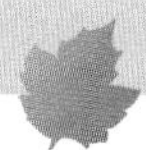

box 18-7

The Older Cardiac Patient

- Assess whether the patient will have assistance in the home with meals, cleaning, self-care, and transportation to medical appointments.
- Closely monitor kidney function before and after PCI because elderly patients may be sensitive to small amounts of radiocontrast.
- Monitor vital signs frequently, including temperature, because elderly patients are prone to excessive body heat loss.
- Assess all preexisting comorbidities: arthritis, peripheral vascular disease, diabetes, and so forth.
- Provide clear, precise, written instructions in preparation for discharge.

dilation at the culprit lesion site. All patients should be routinely sent home on aspirin for the antiplatelet effect. Aspirin is continued indefinitely. Clopidogrel should be administered to hospitalized patients who are unable to take aspirin because of hypersensitivity or major gastrointestinal intolerance. Clopidogrel should be continued for at least 1 month and may be administered for a maximum of 9 months.[14] In patients taking clopidogrel in whom elective CABG is planned, however, the drug should be withheld for 5 to 7 days. Often, long-acting nitrates, calcium channel blockers, and lipid-lowering agents are added to the medical regimen. The nurse may be responsible for explaining to the patient the indications for the specific medications ordered by the physician, including side effects and signs of overdose, and should answer any questions that the patient may have regarding his or her follow-up care. Box 18-8 summarizes medications currently associated with PTCA.

Four to 6 weeks after the patient's discharge, an exercise treadmill stress test and a thallium imaging study may be performed to test the efficacy of the PCI. Compared with the pre-PCI tests, an increase in exercise capacity and a decrease in or disappearance of exercise-induced chest pain (without ST segment changes) suggest improved blood flow and normalization of cardiac function in the previously hypoperfused muscle. Treadmill stress testing should be repeated at 6 months and 1 year after PCI.

Complications

The indications for PCI have expanded to include patients with more severe CAD (i.e., total occlusions, multivessel disease, recent or ongoing myocardial infarction, poor left ventricular function). The rate of complications associated with PCI has not increased. Major complications that can result in ischemia and possible severe left ventricular dysfunction necessitating emergent CABG include angina unrelieved by maximal administration of nitrates and calcium channel blockers (see Box 18-8), myocardial infarction, coronary artery spasm, abrupt closure of a dilated segment, coronary artery dissection leading to occlusion, and restenosis. See Box 18-6 for nursing diagnoses and collaborative problems for the patient having PCI or percutaneous balloon valvuloplasty.

ANGINA, MYOCARDIAL INFARCTION, AND VASOSPASM

Some degree of angina is anticipated during the PCI procedure due to the temporary occlusion of the involved vessel during dilation. This angina is handled with intracoronary nitroglycerin or removal of the balloon dilation catheter while the guidewire is left across the lesion. Evidence of persistent chest pain after PCI, reflected in changes in heart rate and blood pressure and elevated ST segments, indicates ischemia predisposing to an insult to the myocardium and requiring immediate intervention. Coronary artery spasm sometimes requires emergent surgical intervention (CABG) when the vasoconstriction, occlusion, or ischemia cannot be reversed through the administration of nitrates.

ABRUPT CLOSURE OF DILATED SEGMENT

Abrupt closure is a serious complication of coronary artery dilation that occurs in approximately 3% of those undergoing angioplasty.[15] An estimated 70% to 80% of abrupt closures occur while the patient is still in the cardiac catheterization laboratory. Approximately one third to one half of those patients whose vessel abruptly closes undergo a successful repeat dilation. Abrupt closure can be caused by coronary artery dissection, coronary artery spasm, and thrombus formation. Treatment options include immediate repeat dilation, emergent CABG surgery, or pharmacological therapy. To maintain blood flow through the occlusion while the patient is being prepared for emergent CABG surgery, the physician can use a perfusion balloon catheter, which has side holes along its shaft to allow blood to flow through the catheter at the site of occlusion and perfuse the distal myocardium.

CORONARY ARTERY DISSECTION

Coronary artery dissection or an intimal tear in the coronary artery can be visualized in the form of intraluminal filling defects or extraluminal extravasation of contrast material. Mild interruptions in the intraluminal wall are an expected result of the splitting and stretching of the intima on inflation of the balloon dilation catheter at the lesion site. A dissection may cause a major luminal obstruction associated with coronary artery occlusion, however, leading to a deterioration in blood flow with resultant severe ischemia or myocardial infarction that requires emergent bypass surgery.

RESTENOSIS

Restenosis of a dilated lesion occurs in approximately 20% to 30% of PTCA cases within the first 6 months after angioplasty. Over-the-counter remedies such as fish oil derivatives have proven unbeneficial. Pharmacological agents to reduce restenosis are currently being investigated (prostacyclins, new anticoagulants, platelet antibodies, and corticosteroids), but have shown little benefit to date.

The development of new devices to remove atherosclerotic plaque (atherectomy catheters) and implantable devices to maintain the opening mechanically (stents) may provide effective adjuncts or alternatives to PTCA for the problem of recurring lesions. Restenosis of de novo lesions

box 18-8
Summary of Medications Most Often Associated With PCI

Anticoagulants/Antiplatelets

Aspirin

Indications: Prophylaxis of coronary and cerebral arterial thrombus formation
Actions: Blocks platelet aggregation
Dosage: 80–325 mg qd, PO
Adverse effects: Well tolerated; nausea, vomiting, diarrhea, headache, and vertigo occasionally

Heparin (fractionated)

Indications: Prophylaxis of impending coronary occlusion and prophylaxis of peripheral arterial embolism
Actions: Inhibits clotting of blood and formation of fibrin clots; inactivates thrombin, preventing conversion of fibrinogen to fibrin; prevents formation of a stable fibrin clot by inhibiting the activation of fibrin stabilizing factor; inhibits reactions that lead to clotting but does not alter normal components of blood; prolongs clotting time but does not affect bleeding time; does not lyse clots
Dosage: Varies with indications; IV or intra-arterial: 10,000 U at start of PCI
Adverse effects: Uncontrollable bleeding, hypersensitivity

Low-Molecular-Weight Heparin (Enoxaparin Sodium, Dalteparin Sodium)

Indications: Treatment of unstable angina and myocardial ischemia, complete and non–Q wave myocardial infarction.
Action: Prevents clotting of blood and formation of thrombin.
Dosage
- Enoxaprin: 1 mg/kg SC q12h for 2–8 days
- Dalteparin sodium: 120 µg/kg SC q12h for 5–8 days

Adverse effects: Thrombocytopenia, hematoma, pain or reaction at the injection site, rash, hemorrhage, fever.

Glycoprotein IIb/IIIa Antagonists (Abciximab, Eptifibatide, Tirofiban)

Indications: Prevention of clotting and abrupt closure during interventional procedures and to prevent restenosis.
Action: Block the receptor on the platelet membrane that leads to the final common pathway of platelet aggregation.
Dosage
- Abciximab: 0.25 mg/kg IV bolus followed by 0.125 µg/kg/min infusion for 12–24 h after PCI
- Eptifibatide: 135 µg/kg IV administered immediately before PCI followed by 0.5 µg/kg/min for 20–24 h
- Tirofiban: 180 µg/kg IV bolus followed by 1.2–2 µg/kg/min infusion for 72–96 h after PCI

Adverse effects: Thrombocytopenia, hemorrhage, nausea, hematoma

Clopidogrel (Plavix)

Indications: Reduction of atherosclerotic events (AMI, stroke, and vascular death) in patients with atherosclerosis documented by a recent stroke or AMI or established peripheral arterial disease
Action: Blocks platelet aggregation
Dosage: 75 mg once daily
Adverse effects: Diarrhea, rash, gastrointestinal disturbances, hemorrhage, neutropenia.

Coronary Vasodilators

Isosorbide Dinitrate (Isordil, Sorbitrate)

Indications: Prophylaxis of angina
Actions: A nitrate that acts as a smooth muscle relaxant; causes coronary vasodilation without increasing myocardial oxygen consumption; secondary to general vasodilation, blood pressure decrease
Dosage
- Sublingual: 2.5–10 mg q2–3h PRN angina
- Oral: 5–40 mg qid
- Sustained-action oral: 40 mg q6–12h

Adverse effects: Cutaneous vasodilation that can cause flushing; headache, transient dizziness, and weakness; excessive hypotension

Nitroglycerin

Indications: Control of blood pressure and angina pectoris
Actions: Potent vasodilator that affects primarily the venous system; selectively dilates large coronary arteries increasing blood flow to ischemic subendocardium
Dosage
- Sublingual: 0.3–0.4 mg PRN chest pain
- Topical (patch): 2.5–10 mg/day; indicated for primary, secondary, or nocturnal angina due to more sustained effect
- IV: 5 µg/min to start—titrate to patient response (no fixed dose due to variable response in different patients)

Adverse effects: Excessive and prolonged hypotension; headache; tachycardia, palpitations; nausea, vomiting, apprehension; retrosternal discomfort

Calcium Channel Blockers

Nifedipine (Procardia), Diltiazem (Cardizem)

Indications: Angina pectoris due to coronary artery spasm and fixed vessel disease; hypertension; dysrhythmias
Actions: Inhibit calcium ion flux across the cell membrane of the cardiac muscle and vascular smooth muscle without changing serum calcium concentration; decrease afterload through peripheral arterial dilation and

1. Reduce systemic and pulmonary vascular resistance
2. Vasodilate coronary circulation
3. Decrease myocardial oxygen demands and increases myocardial oxygen supply

Dosage
- Nifedipine: 10–30 mg tid–qid, PO
- Diltiazem: 30–90 mg tid–qid, PO

Adverse effects: Contraindicated in patients with sick sinus syndrome; hypertension after IV use; gastrointestinal distress; headache, vertigo, flushing; peripheral edema, occasional increase in angina, tachycardia
See text for full discussion of antidysrhythmics.

after atherectomy is similar in character and prevalence to that in PTCA; however, intracoronary stenting may result in a lower restenosis rate in native and vein graft lesions of approximately 10%.

The cause of restenosis still is unclear. It appears to be the result of an excessive healing response to balloon dilation that exposes the subintimal structures of the vessel to circulating blood. These exposed areas are then potential sites for platelet adhesion and aggregation and for thrombus formation. The degree of this "healing" response varies from lesion to lesion and may be influenced by the clinical and angiographic factors associated with restenosis that were discussed previously. Factors associated with increased incidence of restenosis are listed in Box 18-9.

OTHER COMPLICATIONS

Other major complications of PCI requiring medical intervention are bradycardia, which requires temporary pacing; ventricular tachycardia or ventricular fibrillation, which requires immediate defibrillation; and a central nervous system event causing transient or persistent neurological deficit.

Peripheral vascular complications occurring primarily at the catheter site include arterial thrombosis, excessive bleeding that causes a significant hematoma, pseudoaneurysm, femoral arteriovenous fistula, and arterial laceration. If any of these complications persists or compromises distal blood flow to the involved extremity, surgical intervention may be required.

Table 18-10 summarizes the complications that may result from PCI, including general signs of the complications and possible interventional actions.

Box 18-10 provides a Collaborative Care Guide for a complete outline of care for the patient undergoing PCI.

Other Interventional Cardiology Techniques

The immediate and long-term efficacy of PCI in treating symptomatic patients with single-vessel disease has been well established. In many centers, PTCA also is routinely and successfully applied to patients with multivessel disease. The safety and efficacy with which angioplasty has been applied have fostered research into treating patients with unstable angina, AMI, and cardiogenic shock.

New technologies are being developed to address the challenges associated with complex PCI. These include laser angioplasty, atherectomy, and intracoronary stents. Percutaneous removal of plaque using directional or rotational atherectomy catheters has been used in coronary arteries with good results. Laser technology has progressed and is being used to ablate plaque or as an adjunct to PTCA to make a pathway in total occlusions. Implantations of intravascular stents to reinforce arterial walls have been successful and are well suited for repairing acute occlusive dissection.

LASER ANGIOPLASTY

Laser angioplasty has become an exciting addition to the interventional cardiology arsenal. A laser is a device that generates a directional beam of monochromatic light. The acronym LASER stands for "light amplification through stimulated emission of radiation." Through a series of mirrors and lenses, the laser beam is directed into a catheter containing numerous glass fibers. These fibers transmit the light energy through the catheter to the plaque that is to be ablated.[16]

Laser angioplasty is performed much like a standard balloon angioplasty procedure. The guide catheter is advanced to the ostium of the coronary artery targeted by fluoroscopy. Once the lesion location is ascertained through contrast injection, a guidewire is advanced up and through the lesion. Before the laser is activated, everyone in the room (including the patient) must don protective eyewear. The laser catheter is then advanced through the guidewire and brought into contact with the lesion. Depending on anticipated lesion morphology, energy settings are chosen that will presumably suffice to ablate the plaque. The laser settings include the fluency (millijoules per square millimeter) to be delivered and the repetition rate (pulses per second). The plaque is then vaporized by the laser energy. Several passes down the length of the lesion may be performed. Laser success is determined by fluoroscopy and coronary injections with contrast dye. If there is residual stenosis after use of the laser, adjunctive angioplasty balloon inflations can be performed to achieve an optimal final result.

Stenotic lesions best suited for laser angioplasty include those that are long and diffuse (longer than 15 to 20 mm), ostial in location, highly calcified, in vein grafts, and totally occluded. Risks associated with laser angioplasty include perforation of the coronary artery, dissections, and aneurysms.

ATHERECTOMY

Atherectomy is the process of removing atherosclerotic plaque from the coronary artery by cutting or ablating and thus "debulking" the lesion. Atherectomy devices include directional coronary atherectomy (DCA), transluminal extraction catheter (TEC), or rotational ablation (Rotablator).

Potential complications of all atherectomy devices include perforation of the coronary artery, abrupt closure, embolization distal to the lesion site, and myocardial infarction. The rate of restenosis and other complications is comparable to that with PTCA.

box 18-9
Factors Associated With Increased Incidence of Restenosis

Clinical Factors
- Severe angina
- Absence of prior myocardial infarction
- Diabetes
- Smoking cigarettes

Angiographic Factors
- Lesion location
- Lesion length
- Lesion severity before and after PCI
- Adjacent arterial diameter

table 18-10 Complications of PCI

Complications	General Signs/Symptoms	Possible Interventions
Prolonged angina	Angina pectoris	CABG
Myocardial infarction	Dysrhythmias: tachycardia, bradycardia, ventricular tachycardia/fibrillation	Redo PTCA Oxygen
Abrupt reclosure Dissection/intimal tear Hypotension	Marked hypotension Acute ECG changes (ST segment change) Nausea/vomiting	Medications: vasodilators (nitrates), calcium channel blockers, analgesics, anticoagulants, vasopressors
Coronary branch occlusion	Pallor	Complete bed rest
Coronary thrombosis	Restlessness Cardiac/respiratory arrest	Increase IV fluid volume within patient tolerance
Restenosis	Angina pectoris Positive exercise test	Redo PTCA CABG
Marked change in heart rate: bradycardia, ventricular tachycardia, ventricular fibrillation	Rate below 60 beats/min Rate above 250 beats/min No discernible cardiac rhythm Pallor Loss of consciousness Hypotension	Temporary pacemaker Defibrillation Medications: antidysrhythmics, vasopressors
Vascular: excessive blood loss	Hypotension Decreased urine output (from hypovolemia) Decreased hemoglobin/hematocrit Pallor	Possible surgical repair Fluids Transfusion Oxygen
	Hematoma at puncture site	Flat in bed or in Trendelenburg position
Allergic	Hypotension, urticaria, nausea/vomiting, hives, laryngospasm, erythema, shortness of breath	Medications: antihistamines, steroids, antiemetics Clear liquids/NPO Oxygen With anaphylaxis: fluids for volume expansion, epinephrine, vasopressors for hypotension
Central nervous system events	Changes in level of consciousness Hemiparesis Hypoventilation/respiratory depression	Oxygen Discontinue/hold sedatives Medication: narcotic antagonist as a respiratory stimulant

Miscellaneous complications: conduction defects, pulmonary embolism, pulmonary edema, coronary air embolism, respiratory arrest, febrile episode, nausea, minor bleeding.

Directional Coronary Atherectomy

The DCA device is a cutting catheter that is inserted over a guidewire into the coronary artery across the stenotic lesion. It is positioned so that the opening for the blade faces the lesion. A low-pressure balloon on the opposite side of the catheter is inflated, thus forcing the atherosclerotic plaque into the opening near the cutting blade. The cutting blade turns at approximately 1,200 revolutions per minute (rpm) and is then slowly advanced along the length of the lesion, cutting the plaque and collecting it in the catheter nosecone. The DCA catheter is turned a complete 360 degrees in the artery to shave all sides of the atherosclerotic plaque with repeated passes. The procedure is repeated until the atherosclerotic plaque is sufficiently removed. The catheter, laden with plaque, is then withdrawn from the patient (Fig. 18-12).

Transluminal Extraction Catheter

The TEC device is a percutaneous, over-the-wire, motor-driven cutting and aspiration system.[17] The TEC device is unique in that it has a detachable vacuum bottle. The TEC device simultaneously cuts the atherosclerotic

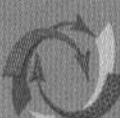

box 18-10 collaborative care guide *for the Patient Undergoing PCI*

OUTCOMES	INTERVENTIONS
Oxygenation/Ventilation	
Patient will maintain normal arterial blood gases, or pulse oximeter reading.	■ Provide supplemental oxygen per face mask or nasal cannula per hospital post-PCI protocol. ■ Monitor blood gases/pulse oximeter per protocol. ■ Auscultate breath sounds when taking vital signs. ■ Monitor for signs of pulmonary edema or respiratory distress.
Circulation/Perfusion	
The patient will have stable vital signs following PCI.	■ Monitor blood pressure, heart rate, respiration rate, arterial puncture site, distal pulses, and distal motor function and sensation: q15min × 4, q30min × 4 q1h × 4, then q4h
There is no evidence of post-PCI myocardial ischemia or infarction due to coronary reocclusion (e.g., no ECG changes or angina).	■ Monitor cardiac rhythm in leads specific to myocardium most affected by PCI location. ■ Administer medications to treat coronary artery spasms (e.g., nifedipine and nitroglycerin). ■ Administer heparin per protocol.
There is no evidence of cardiac dysrhythmias post-PCI.	■ Report type and frequency of dysrhythmias. ■ Administer antidysrhythmic medication as indicated and ordered. ■ Temporary transvenous or external pacemaker and defibrillator are readily available.
There is no evidence of bleeding at the puncture site.	■ Monitor site for hematoma as above with vital signs. ■ Assess for tenderness, ecchymosis, warmth over puncture site. ■ Apply direct pressure to puncture site for 15 to 30 min after sheath is removed. ■ Apply sandbag to puncture site if oozing continues, per hospital protocol. ■ Apply a pressure dressing to puncture site when oozing has stopped. ■ Monitor ACT, prothrombin time, partial thromboplastin time, and platelets, reporting coagulopathies per protocol.
There is no evidence of arterial occlusion at puncture site.	■ Monitor involved extremity with vital signs for mottling, coolness, pallor, diminished pulses, numbness, tingling, pain, and so forth.
Fluids/Electrolytes	
Patient is euvolemic.	■ Monitor intake and output. ■ Obtain type and cross-match, complete blood count, electrolytes prior to PCI. ■ Maintain IV patency.
Renal function is maintained after administration of radiographic IV contrast.	■ Obtain pre-PCI and post-PCI BUN, creatinine, and electrolytes. ■ Closely monitor urine output; report if less than 30 mL/h. ■ Monitor urine specific gravity or osmolarity for clearance of IV contrast. ■ Administer diuretic agents as ordered.
Mobility/Safety	
	■ The patient is on bed rest for 4 to 6 hours post-PCI per hospital protocol. ■ While sheath is in place and while on bed rest, keep head of bed less than 45 degrees.

(continued)

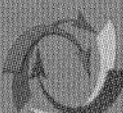

box 18-10 collaborative care guide *for the Patient Undergoing PCI (Continued)*

OUTCOMES	INTERVENTIONS
Skin Integrity	
Patient's skin will remain intact.	■ Assess skin immediately post-PCI for pressure areas. ■ Reposition to relieve pressure from bony prominences, maintaining alignment of extremity involved in procedure. ■ Consider pressure relief/reduction mattress.
Nutrition	
Nutritional intake is reestablished.	■ Resume PO fluids and diet per protocol. ■ Monitor swallowing and protective airway reflexes while patient is receiving sedatives or narcotics.
Patient does not experience nausea or vomiting post-PCI.	■ Monitor nausea and vomiting. ■ Administer antiemetic medication as appropriate.
Comfort/Pain Control	
Patient will not experience anginal pain.	■ Instruct patient to verbalize discomfort and pain. ■ Evaluate severity and location of pain, distinguishing angina from other causes of discomfort. ■ Administer nitrates or narcotics per order or protocol for angina. ■ Evaluate patient response to medication.
Patient will not experience pain from mobility restrictions.	■ Reposition patient frequently, keeping involved extremity straight. ■ Use mattress overlay or egg crate for comfort. ■ Administer analgesics as appropriate, after distinguishing joint or muscular pain from angina.
Psychosocial	
Patient and family state risks associated with PCI.	■ Provide information for informed procedural consent. ■ Encourage verbalization of questions, concerns, and fears.
Patient uses personal support systems to reduce anxiety.	■ Encourage significant other to visit in early postprocedural recovery phase. ■ Validate patient/significant others' understanding of surgery and illness. ■ Initiate referrals to social services, clergy, and so forth as necessary.
Teaching/Discharge Planning	
Patient and family are prepared for possibility of emergent repeat PCI or cardiac surgery.	■ Preprocedure teaching includes discussion regarding causes for coronary reocclusion or perforation and rationale for surgery or repeat PCI.
Patient cooperates with post-PCI mobility restrictions.	■ Provide preprocedure and postprocedure instruction and rationale for bed rest and limited movement of involved extremity.
Patient states lifestyle changes required to reduce risk of worsening coronary artery disease.	■ Provide verbal and written instruction/information regarding risk factors and pathophysiology, activity, diet, stress reduction, medication administration, and appropriate times/indications to seek medical attention.

plaque and then sucks the plaque and thrombus into the vacuum bottle. The cutting device is advanced over the guidewire and positioned 1 to 2 mm proximal to the stenotic lesion. The cutting blade and the vacuum suction are then activated. The cutting blade rotates at 750 rpm and is manually advanced along the length of the stenotic lesion, pulling excised plaque and thrombus through the TEC catheter and into the vacuum bottle. Several passes across the lesion are performed. Adjunctive balloon angioplasty may be performed after use of the TEC device (Fig. 18-13).

Rotational Ablation Device

The Rotablator device is a high-speed rotating, abrasive burr-tipped catheter that ablates the atherosclerotic plaque in the coronary artery. The Rotablator has proved to be especially effective in complex stenotic lesions that

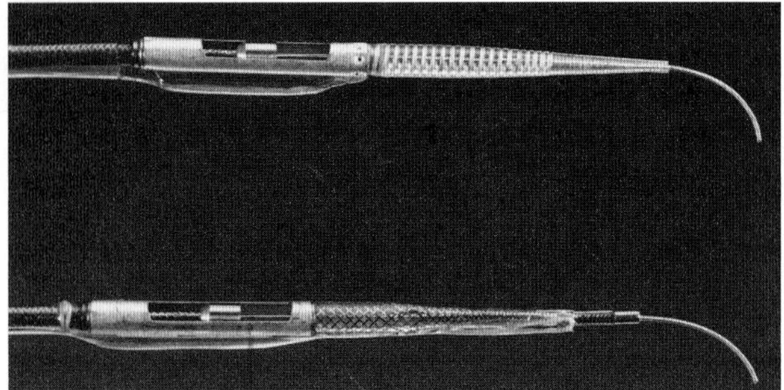

figure 18-12 Directional coronary atherectomy catheters: Simpson Coronary AtheroCaths. (Courtesy of Guidant/Advanced Cardiovascular Systems, Santa Clara, CA.)

are calcified, tortuous, small in diameter, ostial, or diffuse in character. The device consists of a football-shaped, diamond-studded burr attached to a drive shaft. The Rotablator is advanced over a guidewire to the lesion site. The burr rotates at 160,000 to 190,000 rpm and pulverizes the atherosclerotic plaque into microparticles that are absorbed into the patient's circulatory system. The spinning burr is advanced across the lesion several times to debulk the stenotic lesion. Adjunctive balloon angioplasty may be performed after use of the Rotablator device (Fig. 18-14).

STENTS

Intracoronary stents are hollow stainless steel tubes that act as "scaffolding" in the coronary artery. There are currently over a hundred different stents that have received U.S. Food and Drug Administration (FDA) approval (Fig. 18-15). After predilation with a PTCA balloon catheter, most stents are premounted on a balloon catheter and inserted through the guide catheter along a guidewire to the lesion site. Once placed across the stenotic lesion, the balloon is inflated, and the stent is expanded and left in the coronary artery.

Because many stent designs are stainless steel, they are potent thrombogenic prostheses. Stent thrombus is a major short- and long-term complication. Success of the stenting procedure depends on endothelialization of the stent to provide a smooth flow of blood in the coronary artery and through the stent, yet controlled to prevent stent thrombosis. Anticoagulation and antiplatelet medication regimens are crucial to successful stenting and long-term prognosis. Stenting has been shown in numerous trials to reduce restenosis rates and improve long-term prognosis. Stents made of newer alloys and compounds are currently undergoing investigation. Drug-eluting stent trials are underway to improve the restenosis rates. Drug-eluting stents are coated with drugs such as heparin, paclitaxel, actinomycin D, or rapamycin. It is hoped that the gradual release of these drugs into the coronary vasculature at the site of the atherosclerotic plaque will inhibit restenosis by limiting smooth muscle cell proliferation and inflammation but allowing re-endothelialization to proceed normally. At this time, there are no drug-eluting stents approved for use in the United States. The Cordis/Johnson & Johnson Cypher stent has been approved in Europe. Complications of stenting may include bleeding at the access site, stent migration, coronary artery dissection, and abrupt closure.

A major factor limiting the expansion and long-term efficacy of PTCA is the problem of restenosis. Pharmacological treatment before and after dilation, procedure techniques, and patient identification continue to be investigated as ways to reduce the recurrence rate.

BRACHYTHERAPY

Intracoronary radiation (brachytherapy) is potentially a potent antiproliferative therapy that is currently being investigated for use in conjunction with PCI and might therefore provide a means for effective reduction of restenosis. The radiation therapy is emitted in the form of temporarily implanted or inserted radioactive sources, such as seeds, radioactive stents, or radioactive liquid–filled balloons. Radiation works particularly well in inhibiting new growth by attacking the newer, more aggressive neoplastic cells, while often having little effect on normal tissue.[18] In brachytherapy, endovascular low-dose radiation is applied at the site of balloon dilation or stent implantation by a catheter system. Two types of radiation are used to treat restenosis: gamma and beta emitters. Gamma emitters create a radiation field for a considerable distance away from their source. This requires the treatment to be conducted in a heavily lead-shielded cardiac catheterization laboratory. Gamma emitter intensity is lower than that of beta emitters, and they must be left in place 14 to 45 minutes, depending on the strength of the source used. Beta sources,

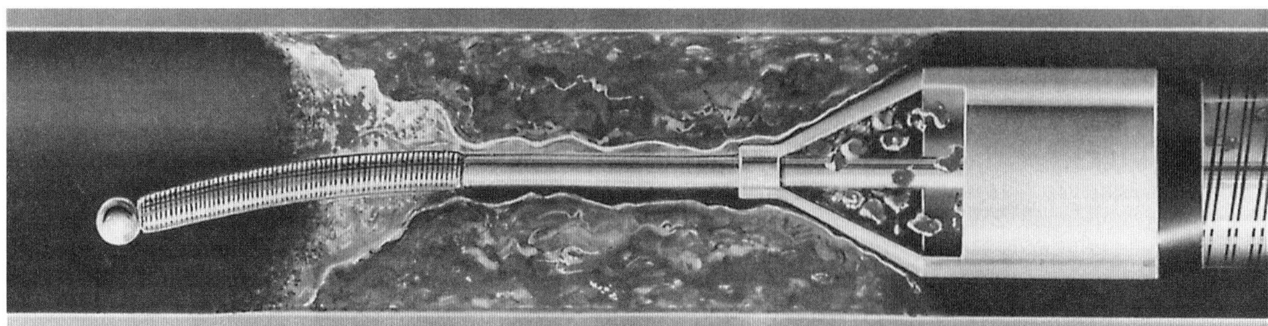

figure 18-13 Distal end of the Transluminal Extraction Catheter (TEC) coaxially placed over the TEC guide wire. (Courtesy of InterVentional Technologies, Inc., San Diego, CA.)

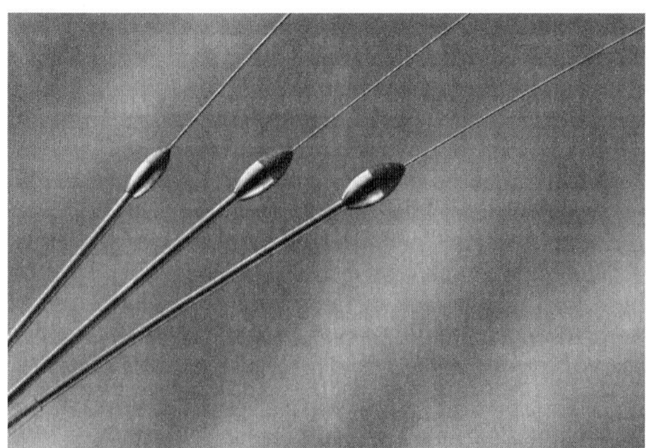

figure 18-14 Rotational ablation catheters in different sizes. (Courtesy of SCIMED/Boston Scientific Corporation, Maple Grove, MN.)

with a higher intensity of radiation near the source, can be more concentrated, enabling the brachytherapy to last only 3 to 10 minutes. The beta source can be shielded with only approximately 0.5 inch of Lucite. The FDA currently approves the use of brachytherapy only for in-stent restenosis.

PERCUTANEOUS MYOCARDIAL REVASCULARIZATION

Percutaneous myocardial revascularization (PMR) is an investigational procedure that uses a laser to create channels in the heart muscle in an effort to improve myocardial perfusion. A laser catheter is used to create 10 to 30 transmural channels from the epicardial layer of the heart into the myocardium, extending into the left ventricular chamber. It is hoped that angiogenesis, or the formation of new blood vessels in the area surrounding the channels, will alleviate symptoms of myocardial ischemia. This procedure is typically performed in the cardiac catheterization laboratory. Arterial access is gained through the brachial or femoral artery. The laser catheter is then advanced through the left ventricle to the areas of the myocardium that have been shown by nuclear testing (dipyridamole [Persantine] thallium scans) to be ischemic, and is used to create transmural channels as described previously. The channels are approximately 1 mm wide, 5 to 7 mm deep, and 1 cm apart. The potential complications include dysrhythmias, those risks associated with cardiac catheterization, left ventricular perforation, pericardial effusion, new left bundle branch block, and cardiac tamponade. The treatment for these complications includes pericardiocentesis or emergent CABG.

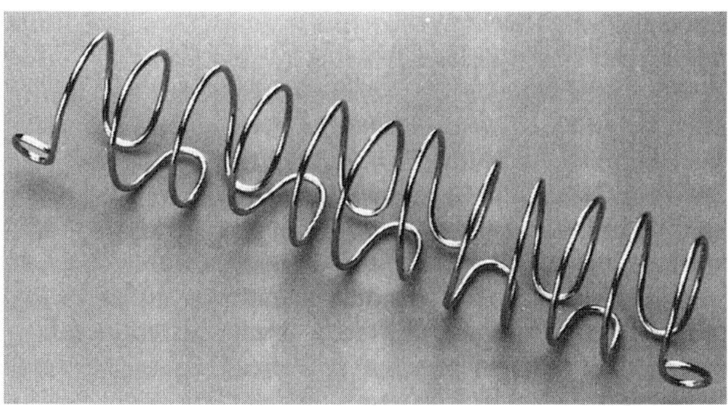

figure 18-15 The Gianturco-Roubin Flex-Stent. (Courtesy of Cook, Inc., Bloomington, IN.)

Post-PCI management is appropriate in patients undergoing PMR. Patients are typically discharged within 24 hours of the procedure. Patients typically do not notice an improvement in their angina until approximately 2 to 3 months after the procedure, when collateral circulation develops. The Blinded Evaluation of Laser PMR Intervention Electively for Angina Pectoris (BELIEF) trial revealed that 40% of patients improve two or more classes in their angina assessment after PMR, compared with only 13% in the control group.[19]

GENE THERAPY FOR MYOCARDIAL ANGIOGENESIS

The goal of gene therapy is to insert normal or modified genes into the cells of patients to prevent or treat disorders caused by the absence or malfunction of the corresponding gene. Intramyocardial transfection of genes encoding angiogenic cytokines may constitute an alternative treatment strategy for patients with severe myocardial ischemia. This strategy is designed to promote the development of supplemental collateral blood vessels (angiogenesis). Gene therapy can be accomplished in one of three ways: gene insertion, gene addition, or gene replacement. Gene insertion is accomplished by adding the gene randomly into the host cell. Gene addition allows replication of the host cell DNA independently. Gene replacement is accomplished when the therapeutic gene is added into the host cell of DNA at the exact location of the abnormal gene.

Gene transfer and gene therapy can use ex vivo and in vivo methods. In the ex vivo method, genetic material is placed into cells that have been taken from the patient and then are readministered. In the in vivo method, genetic material is administered directly into the patient's tissues or blood vessels.

Gene therapy can be delivered in one of two ways: physical methods (microinjection or electroporation) or virus-based vector systems. Microinjection involves the injection of plasmid DNA directly into the cells of the host, one cell at a time. Electroporation is the transfer of genetic DNA material directly across the host cell membrane by means of an electrical current. Viral vectors work by incorporating the gene therapy into the host cell of the patient. Viruses used as vectors for gene therapy include adenoviruses and other DNA viruses, and RNA viruses.[20]

Gene therapy for CAD is usually performed in the cardiac catheterization laboratory and administered directly into the coronary arteries through arterial access obtained by the brachial or femoral approach. Patients are typically hospitalized for 24 hours.

OTHER TECHNOLOGY

Devices for viewing the vasculature directly, such as angioscopy and intravascular ultrasonography, are used to assess lesion severity and type before inflation and to determine change in lesion diameter and arterial structure after deflation. Angioscopy and ultrasonography also may provide information to help determine which interventional technology (i.e., PTCA, atherectomy, stent implantation) is best suited to the lesion.

Magnetic Resonance Coronary Angiography

Noninvasive techniques are being developed and refined that could reliably provide both anatomical and functional information about the coronary circulation. Magnetic resonance coronary angiography (MRA) is one such technique. MRA has made possible the visualization of the major epicardial coronary vessels by noninvasive assessment. It has allowed for assessment of coronary blood flow and imaging of the left and right ventricles in one complete, low-risk, low-discomfort, cost-saving method. Current methods for MRA combine fast imaging sequences with techniques for suppressing cardiac and respiratory motion.

With the various tools and technologies available to the interventional cardiologist and improved pharmacological adjunctive therapy, the future should bring further improvement in the efficacy and predictability of PTCA and in the long-term patency of involved atherosclerotic vessels.

PERCUTANEOUS BALLOON VALVULOPLASTY

Percutaneous balloon valvuloplasty (PBV) is a nonsurgical technique for increasing blood flow through stenotic cardiac valves using dilation catheters. This relatively new procedure is similar to PTCA in that a catheter system is inserted percutaneously and advanced to the region of narrowing using fluoroscopic guidance. A dilation catheter then is inflated to increase the valvular opening and improve blood flow.

Historical Background

The first cases of balloon dilation of stenotic cardiac valves were reported in 1979 and 1982, when physicians successfully dilated pulmonary valve stenoses. This technique was considered an effective alternative to open heart surgery, although long-term results could not yet be evaluated. Because surgical commissurotomy was successful in treating mitral valve stenoses and because of the initial success with pulmonary valve dilation, physicians began percutaneous dilation of mitral valves in 1984 to avoid the need for thoracotomy. In 1984 and 1985, physicians successfully dilated congenital aortic valve stenoses (AVS). A calcific AVS was first dilated in 1985. These procedures improved cardiac function with no serious procedural complications.

The number of PBVs does not approach the volume of coronary angioplasty. This is due partly to the lesser incidence of valve disease compared with CAD.

Assuming patients have long-term clinical improvement associated with PBV, the advantages compared with surgery are similar to those of PTCA versus CABG. PBV is less traumatic, requires no anesthesia, is associated with lower morbidity and a shorter hospital stay, causes no scarring, and is less expensive.

Pathophysiology of Stenotic Valves

Stenotic valves are caused by calcific degeneration, congenital abnormalities, or rheumatic heart disease. Calcific aortic and mitral valve degeneration now appears to be the most frequent causes of valve disease requiring surgical treatment. Refer to Chapter 19 for a discussion of the pathophysiology and clinical manifestations of specific stenotic valves.

Diagnostic Tests for Percutaneous Balloon Valvuloplasty and Valve Replacement

Before deciding on the appropriate intervention, the physician evaluates the patient for evidence and severity of valvular stenosis. A variety of noninvasive tests allow the physician to determine the degree of left atrial or left ventricular hypertrophy, pulmonary venous congestion or hypertension, valvular rigidity, and transvalvular gradient. In a 12-lead ECG, the magnitude of the R wave in the precordial leads reflects the presence of left ventricular hypertrophy associated with AVS. The presence of broad, notched P waves reflects left atrial hypertrophy associated with mitral valve stenosis. A chest radiograph illustrates the presence of calcium in or around the valve, left ventricular or atrial hypertrophy, and pulmonary venous congestion or CHF. A two-dimensional echocardiogram is used to scan the cardiac valves and chambers. A Doppler ultrasound study allows measurement of the transvalvular gradient, indirect calculation of valve area, and assessment of valvular regurgitation. With this information, the physician is able to (1) estimate the size of the valve orifice, (2) visualize the degree of valve leaflet movement, and (3) determine the extent of left ventricular or atrial hypertrophy.

Right and left heart catheterization is done if the previous tests indicate valvular disease. Although this procedure is invasive, it is required to determine the pressures within each of the cardiac chambers and to confirm transvalvular gradients. Once the pressures and gradients are obtained, a series of radiographs may be taken by injecting radiopaque contrast medium, either in the aorta to visualize aortic regurgitation or in the left ventricle to visualize mitral regurgitation. This procedure yields a cineangiogram illustrating the function of the cardiac valves and chamber sizes.

After this series of tests, the physician can analyze the valves closely, gaining precise information with which to decide the mode of treatment. The nurse should be familiar with the results of these tests because a better understanding of the patient's diagnosis and related symptoms, and thus of the reasons for intervention, promotes better care.

Equipment Features

Although PBV and PTCA catheters are based on similar designs, there are important differences, primarily because of the larger diameters of heart valves compared with coronary arteries. One major difference is the outer diameter of the catheters. PBV catheter shafts range from 7 to 9 Fr. PBV balloons range from 15 to 25 mm in diameter when inflated. A 10- to 14-Fr introducing sheath may be used at the arterial or venous puncture site to allow for introduction of the valve dilation catheter. A large guidewire, 0.035 to 0.038 in, also is used to provide the added stiffness and support required to introduce the dilatation catheter. PBV dilation catheters have radiopaque markers similar to PTCA dilation catheters for fluoroscopic imaging.

Indications for and Contraindications to Percutaneous Balloon Valvuloplasty

The use of PBV initially was limited by the fear of embolization of calcific debris, disruption of the valve ring, acute valvular regurgitation, and valvular restenosis. The incidence of these complications continues to be a concern. Both major and minor complications have been reported in numerous early studies; however, these complications must be assessed in terms of the patient population in which the procedure is performed.

Although surgical valve replacement is an effective treatment for those with AVS and operative mortality rates are low, the operative mortality rate significantly increases in patients with multisystem disease (who often are older). PBV initially has proven to be a safe and efficacious alternative for these patients. It also is an effective therapy for children who are high surgical risks because it delays the need for surgery until the child is older and can better tolerate an operation. In addition, the longevity of both mechanical and bioprosthetic valves is approximately 10 years, so PBV delays or prevents the need for a second operation. Also, the long-term anticoagulation therapy required with mechanical valve prostheses is undesirable in younger patients and pregnant women. PBV also is effective for stabilizing those with poor left ventricular function before surgery; it is contraindicated in patients with moderate to severe valvular regurgitation due to a small but significant risk of increasing valvular insufficiency with the procedure (Box 18-11).

A complication associated with PBV is excessive bleeding at the puncture site due to the large catheters required to perform dilation. The development of smaller catheters may reduce the incidence of bleeding. As with PTCA, PBV catheters are being refined continually to increase procedural safety, time, and efficacy.

Procedure

The procedure is performed in the cardiac catheterization laboratory and involves many of the same steps as PTCA (see earlier section on PTCA procedure). Right and left heart catheterization is repeated to evaluate hemodynamic status and to obtain baseline transvalvular gradients. Coronary angiography, when indicated, is repeated to determine whether the patient still meets the criteria for valvuloplasty. Thorough repeat evaluation is necessary because a patient's status can change, precluding treatment with this intervention.

box 18-11
Indications and Contraindications for PBV

Clinical Indications

High-risk surgical patients (advanced age, severe pulmonary hypertension, renal failure, pulmonary dysfunction, left ventricular dysfunction)
Unstable presurgical patients
Patients not candidates for chronic anticoagulation

Anatomical Indications

Moderate to severe valvular narrowing
Moderate to severe valvular calcification
Mild valvular regurgitation

Anatomical Contraindications

Inability to access vasculature
Thrombus
Severe valvular regurgitation
History of embolic events

The angiographic catheter is replaced either by an introducing sheath or a dilation catheter. In mitral PBV, a venous puncture is made in the right femoral vein. During both aortic and mitral PBV, maintaining patent IV and radial or femoral arterial lines is important to administer medications and draw blood samples.

In aortic PBV, once the sheaths are in place, the patient is anticoagulated with 5,000 to 10,000 U heparin to prevent clot formation in the catheter system. The dilation catheter and guidewire then are advanced to the root of the ascending aorta. The guidewire is advanced across the stenotic aortic valve, and the dilation catheter is advanced over the guidewire (Fig. 18-16). Exact placement of the dilation catheter is facilitated by fluoroscopy and radiopaque markers on the balloon.

In mitral PBV, a pacing catheter may be positioned through a separate venous sheath at the level of the inferior vena cava or right atrium and placed on standby. The mitral valve then is approached either by way of the femoral artery

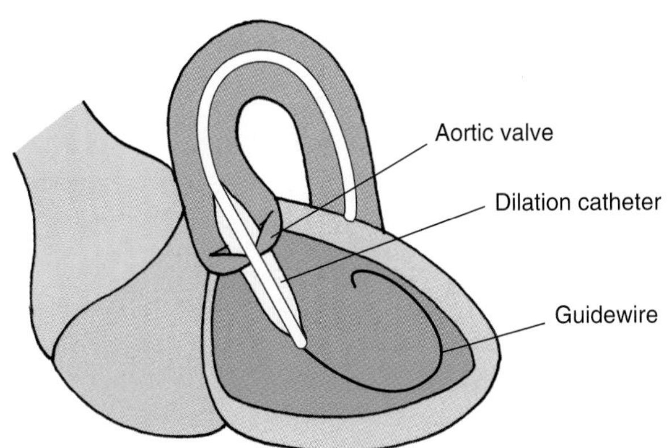

figure 18-16 Cross-sectional view of heart illustrating guidewire and dilation catheter positions across the aortic valve. The guidewire is curved to prevent ventricular dysrhythmias or puncture.

and aortic valve or, in most cases, through the right heart by perforating the atrial septum to enter the left atrium. Once the mitral valve has been accessed, the patient is anticoagulated with 5,000 to 10,000 U heparin. The dilation catheter is then advanced over the guidewire through the atrial septal puncture and across the mitral valve (Fig. 18-17). Again, exact placement of the dilation catheter in the valve is facilitated by fluoroscopy and radiopaque markers on the balloon.

Average inflation time of the dilation catheter is 15 to 60 seconds in aortic valvuloplasty and 10 to 30 seconds in mitral valvuloplasty. During dilation of either valve, the nurse monitors blood pressure closely because of the imposed decrease in cardiac output. Once the dilation catheter has been deflated, blood pressure should return to normal. During dilation of the mitral valve, there is a temporary increase in the pulmonary artery wedge pressure (PAWP). Once the dilation catheter has been deflated, the PAWP should return to baseline. Dysrhythmias such as ventricular tachycardia, ventricular fibrillation, or sinus bradycardia also may occur during dilation.

Once maximum dilation has been obtained, the catheter is removed. Hemodynamic measurements, including transvalvular gradients, are repeated to determine efficacy of the procedure. Repeat angiography is done to assess for valvular regurgitation. When the procedure is complete, to prevent bleeding complications associated with the large puncture site, the anticoagulant effects of heparin are reversed.

Results

Aortic PBV is associated with a decrease in pressure gradient and end-systolic volume and an increase in aortic valve area, ejection fraction, and cardiac output. In-hospital mortality rates range from 1% to 3%. Although there is an increase in the aortic valve area, it is not as great as with surgical valve replacement. In addition, the restenosis rate associated with PBV is high. Therefore, aortic valvuloplasty is indicated primarily for older and high-risk surgical patients and generally is considered a palliative, not a curative, procedure.

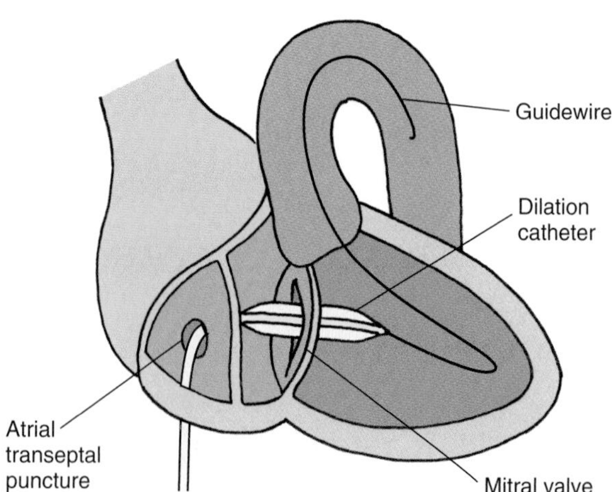

figure 18-17 Cross-sectional view of heart illustrating guidewire and dilation catheter placed through an atrial transseptal puncture and across the mitral valve. The guidewire is extended out the aortic valve into the aorta for catheter support.

Results of mitral valvuloplasty are more dramatic. There is a more significant increase in valve area and cardiac output and a decrease in valve gradient, PAWP, and mean pulmonary arterial pressure. The operative mortality rate has been reported as 1.5%, and sustained clinical improvement has been reported in 63% to 90% of cases. Late deaths occur in approximately 5% to 10%.

Three mechanisms have been postulated for the improvement of valvular function due to PBV: (1) fracture of calcific nodules adherent to leaflets (most frequent); (2) separation of fused commissures; and (3) stretching of the anulus and leaflet structure.

Assessment and Management

PATIENT PREPARATION

The patient is admitted to the hospital the day of the PBV procedure. The goal of nursing care is to reduce the cardiac workload, monitor fluid and electrolyte balance, and reduce psychological stress so the patient remains hemodynamically stable.

In most cases, the patient does not have invasive pressure monitoring lines in place before the procedure. The nurse therefore carefully monitors signs and symptoms of CHF: narrowing in the arterial pulse pressure, more frequent increases in heart rate during activity, peripheral edema, presence of a cough, complaints of dyspnea, or rales in lung fields. The nurse also must note any changes in sensorium, color, skin temperature, and pulse volume, and any decrease in urinary output. To monitor fluid and electrolyte balance, the nurse obtains a baseline serum electrolyte level and baseline body weight. In addition, daily fluid intake and output are recorded.

The patient's medications before admission may have included diuretics, digoxin, and anticoagulants. Before the procedure, any anticoagulant medication is discontinued because of the possibility of emergency surgery. Therefore, patients with chronic atrial fibrillation who have the potential for systemic embolization due to thrombus should be monitored closely. The nurse also monitors preliminary laboratory tests and notifies the physician of any abnormalities. (See the section on Patient Preparation for PTCA for further information on these tests.)

After the patient fully understands the procedure, the physician must obtain an informed consent for PBV, anesthesia, and surgery. Surgical standby usually is provided during PBV due to possible complications requiring emergency valve replacement.

NURSING ASSESSMENT AND MANAGEMENT

During Percutaneous Balloon Valvuloplasty

The nurse continuously monitors pulmonary artery pressure and PAWP and is aware of changes in tracings that may suggest symptoms of CHF or pulmonary edema. In the presence of severe hypotension, the nurse should be prepared to start an IV infusion of dopamine or norepinephrine (Levophed). In the case of ventricular dysrhythmias, a lidocaine drip should be available for infusion.

After Percutaneous Balloon Valvuloplasty

The nurse is important in the patient's recovery. The goal of postvalvuloplasty nursing care is to maintain adequate cardiac output, maintain fluid and electrolyte balance, and verify hemostasis at the puncture site. Alterations in cardiac output can be caused by dysrhythmias secondary to valve manipulation, resulting in edema near the bundle of His; left-to-right atrial shunt through the transseptal puncture created during mitral valvuloplasty; cardiac tamponade; alteration in circulating fluid volume; or blood loss. Alteration in fluid and electrolyte balance results from diuretic therapy and contrast medium used during catheterization. Bleeding at the puncture site is secondary to the combined effect of systemic anticoagulation and the large diameter of catheters used.

Because fluids are important in the hemodynamic balance of the patient with valvular disease, the volume of IV fluids is recorded to establish an accurate intake and output. The decreased circulating volume from diuretic medications given before PBV combined with improved stroke volume after successful PBV can be reflected as a decrease in cardiac output. Therefore, careful monitoring of central venous pressure, pulmonary artery pressure, PAWP, and blood pressure, in addition to heart rate, urinary output, and electrolyte balance, is essential in the evaluation and assessment of circulating fluid volume and cardiac pumping status.

In addition, the nurse assesses the patient's status from head to toe, noting overall skin color and temperature and carefully observing the level of consciousness and neurological signs. The nurse also listens closely to heart and breath sounds. Circulation distal to the puncture site is evaluated by noting peripheral skin color and temperature in addition to the presence and quality of the dorsalis pedis and posterior tibial pulses.

Finally, the presence of any drainage on the puncture site dressing or tenderness during palpation should be noted to establish a baseline for the possibility of increased pericatheter bleeding. The nurse reports immediately any changes that may indicate excessive bleeding. Bleeding at the sheath site may result in a hematoma requiring surgical evacuation. To prevent excessive bleeding and to aid hemostasis, the physician may order a sandbag or clamp placed over the puncture site.

If the patient has documented CAD, the physician also may request a serum cardiac enzyme panel. Particular attention should be paid to creatine kinase (CK) and CK isoenzymes (see section on Nursing Management After Percutaneous Coronary Interventions). The nurse should be aware of the signs and symptoms of myocardial ischemia in addition to the appropriate interventions.

The nurse instructs the patient about the importance of keeping the involved leg straight for the first few hours after valvuloplasty.

Post-PBV laboratory evaluation may include prothrombin time, hemoglobin and hematocrit, coagulation studies, serum electrolytes, CK, ECG, and chest x-ray. Box 18-6, in the section on Nursing Management During Percutaneous Transluminal Coronary Angioplasty, lists nursing diagnoses and collaborative problems for patients undergoing PBV. Implications for home care for the patient after PCI or PBV are described in Box 18-12.

COMPLICATIONS

A common in-hospital complication associated with PBV is bleeding at the arterial puncture site due to the large diameter of the catheters needed to dilate the valve anulus. In addition, in mitral PBV, a common complication is left-to-right shunting secondary to septal dilation, again due to the large diameter of the dilation catheters. Systemic embolization in both mitral and aortic PBV is a potential and significant complication, although its incidence is low. There have been few reports of significant increases in valvular regurgitation. Complications associated with PBV are listed in Box 18-13.

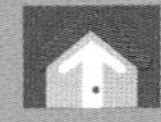

box 18-12 *The Cardiac Patient After PCI or PBV*

Physiological

- Restrict physical activities first week post-PCI/PBV
- No lifting over 10 pounds the first 2 weeks after PCI
- May resume exercise program after exercise stress test
- Follow prescribed low-fat diet
- Consider cardiac rehabilitation
- Limit alcohol to three drinks per week
- Notify physician of any oozing, bleeding, or pain at puncture site
- Notify physician of fever or other signs of infection
- Notify physician or call 911 for any chest discomfort not relieved with three nitroglycerin tablets taken 5 minutes apart
- Weight loss if indicated

Psychosocial

- No smoking or exposure to second-hand smoke
- May resume sexual activities after exercise stress test
- Stress management
- Recognize signs of depression
- Compliance with medication regimen
- Compliance with medical appointments

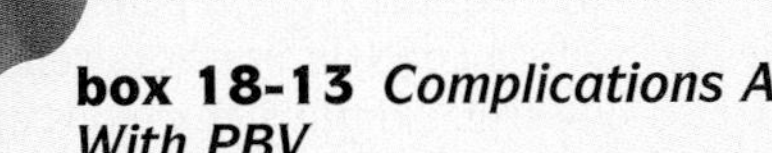

box 18-13 *Complications Associated With PBV*

- Embolization of calcific debris
- Valve ring disruption
- Valvular regurgitation
- Valvular restenosis
- Bleeding at arterial puncture site
- Left ventricular perforation
- Severe hypotension
- Transient ischemia
- Vascular trauma
- Atrial septal defect (with mitral PBV)
- Aortic dissection
- Aortic rupture
- Cardiac tamponade
- Chordae tendineae rupture

Intra-aortic Balloon Pump Counterpulsation and Mechanical Circulatory Support

INTRA-AORTIC BALLOON PUMP COUNTERPULSATION

Harken and colleagues of Boston originally described the concept of counterpulsation in 1958 when, in an attempt to increase coronary artery perfusion, they used femoral access to remove blood during systole and replace it during diastole. Intra-aortic balloon pump (IABP) counterpulsation was first introduced clinically by Kantrowitz and associates in 1967. This therapeutic approach was instituted for treatment of two patients with left ventricular failure after AMI. Since that time, IABP has become a standard treatment for medical and surgical patients with acute left ventricular failure that is unresponsive to pharmacological and volume therapy.

Therapeutic goals are directed toward increasing oxygen supply to the myocardium, decreasing left ventricular work, and improving cardiac output. Before IABP, no single therapeutic agent was capable of meeting these three goals.

IABP counterpulsation is designed to increase coronary artery perfusion pressure and blood flow during the diastolic phase of the cardiac cycle by inflation of a balloon in the thoracic aorta. Deflation of the balloon, just before systolic ejection, decreases the impedance to ejection (afterload) and thus left ventricular work, with subsequent decreased myocardial oxygen consumption. Inflation and deflation counterpulse each heart beat. With improved blood flow and effective reduction in left ventricular work, the desired results are increased coronary artery perfusion and decreased afterload with subsequent increase in cardiac output.

Physiological Principles

Greater work is required to maintain cardiac output in the failing heart. With this added work requirement, oxygen demand increases. These circumstances may occur at a time when the myocardium already is ischemic and coronary artery perfusion is unable to meet the oxygen demands. As a result, left ventricular performance diminishes even further, resulting in decreased cardiac output. A vicious cycle ensues that is difficult to interrupt (Fig. 18-18). Without interruption of the cycle, cardiogenic shock may be imminent. This cycle can be broken with IABP therapy by increasing aortic root pressure during diastole through inflation of the balloon. With increased aortic root pressure, the perfusion pressure of the coronary arteries is increased.

Effective therapy for the patient in left ventricular failure also involves decreasing myocardial oxygen demand. Four major determinants of myocardial oxygen demand are afterload, preload, contractility, and heart rate. IABP counterpulsation therapy can have an effect on all these factors. It decreases afterload directly and affects the other three determinants indirectly as cardiac function improves. Because IABP therapy assists the left heart, only the left ventricle is discussed here.

AFTERLOAD AND PRELOAD

The greatest amount of oxygen required during the cardiac cycle is for the development of afterload (see Chapter 16). With greater impedance to ejection, afterload increases, thus resulting in increased myocardial oxygen demand. Impedance to ejection is caused by the aortic valve, aortic end-diastolic pressure, and vascular resistance. Greater aortic end-diastolic pressures require higher afterload to overcome impedance and ejection. Vascular resistance increases impedance when vessels become vasoconstricted. Vasodilation or lower vascular resistance decreases afterload by decreasing impedance to ejection. Deflation of the balloon in the aorta just before ventricular systole lowers aortic end-diastolic pressure. This decreases impedance to ejection and decreases left ventricular workload. In this way, IABP can effectively decrease the oxygen demand of the heart.

A person in acute left ventricular failure has increased volume in the ventricle at end-diastole (preload; see Chapter 16) as a result of the heart's inability to pump effectively. This excessive increase in preload increases the workload of the heart. IABP therapy helps to decrease excessive preload by decreasing impedance to ejection. With decreased impedance, there is more effective forward flow of blood and more efficient emptying of the left ventricle.

CONTRACTILITY

Contractility refers to the velocity and vigor of contraction during systole. Although vigorous contractility requires more oxygen, it is a benefit to cardiac function because it ensures good, efficient pumping, which increases cardiac output. In failure, contractility is depressed. The biochemical status of the myocardium directly affects contractility. Contractility is depressed when calcium levels are low, catecholamine levels are low, and ischemia is present with resultant acidosis.

IABP counterpulsation can increase oxygen supply, thereby decreasing ischemia and acidosis. In this way, IABP therapy contributes to improved contractility and better cardiac function (see Fig. 18-18).

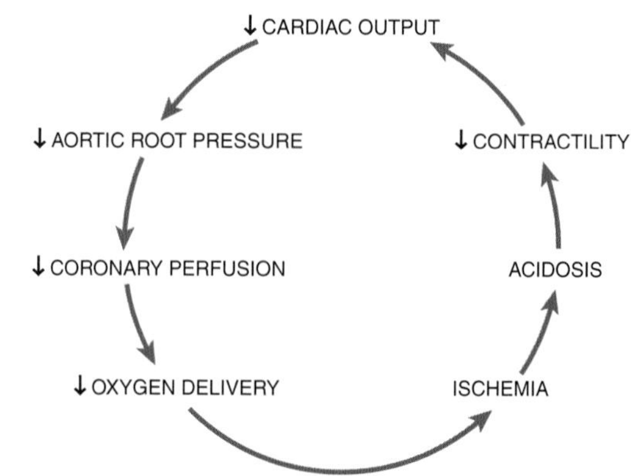

figure 18-18 Cycle leading to cardiogenic shock.

HEART RATE

Heart rate is a major determinant of oxygen demand because the rate determines the number of times per minute the high pressures must be generated during systole. Normally, myocardial perfusion takes place during diastole. Coronary artery perfusion pressure is determined by the gradient between aortic diastolic pressure and myocardial wall tension. Pulmonary artery wedge pressure (PAWP) estimates wall tension and resistance to perfusion by approximating left ventricular end-diastolic volume. It can be expressed by the following equation:

$$\text{Coronary perfusion pressure} = \text{aortic diastolic pressure} - \text{myocardial wall tension}$$

Tension in the muscle retards blood flow, which is why approximately 80% of coronary artery perfusion occurs during diastole. With faster heart rates, diastolic time becomes shortened, with very little change occurring in systolic time. A rapid heart rate not only increases oxygen demand but decreases the time available for oxygen delivery. In acute ventricular failure, a person may not be able to maintain cardiac output by increasing the volume of blood pumped with each beat (stroke volume) because contractility is depressed. Cardiac output is a function of both stroke volume and heart rate:

$$\text{Cardiac output} = \text{stroke volume} \times \text{heart rate}$$

If stroke volume cannot be increased, heart rate must increase to maintain cardiac output. This is very costly in terms of oxygen demand.

By improving contractility, IABP therapy helps improve myocardial pumping and the ability to increase stroke volume. Decreasing afterload also increases pumping efficiency. With improved myocardial function and cardiac output, the need for compensatory tachycardia diminishes. IABP counterpulsation increases coronary artery perfusion pressure by increasing aortic diastolic pressure during inflation of the balloon, resulting in improved blood flow and oxygen delivery to the myocardium.

The physiological effects of IABP therapy are summarized in Box 18-14. Proper inflation of the balloon increases oxygen supply, and proper deflation of the balloon decreases oxygen demand. Timing of inflation and deflation is crucial and must coincide with the cardiac cycle.

box 18-14
Direct Physiological Effects of IABP Therapy

Inflation

↑ Aortic diastolic pressure
↑ Aortic root pressure
↑ Coronary perfusion pressure
↑ Oxygen supply

Deflation

↓ Aortic end-diastolic pressure
↓ Impedance to ejection
↓ Afterload
↓ Oxygen demand

table 18-11 IABP Balloon Size Guidelines

Patient Height	Balloon Volume	Body Surface Area
<5′4″	30 mL	≤1.8 m²
5′4″–6′0″	40 mL	>1.8 m²
>6′0″ (or aortic diameter >20 cm)	50 mL	>1.8 m²

Equipment Features

The intra-aortic balloon catheter and the balloon mounted on the end are constructed of a biocompatible polyurethane material. Filling of the balloon is achieved with a pressurized gas that enters through the catheter. Because of its low molecular weight, helium is the pressurized gas of choice. Balloon size should be determined by the patient's physical stature to optimize counterpulsation (Table 18-11). With inflation, the addition of the balloon volume into the aorta acutely increases aortic pressure and retrograde blood flow back toward the aortic valve. With deflation, the sudden evacuation of the balloon volume acutely decreases aortic pressure. Catheters have a central lumen with which aortic pressure can be measured from the tip of the balloon.

Indications for Intra-aortic Balloon Pump Counterpulsation

Two major applications of IABP therapy are for treatment of cardiogenic shock after myocardial infarction and for acute left ventricular failure after cardiac surgery. Other applications of IABP therapy for patients with cardiac pathophysiological conditions are noted in Box 18-15.

CARDIOGENIC SHOCK

Treatment of cardiogenic shock is complicated, and the mortality rate remains high. Cardiogenic shock develops in approximately 15% of patients with myocardial infarction.

Patients initially are treated with various inotropic drugs, vasopressors, and volume. A lack of, or minimal response in, cardiac output, arterial pressure, urine output, and mental status after this therapy indicates a need for assisted circulation with IABP therapy. Once hypotension is present, the self-perpetuating process of injury is in effect. Control

box 18-15
Indications for IABP Therapy

- Cardiogenic shock after acute infarction
- Left ventricular failure in the postoperative cardiac surgery patient
- Severe unstable angina
- Postinfarction ventricular septal defect or mitral regurgitation
- Short-term bridge to cardiac transplantation

of further injury and improvement in survival require early reversal of the shock state.

Once IABP therapy is instituted, improvement should be observed within 1 to 2 hours. At this time, steady improvement should be seen in cardiac output, peripheral perfusion, urine output, mental status, and pulmonary congestion. With improved cardiac function, a decrease in central venous pressure and PAWP also should be seen. Average peak effect should be achieved within 24 to 48 hours.

POSTOPERATIVE LEFT VENTRICULAR FAILURE

Although the best outcomes result when IABP counterpulsation is initiated at least 2 hours before cardiac surgery, a successful reduction in the mortality rate has been achieved by using IABP therapy for patients with acute left ventricular failure after cardiac surgery.[1] Two major conditions might lead to postoperative pump failure: severe preoperative left ventricular dysfunction and intraoperative myocardial injury.

IABP counterpulsation therapy can be used to wean patients from cardiopulmonary bypass and to provide postoperative circulatory assistance until left ventricular recovery occurs. In these situations, early recognition of failure is evidenced by the heart's inability to support circulation after cardiopulmonary bypass. Early recognition and treatment are crucial if left ventricular failure is to be reversed.

UNSTABLE ANGINA

IABP counterpulsation therapy may be used during PCI for patients with unstable angina or mechanical problems. In this situation, PCI procedures usually are followed by emergency cardiac surgery. Patients in this category include those with unstable angina, postinfarction angina and postinfarction ventricular septal defects, or mitral regurgitation from papillary muscle injury with resultant cardiac failure. IABP counterpulsation therapy has been used successfully to control the severity of angina in patients in whom previous medical therapy has failed. The use of IABP therapy for patients with cardiac failure after ventricular septal rupture or mitral valve incompetence aids in the promotion of forward blood flow, which decreases shunting through the septal defect and decreases the amount of mitral regurgitation.

Contraindications to Intra-aortic Balloon Pump Counterpulsation

There are few contraindications to the use of IABP therapy. A competent aortic valve is necessary if the patient is to benefit from IABP therapy. With *aortic insufficiency*, balloon inflation would only increase aortic regurgitation and offer little, if any, augmentation of coronary artery perfusion pressure. In fact, the patient's heart failure could be expected to become worse.

Severe peripheral vascular occlusive disease also is a relative contraindication to the use of IABP therapy. Occlusive disease would make insertion of the catheter difficult and possibly interrupt blood flow to the distal extremity or cause dislodgement of plaque formation along the vessel wall, resulting in potential emboli. In patients who absolutely require IABP therapy, insertion can be achieved through the thoracic aorta, thus bypassing diseased peripheral vessels. Any previous aortofemoral or aortoiliac *bypass graft* contraindicates femoral artery insertion.

The presence of an *aortic aneurysm* also is a contraindication to the use of IABP therapy. A pulsating balloon against an aneurysm may predispose the patient to dislodgement of aneurysmal debris with resultant emboli. A more serious complication is rupture of the aneurysm; it is possible for the catheter to perforate the wall of the aneurysm during insertion.

Procedure

INSERTION

Proper positioning of the balloon is in the thoracic aorta just distal to the left subclavian artery and proximal to the renal arteries (Fig. 18-19). The most commonly used method of catheter placement is percutaneous insertion using a Seldinger technique, although other approaches have been described. The most common alternative is direct insertion into the thoracic aorta. Because this requires a median ster-

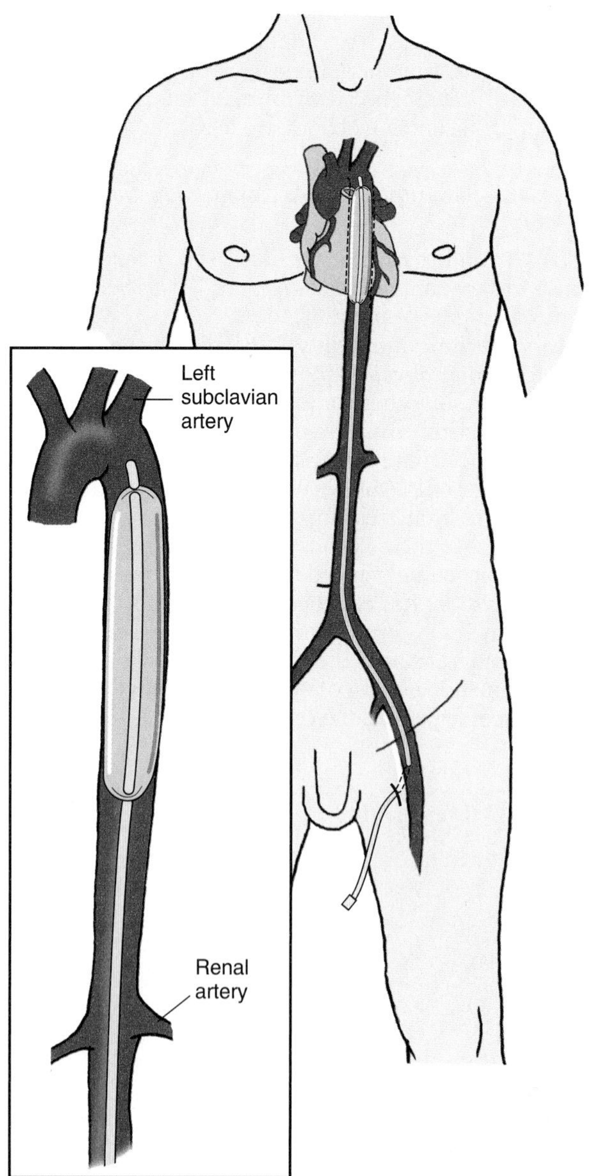

figure 18-19 Proper position of the balloon catheter; illustrating percutaneous insertion.

notomy incision, it is restricted to cardiac surgical patients whose chests have been opened for the surgery.

Once in place, the catheter is attached to a machine console that has three basic components: a monitoring system, an electronic trigger mechanism, and a drive system that moves gas in and out of the balloon. Monitoring systems have the capability of displaying the patient's ECG and an arterial waveform showing the effect of balloon inflation–deflation. Consoles also are capable of displaying a balloon waveform that illustrates the inflation and deflation of the balloon itself. The standard trigger mechanism for the balloon pump is the R wave that is sensed from the patient's ECG. This trigger signals the beginning of each cardiac cycle for the drive system. Other possible triggers include systolic arterial pressure or pacemaker spikes on the ECG. Adjustment of exact timing is controlled on the machine console. The drive system is the actual mechanism that drives gas into and out of the balloon by alternating pressure and vacuum.

TIMING

Two methods of timing can be used with IABP therapy: conventional timing and real timing. Conventional timing uses the arterial waveform as the triggering mechanism to determine both inflation and deflation of the balloon. Real timing uses the same point of reference (the dicrotic notch on the arterial waveform) for balloon inflation but uses the ECG signal as the trigger for balloon deflation. Real timing is discussed briefly after conventional timing.

Conventional Timing

The first step to proper timing of the balloon pump using conventional timing is the identification of the beginning of systole and diastole on the arterial waveform. Systole begins when left ventricular pressure exceeds left atrial pressure, forcing the mitral valve closed.

There are two phases of systole: isovolumetric contraction and ejection. Once the mitral valve is closed, isovolumetric contraction begins and continues until enough pressure is generated to overcome impedance to ejection. When ventricular pressure exceeds aortic pressure, the aortic valve is forced open, initiating ejection, or phase two. Ejection continues until pressure in the left ventricle falls below pressure in the aorta. At this point, the aortic valve closes, and diastole begins.

Closing of the aortic valve creates an artifact on the arterial waveform that is called the dicrotic notch. The dicrotic notch is used as a timing reference to determine when balloon inflation should occur. Inflation should not occur before the notch because systole has not been completed.

After aortic valve closure, two phases of diastole begin: isovolumic relaxation and ventricular filling. After aortic valve closure, there is a period in which neither the aortic nor mitral valve is open. The mitral valve remains closed because left ventricular pressure still is higher than left atrial pressure. This phase is isovolumic relaxation. When left ventricular pressure falls below left atrial pressure, the mitral valve is forced open by the higher pressure in the left atrium. This begins the filling phase of diastole. Balloon inflation should continue throughout diastole. Deflation should be timed to occur at end-diastole, just before the next sharp systolic upstroke on the arterial waveform.

Figure 18-20 illustrates the cardiac cycle with left atrial, left ventricular, and aortic pressures superimposed on one another. Figure 18-21 illustrates a radial artery waveform with the beginning of systole and diastole marked.

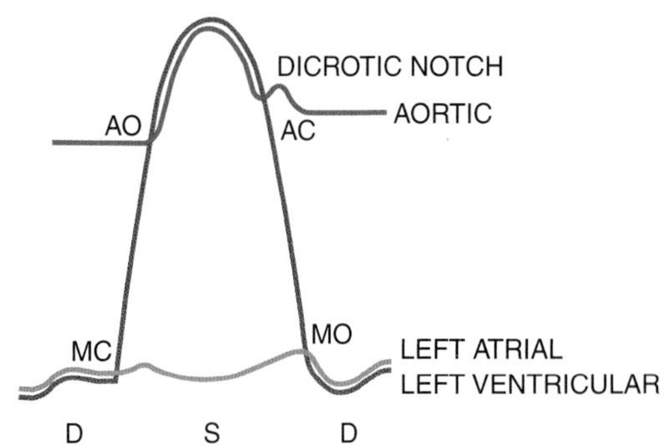

figure 18-20 Cardiac cycle of the left heart with aortic, left ventricular, and left atrial pressure waveforms. AO, aortic valve opening; AC, aortic valve closure; D, diastole; MO, mitral valve opening; MC, mitral valve closure; S, systole.

Real Timing

The main difference between the two timing methods is balloon deflation and the triggering mechanism used. Real timing uses the ECG as the trigger signal for balloon deflation. The QRS complex is recognized as the onset of ventricular systole, and balloon deflation occurs at this time. Triggering off of the R wave allows for balloon deflation to occur at the time of systolic ejection and not before (as with conventional timing). This timing mechanism is more effective in patients with irregular heart rhythms because balloon deflation occurs on recognition of the R wave (systolic ejection). It does not need to be approximated by the operator or an algorithm, as in conventional timing. Both a rapid deflation mechanism and a reliable ECG signal are necessary for IABP using real timing to augment blood pressure effectively. Balloon inflation with real timing occurs at the onset of diastole as triggered by the dicrotic notch on an arterial waveform, just as in conventional timing.

Interpretation of Results

WAVEFORM ASSESSMENT

Analysis of the arterial pressure waveform and the effectiveness of IABP therapy is an important nursing function. Nurses must be able to recognize and correct problems in balloon pump timing.

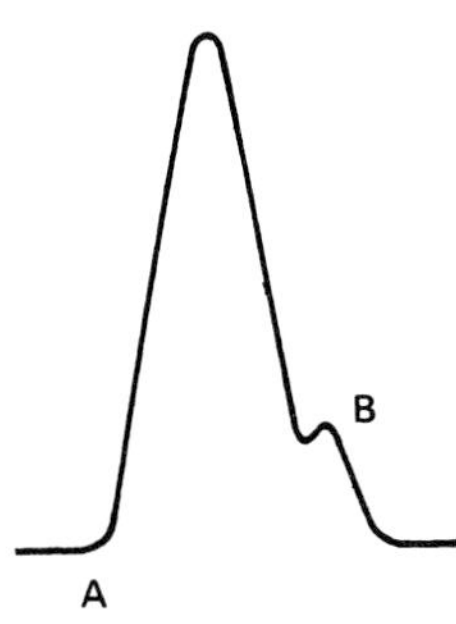

figure 18-21 Arterial waveform, with *A* representing the point of balloon deflation before the systolic upstroke, and *B* representing balloon inflation at the dicrotic notch, at diastole.

Step 1

The first step in timing assessment is the ability to recognize the beginnings of systole and diastole on the arterial waveform, as shown in Figure 18-21. Systole begins at point A, where the sharp upstroke begins. Point B marks the dicrotic notch, which represents aortic valve closure. At this point, diastole begins and the balloon should be inflated. Balloon deflation occurs just before point A, at end-diastole.

Box 18-16 lists five criteria that can be used to measure the effectiveness of IABP therapy on the arterial pressure waveform. To evaluate the waveform effectively, the patient's unassisted pressure tracing must be viewed alongside the assisted pressure tracing. This can be accomplished through adjustment of the console so that the balloon inflates and deflates on every other beat (i.e., a 1:2 assist ratio). Most patients tolerate this well for a brief period of time. Machine consoles are capable of freezing the waveform on the console monitor so that it would be necessary to assist at a 1:2 ratio only for one screen. Another alternative would be to obtain a strip recording of the 1:2 assistance for analysis.

Step 2

After identification of the patient's dicrotic notch, a comparison is made with the assisted tracing to see that inflation occurs at the point of the dicrotic notch. Inflation before the dicrotic notch shortens systole abruptly and increases ventricular volume as ejection is interrupted. Late inflation, past the dicrotic notch, does not raise coronary artery perfusion pressure. The peak-diastolic pressure may not be as high as it would be with proper timing.

Step 3

Next, the slopes of systolic upstroke and diastolic augmentation should be compared. The diastolic slope should be sharp and parallel the systolic upstroke. The slope always should be a straight line. The greater the peak in diastolic pressure, the greater the increase in aortic root pressure. For this reason, balloon assistance is adjusted until the highest peak possible is achieved.

Step 4

Deflation should occur just before systole, causing an acute drop in aortic end-diastolic pressure. This quick deflation displaces approximately 40 mL of volume. The result is an end-diastolic dip in pressure that reduces the impedance to the next systolic ejection. The end-diastolic pressure without the balloon assistance should be compared with the end-diastolic pressure with the dip created by balloon deflation. Optimally, a pressure difference of at least 10 mm Hg should be obtained. Better afterload reduction is achieved with the lowest possible end-diastolic dip.

The point of deflation also is crucial. Deflation that is too early allows pressure to rise to normal end-diastolic levels preceding systole. In this situation, there is no decrease in afterload. Late deflation encroaches on the next systole and actually increases afterload owing to greater impedance to ejection from the presence of the still-inflated balloon during systolic ejection.

Step 5

Finally, if afterload has been reduced, the next systolic pressure peak will be lower than the unassisted systolic pressure peak. This implies that the ventricle did not have to generate as great a pressure to overcome impedance to ejection. This may not always be seen because the systolic pressure peak also represents the compliance of the vasculature. If the vasculature is noncompliant due to atherosclerotic disease, the systolic peak may not change very much. Figure 18-22 illustrates the five points that are assessed on the waveform, whereas Figure 18-23 demonstrates possible errors in timing.

Balloon Fit

The fit of the balloon to any particular patient's aorta determines how well these criteria are met. Ideally, approximately 80% of the aorta is occluded with balloon inflation. In a dilated aorta, in which less than 80% occlusion occurs, the effect of inflation and deflation is not as dramatic on the waveform. When a patient is hypotensive or hypovolemic, the balloon does not have as pronounced an effect on the waveform because there is less volume displacement as the balloon inflates or deflates.

Assessment and Management

Patients requiring IABP are managed much like any other critically ill patient in cardiogenic shock or acute left ventricular failure. Nursing assessment and management of

box 18-16
Criteria for Assessment of Effective IABP Therapy on the Arterial Pressure Waveform

- Inflation occurs at the dicrotic notch.
- Inflation slope is parallel to the systolic upstroke and is a straight line.
- Diastolic augmentation peak is greater than or equal to the preceding systolic peak.
- An end-diastolic dip in pressure is created with balloon deflation.
- The following systolic peak (assisted systole) is lower than the preceding systole (unassisted systole).

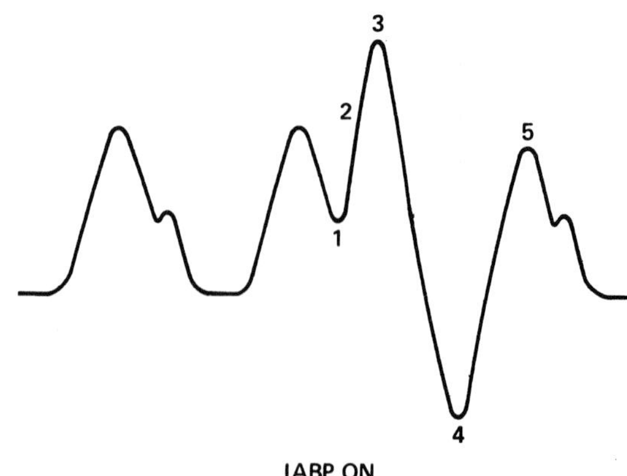

figure 18-22 Inspection of the arterial waveform with intra-aortic balloon assistance should include observation of (1) inflation point; (2) inflation slope; (3) diastolic peak pressure; (4) end-diastolic dip; and (5) next systolic peak.

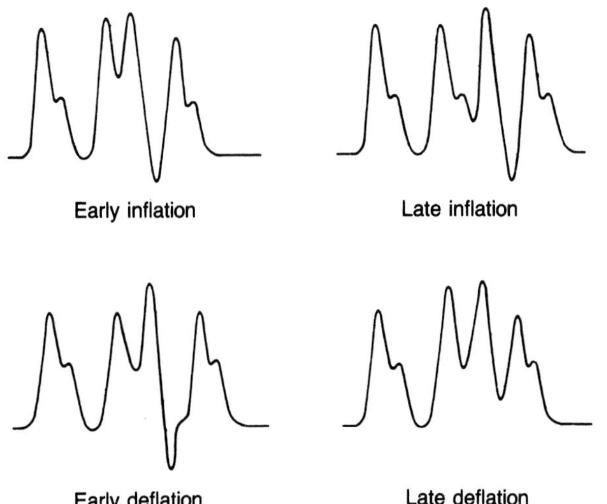

figure 18-23 Illustration of possible errors occurring with timing.

these conditions are discussed in Chapter 50. Additional nursing skills and assessment considerations specific to IABP therapy must be included in the care of these patients. These are summarized in Box 18-17.

SYSTEM MONITORING

Cardiovascular System

Monitoring the cardiovascular system is extremely important in determining the effectiveness of balloon pump therapy. The basis for this assessment includes vital signs, cardiac output, heart rhythm and regularity, urine output, color, perfusion, and mentation.

Vital Signs. Three important vital signs with respect to IABP therapy are heart rate, mean arterial pressure (MAP), and PAWP. Effective IABP therapy causes a decrease in all three parameters. Acute changes in the MAP may indicate volume depletion. Critically ill patients tolerate little change in their volume status. The PAWP is an important parameter for monitoring volume and provides the clinician with an early indication of volume depletion or overload.

Blood pressure readings require special consideration. Because the balloon inflates during diastole, peak-diastolic pressure may be higher than peak-systolic pressure. Most IABP consoles have monitoring systems capable of distinguishing systole from peak diastole; however, some monitoring equipment can distinguish only peak pressures from low-point pressures. For this reason, a monitor's digital display of systolic pressure actually may represent peak-diastolic pressure. It is advisable to record blood pressure as systolic, peak-diastolic, and end-diastolic—that is, 100/110/60. These pressures can be read from a strip recording of the arterial waveform.

Heart Rhythm and Regularity. Heart rhythm and regularity are important considerations. Early recognition and treatment of dysrhythmias are crucial for effective IABP support. Irregular dysrhythmias may inhibit efficient IABP therapy with some types of consoles because timing is set by the regular R-R interval on the ECG. A safety feature of all balloon pump consoles is automatic deflation of the balloon for premature QRS complexes. One particular IABP model tracks real time versus any average of beats so it more effectively tracks dysrhythmias. If the dysrhythmia persists and timing is ineffective, another alternative might be use of the systolic peak on the arterial waveform as the trigger mechanism for balloon inflation. The primary goal in dysrhythmias is to treat the dysrhythmia.

Other Observations. Urine output, color, perfusion, and mentation all are important assessment parameters for determining the adequacy of cardiac output. All should improve in patients responsive to IABP therapy. Any deterioration in these signs also might indicate a fall in cardiac output. Cardiac output measurement is indicated when deterioration is evident, when a major change in volume or pharmacological therapy has been instituted, and during weaning from IABP support.

The left radial pulse and the cannulated extremity should be frequently assessed. A decrease, absence, or change in character of the left radial pulse may indicate that the balloon has advanced up the aorta and may be partially obstructing or has advanced into the left subclavian artery.

The presence of the balloon catheter in the femoral or iliac artery predisposes the patient to impaired circulation of the involved extremity. The affected extremity needs to be kept relatively immobile. Because flexion of the hip may kink the catheter and impair balloon pumping, it may be helpful to use a knee immobilizer to remind the patient to avoid hip flexion. The head of the bed also should not be elevated more than 30 degrees. Hip flexion also contributes to decreased perfusion to the distal extremity. Extremities should be checked hourly for pulses, color, and sensation. Any deterioration in the affected extremity should be reported to the physician. Severe arterial insufficiency necessitates removal of the catheter.

Physicians advocate the use of heparin therapy to prevent possible thrombus formation around the catheter and vascular insufficiency, especially in medical patients. Each physician will determine whether the risks of anticoagulation outweigh the benefits for the specific patient. Low–molecular-weight dextran is another possible choice of therapy to prevent thrombus formation. This agent impairs platelet function and prevents triggering of the coagulation cascade. It is usually preferred in the cardiac surgical patient for the first 24 hours.

Pulmonary System

Many patients on IABP therapy require intubation and ventilatory assistance. Some of these patients may have respiratory insufficiency secondary to fluid overload associated with CHF. The immobile, intubated patient is always at risk for respiratory infections and the development of atelectasis. Turning the patient is appropriate provided modifications are implemented to keep the extremity cannulated by the balloon catheter straight. Daily chest roentgenograms are needed to follow pulmonary status and to inspect IV catheter placement. The position of the balloon catheter also can be determined in this manner.

Renal System

Patients in cardiogenic shock or severe left ventricular failure are at risk for the development of acute renal failure. In the shock state, the kidneys suffer the consequences of hypoperfusion; therefore, urine output and quality should

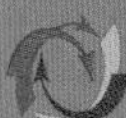

box 18-17 nursing interventions for *IABP Counterpulsation and Ventricular Assist Devices*

IABP Nursing Interventions

- Verify correct timing using assist ratio of 1:2 and document settings hourly.
- Reevaluate timing for any change in the heart rate greater than 10 beats/minute.
- Maintain proper balloon volume and refill as needed every 2 to 4 hours. Use automatic filling mode if available. Avoid hip flexion, which may impair gas movement in and out of IABP catheter.
- Maintain good arterial waveform and adequate ECG signal for evaluation of timing.
- Transduce aortic arterial line to the IABP per unit protocol.
- Reduce or eliminate situations that will interfere with the IABP's ability to maintain proper assist ratio. Notify physician of the development of tachycardias or irregular rhythms, and treat dysrhythmias with drug therapy or pacing as ordered. Use appropriate trigger (i.e., ECG, arterial pressure, pacing).
- Use pacer modes only if the patient is 100% paced.
- Notify physician of significant changes in balloon pressure waveform.

VAD Nursing Interventions

- Assess and maintain adequate filling pressures during immediate postoperative phase.
- Monitor and assess heart rate, blood pressure, mean arterial pressure, pump flow, urine output, and neurological status hourly. Treat changes as ordered.
- Assess and change equipment level for devices that require specific placement of equipment for adequate pump flow.
- Evaluate pump flow and rate of VAD in relation to native heart rate and activity level of patient.
- Manage VAD function and volume status as ordered to maintain adequate device output.

General Nursing Interventions

- Monitor and record temperatures every 4 hours and PRN.
- Observe all insertion sites and incisions for signs of infection. Maintain sterile technique with dressing changes.
- Change any dressing that is wet or not intact.
- Change all infusion lines and infusion bags per unit protocol.
- Culture any site with suspicious drainage, redness, or swelling.
- Notify physician of elevation in white blood cell count.
- Treat patient with antibiotics as ordered.
- Auscultate and document breath sounds every 2 to 4 hours.
- Assist patient with pulmonary toilet (i.e., coughing, deep breathing, frequent turning). Suction intubated patients as needed.
- Use pulse oximeter to monitor patients with abnormal blood gases, excessive secretions, or respiratory difficulty.
- Extubate patient and increase activity level as tolerated—particularly those with VADs.
- Document quality of peripheral pulses and neurological status before AIBP or VAD insertion. Assess and document quality of pulses, skin perfusion, and neurological status per protocol. Evaluate peripheral perfusion with any complaints of leg/foot pain by patient.
- Notify physician of any changes in pulses or neurological status.
- Maintain anticoagulation as ordered.
- Avoid hip flexion, which might obstruct flow to the affected extremity, by keeping the cannulated leg straight and the bed at angle less than 30 degrees.
- Always maintain balloon motion to avoid thrombus formation on the balloon.
- Assess skin integrity, and document any redness and ulcerations over bony prominences.
- Use sheepskin, foam pads, and specialty beds as needed. Turn patient every 2 hours.
- Ensure that skin remains clean and dry.
- Maintain adequate nutrition by encouraging oral intake or implementing use of parenteral or enteral nutrition when necessary.
- Maintain alarm volumes, monitor noise at lowest level possible, and minimize unnecessary noise in the room.
- Talk with patient and reorient to date and time frequently.
- Encourage family visits.
- Explain all procedures and activities to the patient.
- Organize care to allow for periods of uninterrupted sleep. Turn the lights off in room at night if possible.
- Sedate patient if necessary and as tolerated per physician orders.

be monitored closely. Serum BUN, creatinine, and creatinine clearance should be monitored daily to assess renal function. Creatinine clearance indicates renal dysfunction and possible failure much earlier than elevated serum creatinine. Any acute, dramatic drop in urine output might be an indication that the catheter has slipped down the aorta and is obstructing the renal arteries.

WEANING

Indications for Weaning

Weaning patients from balloon assistance usually can begin 24 to 72 hours after insertion. Some patients require longer periods of support. Weaning can begin when there is evidence of hemodynamic stability that does not require excessive vasopressor support. Ideally, vasopressor support is minimal when weaning begins. After the balloon is removed, it is much easier to increase vasopressor support than to reinsert a balloon catheter for hemodynamic support.

The patient should exhibit signs of *adequate cardiac function*, demonstrated by good peripheral pulses, adequate urine output, absence of pulmonary edema, and improved mentation. *Good coronary artery perfusion* will be evidenced by an absence of ventricular ectopy and no evidence of ischemia or injury on the ECG.

Complications may require abrupt cessation of IABP. This may or may not result in reinsertion of another balloon catheter. Severe arterial insufficiency evidenced by a loss of pulses in the distal extremity, pain, and pallor is definitely an indication to remove the balloon catheter from that particular insertion site. Any balloon that develops a leak also requires removal. The physician may choose to reinsert the balloon catheter in another extremity or to replace the faulty balloon if the patient is hemodynamically unstable. Depending on the philosophy of the institution and physician, a deteriorating, irreversible situation also might be an indication for weaning or discontinuing balloon pump support. Box 18-18 lists major indications for weaning from IABP therapy.

Approaches to Weaning

Weaning is commonly achieved by decreasing the assist ratio from 1:1 to 1:2 and so on until the minimum assist ratio is achieved on any particular console. A patient might be assisted at the first decrease for up to 4 to 6 hours. The minimum amount of time should be 30 minutes. During this time, the patient must be assessed for any change in hemodynamic status. An increase in heart rate, a decrease in blood pressure, and a decrease in cardiac output indicate a deterioration in hemodynamic status. Weaning should be discontinued temporarily and therapy should be adjusted before another weaning attempt. If the first decrease in assist ratio is tolerated, the assist ratio is decreased to minimum, with 1 to 4 hours allowed for each new assist ratio. The patient must be assessed continually for any indications of intolerance to the process. Although less common, weaning can also occur by decreasing balloon volume, which in many models is controlled from the console.

Complications Specific to Intra-aortic Balloon Pump Therapy

Patients with IABP counterpulsation need to be monitored for development of poor blood flow to the cannulated extremity, which could lead to compartment syndrome. It may occur within the first 24 hours of support or not until several days after catheter insertion. Compartment syndrome is caused by a rise in the tissue pressure in one of the compartments of the affected lower extremity. Bone, muscle, nerve tissue, and blood vessels all are enclosed by a fibrous membrane called the *fascia*, and this enclosed space is called a *compartment*. It is nonyielding, so a rise in volume in the compartment increases the pressure in the compartment. The patient with IABP in whom limb ischemia develops from decreased capillary flow can suffer cellular and capillary damage that leads to increased capillary permeability. The resultant transudation of fluid into the closed compartment space increases tissue pressure to a level that can interfere with capillary blood flow. When this degree of tissue pressure is reached, tissue viability may be threatened. Treatment is directed at improving blood flow. Pressure release by fasciotomy may be needed to prevent tissue death.

Decreased circulating platelets in the first 24 hours of IABP therapy and a minimal decrease in red blood cell count have been reported; however, they are not thought to be significant problems. There is a low incidence of balloon leakage and rupture. These complications might result from balloon inflation against a calcific, atherosclerotic plaque in the aorta. This disruption in the balloon surface may be as small as a pinhole or may be a large tear. The associated danger is gas embolism. In addition, the risk of entrapment is minimal but still exists. Table 18-12 provides additional details about injury secondary to balloons.

Insertion of the catheter in the face of severe atherosclerotic vascular disease might result in arterial perforation or occlusion. Any leak is an indication for immediate balloon removal. Iatrogenic dissection of the aorta is rare but has been reported. Arterial insufficiency is the most common complication of IABP therapy. Arterial insufficiency may be permanent, or it may be relieved by aortofemoral or ileofemoral bypass grafting. Neuropathy in the catheterized extremity is another reported complication.

box 18-18 ***Indications for Weaning From IABP***

- Hemodynamic stability
  - Cardiac index >2 L/min
  - PAWP <20 mm Hg
  - Systolic blood pressure >100 mm Hg
- Minimal requirements for vasopressor support
- Evidence of adequate cardiac function
  - Good peripheral pulses
  - Adequate urine output
  - Absence of pulmonary edema
  - Improved mentation
- Evidence of good coronary perfusion
  - Absence of ventricular ectopy
  - Absence of ischemia on the ECG
- Severe vascular insufficiency
- Deteriorating, irreversible condition

MECHANICAL CIRCULATORY SUPPORT

When there is profound myocardial injury, the augmentation of systemic blood pressure by IABP counterpulsation may not be adequate for patient survival. Use of IABP for circulatory support requires that a patient have a functioning left ventricle because IABP augments cardiac output only by 8% to 10%. Patients with severe, acute left ventricular failure after a myocardial infarction, after a surgical procedure, or from end-stage CHF may need a mechanism for replacing left ventricular function. Circulatory support with a ventricular assist device (VAD) has become a successful treatment for patients with cardiac failure refractory to pharmacological therapies, revascularization procedures, and IABP counterpulsation. These devices are capable of supporting circulation until the heart recovers or a donor heart is obtained for transplantation. As of 2003, left ventricular devices have been used as a bridge to transplantation in over 3,500 patients. Nearly 50% of recent implantable device recipients are discharged home.[2]

Interest in the research and development of artificial circulatory support devices has existed since the 1930s. Cardiopulmonary bypass, an early example of these efforts, was successfully implemented in the 1950s. In 1964, a National

table 18-12 Injuries Secondary to Balloons

Injury	Assessment Findings	Nursing Intervention
Balloon rupture	Presence of bright red blood or flecks of dried blood in the catheter or helium delivery line Gas alarm sounds Decreased augmentation Signs of embolic event Entrapment (may be the first indication)	Immediate removal of the catheter by the appropriate personnel Before removal: Turn pump off Clamp the line Place the patient on left side in Trendelenburg position
Balloon entrapment	Balloon pressure waveform indicates leaks Small amounts of blood in tubing or flecks of dried blood in tubing	Surgical removal is usually indicated Physician may consider pharmacological dissolution of clot with thrombolytics Physician may consider use of Fogerty embolectomy to remove fresh clot

Institutes of Health initiative helped to organize and support these efforts on a national level. Michael DeBakey became the first clinician to support successfully a postcardiotomy patient with a left ventricular bypass pump in 1966. An impetus for continued research during the 1960s and 1970s was the limited early success with heart transplantation. The focus of research at that time was to develop a device that could support the failing heart until sufficient cardiac function had returned. Current research focuses on the use of these devices as a bridge to heart transplantation and as a method of permanent cardiac support for patients with end-stage cardiac disease.

Physiological Principles

Patients who are candidates for ventricular assistance suffer from heart failure resulting from ischemic or myopathic heart disease. Both disease processes lead to a reduction in cardiac output and oxygen delivery. The physiological response of the body to this low output state is vasoconstriction and increased systemic vascular resistance. Although these compensatory mechanisms are meant to protect and preserve cardiovascular function in the short term, a vicious cycle develops that is characterized by compromised cardiac contractility and a low ventricular ejection fraction. Hypotension ensues, leading to hemodynamic instability requiring the use of pharmacological agents and possibly IABP therapy for cardiovascular support. Should the patient continue to deteriorate despite drug therapy and IABP, a VAD may be necessary for survival. Hemodynamically, these patients usually demonstrate a cardiac index of less than 2 L/minute/m^2, a PAWP of greater than 20 mm Hg, and a systolic blood pressure of less than 80 mm Hg despite pharmacological therapies and the use of IABP counterpulsation.

Restoration of adequate blood flow and preservation of end-organ function are the fundamental goals of short- or long-term VAD use. Hemodynamics and perfusion improve as the VAD(s) assumes the workload of the failing ventricle(s). Ventricular assistance may involve supporting one or both ventricles depending on the extent of myocardial damage and ventricular failure.

Left ventricular support usually requires cannulation of the left ventricle with a conduit that leads to the device. The ascending aorta, which receives the output from the device, is also cannulated with a conduit. In certain situations, the left atrium may be cannulated instead of the left ventricle. Circulation in the patient supported by a left ventricular assist device (LVAD) is similar to the normal circulatory process. Venous blood returns to the right heart, passes through the lungs to be oxygenated, and then returns to the left atrium through the pulmonary veins. Blood then passes from the left atrium through the left ventricle and into the LVAD. The LVAD then ejects blood into the ascending aorta during pump systole.

In situations that necessitate biventricular support, two pump units function in synchrony to assume the roles of the native right and left ventricles. One pump supports right heart circulation while the other supports left heart circulation. The addition of right ventricular assistance requires cannulation of the right atrium for inflow to the pump and the pulmonary artery for outflow from the right ventricular assist device (RVAD). During biventricular assistance, blood is diverted from the right atrium to the lungs through the RVAD, bypassing the right ventricle. Circulation continues to the left heart, where the LVAD undertakes support of systemic circulation. Univentricular or biventricular assistance relieves the ventricle(s) of its workload by acting as the primary pump supporting pulmonary circulation or systemic blood pressure. Reducing ventricular workload decreases cardiac oxygen demand.

Devices

Several VADs are available for use. Certain devices are commercially available, whereas others require special exemption for investigational purposes. Although no universal classification system exists, the devices can be categorized according to four general functional characteristics: the intended duration of support (short term versus long term), the type of support provided (univentricular versus biventricular), the actual physical placement of the device (internal versus external), and the type of blood flow produced (pulsatile versus nonpulsatile). Short-term support usually refers to assistance for patients expected to recover from episodes of acute left ventricular failure secondary to myocardial infarction or surgical procedures. Long-term ventricular assistance may be an option for individuals awaiting heart transplantation, or it may provide an alternative method of permanent cardiac support.

NONPULSATILE PUMPS

Centrifugal and roller pumps are examples of nonpulsatile VADs capable of providing univentricular (to either ventricle) or biventricular support. They are primarily used for short-term ventricular assistance when myocardial recovery is expected. These devices have been used, infrequently, as bridges to transplantation. Both types are approved by the FDA and are commercially available. Centrifugal and roller pumps are extracorporeal devices designed to support circulation of the patient's blood. Because these devices do not generate pulsatile blood flow, IABP is often used in conjunction with them to create a pulse. Blood is transported from the cannulated chamber to an external pump console that circulates the blood back to the corresponding great vessel by a separate cannula. Should right ventricular failure be identified after placement of an LVAD, an RVAD can be added for additional support with these devices.

These devices can be inserted relatively quickly and are adequate methods of deploying short-term circulatory assistance. Methods of cannulation and physical placement of the equipment limit the mobility and activity level of the patient. Patients supported by these VADs are often sedated and paralyzed. A commonly used centrifugal pump is the BioMedicus.

Extracorporeal membrane oxygenation (ECMO) or cardiopulmonary bypass (CPB) systems are alternative methods of temporary CPR involving circulatory support and oxygenation of the patient's blood. CPB is primarily used for operative situations but has demonstrated effectiveness as a mechanism of support for patients unable to wean from the pump perioperatively or for those requiring cardiopulmonary support refractory to conventional efforts. Circulation of blood between the patient and an external pump is supported by cannulation of the femoral vessels. Venous blood is diverted from central venous circulation; pumped through a membrane oxygenator, where oxygen and carbon dioxide are exchanged; and returned to the arterial circulation through the femoral artery cannula. A heating mechanism in the pump console helps to maintain body temperature during circulatory support.

Rapid deployment without the need for surgical intervention and the ability to provide hemodynamic stabilization for a brief period are the major advantages of these resuscitative devices. CPB and ECMO allow time for further assessment and intervention during episodes of acute hemodynamic decompensation. Disadvantages include the need for continuous anticoagulation and the inability to provide extended circulatory support. The presence of occlusive peripheral vascular disease could be a contraindication to use of these devices.

PULSATILE PUMPS

Implantable Pumps

Implantable pumps were designed with the intention of providing long-term left ventricular support while allowing the patient a certain amount of physical independence. A few devices have successfully supported a patient for greater than 1 year while awaiting heart transplantation. Many patients with the implantable devices have been physically rehabilitated by participating in regular physical therapy programs and normal activities of daily living while being supported with a VAD. This might better prepare them physically to endure the transplantation process. Examples of the implantable devices are the HeartMate IP, and the Novacor left ventricular assist system (LVAS). The Novacor device operates on electricity, whereas the HeartMate IP operates as a pneumatic unit.

Surgical implantation of the VAD necessitates a sternotomy and the use of CPB. Device placement is in an abdominal pocket just below the left diaphragm. Typically, the inflow conduit is tunneled through the diaphragm and anastomosed to the apex of the left ventricle. The outflow conduit is brought around the diaphragm and is anastomosed to the ascending aorta. Drivelines extending from the implanted device are tunneled through the patient's skin and connected to a portable, external power source. This power source may be a portable console or battery pack that is worn by the patient (Fig. 18-24). Either situation allows the patient mobility and independence during the recovery period.

Pump units of the implantable VADs are encapsulated in rigid housing and consist of a blood pump sac and single or dual pusher plates (depending on the particular device). Inflow and outflow conduits have valves that

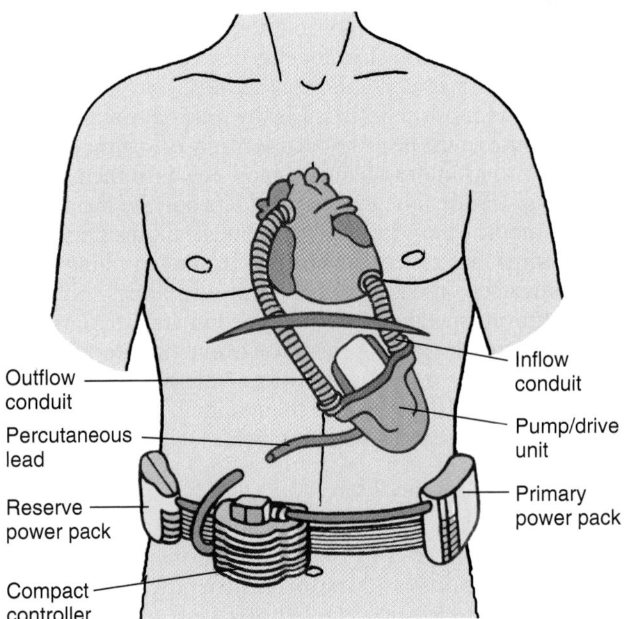

figure 18-24 Portable, implantable left ventricular assist device. (Artwork courtesy of the Novacor Division, Baxter Healthcare Corporation, Oakland, CA.)

support unidirectional blood flow. These devices work on the principle of converting electrical or pneumatic energy to mechanical energy. This mechanical energy activates the pusher plates, causing them to compress the blood sac at the appropriate time. Blood sac compression causes ejection of the blood out of the pump sac and into the ascending aorta through the outflow conduit. These devices have stroke volumes of 70 to 83 mL and can support pump outputs of greater than 10 L/minute. Depending on the device implanted, long-term anticoagulation may be necessary to prevent thromboembolic events.

External Pumps

Two commonly used external pulsatile devices are the Thoratec VAD and the Abiomed pump. Both devices have successfully supported patients postcardiotomy and patients bridged to heart transplantation.

The Thoratec VAD is a pneumatically driven device that is positioned externally on the recipient's upper abdomen. Placement of this device requires a sternotomy incision and use of CPB. The structure of the pump drive, the inflow and outflow conduits, and the cannulation techniques of the chambers and great vessels are all similar to that of the implantable devices. A major difference is that the cannulas supporting the blood flow pass through the patient's chest wall to the externally positioned pump. One advantage of this device is the ability to provide univentricular or biventricular support, depending on the extent of heart failure. Figure 18-25 is an example of biventricular support. Another advantage is that due to its external placement, small patient body size is less of a contraindication when considering the need for ventricular assistance.

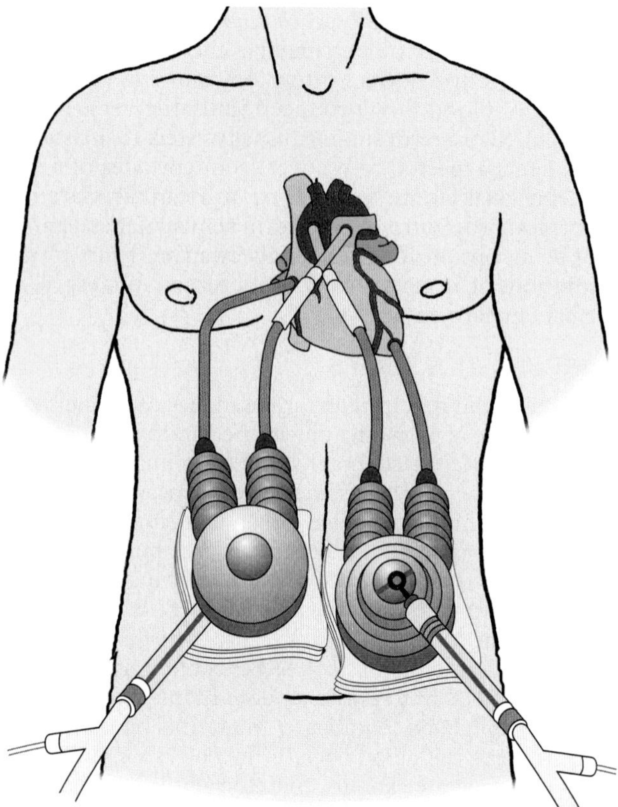

figure 18-25 Thoratec pneumatic ventricular assist device. External placement with biventricular assist capabilities. (Courtesy of Kathy J. Vaca, RN; Department of Surgery, St. Louis Health Sciences Center, St. Louis, MO.)

Another external VAD, the Abiomed pump, is designed for short-term univentricular or biventricular support. It has been used in patients when myocardial recovery is expected and as a bridge to transplantation. Components consist of cannulas for venous and arterial access, blood pumps to support unidirectional blood flow and systemic circulation, and a pneumatically driven console that provides the power source. Cannulation sites for this device are either atria, the pulmonary artery, and the ascending aorta. Filling of the blood pumps occurs passively by gravity; therefore, the blood pumps must be positioned securely below the level of the heart to promote adequate blood flow into their chambers (Fig. 18-26). The internal bladders operate in a fill-to-empty mode. Pumps positioned too high fill insufficiently, and pumps that are too low have a prolonged filling time, each adversely affecting patient hemodynamics. Nursing interventions specific to the Abiomed include monitoring and adjusting the level of the blood pumps and monitoring filling pressures to ensure adequate volumes necessary to support optimal flow through the system. Use of this device significantly impairs patient mobility.

Advances in Mechanical Circulatory Support

In November 2002, the FDA approved the Thoratec HeartMate SNAP-VE LVAS for permanent implantation, also known as "destination therapy," in patients with end-stage heart failure who are not candidates for traditional heart transplantation. Since October 2003, the Centers for Medicare and Medicaid Services have provided coverage for patients who meet specific criteria. The HeartMate SNAP-VE LVAS is an implantable electric pump that allows patients to ambulate and participate in cardiac rehabilitation programs, making it an appropriate system for in-home use by specific heart failure populations.

Additional improvements in mechanical circulatory support are on the horizon. In February 2001, the FDA approved the first series of clinical trials for the Arrow LionHeart, which was developed by researchers at Pennsylvania State University.[3] The LionHeart is one of the first totally implantable assist devices powered by wireless electrical transmission. World Heart Corporation of Ottawa, Canada has also developed a totally implantable device known as HeartSaver.[4] HeartSaver, like LionHeart, uses principles of transcutaneous energy transfer in its wireless design. Both models are undergoing trials not as a bridge to transplantation, but rather as a form of destination therapy much like the aforementioned HeartMate VE. Clinical trials are expected to take several years. The devices are referred to as "heart helpers," and are not artificial hearts.

Artificial hearts have been approved in the United States by the FDA for investigational use. Abiomed has developed the first fully implantable replacement heart known as the AbioCor TAH (totally artificial heart).[4] Devices such as the

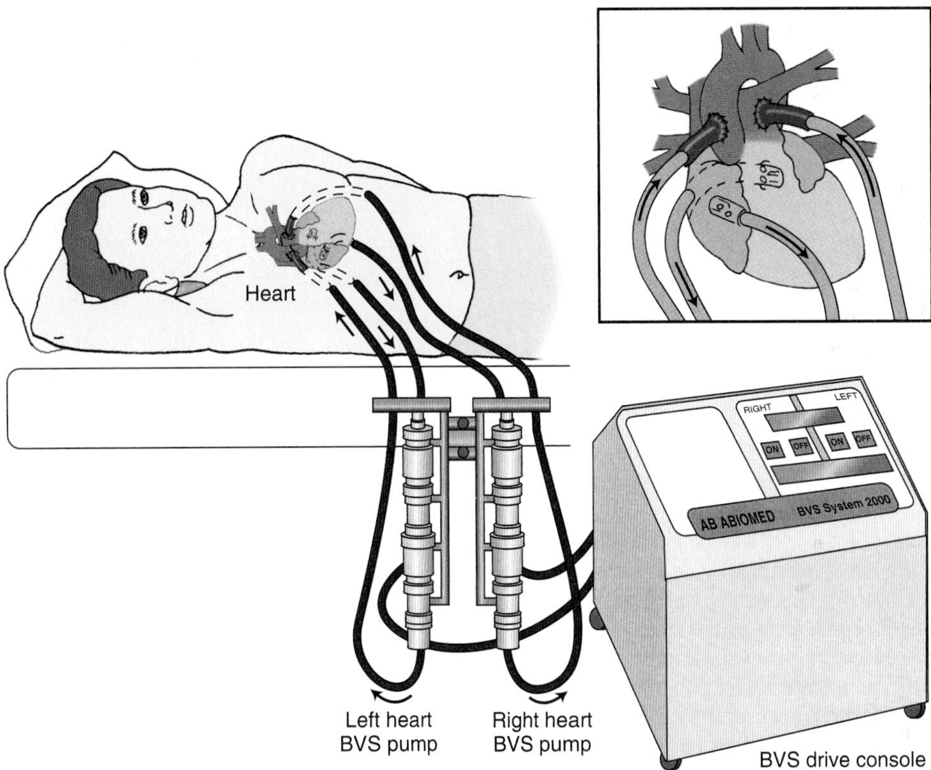

figure 18-26 Abiomed biventricular support system. (Artwork courtesy of ABIOMED Cardiovascular, Inc., Danvers, MA.)

AbioCor are designed for use in patients ineligible to receive a VAD, such as those with both right- and left-sided heart failure. Table 18-13 provides a comprehensive review of VADs.

Modes of Operation

With the exception of the Abiomed device, the pulsatile pumps have several modes of operation. Two primary modes depend on the patient's ECG or the rate of blood flow through the pump during each cardiac cycle. In the ECG trigger mode, the pump initiates blood ejection in conjunction with the patient's QRS complex; the R wave acts as the trigger for pump systole. The second mode is a dynamic mode that allows the pump to respond to the changing heart rate, depending on patient activity level. Pump systole and cardiac output depend on the blood flow sensed by the device, which is programmed to respond to changes in pump filling rate as blood passes from the left ventricle into the blood sac of the pump drive. This ability is particularly important as a patient's level of activity increases during the recovery phase after implantation. A third mode of operation, rarely used clinically, is a fixed-rate mode that functions independently of the native heart.

Nursing Implications

Historically, VAD recipients have received care in the ICU, usually intubated and sedated. Evolution of the technology and the use of portable devices as bridges to transplantation have changed the mode of care. Now, patients are encouraged to be independent, pursue physical rehabilitation, and engage in normal activities of daily living when possible (Fig. 18-27). Certain patients may even be discharged from the hospital. Nursing has an opportunity to be instrumental in the coordination of patient care and outcomes management with this new patient population.

During the immediate postoperative phase, the critical care nurse must be cognizant of the physiological responses expected and the common postoperative complications associated with device implantation. The nurse determines whether the equipment is functioning appropriately by monitoring parameters associated with adequate tissue perfusion and improved end-organ function because these are the primary goals of VAD implantation. Hemodynamic instability and the maintenance of adequate filling pressures are critical issues in the immediate postoperative period. Other issues the critical care nurse encounters include, but are not limited to, dysrhythmias, bleeding complications, infections, thromboembolic events, and possible mechanical problems associated with the devices.

Psychosocial issues and patient education dominate the nursing focus during periods of extended support with a VAD; most of these patients require minimal direct nursing care once stabilized and discharged from the ICU. Increased independence in activities of daily living, continued physical rehabilitation, and patient education are emphasized. All aspects of the rehabilitation phase should include the recipient's family members or identified support person. As patients are discharged, they and their primary caregivers need to be educated on the operation of the equipment and how to troubleshoot malfunctions. An individual capable of operating the VAD needs to accom-

table 18-13 Ventricular Assist Devices

Manufacturer/Device	Type	Approved Use	Comments
Abiomed BVS 5000	Pneumatic	Univentricular or biventricular support Bridge to transplantation	External pulsatile pump Cannulation sites Atria Pulmonary artery Ascending aorta
Thoratec VAD	Pneumatic	Univentricular or biventricular support Bridge to transplantation	External pulsatile pump Paracorporeal (blood flows though cannulas that pass through chest wall to external pump) Biventricular assist device can be used to support both ventricles
Novacor	Electric	Left ventricular assist device	Implantable pulsatile pump Implanted in the upper abdomen Cannulation sites Left ventricular apex Ascending aorta
BioMedicus	Centrifugal	Univentricular or biventricular support	External nonpulsatile pump Cannulation sites Left atrium (LVAD) Right atrium Aorta (by way of femoral artery)
HeartMate IP	Pneumatic	Left ventricular assist device	Implantable pulsatile pump Cannulation site Left ventricular apex
HeartMate VE	Electric	Left ventricular assist device Permanent implantation (destination therapy)	Implantable pulsatile pump Cannulation site Left ventricular apex Approved for coverage by CMS
Arrow LionHeart	Electric—wireless (transcutaneous energy transfer)	Left ventricular assist "heart helper" in clinical trial only	Implantable pulsatile pump Uses wireless technology for recharging Cannulation site Left ventricular apex
World Heart HeartSaver	Electric—wireless (transcutaneous energy transfer)	Left ventricular assist "heart helper" in clinical trial only	Implantable pulsatile pump Uses wireless technology for recharging Cannulation site Left ventricular apex

pany the patient at all times. Nursing must facilitate the integration of the patient's lifestyle with the boundaries created by having a VAD implanted for extended support. Feelings of isolation may unfold because investigational device protocols governed by the FDA may restrict the patients' social activity and geographical mobility.

An advanced-practice nurse is in a pivotal position to assume the role of case manager facilitating the implementation of clinical paths, protocols, and procedures related to patient progress from the acute to chronic phases of rehabilitation. Nursing education facilitated by a clinical nurse specialist will be vital to patient care as increasing numbers of nurses on the general floors, and possibly the outpatient setting, are exposed to this patient population. As more patients receive the portable devices and approach the possibility of hospital discharge, case management will be a principal facet of patient care.

COMPLICATIONS ASSOCIATED WITH INTRA-AORTIC BALLOON PUMP THERAPY AND CIRCULATORY SUPPORT

Bleeding

Prolongation of bleeding times is a side effect of exposure to CPB, which is normally reversed in the early postoperative period. With the use of mechanical circulatory support, the continued exposure of blood to an artificial surface causes trauma to platelets. A cascade of events involving the platelets, white blood cells, fibrinolytic system, and complement system occurs. The frequency and severity of bleeding associated with artificial circulatory devices have been reduced by improved surgical techniques and meth-

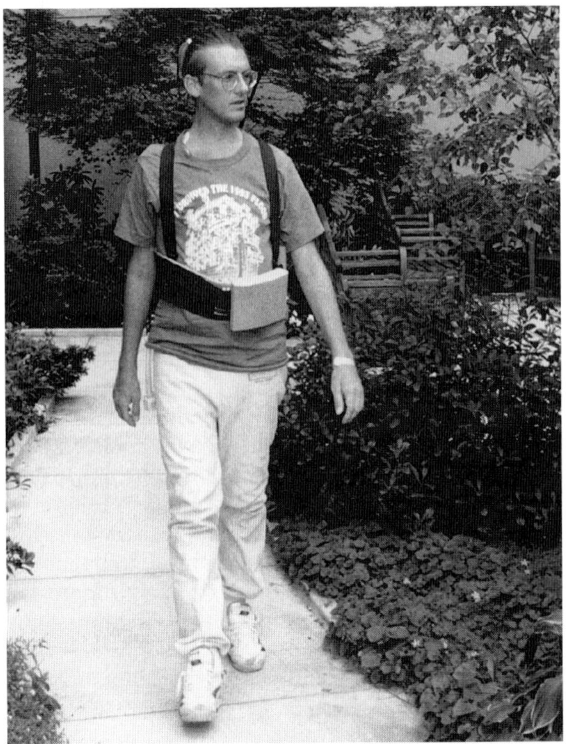

figure 18-27 Wearing the portable left ventricular assist system, a patient is able to enjoy the independence of outdoor activities. Some patients may take day trips or be discharged from the hospital. (Photograph courtesy of Stanford Health Services, Stanford, CA.)

ods of maintaining hemostasis, the reversal of heparin, the infusion of coagulation factors (platelets, fresh frozen plasma), and continued experience with the equipment. Episodes of severe bleeding are usually corrected within the first 24 hours after surgical implantation of a VAD.

Factors associated with increased postoperative bleeding in VAD recipients are preoperative and postoperative use of anticoagulants; coagulopathies secondary to cardiogenic shock, CHF, and extended CPB exposure; and the use of multiple cannulation sites. Hemodynamic instability, a reduction in native cardiac output and device output, a risk of ischemia to target organs, and possible cardiac tamponade are all deleterious events associated with uncontrolled bleeding in the patient supported with a VAD. In the patient receiving IABP therapy, bleeding is usually related to use of continuous anticoagulation or the development of coagulopathies. Bleeding commonly occurs at the insertion site of the balloon catheter. In both patient populations, nursing interventions include observing external cannulation sites for oozing, monitoring changes in vital signs (particularly hemodynamic parameters, such as filling pressures for VAD recipients) and laboratory values, and regularly assessing adequate tissue perfusion.

Thromboembolic Events

Placement of IABP puts a patient at risk for thromboembolic events. At the time of insertion, plaque may become dislodged from the vessel wall or emboli may break off a thrombus that has formed on the indwelling catheter or balloon. Both situations can impair circulation to distal extremities and other vital organs or cause a CVA. Continuous anticoagulation with a heparin infusion is required during IABP therapy; dextran infusions may also be used.

The development of a thrombus and the migration of emboli have been reported with the use of mechanical circulatory support. Anticoagulation regimens and the prevention of embolic events are unresolved issues in the clinical management of VAD recipients. Currently, anticoagulation therapy is managed differently depending on the device that is inserted. Devices used for short-term support require prophylactic use of low-dose heparin infusions. Similar to IABP, dextran infusions may be used in conjunction with heparin. Patients supported with the Novacor, HeartMate, and Thoratec devices who require long-term support are at greater risk secondary to extended periods of exposure to the device. These patients are usually managed with heparin infusions in the immediate postoperative phase. During the extended support period, the heparin is weaned and warfarin (Coumadin) therapy is initiated to maintain the prothrombin time at an INR of 3 to 4.[5] Antiplatelet agents, such as dipyridamole, may be used in conjunction with warfarin therapy. Obtaining baseline and postimplantation neurological assessments; monitoring peripheral pulses, especially those distal to cannulation sites; and assessing tissue perfusion are critical to the early recognition and intervention of any embolic event.

Right Ventricular Failure

Right ventricular failure continues to be a significant problem associated with LVAD implantation. Right ventricular failure develops in 20% to 25% of LVAD recipients after device implantation secondary to the physiological effects of the LVAD on systemic circulation.[6,7] Because the pumping capabilities of the device exceed those of the impaired left ventricle, systemic circulation and right ventricular preload increase, subsequently increasing right ventricular workload. Right ventricular output is increased in a patient with a healthy right ventricle. A patient with underlying right ventricular failure, however, may not be able to handle this augmentation in circulatory volume. Evidence of primary right ventricular dysfunction may not become apparent until the right heart is challenged by the cardiac output of the LVAD.[7,8] When right ventricular failure develops after LVAD implantation, vasodilators and IV inotropes, such as prostaglandin E_1, isoproterenol, and epinephrine, are used to reduce pulmonary pressures and improve right ventricular contractility. It may be possible to add an RVAD for additional support if pharmacological intervention is unsuccessful. Clinical practice has shown that the addition of an RVAD after LVAD placement is a poor prognostic indicator.[6]

Infection

Individuals requiring mechanical circulatory assistance and IABP therapy are at increased risk for infection secondary to the surgical procedures and the presence of external cannulas, pumps, drivelines, and so forth. Many of these patients suffer from chronic illness that render them more immunocompromised. Infection may be related to surgical wounds after device insertion, invasive monitoring lines, drain placement, pulmonary status, or nutritional status. Early recognition of signs and symptoms of infection and early intervention can prevent the development of sepsis. Early detection is particularly important because some of these patients await heart transplantation, and an infection could preclude transplantation. Diligent handwashing, changing or removing invasive lines or drainage tubes when appropriate, adherence to sterile dressing techniques and schedules, and the use of appropriate prophylactic antibiotics are effective barriers to the development of infection. Early extubation and mobilization are goals for patients with the implanted devices. Primary nursing interventions include monitoring invasive sites for signs of infection, encouraging good pulmonary toilet, increasing activity level as tolerated, and promoting adequate nutrition.

Dysrhythmias

Most patients with cardiomyopathy who require some form of circulatory assistance experience dysrhythmias before insertion of a device. These dysrhythmias often continue after device implantation and may hinder device function depending on the rhythm. Dysrhythmias should be treated when they occur, and attempts should be made to restore sinus rhythm.

Circulatory assistance with IABP is affected by dysrhythmias. Diastolic augmentation and systolic assistance decrease in the presence of irregular rhythms, such as atrial fibrillation or sinus rhythm with frequent ectopy. These rhythm changes make it difficult to manage the timing of balloon inflation and deflation. Lethal ventricular dysrhythmias need to be treated conventionally because IABP is designed only to augment existing cardiac output.

Right ventricular function and the maintenance of adequate pump output are of primary concern in LVAD recipients with lethal ventricular dysrhythmias. These patients may lack sufficient right ventricular function to support cardiac output during ventricular dysrhythmia even though left ventricular function has been assumed by the LVAD. Although LVAD flow and mean blood pressure have been known to decrease by approximately 20%, it has been demonstrated that patients with LVADs do tolerate sustained lethal ventricular dysrhythmias without the need for RVAD support. Symptoms associated with these rhythms and low-flow states are usually weakness and palpitations.[9] Patients receiving biventricular support should be able to maintain adequate device outputs despite the dysrhythmia because left and right ventricular function has been taken over by the VAD. Atrial fibrillation is usually tolerated by these patients even though it may have some effect on right heart function. Severe bradycardia and tachydysrhythmia need to be addressed because they will change pump flow and output. Cardiac rhythms require close monitoring for any acute changes.

Nutritional Deficits

Nutritional status is an important element of any recovery process. Many patients have had end-stage CHF and are nutritionally depleted before any surgical intervention, placing them at a higher risk for nutritional deficits during the postoperative phase. Adequate nutrition is necessary for wound healing. Obtaining dietary consultation, encouraging increased oral intake, and providing flexibility with meals will assist these patients in meeting their nutritional goals. Patients supported by IABP and VADs that require intubation and sedation require parenteral or enteral feedings. Those with implanted devices eventually progress to a regular diet but may need smaller, more frequent meals. Experiencing feelings of fullness or early satiety is not uncommon for these patients due to the abdominal placement of the device.

Psychosocial Factors

Balloon and VAD insertion are usually unplanned, emergent interventions for a deteriorating condition. Abundant monitoring is frightening for both patient and family; therefore, explanations of procedures and surroundings are very important. Family members need to be prepared before visiting their loved one immediately after device insertion. The goal is to alleviate anxiety and to help the patient and family feel more secure in a foreign environment. Honest communication is important. This helps the family members recognize changes in their loved one's condition and make informed, realistic decisions regarding the patient's care. Putting the family in contact with nonmedical personnel who can objectively provide emotional support is often beneficial. Issues that families and patients struggle with are fear, hopelessness, and death.

Critically ill patients often suffer from disorientation and sleep deprivation. Immobility and unfamiliar noises of the ICU tend to increase stress and anxiety. Mechanisms to help alleviate this stress and anxiety include frequent reorientation by the nursing staff and contact with family members. Better organization of time and procedures also reduces stress because it allows the patient longer periods of uninterrupted rest.

Management of Dysrhythmias

CARDIOVERSION

Electrical countershock therapy is useful in converting supraventricular and ventricular dysrhythmias to sinus rhythm, especially when the patient becomes hemodynamically unstable or does not convert to a normal rhythm with pharmacological agents. As opposed to defibrillation, which delivers an unsynchronized current to the heart through the chest wall in an attempt to convert pulseless ventricular tachycardia/fibrillation to sinus rhythm (see section on Cardiopulmonary Resuscitation, later), cardioversion delivers a shock that is synchronized with the heart's activity. By setting the defibrillator to the synchronized mode, the device detects the patient's R wave and delivers the shock during ventricular depolarization. As a result, there is no danger of the shock

table 18-14 Indications and Energy Requirements for Cardioversion

Indications	Energy in Joules (J)
Monomorphic ventricular tachycardia with a pulse	100–360
Supraventricular tachycardia	100
Atrial flutter	50 initially
Atrial fibrillation	200 initially

being delivered during ventricular repolarization (T wave), which could result in spontaneous ventricular fibrillation. Indications for cardioversion and recommendations for initial joules used are listed in Table 18-14.[1–3] Precautions, relative contraindications, and resulting complications for cardioversion are described in Table 18-15.

The energy needed to convert monomorphic ventricular tachycardia with a pulse may be as low as 100 J initially, followed by 200, 300, or 360 J, as necessary for conversion. The energy required for conversion of paroxysmal supraventricular tachycardia (PSVT) and atrial flutter starts at 50 J initially. Further increases in energy may be needed for conversion. The energy required to convert atrial fibrillation is greater, starting at 200 J with increases to 400 J if necessary.[3] After conversion to sinus rhythm, further antidysrhythmic therapy should be initiated. Although recommendations are made for the number of joules needed to convert various rhythms, the actual energy needed varies with the duration of the dysrhythmia, rate, morphology, and underlying cause of the dysrhythmias, as well as transthoracic impedance.

Procedure

The steps for cardioversion are as follows:

1. Restrict the patient's food and water for 6 to 8 hours before cardioversion, unless emergency cardioversion is required.
2. If the patient is on chronic digitalis, confirm that digoxin levels are therapeutic. Patients with digitalis toxicity should not undergo elective cardioversion until levels are normalized.
3. Explain the procedure to the patient, and obtain informed consent.
4. Record a 12-lead ECG and vital signs, establish an IV line, and ready all necessary resuscitation equipment.
5. Turn on the defibrillator and monitor, and attach the monitoring electrodes to the patient's chest. Avoid placing the electrodes in the area where the defibrillation paddles will be positioned. Some devices permit both monitoring and defibrillation through disposable defibrillation patches.
6. Select a monitoring lead that provides a good ECG pattern with a tall R wave. If monitoring by way of the disposable defibrillator patches, select "paddles" lead.
7. Turn on the synchronizer mode button. The size of the R wave or the monitored lead may need to be adjusted until the synchronization marker appears on each R wave.
8. Sedate the patient, and maintain an adequate airway (see Conscious Sedation, Chapter 14).
9. Remove paddles and apply a generous amount of electrode jelly to them, or apply gel pads to the chest wall. This is done to prevent skin burns and decrease electrical resistance. Care should be taken not to smear electrode gel between the two paddles on the chest. Disposable pregelled defibrillator patches may be selected rather than using standard paddles. When using patches, be sure that there are no air pockets by applying the patches firmly from the center to the periphery. Air pockets can cause skin burns.
10. Apply paddles, one just below the right clavicle and the other over the apex of the heart. If anterior-posterior patches are used, place the anterior patch over the left precordium and the posterior one behind the heart in the left infrascapular location. Make sure the paddles/patches are away from electrode wires or from an implanted pacemaker or implantable cardioverter–defibrillator generator.
11. Set the desired energy level.
12. Press the charge button. A light will flash until paddles are fully charged.
13. Reconfirm the synchronization markers on the R waves on the monitor.
14. Call out "clear" to make sure no one is touching the patient or the bed.
15. Discharge the paddles while applying firm pressure. Push and hold both paddle discharge buttons until the defibrillator discharges. Maintain contact on the chest wall until the machine has delivered the shock. There will be a momentary delay from the pressing of the discharge button to delivery of the shock because of the synchronization with the R wave. Failure to keep the paddles on the chest can result in failure to cardiovert and burns to the chest.

table 18-15 Precautions/Relative Contraindications to Cardioversion

Condition	Complications
Digitalis toxicity	Ventricular irritability, asystole
Hypokalemia	Ventricular irritability/fibrillation
Atrial fibrillation with slow ventricular response	Postcardioversion asystole
Atrial fibrillation of unknown duration with inadequate anticoagulation	Thromboembolization
Pacemaker dependency	Rise in thresholds with loss of capture
Low-amplitude R wave	Synchronization on T wave leading to ventricular fibrillation

16. Remove the paddles, and assess the patient's rhythm and vital signs.
17. Subsequent shocks may need to be delivered. If so, be certain to select the synchronized mode.
18. If the patient's rhythm deteriorates to ventricular fibrillation, turn off the synchronizer and immediately defibrillate the patient, starting with 200 J and increasing to 360 J as needed.
19. After cardioversion, observe the patient for changes in rhythm, blood pressure, and respirations. Patients with atrial fibrillation with slow ventricular rates in the absence of AV nodal blocking agents may have underlying sinus node dysfunction. Be prepared for transcutaneous pacing if needed, or have atropine sulfate readily available. If a patient has a pacemaker, the pacemaker may need to be interrogated or reprogrammed because a temporary rise in capture thresholds may follow cardioversion. Older pacemaker models may revert to a reset or backup mode.
20. Further antidysrhythmic agents may need to be administered to maintain sinus rhythm.
21. Monitor the patient's respiratory status and level of consciousness because sedation was delivered before the procedure. Inspect the chest wall for any signs of burns and treat appropriately.
22. Clean the paddles thoroughly before storing them in the device.
23. Document the procedure, the outcomes of the procedure, and the patient's status in the medical record.

RADIOFREQUENCY CATHETER ABLATION

Radiofrequency catheter ablation is an invasive procedure used for the treatment of dysrhythmias. The technique uses an endovascular catheter to isolate and achieve localized destruction of cardiac tissue responsible for the initiation or conduction of the dysrhythmia.

Clinical use of catheter ablation of cardiac tissue began in 1982. Direct current shocks were delivered to the cardiac tissue through a catheter attached to a defibrillator. Because this technique was associated with significant complications, safer means to ablate tissue were investigated.

Radiofrequency energy is now used as the means to ablate cardiac tissue. A form of electrical energy, radiofrequency energy is produced by alternating current delivered at 300 to 750 kHz that is passed through tissue. Heat is created as the energy dissipates, which results in a small, localized lesion in cardiac tissue. If properly targeted, this localized area of damage can prevent the initiation of the dysrhythmia or interrupt the conduction of the dysrhythmia. The amount of heat produced and the size of the resulting lesion depend on the frequency, amount, and duration of the alternating current used. The size and shape of the ablating electrode also influence the resulting lesion.

Indications for Ablation

A PSVT can be treated with radiofrequency ablation. Most PSVTs are caused by either AV nodal reentrant tachycardia (AVNRT) or by AV reentrant tachycardia (AVRT). PSVT also can be caused by intra-atrial reentrant tachycardia. Recurrent symptomatic or life-threatening ventricular dysrhythmias may also be indications for ablation. Indications for intracardiac electrophysiological and catheter ablation procedures are included in the 1995 guidelines developed by the American College of Cardiology (ACC) and American Heart Association (AHA) in collaboration with the North American Association of Pacing and Electrophysiology (NASPE/Heart Rhythm Society).[4]

Reentry occurs when conduction of an impulse through myocardial tissue is blocked (or functionally refractory, unresponsive to stimuli) in one direction. The advancing wavefront proceeds through an alternate slower route. Slow conduction allows recovery of excitability of the previously refractory pathway/tissues and the impulse reenters where it started. As a result, a circular reentrant pattern of conduction occurs, which is the most common mechanism associated with PSVTs.

ATRIOVENTRICULAR NODAL REENTRANT TACHYCARDIA

Two functional pathways for conduction can exist in the AV node: a slow pathway and a fast pathway. When both are present, the AV node is described as having dual physiology. AVNRT, the most common type of PSVT, occurs when an AV node with dual physiology is stimulated by a premature atrial contraction. The fast pathway, which is preferentially used in normal sinus rhythm, has not recovered, so the impulse travels down the slow pathway and activates the ventricles. On surface ECG, this initiating rhythm would be viewed as a premature atrial contraction with a long PR interval. The impulse then returns back up to the atria through the fast pathway, which has now recovered excitability, then back down to the ventricles by the slow pathway, causing the reentrant circuit to perpetuate. Selective ablation of the slow pathway is the preferred method of treating AVNRT. The fast-pathway ablation sites are closer to the compact AV node, and ablation of the fast pathway may be complicated by high-grade AV block.

ATRIOVENTRICULAR REENTRANT TACHYCARDIA

In the normal heart, the AV node and the bundle of His serve as the connection between the atria and the ventricles for the conducting system. AVRT rhythms are characterized by the presence of additional accessory pathways that link conduction between the atria and the ventricles. Conduction through accessory pathways may be from the atria to the ventricles (antegrade conduction), from the ventricles to the atria (retrograde conduction), or in both directions. AVRT rhythms result when circular movement of the impulse occurs because of the ability of the accessory pathways to conduct signals in either direction.

In WPW syndrome, an ECG pattern associated with PSVT and sometimes with Ebstein's anomaly of the tricuspid valve, the person has an anomalous conduction accessory pathway or pathways linking the atria and the ventricles. Because of the presence of these accessory pathways, the person with WPW syndrome is prone to AVRT and atrial fibrillation.

When rapidly conducting, these PSVTs may deteriorate into ventricular fibrillation. Ablation of the accessory pathway(s) is used to interrupt the rapid limb of the reentrant circuit and eliminate the offending dysrhythmias.

ATRIAL FIBRILLATION OR FLUTTER

Ablation therapy may be indicated for patients with atrial fibrillation/flutter with a rapid ventricular response that has not been controlled by pharmacological therapy. The AV junction may be ablated to control the ventricular response. Successful ablation usually results in complete heart block with a nodal escape rhythm at a rate of 40 to 60 beats/minute. A permanent pacemaker is inserted to ensure the presence of a reliable rhythm and adequate rate, and to reduce the risk of bradycardia-dependent torsades de pointes.

Ablation therapy for primary atrial flutter is indicated in those patients who have reentrant circuits in the right atrium. Ablation lesions are directed at creating a line of block along a narrow isthmus between the inferior vena cava and tricuspid annulus to interrupt the circuit. When successful, atrial flutter ablation can provide a permanent cure for atrial flutter. Unlike AV node ablation, atrial flutter ablation does not require permanent pacemaker implantation.

VENTRICULAR DYSRHYTHMIAS

The success of ablation for the treatment of ventricular tachycardia depends on the cause of the dysrhythmia. Radiofrequency ablation has been shown to be effective in patients with ventricular tachycardia in structurally normal hearts and in patients with ventricular tachycardia due to bundle branch reentry. The technique also has had some limited success in patients with hemodynamically stable, monomorphic ventricular tachycardia associated with a healed myocardial scar. It is, however, not unusual to have multiple morphologies (forms) of ventricular tachycardia in this population, and some unstable morphologies may not be amenable to ablation.

Procedure

Several days or just before an ablation, the patient undergoes an electrophysiological study (EPS) to evaluate the electrical activity of the heart. The EPS is an invasive test in which catheters are placed in the heart to record intracardiac ECGs. The test provides information about the sequence of activation of the heart during sinus rhythm and any abnormal sequence of activation during a dysrhythmia. (For a more detailed discussion of EPS, see Chapter 17).

Once a diagnosis of the dysrhythmia is made by EPS, an ablating catheter is positioned in the targeted area of the heart. Additional catheters are positioned in the right heart to stimulate atrial and ventricular tissue and to help localize the target area. The ablation catheter contains multiple electrodes designed to localize the site of the dysrhythmia and to deliver the ablation current. The shaft of the catheter can be extended or flexed at the tip to provide access to the abnormal tissue and to ensure direct contact with the tissue. Fluoroscopy and the electrogram pattern from the catheter help the physician determine the appropriate target area.

After the catheters are positioned, ECG recordings are made from the surface electrodes on the patient's chest and from the intracardiac electrodes. Programmed electrical stimulation (PES) is then performed to induce the dysrhythmia so that its mechanism and pathway can be evaluated. The clinical ECG of the tachycardia is sometimes used as a template when several morphologies of the dysrhythmia are induced. When the appropriate site is identified, the radiofrequency current is applied for about 30 seconds. Enough lesions are created until the abnormal conducting tissue is eliminated. Successful elimination of the target site is determined by examining the surface and intracardiac tracings and confirmed when the dysrhythmia is no longer inducible. When the procedure is finished, the intracardiac catheters and venous sheaths are removed, and efforts to attain hemostasis at the insertion site are implemented.

Nursing Management

The nurse plays a vital role in the care of the patient undergoing radiofrequency ablation. In collaboration with the physician, the nurse provides information to the patient and family about what to expect before, during, and after the procedure. The psychosocial support provided by the nurse may be crucial in helping the patient and family cope with the uncertainties of dysrhythmia management.

PREABLATION

The nurse participates in educating the patient and family about radiofrequency ablation. Box 18-19 provides a

box 18-19
Preablation Teaching

- Purpose of the procedure
- The patient's dysrhythmia and how the procedure will help
- Interventions before transport to the electrophysiology laboratory
- The electrophysiology laboratory:
  - The appearance of the laboratory
  - The equipment in the laboratory
  - The personnel in the laboratory
- The use of IV conscious sedation
- The amnesic/analgesic effect of conscious sedation:
  - Possible side effects such as nausea, vomiting, or hypotension
- Sensations associated with the procedure:
  - Cool sensation from cleansing agents
  - Pressure sensation from catheter insertion
  - Palpitations, dizziness, or other sensations when the patient's dysrhythmia is induced
  - Possible mild burning sensation during ablation
  - Restlessness or back discomfort from lying immobilized
  - Anticipated length of the procedure
  - Potential for placement of a permanent pacemaker
- Anticipated after effects:
  - Skipped beats or faster than usual resting rate may be felt initially
  - Mild chest discomfort or burning may occur for a few days
  - "Skin effect," which is a dark outline of the grounding or defibrillation pad, may be noticeable and may persist for a few months

guide for patient and family education. During the preablation period, the nurse records a 12-lead ECG, continuously monitors the patient's cardiac rhythm, and treats any dysrhythmias per the physician's orders. Other baseline data obtained include vital signs, breath sounds, fluid status, serum chemistries, prothrombin time, and complete blood counts. Antidysrhythmic drugs are usually stopped 2 to 3 days before the procedure. The patient receives nothing by mouth for about 8 hours before the procedure. Because of x-ray exposure during the test, it is important to verify that a female patient is not pregnant. No activity restrictions are imposed before the procedure.

DURING ABLATION

The nurse in the electrophysiology laboratory is responsible for monitoring of the patient throughout the procedure and assisting the physician with necessary interventions. The nurse must be competent in advanced cardiac life support so that an emergency situation can be handled appropriately.

Once the patient arrives in the laboratory, the nurse explains all procedures to the patient and helps to put the patient at ease. The nurse connects the patient to an automatic external defibrillator, a grounding pad, physiological recorder, cardiac monitor, automatic blood pressure device, and pulse oximeter. Oxygen is provided by a nasal cannula. If not already in place, an IV line is inserted. IV conscious sedation is administered to ensure patient comfort. A urinary catheter is inserted if the procedure is anticipated to be lengthy. Both groins and the right subclavian vein sites are shaved and the skin prepared. A sterile field is established and maintained throughout the procedure. A lead apron is placed under the patient's lower back to block fluoroscopy radiation from penetrating the reproductive system.

Throughout the procedure, the nurse monitors hemodynamic status, activated clotting time (ACT) if heparin is used, sedation level, and patient comfort. Communication with the patient is essential so that the patient is kept informed about the progress of the procedure, and anxiety and fear are minimized. The nurse also warns the patient that a burning sensation may be felt for a very brief time during the actual ablation.

POSTABLATION

Thorough assessment and monitoring of the patient are continued after the ablation procedure. Essential components of the assessment include vital signs, cardiac rhythm, catheter insertion sites, peripheral pulses, and level of consciousness. The patient may remain drowsy for several hours and experience nausea and vomiting as a result of the medications. When an arterial site has been used, leg immobilization and bed rest are maintained for about 6 hours. If only venous sites were used, the patient may begin ambulation in about 4 hours. The nurse assesses the patient for any pain or discomfort and provides comfort measures if indicated. Fluid volume status is checked, and when stable, the urinary catheter is removed.

During the postablation period, the nurse carefully assesses the patient for any evidence of complications. Table 18-16 lists potential complications of radiofrequency ablation and associated signs and symptoms.

table 18-16 Potential Complications of Radiofrequency Ablation and Associated Signs and Symptoms

Complications	Signs and Symptoms
Cardiac perforation	Tachycardia, hypotension, dyspnea, pleuritic chest pain
Cardiac tamponade	Hypotension, distended neck veins, muffled heart sounds, pulsus paradoxus, change in level of consciousness
Coronary artery spasm	Chest pain, ECG changes
Pneumothorax	Dyspnea, decreased oxygen saturation decreased breath sounds
Cerebral embolus	Slurred speech, blurred vision, headache, seizures
Pulmonary embolus	Chest pain, dyspnea, tachycardia
Deep venous thrombosis	Swelling of leg at site of catheter insertion, calf pain

CARDIAC PACEMAKERS

Electrical stimulation of the heart was tried experimentally as early as 1819. In 1930, Hyman noted that he could inject the right atrium with a diversity of substances and restore a heart beat. He devised an "ingenious apparatus" that he labeled an artificial pacemaker, which delivered a rhythmical charge to the heart. In 1952, Zoll demonstrated that patients with Stokes-Adams syndrome could be sustained by the administration of current directly to the chest wall. In 1957, Lillehei affixed electrodes directly to the ventricles during open heart surgery.

From 1958 to 1961, implantable pacemakers became accepted treatment for complete heart block. In the 1970s and 1980s, AV synchrony and "physiological" pacing became available. The start of the decade 2000 introduced right and left ventricular (biventricular) synchronization with AV synchrony. Currently, technological advances have resulted in smaller pacemakers with longer battery life and numerous programmable options. The goal of individualized, physiological pacing has been achieved with more recent types of pacemakers.

Indications for Cardiac Pacing

Cardiac pacing is indicated for conditions that result in failure of the heart to initiate or conduct an intrinsic electrical impulse at a rate adequate to maintain perfusion. Pacemakers are necessary when dysrhythmias or conduction defects compromise the electrical system and the hemodynamic response of the heart. The original pacemakers were designed to treat bradydysrhythmias, whereas today's pacemakers are intended to treat bradydysrhythmias and tachydysrhythmias. Further research and advances in technology have allowed for the use of pacemakers in heart conditions such as congestive heart failure (cardiac resynchronization therapy), hypertrophic cardiomyopathy, and vasovagal syncope.[5]

Critical care nurses work with members of the health care team to assess potential pacemaker patients who may exhibit dysrhythmias, atherosclerotic heart disease, AMI, or other conditions that alter the conduction of the heart. To assist medical professionals in determining the clinical criteria for pacemaker implantation, a Joint Committee of the American College of Cardiology and the American Heart Association was formed to establish uniform criteria for pacemaker implantation.[6] The Committee divided its recommendations for implantation into three classes. Class I includes conditions when a pacemaker implantation is considered necessary. Class II includes conditions when pacemaker implantation may be necessary, but there is some divergence of opinion. Class III includes conditions when pacemaker implantation is not effective or may be harmful. The revised 1998 Committee recommendations for pacemaker implantation are summarized in Box 18-20.[6]

The Pacemaker System

Consisting of a pulse generator and a lead with electrodes, a pacemaker system performs two main functions: diagnosis and treatment. The diagnostic function is to sense intrinsic cardiac activity; the treatment function is to emit an electrical impulse that excites endocardial cells and produces a wave of depolarization in the myocardium. Clinical terminology regarding pacemakers can be found in Box 18-21.

THE PULSE GENERATOR

The pulse generator for a permanent pacemaker is composed of a lithium iodide battery source and electronic circuits enclosed in a hermetically sealed metal container. The generator weighs 20 to 30 g and is 5 to 7 mm thick (Fig. 18-28). The longevity of most permanent pacemakers is about 6 to 12 years, depending on the percentage of pacing the heart requires over time. Most permanent pulse generators are inserted in a subcutaneous pocket in the pectoral region below the clavicle (Fig. 18-29).

THE LEAD SYSTEM

The lead is a wire that provides the communication network between the pulse generator and the heart muscle. One or more electrodes are at the distal end of the lead and provide sensing and pacing of the heart muscle. In a bipolar lead, the negative electrode (cathode) is at the tip and

box 18-20
Indications for Permanent Cardiac Pacing

Atrioventricular Block

Class I: Symptomatic second-degree AV block; symptomatic complete heart block; asymptomatic complete heart block with a heart rate <40 beats/minute or asystolic pause ≥3.0 seconds while awake or after AV node ablation

Class II: Asymptomatic second-degree type II heart block; complete heart block with average awake heart rate ≥40 beats/minute, symptomatic first-degree AV block with documented hemodynamic improvement by temporary AV pacing studies

Class III: Asymptomatic first-degree AV block and type I second-degree AV block, transient AV block

Chronic Bifascicular or Trifascicular Block

Class I: Bifascicular block with intermittent complete heart block; bifascicular or trifascicular block with type II second-degree AV block

Class II: Bifascicular or trifascicular block associated with syncope not proved to be due to AV block when other likely causes have been excluded; prolonged His–ventricular (HV) interval on electrophysiological study in asymptomatic patients

Class III: Fascicular block without AV block or symptoms and asymptomatic fascicular block with first-degree AV block

Sinus Node Dysfunction

Class I: Sinus node dysfunction with documented symptomatic bradycardia and symptomatic chronotropic incompetence

Class II: Sinus node dysfunction with chronic awake heart rate <30 beats/minute with minimal or no symptoms

Class III: Sinus node dysfunction in asymptomatic patients; sinus node dysfunction in patients in whom symptoms are clearly documented not to be associated with bradycardia; sinus node dysfunction with symptomatic bradycardia due to nonessential drug therapy

Hypersensitive Carotid Sinus Syndrome and Neurocardiogenic Syncope

Class I: Recurrent syncope associated with clear, spontaneous events provoked by carotid sinus stimulation; asystole of >3 seconds induced by minimal carotid sinus pressure in the absence of any medication that depresses sinus and AV node conduction

Class II: Recurrent syncope without clear, provocative events and a hypersensitive cardioinhibitory response; syncope associated with bradycardia reproduced by a head-up tilt

Class III: Recurrent syncope in the absence of a cardioinhibitory response; a hyperactive cardioinhibitory response in the absence of symptoms; situational vasovagal syncope improved by avoidance behavior

Tachydysrhythmias

Class I: Symptomatic recurrent supraventricular tachycardia refractory or intolerant to drugs and failing ablation

Class II: An alternative to drug therapy or ablation in patients with recurrent pace-terminable supraventricular tachycardia

Class III: Tachycardias that are accelerated or converted to fibrillation by pacing or in the presence of rapidly conducting AV pathways

Adapted from Gregoratos G, Cheitlin MD, Conill A, et al: ACC/AHA guidelines for implantation of cardiac pacemakers and antiarrhythmia devices. A report of the American College of Cardiology/American Heart Association Task Force on Practice Guidelines (Committee on Pacemaker Implantation). J Am Coll Cardiol 31:1175–1209, 1998.

box 18-21
Clinical Terminology Regarding Pacemakers

Active fixation lead: A pacing lead with some design at the lead tip (corkscrew, coil) that allows the tip to be embedded in heart tissue, thus decreasing the likelihood of dislodgement.

Asynchronous pacing: The pacemaker releases a pacing stimulus at the programmed rate regardless of the heart's intrinsic activity. No sensing occurs, so the pacemaker fires in competition with the heart's natural rhythm.

Base rate: The rate at which the pacemaker paces when no intrinsic cardiac activity is present. Also is called the *minimum rate* or *lower rate*.

Bipolar lead: Having two poles. (1) A pacing lead with two electrical poles. The negative pole is the distal tip of the lead and the positive pole is a metal ring located a few millimeters proximal to the distal tip. The stimulating pulse is delivered through the distal-tip electrode. (2) A pacing system with both electrical poles in or on the heart.

Capture: Ability of the pacing stimulus to depolarize the chamber being paced. Capture is recognized on the electrocardiogram whenever the pacing spike is followed immediately by the appropriate waveform: an atrial spike followed by a P wave or a ventricular spike followed by a wide QRS complex.

Chronotropic incompetence: Inability of the sinus node to accelerate in response to exercise.

Demand pacing: The pacemaker paces only when the heart's intrinsic rate is below the pacemaker's programmed rate (only when necessary, or on demand). This mode means that the pacemaker senses intrinsic cardiac activity and inhibits its output when intrinsic activity is present.

Dual-chamber pacing (physiological pacing): Pacing in both the atria and the ventricles to restore artificially atrioventricular synchrony.

Electromagnetic interference: Electrical signals from the environment (i.e., radiofrequency waves) that can be sensed by the pacemaker and interfere with pacer function; abbreviated as EMI.

Escape interval: The period between a sensed cardiac event and the next pacemaker output. The escape interval is usually equal to the basic pacing rate, but it can be programmed longer in some pacemakers (hysteresis).

Fusion beat: A cardiac depolarization (either atrial or ventricular) that results from two foci both contributing to depolarization of the chamber. In pacing, a fusion beat results when an intrinsic depolarization and a pacing stimulus occur simultaneously and both contribute to depolarization (usually seen in the ventricle.)

Hysteresis: A programmable feature in some pacemakers that allows the escape interval to be programmed longer than the basic pacing interval (the pacing interval after a sensed beat is longer than the basic pacing interval). This allows more time for the heart's intrinsic activity to occur.

Inhibited response: A type of response to sensing that inhibits pacemaker output when an intrinsic beat is sensed. This results in demand pacing, or pacing only when the heart's intrinsic activity is slower than the basic pacing rate.

Lead: The insulated wire and its electrode that transmits the pacing stimulus from the pulse generator to the heart and relays sensed intrinsic activity back to the pulse generator. A single-chamber pacemaker uses one lead and a dual-chamber pacemaker usually uses two leads, one in the atrium and one in the ventricle.

Magnet mode: The pacemaker's response when a magnet is placed over the pulse generator. A magnet inactivates the sensing circuitry and causes the pacemaker to function asynchronously at a predetermined rate and in a preset manner. The magnet mode differs among manufacturers in pacing rate and number of impulses delivered with the magnet in place. A change in magnet-induced pacing rate is often an indicator of battery depletion and warrants pulse generator replacement.

Milliamperage (mA): The unit of measure used for the electrical stimulus (output) generated by the pacemaker.

Output: The electrical stimulus delivered by the pulse generator, usually defined in terms of pulse amplitude (volts) and pulse widths (milliseconds).

Overdrive pacing: A method to suppress a tachycardia by pacing the heart at a rate faster than the patient's intrinsic rate.

Oversensing: Detection of inappropriate electrical signals by the pacemaker's sensing circuit, resulting in inappropriate inhibition of pacer output. Sources of oversensing can include electromagnetic interference, myopotential, T waves, or cross-talk between atrial and ventricular channels in dual-chamber pacemakers.

Pacing interval: The time between two consecutive paced events without an intervening sensed event. Measured in milliseconds. AA interval = atrial pacing interval; VV interval = ventricular pacing interval.

Pacing spike: The small vertical "blip" recorded on the electrocardiogram with every pacemaker output response. The presence of a pacing spike indicates that a stimulus was released by the pacemaker.

Pacing threshold: The minimum electrical stimulation required to initiate atrial or ventricular depolarization consistently.

Passive fixation lead: A pacing lead that lodges in the trabeculae of the heart without actually penetrating the cardiac wall.

Pulse generator: The device that contains the power source (battery) and the electronic circuits that control pacemaker function. The term *pacemaker* is commonly used for the pulse generator.

Rate modulation: The ability of a pacemaker to increase the pacing rate in response to physical activity or metabolic demand. The pacemaker uses some type of physiological sensor to determine the need for increased pacing rate. The most commonly used sensors are motion sensors and minute ventilation sensors. Also called *rate adaptation* or *rate response*.

(continued)

box 18-21
Clinical Terminology Regarding Pacemakers (Continued)

Refractory period: (1) In the heart, the period of time during which the myocardium is incapable of responding to a stimulus. (2) In the pacemaker, an interval or timing cycle after a sensed or paced event during which the pacemaker does not respond to incoming signals. A single-chamber pacemaker has one refractory period, and a dual-chamber pacemaker has an atrial refractory and a ventricular refractory period.

Sensing: The ability of the pacemaker to detect intrinsic cardiac activity and respond appropriately. How the pacemaker responds depends on the programmed mode of pacing.

Sensing threshold: The smallest intrinsic atrial or ventricular signal (measured in millivolts) that can be consistently sensed by the pacemaker.

Situational vasovagal syncope: Syncope associated with bradycardia by vagal stimulation during coughing, micturition, or severe pain.

Stimulation threshold: The minimum amount of voltage necessary to capture the heart consistently. Also called *capture threshold* or *pacing threshold.*

Triggered: A response to sensing in which the pacemaker fires a stimulus in response to intrinsic cardiac activity. In pacemaker terms, *triggered* is the opposite of *inhibited.*

Undersensing: Failure of a pacemaker to sense intrinsic cardiac depolarization. This can result in competition between the pacemaker and the intrinsic rhythm.

Unipolar: Having one pole. (1) A unipolar lead has only one pole, located at the distal tip. (2) A unipolar pacing system is one with one pole in or on the heart and the second pole located remote from the heart to complete the circuit. Permanent unipolar systems use the back of the pulse generator as the second pole. Temporary epicardial pacing systems use a ground wire in subcutaneous tissue as the second pole.

Adapted from Woods S, Froelicher ES, Motzer SU. Cardiac Nursing (4th Ed). Philadelphia, Lippincott Williams & Wilkins, 2000.

the positive electrode (anode) is approximately 1 to 3 cm proximal to the tip (Fig. 18-30).

The permanent pacemaker lead is typically inserted either through a subclavian vein or a cephalic vein through the chest wall. Alternate insertion sites include the external jugular, internal jugular, and, rarely, femoral vein. The lead is then positioned with fluoroscopic guidance and affixed in the right atrial appendage or into the apex of the right ventricle. A third lead may be inserted in a coronary sinus branch to stimulate the left ventricle for cardiac resynchronization. The lead(s) must provide adequate electrical conduction, be sufficiently insulated, and have the endurance to withstand pulsatile turbulence.

The permanent pacemaker lead can be affixed to the myocardium with a lead fixation device. Called *active fixation*, these devices include screws or coils. Another alternative is to use passive (tines) and steroid-eluting electrodes (tips designed to reduce cardiac inflammation) placed in the trabeculae of the heart (Fig. 18-31). Over time, fibrous tissue forms around the tip to secure placement and ensure proper function of the electrode.

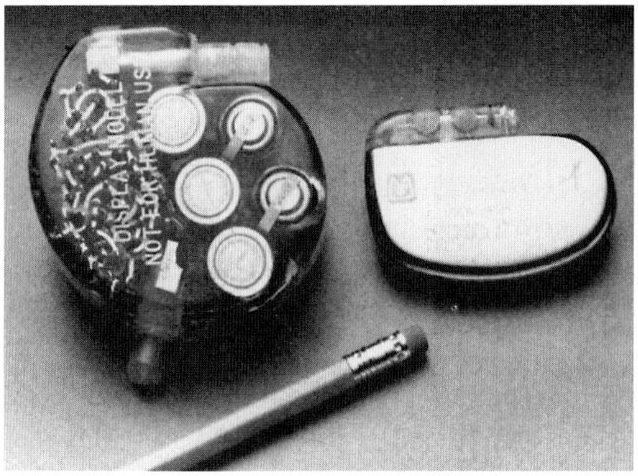

Temporary Pacing Systems

Temporary pacemaker systems are used in emergency and elective situations. In life-threatening situations, temporary pacemakers can be used for asystole, complete heart block, severe bradydysrhythmias, or during cardiac arrest. Electively, temporary pacemakers are used while evaluating the need for permanent pacing, after cardiac surgery, or for pace-terminating rapid supraventricular tachydysrhythmias. Temporary pacing systems can be transvenous, epicardial, transcutaneous, or transthoracic.

figure 18-28 Permanent pulse generators, old and new models. Note the decrease in size and weight that has been achieved over the years. The smaller unit is an example of an activity-responsive pulse generator and is four times smaller than the larger 1968 unit.

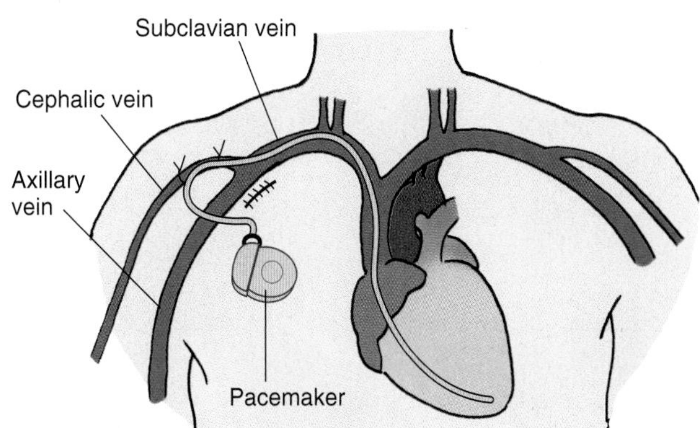

figure 18-29 Transvenous installation of a permanent pacemaker. For dual-chamber pacing, a separate pacing wire would be in the atrium.

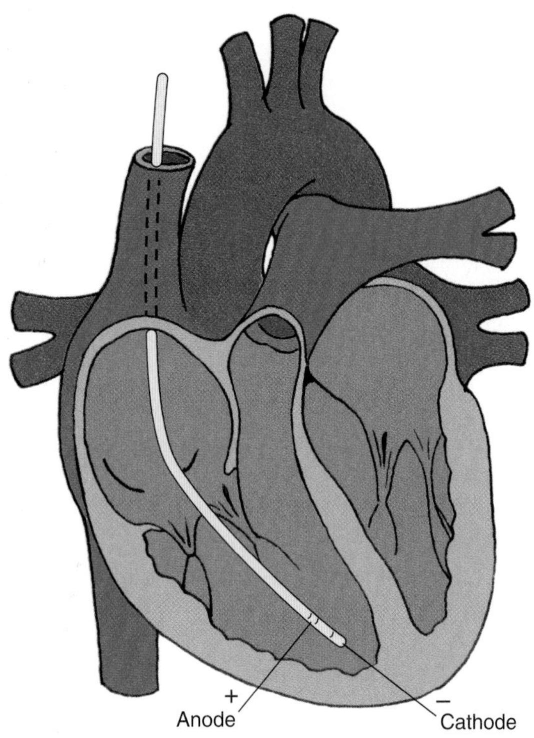

figure 18-30 Transvenous bipolar pacing catheter in place.

METHODS OF TEMPORARY PACING

A transvenous pacemaker system consists of an external pulse generator and a temporary transvenous pacing wire. The temporary transvenous lead system usually includes the use of a bipolar catheter. A bipolar catheter contains a negative (distal) electrode attached to the negative generator terminal on the pulse generator and the positive proximal electrode attached to the positive generator terminal on the pulse generator.

For temporary transvenous pacing, the catheter is introduced into a superficial vein, using local anesthesia. The brachial, internal or external jugular, subclavian, and femoral veins may be used. The subclavian and internal jugular sites afford catheter stability and allow for patient mobility. The pacing catheter is threaded through a sheath in the vein, into the vena cava and the right atrium, through the tricuspid valve, and into the right ventricle. The catheter tip is placed in contact with the endocardial surface of the right ventricular apex for stability and reliability (Fig. 18-30). For atrial pacing, an atrial bipolar catheter is placed in the right atrial appendage. There are also pulmonary artery balloon flotation catheters with atrial and ventricular pacing ports for dual-chamber pacing. Balloon flotation catheters are useful in the critical care setting because they provide thermodilution cardiac output determination and do not require fluoroscopy for positioning.

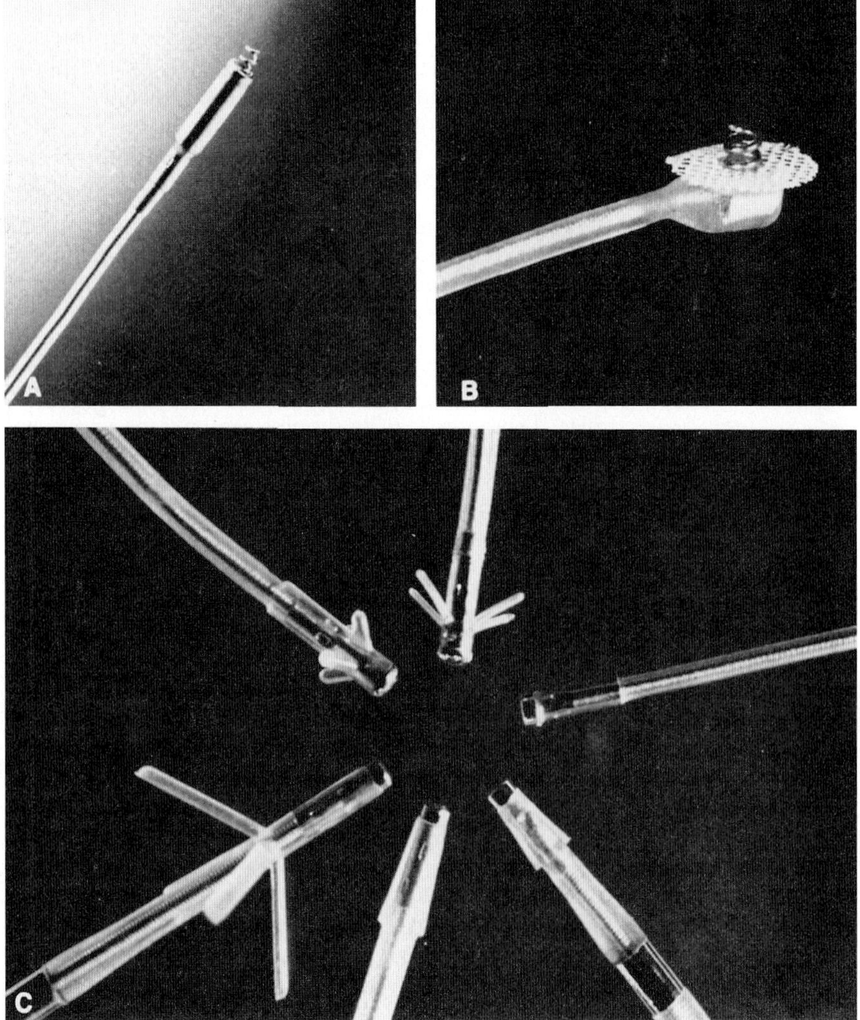

figure 18-31 Permanent pacemaker leads. (**A**) Active fixation, endocardial. (**B**) Active fixation, myocardial. (**C**) Passive fixation, endocardial.

After catheter placement, the leads are affixed at the skin entry site with nonabsorbable sutures. The sheath should be sutured and attached to a continuous drip if used for drawing blood or administering drugs. To enhance sterility at the connection site and terminal tip of the catheter, a sterile protective sleeve over the catheter can be used before insertion, and is connected to the end of the sheath after satisfactory position is confirmed. The sheath entry site should be covered with an antiseptic ointment and a self-adhesive, semipermeable transparent dressing. A small label above the dressing, initialed by the nurse, should indicate time and date of application.

Placement of epicardial wires provides another method for temporary pacing. This method can be accomplished by thoracotomy or through a subxiphoid incision with the placement of pacing electrodes directly on the surface of the heart. Epicardial wires often are used as a temporary adjunct during and after open heart surgery. The pacing wires are sutured or screwed to the epicardial surface of the heart, brought outside through the chest incision, and either connected to a temporary pacemaker generator or capped and then connected if the need arises. In a screw-in type electrode, the wires are extracted without reopening the incision, even after scar tissue has formed over the tips.

Another method of temporary pacing is known as *external transcutaneous pacing*. This method involves placing large gelled electrode patches directly on the chest wall. The cathode or negative electrode is applied anteriorly to the left of the sternum and the anode or positive electrode is applied posteriorly behind the anterior electrode, and then connected to an external transcutaneous pacemaker (Fig. 18-32). When first developed, transcutaneous pacing required higher amounts of electricity for pacing, resulting in pain, burns, and skeletal muscle twitching. Because of these problems, the method was abandoned. Today's technology has permitted the use of lower amounts of electrical current delivered through longer pulse widths, eliminating the skin burns. Transcutaneous pacing can still cause significant discomfort and the patient should be informed and adequately sedated, if necessary. Transcutaneous pacing is used when temporary transvenous pacing is not immediately available. It should not be relied on indefinitely, however, in patients with profound asystolic arrest.

Transthoracic pacing is a temporary pacing method used as a last resort in an emergency situation. This method involves introduction of a pacing lead into the heart through a needle in the anterior wall. Transthoracic pacing has limited success rates and a high potential for complications.

The pulse generator for a temporary transvenous, epicardial, or transthoracic pacing system is an external device powered by a 9-V alkaline or lithium replaceable battery (Fig. 18-33). Often called a *temporary pacemaker*, the device contains several controls that regulate the current output, rate, sensitivity, and the mode of pacing; for dual-chamber pacing, base and upper rate, AV interval, and refractory period settings can be chosen. A dual-chamber pulse generator has separate terminals for the atrial and ventricular inputs. The wires should be labeled appropriately in the distal portion: atrial or ventricular. Care should be taken not to interchange the electrode positions when attaching leads to the pulse generator. Care of the patient after placement of a temporary transvenous pacemaker is summarized in Box 18-22.[7]

Pacemaker Functioning

When the pacemaker system functions appropriately, it diagnoses and treats the heart rhythm dysfunction. To diagnose appropriately, the pacemaker wire must sense intrinsic cardiac impulses. This ability of the pacemaker to detect the heart's intrinsic activity is known as the *sensing function* of the pacemaker system. Once proper sensing occurs, the pacemaker usually responds by inhibiting a pacing stimulus if the intrinsic activity of the heart is adequate. If the intrinsic rate is not adequate, the pacemaker delivers an impulse through the lead. When the pacemaker fires, a pacemaker artifact known as a *pacing spike* appears on the ECG, as shown in Figure 18-34. As a result of the firing,

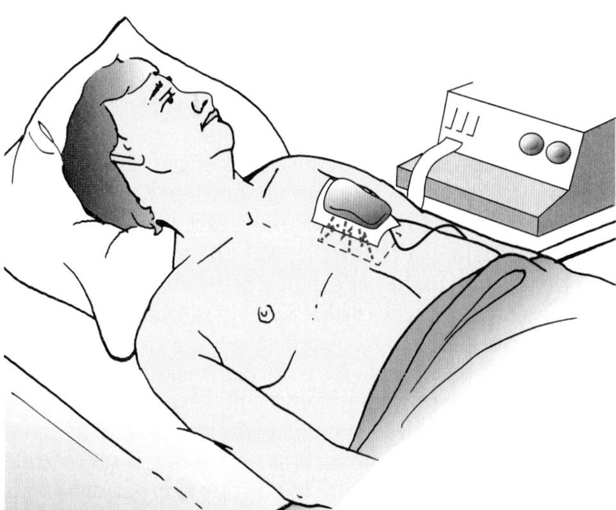

figure 18-32 Transcutaneous pacing. Electrodes are placed on anterior and posterior chest walls and attached to the external pacing unit.

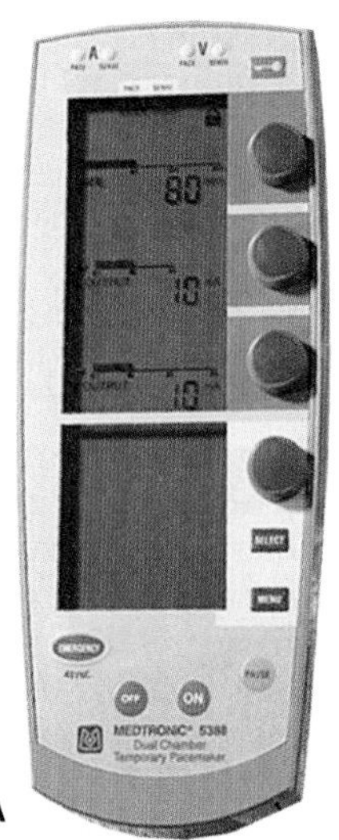

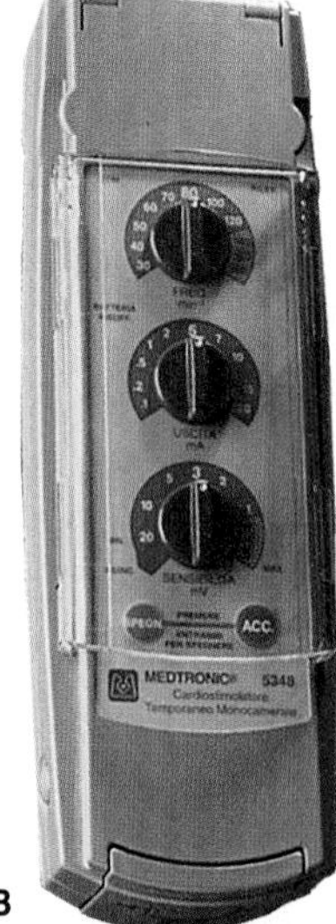

figure 18-33 Two types of temporary pacemakers. (**A**) Dual-chamber. (**B**) Single-chamber. (Courtesy of Medtronic, Minneapolis, MN.)

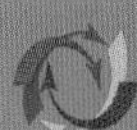

box 18-22 nursing interventions for the Patient With a Temporary Transvenous Pacemaker

Assessment

- After insertion:
  - Date, time, method and site of insertion
  - Location of wire inserted (atrial, ventricular, atrial and ventricular)
  - Sensitivity (mV) and capture (mA) thresholds at insertion
  - Rate setting, mV setting, mA setting, mode of operation (demand, asynchronous) and AV interval (if appropriate)
  - Pacemaker turned off or on
  - Patient's tolerance of procedure
  - Rhythm strip, capture and intrinsic, if appropriate; 12-lead ECG
  - Status on insertion site and sutures (if present)
  - Chest x-ray done, results on chart
- Every change of shift:
  - Pacemaker turned off or on
  - Setting for rate, mA, sensitivity, mode of operation, AV interval (if appropriate)
  - Rhythm strip (and with any clinical change or intervention)
  - Sensing and capture
  - Pulse perfusion distal to insertion site (if appropriate)
  - Presence/absence of hiccupping or muscle twitching
  - All connections are secure
  - Pacemaker secured appropriately to patient
  - Status of insertion site and sutures (if present)
  - Connective ends of pacer wires covered (as appropriate)

Intervention

- Continuous cardiac monitoring
- Pacemaker generator:
  - Verify replacement 9-volt battery available.
  - Verify connections are intact.
- Rubber/latex gloves will be worn when handling the connective ends of pacer wires.
- At all times, connective ends of pacer wires will be covered to prevent microshock hazard.
- Label epicardial pacer wires *atrial* or *ventricular*.
- Pacer wire insertion site(s) will be cleaned and dressed daily with gauze dressing or transparent dressing per institutional protocol. Label time and date of dressing change and initial.

Documentation

- Document in Critical Care Flow Sheet/Nursing Notes:
  - Assessment
  - Pacing wire insertion site care
  - Pacing thresholds as determined by physician
  - Pacing problems, nursing interventions, and results of interventions

Adapted from NIH Clinical Center Nursing Department: SOP: Care of the patient with a temporary transvenous pacemaker. Available at http://www.cc.nih.gov/nursing/pacemakt.html.

the cardiac chamber containing the pacemaker lead is depolarized. *Capture* is the term used to indicate depolarization of the atrium or ventricle in response to a pacing stimulus. The minimal amount of voltage required from the pacemaker to initiate consistent capture is known as the *pacing threshold.* This threshold level is determined by establishing successful pacing at higher energy and then gradually decreasing the energy output of the generator until capture ceases. The pacing threshold is expressed as milliamperage (mA) in the temporary generator and voltage (V) in the permanent pulse generator, within a given pulse width duration. The generator output is then set at twice or three times the threshold level to allow for an adequate safety margin.

Many factors affect the pacing threshold. These include hypoxia, hyperkalemia, antidysrhythmic drugs, catecholamines, digoxin toxicity, and corticosteroids.

The sensing amplitude is the largest atrial or ventricular intrinsic signal that is consistently sensed by the pacemaker. The amplitude of the intrinsic depolarization wave at the site of the sensing electrode is measured in millivolts. The smallest number on the sensor control represents the most sensitive setting. The sensitivity setting, in millivolts, indicates the smallest signal the pacemaker will sense. If the heart's intrinsic amplitude is smaller than the sensitivity setting, undersensing occurs. However, when the pacemaker is set to the most sensitive setting, the pacemaker could sense extraneous signals, such as the T wave or signals from the other chamber, and oversensing occurs.

The Pacemaker Code

Since the initial use of cardiac pacemakers, the technology has become so complex and diverse that a coding system has been formed to identify the various modes of pacemaker operation. Initially developed in 1974, the pacemaker coding system has undergone several revisions. The most recent version of the code was developed in 2002 through the joint efforts of the North American Society of Pacing and Electrophysiology (NASPE) and the British Pacing and Electrophysiology Group (BPEG).[8] The NASPE/BPEG Generic Pacemaker Code is shown in Table 18-17 and is simply called the NBG pacemaker code.

The first three letters of the code indicate the chambers in which pacing and sensing occur. The first letter describes the chamber or chambers of the heart in which pacing occurs: A, atrium; V, ventricle; and D, dual chamber. The second position of the code indicates the chamber or chambers in which intrinsic cardiac activity is sensed: A, atrium; V, ventricle; and D, dual chamber.

The third position denotes the pacemaker's response to sensed intrinsic cardiac activity. The letter "I" means the pacemaker is inhibited from firing in response to a sensed intrinsic beat. For example, if the pacemaker is set to a rate of 70, the pacemaker will not fire if the patient's rate exceeds 70 beats/minute. The pacemaker will fire only if the patient's intrinsic rate drops below the paced rate. Thus, the pacemaker functions on demand and is known as a *demand pacemaker*. Because the pacemaker is inhibited

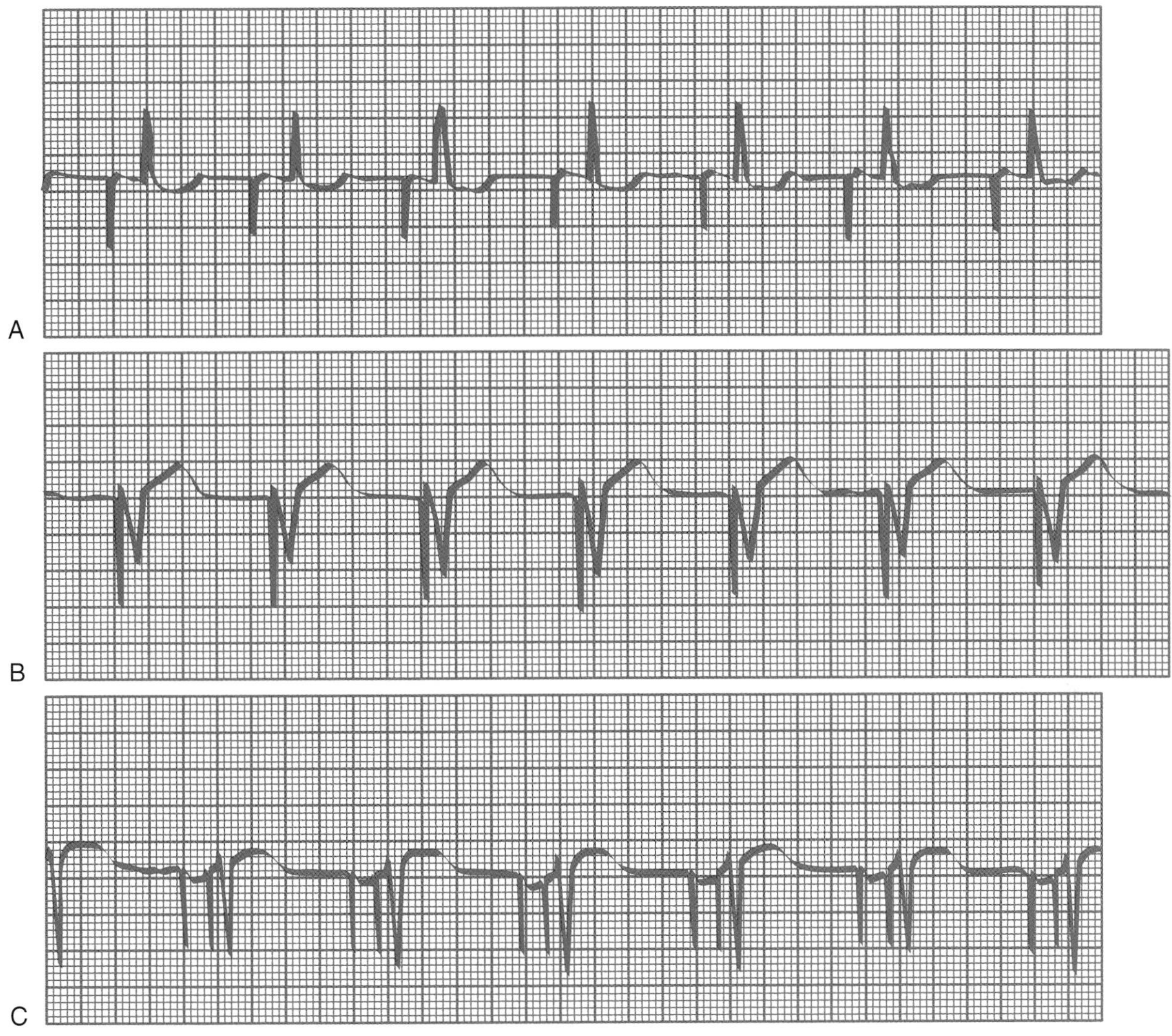

figure 18-34 **Strip A** shows an atrial pacemaker. Note that each pacing stimulus is followed by a P wave. **Strip B** shows a ventricular pacemaker. Note that each pacing stimulus is followed by a wide QRS complex. **Strip C** shows a dual-chamber pacemaker. Note that the first spike is followed by a P wave and the second spike is followed by a QRS complex. All strips show 1:1 capture.

table 18-17 **The NASPE/BPEG Generic Pacemaker Code: the Revised NASPE/BPEG Generic Code for Antibradycardia Pacing**

Position—Category				
I—Chamber(s) Paced	***II—Chamber(s) Sensed***	***III—Response to Sensing***	***IV—Rate Modulation***	***V—Multisite Pacing***
O = None	**O** = None	**O** = None	**O** = None	**O** = None
A = Atrium	**A** = Atrium	**T** = Triggered	**R** = Rate modulation	**A** = Atrium
V = Ventricle	**V** = Ventricle	**I** = Inhibited		**V** = Ventricle
D = Dual (A+V)	**D** = Dual (A+V)	**D** = Dual (T+I)		**D** = Dual (A+V)
S = Single* (A or V)	**S** = Single* (A or V)			

*Manufacturer designation only.

From Bernstein AD, Daubert JC, Fletcher RD, et al: The revised NASPE/BPEG generic code for antibradycardia, adaptive-rate, and multisite pacing. Pacing Clin Electrophysiol 25:260–264, 2002.

by intrinsic heart activity, there is no danger of the pacemaker firing at a time that could initiate a dangerous cardiac dysrhythmia, such as ventricular tachycardia. The letter "T" in the third position of the code indicates a pacemaker that triggers pacing stimuli in response to a sensed intrinsic beat. In a patient with sinus rhythm and complete AV block, a dual-chamber pacemaker is capable of sensing intrinsic sinus activity, which results in a triggered ventricular pacing stimulus for each sensed atrial event. The letter "D" in the third position designates a dual response (inhibited pacing output and triggered pacing after sensed event). The letter "O" in the third position designates a mode in which the pacemaker does not respond to sensed intrinsic activity. The inability of the pacemaker to respond to sensed intrinsic activity is known as *asynchronous pacing*. Permanent pacemakers may be switched to an asynchronous mode temporarily by placing a large magnet over the pulse generator. This maneuver causes the pacemaker to fire in an asynchronous mode, allowing the physician to assess for appropriate firing and capture.

The fourth position of the pacemaker code indicates the presence (R) or absence (O) of an adaptive-rate mechanism known as *rate modulation*. This is a feature in which the pacing rate varies in response to a physiological variable rather than being set at a fixed pacing rate. The physiological variable used most often is muscle motion. When patients increase their activity, the pacer detects vibrations from muscle and increases the pacing rate to meet increased metabolic demands.

The fifth position of the code indicates if multisite pacing is present. The letter "A" indicates either stimulation sites in both atria, more than one stimulation site in either atrium, or any combination of the two. A letter "V" in the fifth position indicates either stimulation sites in both ventricles, more than one stimulation site in either ventricle, or any combination of the two. The letter "D" represents any combination of A or V. If multisite pacing is not a feature, the letter "O" is used in the fifth position of the code.

Pacing Modes

Knowledge of the five-letter pacemaker code helps the critical care nurse determine the type of implanted device, the intended mode of operation, and the actual mode of operation. Modes of operation can be classified as single- and dual-chamber modes.

SINGLE-CHAMBER MODES OF OPERATION

A VVIRO mode is a commonly used mode of operation for permanent ventricular pacemakers. Devices with this mode of operation are characterized by ventricular demand pacing, ventricular sensing with inhibited ventricular response to sensing, rate modulation, and no multisite pacing. The rate modulation feature offers the benefit of adjusting the paced rate in response to metabolic demand. This rate modulation feature is not used in temporary pacing, so the mode would be designated as VVI. A disadvantage of the VVIR and the VVI modes is the lack of hemodynamic benefit from AV synchrony provided by dual-chamber pacing. However, in chronic atrial fibrillation with slow ventricular response rates, VVIR is the appropriate mode to use.

An AAIOO is a mode of operation for permanent atrial pacemakers. With this mode of operation, there is atrial demand pacing, atrial sensing with inhibited atrial response to sensing, and no rate modulation or multisite pacing. Temporary atrial pacemakers most often are set to an AAI mode and are particularly useful in overdrive pacing of atrial dysrhythmias. These modes of pacing can be used only for patients with normal functioning of the AV node and intraventricular conduction system. If needed, the pacemaker provides atrial depolarization, but the patient's AV node must conduct the signal to the ventricles. An advantage of these modes is the presence of AV synchrony.

DUAL-CHAMBER MODES OF OPERATION

Temporary and permanent dual-chamber pacemakers can operate in a variety of modes. The most common mode is DDD for temporary pacemakers and DDDRO for permanent pacemakers. A DDDOO mode provides dual-chamber pacing, dual-chamber sensing with both inhibited and triggered responses to sensing, and no rate modulation or multisite pacing. The DDDRV mode has the additional feature of rate modulation and multisite ventricular pacing. A VDDOO mode senses in both atria and ventricles but paces only in the ventricles. This mode is particularly useful in patients with intact sinus node function but high-grade AV block. Ventricular pacing is triggered by a sensed P wave.

Pacemaker Malfunction

Pacemaker malfunction can be a result of a programmed function (pseudomalfunction) or can be due to true component malfunction. Whereas pacemakers are now manufactured to provide more complex capabilities, unanticipated pacemaker malfunctions have increased in prevalence.[9] For this reason, it is important for the patient to know the manufacturer, model, and serial number of their pacemaker components (pulse generator and leads) and to ascertain that they have been appropriately registered with the manufacturer. Most manufacturers have toll-free numbers that can provide information on safety alerts. It is important, however, for patients to contact their physician to advise them on the implications of such recalls or safety alerts. At times, programming may correct the problem.

Temporary pacemaker malfunction should be addressed systematically. First and most important, immediate action to restore pacemaker capture in patients with no underlying rhythm requires the following steps:

1. Increase pulse generator output (in milliamperes) to the highest setting, asynchronous mode.
2. Check patient hemodynamics, simultaneous multiple ECG lead recordings; intervene if appropriate with transcutaneous pacing, atropine sulfate, or isoproterenol.
3. Check all connections.
4. Replace pulse generator or battery; be prepared for transcutaneous pacing backup during change.

Proceed with troubleshooting if the patient is stable. Table 18-18 describes troubleshooting strategies for temporary pacemaker malfunction.

table 18-18 Troubleshooting a Temporary Pacemaker

Problem	Cause	Intervention
Failure to discharge: No evidence of pacing stimulus, patient's heart rate below programmed rate	Due to battery depletion or pulse generator failure, output or timing circuit failure	Replace battery or generator.
	Due to loose cable connection	Check all connections for tightness.
Failure to capture: Pacing stimulus not followed by ECG evidence of depolarization	Due to lead dislodgement	Review chest film, turn patient to left lateral decubitus position until lead can be replaced.
	Due to broken connector pins or fractured extension connecting cable	Connect wire directly to generator to diagnose cable problem, replace connecting cable.
	Due to incompatibility of wire pins with cable or with generator	Ascertain a secure fit of the exposed pin to the cable or the generator, adjust connection or replace pulse generator.
	Due to output setting (mA) too low	Check capture thresholds and adjust output to a two- to threefold safety margin.
	Due to perforation	Review 12-lead ECG, report signs of perforation, stabilize hemodynamics.
	Due to lead fracture without insulation break	Check intracavitary ECG; if evidence of fracture in one pole, unipolarize lead; if total fracture, lead replacement needed.
	Due to increase in pacing threshold from medication or metabolic changes	Check laboratory test results, correct metabolic alterations, review medications and vital signs, increase output.
Oversensing: Device detects noncardiac electrical events and interprets them as depolarization	Due to oversensitive setting	Reduce sensitivity (value [in millivolts] should be larger to make pacer less sensitive); if patient is pacer dependent (no intrinsic R wave), program to asynchronous mode until problem is corrected.
	Due to device detecting tall T waves and interpreting them as R waves	Increase ventricular refractory period beyond T wave.
In dual-chamber pacing, cross-talk is a form of oversensing: The device detects signals from the other chamber and inhibits; in atrial channel, R waves are detected as P waves.	Caused by atrial lead dislodgement	Recheck atrial capture thresholds; if high, dislodgement is probable.
In ventricular channel, atrial pacing stimulus afterpotential is detected as an R wave, with V pacing inappropriately inhibited	Due to high output from atrial channel	Reduce output from atrial channel, decrease ventricular channel sensitivity (higher millivolt value).
	Due to electrical interference, improperly grounded electrical devices	Remove nongrounded equipment.
Undersensing: Device fails to detect intrinsic cardiac activity and fires inappropriately	Due to asynchronous mode setting (VOO, DOO, AOO)	Reprogram to synchronous mode (VVI, DDD, AAI).
	Due to small intrinsic amplitude	Increase sensitivity (turn sensitivity dial toward lower millivolt value).
	Due to lead dislodgement	Recheck capture thresholds; if high, lead probably dislodged and needs repositioning.
	Due to lead insulation break	Check lead with pacing system analyzer, if impedance too low (<200 ohms), insulation break is likely, and lead needs to be replaced or can be temporarily placed in unipolar configuration.

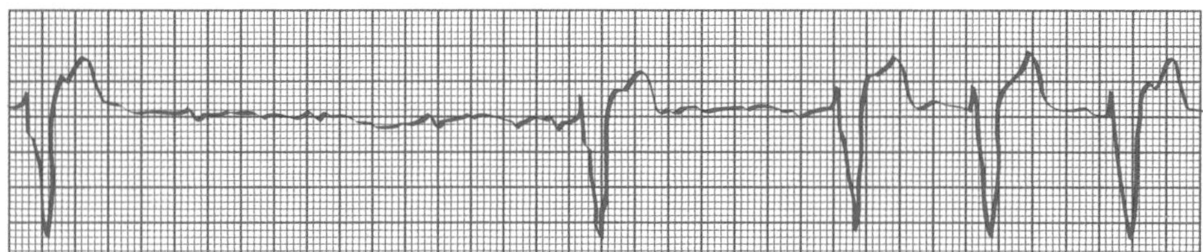

figure 18-35 Failure to discharge or oversensing with pacing inhibition. Note pacemaker spikes are missing at appropriate intervals.

FAILURE TO DISCHARGE

Because stimulus discharge from the pacemaker causes an artifact, or "spike," to appear on the ECG, failure to discharge results in absence of the artifact and unexplained loss of pacing (Fig. 18-35). The cause of this failure may be within the generator itself, either processor or battery failure. Processor failure is not common, but battery failure is more prevalent among patients who are noncompliant to follow-up or unaware of the longevity of their pacemaker battery. This may be evaluated by measuring the output values of the generator through a programmer. In extreme cases, the generator fails to communicate with the programmer. Replacement of the generator must be done immediately. If the situation is emergent, the physician may insert a temporary transvenous pacemaker to support the patient hemodynamically until the permanent pacemaker problem can be corrected.

FAILURE TO CAPTURE

Failure of the pacing stimulus to capture the ventricles or atria is noted by the absence of the QRS or P wave immediately after the pacemaker artifact on the ECG (Fig. 18-36). Impending battery depletion may also cause failure to capture. When the battery is low, the output may not be sufficient to meet the capture threshold. If the patient is pacemaker dependent and becomes symptomatic, drug therapy (atropine, isoproterenol), transcutaneous pacing, or CPR may be required until the cause of the problem is found and corrected.

OVERSENSING

Oversensing is the term used to describe a sensing malfunction when the pacemaker detects events other than those it was programmed to sense. For example, if tall T waves are present on the ECG, they may be mistaken for QRS complexes, causing the pacemaker to be inhibited. Similarly, electromagnetic interference may result in inappropriate sensing and, as a result, incorrectly activate the inhibited or triggered mode of the pacemaker. Oversensing may be due to electrode displacement, inappropriate sensitivity settings, or impending lead fracture. A partially fractured lead often allows signals to saturate the generator, causing oversensing and inhibition of pacing output in demand mode. On surface ECG, oversensing mimics failure to discharge because of the inhibition of pacing stimuli (see Fig. 18-35). The only way to confirm oversensing is to examine the intracardiac electrogram (EGM) through a programmer. If noise is recorded on the EGM, then the problem is due to oversensing.

To correct oversensing problems in a temporary pacemaker system, the nurse checks the connection between the temporary pacemaker and the lead. A thorough assessment of potential sources of electromagnetic interference is made. The grounding wires of all electrical equipment should be checked. The sensitivity may be decreased by turning the dial toward *asynchronous*, which is toward a higher millivolt (mV) value. Oversensing due to partial wire fracture in a temporary transvenous bipolar catheter may also be corrected by conversion to a unipolar system. To diagnose, an intracavitary ECG is obtained by connecting a single pole to a surface V lead by alligator clamp connector and obtaining a V1 precordial recording. The recording should show a large voltage artifact amplitude and an elevated ST segment. A complete fracture shows a flat tracing. Noise on the recording that is not related to the intrinsic ECG, or diminished artifact amplitude demonstrates partial fracture. If one of the poles is intact, this lead can be unipolarized by inserting the terminal tip of the intact pole into the negative port of the generator terminal. The unused pole terminal of the lead is shielded with rubber tubing. The tip of an external ECG single-wire electrode applied on the skin is inserted into the positive port of the generator, serving as the ground (Fig. 18-37). This is, how-

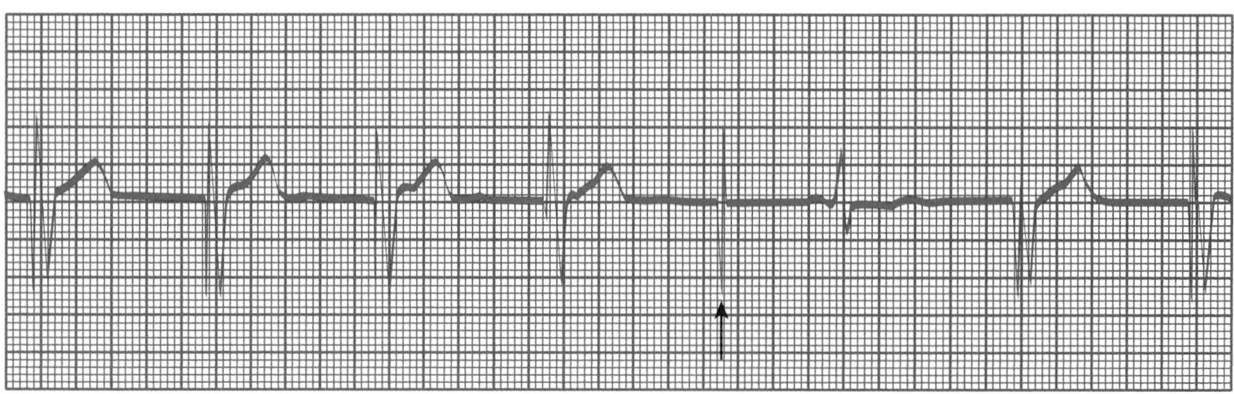

figure 18-36 ECG strip showing evidence of failure to capture. Note pacing stimulus is not followed by a QRS complex.

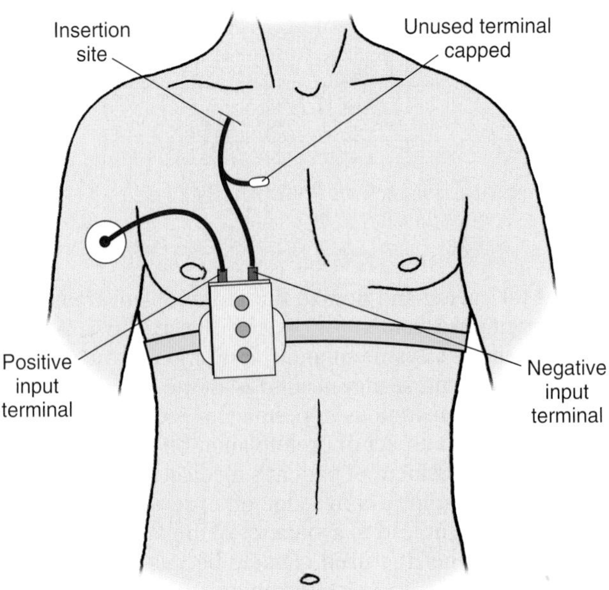

figure 18-37 Unipolarizing a temporary bipolar lead.

ever, a temporary and unsafe measure and may be subject to electromagnetic interference. The safest intervention for a fractured lead is lead replacement.

UNDERSENSING

Failure of the pacemaker to sense intrinsic beats is known as *undersensing* and results in inappropriately placed pacemaker artifacts on the ECG (Fig. 18-38). Undersensing may be caused by lead dislodgement, capacitor failure, lead insulation defect, or lead wire fracture. Ventricular dysrhythmia caused by the pacemaker firing during the vulnerable phase of the T wave is of concern with undersensing. The most likely cause for sensing failure in the temporary pacemaker is lead displacement.

To correct undersensing problems in the temporary pacemaker, the nurse must first ascertain that the lead is properly connected to the temporary pacer. Undersensing may also be corrected by increasing the sensitivity of the device, which is done by turning the dial to a lower millivolt value. If problems persist, the physician may need to reposition or replace the lead. In permanent pacemakers, undersensing can sometimes be corrected by reprogramming to a more sensitive setting or by switching from bipolar to unipolar mode.

Pacemaker Complications

Numerous possible complications are associated with cardiac pacemakers. The critical care nurse plays a vital role in the early detection and management of these complications.

PNEUMOTHORAX

Insertion of a transvenous lead through the subclavian vein can be complicated by traumatic injury to the lung by the exploring needle because of the proximity of the subclavian vein to the apex of the lung. The symptoms may occur suddenly or may insidiously present up to 48 hours after the procedure. The symptoms include pleuritic pain, hypotension, respiratory distress, or hypoxia. A chest x-ray can reveal the extent of the trauma. When severe, a chest tube allows for lung reexpansion.

VENTRICULAR IRRITABILITY

Ventricular irritability at the site of the endocardial catheter tip is occasionally encountered in temporary pacing systems after initial catheter insertion. The premature ventricular complexes usually appear similar in configuration to the pacemaker complexes. Irritability from the catheter as a foreign body usually disappears after a few hours (Fig. 18-39). Persistent ventricular irritability may indicate lead dislodgement in both temporary and permanent pacing systems.

PERFORATION OF VENTRICULAR WALL OR SEPTUM

Perforation of the ventricular free wall or septum by the transvenous catheter occurs in a small number of patients. This may or may not result in cardiac tamponade. Elderly patients and patients on chronic corticosteroid or anticoagulant therapy are at highest risk. Perforation can be suspected if the patient demonstrates a change in precordial lead morphology on cardiac monitoring. Right ventricular apical pacing often results in a negative QRS complex in a V1 lead. Ventricular perforation may result in pacing from the left ventricle, and the QRS complex becomes positive in polarity. (Newer methods of biventricular pacing can, however, confound this finding because a positive narrow QRS polarity is not abnormal in biventricular pacemaker morphology.) When ventricular wall perforation is suspected, pericardial tamponade, causing a decrease in blood pressure and an increase in sinus rate, can be confirmed by echocardiography.

CATHETER OR LEAD DISLODGEMENT

Dislodgement of the pacing catheter or lead may occur, resulting in oversensing, undersensing, or failure to capture. A chest x-ray usually confirms the findings. Catheter or lead dislodgement usually requires repositioning.

INFECTION AND PHLEBITIS/ HEMATOMA FORMATION

Infection and phlebitis can occur at the temporary pacemaker insertion site, and infection or hematoma may occur at the site of permanent generator implantation. These sites must be inspected for swelling and inflammation and kept dry. In temporary pacing sites, sterile technique must be used when dressings are changed.

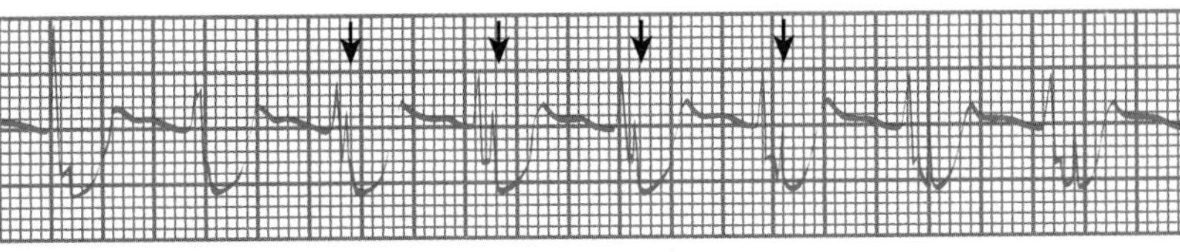

figure 18-38 ECG strip showing evidence of undersensing. Failure of the ventricular demand pacemaker to detect the intrinsic rhythm is shown by pacemaker spikes at inappropriate intervals after spontaneous QRS complexes.

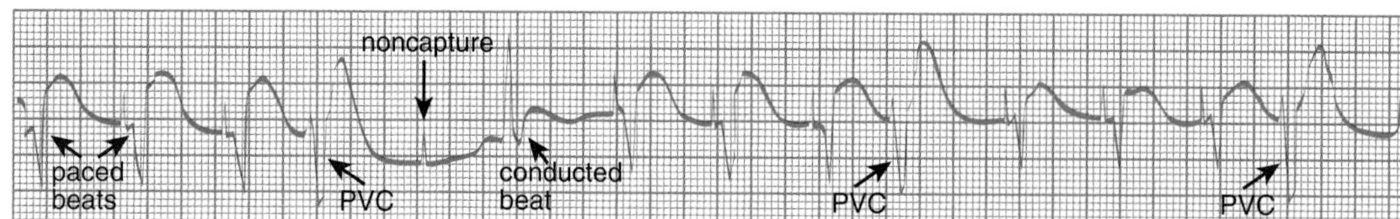

figure 18-39 Ventricular demand pacemaker with premature ventricular contractions (PVCs). This strip also shows one noncaptured pacemaker spike followed by a spontaneous conducted beat.

ABDOMINAL TWITCHING OR HICCUPS

Abdominal twitching or hiccups occur occasionally as a result of electrode placement against a thin right ventricular wall and resultant electrical stimulation of the abdominal muscles or diaphragm. This complication usually is very uncomfortable for the patient, but can sometimes be corrected by programming the output of the generator to a lower level. Diaphragmatic stimulation can sometimes be associated with perforation. A drop in the patient's blood pressure and high capture thresholds accompanying diaphragmatic stimulation warrant critical observation and evaluation.

POCKET EROSION

Erosion at the implantation site occurs rarely in the early postimplantation period and is more often regarded as a late complication of permanent pacemaker implantation. At times, erosion heralds a fulminant infection. At other times, however, erosion may be due to poor skin integrity or cachexia. In the latter case, early detection of pre-erosion with prompt reoperation for pocket relocation can protect the patient from a potentially malignant cause of systemic infection. When a pacemaker system erodes, an aggressive infection may occur throughout the lead system into the heart, making lead extraction necessary.

Nursing Management

Critical care nurses play a key role in caring for patients with a pacemaker. The nurse is responsible for comprehensively assessing the patient, educating the patient and family, monitoring the ECG, and maintaining patient safety. Box 18-23 lists nursing diagnoses for patients with a cardiac pacemaker.

PATIENT ASSESSMENT

The critical care nurse may be the first to detect the patient's dysrhythmia that will necessitate pacing. Knowing the indications for pacing and how to initiate emergent transcutaneous pacing is essential for the critical care nurse. After a comprehensive assessment and stabilization of the patient, the critical care nurse may need to assist the physician in the insertion of a transvenous or permanent pacing system.

An important aspect of preimplantation of a pacemaker includes an assessment of patient's medical as well as social history. For example, knowledge of a previous fracture to the clavicle might lead to avoidance of implantation on the same side as the fractured clavicle because of potential anatomical distortion. A subclavian approach might be avoided in a person with a history of a collapsed lung or previous lobectomy. A patient with a right arm arteriovenous fistula would be best served with a left-sided implant. For social history, avocations such as hunting, professional sport activities, and even simply preferential arm dexterity come into consideration. For example, the right pectoral region should not be used in the right-handed tennis player.

To assess patients with pacemakers accurately, the nurse must understand the pacemaker code to know the type of pacer used and the intended mode of the device.[10] The nurse must be aware of the patient's underlying rhythm so that if the pacemaker fails, the nurse will be prepared to treat any life-threatening dysrhythmias.

A thorough assessment also helps the nurse determine the patient's physiological response to pacing therapy. Important parameters to assess include pulse rate, underlying cardiac rhythm, blood pressure, activity tolerance, and evidence of dizziness, syncope, dyspnea, palpitations, or edema. The nurse should be attentive to results of chest radiographs, blood tests, and other relevant laboratory tests. If a permanent pacemaker has been implanted, the incision should be examined for swelling, redness, drainage, hematoma, and tenderness.

A psychosocial assessment is another essential component of comprehensive care of the patient with a cardiac pacemaker. Patients' psychosocial responses to the need for cardiac pacing may differ. Some may be relieved to have a device that supports the functioning of their heart, whereas others may be anxious about the technology and express fears of dying. If a permanent pacemaker is implanted, patients and families should be encouraged to join support groups where they can share their fears and concerns with others who are dependent on pacing technology.

PATIENT AND FAMILY EDUCATION

A planned and systematic approach to teaching the patient and family about cardiac pacing is a vital part of nursing care. Teaching a patient about pacemakers begins at the time the decision for pacemaker insertion is made. The nurse can begin by eliciting the patient's previous knowledge of pacemakers and clarifying any misconceptions.

box 18-23 *Examples of Nursing Diagnoses and Collaborative Problems for the Patient With a Pacemaker*

- Anxiety related to life-threatening cardiac disease requiring pacemaker
- Deficient Knowledge related to newly diagnosed condition
- Risk of Infection related to invasive procedure and presence of foreign body
- Decreased Cardiac Output related to pacemaker syndrome or absence of AV synchrony

Nothing is assumed about the patient's understanding. If appropriate, the difference between heart block and heart attack is clarified. The patient may confuse cardiac monitoring with pacing and become anxious when the monitoring electrodes are removed.

The patient and family should be told why the pacemaker is necessary. The anatomy of the heart should be discussed in general terms when explaining the need for pacing and how the pacemaker takes the place of or complements spontaneous rhythm. The insertion procedure and the immediate postinsertion care that can be expected should be explained.

Many booklets and media presentations are available to aid the nurse in teaching the pacemaker recipient. Visual and written guidelines are helpful for the patient and family to review after discharge from the hospital.

The depth of teaching that is appropriate and the teaching tools used depend on such variables as the patient's age, intellect, attention span, vision, and interest in learning. Initial teaching should be confined to the positive aspects of life with a pacemaker. Knowledge of the function and care of the pacemaker are of no interest until this patient is able to accept it as part of life. Box 18-24 provides a guide for teaching patients and families about pacemakers.

ELECTROCARDIOGRAM MONITORING

Careful monitoring of the ECG of the patient with a cardiac pacemaker is an essential component of comprehensive patient assessment. The first step in the analysis involves examining the strip for evidence of discharge. This evidence is noted by the presence of pacing spikes on the strip. Unipolar pacing spikes are usually tall and visible, but bipolar pacing spikes may not be visible in certain leads. Each pacing spike should result in capture. If the pacing lead is in the atrium, a pacing spike is followed by a P wave. If the pacing wire is in the ventricle, the spike is followed by a wide QRS complex. A narrow QRS complex, however, after a pacing spike does not necessarily mean there is pacemaker malfunction. When fusion is present, the pacing spike appears right before the intrinsic QRS complex (Fig. 18-40). Biventricular pacing (pacing both ventricles) for cardiac resynchronization in congestive heart failure also results in narrow QRS.

The sensing function of the pacemaker is evaluated next. If the pacemaker does not sense intrinsic cardiac activity (undersensing), inappropriate pacemaker spikes may appear throughout the underlying rhythm. An oversensing problem can be detected when the pacemaker senses events other than the intrinsic rhythm and is inappropriately inhibited in that chamber or causes a triggered response in the other chamber.

The third step in evaluating the ECG is to measure various intervals in milliseconds (msec). Each small box on the ECG paper represents 40 msec, and one large box represents 200 msec. The duration of each interval is compared with the programmed setting for that interval.

The first interval, the pacing interval, is the amount of time between two consecutive atrial pacing spikes or two consecutive ventricular pacing spikes. This interval is used to determine the pacing rate. To calculate the pacing rate, the nurse counts the number of milliseconds between two consecutive atrial spikes or two consecutive ventricular spikes (Fig. 18-41). To convert from milliseconds to beats per minute, the following formula is used: 60,000 msec/minute divided by the number of milliseconds between pacing spikes equals the pacing rate.

The next interval to measure is the AV interval, also known as the AV delay. This interval is analogous to the PR interval on the ECG. The AV interval is measured from the beginning of an intrinsic P wave or an atrial pacing spike to the beginning of the intrinsic QRS complex or the ventricular pacing spike (see Fig. 18-41).

The third interval to measure is the ventriculoatrial (VA) interval, also called the atrial escape interval. The VA interval is the amount of time from a ventricular paced or sensed event to the next atrial paced stimulus (see Fig. 18-41). The sum of the AV and the VA intervals equals the pacing interval.

PATIENT SAFETY

Electrical safety precautions must be observed when the patient has a temporary pacemaker. Electrical equipment in the room is kept at a minimum and must be properly grounded. Use of a nonelectric bed is preferable. If an electric bed is used, it must be properly grounded or remain disconnected from alternating current (AC). Only battery-operated electric shavers, toothbrushes, or radios are recommended. An AC-powered television may be used if it is operated by someone who is not in contact with the patient. The nurse should avoid simultaneous contact with the patient and any electrical equipment. The patient's bed must be kept dry at all times. Diathermy and electrocautery equipment should not be used because their waves may be sensed by and inhibit the demand pacemaker.

The literature on ensuring electrical safety in temporary pacemaker wires has been sparse; however, manufacturers have been guided by the FDA to increase vigilance over patient safety. Currently manufactured leads have no exposed areas after they are inserted tightly into the connecting cable. The use of rubber gloves to handle temporary pacing lead terminal pins is often recommended. Most manufacturers supply connecting cables with the pulse generator to ensure compatibility. Some connecting cables are nonsterilizable, and integrity may be compromised by resterilization. Care should also be taken to ensure that nonsterile cables are not in close proximity with the sterile field during insertion.

When using the older pulse generator model, the hard plastic cover over the dials of the temporary generator must be secured in place to prevent inadvertent change in settings. The generator should be attached to the patient's arm or visibly pinned to the patients' gown. The catheter should be taped securely to the patient's skin without direct tension on the catheter. Motion of the extremity nearest the catheter entry site should be minimized, especially if the femoral site has been used.

According to manufacturers of permanent pacemaker generators, there are very few electrical hazards associated with the permanent generators currently in use. These generators are shielded from external electrical sources and usually are not affected by microwave ovens or small appliances. There have been rare reports of unipolar pacemakers being affected by large electromagnetic fields and radiofrequency signals, such as radio transmitters.

box 18-24
Living With a Pacemaker

Patient Activity

- Start passive and active range-of-motion exercises on the affected arm 48 hours after implantation to avoid "frozen shoulder." For those with new leads implanted, avoid abduction of the affected arm above the shoulder level for 4 to 6 weeks to prevent lead dislodgement.
- Avoid activities that may result in high impact or stress at the implantation site.
- Return to work at the discretion of your physician after discussing the type of work you do and what your job entails.
- Return to whatever degree of sexual activity you prefer.
- Your pacemaker will set off the alarm on metal-detector devices in airports, so avoid going through the detector gates. Show your pacemaker identification card. A manual search may be done or a magnetic wand may be used. Do not allow the wand to linger at the pacemaker site for an indefinite amount of time because the magnet in the wand may temporarily put the pacemaker in asynchronous mode. The metal detector or wand will not cause any permanent damage to your pacemaker.

Signs of Pacemaker Malfunction

- Be alert for symptoms of pacemaker malfunction: those associated with decreased perfusion of the brain, heart, or skeletal muscles. Be particularly mindful of return of symptoms you experienced before pacemaker implantation.
- Report any dizziness, fainting, shortness of breath, undue fatigue, or fluid retention. Fluid retention includes sudden weight gain, "puffy ankles," "tightness of rings," and so forth.
- Take pulse once daily upon awakening. Report a pulse rate more than 5 beats/minute slower than that at which pacemaker is set.
- Be aware that pulse may be somewhat irregular if it is a demand pacemaker and has some spontaneous beats and paced beats. This does not signify pacemaker malfunction.

Signs of Infection

- Report any redness, swelling, warmth, drainage, or increase in soreness at the implantation site.

Medications

- Antibiotics are usually given within 24 hours of pacemaker implantation. Report any unusual reactions.
- Medications that were withdrawn before pacemaker implantation may need to be restarted. Check with your physician about beta blockers, digitalis, or blood thinners. Know the name of the medication and the dose, frequency of administration, side effects, and use of each medication.
- If warfarin is restarted, levels should be rechecked after reinitiation of drug.

Considerations for Home Care

- Carry a pacemaker identification card at all times. This card shows the brand and model of pacemaker, the date of insertion, and the implanting physician.
- Wear a medical alert bracelet or necklace stating a pacemaker is worn.
- Adhere to schedule of follow-up visits with your physician or clinic. The follow-up visit will include an interval history and ECG recording. Many pacemaker clinics have specialized equipment available to determine pacemaker and lead performance and to predict battery longevity. Some clinics have the capability for obtaining some of this information by telephone, reducing the necessity for travel to the clinic. However, when pacemaker follow-up is done by phone transmission, have the pacemaker checked at least once a year in the pacemaker clinic. Many problems related to the pacemaker pocket or intermittent failure of components cannot be picked up through telephone transmission tests.
- If you have any symptoms similar to those before pacemaker insertion, have the pacemaker checked. Be alert for other symptoms of malfunction such as unexplained dizzy spells, fatigue, or slow pulse.
- Inform any physician or dentist of the pacemaker and of the medications being taken.

Pulse Generator Replacement

- Follow-up is intensified when the pacemaker battery approaches its elective replacement indicator. Avoid extended absences or vacations without consulting your physician at this time.
- Be aware that when the battery depletes, the generator stops working.
- The battery cannot be removed from the generator, so the entire generator is replaced when the battery is low.
- Generator replacement can be done within a 24-hour stay, as long as the leads are in good condition. Usually only the generator needs to be replaced.

Considerations for the Older Patient

- Report any changes in skin condition at the pacemaker site. Sudden weight loss or poor nutritional status may predispose elderly patients to pocket erosion.
- Report symptoms such as fatigue, neck pulsations, and lack of energy. Loss of AV synchrony in patients with single-chamber VVI pacemakers may result in pacemaker syndrome.
- If the pacemaker feels like it is "flipping" inside the pocket, report it to your doctor and do not reposition it. When the skin is loose or when the patient "twiddles" with the pacemaker, the leads can become tangled and coiled and may fracture.

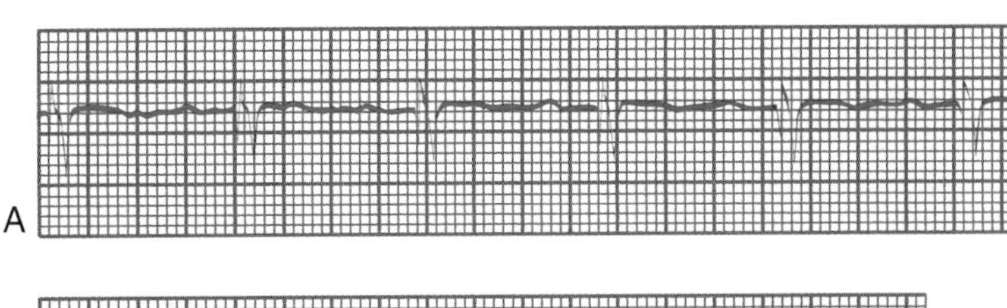

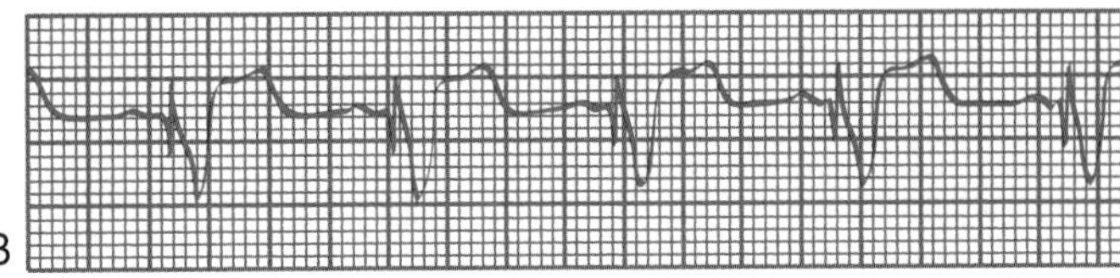

figure 18-40 Pacemaker fusion beats. (**A**) The pacemaker artifact is followed by intrinsic QRS complex deflection. (**B**) Pacemaker capture (ventricular capture) beats with typical widening of QRS complex.

IMPLANTABLE CARDIOVERTER–DEFIBRILLATORS

In the United States, about 250,000 people die each year of coronary heart disease without being hospitalized.[11] Most of these are sudden death due to cardiac arrest. This sudden rapid loss of heart function, the result of an unresuscitated cardiac arrest, may be due to heart disease, AMI, and possibly other factors. Most cardiac arrests are caused by ventricular fibrillation. Ventricular tachycardia and fibrillation can be reversed when treated within minutes with electrical cardioversion or defibrillation.

In the late 1960s, Dr. Michel Mirowski and Dr. Morton Mower developed a device called an *implantable cardioverter–defibrillator* (ICD) to treat patients at risk for sudden death due to ventricular dysrhythmia. In 1980, the first device was implanted successfully in a person. The device was found to be safe and effective and, as a result, received FDA approval in 1985. Since its initial use in 1980, the ICD generator and lead technology have undergone many improvements in design and function. With these improvements, as well as with expanded indications and increased understanding of patients at risk, implantation of ICDs has rapidly increased. From 1993 to 1999, the number of ICDs implanted in the United States alone increased by 227%. In the year 2000, it was projected that 61,000 ICDs would be implanted in the United States, with a total of approximately 81,000 worldwide.[12]

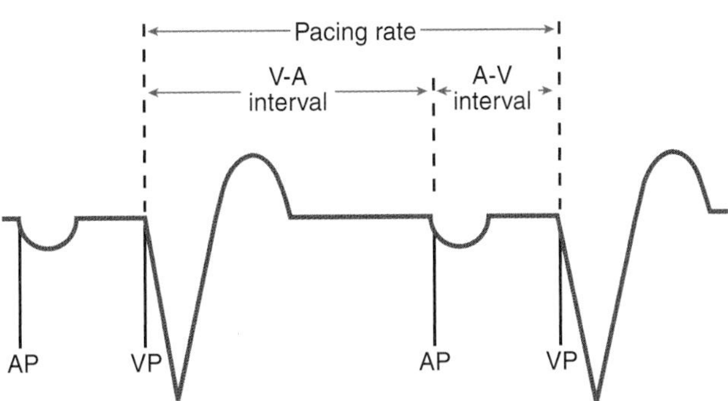

figure 18-41 The intervals measured on an ECG strip for a patient with a pacemaker. The pacing interval is the amount of time between two consecutive atrial pacing spikes or two consecutive ventricular pacing spikes. The atrioventricular (AV) interval is measured from the beginning of a P wave or an atrial pacing spike to the beginning of an intrinsic QRS complex or the ventricular pacing spike. The ventriculoatrial (VA) interval is measured from a ventricular pacing or sensed beat to the next atrial pacing spike. The sum of the AV and VA interval equals the pacing interval.

Indications for Implantable Cardioverter–Defibrillators

A joint committee of the American College of Cardiology and the American Heart Association developed guidelines for the use of ICDs.[6] Class I include indications for which there is general agreement that the device should be implanted. Class II consists of conditions for which ICDs are frequently used, but there are differences of opinion regarding the necessity of insertion. Conditions for which there is general agreement that ICDs are unnecessary are considered class III. Box 18-25 lists the indications for use of ICD therapy.

The Implantable Cardioverter–Defibrillator System

The purpose of an ICD is to monitor continuously the patient's rhythm, diagnose rhythm changes, and treat life-threatening ventricular dysrhythmias. Similar to a pacemaker, the ICD consists of a lead system and a pulse generator containing the battery, capacitors, and circuits. The lead system and the pulse generator have undergone significant changes in design and function since their initial use in 1980.

THE PULSE GENERATOR

Early ICD pulse generators were large and heavy compared with the pacemaker pulse generator. Because of their size and weight, these ICD pulse generators required implantation in the patient's abdomen. Currently used ICD pulse generators are not much larger than the earlier models of pacemakers and can be implanted in the pectoral area. The size of the device is shown in Figure 18-42. Lithium-silver-vanadium oxide (Li/SVO) batteries provide the power source for ICDs and last 4 to 7 years. Improved circuit design has expanded the capabilities and functions of the ICD.

THE LEAD SYSTEM

Lead systems sense the life-threatening ventricular rhythm and deliver a shock to convert the rhythm. At its inception,

box 18-25
Indications for Implantable Cardioverter–Defibrillators

Class I
- Cardiac arrest due to VF or VT, not due to transient or reversible cause.
- Spontaneous sustained VT.
- Syncope of undetermined origin with induced sustained VT at electrophysiological study when drug therapy is ineffective, not tolerated, or not preferred.
- Nonsustained VT with coronary artery disease, prior MI, LV dysfunction, and inducible VF or sustained VT at electrophysiological study that is not suppressible by a class I antidysrhythmic drug.

Class II
- Cardiac arrest presumed to be due to VF when electrophysiological testing is not feasible.
- Severe symptoms attributable to sustained ventricular tachydysrhythmias while awaiting cardiac transplantation.
- Familial or inherited conditions with a high risk for life-threatening ventricular tachydysrhythmias such as the long QT syndrome or hypertrophic cardiomyopathy.
- Recurrent syncope of undetermined etiology with ventricular dysrhythmias and left ventricular dysfunction, when other causes of syncope have been excluded.
- Spontaneous sustained VT in an individual with a nonischemic cardiomyopathy, severe LV systolic dysfunction; not inducible with electrophysiological testing.
- Nonsustained VT with coronary artery disease, prior MI, LV dysfunction, and inducible sustained VT or VF at electrophysiological study.

Class III
- Syncope of undetermined etiology without inducible ventricular tachydysrhythmias without sufficient evidence to suspect dysrhythmia as a possible etiology.
- Incessant ventricular tachydysrhythmias.
- Ventricular tachydysrhythmias arising from rhythm disturbances that are amenable to surgical or catheter ablation.
- Ventricular tachydysrhythmias due to a transient or reversible etiology.
- Significant psychiatric illnesses that may be aggravated by device implantation or may preclude systematic follow-up.
- Terminal illnesses with projected life expectancy <6 months.
- Patients with coronary artery disease, LV dysfunction, and prolonged QRS complex duration without spontaneous or inducible VT undergoing coronary artery bypass surgery.
- Patients with class IV heart failure who are not candidates for cardiac transplantation.

VF, ventricular fibrillation; LV, left ventricular.
Adapted from Gregoratos G, Cheitlin MD, Conill A, et al: ACC/AHA guidelines for implantation of cardiac pacemakers and antiarrhythmia devices: A report of the American College of Cardiology/American Heart Association Task Force on Practice Guidelines (Committee on Pacemaker Implantation). J Am Coll Cardiol 31:1175–1209, 1998.

the lead system consisted of two epicardial patches for energy delivery and epicardial coils for sensing. The leads were often implanted at the time of CABG, when indicated, or by a subxiphoid approach. The sensing coils were later replaced with a long transvenous lead positioned in the right ventricular endocardium and tunneled down from the subclavian insertion site to the generator in the abdomen. Improved lead design and smaller generators paved the way for prepectoral implantation. At this time, previously implanted epicardial leads are used only with replacement of ICD generators, when the leads are deemed to be usable. Newer implants use bipolar or tripolar transvenous leads for sensing and defibrillation. The sensing electrodes are bipoles at the tip of the lead. One unipolar coil in the distal portion of the ventricular lead serves as the defibrillation cathode, whereas another coil in the mid-proximal portion or the ICD generator serve as the defibrillation anode, giving rise to the term *active can* or *hot can*. With dual-chamber ICDs, an additional bipolar electrode in the right atrium provides atrial sensing and pacing. In biventricular ICDs, a third lead is inserted in the coronary sinus and positioned in the lateral vein for left ventricular stimulation and resynchronization of the ventricles. Ideally, the generator is implanted in the left pectoral area so that the heart is central to the vector of the defibrillation current. The improvements in lead design have allowed an ease of implantation not unlike that with permanent pacemaker implantation. It is no longer unusual for a patient to be discharged the day after ICD implantation (Fig. 18-43).

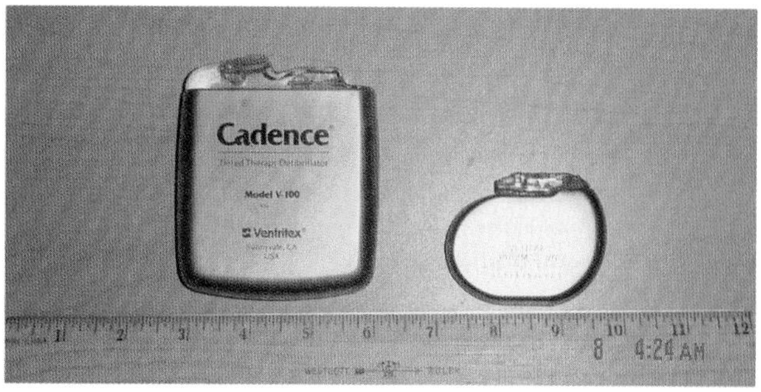

figure 18-42 Implantable cardioverter–defibrillator, old and new models. Note the decrease in size and weight that has been achieved with the newer generation, allowing pre-pectoral implantation. (Courtesy of St. Jude Medical, Sunnyvale, CA and Guidant Corp., Minneapolis, MN.)

Implantable Cardioverter–Defibrillator Functioning

Based on their functioning, ICDs have been categorized into "generations." The first-generation ICDs were nonprogrammable devices that used a preset rate criterion to detect ventricular dysrhythmias and deliver a shock at a

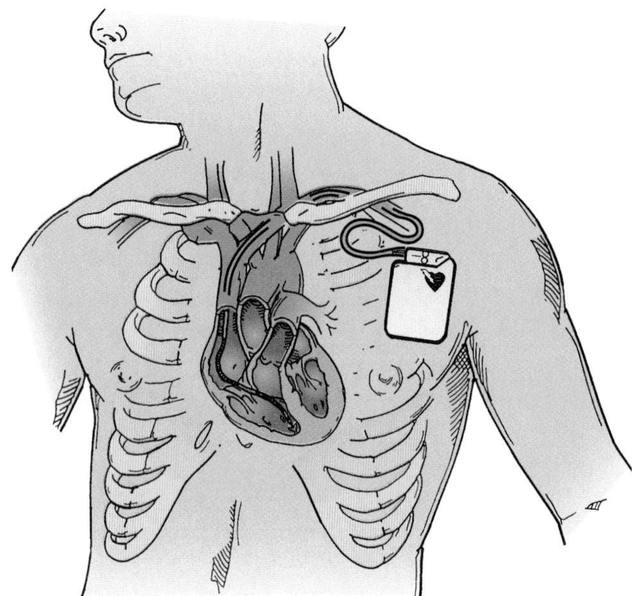

figure 18-43 The implantable cardioverter defibrillator (ICD) mechanical system consists of a generator and a sensing/pacing/defibrillating electrode.

preset energy level. In the mid-1980s, the second generation of the device became available and included more programmable features, among them bradycardia and antitachycardia pacing and synchronized cardioversion. These features allow the use of tiered therapy; the term is used to describe different levels of therapy to terminate a dysrhythmia. The first tier of therapy is usually antitachycardia pacing, which involves the carefully timed delivery of pacing stimuli. If antitachycardia pacing is not successful, the second tier of therapy is initiated by the device. With the second tier, a low-energy synchronized cardioversion is delivered. The energy level for cardioversion can be programmed anywhere from 0.1 to 35 J, depending on the specific device. Some devices allow multiple attempts at cardioversion. If cardioversion is not successful, the third tier of therapy, defibrillation, is used. The energy delivered for defibrillation can be programmed to a maximum of 35 J, again depending on the model and capacity of a device. The number of defibrillation attempts varies with different devices, but six attempts is usually the maximum. If the patient is successfully converted to a life-compatible rhythm, but the rate is slow, ventricular demand pacing is initiated. This fourth tier of therapy is usually intended for brief periods of pacing until normal rhythm resumes.

Today's ICDs are known as third-generation devices and have many programmable features that allow the physician to tailor the device to the patient's needs. Bradycardia pacing therapies with dual-chamber defibrillators are common features of current ICDs. In addition, the availability of an atrial sensing lead allows for a more specific SVT discrimination algorithm. To improve discrimination of tachydysrhythmias, the device allows programming of discrimination algorithms, which withhold ventricular tachycardia therapy when PSVT is confirmed. Some devices also have separate tiers of therapy for atrial tachycardia and atrial fibrillation/flutter. All of the current devices are "noncommitted," that is, therapy is aborted if the tachycardia terminates even while the ICD is charging up. Patients with nonsustained VT need not suffer the discomfort of an inappropriate shock. Third-generation defibrillators have additional features, including memory and event retrieval. Event retrieval may involve R-wave-to-R-wave analysis or the recording of an electrogram. These methods document the dysrhythmia before and after the therapy, allowing the physician to analyze the problematic rhythm. Ideally, these data can be correlated to the patients' symptoms to help further diagnose the dysrhythmia.

Current devices also have the ability to deliver a programmed electrical stimulation (PES) through a programmer. PES is a noninvasive testing method similar to an electrophysiological test. It is used to induce a suspected dysrhythmia to determine the device's ability to terminate it with programmed antitachycardia therapies. It can also be used to ascertain the integrity of the shocking coil, if a lead problem is suspected, and for defining the defibrillation threshold (DFT) of a patient after antidysrhythmia therapy is initiated. The DFT is the lowest amount of energy tested that successfully converts ventricular fibrillation. Certain antidysrhythmic drugs can increase DFTs. For the sake of patient safety, the device should be capable of delivering at least 10 J above the patient's DFT.

PES minimizes the need to test the device in a laboratory situation where catheters are placed in the patient's heart to induce the rhythm disturbance. Testing is done in the device itself, thus reducing the risk associated with the invasive procedure.

The Implantable Cardioverter–Defibrillator Code

The cardiac pacemaker code previously discussed has limited ability to describe modes of ICD function. As a result, in 1993, NASPE and BPEG developed the NASPE/BPEG Defibrillator Code.[13] Known as the NBD defibrillator code, it describes ICD capabilities and operation.

Nursing Management

The critical care nurse plays a key role in the preimplantation and postimplantation management of patients with an ICD. Patient teaching is one of the most important roles for the critical care nurse. Topics for discussion are included in Box 18-26. Patients and families need to understand why an ICD is indicated, the purpose of an ICD, the basic parts of the ICD system, and how the ICD functions. Once the physician has determined the type of system to be used, the nurse reinforces the physician's explanation of how the device will be implanted and where the leads and pulse generator will be placed. The patient and family should be informed of the expected length of hospitalization and plans for follow-up care. Many resources for patient education are available from manufacturers of ICDs, including printed materials and videotapes. In addition, the patient and family may find it helpful to meet with a person who has an ICD. This person may be able to allay any fears or clarify misconceptions about living with an ICD.

In the postimplantation period, the nurse continuously monitors the patient for the development of any ventricular dysrhythmias and intervenes immediately if necessary. If the patient experiences a sustained VT and no therapy is

box 18-26
Using an Implantable Cardioverter–Defibrillator (ICD)

- Why an ICD is indicated
- Purpose of an ICD
- Components of an ICD
- How the ICD works
- How a shock feels
- How the ICD will be implanted
- Expected length of hospitalization
- Postimplant activities of daily living
- Rate cutoff and therapies programmed in the ICD
- Plans for follow-up care
- When to call the doctor
- Importance of an ICD identification card and medical alert bracelet or necklace
- What the patient and family should do if a shock occurs
- Safety precautions
- Support groups

delivered, it is an indication that the programmed detection rate may be above the rate of the tachycardia. A patient with an ICD who has a sustained, hemodynamically unstable rhythm should not be treated any differently from one without an ICD. External cardioversion can be given in an emergency in the absence of therapy from the patient's ICD. Care should be taken not to apply paddles near or above the ICD generator.

The nurse must be aware of the programmed settings and features of the patient's ICD to provide safe and competent care. Device information should be readily available at the bedside and clearly documented in the patient's chart. If the device fires, the status of the patient and the patient's rhythm is assessed and documented. When a device fires in the absence of dysrhythmias, there is a high probability of oversensing due to a dislodged lead, loose connection at the header or an oversensitive setting. Immediate intervention by the electrophysiology service is necessary to avoid further discomfort to the patient.

box 18-27 ***Considerations for Home Care for Patients With an ICD***

- Carry an ICD identification card.
- Wear a medical alert necklace or bracelet.
- Carry a list of your medications and dosages.
- Keep emergency phone numbers readily available.
- Call your physician after receiving a shock if you do not feel completely recovered.
- Call your physician immediately if you receive more than one shock or several in succession.
- Inform family, significant others, coworkers, and traveling companions about your ICD.
- When traveling by air, inform airline security personnel of your ICD.
- Encourage your family members to take a CPR course.

Other immediate postoperative care (wound care, activity instructions) is very similar to that of the patient after pacemaker implantation. Furthermore, because the operative approach is almost identical to that of pacemaker implantation, the complications that might be expected with pacemaker implantation can also be encountered after ICD implantation.

In collaboration with the physician, the nurse provides discharge instructions about resuming daily activities. Patients are usually cautioned against swimming or boating alone or climbing ladders, and to avoid operating equipment that may produce sparks or cause electromagnetic interference. Considerations for home care, listed in Box 18-27, should be reviewed with the patient and family.

Discussion of psychosocial issues regarding living with an ICD also should be part of the discharge preparation. Although the emotional adjustment varies with each patient, many have fears about receiving their first shock. Other potential patient concerns the nurse should discuss include alterations in body image, return to work, participation in recreational activities, and reaction of family and friends to the device. If support groups are available, the patient and family should be encouraged to join.

Cardiopulmonary Resuscitation

In any ICU, there is an increased chance that the patient's condition will deteriorate. The cessation of breathing and circulation is known as *cardiopulmonary arrest*. When a patient is determined to be in cardiopulmonary arrest, seconds matter. Unless definitive action is taken within 4 to 6 minutes, the patient will suffer irreversible brain injury. Prompt intervention is necessary if the patient is going to have a chance of survival. Immediate and effective cardiopulmonary resuscitation (CPR) often prevents fatal complications. CPR is divided into basic life support (BLS), which is discussed in this chapter, and advanced cardiac life support (ACLS).[1,2] The ACLS guidelines developed by the American Heart Association can be found in Appendix A. This section of the chapter outlines assessment, procedures, interventions, and roles of the nurse in the cardiopulmonary arrest situation. Box 18-28 defines some common terms used during CPR.

CAUSES OF CARDIOPULMONARY ARREST

Box 18-29 outlines some of the causes of cardiopulmonary arrest. There are many additional causes of cardiopulmonary arrest. Determination of the cause of the arrest is secondary to rapid intervention. Once intervention to preserve life has been initiated, the cause of the arrest can then be ascertained, and any specific interventions designed

box 18-28
Common Terms in Cardiopulmonary Resuscitation

Cardiac arrest: Abrupt cessation of effective cardiac pumping activity, resulting in cessation of circulation.
Code: Informal term for emergency resuscitation.
Crash cart: Emergency cart (see Table 18-19).
Resuscitation: Restoration of vitals signs by mechanical, physiological, and pharmacological means.
Clinical death: Absence of vital signs.
Biological death: Irreversible cellular changes.

to correct the underlying cause can be added to the BLS and ACLS measures.

ASSESSMENT AND MANAGEMENT OF THE PATIENT IN CARDIOPULMONARY ARREST

Before implementing the resuscitative measures in a code situation, the patient must first be assessed. A myriad of technological monitoring devices are used in the ICU, but it is the everyday physical assessment skills used by nurses that are most accurate in determining a patient's status.

box 18-29
Causes of Cardiopulmonary Arrest

Cardiac Causes
- Myocardial infarction
- Heart failure
- Dysrhythmia
- Coronary artery spasms
- Cardiac tamponade

Pulmonary Causes
- Respiratory failure secondary to respiratory depression
- Airway obstruction
- Impaired gas exchange, such as in acute respiratory distress syndrome
- Impaired ventilation, such as pneumothorax
- Pulmonary embolus
- Electrolyte imbalances
- Hyperkalemia
- Hypomagnesemia
- Hypercalcemia/hypocalcemia

Procedures
- Pulmonary artery catheterization
- Cardiac catheterization
- Surgery

Miscellaneous
- Drug toxicity
- Drug side effects

Determine Responsiveness

The nurse first determines the patient's responsiveness before initiating CPR. If the patient is unresponsive, the nurse calls for help ("initiate a code"), and initiates BLS measures following the acronym *ABC* (airway–breathing–circulation). Box 18-30 summarizes the ABCs of resuscitation.

Position the Patient

The patient should be placed in a supine position on a firm, flat surface. This position enables the rescuer to open the airway and assess for the presence and effectiveness of any spontaneous breathing. If the patient is in a standard hospital bed, a resuscitation board is placed under his or her torso when help arrives. If the patient is in a specialty bed, the CPR setting on the bed is selected.

If the patient is found to be breathing effectively and there is no evidence of trauma, the patient is placed in the recovery position. The recovery position is used to reduce the possibility of airway obstruction by the tongue or by secretions or emesis. To place the patient in the recovery position, the rescuer kneels next to the shoulder of the patient. The rescuer lifts the arm of the patient nearest the rescuer and bends it at the elbow. The arm is then positioned so that the patient's palm of the hand is turned upward and moved toward the patient's face. The rescuer then lifts the leg of the patient furthest from the rescuer and crosses it over the patient's body, moving it toward the res-

box 18-30
Airway, Breathing, and Circulation

Airway
- Open patient's airway using head tilt–chin lift maneuver (jaw thrust for cervically injured patients).
- Observe for spontaneous breathing.
- If patient is not breathing:
  - Place oropharyngeal airway (if possible).
  - Suction as necessary.

Breathing
- Connect Ambu-bag to 100% oxygen.
- Deliver two slow, initial breaths (2 seconds per breath).
- Maintain seal around patient's mouth and nose.
- Observe for chest rise and fall.
- Monitor pulse oximeter.
- Auscultate for bilateral breath sounds.

Circulation
- Check for carotid pulse and other signs of circulation.
- If no signs of circulation are present:
  - Perform chest compressions at rate of 100/minute followed by two slow breaths using a 15:2 ratio for compressions to breaths.
  - After four cycles, recheck the carotid pulse.
- Continue to assess the effectiveness of CPR by:
  - Watching the ECG monitor to assist with ensuring rate.
  - Palpating pulses (radial, femoral, pedal) to determine effectiveness.

cuer. One hand of the rescuer supports the patient's head during turning and the second hand is used to turn the patient's hips toward the rescuer[3] (Fig. 18-44).

Airway

The nurse assesses for an adequate airway. The patient is positioned to ensure an open, patent airway. The patient is placed in the supine position and the airway is opened using the head tilt–chin lift method. In this method, the head is tilted back and the chin is raised to stretch the airway and advance the tongue in preparation for ventilation (Fig. 18-45).

In the case of patients with confirmed or suspected cervical spine injuries, the jaw thrust method is used. The patient's head and neck must not be moved in an effort to ensure that no damage is done to the cervical spinal cord. Keeping the head in a neutral position, the rescuer places a hand on each side of the patient's head behind the temporomandibular joint, and gently pushes the jaw forward. This will open the airway enough to allow for ventilation.

If spontaneous respirations have not returned once a patent airway has been established, then the patient must be assisted with breathing.

Breathing

Using a bag-valve device (BVD), also known as an "Ambubag," oxygen is delivered as rescue breaths. The BVD is connected to 100% high-flow oxygen, and the mask portion is placed over the patient's mouth and nose. If the patient has an endotracheal tube or tracheostomy tube, there is an adapter that allows for delivery of breaths through an artificial airway. The bag reservoir is then squeezed to deliver the breaths. Observation of the patient's chest is necessary to determine whether the delivered breaths are actually ventilating the lungs. A second person assisting with CPR should auscultate all lung fields to confirm that the delivered breaths are reaching the lungs. Pulse oximetry is used to determine oxygenation.

When one person is performing CPR, two slow breaths are delivered initially, after which the ratio is 15 compressions to 2 slow breaths. This is done at a rate of 100 compressions per minute and about 10 to 12 breaths per minute.[1]

Since the advent of the new American Heart Association CPR Guidelines in 2000, two-rescuer CPR now uses the same 15:2 ratio, at the same rate, with rescuer number one giving the breaths and rescuer number two performing the compressions. Once the airway is secure and ACLS has been started, a ratio of 5:1 may be used.[1]

Circulation

Once it has been determined that adequate ventilation is taking place, a rescuer should palpate for a carotid pulse. If no pulse is palpated, chest compressions must be initiated per BLS protocol. External cardiac compression is a simple technique performed by standing at either side of the patient, placing the heel of one hand two to three finger breadths above the xiphoid process, and placing the heel of the other hand over the first. Firm compressions are applied directly downward, and the sternum is depressed between 1½ and 2 inches and released abruptly. This rhythm is maintained at the rate of approximately 100 times per minute. A 15:2 compression–ventilation ratio is used, with a pause to provide the ventilation. To be effective, this technique must be learned correctly and applied skillfully[1] (Fig. 18-46).

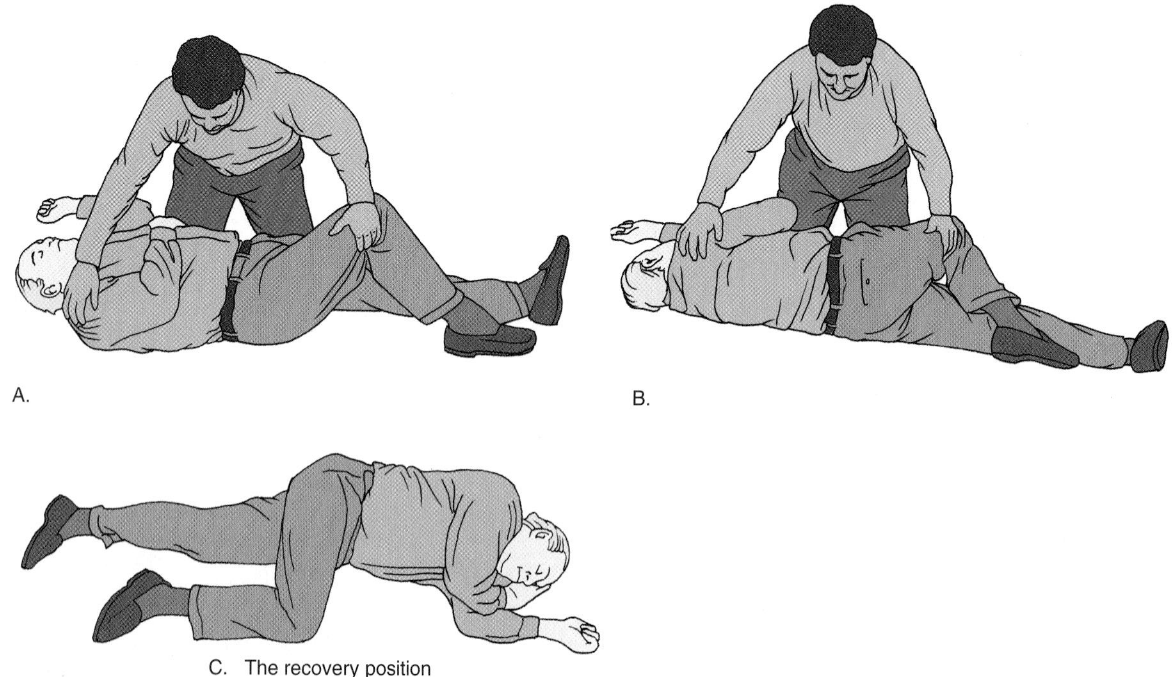

figure 18-44 BLS—The recovery position. How to place a person in the recovery position if unresponsive but breathing. (From Hazinski MF, Cummins RO, Field JM [eds]: 2000 Handbook of Cardiovascular Care for Healthcare Providers. Dallas, TX, American Heart Association, 2000.)

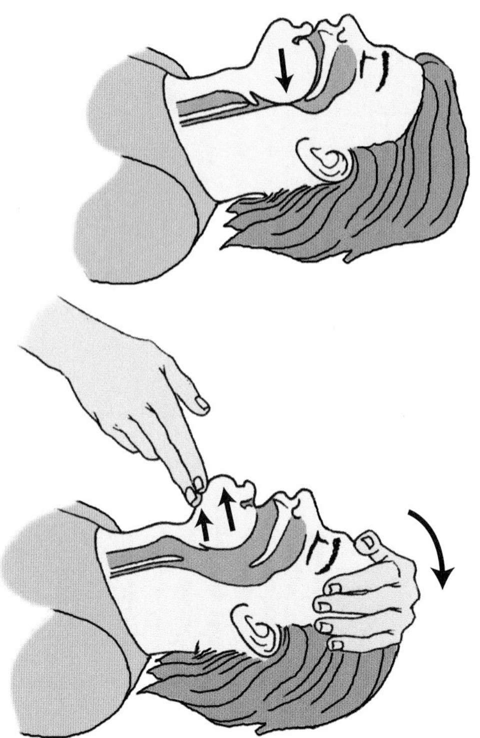

figure 18-45 Opening the airway with back head tilt and chin lift.

If one person must apply both ventilation and compression, it is best to give two complete ventilations mouth-to-mouth or by other readily available means, followed by 15 external cardiac compressions. This routine may be maintained until additional members of the team arrive. When help arrives, one person delivers breaths using the BVD, while another performs chest compressions. The patient's radial, carotid, or femoral pulse is checked at regular intervals to determine the adequacy of compressions. If compressions are being delivered effectively, a pulse should be felt in these regions.

CPR considerations for the pediatric patient and the older patient are found in Boxes 18-31 and 18-32.

ROLE OF RESUSCITATION TEAM MEMBERS

When a cardiopulmonary arrest ("code") is called, various members of the emergency response team are notified. Each institution has its own policies regarding who will respond. In many teaching hospitals, there are residents, medical students, and other students who may respond. Box 18-33 outlines the roles and responsibilities of the code team members.

EQUIPMENT USED IN CARDIOPULMONARY ARREST

The equipment used in resuscitative efforts is kept in a central location in what is commonly referred to as the "crash cart." Most hospitals have rolling carts in easy-to-access locations throughout the hospital. These carts are stocked in a standard way so that all hospital personnel are familiar with the contents and layout of the equipment. The carts must be inventoried daily to ensure their contents are complete and available in the event of a cardiopulmonary arrest. The cart consists of several drawers, a flat top for the storage of larger equipment, an oxygen tank rack, and space for the storage of a backboard. The drawers and intubation tray are locked with a numbered lock in most cases to ensure that all vital equipment remains in place and undisturbed unless needed for an emergency situation. When any of the locks are broken to access the equipment, resupply must be performed at the earliest convenience.

The drawers are labeled to assist personnel in locating specific equipment. The intubation tray is separate from the rest of the crash cart because intubation may be the only measure required to treat an individual in respiratory

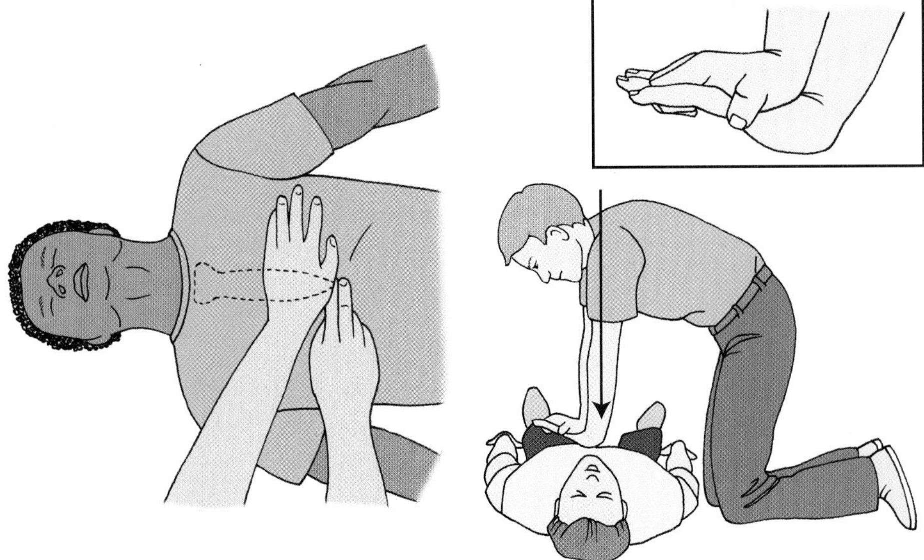

figure 18-46 External chest compression. *Left,* proper hand position over lower portion of sternum; *Right,* correct rescuer position.

box 18-31

CPR Considerations for the Pediatric Patient

- Calculate pediatric dosages of medications.
- Use decreased joules in defibrillation.
- Determine appropriateness of parental presence.
- Consider susceptibility to hypothermia.
- Obtain training in a pediatric advanced life support (PALS) course.
- Remember respiratory arrest is more common than cardiac arrest in children.
- Keep in mind that anatomical differences require specific equipment:
  Smaller endotracheal tubes
  Smaller IV catheters
  Smaller Ambu-bags (adult size may cause barotrauma)
- Note that asystole rather that ventricular fibrillation is the terminal rhythm.
- Keep in mind the normal parameters of vital signs for children.
- Use higher respiratory and pulse rates.
- Adjust depth of compression.
- Adjust techniques of compression (two fingers for infants, one hand for children younger than 12 years).
- Adjust communication technique based on age of child
- Keep separate pediatric emergency equipment cart (Peds Crash Cart).

distress, or in whom there is the potential for a compromised airway. In addition to the intubation tray, a cardiac monitor/defibrillator (preferably with transcutaneous pacing capabilities) is on the top of the cart. An oxygen tank, oxygen tubing, and a BVD (Ambu-bag) are found on the outside of the cart for the same reason, as is portable suctioning equipment. Table 18-19 details the contents and the rationale for the equipment and medications found inside the cart.

MEDICATIONS

There are numerous pharmacological interventions that are used during and immediately after a cardiopulmonary arrest situation. These drugs should be readily available in the crash cart and include antidysrhythmics, inotropes, vasoconstrictors, and electrolyte replacements. Table 18-20 lists these medications, the indications for their use, and their dosages.

box 18-32

CPR Considerations for the Older Patient

- Assess for fractured sternum after CPR. Continue with CPR even if fracture occurs.
- Be certain the health care team implements the patient's desire for Do Not Resuscitate (DNR) or Do Not Intubate (DNI) orders.
- Consider family presence during code.
- Keep in mind the effect of medications due to delayed clearance and altered metabolic response.

box 18-33

Roles and Responsibilities of Code Team Members

Director of the Code (Physician/ Nurse Practitioner/ACLS Qualified Personnel)
- Make diagnosis.
- Direct treatment.

Primary Nurse
- Provide information to code director.
- Contact attending physician.

Second Nurse
- Coordinate use of emergency cart.
- Prepare medications.
- Assemble/pass equipment.
- Defibrillate.

Medication Nurse
- Administer medications.

Charge Nurse
- Coordinate personnel performing CPR.

Nursing Supervisor
- Control crowd.

Anesthesiologist/Nurse Anesthetist
- Intubate patient.
- Manage airway/oxygenation.

Respiratory Therapist
- Assist with manual ventilation.
- Draw arterial blood gas.
- Assist with intubation.
- Set up mechanical ventilator.

Recorder
- Record events, personnel involved.

DEFIBRILLATION

All patients in an ICU are connected to a cardiac monitor that provides useful information during a cardiopulmonary arrest. Once BLS procedures have been initiated, further intervention may be necessary. The nurse assesses the ECG rhythms on the monitor throughout the resuscitation. If the patient is in ventricular fibrillation or pulseless VT, preparations for defibrillation need to be started immediately to avoid death. The delivery of an electrical impulse by an external defibrillator simultaneously depolarizes a majority of the ventricular cells during ventricular fibrillation and the reentry abnormalities of VT. If the conditions are right, and there has not been too much damage to the heart's intrinsic electrical conduction system, the sinoatrial node may resume its function as the pacemaker of the heart.

If indicated, an external countershock should be applied as soon as the instrument is available. The defibrillator pad-

table 18-19 Resuscitation Equipment Cart

Equipment	Rationale
Intubation equipment (usually a separate locked container) Straight and curved blades Endotracheal tubes Syringes Oropharyngeal airways Nasopharyngeal airways Suction catheters	• Provides adequate, patent airway, thus ensuring oxygenation of the lungs during resuscitation • Allows for patient to be placed on mechanical ventilation • Reduces chances for gastric distention, aspiration, or vomiting • Permits suctioning • Allows for the administration of oxygen in high concentrations • Provides route for certain medications (NAVEL)*
Oxygen source (separate tank)	• Ensures that oxygen is available if wall oxygen unavailable
Bag-Valve Device (Ambu-bag)	• Provides seal over patient's mouth and nose; reduces risk to rescuer
Suctioning Equipment Suctioning source Suctioning catheters Suction tubing	• Ensures suctioning available if wall suction unavailable • Clears oropharyngeal (nasopharyngeal) airway before intubation
Intravenous (IV) fluids and tubing	• Improves hypotension
Nitroglycerin tubing	• Prevents precipitation of IV nitroglycerin
Medications (ACLS drugs as a minimum)	• Amiodarone • Lidocaine • Atropine • Epinephrine • Sodium bicarbonate • Calcium chloride • D_{50} • Premixed dopamine infusion
Drip chart (attached to outside of cart)	• Allows for rapid titration of ACLS/Critical Care drugs during and after resuscitation without having to perform complex calculations
Blood tubes	• Allows for the rapid drawing and sending of blood for analysis • Red—chemistries • Blue—coagulation studies • Purple—hematology (complete blood count) • Green—troponin
Arterial blood gas kits	• Allows for rapid drawing and sending of arterial blood gasses
Peripheral IV supplies	• Ensures access for fluid and IV drug administration
Prefilled flush syringes (normal saline)	• Allows for faster flushing of IV lines
Needles	• Allows for drawing up of medications
Decompression (cardiac) needles	• Used in cardiac tamponade
Clipboard with paper and pen; code sheets	• Used to document the arrest
Pressure bags	• Used for rapid infusion of fluid boluses
Manual blood pressure cuff	• Provides dedicated equipment to monitor resuscitative effectiveness
Gloves (latex, nonlatex, sterile)	• Provides protection for rescuers • Provides sterile gloves for invasive/sterile procedures
Defibrillator/transcutaneous pacemaker	• Used in defibrillation, cardioversion, and temporary transcutaneous pacing

*NAVEL is a mnemonic for drugs that may be administered by endotracheal tube: naloxone, atropine, valium, epinephrine, lidocaine.

dles are positioned so that the heart is in the current pathway. The anterior apex, also known as the anterolateral or sternum-apex position, is used most often. The anterior paddle is placed firmly on the patient's upper right chest below the clavicle and to the right of the sternum. The apex paddle is positioned firmly on the patient's lower left chest in a mid-axillary line (Fig. 18-47). The initial shock is delivered at 200 J. If subsequent shocks are needed, a second shock is administered at 200 to 300 J, and a third shock is administered at 360 J.[1] All personnel are advised to avoid touching the patient or bed when the shock is delivered. Immediate resumption of artificial circulation and ventilation (CPR) should occur after each countershock if no pulse returns. Box 18-34 outlines the procedure for defibrillation.

table 18-20 ■ Medications Used to Treat a Patient in Cardiopulmonary Arrest

Drug	Class	Uses	Dosages
Adenosine	Antidysrhythmic	SVT, AF	6 mg rapid IV followed by 10 mL NS flush Repeat twice with 12 mg Max. dose: 30 mg
Amiodarone	Antidysrhythmic	VT, SVT, AF, VF	150–300 mg bolus, 1 mg/min for 6 h, then 0.5 mg/min for 18 h
Atropine	Anticholinergic	Bradycardia, PEA	0.5–1.0 mg IV Max. dose: 3 mg
Bretylium tosylate	Antidysrhythmic	VT, VF	
Calcium chloride	Electrolyte	Hyperkalemia, hypocalcemia, calcium channel blocker toxicity	Syringe 10 mL of 10% solution (100 mg/mL), 2–4 mg/kg
Dobutamine	Inotrope; $beta_1$ agonist	Decreased cardiac output	5–20 μg/kg/min
Dopamine	Inotrope; $beta_1$ agonist	Hypotension	5–20 μg/kg/min
Epinephrine	Catecholamine	VF	Syringe 1:10,000, 1-mg bolus IV Repeat q3–5min
Isoproterenol	Catecholamine; beta agonist	VT, VF	Drip 0.5–5 μg/min
Lidocaine	Antidysrhythmic	VT, VF	Bolus 1–1.5 mg/kg Drip 20–50 μg/kg/min
Magnesium sulfate	Electrolyte	Torsades de pointes	Drip 1–2 g/50 mL NS
Nitroglycerin	Coronary vasodilator	Myocardial infarction, angina	5–100 μg/min
Procainamide	Antidysrhythmic	VT, VF	Bolus 5–10 mg/kg over 8–10 min Drip 20–30 mg/min
Sodium bicarbonate	Alkalinizer	Acidosis	50 mEq syringe Normal dose is 1 mEq/kg
Verapamil	Calcium channel blocker	SVT	2.5–5 mg IV over 2 min Repeat 5–10 mg in 15–30 minutes

AF, atrial fibrillation; NS, normal saline; PEA, pulseless electrical activity; VF, ventricular fibrillation.

Defibrillators are classified based on the type of waveform used by the defibrillator. Since the early 1970s, monophasic defibrillators have been used. This type of defibrillator provides a shock that flows in one direction from one paddle or electrode pad to the other. In more recent years, newer technology has been developed that changes the way the electrical current flows during defibrillation. Known as a biphasic defibrillator, this newer type delivers the current in two phases. The current initially flows in one direction, then flows in the opposite direction. The biphasic wave uses less peak current, so there is less damage to the heart during defibrillation.[4] ICDs have used biphasic technology for over a decade, but it is only recently that transthoracic biphasic defibrillation has been made possible. Clinical trials continue to standardize the amount of energy needed for biphasic defibrillation. The American Heart Association and the International Liaison Committee on Resuscitation (ILCOR) continue to research the applicability of biphasic technology in resuscitation.

AUTOMATED EXTERNAL DEFIBRILLATOR

Studies have shown that the sooner a patient in ventricular fibrillation is defibrillated, the greater the chance for survival. The development of the automated external defibrillator (AED) has improved the survivability of individuals suffering from potentially life-threatening dysrhythmias. The AED allows for defibrillation to be performed in a variety of settings by personnel trained in the use of the AED, but not trained in BLS/ACLS.

The AED consists of a computerized detection system that recognizes the patient's inherent heart rhythm and delivers a defibrillatory countershock when necessary. This cycle of rhythm analysis followed by countershock lasts approximately 30 seconds. AEDs are now found in airports, train stations, sports stadiums, and shopping malls. AEDs are also available in most hospitals in common areas, general floors, and laboratories. The wide-

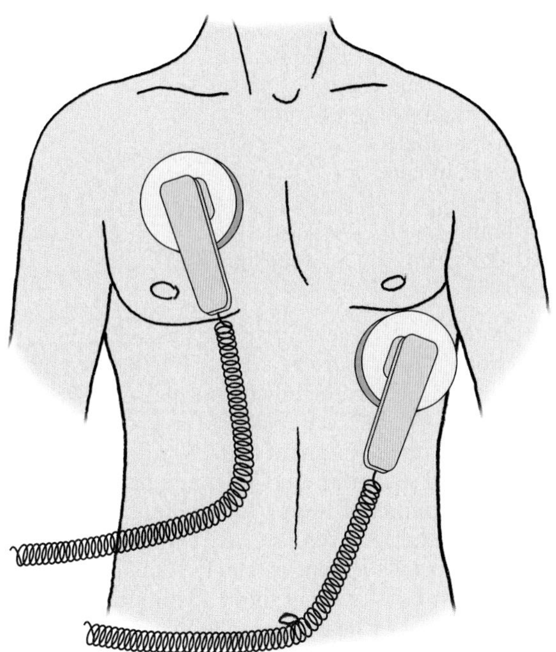

figure 18-47 Standard positioning of defibrillator paddles.

spread availability of these devices allows for a much quicker response time when a person experiences cardiac arrest.[5]

TRANSCUTANEOUS PACING

A combination defibrillator/transcutaneous pacemaker is usually found on top of the crash cart. The large pacing electrodes ("combination pads") used in defibrillation can also be used to pace a patient transcutaneously. Transcutaneous pacing may be used as a "bridge" (temporary measure) until either a transvenous or permanent pacemaker can be placed. The combination pads are placed in an anterior-posterior configuration for more effective pacing.

A nurse, nurse practitioner, or physician quickly and easily initiates transcutaneous pacing. This procedure is noninvasive and therefore is low risk and saves time during an arrest situation. Indications for transcutaneous pacing include new complete (third-degree) heart block, bradycardia (unresponsive to drug therapy), or asystole. The pacing electrodes are also placed when the patient's rhythm changes to a new second-degree, Mobitz II heart block. Transcutaneous pacing also is used when invasive (transvenous) pacing is unsuccessful or contraindicated, such as after the use of thrombolytics and for the patient with sepsis.

The transcutaneous pacemaker is used in a "demand mode" for bradycardia and asystole; it paces the heart only when needed. This mode is safer because the chance of firing on the T wave (R-on-T phenomenon) is greatly reduced. When the pacemaker is used in an asynchronous mode, the heart is paced at a fixed rate, regardless of the heart's intrinsic rate or rhythm. The pacemaker may fire on the T wave, producing either atrial fibrillation or VT. Box 18-35 outlines the procedures for transcutaneous pacing.

THERAPEUTIC HYPOTHERMIA

Unconscious adult patients who suffer out-of-hospital cardiac arrest due to ventricular fibrillation and are resuscitated in the field may benefit from induced mild hypothermia. During cardiac arrest, blood flow to the brain is compromised, and even prompt interventions may not

box 18-34
Indications and Procedure for Defibrillation

Indications

- Pulseless ventricular tachycardia
- Ventricular fibrillation

Procedure

1. Apply defibrillator pads to patient.
2. Turn on defibrillator.
3. Charge defibrillator to 200 joules.
4. Ensure all personnel are not touching patient or bed.
5. Deliver shock.
6. Determine effectiveness of treatment. Check pulse and observe patient's rhythm.
7. Be prepared to deliver subsequent shocks per ACLS protocol.

box 18-35
Indication and Procedure for Transcutaneous Pacing

Indication

- Complete (third-degree) heart block

Procedure

1. Explain procedure to patient.
2. Clip excess hair from chest. Ensure skin is dry.
3. Apply anterior electrode to chest at the fourth intercostal space to the left of the sternum.
4. Apply posterior electrode to patient's back in the area of the left scapula.
5. Connect pacing electrodes to transcutaneous pacemaker.
6. Set pacemaker mode, heart rate, and output.
7. Turn unit on.
8. Assess for effectiveness of pacing:
   - Observe for pacemaker spike with subsequent capture.
   - Assess heart rate and rhythm.
   - Assess blood pressure.
   - Check level of consciousness.
   - Observe for patient anxiety/pain and treat accordingly.

counteract the deleterious effects of this hemodynamic compromise. The cerebral metabolic rate for oxygen ($CMRO_2$) is reduced when the body temperature is reduced. Apoptosis (programmed cell death) and the production of free radicals are reduced in a hypothermic state. Studies have shown that the cooling of the patient after cardiac arrest may preserve neurological function. This therapy is currently contraindicated in children of any age, although research continues. There is evidence that supports hypothermic therapy for cardiac arrest caused by dysrhythmias.[6]

FAMILY PRESENCE IN CARDIAC ARREST SITUATIONS

One aspect of the treatment of cardiopulmonary arrest that has gained attention in recent years is the issue of family presence during a code. Nurses have voiced strong opinions for both sides of the issue. Health care institutions have become more flexible and accommodating for families and visitors. Some emergency departments and ICUs have protocols in place regarding having loved ones at the bedside while resuscitation efforts are taking place. Every effort must be made to have a knowledgeable person explain to the family what measures are being implemented and the rationale. By involving the family in this manner, they can make more informed decisions about the continuation of resuscitation.[7]

Many family members express a desire to be with the patient during CPR for various reasons. Some want to be reassured that all resuscitative efforts were attempted. There are those who want to have a chance to say goodbye at the moment of death, rather than in the hours or days after death. One of the most often cited reasons for wanting to be with the patient is to make sure that the death is painless.

When discussing advanced directives with patients and their families, the techniques of resuscitation are often described. In the event of a cardiac arrest situation, some family members have seen these measures taking place, and make the determination to terminate resuscitation.

The recognition of families after a successful resuscitation must be experienced in order to appreciate it. When the family sees a team of health care professionals working against time to save a patient, they express the realization that nurses, physicians, respiratory therapists, and others combine to provide excellent and compassionate care.

Many nurses and physicians feel that family presence during CPR detracts from their performance, and that individuals who have an emotional attachment to the patient hinder their efforts. Rules must be in place to escort family members from the room if the rescuers cannot effectively perform resuscitative measures.

case study ■ MYOCARDIAL INFARCTION

Mrs. J is a 76-year-old white women currently recovering from an inferior wall myocardial infarction. Her prior medical history includes hypertension, heart failure, chronic obstructive pulmonary disease, type 2 diabetes, and morbid obesity. She is currently on the following medications:

Lisinopril 40 mg orally (PO) qd
Metoprolol 25 mg PO qd
Digoxin 250 μg PO qd
Furosemide 40 mg PO qd
Atrovent inhaler
Serevent inhaler
NPH insulin 20 U subcutaneously (SC) qAM
NPH insulin 10 U SC qPM
Nitroglycerin drip at 30 μg/minute
Heparin drip at 700 units/hour

In addition, she is receiving oxygen by nasal cannula with 2 L fraction of inspired oxygen (FIO_2). She has a right antecubital peripheral IV catheter with normal saline at 84 mL/hour. A Foley catheter is in place. Mrs. J's urine has been clear yellow, with an output of 50 to 60 mL/hour. She has been in normal sinus rhythm with a rate of 70 to 80 beats per minute (bpm). She is on a low-sodium, 2,000-calorie American Dietetic Association (ADA) diet. Her husband visits every morning at approximately 1000, but called this morning to say he is running about 30 minutes late.

Mrs. J's morning laboratory results include the following:

Sodium	133 mEq/L	WBC	7.4 × 10³ mL
Potassium	2.8 mEq/L	Hemoglobin	11.3 g/dL
Chloride	99 mEq/L	Hematocrit	33.4%
CO_2 (venous)	24 mEq/dL	Platelet count	220 × 10³ mL
BUN	22 mg/dL	PT	14.5 sec
Creatinine	1.3 mg/dL	INR	1.1
Glucose	212 mg/dL	PTT	35 sec
Calcium (total)	8.4 mg/dL		
Magnesium	1.4 mEq/L		
Phosphate	4.2 mg/dL		

Mrs. J received her morning medications at 0910. It is now 1015. While at the nurses' station, you observe that Mrs. J's heart rate is now 40 bpm, and appears to be sinus bradycardia. You immediately move to her room, and as you enter the room, you note on the bedside monitor that she is now in severe bradycardia, with a rate of approximately 20 bpm.

You observe Mrs. J take a deep sighing breath. You then place two fingers on her carotid artery. There is a faint pulse, but no respiratory effort. ■

clinical applicability challenges

Self-Challenge: Critical Thinking Questions

1. *Refer to the Case Study at the end of the chapter and answer the following questions.*
   a. *What additional information do you need about Mrs. J?*
   b. *What is your first response?*
   c. *What are your priorities?*
   d. *What has probably happened?*
   e. *What equipment is needed?*
   f. *What are the priority nursing actions after a successful resuscitation?*
   g. *What will you tell Mr. J?*

2. *Mr. King suddenly experiences mid-sternal chest pain, shortness of breath, and diaphoresis. An electrocardiogram reveals ST segment elevation in the anterior leads. List the cardiovascular drugs that you might give Mr. King within the first 30 minutes. Describe the purpose of each drug and how you would evaluate whether the drug produced the intended effect.*
3. *Describe the postprocedure care of patients undergoing a PCI or PBV.*
4. *Many different interventional devices are available for the treatment of CAD. Categorize these devices by the specific lesion types that are best suited for each device.*
5. *Effective timing is critical for achieving successful outcomes with IABP therapy. Describe the implications of tachydysrhythmias on effective diastolic augmentation for patients requiring IABP therapy.*
6. *Compare and contrast the features of internal and external ventricular assist devices.*
7. *Physical assessment is a key nursing function in caring for patients receiving IABP therapy. Describe the abnormal findings you detect when assessing a patient receiving IABP therapy.*
8. *Examine the ethical issues faced by the family of a patient without advance directives when the patient is terminally ill and has an ICD.*
9. *Mr. L has an ICD and reports multiple shocks. What information would you need to assess this patient? What nursing interventions are required?*
10. *A patient who is pacemaker dependent is admitted to the unit with impending battery depletion. You find out that the patient lives alone and has not been compliant with clinic visits. As you prepare your patient for pacemaker generator replacement, formulate a teaching plan encompassing follow-up care.*

Study Questions

1. *Which of the following fibrinolytic drugs is given as a single bolus over 5 seconds?*
   a. *Alteplase*
   b. *Lidocaine*
   c. *Tenecteplase*
   d. *Streptokinase*
2. *Which of the following would amiodarone be used to treat?*
   a. *Ventricular dysrhythmias only*
   b. *Atrial dysrhythmias only*
   c. *Asystole only*
   d. *Both ventricular and atrial dysrhythmias*
3. *Which of the following are actions involving inotropic drugs?*
   a. *Increase myocardial contractility and cardiac output*
   b. *Decrease myocardial oxygen requirements*
   c. *May all be given through an endotracheal tube when the patient does not have IV access*
   d. *Can stop a myocardial infarction*
4. *Angiotensin-converting enzyme inhibitors are used to treat all of the following except*
   a. *congestive heart failure.*
   b. *acute myocardial infarction.*
   c. *hypertension.*
   d. *ventricular tachycardia.*
5. *Coronary stenting as an adjunct may be advantageous over stand-alone PTCA in terms of*
   a. *cost.*
   b. *restenosis rate.*
   c. *risk.*
   d. *length of hospitalization.*
6. *Primary angioplasty refers to*
   a. *PTCA within 1 hour after administration of a thrombolytic in AMI.*
   b. *PTCA within 4 to 6 hours after administration of a thrombolytic in AMI.*
   c. *PTCA without prior administration of a thrombolytic in AMI.*
   d. *PTCA only after a thrombolytic has failed to open the vessel in AMI.*
7. *Restenosis is defined as*
   a. *a reoccurrence of the blockage in a coronary artery.*
   b. *platelet adhesion on the coronary valves.*
   c. *excision of plaque from the coronary artery.*
   d. *dissolving the thrombus in the coronary artery.*
8. *The signs and symptoms of an acute closure after an interventional cardiology procedure are*
   a. *ST segment elevation, chest pain, dysrhythmias.*
   b. *fever, headache, and chest pain.*
   c. *shortness of breath, chest pain, headache.*
   d. *chest pain, sudden cardiac death, and oozing from the puncture site.*
9. *Complications associated with an interventional cardiology procedure include all except which of the following?*
   a. *Bleeding at the catheter insertion site*
   b. *Myocardial infarction*
   c. *Hyperlipidemia*
   d. *Restenosis*
10. *Which of the following are FDA-approved treatments for CAD?*
    a. *PTCA, laser, gene therapy, and directional coronary atherectomy*
    b. *PTCA, stents, laser, and directional coronary atherectomy*
    c. *Medication, PTCA, and magnet resonance angiography*
    d. *PTCA, gene therapy, PMR, and PBV*
11. *Coronary artery perfusion occurs during which phase of the cardiac cycle?*
    a. *Diastole*
    b. *Isovolumetric contraction*
    c. *Systole*
    d. *Isovolumetric relaxation*
12. *The dicrotic notch on the arterial IABP waveform represents which of the following?*
    a. *Closure of the pulmonic valve*
    b. *Closure of the aortic valve*
    c. *Closure of the tricuspid valve*
    d. *Closure of the mitral valve*
13. *Inflation of the intra-aortic balloon occurs at which point of the IABP waveform?*
    a. *Dicrotic notch*
    b. *End-diastolic dip*
    c. *Inflation slope*
    d. *Systolic peak*

14. *Ensuring proper nutritional support for patients requiring ventricular assist device (VAD) support includes all but which one of the following?*
   a. *Obtaining dietary consult*
   b. *Discouraging family visits at mealtime*
   c. *Providing mealtime flexibility*
   d. *Encouraging oral intake*
15. *Which deployed pacemaker mode allows intrinsic AV conduction?*
   a. *VDDRO*
   b. *AAIRO*
   c. *DOOMS*
   d. *VOOCO*
16. *Mr. Wood has an ICD implanted in the left lower quadrant of his abdomen. When obtaining his history, you find out that the patient also had CABG surgery at the time of ICD lead implant. You do not see any incision lines at the subclavicular area. What kind of leads does Mr. Wood have?*
   a. *Transvenous sensing with "hot can"*
   b. *Transvenous sensing and epicardial patches*
   c. *Epicardial patches and myocardial sensing leads*
   d. *Abdominal patches and transvenous sensing*
17. *Ms. Roth returns to the unit after ablation of AVNRT. The patient complains of palpitations and the monitor shows sinus rhythm with premature atrial contractions. What do you tell the patient?*
   a. *The ablation failed and needs to be redone.*
   b. *It is normal to have some skipped beats after ablation and does not necessarily mean failure of intervention.*
   c. *She will probably develop a different kind of rhythm disorder.*
   d. *She needs to avoid all caffeinated products from now on.*
18. *Mrs. Taylor is undergoing cardioversion for atrial fibrillation. She is on amiodarone, digoxin, and warfarin (Coumadin). Her creatinine level was reported above the upper limits of normal. What other laboratory test(s) would be needed to ensure safe cardioversion?*
   a. *Potassium, digoxin levels*
   b. *BUN*
   c. *Amiodarone levels*
   d. *Liver function tests*
19. *Programmed electrical stimulation (PES) performed through an ICD is indicated in which of the following conditions?*
   a. *After initiation of amiodarone*
   b. *Nonsustained VT without device firings*
   c. *Sustained VT with appropriate device firings*
   d. *New-onset atrial fibrillation*
20. *You are caring for Mr. Smith, who has a temporary transvenous VVI pacemaker. You note some pauses on the monitor, without pacemaker spikes. The patient is in no acute distress. After verifying tight connections, you note that the sensitivity setting is at 0.5 mV, output at 10 mA. What adjustment do you make with to the pacemaker setting?*
   a. *Increase sensitivity to 0.1 mV.*
   b. *Decrease sensitivity to 2.5 mV.*
   c. *Increase output 15 mA.*
   d. *Decrease output to 5 mA.*
21. *As you enter your patient's room, you note that the patient's monitor indicates sustained ventricular tachycardia. The first action is to*
   a. *activate the code system.*
   b. *defibrillate using 200 J.*
   c. *begin cardiopulmonary resuscitation.*
   d. *assess the patient's responsiveness, airway, breathing, and circulation.*
22. *Compressions are started on an elderly woman with osteoporosis and cracking of the sternum occurs after the third compression. What does the person performing compressions do?*
   a. *Cease compressions until a chest x-ray is obtained.*
   b. *Continue with compressions.*
   c. *Call for IV epinephrine.*
   d. *Cease compressions because the patient is deceased.*
23. *Automated external defibrillators (AEDs) are now being used in may public access areas such as airports, sports stadiums, and shopping malls. The rationale for this is*
   a. *many more victims of potentially lethal dysrhythmias can be treated, thus increasing the chance of survival.*
   b. *people with pacemakers need these special devices.*
   c. *emergency response workers will not have to carry as much equipment.*
   d. *more cardiac arrests occur in these areas.*
24. *During a cardiac arrest situation, a patient's family member requests to be present during cardiopulmonary resuscitation. As the nurse at the bedside, what is the paramount concern while the family member is in the room?*
   a. *Staff safety*
   b. *Family member comfort*
   c. *Lack of interference in resuscitation efforts*
   d. *Allowing the family member to participate*

REFERENCES

Pharmacological Therapy

1. White HD, Wan de Werf FJ: Thrombolysis for acute myocardial infarction. Circulation 97:1632–1646, 1998
2. White HD, Gersh BJ, Opie LH: Antithrombotic agents: Platelet inhibitors, anticoagulants, and fibrinolytics. In Opie LH, Gersh BJ (eds): Drugs for the Heart (5th Ed), pp 273–322. Philadelphia, WB Saunders, 2001
3. Cannon CP, Gibson CM, McCabe CH, et al: TNK-tissue plasminogen activator compared with front-loaded alteplase in acute myocardial infarction: Results of the TIMI 10B trial. Circulation 98:2805–2814, 1998
4. Assessment of the Safety and Efficacy of a New Thrombolytic (ASSENT-2) Investigators: Single-bolus tenecteplase compared with front-loaded alteplase in acute myocardial infarction: The ASSENT-2 double-blind randomised trial. Lancet 354:716–722, 1999
5. The GUSTO V Investigators: Reperfusion therapy for acute myocardial infarction with fibrinolytic therapy or combination reduced fibrinolytic therapy and platelet glycoprotein IIb/IIIa inhibition: The GUSTO V randomised trial. Lancet 357:1905–1914, 2001
6. Ryan TJ, Antman EM, Brooks NH, et al: ACC/AHA guidelines for the management of patients with acute myocardial infarction: 1999 update: A report of the American College of Cardiology/American Heart Association Task Force on Practice Guidelines (Committee on Management of Acute Myocardial Infarction). Available at www.acc.org. Accessed on August 18, 2001
7. Cohen M, Demers C, Gurfinkel EP, et al., for the ESSENCE Study Group: A comparison of low-molecular-weight heparin with unfractionated heparin for unstable coronary artery disease. N Engl J Med 337:447–452, 1997
8. Goodman SG, Cohen M, Bigonzi F, et al., for the ESSENCE Study Group: Randomized trial of low molecular weight heparin (Enoxaparin) versus unfractionated heparin for unstable coronary artery disease. J Am Coll Cardiol 36:693–698, 2000

9. Antman E, McCabe CH, Gurfinkel EP, et al: Enoxaparin prevents death and cardiac ischemic events in unstable angina/non-Q-wave myocardial infarction: Results of the Thrombolysis in Myocardial Infarction (TIMI) 11B trial. Circulation 100:1593–1601, 1999
10. Antman E, Cohen M, Radley D, et al: Assessment of the treatment effect of enoxaparin for unstable angina/non-Q-wave myocardial infarction: TIMI 11B-ESSENCE meta-analysis. Circulation 100: 1602–1608, 1999
11. The Coumadin Aspirin Reinfarction Study (CARS) Investigators: Randomised double-blind trial of fixed low-dose warfarin with aspirin after myocardial infarction. Lancet 350:389–396, 1997
12. CAPRIE Steering Committee: A randomised, blinded trial of clopidogrel versus aspirin in patients at risk of ischemic events (CAPRIE). Lancet 348:1329–1339, 1996
13. O'Shea JC, Hafley GE, Greenberg S, et al: Platelet glycoprotein IIb/IIIa integrin blockade with eptifibatide in coronary stent intervention. JAMA 285:2468–2473, 2001
14. The ESPRIT Investigators: Novel dosing regimen of eptifibatide in planned coronary stent implantation (ESPRIT): A randomised, placebo-controlled trial. Lancet 356:2037–2044, 2000
15. The EPISTENT Investigators: Randomised placebo-controlled and balloon-angioplasty-controlled trial to assess safety of coronary stenting with use of platelet glycoprotein-IIb/IIIa blockade. Lancet 352:87–92, 1998
16. Schömig A, Kastrati A, Dirschinger J, et al., for the STOPAMI Study Investigators: Coronary stenting plus platelet glycoprotein IIb/IIIa blockade compared with tissue plasminogen activator in acute myocardial infarction. N Engl J Med 343:385–391, 2000
17. Antman E, Giugliano RP, Gibson CM, et al: Abciximab facilitates the rate and extent of thrombolysis: Results of the Thrombolysis in Myocardial Infarction (TIMI) 14 trial. Circulation 99:2720–2732, 1999
18. The Platelet Receptor Inhibition in Ischemic Syndrome Management (PRISM) Study Investigators: A comparison of aspirin plus tirofiban with aspirin plus heparin for unstable angina. N Engl J Med 338:1498–1505, 1998
19. The Platelet Receptor Inhibition in Ischemic Syndrome Management in Patients Limited by Unstable Signs and Symptoms (PRISM-PLUS) Investigators: Inhibition of the platelet glycoprotein IIb/IIIa receptor with tirofiban in unstable angina and non-Q-wave myocardial infarction. N Engl J Med 338:1488–1497, 1998
20. Woosley RL: Antiarrhythmic drugs. In Fuster V, Alexander RW, O'Rourke FA (eds): Hurst's The Heart (10th Ed), pp 899–924. New York, McGraw-Hill, 2001
21. Camm AJ, Al-Saady NM, Opie LH: Antiarrhythmic agents. In Opie LH, Gersh BJ (eds): Drugs for the Heart (5th Ed), pp 221–272. Philadelphia, WB Saunders, 2001
22. The CAPRICORN Investigators: Effect of carvedilol on outcome after myocardial infarction in patients with left-ventricular dysfunction: The CAPRICORN randomised trial. Lancet 357:1385–1390, 2001
23. Packer M, Coats AJS, Fowler MB, et al., for the COPERNICUS Study Group: Effects of carvedilol on survival in severe chronic heart failure. N Engl J Med 344:1651–1658, 2001
24. MERIT-HF Study Group: Effect of metoprolol CR/XL in chronic heart failure: Metoprolol CR/XL randomised intervention trial in congestive heart failure (MERIT-HF). Lancet 353:2001–2007, 1999
25. The CIBIS-II Investigators and Committees: The cardiac insufficiency bisoprolol study II (CIBIS-II): A randomised trial. Lancet 353:9–13, 1999
26. Braunwald E, Antman EM, Beasley JW, et al: ACC/AHA guidelines for the management of patients with unstable angina and non-ST-segment elevation myocardial infarction: A report of the American College of Cardiology/American Heart Association Task Force on Practice Guidelines. J Am Coll Cardiol 36:970–1062, 2000
27. O'Rourke RA: Optimal medical management of patients with chronic ischemic heart disease. Curr Probl Cardiol 26:195–238, 2001
28. Sra J, Dhala A, Blanck Z, et al: Atrial fibrillation: Epidemiology, mechanisms, and management. Curr Probl Cardiol 25:413–524, 2000
29. Cairns JA, Connolly SJ, Roberts R, et al., for the Canadian Amiodarone Myocardial Infarction Arrhythmias Trial Investigators: Randomised trial of outcome after myocardial infarction in patients with frequent or repetitive ventricular premature depolarisations: CAMIAT. Lancet 349:675–682, 1997
30. Roy D, Talajic M, Dorian P, et al: Amiodarone to prevent recurrence of atrial fibrillation. N Engl J Med 342:913–920, 2000
31. Giri S, White CM, Dunn AB, et al: Oral amiodarone for prevention of atrial fibrillation after open heart surgery, the Atrial Fibrillation Suppression Trial (AFIST): A randomised placebo-controlled trial. Lancet 357:830–836, 2001
32. Hazinski MF, Cummins RO, Field JM (eds): 2000 Handbook of Emergency Cardiovascular Care for Healthcare Providers. Dallas, American Heart Association, 2000
33. Freher M, Challapalli S, Pinto JV, et al: Current status of calcium channel blockers in patients with cardiovascular disease. Curr Probl Cardiol 24:236–340, 1999
34. Chai AU, Crawford MH: "Traditional" medical therapy for unstable angina: How important? How to use? Cardiol Clin 17:359–372, 1999
35. Opie LH, Gersh BJ: Digitalis, acute inotropes, and inotropic dilators. In Opie LH, Gersh BJ (eds): Drugs for the Heart (5th Ed), pp 154–186. Philadelphia, WB Saunders, 2001
36. The Digitalis Investigation Group: The effect of digoxin on mortality and morbidity in patients with heart failure. N Engl J Med 336:525–533, 1997
37. Hauptman PJ, Kelly RA: Digitalis. Circulation 99:1265–1270, 1999
38. Opie L, Frishman WH: Adverse cardiovascular drug interactions and complications. In Fuster V, Alexander RW, O'Rourke FA (eds): Hurst's The Heart (10th Ed), pp 2251–2269. New York, McGraw-Hill, 2001
39. Opie LH, Yusuf S, Poole-Wilson PA, et al: Angiotensin-converting enzyme (ACE) inhibitors, angiotensin-II receptor blockers (ARBs), and aldosterone antagonism. In Opie LH, Gersh BJ (eds): Drugs for the Heart (5th Ed), pp 107–153. Philadelphia, WB Saunders, 2001
40. Frishman WH, Cheng A: Secondary prevention of myocardial infarction: Role of β-adrenergic blockers and angiotensin-converting enzyme inhibitors. Am Heart J 137:S25–S34, 1999
41. ACE Inhibitor Myocardial Infarction Collaborative Group: Indications for ACE inhibitors in the early treatment of acute myocardial infarction: Systematic overview of individual data from 100,000 patients in randomized trials. Circulation 97:2202–2212, 1998
42. Domanski MJ, Exner DV, Borkowf CB, et al: Effect of angiotensin converting enzyme inhibition on sudden cardiac death in patients following acute myocardial infarction: A meta-analysis of randomized clinical trials. J Am Coll Cardiol 33:598–604, 1999
43. The Heart Outcomes Prevention Evaluation Study Investigators: Effects of an angiotensin-converting enzyme inhibitor, ramipril, on cardiovascular events in high-risk patients. N Engl J Med 342:145–153, 2000
44. Aronow HD, Topol EJ, Roe MT, et al: Effect of lipid-lowering therapy on early mortality after acute coronary syndromes: An observational study. Lancet 357:1063–1068, 2001
45. Expert Panel on Detection, Evaluation, and Treatment of High Blood Cholesterol in Adults: Executive summary of the third report of the National Cholesterol Education Program (NCEP) Expert Panel on detection, evaluation, and treatment of high blood cholesterol in adults (Adult Treatment Panel III). JAMA 285:2486–2497, 2001

Percutaneous Coronary Interventions and Percutaneous Balloon Valvuloplasty

1. American Heart Association: 2004 Heart and Stroke Facts. Dallas, TX, American Heart Association, 2004
2. Bain DS: Coronary angioplasty. In Grossman W, Bain DS (eds). Cardiac Catheterization, Angiography and Intervention (p 441). Philadelphia, Lee & Febiger, 1991
3. Society of Thoracic Surgeons: National Adult Cardiac Surgical Database Report 2000–2001. Chicago, author, 2004
4. Detre K, et al: New approaches to coronary interventions. J Am Coll Cardiol 35:1122–1129, 2000
5. Bentivoglio LG, Holubkov R, Kelsey SF, et al: Short and long term outcome of percutaneous transluminal coronary angioplasty in unstable versus stable angina pectoris: A report of the 1985/1986 NHLBI PTCA registry. Cathet Cardiovasc Diagn 23:227–238, 1991
6. O'Keefe JH Jr, Rutherford BD, McConahay DR, et al: Multi-vessel coronary angioplasty from 1980 to 1989: Procedural results and long-term outcome. J Am Coll Cardiol 16:1097–1102, 1990
7. Dorros G, Iyer SS, Hall P, et al: Percutaneous coronary angioplasty in 1001 multi-vessel coronary disease patients: An analysis of different patient subsets. J Interv Cardiol 4:71–80, 1991
8. Alderman EL, Bourassa MG, Cohen LS, et al., for the CASS Investigators: Ten-year follow-up of survival and myocardial infarction

in the randomized coronary artery surgery study. Circulation 82: 1629–1646, 1990
9. Meyer J, Merx W, Schmitz H, et al: Percutaneous transluminal coronary angioplasty immediately after intracoronary streptolysis of transmural myocardial infarction. Circulation 66:905–913, 1982
10. Grines CL: Primary angioplasty in myocardial infarction. J Am Coll Cardiol 33: 640–646, 1999
11. Coombs VJ, Brinker JA: Primary angioplasty in the acute myocardial infarction setting. AACN Clin Issues 6:387–397, 1995
12. Simari RD, et al: Coronary angioplasty in acute myocardial infarction: Primary, immediate, adjunctive, rescue or deferred adjunctive approach? Mayo Clin Proc 69:346–358, 1994
13. Aversano T, Aversano LT, Passamani E, et al: Thrombolytic therapy versus primary percutaneous coronary intervention for myocardial infarction in patients presenting to hospitals without on-site cardiac surgery: A randomized controlled trial. JAMA 287:1943–1951, 2002
14. Braunwald E, Antman EM, Beasley JW, et al: ACC/AHA Guideline Update for the Management of Patients with Unstable Angina and Non-ST Segment Elevation Myocardial Infarction-2002: Summary article. Circulation 106:1893–1900, 2002
15. Banks A, Drew B, Ide B: Does recording of a patient's ST segment "fingerprint" during percutaneous transluminal coronary angioplasty (PTCA) help to exclude coronary artery reocclusion as the cause of transient ischemia following the procedure? Prog Cardiovasc Nurs 14(3):115–116, 1999
16. Goodkind J, Coombs VJ, Golobic RA: Excimer laser angioplasty. Heart Lung 22:26–35, 1993
17. U.S. Food and Drug Administration: Center for Devices and Radiological Health. PMA Final Decisions. Publication No. P880047/S005, 1998
18. Waksman R, Robinson KA, Crocker IR, et al: Intracoronary radiation before stent implantation inhibits neointima formation in stented porcine coronary arteries. Circulation 92:1383–1386, 1995
19. Oesterle SN, et al: Percutaneous transmyocardial revascularization for severe angina: The PACIFIC trial. Lancet 356:1705–1710, 2000
20. Coombs VJ: Gene therapy for the treatment of cardiovascular disease. Crit Care Clin North Am 11(3), 349–353, 1999

Intra-aortic Balloon Pump Counterpulsation and Mechanical Circulatory Support

1. Marra C, DeSanto LS, et al: Coronary artery by-pass grafting in patients with severe left ventricle dysfunction: A prospective randomized study. Int J Artif Organs 25:141, 2002
2. Stevenson LW, Kormos RL: Mechanical cardiac support 2000: Current applications and future trial design. J Am Coll Cardiol 37:340–370, 2001
3. Heart Assist Pump. The Penn State Heart Devices page. Available at http://www.psu.edu/ur/heartdevices/asstpump.htm. Accessed November 1, 2003
4. Delagado DH, Rao V, Ross HJ, et al: Mechanical circulatory assistance: State of the art. Circulation 106:2046–2050, 2002
5. Holman WL, Bourge RC, McGriffin DC, et al: Ventricular assist: Experience with a pulsatile heterotopic device. Semin Thorac Cardiovasc Surg 6(3):147–153, 1994
6. McCarthy PM, Sabik JF: Implantable circulatory support devices as a bridge to heart transplantation. Semin Thorac Cardiovasc Surg 6(3):174–180, 1994
7. Farrar DJ: Ventricular interactions during mechanical circulatory support. Semin Thorac Cardiovasc Surg 6(3):163–168, 1994
8. Dasse KA, Frazier OH, Graham TR: The physiology of left ventricular assistance. In Lewis T, Graham TR (eds): Mechanical Circulatory Support, pp 13–25. London, Edward Arnold, 1995
9. Oz MC, Rose EA, Slater J, et al: Malignant ventricular rhythms are well tolerated in patients receiving long-term left ventricular assist devices. J Am Coll Cardiol 24:1688–1691, 1994

Management of Dysrhythmias

1. Cummins RO: Textbook of Advanced Cardiac Life Support. Dallas, American Heart Association, 2001
2. ACLS.net Synchronized Cardioversion Algorithm 2001. Available at http://www.acls.net/newalgo/cardioversion.htm. Accessed August 30, 2001
3. Fuster V, Ryden LE, Asinger RW, et al: ACC/AHA/ESC guidelines for the management of patients with atrial fibrillation: A report of the American College of Cardiology/American Heart Association Task Force on Practice Guidelines and the European Society of Cardiology Committee for Practice Guidelines and Policy Conferences (Committee to Develop Guidelines for the Management of Patients With Atrial Fibrillation). J Am Coll Cardiol 38:1231–1266, 2001
4. Zipes D, DiMarco J, Gillette P, et al: ACC/AHA guidelines for the clinical intracardiac electrophysiological and catheter ablation procedures: A report of the American College of Cardiology/American Heart Association Task Force on Practice Guidelines (Committee on Clinical Intracardiac Electrophysiologic and Catheter Ablation Procedures) 1. Circulation 92:673–691, 1995
5. Obias-Manno D: Unconventional applications in pacemaker therapy. AACN Clin Issues 12:127–139, 167–169, 2001
6. Gregoratos G, Cheitlin MD, Conill A, et al: ACC/AHA guidelines for implantation of cardiac pacemakers and antiarrhythmia devices: A report of the American College of Cardiology/American Heart Association Task Force on Practice Guidelines (Committee on Pacemaker Implantation). J Am Coll Cardiol 31:1175–1209, 1998
7. NIH Clinical Center Nursing Department: SOP: Care of the patient with a temporary transvenous pacemaker. Available at http://www.cc.nih.gov/nursing/pacemakt.html. Accessed August 30, 2001
8. Bernstein AD, Daubert JC, Fletcher RD, et al: The revised NASPE/BPEG generic code for antibradycardia, adaptive-rate, and multisite pacing. Pacing Clin Electrophysiol 25:260–264, 2002
9. Maisel WH, Sweeney MO, Stevenson SG, et al: Recalls and safety alerts involving pacemakers and implantable cardioverter-defibrillator generators. JAMA 286:793–799, 2001
10. Morton PG: The pacemaker and defibrillator codes: Implications for critical care nursing. Crit Care Nurse 17(1):50–59, 1997
11. American Heart Association: Heart and Stroke Statistical Update, 2001. Available at http://www.Americanheart.org/statistics/index.html. Accessed November, 2003
12. Winters S, Packer D, Marchlinski F, et al: Consensus statement on indications, guidelines for use, and recommendations for follow-up of implantable cardioverter defibrillators. Pacing Clin Electrophysiol 24:262–269, 2001
13. Bernstein AD, Camm AJ, Fisher JD, et al: The NASPE/BPEG defibrillator code. Pacing Clin Electrophysiol 16:1776–1780, 1993

Cardiopulmonary Resuscitation

1. American Heart Association: Instructor's Manual: Basic Life Support. Dallas, American Heart Association, 2000
2. American Heart Association: Advanced Cardiac Life Support. Dallas, American Heart Association, 2001
3. Hazinski MF, Cummins RO, Field JM: 2000 Handbook of Emergency Cardiovascular Care for Healthcare Providers. Dallas, American Heart Association, 2000
4. Mair M: Monophasic and biphasic defibrillators: The evolving technology of cardiac defibrillation. Am J Nurs 103(8):58–60, 2003
5. Powers C, Martin K: When seconds count, use an AED. Am J Nurs 102(May Suppl):8–10, 2002
6. Nolan JP, Morley PT, Vander Hoek TL, et al: Therapeutic hypothermia after cardiac arrest: An advisory statement by the Advanced Life Support Task Force of the International Liaison Committee on Resuscitation. Circulation 108:118–121, 2003
7. Tucker T: Family presence during resuscitation. Crit Care Nurs Clin North Am 14:177–185, 2002

OTHER SELECTED READING

Pharmacological Therapy

Haugh KH: Antidysrhythmic agents at the turn of the twenty-first century: A current review. Crit Care Nurs Clin North Am 14:53–70, 2002
Kee V: Hemodynamic pharmacology of intravenous vasopressor. Crit Care Nurse 23(4):79–82, 2003
Kuhn M: Herbal remedies: Drug-herb interactions. Crit Care Nurse 22(2):22–32, 2002
Moore LA, Blount KA: Medications and the elderly in critical care settings. Crit Care Nurs Clin North Am 14:111–120, 2002
Moser D, Biddle M: Angiotensin-converting enzyme inhibitors and angiotensin II receptor blockers: What we know and current controversies. Crit Care Nurs Clin North Am 15:223–237, 2003
Stewart-Amidei C: Pharmacology advances in neuroscience intensive care units. Crit Care Nurs Clin North Am 14:31–38, 2002

Wedekind C, Fidler B: Compatibility of commonly used intravenous infusions in a pediatric intensive care unit. Crit Care Nurse 21(4):45–51, 2001

Percutaneous Coronary Interventions and Percutaneous Balloon Valvuloplasty

Apple S, Lindsay J: Principles and Practice of Interventional Cardiology. Philadelphia, Lippincott Williams & Wilkins, 2000

Bally K, Campbell D, Chesnick K, et al: Effects of patient-controlled music therapy during coronary angioplasty on procedural pain and anxiety distress syndrome. Crit Care Nurse 23(2):50–58, 2003

Smith SC, Dove JT, Jacobs AK, et al: ACC/AHA guidelines for percutaneous coronary interventions: A report of the American College of Cardiology/American Heart Association Task Force on Practice Guidelines (Committee to Revise the 1993 Guidelines for Percutaneous Transluminal Coronary Angioplasty). J Am Coll Cardiol 37:2239i–lxvi, 2001

Ronnevig M, Bjorsvik E, Gullestad L, et al: A descriptive study of early nonspecific chest pain after PTCA: Important area for the acute health care personnel. Heart Lung 32:241–249, 2003

Serruys PW, Kutryk MJB (eds): Handbook of Coronary Stents. Malden, MA, Blackwell Science, 2000

Sulzbach-Hoke L, Cupich D: Capping arterial sheaths in patients undergoing percutaneous coronary intervention: Evidence-based practice. Crit Care Nurse 22(3):64–68, 2001

Thompson EJ, King SL: Acetylcysteine and fenoldopam: Promising new approaches for preventing effects of contrast nephrotoxicity. Crit Care Nurse 23(3):39–46, 2003

Topol EJ (ed): Textbook of Interventional Cardiology (4th Ed). Philadelphia, WB Saunders, 2002

Intra-aortic Balloon Pump Counterpulsation and Mechanical Circulatory Support

Andrus S, Dubois J, Jansen C, et al: Teaching documentation tool: Building a successful discharge. Crit Care Nurse 23(2):39–48, 2003

Bond AE, Nelson K, Germany CL, et al: The left ventricular assist device. Am J Nurs 103(1):32–40, 2003

Christenson JT, Simonet F, Badel P, et al: Optimal timing of preoperative intra-aortic balloon pump support in high-risk coronary patients. Ann Thorac Surg 68:934–939, 1999

French JK, Feldman HA, Assmann SF, et al: Influence of thrombolytic therapy, with or without intra-aortic balloon counterpulsation, on 12-month survival in the SHOCK trial. Am Heart J 145:805–810, 2003

McCafferty M, Sorbellini D, Cianci P: Telemetry to home: Successful discharge of patients with ventricular assist devices. Crit Care Nurse 22(3):43–51, 2002

McNamara NS, Wharton TP, LaRochelle T, et al: Use of intraaortic balloon counterpulsation in patients with acute myocardial infarction who present to community hospitals. Crit Pathways Cardiol 1(3):159–179, 2002

Savage L: Quality of life among patients with a left ventricular assist device: What is new? AACN Clin Issues 14(1):64–72, 2003

Warner Stevenson L, Rose EA: Left ventricular assist devices: Bridges to transplantation, recovery, and destination for whom? Circulation 108:3059–3063, 2003

Management of Dysrhythmias

Abrams J, Epstein AE, Freedman R, et al: ACC/AHA/NASPE 2002 guideline update for implantation of cardiac pacemakers and antiarrhythmic devices. Available at www.acc.org/clinical/guidelines/pacemaker/pacemaker.pdf

Bubien RS: A new beat on an old rhythm. Am J Nurs 100(1):42–51, 2000

Boyle J, Rost MK: Present status of cardiac pacing: a nursing perspective. Crit Care Nurs Q 23(1):1–19, insert 2p, 2000

Dimarco JB: Implantable cardioverter-defibrillators. N Engl J Med 349:1836–1847, 2003

Ezkowitz JA, Armstrong PW, McAlister FA: Implantable cardioverter defibrillators in primary and secondary prevention: A systematic review of randomized, controlled trials. Ann Intern Med 138:445–452, 2003

Fenton JM: The clinician's approach to evaluating patients with dysrhythmias. AACN Clin Issues 12(1):72–86, 2001

Gilbert CJ: Common supraventricular tachycardias: mechanisms and management. AACN Clin Issues 12(1):100–113, 2001

Kelly A: Does pre-hospital transcutaneous cardiac pacing improve patient outcome? Prehosp Immed Care 4(4):194–195, 2000

Mansfield R: Current practice and complications of temporary cardiac pacing. Care Crit Ill 16(5):184–188, 2000

Reynolds J, Apple S: A systematic approach to pacemaker assessment. AACN Clin Issues 12(1):114–126, 2001

Ross RA, Kenny RA: Pacemaker syndrome in older people. Age Ageing 29(1):13–15, 2000

Shaffer R: ICD therapy: The patient's perspective. Am J Nurs 102(2): 46–49, 2002

Steinke E: Sexual concerns of patients and partners after an implantable cardioverter defibrillator. Dimens Crit Care Nurs 22(2):89–96, 2003

Thomas SA, Friedmann E, Kelley FJ: Living with an implantable cardioverter-defibrillator: A review of the current literature related to psychosocial factors. AACN Clinical Issues 12(1):156–163, 2001

Van Orden Wallace CJ: Diagnosing and treating pacemaker syndrome. Crit Care Nurse 21(1):24–31, 35–37, 2001

Radiofrequency Catheter Ablation

Bubien RS, Sanchez JE: Atrial fibrillation: Treatment rationale and clinical utility of nonpharmacologic therapies. AACN Clinical Issues 12(1):140–155, 2001

Larson MS, McDonald K, Young C, et al: Quality of life before and after radiofrequency catheter ablation in patients with drug refractory atrioventricular nodal reentrant tachycardia. Am J Cardiol 84:471–473, 1999

Natale A, Zimerman L, Tomassoni G, et al: AV node ablation and pacemaker implantation after withdrawal of effective rate-control medications for chronic atrial fibrillation: Effect on quality of life and exercise performance. Pacing Clin Electrophysiol 22):1634–1639, 1999

Teplitz L: Treating tachyarrhythmias with radiofrequency catheter ablation. Dimens Crit Care Nurs 19(3):28–31, 2000

Teplitz L: Zapping tachyarrhythmias with radiofrequency catheter ablation. Nursing 2000 30(2 Crit Care):32cc1–32cc2, 32cc4, 32cc6, 2000

Cardiopulmonary Resuscitation

Bourdreaux ED, Francis JL, Loyacano T: Family Presence during invasive procedures and resuscitations in the emergency department critical review and suggestions for future research. Am J Emerg Med 40:193–205, 2002

Clark AP, Calvin AO, Meyers TA, et al: Family presence during cardiopulmonary resuscitation and invasive procedures: A research based intervention. Crit Care Nurs Clin North Am 13:569–575, 2001

Cummins RO, Hazinski MF, Kerber RE, et al: Low-energy biphasic waveform defibrillation: Evidence-based review applied to emergency cardiovascular care guidelines. Circulation 97:1654–1667, 1998

Eichhorn DJ, Meyers TA, Guzzetta CE, et al: During invasive procedures and resuscitation: Hearing the voice of the patient. Am J Nurs 101(5):48–55, 2001

Ellison S: Nurses' attitudes toward family presence during resuscitative efforts and invasive procedure. J Emerg Nurs 29:515–521, 2003

Maclean SL, Guzzette CE, White C, et al: Family presence during cardiopulmonary resuscitation and invasive procedures: Practices of critical care and emergency nurses. Am J Crit Care 12:246–257, 2003

McClenathan BM, Torrington KG, Uyehara CF: Family member presence during cardiopulmonary resuscitation: A survey of US and international critical care professionals. Chest 122:2204–2211, 2002

Meischke HW, Rea TD, Eisenberg MS, et al: Intentions to use an automated external defibrillator during a cardiac emergency among a group of seniors trained in its operation. Heart Lung 31:25–29, 2002

Meyers TA, Eichhorn DJ, Guzzetta CE, et al: Family presence during invasive procedures and resuscitation. Am J Nurs 100(2):32–42, 2000

Samson RA, Berg RA, Bingham R, et al: Use of automated external defibrillators for children: An update. Pediatrics 112:163–168, 2003

Sanford M, Pugh D, Warren NA: Family presence during CPR: New decisions in the twenty-first century. Crit Care Nurs Q 25(2):61–66, 2002

Swor R, Compton S, Farr L, et al: Perceived self-sufficiency in performing and willingness to learn cardiopulmonary resuscitation in an elderly population in a suburban community. Am J Crit Care 12:65–70, 2003

Wenzel V, Krismer AC, Arntz R, et al: A comparison of vasopressin and epinephrine for out-of-hospital cardiopulmonary resuscitation. N Engl J Med 350:105–113, 2004

Williams JM: Family presence during resuscitation: To see or not to see? Nurs Clin North Am 37:211–220, 2002

chapter 19

Common Cardiovascular Disorders

M. SUE APPLE

objectives

Based on the content in this chapter, the reader should be able to:

- Differentiate between pericarditic and ischemic chest pain.
- Explain the underlying disease process in myocarditis.
- Explain the long-term effect of endocarditis on the heart valves.
- Differentiate dilated cardiomyopathy from hypertrophic cardiomyopathy.
- Analyze the similarities in clinical management between the three types of cardiomyopathies.
- Analyze the differences between arterial and venous peripheral vascular disease.
- Compare and contrast the clinical findings of aortic aneurysm with acute aortic dissection.
- Compose a plan of care for the patient in hypertensive crisis covering the first hour of treatment.

The first intensive/coronary care units were developed in the mid-1960s to treat patients suffering from acute myocardial infarction. Since those early days, critical care nurses have expanded their focus to include a wide spectrum of cardiovascular diseases. In addition to acute myocardial infarction, these disorders include inflammation and infections of the heart, pericardium, and valves, as well as diseases involving the aorta and peripheral vascular system. This chapter reviews several common cardiovascular disorders, including pericarditis, myocarditis, endocarditis, cardiomyopathy, peripheral vascular disease, aortic diseases, and hypertensive crisis.

INFECTION AND INFLAMMATION OF THE HEART

Infectious and inflammatory diseases of the heart have multiple etiologies, making diagnosis and treatment a clinical challenge. Patients may present with acute pain mimicking myocardial infarction, or may seek medical attention because of fatigue and vague, "flulike" symptoms that fail to resolve over a period of weeks. Because of the permanent damage these diseases can cause to structures of the heart, patients often face serious long-term cardiac disability.

Pericarditis

PATHOPHYSIOLOGY

A double-walled membranous sac, the pericardium, surrounds the heart and the roots of the great vessels.[1] The outer tough fibrous pericardium is bound to the diaphragm by tendons. Lining the internal surface of the fibrous pericardium is the parietal layer. This layer then folds over on itself to form the inner visceral layer. Between these two layers is 10 to 50 mL of clear pericardial fluid, which acts as a lubricant. The pericardium helps to support the heart and isolate it from infections in the surrounding structures.[2]

Pericarditis refers to inflammation of the layers of the pericardium (Fig. 19-1). This inflammation often involves the adjoining diaphragm. It can be a primary disease or occur secondarily as the result of some other disorder, such as acute myocardial infarction or renal failure.[2] Dressler's syndrome refers to the development of pericarditis, malaise, fever, and elevated white blood cell count appearing weeks to months after a myocardial infarction. This syndrome is believed to be the result of an autoimmune reaction that occurs after the infarct.[3] Infectious pericarditis is an increasing problem in the immunocompromised patient.[4] Causes of pericarditis are listed in Box 19-1.

Repeated episodes of pericarditis can lead to the formation of adhesions between the layers of the pericardium or between the pericardium and adjacent structures, resulting in constrictive pericarditis. In constrictive pericarditis, the primary problem is failure of the heart to fill during diastole owing to its inability to stretch.[3] Unless the diseased pericardium is removed surgically, diastolic filling will continued to be impaired, eventually leading to a decrease in cardiac output and systemic signs of heart failure.

ASSESSMENT

History and Physical Examination

Important clues to the diagnosis of pericarditis can be obtained from the history and physical examination. The primary symptom in acute pericarditis is chest pain. This pain tends to be pleuritic and classically is made worse by breathing deeply or lying supine. Because of pain from breathing, patients often complain of dyspnea. Relief is often obtained by sitting up, leaning forward, and taking shallow breaths. The chest pain of pericarditis may be difficult to distinguish from ischemic chest pain.[5] Differential diagnoses of chest pain are summarized in Table 19-1. One clue in the differentiation is that ischemic chest pain is not relieved by a change in the patient's position.

There may also be general symptoms of an infection, such as a low-grade fever, cough, or malaise. The presence of a pericardial friction rub confirms the diagnosis; however, absence of a rub does not rule out pericarditis. The classic friction rub produces a "rasping" or "scraping," high-pitched sound that varies with the cardiac cycle. The rub may wax and wane, and may even transiently disappear during the course of the illness. It is best heard with the diaphragm of the stethoscope placed over the lower to middle left sternal edge.[2]

Laboratory and Diagnostic Studies

The chest x-ray may not be helpful; however, the electrocardiogram (ECG) may show diffuse ST segment elevation with an upward concavity and PR segment depression[6] (Fig. 19-2). This contrasts with the ECG seen in acute myocardial injury, which typically shows upward convexity in leads facing the infarct zone (Fig. 19-3).

Laboratory tests include complete blood count (CBC), cardiac enzymes (which may be elevated if the inflammation extends to the myocardium), rheumatoid factors, and antinuclear antibody (ANA) titers. Blood cultures may be indicated if there is evidence of infection. Viral studies may be obtained if the rest of the diagnostic workup is negative.

MANAGEMENT

Treatment goals for the patient with pericarditis are to relieve symptoms and eliminate any possible causative agents. Symptom relief includes the use of nonsteroidal anti-inflammatory agents (NSAIDs), such as aspirin or ibuprofen. Steroids may be indicated in resistant cases in which infectious causes have been excluded. Anticoagulants should be avoided in the patient recovering from myocardial infarction. The goal of nursing management is pain relief and patient/family education concerning possible etiologies.

Most episodes of pericarditis abate over 2 to 6 weeks. Rarely do patients experience recurrent episodes. Pericardial effusion with the potential for cardiac tamponade is a rare complication.

Myocarditis

PATHOPHYSIOLOGY

Myocarditis is an inflammation of the myocardium and the conduction system of the heart in the absence of myocardial infarction.[7] This disease can be caused by many infectious agents, as listed in Box 19-2, and can occur in any age group. In some cases, damage to the myocardium results from either toxins or from an immunological reaction.[7,8] The prevalence is unknown because the clinical presentation is so varied and often subacute; however, several postmortem studies suggest that myocarditis may be a major cause of sudden death in young adults.[9] Myocarditis can be a devastating illness that evolves into a chronic, progressive disease with a poor prognosis. This disorder may result in dysrhythmias, congestive heart failure, or death.[7]

ASSESSMENT

The clinical presentation of myocarditis is variable, although unexplained heart failure is a common manifestation.[7] Chest pain, often pleuritic, is a frequent complaint. The presence of vague symptoms, such as fatigue, dyspnea, palpitations, and precordial discomfort, accompanied by a slight rise in serum enzymes and nonspecific ST-T wave changes on the ECG, may point to the diagnosis of myocarditis. Definitive diagnosis requires a positive endomyocardial biopsy.[9,10]

MANAGEMENT

Management of myocarditis depends on the etiology and clinical presentation; however, treatment is largely supportive.[7] Although myocarditis evokes a severe inflammatory response, treatment with corticosteroids or immunosuppressive agents has not been effective in changing the clinical course.[9,10]

Box 19-3 lists sample nursing diagnoses for a patient with myocarditis. Many of the skills required by the nurse to care for the patient with myocarditis are similar to those needed in the care of the patient with heart failure. In addition, the nurse must be prepared to help the patient and family deal with the unexpected reality of a potentially lethal disease that often has no cure and may require heart transplantation.

Some episodes of myocarditis resolve without further sequelae. In other patients, a subacute disease develops with persistent laboratory findings of inflammation (e.g., an

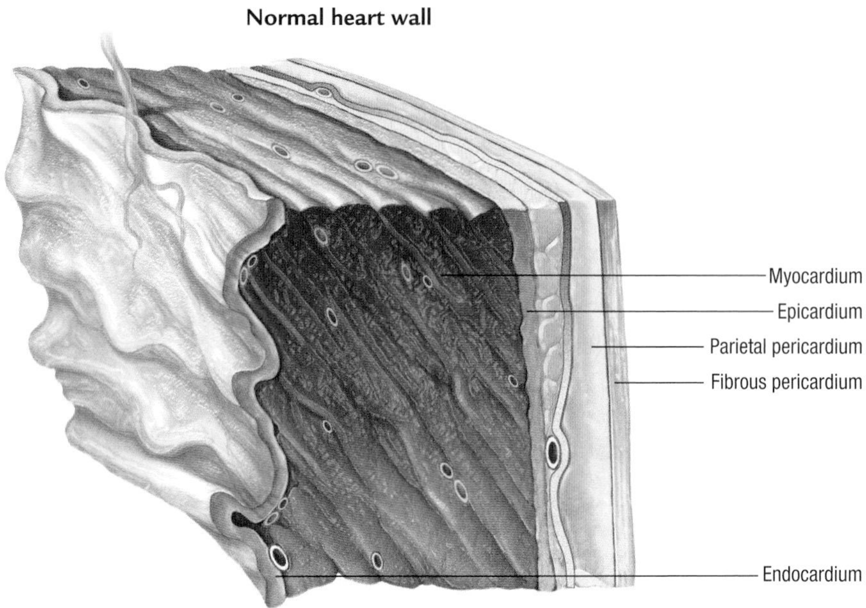

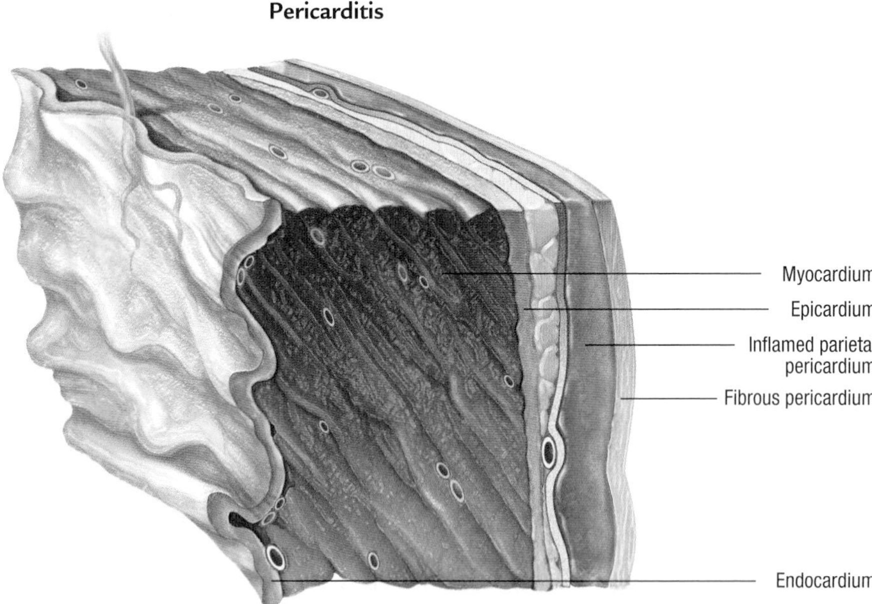

figure 19-1 Tissue changes in pericarditis. (Reprinted with permission from the Anatomical Chart Company: Atlas of Pathophysiology, p 65. Springhouse, PA, Springhouse, 2001.)

box 19-1
Causes of Pericarditis

- Idiopathic
- Bacteria and viruses
- Immunological disorders
- Connective tissue diseases
- Neoplasms
- Renal failure
- Myocardial and pericardial injury
- Radiation
- Drugs

increased white blood cell count or an elevated sedimentation rate). Idiopathic dilated cardiomyopathy may be the result of past episodes of viral myocarditis.

Endocarditis

PATHOPHYSIOLOGY

Endocarditis is an infection of the endocardial surface of the heart, including the valves. Infective endocarditis is a serious illness with mortality rates of 20% to 30%. These rates are higher in individuals older than 60 years.[3,11] Rapid diagnosis, initiation of appropriate treatment, and early identification of complications are the keys to good patient outcomes.

In the past, rheumatic heart disease caused most cases of endocarditis. Currently, endocarditis is more likely to be found in patients with prosthetic valves, those who abuse intravenous (IV) drugs, or patients with mitral valve prolapse or other nonrheumatic abnormalities, as detailed in Box 19-4.[12] Common infectious organisms include streptococci, enterococci, and *Staphylococcus aureus*.

The development of infective endocarditis is a complex process that requires the occurrence of several critical elements.[3,11] First, there must be endothelial damage that exposes the basement membrane of the valve to turbulent blood flow. This exposure leads to the development of a clot on the valve leaflet, composed of platelets and fibrin. Second, these clots, or vegetations, must be exposed to bacteria by way of bloodstream transport, such as occurs after dental manipulations or urological procedures. Bacteria proliferate on these vegetations for two reasons: (1) the turbulent blood flow across the valves helps to concentrate the numbers of bacteria near the vegetation; and (2) the vegetation itself covers the bacteria with layers of platelets and fibrin, protecting the bacterial colony from the body's natural defense mechanisms.[3,11] The infected vegetation interferes with normal valve function and eventually damages the valve structure. These incompetent valves eventually lead to severe heart failure. Particles from the infected vegetation or severely damaged valve can break loose and cause peripheral emboli (Osler nodes).

ASSESSMENT

Symptoms of endocarditis usually occur within 2 weeks of the precipitating bacteremia (Box 19-5). Nonspecific complaints, such as general malaise, anorexia, fatigue, weight loss, and night sweats, are common. Fevers and heart murmurs are present in almost all patients.[11] Because symptoms are nonspecific, a careful history and physical examination are needed to alert the nurse to the potential diagnosis of endocarditis.[12] Look carefully for the presence of Osler nodes (small, tender, purplish, erythematous skin lesions, occurring most frequently in the pads of the fingers or toes and in the palms of the hands or soles of the feet).[11]

MANAGEMENT

Cure of infectious endocarditis is difficult and requires complete eradication of the bacterial colony from the vegetation. This usually involves a prolonged course of antibiotics. Treatment should not be delayed while waiting for identification of the specific organism but should begin as soon as blood cultures are drawn. Antibiotic therapy is often continued in the home after discharge.[12]

Immediate surgical intervention is indicated in the presence of severe congestive heart failure secondary to valve dysfunction, uncontrolled infections, and prosthetic

table 19-1 Differential Diagnosis of Chest Pain

Diagnosis	Onset of Pain	Quality of Pain	Relieved by
Angina pectoris	Sudden, after heavy meal or exertion	Crushing Squeezing Choking	Rest, nitrates
Acute myocardial infarction	Varies, may be associated with feeling of doom	Similar to angina, but more severe	No relief with rest
Pericarditis	Varies, may be preceded by "flu-like" symptoms for several days to weeks	Pleuritic Sharp, stabbing	Sitting up Shallow breathing NSAIDs
Acute aortic dissection	Sudden, may be associated with syncope Intense from the onset	Ripping Tearing Worst pain in patient's life	No relief

NSAIDs, nonsteroidal anti-inflammatory drugs.

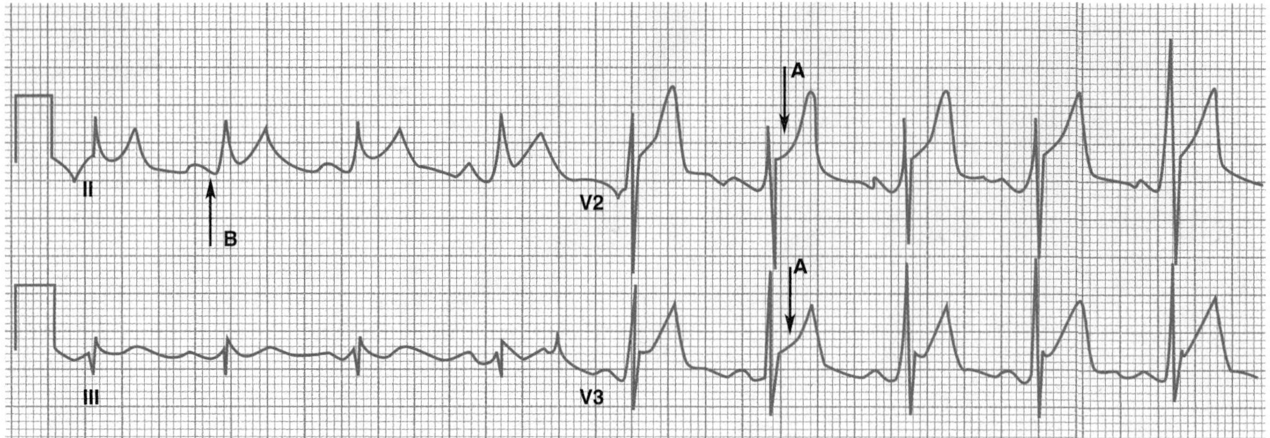

figure 19-2 The 12-lead electrocardiogram (ECG) in acute pericarditis. Note the diffuse upward concavity ST changes (**A**) and the PR segment depression (**B**).

valve dysfunction or dehiscence. Box 19-6 outlines considerations for discharge planning for the patient with endocarditis.

CARDIOMYOPATHIES

Cardiomyopathy refers to diseases of unknown etiology involving heart muscle. Cardiomyopathies are classified according to the World Health Organization (WHO) and the International Society and Federation of Cardiology (ISFC) to include three types of functional abnormalities: dilated, hypertrophic, and restrictive[13] (Table 19-2). Of the three types, dilated cardiomyopathy accounts for over 60% of the cases.[14]

The other forms of cardiomyopathy include arrhythmogenic right ventricular dysplasia and unclassified. Right ventricular dysplasia involves progressive fibrofatty replacement of the right ventricle. Familial disease is common. The "unclassified" category includes diseases that do not readily fit into other categories, such as systolic dysfunction with minimal chamber dilation.[13]

Ventricular dysfunction leading to cardiomyopathy can be the result of specific disorders, such as ischemic coronary artery disease (CAD), or failure to correct pressure or volume overload, such as severe valvular dysfunction or hypertension. Other forms of cardiomyopathy are the result of intrinsic disorders of the heart muscle itself.[15]

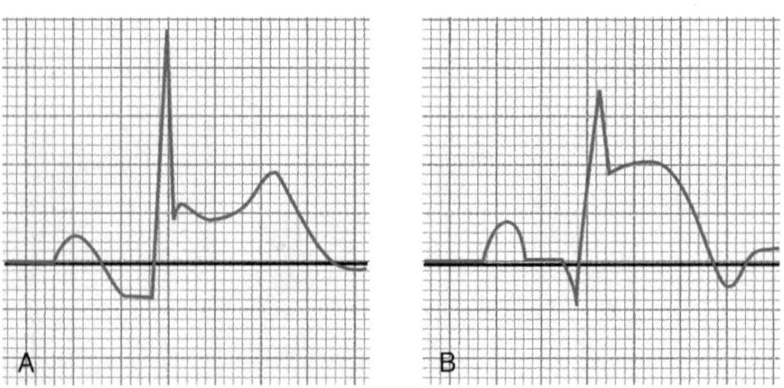

figure 19-3 ST segment changes seen in (**A**) acute pericarditis and (**B**) myocardial infarction.

Pathophysiology

DILATED CARDIOMYOPATHY

Dilated cardiomyopathy is characterized by increased ventricular cavity size in the face of normal or reduced left ventricular wall thickness, and impaired systolic function.[4,14] In most instances, the cause is unknown. Current investigations are focusing on three basic mechanisms of damage: (1) familial and genetic factors, (2) viral infections, and (3) immunological defects.[14] Some researchers believe that alcohol is the most prevalent toxic cause of dilated cardiomyopathy.[15]

Regardless of the etiology, the natural history of dilated cardiomyopathy is not well defined.[14] Some patients remain asymptomatic or have minimal signs of heart failure. However, in symptomatic patients the clinical course is usually marked by progressive dilation of the heart chambers. As ventricular dilation increases, mitral and tricuspid insufficiency occur as the valve leaflets are stretched and separated. Left ventricular failure becomes a major clinical problem. Dysrhythmias, such as ventricular tachycardia and fibrillation, also make management of this condition difficult.

HYPERTROPHIC CARDIOMYOPATHY

Hypertrophic cardiomyopathy is distinguished by excessive myocardial hypertrophy out of proportion to the hemodynamic load.[14] The most characteristic feature of hypertrophic cardiomyopathy is diastolic dysfunction.

box 19-2
Potential Causes of Myocarditis

- Viruses (especially in North America and Europe)[9]
- Bacteria
- Protozoa
- Helminths
- Toxins
- Hypersensitivity
- Systemic disease

box 19-3 *Examples of Nursing Diagnoses for the Patient With Myocarditis*

- Fatigue related to acute myocarditis
- Ineffective Individual or Family Coping related to sudden onset of a critical disease
- Powerlessness related to medical regimen
- Anticipatory Grieving related to loss of former lifestyle

The heart is able to contract but is not able to relax and remains abnormally stiff in diastole. Hypertrophic cardiomyopathy appears to be a common genetic malformation of the heart, with an incidence in the general population of approximately 1 in 500.[16] Sudden death is a catastrophic outcome of hypertrophic cardiomyopathy that occurs in asymptomatic or mildly symptomatic people of any age group, usually from a ventricular dysrhythmia.[17] The risk of sudden death is constant; mortality is higher in younger patients. Early identification of patients at risk for hypertrophic cardiomyopathy (and therefore, sudden death) is imperative. However, how best to identify people at high risk is not known at this time. The increase in ventricular muscle mass does not occur until early adolescence, making it impossible to identify gene carriers of hypertrophic cardiomyopathy by simple screening methods in children.[15]

box 19-4 *Risk Factors for Endocarditis*

Native Valve Endocarditis

- Mitral valve prolapse
- Degenerative lesions of the mitral and aortic valves
- Congenital heart disease
- Rheumatic heart disease
- Intravenous (IV) drug abuse
- Age greater than 60 years (especially in people with prosthetic valves or degenerative lesions)
- Diabetes (because of accelerated atherosclerosis and a predisposition to infections)
- Pregnancy (rare), associated with underlying cardiac disease, dental procedures, premature labor, prolonged rupture of membranes, prolonged third stage of labor, and manual removal of the placenta

Prosthetic Valve Endocarditis

Early (Within 60 Days of Surgery)

- Nosocomial infections
- Central IV catheters
- Arterial catheters
- Cardiac pacing wires
- Endotracheal tubes

Late (After 60 Days)

- Dental, genitourinary, or gastrointestinal manipulations

Adapted from Karchmer AW: Infective endocarditis. In Braunwald E, Zipes DP, Libby P (eds): Heart Disease (6th Ed), pp 1723–1750. Philadelphia, WB Saunders, 2001.

box 19-5 *Signs and Symptoms of Endocarditis*

- Fever
- Heart murmurs
- Splenomegaly
- Petechiae
  - Splinter hemorrhages
  - Osler's nodes (small, raised, tender nodules that occur on the fingers or toes)
  - Janeway lesions (small erythematous or hemorrhagic lesions on the palms or soles)
- Musculoskeletal complaints
- Systemic or pulmonary emboli
- Neurological manifestations
  - Headache
  - Mycotic aneurysms

RESTRICTIVE CARDIOMYOPATHY

The least common of the three types of functional cardiomyopathy in the United States is restrictive cardiomyopathy. Its hallmark is also a "stiff" ventricle, or diastolic dysfunction. Myocardial hypertrophy, fibrosis, or infiltration of the muscle can be the underlying pathological process. Classically, restrictive cardiomyopathy presents as congestive heart failure with only a small or slightly enlarged heart.[14]

Assessment

Clinical findings depend on the type of cardiomyopathy and the extent of the disease. See Table 19-2 for details regarding the clinical manifestations and major management issues in cardiomyopathy.

Management

Nursing management of cardiomyopathy is similar to the care of patients with severe congestive heart failure and their families. Refer to Chapter 20 for a detailed discussion of heart failure and the associated medical and nursing management. The nurse must incorporate the type of cardiomyopathy, the current level of physical functioning,

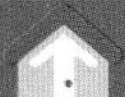

box 19-6 *Endocarditis*

- Ensure that the patient's condition is stabilized and without complications, and that the patient is able to comply with the medical regimen.
- Plan for daily nursing follow-up.
- Make arrangements for intravenous (IV) administration of antibiotics (the preferred route).
- Teach the patient or family member how to care for the vascular access site to avoid repeat infections.
- Identify the original infectious source.
- Anticipate the future need for endocarditis prophylaxis.

table 19-2 Types of Functional Cardiomyopathy

Cardiomyopathy	Description	Clinical Manifestations	Management
Dilated (congestive) Increased atrial chamber size Increased ventricular chamber size Decreased muscle size	Dilation and impaired contraction of the left ventricle, or both ventricles	• Fatigue, weakness • Congestive heart failure, especially left ventricular failure • Dysrhythmias • Mitral valve regurgitation, sometimes tricuspid	• Symptomatic treatment • Control heart failure • Control dysrhythmias
Hypertrophic Thickened interventricular septum Left ventricular hypertrophy	Marked hypertrophy of left ventricle, occasionally also of right ventricle, and usually (but not always) disproportionate hypertrophy of septum	• Dyspnea • Angina • Fatigue • Syncope • Palpitations • Atrial fibrillation • Ventricular dysrhythmias • Congestive heart failure • Sudden death	• Symptomatic treatment • Beta blockers • Pacemaker • Surgery
Restrictive Left ventricular hypertrophy Decreased ventricular chamber size	Restrictive filling and reduced ventricular compliance of either or both ventricles, normal or near-normal systolic function; usually caused by infiltration of myocardium (e.g., amyloidosis or endomyocardial disease)	• Dyspnea • Fatigue • Congestive heart failure • Tricuspid and mitral valve regurgitation • Heart blocks • Emboli	• Symptomatic treatment • Control hypertension • Exercise restrictions

Images reprinted with permission from the Anatomical Chart Company: Atlas of Pathophysiology. Springhouse, PA, Springhouse, 2001.

and family needs into the plan of care. Psychosocial concerns are important as patients and families try to cope with this debilitating and potentially fatal illness. They must deal with feelings of uncertainty and loss of control as well as the financial impact of a serious chronic illness. Genetic counseling and screening, indicated for some types of cardiomyopathy, also add to the emotional impact of the diagnosis.

PERIPHERAL VASCULAR DISEASE

Peripheral vascular disease includes a group of distinct disorders involving the arteries, veins, and lymphatic vessels of the peripheral circulation. Atherosclerosis is the most common cause. Risk factors include smoking, diabetes, lipid disorders, hypertension, and elevated homocysteine levels. Age, heredity, obesity, and stress are also linked to peripheral vascular disease.[18] As the population of the United States ages, management of peripheral vascular diseases is becoming a major focus in terms not only of prevention and cure, but of maintaining the quality of life and independence of the elderly (Box 19-7).

Arterial Disease

PATHOPHYSIOLOGY

The term *peripheral arterial disease* is used to refer to atherosclerosis when it obstructs blood supply to the lower or upper extremities.[19] The incidence of peripheral arterial disease depends on the population studied and the type of method used to establish the diagnosis. In general, symptomatic peripheral arterial disease is found more commonly in men between the ages of 50 and 75 years, with the incidence increasing steadily with age.[20] Peripheral arterial disease develops in major bifurcations and areas of acute angulations (Fig. 19-4). In people with diabetes, there is greater involvement of the smaller and more distal vessels.[18] Upper extremity involvement is less common than lower extremity involvement.[21]

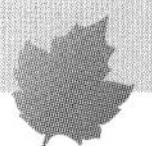

box 19-7

Peripheral Arterial Disease: Implications for the Older Patient

- Management of peripheral arterial disease in older adults is often more complicated because of the presence of comorbidities, polypharmacy, financial concerns, physical and cognitive limitations, inadequate social support or isolation, and depression and anxiety.
- The incidence of symptomatic peripheral arterial disease increases with age, directly affecting quality of life.
- Conservative management (e.g., smoking cessation, walking, foot care) can reduce symptoms and significantly improve quality of life in people of any age.

Thromboangiitis obliterans, or Buerger's disease, is a severe, chronic inflammatory disease affecting the intermediate and small arteries of the extremities. It may also involve adjacent veins and nerves. The etiology is unknown, but it is associated with heavy smoking, especially in young people. The chronic inflammatory process is often followed by thrombosis, with vascular lesions and fibrous obliteration of the vessel.[18]

ASSESSMENT

History and Physical Examination

Clinical signs of peripheral arterial disease reflect the blood's inability to circulate freely to the extremity. Symptoms depend on the extent of the disease and the presence of collateral circulation.[21] The classic symptom of peripheral arterial disease, intermittent claudication, is experienced as a cramping, burning, or aching pain in the legs or buttocks that is relieved with rest. Symptoms do not correlate with the extent of the disease. For example, patients may experience severe claudication but still have strong peripheral pulses. If the peripheral arterial disease is extensive and multilevel, the patient may present with "rest pain," that is, a sensation of burning or numbness in the foot or toes.[18,21] Patients also experience trophic changes, such as hair loss on the extremities, thickening of the nails, and drying of the skin. Acute arterial obstruction, such as occurs with an embolism, results in the sudden onset of extreme pain and other signs of acute arterial obstruction (Box 19-8).

In addition to a careful vascular examination that includes examination of the extremities and assessment of all peripheral pulses, most clinicians include the measurement of the ankle/brachial index (ABI) to diagnosis peripheral arterial disease.[18,19,21] The ABI is the ratio of ankle to brachial systolic blood pressure. A normal ABI should be 1.0 or greater. Patients with critical limb ischemia may have an ABI of less than 0.5[18,21] (see Fig. 19-5).

Management

Treatment of peripheral arterial disease is focused on modifying or eliminating risk factors, especially smoking. Medications, such as peripheral vasodilators, are controversial and have not been shown to improve clinical outcome.[22] Peripheral interventional procedures, such as balloon angioplasty, are successful in restoring circulation in many cases.[23] Surgical bypass may be required when severe or diffuse arterial obstruction is present. Implications for home care of a patient with peripheral arterial disease are given in Box 19-9.

insights into clinical research

Froelicher ES, Christopherson DJ: Women's initiative for nonsmoking (WINS) I: Design and methods. Heart Lung 29(6):429–437, 2000

The Women's Initiative for Nonsmoking (WINS) is a nurse-managed intervention for smoking cessation and prevention of relapse in women with coronary artery disease (CAD). This article reports on the design and methods; the trial is ongoing.

Two hundred seventy-eight women have been enrolled from 10 hospitals in the San Francisco area. Women admitted with a variety of cardiovascular diseases were screened for smoking. Participants had to be older than 18 years of age, have a history of tobacco use in the past month, show evidence of a willingness to quit, and have a hospitalization long enough to allow baseline assessment and the initial interview to be completed. Patients who could not understand English, were medically unstable, or had polysubstance abuse were not eligible for the WINS trial.

Clinical nurse specialists who had undergone special training interviewed potential candidates and obtained informed consent. Baseline data consisted of seven different tools that assess a variety of physical and psychosocial factors that influence a person's decision to smoke. After baseline data are collected, subjects were randomized to usual care (physician counseling) or the WINS protocol (inpatient counseling by the clinical nurse specialist). In addition to counseling from the clinical nurse specialist, participants viewed an educational video, received follow-up phone calls, and were assessed for nicotine replacement therapy. Telephone interviews continued at 6, 12, 24, and 30 months after enrollment. The hypothesis is that women enrolled in the clinical nurse specialist protocol will have a significant reduction in smoking behaviors compared with women in the standard care arm at the completion of this trial. Although the final results have not yet been released, the investigators have published additional information about the women enrolled in the study (Froelicher ES, et al: Heart Lung 31:3–14, 2002) and the use of nicotine replacement therapy in this population (Mahrer-Imhof R, et al: Heart Lung 31:368–373, 2002).

Venous Disease

Disease of the veins involves obstruction of blood flow or disruption of the venous valves. The most common form of venous disease is thrombophlebitis. Phlebitis is an inflammation of the vessel wall as the result of direct

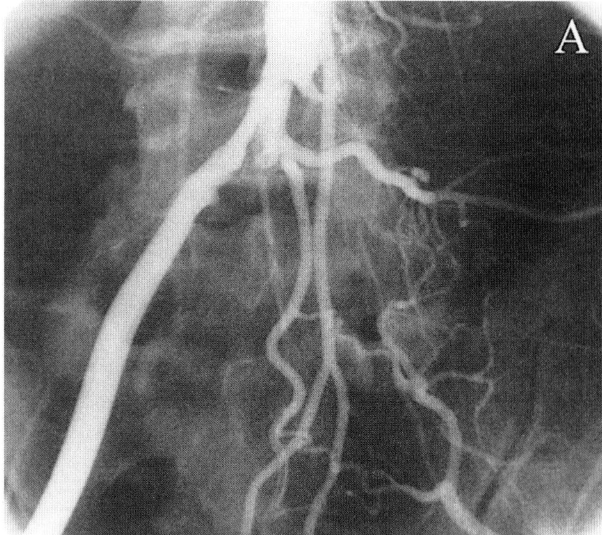

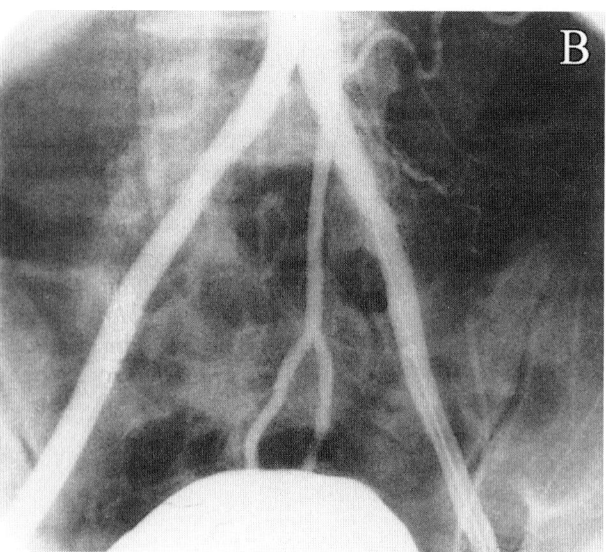

figure 19-4 (**A**) A baseline angiogram demonstrating a total occlusion of the left iliac artery. In addition, there is a significant stenosis of the right common iliac artery and occlusion of the internal iliac arteries. (**B**) The final result following angioplasty and stenting of the right and left common iliac arteries with Palmaz stents. (Reprinted with permission from Laird JR, Lansky AJ: Percutaneous transluminal angioplasty for the treatment of peripheral vascular disease. In Apple S, Lindsay J Jr (eds): Principles and Practice of Interventional Cardiology, p 196. Philadelphia, Lippincott Williams & Wilkins, 2000.)

injury to the vein or as a complication of varicose veins. Vessel wall injury, stasis of blood, and increased blood coagulability are known as *Virchow's triad.* These three conditions have been recognized as causative factors in the development of thrombophlebitis since 1846.[24] Two of the three factors must be present for phlebitis to develop.

Venous insufficiency is another form of venous disease. The cause of venous insufficiency is incompetence of the valves. Veins become overstretched owing to persistent excessive venous pressure, such as occurs with episodes of deep venous thrombosis (DVT). Over time, this condition may lead to stasis ulcers.

box 19-8 ***Symptoms of Vascular Obstruction***

Acute Arterial Occlusion

- Pain
- Pulselessness
- Pallor
- Paresthesia
- Paralysis

Deep Venous Thrombosis (DVT)

- Pain in calf with dorsiflexion of foot (Homans' sign)
- Pain when standing
- Inflammation
- Swelling
- Tenderness
- Redness, soreness

ASSESSMENT

Clinical signs of peripheral venous disease reflect the inability of the blood to drain from the extremity. Patients with venous insufficiency complain of dull aching in the affected leg. Swelling increases throughout the day but is usually relieved by lying down or elevating the legs. DVT is characterized by pain, swelling, tenderness, and increased temperature over the affected area (see Box 19-8). The patient also exhibits a positive Homans' sign (pain in the calf with passive dorsiflexion of the foot).

MANAGEMENT

The focus of care for the patient with venous disease is to increase blood flow and prevent complications. Patients with DVT are at high risk for the development of pulmonary emboli. Treatment strategies include anticoagulant therapy to prevent the formation of emboli, bed rest, and analgesics. Warm, moist compresses may be applied. Calf or thigh measurements should be obtained daily. Elastic stockings or Ace wraps may also be used.[25]

AORTIC DISEASE

Aortic Aneurysm

Aortic aneurysms are defined as a localized dilation of the aorta to a size greater than 1.5 times its normal diameter.[26,27] Most aneurysms are arteriosclerotic in origin. Other causes include syphilis, infection, inflammatory diseases, medial degeneration, aortic dissection, and trauma. Aneurysms tend to occur mostly in men. Frequently hypertension is present, and most patients have a history of smoking.

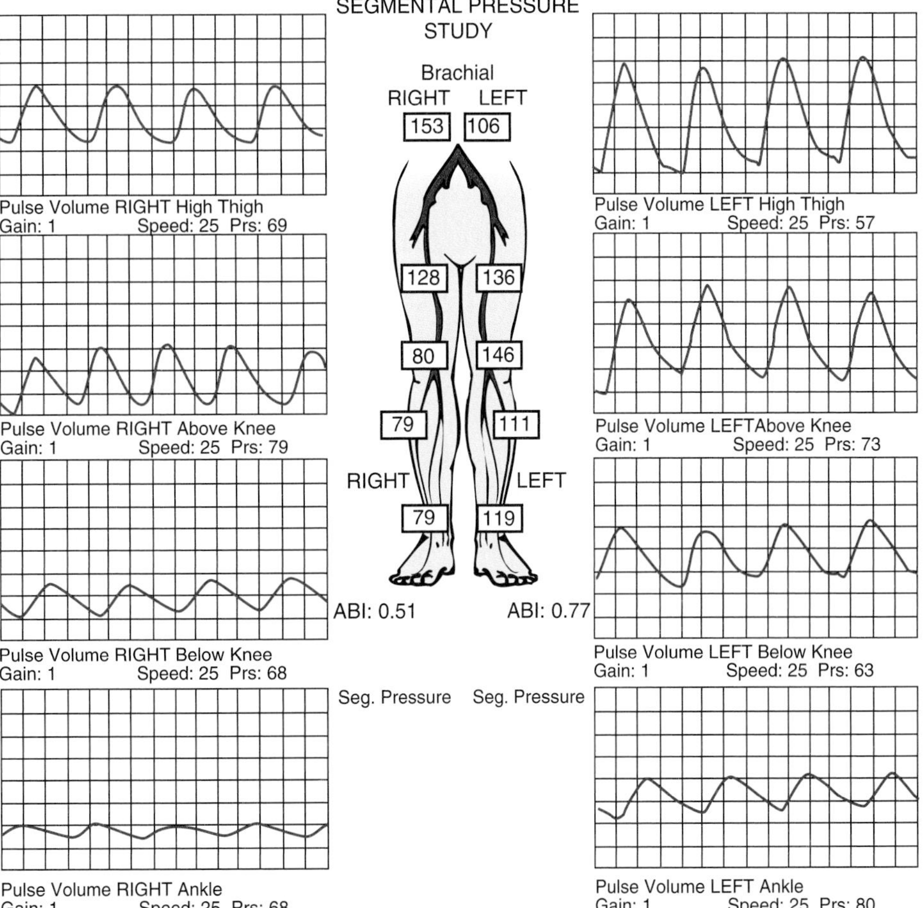

figure 19-5 Segmental pressures and ankle/brachial indices (ABIs) indicating bilateral lower extremity occlusive disease with more severe involvement of the right lower extremity. There is also a probable significant stenosis of the left subclavian artery, which explains the difference between the right and left brachial pressures (*Prs* = pressures). (Reprinted with permission from Saucedo JF, Laird JR: Peripheral vascular disease. In Apple S, Lindsay J Jr (eds): Principles and Practice of Interventional Cardiology, p 47. Philadelphia, Lippincott Williams & Wilkins, 2000.)

Aneurysms are classified according to their shape (Fig. 19-6). Fusiform aneurysms are diffuse dilations of the entire circumference of the artery. Saccular aneurysms are localized balloon-shaped outpouchings. True aneurysms involve the entire vessel wall. A false aneurysm is formed when blood leaks outside of the artery but is contained by the surrounding tissues.

Aneurysms may be thoracic or abdominal. Thoracic aneurysms occur relatively infrequently and are most often atherosclerotic and fusiform.[28] Like abdominal aneurysms, many thoracic aneurysms are asymptomatic at the time of diagnosis. Symptoms may include aortic insufficiency and signs of pericardial tamponade if the aneurysm involves the aortic root.

ASSESSMENT

In most patients, aneurysms are asymptomatic. Improvements in noninvasive testing with ultrasonography have led to the incidental discovery of many small (3 to 5 cm), asymptomatic aneurysms. Symptoms are usually related to expansion or rupture of the aneurysm.

Detection of aortic aneurysms by physical examination is difficult, especially in obese patients. The abdomen should be examined for the presence of bruits or masses, and peripheral pulses should be carefully evaluated.

MANAGEMENT

Management of aortic aneurysm includes control of hypertension and elimination of risk factors, such as smoking.[28,29] The patient should be followed with serial noninvasive tests, such as ultrasonography. Treatment for aneurysms involves surgical repair, which is usually indicated in aneurysms larger than 5 cm (Box 19-10). Management of aneurysms between 4 and 5 cm remains controversial.[30] Patients who are healthy with no other morbidity may elect to have 4-cm aneurysms repaired.

In addition to surgery, abdominal aneurysms may be repaired by a minimally invasive approach using an endovascular graft.[29,31] This approach involves placement of a graft

box 19-9 *Peripheral Arterial Disease*

- Ensure that the patient has a prescription for exercise based on current assessment of the patient's physical ability.
- Develop a smoking cessation plan with the patient based on current assessment of the patient's willingness to quit.
- Arrange for adjunct pharmacotherapy as indicated.
- Follow-up is crucial to success in permanently changing behaviors.

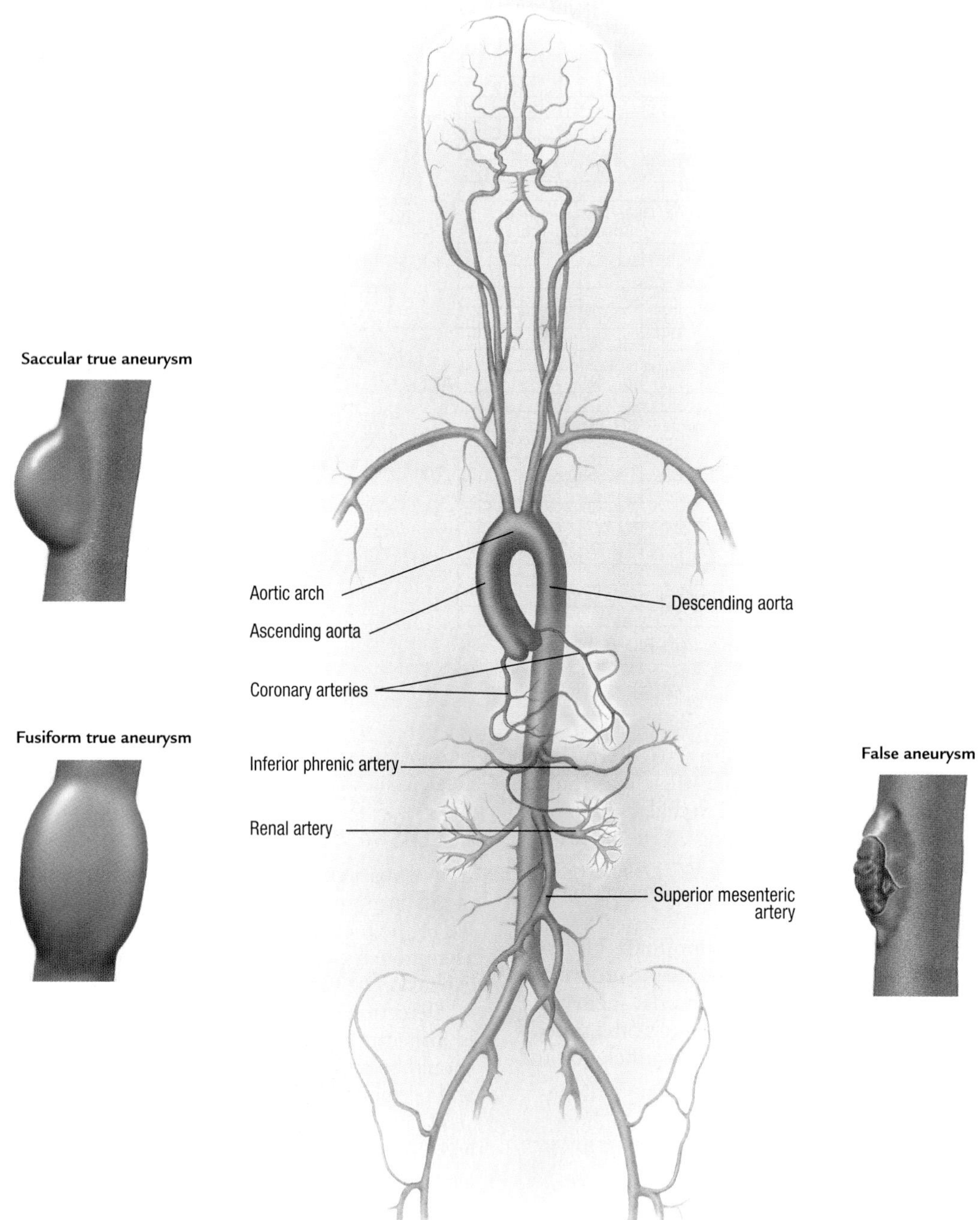

figure 19-6 Types of aortic aneurysms. (Reprinted with permission from the Anatomical Chart Company: Atlas of Pathophysiology, p 37. Springhouse, PA, Springhouse, 2001.)

box 19-10
Indications for Surgical Repair of Aortic Aneurysms

Thoracic
- Diameter 6 cm (5 cm in patients with Marfan's syndrome)
- Symptoms suggesting expansion or compression of surrounding structures

Abdominal
- Diameter 5 cm or more
- Diameter 4 cm or less, need regular follow-up
- Diameter 4–5 cm, management is controversial

Other
- Rapidly expanding aneurysms (growth rate >0.5 cm over a 6-month period)
- Symptomatic aneurysm regardless of size

through the femoral artery. The graft is then anchored to the wall of the aorta by means of self-expanding or balloon-expanded stents. Although this new treatment for abdominal aneurysms holds much promise, long-term results are not yet available.

case study ■ ABDOMINAL ANEURYSM

Mr. Smith, a 57-year-old father of three, went to the local hospital emergency department complaining of "chest tightness progressing to my back." The emergency department nurse noted that the patient had a history of hypertension (for which he was taking no medications) and that he was a heavy smoker.

On admission to the emergency department, the patient appeared to be in moderate distress. His vital signs were as follows: blood pressure 170/120 mm Hg, equal in both arms; heart rate 65 beats/minute and regular; respiratory rate 28 breaths/minute; temperature 99.0°F (37.2°C). Pulses were equal throughout. His skin was cool and diaphoretic.

While the emergency department staff was obtaining IV access, the patient suddenly complained of worsening chest pain and weakness in his legs. This weakness rapidly developed to paralysis of his lower extremities. The patient was given morphine sulfate (2 mg IV) to relieve his pain and placed on IV nitroglycerin to control his blood pressure. He was also started on oxygen (2 L by nasal cannula), which increased his oxygen saturation to 95%. The bedside ECG monitor displayed sinus tachycardia with no ectopy.

The ECG revealed nonspecific ST-T wave changes. The chest x-ray was nondiagnostic. A transesophageal echocardiogram (TEE) was suspect for an aortic tear near the arch, but this was not confirmed by computed tomography (CT) scan.

The patient was stabilized and transferred to a tertiary care hospital for further management and possible surgery for acute aortic dissection. On arrival to the cardiac critical care unit, the patient's paralysis had resolved. The patient's blood pressure remained at 160 to 170/120 mm Hg, so the decision was made to start nitroprusside. Labetalol was also started to decrease the stress on the wall of the aorta. Despite repeated reassurances and explanations of the procedures from the nurse, the patient became increasingly agitated. The oxygen saturation remained normal. Lorazepam (Ativan) was administered IV to decrease Mr. Smith's agitation and help control his blood pressure.

A repeat TEE found no evidence of acute dissection. However, the TEE did find a bicuspid aortic valve and a diffusely dilated thoracic aorta, varying from 4.3 to 4.8 cm (normal is 2.5 to 3.5 cm). In addition, a 6.5-cm abdominal aortic aneurysm was noted. Because of the size of the aneurysm, urgent surgical repair was recommended. ■

Aortic Dissection

Acute aortic dissection is the most common and the most lethal process involving the aorta. Mortality rates are very high, with death usually occurring from rupture of the aorta.[32] The incidence is highest in men older than 40 years of age with a history of hypertension.

PATHOPHYSIOLOGY

Dissection involves a longitudinal separation of the medial layers of the aorta by a column of blood, as illustrated in Figure 19-7. The dissection begins at a tear in the aortic wall, usually at the proximal end of the dissection. Blood pumped

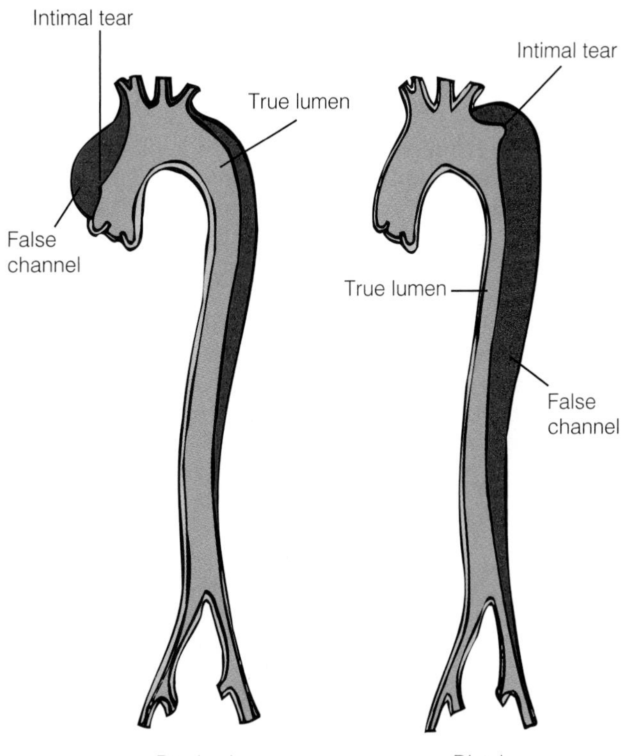

figure 19-7 Two major patterns of aortic dissection. Blood pumps through a tear in the wall, creating a false channel or lumen. The false channel rapidly becomes larger than the true lumen.

through this tear creates a false channel, or lumen, that rapidly becomes larger than the true aortic lumen. In most patients, the plane of the dissection involves the ascending aorta. The false lumen typically extends all the way to the iliac bifurcation.[28]

ASSESSMENT

Over 90% of patients present with sudden, intense chest pain. Frequently the pain is described as "ripping" or "tearing" and may be accompanied by syncope (see Table 19-1). In most patients, the diagnosis can be determined with a careful history and physical examination. The clinician should look for the murmur of aortic regurgitation or alteration of the peripheral pulses in patients with known risk factors, such as hypertension. The chest x-ray may show a widened mediastinum. Cardiac ischemia may be present if the dissection involves the coronary arteries. Cardiac tamponade may be another complication of dissection involving the aortic root. Neurological deficits may occur if the aortic arch vessels are involved. Dissections involving the renal arteries result in elevated serum creatinine, decreased urine output, and severe hypertension that is difficult to manage.

To confirm the diagnosis of acute aortic dissection, TEE or contrast medium–enhanced CT may be ordered.

MANAGEMENT

Survival of the acute phase depends on the location of the dissection, the severity of the complications, and the rapidity with which the diagnosis is confirmed. Clinical management focuses on controlling the blood pressure and on pain management. Surgery is the treatment of choice when the dissection involves the ascending aorta.

HYPERTENSIVE CRISIS

Hypertension affects approximately 50 million people in the United States and is a major controllable risk factor for the development of cardiovascular diseases.[33,34] Recognition of the extent of this risk led to the inclusion of a new category in the classification of hypertension, prehypertension, which includes individuals with a systolic blood pressure of 120 to 139 mm Hg or a diastolic blood pressure of 80 to 89 mm Hg (Table 19-3). People with prehypertension should be counseled to adopt healthy lifestyle modifications to reduce their risk for development of cardiovascular disease.

Pathophysiology

Patients who are known to have high blood pressure are also at risk of experiencing a hypertensive crisis. A hypertensive crisis or emergency can be defined as an acute elevation of blood pressure (systolic pressure usually greater than 240 mm Hg, diastolic pressure usually greater than 140 mm Hg) that is associated with acute or imminent target organ damage.[34,35] This rare but potentially fatal condition strikes about 1% to 2% of hypertensive patients, occurring more frequently in African-American men and the elderly. It is characterized by a marked rapid increase in blood pressure leading initially to intense vasoconstriction as the body attempts to protect itself from the elevated pressure. If the blood pressure remains critically high, compensatory vasoconstriction fails, resulting in increased pressure and blood flow throughout the vascular system. In the cerebral circulation this may quickly lead to hypertensive encephalopathy.[34,35] Hypertensive crisis is associated with a variety of clinical situations, as outlined in Box 19-11.

Assessment

Most patients who present with hypertensive crisis are critically ill and in need of immediate treatment. Clinical findings depend on the degree of vascular injury.[36] Signs of encephalopathy include headache, visual disturbances, confusion, nausea, and vomiting. Examination of the eyes may reveal cotton-wool exudates and hemorrhages, indicating damage to retinal nerves and rupture of retinal blood vessels; papilledema is diagnostic of increased intracranial pressure (ICP). Chest pain may represent acute coronary syndrome or aortic dissection. Depending on the damage to the kidneys, the patient may present with decreased urine output (oliguria) or azotemia (excess urea in the blood).[34,35]

Management

The goal is to reduce the mean blood pressure within 1 to 2 hours of starting treatment, and to prevent or reverse target organ damage.[36] Several IV medications are indicated in the treatment of hypertensive crises; the choice depends on availability and the clinical situation (Table 19-4). Constant monitoring is necessary to avoid lowering the blood pressure too quickly. This is best accomplished with an intra-arterial catheter.

Once the blood pressure has been stabilized, treatment goals depend on the etiology of the crisis. All patients require careful long-term management to control their blood pressure and prevent future episodes.

table 19-3 Classification of Blood Pressure for Adults

Blood Pressure Classification	Systolic (mm Hg)	Diastolic (mm Hg)
Normal	<120	and <80
Prehypertension	120–139	or 80–89
Stage 1 Hypertension	140–159	or 90–99
Stage 2 Hypertension	≥160	or ≥100

Adapted from the Seventh Report of the Joint National Committee on Prevention, Detection, Evaluation, and Treatment of High Blood Pressure (JNC 7). May 2003. Available at: www.nhlbi.nih.gov/guidelines/hypertension.

box 19-11
Summary of Hypertensive Crisis

Causes

- Acute or chronic renal disease
- Exacerbation of chronic hypertension
- Sudden withdrawal of antihypertensive medications

Associated Clinical Situations

- Acute cerebrovascular syndrome
  - Acute stroke
  - Hypertensive encephalopathy
- Acute cardiovascular syndromes
  - Myocardial infarction
  - Unstable angina
  - Pulmonary edema
- Aortic dissection
- Extensive burns
- Postoperative period
- Pheochromocytoma
- Eclampsia

Management

- Intravenous (IV) medications with continuous arterial pressure monitoring
- Goal is to reduce blood pressure over 1 to 2 hours to a mean of 120 mm Hg, or a 20% reduction in mean arterial pressure while avoiding hypoperfusion

clinical applicability challenges

Self-Challenge: Critical Thinking

1. *Examine critical differences in the clinical assessment between a patient presenting with an acute aortic dissection and the patient with acute pericarditis.*
2. *Compare and contrast the similarities and differences in the nursing management of the patient with acute myocarditis and acute endocarditis.*
3. *Management of patients with a suspected acute aortic dissection, such as Mr. Smith (the subject of the case study), requires rapid interventions from the health care team. Formulate a plan of care for these patients, classifying nursing actions in order of importance.*

Study Questions

1. *Signs and symptoms of endocarditis include*
   a. *fever, cough, peripheral edema.*
   b. *fever, urinary frequency, peripheral edema.*
   c. *fever, heart murmurs, petechiae.*
   d. *fever, petechiae, urinary frequency.*
2. *Pain on inspiration associated with pericarditis is due to*
   a. *contact between the inflamed pericardium and the diaphragm.*
   b. *contact between the inflamed pericardium and the trachea.*
   c. *inflammation of the mediastinum.*

table 19-4 ■ Intravenous Medications in Hypertensive Emergencies*

Drug	Class	Onset of Action	Adverse Effects
Sodium nitroprusside	Vasodilator	Immediate	Hypotension, nausea, vomiting, muscle twitching, thiocyanate and cyanide toxicity, methemoglobinemia
Nitroglycerin	Vasodilator	1–2 min	Hypotension, reflex tachycardia, headache, tolerance with prolonged use
Labetalol	Adrenergic blocker	<5 min	Nausea, vomiting, bronchospasm, heart block
Fenoldopam	Vasodilator	<5 min	Reflex tachycardia, headache, nausea
Esmolol	Adrenergic blocker	Immediate	Hypotension, heart block
Nicardipine	Calcium channel blocker	5–6 min	Reflex tachycardia, headache, nausea, vomiting, flushing
Enalaprilat	Angiotensin-converting enzyme inhibitor	10–15 min	Hypotension, renal failure
Hydralazine	Vasodilator	15–30 min	Reflex tachycardia, headache, exacerbation of angina pectoris

*Choice of agent depends on the etiology of the hypertensive emergency and the clinical setting.
Adapted from Mansoor GA, Frishman WH: Comprehensive management of hypertensive emergencies and urgencies. Heart Dis 4:358, 2002; and Tuncel M, Ram VCS: Hypertensive emergencies: Etiology and management. Am J Cardiovasc Drugs 3(1):21–31, 2003.

d. *contact between the inflamed pericardium and the pancreas.*

3. *Key clinical findings in the assessment of the patient with suspected acute arterial occlusion include*
   a. *pain, pallor, polydipsia, polyphagia.*
   b. *unequal peripheral pulses, pain, swelling.*
   c. *pain with dorsiflexion of the foot, inflammation, tenderness.*
   d. *pain, absent distal pulses, pallor, paresthesia.*
4. *Risk factors for the development of aortic aneurysms include*
   a. *smoking, hypertension, pericarditis.*
   b. *smoking, myocarditis, pericarditis.*
   c. *diabetes, hypertension, family history.*
   d. *family history, hypertension, pericarditis.*
5. *Factors that contribute to complicated management of the elderly with PVD include*
   a. *confusion, limited mobility, lack of effective therapies.*
   b. *presence of family support, confusion, lack of effective therapies.*
   c. *difficulty in establishing a medical diagnosis, confusion, presence of financial support.*
   d. *lack of family support, confusion, presence of comorbidities.*

REFERENCES

1. Moore KL, Dalley AF (eds): The thorax. In Clinically Oriented Anatomy (4th Ed). Philadelphia, Lippincott Williams & Wilkins, 1999
2. Spodick DH: Pericardial diseases. In Braunwald E, Zipes DP, Libby P (eds): Heart Disease (6th Ed), pp 1823–1876. Philadelphia, WB Saunders, 2001
3. McNeill MM: Pericardial, myocardial, and endocardial disease. In Woods S, Froelicher E, Motzer S (eds): Cardiac Nursing (4th Ed), pp 719–735. Philadelphia, Lippincott Williams & Wilkins, 2000
4. Krasuski RA, Bashmore TM: Cardiac involvement in HIV: Four common presentations. Emerg Med 32(1):28–30, 33–34, 37, 2000
5. Fallon EM, Roques J: Acute chest pain. AACN Clin Issues 8(3):383–397, 1997
6. Chan TC, Brady WJ, Pollack M: Electrocardiographic manifestations: Acute myopericarditis. J Emerg Med 17(5):865–872, 1999
7. Oakley CM: Myocarditis, pericarditis, and other pericardial diseases. Heart 84(4):449–454, 2000
8. Sparacino PS: Cardiac infections: Medical and surgical therapies. J Cardiovasc Nurs 13(2):49–65, 1999
9. Feldman AM, McNamara D: Myocarditis. N Engl J Med 343: 1388–1398, 2000
10. Wynne J, Braunwald E: The cardiomyopathies and myocarditides. In Braunwald E, Zipes DP, Libby P (eds): Heart Disease (6th Ed), pp 1751–1806. Philadelphia, WB Saunders, 2001
11. Karchmer AW: Infective endocarditis. In Braunwald E, Zipes DP, Libby P (eds): Heart Disease (6th Ed), pp 1723–1750. Philadelphia, WB Saunders, 2001
12. Bayer AS, Bolger AF, Taubert KA, et al: Diagnosis and management of infective endocarditis and its complications. Circulation 98(25):2936–2948, 1998
13. Richardson P, McKenna W, Bristow M: Report of the 1995 World Health Organization/International Society and Federation of Cardiology Task Force on the definition and classification of cardiomyopathies. Circulation 93:841–842, 1996
14. Wynne J, Braunwald E: The cardiomyopathies and myocarditides. In Braunwald E, Zipes DP, Libby P (eds): Heart Disease (6th Ed), pp 1751–1806. Philadelphia, WB Saunders, 2001
15. Davies MJ: The cardiomyopathies: An overview. Heart 83(4):469–474, 2000
16. Spirito P, Seidman CE, McKenna WJ, et al: The management of hypertrophic cardiomyopathy. N Engl J Med 336(11):775–785, 1997
17. Beery TA: The evolving role of genetics in the diagnosis and management of heart disease. Nurs Clin North Am 35(4):963–973, 2000
18. Creager MA, Libby P: Peripheral arterial diseases. In Braunwald E, Zipes DP, Libby P (eds): Heart Disease (6th Ed), pp 1457–1484. Philadelphia, WB Saunders, 2001
19. Lewis CD: Peripheral arterial disease of the lower extremity. J Cardiovasc Nurs 15(4):45–63, 2001
20. Belch JJF, Topol EJ, Agnelli G, et al: Critical issues in peripheral arterial disease detection and management. Arch Intern Med 163:884–892, 2003
21. Saucedo JF, Laird JR: Peripheral vascular disease. In Apple S, Lindsay J (eds): Principles and Practice of Interventional Cardiology, pp 41–62. Philadelphia, Lippincott Williams & Wilkins, 2000
22. Hiatt WR: Medical treatment of peripheral and arterial disease and claudication. N Engl J Med 344(21):1608–1621, 2001
23. Laird JR, Lansky AJ: Percutaneous transluminal angioplasty for the treatment of peripheral vascular disease. In Apple S, Lindsay J (eds): Principles and Practice of Interventional Cardiology, pp 191–209. Philadelphia, Lippincott Williams & Wilkins, 2000
24. Lea H, Zierler BK: Hematopoiesis and coagulation. In Woods S, Froelicher E, Motzer S (eds): Cardiac Nursing (4th Ed), pp 109–131. Philadelphia, Lippincott Williams & Wilkins, 2000
25. Wennberg PW, Rooke TW: Diagnosis and management of disease of the peripheral arteries and veins. In Fuster V, Alexander RW, O'Rourke RA (eds): Hurst's The Heart (10th Ed), pp 2421–2441. New York, McGraw-Hill, 2001
26. Isselbacher EM: Diseases of the aorta. In Braunwald E, Zipes DP, Libby P (eds): Heart Disease (6th Ed), pp 1422–1456. Philadelphia, WB Saunders, 2001
27. Anderson LA: Abdominal aortic aneurysm. J Cardiovasc Nurs 15(4):1–14, 2001
28. Lindsay J: Diagnosis and treatment of diseases of the aorta. In Fuster V, Alexander RW, O'Rourke RA (eds): Hurst's The Heart (10th Ed), pp 2375–2395. New York, McGraw-Hill, 2001
29. Anderson LA: Abdominal aortic aneurysm. J Cardiovasc Nurs 15(4):1–14, 2001
30. Lederle FA, Wilson SE, Johnson GR, et al: Immediate repair compared with surveillance of small abdominal aortic aneurysms. N Engl J Med 346(19):1437–1444, 2002
31. Hall SW: Endovascular repair of abdominal aortic aneurysms. AORN 77(3):630–648, 2003
32. Finkelmeier BA, Marolda D: Aortic dissection. J Cardiovasc Nurs 15(4):15–24, 2001
33. Seventh Report of the Joint National Committee on the Prevention, Detection, Evaluation, and Treatment of High Blood Pressure (JNC 7). Available at: www.nhlbi.nih.gov/guidelines/hypertension. Accessed October 27, 2003
34. Kaplan NM: Systemic hypertension: Mechanism and diagnosis. In Braunwald E, Zipes DP, Libby P (eds): Heart Disease (6th Ed), pp 941–971. Philadelphia, WB Saunders, 2001
35. Mansoor GA, Frishman WH: Comprehensive management of hypertensive emergencies and urgencies. Heart Dis 4(6):358–371, 2002
36. Tuncel M, Ram VCS: Hypertensive emergencies: Etiology and management. Am J Cardiovasc Drugs 3(1):21–31, 2003

OTHER SELECTED READING

Braunwald E, Zipes DP, Libby P (eds): Heart Disease (6th Ed). Philadelphia, WB Saunders, 2001

Fahey VA (ed): Vascular disease. J Cardiovasc Nurs 15:2001

Fuster V, Alexander RW, O'Rourke RA (eds): Hurst's The Heart (10th Ed). New York, McGraw-Hill, 2001

Woods SL, Froelicher ESS, Motzer SU (eds): Cardiac Nursing (4th Ed). Philadelphia, Lippincott Williams & Wilkins, 2000

chapter 20

Heart Failure

KAY BLUM

objectives

Based on the content in this chapter, the reader should be able to:

- Define heart failure.
- Identify the physiological basis for the clinical manifestations of heart failure.
- Describe expected clinical assessment findings for patients with heart failure.
- Define expected outcomes for therapeutic management of patients with heart failure.
- Explain the standard pharmacological therapies for chronic heart failure and acute exacerbation of chronic heart failure, and their rationale.
- Describe the nonpharmacological therapies for management of heart failure.
- Formulate a teaching plan for patients and families regarding heart failure.

Approximately 4.6 million Americans live with heart failure. About 550,000 new individuals receive the diagnosis of heart failure each year. The incidence of heart failure approaches 10 per 1,000 population after age 65 years, and 75% of patients have antecedent hypertension. Incidence and prevalence statistics indicate heart failure is a common occurrence in certain patient populations, most notably the elderly and patients with a history of hypertension, myocardial infarction, or both. Although other cardiovascular mortality and morbidity statistics have decreased, the incidence of new-onset heart failure has continued to increase.

The 5-year mortality rate for heart failure is about 50%. Sudden cardiac death occurs six to nine times as often in patients with heart failure compared with the general population. An estimated 957,000 patients were discharged with heart failure in 1997.[1] Heart failure is a common diagnosis in the intensive care unit (ICU) because the onset is sudden. An acute myocardial infarction (MI) or an acute exacerbation of chronic heart failure is often life-threatening. Hospitalization is associated with high financial costs, and the physical and emotional burdens of inpatient care are great for both patients and their families.

Management of patients with heart failure requires a collaborative effort on the part of physicians, nurses, pharmacologists, and dietitians as well as other allied health professionals. The care of patients with heart failure extends across all parts of the medical system. Patients with heart failure may be located in ambulatory care, acute care, critical care, and rehabilitation care facilities. As patients take charge of their own disease prevention, they are also found in the home.

This chapter reviews the key points of cardiovascular physiology and pathophysiology that are critical to understanding heart failure, and the principles of management for patients admitted for treatment. It also presents the current evidence-based guidelines for the management of heart failure, with special attention to the pharmacological agents used for both chronic heart failure and those medications used in the ICU for treatment of acute episodes. Key points for discharge planning, teaching, and special populations are also included.

DEFINITION

Heart failure is a clinical syndrome characterized by shortness of breath, dyspnea on exertion, paroxysmal nocturnal dyspnea, orthopnea, and peripheral or pulmonary edema. Not all patients have all these clinical indicators. *Heart failure* is a general term used to describe the general clinical syndrome regardless of the kind of heart failure or the etiology that produces the symptoms. *Congestive heart failure* is so named because the interruption in circulation related to failure of the heart to function normally leads to congestion in the vascular beds of the lungs and peripheral tissues, resulting in respiratory symptoms and peripheral edema. The revised guidelines recently published by a joint American College of Cardiology (ACC) and American Heart Association (AHA) task force[2] use the preferred term *heart failure* rather than *congestive heart failure* because patients with chronic heart failure rarely demonstrate the rales and alveolar edema associated with congestion. For this reason, it is important to look at the way heart failure is classified, because the pathophysiology and etiology are keys to appropriate management.

CLASSIFICATION

Heart failure is more difficult to understand when signs and symptoms are common to more than one type of failure and when types of heart failure are used interchangeably. Several categories are used to describe and classify heart failure. Using these categories to organize information about heart failure and for discussion of any individual patient case makes diagnosis, management, and outcome evaluation clearer.

Acute Versus Chronic

The terms *acute* and *chronic* are used to describe both the onset of symptoms of heart failure and the intensity of symptoms. Heart failure of acute onset refers to the sudden appearance of symptoms, usually over days or hours. Acute symptoms have progressed to a point at which immediate or emergency intervention is necessary to save the patient's life. Heart failure of chronic onset refers to the development of symptoms over months to years. Chronic symptoms represent the baseline condition, the limitations the patient lives with on a daily basis. If the cause of the acute onset or the acute symptoms is not reversible, then the heart failure may become chronic. For example, a patient who has an acute MI with severe damage to the left ventricle has acute heart failure with pulmonary edema, causing lasting damage to the left ventricle. As a result, the patient has poor contractility (and, therefore, dyspnea on exertion) after the MI has resolved. The patient's acute onset of heart failure has left him with chronic symptoms.

Left-Sided Heart Failure Versus Right-Sided Heart Failure

LEFT-SIDED HEART FAILURE

Left-sided heart failure refers to failure of the left ventricle to fill or empty properly. This leads to increased pressures inside the ventricle and congestion in the pulmonary vascular system. Left-sided heart failure may be further classified into systolic and diastolic dysfunction.

Systolic Dysfunction

Systolic dysfunction is usually estimated by ejection fraction, or the percentage of the left ventricular end-diastolic volume (LVEDV) that is ejected from the ventricle in one cycle. If the LVEDV is 100 mL and the stroke volume is 60 mL, the ejection fraction is 60%. Normal ejection fraction is 50% to 70%. Systolic dysfunction is defined as an ejection fraction of less than 40% and is caused by a decrease in contractility. The ventricle is not emptied adequately because of poor pumping, and the end result is decreased cardiac output.

Diastolic Dysfunction

Diastolic dysfunction is less well defined and more difficult to measure, and it is often referred to as *heart failure with preserved left ventricular function.* Pumping is normal or even increased, with an ejection fraction as high as 80% at times. Diastolic dysfunction is caused by impaired relaxation and filling. Left ventricular filling, a complex process that takes place during diastole, is a combination of passive filling and atrial contraction. If the ventricle is stiff and poorly compliant (due to aging, uncontrolled hypertension, or volume overload), relaxation is slow or incomplete. If the heart rate is fast, diastole is short, or if the patient has atrial fibrillation, there is no organized atrial contraction. These mechanisms all reduce filling of the ventricle and contribute to diastolic dysfunction, therefore decreasing cardiac output.

RIGHT-SIDED HEART FAILURE

Right-sided heart failure refers to failure of the right ventricle to pump adequately. The most common cause of right-sided heart failure is left-sided heart failure, but right-sided heart failure can exist in the presence of a perfectly normal left ventricle and does not lead to left-sided heart failure. Right-sided heart failure can also result from pulmonary disease and primary pulmonary artery hypertension (where it is referred to as *cor pulmonale*). Acute onset of right-sided heart failure is often caused by pulmonary embolus.

Classification Systems

NEW YORK HEART ASSOCIATION FUNCTIONAL CLASSIFICATION

The New York Heart Association (NYHA) Functional Classification is a measure of how much the symptoms of heart failure limit the activities of patients (Box 20-1). Although ejection fraction is used to define left ventricular function, ejection fraction is poorly correlated with the patient's functional capacity or prognosis.[3]

AMERICAN COLLEGE OF CARDIOLOGY/AMERICAN HEART ASSOCIATION GUIDELINES

The ACC/AHA Guidelines[2] outline four stages of heart failure that are useful for organizing the prevention, diagnosis, management, and prognosis for patients with heart failure (Box 20-2). These stages are not meant to replace the NYHA functional classification but rather to augment it. Only stages C and D are applicable to the NYHA functional classification system.

FACTORS THAT DETERMINE CARDIAC OUTPUT

The underlying result of all types of heart failure is insufficient cardiac output. That is, the volume of blood pumped by the heart in 1 minute is inadequate. Some patients may have a normal cardiac output at rest, but they do not have the reserve function to increase cardiac output to meet the increased demands of exercise, hypoxemia, or anemia. Therefore, it is important to understand the physiological basis of cardiac output and review the mechanisms of compensation of decreased cardiac output. (See Chapter 16 for a review of cardiovascular physiology.)

box 20-1
New York Heart Association (NYHA) Functional Classification of Heart Failure

Class I: No limitation of physical activity. Ordinary physical activity does not cause undue fatigue or dyspnea.
Class II: Slight limitation of physical activity. Comfortable at rest, but ordinary physical activity results in fatigue or dyspnea.
Class III: Marked limitation of physical activity without symptoms. Symptoms are present even at rest. If any physical activity is undertaken, symptoms are increased.
Class IV: Unable to carry on any physical activity without symptoms. Symptoms are present even at rest. If any physical activity is undertaken, symptoms are increased.

box 20-2
American College of Cardiology (ACC)/American Heart Association (AHA) Guidelines for Stages of Heart Failure*

A Patients at high risk for heart failure because of the presence of conditions that are strongly associated with the development of heart failure. Such patients have no identified structural or functional abnormalities of the pericardium, myocardium, or cardiac valves and have never shown signs or symptoms of heart failure.
B Patients who have structural heart disease that is strongly associated with the development of heart failure but who have never shown signs or symptoms of heart failure.
C Patients who have current or prior symptoms of heart failure associated with underlying structural heart disease
D Patients with advanced structural heart disease and marked symptoms of heart failure at rest despite maximal medical therapy and who require specialized interventions.

*New York Heart Association classification is applicable only to stages C and D.

Oxygen Demand

The required cardiac output is determined by the body's metabolic demand for oxygen. At rest, the body needs sufficient oxygen to burn calories to support cellular function, as measured by basal metabolic rate. Oxygen delivery to the tissues depends on arterial oxygen content (CaO_2) and cardiac output. CaO_2, a combination of arterial oxygen saturation (SaO_2) and hemoglobin, is constant in healthy people. Any factor that increases metabolic demand for oxygen, such as exercise, fever, hyperthyroidism, or trauma, increases cardiac output. If CaO_2 is decreased, as it is in hypoxemia or anemia, then cardiac output increases to ensure sufficient oxygen to meet the metabolic demand. Exercise or fever in a patient with anemia puts a tremendous burden on the heart to supply sufficient oxygen to meet the metabolic demands.

A person with a healthy heart has sufficient reserve to meet this increased metabolic demand and increase cardiac output. At best, a patient with myocardial ischemia, cardiomyopathy, valvular disease, dysrhythmia, or lung disease may not be able to meet the metabolic demand for oxygen associated with exercise. At worst, the patient with one or more of these problems may not be able to meet the basal metabolic demand for oxygen and becomes symptomatic, even at rest.

Mechanical Factors

Cardiac output equals stroke volume multiplied by heart rate.

STROKE VOLUME

Stroke volume results from the complex interaction of preload, afterload, and contractility. Preload stretches the ventricle and, as the ventricle begins to contract, the volume of blood pumped is equally dependent on both the loading and the efficiency and force of the contraction. Approximately 60% of resting blood volume is located in the venous reservoir. This stored volume can be recruited to increase preload and therefore contractility and stroke volume.

To optimize stroke volume, these factors must be balanced; they must increase and decrease in relation to each other. Resting stroke volume can be increased by increasing preload, increasing contractility, and decreasing afterload. This happens with exercise, as does an increase in blood pressure and a neurohormonally regulated decrease in afterload. All of these processes produce an increase in stroke volume. However, increased heart rate raises cardiac output much more than increased stroke volume because the ability to increase stroke volume is limited, even in a healthy heart.

Preload

Preload is the volume of blood in the ventricle at the end of diastole.[4] Because of the curvilinear relationship of volume and pressure in the heart, volumes are often estimated using pressure. Volume in the heart is difficult to measure, and left ventricular end-diastolic pressure is used to estimate left ventricular end-diastolic volume and therefore preload. However, it is impossible to measure left ventricular end-diastolic pressure on a regular basis outside the catheterization laboratory; pulmonary artery wedge pressure is used to estimate left ventricular end-diastolic pressure. Central venous pressure and right atrial pressure are used to estimate right ventricular end-diastolic pressure. In a person with a healthy heart, central venous pressure is an adequate estimate of left ventricular end-diastolic pressure because variation is most often related to total body volume that affects the right and left ventricles equally. In a patient with heart or lung disease, central venous pressure does not reliably reflect left ventricular end-diastolic pressure; in these patients, many factors in addition to total body volume may affect left ventricular end-diastolic pressure.

Afterload

Afterload is the resistance to the flow of blood from the heart. Afterload depends on the competency of the heart valves, especially the aortic valve, and vascular resistance. Vascular resistance is a major contributor to blood pressure, which equals resistance multiplied by the volume or flow through the artery. Resistance is a function of both the compliance and the diameter of the artery. The ventricle must overcome resistance to open the aortic valve before any blood is pumped. A high resistance may decrease stroke volume; there is less energy to pump blood after the aortic valve is opened. Similarly, a stenotic aortic valve reduces stroke volume because stenosis restricts the opening and therefore increases the resistance to blood flow.

Contractility

Contractility is the force and velocity with which the ventricle contracts. Contractility involves the alignment of actin and myosin fibers in the cardiac muscle fibers. Starling described the relationship between stretch of the muscle fibers and the velocity with which they contract. The filling of the ventricular cavity with blood stretches the muscle fibers, and the fuller the ventricle, the more stretch it has, and the more energy is has to overcome resistance and pump blood. This relationship is referred to as the *Frank-Starling curve* or the *Frank-Starling law.*

An increase in muscle mass increases the number of fibers available for contraction and therefore increases contractility. Sufficient oxygen is also necessary for normal contraction. Calcium plays a critical role in the alignment of actin and myosin. The alignment of the fibers and the connective tissues contributes to the elliptical shape of the ventricle that makes the contraction more efficient.

HEART RATE

As stated earlier, cardiac output equals stroke volume multiplied by heart rate. Therefore, just doubling the heart rate doubles cardiac output without changing stroke volume. The immediate response to a decrease in stroke volume, a decrease in arterial oxygen content, or an increase in metabolic demand is an increase in heart rate. However, at a certain point, increasing heart rate can actually decrease stroke volume and therefore cardiac output as well. Because the ventricle fills during diastole, preload becomes compromised at higher heart rates because of the shortened diastolic filling time. A decrease in preload compromises contractility.

The physiological role of heart rate in the regulation of cardiac output involves more than just the absolute rate. Cardiac rhythm is important. As previously stated, rapid tachycardia can compromise stroke volume. Any rhythm that does not include a rhythmic atrial contraction, such as atrial fibrillation/flutter, junctional rhythms, ventricular rhythms, and ventricular pacing, can compromise filling and therefore stroke volume and cardiac output. A heart rate that is too slow, such as that which occurs in third-degree atrioventricular (AV) block or sick sinus syndrome, may compromise cardiac output, not by decreasing stroke volume, but by decreasing overall cardiac output.

Neurohormonal Mechanisms

Metabolic demand for oxygen is the primary factor in the regulation of cardiac output, and the mechanical relationships between loading and contractility provide a means to regulate it. Neurohormones, therefore, are the messengers that initiate, coordinate, and mediate the complex processes that meet the dynamic need for cardiac output.

CATECHOLAMINES

Catecholamines are released from the adrenal medulla as part of the primitive "fight or flight" response to any stressor. Stressors can be physiological or psychological. Epinephrine and norepinephrine as well as cortical hormones, such as cortisol and aldosterone, are released.

Epinephrine and norepinephrine are the key catecholamines involved in the regulation of the cardiovascular system. The heart and blood vessels contain alpha- and beta-adrenergic receptors that bind with these hormones to support cardiac output and blood pressure. Norepinephrine has almost exclusively alpha-adrenergic properties that increase vascular resistance and therefore blood pressure. Epinephrine has both alpha- and beta-adrenergic properties. Beta-agonist effects include increased heart rate, increased contractility, and vasodilation. The net effect of epinephrine is increased cardiac output; it increases stroke volume by increasing contractility and decreasing afterload. The increase in heart rate and stroke volume together produce a greater increase in cardiac output than either would alone.

RENIN–ANGIOTENSIN–ALDOSTERONE SYSTEM

One of the most important mechanisms of blood pressure control in relation to heart failure is the renin–angiotensin–aldosterone system. Fluids such as blood flow down pressure gradients (i.e., from higher pressure to lower pressure). Consequently, pressure in the aorta is higher than pressures distal to it, including the arteriolar and capillary levels. Arterial blood pressure is critical to the delivery of blood (and therefore oxygen) to the cells to support cellular function. Several mechanisms are in place to maintain normal blood pressure across variable body fluid volumes, different positions (sitting or standing versus supine), and cardiac output demands.

Renin is an enzyme produced in the kidney in response to even small decreases in blood pressure. Renin has a direct effect on the kidney, causing increased reabsorption of salt and water. Much of the renin travels to the lung to act enzymatically on angiotensinogen to form angiotensin I. In the presence of angiotensin-converting enzyme (ACE) in the lung, angiotensin I is converted to angiotensin II.

A powerful vasoconstrictor, angiotensin II increases arterial resistance quickly and profoundly, providing immediate support for blood pressure and maintaining perfusion in the short term until a longer-term strategy can be implemented. Angiotensin II has a much more modest effect on venous resistance, but does increase venous resistance and therefore venous return. Angiotensin II also stimulates the adrenal cortex to release aldosterone. Aldosterone then acts on the kidney to increase salt reabsorption in the distal tubule, and this salt increases water reabsorption in the kidney, resulting in increased circulating volume. Increased circulating volume is the longer-term strategy. The renin–angiotensin–aldosterone system initiates a process that assumes any decrease in blood pressure is a volume loss (e.g., hemorrhage), and the long-term strategy is to replace that loss.

box 20-3
Causes of Heart Failure

Impaired Cardiac Function
- Myocardial disease
  - Cardiomyopathies
  - Myocarditis
  - Coronary insufficiency
  - Myocardial infarction
- Valvular heart disease
  - Stenotic valvular disease
  - Regurgitant valvular disease
- Congenital heart defects
- Constrictive pericarditis

Excess Work Demands
- Increased pressure work
  - Systemic hypertension
  - Pulmonary hypertension
- Increased perfusion work
  - Thyrotoxicosis

Modified with permission from Porth CM: Pathophysiology: Concepts of Altered Health States, (6th Ed), p 551. Philadelphia, Lippincott Williams & Wilkins, 2002.

PATHOPHYSIOLOGY

The physiological principles discussed in the previous section form the basis for understanding the patient's signs, symptoms, responses, and compensation for the disease process as well as the basis for management strategies. Heart failure has many causes (Box 20-3).

Cardiomyopathy

The distinguishing pathophysiological factor in heart failure is the presence of a cardiomyopathy, but cardiomyopathy is not synonymous with heart failure.[2] Literally, cardiomyopathy is a progressive pathological process in the heart muscle. Cardiomyopathy may be congenital or acquired; this discussion is limited to acquired cardiomyopathy. Hypertrophic, nonobstructive cardiomyopathy and dilated cardiomyopathy are the two most common forms.

Exactly how cardiomyopathy develops is not completely understood. Current theories under investigation suggest that ischemic, immune, mechanical, and neurohormonal effects on the pericardium, myocardium, and endothelium lead to structural changes that result in functional changes. Structural changes at the cellular level include replacement of contractile and elastic muscle cells with fibrotic elements, which leads to stiffness of the ventricles and smooth muscle layers in the arteries. In hypertrophic cardiomyopathy, the heart muscle becomes thickened, with increased mass and poor relaxation. In dilated cardiomyopathy, the ventricular chamber dilates, thins, and changes from a normally elliptical shape to a less efficient spherical shape, reducing contractility and impairing emptying. Both stiffness and spherical remodeling may occur in the same heart, leading to a compromised cardiac output from impaired relaxation and impaired emptying. Stiffening of arteries seen in aging, atherosclerosis, and arteriosclerosis decreases stroke volume and exacerbates the ventricular wall stress by overfilling the ventricle. The heart attempts to maintain cardiac output in the face of a decreased stroke volume by increasing heart rate, which decreases relaxation time and impairs filling. This endless spiral of dysfunction is manifested by the progressive nature of heart failure.

The resulting decrease in cardiac output leads to activation of the renin–angiotensin–aldosterone system and the release of catecholamines. As previously described, these neurohormones were meant to respond to temporary decreases in blood pressure such as hemorrhage, but in cardiomyopathy the problem is chronic. Consequently, the neurohormonal effects, which were intended to be temporary, become permanent and become part of the problem instead of the solution to a decreased cardiac output.

The persistence of these neurohormones is hypothesized to be the mechanism by which the ventricle remodels from an elliptical shape to spherical, further decreasing its pumping efficiency. The realignment of the muscle fibers has been attributed to long-term exposure to aldosterone. Furthermore, long-term exposure to catecholamines leads to downregulation of beta-adrenergic receptors and contributes to decreased contractility.[5,6]

HYPERTROPHIC CARDIOMYOPATHY

Hypertrophic cardiomyopathy is caused by an increase in muscle mass in the ventricle. The result is a measurable increase in the thickness of the ventricular wall. Hypertrophy is the response to a prolonged increase in resistance (afterload). Hypertrophy may result from prolonged or uncontrolled hypertension; it may also occur in patients with aortic stenosis, mitral stenosis, or primary pulmonary artery hypertension. Increased muscle mass results in increased energy and therefore increased contraction. However, the increase in mass decreases compliance of the ventricle and slows relaxation. The decreased compliance and slower relaxation make ventricular filling more difficult, resulting in a decrease in cardiac output even though contractility may be normal or actually increased.

DILATED CARDIOMYOPATHY

Dilated cardiomyopathy is an increase in the size of the ventricular chamber without an increase in wall size, and is a response to decreased contractility. A decrease in contractility may occur for many reasons, including ischemia, alcohol abuse, endocrine disorders, pregnancy, viral infections, and valvular disease. The result of the decrease in contractility (ejection fraction <40%) is an increase in end-systolic volume. Over time, the ventricle dilates to accommodate the increased intraventricular volumes (preload). The increased preload in a normal heart would lead to an increase in stroke volume, but in the dilated heart, the increased volume leads to a decreasing stroke volume. Dilated cardiomyopathy can be further divided into two types: ischemic and nonischemic.

Ischemic Cardiomyopathy

Ischemic cardiomyopathy is the result of oxygen levels that are inadequate to meet the metabolic demands of the myocardial cells. It occurs when there is obstruction in the coronary arteries and may be acute or chronic. Oxygen is essential to the function of cells. It is necessary for the metabolism of nutritional substrates and the formation of adenosine triphosphate (ATP), which powers all intracellular processes. When oxygen is inadequate, ATP becomes insufficient, and the calcium, sodium, and potassium pumps fail, leading to interruptions in both the mechanical and electrical function of the cells. The net result is a decrease in contractility and dysrhythmia. If oxygen is restored to the muscle cells, then function returns and the dysrhythmia disappears.

If the ischemia is severe or persists, the muscle tissue dies, causing an MI. Dead muscle cannot regenerate and is replaced with scar tissue. The larger the scar, the larger the dysfunction. The decrease in muscle mass leads to decreased energy for pumping blood and therefore decreased cardiac output. The goal in treatment of unstable angina and acute MI is preservation of muscle mass to prevent systolic dysfunction.

If an MI is small, the damage may be insufficient to cause heart failure because there is still enough muscle to meet the body's demands for oxygen at rest and with exercise. The ejection fraction may still be within the normal range, although it may be decreased somewhat due to the myocardial damage. However, repeated damage from subsequent infarctions or persistent ischemia in other areas of the heart muscle may exhaust the reserve function. "Hibernating" myocardium is an area of myocardial cells that are not dead (MI), but lack sufficient oxygen and nutrient substrates to contract. Once a patient is stable after an MI, it is important to identify any viable myocardium that may be "hibernating" because of reversible ischemia. If perfusion can be restored to this viable but underperforming myocardium, ventricular function can be improved.

If an MI is very large, or critical structures such as the chordae tendineae are involved, then the consequences may be life-threatening. Damage or rupture of the chordae may lead to acute, severe mitral regurgitation and profound heart failure. The loss of ventricular pumping function that results from a massive MI or smaller repeated MIs may produce such an acute loss of pump function that all the body's compensatory mechanisms are not effectively able to overcome the deficit in cardiac output.

This condition represents cardiogenic shock, in which cardiac output is severely inadequate and the left ventricle empties poorly (see Chapter 50). Consequently, left ventricular end-diastolic pressure increases, pulmonary artery pressures increase, and pulmonary edema results. End-organ damage due to inadequate oxygen begins to occur depending on the function of the organ. The skin becomes cool, perhaps clammy and pale. The respiratory rate increases to supply as much oxygen as possible to the blood being pumped because the pulmonary edema severely decreases the effective area for gas transport. The pulmonary edema makes the lungs heavy and less compliant and reduces the effective tidal volume. Increases in respiratory rate are necessary to maintain minute volume. In addition, the tissues that are not adequately supplied with oxygen begin to produce lactic acid, leading to metabolic acidosis. The short-term compensation for metabolic acidosis is an increase in minute volume, or hyperpnea. The patient complains of feeling short of breath even at rest and may not be able to breathe in any recumbent position.

The hierarchy of protection in times of inadequate perfusion preserves most of the cardiac output for the brain, heart, and kidneys. Autoregulation mechanisms are present in all these organs to preserve pressure gradients and blood flow even when blood pressure and flow are compromised in other areas such as the skin, muscle, and gut. Indications that the brain is inadequately perfused are confusion, disorientation, somnolence, and agitation. Early indications of inadequate renal flow are an increase in blood urea nitrogen (BUN) and creatinine. Early on, the normal 10 to

20:1 ratio of BUN to creatinine increases to greater than 20:1; this signals the onset of prerenal azotemia. If perfusion is restored to the kidney at this time, the BUN and creatinine levels return to normal, as does kidney function. If the poor perfusion is profound or prolonged, the kidneys become damaged, and the BUN and creatinine continue to increase, although the ratio returns to normal. This ischemic damage to the kidneys is known as *acute tubular necrosis* (ATN) and may be reversible.

If cardiogenic shock persists uncorrected for an extended period, the damage cannot be reversed and the patient will die. Even if the patient is treated appropriately, further damage may occur in areas where the oxygen demand is lower than that of the brain and kidneys. Prolonged episodes of low cardiac output may lead to ileus, bowel infarction, liver failure, and increased risk of pneumonia and skin breakdown.

Patients who survive the initial episode of acute heart failure may recover completely if an intervention such as angioplasty or coronary artery bypass restores perfusion to the heart muscle and the damage to the remaining muscle is not severe. Chronic heart failure eventually develops in many patients and is characterized by the same symptoms as acute heart failure, but usually at a lower intensity; the body has had time to compensate for the decreased cardiac output. Usually, chronic heart failure does not have the intense limitations associated with acute heart failure. Patients often modify their activity to match the limited reserve of cardiac output available.

Nonischemic Cardiomyopathy

Nonischemic cardiomyopathy results from several causes. A large number of people have idiopathic dilated cardiomyopathy. For some as yet unknown reason, their hearts dilate, remodel, and become ineffective pumps. Others have myocarditis, often due to viral infection of the myocardium, hypothyroidism or hyperthyroidism, valvular disease, human immunodeficiency virus (HIV), or hemochromatosis. In addition, myocarditis may be bacterial or idiopathic. Nonischemic cardiomyopathy may also result from pregnancy, heavy alcohol use, hypertension, and tachycardia. Heart failure that results from hypothyroidism or hyperthyroidism, hemochromatosis, valvular disease, and tachycardia is reversible and disappears when these problems are corrected.

Nonischemic cardiomyopathy, like ischemic cardiomyopathy, may be acute or chronic. Patients with chronic disease are often quite limited in their ability to carry out everyday activities. The mechanism by which the dilation is triggered and progresses is not well understood. Dilated cardiomyopathy, whether ischemic or nonischemic, produces symptoms after all the compensatory mechanisms have been exhausted.

Consequently, unless the onset of symptoms is acute, pathological changes may be quite advanced before activity is sufficiently limited and the patient seeks medical care. However, myocarditis frequently has an acute onset. The patient feels fine and is free of symptoms before fatigue and dyspnea on exertion, or, occasionally, pulmonary edema, suddenly develop. Dysfunction results from inflammation of the heart muscle. Metabolic function of inflamed muscle cells is impaired; the cells do not contract properly, leading to decreased cardiac output. Severity of the condition ranges from cardiogenic shock to mild limitation of activity. Once the initial acute phase passes, the patient has a low ejection fraction, with varying levels of physical limitation of activity and shortness of breath, or chronic heart failure.

Alcoholism, hypertension, and idiopathic etiologic factors are nonischemic conditions that may lead to dilated cardiomyopathy over longer periods—months to years as opposed to days to weeks with acute onset. As the ventricle begins to dilate, compensatory mechanisms, including the previously described catecholamines and other neurohormonal factors, begin to work. The proposed mechanism by which the ventricle remodels from the normal, efficient elliptical dimensions to a thin-walled, inefficient spherical shape involves constant exposure of the myocardium to these neurohormones. The natural progression is from dilation without symptoms, to compensated heart failure, to uncompensated heart failure, to refractory heart failure. Patients most often present when their heart failure is no longer compensated and symptoms interfere with normal daily activities. At this point, medication may relieve all or most symptoms. However, the structural changes that occur are progressive, and, even with medication, symptoms worsen over time. Medication can be adjusted to treat the worsening symptoms, but eventually, the medications will not be enough and the patient dies. Mortality is usually due to worsening of the cardiac output, leading to system failure or sudden death from ventricular dysrhythmia. Before the stage of refractory heart failure is reached, much can be done to control the patient's symptoms, improve activity tolerance, control the progression of the disease, and improve quality of life.

Dysrhythmia

Heart failure is commonly associated with dysrhythmias, both atrial and ventricular. The structural and metabolic changes that occur in heart failure frequently lead to dysrhythmia, and the dysrhythmia itself may lead to heart failure.

ATRIAL DYSRHYTHMIAS

Atrial tachycardias may cause heart failure in two ways. First, the shortened diastole leads to decreased filling and may cause or aggravate diastolic dysfunction, resulting in decreased cardiac output and the symptoms of heart failure. When the tachycardia is caused by atrial fibrillation, the loss of atrial kick increases the impact of the atrial dysrhythmia on left ventricular dysfunction. In one study, systolic dysfunction developed in 11% of patients with atrial fibrillation, and 6% of the patients died.[7]

Atrial fibrillation is a significant problem in patients with heart failure. The most common sustained dysrhythmia, atrial fibrillation, affects 2.2 million Americans. The median age for atrial fibrillation is 75 years; it affects 8.8% of Americans older than 80 years. (The risk of stroke is increased five times in patients who have this dysrhythmia.[8]) The incidence of both atrial fibrillation and heart failure increases with age, increasing the likelihood that patients with heart failure will also have atrial fibrillation at some time.

VENTRICULAR DYSRHYTHMIAS

Ventricular dysrhythmias, in particular premature ventricular beats and nonsustained ventricular tachycardia (NSVT), are common in patients with dilated cardiomyopathy, whether ischemic or nonischemic. Sudden death from ventricular dysrhythmia or bradycardia accounts for 30% to 40% of deaths associated with heart failure.[9] The presence of premature ventricular beats or even NSVT has not been shown to be reliably predictive of risk of sudden death for any particular patient. However, the presence of these dysrhythmias does seem to reliably reflect a globally impaired myocardium.

Several mechanisms play a role in the development of ventricular dysrhythmias. The low ejection fraction leads to stretch of the myocardial fibers, thus increasing excitability. Excitability is also affected by the presence of increased catecholamines; increased sympathetic tone; and, on occasion, antiarrhythmic drugs. Activation of the renin–angiotensin–aldosterone system contributes to the overall environment that generates dysrhythmia. Ischemia leads to failure of the sodium–potassium pump, and the loss of potassium from the cell increases the risk of premature ventricular beats. Scar tissue from previous infarctions and surgery can stimulate dysrhythmia. Electrolyte shifts involving potassium, calcium, and magnesium are often associated with prolonged or aggressive diuretic use. Lung disease such as emphysema or chronic bronchitis is often comorbid with heart failure, and the lung disease may lead to hypoxemia, which contributes to the genesis of ventricular dysrhythmias. The traditional sources of ventricular dysrhythmia that occur in patients without heart failure, such as reentry, enhanced automaticity, and delayed after-potentials, may also be involved.

Acute Exacerbation of Chronic Heart Failure

Patients with chronic heart failure may live from day to day with no symptoms of heart failure, or well-controlled symptoms. Chronic heart failure may become acutely worse, however, resulting in an increase in symptoms and limitations associated with left ventricular dysfunction. Several factors may lead to an exacerbation.

Alcohol, anemia, hypoxemia, hypertension, ischemia, and worsening left ventricular function may trigger an acute exacerbation. Any factor that increases oxygen demand, and therefore demand for increased cardiac output beyond the ability of the ventricle to function (e.g., hypertension, tachycardia, anemia, exercise), causes an exacerbation. Similarly, any factor that depresses the function of the already compromised ventricle leads to exacerbation (e.g., alcohol, drugs that exert a negative inotropic effect such as calcium channel blockers and beta blockers). As the ventricle is called on to work harder, it works less efficiently, and the left ventricular end-diastolic pressure increases, leading to increased pulmonary artery pressures. The increased pulmonary artery pressures, in turn, lead to orthopnea, possibly pulmonary edema, elevated venous pressures, liver congestion, lower extremity edema, and paroxysmal nocturnal dyspnea. Patients may also present with lower blood pressures, more rapid heart rates, and prerenal azotemia. Potentially, the acute decompensation is reversible if treated quickly and aggressively.

ASSESSMENT

Heart failure has long been defined by the presence of pulmonary edema characterized by bibasilar rales or crackles. Once, the absence of crackles ruled out heart failure. However, chronic heart failure is a persistent, not episodic, condition, and it rarely includes pulmonary edema and crackles. History, physical examination, diagnostic procedures, and hemodynamic evaluation all contribute to diagnosing heart failure, perhaps determining its cause, and evaluating the success of therapy.

History

The symptoms of heart failure are nonspecific (i.e., they are common to many disease processes). The history is used to put the symptoms into a context that may lead to their interpretation as heart failure and not pulmonary disease, deconditioning, or other conditions that produce shortness of breath, dyspnea on exertion, fatigue, and swelling of the lower extremities. History alone does not confirm the diagnosis, but helps determine what follow-up examination and diagnostic tests may be appropriate.

ONSET

The basic question is, "When did the symptoms start?" The answer to this question helps categorize the condition as acute or chronic. Most patients indicate an acute onset of 2 weeks or less if this is their first visit for their symptoms. If they are asked additional questions about their activity tolerance for the past year or so, patients with chronic heart failure note a gradual slowing of activity to match the amount of energy available or to control symptoms. The recent identification of symptoms indicates that the patient is now aware of them or they have become unbearable. Acuity is important because reversible ischemia is a potentially life-threatening etiology that may present acutely. When identified and treated, chronic heart failure can be avoided, and perhaps a patient's life may be saved.

DURATION

It is important to know whether the symptoms are persistent and independent of activity or come and go with activity, change of position, food ingestion, or other events. This helps differentiate between heart failure and other conditions that can cause the same symptoms. Heart failure symptoms typically worsen with activity and improve with rest. Cough and shortness of breath may increase when lying down and improve with sitting up. Hiatal hernia and gastric reflux may produce shortness of breath, chest pain, and cough but typically occur after eating and more often in the evening. Lung disease or sleep apnea may also cause the shortness of breath that occurs at rest or awakens the patient at night, characteristic of heart failure. History alone will not differentiate the diagnosis, but it will help to determine what follow-up examination and diagnostic tests may be appropriate.

SEVERITY

Severity of symptoms is important to determine because it is the basis for establishing functional class (see Box 20-1). Severity of symptoms is also an important standard for the evaluation of the success of therapy. A major goal of therapy is symptomatic improvement or, if possible, elimination of symptoms. The evaluation of severity requires that patients be asked certain questions about their symptoms (Table 20-1).

COMORBID DISEASES

Many patients with heart failure have comorbid disorders that contribute to or aggravate their heart failure. The most common of these diseases are coronary artery disease (CAD), hypertension, diabetes mellitus, chronic obstructive pulmonary disease (COPD), and chronic renal insufficiency. Worsening of one or more comorbid diseases may lead to an exacerbation of stable chronic heart failure. In the case of CAD, hypertension, and diabetes, heart failure may be the long-term result of complications of these disease processes. Identification and tight control of these comorbid diseases contribute to the control and treatment of the symptoms of heart failure.

MEDICATIONS

It is very important to obtain a complete list of medications taken by the patient, with dosages. The list should include both prescription and nonprescription medications. In cases of new-onset heart failure, even old medications may contribute to the severity of symptoms. For example, patients who have been treated with a calcium channel blocker for hypertension and now present with a decreased ejection fraction and heart failure may improve when the medication is changed and does not depress myocardial function. Other medications may contribute to heart failure. Patients taking over-the-counter medications such as nonsteroidal anti-inflammatory drugs (NSAIDs) may present with worsening heart failure and renal function because of the effect of the NSAIDs on renal blood flow. NSAIDs block the effect of prostaglandins, which the body secretes to maintain renal blood flow in the context of decreased cardiac output. Cold medicines with systemic decongestants can lead to increased blood pressure that precipitates worsening symptoms of heart failure.

PSYCHOSOCIAL FACTORS

Noncardiac factors may also affect patients with heart failure. Because many affected patients are elderly, they may have problems remembering to fill prescriptions or take medications. Financial hardships may force them to choose between buying medication and buying food. Transportation may depend on friends or family who may be unreliable. Housekeeping may be difficult or impossible because of fatigue and shortness of breath. Patients

table 20-1 Assessment of Severity of Heart Failure

Symptom	Measure(s)	Questions
Orthopnea	Number of pillows patient sleeps on regularly	How many pillows do you sleep on at night? If more than one, is it for comfort or because you cannot breathe with one or two?
Dyspnea on exertion	Number of blocks patient can walk without stopping to rest or catch breath Number of flights of stairs patient can climb without stopping to rest or catch breath Number of times patient must rest while doing activities of daily living such as toileting or minor housework	How many blocks and flights of stairs can you walk without stopping to rest or catch your breath? Do you stop because you cannot go further or because you want to avoid getting short of breath? For patients who are limited by peripheral vascular disease or orthopedic problems: Do you stop because you cannot breathe or because of pain? Which comes first?
Paroxysmal nocturnal dyspnea	Average number of times per night or week	After you go to bed, do you ever have to sit up suddenly to catch your breath? How much time passes before you can breathe normally? Do you need to do anything besides sit up to relieve the shortness of breath?
Dizziness or lightheadedness	Presence or absence (of real concern when symptom occurs when the patient is standing and persists or occurs with activity)	Do you ever become dizzy or lightheaded? What are you doing when this occurs?
Chest pain or pressure*	Presence or absence	Do you have chest pain or pressure? Do you become short of breath with the chest pain or pressure? Which comes first, the pain or the shortness of breath?†

*Chest pain should be fully investigated to determine whether active ischemia is present. This is especially true in patients who are presenting for the first time for evaluation of symptoms of heart failure. Once ischemia has been ruled out, patients may still have chest pain, and it should be evaluated by using these assessment questions.

†Chest pain that comes after shortness of breath is often caused by the heart failure.

living on the second or third floor of buildings without elevators may become isolated and lonely. Depression is not uncommon; the exact incidence is not known. Ongoing family dysfunction and family members who depend on the patient for care and financial support (e.g., grandchildren, dependent adult children) add a burden to the patient's management. Illiteracy is still prevalent; even patients who can read may not read medication instructions correctly. Some patients may skip diuretic doses when visiting places where they are uncertain about access to bathroom facilities; they may not take the diuretic when they return home.

Although many of these factors are significant, they may not be obvious until the patient has visited the same health care facility many times. Early case management and skillful discharge planning depend on recognizing these problems before they lead to repeated hospitalizations and increased mortality.

SUBSTANCE ABUSE

Alcohol and drug (e.g., cocaine) use is also important because it may contribute to the development and progression of heart failure. If alcohol use is the cause of cardiomyopathy, abstinence may lead to complete reversal. Patients who have substance abuse problems often forget to buy or take medication. They may be homeless, which increases the likelihood that they will not return to the health care facility for regular follow-up.

Physical Examination

The physical findings in heart failure differ depending on whether the patient has (1) acute or chronic heart failure or (2) systolic or diastolic dysfunction. When the physiological changes of left ventricular dysfunction occur over a long period, the body adapts and compensates. Consequently, many of the findings on physical examination are normal, despite moderate to severe disease. However, when the problem occurs acutely, there is no time for compensation or adaptation, and the symptoms and consequences are severe. Patients with chronic heart failure due to systolic dysfunction who do have abnormal findings have them persistently. Patients with diastolic dysfunction may have abnormal findings only during an exacerbation.

One or more of the following findings characterizes acute exacerbation. The patient may be volume overloaded by 5 to 50 pounds over dry weight; dry weight is the patient's weight when he or she is euvolemic. Patient self-monitoring is often geared to maintenance of dry weight; maintaining dry weight within 1 to 2 pounds can frequently prevent exacerbation. A second finding is often renal insufficiency characterized by an increase in both BUN and creatinine, with a ratio of BUN to creatinine of greater than 20:1. The third finding is decreased cardiac output manifested by increased dyspnea on exertion and decreased exercise tolerance in general, often described as "fatigue." Patients may also complain of increased orthopnea, paroxysmal nocturnal dyspnea, or both. Some patients have all of the findings, and it is not unusual for patients to be short of breath at rest (NYHA class IV) or demonstrate Cheyne-Stokes respirations. Brain natriuretic peptide (BNP) is elevated in proportion to increases in end-diastolic pressure, and levels may be greater than 1000 pg/mL.

GENERAL FINDINGS

Patients with acute heart failure or acute exacerbation of chronic heart failure appear ill; they are often breathing rapidly, looking anxious, and either sitting up straight or leaning forward and resting their arms on a table or their knees. Patients with stable, chronic heart failure may be quite comfortable but may have evidence of cachexia, muscle wasting, and thin skin.

VITAL SIGNS

Patients with systolic dysfunction may have quite low, but asymptomatic, blood pressures (systolic, 80 to 99 mm Hg; diastolic, 40 to 49 mm Hg). Heart rates may be rapid (90 beats/minute or more), or lower at rest. Patients with diastolic dysfunction may or may not be hypertensive.

Serial weights are very important in following fluid status. Daily weights, when performed properly on a calibrated scale, are more accurate estimates of fluid status than intake and output. Daily weights can be used to evaluate fluid status because 1 L of water weighs 1 kg. Overnight fluctuations in weight are always related to water retention or diuresis.

NECK

Jugular venous pressure is an estimate of right heart filling pressures. When either the total body fluid volume or right atrial pressure increases, the jugular venous pressure increases, and the vein dilates. Jugular venous pressure is estimated by identifying the internal jugular vein and measuring the height of the pulse from the level of the clavicle in centimeters. The patient's head is elevated at 45 degrees. It is important not to use the external jugular vein, which often appears distended and prominent in patients with normal volume and pressure.

LUNGS

It is necessary to determine the respiratory rate and observe the depth of respiration as well as the respiratory rhythm. It is not unusual for patients with severe NYHA class IV heart failure to have a Cheyne-Stokes respiratory pattern. The heart failure may be chronic and persistently class IV, or may represent an acute exacerbation.

Results of auscultation of the chest may be completely normal. Because patients with increased pulmonary artery pressures have increased lymph drainage over time, fluid does not collect in the alveoli. Rales or crackles are sounds made by air bubbling through water in the alveoli, and if no water is present, the sounds are not audible. When pressures increase suddenly, water is forced into the alveoli by increased hydrostatic pressure. Consequently, in acute heart failure and acute exacerbation, in which pulmonary edema is common, bibasilar crackles occur. The presence of unilateral crackles or nondependent crackles is indicative of a pulmonary process, not heart failure. Pulmonary edema can cause wheezing that may be difficult to distinguish from reactive airway disease, such as asthma.

HEART

Progression from left-sided heart failure to left-sided *and* right-sided heart failure or chronic elevations of pulmonary artery pressure often results in a visible, palpable right ventricular or pulmonary artery pulsation at the left sternal border. The point of maximal impulse may be extremely displaced. In advanced heart failure, it may be at the posterior axillary line and at the fifth or sixth intercostal space.

Figure 20-1 shows the areas of cardiac auscultation that are examined in a patient with heart failure. The first (S_1) and second (S_2) heart sounds are expected. The sudden appearance of a third heart sound (S_3) is a warning of impending or worsening heart failure. In chronic heart failure, S_3 is a common and chronic finding. A fourth heart sound (S_4) is common in patients with long-standing hypertension and is not considered ominous. However, in severe heart failure, all four heart sounds may be heard; this is known as a *summation gallop*.

When valvular disease is the cause of heart failure, a heart murmur associated with the diseased valve is heard. In patients with dilated cardiomyopathy, a mitral regurgitation murmur is commonly heard. This holosystolic murmur is best heard at the left sternal border or, in patients with very large hearts, at the apex. The mitral valve is usually structurally intact. The dilation of the left ventricle in chronic heart failure dilates the mitral annulus and prevents the close approximation of the valve leaflets. Consequently, blood regurgitates back across the mitral valve into the left atrium with each systole.

When a mitral regurgitation murmur develops acutely, as when there is damage to the papillary muscles that open and close the mitral valve, severe, acute heart failure results. The sudden appearance of a mitral regurgitation murmur in a patient with MI is a warning of impending heart failure. The disappearance of this murmur in a patient with severe systolic dysfunction suggests a worsening of the heart failure; the ventricle cannot pump enough to generate the turbulence necessary to make the sound of the murmur.

Tricuspid regurgitation develops in patients with right-sided heart failure alone or from left-sided heart failure for the same reasons as mitral regurgitation. This murmur is also a holosystolic murmur and is heard at the right sternal border. It may be increased with inspiration. When both mitral regurgitation and tricuspid regurgitation murmurs are present, it may be impossible to distinguish between them.

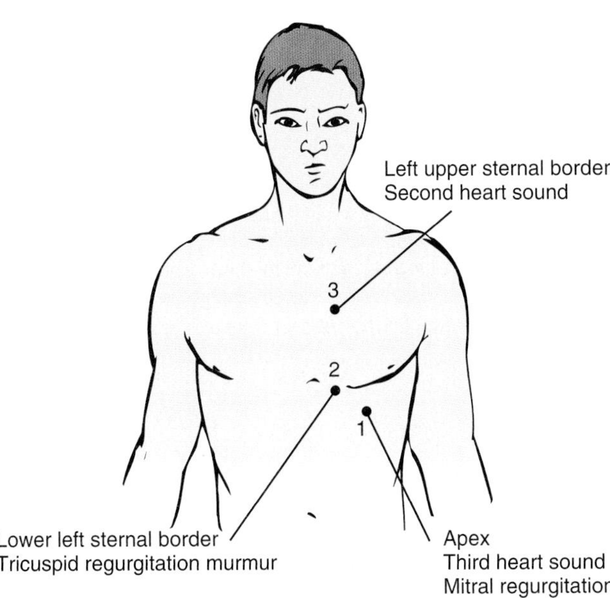

figure 20-1 Cardiac auscultation in the patient with heart failure.

ABDOMEN

It is necessary to palpate and percuss the abdomen to identify any ascites and the lower liver edge. High right atrial pressures that are translated into high venous pressures characterize right-sided heart failure, and the liver becomes a reservoir for the increased venous volume and increases in size (hepatomegaly) when congested. Once the liver becomes engorged, pressure increases in the portal vein and in the capillaries of the intestines. When the lymph system is no longer able to drain off sufficient fluid to relieve the pressure, ascites develops. Ascites is the transudation or third spacing of fluid and sometimes protein into the abdominal cavity. In the absence of hepatomegaly and ascites, a congested liver may conceal significant fluid. Eliciting hepatojugular reflux may identify this concealed fluid. To assess hepatojugular reflux, it is necessary to observe the internal jugular vein while pressing on the liver. When the height of the pulse increases or the vein engorges, hepatojugular reflux is positive.

EXTREMITIES

The lower extremities are inspected for the presence of edema. The edema associated with heart failure is bilateral, dependent, and pitting. Unilateral or nonpitting edema is not related specifically to heart failure, and other causes such as arterial insufficiency, myxedema, or lymphedema should be suspected.

In the ambulatory patient, the edema can be assessed by pressing the skin over the tibia. Pitting here is referred to as *pretibial edema*. The edema is usually graduated and worse in the ankles than at the calf, and is greater than at the thigh if the edema is present that high. In patients who are confined to bed, the edema is dependent posteriorly, and pretibial edema may be absent even in frank fluid overload. The patient must be assessed for pitting edema on the backs of the legs, the buttocks, and back. Occasionally, an ambulatory patient is so volume overloaded that presacral edema develops. To assess presacral edema and the presence of pitting, press the skin over the sacrum against the bone.

There are several schemes for describing the severity of pitting edema. None is superior to another; consistency is the most important factor. It is less important whether a series of pluses on a scale from 0 for no edema to 4+ for severe edema is based on the depth of the pit or the height of the edema on the lower extremity. When in doubt about the scale, a clear description of the depth of the pit and the level of the edema communicates the condition more effectively than a subjective number. A clear description allows for better continuity between clinicians and a better estimate of improvement.

Long-standing venous stasis and the consequent edema produces skin color and texture changes. The skin becomes leathery and discolored and may be hard to assess. These changes always indicate that the edema is chronic and not acute. Acute increases in the chronic edema may also be hard to assess. Pressing the skin firmly to the side of the tibia instead of directly over it may be of some help.

Laboratory Studies

Laboratory studies are used to rule out some reversible causes of systolic dysfunction and to monitor the effects of management strategies. On initial evaluation of a patient presenting with new-onset heart failure, a battery of baseline laboratory studies is ordered (Table 20-2).

In addition to the studies listed in Table 20-2, patients who take digoxin are monitored periodically to determine whether the dose should be adjusted. The initial digoxin level is drawn 2 weeks after initiation of the therapy and then as indicated by signs and symptoms or suspicion of toxic levels. Patients receiving anticoagulation therapy with warfarin are also monitored regularly, using the international normalized ratio (INR) to adjust the dose. Before the initiation of amiodarone, patients have thyroid function and liver function tests performed to obtain baseline values, along with pulmonary function tests. These tests are repeated at least yearly and if any complications occur.

Brain natriuretic peptide (BNP) is a naturally occurring substance secreted by the ventricles when overfilled. Because the BNP level is well correlated with left ventricular end-diastolic pressure and pulmonary capillary wedge pressure (PCWP), it makes an excellent marker of heart failure. Recent approval of laboratory assays for BNP and pro-BNP facilitate the use of BNP in the evaluation of patients with symptoms of heart failure. Patients with BNP levels greater than 80 pg/mL show evidence of elevated PCWP, confirming heart failure decompensation as the source of worsening symptoms.

Although the relationship between BNP level and heart failure is clear, the appropriate use of BNP levels in the management of heart failure is less clear. One important use of BNP levels has been proposed: to distinguish between pulmonary and heart failure–related causes of dyspnea in the emergency department.[10] Many patients have both heart failure and lung disease, and the existence of a test that clearly distinguishes between the two conditions as a cause of acute respiratory problems is a real advantage for individualizing and targeting treatment. In addition, BNP has been proposed as a marker for adequacy of treatment and for acute progression of heart failure, but the reliability of BNP for this use has not been established.[11]

Diagnostic Studies

Diagnostic studies are used to establish baseline values, identify potentially reversible etiologies, evaluate the effectiveness of treatment, and assess changes in condition. Several invasive and noninvasive tests are performed routinely when heart failure is suspected. Some tests are performed initially, when the symptoms of heart failure are first identified; some on a regular basis; and others only if indicated.

ELECTROCARDIOGRAPHY

The electrocardiogram (ECG) is used to assess rate and rhythm, and is also useful in diagnosing dysrhythmias, conduction defects, and MI. In addition, an ECG is often used to identify atrial enlargement and ventricular hypertrophy. However, in such cases an echocardiogram is more helpful because it can quantify these structural changes.

ECGs are useful in the identification of the atrial fibrillation and ventricular dysrhythmias common in patients

table 20-2 Laboratory Studies Used in the Baseline Evaluation of New-Onset Heart Failure

Laboratory Study	Significance	When Performed
Complete blood count	Used to identify any anemia or infection	Yearly if no specific indication With any exacerbation
Iron studies	Anemia workup Used to rule out hemochromatosis	As needed to evaluate any treatment for iron deficiency anemia
Thyroid function tests (thyroid-stimulating hormone [TSH] and free thyroxine [T_4])	To rule out hyperthyroidism or hypothyroidism as a cause of heart failure	No follow-up unless indicated before initiation of amiodarone
Electrolytes	Used to assess the effects of diuresis, in particular on potassium Hyponatremia is common	With changes in diuretic dose, aggressive diuresis, and titration of drugs that affect potassium (ACE inhibitors, angiotensin receptor blockers, spironolactone)
BUN and creatinine	Used to assess renal function; BUN:creatinine ratio distinguishes between prerenal azotemia and kidney disease	With increased edema or an exacerbation With titration of ACE inhibitors
Liver function tests, especially albumin, bilirubin, and alkaline phosphatase (AP)	Bilirubin and AP are often elevated in liver congestion caused by heart failure Low albumin makes peripheral edema more difficult to reduce	With any exacerbation Before initiation of lipid-lowering drugs or amiodarone
HIV	Used to rule out HIV/AIDS as etiologic factor	As indicated by history or change in status
Lipid panel	Used to assess risk of coronary artery disease and nutritional status	Yearly or more often as indicated to evaluate treatment

with heart failure. Sudden exacerbation of symptoms of heart failure often results from new-onset atrial fibrillation, especially when it is associated with a rapid ventricular response. An ECG can also distinguish frequent premature ventricular beats, which are common in acute and chronic heart failure. Episodes of asymptomatic NSVT often occur in patients who are monitored in ICUs, in telemetry units, or with Holter monitors. These asymptomatic dysrhythmias are usually not treated, and their prognostic importance is unclear. In contrast, symptomatic ventricular tachycardia, even if it is nonsustained, requires evaluation and usually results in placement of an implantable cardioverter–defibrillator.

Conduction defects are also common in patients with heart failure. A left bundle branch block is the most common conduction defect in patients with systolic dysfunction and may make interpretation of the ECG very difficult. New anterior ischemia or infarct may be impossible to identify because of this block. Bundle branch blocks and atrioventricular blocks require a 12-lead ECG for diagnosis.

ECGs are also useful in diagnosing ischemia, MI, and prior MI that may explain new-onset heart failure. For patients who do not present with typical chest pain (such as those with diabetes mellitus and women), the ECG may show a prior MI that was never diagnosed. New-onset heart failure may be the first indication of MI. An ECG is completed as part of the workup for new-onset heart failure and then repeated as necessary for any new symptoms that may reflect new ischemia or a rhythm change. In addition, ECGs are performed on inpatients who experience chest pain to rule out ischemia as the source of the pain.

ECHOCARDIOGRAPHY

Echocardiography uses the reflection of sound waves off cardiac structures to recreate a two-dimensional representation of the heart chambers, walls, valves, and large vessels such as the aorta, pulmonary artery, and vena cava. This technique provides information about both structure and function of the heart and is used to measure ejection fraction, evaluate valve structure and competence, and describe wall motion abnormalities. The addition of Doppler to the traditional echocardiogram allows for the evaluation of volume and direction of blood flow through the vessels and the heart. The reliability of echocardiography is greatly influenced by the competence of the echocardiographic technician and the cardiologist who interprets the echocardiograph. Echocardiography is of limited use in patients who are obese, have very large breasts, or have an increased anterior–posterior chest diameter and air trapping (e.g., patients with COPD).

Transesophageal echocardiography may be performed in addition to the transthoracic echocardiography previously described. The limitations of the transthoracic procedure can be remedied by the use of the transesophageal procedure; however, the risks are increased because the transponder must be passed down the esophagus, and conscious sedation is often required. The ability to assess the mitral valve and to identify transmural clots is greatly improved when transesophageal echocardiography is used.

RADIONUCLIDE VENTRICULOGRAPHY

A radionuclide ventriculogram or multigated acquisition (MUGA) scan is a precise means of calculating ejection fraction using a radioactive isotope. A MUGA scan is currently the gold standard for calculation of ejection fraction because it is not based on the subjective analysis of the person who "reads" it. A MUGA scan can describe abnormal wall motion, dilation, and wall thickness, in addition to ejection fraction. Valve function and flow direction cannot be evaluated by MUGA scan.

CHEST RADIOGRAPHY

Chest radiography is useful in screening the patient with shortness of breath or dyspnea on exertion. It allows the clinician to rule out infection or pneumonia, COPD, or a mass as the cause of the patient's symptoms. Chest radiography may also help identify pulmonary edema and chronic congestion. However, because changes in the patient's condition and fluid status may not be apparent on a chest radiograph for several days, this procedure is not helpful in evaluating therapy.

EXERCISE TESTING

When ischemia is suspected as the primary cause of the heart failure, stress testing may be used to confirm or rule out this diagnosis. When the body is physically stressed (i.e., when oxygen demand is increased, such as in exercise), heart rate and cardiac output increase. This increase requires an increased oxygen supply to the heart muscle. If the supply of oxygen is not sufficient, portions of the heart muscle become ischemic and function is decreased. For patients who can exercise, a treadmill or bike is used to provide stress, and function is measured by radioisotope uptake or echocardiography; areas of the heart that are inadequately perfused are indicated. For patients who are unable to exercise, pharmacological agents such as adenosine, dipyridamole, or dobutamine are used to simulate the increased demand for oxygen caused by exercise.

Exercise (or the pharmacological surrogate) combined with radionuclide scanning is more sensitive and specific for the diagnosis of stress-induced myocardial ischemia than exercise testing alone. With a stress thallium test, uptake of a radioactive isotope of thallium is measured with a gamma camera at the time of peak stress or symptom development. Areas of the heart that are underperfused either do not absorb the thallium or absorb it incompletely or more slowly than the well-perfused areas. In some cases, sestamibi is used instead of thallium, and a picture is taken 12 or 24 hours later to determine if more of the marker has been absorbed, suggesting that the heart muscle that appeared nonfunctional at first is still viable and would benefit from revascularization.

A stress echocardiogram may be used instead of a stress thallium test. Instead of the injection of an isotope such as thallium, the patient is stressed with exercise or pharmacological alternatives, and an echocardiogram is performed. The patient with ischemic myocardium may have changes in dilation, ejection fraction, or segmental wall motion that indicate that the dysfunction is related to inadequate perfusion.

In most cases, a positive stress test (i.e., one that shows stress-induced, reversible ischemia) leads to a cardiac catheterization. This procedure involves injecting radiopaque dye into the coronary arteries to evaluate the patency of the coronary arteries. Depending on the size, location, and number of lesions found in the coronary arteries, the patient undergoes balloon angioplasty and possibly receives a stent, or is referred for coronary artery bypass surgery. In many cases, correction of the perfusion abnormality completely reverses the heart failure and systolic dysfunction.

Cardiopulmonary exercise testing is used to determine if dyspnea on exertion is more related to cardiovascular causes (ventricular dysfunction), pulmonary causes (COPD, restrictive lung disease), or deconditioning. Such testing is performed when a precise measure of activity limitation is needed or when a patient is being evaluated for heart transplantation. The patient is exercised on a treadmill or exercise bicycle while a 12-lead ECG is obtained and blood pressure is measured in response to graded exercise. In addition, all the patient's expired gases are collected and carbon dioxide is measured. This allows for the measurement of oxygen consumption, cardiac index, and anaerobic threshold.

Hemodynamics

The basics of hemodynamic monitoring are discussed in Chapter 17. The application of hemodynamic monitoring in the assessment and management of acute heart failure and acute exacerbation of chronic heart failure is discussed here. It may be necessary to obtain more sensitive information about fluid status, cardiac function, and symptom causation to guide evaluation and therapy. For most patients with acute heart failure or acute exacerbation of chronic heart failure, the problem is obvious based on history and physical examination. The problem is a combination of decreased cardiac output and increased left ventricular end-diastolic pressure related to volume overload, added to poor contractility. Precise quantification of the low cardiac output or the estimation of left ventricular end-diastolic pressure by pulmonary artery wedge pressure does not change the basic assessments made on physical examination and does not affect management.

INDICATIONS FOR HEMODYNAMIC MONITORING

The decision to use aggressive diuresis or inotropes is not based on any specific numerical values for pulmonary artery wedge pressure or cardiac output. Pulmonary artery catheters are common in critical care units today, but they are expensive and not without risk. The potential benefit of more specific, guided management must be weighed against the risk associated with pulmonary artery catheter placement.

Three types of patients with heart failure have clear indications for hemodynamic monitoring in the management of their condition. In the first type, the patient has been empirically started on inotropes and intravenous (IV) diuretics but has not responded appropriately by diuresis and improved symptoms. The second type of patient has both COPD and heart failure. At times, only pulmonary artery pressure measurements can differentiate the source of the current decompensation. BNP testing may be as effective in this setting, however. The third type of patient continues to have peripheral edema or ascites and has renal function parameters indicating worsening prerenal azotemia and may benefit from a clearer definition of fluid balance. In this patient, it may be impossible to determine fluid status without the aid of a pulmonary artery catheter.

In summary, a pulmonary artery catheter is indicated in the following situations:

- The patient does not respond to empirical therapy for heart failure.
- Differentiation between pulmonary and cardiac causes of respiratory distress is necessary.
- Complex fluid status needs to be evaluated.

These categories are not mutually exclusive, and there is much overlap. They are discussed separately here, for clarity.

Inadequate Response to Empirical Therapy

Respiratory distress, volume overload, and renal insufficiency are common indicators of acute heart failure or acute exacerbation of chronic heart failure. Typically, the patient needs inotropic support and IV diuresis to resolve the problem. These therapies are usually started empirically and the patient's improvement monitored as a basis for titration of dose. In most patients, improvement follows rapidly, and after 2 to 3 days of therapy, the inotrope is gradually discontinued and the patient is restarted on oral therapy in preparation for discharge.

Cardiac Versus Pulmonary Cause of Symptoms

In the minority of patients who do not respond to empiric therapy, a pulmonary artery catheter may be helpful in identifying any additional factors that have contributed to the persistence of symptoms, especially cardiac and pulmonary causes. It may be particularly difficult to differentiate the cause of worsening dyspnea on exertion, orthopnea, and paroxysmal nocturnal dyspnea in patients with both pulmonary disease and known heart failure. In COPD and in exacerbations of heart failure, results of history and physical examination are often identical. Pulmonary artery pressures, pulmonary artery wedge pressure, and cardiac output or cardiac index can be very useful in distinguishing COPD from acute heart failure and therefore targeting therapy decisions based on the correct diagnosis. In patients with a predominantly pulmonary cause of their respiratory symptoms, pulmonary artery systolic and diastolic pressures are elevated, but pulmonary artery wedge pressure, cardiac output, and cardiac index are normal. In patients with a primarily cardiac cause, pulmonary artery systolic and diastolic pressures are also elevated, but the pulmonary artery wedge pressure is elevated and the cardiac output or cardiac index is decreased.

As with all pulmonary artery wedge pressure readings, the measurement should be recorded on a paper printout and read at end-expiration. Most patients with dilated cardiomyopathy have some degree of mitral regurgitation. Mitral regurgitation causes V waves on the waveform; the greater the mitral regurgitation, the higher the V waves. This makes it even more important to read the pulmonary artery wedge pressure from a tracing because most monitors average the highs and lows and return a falsely elevated pulmonary artery wedge pressure if the value is read from the digital readout of the monitoring system.

Patients with long-standing heart failure due to dilated cardiomyopathy also tend to have higher-than-normal pulmonary artery wedge pressure values even at baseline, and values of 18 to 22 mm Hg are not uncommon, even in patients who are euvolemic. Reducing their volume status to the point of normal wedge pressures usually results in a decrease in cardiac output and an increase in renal insufficiency because the higher pressures are necessary for ventricular filling. Readings of wedge pressure must be evaluated in conjunction with cardiac output and physical findings to determine the optimum pulmonary artery wedge pressure for any individual patient.

Fluid Status

Patients may respond initially to IV diuresis with or without inotropes and low-dose dopamine. After this initial diuresis, they begin to have a decreased urine output associated with increasing BUN and creatinine in the presence of persistent peripheral edema. They are frequently referred to as *intravascularly dry*.

The strategy for dealing with this problem is unclear. Insertion of a pulmonary artery catheter may determine whether high pulmonary artery pressures are the cause and whether those pulmonary artery pressures are elevated because of an elevated left ventricular end-diastolic pressure. The readings can then be evaluated in light of the patient's serum albumin and any comorbid diseases such as primary liver failure, sepsis, or vascular insufficiency.

Pulse Oximetry

Pulse oximetry is frequently monitored in patients with heart failure. Unfortunately, routine intermittent monitoring is of little value. At best, it gives irrelevant information, and at worst it enables a false sense of security over the patient's oxygen delivery status (Box 20-4). The results of pulse oximetry should be normal. Decreased estimates of oxygen saturation are usually not the result of heart failure unless the patient has severe pulmonary edema.

box 20-4
Pulse Oximetry

Pulse oximetry (Spo_2) estimates arterial oxygen saturation (Sao_2) or the percentage of hemoglobin (Hgb) saturated with oxygen. Oxygen saturation and hemoglobin are the two major components of arterial oxygen content (Cao_2). The dissolved oxygen in the arterial blood (Pao_2) contributes only a tiny portion of the arterial oxygen content. Arterial oxygen content multiplied by cardiac output (CO) equals tissue oxygen delivery (DO_2). If arterial oxygen content is decreased for any reason, cardiac output (mostly heart rate) increases to compensate. This is why patients with anemia or hypoxemia are tachycardic. As long as cardiac output can increase to compensate for a decreased Cao_2, tissues have sufficient oxygen to carry out their functions and the patient is asymptomatic. When a patient cannot increase cardiac output, as in heart failure, then even modest decreases in Cao_2 produce symptoms and increase the likelihood of an exacerbation or death.

$$(Sao_2 \times Hgb \times 1.34) + (Pao_2 \times 0.0031) = Cao_2$$

$$Cao_2 \times CO \times 10 = DO_2$$

Most nurses would be concerned about a patient with a pulse oximetry reading of 85%, but not one with 98%. The following examples demonstrate that the patient with normal hemoglobin and a pulse oximetry reading of 85% has more oxygen in the blood and a better oxygen delivery than a person with a 98% saturation and a hemoglobin of 10. The patients in all these examples have a normal cardiac output at rest but cannot increase cardiac output in response to decreasing arterial oxygen content.

A patient with normal blood gases and a 5-L cardiac output would have a calculated oxygen delivery of 1,000 mL O_2/minute:

$$(Sao_2 \times Hgb \times 1.34) + (Pao_2 \times 0.0031) = Cao_2$$

$$(0.98 \times 15 \times 1.34) + (90 \times 0.0031) = \\ 19.7 + 0.3 = 20 \text{ mL } O_2\text{/min}$$

$$Cao_2 \times CO \times 10 = DO_2$$

$$20 \text{ mL } O_2\text{/min} \times 5000 \text{ mL} \times 10 = 1000 \text{ mL } O_2\text{/min}$$

Suppose a patient has a low Sao_2 and normal hemoglobin:

$$(Sao_2 \times Hgb \times 1.34) + (Pao_2 \times 0.0031) = Cao_2$$

$$(0.85 \times 15 \times 1.34) + (60 \times 0.0031) = \\ 17.085 + 0.186 = 17.271 \text{mL } O_2\text{/min}$$

$$Cao_2 \times CO \times 10 = DO_2$$

$$17.271 \text{ mL } O_2\text{/min} \times 5{,}000 \text{ mL} \times 10 = 863.55 \text{ mL } O_2\text{/min}$$

Suppose a patient has a normal Sao_2 and low hemoglobin:

$$(Sao_2 \times Hgb \times 1.34) + (Pao_2 \times 0.0031) = Cao_2$$

$$(0.98 \times 10 \times 1.34) + (98 \times 0.0031) = \\ 13.132 + 0.3 = 13.44 \text{ mL } O_2\text{/min}$$

$$Cao_2 \times CO \times 10 = DO_2$$

$$13.44 \text{ mL } O_2\text{/min} \times 5{,}000 \text{ mL} \times 10 = 672 \text{ mL } O_2\text{/min}$$

Suppose a patient has low Sao_2 and low hemoglobin:

$$(Sao_2 \times Hgb \times 1.34) + (Pao_2 \times 0.0031) = Cao_2$$

$$(0.85 \times 10 \times 1.34) + (60 \times 0.0031) = \\ 11.39 + 0.186 = 11.58 \text{ mL } O_2\text{/min}$$

$$Cao_2 \times CO \times 10 = DO_2$$

$$11.58 \text{ mL } O_2\text{/min} \times 5{,}000 \text{ mL} \times 10 = 579 \text{ mL } O_2\text{/min}$$

A low pulse oximetry reading in patients with heart failure and no pulmonary edema suggests that pulmonary disease is complicating the heart failure. Hypoxemia rarely occurs in the absence of comorbid pulmonary disease. Even patients with Cheyne-Stokes respirations associated with an acute exacerbation may have oxygen saturations greater than 95%. The pulse oximetry reading is only half of the information needed to assess oxygenation accurately. The oxygen saturation is meaningless unless the hemoglobin level is known as well. Even normal arterial oxygen content in a patient with decreased cardiac output and no reserve may lead to tissue hypoxia. If the arterial oxygen content is decreased, as it is in patients with low hemoglobin (patients are rarely transfused unless the hemoglobin is less than 10 g/dL), the patient with heart failure may not be able to increase cardiac output enough to compensate.

Pulse oximetry may be of some value when used continuously in an ICU for patients with acute pulmonary edema. Particularly in patients with ischemic cardiomyopathy and MI, continuous monitoring may alert the nursing staff to impending ischemia or adverse effects of analgesia or conscious sedation.

MANAGEMENT OF CHRONIC HEART FAILURE

Heart failure is not a true disease, but rather a manifestation of disease. Management is based on the same therapeutic principles that apply to any disease. The cause of disease should be identified and then treated. If an etiologic factor cannot be identified or cannot be treated, then its manifestations should be treated. Often, the cause of heart failure is not identified, and even when it is, it may not be reversible. Reversible causes of heart failure have been discussed previously and are not addressed here. Isolated right-sided heart failure (cor pulmonale) also is not addressed here.

Heart failure due to diastolic dysfunction is a complex and poorly defined entity. Few studies of investigational medications or therapies have included patients with diastolic dysfunction, and consequently there is little in the way of evidence-based therapy. In general, treatment strategies are directed toward controlling blood pressure, fluid volume, and heart rate and rhythm. There is no consensus as to how this control should be established and maintained.

Chronic heart failure secondary to dilated cardiomyopathy and systolic dysfunction is better defined. This section discusses the current evidence-based guidelines for the management of chronic heart failure and acute exacerbation. Where appropriate, management of acute heart failure is distinguished from acute exacerbation; the use of IV inotropes, diuresis, and afterload reduction is similar in both conditions.

Pharmacological Treatment

The ACC and the AHA have published a consensus of evidence-based guidelines for the pharmacological management of heart failure[2] (Table 20-3). These guidelines present the most current recommendations based on available clinical trials for the medical management of heart failure. Heart failure in special patient populations has particular management implications (Boxes 20-5 and 20-6).

ANGIOTENSIN-CONVERTING ENZYME INHIBITORS

Angiotensin-converting enzyme (ACE) inhibitors are the mainstay of standard therapy for heart failure today; they represent one-third of the classic three-drug combination of drugs used. The Studies of Left Ventricular Dysfunction (SOLVD) and Cooperative North Scandinavian Enalapril Survival Study (CONSENSUS) trials demonstrated improvement in mortality as well as symptom management and exercise tolerance in even the sickest of patients with heart failure.[12,13] ACE inhibitors are typically started at low doses and titrated to target doses established in clinical trials. When studies showed that ACE inhibitors were being underprescribed for appropriate patients, the Assessment of Treatment with Lisinopril and Survival (ATLAS) trial found that being on the medication alone was not sufficient and that target doses used in the clinical trials were necessary to achieve the optimum results.[14]

ACE inhibitors work by blocking the renin–angiotensin–aldosterone system, resulting in vasodilation and antagonism of aldosterone and decreasing afterload and sodium reabsorption. Blockage of the long-term effects of myocardial cell exposure to the renin–angiotensin–aldosterone system is hypothesized to be the mechanism by which ACE inhibitors decrease mortality and limit the progression of remodeling.[15]

ACE inhibitors do have some side effects. Some patients are allergic to ACE inhibitors and experience angioedema, a potentially fatal reaction that involves edema of the mouth, pharynx, and larynx. There is no way to predict which patients will have this reaction, but when it presents, it is critical that the medication be stopped and a notation be made in the patient record so that it is not prescribed again. Patients should also be educated about the names of potential ACE inhibitors and why they should not be taken.

A troubling but not dangerous cough develops in some patients who take ACE inhibitors. Typically, after starting ACE inhibitors, patients may complain of a persistent, dry, nonproductive cough. The cough is not related to patient position or time of day, and it disappears when the ACE inhibitor is discontinued.

Hyperkalemia develops in some patients who take ACE inhibitors. Like the cough, the hyperkalemia resolves when the drug is discontinued. Serum potassium levels greater than 6.0 mEq/L are potentially dysrhythmogenic and should be treated with exchange resin. Patients with serum creatinine levels greater than 1.5 μg/dL are often denied ACE inhibitors in the mistaken belief that they will develop renal failure if they are given ACE inhibitors. In fact, patients with elevated creatinine levels are no more likely to develop an increased creatinine than patients with a normal creatinine when the ACE inhibitors were started.[16] The two types of patients most likely to show increased creatinine when started on ACE inhibitors are patients with renal artery stenosis and those with hypovolemia.

table 20-3 ■ Medications Used in the Treatment of Heart Failure

Agent	Action	Starting Dose	Target Dose	Indications, Contraindications, Adverse Effects
Chronic Heart Failure				
ACE inhibitors Lisinopril Enalapril Captopril	Block renin–angiotensin–aldosterone system, decrease symptoms and mortality Block conversion of angiotensin I to angiotensin II for afterload reduction	Lisinopril: 2.5–5 mg qd Enalapril: 2.5–5 mg bid Captopril: 6.25–12.5 tid	Lisinopril: 20–40 mg qd Enalapril: 10–20 mg bid Captopril: 50 mg tid	May cause angioedema, hyperkalemia, increased creatinine, symptomatic hypotension
Hydralazine	Pure vasodilator Used to decrease afterload	10–25 mg PO q6–8h	75 mg PO q6h or 100 mg PO q8h	May cause tachycardia Used for intolerance of ACE inhibitors, for additional blood pressure control, or for afterload reduction in severe mitral regurgitation or atrial insufficiency
Nitrates Isosorbide dinitrate Isosorbide mononitrate	Decrease preload, relieve angina, decrease orthopnea	Isosorbide dinitrate: 10 mg q6h (hold midnight dose) Isosorbide mononitrate: 30 mg qd	Isosorbide dinitrate: up to 40 mg q6h (hold midnight dose) Isosorbide mononitrate: up to 120 mg qd	Dose limited by symptoms such as headache or hypotension Use least dose that relieves symptoms
Digoxin	Oral inotrope Blocks neurohormonal bombardment of heart	0.125–0.25 mg PO qd	Same	Limited by renal excretion; smaller doses used when creatinine is >1.3 mg/dL Dose should be decreased in patients receiving amiodarone
Diuretics Furosemide Metolazone	Control fluid volume	Furosemide: 20–40 mg (in patient who has never been on diuretics) Metolazone: 2.5–5 mg qd	Up to 320 mg bid if necessary to control fluid Metolazone 10 mg qd if necessary in addition to furosemide	Diuretic dosage requirements are higher during aggressive diuresis than during maintenance Combination of furosemide and metolazone is very powerful, and loss of potassium, magnesium, and calcium can be dramatic, increasing risk of dysrhythmia
Spironolactone	Blocks effects of aldosterone and protects potassium	25 mg qd	25 mg qd	May cause hyperkalemia, so potassium should be monitored regularly May cause gynecomastia in men
Beta blockers Metoprolol SR Carvedilol Bisoprolol	Improve symptoms, increase exercise tolerance, decrease hospitalizations and mortality	Metoprolol SR: 12.5 mg qd Carvedilol: 3.125 mg bid Bisoprolol: 1.25 mg qd	Metoprolol SR: 100–200 mg qd Carvedilol: 25–50 mg bid Bisoprolol: 10 mg qd	May precipitate exacerbation during initiation and titration Monitor weight and heart rate carefully; do not stop drugs suddenly Benefit is long term and may not be evident for up to 3 months
Acute Heart Failure and Acute Exacerbation of Chronic Heart Failure				
Inodilators Dobutamine Milrinone	Increase contractility, decrease afterload and therefore increase cardiac output	Dobutamine: 2–5 μg/kg/min Milrinone: 0.2–0.3 μg/kg/min (with or without loading dose)	Dobutamine 5–15 μg/kg/min Milrinone: 0.375–0.7 μg/kg/min	Use smallest dose that produces desired hemodynamic effect May cause tachycardia and ventricular dysrhythmias Can be given effectively to patients who are receiving beta blockers

(continued)

table 20-3 ■ Medications Used in the Treatment of Heart Failure (Continued)

Agent	Action	Starting Dose	Target Dose	Indications, Contraindications, Adverse Effects
	Increased forward flow decreases left ventricular end-diastolic pressure			
Dopamine	Increases renal perfusion and improves diuresis	1–3 μg/kg/min	1–3 μg/kg/min	The higher the dose, the more likely dopamine is to increase afterload Do *not* give through a peripheral line
Nitroprusside	Used for afterload reduction and blood pressure control	0.5 μg/kg/min	Up to 1.5 μg/kg/min	High doses or prolonged administration is associated with increased cyanide levels and should be avoided
Nesiritide	Used for afterload reduction	2 μg/kg/min bolus with 0.01 μg/kg/min infusion	Increase by 0.005 μg/kg/min to maximum of 0.3 μg/kg/min	Use caution if systolic blood pressure <90 mm Hg
Hydralazine	Used for afterload reduction and blood pressure control	5–10 mg IV q4h PRN	5–10 mg IV q4h PRN	May cause tachycardia

Patients receiving ACE inhibitors also have decreased blood pressure. It is not uncommon to see asymptomatic systolic pressures of 80 to 99 mm Hg, and diastolic pressures may be 40 to 59 mm Hg. These low pressures are not symptomatic because perfusion of the brain and kidneys is not compromised as it might be in a patient with normal systolic function. The increased flow or stroke volume more than compensates for the decrease in resistance, and the tissues actually receive more blood and therefore oxygen than they would at a higher resistance and pressure. It is unnecessary to hold or decrease ACE inhibitors for *asymptomatic* hypotension.

For patients who truly cannot tolerate ACE inhibitors, other options are available. The use of hydralazine and nitrates preceded the studies on ACE inhibitors and has similar mortality benefits. Hydralazine must be taken three or four times a day, and many patients have trouble complying with a multidose medication regimen. Long-acting nitrates are used in conjunction with the hydralazine. Once-a-day preparations such as isosorbide mononitrate

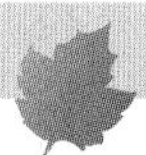

box 20-5

Heart Failure in Older Patients

Most patients with heart failure are elderly and many fit the category of "old old." They have a variety of limitations and comorbid diseases that may or may not relate to heart failure, as well as a remarkable resiliency and adaptability not found in younger patients. Therefore, it is critical to evaluate their limitations and strengths on an individual basis. It is important to treat the comorbid diseases aggressively according to patients' wishes and to include them in the planning and treatment decisions at all levels.

It is also critical to assess fall risk, activity level, visual acuity, manual dexterity, cognitive ability, and memory when administering, evaluating, or teaching about any medication. For some older patients, the assistance of a family member or friend is critical to successful medication adherence. Financial considerations are also important because many older patients are on Medicare and have no drug plan to pay for expensive medications. Having to choose between medication and food is no choice.

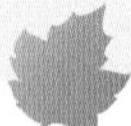

box 20-6

Heart Failure in Children

Most heart failure in children is related to congenital anomalies, and the management is different. Dilated cardiomyopathy in adolescents is often associated with viral infections, although it may be idiopathic. No assumptions can be made about heart failure in children from knowledge of heart failure in adults. With the increase in hypertension in children and adolescents, it is conceivable that more diastolic dysfunction may present. None of the clinical trials described in this chapter has included subjects younger than 18 years of age.

or a nitroglycerin patch may be used if compliance is a problem. Isosorbide dinitrate can be used if a rest period of at least 6 to 8 hours is taken.

Another option for patients who cannot take ACE inhibitors because of cough is an angiotensin II receptor blocker. Losartan, valsartan, and candesartan are currently being studied in the treatment of heart failure. Early results suggest that these agents are effective in patients who are not taking ACE inhibitors.

DIGOXIN

Cardiac glycosides have been used for centuries in the empirical management of heart failure. However, until recently, no objective evidence indicated that digitalis preparations made any actual difference in the management of heart failure. Beginning in 1993, the Prospective Randomized Study of Ventricular Failure and the Efficacy of Digoxin (PROVED) trial and, more recently, the Randomized Assessment of Digoxin on Inhibitors of Angiotensin-Converting Enzyme (RADIANCE) and Digitalis Investigation Group (DIG) trials[17] provided evidence that digoxin is of value in the treatment of heart failure. Although none of the studies has shown that digoxin affects mortality, they all have consistently shown that digoxin leads to improvement in symptom management and exercise tolerance as well as decreased hospitalizations for heart failure.

The benefit of digoxin has long been thought to be due to its inotropic effects. However, it is a very weak inotrope. The long-term benefit of digoxin may be in its proven blockade of neurohormones such as norepinephrine. As discussed previously, long-term exposure of the myocardium to catecholamines is hypothesized to cause progression of heart failure.

Digoxin should be given in daily doses of 0.125 mg. Lower doses are used in patients who have renal insufficiency or also take amiodarone. Digoxin is safe and has few, if any, adverse effects as long as the blood levels remain less than 2.0 ng/mL. No studies have identified a therapeutic level for digoxin in heart failure or guidelines for interpreting drug levels.[2] The traditional therapeutic levels given in studies of atrial fibrillation may be excessively high; lower levels (i.e., 1.0 ng/mL) may be equally beneficial and safer.

DIURETICS

Since furosemide became available in the 1960s, diuretics have become a mainstay of heart failure management. Edema, a common finding in patients with heart failure, is the result of volume expansion in response to neurohormonally mediated salt and water retention. In certain conditions (e.g., ascites, pleural effusions), "third spacing" of fluids is a common result of excess volume and increased hydrostatic pressure. Edema worsens when patients are unwilling or unable to reduce sodium in their diets. Patients who have advanced heart failure are frequently malnourished and may have low serum albumin levels with a consequent decrease in osmotic gradients to pull fluids back into the circulation. Patients who are symptomatic from volume overload feel dramatically better when they are diuresed to their dry weight. Drugs such as ACE inhibitors and beta blockers work best in euvolemic patients.

Loop diuretics such as furosemide are standard therapy for diuresis in patients with heart failure.[18] More expensive loop diuretics are available but have not been shown to be superior to furosemide. Loop diuretics are threshold drugs, and the threshold varies from patient to patient. This means that the appropriate dosage must be determined by the patient's response. In a patient who requires oral doses of 200 mg of furosemide to maintain dry weight, 100 mg twice daily is not sufficient. Doses in excess of 200 mg daily may be necessary. When patients are receiving oral doses of 240 mg or more, yet continue to have edema or increased edema, diuretic resistance must be considered. Loop diuretics should not be abandoned; however, a brief course of IV diuretic or the addition of a thiazide such as metolazone until the edema is controlled may be required.

The combination of loop and thiazide diuretics works more efficiently than either type of diuretic alone. However, this drug combination should be reserved for refractory edema, and when the edema resolves, an appropriate dose of loop diuretic should be determined and continued.

As heart failure progresses or when exacerbations occur, dose adjustments are necessary. Patients should be taught to weigh themselves daily and record their weights. Increases of 2 or more pounds overnight or 5 or more pounds in a week is water weight, which can be controlled with additional doses of diuretic (1 L [1.06 quarts] of water weighs 1 kg [2.2 lbs]). Some patients can manage their fluid balance with a sliding-scale diuretic, much like patients with diabetes mellitus manage their blood glucose with sliding-scale insulin.

SPIRONOLACTONE

Spironolactone is a weak diuretic with potassium-sparing properties. It is not used specifically for its diuretic activity. The Randomized Aldactone Evaluation Study (RALES) trial[19] studied mortality in patients with NYHA class III or IV heart failure who took spironolactone as well as ACE inhibitors, digoxin, and diuretics. The results were a 30% reduction in mortality in patients receiving only 25 mg per day of spironolactone. The reasons for the decreased mortality are unclear, but the hypothetical mechanism is that spironolactone blocks aldosterone and its damaging effects on heart muscle. Of theoretical concern is the addition of another potassium-sparing drug to the regimen of patients who are already taking an ACE inhibitor, which also spares potassium. However, few patients had serum potassium levels high enough to discontinue the spironolactone. Many of those patients tolerated every-other-day administration of spironolactone well, with excellent results.

BETA BLOCKERS

Intuitively, beta blockers, with their negative inotropic properties, ought to be the least likely intervention to benefit patients with systolic dysfunction. For many years, the prevailing standard of care specifically excluded beta blockers for patients with ineffective heart pumps. During the past 30 years, both small studies and large, multicenter, international, randomized, placebo-controlled studies challenged this idea. Meta-analysis of the smaller studies and primary analysis of the recent studies documented a 34% improvement in mortality in NYHA class II and III heart failure. Other long-term benefits of beta blockers include improved exercise tolerance, better symptom control, fewer hospitalizations, and improved ejection fraction.

Short-term use of beta blockers makes heart failure worse. Consequently, beta blockers should be used as a long-term strategy that is begun only when patients are stable using optimum background therapy with ACE inhibitors, digoxin, and diuretics. Beta blockers should not be started when a patient is in the midst of an exacerbation. The specific drug used should be started at a very small dose and gradually increased to the target range. The initiation and titration of beta blockers are beyond the scope of this text, but are outlined in detail elsewhere.[20]

Under no circumstances should beta blockers be stopped suddenly. The rebound tachycardia can be fatal, especially in patients with coronary insufficiency. Patients who come into the hospital because of an exacerbation of heart failure who are on beta blockers should continue taking the beta blocker. If a temporal relationship exists between titration of the beta blocker dose and the onset of the exacerbation, the dose should be reduced to the last well-tolerated dose. Patients who are taking beta blockers may receive inotropes without discontinuing the beta blocker and may respond well because of the upregulation of beta-adrenergic receptors.

CALCIUM CHANNEL BLOCKERS

First-generation calcium channel blockers such as diltiazem, verapamil, and nifedipine should be avoided in patients with systolic dysfunction. These drugs exert a strong negative inotropic effect without the long-term benefits of beta blockers. Second-generation calcium channel blockers such as amlodipine or felodipine have been used in patients with heart failure because they are vasodilators with minimal negative inotropic effects. They are most commonly used to control blood pressure in patients who are on target doses of ACE inhibitors but continue to have blood pressure levels that exceed the recommendations of the Seventh Report of the Joint National Committee on Detection, Evaluation and Treatment of High Blood Pressure (JNC-7).[21] (The JNC-7 recommends that blood pressure in patients with heart failure be less than 130/80 mm Hg.)

NITRATES

Nitrates are venodilators, and their primary effect is to decrease preload. As coronary vasodilators, they are used to treat angina. In very high doses, they may lower blood pressure, but they are not first-line drugs for the treatment of hypertension. When given to patients who are volume depleted or have right ventricular infarctions, nitrates may lead to abrupt hypotension, which is the result of inadequate preload to maintain stroke volume and cardiac output.

Nitrates are used in heart failure to help alleviate the symptoms of orthopnea and dyspnea on exertion.[22] Often, when patients lie down, the increased venous return (preload) leads to increased pulmonary artery pressure because the volume is too great for the weakened left ventricle. This sudden increase in preload and pulmonary artery pressure causes the sensation of dyspnea. Sitting up reduces the preload and relieves the symptoms. Nitrates decrease preload and mediate the volume of blood presented to the left ventricle, thus helping to control dyspnea. For this reason, nitrates may be used for patients who do not have angina specifically for the management of orthopnea and dyspnea on exertion.

insights into clinical research

Meghani S, Becker D: β-Blockers: A new therapy in congestive heart failure. Am J Crit Care 10(6):417–427, 2001

More than 2 million persons in the United States have heart failure. The authors of this study wished to analyze results of major studies to provide recommendations for the treatment of and education about the use of beta blockers in heart failure. MEDLINE and biomedical databases were searched for literature on the use of beta blockers in patients with heart failure. Randomized, controlled trials with reports of mortality and morbidity were reviewed. The evidence suggesting that beta blockers are an important adjunct to conventional therapy is overwhelming. However, beta blockers may have certain side effects in certain patients, particularly bronchospasm in patients with chronic obstructive pulmonary disease. Results of this study were consistent with a meta-analysis of 18 studies and strongly suggest that both cardioselective and nonselective beta blockers significantly reduce mortality and morbidity in patients with heart failure. Strong empirical evidence suggests adding beta blockers to the treatment of heart failure, and points to the need for future efforts toward establishing safe guidelines for the use of beta blockers in patients with NYHA Class IV heart failure with other comorbidities.

Nonpharmacological Treatment

ROLE OF THE PATIENT

Several strategies can be used to manage symptoms and prevent hospitalization of patients with heart failure.[23,24] The participation and commitment of the patient is necessary for success.

Sodium restriction is critical. Patients often believe that if they no longer use a salt shaker, they have eliminated all excess salt from their diet., and they may be surprised to learn that canned soup and canned vegetables are extremely high in salt. Education about the natural salt content of foods and the salt that is added as part of food processing is essential. Patients must be taught to read labels and shop for foods that provide optimum nutrition with minimal salt.

Alcohol use should be stopped. As noted previously, alcohol is a powerful cardiac depressant. Many patients have read that a glass of wine or drink each day decreases the risk of coronary artery disease. Although this may be true, the studies were performed in patients who did not have systolic dysfunction. It is important to clarify this fact and explain to the patient the adverse effects of alcohol.

Exercise should be encouraged. Patients with heart failure have limited stamina, and the goal is to increase stamina with low-level exercise over a longer period of time instead of intense exercise for short periods of time. Obviously, some patients with heart failure start at a higher level of functioning and have a better exercise tolerance than patients with advanced heart failure. Exercise for patients with heart failure is not the same as that for development of cardiovascular fitness, and heart rate is not a good indicator of exercise efficacy.

Patients with heart failure should be encouraged to maintain their level of activity. Walking is by far the best recommended exercise. Neither speed nor distance is important. Patients should aim for 15 to 20 minutes each day without stopping to rest or "catch their breath" at whatever pace they are able to manage. Some patients need to take many rests before they begin to exercise, and it may be quite a while before they can exercise for this length of time even at low levels. Weight-lifting is not recommended because this activity increases afterload and may worsen symptoms.

The most important thing patients can do to stay out of the hospital and control symptoms is to take their medication. The second most important activity is to take their weight every day. An overnight weight change of more than 3 pounds is due to water weight. If patients take and record their weight every day, modest fluid accumulations of 1 quart or less can be identified. Patients can be diuresed before they become so fluid overloaded that hospitalization for IV diuresis is necessary.

Fluid restrictions are punishing, and there is no evidence that water restriction has any value in the absence of significant hyponatremia. Likewise, there is no physiological basis for decreasing or controlling edema by fluid restriction, or any evidence that restricting fluids is effective.[25] The problem for patients with heart failure is the retention of sodium, which "holds on" to water. Restricting sodium does decrease or control edema, as discussed in the section on diuretics.

IMPLANTABLE CARDIOVERTER–DEFIBRILLATOR

In dilated cardiomyopathy, the incidence of sudden death from ventricular tachycardia or ventricular fibrillation is very high. Asymptomatic ventricular tachycardia is common, but its prognostic impact is unknown. For patients who have syncopal episodes or survive sudden death, an implantable cardioverter–defibrillator is usually indicated. An implantable cardioverter–defibrillator interrupts life-threatening dysrhythmias. If this device fires frequently or symptomatic NSVT occurs, amiodarone may be added to the regimen for rhythm control.

BIVENTRICULAR PACING

In a select group of patients with heart failure and intraventricular conduction delays (QRS duration > 130 milliseconds), biventricular pacing or cardiac resynchronization may improve cardiac output and therefore symptoms and exercise tolerance.[26] Pacing both ventricles of the spherically dilated heart reproduces the bottom-to-top contraction of a normal ventricle that is lost with myocardial remodeling and bundle branch block.

MANAGEMENT OF ACUTE EXACERBATIONS OF HEART FAILURE

Acute exacerbations of heart failure are an acute worsening of chronic heart failure and may occur for many reasons. Left ventricular function may deteriorate; heart failure is a progressive disease. If function deteriorates beyond the patient's ability to compensate, then symptoms worsen. Although heart function may be stable, the development of other problems such as pneumonia, anemia, dysrhythmia, hypertension, or trauma may tax the ability of the compromised heart to increase cardiac output to meet the increased metabolic demand. Dietary lapses, medication disruption, or lack of vigilance on the part of the patient regarding progressive water weight gain may all contribute to exacerbation. If possible, it is important to identify the cause of an exacerbation so that a long-term strategy to control the underlying problem can be implemented. However, in the intervening period, an acute exacerbation must be treated aggressively, often to save the life of a patient.

The main concerns for the care of patients with acute exacerbations of chronic heart failure are the same as in any patient with a life-threatening condition. They start with the basic priorities: airway, breathing, and circulation. Once these issues are addressed, etiologic factors and long-term strategies can become the focus of care.

Airway and Breathing

For most patients with acute symptoms of heart failure, airway patency is not a problem. Likewise, oxygenation is not usually compromised unless pulmonary edema is severe or a comorbid pulmonary disease is present. However, when the acute onset of heart failure or the acute exacerbation is accompanied by profound pulmonary edema, such as in MI or flash pulmonary edema, the airway may become compromised. With severe pulmonary edema, surfactant may be washed out of the alveoli, decreasing lung compliance and making ventilation difficult. In patients who also have COPD or restrictive lung disease, the compromise in compliance may make normal minute ventilation difficult if not impossible. An indication that normal minute ventilation is not being maintained is increased partial pressure of arterial carbon dioxide ($Pa{CO_2}$) associated with increased work of breathing and respiratory acidosis. For example, a patient may initially do well but tire as the increased work of ventilating wet lungs is prolonged.

INTUBATION

The usual indications for endotracheal intubation in patients with heart failure are the same as for patients in respiratory distress. Intubation and assisted ventilation are indicated if patients are unable to maintain oxygenation or ventilation. Patients who have pulmonary edema and a persistent oxygen saturation of less than 90% on 100% oxygen should be intubated and supported until they can obtain oxygen on their own. If the increased work of breathing is leading to fatigue of the respiratory muscles and the $PaCO_2$ is rising in association with a falling pH, intubation is indicated even if the patient is able to breathe unaided. The intubation may not be required for more than 12 to 24 hours, but it may be better to protect the airway than to try to intubate a patient after respiratory arrest.

DIURESIS

Once the airway is protected, attention is directed toward reducing the pulmonary edema. In most cases, aggressive IV diuresis is indicated. The presence of bilateral crackles on physical examination is not always an indication of total body volume excess. Evaluation of crackles along with peripheral edema, liver congestion or ascites, and renal function allows for a better assessment of fluid status than crackles alone. If the patient is determined to be volume overloaded, then IV diuretics facilitate the excretion of excess fluid rapidly and quickly make the patient feel better.

Aggressive diuresis usually starts with the patient's oral dose of loop diuretic in IV form. An adequate diuretic response is about 1 L of urine within 2 hours of the IV dose. If urine output is less than 1 L, the dose is doubled until a maximum dose is reached (for furosemide, a 400-mg single dose) or until the 1 L urine output goal is met. If the IV loop diuretic is not sufficient to produce this level of diuresis, a thiazide such as metolazone may be given orally along with the loop diuretic.[18] The desired weight loss is 1 to 2 kg per day until the patient's dry weight is reached. Initial weight loss may be greater. Careful monitoring of potassium and magnesium is indicated. If the creatinine begins to rise in response to the diuresis, then the ACE inhibitor should be held until after the diuresis is complete.

Circulation

Once the airway is protected and breathing is adequate to maintain oxygen and carbon dioxide levels, the circulation of blood to perfuse cells and supply oxygen for cellular function becomes the priority. Two indicators are used to determine the adequacy of perfusion. The first indicator is function of organ systems. Inadequate perfusion affects the brain, leading to confusion and change in level of consciousness; the kidneys, leading to increased BUN and creatinine; and the gastrointestinal system, leading to ileus and liver failure. The second indicator is metabolic acidosis. If perfusion is severely inadequate or prolonged past the capacity of the body to buffer the lactic acid produced, the level of sodium bicarbonate decreases, as does the pH, producing metabolic acidosis. Metabolic acidosis is a system-wide measure of inadequate oxygen to meet the metabolic demands of tissues.

Hypotension alone is not sufficient to diagnose hypoperfusion in patients with heart failure because many such patients are chronically hypotensive. Hypotension associated with hypoperfusion should be treated in a way that increases flow without increasing afterload. The problem is decreased cardiac output caused by decreased contractility. Whether the patient has acute heart failure associated with cardiogenic shock or acute exacerbation of chronic heart failure, the goal of treatment should be to increase cardiac output. Several interventions increase cardiac output.

The normal physiological response to decreased cardiac output is vasoconstriction and increased afterload. In patients with heart failure, afterload may be increased without a dramatic increase in blood pressure, and it is not safe to assume that a low blood pressure means a decreased afterload. Decreasing afterload increases stroke volume, and even in patients with low blood pressures, the increase in stroke volume and perfusion more than compensates for the low blood pressure.

OPTIMIZE HEMODYNAMICS

One way to increase cardiac output is to optimize preload. If a patient is dehydrated or fluid overloaded, contractility is compromised.

Decreased preload is usually related to iatrogenic overdiuresis. However, patients who are on stable doses of diuretics may become dehydrated if they become hyperglycemic or experience vomiting and diarrhea while continuing to take the prescribed diuretic dose. Careful fluid repletion usually corrects this problem and improves cardiac output. The symptomatic hypotension and increased BUN and creatinine that are the hallmarks of decreased preload should quickly return to baseline levels.

More commonly, increased preload is a problem; patients are total body volume–overloaded. The combination of fluid overload and decreased contractility leads to cardiopulmonary congestion with increased pulmonary artery pressures and overfilling of the heart. When the heart is overfilled, it becomes stiff and does not empty or fill well. The result is compromised stroke volume and sometimes localized ischemia. The ischemia further worsens contractility. Patients may present with classic angina even if they have no documented CAD. Diuresis with IV loop diuretics often restores the pressure–volume dynamics that optimize stroke volume. For patients who do not respond to diuresis, increasing contractility may decrease preload.

INCREASE CONTRACTILITY

To increase cardiac output, it is necessary to increase contractility and decrease afterload. Drugs that directly increase contractility are called *inotropes.* All inotropes increase myocardial oxygen consumption. To be useful in patients with heart failure, there must be greater improvement in oxygen delivery than in oxygen consumption. For this reason, inotropes such as epinephrine and isoproterenol are not used.

The following are indications for the use of inotropes:

- Low cardiac output and high PCWP, especially with symptomatic hypotension
- High PCWP with poor response to diuretics in volume-overloaded patients
- Severe right-sided heart failure that is the direct result of left ventricular failure
- Symptoms of heart failure at rest despite excellent maintenance therapy

Dopamine is also an excellent inotrope at mid-level doses. However, because dopamine is also a vasoconstrictor, especially at higher doses, it increases afterload in patients with heart failure and decreases stroke volume or, at the very least, does not increase it. Although there are no data to support its use, so-called "renal-dose dopamine" is used frequently in patients with heart failure.[27] The use of renal-dose dopamine is based on the knowledge that the effects of dopamine are dose related. At low doses of 1 to 3 μg/kg/minute, the main effect of dopamine is stimulation of dopaminergic receptors that dilate renal and splanchnic circulations. Higher doses have inotropic and vasoconstrictor activity. Low-dose dopamine may be used to increase BUN and creatinine in patients who are already taking inodilators or to increase creatinine in patients who respond poorly to diuretics. Even low-dose dopamine should not be used routinely.

Drugs called *inodilators* are used to stimulate beta-adrenergic receptors located in the heart and blood vessels to increase contractility and cause vasodilation.[27] The two inodilators most commonly used in ICUs are dobutamine and milrinone. Although these drugs have different pharmacological mechanisms, they both increase stimulation of beta-adrenergic receptors. Because they stimulate beta receptors, they are also chronotropic (i.e., they increase heart rate), and they must be used carefully and titrated slowly in patients with tachycardia or ventricular dysrhythmia.

The effect of inotropes and inodilators can be measured when a pulmonary artery catheter is in place. As the drugs are titrated to optimum doses, cardiac output increases, and the pulmonary artery wedge pressure decreases. Urine output should increase, and BUN and creatinine should return to baseline levels. Any organ function that was compromised because of inadequate perfusion should improve.

VASODILATION

Sometimes an inodilator alone is not sufficient to decrease afterload adequately. In patients with cardiogenic shock or patients who have an exacerbation related to hypertensive emergency, the afterload is the primary limiting factor. Decreasing and controlling the blood pressure or decreasing the workload of the damaged myocardium requires immediate treatment, and vasodilation with parenteral medications is necessary to maintain life or limit end-organ damage. Nitroprusside has the most rapid onset with the shortest half-life of any of these medications. It provides for rapid, efficient decrease in blood pressure, and the effect is limited to minutes if the medication is stopped because of an exaggerated response. Nitroprusside must be given as a continuous drip and requires reliable monitoring of blood pressure in a setting where emergency resuscitation is available.

Nesiritide, a BNP, has recently been approved as a vasodilator for treatment of acute decompensation of chronic heart failure.[28,29] It is unclear whether this vasodilator has any advantages over nitroprusside or nitroglycerin. Studies are underway to answer remaining questions about nesiritide, such as whether it is more effective than less expensive inodilators or more effective in patients with renal dysfunction.

For intermittent blood pressure control, hydralazine IV or orally provides vasodilation with a decrease in afterload, without any negative inotropic effects. Sublingual nifedipine should *never* be used to control blood pressure.[2] IV nitroglycerin is valuable in decreasing preload and in treating angina associated with hypertensive emergency, but is not a good afterload reducer or antihypertensive.

Intra-aortic balloon counterpulsation has proven very successful in reducing afterload in cardiogenic shock by augmenting perfusion pressure and decreasing the workload of the left ventricle. Intra-aortic balloon counterpulsation is often critical to survival in patients with acute MI who suffer acute left ventricular failure. Intra-aortic balloon counterpulsation is used for a limited time for support of the patient until a revascularization procedure can restore oxygenation and function or until the stunned myocardium has recovered somewhat (in a patient who cannot be revascularized). For a more detailed discussion of intra-aortic balloon counterpulsation, see Chapter 18.

HEART RATE

Heart rate and rhythm must be optimized for adequate cardiac output. If the heart rate is too slow, such as in sick sinus syndrome, second- or third-degree AV block, or sinus bradycardia, stroke volume cannot be increased adequately to compensate, resulting in an exacerbation. A heart rate that is too slow or too fast can compromise filling, and in patients with ischemia, can contribute directly to decreased contractility. A fast rate may be a compensation for a decreased stroke volume and usually responds to increasing stroke volume.

The administration of beta-adrenergic inotropes may improve heart rate along with the inotropic effect and greatly improve cardiac output. However, the reason for the bradycardia must be identified and treated if the improvement is to be sustained. In many cases, problems with bradycardia result from ischemic damage to the conduction system. In this situation, a permanent pacemaker resolves the problem. If the bradycardia is the result of active ongoing ischemia, a temporary pacemaker along with treatment of the ischemia is indicated. If the bradycardia is the result of medication, then the medication should be held or discontinued until the indication for the medication can be reevaluated. In this situation, beta blockers may be held for 24 to 36 hours but should not be discontinued suddenly. If the bradycardia is the result of beta blockers, then temporary pacing may be required while the drug is titrated down.

Sinus tachycardia is usually the result of decreased stroke volume and therefore cardiac output. Treatment of the tachycardia without increasing stroke volume leads to worsening end-organ perfusion. Sinus tachycardia usually resolves if the underlying decrease in stroke volume is corrected.

When the tachycardia is caused by atrial flutter or atrial fibrillation with rapid ventricular response, the heart rate is the cause of the problem, and it is necessary to control this directly. If the patient is unconscious secondary to the heart rhythm, direct-current countershock cardioversion is indicated. Otherwise, mechanical methods such as the Valsalva maneuver or carotid massage may be helpful. If medication is required to slow the rhythm, amiodarone is the least dangerous medication to use in systolic dysfunction. Calcium channel blockers such as verapamil and diltiazem are powerful negative inotropes and may aggravate the low–cardiac-output state. In many cases, the tachycardia is associated with ischemia or hypertensive crisis, and treatment of the underlying problem also treats the tachycardia.

box 20-7 *Examples of Nursing Diagnoses and Collaborative Problems for the Patient With Heart Failure*

- Decreased Cardiac Output related to altered preload
- Decreased Cardiac Output related to altered contractility
- Decreased Cardiac Output related to altered heart rate
- Decreased Activity Tolerance related to decreased cardiac output and deconditioning

Once the patient is stabilized and cardiac output has been supported by inodilators or vasodilators, any uncontrolled comorbid diseases that may have triggered or worsened the exacerbation must be treated. Anemia with a hemoglobin level of less than 10 g/dL should usually be treated with transfusion. Pneumonia or other infection should be diagnosed and treated with the appropriate antibiotics. Blood glucose should be controlled using insulin if necessary. Examples of nursing diagnoses for heart failure are shown in Box 20-7.

Discharge Planning and Patient Education

Many times, severe exacerbations requiring hospitalization can be avoided. If a weight gain of 2 to 3 pounds can be treated with intermittent extra doses of diuretic, then 15- and 20-pound weight gains that require hospitalization will not occur. Helping patients control both their heart failure and their comorbid diseases empowers them instead of victimizing them and gives them a sense of control that also helps to limit hospitalization. There have been many reports of improved quality of life, decreased hospitalizations, and decreased cost of care for patients in disease management programs.[30–32]

Home care provides many opportunities for disease management. As the home care nurse enters the patient's environment, the opportunities for teaching become evident. Even in situations in which the number of visits after a hospital stay is limited, such as with patients covered by Medicare, there are many opportunities for the home care nurse not only to assess but to intervene (Box 20-8).

Discharge planning begins with the first day of hospitalization. A program of education, referral, and follow-up is initiated with the goal of preventing further hospitalization. Patient teaching is necessary (Box 20-9). Clearly, patients must be on target levels of standard medications to reap the benefits of the clinical studies that have been done in heart failure. However, patients must work in collaboration with health care providers to maximize this benefit (Box 20-10).

box 20-8 *Heart Failure*

- Reinforce education about the disease process and lifestyle changes that best match the energy and activity tolerance of an individual patient.
- Teach patients to do daily weights and record them, observe them doing it, and ensure that patients understand their purpose and when to call a health care provider.
- Teach patients about salt restriction and go through kitchen cabinets with the patient to discuss food habits concretely.
- Watch patients prepare medications and formulate solutions for patients who have difficulty seeing or reading.
- Include family and significant others in teaching and demonstrations.
- Arrange for the administration of intravenous diuretics if indicated.

case study ■ CARDIOMYOPATHY AND HEART FAILURE

Mr. Frank is a 58-year-old man with known dilated cardiomyopathy and heart failure. He presents to his primary care provider complaining of not being able to sleep at night. Each time he lies down, he has to sit up immediately because he cannot breathe. Usually he sleeps on two pillows, but for the past week, he has had to sleep on four pillows, and he has awoken suddenly two or three times per night just to sit up and breathe. Last night he had to sit up in a recliner to breathe. Two weeks ago, he could walk four blocks without stopping to catch his breath, but now he becomes short of breath just walking from the chair to the bathroom. In light of these worsening symptoms, Mr. Frank's primary care provider has admitted him to the hospital.

In addition to the cardiomyopathy and chronic heart failure, he has hypertension, type 2 diabetes mellitus, and COPD. He has smoked one pack of cigarettes a day for 45 years, and he drinks one to two six-packs of beer each week. Once he was a carpenter's helper, but he has been unable to work for 2 years and is now on disability. The man's heart failure is clearly worse. He has severe orthopnea and has developed paroxysmal nocturnal dyspnea, which has accelerated over the last 24 hours until he must sleep sitting up. His exercise tolerance has decreased dramatically, and his symptoms indicate that he is now in NYHA class IV.

In spite of his COPD, the man has not stopped smoking. He is also continuing to use alcohol. It is not clear whether alcohol causes his cardiomyopathy or just contributes to it. It is difficult to determine whether his worsening symptoms are an exacerbation of COPD, an exacerbation of heart failure, or some combination.

Currently, he is taking lisinopril (20 mg/day PO), glyburide (5 mg/day), digoxin (0.25 mg/day PO), atorvastatin (10 mg/day), furosemide (80 mg/day PO), and spironolactone (25 mg/day PO). He also uses albuterol/ipratropium inhaled, 2 puffs three times daily and as needed for COPD bronchospasm. He is taking the target doses of these medications, although there is room for titration of some of them if indicated to better control his symptoms and prevent future hospitalization for heart failure exacerbation.

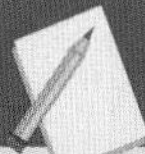

box 20-9
Living With Heart Failure

Medications

- Take all medications as instructed. If you cannot afford them, please let your provider know so that you can be put in touch with someone to help.
- Do not stop taking medication because you feel better. These are lifetime medications in most instances. Some of the medications will need to be adjusted over time, but your health care provider will discuss the changes with you.
- You may be taking several drugs. These medications do not interfere with each other, and they are given together so that they can work together to do more than any one or two of them can do alone.
- Do not let your medication supply run out because stopping some of them suddenly can cause serious problems.
- Take your medications about the same time every day.
- If you are going out for a few hours and will not have easy access to a bathroom when you need it, hold off on your diuretic until you return home. Do not skip a day's dose of diuretic because this could lead to serious water accumulations and worsening of your heart failure.

Diet

- Restrict your salt intake by removing the salt shaker from the table and the food preparation area. Do not add salt to any food you are cooking or any food on your plate.
- Avoid foods that have a high salt content naturally or because of the way they are preserved. Foods such as canned soup, canned vegetables, canned meats, foods frozen in sauces, cold cuts, sauerkraut, dill pickles, cheese, and processed foods of any kind are loaded with salt. Seasonings such as garlic and onion salt, Old Bay, and monosodium glutamate are the same as salt. Avoid salt substitutes because they are made with potassium; in combination with the medications you are taking, they can lead to potassium excesses. Avoid fast food such as hamburgers, french fries, fried chicken, and tacos.
- Seasonings such as pepper, Mrs. Dash, onion and garlic powder, herbs, seeds, and spices are acceptable.
- Fresh or frozen vegetables (frozen without sauces), fresh lean meats and poultry, and fish (not fried) are all good choices.

Daily Weights

- Weigh yourself every day at about the same time and record the value.
- The best time to weigh yourself is in the morning when you first get up and after you go to the bathroom.
- Weigh yourself without clothes if possible.
- Record your weight and the date in a daily diary. Bring this diary with you to the office when you visit your health care provider.
- Call if your weight goes up more than 2 lb overnight and does not go back to baseline the next day, or if you gain more than 3 lb in a week.

Activity

- Stay as active as possible.
- The stronger your skeletal muscles are, the easier it is for your heart.
- Do not use heart rate as a measure of adequacy of exercise effort.
- If you get tired or short of breath, stop and rest and then try again. The goal is 15 to 20 minutes of continuous activity each day.
- There are no speed or distance goals, and walking at whatever pace you can accomplish is a good choice. Homemaking and gardening are good choices as well. Choose an activity that you enjoy.
- Shortness of breath is uncomfortable but not dangerous. It is an indication that you are nearing the end of your exercise tolerance for this period, but once your breathing normalizes you can go again. If you stop before you get short of breath out of fear, you will not be able to increase your activity tolerance.
- If you have any questions about how much exercise you can tolerate, discuss it with your health care provider. That person is the best advisor for you because you are well known.
- Do not lift weights unless your health care provider has specifically said it is an acceptable activity for you.

Call Your Health Care Provider if:

- Your weight increases or decreases suddenly.
- You begin waking up at night short of breath and need to sit up to breathe.
- You start needing more pillows at night to breathe when you lay down or you are unable to lay down.
- You become short of breath at rest.
- You cannot walk up stairs that you used to climb regularly because now it makes you too short of breath or tired.
- Your feet and legs start to swell.
- You faint or feel as though you are going to faint.
- You become dizzy and weak when you stand.

At the time of admission, his vital signs were temperature 98.8°F (37.1°C); respirations 32 breaths/minute; heart rate 116 beats/minute; and blood pressure 92/44 mm Hg. The patient's weight is 195 lbs (usual weight, 180 lbs) and his height is 6′1″. His heart rate is high, and his blood pressure is low. He looks fluid overloaded and may have at least 15 pounds of excess water weight. Stroke volume is decreased, leading to an attempt by the heart to compensate by increasing heart rate. On physical examination, the patient is a thin, anxious-appearing, African-American man who is leaning forward on the overbed table. With the head of the bed elevated 45 degrees, jugular venous pressure at the earlobes with earlobe pulsation is seen. The patient's anterior–posterior diameter is increased. The patient is using accessory muscles to breathe, with clavicular and intercostal retractions. No crackles are heard, and wheezes are scattered. Activity or talking results in Cheyne-Stokes respirations. SpO_2 is 96% on 2 L

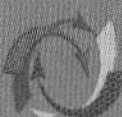

box 20-10 collaborative care guide *for the Patient With Acute Decompensation of Chronic Heart Failure*

OUTCOMES	INTERVENTIONS
Oxygenation/Ventilation	
There will be adequate oxygen to meet the metabolic demands of the tissue. Minimum arterial oxygen content evidenced by: 1. Hgb ≥10 g/dL 2. Spo_2 ≥90%	■ Consider the transfusion of RBCs if Hgb ≤9.0 g/dL. ■ Supplemental oxygen to maintain Spo_2 >90%. ■ Consider intubation and mechanical ventilation if patient develops respiratory acidosis or cannot maintain oxygen saturation on 100% oxygen by mask ■ Consider primary pulmonary problem as cause of hypoxemia and check brain natriuretic peptide (BNP) level.
The patient's symptom of dyspnea will be managed. 1. Patient denies dyspnea at rest 2. Patient reports increased activity before feeling sufficient dyspnea to limit activity 3. NYHA class equal to or better than baseline before decompensation	■ Elevate head of bed or allow patient to select upright position that best relieves dyspnea. ■ Apply damp washcloth to patient's face. ■ Use a fan or other means to create air movement across the patient's face. ■ Encourage the patient to ambulate as soon and as much as possible once dyspnea at rest is relieved.
Circulation/Perfusion	
Cardiac output will be maximized. Optimum cardiac output evidenced by: 1. Cardiac index >2.0 2. $S\bar{v}o_2$>50% 3. Urine output >30 mL/h 4. Baseline level of consciousness and orientation	■ Optimize preload with diuresis, fluid administration, or vasodilation with agent such as nitroglycerin, nitroprusside, or nesiritide. ■ Increase contractility with inotrope such as milrinone or dobutamine. ■ Decrease afterload with diuresis and vasodilation.
Hypotension will be asymptomatic and the patient's blood pressure is at baseline.	■ Determine the patient's baseline blood pressure; systolic pressure may be <90 mm Hg. ■ If blood pressure is less than baseline, assess for orthostatic decreases in blood pressure and increases in heart rate that would suggest dehydration. ■ Continue to give ACE inhibitors and other afterload reducers if hypotension is asymptomatic. ■ If patient is symptomatic on standing keep on bed rest until orthostasis resolves. ■ If patient is orthostatic, symptomatic, and BUN and creatinine levels are elevated, hold diuretics and consider giving IV normal saline.
Fluids/Electrolytes	
Euvolemia will be achieved. Euvolemia evidenced by: 1. Absence of peripheral edema 2. Absence of ascites 3. Documented dry weight 4. Baseline BUN and creatinine 5. Moist mucous membranes	■ Administer loop diuretic sufficient to produce 1 L of urine output within 2 hours of administration. ■ Obtain daily weights. ■ Strive for a weight loss of 1–2 kg/day until dry weight is achieved. ■ Monitor electrolytes at least daily. ■ Replenish potassium, magnesium, and calcium as needed. ■ Measure serum albumin. ■ If inadequate response to loop diuretics add metolazone or inotropes as above ■ Report new or worsened rales to physician.

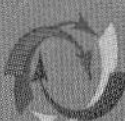

box 20-10 collaborative care guide *for the Patient With Acute Decompensation of Chronic Heart Failure (Continued)*

OUTCOMES	INTERVENTIONS
Teaching/Discharge Planning	
Rehospitalization will be prevented.	■ Assess the patient's understanding of medication regimen. ■ Assess the patient's reading ability before giving written instructions. ■ Include a family member in the discussions if the patient has trouble reading, seeing, or remembering. ■ Consider a means of preparing medications so that the patient has to open only one container each day. ■ Teach the patient the importance of daily weights to follow fluid balance. ■ Have the patient weigh himself each day and record. Call physician if weight is 3–5 lbs over baseline. ■ Have the patient or family member repeat early signs and symptoms of worsening heart failure and when to call physician for them. ■ Teach the patient about foods that have a high sodium content. ■ Encourage the patient to abstain from alcohol. ■ Encourage the patient to walk and stay as active as possible. ■ Consider case management referral or social work referral if the patient has multiple admissions or problems obtaining medications.

by nasal cannula. Right ventricular pulsation is visible and palpable. The heart rhythm is regular with occasional ectopy. There is a summation gallop. A II/VI mitral regurgitation murmur is best heard at the apex, and a II/VI tricuspid regurgitation murmur increases with inspiration. The abdomen is distended, firm, and nontender. It is flat to percussion, and the liver edge is not palpable. The liver span is 10 cm, and it extends 5 cm below the costal margin. There is a positive hepatojugular reflex. The knees show 2+ edema bilaterally.

All aspects of the examination indicate an excess of total body fluid volume. The absence of crackles indicates chronicity of the elevated pulmonary artery pressures. The liver is not enlarged, suggesting that it has been pushed down by a flattened diaphragm. The Cheyne-Stokes respiratory pattern is associated with NYHA class IV heart failure.

Laboratory results are as follows: sodium 120 mEq/L; potassium 3.6 mEq/L; chloride 102 mEq/L; serum carbon dioxide 25 mEq/L; BUN 65 mg/dL; creatinine 2.4 mg/dL; glucose 450 mg/dL; white blood cell count (WBC) 8.2 cells/mm^3; hemoglobin 8.4 g/dL; hematocrit 25.5%; platelets 224 cells/mm^3; alkaline phosphatase 385 IU/L; total bilirubin 2.3 µg/dL; and albumin 2.9 g/dL. The sodium level is quite low; this is not uncommon in patents with severe heart failure. It reflects an excess of water rather than a loss of sodium. This may be related to excess secretion of antidiuretic hormone (ADH). Unlike trauma or surgery patients who acutely develop hyponatremia and life-threatening seizures, hyponatremia in patients with heart failure is often chronic and does not cause acute seizures. Treatment of the exacerbation usually resolves the hyponatremia. The BUN and creatinine are both elevated, with a BUN:creatinine ratio greater than 20. This reflects a low cardiac output as the source of renal hypoperfusion. Improving cardiac output and therefore renal perfusion corrects renal hypoperfusion and returns the BUN:creatinine ratio to normal. The BUN:creatinine ratio does not reflect dehydration as it might in a surgical, trauma, or elderly nursing home patient and should not be treated with IV normal saline. The glucose level is very high, reflecting the physiological stress that the patient is under. The hemoglobin and hematocrit reflect a severe anemia that could have potentially brought on this exacerbation. The alkaline phosphatase and total bilirubin are both elevated, reflecting the liver congestion noted in the physical examination. The hypoalbuminemia makes diuresis more difficult because it reduces osmotic pressure and makes reabsorption of interstitial and third space fluids more difficult.

Echocardiography results are as follows:

From 1 year ago: left ventricle dilated with mild concentric hypertrophy and global hypokinesis; ejection fraction 30%; valves structurally normal; mild mitral regurgitation and moderate tricuspid regurgitation; estimated pulmonary artery systolic pressure 40 to 45 mm Hg. From 1 month ago: left ventricle dilated without hypertrophy and global hypokinesis; ejection fraction 25%; valves structurally normal; moderate to severe mitral regurgitation and severe tricuspid regurgitation; estimated pulmonary artery systolic pressure 65 to 70 mm Hg.

The echocardiogram from 1 month ago shows deterioration in left ventricular function associated with worsened dilation, decreased ejection fraction, and worsened valve regurgitation. Pulmonary artery pressures are increased as well and may reflect the worsened left ventricular function or structural changes secondary to COPD.

The following conclusions can be drawn from the data presented. The patient has acute exacerbation of chronic heart failure with worsening left ventricular systolic dysfunction characterized by worsening orthopnea and dyspnea on exertion and multiple episodes of paroxysmal nocturnal dyspnea. He has right-sided heart failure characterized by jugular venous distension, liver congestion, and ascites. He has severe volume overload, hyponatremia, hyperglycemia, and prerenal azotemia, as well as severe anemia of unknown etiology. Increased anterior–posterior diameter and flattening of the diaphragm, which pushes the liver down into the abdomen, are the result of COPD.

The etiology of the patient's exacerbation is not clear, but several possibilities are suggested by the data. More than one may be contributing to the decline. Alcohol is a powerful myocardial depressant and continued alcohol intake promotes the progression of left ventricular dysfunction, so worsening heart failure may be a factor. The anemia (hemoglobin 8.5 g/dL) alone could have precipitated the exacerbation. The volume excess may be the etiology or the result of worsening function, as could the worsening renal function.

The following treatment plan was implemented, with the goal of effecting an improvement to baseline:

1. Diuresis with an IV loop diuretic with a goal of 1 to 2 kg/day weight loss until the patient is at his dry weight
2. Inotropic support to improve cardiac output and renal perfusion, and to facilitate diuresis
3. Insulin drip to manage hyperglycemia
4. Anemia workup to include iron, total iron-binding capacity, ferritin, and vitamin B_{12} levels with a peripheral smear; consider transfusing with packed red blood cells
5. Counseling and referral for smoking cessation and alcohol abuse
6. Nutrition counseling for better food choices
7. Case management to increase access to services for patient and family, and for continuity of care

After 4 days of inotropic support and aggressive diuresis, the patient was euvolemic at 185 lbs and able to breathe comfortably with his head elevated on two pillows. His BUN level was 48 mg/dL and his creatinine level was 1.9 mg/dL (his baseline values). The patient's anemia was diagnosed as macrocytic, and he was started on vitamin B_{12} and folic acid supplements. The patient was enrolled in a medical assistance program that will cover his medications and 10 visits for home nursing follow-up. He and his wife were counseled by the dietitian, and the patient has agreed to attend Alcoholics Anonymous meetings. He is unwilling to give up his cigarettes at this time. The patient was discharged with a follow-up appointment at a heart failure clinic. ■

clinical applicability challenges

Self-Challenge: Critical Thinking

Refer to the case study at the end of this chapter and answer the following questions regarding Mr. Frank:

1. *Does this patient need to be intubated?*
2. *Does this patient need a pulmonary artery catheter?*
3. *What medications do you anticipate will be ordered for this patient?*
4. *What nursing diagnoses apply to this patient?*
5. *Does this patient need an intra-aortic balloon pump?*
6. *Is his oxygen transport adequate? What, if anything, should be done to support him?*

Study Questions

1. *Which of the following phrases best defines heart failure?*
   a. *Decreased ejection fraction secondary to myocardial infarction*
   b. *Shortness of breath and decreased activity tolerance related to impaired filling or emptying of the heart*
   c. *Shortness of breath and liver congestion associated with high pulmonary pressures*
   d. *Dilated cardiomyopathy*
2. *Which of the following phrases best describes the overall goal in the treatment of heart failure?*
   a. *Restore normal ventricular function.*
   b. *Improve aerobic fitness.*
   c. *Attain overall fluid management, leading to euvolemia.*
   d. *Maximize symptom control.*
3. *The administration of dobutamine to a patient with acute exacerbation of chronic heart failure is likely to produce what result?*
   a. *Decreased cardiac output, decreased pulmonary capillary wedge pressure, decreased afterload*
   b. *Increased cardiac output, decreased pulmonary capillary wedge pressure, decreased afterload*
   c. *Increased cardiac output, increased pulmonary capillary wedge pressure, decreased afterload*
   d. *Decreased cardiac output, increased pulmonary capillary wedge pressure, increased afterload*
4. *Which of the following medications can be used to treat orthopnea in patients with heart failure?*
   a. *Nitroglycerin*
   b. *Angiotensin-converting enzyme (ACE) inhibitors*
   c. *Digoxin*
   d. *Verapamil*
5. *Which of the following combinations of laboratory studies are used to monitor for side effects of angiotensin-converting enzyme (ACE) inhibitors?*
   a. *Blood urea nitrogen (BUN), creatinine, potassium*
   b. *Sodium, potassium, calcium*
   c. *Hemoglobin, sodium, creatinine*
   d. *Magnesium, BUN, chloride*

REFERENCES

1. American Heart Association: 2000 Heart and Stroke Statistical Update. Dallas, American Heart Association, 1999
2. Hunt SA, Baker DW, Chin MH, et al: ACC/AHA Guidelines for the Evaluation and Management of Chronic Heart Failure in the Adult: A Report of the American College of Cardiology/American Heart Association Task Force on Practice Guidelines (Committee to Revise the 1995 Guidelines for the Evaluation and Management of Heart Failure), 2001. Available at: http://www.acc.org/clinical/guide lines/failure/hf_index.htm
3. New York Heart Association: Diseases of the Heart and Blood Vessels: Nomenclature and Criteria for Diagnosis (6th Ed). Boston, Little, Brown and Company, 1964
4. Opie LH: Mechanisms of cardiac contraction and relaxation. In Braunwald E, Zipes D, Libby P (eds): Heart Disease: A Textbook of Cardiovascular Medicine (6th Ed). New York, WB Saunders, 2001
5. Packer M: Evolution of the neurohormonal hypothesis to explain the progression of chronic heart failure. Eur Heart J 16(Suppl f):4–6, 1995
6. Piano MR, Kim SD, Jarvis C: Cellular events linked to cardiac remodeling in heart failure: Targets for pharmacologic intervention. J Cardiovasc Nurs 14(4):1–23, 2000
7. Tuinenburg AE, Van Gelder IC, Van Der Berg MP, et al: Lack of prevention of heart failure by serial electrical cardioversion in patients with persistent atrial fibrillation. Heart 82(4):486–493, 1999
8. Ryder KM, Benjamin EJ: Epidemiology and significance of atrial fibrillation. Am J Cardiol 84(9A):131R–138R, 1999
9. Audrey H, Wu MD, Sunil KD: Sudden death in dilated cardiomyopathy. Clin Cardiol 22:267–272, 1999
10. Maisel A: B-type natriuretic peptide levels: A potential "white count" for congestive heart failure. J Card Fail 7:183–193, 2001
11. Troughton RW, Frampton CM, Yandle TG, et al: Treatment of heart failure guided by plasma aminoterminal brain natriuretic peptide (N-BNP) concentrations. Lancet 355:1126–1130, 2000
12. Garg R, Yusuf S: Overview of randomized trials of angiotensin-converting enzyme inhibitors on mortality and morbidity inpatients with heart failure. Collaborative Group on ACE Inhibitor Trials. JAMA 273(18):1450–1456, 1995
13. Milfred-LaForest SK: Pharmacotherapy of systolic heart failure: A review of recent literature and practical applications. J Cardiovasc Nurs 14(4):57–75, 2000
14. Nicklas JM, Cohn JN, Pitt B: What does ATLAS really tell us about "high" dose angiotensin-converting enzyme inhibition in heart failure? J Card Fail 6(2):165–168, 2000
15. Francis G: Neurohormonal activation and progression of heart failure: Hypothetical and clinical considerations. J Cardiovasc Pharmacol 32(Suppl 1):S16–S21, 1998
16. Gottlieb SS, Robinson S, Weir MR, et al: Determinants of the renal response to ACE inhibition in patients with congestive heart failure. Am Heart J 124:131–136, 1992
17. The Digitalis Investigation Group: The effect of digoxin on mortality and morbidity in patients with heart failure. N Engl J Med 336(8):525–533, 1977
18. Cody RJ, Pickworth KK: Approaches to diuretic therapy and electrolyte imbalance in congestive heart failure. Cardiol Clin 12(1): 37–50, 1994
19. Pitt B, Zannad F, Remme WJ, et al, for the Randomized Aldactone Evaluation Study Investigators: The effect of spironolactone on morbidity and mortality inpatients with severe heart failure. N Engl J Med 341(10):709–717, 1999
20. Branum K: Using beta-blockers in the treatment of heart failure. Nurse Practitioner 24(7):75–83, 1999
21. Chobanian AV, Bakris GL, Black HR, et al: National High Blood Pressure Education Coordinating Committee: The seventh report of the joint national committee for prevention, detection, evaluation, and treatment of high blood pressure. The JNC-7 report. JAMA 289(19):2560–2571, 2003
22. Elkayam U: Nitrates in heart failure. Cardiol Clin 12(1):73–85, 1994
23. Krumholz HM, Butler J, Miller J, et al: Prognostic importance of emotional support for elderly patients hospitalized with heart failure. Circulation 97(10):958–964, 1998
24. Carlson B, Riegel B, Moser DK: Self care abilities of patients with heart failure. Heart Lung 30(5):351–359, 2001
25. Chaney WE, Blaum CS, Bleshe BE, et al: Guidelines for the management of heart failure caused by systolic dysfunction: Part II. Am Fam Physician 64(6):1045–1054, 2001
26. Nelson GS, Berger RD, Fetics BJ: Left ventricular or biventricular pacing improves cardiac function at diminished energy cost inpatients with dilated cardiomyopathy and left bundle-branch block. Circulation 102:3053–3059, 2000
27. Taneja T, Johnson MR, Gheorghiade M: Current status of acute intravenous therapy for chronic heart failure exacerbations. Heart Fail 5:199–207, 215, 1999
28. Colucci WS, Elkayam U, Horton DP, et al: Intravenous nesiritide, a natriuretic peptide, in the treatment of decompensated congestive heart failure. N Engl J Med 343(4):246–253, 2000
29. Kayser SR: The use of nesiritide in the management of acute decompensated heart failure. Prog Cardiovasc Nurs 17(2):89–95, 2002
30. Rich MW: Heart failure disease management: A critical review. J Card Fail 5(1):64–75, 1999
31. Atkinson RC, Branum K: Home-based disease management in congestive heart failure. Home Health Care Manage Pract 13(2): 106–113, 2001
32. Stewart S, Horowitz JD: Home-based intervention in congestive heart failure: Long-term implications on readmission and survival. Circulation 105:2861–2866, 2002

OTHER SELECTED READING

Futterman LG, Lemberg L: Heart failure: Update on treatment and prognosis. Am J Crit Care 10(6):285–293, 2001

Hou N, Chui M, Eckert G, et al: Relationship of age and sex to health-related quality of life in patients with heart failure. Am J Crit Care 13(2):153–161, 2004

MacKlin M: Managing heart failure: A case study approach. Crit Care Nurse 21(2):36, 2001

Meghani SH, Becker D: β-Blockers: A new therapy in congestive heart failure. Am J Crit Care 10(6):417–429, 2001

Paul S: Impact of a nurse-managed heart failure clinic: A pilot study. Am J Crit Care 9(6):140–146, 2000

Riegel B, Bennett JA, Davis A, et al: Cognitive impairment in heart failure: Issues of measurement and etiology. Am J Crit Care 11(6): 520–528, 2002

Rodgers JM, Reeder SJ: Current therapies in the management of systolic and diastolic dysfunction. Dimens Crit Care Nurs 20(6):2–10, 2001

Sneed NV, Paul SC: Readiness for behavioral change in patients with heart failure. Am J Crit Care 12(6):444–453, 2003

Stanley M, Prasun M: Heart failure in older adults: Keys to successful management. AACN Clin Issues 13(1):94–102, 2002

chapter 21

Acute Myocardial Infarction

PATRICIA GONCE MORTON

objectives

Based on the content in this chapter, the reader should be able to:

- Explain the pathophysiology and risk factors for atherosclerosis.
- Describe the classification, assessment, and management of patients with angina pectoris.
- Compare and contrast the pathophysiological principles and assessment findings of a patient with angina pectoris versus a patient with a myocardial infarction.
- Discuss the diagnostic tests used for a patient with a myocardial infarction.
- Summarize principles of patient management in the early phase, intensive care phase, and intermediate care phase of management.
- Describe the complications for a patient with a myocardial infarction.
- Explain the principles of cardiac rehabilitation and patient education.

About 64.5 million Americans have one or more types of cardiovascular disease. Although death rates from cardiovascular disease have declined by 9.2% between 1991 and 2001, cardiovascular disease remains the number one killer and accounts for 38.5% of all deaths in the United States. Approximately 2,600 Americans die each day from cardiovascular disease, which represents an average of 1 death every 34 seconds. More Americans die from cardiovascular disease each year than the next five leading causes of death combined. Of those who died from cardiovascular disease, the majority (54%) died as a result of coronary heart disease (myocardial infarction [MI] and angina pectoris).[1]

Coronary heart disease is the single largest killer of American men and women. About every 26 seconds, an American will have a coronary event, and about every minute, a person will die from one. The death rate from coronary heart disease for black men (262 per 100,000) exceeds that of white men (228.4 per 100,000), and the death rate for black women (176.7 per 100,000) exceeds that of white women (137.4 per 100,000). About 84% of people who die from coronary heart disease are 65 years of age and older. Coronary heart disease is the leading cause of premature, permanent disability in the United States labor force. In 2004, the estimated direct and indirect cost of coronary heart disease was $133.2 billion.[1]

Approximately 565,000 Americans have a new MI each year and about 300,000 have a recurrent MI annually. The average age at the time of the first MI is 65.8 years for men and 70.4 years for women. About 25% of men and 38% of women will die within 1 year of having an initial MI. Women are more likely to die because they have their initial MI at an older age than men. Of those who survive their initial MI, 18% of men and 35% of women will have another MI within 6 years. About half of men and women younger than the age of 65 years who have a MI die within 8 years.[1]

As overwhelming as the mortality and morbidity statistics appear, much progress has been made in the prevention, diagnosis, and management of cardiovascular disease. As a result, the death rates from cardiovascular disease declined 16.5% from 1990 to 2000. During that same decade, the death rate from coronary heart disease declined 24.8%.[1]

Since the Framingham Study of risk factors in 1951 and the development of coronary care units in the 1960s, the critical care nurse has played a major role in helping to reduce the mortality associated with heart disease. The critical care nurse uses advanced assessment skills, rapid decision making, and therapeutic interventions to treat the patient in the acute phase of cardiovascular disease. Patient education and psychological support provided by the nurse have enabled patients and their families to return home and maximize their health status.

ATHEROSCLEROSIS

Atherosclerosis is a major cause of cardiovascular disease. The term *atherosclerosis* comes from the Greek words *athere*, meaning "gruel" or "paste," and *sclerosis*, meaning "hardness."

Pathophysiological Principles

Atherosclerosis is a complex, insidious process, beginning long before symptoms occur. Although the process is not completely understood, scientific evidence suggests that it begins when the inner, protective layer of the artery (endothelium) is damaged. Three known causes of the damage include elevated levels of cholesterol and triglycerides in the blood, hypertension, and cigarette smoking.[2]

Gradually, as fatty substances, cholesterol, cellular waste products, calcium, and fibrin pass through the vessel, they are deposited in the inner lining of an artery. As a result of the deposition of these materials, a lipid plaque with a fibrous covering, also known as an *atheroma*, builds up, and blood flow in the artery becomes partially or completely blocked.

The injury to the vessel and the resulting accumulation of these substances in the inner lining of the artery cause white blood cells, smooth muscle cells, and platelets to aggregate at the site. As a result, a matrix of collagen and elastic fibers form, and the endothelium becomes much thicker. The core of the fibrous plaque can become necrotic, and hemorrhage and calcification may result. A thrombosis may also occur, thus contributing even more to the blockage of the vessel lumen (Fig. 21-1). These fibrous plaques are most often found in the coronary, popliteal, and internal carotid arteries and in the abdominal aorta.

Because of the fibrous plaque, the amount of blood flow through the artery is reduced, resulting in decreased supply of oxygen to tissues. Symptoms often do not occur, however, until 75% or more of the blood supply to the area is occluded. The occurrence of symptoms may depend to an extent on the development of collateral circulation. Collateral vessels are small arteries that connect two larger arteries or different segments of the same artery. Under normal conditions, these collateral arteries carry very little of the blood flow. As the larger artery gradually occludes, pressure builds on the proximal side of the occlusion. As a result, flow is redirected through the collateral vessels, which enlarge and dilate over time (Fig. 21-2). Blood is then allowed to flow around an area of blockage through these alternate routes.

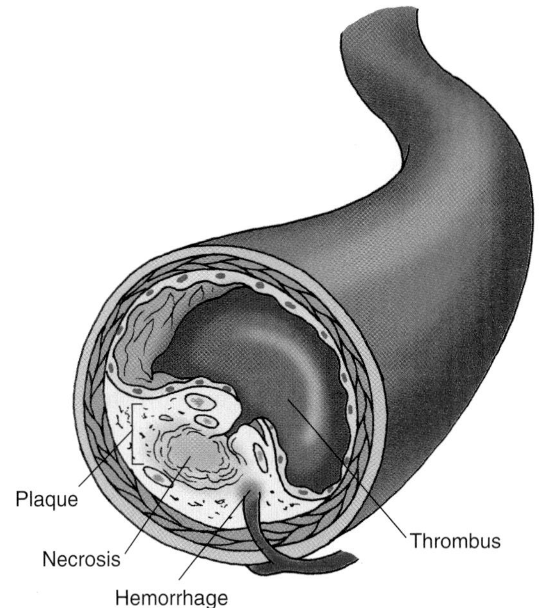

figure 21-1 Thrombosis of an atherosclerotic plaque. It may partially or completely occlude the lumen of the vessel. (Source: Bullock BL: Pathophysiology: Adaptations and Alterations in Function [4th Ed]. Philadelphia, Lippincott-Raven, 1996.)

Scientific advances have highlighted the role of inflammation in the pathophysiological process of atherosclerosis. The classic signs and symptoms of inflammation include redness, pain, heat, and swelling. They indicate that the injured tissue is in the process of restoring homeostasis,

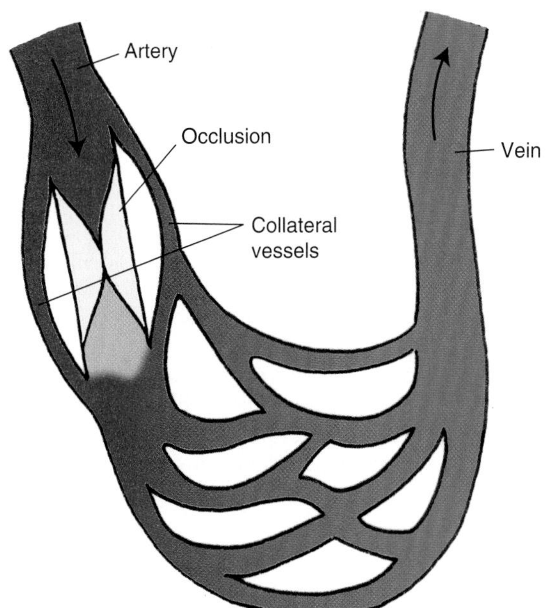

figure 21-2 Collateral circulation can develop for slowly developing lesions to provide myocardial blood flow until the atherosclerosis progresses beyond the limits of collateral supply. (Source: Bullock BL: Pathophysiology: Adaptations and Alterations in Function [4th Ed]. Philadelphia, Lippincott-Raven, 1996.)

which includes three phases: vasodilation and increased permeability of the blood vessels; emigration of phagocytes from the blood into the tissue; and tissue repair. This process of restoring homeostasis is meant to be protective, but in the setting of atherosclerosis, the process has been found to be destructive. The atherosclerotic plaque continues to develop, aided by inflammatory molecules, and a fibrous cap forms over the lipid core. As the cap matures, inflammatory substances weaken the cap and cause it to rupture. Once the cap is ruptured, the coagulation cascade is initiated and a clot is formed, resulting in obstruction of blood flow in the vessel.

Markers of inflammation are now being used to assess the risk of atherosclerosis. C-reactive protein is an inflammatory marker that is predictive of unstable angina and acute MI. C-reactive protein levels greater than 3 mg/L have been found in greater than 65% of patients with unstable angina and in more than 90% of patients with acute MI preceded by unstable angina.[3]

Risk Factors

The cause of atherosclerosis is not clearly known. Through epidemiological studies, risk factors for the development of atherosclerosis have been identified. These risk factors are usually classified into two groups: major risk factors and contributing risk factors. Major risk factors are those that have been shown through research to increase significantly the risk of cardiovascular disease. Contributing risk factors are known to be associated with an increased risk of cardiovascular disease, but their significance and prevalence are still under investigation. Major risk factors are further divided into those that are uncontrollable and those that can be lowered by modification, treatment, or control.

MAJOR UNCONTROLLABLE RISK FACTORS

Age

There is an increased incidence of all types of atherosclerotic disease with aging. About 84% of people who die from coronary heart disease are 65 years of age and older. At older ages, women who have an MI are more likely than men to die from it within a few weeks.[4]

Heredity

The tendency to develop atherosclerosis seems to run in families, although the risk is presumed to be a combination of environmental and genetic influences. Even when other risk factors are controlled, the chance for developing coronary artery disease increases when there is a familial tendency. People with a parent or sibling who developed cardiovascular disease before 55 years of age generally have two to six times the risk for developing cardiovascular disease as those without a family history.[5] Most people with a strong family history of cardiovascular disease also have one or more additional risk factors.

Race

Rates of cardiovascular disease are higher for African Americans, Mexican Americans, Native Americans, Native Hawaiians, and some Asian Americans. These higher rates are partly due to higher rates of hypertension, obesity, and diabetes.[2]

Sex

Men have a greater risk for development of coronary artery disease than woman, and men have MIs at a younger age. After menopause, however, women's death rate from coronary disease rises, but it never reaches the risk level of men.[2]

MAJOR RISK FACTORS THAT CAN BE MODIFIED, TREATED, OR CONTROLLED

Cigarette Smoking

A smoker's risk of an MI is double that of a nonsmoker. Smoking is the biggest risk factor for sudden cardiac death. A smoker's risk of sudden death is two to four times greater than the nonsmoker's risk. Smokers are more likely to die from the infarction and to die within 1 hour than nonsmokers. Exposure to environmental smoke also increases the risk of heart disease for nonsmokers.[4]

High Blood Cholesterol

High cholesterol levels increase the risk of coronary artery disease. Middle-aged adults with a total blood cholesterol level below 200 mg/dL have a relatively low risk of coronary artery disease. A total blood cholesterol level in the range of 200 to 239 mg/dL represents a moderate but increasing risk. When the level rises above 240 mg/dL, the risk of coronary artery disease is about double.[2]

Most cholesterol in the blood is carried in low-density lipoprotein (LDL), often called "bad" cholesterol. This type of cholesterol is deposited in the artery walls, and high blood levels of LDL increase the risk of coronary heart disease. An LDL level of less than 100 mg/dL is optimal.[2]

High-density cholesterol (HDL) removes cholesterol from tissues and transports the excess cholesterol back to the liver, where it is metabolized. For this reason, HDL is often called "good" cholesterol. A low level of HDL (<40 mg/dL) is associated with a higher risk of coronary artery disease.[2]

Hypertension

Hypertension is a major risk factor that is termed the *silent killer* because it has no specific symptoms and no early warning signs. Men have a greater risk for hypertension than women until the age of 55 years. Between 55 and 75 years, the risk for development of hypertension is about the same for men and women. After the age of 75 years, hypertension is more likely to develop in women than in men. Compared with whites, hypertension develops in blacks earlier in life and their average blood pressures are significantly higher.[1]

Physical Inactivity

A lack of physical activity plays a significant role in the development of heart disease. When lack of regular exercise is combined with overeating and obesity, high cholesterol can result and further increase the risk of heart disease. Even moderate levels of regular, low-intensity exercise have been shown to be beneficial in the prevention of heart disease.[4]

Obesity and Overweight

Obesity and excess weight are associated with an increased mortality rate from coronary artery disease and stroke. Excess weight is also linked with an increased incidence of hypertension, insulin resistance, diabetes, and dyslipidemia. Central obesity (intra-abdominal fat) appears to be a stronger predictor of cardiovascular disease than peripheral or subcutaneous obesity. The waist measurement and the body mass index (a measure of weight relative to height) are the recommended means to estimate a person's body fat. A higher risk for cardiovascular disease is found for women with a waist greater than 35 inches and for men with a waist greater than 40 inches.[2]

Diabetes Mellitus

Diabetes mellitus is associated with a markedly increased risk of cardiovascular disease. This increased risk occurs even if the person maintains control of blood glucose levels. About two thirds of people with diabetes die of some form of heart or blood vessel disease.[2,4]

CONTRIBUTING RISK FACTORS

Stress

A person's response to stress may be a contributing factor to cardiovascular disease. The behaviors that a person engages in when under stress (such as smoking, overeating) may contribute to the risk of cardiovascular disease.

Sex Hormones

Sex hormones are known to play a role in the risk for development of cardiovascular disease. Men have a higher incidence of MI than women who are premenopausal. However, the loss of estrogen as women age is believed to be a contributing factor to the marked rise in women's risk of heart disease after menopause. Female hormones are also know to raise HDL and to lower total blood cholesterol levels, whereas male hormones have the opposite effect.[4]

Birth Control Pills

Low-dose oral contraceptives are associated with a lower risk for development of heart disease than are the earlier, higher-dose forms of birth control pills. However, for a woman who takes the low-dose form, the risk of heart disease increases if she also smokes or has hypertension.[4]

Excessive Alcohol Intake

The excessive intake of alcohol has been associated with hypertension, heart failure, stroke, high triglycerides, and dysrhythmias. The risk of heart disease in moderate drinkers is lower than in nondrinkers. Moderate drinking means one drink for a woman per day and two drinks for a man per day. One drink is defined as 1.5 fluid ounces of 80-proof spirits, 1 fluid ounce of 100-proof spirits, 4 fluid ounces of wine, or 12 fluid ounces of beer.[4]

Homocysteine Levels

Homocysteine is a sulfur-containing amino acid that is synthesized during protein catabolism. It depends on vitamin B_6, folate, and vitamin B_{12} to be metabolized. Homocysteine aids in the growth and maintenance of tissue and plays a role in the prevention of skin and nail disorders. Hyperhomocysteinemia can be genetic (rare) or acquired. The acquired form occurs in about 5% to 7% of the population.[6] An association has been shown between elevated levels of homocysteine and cardiovascular disease. Homocysteine causes increased platelet adhesiveness, enhances LDL deposition in the arterial wall, and activates the coagulation cascade.[7,8]

ACUTE CORONARY SYNDROME

Acute coronary syndrome is a relatively new term used to describe patients who have clinical symptoms compatible with acute myocardial ischemia. Acute coronary syndrome includes unstable angina and acute MI. Unstable angina refers to unexpected chest pain or discomfort that usually occurs while at rest. Patients with MI are further classified into one of two groups: those with ST segment elevation MI and those with non–ST segment elevation MI.[1,9]

ANGINA PECTORIS

The term *angina* comes from the Latin word meaning "to choke." *Angina pectoris* is the term used to describe chest pain or discomfort that results from coronary artery disease. The patient may describe the sensation as pressure, fullness, squeezing, heaviness, or pain.

Pathophysiological Principles

Angina pectoris is caused by transient, reversible myocardial ischemia precipitated by an imbalance between myocardial oxygen demand and myocardial oxygen supply. In most cases, angina pectoris is the result of a reduced oxygen supply. The most common cause of a reduced supply of oxygen is from atherosclerotic narrowing of the coronary arteries. A nonocclusive thrombus develops on a disrupted atherosclerotic plaque, resulting in a reduction in myocardial perfusion. As blood flow to the myocardium decreases, autoregulation of coronary blood flow occurs as a compensatory mechanism. The smooth muscles of the arterioles relax, thus decreasing resistance to blood flow in the arteriolar bed. When this compensatory mechanism can no longer meet the metabolic demands, myocardial ischemia occurs, and the person feels pain.

A less common cause of unstable angina is dynamic obstruction resulting from intense focal spasm of a coronary artery. The spasm is caused by hypercontractility of vascular smooth muscle, endothelial dysfunction, or abnormal constriction of small resistance vessels. As a result of the spasm, perfusion to the myocardium is interrupted, thus reducing the supply of oxygen.[9]

Arterial inflammation may be another cause of decreased oxygen supply that results in unstable angina. The inflammatory process may cause arterial narrowing, plaque destabilization, rupture, and thrombogenesis. Numerous investigations are underway to understand better the role of inflammation in acute coronary syndromes.

A marked increase in oxygen demand is another cause of unstable angina. Conditions such as fever, tachycardia, and thyrotoxicosis may result in an increased oxygen demand that is unable to be met, especially if the patient has underlying coronary artery disease.[9]

When the balance between oxygen supply and demand is not met, the myocardial tissue's need for oxygen and nutrients continues. The same work of pumping blood must be accomplished with less available energy and oxygen. The tissue that depends on the blood supply becomes ischemic as it functions with less oxygenated blood. Anaerobic metabolism can provide only 6% of the total energy needed. Glucose uptake by the cells is markedly increased as glycogen and adenosine triphosphate stores are depleted. Potassium rapidly moves out of the myocardial cells during ischemia. An acidotic cellular bath develops, further compromising cellular metabolism.

Classification of Angina

Many terms are used clinically to describe angina. Stable angina (also known as chronic stable angina, classic angina, or exertional angina) is a term used to describe paroxysmal substernal pain that is usually predictable. The pain occurs with physical exertion or emotional stress and is relieved by rest or nitroglycerin.

Unstable angina, also called preinfarction angina or crescendo angina, refers to cardiac chest pain that usually occurs while at rest. The patient with unstable angina has more prolonged and severe chest discomfort than the person with stable angina. Unstable angina is a type of acute coronary syndrome and requires immediate treatment because the patient is at increased risk for acute MI, cardiac dysrhythmias, or cardiac sudden death.

Variant angina, also know as Prinzmetal's angina or vasospastic angina, is a form of unstable angina. Variant angina usually occurs at rest, most often between midnight and 8 AM. It does not usually occur after exertion or emotional stress. Variant angina is the result of coronary artery spasm. Most people who experience variant angina have severe coronary atherosclerosis of at least one major coronary artery and the spasm occurs very near the area of blockage.[2]

The Canadian Cardiovascular Society also has proposed a classification system for grading for angina. Each stage of the four-class system is described in Box 21-1.

box 21-1
Grading of Angina Pectoris by the Canadian Cardiovascular Society Classification System

Class I: Ordinary physical activity does not cause angina, such as walking, climbing stairs. Angina occurs with strenuous, rapid, or prolonged exertion at work or recreation.

Class II: Slight limitation of ordinary activity occurs. Angina occurs when walking or climbing stairs rapidly, walking uphill, walking or climbing stairs after meals, in cold, in wind, under emotional stress, or during the few hours after awakening. Angina occurs when walking more than two level blocks and climbing more than one flight of ordinary stairs at a normal pace and in normal conditions.

Class III: Ordinary physical activity is markedly limited. Angina occurs when walking one to two level blocks and climbing one flight of stairs in normal conditions and at a normal pace.

Class IV: Physical activity without discomfort is impossible; anginal symptoms may be present at rest.

From Campeau L: Grading of angina pectoris [letter]. Circulation 54:522–523, 1976; copyright 1976, American Heart Association, Inc; used with permission.

Assessment

HISTORY

The five most important factors that indicate a likelihood of ischemia due to coronary artery disease are obtained rapidly during the history. These factors include a description of the symptoms, information about a prior history of coronary artery disease, the patient's sex and age, and the number of risk factors present.[9]

The nurse uses the N, O, P, Q, R, S, T method of pain assessment when taking the patient's history. For a review of the assessment questions, see Box 17-1 in Chapter 17. After determining the patient's *normal* baseline, the nurse asks about the time of *onset* of the pain. The nurse determines causes (*provocative*) of the pain and any measures the patient has used to relieve the pain (*palliative*). The pain of angina is often brought on by exertion or emotion. It may also occur after meals, exposure to cold, and at rest. Patients with angina often obtain relief from the pain with rest or by taking sublingual nitroglycerin. As the angina becomes more severe (unstable angina), the pain may occur at rest or be caused by less exertion and is no longer relieved with rest or sublingual nitroglycerin. The *quality* of anginal pain is frequently described as deep, poorly localized chest or arm discomfort. Patients often describe heaviness, squeezing, choking, or smothering sensations. When asked about *region* and *radiation* of the pain, patients report substernal, left-sided chest, or epigastric pain that may radiate to the left arm, neck, back, or jaw. The *severity* of the pain is evaluated by asking the patient to rate the pain on a scale of 1 to 10, with 10 being the worst pain they have experienced. Additional information is obtained related to *time*. The nurse asks how long the pain lasts, how frequently it occurs, and the time of day it occurs. Finally, the nurse asks about associated symptoms such as dyspnea, nausea, vomiting, and diaphoresis. Box 21-2 summarizes the assessment findings for a patient with myocardial ischemia.

The older patient, especially women, who experiences angina may have a different presentation because of changes in neuroreceptors. Considerations for the older patient are described in Box 21-3.

PHYSICAL EXAMINATION

The physical examination helps to determine the cause of the pain, to detect comorbid conditions, and to assess any hemodynamic consequences of the pain. When the vital signs are done, the nurse should measure the blood pressure in both arms of the patient. If the physical examination is done during an anginal episode, the patient may present with tachycardia and pulsus alternans. During the initial phase of an anginal episode, the patient may be hypertensive. The patient may exhibit pallor with cold, clammy skin. On further examination of the skin, the nurse may detect xanthomas, which are yellow nodules or plaques, especially on the skin. Xanthomas may be indications of hypercholesterolemia. Carotid or femoral bruits may be auscultated, indicating the possible presence of obstructive cardiovascular disease. The nurse may hear a paradoxical split

box 21-2
The N, O, P, Q, R, S, T Characteristics of Chest Pain Due to Myocardial Ischemia

N—Normal
- The patient's baseline before the onset of the pain

O—Onset
- The time when the pain/discomfort started

P—Precipitating and Palliative Factors

Precipitating
- Exercise
- Exercise after a large meal
- Exertion
- Walking on a cold or windy day
- Cold weather
- Stress or anxiety
- Anger
- Fear

Palliative
- Stop exercise.
- Sit down and rest.
- Use sublingual nitroglycerin; pain of myocardial infarction is often not relieved by sublingual nitroglycerin.

Q—Quality
- Heaviness
- Tightness
- Squeezing
- Choking
- Suffocating
- Viselike

R—Region and Radiation
- Substernal with radiation to the back, left arm, neck, or jaw
- Upper chest
- Epigastric
- Left shoulder
- Intrascapular

S—Severity
- Pain rated on a scale of 1 to 10, with 10 being the worst pain ever experienced, often rated as 5 or above

T—Time
- Pain lasts from 30 seconds to 30 minutes.
- Pain can last longer than 30 minutes for unstable angina or myocardial infarction.

of S_2 or auscultate an S_3 heart sound. Both sounds are indicators of left ventricular failure. An S_4 may be heard, which is suggestive of decreased left ventricular compliance. Deficits in peripheral pulses may indicate peripheral vascular disease.

DIAGNOSTIC TESTS

A 12-lead electrocardiogram (ECG) is a standard diagnostic test for patients with angina and should be obtained immediately in patients with chest discomfort. During the anginal episode, the ECG may show T-wave inversions and ST segment depressions in the ECG leads associated with the anatomical region of myocardial ischemia (Fig. 21-3). Transient ST segment changes (≥0.05 mV) that occur during a symptomatic episode while at rest and that resolve when the patient is asymptomatic are highly suggestive of severe coronary artery disease.[9] Ectopic beats may also be present during an anginal episode. The ECG should be compared with previous ECGs. Between anginal episodes, the ECG may appear normal. Ambulatory ECG monitoring may be used to assist in the diagnosis of angina, especially for patients who have angina at rest.

Biochemical cardiac markers are useful in determining both the diagnosis and the prognosis of acute coronary syndromes. For a more detailed discussion of cardiac markers, see Chapter 17. A cardiac-specific troponin (troponin T or troponin I) is the preferred marker to obtain in all patients who present with chest discomfort consistent with acute coronary syndrome. The creatine kinase with myocardial bands (CK-MB) is an acceptable marker to use. If the patient has a negative cardiac marker within 6 hours of the onset of chest discomfort, another sample should be drawn in the 6- to 12-hour period after onset of chest discomfort.[9] Additional blood tests include chemistry, complete blood count, and coagulation studies.

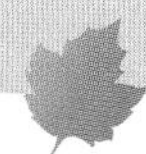

box 21-3
Considerations for the Older Patient With Acute Coronary Syndrome

Coronary artery disease is more common and more severe in the older patient. Older patients often present with special problems because of their numerous comorbidities, such as diminished beta-sympathetic response, increased cardiac afterload due to decreased arterial compliance and arterial hypertension, cardiac hypertrophy, and ventricular diastolic dysfunction.[9]

The older patient is more likely to present with atypical symptoms such as dyspnea, confusion, weakness, or fainting rather than with typical substernal chest pain. Because of differences in amount and distribution of subcutaneous fat, the older person may develop anginal symptoms more quickly when exposed to cold. The older person should be taught to dress in warm clothing and to recognize feelings of weakness, shortness of breath, or fainting as possible indicators of angina.

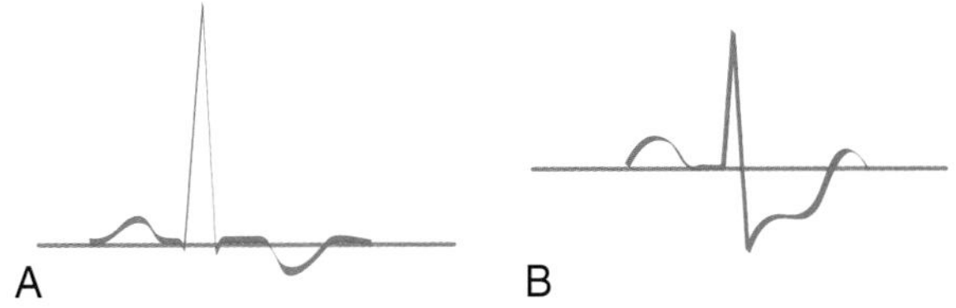

figure 21-3 Inversion of T wave (**A**) and depression of ST segment (**B**). (Source: Bullock BL: Pathophysiology: Adaptations and Alterations in Function [4th Ed]. Philadelphia, Lippincott-Raven, 1996.)

Other diagnostic tests include exercise stress testing in which the ECG and blood pressure are monitored before, during, and after exercise. The exercise stress test is especially useful in risk stratification of patients. For patients who are unable to exercise, pharmacological stress testing may be done in which the medication increases myocardial oxygen demand while the patient remains inactive. Intravenous medications used for pharmacological stress testing include adenosine, dobutamine, and dipyridamole.

Cardiac imaging studies usually start with chest radiographs, although they have limited value in diagnosing coronary heart disease. Thallium-201 or technetium-99m sestamibi perfusion imaging can be used with exercise or pharmacological stress testing to detect perfusion defects. Positron emission tomography (PET) may be helpful in differentiating ischemic from infarcted myocardium. Echocardiography is performed to evaluate wall motion abnormalities and thickness, valvular function, and ejection fraction. Magnetic resonance imaging (MRI) may be used to view structural cardiovascular abnormalities when other diagnostic techniques (e.g., the echocardiogram) are inconclusive or ambiguous.

Coronary angiography is an invasive diagnostic test that provides a definitive diagnosis of coronary artery disease. Results from coronary angiography are used to guide the decision whether to manage the patient medically or surgically. For further discussion of cardiovascular diagnostic tests, see Chapter 17.

Management

The goal of therapy for the patient with angina pectoris is to restore the balance between oxygen supply and oxygen demand. The nurse assesses the patient's vital signs and mental status frequently. The patient is placed on a cardiac monitor for ischemia and dysrhythmia detection. The patient is placed on bed rest until stabilized to minimize oxygen demands. Supplemental oxygen may be given to unstable patients to increase oxygen supply. A pulse oximeter and arterial blood gases are used to evaluate oxygenation status.

PHARMACOLOGICAL THERAPY

Pharmacological therapy is an important component in the management of patients with angina pectoris. The severity of symptoms, hemodynamic status of the patient, and medication history guide the drug regimen.

Nitroglycerin is a mainstay of therapy and is used sublingually or as a spray for acute anginal attacks. If three sublingual tablets (0.4 mg) or spray taken 5 minutes apart does not relieve the pain of angina, intravenous (IV) nitroglycerin may be useful. IV nitroglycerin should be started at a rate of 10 µg/minute by continuous infusion and titrated up by 10 µg/minute every 3 to 5 minutes until some symptom or blood pressure response is noted. If no response is noted at 20 µg/minute, increments of 10 µg/minute, and later 20 µg/minute can be used. If signs and symptoms are relieved, there is no need to continue to increase the dose. However, if relief is not obtained, the dose can be increased until a blood pressure response is noted. Once patients have been pain free and have no other indications of ischemia for 12 to 24 hours, the dosage of IV nitroglycerin should be reduced with a goal of switching to oral or topical nitrates.[9]

Morphine sulfate is indicated for patients whose symptoms are not relieved after three serial sublingual nitroglycerin tablets or whose symptoms recur with adequate anti-ischemic therapy. A dose of 1 to 5 mg IV is recommended and may be repeated every 5 to 30 minutes as needed to relieve symptoms and maintain comfort. The nurse carefully monitors the patient's respiratory rate and blood pressure, especially if the patient continues to receive IV nitroglycerin.[9]

Beta blockers may be used to decrease myocardial oxygen consumption by reducing myocardial contractility, sinus node rate, and atrioventricular (AV) node conduction velocity. The reduction in myocardial contractility reduces the work of the heart and decreases myocardial oxygen demand. The slowing of the heart rate helps to increase the time for diastolic filling, thus improving blood flow to the coronary arteries. Beta blockers are started by an IV route, followed by oral administration.[9]

Calcium antagonists may be beneficial for the patient with unstable angina. Calcium antagonists decrease myocardial oxygen demand by decreasing afterload, contractility, and heart rate. Verapamil or diltiazem can be used as second- or third-choice therapy after the initiation of nitrates and beta blockers. Verapamil or diltiazem can be given as initial therapy when beta blockers are contraindicated.[9]

Antiplatelet therapy should be initiated promptly for the patient with unstable angina. Aspirin is administered as soon as possible and is continued indefinitely unless contraindicated. A second class of antiplatelet drugs known as thienopyridines can be used in patients with unstable angina. Clopidogrel is the preferred drug in this class because of its rapid onset of action and safety profile. Clopidogrel is used for patients who are unable to tolerate aspirin. The drug is also recommended for hospitalized patients in addition to aspirin unless the patient is scheduled for coronary artery bypass grafting surgery. A third group of antiplatelet drugs known as glycoprotein IIb/IIIa antagonists are used for patients with unstable angina who are undergoing percutaneous coronary interventions. Anticoagulation with low–molecular-weight heparin or IV unfractionated heparin should be added to antiplatelet therapy.[9]

INVASIVE THERAPY

Invasive therapy may be indicated for the management of patients with unstable angina. Intra-aortic balloon pump support may be used in a critically ill patient to provide increased coronary artery perfusion and to decrease afterload. Percutaneous transluminal coronary angioplasty and stent placement may be used for treating patients with unstable angina. See Chapter 18 for a more detailed discussion of the intra-aortic balloon pump, percutaneous transluminal coronary angioplasty, and stent placement. Coronary artery bypass grafting is another invasive options for treatment. See Chapter 22 for a more detailed discussion of cardiac surgery.

RISK FACTOR MODIFICATION

Risk factor modification may help prevent an anginal episode or delay the worsening of existing angina. Patients should be encouraged to stop smoking, achieve or maintain optimal weight, and exercise daily. Diet and medications may be prescribed to control hypertension, diabetes, and hyperlipidemia. Patient education, including home care considerations, is essential for patients with angina pectoris. Patient education guidelines and home care considerations are described in Box 21-4.

MYOCARDIAL INFARCTION

Prolonged ischemia caused by an imbalance between oxygen supply and oxygen demand causes MI. The prolonged ischemia causes irreversible cell damage and muscle death. Although multiple factors can contribute to the imbalance between oxygen supply and oxygen demand, the presence of a coronary artery thrombosis characterizes most MIs. In a classic investigation, DeWood and colleagues demonstrated that 87% of patients studied in the first 4 hours after onset of MI symptoms had a thrombotic occlusion. The incidence of thrombotic occlusion decreases to 65% at 12 to 24 hours.[10]

An MI can be determined from several different perspectives, including clinical, electrocardiographic, biochemical, and pathological. The European Society of Cardiology and the American College of Cardiology Committee developed a joint consensus document for the redefinition of MI.[11] Their definition of an acute MI is shown in Box 21-5.

Pathophysiological Principles

Most patients who sustain an MI have coronary atherosclerosis. The thrombus formation occurs most often at the site of an atherosclerotic lesion, thus obstructing blood flow to the myocardial tissues. Plaque rupture is believed to be the triggering mechanism for the development of the thrombus in most patients with an MI. As mentioned previously, the role of inflammatory processes in the development of atherosclerotic plaque is an area of intense scientific investigation. Cardiovascular risk factors play a role in endothelial damage resulting in endothelial dysfunction. The dysfunctioning endothelium contributes to the activation of the inflammatory response and the formation of atherosclerotic plaques. When the plaques rupture, a thrombus is formed at the site that can occlude blood flow, thus resulting in an MI. Figure 21-4 shows the atherosclerotic plaque in stable angina and in acute coronary syndromes.

Irreversible damage to the myocardium can begin as early as 20 to 40 minutes after interruption of blood flow. The dynamic process of infarction may not be completed, however, for several hours. Necrosis of tissue appears to occur in a sequential fashion. Reimer and associates demonstrated that cellular death occurs first in the subendocardial layer and spreads like a "wavefront" throughout the thickness of the wall of the heart. Using dogs, they showed that the shorter the time between coronary occlusion and coro-

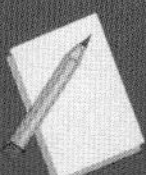

box 21-4
Patient Teaching for Patients With Angina Pectoris

Activity and Exercise

- Participate in a daily program of exercise that does not precipitate pain.
- Alternate activity with periods of rest and moderate activity level as needed.

Diet

- Eat a well-balanced diet with an appropriate caloric intake.
- If obese, participate in a supervised weight-reduction program.
- Avoid activity immediately after meals.
- Restrict intake of caffeine because it can increase heart rate.
- Maintain a diet low in fat.

Smoking

- Participate in a smoking cessation program. Smoking can increase heart rate, blood pressure, and blood carbon monoxide levels.
- Avoid smoke-filled environments.

Cold Weather

- Avoid exposure to cold and windy weather. Exercise indoors when necessary.
- When outdoors, dress in warm clothing, and cover mouth and nose with a scarf.
- Use a moderate pace of walking in cold weather.

Medications

- Carry sublingual nitroglycerin at all times.
- Keep the pills in a dark-colored glass bottle to protect them from sunlight.
- Do not place cotton in the bottle because the cotton will absorb the active ingredients of the medication.
- If pain occurs, place tablet under the tongue, stop activity, and wait for medication to dissolve. Take another tablet in 3 to 5 minutes if pain is not resolved.
- If pain continues, seek immediate care.
- Be aware of side effects of nitroglycerin, including headache, flushing, and dizziness.

box 21-5
Definition of Acute, Evolving, or Recent Myocardial Infarction

Either one of the following criteria satisfies the diagnosis for an acute, evolving, or recent myocardial infarction:

1. Typical rise and gradual fall (troponin) or more rapid rise and fall (CK-MB) of biochemical markers of myocardial necrosis with at least one of the following:
   a. Ischemic symptoms
   b. Development of pathologic Q waves on the electrocardiogram
   c. Electrocardiographic changes indicative of ischemia (ST segment elevation or depression)
   d. Coronary artery intervention (e.g., coronary angioplasty)
2. Pathological findings of an acute myocardial infarction

Adapted from The Joint European Society of Cardiology and the American College of Cardiology Committee: Myocardial infarction redefined: A consensus document of the Joint European Society of Cardiology/American College of Cardiology Committee for the redefinition of myocardial infarction. J Am Coll Cardiol 36(3):967, 2000.

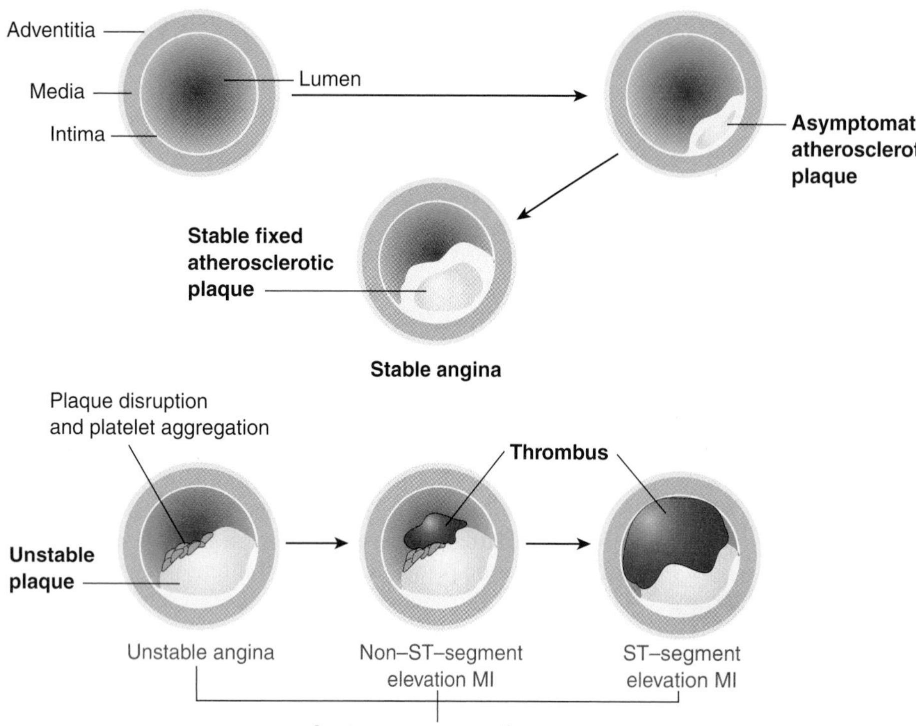

figure 21-4 Atherosclerotic plaque. Stable fixed atherosclerotic plaque in stable angina and the unstable plaque with plaque disruption and platelet aggregation in the acute coronary syndromes. (From Porth CM: Pathophysiology. Concepts of Altered Health States [6th Ed], p 495. Philadelphia, Lippincott Williams & Wilkins, 2002.)

nary reperfusion, the greater the amount of myocardial tissue that could be salvaged. Their classic work indicates that a substantial amount of myocardial tissue can be salvaged if flow is restored within 6 hours after the onset of coronary occlusion.[12] For the clinician, this means time is muscle.

The cellular changes associated with an MI can be followed by the development of infarct extension (new myocardial necrosis), infarct expansion (a disproportionate thinning and dilation of the infarct zone), or ventricular remodeling (a disproportionate thinning and dilation of the ventricle).

SIZE OF THE INFARCTION

Several factors determine the size of the resulting MI. These factors include the extent, severity, and duration of the ischemic episode; the size of the vessel; the amount of collateral circulation; the status of the intrinsic fibrinolytic system; vascular tone; and the metabolic demands of the myocardium at the time of the event.[13] MIs most often result in damage to the left ventricle, leading to an alteration in left ventricular function. Infarctions can also occur in the right ventricle or in both ventricles.

The term *transmural infarction* is used to imply an infarction process that has resulted in necrosis of the tissue in all the layers of the myocardium. Because the heart functions as a squeezing pump, systolic and diastolic efforts can be significantly altered when a segment of the heart muscle is necrotic and nonfunctional. If the area of the transmural infarction is small, the necrotic wall may be dyskinetic, a term meaning "difficulty in moving." If the damage to the myocardial tissue is more extensive, the myocardial muscle may become akinetic, meaning "without motion."

The normal myocardial muscle contracts with systole and relaxes with diastole. When normal motion is not possible because of infarction, diastolic filling and systolic pumping are altered. As a result, cardiac output is compromised. The larger the area of infarction, the greater the impact on ventricular function.

LOCATION OF THE INFARCTION

In addition to size, location of the infarction is an important determinant of ventricular function. MIs can be located in the anterior, septal, lateral, posterior, or inferior walls of the left ventricle. In more recent years, clinicians have acknowledged the presence and clinical significance of MIs occurring in the right ventricle.

Anterior Left Ventricle

Infarctions of the anterior wall of the left ventricle and the interventricular septum result from occlusion of the left anterior descending (LAD) coronary artery. The LAD coronary artery supplies oxygenated blood to the anterior wall of the left ventricle, the interventricular septum, and the ventricular conducting tissue. (See Chapter 16 for a more detailed discussion of coronary artery anatomy and physiology.) Anteroseptal wall MIs are the most frequent type of infarction and have the potential for causing a significant amount of left ventricular dysfunction. Patients with an anteroseptal MI are at high risk for heart failure, pulmonary edema, cardiogenic shock, and death because of an inadequate pump. Anteroseptal wall MIs are also associated with increased risk of intraventricular conduction disturbances, such as bundle branch blocks and fascicular blocks, which are also known as hemi-blocks.

Lateral and Posterior Left Ventricle

Infarctions of the lateral and posterior walls of the left ventricle result from occlusion of the left circumflex vessel. In addition to supplying oxygenated blood to the lateral and posterior walls, the left circumflex vessel is the source of blood supply to the sinoatrial (SA) node in about 50% of the population and to the AV node in about 10% of the population. Infarctions of the lateral and posterior walls are less common than infarctions of the anteroseptal wall. Although muscle necrosis occurs with lateral and posterior wall MIs, the impact on left ventricular function is usually less than for patients with anteroseptal MI. Patients with a lateral or posterior wall MI are also at risk for dysrhythmias associated with dysfunction of the SA or AV nodes. Examples include sinus arrest, wandering atrial pacemaker, sinus pause, or junction rhythm.

Inferior Left Ventricle

Infarctions of the inferior wall result from occlusion of the right coronary artery. The right coronary artery supplies oxygenated blood to the inferior wall and the right ventricle. In addition, it is the source of blood supply to the SA node in about 50% of the population and the AV node in about 90% of the population. Infarctions of the inferior wall are less common than anteroseptal MIs but occur more frequently than MIs of the lateral or posterior walls. The potential impact on left ventricular function usually is less for a patient with an inferior wall MI than for a patient with an anteroseptal wall infarct. Because the right coronary artery supplies oxygenated blood to much of the conducting tissue, patients are at frequent risk for dysrhythmias related to altered function of the SA and AV nodes.

Right Ventricle

The right coronary artery provides the blood supply to the inferior wall and the right ventricle. Consequently, right coronary artery disease causing an inferior wall MI is likely to be associated with concomitant right ventricular infarction. Approximately 33% to 50% of patients with an inferior wall MI have associated right ventricular involvement.[14–16] Patients may experience significant hemodynamic compromise due to biventricular dysfunction. Associated dysrhythmias involve dysfunction of the SA and AV nodes.

TYPE OF INFARCTION

Patients with chest pain may present with or without ST segment elevations on their ECG. In most patients with ST segment elevation, a Q wave ultimately develops on the ECG, and the term *Q-wave MI* is used to describe the type of MI they experience. In a much smaller number of patients who present with ST segment elevation, a Q wave does not develop, and the term *non–Q-wave MI* is used to classify these patients. Patients who present without ST segment elevations are diagnosed with either unstable angina or a non–ST segment elevation MI[17] (Fig. 21-5).

The ST segment is the portion of the ECG tracing from the end of the QRS complex to the beginning of the T wave. Normally, the ST segment is isoelectric, meaning it joins the QRS complex at the baseline. When the ST segment is elevated, the amount of elevation is measured in millimeters on the ECG paper.

A Q wave is a portion of the QRS complex on the ECG. Specifically, the Q wave is the initial downward deflection of the QRS complex. A Q wave is not present on the normal ECG. The presence of significant Q waves indicates an MI. For a review of ECG waveforms, see Chapter 17.

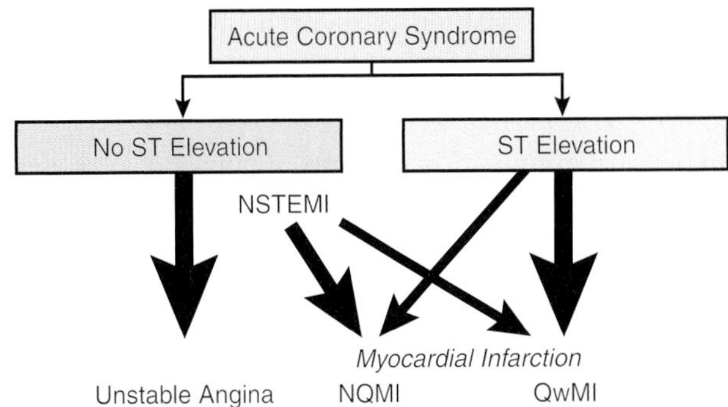

figure 21-5 Acute coronary syndrome. Patients may present with or without ST segment elevation on electrocardiography. Most patients with ST segment elevation (*large arrows*) ultimately develop a Q-wave AMI (QwMI), whereas a minority (*small arrow*) develop a non–Q-wave AMI (NQMI). Patients who present without ST segment elevation are experiencing either unstable angina or NSTEMI (non–ST segment elevation MI). (Redrawn with permission from Braunwald et al: ACC/AHA Practice Guidelines. American College of Cardiology, 2002.)

Assessment

The nursing assessment of a patient with a probable MI must be organized and thorough. It is best to start with the history because this establishes rapport and provides valuable data. The history is followed by the physical examination and evaluation of diagnostic tests. Based on the data, a management plan is developed initially for the acute phase. Once the patient is stabilized, plans for cardiac rehabilitation are initiated.

HISTORY

The most common presenting complaint of a patient with an MI is the presence of chest discomfort or pain. Other assessment findings are similar to those described in Box 21-2. Like patients with angina, patients with MI describe a heaviness, squeezing, choking, or smothering sensation. Patients often describe the sensation as "someone sitting on my chest." The substernal pain can radiate to the neck, left arm, back, or jaw. Unlike the pain of angina, the pain of an MI is often more prolonged and unrelieved by rest or sublingual nitroglycerin. For a review of the assessment questions, see Box 17-1 in Chapter 17.

Associated findings on history include nausea and vomiting, especially for the patient with an inferior wall MI. These gastrointestinal complaints are believed to be related to the severity of the pain and the resulting vagal stimulation. Patients may initially seek relief of the gastrointestinal symptoms through antacids and other home remedies, thus delaying their decision to go the hospital. Additional complaints described during the history include diaphoresis, dyspnea, weakness, fatigue, anxiety, restlessness, confusion, shortness of breath, or a sense of impending death.

After the patient is stabilized, a more comprehensive history is obtained. Information about risk factors, previous cardiac illnesses and surgeries, and family history is important to acquire. This information will be useful in guiding patient education, cardiac rehabilitation, and care at home.

PHYSICAL EXAMINATION

On physical examination, patients usually appear restless and in distress. They often assume a position to promote breathing and alleviate pain. The skin is warm and moist. Breathing may be labored and rapid. Fine crackles, coarse crackles, or rhonchi may be heard when auscultating the lungs. These sounds may indicate the presence of heart failure or pulmonary edema.

The cardiovascular examination may reveal an increased blood pressure related to anxiety or a decreased blood pressure caused by heart failure. The heart rate may vary from bradycardia to tachycardia. Sinus tachycardia that persists more than 24 hours after the infarction is associated with high mortality rates.[5] When the patient is placed in the left lateral decubitus position, abnormalities of the precordial pulsations can be felt. These abnormalities include a lack of a point of maximal impulse or the presence of diffuse contraction. On auscultation, the first heart sound may be diminished as a result of decreased contractility. A fourth heart sound is heard in almost all patients with MI, whereas a third heart sound is detected in only about 10% to 20% of patients. Transient systolic murmurs may be heard because of papillary muscle dysfunction. After about 48 to 72 hours, many patients acquire a pericardial friction rub.[18] Additional findings on physical examination may be related to the development of complications such as heart failure or pulmonary edema.

Patients with right ventricular infarcts may present with jugular vein distension, peripheral edema, and an elevated central venous pressure. Their lungs may be clear because the failing right ventricle has not provided adequate forward flow.

DIAGNOSTIC TESTS

The Electrocardiogram

When a coronary artery becomes about 70% occluded and oxygen demand exceeds oxygen supply, myocardial ischemia may result. If the ischemic state is not corrected, injury to the myocardium may occur. Eventually, if adequate blood flow to the myocardium is not restored, an MI may result. Ischemia and injury are reversible processes; however, infarction is not.

An ECG can be used to detect patterns of ischemia, injury, and infarction. When the heart muscle becomes ischemic, injured, or infarcted, depolarization and repolarization of the cardiac cells are altered, causing changes in the QRS complex, ST segment, and T wave in the ECG leads overlying the affected area of the heart. Table 21-1 shows location of the MI, the artery affected, findings from the ECG, and clinical implications.

table 21-1 Location of Myocardial Infarction, Electrocardiographic (ECG) Findings, and Clinical Implications

Anatomical Location	Coronary Artery	ECG Evidence	Clinical Implications
Anteroseptal wall	Left anterior descending: Supplies blood to the anterior wall of left ventricle, the interventricular septum, and the ventricular conducting tissue	V_1 through V_4. Q waves and ST segment elevations	Potential for significant hemodynamic compromise; congestive heart failure, pulmonary edema, cardiogenic shock; intraventricular conduction disturbances
Lateral wall	Left circumflex: Supplies blood to the left lateral and left posterior walls and to the SA node in 45% of people and AV node in 10% of people	I, aVL, V_5, and V_6. Q waves and ST segment elevations	Evaluation for posterior wall involvement; some hemodynamic changes; dysrhythmias caused by SA and AV node dysfunction
Posterior wall	Left circumflex: Supplies blood to the left lateral and left posterior walls and to the SA node in 45% of people and AV node in 10% of people	V_1 and V_2, tall upright R waves with ST segment depression; Q waves and ST segment elevation in V_7 through V_9	Evaluation for lateral wall involvement; some hemodynamic changes; dysrhythmias caused by SA and AV node dysfunction
Inferior wall	Right coronary artery: Supplies blood to the inferior wall of the left ventricle, the right ventricle, and the SA node in 55% of people and the AV node in 90% of people	Q waves and ST segment elevation in II, III, aVF	Evaluation for right ventricular wall involvement; some hemodynamic changes; potential for significant arrhythmias caused by SA and AV node dysfunction
Right ventricular wall	Right coronary artery: Supplies blood to the inferior wall of the left ventricle, the right ventricle, and the SA node in 55% of people and the AV node in 90% of people	Q waves and ST segment elevations in right precordial chest leads (RV_1 through RV_6)	Evaluation for inferior wall involvement; some hemodynamic changes; potential for significant dysrhythmias caused by SA and AV node dysfunction

Ischemia. Myocardial ischemia may be a transient finding on ECG, or ischemic patterns may be more prolonged due to the presence of ischemic tissue surrounding a region of infarcted tissue. On the ECG, myocardial ischemia results in T-wave inversion or ST segment depression in the leads facing the ischemic area. The inverted T wave representative of ischemia is symmetrical, relatively narrow, and somewhat pointed. In contrast, asymmetrical inversion of the T wave usually does not indicate ischemia. Instead, it may signify ventricular hypertrophy or bundle branch block (Fig. 21-6). ST segment depressions of 1 to 2 mm or more for a duration of 0.08 second may indicate myocardial ischemia. Ischemia also should be suspected when a flat or depressed ST segment makes a sharp angle when joining an upright T wave rather than merging smoothly and imperceptibly with the T wave (Fig. 21-7).

Injury. ECG patterns of myocardial injury indicate a state of cellular damage beyond ischemia. Like ischemia, myocardial injury is a reversible process if interventions are instituted rapidly. As described previously, the injury process begins in the subendocardial layer and moves throughout the thickness of the wall of the heart like a wave. If the injury process is not interrupted, it eventually results in a transmural MI.

On ECG, the hallmark of acute myocardial injury is the presence of ST segment elevations. In the normal ECG, the ST segment should not be elevated more than 1 mm in the standard leads or more than 2 mm in the precordial leads. With an acute injury, the ST segments in the leads facing the injured area are elevated. The elevated ST segments also have a downward concave or coved shape and merge unnoticed with the T wave (Fig. 21-8).

Infarction. When myocardial injury persists, MI is the result. The pattern of the ECG indicative of an MI is seen on the ECG in stages and involves changes in the T wave, the ST segment, and the Q wave in the leads overlying the infarcted area. Figure 21-9 shows the evolution of the ECG in an MI. During the earliest stage of MI, known as the hyperacute phase, the T waves become tall and narrow. This configuration is referred to as hyperacute or peaked T waves. Within a few hours, these hyperacute T waves invert.

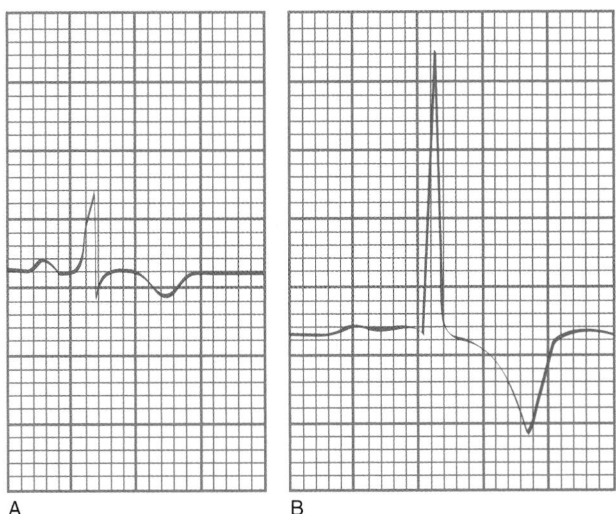

figure 21-6 T-wave inversion seen with ischemia (**A**) versus T-wave inversion seen with left ventricular hypertrophy (**B**).

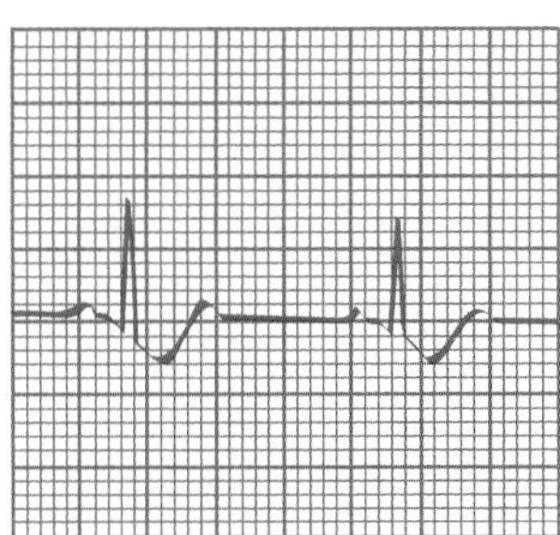

figure 21-7 An ST segment pattern consistent with myocardial ischemia. Notice how the ST segment forms a sharp angle when joining an upright T wave rather than merging smoothly and imperceptibly with the T wave.

Next, the ST segments elevate, a pattern that usually lasts from several hours to several days. In addition to the ST segment elevations in the leads of the ECG facing the injured heart, the leads facing away from the injured area may show ST segment depression. This finding is known as reciprocal ST segment changes. Reciprocal changes are most likely to be seen at the onset of infarction, but their presence on the ECG does not last long.[19] Reciprocal ST segment depressions may simply be a mirror image of the ST segment elevations. However, others have suggested that reciprocal changes may reflect ischemia due to narrowing of another coronary artery in other areas of the heart.[19]

The last stage in the ECG evolution of an MI is the development of Q waves, the initial downward deflection of the QRS complex. Q waves represent the flow of electrical forces toward the septum. Small, narrow Q waves may be seen in the normal ECG in leads I, II, III, aVR,

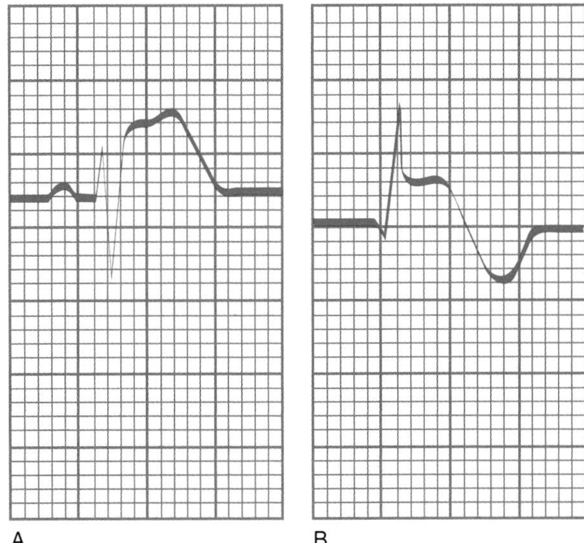

figure 21-8 ST segment pattern consistent with acute myocardial injury. (**A**) ST segment elevation without T-wave inversion. (**B**) ST segment elevation with T-wave inversion. The elevated ST segments have a downward concave or coved shape and merge unnoticed with the T wave.

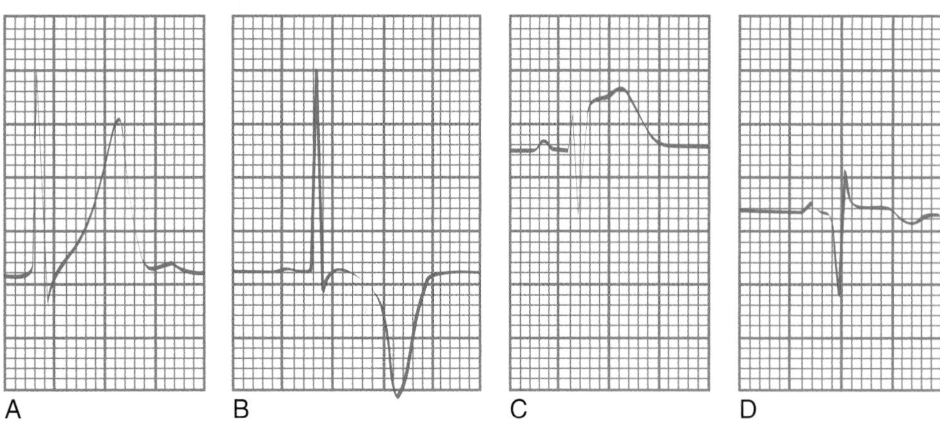

figure 21-9 Evolution of the electrocardiogram in a patient with myocardial infarction. (**A**) Tall peak T waves known as hyperacute T waves; (**B**) symmetrical T wave inversions; (**C**) ST segment elevation; and (**D**) development of the Q wave.

aVL, V_5, and V_6. Q waves compatible with an MI are usually 0.04 second or more in width or one-fourth to one-third the height of the R wave. Q waves indicative of infarction usually develop within several hours of the onset of the infarction, but in some patients may not appear until 24 to 48 hours after the infarction.

Within a few days after the MI, the elevated ST segments return to baseline. Persistent elevation of the ST segment may indicate the presence of a ventricular aneurysm. The T waves may remain inverted for several weeks, indicating areas of ischemia near the infarct region. Eventually, the T waves should return to their upright configuration. The Q waves do not disappear and therefore always provide ECG evidence of a previous MI.

The ECG pattern can be used to distinguish acute MIs from "old" MIs. Abnormal Q waves accompanied by ST segment elevations indicate an acute MI. Abnormal Q waves accompanied by a normal ST segment indicate a previous MI. How long ago the infarction occurred cannot be determined by the ECG. The pattern could signify an infarction that occurred 2 weeks or 20 years before.

The ECG is helpful not only in determining patterns of ischemia, injury, and infarction, but in revealing the anatomical region of the heart where the abnormality has occurred. ECG leads V_1 through V_4 show the anteroseptal wall of the left ventricle. The inferior wall is seen in leads II, III, and aVF. Leads I, aVL, V_5, and V_6 reveal the lateral wall of the left ventricle.

The routine 12-lead ECG does not provide an adequate view of the right ventricle or of the posterior wall of the left ventricle. As a result, additional leads are needed to view these anatomical areas. To attain an accurate view of the right ventricle, right-sided chest leads are recorded by placing the six chest electrodes on the right side of the chest using landmarks analogous to those used on the left side (see Fig. 17-14 in Chapter 17). These six right-sided views are examined for patterns of ischemia, injury, and infarction in the same way left-sided chest leads are evaluated.

Detection of posterior wall abnormalities is also difficult on the standard 12-lead ECG because none of the 6 chest leads provides an adequate view of the posterior wall. To detect posterior wall abnormalities, three of the precordial electrodes are placed posteriorly over the heart, a view known as V_7, V_8, and V_9. V_7 is positioned at the posterior axillary line; V_8 at the posterior scapular line; and V_9 at the left border of the spine. All three posterior leads are positioned along the same horizontal line established by V_6. The recording is examined for evidence of ischemia, injury, or infarction using the same criteria as described previously. If posterior leads were not recorded, it may still be possible to detect posterior wall abnormalities. To do so, the principle of reciprocal change is used. When an infarction in the posterior wall is suspected, the leads anatomically opposite the posterior wall are examined. These include V_1 and V_2 because the anterior wall is anatomically opposite the posterior wall. If tall R waves with ST segment depressions are noted in V_1 and V_2, the pattern is consistent with a posterior wall MI. Figures 21-10 through 21-13 show the 12-lead ECGs of patients with MIs.

Laboratory Tests

When myocardial cells are damaged by an infarction, biochemical markers are released into the bloodstream and can be detected by laboratory tests. The presence of abnormally high levels of biochemical markers, their distribution, and the time pattern for their appearance and disappearance make them very useful in the diagnosis of acute MI. For a more detailed discussion of laboratory tests, see Chapter 17.

Creatine Kinase. Creatine kinase (CK) is an enzyme found mainly in heart and skeletal muscles. When heart muscle is damaged, CK is released into the blood. The level of CK becomes abnormal within 6 to 8 hours after the onset of infarction, peaks within 12 to 28 hours, and returns to normal in 24 to 36 hours. The isoenzymes of CK are measured to determine if the CK came from the heart (MB) or the skeletal muscle. Elevation of CK-MB offers a more definitive indication of myocardial cell damage than total CK alone. For the patient with an MI, CK-MB appears in the serum in 6 to 12 hours, peaks between 12 and 28 hours, and returns to normal levels in about 72 to 96 hours. Serial samplings are performed every 4 to 6 hours for the first 24 to 48 hours after the onset of symptoms.[17]

New assay techniques to measure CK-MB based on monoclonal antibodies offer greater sensitivity and specificity than conventional means. In addition, the results can be available in 30 minutes, which provides a distinct advantage in the diagnosis of a MI, especially in the emergency department.

Creatine Kinase Isoforms. When the myocardial cells release CK-MB, it is quickly transformed into two isoforms,

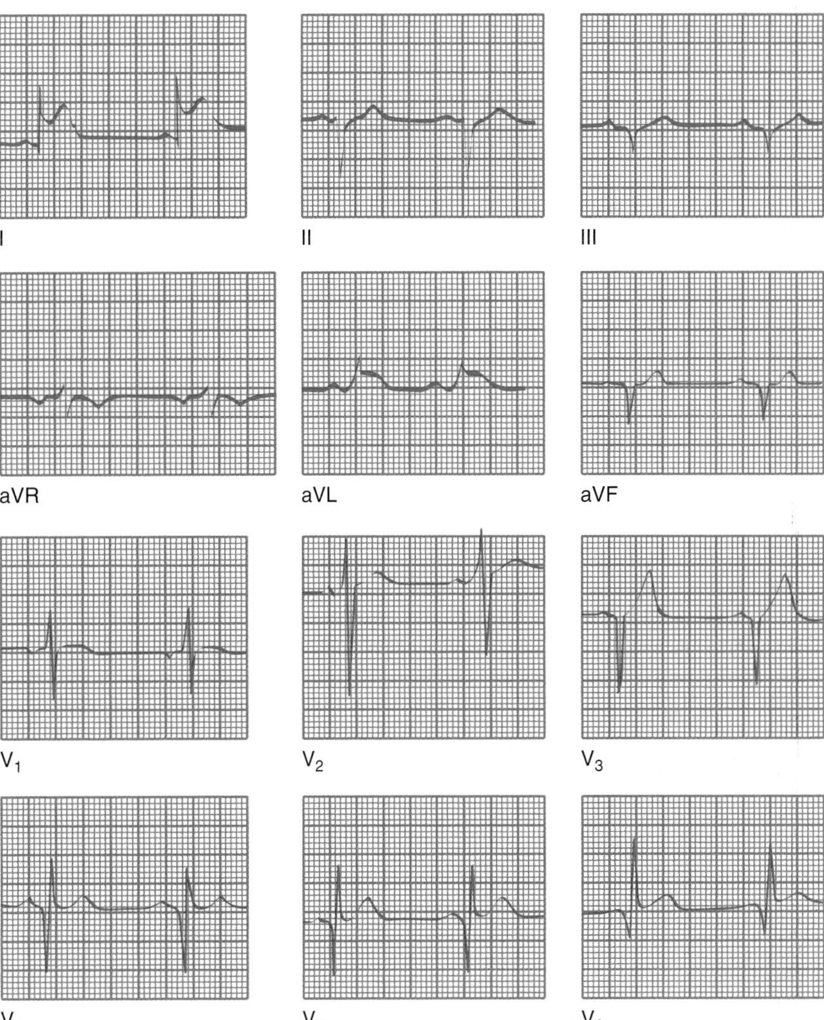

figure 21-10 Twelve-lead ECG showing an acute lateral wall myocardial infarction. ST segment elevations can be seen in leads I, aVL, V_5, and V_6. Note also the deep Q waves in II, III, and aVF and normal ST segments, indicating a previous inferior wall myocardial infarction.

also known as subforms. $CK\text{-}MB_1$ is the isoform found in the plasma, and $CK\text{-}MB_2$ is found in the tissues. In the normal person, these two isoforms are found in about equal amounts, resulting in a ratio of approximately one. In the patient with an MI, the $CK\text{-}MB_2$ level rises, resulting in a $CK\text{-}MB_2$ to $CK\text{-}MB_1$ ratio greater than one. This ratio can be rapidly measured in the laboratory and provides an excellent diagnostic marker for acute MI. The $CK\text{-}MB_2$ to $CK\text{-}MB_1$ ratio has improved sensitivity and specificity for diagnosis of MI within the first 6 hours compared with conventional assays for CK-MB. Isoform $CK\text{-}MB_2$ is also a sensitive test for detecting an early extension of an MI during the first 24 hours.[17]

Myoglobin. Myoglobin is an oxygen-binding protein found in skeletal and cardiac muscle. Myoglobin's release from ischemic muscle occurs earlier than the release of CK. As a result, elevation of serum levels of myoglobin can be detected soon after the onset of symptoms. The myoglobin level can elevate within 1 to 2 hours of acute MI and peaks within 3 to 15 hours. Because myoglobin is also present in skeletal muscle, an elevated myoglobin level is not specific for the diagnosis of MI. Consequently, its diagnostic value in detecting an MI is limited.[17] However, the early release of myoglobin makes it valuable in helping to detect MI. For patients presenting within the first 2 to 3 hours of the onset of symptoms, the two markers that are best to obtain are myoglobin and CK-MB.[9,17]

Troponin. Troponin is a contractile protein with two subforms (troponin T and troponin I) that are highly specific for cardiac muscle. Troponin levels are not detected in the healthy person, and skeletal muscle injury does not affect the level. Troponin has been found to be a sensitive marker during the early hours after an MI. Troponin I levels rise in about 3 hours, peak at 14 to 18 hours, and remain elevated for 5 to 7 days. Troponin T levels rise in 3 to 5 hours and remain elevated for 10 to 14 days.[17] Because the cardiac troponins are detectable in the peripheral circulation 8 to 12 hours after the onset of MI, an initial assay of serum levels of either troponin T or troponin I should be obtained on admission and at least once more in the next 8 to 12 hours.[9,17] Because of the length of time that troponin T and troponin I remain elevated, they are excellent diagnostic markers for patients who present late with symptoms of MI.[9,17]

Management

EARLY MANAGEMENT

When a patient with a possible MI arrives in the emergency department, the diagnosis and initial management of the patient must be rapid because the benefit of reper-

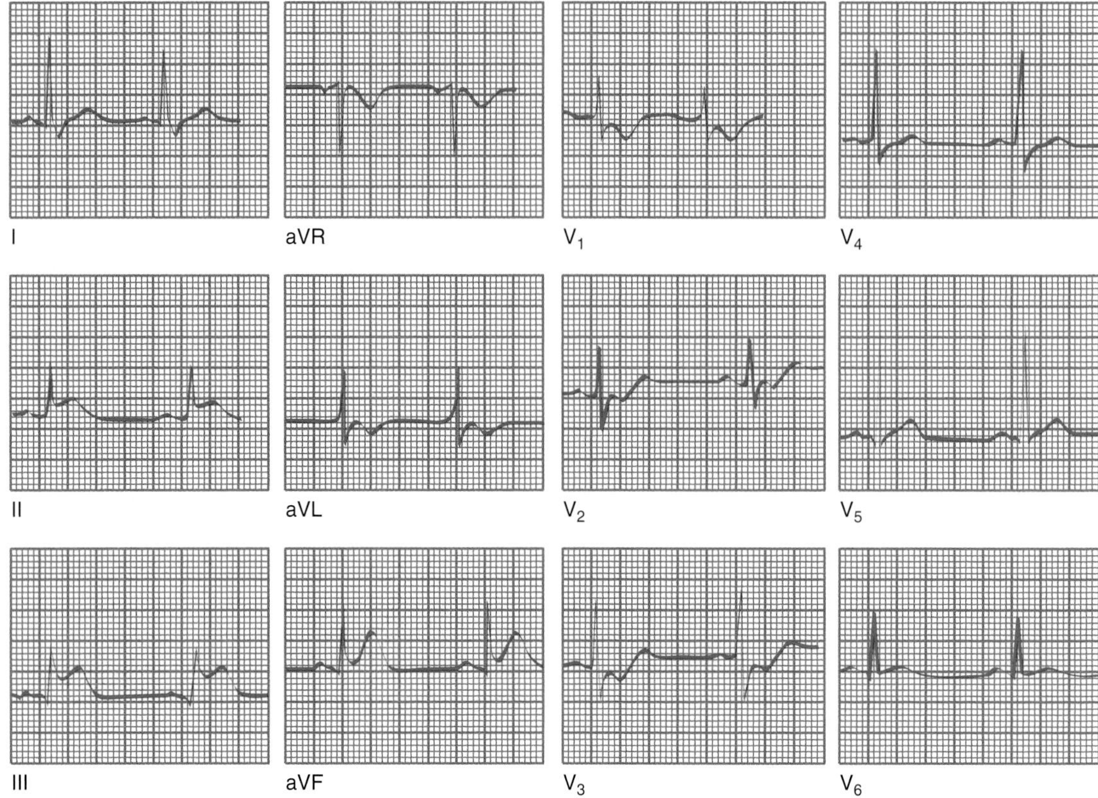

figure 21-11 Twelve-lead ECG showing an acute inferior wall myocardial infarction. Note the ST segment elevations in II, III, and aVF. The posterior wall infarction is evidenced by a tall R wave, ST segment depression, and inverted T wave in V_1 and V_2.

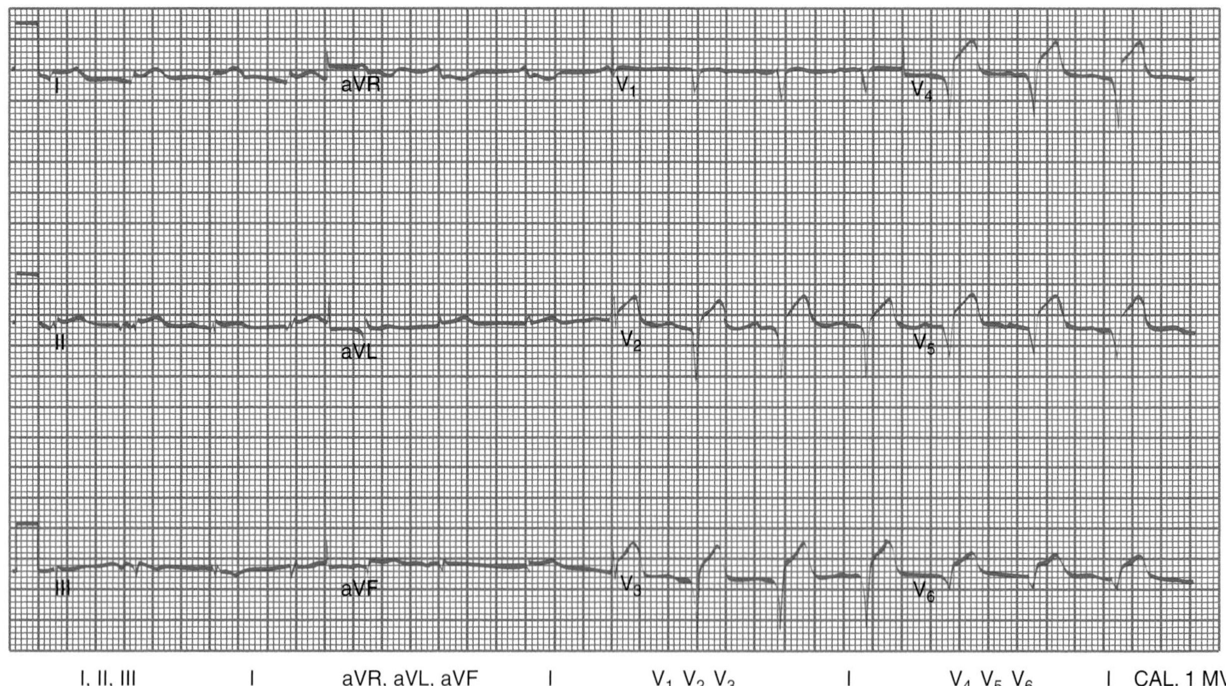

figure 21-12 Twelve-lead ECG showing an acute anterior and lateral wall myocardial infarction. Note the ST segment elevations and Q waves in I, aVL, V_5, and V_6 (lateral), and V_2, V_3, and V_4 (anterior).

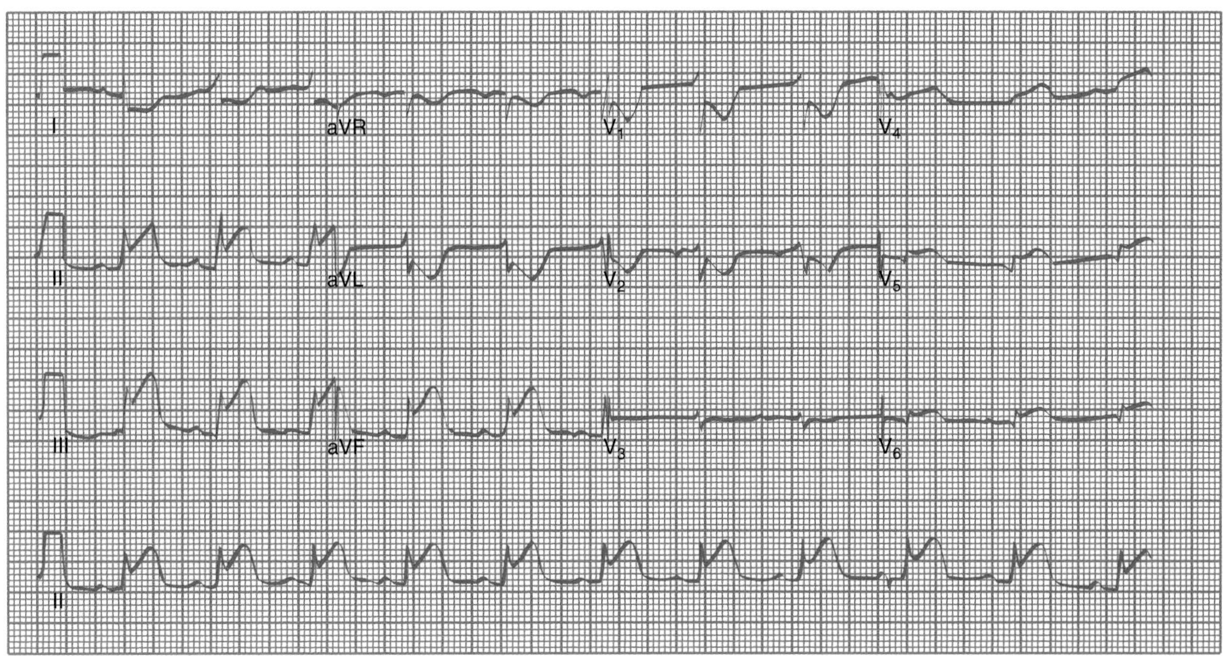

figure 21-13 Twelve-lead ECG showing right ventricular infarction. The six chest leads have been positioned on the right side of the chest. Note the ST segment elevation in RV_4, RV_5, and RV_6. The ECG also shows elevated ST segments in the inferior leads (II, III, aVF). Patients with an inferior wall MI often also have an infarction in the right ventricle.

fusion therapy is greatest if therapy is initiated quickly. An initial evaluation of the patient should occur ideally within the first 10 minutes after arrival, but certainly within the first 20 minutes.[17] The patient's history and 12-lead ECG are the primary methods used to determine initially the diagnosis of MI. The ECG is examined for the presence of ST segment elevations of 1 mm or greater in contiguous leads. This pattern provides evidence of thrombotic coronary arterial occlusion.

If the initial screening suggests an MI, the interventions listed in Box 21-6 are initiated. The nurse checks the vital signs frequently, establishes IV access, and continuously assesses the patient's cardiac rhythm. Blood is drawn for serum cardiac markers, hematology, chemistry, and lipid profile. A chest x-ray and echocardiogram, obtained as soon as possible, are useful in ruling out an aortic dissection and acute pericarditis. During the initial evaluation, the patient and family may be anxious, necessitating brief and clear explanations of the interventions. Reassurance and support are essential components of the nurse's responsibilities.

Thrombolytic Therapy

If the patient is diagnosed with an MI, thrombolytic therapy may be used to establish reperfusion if there are no contraindications to its use. Thrombolytic drugs lyse coronary thrombi by converting plasminogen to plasmin. This conversion causes the degradation of fibrin and fibrinogen, resulting in clot lysis. Box 21-7 lists contraindications to thrombolytic therapy.[17]

The goal is to complete the assessment of the patient and the administration of the thrombolytic drug (if indicated) within 30 minutes of the patient's arrival to the emergency department. Thrombolytic therapy provides maximal benefit if given within the first 3 hours after the onset of symptoms. Significant benefit still occurs if therapy is given up to 12 hours after onset of symptoms. Minimal benefit is realized, however, if thrombolytics are given more than 12 hours after the onset of symptoms. In addition to the thrombolytic agent, the patient should receive heparin and aspirin.[17]

For the patient receiving thrombolytic therapy, two to three 18-gauge peripheral IV lines are usually started. One line is for the thrombolytic, and one to two lines are for the administration of other drugs. Subclavian and jugular sites are avoided because they are noncompressible, and blood could be lost into the chest or neck. Some type of blood sampling device is also inserted so that peripheral venous punctures can be avoided.

The patient is closely monitored during and after the infusion of a thrombolytic agent. The nurse assesses the patient for resolution of chest pain, normalization of elevated ST segments, development of reperfusion dysrhythmias, any allergic reactions, evidence of bleeding, and the onset of hypotension. Commonly seen reperfusion dysrhythmias include an accelerated idioventricular rhythm, ventricular tachycardia, and AV heart block.

Evaluation of complications remains a key nursing intervention. The patient is closely monitored for evidence of reocclusion of the coronary artery. Indicators of reocclusion include chest pain, ST segment elevation, and hemodynamic instability. Close observation for evidence of bleeding also is essential. The patient is carefully assessed for indications of subcutaneous or mucous membrane bleeding. The nurse also monitors the patient for signs of internal bleeding, including positive results of urine and stool for blood or altered levels of consciousness due to intracranial bleeding.

box 21-6
Initial Management of the Patient With a Suspected Myocardial Infarction

Action: Administer aspirin, 160 to 325 mg chewed.
Rationale: Aspirin is used because it diminishes platelet aggregation. This effect is important because platelets are one of the main components in thrombus formation when a coronary plaque is disrupted. Aspirin has been shown to reduce mortality rates independently in patients with acute myocardial infarction. Patients diagnosed with a myocardial infarction should be continued on aspirin indefinitely.

Action: After recording the initial 12-lead ECG, place the patient on a cardiac monitor and obtain serial ECGs.
Rationale: The 12-lead ECG is central in the decision pathway for the diagnosis and treatment of the patient. The patient is placed on a continuous cardiac monitor after the 12-lead ECG is recorded to detect dysrhythmias and to monitor ST segment changes.

Action: Give oxygen by nasal cannula.
Rationale: Hypoxemia often occurs in patients with a myocardial infarction because of pulmonary edema. If severe pulmonary edema is present and the patient is in respiratory distress, intubation may be necessary. A pulse oximeter is often applied, and, when time permits, an arterial blood gas may be drawn.

Action: Administer sublingual nitroglycerin (unless the systolic blood pressure is less than 90 mm Hg or the heart rate is less than 50 or greater than 100 beats/minute).
Rationale: Nitroglycerin helps to promote vasodilation but is relatively ineffective in relieving pain in the early stages of a myocardial infarction. Intravenous nitroglycerin is recommended for the first 24 to 48 hours for patients with acute myocardial infarction and heart failure, large anterior wall infarctions, persistent ischemia, or hypertension.

Action: Provide adequate analgesia with morphine sulfate.
Rationale: Morphine is the drug of choice to relieve the pain of a myocardial infarction. The drug is given intravenously in small doses (2–4 mg) and can be repeated every 5 minutes until the pain is relieved. Close respiratory monitoring is indicated because morphine can depress respirations.

Adapted from Ryan TJ, Anderson JL, Antman EM, et al: ACC/AHA guidelines for the management of patients with acute myocardial infarction: A report of the American College of Cardiology/American Heart Association Task Force on Practice Guidelines (Committee on Management of Acute Myocardial Infarction), 1999. Available at http://www.americanheart.org.

box 21-7
Contraindications to Thrombolytic Therapy

Contraindications

- Previous hemorrhagic stroke at any time; other stokes or cerebrovascular events within 1 year
- Known intracranial neoplasm
- Active internal bleeding (does not include menses)
- Suspected aortic dissection

Cautions/Relative Contraindications

- Severe uncontrolled hypertension on presentation (blood pressure >180/110 mm Hg)
- History of prior cerebrovascular accident or known intracerebral disease not covered in contraindications
- Current use of anticoagulants in therapeutic doses (international normalized ratio [INR] ≥2:3); known bleeding diathesis
- Recent trauma (within 2–4 weeks), including head trauma or traumatic or prolonged (>10 minutes) cardiopulmonary resuscitation (CPR) or major surgery (<3 weeks)
- Noncompressible vascular punctures
- Recent (within 2–4 weeks) internal bleeding
- For streptokinase/anistreplase: prior exposure (especially within 5 days to 2 years) or prior allergic reaction
- Pregnancy
- Active peptic ulcer
- History of chronic severe hypertension

From Ryan TJ, Anderson JL, Antman EM, Brooks NH, et al: ACC/AHA guidelines for the management of patients with acute myocardial infarction: A report of the American College of Cardiology/American Heart Association Task Force on Practice Guidelines (Committee on Management of Acute Myocardial Infarction), p 40, 1999. Available at http://www.americanheart.org.

Primary Percutaneous Transluminal Coronary Angioplasty

Early reperfusion of myocardial tissue is essential to preserve myocardial function. In addition to pharmacological therapy, primary percutaneous transluminal coronary angioplasty (PTCA) is an effective alternative to reestablish blood flow to ischemic myocardium. Primary PTCA is an invasive procedure in which the infarct-related coronary artery is dilated during the acute phase of an MI without prior administration of thrombolytic agents. Primary PTCA is used for patients who present within 12 hours of the onset of symptoms; PTCA also can be done for patients whose ischemic symptoms persist.[17] This therapeutic intervention necessitates the availability of a cardiac catheterization laboratory and skilled personnel at all times. (See Chapter 18 for a more detailed discussion of the PTCA procedure.)

Evaluation of patients for primary PTCA is similar to that of thrombolytic therapy. The accessibility of the lesion in the coronary artery is an additional factor that must be considered. Primary PTCA may be an excellent reperfusion alternative for patients ineligible for thrombolytic therapy. The nurse must carefully monitor the patient after a primary PTCA for evidence of complications. These complications can include retroperitoneal or vascular hemorrhage, other evidence of bleeding, early acute reocclusion, and late restenosis.

INTENSIVE AND INTERMEDIATE CARE MANAGEMENT

The management goal for the patient in the intensive care unit and intermediate care unit continues to be maximizing cardiac output while carefully minimizing cardiac workload. To achieve this goal, the patient will have frequent vital signs taken and continue on a cardiac monitor with ST segment monitoring. The lead selected for monitoring should be based on the infarct location and underlying rhythm. Serial ECGs and serial evaluations of serum cardiac markers of infarction are recorded. Serum hematology and chemistry are monitored.

For the first 12 hours of hospitalization, patients who are hemodynamically stable and free of ischemic-type chest discomfort remain on bed rest with bedside commode privileges. Activity level increases gradually in hemodynamically stable patients. Careful attention is paid to maximal pain relief. Nitroglycerin is not an appropriate substitute for analgesics. A pulse oximeter is used to monitor oxygen saturation continuously and is a good indicator of early hypoxemia.

The patient is often not given anything by mouth until pain free. When pain free, the patient is given clear liquids and progressed to a heart-healthy diet as tolerated. Daily weights are recorded and intake and output are measured to detect fluid retention. Stools softeners are administered so that the patient avoids a Valsalva maneuver. During a Valsalva maneuver, forced expiration against a closed glottis causes sudden and significant changes in systolic blood pressure and heart rate. These changes may influence regional endocardial repolarization and place the patient at risk for ventricular dysrhythmias.[17] Nursing diagnoses and collaborative care problems for patients with acute MI are listed in Box 21-8.

Pharmacological Therapy

Prophylactic antidysrhythmics during the first 24 hours of hospitalization are not recommended. However, easy access to atropine, lidocaine, amiodarone, transcutaneous pacing patches, transvenous pacing wires, a defibrillator, and epinephrine are essential for management of dysrhythmias. IV nitroglycerin is continued for 24 to 48 hours. Daily aspirin is continued on an indefinite basis. Clopidogrel may be used for patients who are intolerant of aspirin.[9,17]

IV beta blocker therapy should be administered within the initial hours of the evolving infarction, followed by oral therapy provided there are no contraindications. Beta blockers are one of the few pharmacological agents that have been shown to reduce morbidity and mortality in the patient with an MI. They reduce oxygen demand by decreasing the heart rate and contractility. They also increase coronary artery filling by prolonging diastole. Calcium channel blockers may be given to patients in whom beta blocker therapy is ineffective or contraindicated.[17]

Angiotensin-converting enzyme (ACE) inhibitors are administered to patients with anterior wall MI and to patients who have an MI with heart failure in the absence of significant hypotension. ACE inhibitors help prevent ventricular remodeling (dilation) and preserve ejection fraction.[17]

Heparin is given to patients undergoing percutaneous or surgical revascularization and for those receiving thrombolytic therapy with alteplase. Low-molecular-weight heparin should be used for patients with non–Q-wave MI.[9,17]

box 21-8 ***Examples of Nursing Diagnoses and Collaborative Problems for Patients With Acute Myocardial Infarction***

- Chest Pain related to myocardial infarction, angina
- Decreased Cardiac Output: Electrical factors affecting rate, rhythm, or conduction
- Decreased Cardiac Output: Mechanical factors related to preload, afterload, or left ventricular failure
- Knowledge Deficit related to illness and impact on patient's future
- Anxiety, stress related to fear of illness, death, and critical care environment
- Activity Intolerance related to decreased cardiac output or alterations in myocardial tissue perfusion
- Risk for Ineffective Tissue Perfusion related to thrombolytic therapy impact on myocardial tissue

Hemodynamic Monitoring

Use of a pulmonary artery catheter for hemodynamic monitoring is indicated in the patient with MI who has severe or progressive congestive heart failure or pulmonary edema, cardiogenic shock, progressive hypotension, or suspected mechanical complications, such as ventricular septal defect, papillary muscle rupture, or pericardial tamponade.[17] The pulmonary artery wedge pressure (PAWP) is closely followed for assessment of left ventricular filling pressures. A PAWP below 18 mm Hg may indicate volume depletion, whereas a PAWP greater than 18 mm Hg indicates pulmonary congestion or cardiogenic shock. Using the thermodilution technique, frequent measurements of cardiac output and cardiac index can be made to evaluate hemodynamic status further. In some situations, monitoring venous oxygen saturation may also be useful. For a more detailed discussion of hemodynamic monitoring, see Chapter 17.

Invasive arterial monitoring is indicated for patients with MI who have severe hypotension or for those receiving vasopressor or vasodilator drugs. The collaborative care guide for the patient with an MI (Box 21-9) provides further information about the care of these patients.

Additional Diagnostic Tests

Radionuclide Imaging. The patient may undergo further diagnostic tests to assess cardiac structure and functions. Radionuclide studies provide information about the presence of coronary artery disease as well as the location and quantity of ischemic and infracted myocardium. A radioactive tracer is injected into the patient and a gamma camera is used to record images.

One agent, thallium-201, is often used because it accumulates rapidly in viable myocardial cells. When myocardial perfusion is normal, the radioactive substance is distributed equally throughout the myocardium. If coronary blood flow is significantly reduced, thallium fails to accumulate in the tissue and forms an area known as a "cold spot" or perfusion defect.[17]

Some tracers, such as technetium pyrophosphate, are taken up by necrotic tissue and form an area known as a "hot spot" on the image. This hot spot image aids in locat-

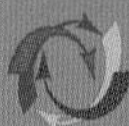

box 21-9 collaborative care guide *for the Patient With Myocardial Infarction*

OUTCOMES	INTERVENTIONS
Oxygenation/Ventilation	
Patient has arterial blood gases within normal limits and pulse oximeter value >90%.	▪ Assess respiratory rate, effort, and breath sounds q2–4h. ▪ Obtain arterial blood gases per order or signs of respiratory distress. ▪ Monitor arterial saturation by pulse oximeter. ▪ Provide supplemental oxygen by nasal cannula or face mask for the first 6 h, then as needed. ▪ Provide intubation and mechanical ventilation as necessary. (Refer to Chapter 25, Mechanical Ventilation Care Guide.)
There is no evidence of pulmonary edema on chest x-ray and by clear breath sounds.	▪ Obtain chest x-ray qd. ▪ Administer diuretics per order. ▪ Monitor signs of fluid overload as described below.
There is no evidence of atelectasis.	▪ Encourage nonintubated patients to use incentive spirometer, cough, and deep breath q4h and PRN. ▪ While on bed rest, turn side to side q2h.
Circulation/Perfusion	
Vital signs are within normal limits, including MAP >70 mm Hg and cardiac index >2.2 L/min/m^2.	▪ Monitor HR and BP q1–2h and PRN during acute failure phase. ▪ Assist with pulmonary artery catheter insertion. ▪ Monitor PAP and PAWP, CVP, or right atrial pressure (RAP) q1h and cardiac output, SVR, and PVR q6–12h if pulmonary artery catheter is in place. ▪ Maintain patent IV access. ▪ Administer positive inotropic agents, and reduce afterload with vasodilating agents guided by hemodynamic parameters and physician orders. ▪ Evaluate effect of medications on BP, HR, and hemodynamic parameters. ▪ Prepare patient for intra-aortic balloon pump assist if necessary.
Patient has no evidence of congestive heart failure due to decreased cardiac output.	▪ Restrict volume administration as indicated by PAWP or CVP values. ▪ Assess for neck vein distension, pulmonary crackles, S_3 or S_4, peripheral edema, increased preload parameters, elevated "a" wave of CVP, RAP, or PAWP waveform. ▪ Monitor 12-lead ECG qd and PRN.
Patient has no evidence of further myocardial dysfunction, such as altered ECG or cardiac enzymes.	▪ Monitor cardiac markers, magnesium, phosphorus, calcium, and potassium as ordered. ▪ Monitor ECG for changes consistent with evolving MI. ▪ Consider obtaining right precordial chest leads, 12-lead ECG, if inferior wall/right ventricle is involved. ▪ Report and treat abnormalities per protocols or orders.
Dysrhythmias are controlled.	▪ Provide continuous ECG monitoring in the appropriate lead. ▪ Document rhythm strips every shift. ▪ Anticipate need for/administer pharmacological agents to control dysrhythmias.
After thrombolytic therapy, patient will have relief of pain; no evidence of bleeding; no evidence of allergic reaction.	▪ Assess, monitor, and treat pain as described below. ▪ Monitor signs of reperfusion, such as dysrhythmias, ST segment return to baseline, early rise and peak in CK. ▪ Monitor for signs of bleeding, including neurological, GI, and GU assessment. ▪ Monitor PT, aPTT, ACT per protocol.

(continued)

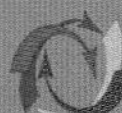

box 21-9 collaborative care guide
for the Patient With Myocardial Infarction (Continued)

OUTCOMES	INTERVENTIONS
	■ Have anticoagulant antidotes available. ■ Assess for itching, hives, sudden onset of hypotension or tachycardia. ■ Administer hydrocortisone or diphenhydramine (Benadryl) per protocol.
There is no evidence of cardiogenic shock, cardiac valve dysfunction, or ventricular septal defect.	■ Monitor ECG, heart sounds, hemodynamic parameters, level of consciousness, and breath sounds for changes. ■ Report and treat deleterious changes as indicated.
Fluids/Electrolytes	
Renal function is maintained as evidenced by urine output >30 mL/h, normal laboratory values.	■ Monitor intake and output q1–2h. ■ Monitor BUN, creatinine, electrolytes qd and PRN. Take daily weights. ■ Administer fluid volume and diuretics as ordered.
Mobility/Safety	
Patient will comply with ADL limitations.	■ Provide clear explanation of limitations. ■ Provide bed rest with bed side commode privileges first 6 h. ■ Progress to chair for meals, bathing self, bathroom privileges. Continually assess patient response to all activities.
Patient will not fall or accidentally harm self.	■ Provide environment to prevent falls, bruising, or injury. ■ Use self-protective devices as indicated and per hospital policy.
Skin Integrity	
Patient has no evidence of skin breakdown.	■ Turn side to side q2h while patient is on bed rest. ■ Evaluate skin for signs of pressure areas when turning. ■ Consider pressure relief/reduction mattress for high-risk patients. ■ Use Braden Scale to monitor risk of skin breakdown.
Nutrition	
Caloric and nutrient intake meet metabolic requirements per calculation (e.g., basal energy expenditure).	■ Provide appropriate diet: oral, parenteral, or enteral feeding. ■ Provide clear or full liquids the first 24 hours. ■ Restrict sodium, fat, cholesterol, fluid, and calories if indicated. ■ Consult dietitian or nutritional support services.
Patient has normal laboratory values reflective of nutritional status.	■ Monitor albumin, prealbumin, transferrin, cholesterol, triglycerides, total protein.
Comfort/Pain Control	
Patient has relief of chest pain. There is no evidence of pain, such as increased HR, BP, RR, or agitation during activity or procedures.	■ Use visual analog scale to assess pain quantity. ■ Assess quality, duration, location of pain. ■ Administer IV morphine sulfate, and monitor pain and hemodynamic response. ■ Administer analgesics appropriately for chest pain and assess response. ■ Monitor physiological response to pain during procedures or after administration of pain medication. ■ Provide a calm, quiet environment.
Psychosocial	
Patient demonstrates decreased anxiety by calm demeanor and vital signs during, for example, procedures, discussions.	■ Assess vital signs during treatments, discussions, and so forth. ■ Provide explanations and stable reassurance in calm and caring manner. ■ Cautiously administer sedatives and monitor response.

(continued)

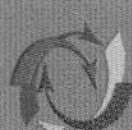

box 21-9 collaborative care guide
for the Patient With Myocardial Infarction (Continued)

OUTCOMES	INTERVENTIONS
Patient/family demonstrate understanding of MI and treatment plan by asking questions and participating in care.	■ Consult social services and clergy as appropriate. ■ Assess coping mechanism history. ■ Allow free expression of feelings. ■ Encourage patient/family participation in care as soon as feasible. ■ Provide blocks of time for adequate rest and sleep.
Teaching/Discharge Planning	
Patient reports occurrence of chest pain or discomfort.	■ Explain importance of reporting all episodes of chest pain.
Family demonstrates appropriate coping during the critical phase of an acute MI.	■ Provide frequent explanations and information to family. ■ Encourage family to ask questions regarding treatment plan, patient response to therapy, prognosis, and so forth.
In preparation for discharge to home, patient understands activity levels, dietary restrictions, medication regimen, what to do if pain recurs.	■ Make appropriate referrals and consults early during hospitalization. ■ Initiate family education regarding heart-healthy diet, cardiac rehabilitation program, stress-reduction strategies, management of chest pain, after crisis phase has passed.

ing the infarction and in determining its size. Hot spot imaging may be especially useful for the diagnosis of MI in patients who present to the hospital several days after the onset of their pain when their cardiac serum markers have returned to normal.[17] (See Chapter 17 for further discussion of radionuclide imaging.)

Echocardiogram. An echocardiogram is a noninvasive ultrasonographic test involving the transmission of high-frequency sound waves into the heart. This commonly used diagnostic test helps determine ejection fraction, segmental wall motion, systolic and diastolic ventricular volumes, valve function, mural thrombi, pericardial fluid, intracardiac tumors, and aortic dissection.[17] Two-dimensional, Doppler, and transesophageal echocardiograms are the most frequently used types of echocardiograms for patients with an MI. (See Chapter 17 for further discussion of echocardiograms.)

Stress Test. Stress testing, also known as exercise electrocardiography, may be performed before discharge or within the first 3 weeks after discharge. The test is intended to assess the patient's functional capacity and ability to perform activities of daily living, to evaluate the efficacy of the patient's medical therapy, and to risk-stratify the patient based on the likelihood of a subsequent cardiac event. Stress testing may be combined with perfusion imaging to determine better the size of the infarction.[17] (See Chapter 17 for further discussion of stress testing.)

Coronary Angiography. During the course of hospitalization, patients may be further evaluated by coronary angiography. Results of the angiography help the physician determine if a PTCA or placement of a stent is indicated, or if the patient is a candidate for coronary artery bypass grafting surgery (CABG). (A more detailed discussion of PTCA can be found in Chapter 18, and a more detailed discussion of CABG can be found in Chapter 22.)

Complications

The nurse closely monitors the patient with MI for evidence of complications. Numerous complications can occur, and a list of possible complications is provided in Box 21-10. Prompt recognition and management of complications are essential in reducing mortality and morbidity.

VASCULAR COMPLICATIONS

Recurrent myocardial ischemia occurs in about 15% to 20% of patients and is often transient.[20] A recurrent MI is another possible complication. If the reinfarction occurs within the first 24 hours, it may be hard to diagnose because the cardiac serum markers have not yet returned to baseline. Early recognition and management are essential for both of these vascular complications. Efforts are made to lower myocardial oxygen demand, to relieve pain. Emergent PTCA or surgical revascularization may be considered.[18]

MYOCARDIAL COMPLICATIONS

Cardiogenic shock is the most serious myocardial complication of MI. Cardiogenic shock occurs because of the loss of contractile forces in the heart. Cardiogenic shock develops in about 5% to 15% of hospitalized patients after an MI, and it is most likely to occur when necrosis involves 40% or more of the left ventricle.[21] Cardiogenic shock is the most common cause of in-hospital death for patients with MI, with a mortality rate of nearly 80%.[18] (For a more detailed discussion of cardiogenic shock, see Chapter 50.)

box 21-10
Complications of Acute Myocardial Infarction

Vascular Complications
- Recurrent ischemia
- Recurrent infarction

Myocardial Complications
- Diastolic dysfunction
- Systolic dysfunction
- Congestive heart failure
- Hypotension/cardiogenic shock
- Right ventricular infarction
- Ventricular cavity dilation
- Aneurysm formation (true, false)

Mechanical Complications
- Left ventricular free wall rupture
- Ventricular septal rupture
- Papillary muscle rupture with acute mitral regurgitation

Pericardial Complications
- Pericarditis
- Dressler's syndrome
- Pericardial effusion

Thromboembolic Complications
- Mural thrombosis
- Systemic thromboembolism
- Deep venous thrombosis
- Pulmonary embolism

Electrical Complications
- Ventricular tachycardia
- Ventricular fibrillation
- Supraventricular tachydysrhythmias
- Bradydysrhythmias
- Atrioventricular block (first, second, or third degree)

From Becker RC: Complicated myocardial infarction. Crit Pathways Cardiol 2(2):125–152, 2003.

insights into clinical research

Cherrington CC, Moser DK, Lennie TA, et al: Illness representation after acute myocardial infarction: Impact of in-hospital recovery. Am J Crit Care 13(2):136–145, 2004.

Heart disease remains the leading cause of death in the United States, and about 1.1 million persons have an acute myocardial infarction (MI) each year. The role of psychosocial factors in the recovery from MI has been investigated and anxiety and depression have been shown to influence a patient's recovery. The purpose of this study was to examine the relationship between illness representation of myocardial infarction and the occurrence of in-hospital complications, and whether anxiety and depression mediate this relationship. The self-regulation model of illness was the theoretical model that guided the study. According to the model, when patients encounter health-threatening illnesses, they form a representation of the illness.

The investigators used a prospective correlational design to measure illness representation, anxiety, and depression 24 to 48 hours after admission to the hospital for a diagnosis of acute MI and to ascertain the frequency of complications. The sample comprised 40 patients with a mean age of 60.8 years. Data were analyzed using logistic regression to determine the likelihood of experiencing a complication. Results of the study indicated that the more negative the representation of the illness, the greater were the odds of experiencing a complication, when demographic and clinical variables were controlled. The researchers concluded that the illness representation was predictive of the likelihood of experiencing a complication after MI.

Clinical manifestations of cardiogenic shock include a rapid, thready pulse; a narrow pulse pressure; dyspnea; tachypnea; inspiratory crackles; distended neck veins; chest pain; cool, moist skin; oliguria; and decreased mentation. Arterial blood gas analysis reveals a decreased PaO_2 and respiratory alkalosis. Hemodynamic findings include a systolic blood pressure less than 85 mm Hg, a mean arterial blood pressure less than 65 mm Hg, a cardiac index less than 2.2 L/minute/m^2, and a PAWP greater than 18 mm Hg. Cardiac enzymes may show an additional rise or a delay in reaching peak values.

The goal of treatment for cardiogenic shock is to minimize myocardial workload and maximize myocardial oxygen delivery. Immediate actions must be taken to improve tissue perfusion and preserve viable myocardium. To improve oxygenation, supplemental oxygen is given to the patient and, if necessary, the patient may be intubated and placed on a mechanical ventilator. Efforts are aimed toward restoring blood pressure. This may require discontinuation of vasodilator drugs and drugs with negative inotropic effects. An IV dopamine drip may be initiated to improve the patient's blood pressure and improve myocardial contractility. Dobutamine may be used to improve contractility, especially in low cardiac output states. Nitroprusside, a vasodilator, may be used with a vasopressor to improve cardiac output by decreasing peripheral vascular resistance and reducing left ventricular preload. Treatment may also require the use of an intra-aortic balloon pump (IABP). This invasive device helps improve coronary artery perfusion and decrease left ventricular afterload. (For a more detailed discussion of IABP therapy, see Chapter 18.)

MECHANICAL COMPLICATIONS

The most catastrophic mechanical complications of MI are intraventricular septal rupture and left ventricular free wall rupture. These clinical situations develop rapidly and result in almost immediate physiological deterioration.

Ventricular Septal Wall Rupture

Ventricular septal rupture occurs in about 2% to 4% of patients with a MI and accounts for approximately 15% of all in-hospital deaths.[18] The greatest risk for ventricular septal wall rupture is within the first 24 hours and continues for up to 5 days.[18] The patient presents with a new, loud, holosystolic murmur associated with a thrill felt in the parasternal area. In addition, the patient has progressive dyspnea, tachycardia, and pulmonary congestion. Oxygen samples taken from the right atrium, right ventricle, and pulmonary artery show a higher PaO_2 in the right ventricle than in the right atrium because the oxygenated left ventricular blood is shunted to the right ventricle. This testing can be accomplished during pulmonary artery catheterization. Urgent cardiac catheterization and surgical correction are needed. The patient can be supported with fluid administration, inotropic support (dopamine and dobutamine), afterload reduction (nitroprusside), and IABP counterpulsation until emergency surgery is possible. Some fibrosis of the tissue is needed for suturing. Often it is impossible to maintain the patient medically until this occurs.

Left Ventricular Free Wall Rupture

Left ventricular free wall rupture occurs in about 1% to 2% of patients with MI and accounts for approximately 10% to 15% of in-hospital deaths.[18] It occurs more frequently than rupture of the intraventricular septum or the papillary muscle. Left ventricular free wall rupture is more likely to occur in patients older than 70 years of age, women, hypertensive patients, and patients with their first MI. The patient experiences prolonged chest pain, dyspnea, sudden hypotension, jugular venous distension, tamponade, and ECG evidence of electrical–mechanical dissociation. This event occurs so suddenly and with such severity that lifesaving efforts are often futile.

PERICARDIAL COMPLICATION

Pericarditis is common after MI and is most likely to occur during the 48- to 72-hour postinfarction period. The patient reports chest pain that may be confused with ischemic pain. The precordial pain of pericarditis intensifies with deep breathing, coughing, swallowing, and lying flat. The pain is lessened when the patient sits up and leans forward. The patient may have a fever, usually less than 38.6°C, that lasts for several days. On auscultation, a friction rub often can be heard along the left sternal border. Some friction rubs are transient; therefore, the absence of such a rub is not conclusive. The ECG often shows concave upward ST segment elevation on five or more leads. Anti-inflammatory agents, such as aspirin, indomethacin, and corticosteroids, are given in usual doses for 7 to 14 days.[18]

THROMBOEMBOLIC COMPLICATIONS

Thromboembolisms occur in about 5% to 10% of patients with MI. These patients are often predisposed to deep venous thrombosis (DVT) because of the systemic inflammatory response associated with infarction, immobility, venous stasis, and reduced cardiac output. Pulmonary embolism develops in about 10% to 15% of patients with DVT. After MI, patients are also at risk for systemic emboli that usually originate in the wall of the left ventricle. These emboli can occlude the cerebral, renal, mesenteric, or iliofemoral artery. Patients are systemically anticoagulated with unfractionated or low–molecular-weight heparin followed by warfarin (Coumadin) for 6 to 12 months.[18]

ELECTRICAL COMPLICATIONS

Cardiac dysrhythmias and conduction disturbances often accompany acute MIs and can be life-threatening. The causes of electrical complications are many and include myocardial ischemia, myocardial necrosis, altered autonomic tone, electrolyte imbalances, acid–base disturbances, and adverse drug effects.[18]

Cardiac Dysrhythmias

Ventricular dysrhythmias that occur in the prehospital phase cause the majority of sudden cardiac deaths. Ischemic myocardium has a lower fibrillatory threshold, and few ventricular dysrhythmias are considered benign after an infarct. Patients may experience tachydysrhythmias or bradydysrhythmias during the hospital phase of treatment. Supraventricular rhythms may be the result of high left atrial pressures caused by left ventricular failure.

Conduction Disturbances

Conduction disturbances after MI can include those caused by SA node, AV node, or ventricular conducting tissue abnormalities. The right coronary artery supplies the SA node in about half of all patients and the left circumflex coronary artery supplies the SA node in the other half. Because the right coronary artery is also the source of oxygenated blood for the inferior, right posterior, and right ventricular walls, patients with inferior, right posterior, or right ventricular wall MIs are at risk for conduction disturbances resulting from poor SA node functioning. Patients with lateral wall MIs also are at risk for SA nodal conduction disturbances because the left circumflex vessel supplies the lateral wall of the heart.

The right coronary artery also is the source of oxygenated blood for the AV node in about 90% of people. Therefore, patients with inferior, right posterior, or right ventricular wall infarctions due to right coronary artery occlusion are at risk for AV nodal conduction disturbances. First-degree heart block and Mobitz type I (Wenckebach) block may appear, but often are transient. These rhythm disturbances may progress to complete heart block and require pacing therapy.

The LAD coronary artery is the primary source of blood supply to the bundle of His and bundle branches. Therefore, patients with an anterior wall MI caused by an LAD occlusion are at risk of ventricular conduction defects. Conduction defects, such as right bundle branch block, left bundle branch block, anterior fascicular block, posterior fascicular block, bifascicular block, or trifascicular block, may occur.

For patients with MI, the nurse continuously monitors the cardiac rate and rhythm, assesses the apical and peripheral pulses, auscultates the heart, and monitors blood pressure and other indicators of hemodynamics such as urine output and level of consciousness. The goals of therapy for cardiac dysrhythmias and conduction disturbances are to restore normal rate, rhythm, and AV synchrony, and to maintain adequate cardiac output. To achieve these goals, pharmacological therapy may be indicated. Cardioversion may be used to treat patients with supraventricular dysrhythmias such as atrial fibrillation or atrial flutter. Transcutaneous pacing may be indicated in an emergent situation for heart block dysrhythmias until a transvenous temporary pacemaker can be initiated. The patient may require permanent pacemaker implantation to maintain an adequate rate and rhythm. Some patients may require an implantable cardioverter–defibrillator to manage ventricular dysrhythmias. (For a more detailed discussion of pacemakers and implanted cardioverter–defibrillators, see Chapter 18.)

Cardiac Rehabilitation

Preparation for discharge must begin early in the patient's course of hospitalization. Patient and family education is an essential component of the process. A severely compromised, critically ill patient may lack the ability to process and retain new information but usually is motivated to learn after the life-threatening event. Guidelines for patient and family education after an acute MI are described in Table 21-2.

Cardiac rehabilitation is recommended for most patients after an MI. Cardiac rehabilitation involves a combination of prescribed exercise, education, and counseling. The goals of cardiac rehabilitation are to limit the adverse physiological and psychological effects of heart disease, modify risk factors, reduce the risk of sudden death or reinfarction, control cardiac symptoms, stabilize or reverse the atherosclerotic process, and enhance the patient's psychosocial and vocational status. Components of cardiac rehabilitation programs include exercise, smoking cessation, lipid management, weight control, blood pressure control, psychological interventions, and guidance for return to work. Cardiac rehabilitation programs have been shown to improve the patient's functional capacity and quality of life, and to decrease emotional distress, risk of subsequent coronary events, and cardiovascular mortality. Although the benefits of cardiac rehabilitation are well known, only 15% of eligible patients participate.[17]

Family members of patients with MI should be included in the educational process so that they can learn about heart disease and help the patient achieve the goals of rehabilitation. Family members also should be given the opportunity to learn cardiopulmonary resuscitation because most episodes of cardiac arrest in patients with MI occur within the first 18 months after discharge from the hospital.[17]

case study ■ ACUTE MYOCARDIAL INFARCTION

Mr. O'Keefe, a 68-year-old black man, was brought to the emergency department (ED) by an ambulance at 10:30 AM. He described substernal chest pain with radiation to his back that began 1 hour ago. The pain is not relieved by rest or sublingual nitroglycerin. He describes the pain as dull and rates it an 8 on a scale of 10. He has a history of hypertension, obesity, and elevated cholesterol. He has no known drug allergies.

On physical examination, he was awake, alert, oriented, and cooperative. His skin was cool and diaphoretic. Blood pressure was 90/42 mm Hg; heart rate, 110 beats/minute and irregular; respiratory rate, 26 breaths/minute on 2 L O_2 per nasal cannula; temperature, 98°F. His cardiac examination revealed S_1, S_2, and an S_3. He had no jugular venous distension. Peripheral pulses were present but thready and there was no peripheral edema. Auscultation

table 21-2 Patient Teaching: Goals After Acute Myocardial Infarction

	When Mastery of Content Is To Be Expected:		
Content	**Acute Phase**	**Before ICU Discharge**	**At Hospital Discharge**
Pathophysiology of heart disease	Can identify angina, using 1–10 pain scale for reference	Can initiate treatment of angina (rest, nitroglycerin, O_2 use)	Knowledgeable about medications, when to seek medical assistance
Environment of hospital	Understands procedures	Asks appropriate questions	Knowledgeable about disease process and therapy
Lifestyle modifications	Complies with activity limitations Complies with dietary limitations	Can state relationship between activity and cardiac workload Begins light activity States risk factors Selects appropriate meals	Can progress activity as tolerated Placement in cardiac rehabilitation program Can state dietary restrictions
Treatment of disease	Accepts medications as ordered	Can identify medications Can identify risk factors	Knowledgeable about medications, dose, timing, action, and side effects Plans for risk factor reduction Begins cardiac rehabilitation program
Emotional adaptation	Able to define support system	Begins to communicate about lifestyle changes Becomes involved with resolving emotions related to surviving a critical illness	Involves self and loved ones in plans for lifestyle changes Expresses feelings Participates in group recovery program

of his lungs revealed bilateral basilar crackles. He had no evidence of cyanosis or clubbing. His abdominal examination showed positive bowel sounds in all four quadrants. His abdomen was soft and nontender with no palpable masses.

The nurse immediately recorded a 12-lead ECG that showed 4-mm ST segment elevation in leads V_1 through V_4. Blood samples were drawn that revealed an elevated CK level positive for MB. His troponin level was also abnormal. Mr. O'Keefe was given an aspirin and an IV line was started. Mr. O'Keefe was diagnosed with an acute anteroseptal wall MI. The plan was to perform a primary percutaneous transluminal coronary angioplasty (PTCA). ■

clinical applicability challenges

Self-Challenge: Critical Thinking

Refer to the case study at the end of this chapter and answer the following questions regarding Mr. O'Keefe:

1. *Role-play an interaction with Mr. O'Keefe's family. Explain the diagnosis of an MI and why an emergent PTCA is being performed.*
2. *When you receive Mr. O'Keefe into your unit after PTCA, what are your priorities for his care?*
3. *Mr. O'Keefe has a successful PTCA with a stent placed in his left anterior descending coronary artery. He is preparing to go home. What discharge instructions and patient education would you provide to him and his family?*

Study Questions

1. *A description of pain that occurs with pericarditis is*
   a. *pain that worsens with leaning or sitting forward.*
   b. *pain that decreases with swallowing.*
   c. *abrupt onset of pain that resolves within a few days.*
   d. *pain that intensifies with a deep breath and often is accompanied by a fever.*
2. *The electrocardiographic finding consistent with an acute injury process is*
   a. *the presence of a Q wave.*
   b. *the presence of an inverted T wave.*
   c. *the presence of an elevated ST segment.*
   d. *the presence of a depressed ST segment.*
3. *The drug of choice for pain relief for a patient with an acute MI is*
   a. *morphine sulfate.*
   b. *aspirin.*
   c. *Tylenol.*
   d. *Demerol.*
4. *When examining the 12-lead ECG of Mr. Lopez, you note a Q wave in leads II, III, and aVF. These three leads on the ECG provide a picture of what wall of the heart?*
   a. *Anterior*
   b. *Lateral*
   c. *Posterior*
   d. *Inferior*
5. *Risk factor modification is an important component of patient education and rehabilitation after MI. Which of the following risk factors is considered a major controllable risk factor?*
   a. *Age*
   b. *Obesity*
   c. *Excessive alcohol intake*
   d. *Stress*

REFERENCES

1. American Heart Association: Heart Disease and Stoke Statistics: 2004 update. Dallas, American Heart Association, 2003
2. American Heart Association: Heart and Stoke Facts. Dallas, American Heart Association, 2003
3. Libby P, Ridker P, Maseri A: Inflammation and atherosclerosis. Circulation 105:1135–1143, 2002
4. American Heart Association: Risk factors and coronary heart disease. Available at www.americanheart.org. Accessed March 27, 2004
5. Roberts R: Acute myocardial infarction. In Kelley WN (ed): Textbook of Internal Medicine (3rd Ed), pp 385–398. Philadelphia, Lippincott-Raven, 1997
6. Welch G, Loscalzo J: Mechanisms of disease: Homocysteine and atherothrombosis. N Engl J Med 338:1042–1050, 1998
7. Reeder SJ, Hoffman RL, Magdic KS, et al: Homocysteine: The latest risk factor for heart disease. Dimens Crit Care Nurs 19(1):22–28, 2000
8. Coffey M, Crowder GK, Cheek D: Reducing coronary artery disease by decreasing homocysteine levels. Crit Care Nurse 23(1):25–30, 2003
9. Braunwald E, Antman EM, Beasley JW, et al: ACC/AHA 2002 guideline update for the management of patients with unstable angina and non-ST-segment elevation myocardial infarction: A report of the American College of Cardiology and the American Heart Association Taskforce on Practice Guidelines (Committee on the Management of Patients With Unstable Angina). 2002. Available at http://www.acc.org/clinical/guidelines/unstable/unstable.pdf. Accessed July 29, 2004.
10. DeWood MA, Spores J, Notske R, et al: Prevalence of total coronary occlusion during the early hours of transmural myocardial infarction. N Engl J Med 303:897–902, 1980
11. The Joint European Society of Cardiology and the American College of Cardiology Committee: Myocardial infarction redefined: A consensus document of the Joint European Society of Cardiology/American College of Cardiology Committee for the Redefinition of Myocardial Infarction. J Am Coll Cardiol 36(3):959–969, 2000
12. Reimer KA, Lower JE, Rasmussen MM, et al: The wave front phenomenon of ischemic cell death: 1. Myocardial infarct size versus duration of coronary occlusion in dogs. Circulation 56:786–794, 1977
13. Cunningham S: Pathophysiology of myocardial ischemia and infarction. In Woods SL, Froelicher ES, Motzer SU (eds): Cardiac Nursing (4th Ed), pp 495–505. Philadelphia, Lippincott Williams & Wilkins, 2000
14. Kinch J, Ryan T: Right ventricular infarction. N Engl J Med 330(17):1211–1216, 1994
15. Levin T, Samaha F, Follman D, et al: Right ventricular MI: When to suspect, what to do. J Crit Illness 10(1):14–22, 1995
16. DelBene S, Vaughan A: Diagnosis and management of myocardial infarction. In Woods SL, Froelicher ES, Motzer SU (eds): Cardiac Nursing (4th Ed), 513–540. Philadelphia, Lippincott Williams & Wilkins, 2000
17. Ryan TJ, Anderson JL, Antman EM, et al: ACC/AHA guidelines for the management of patients with acute myocardial infarction: A report of the American College of Cardiology/American Heart Association Task Force on Practice Guidelines (Committee on Management of Acute Myocardial Infarction), 1999. Available at http://www.americanheart.org. Accessed July 29, 2004.
18. Becker RC: Complicated myocardial infarction. Crit Pathways Cardiol 2(2):125–152, 2003
19. Grauer K: A Practical Guide to ECG Interpretation (2nd Ed). St. Louis, Mosby-Year Book, 1998
20. TIMI Study Group: Comparison of invasive and conservative strategies after treatment with intravenous tissue plasminogen activator in acute myocardial infarction: Results of the Thrombolysis in Myocardial Infarction (TIMI) Phase II Trial. N Engl J Med 320:618, 1989

21. Goldberg RJ, Gore JM, Alpert JS, et al: Cardiogenic shock resulting from acute myocardial infarction: A fourteen year community wide perspective. N Engl J Med 325:1117–1122, 1991

OTHER SELECTED READING

Myocardial Infarction

Adam-Hamoda MG, Caldwell M, Stotts N, et al: Factors to consider when analyzing 12-lead electrocardiograms for evidence of acute myocardial ischemia. Am J Crit Care 12(1):9–18, 2003

An K, DeJong MJ, Riegel BJ, et al: A cross-sectional examination of changes in anxiety early after acute myocardial infarction. Heart Lung 33(2):75–82, 2004

Ashton K, DiMattio MJ: Recruitment and retention of women in two longitudinal studies of recovery from coronary events: A secondary analysis. Heart Lung 33(1):26–32, 2004

Booker KJ, Holm K, Drew BJ, et al: Frequency and outcomes of transient myocardial ischemia in critically ill adults admitted for noncardiac conditions. Am J Crit Care 12(6):508–516, 2003

Fukuoka Y, Dracup K, Kobayashi F, et al: Illness attribution among Japanese patients with acute myocardial infarction. Heart Lung 33(3):146–153, 2004

Futterman LG, Lemberg L: Seminal changes in the management of the acute coronary event: Current concepts. Am J Crit Care 12(1):73–76, 2003

Gassner LA, Dunn S, Piller N: Aerobic exercise and post-myocardial infarction patient: A review of the literature. Heart Lung 22(4): 258–265, 2003

Moruzzi P, Marenzi G, Caallegri M, et al: Circadian distribution of acute myocardial infarction by anatomic location and coronary artery involvement. Am J Med 116(1):24–27, 2004

Pedersen S, Mideel B, Larsen ML: Posttraumatic stress disorder in first-time myocardial infarction patients. Heart Lung 32(5):300–307, 2003

Pelter MM, Adams MG, Drew BJ: Transient myocardial ischemia is an independent predictor of adverse in-hospital outcomes in patients with acute coronary syndromes treated in the telemetry unit. Heart Lung 32(2):71–78, 2003

chapter

22

Cardiac Surgery

NANCY MUNRO

objectives

Based on the content in this chapter, the reader should be able to:

- Compare and contrast the pathophysiological impacts of stenosis and insufficiency in the mitral and aortic valves.
- Explain the cardiopulmonary bypass process.
- Describe five key assessment areas in the early postoperative period.
- Discuss causes of postoperative hypotension in a cardiac surgery patient, and assessments and interventions for same.
- Discuss advantages and disadvantages of off-bypass coronary artery surgery.
- Discuss the indications for transmyocardial laser revascularization.
- Discuss the impact of the inflammatory response on patients after coronary artery surgery.

Despite emphasis on modifying and eliminating risk factors, cardiovascular disease remains a leading cause of disability and death in the United States. Development of new treatments, such as thrombolytic and anticoagulation therapy, balloon and laser angioplasty, and coronary artery stenting, has improved medical management of cardiac disease. These nonsurgical approaches are discussed in Chapter 18. However, surgical intervention remains the treatment of choice in some patients. In particular, cardiac surgery is sometimes necessary in two common conditions, coronary artery disease (CAD) and valvular disease.

INDICATIONS FOR CARDIAC SURGERY

Coronary Artery Disease

PATHOPHYSIOLOGY

A complete discussion of the pathophysiology of coronary artery disease is found in Chapter 21.

SURGICAL TREATMENT

Coronary Artery Bypass Graft Surgery

In coronary artery bypass graft (CABG) surgery, native vessels or conduits are "harvested" during the initial phase of surgery to reroute or bypass blood flow past diseased areas of the coronary arteries. The first saphenous vein aortocoronary bypass graft was performed in 1964. Since then, the use of CABGs has become an acceptable treatment for CAD. Compared with medical treatment, CABG has proved effective in relieving angina and improving exercise tolerance, and it prolongs life in patients with left main CAD and three-vessel disease with poor left ventricular function.[1]

Increased use of percutaneous transluminal coronary angioplasty and stenting has decreased the need for CABG in many cases. Patients selected for CABG today are older; have more advanced coronary disease; have more impaired left ventricular function; and, in many cases, have had previous CABG surgery. To decrease the mortality associated with bypass surgery, it is necessary to consider several factors: urgency of operation, age, previous heart surgery, sex, left ventricular ejection fraction, percentage stenosis of the left main coronary artery, and the number of major coronary arteries with greater than 70% stenosis.[1]

Desired characteristics for a graft or conduit are (1) diameter similar to the coronary arteries, (2) no disease or wall abnormalities, and (3) adequate length. Commonly used grafts include saphenous vein grafts and internal mammary artery grafts, although other potential grafts are being explored.

Saphenous Vein Grafts. Saphenous vein grafts are used to bypass the obstruction in the coronary artery by anastomosing one end of the vein to the aorta (proximal anastomosis) and the other end to the coronary artery just past the obstruction (distal anastomosis). Saphenous vein grafts may be *simple*, with an end-to-side anastomosis to the aorta and the coronary artery, or *sequential* (also called *skip*), with an end-to-side anastomosis to the aorta, a side-to-side anastomosis to one coronary artery, and an end-to-side anastomosis to another coronary artery (Fig. 22-1).

Although the saphenous vein can be taken from above or below the knee, a vein from below the knee is generally preferred because it is close in diameter to the size of the coronary artery. To remove the vein, an incision is made along the inner aspect of the leg. Alternatively, small incisions can be made in the area of the vein, and a flexible fiberoptic scope is inserted to visualize the vessel and remove it. The fiberoptic method of vein removal is associated with improved wound healing and reduced complications involving the incision site.[2]

Fifty percent of saphenous vein grafts are occluded after 10 years. Three main processes account for saphenous vein failure: thrombosis, fibrointimal hyperplasia, and atherosclerosis. Thrombosis is most common in the first month, but may occur for as long as 1 year. Fibrointimal hyperplasia occurs predominantly between 1 month and 5 years and may result in a 25% decrease in luminal vessel diameter. Atherosclerosis begins as early as 1 year after surgery

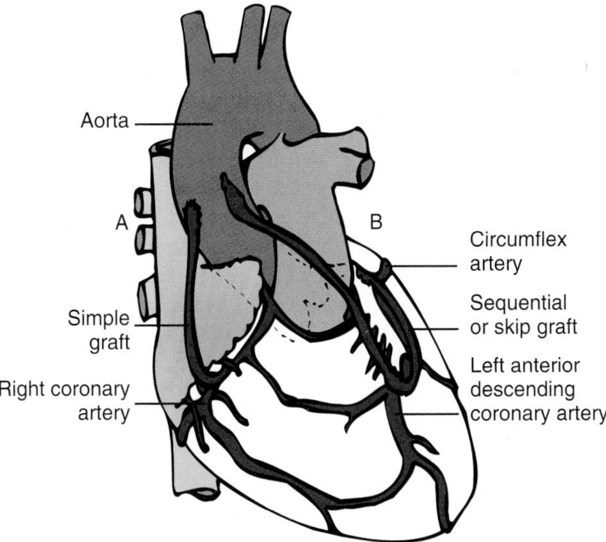

figure 22-1 Aortocoronary bypass grafts using saphenous vein. (**A**) Simple graft from aorta to right coronary artery. (**B**) Sequential graft from aorta to left anterior descending coronary artery to diagonal or circumflex artery.

and is fully developed after 5 years. To decrease the incidence of occlusion of grafts from the saphenous vein, grafts from other vessels are being used.[3]

Internal Mammary Artery Grafts. The internal mammary artery is a preferred alternative to the saphenous vein for surgical revascularization. The internal mammary artery is used as a *pedicle* graft (i.e., the proximal end remains attached to the subclavian artery) to bypass diseased coronary arteries. Both the left and the right internal mammary artery can be used. Because the left internal mammary artery is longer and larger than the right, it is usually used to bypass the left anterior descending coronary artery. The right internal mammary artery is anastomosed to the right coronary artery or the circumflex coronary artery.

The internal mammary artery, the second branch of the subclavian artery, descends down the anterior chest wall just lateral to the sternum behind the costal cartilage. To isolate the internal mammary artery, the pleural space is entered, the internal mammary artery is dissected free from the chest wall, and the intercostal artery branches are cauterized.

Compared with saphenous vein grafts, internal mammary artery grafts have superior graft patency rates; 90% were patent 10 years after surgery. In addition, internal mammary artery grafts exhibit less atherosclerosis over time, and they have been associated with lower long-term morbidity and improved long-term survival.[1] Other advantages and disadvantages of using the internal mammary artery for surgical revascularization are listed in Box 22-1.

Other Grafts. The search for other native vessels to serve as conduits continues as patients return for reoperation. The use of the radial artery has gained popularity; occlusion rates have lowered as harvesting techniques have improved. The radial artery, a thick, muscular artery, is prone to spasm with mechanical stimulation, and to prevent spasm, the artery is perfused with a calcium channel blocker solution during surgery and minimally stimulated. Once the radial artery has been implanted, spasm has not been a major factor, and patency rates of 84% for 5 years have been reported.[4] Initiation of nitroglycerin followed by oral nitrates (isosorbide mononitrate) postoperatively has helped decrease the occurrence of spasm; results have been better than with calcium channel blockers.[5]

Acceptable alternative conduits must have short- and long-term acceptable patency rates. The right gastroepiploic artery, which is harvested by extending the sternotomy incision toward the umbilicus and dissecting the artery off the greater curvature of the stomach, is used for coronary grafting. Patency rates have been acceptable, but long-term data are not available.[1] Homologous (nonnative) conduits using the saphenous vein, umbilical vein, or bovine internal mammary artery have resulted in poor patency rates and therefore are not recommended.[1]

Off-Pump Coronary Artery Bypass Graft Surgery

CABG surgery actually began as a surgical procedure performed on a beating heart because the cardiopulmonary bypass machine was not yet available. Once the cardiopulmonary bypass machine was perfected, "beating heart" surgery was used less often. However, complications asso-

box 22-1
Advantages and Disadvantages of Using the Internal Mammary Artery for Myocardial Revascularization

Advantages
- Improved short- and long-term patency rates over saphenous vein grafts
- Diameter close to diameter of coronary arteries
- Aortic anastomosis not required
- Internal mammary artery retains its nervous system innervation and thus has the ability to adapt size to provide blood flow according to myocardial demands
- No leg incision if only internal mammary artery used
- Vascular endothelium adapted to arterial pressure and high flow, resulting in decreased intimal hyperplasia and atherosclerosis
- May be used as a free or sequential graft with good results

Disadvantages
- Dissection of internal mammary artery takes longer, resulting in longer cardiopulmonary bypass time, but this depends on surgeon's experience.
- Extensive dissection may increase risk of postoperative bleeding.
- Pleural space is entered, so pleural chest tube is required postoperatively.
- Postoperative pain may be increased because of entry into pleural space and extensive dissection.
- Use of bilateral internal mammary arteries can increase the risk of infection and sternal dehiscence, especially in diabetic patients.

ciated with cardiopulmonary bypass have led surgeons to reconsider performing CABG "off pump" (OPCABG)—in other words, on beating hearts—in the hope of improving patient outcome.

Initially, surgeons wanted to avoid using the midline sternotomy incision and use the less invasive "mini" left and right thoracotomy approaches while performing CABG surgery, on or off bypass. This approach, which is known as *minimally invasive direct coronary artery bypass grafting (MIDCABG)*, restricts the number of grafts that can be performed because the small incision does not allow access to the entire heart surface. Grafts to the left anterior descending artery are most frequent. Depending on where the "mini" incision is placed, grafts to the right coronary artery and the posterior descending artery can also be made.[6] Experience with MIDCABG has not been as successful as anticipated, but the technique is still used depending on the patient situation. The trend is toward using the median sternotomy incision but performing the grafting process off bypass.

In the 1990s, as neurological complications associated with the cardiopulmonary bypass machine, especially cognitive dysfunction, became more prominent, OPCABG was reinstituted.[7] The initial results of OPCABG have been promising but sometimes difficult to compare with the large data pool for on-pump CABG. Length of stay in patients after OPCABG has decreased compared with length of stay in patients who have had on-pump CABG.[8] Neurological dysfunction seems less after OPCABG. However, Stamou et al. have demonstrated that the stroke rate is similar in patients who have OPCABG compared with those who have on-pump CABG; after OPCABG, the symptoms of the stroke appear 48 to 72 hours after surgery, and after on-pump CABG, the symptoms of stroke occur immediately after surgery.[9] The explanation for this finding is that systemic inflammatory response syndrome (SIRS; discussed in detail in Chapter 50) causes diffuse microembolic events that take time to develop. The microembolization is the result of the inflammation of the endothelium, which activates the coagulation cascade.

The significance of these differences for patient care after OPCABG is not well documented in the nursing literature because OPCABG is a new procedure. Data from institutions with larger numbers of patients who have had OPCABG seem to suggest that emphasis should be placed on anticoagulation interventions.[9] Traditional agents such as heparin (weight-based protocols), aspirin, clopidogrel (Plavix), and low–molecular-weight heparin are aggressively implemented to prevent platelet activation and suppress activation of the coagulation cascade. Nursing assessment focuses on the detection of embolic events in any body system and monitors for side effects of anticoagulation such as gastrointestinal bleeding and heparin-induced thrombocytopenia. Because the SIRS process can develop in 48 to 72 hours, the critical care nurse must continually reassess the patient who has undergone OPCABG and report any changes that may occur, especially with regard to neurological changes or electrocardiographic (ECG) ST segment monitoring. If the thoracotomy approach is used in OPCABG, the increased need for pain medication may decrease patient compliance to cough and deep breathe postoperatively. A high index of suspicion is the key nursing intervention after OPCABG, and may improve patient outcome.

Transmyocardial Laser Revascularization

Transmyocardial laser revascularization (TMR; TMLR) may be an option for patients who continue to have unstable angina that is refractory to interventions. Eligible patients usually have had prior CABG surgery, multiple cardiac interventions with maximal medication manipulation, or both. A laser probe is inserted into the wall of the left ventricle to create channels that encourage revascularization. The location and number of channels created depends on the patient's preoperative cardiac performance. Revascularization theoretically occurs through two mechanisms: (1) angiogenesis, and (2) direct channel patency and endothelialization.[10] With angiogenesis, the formation of new blood vessels or the modeling of existing blood vessels increases collateral flow to the dysfunctional areas. Direct channel patency with endothelialization may result in direct perfusion to impaired walls of the left ventricle. Although the actual mechanisms are not clearly understood, the clinical outcomes are promising. In TMR, revascularization takes months to develop, which should be emphasized to the patient and family. In TMR, three types of lasers of different wavelengths are used: holmium:YAG, excimer, and carbon dioxide. All produce clean channels with minimal tissue trauma.[10]

Care of patients after TMR is similar to care after cardiovascular surgery, with some special concerns. The life of patients who have had TMR can become relatively normal, but careful observation is required. In TMR, patients have sustained direct myocardial insult that can result in a decrease in left ventricular function 48 to 72 hours after the surgery. Inotropic support using dobutamine or milrinone may be required for several days. Vigilant monitoring of fluid status is necessary because congestive failure tends to occur, although patients have higher filling pressures because the desired effects of TMR develop over time. Antiarrhythmic therapy may also be necessary because there may be irritable foci in the ventricle; amiodarone is frequently used. Angina may occur, but because the channel areas are denervated in TMR, the patient may not be able to perceive anginal pain. Continuous ST segment monitoring is needed to detect any changes that occur. Nitrates are started as part of the medication regimen. Anticoagulation is initiated to prevent myocardial infarction and also to maintain the patency of the channels.[11]

Valvular Disease

Cardiac valves maintain the unidirectional flow of blood. If structural changes occur as a result of disease, this function is disrupted. Disease causes either valvular stenosis or insufficiency (regurgitation; Fig. 22-2). The stenotic valve has a narrowed orifice that creates a partial obstruction to blood flow, resulting in increasing pressure behind the valve and decreasing forward blood flow. The insufficient valve is incompetent or leaky; blood flows backward, increasing the pressure and volume behind the valve. Stenosis and insufficiency can occur alone or in combination, in the same valve, or in more than one valve. Abnormalities can affect the tricuspid, pulmonic, mitral, and aortic valves. This discussion focuses on mitral and aortic abnormalities, which are more common and produce profound hemodynamic changes.

The diagnosis of valvular disease is suggested by the history, clinical signs and symptoms, physical examination, and auscultation of the characteristic murmur (see Chapter 17). Diagnosis is confirmed by echocardiography and catheterization of both sides of the heart, at which time valvular gradients are measured. To determine the gradient across the mitral valve, left atrial and left ventricular pressures are measured during diastole. A gradient of more than 15 to 20 mm Hg (i.e., left atrial diastolic pressure is 15 to 20 mm Hg higher than left ventricular diastolic pressure) means that severe mitral stenosis exists. Valve area is also calculated during cardiac catheterization. The normal mitral valve area is 4 to 6 cm^2. An area less than 1.5 cm^2 signifies critical mitral stenosis, and surgery is indicated.

To determine the gradient across the aortic valve, the left ventricular and aortic root pressures are measured during systole. A gradient of more than 50 mm Hg is associated with clinically significant aortic stenosis. Normal aortic

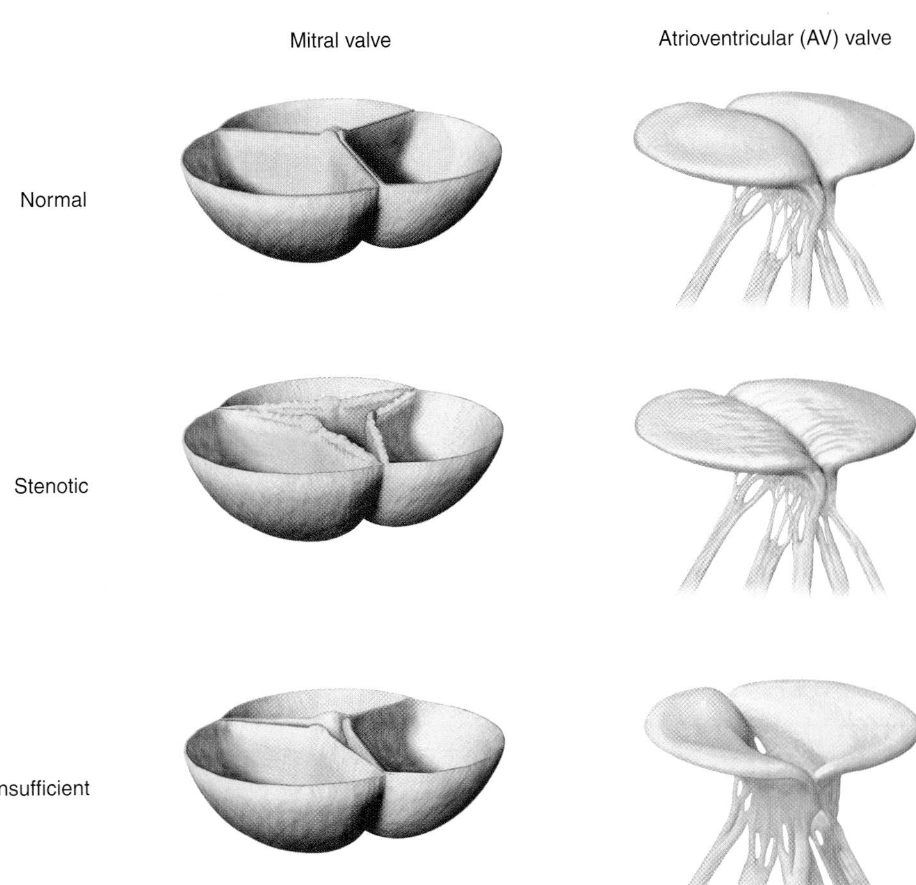

figure 22-2 Normal and diseased heart valves. (Reprinted with permission from Anatomical Chart Company: Atlas of Pathophysiology, pp 74, 75. Springhouse, PA, Springhouse, 2002.)

valve area is 2.6 to 3.5 cm^2. Hemodynamically significant aortic stenosis occurs if the valve area is less than 1 cm^2. Valvular insufficiency is diagnosed by regurgitation of the contrast medium backward through the incompetent valve.

PATHOPHYSIOLOGY

Mitral Stenosis

Mitral stenosis occurs most frequently as a result of rheumatic heart disease. The disease process causes fusion of the commissures and fibrotic contraction of valve leaflets, commissures, and chordae tendineae. As forward flow from the left atrium to the left ventricle decreases, cardiac output falls, creating a decrease in systemic perfusion. Blood backed up behind the stenotic valve causes left atrial dilation and increased left atrial pressure. This is reflected backward into the pulmonary circulation, and with prolonged high pressures, fluid moves from the pulmonary capillaries into the interstitial space and eventually the alveoli. Pulmonary hypertension develops, which can eventually lead to right-sided heart failure (Fig. 22-3A). As a result of this pathophysiology, patients with mitral stenosis present with fatigue, exertional dyspnea, orthopnea, and even pulmonary edema. Left atrial dilation causes atrial fibrillation in 40% to 50% of affected patients.

Mitral Insufficiency

Mitral insufficiency can occur acutely or develop over a period of time. Chronic mitral insufficiency may result from rheumatic heart disease, myxomatous degeneration of the mitral valve, degenerative changes associated with aging, or left ventricular dilation. The basic valve dysfunction is caused by thickening or stretching of the leaflets, resulting in backward blood flow. During ventricular systole, some of the left ventricular blood regurgitates into the atrium rather than being ejected through the aortic valve. This regurgitation decreases the forward cardiac output. Left ventricular hypertrophy occurs in an attempt to improve the cardiac output, but the hypertrophy can actually worsen the regurgitation. Left ventricular volume overload causes left ventricular dilation. Regurgitant flow into the left atrium causes increased left atrial pressure and dilation. This volume overload can be reflected backward to the pulmonary circulation; however, pulmonary and right-sided heart symptoms usually do not develop until late in the disease process (see Fig. 22-3B). As a result of this pathophysiology, patients with chronic mitral insufficiency commonly present with fatigue, palpitations, and sometimes shortness of breath.

Acute mitral insufficiency may result from endocarditis, chest trauma, or myocardial infarction. Endocarditis erodes or perforates the valve leaflets or chordae. Trauma may rupture the chordae. Myocardial infarction may cause papillary muscle rupture, allowing blood to flow backward into the left atrium during ventricular systole. Because of the acute nature of the valve dysfunction, there is inadequate time for dilatation or hypertrophy to compensate. In acute mitral insufficiency, cardiac output decreases dramatically, cascading into pulmonary edema and shock. The treatment of choice for acute mitral regurgitation with hemodynamic compromise is emergent mitral valve replacement.

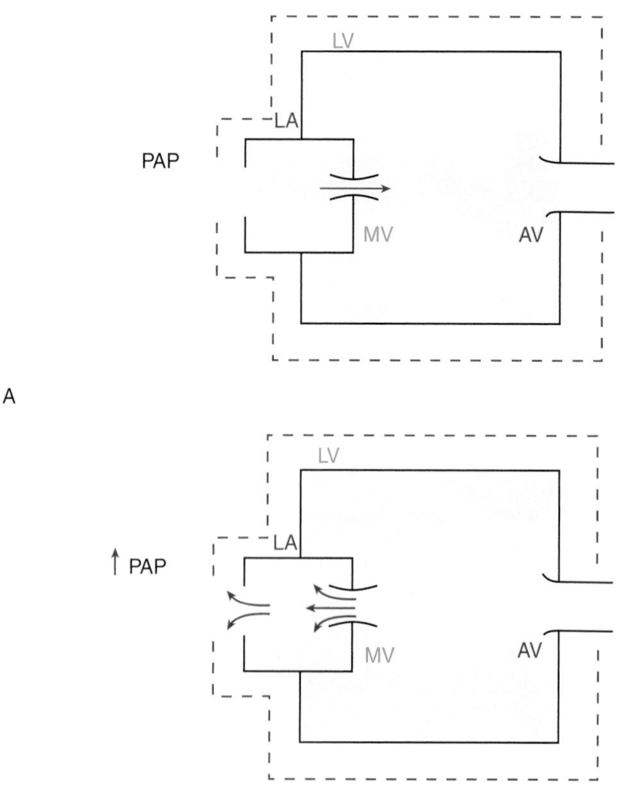

figure 22-3 Mitral valve dysfunction. (**A**) Mitral stenosis. (**B**) Mitral insufficiency. *PAP,* pulmonary artery pressure; *LV,* left ventricle; *MV,* mitral valve; *LA,* left atrium; *AV,* aortic valve.

Aortic Stenosis

Aortic stenosis may develop as a result of rheumatic fever, calcification of a congenital bicuspid valve, or calcific degeneration, especially in the elderly. The resultant fusion of the commissures and fibrous contractures of the cusps leads to obstruction of left ventricular outflow. Forward cardiac output is diminished, and the left ventricle hypertrophies to maintain the cardiac output. As the stenosis worsens, compensation fails, and volume and pressure overload in the left ventricle causes left ventricular dilation. Increased left ventricular pressures are reflected backward through the left atrium and pulmonary vasculature (Fig. 22-4A).

Diminished cardiac output in the person with aortic stenosis may lead to two major problems—angina and syncope. Extreme left ventricular hypertrophy increases myocardial oxygen demand at the same time that cardiac output and coronary artery perfusion are decreased. Ischemic myocardium develops, which may lead to angina. Syncope occurs in the late stages of aortic stenosis, when the forward cardiac output cannot increase to meet the body's demands. As a person with severe aortic stenosis exercises, the blood vessels to the skeletal muscles dilate to increase the blood supply. The normal response to this increased demand is increased cardiac output. However, the person with aortic stenosis is unable to respond in such a way. The vasodilation without a concomitant increase in cardiac output results in insufficient cerebral perfusion and syncope. Patients with aortic stenosis also experience

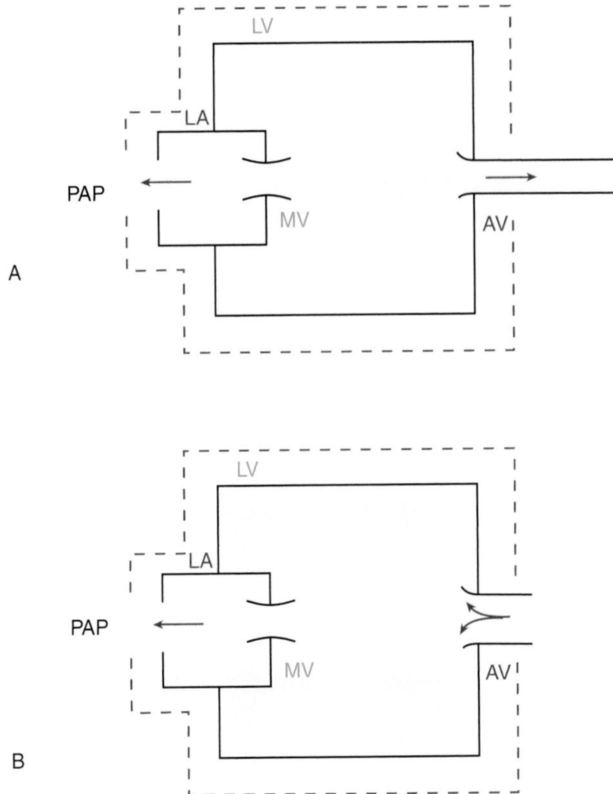

figure 22-4 Aortic valve dysfunction. (**A**) Aortic stenosis. (**B**) Aortic insufficiency. *PAP,* pulmonary artery pressure; *LV,* left ventricle; *MV,* mitral valve; *LA,* left atrium; *AV,* aortic valve.

exertional dyspnea, orthopnea, and paroxysmal nocturnal dyspnea.

Aortic Insufficiency

Like mitral insufficiency, aortic insufficiency can occur acutely or develop over a period of time. Chronic aortic insufficiency is commonly caused by rheumatic fever and aneurysm of the ascending aorta. Rheumatic disease results in thickened and retracted valve cusps, whereas aortic aneurysm causes annular dilation. Both conditions prevent the edges of the valve leaflets from approximating, allowing blood to regurgitate backward from the aorta into the left ventricle during ventricular diastole. Forward cardiac output decreases, and left ventricular volume and pressure increase. Left ventricular hypertrophy ensues. Eventually, the increase in left ventricular pressure is reflected backward into the left atrium and pulmonary circulation (see Fig. 22-4B). Patients with chronic aortic insufficiency present with fatigue, and they have a low diastolic blood pressure and a widened pulse pressure. The pulse may rise rapidly and collapse suddenly (water-hammer or Corrigan's pulse) because of the forceful ventricular contraction and subsequent diastolic regurgitation from the aortic root into the left ventricle. Angina may occur because aortic insufficiency creates an imbalance between left ventricular myocardial oxygen supply and demand. As left ventricular hypertrophy worsens, the oxygen demand increases, but regurgitant flow from the aortic root during diastole decreases coronary artery perfusion.

Acute aortic insufficiency may be caused by blunt chest trauma, ruptured ascending aortic aneurysm, or infective endocarditis. Left-sided heart failure and pulmonary edema develop rapidly in the patient with acute aortic insufficiency because compensatory left ventricular hypertrophy does not have time to develop. In response to the diminished cardiac output, systemic vascular resistance (SVR) increases to maintain the blood pressure. The elevated SVR increases the degree of regurgitation and worsens the situation.

SURGICAL TREATMENT

The goals of valvular surgery are to relieve symptoms and restore normal hemodynamics. Surgery is indicated before left ventricular function deteriorates significantly and the patient's activity becomes severely limited, or before severe signs and symptoms, such as angina or syncope from aortic stenosis or pulmonary hypertension from mitral stenosis, develop. Percutaneous balloon valvuloplasty, a procedure that is indicated primarily for patients considered too high risk for surgery, is discussed in Chapter 18. Surgical intervention consists of either valve reconstruction or valve replacement. Because valve reconstruction is associated with decreased operative mortality and fewer thromboembolic and anticoagulation-related complications than valve replacement, valve reconstruction is gaining popularity.

Valve Reconstruction

With the development of transesophageal echocardiography (TEE) to assess the effectiveness of repair during surgery, the use of valve reconstruction is increasing. Most valve reconstruction procedures are performed on the mitral valve. Compared with mitral valve replacement, reconstruction eliminates the need for long-term anticoagulation, decreases the risks of thromboembolism and endocarditis, decreases the need for reoperation, and increases survival. However, for aortic valve disorders, most attempts at reconstruction have not been successful because of late insufficiency and restenosis.

A common reconstruction technique for mitral stenosis is *commissurotomy.* Although not indicated for patients with severe mitral stenosis, commissurotomy may be effective for patients with moderate stenosis with minimal calcification and regurgitation. During commissurotomy, the fused commissures are surgically divided. Calcified tissue is debrided and fused, and shortened chordae are incised. This procedure improves leaflet mobility and increases the mitral valve area, decreasing the degree of stenosis.

Another technique for treatment of mitral insufficiency is *reconstruction.* If annular dilation causes the regurgitation, annuloplasty can be performed using sutures or a prosthetic ring (e.g., Carpentier-Edwards annuloplasty ring). The ring is sewn around the mitral annulus so that excess annular tissue is drawn up. Suturing and the ring reduce the circumference of the enlarged annulus so that the edges of the leaflets coapt, diminishing regurgitation. If the chordae tendineae are stretched or ruptured, surgical shortening or transposition of chordae to substitute for ruptured chordae can be effective. Redundant mitral leaflets are repaired by resecting a portion of the leaflet, and perforated valve leaflets can be reconstructed by patching. Such repairs are usually supported by an annuloplasty ring.

Reconstruction procedures are more likely to be successful if performed early in the course of the disease, before left ventricular function deteriorates and irreparable damage occurs. Anticoagulation is not usually needed after valve repair unless an annuloplasty ring is used. In such cases, anticoagulants are given for only 3 months until the ring is endothelialized. If reconstruction cannot be accomplished, valves are replaced.

Valve Replacement

The first valve replacement was performed by Harken and Starr in 1960 with a caged ball prosthesis. Since then, many new valve designs have evolved. Valve replacement surgery is done through a median sternotomy incision, and uses cardiopulmonary bypass and myocardial preservation techniques (discussed in detail later in this chapter). The mitral valve is approached through the left atrium. Rather than excising the native valve, the chordae and papillary muscles are preserved when the prosthetic valve is sutured in place. This technique helps maintain left ventricular function and ejection fraction. The aortic valve is approached through the ascending aorta. The native aortic valve is excised, the annulus is sized, and the prosthetic valve of correct size is sutured to the annulus. Once the surgery is completed, the patient is transferred to the intensive care unit (ICU).

Ideally, a prosthetic valve would be durable, last for a patient's life, and perform exactly like a normal human valve. The valve would have normal hemodynamics with unimpeded, nonturbulent blood flow through a central opening, no transvalvular gradient, and no regurgitation when closed. It would be nonthrombogenic and not damaging to blood components, and acceptable to the patient in terms of noise and the need for anticoagulation. Unfortunately, no artificial valve currently meets these criteria, so research continues.

Two major types of prosthetic valves are available—mechanical and biological. Mechanical valves are made entirely of synthetic materials, whereas biological valves combine synthetic materials with chemically treated biological tissues. When choosing an appropriate valve for a particular patient, it is necessary to compare the advantages and disadvantages of the various valve types. The advantages and disadvantages of prosthetic cardiac valves are listed in Box 22-2. Mechanical valves offer the benefits of good long-term durability but pose a significant risk of thromboembolism and require long-term anticoagulation. Biological valves decrease the risk of thromboembolism and can obviate the need for long-term anticoagulation, but are not as durable as mechanical valves. Biological valves studied at autopsy have shown structural deterioration beginning as early as 6 years after implant, and their total useful lifetime is usually considered to be less than 10 years.

Patients with a long life expectancy may receive mechanical valves because they are particularly durable. Older patients may receive biological valves because less calcification and deterioration occur in older people, long-term durability is less important, and the risk of anticoagulation may increase with advancing age. Biological valves are indicated for patients who are unable to comply with an anticoagulation regimen, for those in whom a long-term anticoagulation regimen is contraindicated, and for women of childbearing age who plan to become pregnant (the anticoagulant warfarin crosses the placental barrier).

box 22-2
Advantages and Disadvantages of Prosthetic Cardiac Valves

Mechanical Valves

- Good long-term durability
- Adequate hemodynamics
- High risk of thromboembolism; necessity for long-term anticoagulation
- Increased risk of bleeding complications

Biological Valves

- Poor long-term durability
- Better hemodynamics than mechanical valves (except in small sizes)
- No hemolysis
- Low incidence of thromboembolism; possibly no necessity for anticoagulation
- Fewer bleeding complications

Mechanical Valves. Mechanical valves include the caged ball, tilting disk, and bileaflet designs.

The *caged ball valve* consists of a plastic or metal ball inside of a metal cage attached to a sewing ring. When pressure behind the valve increases, the ball is forced down into the cage, and blood flows around it. When pressure in front of the valve increases, the ball is forced upward against the sewing ring, preventing regurgitant flow. An example of the caged ball valve is the Starr-Edwards valve.

Hemodynamically, the ball in the cage produces a central obstruction to blood flow, which can result in a small stenotic pressure gradient, and ventricular outflow may be partially obstructed because of the cage's size and high profile. Because of the thrombogenicity of the plastic and metal and the turbulent flow around the ball and through the cage, blood clots can form on or around the valve. Thromboembolism is a common problem, and chronic anticoagulant therapy is essential. Caged ball valves have good long-term durability.

The *tilting disk valve* is constructed of a disk held in place by struts attached to a sewing ring. When the pressure behind the valve increases, the disk tilts open approximately 60 to 80 degrees, allowing blood to flow around it. When the pressure in front of the valve increases, the disk tilts back flush with the sewing ring to close. Because of its semicentralized flow and lower profile, the tilting disk valve produces less obstruction to blood flow and has better hemodynamic characteristics than the caged ball valve. The tilting disk valve has good long-term durability, but the risk of thromboembolism requires long-term anticoagulant therapy. Examples of the tilting disk valve are the Medtronic-Hall and the Omniscience valves.

The *bileaflet tilting disk valve*, which consists of two pyrolytic carbon semicircular disks or leaflets hinged to a sewing ring, is the newest type of mechanical valve (Fig. 22-5). When the pressure behind the valve increases, the leaflets open perpendicular to the sewing ring, and blood flows through the central opening with minimal obstruction. When pressure in front of the valve increases, the leaflets return to their flat position against the sewing ring, preventing insufficiency. The bileaf tilting disk valve has good hemodynamic characteristics and durability, but it is thrombogenic and requires long-term anticoagulation. An example of the bileaflet tilting disk valve is the St. Jude Medical valve.

Biological Valves. Biological prostheses, or tissue valves, offer another alternative for valve replacement. The *porcine heterograft* is constructed of an excised pig aortic valve preserved in glutaraldehyde and mounted on a frame attached to a sewing ring. Examples of porcine valves are the Hancock and the Carpentier-Edwards valves. Biological prostheses provide good hemodynamics except in smaller sizes, where obstruction to flow can occur, and a gradient can develop. Their main advantage is the lower risk of thromboembolism compared with mechanical valves. Because most thromboembolic events occur during the first 3 months after implant before the sewing ring is endothelialized, most patients with biological valves receive anticoagulants during that time only. However, the decision regarding anticoagulation must be based on the patient's condition. Patients in chronic atrial fibrillation undergoing mitral valve replacement frequently receive long-term anticoagulation therapy even with a biological prosthesis because of stagnant blood flow in the atria, which predisposes to clot formation.

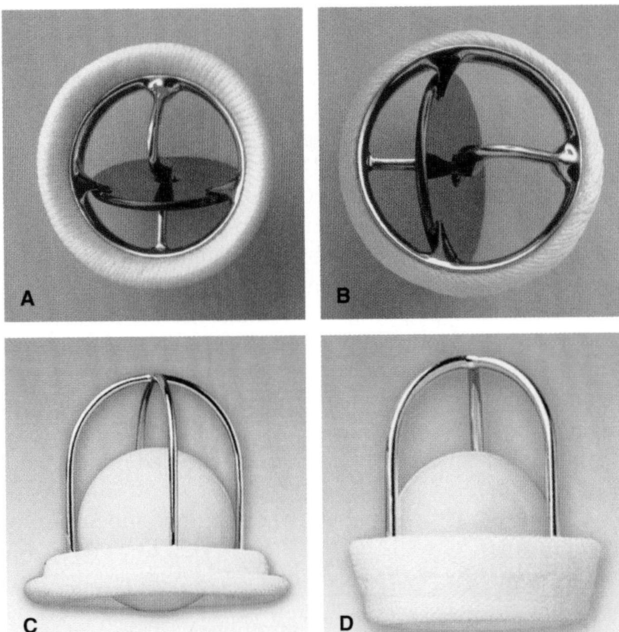

figure 22-5 (**A**) Medtronic Hall Easy-Fit, aortic model. (**B**) Medtronic Hall Easy-Fit, mitral model. (**C**) Starr-Edwards Silastic ball valve, aortic model. (**D**) Starr-Edwards Silastic ball valve, mitral model. A and B courtesy of Medtronic Heart Valves, Minneapolis, MN; C and D courtesy of Edwards Life Sciences, Irvine, CA.

CARDIAC SURGERY

With managed care, rising costs, and the demand for high-quality care, cardiac surgery has come under increased scrutiny. The unique challenge for the critical care nurse is to integrate theoretical knowledge, assessment skills, and problem-solving ability to provide optimal nursing care and maintain high-quality outcomes while decreasing resource consumption, yet always keeping the patient as the focus.

Preoperative Phase

Preoperative preparation for cardiac surgery includes physiological and psychological components. The physiological preparation is similar to that for any preoperative patient and includes history, physical examination, chest radiography, and an ECG. The history and physical examination are extremely important; they can provide information about previous neurological status, current medications, and any other coexisting conditions (e.g., diabetes mellitus, pulmonary disease, renal disease). The chest radiograph can give the surgeon general information about aortic calcification, and the ECG provides baseline information about the patient's heart rhythm. Laboratory tests include complete blood count (CBC), electrolytes, prothrombin time (PT), partial thromboplastin time (PTT), blood urea nitrogen (BUN), and creatinine. Pulmonary function tests and arterial blood gases (ABGs) may be performed if a patient has underlying pulmonary problems. Cost is always a consideration; only necessary tests should be ordered.

Effective preoperative teaching, which reduces anxiety and physiological responses to stress before and after surgery, is an important aspect of psychological preparation. The surgical procedure and the intraoperative and postoperative experiences are explained. The patient usually is not in the ICU before surgery, and a tour of the ICU helps familiarize the patient and family with the specialized equipment and environment. The sight of a patient who is successfully recovering from cardiac surgery helps instill confidence and allay anxiety. Incorporating family members or significant others in the education process is pivotal in patient care. Specific teaching topics related to the patient's stay in the ICU are listed in Box 22-3.

Numerous invasive lines are placed in the patient before surgery and are used for monitoring during and after surgery. These include a thermodilution pulmonary artery catheter, arterial line, and Foley catheter. Use of the pulmonary artery catheter has become controversial recently, and is determined primarily by the patient's preoperative left ventricular function. The patient is intubated, and a nasogastric tube and additional intravenous lines may also be inserted.

Intraoperative Phase

SURGICAL APPROACH

The surgical approach most commonly used for myocardial revascularization and valve surgery is median sternotomy. The sternum is split with a sternal saw from the manubrium to below the xiphoid process, and the ribs are spread to expose the anterior mediastinum and pericardium.

box 22-3
Preoperative Teaching About the Intensive Care Unit Experience for the Patient Undergoing Cardiac Surgery

Equipment to Point Out
- Cardiac monitor
- Arterial line
- Thermodilution catheter
- IV lines and IV infusion pumps
- Endotracheal tube and ventilator
  - Suctioning
  - Explain how to communicate when intubated; unable to talk
  - Explain when extubation can be anticipated
- Foley catheter (increased sensation to urinate)
- Chest tubes (anticipated removal)
- Pacing wires
- Nasogastric tube
- Soft hand restraints

Incisions and Dressings to Expect
- Median sternotomy or other incision
- Leg incision (if saphenous vein is used)

Patient's Immediate Postoperative Appearance
- Skin yellow owing to use of Betadine solution in operating room
- Skin pale and cool to touch because of hypothermia during surgery
- Generalized "puffiness," especially noticeable in neck, face, and hands, because of third spacing of fluid given during cardiopulmonary bypass

Awakening From Anesthesia
- Patient recovers in the intensive care unit (ICU); does not go to the postanesthesia care unit
- Each patient recovers from anesthesia differently
- Patient may feel certain sensations
- Patient may hear certain noises
- Patient may be aware or able to hear but unable to respond

Discomfort
- Amount of discomfort to be expected
- When pain might be expected
- Relief mechanisms
  - Positioning/splinting
  - Medications
  - Patient-controlled analgesia (PCA) and the importance of early administration of pain medication

Postoperative Respiratory Care
- Turning
- Use of pillow to splint median sternotomy incision
- Effective coughing and deep breathing after extubation; have patient practice exercises before surgery
- Incentive spirometry
- Early mobilization

Miscellaneous
- Postoperative activity progression
- Hospital visiting policy in intensive care area

Once the pericardium is opened and the heart and aorta are exposed, the patient is placed on cardiopulmonary bypass.

As myocardial revascularization has become increasingly sophisticated, new interventions to minimize the invasive nature of the surgery have been developed. The number of patients undergoing reoperations using CABG has increased, and if the mediastinal approach is used in a reoperation, injury to old bypass grafts or embolization of debris due to manipulation of diseased grafts may cause problems.[12] A smaller lateral thoracotomy incision is often used to decrease the risks associated with reentry into the mediastinum. The choice of incision is based on the specific needs of each patient and the experience of the surgeon.

CARDIOPULMONARY BYPASS

Cardiac surgery as it is known today was made possible by the development and practical application of cardiopulmonary bypass by Gibbon in 1953.[1] Because the heart must be still (not beating) and empty during the surgery, a cardiopulmonary bypass machine is used. This machine, also called a *pump oxygenator*, assumes the job of oxygenating the patient's blood and circulating it throughout the body.

Before the bypass is implemented, the pump tubing is primed with a balanced electrolyte solution; blood is not used. The patient's deoxygenated venous blood is brought to the pump either through one cannula placed in the right atrial appendage or by two cannulas, one of which is placed directly in the inferior vena cava and the other directly in the superior vena cava. Another cannula is placed in the ascending aorta to return oxygenated blood to the patient's systemic circulation (Fig. 22-6). Heparin is administered throughout cardiopulmonary bypass to prevent massive extravascular coagulation as the blood circulates through the mechanical parts of the bypass system. After bypass is established, the blood is pumped through the circuit by a series of roller-type pumps that, unlike normal heart function, produce a nonpulsatile flow. Venous blood from the patient flows through the venous cannula to the cardiotomy reservoir and then into the oxygenator, where exchange of oxygen and carbon dioxide occurs. The blood then travels through the heat exchanger, where it is cooled initially and later rewarmed.

During bypass, the patient's core body temperature is lowered to 28°C to 32°C (82.4°F to 89.6°F) to decrease metabolism. For each 1°C drop of body temperature, the metabolic demands of the body decrease by 7%. This reduction in metabolic demands helps protect the major organ systems from possible ischemic injury and adverse effects of nonpulsatile perfusion during cardiopulmonary bypass.

Oxygenated blood is filtered and returned to the patient's ascending aorta through the arterial cannula (see Fig. 22-6).

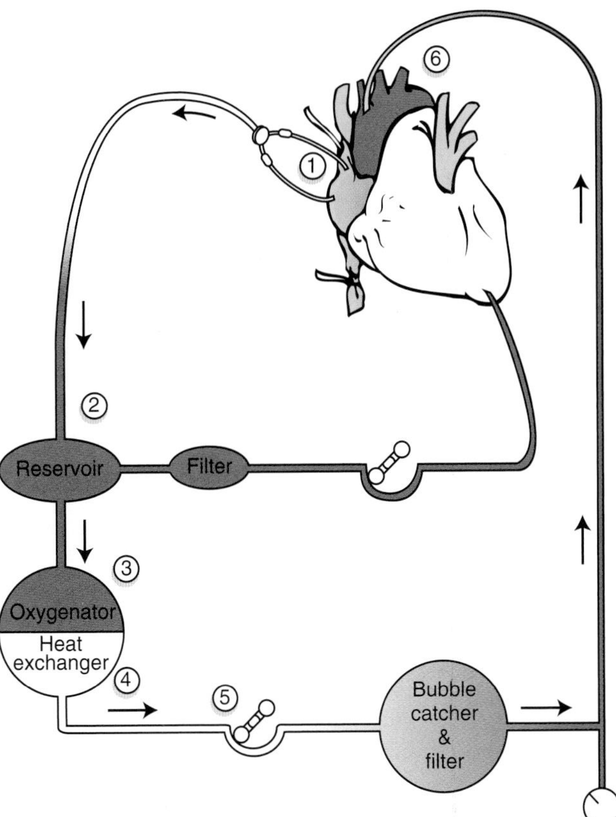

figure 22-6 Blood flow through the circuit of the cardiopulmonary bypass machine: (1): Patient's deoxygenated blood enters the bypass circuit from the venous cannulas in the superior and inferior vena cavae. (2) The reservoir holds the blood temporarily. (3) The oxygenator removes carbon dioxide from and adds oxygen to the patient's blood. (4) The heat exchanger initially cools the blood and then rewarms the blood. (5) Roller pumps pump the blood through the circuit and back to the patient. (6) Oxygenated blood is returned to the ascending aorta by way of the aortic cannula.

Once extracorporeal circulation is established and systemic hypothermia is achieved, the aorta is cross-clamped just above the coronary arteries, and either crystalloid or blood cardioplegia solution is infused into the aortic root. The formula varies, but cardioplegia solution is a balanced electrolyte solution high in potassium. Oxygenated blood from the bypass circuit or oxygenated crystalloid can be added to the cardioplegia solution.

After the aorta is cross-clamped, no blood circulates through the coronary arteries, so the myocardium becomes ischemic. Cold cardioplegia solution at 4°C (39.2°F) is infused into the aortic root under pressure. As it circulates through the coronary arteries, the high potassium concentration causes immediate asystole and relaxation, and the cold produces myocardial hypothermia. Asystole and hypothermia protect against myocardial ischemia by decreasing the metabolic needs of myocardial tissue. The cardioplegia solution provides a substrate for ongoing cellular metabolism and ensures appropriate pH and calcium ion levels for myocardial preservation.[13] The inclusion of blood or oxygenated crystalloid in the cardioplegia solution lessens myocardial ischemia by supplying oxygen. Cardioplegia solution may be infused into the aortic root continuously or intermittently every 15 to 30 minutes and whenever cardiac electrical activity recurs. This process varies, depending on surgeon preference.

Because perfusion of cardioplegia solution through occluded or diseased coronary arteries may not produce an even myocardial cooling, inadequately cooled areas risk ischemic damage. Therefore, hypothermia is also created topically by pouring iced normal saline slush over the heart into the pericardial well. Cardioplegia with concomitant topical hypothermia cools the heart evenly while maintaining the myocardial temperature at 8° to 15°C (46.4°F to 59°F). Thus, throughout surgery, a threefold approach protects the patient against possible detrimental effects: systemic hypothermia, cold cardioplegia, and topical cardiac hypothermia.

Several disadvantages to cold cardioplegia have been identified, including postoperative myocardial depression, ventricular arrhythmias, decreased cerebral blood flow, irreversible platelet dysfunction, and shifts of the oxygen–hemoglobin dissociation curve to the left so that blood delivers oxygen to the tissues less readily. A heart receiving cold crystalloid cardioplegia must have blood reintroduced into the coronary circulation (reperfusion). This reintroduction of oxygen may cause release of toxic substances that injure myocardial cells (reperfusion injury). To avoid these disadvantages, some cardiac surgeons use normothermic blood cardioplegia delivered at 37°C (98.6°F), which keeps the heart at a normal temperature. With the warm technique, topical cardiac hypothermia is not used, and systemic hypothermia may or may not be used. Advantages of warm cardioplegia include more frequent spontaneous return of normal sinus rhythm after surgery, better postoperative left ventricular function and cardiac index, less use of inotropic agents, and less postoperative bleeding. Patients who have undergone warm cardioplegia require less time on the ventilator and almost no rewarming technology in the ICU.

After surgery is completed, the heat exchanger rewarms the blood to return the patient's core temperature to 37°C (98.6°F) if hypothermic techniques were used. After air is vented from the heart chambers and the aortic root, the aortic cross-clamp is removed so that blood again perfuses the coronary arteries, warming the myocardium. As perfusion and rewarming continue, a spontaneous cardiac rhythm may resume, ventricular fibrillation may develop (necessitating internal defibrillation), or pacing may be used to initiate a rhythm. After a reliable rhythm with a rate adequate to maintain the cardiac output and blood pressure is established, total cardiopulmonary bypass is reduced to partial bypass. During partial bypass, some of the patient's blood circulates through the heart and lungs, while some continues to circulate through the pump. If adequate arterial pressures are maintained, the patient's heart then assumes total responsibility for the cardiac output, and bypass is discontinued.

After the heart can maintain an adequate cardiac output, the cannulas are removed from the right atrium and aorta. Heparinization is reversed by the administration of protamine sulfate. If adequate cardiac output cannot be maintained during the weaning process, positive inotropic agents or intra-aortic balloon counterpulsation can be instituted (see Chapter 18).

COMPLETION OF SURGERY

If the need for postoperative cardiac pacing is anticipated, temporary pacing electrodes are placed on the epicardial surface of the heart and brought out through the chest wall on either side of the median sternotomy incision. Ventricular pacing electrodes are typically located to the left and atrial wires to the right of the sternum (Fig. 22-7).

Chest tubes placed in the mediastinum and pericardial space for drainage are brought out through stab wounds just below the median sternotomy. If the pleural space has been entered, pleural tubes are also placed. Smaller, more flexible chest drains are being used instead of the stiff, larger-bore tubes to enhance drainage of the pleural and mediastinal space.[14] After adequate hemostasis is obtained, the edges of the sternum are approximated with stainless steel wires, the incision is closed, and dressings are applied.

Postoperative Phase

Patients are transported directly to the ICU, where they recover from anesthesia and usually remain for 24 hours after surgery. Patients arrive in the ICU with numerous lines and tubes (e.g., endotracheal tube, hemodynamic monitoring lines). Immediate postoperative care involves cardiac monitoring and maintenance of oxygenation/hemodynamic stability, as described in Box 22-4. Because cardiopulmonary bypass produces abnormal blood interface and altered blood flow patterns, it has profound physiological effects (Table 22-1).

The postoperative course depends on the patient's preoperative condition. Factors that may increase mortality include age; sex; previous similar surgery (resurgery); preoperative occurrence of acute myocardial infarction; and concomitant conditions such as diabetes mellitus, peripheral vascular disease, renal insufficiency, and chronic obstructive pulmonary disease (COPD).[1] Whether the surgery is elective or emergent may also influence outcome. Awareness of these conditions helps the critical care nurse anticipate problems. Accurate assessments, vigilant monitoring, and proper interventions are critical in stabilizing patients who have just undergone cardiac surgery. Box 22-5 lists some nursing diagnoses and collaborative problems in cardiac surgery. Box 22-6 presents a collaborative care guide for the patient after such surgery. Certain patient populations present special problems. Box 22-7 lists factors to consider in management of the older cardiac patient.

box 22-4
Nursing Responsibilities in Caring for the Cardiac Surgery Patient in the Immediate Postoperative Period

Priority Interventions Performed by the Critical Care Team on Arrival

- Attach patient to bedside cardiac monitor and note rhythm.
- Attach pressure lines to bedside monitor (arterial and pulmonary artery); level and zero transducers and note pressure values and waveforms.
- Obtain cardiac output/index and note existing inotropic or vasoactive drips.
- Connect ventilator and auscultate breath sounds bilaterally.
- Apply end-tidal carbon dioxide ($ETCO_2$) device to ventilator circuit and note waveform and value (best indicator of endotracheal tube placement).
- Apply pulse oximetry device to patient and note Spo_2 value and waveform.
- Check peripheral pulses and perfusion signs.
- Monitor chest tubes and character of drainage: amount, color, flow. Check for air leaks.
- Measure body temperature and initiate rewarming if temperature <96.8°F (36°C).

Once the Patient Is Determined to Be Hemodynamically Stable

- Measure urine output and note characteristics.
- Obtain clinical data (within 30 minutes of arrival).
- Obtain chest radiograph.
- Obtain 12-lead electrocardiogram (ECG).
- Obtain routine blood work within 15 minutes of arrival; tests may include ABGs, potassium, glucose, PTT, hemoglobin (varies with institution).
- Assess neurological status.
- Test pacemaker function by assessing capture and sensing.

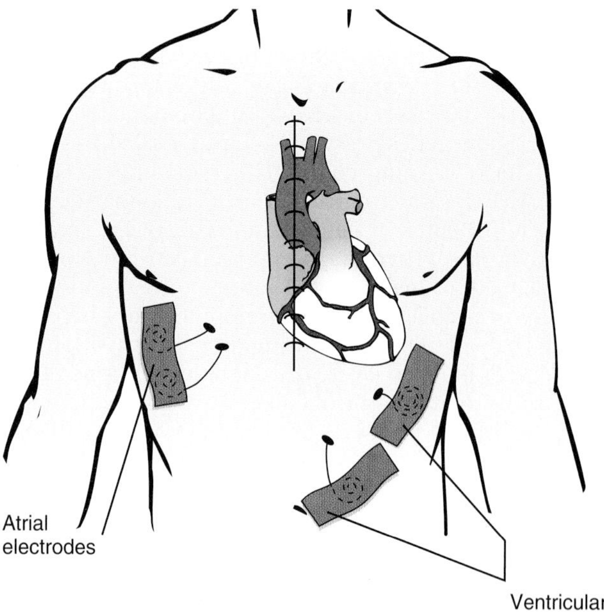

figure 22-7 Temporary epicardial pacing wires: position of atrial and ventricular wires on chest wall.

PREVENTION OF HYPOTHERMIA

Whether the cardiac procedure is performed on or off bypass, hypothermia is a common side effect. During rewarming on cardiopulmonary bypass, the patient's core temperature is returned to 98.6°F (37°C). However, as this warmed blood begins to circulate to the periphery, heat transfer to the surrounding tissues again causes the core temperature to decline. Patients frequently enter the

table 22-1 Effects of Cardiopulmonary Bypass

Causes	Clinical Implications
Increased Capillary Permeability	
Interface between blood and nonphysiological surfaces or bypass circuit leads to • Complement activation that increases capillary permeability • Platelet activation—platelets secrete vasoactive substances that increase capillary permeability • Release of other vasoactive substances that increase capillary permeability	Large amounts of fluid move from the intravascular to the interstitial space during and up to 6 h after cardiopulmonary bypass. Patient becomes edematous.
Hemodilution	
Solution used to prime extracorporeal circuit dilutes patient's blood. Secretion of vasopressin (ADH) is increased. Levels of renin–angiotensin–aldosterone are increased because of nonpulsatile renal perfusion. Total body water is increased.	Decreased blood viscosity improves capillary perfusion during nonpulsatile flow and hypothermia. Hgb and Hct decrease. Levels of coagulation factors are decreased because of dilution. Intravascular colloid osmotic pressure is decreased, contributing to movement of fluid from intravascular to interstitial spaces. Water is retained at collecting tubule of kidney. Aldosterone causes retention of sodium and water at renal tubule. Weight gain occurs.
Altered Coagulation	
Procoagulant effects: • Interface between blood and nonendothelial surfaces of bypass circuit activates intrinsic coagulation cascade. • Platelet damage activates intrinsic pathway.	Risk of microemboli is increased.
Anticoagulant effects: • Interface between blood and nonendothelial surfaces of bypass circuit causes platelets to adhere to tubing and to clump; abnormal platelet function; activation of coagulation cascade, which depletes clotting factors; denaturization of plasma proteins, including coagulation factors. • Coagulation factors are decreased as a result of hemodilution.	Platelet count decreases by 50% to 70% of baseline. Abnormal postoperative bleeding occurs. Possibility of bleeding diathesis exists.
Damage to Blood Cells	
Exposure of blood to nonendothelial surfaces causes mechanical trauma and shear stress. • Platelet damage occurs. • Red blood cell hemolysis occurs. • Leukocytes are damaged.	Platelet count is decreased. Free hemoglobin and hemoglobinuria are increased. Hct is decreased. Immune response is diminished.
Microembolization	
Emboli form from tissue debris, air bubbles, platelet aggregation.	Microemboli to body organs (brain, lungs, kidney) are possible.
Increased Systemic Vascular Resistance (SVR)	
Catecholamine secretion is increased when cardiopulmonary bypass is initiated. Renin secretion is due to nonpulsatile flow to kidney. Hypothermia develops.	Hypertension is possible. Increased SVR may decrease cardiac output.
Increased Capillary Permeability	
Interface between blood and nonphysiological surfaces or bypass circuit leads to • Complement activation that increases capillary permeability • Platelet activation—platelets secrete vasoactive substances that increase capillary permeability	Large amounts of fluid move from the intravascular to the interstitial space during and up to 6 h after cardiopulmonary bypass. Patient becomes edematous.

ICU with a temperature in the 95°F to 96.8°F (35°C to 36°C) range. OPCABG causes hypothermia because of heat loss secondary to prolonged exposure to cool operating room temperatures. Hypothermia causes peripheral vasoconstriction and a shift of the oxygen–hemoglobin dissociation curve to the left, which means that less oxygen is released from the hemoglobin to the tissues. Hypothermia can also impair coagulation because all enzyme systems in the body depend on a tight temperature range for optimum performance.[15]

The nurse assesses the patient's temperature on ICU admission using pulmonary artery or tympanic membrane

box 22-5 *Examples of Nursing Diagnoses and Collaborative Problems for Cardiac Surgery Patients*

- Decreased Cardiac Output related to changes in left ventricular preload, afterload, and contractility
- Decreased Cardiac Output related to cardiac dysrhythmias
- Impaired Tissue Perfusion related to cardiopulmonary bypass, decreased cardiac output, hypotension
- Impaired Tissue Perfusion related to microembolization secondary to the SIRS process
- Impaired Gas Exchange related to cardiopulmonary bypass, anesthesia, poor chest expansion, atelectasis, retained secretions
- Impaired Comfort related to endotracheal tube, surgical incision, chest tubes, rib spreading
- Anxiety related to fear of death, intensive care unit environment
- Risk for Fluid Volume Deficit related to abnormal bleeding
- Risk for Infection related to surgical procedure, invasive lines, drainage tubes, hypoventilation, retained secretions

temperature; if performed properly, both are considered accurate indicators of core temperature. Rectal temperature does not correlate with core temperature measurements until 8 hours after surgery, and bladder temperature differs significantly from core temperature with rapid cooling and rewarming. Increasing the room temperature and using radiant heat, blankets, or a warming blanket are effective techniques for increasing core temperature. Rewarming should occur slowly to prevent hemodynamic instability due to rapid vasodilation.

It is important to prevent shivering, which occurs most often from 90 to 180 minutes after ICU admission, because it increases metabolic rate, oxygen consumption, carbon dioxide production, and myocardial workload. If left ventricular function is compromised, shivering should be managed with a neuromuscular blocker in combination with simultaneous sedation to avoid further cardiac compromise. In unusual situations, the patient may experience discomfort with shivering, which can be treated with meperidine (Demerol).

After rewarming, many patients experience an overshoot in body temperature. One etiological theory is that narcotics and anesthetics administered during surgery reset the hypothalamic regulatory center, altering peripheral blood flow and feedback.[16] A cold, constricted peripheral vascular bed may also be a factor in preventing heat dissipation. If the patient is bleeding after surgery, correction of temperature is imperative to aid in the return of normal coagulation enzyme function and clotting ability.

MONITORING FOR SYSTEMIC INFLAMMATORY RESPONSE SYNDROME

Any process, including surgery, initiates the inflammatory process called SIRS. In recent years, research in critical care medicine has focused on SIRS because it may be the cause of many patient problems. An entire "body" inflammatory response may occur after CABG surgery that appears to be an infection. Symptoms and signs include fever, tachycardia, tachypnea, and an increased white blood cell count. To attempt to differentiate between SIRS and infection or sepsis, the American College of Chest Physicians (ACCP) convened a consensus conference in 1997.[17] The conference developed definitions differentiating the two conditions (Box 22-8) that are now used frequently by critical care experts.

SIRS is a natural defense mechanism that is initiated when tissue or vessels are injured. A vascular injury, the inflammatory response, and the coagulation cascade are interrelated. An event that disrupts the integrity of the endothelium, such as trauma from cutting the vessel or hypoxia in a few endothelial cells, triggers the process. Once the injury occurs, a local inflammatory reaction begins with the release of mediators called *cytokines* from "protector" cells (e.g., lymphocytes, macrophages). These mediators signal other cells (e.g., neutrophils, monocytes) to the injured area, which release other mediators. The endothelium then releases vasodilating mediators (e.g., nitric oxide), which increase blood flow to the area, thereby increasing oxygen delivery. Counter-regulatory mediators cause vasoconstriction to balance vasodilatory actions. Platelets are attracted to the area to start the coagulation process. As a result of the endothelial damage, increased capillary permeability inevitably occurs.[18] This highly complex process is discussed in more detail in Chapter 50.

It was once believed that the cardiopulmonary bypass machine was the major trigger of SIRS; this prompted experts to reconsider the use of the bypass machine. However, Vallely and colleagues have demonstrated that OPCABG also initiates a SIRS response involving the release of different mediators from the on-pump procedure.[7] Few interventions limit SIRS; the inflammatory process is so complex that it has been difficult to develop medications to counter all the numerous reactions. Steroids have been shown to decrease SIRS somewhat if given before surgery, but they should be used with caution, especially in patients with diabetes mellitus.[1] Nursing responsibilities focus on refining assessment skills to increase early detection of embolic events in any system, especially the nervous, cardiovascular, pulmonary, and renal systems. It is important to have a high degree of suspicion when assessing patients and providing postoperative care.

CONTROLLING PAIN

After cardiac surgery, the patient may experience pain resulting from the chest or leg incision, the chest tubes, rib spreading during surgery, and care activities. The ICU environment may accentuate the pain physiologically because of light and noise, and psychologically because of separation and fear. Pain often stimulates the sympathetic nervous system, increasing heart rate and blood pressure, which can be detrimental to the patient's hemodynamics. Discomfort can also result in diminished chest expansion, increased atelectasis, and retention of secretions.

Although pain perception varies from person to person, a median sternotomy incision is usually less painful than a thoracotomy incision, and most people report that the pain is most severe the first 3 to 4 days after surgery. Discomfort from the leg incision often worsens after the patient is ambulatory, especially if leg swelling occurs. Stretching of back and neck muscles as the ribs are spread and immobilization

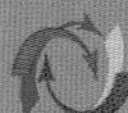

box 22-6 collaborative care guide
for the Patient After Cardiac Surgery

OUTCOMES	INTERVENTIONS
Oxygenation/Ventilation	
Patient will have arterial blood gases within normal limits and pulse oximeter value >92%. Pulmonary edema will be minimized on chest x-ray and demonstrated by improved breath sounds.	■ Obtain arterial blood gases per protocol. ■ Correlate pulse oximeter and end-tidal CO_2 with arterial blood gas results. ■ Adjust ventilator settings after consulting with the respiratory therapist and physician. ■ Wean from mechanical ventilation per protocol using the expertise of respiratory therapy. ■ Extubate when patient is hemodynamically stable; able to protect airway. ■ Provide supplemental oxygen after extubation.
Atelectasis will be improved.	■ Encourage use of incentive spirometer, cough and deep breath q 2 to 4 hours after extubation.
Chest tubes will remain patent.	■ Milk chest tubes if necessary to facilitate forward clot movement.
Circulation/Perfusion	
Patient will maintain adequate clinical perfusion. Vital signs will be within normal limits, including MAP >70 mm Hg; cardiac index will be in a suitable range for the patient's left ventricular function.	■ Monitor PA and PAWP, CVP or RAP, cardiac output, SVR, and PVR per protocol if pulmonary artery catheter is in place. ■ Monitor ECG, ST segments, and arterial blood pressure continuously. ■ Administer positive inotropic agents and reduce afterload with vasodilating agents guided by hemodynamic parameters and physician orders. ■ Regulate volume administration as indicated by PAWP or CVP values. ■ Evaluate effect of medications on BP, HR, and hemodynamic parameters. ■ Monitor and treat dysrhythmias per protocol and physician orders. ■ Anticipate need for temporary cardiac pacing; wires will be properly isolated for electrical safety. ■ Prepare patient for intra-aortic balloon pump assist if necessary. ■ Congestive heart failure due to decreased cardiac output or perioperative MI will be minimized by collaborating with a physician. ■ Assess for neck vein distension, pulmonary crackles, S_3 or S_4, peripheral edema, increased preload parameters, elevated "a" wave of CVP, RAP, or PAWP waveform. ■ Monitor 12-lead ECG if ECG changes observed.
Patient will be euthermic.	■ Assess temperature q 1 h. ■ Warm patient 1°C per hour by using warming blankets, lights, and fluid warmer.
Hematological Issues	
Patient will have minimal bleeding and avoid cardiac tamponade.	■ Chest tube drainage will be <200 mL/h. ■ Monitor for signs of cardiac tamponade (hypotension, pulsus paradoxus, tachycardia, PA pressure equalization). ■ Evaluate chest x-ray for widened mediastinum, consulting with a physician as needed. ■ Monitor PT, PTT, ACT, CBC per protocol. ■ Administer protamine, blood products, and other procoagulants per order or protocol.

(continued)

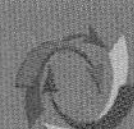

box 22-6 collaborative care guide
for the Patient After Cardiac Surgery (Continued)

OUTCOMES	INTERVENTIONS
	■ Monitor vasoactive drug need and report marked increase of drugs to physician immediately because this change may indicate possible tamponade.
Fluids/Electrolytes	
Patient will maintain or improve preoperative renal function.	■ Renal function will be maintained as evidenced by urine output of approximately 0.5 mL/kg/h. ■ Potassium will be replaced to maintain K^+ >4.0 mEq/L. ■ Monitor intake and output q 1–2 h. ■ Monitor BUN, creatinine, electrolytes, Mg, PO_4. ■ Record daily weights. ■ Administer fluid volume or diuretics as ordered.
Mobility/Skin Integrity	
Patient will maintain range of motion and muscle strength and will have intact skin integrity.	■ Turn patient side to side every 2 hours while on bed rest and evaluate skin closely. ■ Mobilize out of bed after extubation. ■ Progress activity to chair for meals, bathroom privileges, increased distance walking, delegating to assistive personnel as indicated. ■ Monitor vital signs, respiratory effort during activity.
Incisions will heal without evidence of infection.	■ Check stability of sternotomy incision daily, especially with diabetic patients. ■ Assess sternotomy and leg incision for redness, swelling, drainage. ■ Apply TED hose and elevate legs to reduce edema. ■ Caloric and nutrient intake meet metabolic requirements per calculation for long-term patients. ■ Monitor prealbumin for trends on long-term patients.
Comfort and Pain Control	
Patient will have relief of surgical pain. Patient will demonstrate no evidence of pain or anxiety such as increased HR, BP, RR, or agitation during activity or procedures. Timely administration of pain medication will be a priority.	■ Assess quality, duration, location of pain. Use visual analog scale to assess pain quantity. ■ Provide a calm environment. Provide for adequate periods of rest and sleep.
Teaching/Discharge Planning	
Patient and family will understand need for: Tests, procedures, treatments. Self-protective devices as indicated and per hospital policy. In preparation for discharge to home, patient will understand activity levels, dietary restrictions, medication regimen, incision care.	■ Consult nutritional support services. ■ Make appropriate social work referrals early during hospitalization. ■ Initiate family education regarding heart-healthy diet, physical activity limitations (e.g., lifting over 10–15 lbs, driving restrictions), stress reduction strategies, management of pain, incision care.

for several hours during surgery can cause back and neck discomfort. Patients who have internal mammary artery grafts may have increased pain because of increased stretching of the intercostal muscles and the incision into the parietal pleura, which is richly innervated.

Angina after CABG may indicate graft failure; therefore, the nurse must be able to differentiate angina from incisional pain. Typical median sternotomy pain is localized; does not radiate; and can be sharp, dull, aching, or burning. It is often worse with deep breathing, coughing, or movement. Angina is usually precordial or substernal; not well localized; and frequently radiates to arms, neck, or jaw. It is often described as a pressure sensation and is not affected by respiration or movement.

One of the goals of nursing management is a thorough assessment of the patient's pain using a pain scale; administration of analgesics based on the reported pain intensity; provision of adequate pain relief as reported by the patient; and alleviation of factors that enhance pain perception, such as anxiety and fear. The common analgesic agents

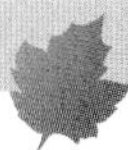

box 22-7

Considerations for the Older Patient After Cardiac Surgery

Physiological Changes

Cardiovascular System

- Increased stiffness of myocardial muscle
- Increased stiffness of peripheral vasculature and decreased ability to adjust to changes in blood volume
- Replacement of cells in conduction system with collagen and elastin
- Decreasing number of pacemaker cells in the sinoatrial (SA) and atrioventricular (AV) nodes
- Decreased cardiac responsiveness to beta-adrenergic stimulation

Pulmonary System

- Breakdown of elastin and collagen, which impairs elastic recoil of lung
- Thoracic cage less compliant
- Decreased expiratory muscle strength and mucociliary clearance

Renal System

- Progressive loss of cortical nephrons and decrease in corticomedullary concentration gradient
- Impaired renal concentrating ability
- Decreased clearance of medications excreted by the kidneys (may be reduced by up to 40% by 80 years of age)

Gastrointestinal System

- Decreased and more variable gastrointestinal absorption of medications
- Decline in liver function, resulting in decreased hepatic breakdown of medications

Musculoskeletal System

- Skeletal osteoporosis

Immune System

- Immune response may be decreased, especially if concomitant malnutrition and decrease in serum proteins

Neurological System

- Decline in neurotransmitters
- Increased risk of acute confusion

Response to Medications

- Decreased percentage of lean body tissue
- Increased percentage of body fat
- Decrease in body water

Clinical Effect

- Higher filling pressures (pulmonary artery diastolic [PAD] pressure and pulmonary artery wedge pressure [PAWP])
- Decreased ability for vasoconstriction with position change, leading to orthostatic hypotension
- SA and AV node impairment
- Cardiac output maintained by increase in stroke volume
- Slowing of renal response to dehydration
- Decreased effectiveness of fluid conservation
- Toxic medication levels or abnormally prolonged duration of action
- Sensitive to drugs with narrow therapeutic range, such as digoxin
- More intense medication effect and longer duration of action for medications broken down in liver (e.g., benzodiazepines)
- As a result of decreased body water, water-soluble medications concentrated in the bloodstream, resulting in higher serum drug levels
- Fat-soluble medications stored in fat; increase in fat tissue may result in slower therapeutic response and longer duration of action as drug is released slowly from fat

Patient Teaching

- Accommodate sensory deficits.
  - Ensure hearing aids are in and functional.
  - Speak loudly and face patient.
  - Use large print, easy-to-read materials.
- Teach one thing at a time, and ensure patient understands before moving on.
- Start with simple and progress to more complex information.
- Teach both patient and caregiver.

Adapted from Dixon V: Effects of vascular surgery on the elderly vascular patient. J Vasc Nurs 17:86–88, 1999.

box 22-8

Definition of Systemic Inflammatory Response Syndrome (SIRS)

SIRS is defined by the presence of two or more of the following conditions:

Temperature	>100.4°F (38°C) or <96.8°F (36°C)
Heart rate	>90 beats/minute
Respiratory rate	>20 breaths/minute or $Paco_2$ <32 mm Hg
White blood cell count	>12,000 cells/m³, <4000 cells/m³, or >10% immature (bands) cells

Sepsis is a systemic response to documented infection and is determined by the same criteria as SIRS.

used are morphine sulfate, fentanyl, and hydromorphone (Dilaudid), as needed. These drugs can be supplemented with nonsteroidal anti-inflammatory drugs (NSAIDs), such as ketorolac (Toradol), which decrease pain through a different mechanism. Caution should be used in administering NSAIDs to patients with compromised renal function. Patient-controlled analgesia (PCA) pumps are frequently used to allow the patient to control administration of pain medication. Interventions such as intercostal nerve blocks and spinal analgesia are less common. Regardless of the mechanism used, pain control is aggressively pursued to ensure comfort and rapid mobilization, which in turn can lessen complications. Alternative therapies such as music therapy and guided imagery may also be useful in controlling pain.

PREVENTING CARDIOVASCULAR COMPLICATIONS

Volume Resuscitation

Adequate intravascular volume to provide preload is a primary concern. Increased capillary permeability due to SIRS causes intravascular volume to shift into the interstitial spaces. To maintain optimal cardiac performance and blood pressure, proper volume resuscitation is imperative. A variety of fluids may be used, including normal saline, hetastarch, and hyperosmolar fluids (e.g., 3% saline).[19] No fluid is definitively recommended. If the patient is bleeding, blood products should be the fluid of choice. If the patient's blood pressure is unresponsive to moderate infusion rates, usually 500 mL is infused using a pressure bag and a large-bore catheter. Hemodynamic parameters, including a low central venous pressure (CVP) (<8 to 10 mm Hg), low pulmonary artery diastolic pressure, and low pulmonary artery wedge pressure (<14 to 18 mm Hg), in combination with a low cardiac index (<2.5 L/minute/m^2), help guide interventions.[15] Caution should be exercised in using these numerical values as absolute goals.

The preoperative condition of the heart is important to consider. If the patient has had a recent myocardial infarction or poor left ventricular performance, higher pressures may be required to maintain optimal cardiac work. The patient with a hypertrophied left ventricle, especially with valvular disease, is heavily dependent on volume resuscitation.

The effectiveness of all interventions must be assessed against the patient's response. Mottling of the extremities, especially the knees, as well as the character of the peripheral pulses (especially dorsalis pedalis) are clinical indications of perfusion.[20] The combination of weak pulses and mottled knees may indicate hypoperfusion. Resolution of these clinical findings, as well as improved pressure values, signal the return of adequate perfusion. The astute critical care nurse continually monitors the appearance of the extremities and the pulses.

Monitoring for Arrhythmias

Arrhythmia is a major issue after CABG surgery. The hemodynamic response to a change in cardiac rhythm dictates the speed of the intervention in patients who have undergone CABG surgery, as in all critical care patients. In emergent situations, Advanced Cardiac Life Support (ACLS) algorithms are used. Knowledge of the patient's baseline rhythm is important. The types of arrhythmias that may occur range from premature atrial contractions to ventricular fibrillation and asystole.

Sinus tachycardia is very common and may result from many factors. Some of the more common causes are sympathomimetic drugs, SIRS, hypovolemia, fever, and pain. Prolonged periods of tachycardia may be harmful due to decreased coronary artery filling time. Sinus bradycardia may occur, but it is not anticipated because patients are in a sympathetically responsive state. In many cases, preoperative beta blockade may be the cause.

Causes of premature atrial contractions are usually electrolyte disturbances, ischemia or infarction, or hypoperfusion. Frequent premature atrial contractions may be a precursor to atrial fibrillation and occur very commonly, especially in patients with a previous history of pulmonary or valve disease in which the atria can be distended. The simple treatment for premature atrial contractions is repletion of potassium and magnesium. Maintenance of adequate potassium (range, 4 to 4.5 mEq/L) and intravenous (IV) infusion of 2 g magnesium may minimize premature atrial contractions.

Atrial fibrillation may occur after CABG, and prevention is a high priority. For new-onset atrial fibrillation, the goal is conversion to sinus rhythm using procainamide or amiodarone. For procainamide, the loading dose is up to 1 g IV at a rate of 20 mg/minute, followed by a 2 mg/minute drip until the arrhythmia is corrected. For amiodarone, the loading dose is 150 mg IV over 10 minutes followed by a 1 mg/minute drip for 6 hours, then a 0.5 mg/minute drip for 18 hours. Additional loading may be necessary. For chronic atrial fibrillation, conversion is not a goal unless the patient has been anticoagulated because of the risk of atrial thrombus and possible embolization. Control of the ventricular response is the goal and can be achieved using diltiazem, starting with a loading dose up to 0.75 mg/kg IV followed by a drip, which is usually started at 5 mg/hour. If emergent cardioversion is required in the immediate postoperative period and anticoagulation is not an option, echocardiography, either Doppler or transesophageal, may be performed to check for thrombus formation in the left atrium.

Heart block arrhythmias occur in patients with valve surgery secondary to the edema at the surgical site, near the conduction system. Resolution of this rhythm is usually attained 48 to 72 hours after surgery once the edema has decreased. Myocardial ischemia and infarction also cause the heart block. Patients who have had cardiac surgery have an advantage with the placement of epicardial pacing wires. Use of these wires allows better control of ventricular response compared with the use of drugs such as atropine and isoproterenol. Atrial pacing is preferred if the atrioventricular (AV) node is intact because it allows optimal hemodynamics with an atrial contraction. If the AV node is not functioning properly, AV sequential pacing may be required. Ventricular pacing is the last choice. If pacing is required for more than 72 hours, permanent pacemaker placement should be considered, especially in patients who have had valve surgery. An in-depth discussion of pacing can be found in Chapter 18.

The occurrence of tachyarrhythmias may lead to emergent situations. If the patient is hemodynamically unstable in a fast rhythm, the first intervention is cardioversion, following ACLS guidelines. If ventricular arrhythmias develop, electrical or pharmacological interventions are necessary. If premature ventricular contractions (PVCs) appear after surgery, magnesium 2 to 4 g IV may help resolve this problem. The new ACLS guidelines de-emphasize the use of lidocaine and recommend amiodarone as the drug of choice, especially in patients with poor left ventricular function. If ventricular tachycardia deteriorates into ventricular fibrillation or other rhythms with no pulse, cardiopulmonary resuscitation should be started immediately; medical personnel should be prepared to open the chest at the bedside to determine and correct the cause of arrest.

Improving Cardiac Contractility

Contractility may be depressed because of the exposure of the heart muscle to manipulation, temperature change, and possible hypoperfusion. The first step taken to improve performance is to ensure optimal volume resuscitation; it will quickly become clear if volume does not increase the cardiac output and index. The addition and titration of sympathomimetic drugs is a common part of the care of patients with decreased contractility. Various drugs, including epinephrine, dobutamine, and milrinone, may be used. Dopamine is another drug that can increase contractility but may cause unwanted tachycardia. The choice of drug varies with institution and health care provider.

As the drug of choice is added, the cause of the ventricular dysfunction should be pursued. Myocardial ischemia and infarction typically cause decreased cardiac function, but other factors may be sources of the problem. *Stunned myocardium*, the transient depression of left ventricular function due to a temporary reduction of myocardial blood flow,[21] may cause transient dysfunction; it is usually associated with normally functioning myocardium. *Hibernating myocardium* is chronically impaired yet viable myocardial tissue, which results in left ventricular dysfunction at rest because of persistently hypoperfused myocardium or repeated stunning.[21] This state can lead to more chronic dysfunction.

Evaluation of cardiac work is not limited to cardiac output and cardiac index. In the more complicated cases, sampling of mixed venous blood gases/mixed venous saturation ($S\bar{v}O_2$) and the arterial–venous difference in oxygen may be useful. These values are indicators of oxygen transport and consumption and can help direct therapy. Although continuous $S\bar{v}O_2$ monitoring may be used in patients with severe myocardial dysfunction, it is not a standard intervention; it is costly and has not proved to make a difference in outcomes.

The intra-aortic balloon pump (IABP) is a mechanical method used to improve coronary perfusion in any of the previously mentioned situations. For a complete discussion of IABP, see Chapter 18. Mechanical factors may lead to depressed cardiac function. Cardiac tamponade, the most common such factor, may require surgical correction. This topic is discussed later in the chapter. Whatever the cause, time and support of function are usually the major factors that improve cardiac performance. However, protracted periods of time with mechanical or pharmacological support may be the signal to start to consider the placement of a ventricular assist device, usually as a bridge to heart transplantation.

Controlling Blood Pressure

A reduction in SVR is another clinical maneuver that can increase cardiac performance. If the patient has an adequate blood pressure (mean arterial pressure [MAP] >70 mm Hg or systolic blood pressure >120 mm Hg) without pharmacological support (alpha-agonist agents to increase blood pressure), afterload reduction should be started even if the patient is on inotropic support. Various agents, including nitroprusside, nitroglycerin, hydralazine, labetalol, and angiotensin-converting enzyme (ACE) inhibitors such as captopril, can be used. The necessary speed of response dictates the choice of drug. For example, IV drugs, especially nitroprusside, rapidly cause a reduction in afterload. Other agents, such as hydralazine and ACE inhibitors, can then be used to augment this effect. ACE inhibitors should be used with caution in patients with impaired renal function because this drug category can exacerbate renal dysfunction. The previously named drugs also reduce blood pressure; in the immediate postoperative period, this is very important in maintaining the integrity of the grafts. A discriminating clinician can easily achieve a clinical goal of well-controlled blood pressure.

PREVENTING PULMONARY COMPLICATIONS

Postoperative pulmonary function depends on preoperative function. The degree of preoperative evaluation in preparation for surgery has changed in the current era of cost containment. If the patient has a significant pulmonary history (e.g., COPD, pulmonary hypertension), baseline pulmonary function tests and ABGs can be very helpful in setting goals in the postoperative period. These tests may help predict how the patient will respond to mechanical ventilation.

The causes of pulmonary dysfunction after cardiac surgery can be attributed to changes that occur with the inflammatory response. Various triggers, such as surgical trauma and regional myocardial ischemia, activate the complement system and release cytokines, leading to an egress of neutrophils and fluid across endothelium. These triggers can also cause end-organ dysfunction, including organs such as the lungs.[7] Such changes in the lungs can lead to alteration in microcirculation and gas exchange that ultimately result in ventilation–perfusion mismatching, shunting, and atelectasis.[15]

Mechanical ventilation is required to achieve adequate oxygenation and ventilation. Adequate oxygenation is achieved by adjusting the level of oxygen delivered by the ventilator; the usual starting point is 40% to 50% oxygen. Effective oxygenation is monitored using pulse oximetry with intermittent ABG sampling. Positive end-expiratory pressure (PEEP) is a standard intervention used to help keep the alveoli open and improve oxygenation. PEEP usually starts at 5 cm H_2O but can be increased to 10 cm H_2O or more if hypoxemia is present. Care must be taken when increasing PEEP because it can decrease preload, thereby decreasing cardiac output and blood pressure. The initial mode for the ventilator is usually assist-control or synchronized intermittent mandatory ventilation (SIMV) and is changed to continuous positive airway pressure (CPAP) when the patient is ready to be weaned for extubation.

Adequate ventilation is maintained by selecting tidal volumes that are appropriate for body size as well as setting a sufficient rate for the ventilator tidal volumes. Monitoring of ventilation should include end-tidal CO_2 monitoring, which should be correlated with the partial pressure of carbon dioxide ($PaCO_2$) on an ABG. End-tidal carbon dioxide ($ETCO_2$) monitoring is also used to confirm proper endotracheal tube placement.

The recent implementation of newer techniques in cardiac anesthesia, which allow for faster recovery times, have led to shorter times on mechanical ventilation. Weaning from mechanical ventilation is a quick process in patients who have undergone CABG surgery. Once the patient has displayed the ability to follow commands and the strength to protect the airway, a short CPAP trial is instituted. The patient can be extubated if (1) cardiac performance is good (cardiac index >2.2 L/minute/m^2), (2) adequate oxygenation and ventilation is achieved without acidosis, and (3) chest tube bleeding is minimal. Aggressive use of incentive spirometry and physical mobility ensures proper pulmonary function. Continual assessment by the critical care nurse is very important. Auscultation of breath sounds should be performed at frequent intervals and as the patient's condition dictates. Diminished breath sounds, especially in the left lower lobe, are common because left lower lobe atelectasis is an expected postoperative outcome. Observation of the work of breathing is also important, and signs such as tachypnea, use of accessory muscles, and prolonged expiratory time can indicate compromised pulmonary function. Bronchodilator therapy may be indicated and should be continued if the patient was using bronchodilators at home.

Prolonged mechanical ventilation may be a complication of cardiac surgery. Protracted poor cardiac function requires continued mechanical ventilation. Phrenic nerve damage due to cold preservation techniques for myocardial protection or physical transection is another cause of ventilatory failure due to diaphragm dysfunction. Acute respiratory distress syndrome (ARDS) associated with SIRS, a hypoperfusion state, or both can also be a reason for prolonged ventilator days. A tracheostomy should be considered in patients with compromised pulmonary function because it can enhance the ventilator weaning process and promote patient comfort. Expert nursing and multidisciplinary care of the patient in ventilatory failure using weaning protocols may make a difference in patient outcome.[22,23]

PREVENTING NEUROLOGICAL COMPLICATIONS

Neurological recovery of the cardiac surgery patient depends on several factors, such as preoperative neurological state; age (older than 70 years); presence of conditions such as aortic atherosclerosis, hypertension, and diabetes mellitus; and use of the IABP.[1] The usual course of neurological recovery is much faster since anesthetic agents have changed. Narcotics and benzodiazepines, with neuromuscular blockade, are used now, and gases are used less.[15] There is little need for sedation when the patient is transported from the operating room unless hemodynamic instability is present. The patient is allowed to wake up and recover from the anesthesia as soon as possible. There may be some barriers to this process, including age and renal failure. The elderly patient is not able to metabolize narcotics and paralytics as quickly as a younger patient and may require a longer recovery time. If the patient is difficult to arouse and has pinpoint pupils, reversal of narcotics with naloxone (Narcan) may be indicated. Naloxone diluted 0.4 mg in 10 mL normal saline and given 1 to 2 mL IV every 5 minutes is a delicate method of regaining level of consciousness that does not reverse pain control. If the patient does not have good muscle strength, reversal of neuromuscular blockade is indicated. Glycopyrrolate 0.6 mg IV and neostigmine 3 mg IV (or more) are used. The patient in renal failure is not able to clear these drugs and probably needs reversal of both narcotics and neuromuscular blockade agents to expedite extubation.

Once the patient is awake, continual evaluation using the standard neurological examination that assesses the level of consciousness and motor and sensory ability is mandatory. Postoperative neurological deficits are divided into two categories: (1) major focal deficits (stroke), stupor, or coma; and (2) deterioration in intellectual function.[1] The best predictor of stroke is proximal aortic atherosclerosis, which is the source of emboli that are released with the manipulation of the aorta, especially during cannulation or cross clamping. Hypoxia, hypoperfusion, hemorrhage, or metabolic abnormalities may also cause strokes.[1] Cognitive changes are more difficult to detect, because there may be deficits in memory, language, and psychomotor function. The family of the patient may be helpful in detecting any subtle changes. These changes are most noticeable immediately after surgery but may still be present 12 to 36 months after the procedure.[24] Confirmation of a stroke can be performed with computed tomography (CT) or magnetic resonance imaging (MRI) of the head, but these studies may need to be repeated; embolic events do not immediately appear on scans. Prevention of such a catastrophic event is difficult, but the risk can be reduced by patient selection and procedure selection.[24] If a patient has known carotid disease, maintaining higher blood pressure may help increase perfusion of the cerebral tissues. Thrombolytic therapy, which is used successfully in other patients with emboli, cannot be used after surgery in the patient who has just had CABG surgery because of bleeding concerns.

MONITORING POSTOPERATIVE BLEEDING

Postoperative bleeding is expected; the challenge is to know when and how to intervene. Anticoagulation interventions that have improved outcomes for the cardiac patient in general confound bleeding problems. Timely correction of bleeding problems can decrease both the occurrence of complications and the cost of patient care. Postoperative thrombolytics, such as warfarin (Coumadin), and antiplatelet therapy hamper coagulation, and their effects are difficult to reverse; reversal may not even be an option, and postoperative bleeding may increase.

Drainage and decompression of the pericardial and pleural spaces is required after cardiac surgery. Traditionally, the chest tubes were large, rigid tubes, which were very uncomfortable for patients. Recently, smaller, more flexible chest tubes with bulb suction have been introduced to decrease discomfort, increase early ambulation, and decrease the accumulation of pleural effusions. Large postoperative pleural effusions may require increased hospital days or rehospitalization. These tubes are longer and more flexible to enhance pleural drainage; they have been found to decrease clinically significant pleural effusions at 6-week follow-up.[14]

Vigilant monitoring of chest tube drainage is imperative to anticipate impending problems. Chest tube drainage is monitored hourly. The usual chest tube output can range from 100 to 200 mL/hour, with periods of increased drainage due to a change in position or temperature. Measurement of drainage may be required at more frequent intervals (every 15 or 30 minutes) if drainage is high. If the chest tube output continues to be greater than 200 mL/hour, then intervention is necessary. Protamine, the first level of intervention, is given at 1 mg for every

100 units of heparin to reverse the effects of heparin, which is used in the surgical process (both on and off bypass).[25] PTT is commonly used to monitor the intrinsic pathway of the coagulation cascade, which heparin affects. Additional protamine may be necessary, especially if the patient is hypothermic, because a "rebound" phenomenon may occur. Aggressive rewarming is very important in a patient who has increased bleeding because the coagulation cascade, with its enzymatic reactions, cannot function properly at hypothermic temperatures. However, as the patient's temperature rises, heparin is reactivated, causing increased bleeding. Platelet infusion (usually 6 units per infusion) is used next to help decrease bleeding. It is important to remember that a platelet infusion can cause a blood product reaction because each infusion may be from multiple donors. Before surgery, patients require therapy to make platelets dysfunctional, thus preventing thrombus formation in the coronary arteries. Causes of platelet dysfunction and postoperative bleeding include medications such as aspirin; the bypass machine itself; the IABP, which mechanically destroys platelets; and heparin-induced thrombocytopenia, a recent phenomenon in which heparin exposure disables platelet function.

Follow-up coagulation studies act as a guide for the need for further infusions as well as monitoring blood loss, but they are not absolute parameters. If bleeding is increasing, a PT can be ordered to monitor the extrinsic pathway of the coagulation cascade and see if other factors need to be replaced. An elevated PT (>15 seconds) may indicate that bleeding is due to a lack of factors such as fibrinogen that can be replaced using fresh frozen plasma, usually 4 to 6 units/infusion. The overall goal is to determine if bleeding is due to a coagulopathy or surgical bleeding. Chest tube bleeding that exceeds 500 mL/hour is considered to be surgical bleeding and mandates surgical reexploration.

Other therapeutic interventions may also be used to decrease bleeding. Coagulation factors such as cryoprecipitate (factors I and VIII) and factor VII are indicated in severe bleeding. Various drugs such as aminocaproic acid (Amicar), a potent inhibitor of fibrinolysis; aprotinin, a serine-protease inhibitor that blocks kallikrein at the beginning of the coagulation cascade; and desmopressin acetate (DDAVP), which influences factor VIII and enhances platelet adhesion, can be administered to promote coagulation.[25] Autotransfusion of mediastinal chest tube drainage using special drainage systems has been used to decrease blood transfusion requirements. However, the possibility that reinfusion can stimulate fibrinolysis and exacerbate bleeding is a concern, and therefore this treatment method is not recommended for routine use (especially in low-risk patients).[1]

Intraoperative measures to prevent bleeding include minimizing hemodilution, minimizing autologous losses, and optimizing coagulation status with full rewarming and antifibrinolytics.[26] Blood loss requires replacement, which should be considered carefully. Transfusion of red blood cells not only can increase exposure to infectious diseases, especially hepatitis and human immunodeficiency virus (HIV), but is associated with increased immunosuppressive and microcirculatory complications.[27] The hemoglobin level indicated for transfusion is a controversial issue. Recent research has indicated that a restrictive transfusion strategy (hemoglobin <7 g/dL) has demonstrated a lower mortality rate in patients who are less critically ill.

Cardiac tamponade is a serious complication of increased postoperative bleeding that occurs when excessive fluid or blood accumulates in the pericardial space, resulting in increasing pressure on the right atrium and ventricle that can lead to collapse of those structures. Tamponade may develop rapidly or slowly, depending on how fast blood accumulates in the pericardial sac. When a patient is treated for excessive bleeding, it is important to monitor the chest tube drainage closely and maintain patency. Decreasing cardiac output and blood pressure and significant increases in pharmacological support (especially norepinephrine [Levophed]) are important warning signs. The mechanism of cardiac tamponade is the collapse of the lower pressure chambers of the right heart as a result of the increasing and equalizing of the CVP, pulmonary artery diastolic pressure (PAD), and the PAWP. This increase and equalization of the three values is classic evidence of cardiac tamponade. However, the clinical situation can be a late finding, and decreasing cardiac performance and blood pressure, despite volume resuscitation, is an earlier indicator. An arterial line waveform with significant respiratory variation (best illustration of an increased pulsus paradoxus) is another warning sign that cardiac tamponade is pending.[28] Definitive diagnosis is made with an echocardiogram (two-dimensional or transesophageal).

Interventions to prevent tamponade include stripping and milking chest tubes when the blood begins to clot, although stripping the tubes can generate increased negative pressure. Because the chambers (atria and ventricles) are being compressed, cardiac pressures may be elevated, especially CVP. Another useful intervention involves the infusion of volume even with increased pressure to keep the structures from collapsing. Performing a pericardial window is the best surgical intervention.

PREVENTING RENAL COMPLICATIONS

The postoperative course of renal function is influenced by preoperative function. Preoperative risk factors are age; history of moderate to severe congestive heart failure; prior CABG; and pre-existing conditions, including type 1 diabetes mellitus and renal disease (serum creatinine 1.4 to 2.0 mg/dL).[1] The usual postoperative course also depends on whether the surgery was performed on or off bypass. After on-bypass CABG, brisk initial urine output is expected because of the priming of the bypass circuit with mannitol and the possible use of diuretics. The output diminishes as these effects decrease with time. After OPCABG, there is a smaller urine volume because patients are not exposed to these interventions. Some patients are able to autodiurese excess volume, but as the inflammatory response diminishes within 24 to 48 hours, the leaky capillary membranes seal and extra interstitial fluid shifts into the intravascular space, increasing the need for pharmacological diuresis with agents such as furosemide. Electrolyte repletion with potassium and magnesium after diuresis is also important to maintaining a regular cardiac rhythm. A slight metabolic acidosis may be present in the patient with existing renal failure and may persist after surgery. If acidosis is present, the source (respiratory, metabolic, or combined) should be determined to intervene appropriately.

The focus of interventions is to remove excess fluid while protecting metabolic and cardiac function.

Oliguria

Decreasing urine output (<0.5 mL/kg/hour) is usually caused by decreased renal perfusion. Obvious causes such as Foley catheter obstruction or malposition may often be overlooked and should be considered initially, so that mechanical problems may be ruled out. Decreased cardiac function might also be causing a decrease in urine output. Hypovolemia is a very common problem that can be addressed with fluid boluses, and monitoring pulmonary artery pressures and cardiac output/cardiac index shortly after fluid infusions indicates whether the intervention was therapeutic. Caution must be exercised when adding volume because excess fluid can cause decreased function in compromised myocardial muscle. In that situation, inotropic agents or vasoactive drugs may be required. Determining the patient's baseline blood pressure is important so that control of vasoactive drugs can be titrated according to a perfusion pressure (MAP or systolic blood pressure) that the patient's kidneys require.

If none of these interventions is successful, diuresis may be necessary. Loop diuretics (e.g., furosemide) are the usual first-line drugs. If urine output does not increase, larger doses may be indicated or other diuretics that act on other areas of the renal tubular system, such as thiazides, may be added. Creatinine and BUN should be closely monitored.

Renal Failure

If acute renal failure develops, dialysis is necessary. The method used depends on patient condition and practitioner preference. Continuous venovenous hemofiltration (CVVH) and hemodialysis are among the several methods that may be used. CVVH is preferred in the patient who is severely hemodynamically compromised because it is more gradual and minimizes preload compromise, which could decrease cardiac performance. Patients who undergo dialysis require fluid restriction, nutrition modification for prolonged renal dysfunction, and other standard interventions, such as dietary modifications to decrease protein and potassium intake. Chapter 31 provides a further discussion about renal failure. Unfortunately, the mortality rate due to acute renal failure in postoperative cardiac surgery patients is greater than 60%.[1]

PREVENTING ENDOCRINE COMPLICATIONS

Diabetes mellitus is one of the major risk factors for the development of cardiovascular disease. This disease affects almost all systems in the body and requires that the vigilant clinician continually monitor blood sugar and maintain strict glucose control. In the initial postoperative period, a blood glucose level less than 200 mg/dL is particularly important in managing wound healing. Aggressive intervention using an insulin drip initially has reduced the incidence of deep sternal wound infections by 50%.[1] Once good glucose control has been achieved, insulin is given subcutaneously, and glucose levels are followed closely. Such insulin therapy also decreases the incidence of diabetic ketoacidosis or hyperosmolar coma. It is important to remember that whereas hyperglycemia is detrimental, severe hypoglycemia can be fatal. The need for vigilant blood glucose monitoring cannot be overemphasized.

Adrenal insufficiency may occur, especially in patients who were receiving steroids at regular intervals before surgery. The administration of steroids can suppress adrenal function. To prevent suppression, postoperative stress doses of hydrocortisone (100 mg every 8 hours) should be given, and the patient's regular dose should be restarted. If the patient is taking vasoactive drugs and is not weaning off the drips, adrenal insufficiency should be considered; this condition may be the result of hypoperfusion of the adrenal gland. Cortisol levels are low and confirm adrenal insufficiency.

Thyroid dysfunction, especially hypothyroidism, is common in elderly persons and women. Although perioperative effects do not result in dysfunction, preoperative function is an important consideration, and undiagnosed dysfunction may become apparent in the postoperative period because the thyroid hormones, especially triiodothyronine (T_3), can have cardiovascular effects.

PREVENTING GASTROINTESTINAL COMPLICATIONS

Fortunately, the gastrointestinal aspects of the postoperative course are uneventful and similar to those of general surgery. After extubation, the patient remains NPO for up to the first 8 hours, with a nasogastric tube in place to decompress the stomach. The patient is then allowed to have small amounts of ice or water. This relatively simple aspect of nursing care is very important for the postoperative patient, who may experience significant thirst because of the anticholinergic drugs that were received before surgery. The use of ice pops and ginger ale can help with compliance and decrease the possibility of nausea, vomiting, and aspiration.

Complications such as cholecystitis, pancreatitis, and bowel infarction rarely occur. Their pathogenesis is not always clear but is attributed to splanchnic hypoperfusion and general gastrointestinal ischemia. Thorough assessment of the abdomen looking for pain, distension, or tympany may help discover subtle abnormalities. Lactate levels greater than 2.5 mmol/L may indicate splanchnic hypoperfusion. However, they may also be the result of nonpulsatile flow of the bypass machine, which may cause a release of angiotensin II, exacerbating splanchnic ischemia.[15] The need for further evaluation is dictated by the clinical presentation.

MONITORING FOR INFECTION

In the early postoperative period, hypothalamic resetting is the cause of temperature derangement. Febrile reactions are usually attributed to SIRS and to overshoot from rewarming. If the fever (temperature >100.4°F [38°C]) persists for more than 48 to 72 hours, infection should be considered. Prevention of infection is the major goal of all programs. This goal is achieved through the prudent use of antibiotics, vancomycin and a cephalosporin (e.g., cefazolin, ceftazidime). Timing of antibiotic administration is pivotal. For optimal results, preoperative doses should be completely infused before the skin is cut. Antibiotic dosing depends on preoperative renal function. A short postoperative course should also be anticipated.

Mediastinitis is the major infection in patients who have undergone CABG surgery and may be a devastating complication that increases the length of hospital stay and mortality. Risk factors associated with mediastinitis are obesity; prior cardiac surgery; pre-existing type 1 diabetes mellitus; and perioperative factors such as excessive electrocautery use and use of both internal mammary arteries, resulting in compromised blood flow to the chest wall. Therapy is an extended antibiotic course and plastic surgery. The aggressive regulation of blood sugar using insulin drips initially instead of subcutaneous administration has been shown to decrease the occurrence of mediastinitis. This intervention is also used in cases that do not involve CABG; a decrease in mortality has been demonstrated.[29] It is very important to instruct the patient not to use the arms excessively when moving and to use a "cough pillow" with coughing (a small pillow that is placed on the sternal incision and squeezed when coughing). Other interventions, such as having the patient sleep on his or her back, are also important. Following these instructions may help maintain the stability of the sternum.

PATIENT TEACHING AND DISCHARGE PLANNING

With managed care, capitation, rising costs, and limited resources, the usual length of hospitalization after cardiac surgery is 4 to 7 days. Discharge planning that begins at admission is imperative because of the short length of hospital stays. Box 22-9 summarizes patient teaching about cardiac postoperative care, and Box 22-10 contains a discharge planning guide for the post-cardiac surgery patient.

box 22-9 *Recovering From Cardiac Surgery*

General Instructions

- Avoid lifting heavy objects (10–15 lbs or more) for first 3 months.
- Avoid strenuous arm movement such as golf or tennis. When getting in and out of chair or bed, use legs. Arms should not bear weight and should be used only for balance.
- Do not drive for 6 weeks after surgery. (May ride in automobile.)
- Follow physician's instructions for activity progression.
- Resume sexual activity when you can climb two flights of stairs without stopping (with physician's recommendations).
- Use alternative positions for 3 to 4 months to decrease stress on sternum; avoid side-lying and prone positions.
- Inspect and cleanse surgical incisions daily with soap and water.
- Understand medications, including reason for taking, dosage, frequency, and side effects.
- Follow dietary restrictions.
- Understand how much pain to expect and how to manage it.

Risk Factors

- Follow instructions on individual risk factors, their impact on health after cardiac surgery, and how to modify them.
- Seek referrals as appropriate (e.g., for a weight loss program or a smoking cessation program).

Follow-up With Physician

- Know how and when to schedule follow-up appointments.
- Be alert for signs and symptoms of infection, such as fever, increased redness, tenderness, drainage, or swelling of incisions.
- Report palpitations, tachycardia, or an irregular pulse (if normally regular) to the physician immediately.
- Seek follow-up care if you experience dizziness or increased fatigue, sudden weight gain or peripheral edema, shortness of breath, or chest pain.

case study ■ CORONARY ARTERY BYPASS GRAFT SURGERY

Mr. Carter, a 62-year-old man, has just returned to the ICU after CABG surgery. An internal mammary artery graft to the left anterior descending (LAD) coronary artery and saphenous vein graft to the right coronary artery (RCA) and diagonal artery was performed off bypass. The patient's history is significant for an anterior myocardial infarction 2 years ago and hypertension controlled with captopril. He stopped smoking 10 years ago. Before surgery, he took aspirin (325 mg orally each day).

The patient is now mechanically ventilated on 50% fraction of inspired oxygen (FIO_2) with 5 cm positive end-expiratory pressure (PEEP). Breath sounds are clear and equal bilaterally, and the saturation of peripheral oxygen (SpO_2) is 98%. Neurologically, the patient is unresponsive with pinpoint pupils. The monitor shows sinus tachycardia at 110 beats/minute with occasional premature ventricular contractions (PVCs). Atrial and ventricular epicardial pacing wires are in place, but they are not connected to a pacemaker. Important clinical parameters are as follows: core temperature 96.6°F (35.9°C); blood pressure (BP) 90/60 mm Hg; cardiac index (CI) 1.6 L/minute/m^2; and pulmonary artery wedge pressure (PAWP) 8 mm Hg. Chest tube drainage is 250 mL, and urine output is 75 mL. Assessment indicates that neurological and respiratory status are as expected immediately after surgery. The low blood pressure and cardiac index, together with the PAWP and tachycardia, indicate hypovolemia. According to protocol, the nurse initiates volume resuscitation with 500 mL hetastarch (Hespan) and provides radiant heat and blankets to increase the core temperature. The chest tube drainage is high normal, and close monitoring is warranted.

One hour after surgery, the patient is beginning to awaken. He opens his eyes and moves all his extremities weakly. His clinical parameters are core temperature 97.2°F (36.2°C); BP 170/90 mm Hg, with a mean arterial pressure (MAP) of 100 mm Hg; CI 2.1 L/minute/m^2; and PAWP 10 mm Hg. Chest tube drainage is 200 mL over the past 30 minutes, and urine output is 50 mL. The CI, PAWP, and urine output are low normal, and the chest tube drainage is rapidly increasing. The BP is high because the patient is awakening. Bleeding is the major problem, and the immediate interventions are (1) volume replace-

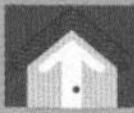

box 22-10 *Cardiac Surgery*

- Assess home environment and family support system; this is essential to planning. If the patient cannot care for self, or family cannot provide convalescent care, consider home care referral for a registered nurse, home health aide, or homemaker as appropriate.
- Provide resources to take home (e.g., written materials, video discharge instructions). Transient cognitive dysfunction, common after cardiac surgery, results in poor concentration, confusion, memory loss, and emotional instability at the time when the patient must assimilate a vast amount of information about postoperative care. Teach both the patient and the caregiver. Caregivers are often instrumental in ensuring that the patient follows the plan of care. They can identify unexpected complications that require medical attention, and they may be responsible for transporting the patient to follow-up appointments.
- Ensure that information/skills needed for postoperative self-care are provided (see Box 22-9).
- Consider referring patients to cardiac rehabilitation programs. Patients benefit from such referrals. However, insurance plans may limit this intervention.
- Ensure that before discharge, the patient is able to verbalize the following: disease process and surgical procedure; rehabilitation and treatment goals and how to achieve these goals; and signs, symptoms, and complications to report.

ment, (2) initiation of bleeding protocol, and (3) control of MAP. Additional volume is infused, and laboratory values are checked. The partial thromboplastin time (PTT) is 45 seconds, and the hemoglobin is 7 g/dL. After consulting with a physician, the nurse administers protamine 50 mg IV for the prolonged PTT and transfuses 1 unit of red blood cells. The MAP is controlled by initiating a propofol drip to sedate the patient while bleeding is an issue. The chest tube drainage 30 minutes later is 200 mL. Six units of platelets are ordered and quickly infused.

Two hours after surgery, the patient's parameters have improved. They are BP 120/60 mm Hg; CI 2.5 L/minute/m^2; PAWP 14 mm Hg; MAP 70 mm Hg; and heart rate 90 beats/minute. Chest tube drainage has decreased to 125 mL, and urine output is 150 mL. The propofol drip is now discontinued. The patient is awake and following commands. ■

CAROTID ENDARTERECTOMY

Stenosis or occlusion of the carotid arteries is usually due to atherosclerotic disease and may cause stroke, a leading cause of morbidity and mortality in the United States. Carotid endarterectomy is the most common noncardiac vascular procedure performed to restore flow to the carotid arteries and is designed to decrease the risk of stroke and stroke-related death.[30]

The right carotid artery is a branch of the innominate artery that arises from the right side of the aortic arch. The left common carotid artery arises directly from the aortic arch. At the level of the thyroid, the common carotids bifurcate into the external and internal carotids. Located near this bifurcation, in the carotid sinus, are the carotid chemoreceptors, which are sensitive to blood carbon dioxide and oxygen levels, and the baroreceptors, which help regulate blood pressure. The external carotid arteries supply blood to the structures in the head and neck, excluding the eyes and brain. The internal carotid arteries give rise to the ophthalmic arteries and the posterior communicating, anterior cerebral, and middle cerebral arteries, which help supply blood to the brain.

Patients with carotid artery occlusive disease may have sudden dysphagia, unilateral motor weakness, expressive aphasia, dizziness, memory deficits, or monocular blindness.[31] They often exhibit signs of vascular disease in other parts of the body, such as the heart (CAD) or the legs (peripheral arterial disease). Risk factors for carotid artery occlusive disease are associated with stroke and should guide patient care. Hypertension is the most important risk factor for stroke, and blood pressure regulation is essential in the postoperative period. Issues such as cigarette smoking, hyperlipidemia, alcohol consumption, and postmenopausal use of estrogen may also affect patient care.[30]

Patients with risk factors for carotid artery occlusive disease must be examined carefully. A carotid bruit can usually be auscultated over the artery due to turbulent flow through the narrowed artery. Carotid Doppler ultrasonography is usually performed to estimate the presence and amount of stenosis, but angiography is the most reliable method to determine the exact amount of stenosis. Magnetic resonance angiography, which is less invasive, may also be used.

Indications for Carotid Endarterectomy

Carotid artery occlusive disease is part of the systemic atherosclerotic process, which is reviewed in Chapter 19. Carotid endarterectomy is indicated for symptomatic patients with ipsilateral 70% to 90% carotid artery stenosis who have had recent nondebilitating carotid artery ischemic events. Recently, it has been shown that asymptomatic patients with greater than 60% carotid artery stenosis and other factors such as need for CABG surgery can also benefit from carotid endarterectomy.[30]

Surgical Procedure

A skin incision is made along the lower anterior border of the sternocleidomastoid muscle just below the angle of the jaw, and the common, internal, and external carotid arteries are isolated. The carotid arteries on the operative side must be clamped. Clamping puts the ipsilateral cerebral hemisphere and eye at risk of ischemia and infarct because the only perfusion to these areas occurs through the circle of Willis and collaterals, which may be inadequate. To prevent thromboembolus formation while the arteries are clamped, a heparin bolus may be given before clamping. Adequacy of circulation is determined by continuous electroencephalographic monitoring in the operating room. If circulation is determined to be inadequate, a temporary bypass or shunt may be placed from the common carotid artery to the distal portion of the internal carotid to provide continued intraoperative perfusion. Patients treated with shunts often include those with contralateral carotid stenosis, neurological deficits, history of cerebrovascular accidents, and stroke in evolution.

Endarterectomy or removal of the ulcerated or stenotic atheromatous plaque is then performed, and the artery is closed. If primary closure will cause a narrowing, a patch may be used.

Postoperative Care

After extubation in the recovery room, patients are transferred to the ICU with ECG monitoring, an arterial line, CVP monitoring, and oxygen. Traditionally, patients usually stay in the ICU for 24 hours. However, cost concerns have led to monitoring patients in an intermediate care unit and reducing the hospital stay to 1 day.[32]

CONTROLLING BLOOD PRESSURE

Blood pressure is commonly labile up to 24 hours after surgery because of surgically induced abnormalities of the carotid baroreceptor sensitivity. This is characterized as baroreflex failure syndrome and is usually associated with bilateral surgical procedures.[30] Preoperative hypertension is thought to be the most important determinant of postoperative hypertension, which means that the critical care nurse must be aware of the patient's preoperative blood pressure range. Increased blood pressure may also increase the risk of wound bleeding and possible hematoma formation. The goal of blood pressure regulation is a systolic blood pressure between 120 and 170 mm Hg. A systolic blood pressure greater than 170 mm Hg should be treated with nitroprusside or other IV agents, whereas one less than 120 mm Hg should be treated with IV fluid or with a phenylephrine drip if the patient is unresponsive to volume.

WOUND CARE

To minimize stress on the operative site, the patient's head and neck should be kept in alignment. The dressing and the area behind the patient's neck and shoulders are assessed for the presence of blood. Persistent oozing from deep tissue, coughing, straining during extubation, and disruption of suture lines may all lead to bleeding into the operative site. The risk of bleeding can be further aggravated by anticoagulation with heparin, aspirin, or antiplatelet therapy. The nurse assesses the neck size, comparing the operative side with the nonoperative side. Swelling could indicate hematoma formation. Any patient complaints of difficulty talking, swallowing, or breathing should be reported to the physician immediately. If a hematoma is suspected because of tracheal compression by a hematoma, surgical evacuation could be indicated. Wound hematomas occur in about 5.5% of patients.[30]

PREVENTING NEUROLOGICAL COMPLICATIONS

Brain injury, local nerve injury, or both may occur. Perioperative stroke occurs in approximately 3% of patients and may be due to embolization of atheromatous debris, air from the operative site, or low flow during carotid artery clamping.[30] Neurological assessment includes level of consciousness, pupil reactivity, eye movement, orientation, appropriateness of response, and motor function (flexion, extension, and hand grips) for the first 24 hours. Abnormalities should be reported to the physician immediately.

Hyperperfusion syndrome occurs in patients with high-grade stenosis. Theoretically, the hemisphere distal to the stenotic area has suffered hypoperfusion that causes the small blood vessels to remain maximally dilated with a loss of autoregulation. Once the stenosis is repaired, autoregulation is still paralyzed, but a marked increase in blood flow occurs that cannot be controlled with vasoconstriction to protect the capillaries. Edema or hemorrhage to the area results.[30] Strict blood pressure control is imperative.

Several cranial nerves (CN) traverse the surgical area and can be exposed to trauma. The most commonly affected are CN VII (the facial nerve), CN X (the vagus nerve), CN XIII (the hypoglossal nerve), and CN XI (the spinal accessory nerve). Specific functional assessment for each nerve should be performed after surgery, including those listed in Table 22-2. If a deficit is present, the nurse should notify the physician and explain to the patient how it occurred and that the deficit is usually temporary.

table 22-2 Postoperative Functional Assessment of Cranial Nerves Following Carotid Endarterectomy

Nerve	Nerve Intervention	Functional Assessment	Functional Damage
Facial nerve (VII)	Motor function of facial muscles	Ability to smile and frown	Asymmetrical contraction of the mouth
Vagus nerve (X)	Motor and sensory function of larynx and throat	Quality and tone of voice and ability to swallow	Difficult swallowing, hoarseness, speech problems, loss of gag reflex
Hypoglossal nerve (XII)	Muscles to tongue	Movement of tongue	Difficult swallowing, speech problems, deviation of tongue, sometimes airway damage
Spinal accessory nerve (XI)	Trapezius and sternocleido-mastoid muscles	Ability to shrug shoulders and raise arm to horizontal position	Shoulder may sag, difficulty raising shoulder against resistance, difficulty raising arm to horizontal position

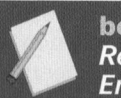

box 22-11
Recovering From Carotid Endarterectomy

Risk Factor Reduction
- Stop smoking.
- Eat a low-fat diet.
- Control hypertension if present.

Activity
- There are usually no restrictions on activity. It is all right to move your neck in a normal manner.

Incision Care
- Bruising and discoloration are common.
- Wash the incision site with soap and water.

General
- Be familiar with signs and symptoms of incisional infection.
- Notify your physician of visual defects, changes in memory or sensation, or an inability to swallow or speak.
- Be knowledgeable about medication indications, including reason for taking, dosage, frequency, and side effects.
- Keep physician appointments.

Home Care Considerations

Patients are usually discharged on the first or second postoperative day. The critical care nurse plays an essential role in the care of the patient who has had an endarterectomy. Although considered a vascular surgical procedure, postoperative complications of carotid endarterectomy usually manifest as neurological symptoms, and the nurse must assess the patient for subtle neurological changes. Patient education is also a key component of care. Patients and their families should understand that the patient has an underlying cardiovascular disease and that risk factor modification is necessary. Education should include the items listed in Box 22-11.

clinical applicability challenges

Self-Challenge: Critical Thinking

Mr. A, a 58-year-old man who has had OPCABG surgery with two grafts and moderate left ventricular dysfunction, has arrived in the ICU from the operating room after surgery. He is receiving epinephrine at 1 μg/minute to improve cardiac performance. Past medical history is significant for chronic atrial fibrillation, for which he is taking warfarin (Coumadin). The anticoagulation medication was stopped several days before CABG surgery. To maintain a cardiac index greater than 2.2 L/minute/m^2, he requires epinephrine and aggressive volume resuscitation. Norepinephrine (Levophed) was started to maintain a mean arterial pressure of greater than 70 mm Hg, despite the adequate volume resuscitation. His chest tube output was less than 50 to 75 mL/hour for the past 3 to 4 hours and has now increased to 130 mL in the past hour.

1. *What do you think was occurring in this patient situation?*
2. *What would be your immediate interventions?*
3. *What interventions would be the most important to make the physician aware of?*
4. *For what emergency situation would you need to prepare?*

Study Questions

1. *The internal mammary artery graft is preferred over the saphenous vein graft (SVG) because*
   a. *it remains patent longer.*
   b. *it is easier to do.*
   c. *fibrointimal hyperplasia does not occur with the SVG.*
   d. *postoperative pain is less with the internal mammary artery.*
2. *Acute mitral insufficiency can occur because of*
   a. *rheumatic heart disease.*
   b. *myocardial infarction.*
   c. *myxoma.*
   d. *left ventricular dilatation.*
3. *Syncope occurs in later stages of aortic stenosis because of*
   a. *myocardial ischemia.*
   b. *stroke.*
   c. *left ventricular hypertrophy.*
   d. *forward cardiac output that cannot increase to meet the body demands of activity or exercise.*
4. *The most important issue when caring for a patient who has a mechanical valve versus a tissue valve is*
   a. *there is no need for anticoagulation.*
   b. *the mechanical valve is not as durable.*
   c. *there is a need for anticoagulation for life.*
   d. *there is no difference between valve types.*
5. *The bypass machine alters the coagulation process. Which of the following effects is not caused by the bypass machine?*
   a. *Platelet damage that activates the intrinsic pathway*
   b. *Decreased coagulation factors*
   c. *Denaturation of plasma proteins*
   d. *Minimal endothelial damage and activation*
6. *The off-pump coronary artery bypass graft (OPCABG) procedure was developed to decrease the harmful effects of the bypass machine, especially because of*
   a. *the changes in cognitive function that occur after surgery.*
   b. *increased systemic vascular resistance.*
   c. *tendency toward hemodilution.*
   d. *increase in activation of antidiuretic hormone (ADH) and the renin system.*
7. *One of the major nursing interventions in this patient population is volume resuscitation. Which step is not helpful in volume resuscitation?*
   a. *Infusing volume through a large-bore access*
   b. *Using a pressure bag to infuse volume*
   c. *Always using a central line*
   d. *Infusing the volume through a short access line*
8. *Cardiac tamponade is a complication of cardiac surgery that needs to be recognized early. Which of the following is a more sensitive finding when trying to recognize tamponade?*
   a. *Equalization of the pulmonary artery pressures*
   b. *Elevated central venous/right atrial pressure*
   c. *Decreased cardiac output*
   d. *Sudden increase in requirement for vasoactive drugs*

9. *After right-sided carotid endarterectomy, you assess that the patient has an uneven smile. One side of the mouth turns up, and one does not. The most likely cause is*
   a. *stroke affecting the left side of the brain.*
   b. *stroke affecting the right side of the brain.*
   c. *surgical damage to the facial nerve (CN VII).*
   d. *surgical damage to the vagus nerve (CN X).*
10. *Systemic inflammatory response syndrome (SIRS) can occur in patients who have undergone either on-pump or off-pump CABG. How do you differentiate between infection and inflammation?*
   a. *Fever that continues for greater than 48 hours*
   b. *Bands in the complete blood count (CBC) differential greater than 2%*
   c. *Documentation of infection*
   d. *All of the above*

REFERENCES

1. Eagle K, Guyton R, Davidoff R, et al: ACC/AHA guidelines for coronary bypass graft surgery. J Am Coll Cardiol 34:1262–1342, 1999
2. Felisky C, Paull D, Hill M, et al: Endoscopic greater saphenous vein harvesting reduces the morbidity of coronary artery bypass surgery. Am J Surg 183:576–579, 2002
3. Nwasokwa O: Coronary artery bypass graft disease. Ann Intern Med 123:528–545, 1995
4. Acar C, Ramshey A, Pagny JY: The radial artery for coronary artery bypass grafting: Clinical and angiographic results at five years. J Thorac Cardiovasc Surg 116:981–989, 1998
5. Shapira O, Xu A, Vita J, et al: Nitroglycerin is superior to diltiazem as a coronary bypass conduit vasodilator. J Thorac Cardiovasc Surg 117:906–911, 1999
6. Emery RW, Arom KV, Holter AR, et al: Advances in coronary artery surgery. In Franco KL, Verrier E (eds): Advanced Therapy in Cardiac Surgery (2nd Ed), pp 124–130. Hamilton, Ontario, BC Decker, 2003
7. Vallely M, Bannon P, Kritharides L: The systemic inflammatory response syndrome and off-pump cardiac surgery. Heart Surg Forum 4(Suppl):S7–S13, 2001
8. Magee M, Jablouski K, Stamou S, et al: Elimination of cardiopulmonary bypass improves early survival for multivessel coronary artery bypass patients. Ann Thorac Surg 73:1196–1202, 2002
9. Peel GK, Stamou SC, Dullum MK, et al: Chronological distribution of stroke after minimally invasive versus conventional coronary artery bypass. J Am Coll Cardiology 43(5):752–756, 2004
10. Horvath KA: Transmyocardial laser revascularization. In Franco KL, Verrier E (eds): Advanced Therapy in Cardiac Surgery (2nd Ed), pp 131–137. Hamilton, Ontario, BC Decker, 2003
11. Lynn-McHale D, Hambach C, Carter T, et al: Transmyocardial laser revascularization. J Cardiovasc Nurs 12:17–28, 1998
12. Lytle BW: Coronary artery reoperations. In Cohn LH, Edmunds LH (eds): Cardiac Surgery in the Adult (2nd Ed), pp 659–679. New York: McGraw-Hill Medical Publishing Division, 2003
13. Kaiser L, Kron I, Spray T: Mastery of Cardiothoracic Surgery. Philadelphia, Lippincott-Raven, 1998
14. Lancey R, Gaca C, Vander Salm T: The use of smaller, more flexible chest drains following open heart surgery. Chest 119:19–24, 2001
15. Corso P, Hockstein M: New techniques in management of the cardiac surgery patient. In Shoemaker W, Ayres S, Grenvik A, et al (eds): Textbook of Critical Care, pp 1130–1155. Philadelphia, WB Saunders, 2002
16. Sladen R, Berend J, Fassero J, et al: Comparison of vecuronium and meperidine on the clinical and metabolic effects of shivering after hypothermic cardiopulmonary bypass. J Cardiothorac Vasc Anesth 9:147–153, 1995
17. Muckart D, Bhagwanjee S: American College of Chest Physicians/Society of Critical Care Medicine Consensus Conference: Definitions of the systemic inflammatory response syndrome and allied disorders in relation to critically injured patients. Crit Care Med 25:1789–1795, 1997
18. Harvey M: Systemic inflammatory response syndrome and multi-organ dysfunction syndrome. In Kinney M, Dunbar S, Brooks-Braun J, et al (eds): AACN Clinical Reference for Critical Care Nursing. St. Louis, Mosby, 1998
19. Sirieix D, Hongnat M, Delayaance M, et al: Comparison of the acute hemodynamic effects of hypertonic or colloid infusions immediately after mitral valve repair. Crit Care Med 27:2159–2165, 1999
20. Le Conte P, Coutaut V, N'Guyeu J, et al: Prognostic factors in acute cardiogenic pulmonary edema. Am J Emerg Med 17:329–332, 1999
21. Brown T: Hibernating myocardium. Am J Crit Care 10:84–90, 2001
22. Ely E, Meade M, Haponik E, et al: Mechanical ventilator weaning protocols driven by non-physician health-care professionals: Evidence-based clinical practice guidelines. Chest 120(6 Suppl):454S–463S, 2001
23. Burns S, Dempsey E: Long-term ventilator management strategies: Experiences in two hospitals. AACN Clin Issues 11:424–441, 2000
24. Jarcia JP, Venkataramana V, Gold JP: Prevention of neurologic injury during cardiac and great vessel surgery. In Franco KL, Verrier E (eds): Advanced Therapy in Cardiac Surgery (2nd Ed), pp 74–82. Hamilton, Ontario, BC Decker, 2003
25. Limbird L, Hardin J (eds): Goodman & Gilman's the Pharmacological Basis of Therapeutics. New York, McGraw-Hill, 2001
26. Rosengart TK: Blood conservation for open heart surgery. In Franco KL, Verrier E (eds): Advanced Therapy in Cardiac Surgery (2nd Ed), pp 37–45. Hamilton, Ontario, BC Decker, 2003
27. Hebert P, Wells G, Blajchman M, et al, and the Transfusion Requirements in Critical Care Investigators for the Canadian Critical Care Trials Group: A multicenter, randomized, controlled clinical trial of transfusion requirements in critical care. N Engl J Med 340:409–417, 1999
28. Shoemaker WC: Pericardial tamponade. In Shoemaker W, Ayres S, Grenvik A, et al (eds): Textbook of Critical Care, pp 1097–1101. Philadelphia, WB Saunders, 2002
29. Van den Berghe G, Vounters P, Weekers F, et al: Intensive insulin therapy in the critically ill patients. N Engl J Med 345:1359–1367, 2001
30. Bettmann M, Katzen B, Whisnant J, et al: A Statement for healthcare professionals from a special writing group of the Stroke Council, American Heart Association. Circulation 97:121–123, 1998
31. Brown M, Fitzgerald C, Morse K, et al: Cardiovascular surgery. In Kinney M, Dunbar S, Brooks-Brunn J, et al (eds): AACN Clinical Reference for Critical Care Nursing, pp 383–428. St. Louis, Mosby, 1998
32. Marwitz Kallenbach A, Rosenblum J: Carotid endarterectomy: Creating the 1-day stay. Crit Care Nurse 20:23–36, 2000

OTHER SELECTED READING

Baumgarter W, Stuart R, Gott V, et al: Atlas of Cardiac Surgery. Philadelphia, Hanley & Belfus, 2000

Ferguson T, Coombs L, Peterson E: Preoperative beta blocker use and mortality and morbidity following CABG surgery in North America. JAMA 287:2221–2227, 2002

King K: Gender and short term recovery from cardiac surgery. Nurs Res 49:29–36, 2000

Ley S: Quality care outcomes in cardiac surgery: The role of evidence-based practice. AACN Clin Issues 12:606–617, 2001

Peterson D: Managing hypotension after cardiac surgery: An algorithm for treatment. Crit Care Nurse 20:36–41, 43–46, 48–49, 2000

Salazar J, Wityk R, Grega M, et al: Stroke after cardiac surgery: Short and long term outcomes. Ann Thorac Cardiovasc Surg 72:1195–1201, 2001

PART
one
two
three
four
five
six
seven
eight
nine
ten
eleven
twelve

Respiratory System

INTERNET RESOURCES

Topic	Web Page Address
Acute Respiratory Distress Syndrome Support Group	www.ards.org
Allergy and Asthma Network Mothers of Asthmatics	www.aanma.org
American Association for Respiratory Care (AARC)	www.aarc.org
American College of Chest Physicians	www.chestnet.org
American Lung Association	www.lungusa.org
American Thoracic Society	www.thoracic.org
Auscultation Assistant	www.wilkes.med.ucla.edu/index.htm
British Thoracic Society	www.brit-thoracic.org.uk
Canadian Thoracic Society	www.lung.ca/cts
Club for Kids With Asthma	www.asthmabusters.org
Emphysema Foundation for Our Right to Survive	www.emphysema.net
European Federation of Allergy and Airways Diseases Patients' Association	www.efanet.org
Educational Website Dedicated to Patient Safety	www.capnography.com
Global Initiative for Chronic Obstructive Lung Disease	www.goldcopd.com
Grafxsman's Pulmonary Monitoring With Graphics	www.hometown.aol.com/grafxsman/index.html
National Heart, Lung, and Blood Institute	www.nhlbi.nih.gov/index.htm
National Institute of Allergy and Infectious Diseases	www.niaid.nih.gov
National Lung Health Education Program	www.nlhep.org
Network ARDS in Children	www.meb.uni-bonn.de/ards
Respiratory Nursing Society	www.respiratorynursingsociety.org
Second Wind Lung Transplant Association, Inc.	www.2ndwind.org
Society of Thoracic Surgeons	www.sts.org
Ventworld Website	www.ventworld.com
Virtual Hospital Website	www.vh.org
World Health Organization	www.who.int

chapter

23

Anatomy and Physiology of the Respiratory System

KAREN JOHNSON

objectives

Based on the content of this chapter, the reader will be able to:

- Identify the major structures of the respiratory system that are located in the thorax.
- Describe the movement of air through the airways from the nose to the alveoli.
- Discuss the function of surfactant in maintaining alveolar inflation.
- Differentiate the function of bronchial and pulmonary circulations.
- Describe the mechanics of ventilation in terms of air movement into and out of the lungs, lung compliance, and airway resistance.
- Explain four factors that affect the diffusion of gases across the alveolar–capillary membrane.
- Identify physiological and pathophysiological conditions that produce a ventilation–perfusion mismatch.
- Identify conditions that affect the relationship described in the oxyhemoglobin dissociation curve and how these conditions affect oxygen exchange.
- Describe the function of the chemoreceptors and lung receptors.

The structures of the respiratory system allow gases to move between the external environment and the internal environment. The cardinal function of the respiratory system is gas exchange, a process by which oxygen moves from the air into the blood and carbon dioxide moves out of the blood and is exhaled to the external environment. The respiratory system also has several other functions, including regulation of acid–base balance, metabolism of some compounds, and filtration of inhaled unwanted materials. Intact respiratory structures and proper functioning of the respiratory system are necessary for transport of gases in and out of the body. This chapter offers a review of anatomy and physiology of the respiratory system. Knowledge of respiratory anatomy and physiology helps the nurse understand respiratory assessment techniques, principles of respiratory system management, and common disorders of the respiratory system.

ANATOMY OF THE RESPIRATORY SYSTEM

The Thorax

The thorax contains the major structures of the respiratory system. These structures include the thoracic cage, the muscles of ventilation, the lungs, the pleural space, and the mediastinum (Fig. 23-1). The thoracic cage is a rigid, yet

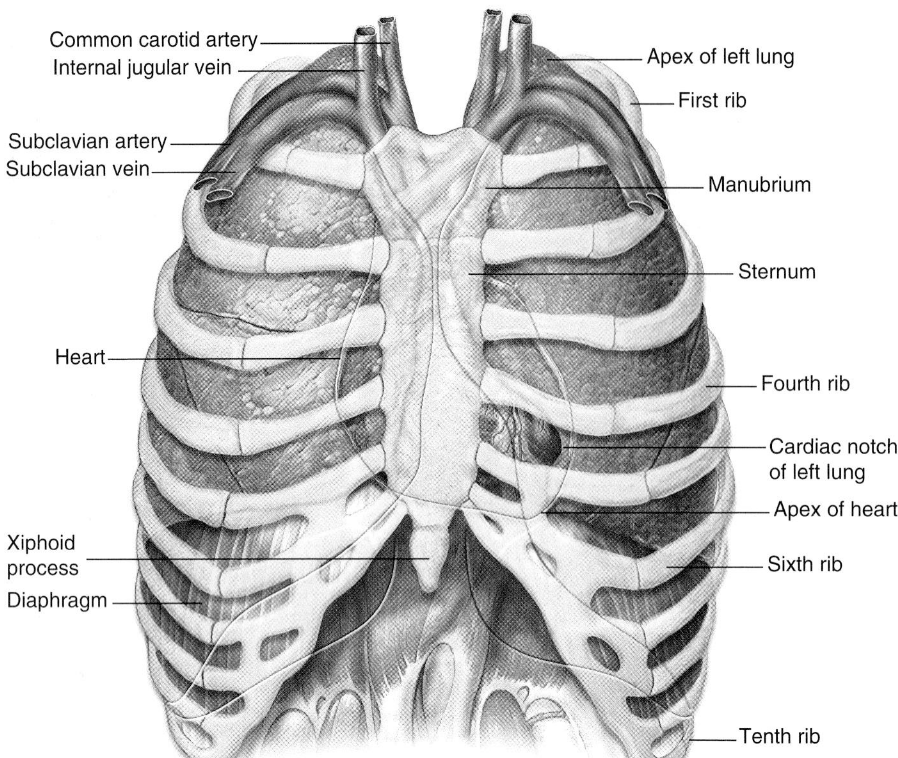

figure 23-1 Thoracic contents. (Source: Anatomical Chart Company: Atlas of Human Anatomy, p 149. Springhouse, Springhouse, PA, 2001.)

flexible structure. Its bony structure protects the major organs in the thoracic cavity. Flexibility allows for inhalation/inflation and exhalation/deflation of the lungs. The thoracic cage consists of 12 vertebrae, each with a pair of ribs. Posteriorly, each rib is attached to a vertebra (Fig. 23-2). Anteriorly, the first seven ribs are attached to the sternum (Fig. 23-3). The 8th, 9th, and 10th ribs are attached by cartilage to the ribs above them. The 11th and 12th ribs are called "floating ribs" because they are not attached anteriorly to another structure.

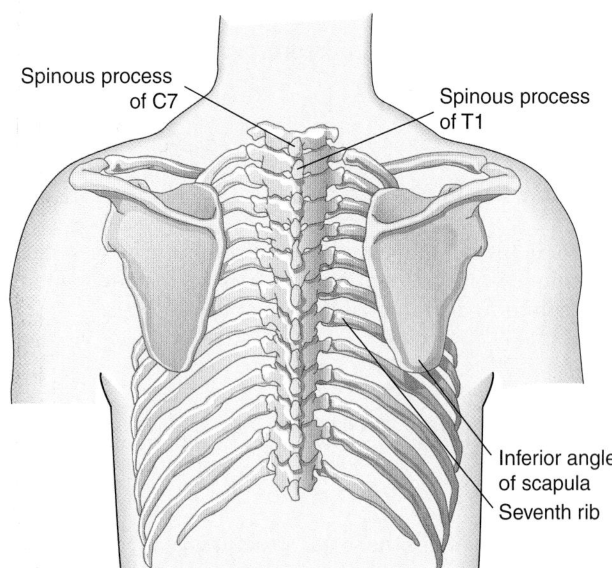

figure 23-2 Posterior thoracic cage. (Source: Bickley LS: Bates' Guide to Physical Examination and History Taking [8th Ed], p 211. Philadelphia, Lippincott Williams & Wilkins, 2003.)

THE LUNGS, MEDIASTINUM, AND PLEURAL SPACE

Positioned within, and protected by, the thoracic cage, the lungs are located on either side of the chest. These air-filled, spongy structures are attached to the body only at

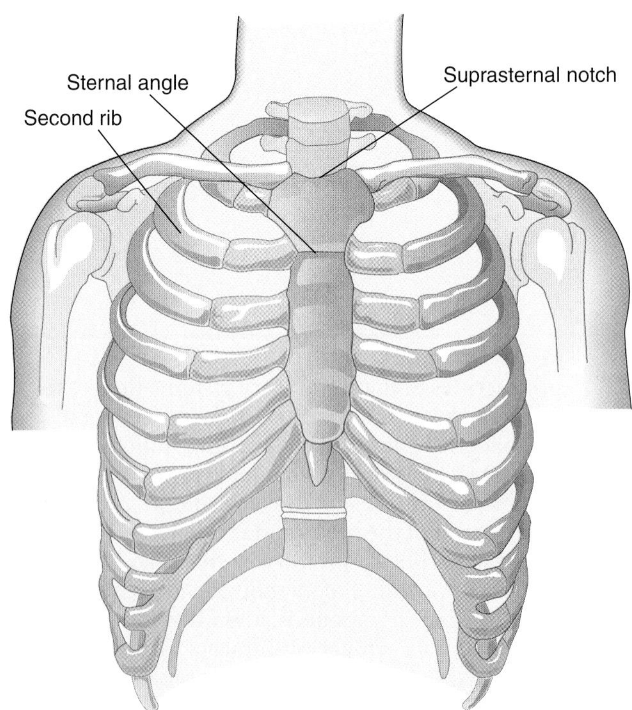

figure 23-3 Anterior thoracic cage. (Source: Bickley LS: Bates' Guide to Physical Examination and History Taking [8th Ed], p 210. Philadelphia, Lippincott Williams & Wilkins, 2003.)

the pulmonary ligament at the mediastinum. The right lung contains three lobes, and the left lung contains only two lobes because of the space limitation imposed by the heart. The base of each lung rests anteriorly at the level of the sixth rib at the mid-clavicular line and at the eighth rib at the mid-axillary line. The apices extend 2 to 4 cm above the inner aspects of the clavicles.

The space between the two lungs is the mediastinum. The mediastinum contains the heart, blood vessels, lymph nodes, thymus gland, nerve fibers, and the esophagus.

Pleural membranes surround the lungs and line the thoracic wall. The parietal pleura is the membrane lining the chest wall, and the visceral pleura overlays the lung parenchyma (Fig. 23-4). A thin layer of serous fluid in the small space between these two pleurae allows the parietal and visceral pleurae to slide over each other during inspiration and expiration. The pressure within the pleural space is called the *intrapleural pressure.* The intrapleural pressure is normally less than the pressures within the lung. It is this negative pressure that keeps the lungs inflated. If the intrapleural space loses its negative pressure (by exposure to atmospheric pressure), the lung collapses, a condition known as a *pneumothorax.* The pleural space is also a potential space for the accumulation of fluid. An abnormal collection of fluid in the pleural space is a *pleural effusion.*

THE RESPIRATORY MUSCLES

The muscles that elevate the thoracic cage are classified as *muscles of inspiration.*[1] The major muscle involved with inspiration is the diaphragm. The diaphragm is a thin, dome-shaped muscle that is innervated by the phrenic nerves. When it contracts, the abdominal contents are forced downward and the chest expands vertically (Fig. 23-5). In normal breathing, the level of the diaphragm moves about 1 cm, but on forced inspiration a total excursion of up to 10 cm may occur.[2] The external intercostal muscles also aid in inspiration (Fig. 23-6). These muscles attach to adjacent ribs and slope downward and forward. When the external muscles contract, the ribs are pulled forward and upward, and this increases the lateral and anterior–posterior diameters of the thoracic cage. The accessory muscles of inspiration include the scalene and sternomastoid muscles. The scalene muscles elevate the first two ribs and the sternomastoid muscles raise the sternum.[2] During normal breathing, these muscles are not used, but during exercise these muscles contract to aid in inspiration.

Muscles that depress the thoracic cage are classified as *muscles of expiration.*[1] Expiration is a largely passive process during normal breathing. During expiration, the diaphragm relaxes, and the elastic recoil of the lungs, chest wall, and abdominal structures compresses the lungs. Expiration can

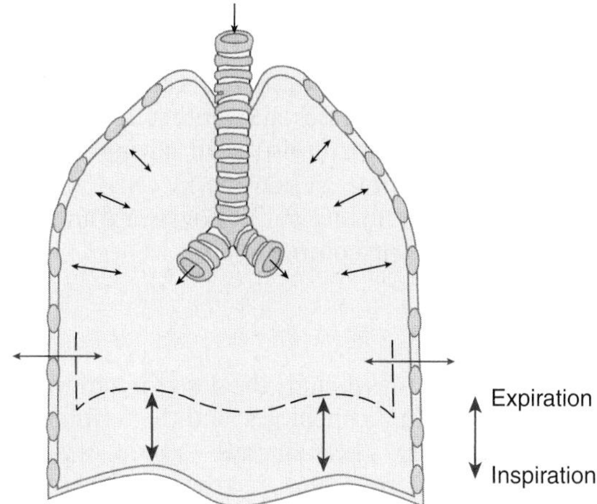

figure 23-5 Frontal section of the chest showing the movement of the rib cage and diaphragm during inspiration and expiration. (Source: Porth CM: Pathophysiology: Concepts of Altered Health States [6th Ed], p 585. Philadelphia, Lippincott Williams & Wilkins, 2002.)

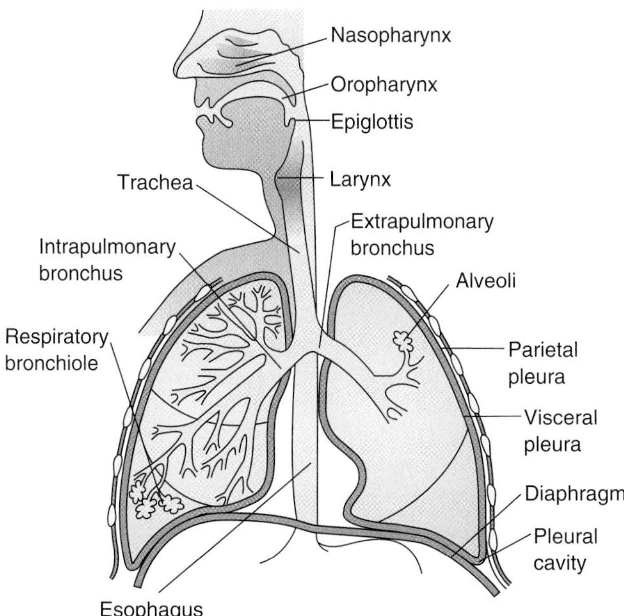

figure 23-4 Structures of the respiratory system. (Source: Porth CM: Pathophysiology: Concepts of Altered Health States [6th Ed], p 578. Philadelphia, Lippincott Williams & Wilkins, 2002.)

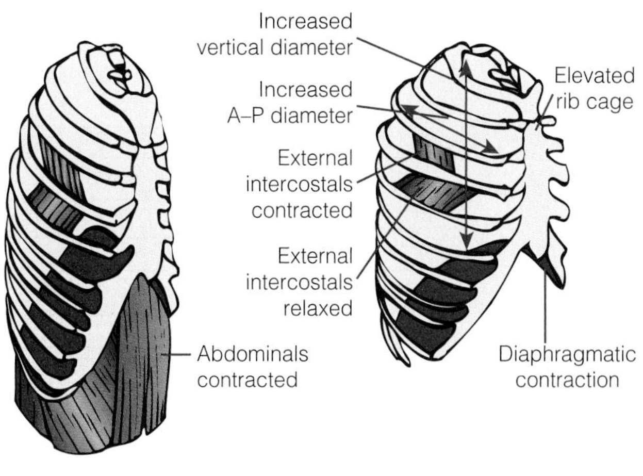

figure 23-6 Contraction and expansion of the thoracic cage during expiration and inspiration, demonstrating diaphragmatic contraction, function of the intercostals, and elevation and depression of the rib cage. *A–P diameter,* anterior–posterior diameter. (Source: Guyton AC, Hall JE: Textbook of Medical Physiology [10th Ed], p 433. Philadelphia, Elsevier Science, 2000.)

become an active process during exercise. The abdominal and intercostal muscles can increase expiratory effort (see Fig. 23-5). When the abdominal muscles contract, the intra-abdominal pressure increases and pushes the diaphragm upward. These muscles are also used during defecation, vomiting, and coughing. When the internal intercostal muscles contract, the ribs are pulled downward and inward, decreasing the thoracic volume.

The Conducting Airways

The conducting airways include the nasopharynx, oropharynx, trachea, bronchi, bronchioles, and the terminal bronchioles (see Fig. 23-4). These airways—a series of tubes that become more numerous and narrow as they penetrate deeper into the lungs (Fig. 23-7)—warm, humidify, and filter air that is inhaled as it is channeled to the gas exchange region. Because the conducting airways contain no alveoli and do not participate in gas exchange, they constitute the *anatomic dead space.* The volume in the anatomic dead space is approximately 150 mL.[2]

THE NASOPHARYNX AND OROPHARYNX

The nasopharynx is the preferred route for entrance of air into the respiratory tract during normal breathing because it filters and warms inspired air.[3] The outer passages are lined with coarse hairs that filter large particles. The upper portion of the nasal cavity supplies warmth and moisture to the air inhaled. If nasal passages are plugged or when larger volumes of gases need to be exchanged (e.g., during exercise), the oropharynx provides an alternate route. Obstruction of the oropharynx leads to immediate cessation of ventilation ("choking"). Foreign bodies and swelling of the pharyngeal airways due to infection, injury, or allergic reaction can also cause airway obstruction.

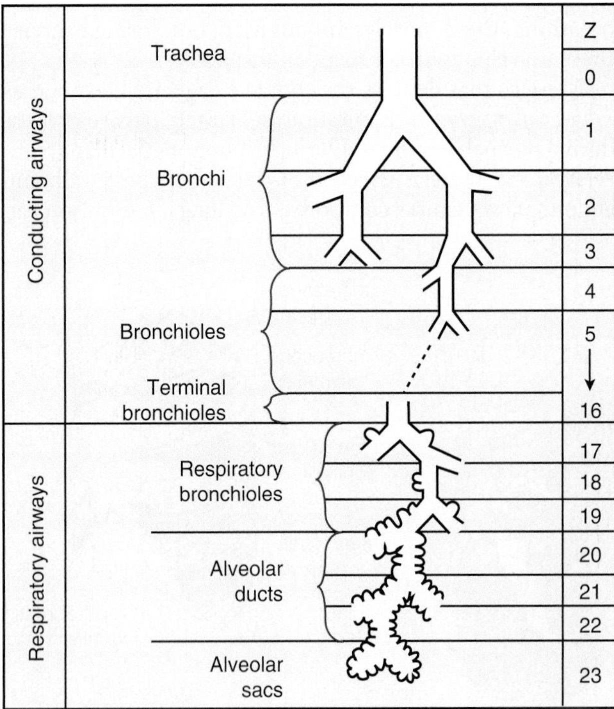

figure 23-7 Idealization of the human airways. Note that the first 16 generations (*Z*) make up the conducting airways, and generations 17 to 23 make up the respiratory airways. Throughout childhood, the airways increase in diameter and length, and the number and size of the alveoli increase until adolescence, when respiratory development matures to that of an adult. (Source: West JB: Respiratory Physiology: The Essentials [6th Ed], p 6. Philadelphia, Lippincott Williams & Wilkins, 2000.)

THE EPIGLOTTIS

The epiglottis is located posterior to the root of the tongue (see Fig. 23-4). It is a leaf-shaped piece of cartilage that moves up and down. During inhalation, the epiglottis moves upward to allow air to move through the trachea. During swallowing, it moves downward to cover the larynx and allow food and liquid to pass into the esophagus. During defecation, especially during defecation associated with straining and constipation, inhaled air is temporarily held in the lungs by closure of the glottis. Contraction of the intra-abdominal muscles causes an increase in the intra-abdominal and intrathoracic pressures. These collective processes are called the *Valsalva maneuver.*

THE TRACHEOBRONCHIAL TREE

The tracheobronchial tree consists of the trachea, bronchi, and bronchioles. The trachea is a hollow tube, or "windpipe," that connects the larynx and the major bronchi of the lungs (see Fig. 23-4). The trachea is primarily smooth muscle and is supported by horseshoe-shaped rings of cartilage that prevent the trachea from collapsing during coughing or bronchoconstriction of the smooth muscle.

The end of the trachea divides, forming the two large mainstem bronchi. The point at which the trachea divides is called the *carina.* The carina is innervated with sensory neurons. When the carina is stimulated (for example, during tracheal suctioning), the cough reflex and bronchoconstriction are elicited. The right mainstem bronchus is wider and shorter than the left bronchus. Thus, the right mainstem bronchus is the most common site of aspiration of foreign bodies. The right and left mainstem bronchi divide into branches that become smaller and more numerous as they divide (Fig. 23-8). The right and left mainstem bronchi divide into lobar and segmental bronchi, which divide into bronchioles, which become terminal bronchioles. The terminal bronchioles are the smallest airways without alveoli. The mainstem bronchi are similar in structure to the trachea, in that they are airways supported by cartilage rings. However, as the bronchi extend into the lungs, the cartilage rings become irregular and smaller until they disappear at about the level of the respiratory bronchioles. Here, smooth muscle wraps around the bronchioles. Contraction of these muscles (*bronchospasm*) causes narrowing of the bronchioles and impairs gas flow.[3]

The Respiratory Airways

The terminal bronchioles branch into the respiratory airways. These airways include the respiratory bronchioles, the alveolar ducts, and the alveolar sacs (see Fig. 23-7). The respiratory zone makes up most of the lung, its volume being about 2.5 to 3 L.[2]

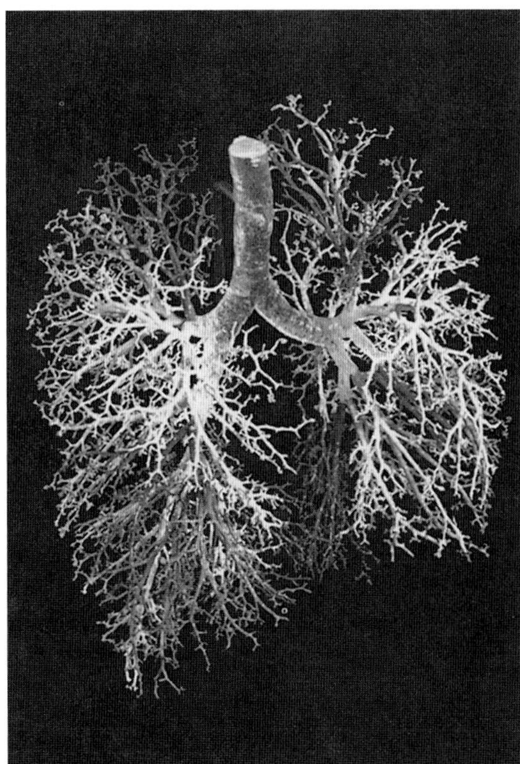

figure 23-8 Cast of the airways of a human lung. The alveoli have been pruned away, allowing the conducting airways from the trachea to the terminal bronchioles to be seen. (Source: West JB: Respiratory Physiology: The Essentials [6th Ed], p 5. Philadelphia, Lippincott Williams & Wilkins, 2000.)

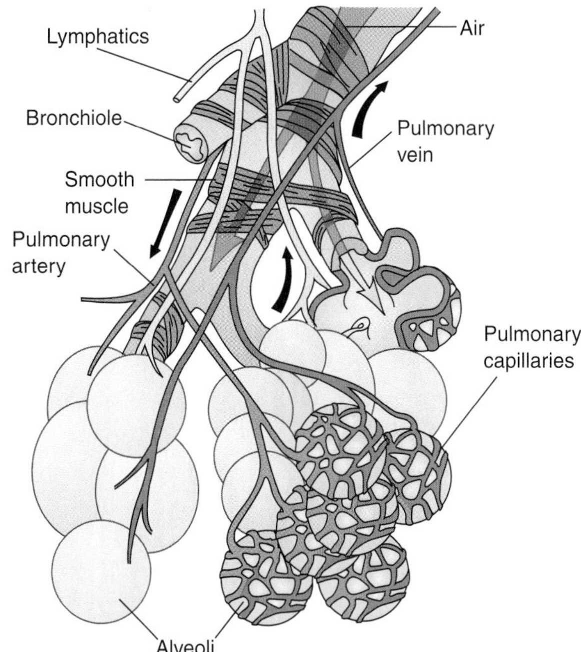

figure 23-9 Lobule of the lung, showing the bronchial smooth muscle fibers, pulmonary blood vessels, and lymphatics. (Source: Porth CM: Pathophysiology: Concepts of Altered Health States [6th Ed], p 581. Philadelphia, Lippincott Williams & Wilkins, 2002.)

THE RESPIRATORY BRONCHIOLES

Each respiratory bronchiole forms a lobule. The lobule is the smallest functional unit of the lung and is where gas exchange takes place. A lobule consists of an arteriole, the pulmonary capillaries, and a venule (Fig. 23-9). Blood enters through a pulmonary artery and exits through a pulmonary vein. This is the only place in the body where highly oxygenated blood flows through a vein.

THE ALVEOLI

Each respiratory bronchiole gives rise to several alveolar ducts that terminate in a cluster of alveoli, as shown in Figure 23-9. The alveolus is the end point of the respiratory tract and it is here where gas exchange takes place. The alveoli are thin-walled, cup-shaped structures. There are approximately 300 million alveoli in the adult lung, with a total surface area of 85 square meters.[2] The alveoli also contain macrophages that perform a phagocytic role. These cells move from alveolus to alveolus, removing foreign substances and keeping the alveoli sterile.

Alveolar structures are composed of two types of cells: type I alveolar cells and type II alveolar cells. *Type I alveolar cells* are flat squamous epithelial cells and comprise approximately 90% of the total alveolar surface area. Gas exchange takes place along these cells. *Type II alveolar cells* secrete pulmonary surfactant. Surfactant is a lipoprotein that decreases surface tension in the alveoli. This prevents collapse of the smaller airways during expiration and makes it easier to inflate the alveoli during inspiration. Therefore, injury to type II alveolar cells leads to alveolar collapse and impaired pulmonary gas exchange.

The Lung Circulation

The lungs have a dual blood supply, the bronchial circulation and the pulmonary circulation. The bronchial circulation distributes blood to the airways and the pulmonary circulation contributes to gas exchange.

THE BRONCHIAL CIRCULATION

The bronchial arteries that perfuse the left side of the thorax arise from the aorta, and the arteries that perfuse the right side of the thorax branch from the internal mammary, subclavian, and intercostal arteries. The capillaries of the bronchial circulation drain into the bronchial veins and eventually empty into the vena cava or the pulmonary vein. The bronchial circulation does not participate in gas exchange. Blood that is emptied into the pulmonary vein is unoxygenated blood and mixes with oxygenated blood flowing to the left side of the heart. This contributes to the "anatomic shunt" and is why arterial oxygen saturation is always less than 100%. The flow through the bronchial circulation is minimal and the lung can function fairly well without it, such as after lung transplantation.[2]

THE PULMONARY CIRCULATION

The pulmonary circulation arises from the pulmonary artery and provides for the gas exchange function of the lung (Fig. 23-10). As shown in Figure 23-10, deoxygenated blood leaves the right ventricle and enters the pulmonary artery. The blood passes from the pulmonary artery through a series of branching arteries to the capillaries, and then back through a series of venules to the pulmonary vein.

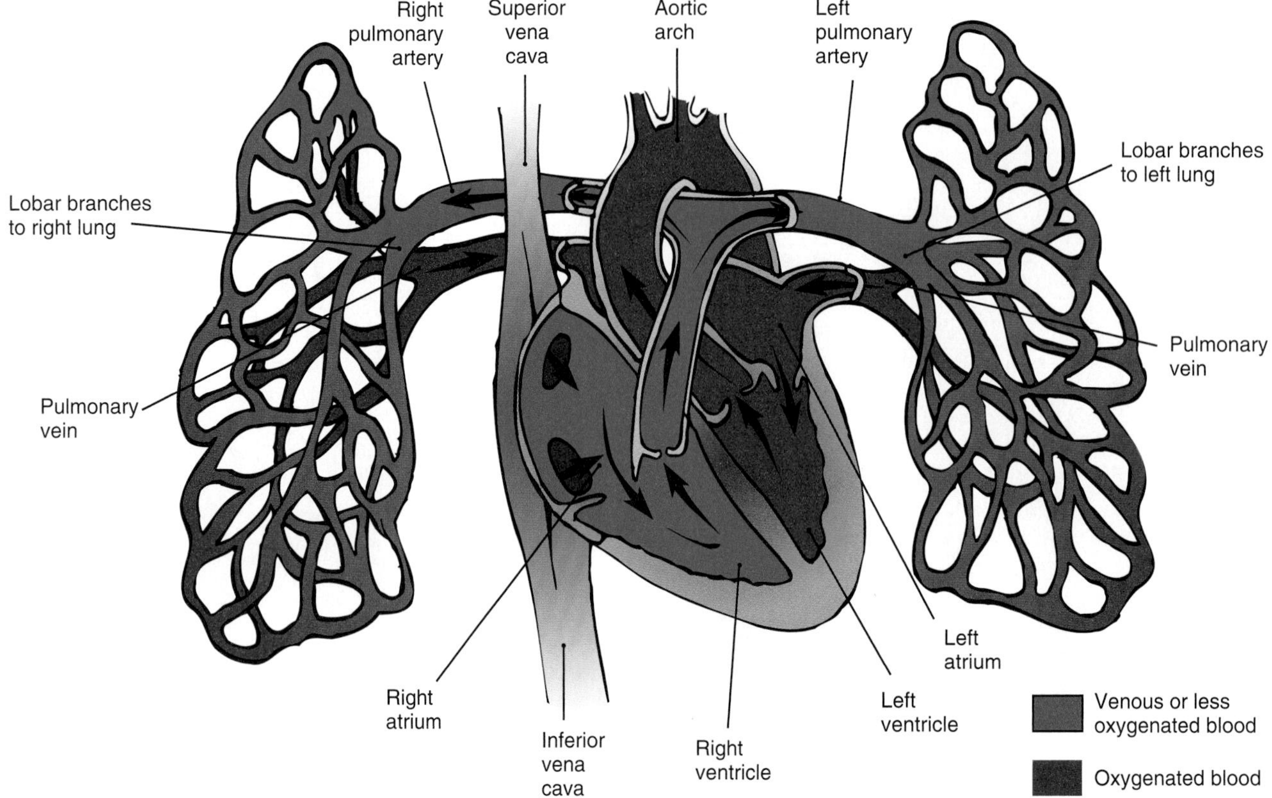

figure 23-10 Circulation from the right heart to the lungs and left heart.

In the walls of the alveoli, the capillaries form a dense network (see Fig. 23-9). The diameter of a capillary segment is about 10 μm, just large enough for one red blood cell.[2] The extreme thinness of the blood–gas barrier is extremely efficient for gas exchange but also means these capillaries are easily damaged. Increasing pressure in the alveoli (such as occurs with pulmonary hypertension) or increasing volume in the alveoli (such as occurs with mechanical ventilation with large tidal volumes) can damage capillaries, causing them to leak plasma into the alveolar spaces. Each red blood cell spends about 0.75 second in the capillary network, and during this time probably transverses two or three alveoli.[2] Almost complete equilibrium of oxygen and carbon dioxide between alveolar gas and capillary blood can occur during this very brief time.

The pulmonary artery receives the whole output from the right ventricle. However, the resistance of the pulmonary circuit is extremely low, compared with the systemic vascular resistance. This is because the pulmonary vascular structures do not have vascular smooth muscle like the systemic vascular structures do. Thus, systolic and diastolic pressures in the pulmonary circulatory system are much lower. Normal pulmonary artery pressures are 20 to 30/8 to 15 mm Hg. Just as hypertension can develop in the systemic circulatory system, hypertension can occur within the pulmonary circulatory system and is called *pulmonary hypertension.*

The Pulmonary Lymphatics

The lungs represent the largest surface area of the body that is exposed to an increasingly hostile environment.[2] Fortunately, the lungs have multiple mechanisms to handle inhaled particles. The nose filters large particles. Particles that deposit in the conducting airways are removed by cilia that line the airways. The cilia brush the particles up toward the epiglottis, where they are then swallowed. Particles in the alveoli are phagocytosed by macrophages or leukocytes. Foreign materials are then removed from alveoli by lymphatic tissue. The lungs have a vast supply of lymphatic tissue. The lymphatic vessels parallel the pulmonary vasculature (see Fig. 23-9). They surround the lobule and aid in the removal of particles and protein from the interstitial spaces. These vessels eventually drain into lymph nodes located at the hila of the lungs.

PHYSIOLOGY OF THE RESPIRATORY SYSTEM

The goals of respiration are to provide oxygen to tissues and to remove carbon dioxide.[1] The physiology of respiration involves the following three processes: (1) *ventilation*, or the movement of air between the atmosphere and the alveoli; (2) *diffusion* of oxygen and carbon dioxide between the pulmonary capillaries and the alveoli; and (3) *transport* of oxygen and carbon dioxide in the blood to and from the cells.

Ventilation

During ventilation, the movement of air into the lungs is known as *inhalation* and the movement of air out of the lungs is known as *exhalation.* Air flows from a region of higher pressure to a region of lower pressure. To initiate a breath, a drop in pressure in the alveoli must precipitate airflow into the lungs.

THE MECHANICS OF VENTILATION

Ventilation is a complex process with multiple variables, including the change in pressures and the integrity of the muscles responsible for moving air in and out of the lungs, the compliance of the lungs, and the resistance afforded by the airways. Collectively, these variables are referred to as the *mechanics of ventilation.*

Movement of Air Into and Out of the Lungs

The movement of air in and out of the lungs requires muscles to expand and contract the chest cavity and a change in gas pressures to facilitate movement of air from one compartment to another. The lungs can be expanded and contracted in two ways: (1) by downward and upward movement of the diaphragm to lengthen and shorten the chest cavity, and (2) by elevation and depression of the ribs to increase and decrease the anterior–posterior diameter of the chest cavity.[1]

According to the laws of physics, the movement of gases is always from an area of higher pressure to lower pressure. There are several pressures involved in the process of respiration: airway pressure, intrapleural pressure, intra-alveolar pressure, and intrathoracic pressure (Fig. 23-11). The *airway pressure* is the pressure in the conducting airways. The *intrapleural pressure* is the pressure in the narrow space between the visceral and parietal pleurae. The *intra-alveolar pressure* is the pressure inside the alveoli. The pressure difference between the intra-alveolar pressure and the intrapleural pressure is called the *transpulmonary pressure.* The *intrathoracic pressure* is the pressure within the entire thoracic cavity.

Figure 23-12 illustrates the mechanics involved in ventilation. Figure 23-12A shows the pressures in the resting state. Pleural pressure, a slightly negative pressure, creates a suction that holds the lungs open to their resting level.

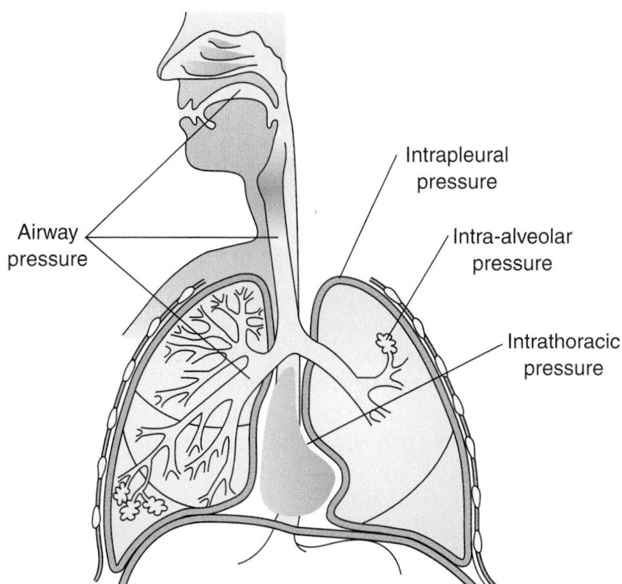

figure 23-11 Partitioning of respiratory pressures. (Source: Porth CM: Pathophysiology: Concepts of Altered Health States [6th Ed], p 585. Philadelphia, Lippincott Williams & Wilkins, 2002.)

Without this negative pressure to hold the lungs against the chest wall, the elastic recoil properties of the lungs would cause them to collapse. When the glottis is open and no air is flowing, the pressure in the conducting airways and alveoli equals atmospheric pressure. Figure 23-11B shows the pressures during inspiration. During inspiration, as the diaphragm and intercostal muscles contract, the volume of the chest cavity increases. Expansion of the chest wall pulls outward on the lungs and the intrapleural pressure becomes more negative. As the alveolar pressure becomes more negative, air flows in from the atmosphere through the conducting airways to the alveoli. After inspiration, the muscles relax, and the chest cavity returns to its resting position. With this decrease in chest size and resultant compression of the lungs, the intra-alveolar pressure builds and forces air out of the lungs during expiration. One respiratory cycle consists of one inhalation and one exhalation. At rest, inhalation requires 1 second and exhalation lasts 2 seconds.

Lung Compliance

The extent to which the lungs expand is called *compliance.* Compliance is a measurement of distensibility, or how easily a tissue is stretched. If compliance is reduced, it is more difficult to expand the lungs for inspiration. And conversely, if compliance is increased, it is easier to expand lung tissue. Compliance is expressed as the ratio of the change in lung volume to the change in lung pressure.

$$\text{Compliance} = \frac{\text{Change in lung volume (L)}}{\text{Change in lung pressure (cm } H_2O)}$$

Compliance can be appreciated by comparing the ease of blowing up a new balloon that is stiff and resistant with one that has been previously blown up and is more compliant. Lung compliance is determined by the elastin and collagen fibers of the lung and the surface tension in the alveoli.

Lung tissue is made up of elastin and collagen fibers. Collagen fibers resist stretching and make lung inflation difficult, whereas elastin fibers are easily stretched and increase the ease of lung inflation. When elastin fibers are replaced with scar tissue, such as that which occurs with pulmonary fibrosis or interstitial lung disease, the lungs become stiff and noncompliant.

The fluid lining the alveoli has a high surface tension. When the surface tension is high, the moist interior surfaces of an alveolus are difficult to separate from one another, and more energy is required to open and fill the alveolus with air during inspiration. When the surface tension is low, the alveoli walls separate more easily, requiring less effort for alveolar filling during inspiration. Recall that a lipoprotein substance called *surfactant,* which is secreted by type II alveolar cells, decreases the surface tension of these fluids in the alveoli.

Surfactant exerts four important effects on lung inflation: it lowers the surface tension; increases lung compliance and ease of inflation; provides for stability and more even inflation of the alveoli; and assists in preventing pulmonary edema by keeping the alveoli dry.[3] Without surfactant, lung inflation is extremely difficult. The type II alveolar cells that produce surfactant do not mature until the 26th to 28th weeks of gestation.[3] Premature infants do not have sufficient amounts of surfactant, which leads to alveolar collapse and severe respiratory distress, a condition

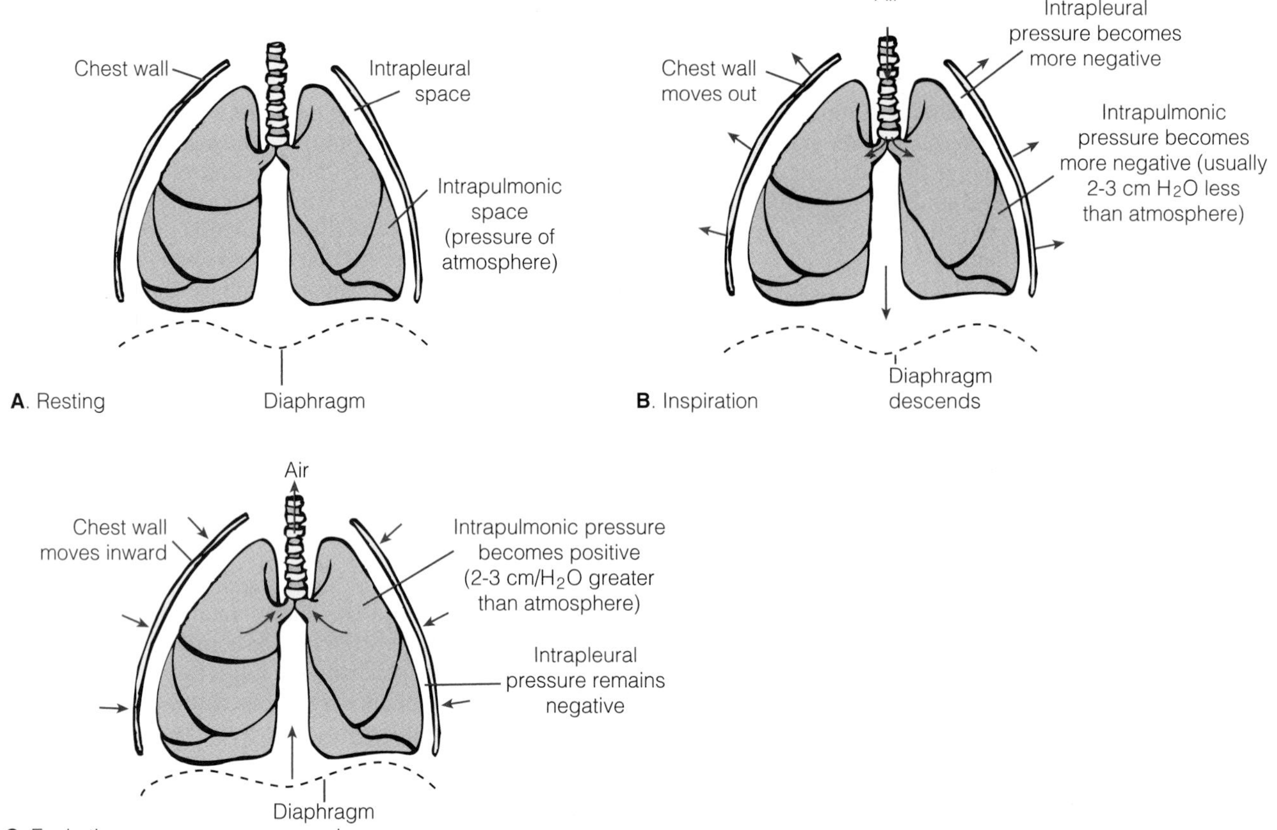

figure 23-12 Phases of ventilation. (**A**) No air movement (resting). (**B**) Air moves from the environment to the intrapulmonic space (inspiration). (**C**) Air moves from the intrapulmonic space to the environment (expiration).

known as *infant respiratory distress syndrome.* Lack of surfactant or inefficient surfactant production may also play a role in the development of *acute respiratory distress syndrome* (ARDS) in adults.

Airway Resistance

Airflow in the conducting airways is affected not only by pressure differences between the atmosphere and alveoli; it is also affected by the resistance that air encounters as it moves through the airways. According to Poiseuille's law, the resistance to flow is inversely proportional to the fourth power of the radius ($R = 1/r^4$). If the radius of the tube that gas is flowing through is cut in half, the resistance is increased 16-fold ($2 \times 2 \times 2 \times 2 = 16$). In the respiratory airways, this means small changes in airway diameter can have enormous effects on airflow resistance. Normally, airway resistance is so small that only small changes in pressure are needed to move large volumes of air into the lungs. But in conditions that decrease airway diameter, such as those caused by pulmonary secretions or bronchospasm, marked increases in airway resistance occur. To maintain the same rate of airflow as before the onset of increased airway resistance, people with these conditions must increase the driving pressure (or respiratory effort) to move air.

ASSESSMENT OF VENTILATION

Minute ventilation is the volume of air inhaled and exhaled per minute. It is calculated by multiplying tidal volume (V_T) and respiratory rate. At rest, minute ventilation is approximately 7,500 mL/minute.

Not all the air that enters the airways reaches the alveoli where gas exchange takes place. The part of tidal volume that does not participate in alveolar gas exchange is called *dead space ventilation.* Dead space ventilation includes anatomical dead space volume and physiological dead space volume. Anatomical dead space is the amount of air in the conducting airways and is normally about 2 mL/kg, or about 150 mL.[4] Anatomical dead space depends on body posture and disease states. In certain disease states, such as chronic obstructive pulmonary disease (COPD), anatomical dead space is larger than normal. Physiological dead space occurs when ventilation is normal, but perfusion to the alveoli is reduced to absent. This can occur with certain disease states, such as reduced cardiac output or pulmonary embolism. Dead space increases the partial pressure of arterial carbon dioxide ($Pa{CO_2}$) because blood that is carrying carbon dioxide back from the tissues cannot reach the alveoli.

The *alveolar ventilation* is the volume of fresh gas entering the respiratory zone each minute. Alveolar ventilation is of key importance because it represents the amount of fresh inspired air available for gas exchange.[2] Alveolar ventilation is a product of minute ventilation minus dead space. It is inversely proportional to $Pa{CO_2}$ levels. If one breathes excessively, alveolar ventilation is increased and $Pa{CO_2}$ decreases. If alveolar ventilation is decreased, $Pa{CO_2}$ levels will increase.

PULMONARY VOLUMES AND CAPACITIES

The flow of air in and out of the lungs provides tangible measures of lung volumes. Although referred to as "pulmonary function" measures, in reality these volumes represent "pulmonary anatomy" measures. In the evaluation of ventilation, structure or anatomy often determines function.

Ventilatory or pulmonary function tests measure the ability of the chest and lungs to move air into and out of the alveoli. Pulmonary function tests include volume measurements, capacity measurements, and dynamic measurements. These measurements are influenced by exercise and disease. Age, sex, body size, and posture are other variables that are taken into consideration when the test results are interpreted. (For a summary of age-related changes affecting the anatomy and physiology of the respiratory system, see Box 23-1). Figure 23-13 illustrates pulmonary function tests showing normal lung volumes and capacity. Volume measurements show the amount of air contained in the lungs during various parts of the respiratory cycle. Measures of lung volume include V_T, inspiratory reserve volume (IRV), expiratory reserve volume (ERV), and residual volume (RV), as shown in Table 23-1. Capacity measurements quantify a part of the pulmonary cycle. They are measured as a combination of the previous volumes and include inspiratory capacity (IC), functional residual capacity (FRC), vital capacity (VC), and total lung capacity (TLC; see Table 23-1).

THE "WORK" OF BREATHING

During normal quiet breathing, muscle contraction occurs during inspiration while expiration is a passive process caused by elastic recoil of the lung. Thus, under normal resting conditions, muscle contraction (or work) is required only during inspiration. The work of inspiration can be divided into three categories: (1) that required to expand the lungs against lung and chest wall elastic forces, called *compliance work* or *elastic work;* (2) that required to overcome the viscosity of the lung and chest wall structures, called *tissue resistance work;* and (3) that required to overcome airway resistance during the movement of air into the lungs, called *airway resistance work.*[1] Normally during quiet respiration, only a small percentage of the total work is used to overcome tissue resistance and a little more is used to overcome airway resistance. However, during heavy breathing when air must flow through the airways at a higher velocity, more work is used to overcome airway resistance. All three types of work are frequently increased in pulmonary disease. Fibrosis of the lungs increases compliance work and tissue resistance work. Diseases that obstruct the airways increase airway resistance work. During normal quiet respiration, only 3% to 5% of the total energy expended by the body is required for ventilation; however, during heavy exercise, the amount of energy required can increase as much as 50-fold, especially if the person has any degree of increased airway resistance or decreased pulmonary compliance.[1]

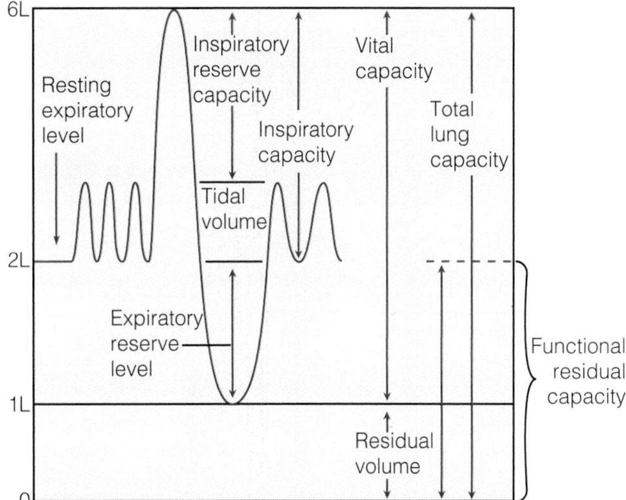

figure 23-13 Pulmonary volumes and capacities. (Source: Bullock BL: Pathophysiology: Adaptations and Alteration in Function [4th Ed], p 566. Philadelphia, Lippincott Williams & Wilkins, 1996.)

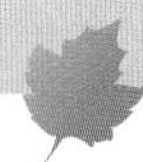

box 23-1

Anatomical and Physiological Changes in the Respiratory System That Occur With Aging

- The anterior–posterior diameter increases.
- Compliance is increased.
- Anatomical dead space is increased.
- The residual volume (RV) increases.
- Respiratory muscle strength decreases.
- The number of alveoli is reduced, resulting in decreased surface area for diffusion.
- Alveolar elasticity is decreased.
- Chest wall motility is decreased.
- The vital capacity (VC) decreases.
- Blood oxygen levels are decreased—subtract 1 mm Hg from a baseline arterial oxygen tension (PaO_2) of 80 mm Hg for every year over age 60.
- Anemia is common due to decreased hemoglobin and oxygen carrying capacity.

Diffusion

After the alveoli are ventilated with fresh air, the next step in the respiratory process is "diffusion" of oxygen from the alveoli to the pulmonary capillaries and diffusion of carbon dioxide from the pulmonary capillaries to the alveoli. Diffusion, or movement of molecules, occurs from an area of high to low concentration. Fick's law describes the diffusion of gases through the alveolar–capillary membrane (Fig. 23-14). Fick's law states that the rate of transfer of gas through a semipermeable membrane is proportional to the tissue surface area and the difference in gas pressures between the two sides, and inversely proportional to the tissue thickness. Recall that the surface area of the alveoli is very large (50 to 100 m^2), and the thickness of the alveolar membrane is 0.3 μm, so the dimensions of the blood–gas barrier are ideal for diffusion of gases.[2] Different gases also cross the barrier at different rates depending on their molecular characteristics. Carbon dioxide diffuses about

table 23-1 Lung Volumes and Lung Capacities

Term Used	Symbol	Description	Remarks	Normal Values
Lung Volumes				
Tidal volume	V_T	Volume of air inhaled and exhaled with each breath	Tidal volume may not vary, even with severe disease.	500 mL
Inspiratory reserve volume	IRV	Maximum volume of air that can be inhaled after a normal inhalation		3,000 mL
Expiratory reserve volume	ERV	Maximum volume of air that can be exhaled forcibly after a normal exhalation	Expiratory reserve volume is decreased with restrictive disorders, such as obesity, ascites, pregnancy.	1,100 mL
Residual volume	RV	Volume of air remaining in the lungs after a maximum exhalation	Residual volume may be increased with obstructive diseases.	1,200 mL
Lung Capacities				
Vital capacity	VC	Maximum volume of air exhaled from the point of maximum inspiration	Decrease in vital capacity may be found in neuromuscular disease, generalized fatigue, atelectasis, pulmonary edema, and chronic obstructive pulmonary disease (COPD).	4,600 mL
Inspiratory capacity	IC	Maximum volume of air inhaled after normal expiration	Decrease in inspiratory capacity may indicate restrictive disease.	3,500 mL
Functional residual capacity	FRC	Volume of air remaining in lungs after a normal expiration	Functional residual capacity may be increased with COPD and decreased in acute respiratory distress syndrome (ARDS).	2,300 mL
Total lung capacity	TLC	Volume of air in lungs after a maximum inspiration and equal to the sum of all four volumes (V_T, IRV, ERV, RV)	Total lung capacity may be decreased with restrictive disease (atelectasis, pneumonia) and increased in COPD.	5,800 mL

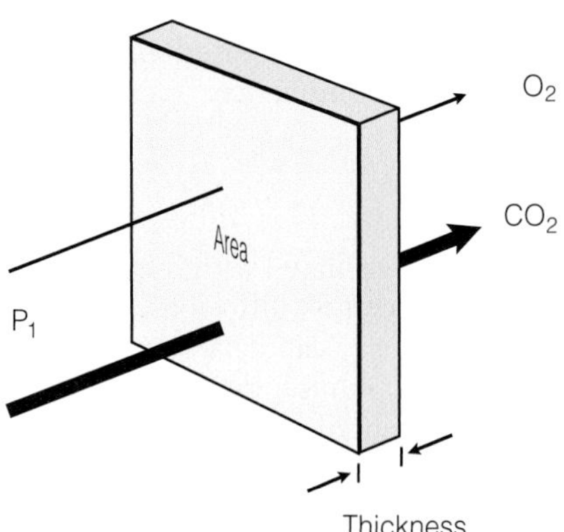

figure 23-14 Fick's law describes diffusion through a tissue sheet. The amount of gas diffused is directly proportional to the surface area and the difference in partial pressures between the tissue sheet (P_1 to P_2). The amount of gas diffused is inversely proportional to the thickness of the tissue sheet. The molecular characteristics of carbon dioxide (CO_2) allow it to diffuse about 20 times more rapidly than oxygen (O_2). (Source: West JB: Respiratory Physiology: The Essentials [6th Ed], p 22. Philadelphia, Lippincott Williams & Wilkins, 2000.)

20 times more rapidly than does oxygen. Thus, there are four factors that affect alveolar–capillary gas exchange: (1) the surface area available for diffusion, (2) the thickness of the alveolar–capillary membrane, (3) the partial pressure of gas across the membrane, and (4) solubility and molecular characteristics of the gas (Table 23-2). Any condition or disease that affects one or more of these factors may impair diffusion of oxygen and carbon dioxide across the alveolar–capillary membrane.

Perfusion

Once oxygen has diffused from the alveolus to the pulmonary capillary, it is carried away from the lung by the bloodstream. This gas exchange function of the lungs requires a constant flow of blood through the respiratory airways. The term *perfusion* is used to describe the flow of blood through the pulmonary capillary bed. As previously described in this chapter, pulmonary capillaries form a dense network around the alveolar wall, making an extremely efficient structure for gas exchange to take place

table 23-2 Factors Affecting Alveolar–Capillary Gas Exchange

Factors Affecting Gas Exchange	Examples
Surface area available for diffusion	Removal of a lung or diseases such as emphysema and chronic bronchitis, which destroy lung tissue or cause mismatching of ventilation and perfusion
Thickness of the alveolar–capillary membrane	Conditions such as pneumonia, interstitial lung disease, and pulmonary edema, which increase membrane thickness
Partial pressure of alveolar gas	Decreasing the partial pressure of a gas in the inspired air (e.g., ascent to high altitudes) decreases the gradient for diffusion; increasing the partial pressure of a gas in the inspired air (e.g., oxygen therapy) increases the gradient for diffusion
Solubility and molecular weight of the gas	Carbon dioxide, which is more soluble in the cell membranes, diffuses across the alveolar–capillary membrane more rapidly than oxygen

From Porth CM: Pathophysiology: Concepts of Altered Health States (6th Ed), p 594. Philadelphia, Lippincott Williams & Wilkins, 2002.

(see Fig. 23-9). The meshwork of the capillaries in the respiratory portion of the lungs is so dense that the flow in these vessels often is described as being similar to a "sheet" of blood.[3] When these blood vessels sense a low oxygen content in the alveoli, they vasoconstrict. The precise mechanism of this response, called *hypoxic vasoconstriction*, is not known.[2] Hypoxic vasoconstriction has the effect of directing blood flow away from hypoxic areas of the lung. By diverting blood flow from these areas, the deleterious effects on gas exchange are reduced.

Relationship of Ventilation to Perfusion

DISTRIBUTION OF VENTILATION

Not all areas of the lung have the same ventilation. Body position affects distribution of ventilation. In a seated or standing position, lower regions of the lung ventilate better than do upper zones. In a supine position, the apex and base of the lung ventilate about the same; however, ventilation in the lowermost (posterior) lung is greater than that of the uppermost (anterior) lung. In a lateral position, the dependent lung is best ventilated.[2]

DISTRIBUTION OF PERFUSION

As with ventilation, the distribution of pulmonary blood flow is affected by body position and gravity. In the upright position, blood flow is better at the base of the lungs than the apex of the lungs. In the supine position, the blood flow from apex to base is almost uniform, but blood flow in the posterior (dependent) regions of the lung exceeds that of the anterior regions. In the prone position, the same would hold true: blood flow in the dependent (now the anterior chest) exceeds that of the posterior chest.

Considerable inequality of blood flow exists within the human lung (Fig. 23-15). The uneven distribution of blood flow can be explained by the hydrostatic pressure differences in the blood vessels. In zone 1, alveolar pressures exceed pulmonary arterial and pulmonary venous pressures. The capillaries are basically squashed flat by the pressure in the alveoli and there is no blood flow. In zone 2, pulmonary arterial pressures are greater than alveolar pressures, so some blood flow occurs. Blood flow here is determined by the differences in arterial and alveolar pressures. In zone 3, there is minimal alveolar pressure influence on

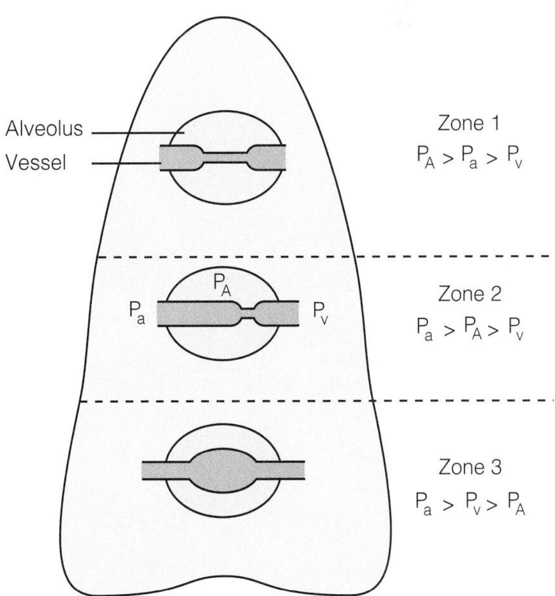

figure 23-15 Explanation of the uneven distribution of blood flow in the lung, based on the pressures affecting the capillaries. *PA*, alveolar pressure; *Pa*, arterial pressure; *Pv*, venous pressure. (Source: West JB: Respiratory Physiology: The Essentials [6th Ed], p 37. Philadelphia, Lippincott Williams & Wilkins, 2000.)

the pulmonary vasculature and blood flow is determined in the usual way by the arteriovenous pressure difference.

MATCHING OF VENTILATION TO PERFUSION

Effective pulmonary gas exchange depends on a balance, or matching of ventilation to perfusion (Fig. 23-16A). Two factors may interfere with the matching of ventilation to perfusion: dead space and shunt. As previously described in this chapter, dead space refers to areas in the respiratory system that do not participate in gas exchange. The air in the conducting airways (about 150 mL) does not participate in gas exchange and is referred to as *anatomical dead space.* Anatomical dead space increases with intubation. In zone 1 of the lung, the region is ventilated but not perfused and this is referred to as *alveolar dead space.* Other areas of the lung may also contain alveolar dead space, such as that which occurs with collapsed alveoli from atelectasis or pneumonia. Shunt refers to blood that bypasses, or shunts by, alveoli without picking up oxygen. There are two types of shunts: anatomical and physiological. With an anatomical shunt, blood moves from the right side to the left side of the heart without passing through the lungs. Anatomical shunts occur with congenital heart diseases. With a physiological shunt, blood is shunted past alveoli without picking up sufficient amounts of oxygen.

A ventilation–perfusion imbalance, known as a ventilation–perfusion mismatch, occurs when there is inadequate ventilation, inadequate perfusion, or both. Three types of ventilation–perfusion imbalances may occur:

- *Physiological shunt (low ventilation–perfusion ratio).* When perfusion exceeds ventilation, the ratio is low and a shunt is present. A shunt means that blood passes by alveoli without gas exchange occurring. Severe hypoxia results when the amount of shunted blood exceeds 20%.[5] A low ventilation–perfusion ratio is seen with pneumonia, atelectasis, tumor, or a mucous plug (see Fig. 23-16B).
- *Alveolar dead space (high ventilation–perfusion ratio).* When ventilation exceeds perfusion, the ratio is high and an alveolar dead space develops. The alveolus has inadequate perfusion available, and gas exchange cannot occur. A high ventilation–perfusion ratio is seen with a pulmonary embolus, pulmonary infarction, cardiogenic shock, and mechanical ventilation associated with high tidal volumes (see Fig. 23-16C).
- *Silent unit.* When both ventilation and perfusion are decreased, a silent unit occurs. A silent unit is seen with pneumothorax and severe ARDS (see Fig. 23-16D).

Gas Transport

OXYGEN

Oxygen is carried in the blood in two forms: dissolved and attached to hemoglobin. The partial pressure of oxygen in arterial blood (PaO_2) represents the level of dissolved oxygen in plasma. Less than 3% of all oxygen is carried in this form. Ninety-seven percent of oxygen carried in the blood is bound to hemoglobin and is called *oxyhemoglobin.* Each

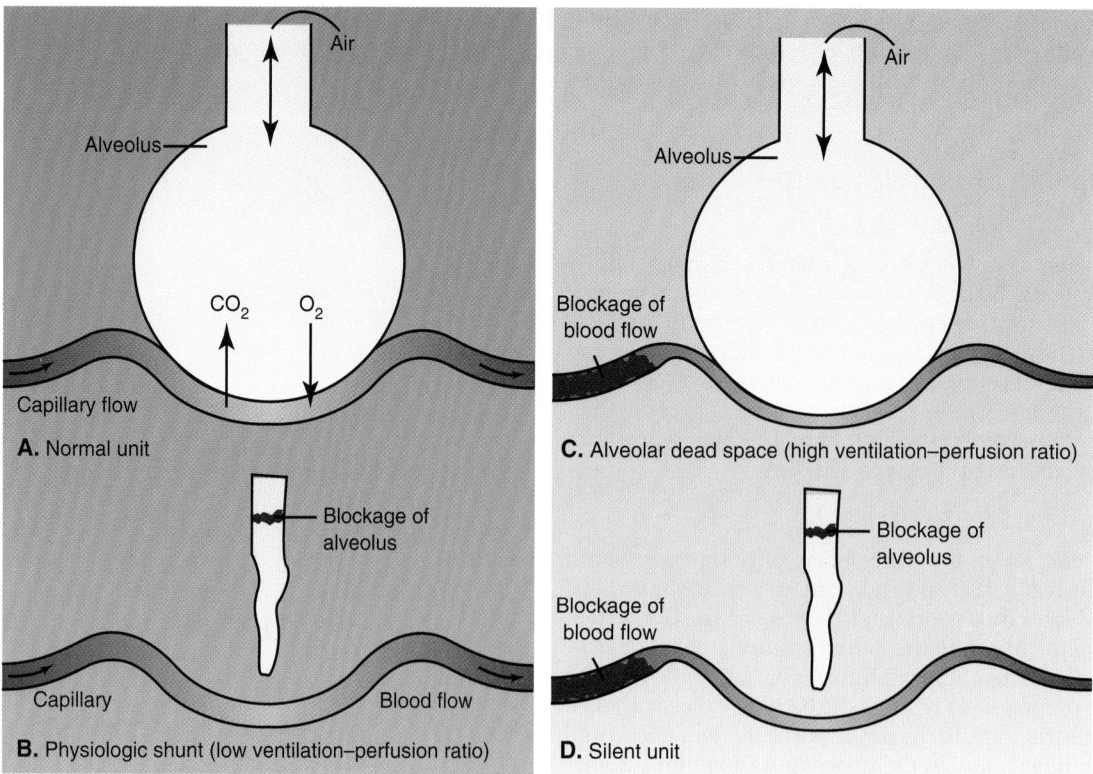

figure 23-16 A schematic representation of various ventilation–perfusion situations. (**A**) Normal unit with normal ventilation and normal perfusion. (**B**) Low ventilation–perfusion ratio—alveoli with no ventilation but normal perfusion. (**C**) High ventilation–perfusion ratio—alveoli with normal ventilation but no perfusion. (**D**) Silent unit—alveoli with no ventilation and no perfusion. CO_2, carbon dioxide; O_2, oxygen. (Source: Smeltzer SC, Bare BG: Brunner and Suddarth's Textbook of Medical Surgical Nursing [9th Ed], p 380. Philadelphia, Lippincott Williams & Wilkins, 2000.)

gram of hemoglobin carries approximately 1.34 mL of oxygen when it is completely saturated. As oxygen diffuses across the alveolar–capillary membrane, it combines with hemoglobin in the red blood cell where it forms a reversible bond. Oxyhemoglobin is transported in arterial blood and made available to the tissues for use in cell metabolism. The saturation of oxygen in arterial blood (SaO_2) represents the percentage of hemoglobin molecules that are bound with oxygen.

The hemoglobin molecule is said to be fully saturated when oxygen is bound to all four of its oxygen-binding sites, and only partially saturated when less than four molecules are bound to it. The term *affinity* is used to refer to the capacity of hemoglobin to combine with oxygen. When the affinity is high, hemoglobin binds readily with oxygen at the alveolar–capillary membrane. But at the tissue level, hemoglobin does not readily release oxygen. When the affinity is low, hemoglobin does not bind readily with oxygen at the alveolar–capillary membrane. Instead, when affinity is low, hemoglobin releases oxygen more readily at the tissue level. The affinity of hemoglobin and oxygen is described by the oxyhemoglobin dissociation curve (Fig. 23-17).

The oxyhemoglobin dissociation curve is a graphic depiction of the relationship between oxyhemoglobin saturation (the percentage of hemoglobin combined with oxygen, or the SaO_2) and the arterial oxygen tension (PaO_2) to which it is exposed. The initial part of the curve is very steep and then flattens at the top. The flat portion represents the binding of oxygen to hemoglobin in the lungs. The steep portion of the curve (between 40 and 60 mm Hg) represents the release of oxygen from the hemoglobin that occurs in the capillaries. At an arterial oxygen tension (PaO_2) of 40 mm Hg, hemoglobin molecules are still about 70% to 75% saturated with oxygen. This provides a reserve supply of oxygen that can be given to the tissues in cases of emergency or strenuous exercise.

Hemoglobin's affinity for oxygen is influenced by pH, carbon dioxide concentration, temperature, and 2,3-diphosphoglycerate (2,3-DPG). 2,3-DPG is a metabolically important phosphate compound found in the blood but in different combinations under different metabolic conditions.[1] Hemoglobin binds more readily with oxygen under conditions of increased pH, decreased carbon dioxide, decreased body temperature, and decreased 2,3-DPG. This is represented on the oxyhemoglobin dissociation curve as a shift to the left (see Fig. 23-17). With a shift to the left, there is higher oxygen saturation for any given PaO_2, increased affinity of hemoglobin for oxygen, and decreased release of oxygen to tissues. Hemoglobin more readily releases oxygen under conditions of decreased pH, increased carbon dioxide, increased body temperature, and increased 2,3-DPG. This relationship is represented on the curve by a shift to the right (see Fig. 23-17). With a shift to the right, there is lower oxygen saturation for any given arterial oxygen tension PaO_2, decreased affinity of hemoglobin for oxygen, and increased release of oxygen to the tissues.

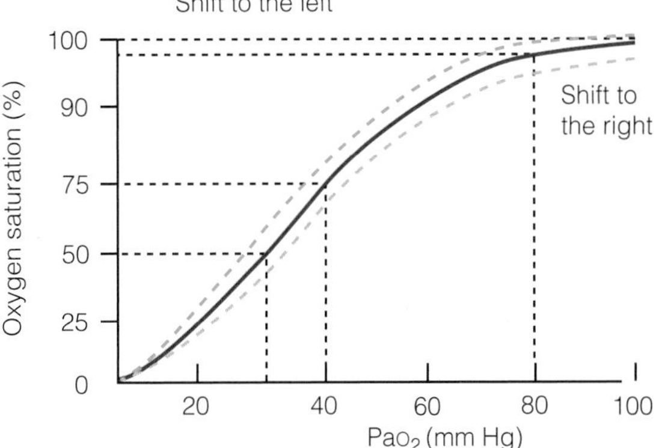

figure 23-17 Oxyhemoglobin dissociation curve. The shift to the left indicates a higher oxygen saturation at any given arterial oxygen tension (*PaO_2*), an increased affinity of hemoglobin for oxygen, and a decreased release of oxygen to the tissues. A shift to the right indicates a lower oxygen saturation at any given PaO_2, a decreased affinity of hemoglobin for oxygen, and an increased release of oxygen to the tissues.

CARBON DIOXIDE

Carbon dioxide is carried in the blood in three forms: as dissolved carbon dioxide (10%), attached to hemoglobin (30%), and as bicarbonate (60%).[3] Carbon dioxide is formed as a metabolic byproduct. It diffuses out of the cell and into the capillaries. Most of it diffuses into red blood cells where it attaches to hemoglobin, and most of that is released from the red blood cell as bicarbonate. In the pulmonary capillaries, the concentration of carbon dioxide is greater in the capillaries than in the alveoli, so the carbon dioxide moves down this concentration gradient and diffuses into the alveoli and is exhaled. An increased rate of exhalation leads to greater elimination of carbon dioxide. The transport of carbon dioxide has a profound effect on the acid–base status of the blood and the body as a whole. The lung excretes over 10,000 mEq of carbonic acid per day, compared with the kidney, which excretes less than 100 mEq of fixed acids per day.[2] Therefore, by altering alveolar ventilation (and subsequently, the elimination of carbon dioxide), the body is able to exert precise control over its acid–base balance.

Regulation of Respiration

Breathing is controlled by both the nervous system and chemical regulation. Nervous system regulation is achieved by the respiratory centers, which are located in the medulla and pons (i.e., the brainstem). Chemical regulation of breathing occurs through chemoreceptors, which respond to blood pH and the levels of oxygen and carbon dioxide in the blood.

BRAINSTEM CENTERS AND THE RESPIRATORY CYCLE

Unlike the heart, the lungs have no spontaneous rhythm. Ventilation depends on rhythmic operation of brainstem centers and intact pathways to the respiratory muscles. There are two centers in the medulla: a center that stimulates inspiration by diaphragmatic contraction (by way of phrenic nerves) and another center that innervates both inspiratory and expiratory intercostal and accessory muscles (Fig. 23-18). The pons also contains two centers involved in controlling respiration, the pneumotaxic

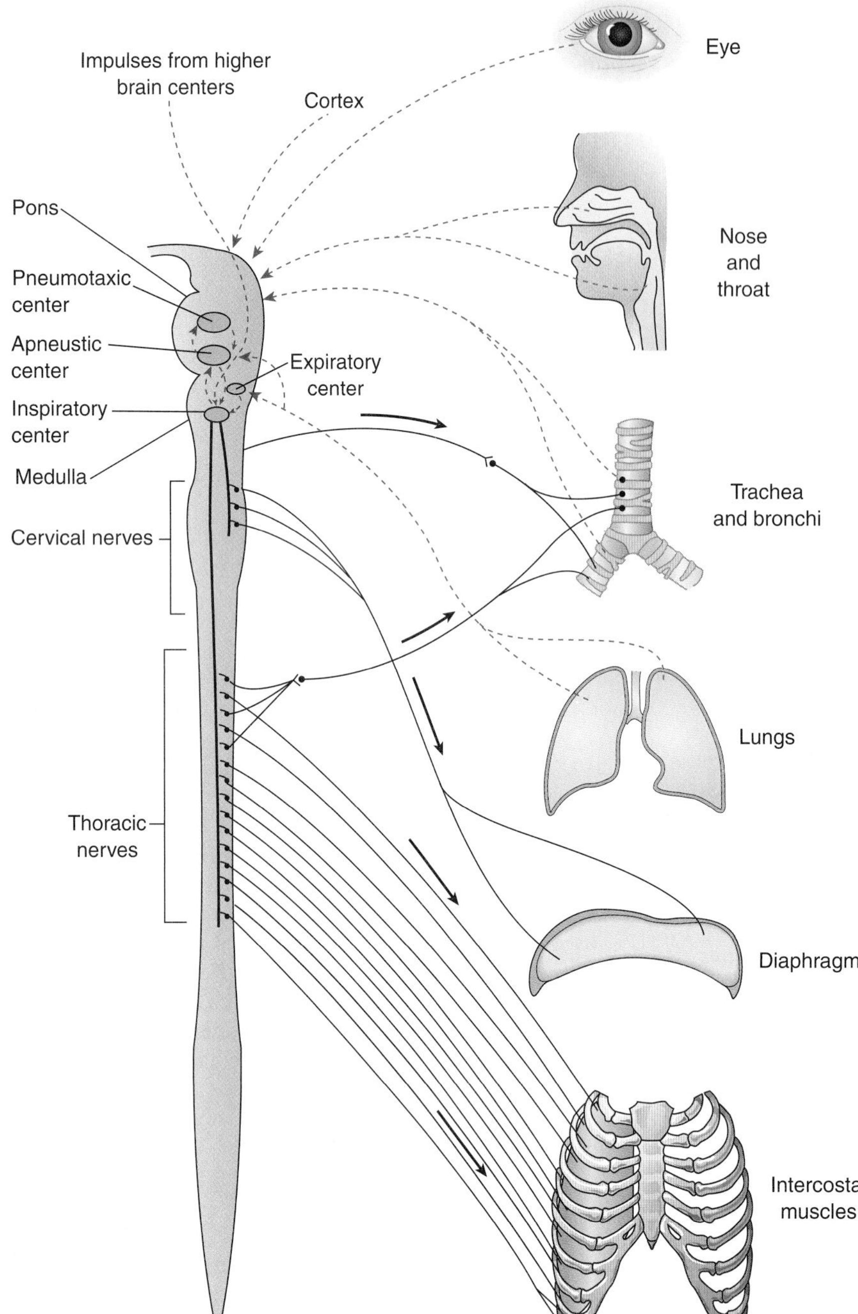

figure 23-18 Schematic representation of activity in the respiratory center. Impulses traveling over afferent neurons activate central neurons, which activate efferent neurons that supply the muscles of respiration. Respiratory movements can be altered by a variety of stimuli.

center and the apneustic center. The apneustic center produces sustained inspiration if stimulated. Voluntary control and involuntary control are further established by descending fibers from other brain centers. Neural control of ventilation is illustrated in Figure 23-18. In breathing at rest, the following sequence is thought to occur. The neurons innervating the inspiratory muscles fire bursts of impulses to these muscles, leading to inspiration. These neurons also stimulate the pneumotaxic center. This center, in turn, fires inhibitory impulses back to the inspiratory neurons, causing a halt in inspiration. Expiration follows passively. After expiration, the inspiratory neurons are again stimulated to fire automatically. During exercise or other occasions when more vigorous ventilation occurs, the expiratory neurons of the medulla are postulated to participate in this sequence, causing active exhalation.

CHEMORECEPTORS

Chemoreceptors are like radar screens planted in the body to monitor blood levels of carbon dioxide and oxygen. Signals from these receptors are transmitted to the respiratory center and ventilation is adjusted to maintain these gases in a normal range. There are two types of chemoreceptors: central chemoreceptors and peripheral chemoreceptors.

Central chemoreceptors sense changes in carbon dioxide content. They are located near the respiratory center in the medulla and are in close contact with cerebrospinal fluid (CSF). Carbon dioxide freely diffuses across the blood–brain barrier into the CSF. As the level of carbon dioxide in the CSF increases and the pH decreases, the nearby respiratory center is stimulated to increase respirations to "blow off" more carbon dioxide.

Peripheral chemoreceptors are located in the arch of the aorta and in the carotid arteries. These chemoreceptors are sensitive to changes in oxygen content in arterial blood. These receptors exert little control over respirations until the PaO_2 is below 60 mm Hg.[3] When this occurs, the respiratory center is stimulated to increase the rate and depth of respirations to inhale more oxygen.

LUNG RECEPTORS

Recall the importance of airway resistance and lung expansion on the respiratory process. Lung and chest wall receptors provide information to the respiratory center on the status of these processes. There are three types of lung receptors: stretch, irritant, and juxtacapillary receptors. Stretch receptors, located in the smooth muscle layers of the conducting airways, respond to pressure changes in the airways. When the lungs are fully inflated, they inhibit further inspiration and trigger exhalation. These receptors are important because they establish respiratory patterns by adjusting respiratory rate and tidal volume in an attempt to respond to changes in airway resistance and lung compliance.

Irritant receptors, located in the airways, are stimulated by inhaled dust, smoke, chemicals, and cold air. Stimulation of these receptors triggers airway constriction and more rapid, shallow breathing. It is possible that these receptors play a key role in the bronchoconstriction that occurs with asthma.[3]

Juxtacapillary receptors are located in the alveolar wall close to the pulmonary capillaries. These receptors sense lung congestion. It may be stimulation of these receptors that produces the rapid, shallow breathing that is characteristic in patients with pneumonia and pulmonary edema.

clinical applicability challenges

Self-Challenge: Critical Thinking

1. *Describe how a pneumothorax would affect the mechanics of ventilation in terms of air movement into and out of the lungs, lung compliance, and airway resistance.*
2. *Identify a pathological condition that affects each of the four factors that affect diffusion of oxygen across the alveolar–capillary membrane.*
3. *Analyze the impact of hypothermia on the oxyhemoglobin dissociation curve. Include in your analysis the binding of oxygen to hemoglobin in the pulmonary capillary and the release of oxygen from hemoglobin at the tissue level.*

Study Questions

1. *Which of the following pressures keeps the lungs inflated?*
   a. *Intrapleural pressure*
   b. *Intra-alveolar pressure*
   c. *Intrathoracic pressure*
   d. *Transpulmonary pressure*
2. *The conducting airways include all of the following except the*
   a. *trachea*
   b. *bronchi*
   c. *terminal bronchioles*
   d. *respiratory bronchioles*
3. *Which of the following statements is true about lung compliance?*
   a. *If lung compliance is reduced, it is easy to expand the lungs for inspiration.*
   b. *If lung compliance is reduced, it is very difficult to expand the lungs for inspiration.*
   c. *If lung compliance is increased, it is very difficult for the lungs to expand for inspiration.*
   d. *If lung compliance is increased, it is very difficult for the lungs to expand for expiration.*
4. *The rate of diffusion across the alveolar capillary membrane depends on all of the following except the*
   a. *pressure gradient of oxygen across the alveolar capillary membrane.*
   b. *thickness of the alveolar walls.*
   c. *radius of the airways.*
   d. *surface area of the lungs.*
5. *A low ventilation–perfusion ratio can occur with which of the following conditions?*
   a. *Atelectasis*
   b. *Pulmonary embolus*
   c. *Pulmonary infarct*
   d. *Cardiogenic shock*

REFERENCES

1. Guyton AC, Hall JE: Textbook of Medical Physiology (10th Ed). Philadelphia, WB Saunders, 2000
2. West JB: Respiratory Physiology: The Essentials (6th Ed). Philadelphia, Lippincott Williams & Wilkins, 2000
3. Porth CB: Pathophysiology: Concepts of Altered Health States (6th Ed). Philadelphia, Lippincott Williams & Wilkins, 2002
4. Pierce LNB: Guide to Mechanical Ventilation and Intensive Respiratory Care. Philadelphia, WB Saunders, 1995
5. Ahrens T, Rutherford K: Essentials of Oxygenation. Boston, Jones & Bartlett, 1993

OTHER SELECTED READING

Berry BE, Pinard AE: Assessing tissue oxygenation. Crit Care Nurse 22(3):22–42, 2002

Bickley LS, Hoekelman RA: Bates' Guide to Physical Examination (8th Ed). Philadelphia, Lippincott Williams & Wilkins, 2003

Johnson LR: Essential Medical Physiology (2nd Ed). Philadelphia, Lippincott Williams & Wilkins, 1998

Lamb AB: Nunn's Applied Respiratory Physiology (5th Ed). Oxford, Butterworth-Heinemann, 2000

Smeltzer SC, Bare BG: Brunner & Suddarth's Textbook of Medical-Surgical Nursing (10th Ed). Philadelphia, Lippincott Williams & Wilkins, 2004

Pilbeam SP: Mechanical Ventilation: Physiology and Clinical Applications (3rd Ed). St. Louis, Mosby, 1998

chapter

24

Patient Assessment: Respiratory System

KENNETH REMPHER ■ PATRICIA GONCE MORTON

objectives

Based on the content in this chapter, the reader should be able to:

- Describe the components of the history for respiratory assessment.
- Explain the use of inspection, palpation, percussion, and auscultation for respiratory assessment.
- Discuss the purpose of pulse oximetry.
- Compare and contrast the arterial oxygen saturation and the partial pressure of oxygen dissolved in arterial blood.
- Describe the purpose of end-tidal carbon dioxide monitoring.
- Explain the components of an arterial blood gas and the normal values for each component.
- Compare and contrast the causes, signs, and symptoms of respiratory acidosis, respiratory alkalosis, metabolic acidosis, and metabolic alkalosis.
- Analyze examples of an arterial blood gas result.
- Describe the purpose of mixed venous oxygen saturation monitoring.
- Discuss the purpose of respiratory diagnostic studies and associated nursing implications.

Nurses contribute significantly to the care of patients with respiratory problems by taking a comprehensive history and performing a thorough physical examination. This information allows the nurse to establish a baseline level of assessment of the patient's status and provides a framework for detection of rapid changes in the patient's condition. Assessments are valuable if made before, during, and after interventions that are likely to alter or improve respiratory status. Because the nurse is with the patient more consistently than most other health care professionals, it is often the nurse who detects the patient's changing condition. High-quality assessments often uncover complications or changes that precede the information provided by other diagnostic tests.

HISTORY

A thorough review of the patient's clinical history is an essential component of the overall physical assessment process. A properly conducted review of the patient's clinical history should serve as a guide for the remainder of the physical examination. In many cases, obtaining a clinical history is the first step in developing a relationship with the patient. Patients often suppress information or under-report personal experiences that may be essential in identifying the underlying cause of illness. As a result, constant subjective evaluation of the patient's report should also serve to guide the procurement of the clinical history. The interviewer must conduct the examination in such a way that the patient feels as comfortable as possible.

The clinical history of the respiratory system is divided into six components, including: (1) chief complaint, (2) history of present illness, (3) past medical history, (4) family history, (5) personal and social history, and (6) review of the respiratory system (Box 24-1). The patient's history starts with the chief complaint and information about the present illness. Often, if the patient is very ill, a relative or friend provides more information. Data about the present illness should include onset of the problem, its manifestations, and the outcomes of any attempts to treat the problem. Principal symptoms that should be investigated in more detail commonly include dyspnea, chest pain, sputum production, and cough. An overview of the patient's past medical history and family's respiratory history, as well as personal and social history, may uncover elements that are contributing to the patient's current medical problem. Because smoking has a significant impact on the patient's respiratory health, the patient's use of tobacco should be quantified by amount and how long the patient has smoked. Box 24-2 demonstrates the process for calculating this quantity, which is known as *pack years*.

Dyspnea

Dyspnea is commonly seen in patients with pulmonary or cardiac compromise. Information about the onset of symptoms gives clues as to the source and duration of the problem. The nurse asks questions such as the following:

- Does the dyspnea occur when the patient is lying flat (therefore requiring the patient to sit up, as is seen more commonly in heart failure)?
- Does the dyspnea awaken the patient at night (paroxysmal nocturnal dyspnea)?
- Does the dyspnea occur only with exertion?

Paroxysmal nocturnal dyspnea and orthopnea often signify heart failure but may occur in a variety of pulmonary disorders. Description of the entire course of dyspnea, including exacerbating factors, length of episodes, and any relief measures attempted, is warranted.

Chest Pain

Dyspnea that occurs with primary lung disease is associated with an anterior chest discomfort that must be distinguished from angina. First, the nurse determines if the patient experiences more than one type of pain. For each type of chest pain, the nurse asks the patient to describe what makes the pain better or worse. For example, the pain may be worsened by breathing or movement (e.g., in pleurisy) or be relieved by position changes or movement. The nurse inquires about the outcome of relief measures that have been used (e.g., over-the-counter drugs, prescription drugs, rest, nitroglycerin, antacids, or belching). In addition, the nurse asks about the quality of the pain, where the pain radiates, the severity of the pain, the duration of the pain, and other associated symptoms.

Mnemonics are helpful in the assessment of any pain, including chest pain. In the mnemonic "PQRST," "P" stands for *provoking* (activities that cause or exacerbate the pain) and *palliative* (what helps the pain decrease or go away?); "Q" stands for *quality* of pain (e.g., throbbing, stabbing, crushing); "R" stands for *region and radiation* (where is the pain; does the pain go to another area of the body such as the neck, left arm, or jaw?); "S" stands for *severity* (quantifying the pain on a 0 to 10 scale, where "0" represents no pain at all and "10" represents the worst pain imaginable); and "T" stands for *timing* (when did the pain start and stop?).

Sputum Production

A pulmonary illness often results in the production (or a change in the production) of sputum. The nurse questions the patient about the amount (e.g., tablespoonful, one-half cup) and color of the sputum produced in 24 hours. The color of the sputum provides important information about infection. An increase in either the color or the amount of sputum often means infection. Yellow, green, or brown sputum typically signifies bacterial infection; clear or white sputum may signify absence of bacterial infection. The color comes from white blood cells in the sputum. However, a yellow color may occur if there are many eosinophils in the sputum, thereby signifying allergy rather than infection. Rust-colored sputum (yellow sputum mixed with blood) may signify tuberculosis. Mucoid, viscid, or blood-streaked sputum is often a sign of a viral infection. Persistent slightly blood-streaked sputum is present in patients with carcinoma. Large amounts of clotted blood are present in the sputum of patients who have suffered a pulmonary infarct.

Occasionally, coughing does not yield sputum. Sometimes, the patient with an infection is unable to cough up sputum. For example, a decrease in sputum production associated with worsening hypoxemia may signify bronchiolitis. A cough without sputum production usually means that the problem is not bacterial in origin.

It is important to know whether the sputum comes from the nose, the chest, or sinus postnasal drainage. Chronic sputum production may indicate chronic obstructive pulmonary disease (COPD).

Sometimes, the patient is afraid to mention if there has been blood in the sputum; it is essential to ask the patient, family members, or caregivers about the presence of blood. The amount of blood should be evaluated. Was it just streaks or specks, blood-colored mucus, or pure blood (bright red or dark)? Through careful questioning, the nurse determines whether the blood is associated with retching and vomiting or sputum production, as it often is in bronchitis and pneumonia, or whether it occurs alone, as is often true with a pulmonary embolus.

Cough

A cough is a frequent respiratory symptom with varying significance. A cough can be stimulated by external agents, by inflammation of the respiratory mucosa, or by pressure on an airway caused by a tumor. Specifically, a cough can be caused by smoking, allergies, heartburn, asthma, and certain medications, including angiotensin-converting enzyme (ACE) inhibitors and beta-blockers. Information obtained from the patient about the cough should include onset, precipitating factors, timing, frequency, and whether the cough is productive.

box 24-1
Major Components of Clinical History

Chief Complaint and History of Present Illness

Dyspnea

- Onset and duration (when did you last feel well?)
  - Sudden or gradual
  - Episodic or continuous
- Characteristics
  - Related to position
    Flat versus upright (improves if patient is upright or with head elevated, number of pillows used for sleeping)
  - Related to time of day
    Nighttime (paroxysmal nocturnal dyspnea or PND) versus daytime
  - Related to activity
    At rest versus exertion (disrupts activities of daily living, unable to climb stairs, worsens with eating)
  - Related to miscellaneous factors
    Environment
    Stress
    Season of the year
- Acuity
  - Extent to which activities of daily living are affected
  - Ability to complete sentences
  - Anxiety about getting air
- Provoking factors
  - Anxiety
  - Exercise
  - Environment
- Relieving factors
  - Rest
  - Repositioning to upright when recumbent
  - Addition of pillows when sleeping
- Associated symptoms
  - Pain or discomfort
  - Cough
  - Diaphoresis
  - Ankle edema
- Self-treatment and effectiveness
  - Prescription or over-the-counter medications
  - Oxygen
  - Nonpharmacologic interventions (e.g., guided imagery)

Chest Pain (PQRST Process)

- Provoking factors
  - Activity
  - Anxiety
- Quality
  - Dull
  - Stabbing
  - Sharp
  - Aching
  - Crushing
  - "Weight on chest"
- Radiation
  - Arm pain
  - Jaw pain
  - Neck pain
  - Back pain
- Severity
  - Rate pain on a scale of 0–10 (0 meaning no pain at all and 10 meaning the worst pain imaginable)
- Timing
  - When did the pain start? (and what was the patient doing at that time?)
  - When did the pain stop?
  - How long did it last?
- Associated symptoms
  - Nausea/vomiting
  - Shortness of breath
  - Diaphoresis
  - Cough
  - Fever
- Self-treatment and effectiveness
  - Prescription and over-the-counter medications
  - Splinting
  - Changes in position
  - Heat

Sputum Production

- Onset and duration (When did you first notice a change in your sputum?)
  - Sudden or gradual
  - Episodic or continuous
- Characteristics
  - Color
    Yellow, green, rust, clear, blood-streaked
  - Mucoid
  - Viscid
  - Purulent
  - Amount
- Associated symptoms
  - Vomiting
  - Retching
  - Fever
  - Shortness of breath
  - Chest pain
- Self-treatment and effectiveness
  - Prescription or over-the-counter medications
  - Vaporizer

Cough

- Onset and duration (When did you first notice a change in your cough?)
  - Sudden or gradual
  - Episodic or continuous
  - Gagging or choking a few days before onset
- Characteristics
  - Dry versus moist
  - Productive versus nonproductive
  - High-pitched versus low-pitched
  - Barking, hoarse, brassy, or congested
  - Postural influences
    Reclining position (postnasal drip)
    Erect position
- Pattern
  - Paroxysmal

(continued)

box 24-1
Major Components of Clinical History (Continued)

- Related to environment, time of day, season, talking, or body position
- Change over time

- Associated symptoms
  - Chest pain
  - Dyspnea
  - Fever
  - Signs of upper respiratory infection
    Sore throat
    Congestion
    Increased mucus production
    Muscle aches
    Ear pain
    Loss of appetite
    Malaise
  - Anxiety
- Self-treatment and effectiveness
  - Prescription and over-the-counter medications
  - Vaporizer

Past Medical History

- Major acute adult illnesses (treatment dates and dates of hospitalization)
  - Upper respiratory infection
  - Strep throat
  - Mumps
  - Tonsillitis
- Major chronic adult illnesses (treatment dates and dates of hospitalization)
  - Tuberculosis
  - Bronchitis
  - Emphysema
  - Asthma
  - Cystic fibrosis
  - Bronchiectasis
  - Sinus infection
  - Heart failure
  - Cancer/malignancy
  - Musculoskeletal disease
  - Neurological disease
- Previous medical tests
  - Tuberculosis skin test
  - Allergy tests
  - Pulmonary function tests
  - Chest x-ray or computed tomography (CT) scan
  - Magnetic resonance imaging (MRI)
  - Magnetic resonance angiography (MRA)
  - Cardiac stress test
- Past surgeries
  - Thoracic surgery
    Coronary artery bypass surgery
    Cardiac valve surgery
    Aortic aneurysm surgery
  - Trauma surgery
- Use of oxygen or ventilatory assist devices
- Immunizations
- Serious injuries
- Medications
- Transfusions
- Emotional status
- Second-hand smoke exposure

Family History

- Health status (or cause of death) of parents and siblings
- Similarity of this illness to any illness in family
- Family history of pulmonary disease
- Family history of cardiac disease
- Tuberculosis
- Cystic fibrosis
- Emphysema
- Asthma
- Atopic dermatitis
- Malignancy

Personal and Social History

- Tobacco use
  - Smoking (cigarette, cigar, pipe)
  - Smokeless
  - Smoking start date
  - Pack-year history (number of packs per day times number of years smoking)
- Illicit drug use
  - Marijuana use
  - Inhaled narcotics or other drugs
- Work environment
  - Nature of work
  - Exposure to environmental hazards
    Chemicals
    Poison gas/vapors
    Dust
    Allergens
    Asbestos
  - Work hours
  - Exposure to extreme heat or cold
- Home environment
  - Location
  - Exposure to allergens
  - Pets
  - Plants
  - Chemicals
    Cleaning agents
    Pesticides
    Fertilizers
  - Type of heating and ventilation system
  - Air-conditioning system
  - Stairs
- Military history
- Postal work history
- Health care worker
- Recent traveling

box 24-2
Steps for Calculating Pack Years

Pack years = (Number of packs smoked per day) × (Number of years smoking)

Example: The patient reports during the physical assessment that he has smoked 2 packs per day for 15 years.

(2 packs per day) × (15 years) = 30 pack years

PHYSICAL EXAMINATION

Physical assessment of the respiratory system is a reliable means of gathering essential data and is guided by the information obtained through the history. A thorough physical assessment includes inspection, palpation, percussion, and auscultation.

Inspection

Inspection of the patient involves checking for the presence or absence of several factors (Box 24-3).

Cyanosis refers to a bluish discoloration of the skin or mucous membranes. Cyanosis is notoriously difficult to detect in a patient with anemia. The patient with polycythemia may have cyanosis in the extremities even if oxygen tension is normal. Peripheral cyanosis occurs in the extremities or on the tip of the nose or ears. Even with normal oxygen tensions, peripheral cyanosis may appear if there is diminished blood flow to these areas, particularly if they are cold or in a dependent position. Central cyanosis is observed on the tongue or lips and usually means the patient has low oxygen tension. Unfortunately, the presence of cyanosis is a late and often ominous sign.

Labored breathing is an important marker of respiratory distress. As part of the inspection, the nurse determines whether the patient is using the accessory muscles of respiration (the scalene and sternocleidomastoid muscles). *Intercostal retractions* (i.e., sucking in of the muscles and skin between the ribs during inspiration) usually mean that the patient is making a larger effort at inspiration than normal. The nurse also observes the patient for use of the abdominal muscles during the usually passive expiratory phase. Labored breathing may be accompanied by staccato speech, in which the patient's speech pattern is frequently interrupted as he or she gulps for air. Sometimes, the number of words a patient can say before having to gasp for another breath is a good measure of the degree of labored breathing.

The *anterior–posterior diameter of the chest* (i.e., the size of the chest from front to back) is also checked (Fig. 24-1). An increased anterior–posterior diameter is often caused by overexpansion of the lungs from obstructive pulmonary disease. An increase in anterior–posterior diameter may also be found in patients with kyphosis (curvature of the spine).

Chest deformities and scars are important in helping to determine the reason for respiratory distress. A chest deformity, such as kyphoscoliosis or flail chest from trauma, may indicate why the patient has respiratory distress. A scar may signify recent or old injuries to the chest and provide clues to possible sources of distress. For example, evidence of recent trauma to the chest, such as a stabbing or compression injuries from an automobile collision, could be responsible for the present distress.

The *patient's posture* must be observed. Patients with obstructive pulmonary disease often sit and prop themselves up on outstretched arms or lean forward with their elbows on a table in an effort to elevate their clavicles. This posture gives the patient a slightly greater ability to expand the chest.

It is important to observe the *position of the trachea.* The nurse determines if the trachea is in the midline as it should

box 24-3
Components of the Inspection Process in the Physical Assessment of the Respiratory System

General
- Mentation
- Anxiety level
- Speech
  - Staccato
  - Coherence
  - Aphasia
  - Articulation
  - Hoarseness
- Skin turgor
- Skin integrity
  - Scars
  - Rash
  - Wounds
- Skin color
  - Pallor
  - Cyanosis
- Weight
  - Obese
  - Malnourished
- Body position
  - Leaning forward
  - Arms elevated

Thorax
- Symmetry of thorax
- Position of sternum
- Anterior–posterior diameter less then transverse by at least half
- Rate, pattern, rhythm, and duration of breathing
- Use of accessory muscles
- Synchrony of chest and abdomen movement
- Alignment of spine
- Supernumerary nipples
- Superficial venous patterns

Head and Neck
- Nasal flaring
- Pursed-lip breathing
- Mouth breathing versus nose
- Use of neck and shoulders
- Tracheal position

Extremities
- Clubbing
- Edema
- Peripheral cyanosis

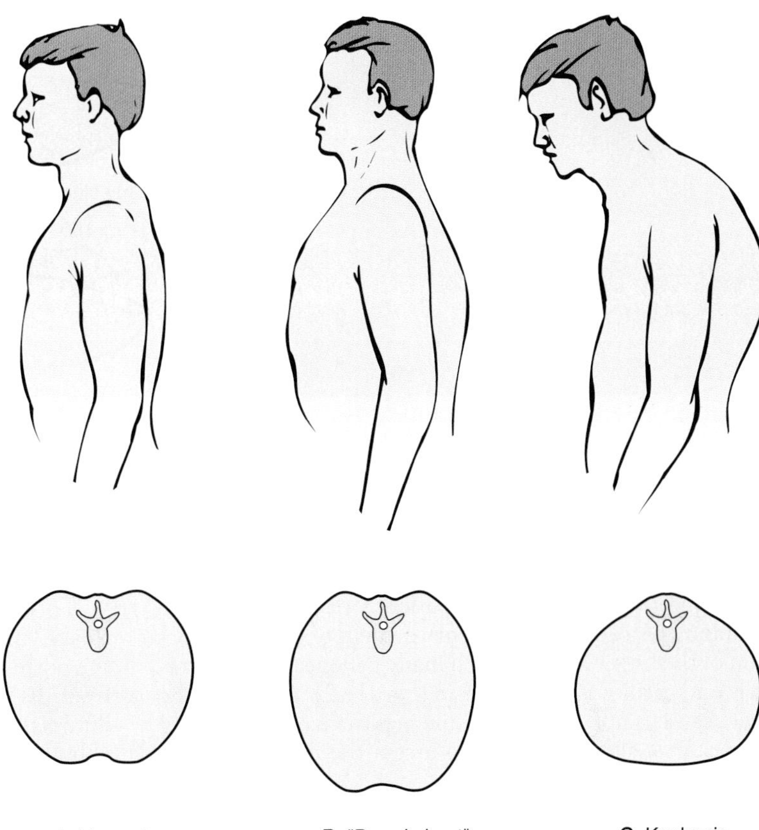

figure 24-1 Deformities and configurations of the human thorax. (**A**) Normal chest. (**B**) "Barrel chest," a chest deformity that typically results from emphysema. (**C**) Kyphosis, a chest deformity that is most common in older adults.

be, or if it is deviated off to one side. Pleural effusion, hemothorax, pneumothorax, or a tension pneumothorax can deviate the trachea away from the affected side (toward the opposite side). However, with atelectasis, fibrosis, tumors, and phrenic nerve paralysis, the trachea often is pulled toward the affected side.

The *respiratory rate* is an important parameter to follow. It should be counted over at least a 15-second period for stable patients and over a full minute for critically ill patients. The patient's rate must be compared with his or her usual rate. Breathing 24 to 26 times a minute may be normal in one patient but abnormal in another. The patient's family or friends may provide additional important information about the patient's usual rate of breathing.

The *depth of respiration* is often as meaningful as the respiratory rate. For instance, if a patient is breathing 40 times per minute, the nurse might think a severe respiratory problem is the source of patient distress. However, the rate may be the result of Kussmaul respirations caused by diabetic acidosis. If a patient's respiration is shallow at a rate of 40 breaths/minute, the indication may be severe respiratory distress from a primary pulmonary problem. Deep, rapid respirations may indicate compensation for acidosis. The pattern of respirations should also be noted because it may correlate with various disease processes.

The *duration of inspiration versus the duration of expiration* helps determine the presence of obstructive lung disease. In patients with any of the obstructive lung diseases, expiration is more than 1½ times as long as inspiration.

Observation of *thoracic expansion* is an integral part of examining a patient. Normally, chest expansion of about 3 inches occurs from maximal expiration to maximal inspiration. Motion of the abdomen in breathing efforts (more likely to be normal in men than women) may be observed. Ankylosing spondylitis may be present; general chest expansion is limited in this condition. During the inspection, the nurse compares the expansion of the upper chest with that of the lower chest. The nurse also observes the movement of the diaphragm to determine whether the patient with obstructive pulmonary disease is concentrating on expanding the lower chest and using the diaphragm properly. Expansion of one side of the chest versus the other side is important to note because atelectasis, especially that caused by a mucus plug, may cause unilaterally diminished chest expansion because the air is unable to move equally through the pulmonary bed. Abnormal chest expansion may also occur with flail chest, in which the chest collapses instead of expanding during inspiration. Flail chest may result from broken or fractured ribs that are unable to maintain the integrity of the chest wall during respiration. The nurse also notes whether the abdomen and chest rise and fall together as they should or if the effort is not coordinated; is there symmetry of respiratory effort? Asynchronous respiratory effort decreases the quality of respiration at the cost of increased work of breathing and often precedes the need for ventilatory support.

A pulmonary embolus, pneumonia, pleural effusion, pneumothorax, or any problem associated with chest pain, such as fractured ribs, may lead to diminished chest expansion. An endotracheal or nasotracheal tube positioned beyond the trachea into one of the mainstem bronchi (usually the right) is a serious cause of diminished expansion of

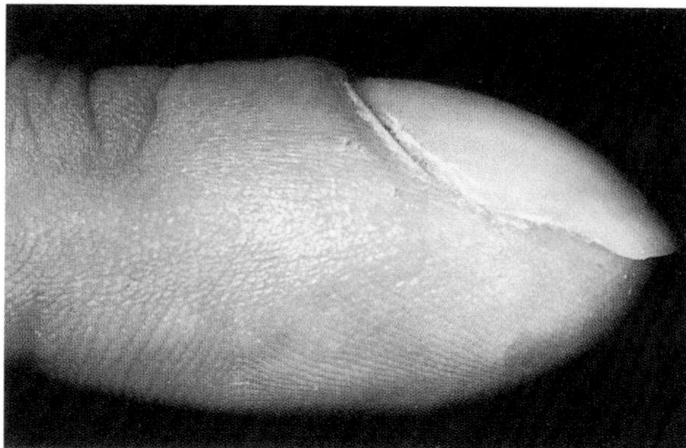

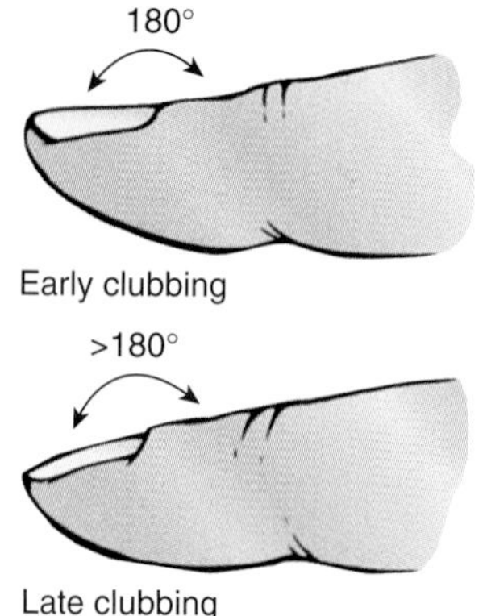

figure 24-2 In clubbing, the angle between the nail plate and the proximal nail fold increases to 180° or more. Clubbing of the fingers is seen in patients with respiratory and cardiovascular disease. (Photo used with permission from Bickley LS: Bates' Guide to Physical Examination and History Taking [8th Ed], p 110. Philadelphia, Lippincott Williams & Wilkins, 2003. Line art used with permission from Weber J, Kelley J: Health Assessment in Nursing [2nd Ed], p 144. Philadelphia, Lippincott Williams & Wilkins, 2003.)

one side of the chest. If the tube slips into the right mainstem bronchus, the left lung is not expanded, and the patient may experience atelectasis on the left side and hypoxemia.

Examination of the *patient's extremities* may provide additional information about the patient's respiratory status. Clubbing of the fingers is an enlargement of the distal portion of the finger and is seen in many patients with respiratory and cardiovascular diseases (Fig. 24-2). Although the exact cause is not known, chronic hypoxia is a contributing factor. It is also important to assess the extremities for edema and peripheral cyanosis.

Palpation

Chest palpation may indicate lung or chest abnormalities. To palpate the chest, the nurse places his or her hand flat against the patient's chest. When the patient speaks, sounds are generated by the larynx, and these sounds travel along the bronchial tree, resulting in a resonant motion of the chest wall. *Tactile fremitus* is the ability to feel the sound on the chest wall. Tactile fremitus is more easily palpated over the large bronchi and is more difficult to palpate over the distant lung fields.

To assess tactile fremitus, the nurse asks the patient to say "ninety-nine" while moving his or her hands over the posterior surfaces of the chest wall (Fig. 24-3). Tactile fremitus should be symmetrical. Tactile fremitus may be diminished or absent if there is an increase in air per unit volume of lung, because air impedes the transmission of sound. For example, patients with emphysema have little or no tactile fremitus on physical examination. Tactile fremitus is slightly increased by the presence of solid substances, such as the consolidation of a lung due to pneumonia. Other respiratory conditions causing an alteration in tactile fremitus are listed in Table 24-1.

Palpation is also used to assess for subcutaneous emphysema, a condition in which air "leaks" out of the alveolus and moves through the subcutaneous tissue. By moving the

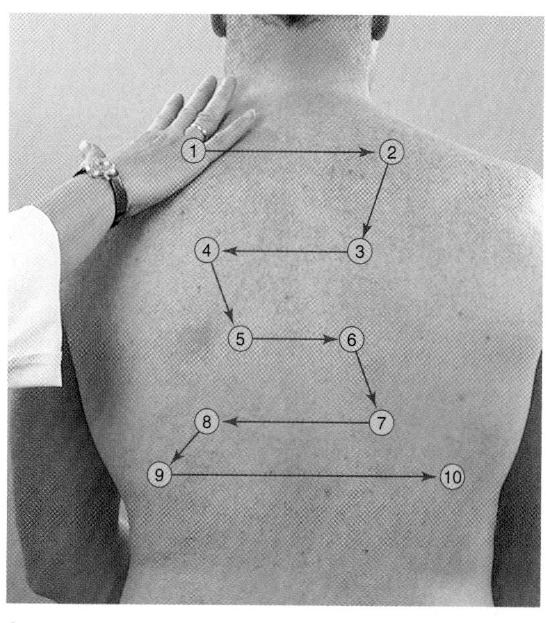

A

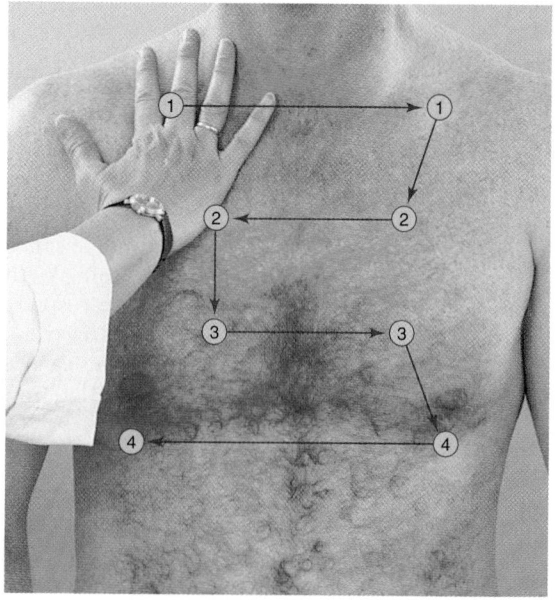

B

figure 24-3 Palpating the thorax is performed in a sequential fashion, starting near the neck and moving systematically downward. (**A**) Posterior thorax. (**B**) Anterior thorax. (Used with permission from Weber J, Kelley J: Health Assessment in Nursing [2nd Ed], p 274. Philadelphia, Lippincott Williams & Wilkins, 2003.)

fingers in a gentle rolling motion across the chest and neck, it is possible to feel the pockets of air underneath the skin. Feeling subcutaneous emphysema is often likened to the "crunch" of Rice Krispies under the skin. Subcutaneous emphysema may result from a pneumothorax, small pockets of alveoli that have burst with increased pulmonary pressure, or the use of positive end-expiratory pressure (PEEP). In severe cases, the subcutaneous emphysema may spread into the lower thorax, arms, and face.

Evaluation of thoracic expansion during respiration also requires palpation (Fig. 24-4). To perform this procedure, the nurse stands behind the patient, identifies the level of the 10th rib, and places his or her thumbs along the spine using the bony processes as a guide, letting the palms come in light contact with the posterolateral surface. The nurse asks the patient to breath normally and then deeply, both times watching as the thumbs diverge. Expansion of the chest wall should be symmetrical. Asymmetrical expansion may be indicative of a collapsed lung or unilateral disease. Retractions may be a sign of obstruction to inspiration and require immediate attention.

Palpation of the patient's trachea is an important element in the physical assessment of the respiratory system. To palpate the trachea to evaluate the midline position, the nurse positions his or her index finger in the suprasternal notch, feeling each side of the notch and palpating the tracheal rings (Fig. 24-5). The trachea should be in the midline position directly above the suprasternal notch.

Percussion

Percussion of the chest results in slight motion of the chest wall and underlying structures, causing audible and tactile vibrations. To percuss a patient's chest, the nurse presses one finger from the nondominant hand flat against the chest and uses a fingertip from the dominant hand to strike the knuckle pressed against the chest (Fig. 24-6). Normally, the chest has a resonant or hollow percussion note. In diseases in which there is increased air in the chest or lungs, such as pneumothorax and emphysema, there can be hyperresonant percussion notes. However, these loud, low-pitched sounds are sometimes difficult to detect.

More important is a flat percussion note (e.g., the sound that is heard when percussing over a part of the body that contains no air). A flat percussion note is a soft, high-pitched sound that is more easily distinguished by noting the change in sound when one moves from percussing an area with air to an area with no air. It is more likely to be heard if a large pleural effusion is present in the lung beneath the examining hand. A dull percussion note is medium in intensity and pitch. It is heard if atelectasis or consolidation due to pneumonia, pulmonary edema, or pulmonary hemorrhage is present. A tympanic drumlike sound is a high-pitched noise heard if asthma or a large pneumothorax is present. See Table 24-1 for a description of percussion sounds associated with various respiratory pathologies.

Auscultation

In chest auscultation, the diaphragm of the stethoscope is pressed firmly against the chest wall. The sequence for auscultating the posterior and anterior thorax is given in Fig. 24-7. The nurse listens to the intensity or loudness of breath sounds. Normally, there is a fourfold increase in loudness of breath sounds when a patient takes a maximum deep breath as opposed to quiet breathing. Sounds are louder in the upper and central chest when listening to the larger bronchus and become quieter as the smaller airways are auscultated. The intensity of the breath sounds may be diminished because of decreased flow through the airways or the presence of substances between the lungs and the stethoscope. In pleural thickening, pleural effusion, pneumothorax, and obesity, an abnormal substance (fibrous tissue, fluid, air, or fat) lies between the stethoscope and the underlying lung; this substance insulates the breath sounds from the stethoscope, making the breath sounds seem less loud. In airway obstruction, such as COPD or atelectasis, the intensity of breath sounds is diminished. With shallow breathing, there is diminished air movement through the airways, and the breath sounds are not as loud. With restricted movement of the thorax or diaphragm, there are diminished breath sounds in the restricted areas.

In general, four types of sounds are heard in the normal chest (Table 24-2). *Vesicular breath sounds* are quiet, low-pitched sounds, and the inspiratory phase is longer than the expiratory phase. *Bronchovesicular breath sounds* are medium in pitch, and the inspiratory and expiratory phases are of equal length. *Bronchial breath sounds* are higher pitched and louder compared with vesicular sounds, and the expiratory phase is longer than the inspiratory phase. *Tracheal breath sounds* are loud, high-pitched sounds, and the inspiratory and expiratory phases are about equal in length.

Bronchial breath sounds are heard over the manubrium not only in the normal state but when consolidation is present, as in pneumonia. Bronchial breath sounds are also heard above a pleural effusion in which the normal lung is compressed and sounds are transmitted through the tissue, which is not participating in airflow. Wherever there is bronchial breathing, there also may be two associated changes: E to A changes and whispered pectoriloquy.

An *E to A change* occurs when the patient says "E" and the nurse listening with a stethoscope actually hears an "A" sound rather than an "E" sound. This occurs if consolidation is present. *Egophony* is the term used to describe voice sounds that are distorted.

Whispered pectoriloquy is the presence of loud, clear sounds heard through the stethoscope when the patient whispers. Normally, the whispered voice is heard faintly and indistinctly through the stethoscope. The increased transmission of voice sounds indicates that air in the lungs has been replaced by fluid as a result of pneumonia, pulmonary edema, or hemorrhage.

Adventitious sounds are additional breath sounds heard with auscultation and include discontinuous sounds, continuous sounds, and rubs. Discontinuous sounds are brief, nonmusical, intermittent sounds and include fine and course crackles. (Crackles were formerly known as *rales.*) Fine crackles are soft, high-pitched, very brief popping sounds that occur most commonly during inspiration. Crackles result from fluid in the airways or alveoli, or from the opening of collapsed alveoli. Restrictive pulmonary

(text continues on page 505)

table 24-1 Physical Examination Signs in Selected Respiratory Disorders

Condition	Trachea	Percussion Note
Normal 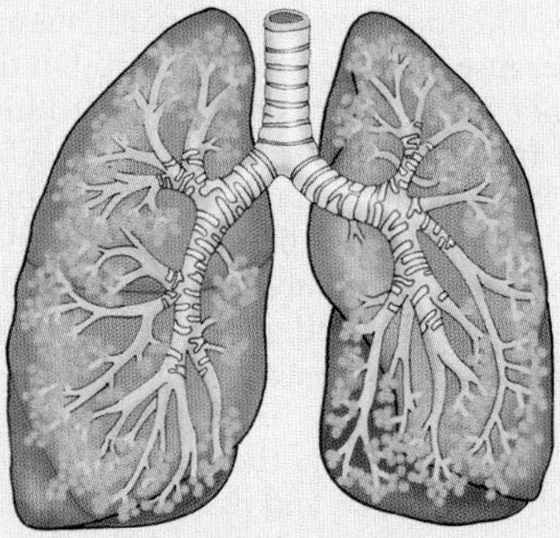	Midline	Resonant
Bronchitis 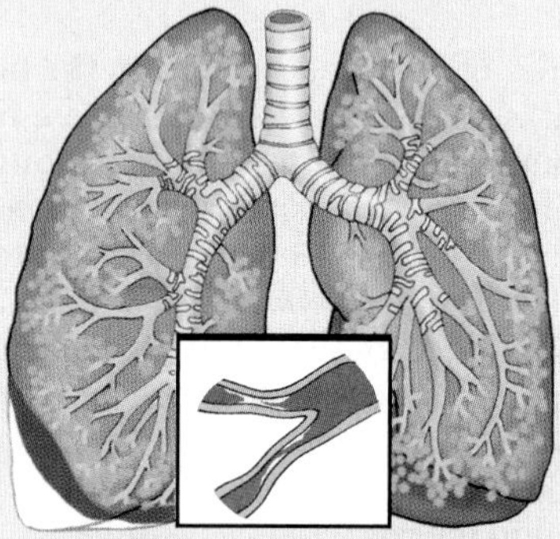 Bronchial inflammation and constriction with mucus	Midline	Resonant
Consolidation Consolidation 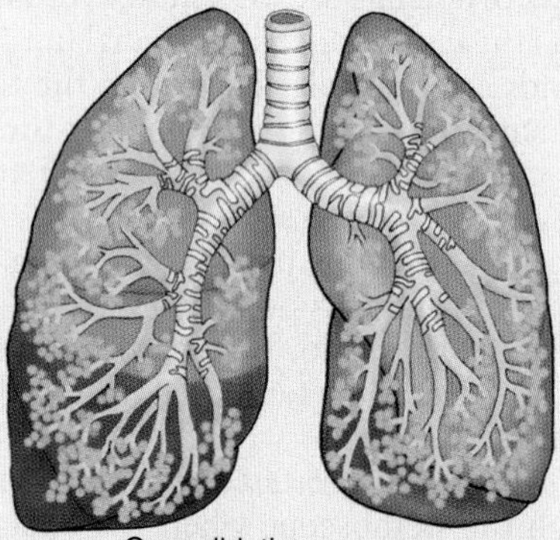	Midline	Dull over the airless area
Atelectasis 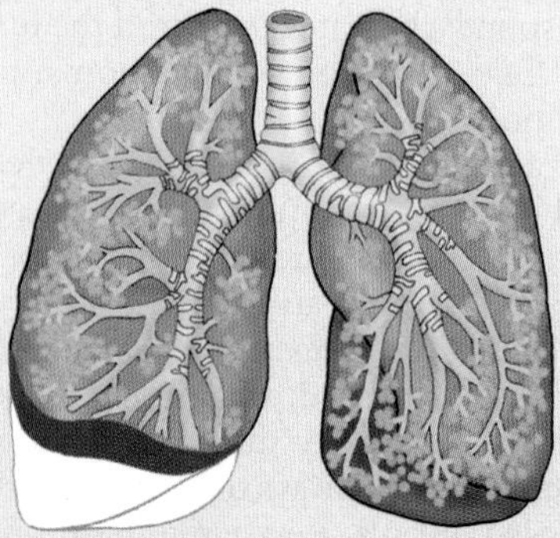 Collapsed portion of lung	May be shifted toward the involved side	Dull over the airless area

Breath Sounds	Tactile Fremitus and Transmitted Voice Sounds	Adventitious Sounds
Vesicular, except perhaps bronchovesicular and bronchial sounds over the large bronchi and trachea, respectively	Normal	None, except perhaps a few transient inspiratory crackles at the bases of the lungs
Normal	Normal	None or scattered coarse crackles in early inspiration and perhaps expiration; or wheezes or rhonchi
Bronchial over the involved area	Increased over the involved area with bronchophony, egophony, and whispered pectoriloquy	Late inspiratory crackles over the involved area
Usually absent when the bronchial plug persists; exceptions—right upper lobe atelectasis, where adjacent tracheal sounds may be transmitted	Usually absent when the bronchial plug persists; exceptions (e.g., right upper lobe atelectasis), may be increased	None

(continued)

table 24-1 Physical Examination Signs in Selected Respiratory Disorders (Continued)

Condition	Trachea	Percussion Note
Pleural effusion 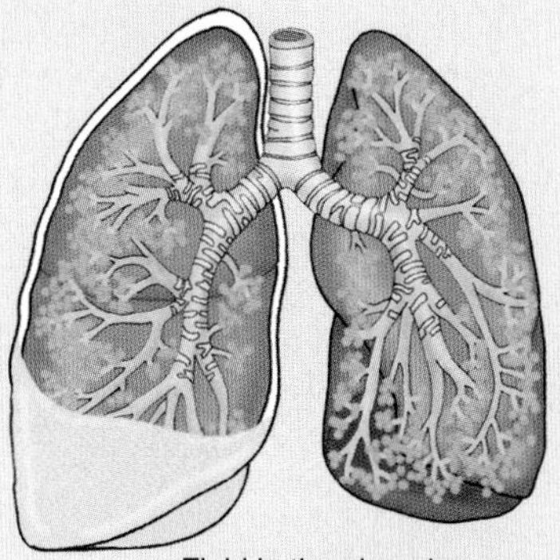 Fluid in the pleural space	Toward the opposite side in a large effusion	Dull to flat over the fluid
Pneumothorax 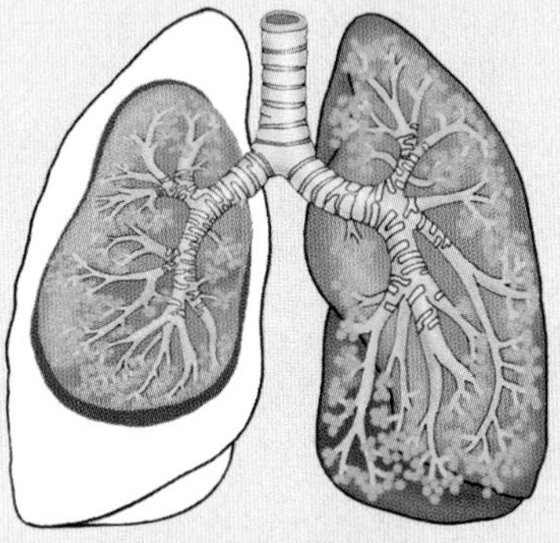 Air in the pleural space	Toward the opposite side if much air	Hyperresonant or tympanitic over the pleural air
Emphysema 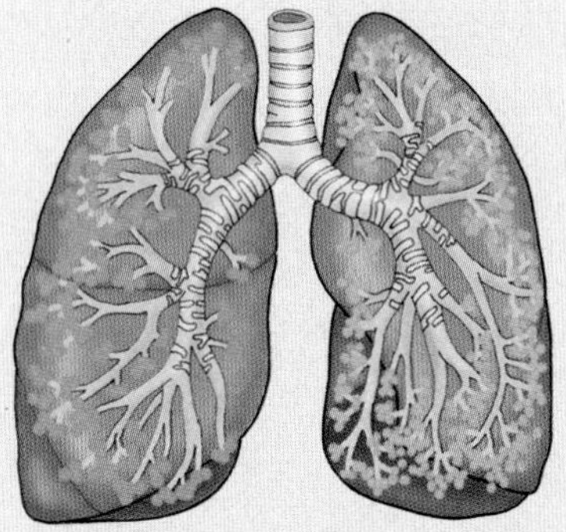 Abnormally distended alveoli	Midline	Diffusely hyperresonant
Asthma 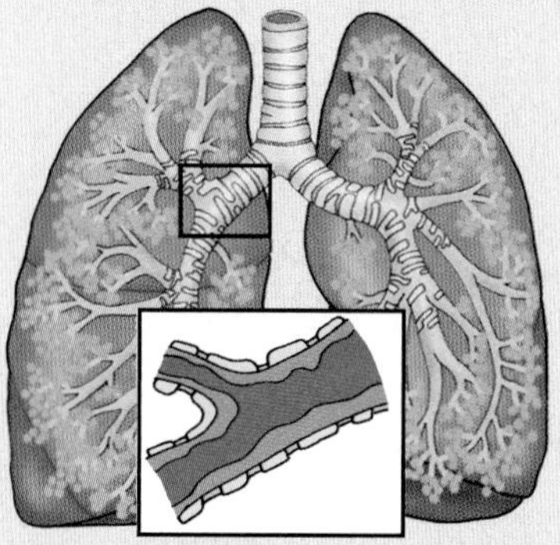 Bronchospasm	Midline	Normal to diffusely hyperresonant

Adapted from Bickley LS: Bates' Guide to Physical Examination and History Taking (8th Ed), pp 242–243. Philadelphia, Lippincott Williams & Wilkins, 2003.

Breath Sounds	Tactile Fremitus and Transmitted Voice Sounds	Adventitious Sounds
Decreased to absent, but bronchial breath sounds possibly heard near the top of a large effusion	Decreased to absent, but may be increased toward the top of a large effusion	None, except a possible pleural rub
Decreased to absent over the pleural air	Decreased to absent over the pleural air	None, except a possible pleural rub
Decreased to absent	Decreased	None, or the crackles, wheezes, and rhonchi of associated chronic bronchitis
Often obscured by wheezes	Decreased	Wheezes, possibly crackles

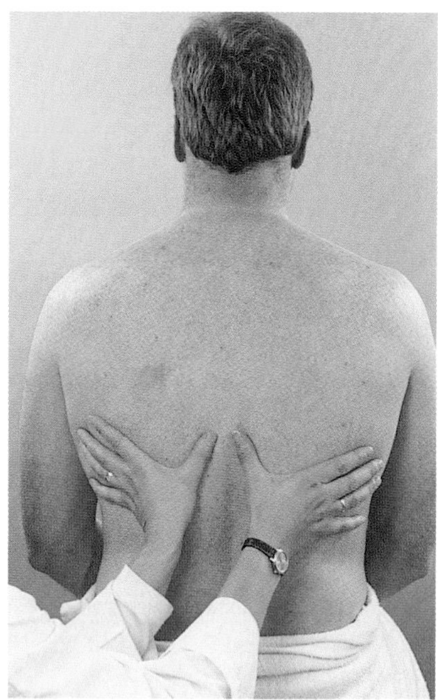

figure 24-4 Palpating chest expansion. The thumbs are positioned at the level of the 10th rib. (Used with permission from Weber J, Kelley J: Health Assessment in Nursing [2nd Ed], p 263. Philadelphia, Lippincott Williams & Wilkins, 2003.)

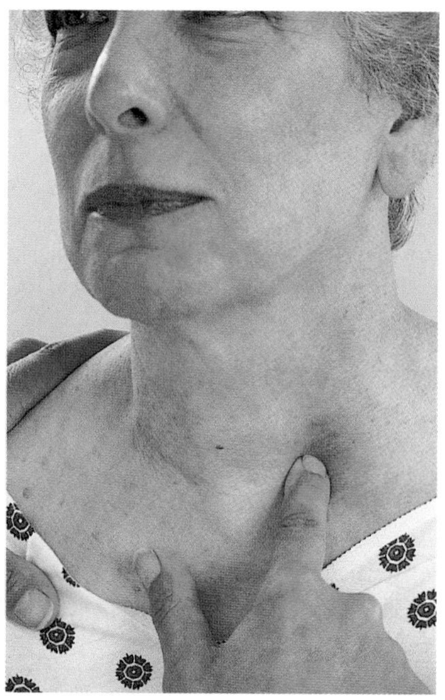

figure 24-5 Palpating the trachea. The trachea should be midline, above the suprasternal notch. Photograph © B. Proud. (Used with permission from Weber J, Kelley J: Health Assessment in Nursing [2nd Ed], p 161. Philadelphia, Lippincott Williams & Wilkins, 2003.)

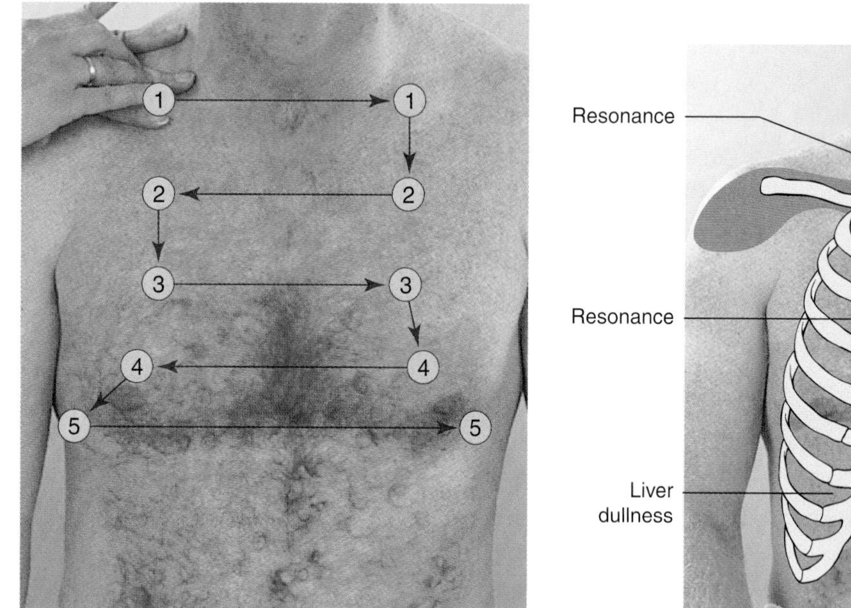

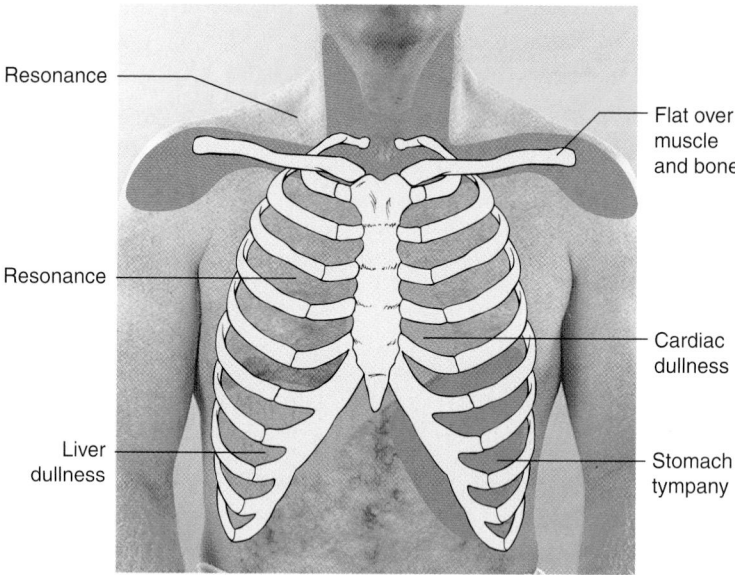

figure 24-6 Percussing the thorax is performed in a sequential fashion, starting near the neck and moving systematically downward. (**A**) Anterior thorax. (**B**) Posterior thorax. (Used with permission from Weber J, Kelley J: Health Assessment in Nursing [2nd Ed], pp 264, 270. Philadelphia, Lippincott Williams & Wilkins, 2003.) (*continued*)

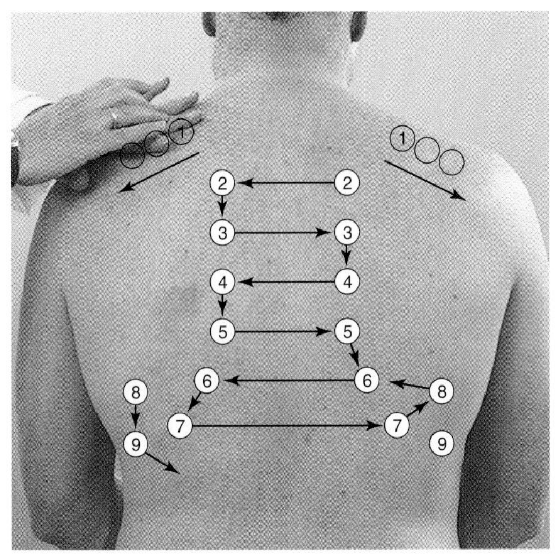

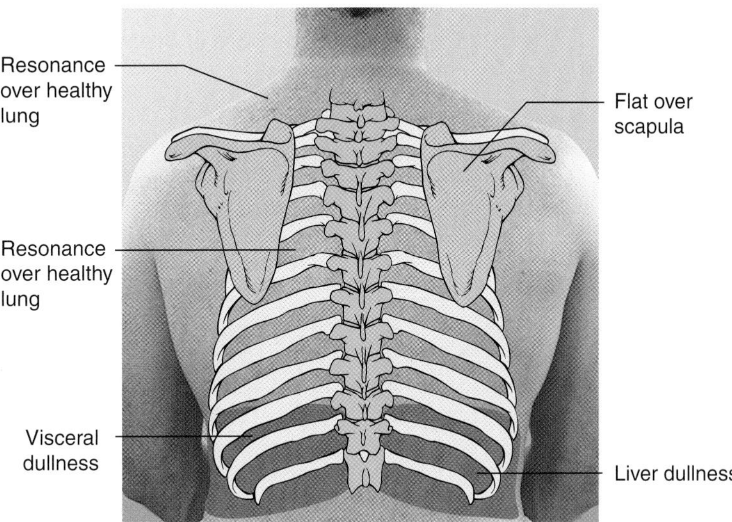

B.

figure 24-6 Continued.

disease results in crackles during late inspiration, whereas obstructive pulmonary disease results in crackles during early inspiration. Crackles become more coarse as the air moves through larger fluid accumulations, such as in bronchitis or pneumonia. Crackles that clear with coughing are not associated with significant pulmonary disease. When assessing crackles, the nurse also notes their loudness, pitch, duration, amount, location, and timing in the respiratory cycle.[1]

Continuous adventitious breath sounds are longer in duration than crackles and include wheezes and rhonchi. Wheezes are continuous musical sounds that are longer than crackles in duration and persist throughout the respiratory cycle. Wheezes (also known as sibilant wheezes) are continuous, high-pitched adventitious sounds that have a shrill quality. They are caused by the movement of air through a narrowed or partially obstructed airway, such as in asthma, COPD, or bronchitis.

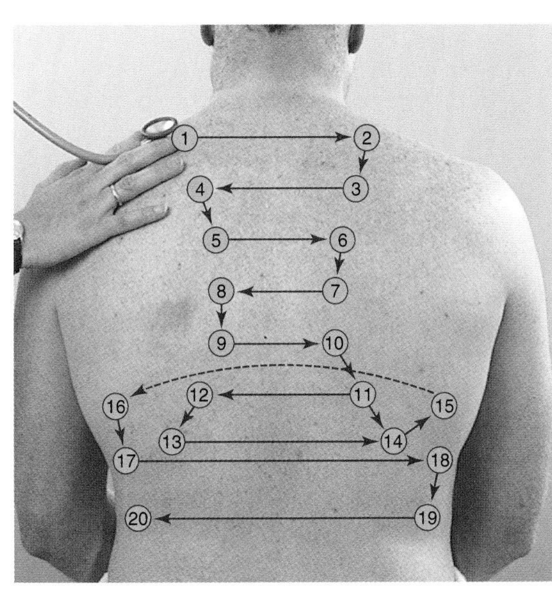

A

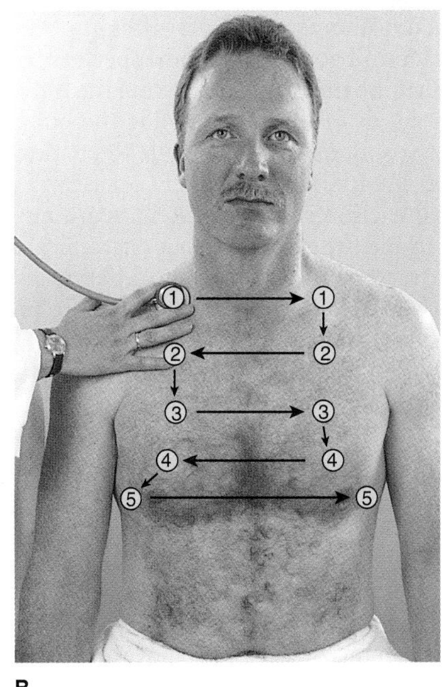

B

figure 24-7 Auscultating the chest is performed in a sequential fashion, starting near the neck and moving systematically downward. (**A**) Posterior thorax. (**B**) Anterior thorax. (Used with permission from Weber J, Kelley J: Health Assessment in Nursing [2nd Ed], p 275. Philadelphia, Lippincott Williams & Wilkins, 2003.)

table 24-2 Characteristics of Breath Sounds

	Duration of Sounds	Intensity of Expiratory Sound	Pitch of Expiratory Sound	Locations Where Heard Normally
Vesicular*	Inspiratory sounds last longer than expiratory ones.	Soft	Relatively low	Over most of both lungs
Bronchovesicular	Inspiratory and expiratory sounds are about equal.	Intermediate	Intermediate	Often in the first and second interspaces anteriorly and between the scapulae
Bronchial	Expiratory sounds last longer than inspiratory ones.	Loud	Relatively high	Over the manubrium, if heard at all
Tracheal	Inspiratory and expiratory sounds are about equal.	Very loud	Relatively high	Over the trachea in the neck

*The thickness of the bars indicates intensity; the steeper their incline, the higher the pitch.
Source: Bickley LS: Bates' Guide to Physical Examination and History Taking (8th Ed), p 227. Philadelphia, Lippincott Williams & Wilkins, 2003.

Rhonchi, another type of continuous adventitious breath sound, are deep, low-pitched rumbling noises that are sometimes referred to as sonorous wheezes or gurgles. The presence of rhonchi indicates the presence of secretions in the large airways.[1] Conditions such as bronchitis cause sonorous wheezing. These sounds may clear somewhat with coughing.

A friction rub is a crackling, grating sound heard more often with inspiration then expiration. The sound of friction results from the visceral and parietal pleura rubbing against each other. A friction rub can be heard with pleural effusion, pneumothorax, or pleurisy. It is important to distinguish a pleural friction rub from a pericardial friction rub. To determine the origin of the rub, the nurse asks the patient to hold his or her breath while the lungs are auscultated. If the sounds continue while the patient is holding his or her breath, it is most likely a pericardial friction rub; a pleural friction rub stops when breathing stops.

In children and the elderly, unique anatomical and physiological characteristics manifest in different assessment findings. Boxes 24-4 and 24-5 show specific respiratory assessment findings in both pediatric and elderly patients.

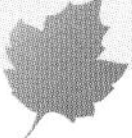

box 24-4

Respiratory Assessment of the Pediatric Patient

- Use of intercostals musculature for breathing by 6 or 7 years of age
- Respiratory rate (breaths/minute)
  Newborn: 30–80
  1–4 years of age: 20–35
  5–16 years of age: 16–22
  ≥17 years of age: 12–20
- Thinner chest
  More resonant
  Increased harshness
- Hyperresonance more likely
- More difficult to identify underlying consolidation
- Bronchovesicular breath sounds heard throughout the chest
- Vesicular breath sounds are accentuated

RESPIRATORY MONITORING

Pulse Oximetry

Approximately 3% of oxygen is dissolved in the plasma (Box 24-6). The partial pressure of oxygen dissolved in the arterial blood is measured by the PaO_2. The normal PaO_2 is 80 to 100 mm Hg at sea level. The remaining 97% of oxygen is attached to hemoglobin molecules in red blood cells. Each gram of hemoglobin can carry a maximum of 1.34 mL of oxygen. The percentage of saturation of hemoglobin is defined as the amount of oxygen that hemoglobin is carrying compared with the amount of oxygen that hemoglobin (Hgb) can carry, expressed as a percentage:

$$\text{Percentage } O_2 \text{ saturation of Hgb} = \frac{\text{Amount } O_2 \text{ Hgb is carrying}}{\text{Amount } O_2 \text{ Hgb can carry}} \times 100$$

Because the amount of oxygen that hemoglobin can carry is a constant 1.34 mL/g,

$$1.34 \text{ mL/g} \times \text{g Hgb} \times \% \text{ saturation Hgb} = \text{mL of } O_2 \text{ that Hgb is carrying}$$

The arterial oxygen saturation of hemoglobin is known as the SaO_2. The normal SaO_2 ranges from 93% to 99%.

The relationship between PaO_2 and SaO_2 is depicted by the oxyhemoglobin dissociation curve (Fig. 24-8). The

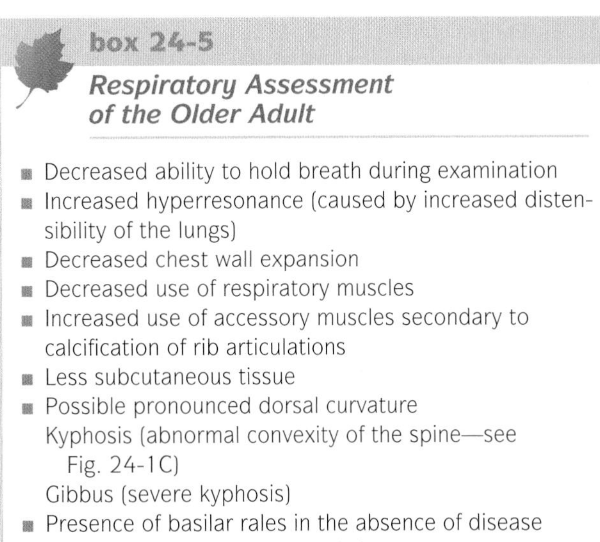

box 24-5

Respiratory Assessment of the Older Adult

- Decreased ability to hold breath during examination
- Increased hyperresonance (caused by increased distensibility of the lungs)
- Decreased chest wall expansion
- Decreased use of respiratory muscles
- Increased use of accessory muscles secondary to calcification of rib articulations
- Less subcutaneous tissue
- Possible pronounced dorsal curvature
  Kyphosis (abnormal convexity of the spine—see Fig. 24-1C)
  Gibbus (severe kyphosis)
- Presence of basilar rales in the absence of disease (should clear after a few coughs)

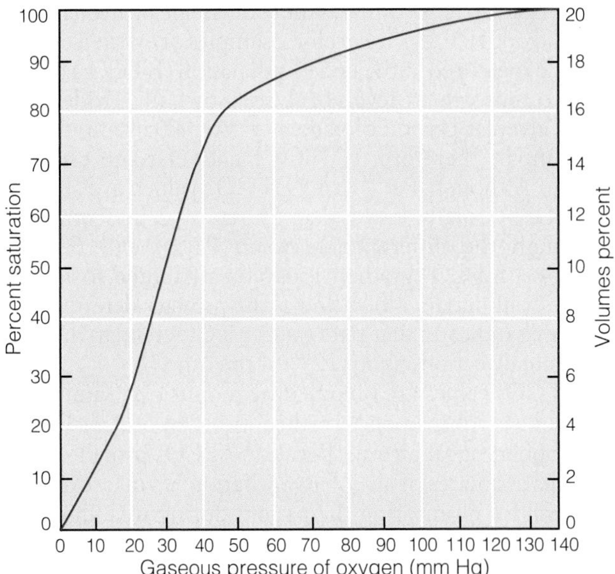

figure 24-8 Oxyhemoglobin dissociation curve.

initial part of the curve is very steep and flattens at the top. The flattened part means that large changes in the PaO_2 result in only small changes in SaO_2. A critical point of the curve occurs when the PaO_2 drops below 60 mm Hg. At this point, the curve drops sharply, signifying that a small decrease in PaO_2 is associated with a large decrease in SaO_2.

When the curve shifts to the right, there is a reduced capacity for hemoglobin to combine with oxygen, resulting in more oxygen released to the tissues. When the curve shifts to the left, there is an increased capacity for hemoglobin to combine with oxygen, resulting in less oxygen released to the tissues. See Chapter 23 for a more detailed discussion of the oxyhemoglobin dissociation curve.

A pulse oximeter, illustrated in Figure 24-9, is a device used to measure a value known as SpO_2 (oxygen saturation as measured by pulse oximetry). The SpO_2 reflects the arterial oxygen saturation of hemoglobin. Through oximetry, light-emitting and light-receiving sensors quantify the amount of light absorbed by oxygenated/deoxygenated hemoglobin in arterial blood. The value displayed on the pulse oximeter is an average of numerous readings taken in a 3- to 10-second period.[2] This reduces the effects of pressure waveform variation caused by patient activity.[2] Usually, the sensors are in a clip placed on a finger or ear lobe, and allow for evaluation of the quality of the pulsatile waveform. For assessment of pulse oximetry in infants, flexible probes can measure saturation when placed on the palm, arm, penis, or foot.[3]

Oximetry should not be used in place of arterial blood gas (ABG) monitoring. Instead, pulse oximetry may be used to assess trends in oxygen saturation when the correlation between arterial blood and pulse oximetry readings has been established. Values obtained by pulse oximetry are unreliable when vasoconstricting medications or intravenous dyes are used and when shock, cardiac arrest, or severe anemia are present. Pulse oximetry has limited usefulness in patients with known dyshemoglobins, such as carboxyhemoglobin, which is elevated in smokers, and methemoglobin, which is seen in patients undergoing nitrate and lidocaine therapy.[4–7] These limitations should be considered when interpreting pulse oximetry readings in certain patients.

box 24-6

How Oxygen Is Carried in the Blood

Oxygen dissolved in the plasma measured as PaO_2	0.3 mL/100 mL of blood
Oxygen combined with hemoglobin measured as SaO_2	19.4 mL/100 mL of blood
Total oxygen in blood	19.7 mL/100 mL of blood

End-Tidal Carbon Dioxide Monitoring

End-tidal carbon dioxide ($ETCO_2$) monitoring measures the level of carbon dioxide at the end of exhalation, when the percentage of carbon dioxide dissolved in the arterial

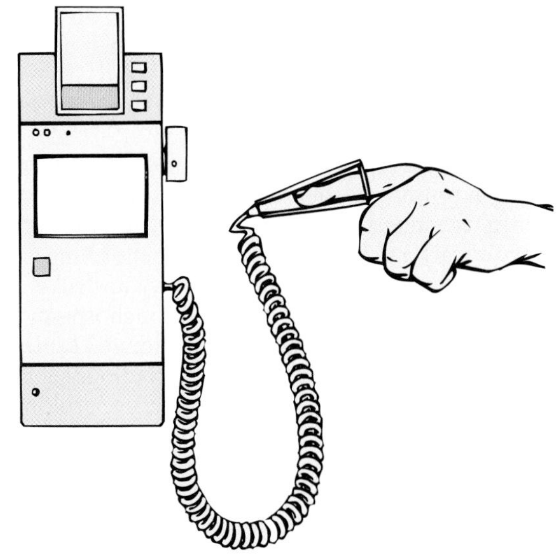

figure 24-9 Pulse oximetry monitor.

blood ($Paco_2$) approximates the percentage of alveolar carbon dioxide ($PACO_2$). Therefore, samples of exhaled carbon dioxide measured at the end of exhalation ($ETCO_2$) can be used to approximate levels of alveolar carbon dioxide. Levels of alveolar carbon dioxide and arterial carbon dioxide are similar; therefore, $ETCO_2$ can be used to estimate $Paco_2$. Although $Paco_2$ and $ETCO_2$ values are similar, $ETCO_2$ is usually lower than $Paco_2$ by 2 to 5 mm Hg. Although the difference between $Paco_2$ and $ETCO_2$ ($Paco_2$ – $ETCO_2$ gradient) may be attributed to several factors, pulmonary blood flow is the primary determinant. Research indicates that $Paco_2$ and $ETCO_2$ tend to move in opposite directions about 22% of the time.[8]

$ETCO_2$ values are obtained by monitoring samples of expired gas from an endotracheal tube, an oral airway, or a nasopharyngeal airway. Because $ETCO_2$ provides continuous estimates of alveolar ventilation, its measurement is useful for monitoring the patient during weaning from a ventilator, in cardiopulmonary resuscitation, and in endotracheal intubation.

The accuracy of the $ETCO_2$ readings may be affected by high concentrations of oxygen and water vapor. The nurse using $ETCO_2$ technology must be aware of these conditions and their effect on the monitor being used. Impaired infrared absorption due to the interaction of carbon dioxide and oxygen in high concentrations may cause falsely low $ETCO_2$ measurements, and the interference of water vapor with the absorption of infrared light may cause falsely elevated measurements. The nurse must combine $ETCO_2$ readings with a variety of other clinical data.

The exhaled carbon dioxide waveform is displayed on the monitor as a plot of $ETCO_2$ versus time called a *capnogram*, which provides the nurse with a continuous graphic reading of the patient's $ETCO_2$ level with each exhaled breath. Changes in the waveform indicate clinical abnormalities, mechanical abnormalities, or both, and require immediate assessment by the nurse or other trained professional.

On a capnogram, the waveform is composed of four phases, each one representing a specific part of the respiratory cycle (Fig. 24-10):

1. The first phase is the baseline phase, which represents both the inspiratory phase and the very beginning of the expiratory phase, when carbon dioxide–free air in the anatomical dead space is exhaled. This value should be zero in a healthy adult.
2. The second phase is the expiratory upstroke, which represents the exhalation of carbon dioxide from the lungs. Any process that delays the delivery of carbon dioxide from the patient's lungs to the detector prolongs the expiratory upstroke. Conditions such as COPD and bronchospasm are known physiological causes of prolonged expiratory upstroke.[9,10] Mechanical obstructions such as kinked ventilator tubing may also cause prolonged expiratory upstroke.
3. The third phase begins as carbon dioxide elimination rapidly continues; a plateau on the capnogram indicates the exhalation of alveolar gases. The $ETCO_2$ is the value generated at the very end of exhalation, indicating the amount of carbon dioxide exhaled from the least ventilated alveoli.
4. The fourth phase is known as the inspiratory downstroke. The downward deflection of the waveform is caused by the washout of carbon dioxide that occurs in the presence of the oxygen influx during inspiration.

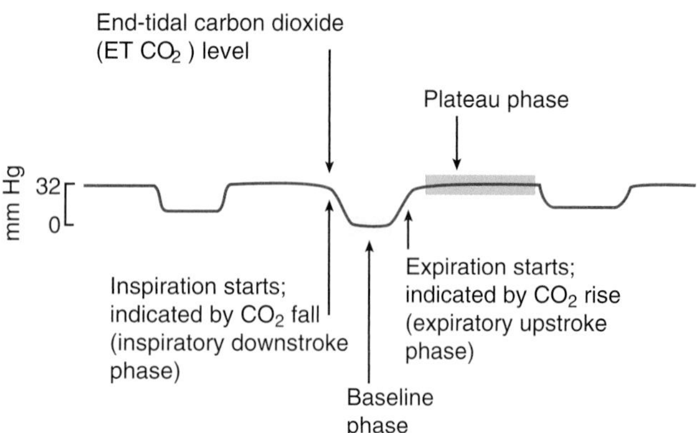

figure 24-10 Capnogram tracing, with four phases labeled. *CO_2*, carbon dioxide.

Arterial Blood Gases

In an ABG test, a sample of arterial blood is drawn and analyzed to help determine the quality and extent of pulmonary gas exchange and acid–base status. The ABG test measures Pao_2, Sao_2, $Paco_2$, pH, and the bicarbonate (HCO_3) level. The procedure involves obtaining arterial blood from a direct arterial puncture or from an arterial line often placed in the radial artery. More recent technology allows the continuous monitoring of ABGs using a fiberoptic sensor placed in the artery. Normal ABG values are given in Box 24-7.

MEASURING OXYGEN IN THE BLOOD

Oxygenation may be measured using an ABG by evaluating the Pao_2 and the Sao_2. As mentioned previously, only 3% of oxygen is dissolved in the arterial blood, and the remaining 97% is attached to hemoglobin in the red blood cells.

The normal Pao_2 is 80 to 100 mm Hg at sea level (barometric pressure of 760 mm Hg). For people living at higher altitudes, the normal Pao_2 is lower because of the lower barometric pressure. Pao_2 tends to decrease with age. For

box 24-7
Normal Values for an Arterial Blood Gas

Pao_2: 80–100 mm Hg
Sao_2: 93%–99%
pH: 7.35–7.45
$Paco_2$: 35–45 mm Hg
HCO_3: 22–26 mEq/L

patients who are 60 to 80 years of age, a Pa_{O_2} of 60 to 80 mm Hg is normal. An abnormally low Pa_{O_2} is referred to as *hypoxemia*. Hypoxemia may result from many conditions, which are most commonly grouped according to their origin: intrapulmonary (disturbances in the lung), intracardiac (disturbance of flow to or from the heart, which impedes pulmonary flow or function), or perfusion deficits (inadequate perfusion of the lung tissues, which causes decreased oxygen uptake from the alveoli).

The normal Sa_{O_2} ranges between 93% and 97%. Sa_{O_2} is an important oxygenation value to assess because most oxygen supplied to tissues is carried by hemoglobin.

MEASURING pH IN THE BLOOD

The pH is a measure of the hydrogen ion concentration in the blood and provides information about the acidity or alkalinity of the blood. A normal pH is 7.35 to 7.45. As hydrogen ions accumulate, the pH drops, resulting in acidemia. Acid*emia* refers to a condition in which the *blood* is too acidic. Acid*osis* refers to the *process* that caused the acidemia.

A decrease in hydrogen ions results in an elevation of the pH and alkalemia. Alkalemia refers to a condition in which the blood is too alkaline. Alkal*osis* refers to the *process* that causes the alkal*emia*. Box 24-8 reviews the terms used in acid–base balance.

Acids

An acid is a substance that can donate a hydrogen ion (H^+) to a solution. There are two different types of acids, volatile acids and nonvolatile acids.

Volatile acids are those that can move between the liquid and gaseous states. Once in the gaseous state, these acids can be removed by the lungs. The major acid in the blood serum is carbonic acid (H_2CO_3). This acid is broken down into carbon dioxide and water by an enzyme produced in the kidneys.

Nonvolatile acids are those that cannot change into a gaseous form and therefore cannot be excreted by the lungs. They can only be excreted by the kidneys (a metabolic process). Examples of nonvolatile acids are lactic acid and ketoacids.

An acid–base disorder may be either respiratory or metabolic in origin. Table 24-3 lists the possible causes and signs and symptoms of acid–base disorders. An excess of either kind of acid results in acidemia. If carbon dioxide accumulates, then respiratory acidosis exists. If nonvolatile acids accumulate, then metabolic acidosis exists.

Alkalemia may be the result of losing too many acids from the serum. If too much carbon dioxide is lost, the result is respiratory alkalosis. If there are less than normal amounts of nonvolatile acids, the result is metabolic alkalosis.

Bases

A base is a substance that can accept a hydrogen ion (H^+), thereby removing it from the circulating serum. The main base found in the serum is bicarbonate (HCO_3). The amount of bicarbonate that is available in the serum is regulated by the kidney (a metabolic process). If there is too little bicarbonate in the serum, the result is metabolic acidosis. If there is too much bicarbonate in the serum, the result is metabolic alkalosis.

Conditions leading to acidemia or alkalemia are influenced by a multitude of physiological processes (see Table 24-3). Some of these processes include respiratory and renal function or dysfunction, tissue oxygenation, circulation, lactic acid production, substance ingestion, and electrolyte loss from the gastrointestinal tract. The identification of a pH abnormality should lead to the investigation of possible contributing factors.

MEASURING CARBON DIOXIDE IN THE BLOOD

The Pa_{CO_2} refers to the pressure or tension exerted by dissolved carbon dioxide gas in arterial blood. Carbon dioxide is the natural byproduct of cellular metabolism. Carbon dioxide levels are regulated primarily by the ventilatory function of the lung. The normal Pa_{CO_2} is 35 to 45 mm Hg. In interpretation of ABGs, Pa_{CO_2} is thought of as an "acid." Elimination of carbon dioxide from the body is one of the main functions of the lungs, and an important relationship exists between the amount of ventilation and the amount of carbon dioxide in blood.

If a patient hypoventilates, carbon dioxide accumulates, and the Pa_{CO_2} value increases above the upper limit of 45 mm Hg. The retention of carbon dioxide results in respiratory acidosis. Respiratory acidosis may occur even with normal lungs if the respiratory center is depressed and the respiratory rate or quality is insufficient to maintain normal carbon dioxide concentrations.

If a patient hyperventilates, carbon dioxide is eliminated from the body, and the Pa_{CO_2} value decreases below the lower limit of 35 mm Hg. The loss of carbon dioxide results in respiratory alkalosis.

MEASURING BICARBONATE IN THE BLOOD

Bicarbonate (HCO_3), the main base found in the serum, helps the body regulate pH because of its ability to accept a hydrogen ion (H^+). The concentration of bicarbonate is regulated by the kidneys and is referred to as a metabolic process of regulation. The normal bicarbonate level is 22 to 26 mEq/L. Bicarbonate may be thought of as a "base" (alkaline). When the bicarbonate level increases above 26 mEq/L, a metabolic alkalosis exists.

box 24-8
Clinical Terminology: Acid–Base

Acid: A substance that can donate hydrogen ions (H^+). Example: H_2CO_3 (an acid) $\rightarrow H^+ + HCO_3$

Base: A substance that can accept hydrogen ions, H^+; all bases are alkaline substances. Example: HCO_3 (base) $+ H^+ \rightarrow H_2CO_3$

Acidemia: Acid condition of the blood in which the pH is <7.35

Alkalemia: Alkaline condition of the blood in which the pH is >7.45

Acidosis: The process causing acidemia

Alkalosis: The process causing alkalemia

table 24-3 Possible Causes and Signs and Symptoms of Acid–Base Disorders

Condition	Possible Causes	Signs and Symptoms
Respiratory Acidosis		
$Paco_2$ >45 mm Hg	Central nervous system depression	Dyspnea
pH <7.35	Head trauma	Restlessness
	Oversedation	Headache
	Anesthesia	Tachycardia
	High cord injury	Confusion
	Pneumothorax	Lethargy
	Hypoventilation	Dysrhythmias
	Bronchial obstruction and atelectasis	Respiratory distress
	Severe pulmonary infections	Drowsiness
	Heart failure and pulmonary edema	Decreased responsiveness
	Massive pulmonary embolus	
	Myasthenia gravis	
	Multiple sclerosis	
Respiratory Alkalosis		
$Paco_2$ <35 mm Hg	Anxiety and nervousness	Light-headedness
pH >7.45	Fear	Confusion
	Pain	Decreased concentration
	Hyperventilation	Paresthesias
	Fever	Tetanic spasms in the arms and legs
	Thyrotoxicosis	Cardiac dysrhythmias
	Central nervous system lesions	Palpitations
	Salicylates	Sweating
	Gram-negative septicemia	Dry mouth
	Pregnancy	Blurred vision
Metabolic Acidosis		
HCO_3 <22 mEq/L	***Increased acids***	Headache
pH <7.35	Renal failure	Confusion
	Ketoacidosis	Restlessness
	Anaerobic metabolism	Lethargy
	Starvation	Weakness
	Salicylate intoxication	Stupor/coma
	Loss of base	Kussmaul respiration
	Diarrhea	Nausea and vomiting
	Intestinal fistulas	Dysrhythmias
		Warm, flushed skin
Metabolic Alkalosis		
HCO_3 >26 mEq/L	***Gain of base***	Muscle twitching and cramps
pH >7.45	Excess use of bicarbonate	Tetany
	Lactate administration in dialysis	Dizziness
	Excess ingestion of antacids	Lethargy
	Loss of acids	Weakness
	Vomiting	Disorientation
	Nasogastric suctioning	Convulsions
	Hypokalemia	Coma
	Hypochloremia	Nausea and vomiting
	Administration of diuretics	Depressed respiration
	Increased levels of aldosterone	

Metabolic alkalosis results from a gain of base (alkaline) substances or a loss of metabolic acids. When the bicarbonate level decreases below 22 mEq/L, a metabolic acidosis exits. Metabolic acidosis results from a loss of base (alkaline) substances or a gain of metabolic acids.

ALTERATIONS IN ACID–BASE BALANCE

Disturbances in acid–base balance result from an abnormality of the metabolic or respiratory system. If the respiratory system is responsible, it is detected by the carbon dioxide in the serum. If the metabolic system is responsible, it is detected by the bicarbonate in the serum.

Respiratory Acidosis

Respiratory acidosis is defined as a $Paco_2$ greater than 45 mm Hg and a pH of less than 7.35. Respiratory acidosis is characterized by inadequate elimination of carbon dioxide by the lungs and may be the result of inefficient pulmonary function or excessive production of carbon dioxide.

Respiratory Alkalosis

Respiratory alkalosis is defined as a $Paco_2$ less than 35 mm Hg and a pH of greater than 7.45. Respiratory alkalosis is characterized by excessive elimination of carbon dioxide from the serum.

Metabolic Acidosis

Metabolic acidosis is defined as a bicarbonate level of less than 22 mEq/L and a pH of less than 7.35. Metabolic acidosis is characterized by an excessive production of nonvolatile acids or an inadequate concentration of bicarbonate for the concentration of acid within the serum.

Metabolic Alkalosis

Metabolic alkalosis is defined as a bicarbonate level of greater than 26 mEq/L and a pH of greater than 7.45. Metabolic alkalosis is characterized by excessive loss of nonvolatile acids or excessive production of bicarbonate.

INTERPRETING ARTERIAL BLOOD GAS RESULTS

When interpreting ABG results, three factors must be considered: (1) oxygenation status, (2) acid–base status, and (3) degree of compensation. A suggested approach for interpreting ABG results is presented in Box 24-9, along with sample values for interpretation.

Evaluating Oxygenation

It is necessary to examine the patient's oxygenation status by evaluating the Pao_2 and the Sao_2. If the Pao_2 value is less than the patient's norm, hypoxemia exists. If the Sao_2 is less than 93%, inadequate amounts of oxygen are bound to hemoglobin.

Evaluating Acid–Base Status

The first step in evaluating acid–base status is the examination of the arterial pH. If the pH is less than 7.35, acidemia exists. If the pH is greater than 7.45, alkalemia exists.

The second step in evaluating acid–base status is examination of the $Paco_2$. A $Paco_2$ of less than 35 mm Hg indicates a respiratory alkalosis, whereas a $Paco_2$ of greater than 45 mm Hg signifies a respiratory acidosis.

The third step in evaluating acid–base status is examination of the bicarbonate level. If the bicarbonate value is less than 22 mEq/L, metabolic acidosis is present. If the bicarbonate value is greater than 26 mEq/L, metabolic alkalosis exists.

Occasionally, patients present with both respiratory and metabolic disorders that *together* cause an acidemia or alkalemia. For example, alkalosis could result from an increase in bicarbonate and a decrease in carbon dioxide, or an acidosis could result from a decrease in bicarbonate and an increase in carbon dioxide. A patient with metabolic acidosis from acute renal failure could also have a very slow respiratory rate that causes the patient to retain carbon dioxide, creating a respiratory acidosis. Therefore, the ABG reflects a *mixed respiratory and metabolic acidosis.* Box 24-10 lists examples of mixed gases.

Determining Compensation

If the patient presents with an alkalemia or acidemia, it is important to determine if the body has tried to compensate for the abnormality. If the buffer systems in the body are unable to maintain normal pH, then the renal or respiratory systems attempt to compensate. *If the problem is respiratory in origin, the kidneys will work to correct it. If the*

box 24-9
Interpretation of Arterial Blood Gas (ABG) Results

Approach

1. Evaluate oxygenation by examining the Pao_2 and the Sao_2.
2. Evaluate the pH. Is it acidotic, alkalotic, or normal?
3. Evaluate the $Paco_2$. Is it high, low, or normal?
4. Evaluate the HCO_3. Is it high, low, or normal?
5. Determine if compensation is occurring. Is it complete, partial, or uncompensated?

Examples

Sample blood gas: Case 1

Pao_2	80 mm Hg	Normal
Sao_2	95%	Normal
pH	7.30	Acidemia
$Paco_2$	55 mm Hg	Increased (respiratory cause)
HCO_3	25 mEq/L	Normal

Conclusion: Respiratory acidosis (uncompensated)

Sample blood gas: Case 2

Pao_2	85 mm Hg	Normal
Sao_2	90%	Low saturation
pH	7.49	Alkalemia
$Paco_2$	40	Normal
HCO_3	29 mEq/L	Increased (metabolic cause)

Conclusion: Metabolic alkalosis with a low saturation (uncompensated)

box 24-10
Arterial Blood Gases in Mixed Respiratory and Metabolic Disorders

MIXED ACIDOSIS	MIXED ALKALOSIS
pH: 7.25	pH: 7.55
$Paco_2$: 56 mm Hg	$Paco_2$: 26 mm Hg
Pao_2: 80 mm Hg	Pao_2: 80 mm Hg
HCO_3: 15 mEq/L	HCO_3: 28 mEq/L

problem is renal in origin, the lungs will try to correct it. It may take as little as 5 to 15 minutes for the lungs to recognize a metabolic presentation and start to correct it. It may take up to 1 day for the kidneys to correct the respiratory-induced problem. One system will not overcompensate; that is, a compensatory mechanism will never make an acidotic patient alkalotic or an alkalotic patient acidotic.

The respiratory system responds to metabolic-based pH imbalances in the following manner:

- *Metabolic acidosis:* increase in respiratory rate and depth
- *Metabolic alkalosis:* decrease in respiratory rate and depth

The renal system responds to respiratory-based pH imbalances in the following manner:

- *Respiratory acidosis:* increase in hydrogen secretion and bicarbonate reabsorption
- *Respiratory alkalosis:* decrease in hydrogen secretion and bicarbonate reabsorption

ABGs are defined by their degree of compensation: uncompensated, partially compensated, or completely compensated. To determine the level of compensation, the pH, carbon dioxide, and bicarbonate are examined. First, it is determined whether the pH is acidotic or alkalotic. In some cases, the pH is not within the normal range, indicating an acidosis or alkalosis. If it is within the normal range, it is important to determine on which side of 7.40 (midpoint of the normal pH range) the pH lies. For example, a pH of 7.38 is *tending toward* acidosis, whereas a pH of 7.41 is *tending toward* alkalosis. Next, an evaluation is made to see whether carbon dioxide or bicarbonate has changed to account for the acidosis or alkalosis. Finally, it is determined whether the opposite system (metabolic or respiratory) has worked to try to shift back toward a normal pH. The primary abnormality (metabolic or respiratory) is correlated with the abnormal pH (acidotic or alkalotic). The secondary abnormality is an attempt to correct the primary disorder. By using the rules for defining compensation in Box 24-11, it is possible to determine the compensatory status of the patient's ABGs.

box 24-11
Compensatory Status of Arterial Blood Gases

Uncompensated: pH is *abnormal*, and *either* the CO_2 or HCO_3 is also abnormal. There is no indication that the opposite system has tried to correct for the other.

In the example below, the patient's pH is alkalotic as a result of the low (below the normal range of 35–45 mm Hg) CO_2 concentration. The renal system value (HCO_3) has not moved out its normal range (22–26 mEq/L) to compensate for the primary respiratory disorder.

Pao_2:	94 mm Hg	Normal
pH:	7.52	Alkalotic
$Paco_2$:	25 mm Hg	Decreased
HCO_3:	24 mEq/L	Normal

Partially compensated: pH is *abnormal,* and *both* the CO_2 and HCO_3 are also abnormal; this indicates that one system has attempted to correct for the other but has not been completely successful.

In the example below, the patient's pH remains alkalotic as a result of the low CO_2 concentration. The renal system value (HCO_3) has moved out its normal range (22–26 mEq/L) to compensate for the primary respiratory disorder but has not been able to bring the pH back within the normal range.

Pao_2:	94 mm Hg	Normal
pH:	7.48	Alkalotic
$Paco_2$:	25 mm Hg	Decreased
HCO_3:	20 mEq/L	Decreased

Completely compensated: pH is *normal* and *both* the CO_2 and HCO_3 are abnormal; the normal pH indicates that one system has been able to compensate for the other.

In the example below, the patient's pH is normal but is tending toward alkalosis (>7.40). The primary abnormality is respiratory because the $Paco_2$ is low (decreased acid concentration). The bicarbonate value of 18 mEq/L reflects decreased concentration of base and is associated with acidosis, not alkalosis. In this case, the decreased bicarbonate has completely compensated for the respiratory alkalosis.

Pao_2:	94 mm Hg	Normal
pH:	7.44	Normal, tending toward alkalosis
$Paco_2$:	25 mm Hg	Decreased, primary problem
HCO_3:	18 mEq/L	Decreased, compensatory response

Mixed Venous Oxygen Saturation

Mixed venous oxygen saturation ($S\bar{v}O_2$) is a parameter that can be measured to evaluate the balance between oxygen supply and oxygen demand. Blood obtained from a vein in an extremity gives information mostly about that extremity; it can be quite misleading if the metabolism in the extremity differs from the metabolism of the body as a whole. This difference is accentuated if the extremity is cold or underperfused (e.g., in shock), if the patient has performed local exercises with the extremity (e.g., opening and closing the fist), or if there is local infection in the extremity.

Sometimes blood is sampled through a central venous pressure (CVP) catheter in the hope of obtaining mixed venous blood, but even in the superior vena cava or right atrium where a CVP catheter ends, there is usually incomplete mixing of venous return from various parts of the body. For complete mixing of the blood, it is necessary to obtain a blood sample from a pulmonary artery catheter. Use of the pulmonary artery catheter provides a sample of blood that has returned from the extremities and has been mixed in the right ventricle.

Oxygen measurements of mixed venous blood indicate whether the tissues are being oxygenated, but $S\bar{v}O_2$ does not distinguish the independent contributions of the heart and the lungs. $S\bar{v}O_2$ indicates the adequacy of the supply of oxygen relative to the demand for oxygen at the tissue levels. Normal mixed venous oxygen saturation is 60% to

80%. A normal $S\bar{v}O_2$ means that supply of oxygen to the tissues is adequate to meet the tissue's demand. However, a normal value does not indicate if compensatory mechanisms were needed to maintain the perfusion. For example, in some patients, an increase in cardiac output is needed to compensate for a low supply of oxygen.

A low $S\bar{v}O_2$ may be caused by a decrease in oxygen supply to the tissues or an increase in oxygen use due to a high demand. A decrease in oxygen supply results from low hemoglobin, hemorrhage, or low cardiac output. An increase in oxygen demand results from hyperthermia, pain, stress, shivering, or seizures. An $S\bar{v}O_2$ of 40% to 60% may occur in heart failure, and values less than 40% may indicate profound shock. A decrease in $S\bar{v}O_2$ often occurs before other hemodynamic changes and, therefore, is an excellent clinical tool in the assessment and management of critically ill patients. The goals of interventions for a low $S\bar{v}O_2$ include increasing the oxygen supply by blood transfusions or by increasing cardiac output. Treatment may also be aimed at eliminating the cause of the high demand.

A high $S\bar{v}O_2$ value indicates that oxygen supply exceeds demand or a decrease in the demand. Elevated $S\bar{v}O_2$ values are associated with increased delivery of oxygen (high fraction of inspired oxygen [FIO_2]) or with decreased demand from hypothermia, hypothyroidism, or anesthesia. An elevated $S\bar{v}O_2$ also is seen in the early stages of septic shock when the tissues are unable to use the oxygen. Table 24-4 summarizes possible causes of abnormalities in $S\bar{v}O_2$.

A pulmonary artery catheter with an oximeter built into its tip that allows continuous monitoring of $S\bar{v}O_2$ provides ongoing assessment of oxygen supply and demand imbalances. If a catheter with a built-in oximeter is not available, the nurse can draw blood from the pulmonary artery through a regular pulmonary artery catheter, send the sample to the laboratory for blood gas and $S\bar{v}O_2$ analysis, and use the information in the same manner.

table 24-4 Possible Causes of Abnormalities in Mixed Venous Oxygen Saturation ($S\bar{v}O_2$)

Abnormality	Possible Cause
Low $S\bar{v}O_2$ <60%	***Decreased oxygen supply***
	Low hematocrit from anemia or hemorrhage
	Low arterial saturation and hypoxemia from lung disease, ventilation–perfusion mismatches
	Low cardiac output from hypovolemia, heart failure, cardiogenic shock, myocardial infarction
	Increased oxygen demand
	Increased metabolic demand, such as hyperthermia, seizures, shivering, pain, anxiety, stress, strenuous exercise
High $S\bar{v}O_2$ >80%	***Increased oxygen supply***
	Supplemental oxygen
	Decreased oxygen demand
	Anesthesia, hypothermia, early stages of sepsis
	Technical problems
	False high reading because of wedged pulmonary artery catheter
	Fibrin clot at end of catheter

RESPIRATORY DIAGNOSTIC STUDIES

Chest Radiography

Chest radiography is a valuable diagnostic tool frequently used to assess anatomical and physiological features of the chest and to detect pathological processes. As x-rays are passed through the chest wall, various structures are visualized. Dense tissues, such as bones, absorb the x-ray beam and appear as opaque or white on the radiograph. Blood vessels and blood-filled organs, such as the heart, are moderately dense structures and appear as gray areas on the radiograph. During inspiration, normal lungs are filled with air and appear black on the radiograph. When parts of the lungs are filled with fluid, which is a more dense material, the lungs appear white.

The radiograph is used by the nurse as an assessment parameter to validate clinical findings and suspected abnormalities. Using a systematic approach, the nurse examines the radiograph by comparing the film with previous films. One recommended approach is to examine the film by moving from external to internal, side to side, and top to bottom.[11] The nurse scrutinizes the soft tissue areas, the bony structures, the inner layers just under the bone, and the internal structures.

Soft tissues are examined on the radiograph by looking for homogeneity, beginning with lateral areas and moving medially. Air visualized in the lateral soft tissue may indicate the presence of a pneumothorax.

Bony structures inspected on the chest film include the ribs, clavicles, sternum, manubrium, spine, and vertebrae. Approximately eight to nine ribs should overlie lung tissue on the normal chest film. The ribs are examined for the presence of fractures by following the curve of each rib, beginning anteriorly and moving around posteriorly. Like the ribs, the other bony structures are examined for correct position and intactness.

The contour of the diaphragm is also examined on the radiograph. Normally, the diaphragm is rounded with sharp, pointed costophrenic angles. Pleural effusions may cause the angles to become blunted. The top of the diaphragm is visualized at about the sixth rib. A lowered diaphragm may indicate hyperinflation caused by emphysema.

The lung parenchyma is assessed by comparing right and left sides, moving top to bottom. Normal air-filled lungs should appear black or very dark compared with the bones and heart. It is important in the evaluation to look for symmetry. Abnormally high density on one side of the chest may indicate edema, a mass, pleural effusion, or pneumonia.[12]

Interlobar fissures separate the lobes of the lungs. The minor fissure in the right lung is usually visible in the frontal film. Displacement of the normal fissures seen on the film may indicate the presence of atelectasis or lobar collapse.

The trachea should appear midline over the thoracic vertebrae. The trachea can shift toward areas of atelectasis and away from areas of pneumothorax, pleural effusion, or tumors.

Ventilation–Perfusion Scanning

Ventilation–perfusion scanning is a nuclear imaging test used to evaluate a suspected alteration in the ventilation–perfusion relationship. (See Chapter 23 for a discussion of ventilation–perfusion relationships.) A ventilation–perfusion scan is helpful in detecting the percentage of each lung that is functioning normally, diagnosing and locating pulmonary emboli, and assessing the pulmonary vascular supply.[13]

The ventilation–perfusion scan consists of two parts: a ventilation scan and a perfusion scan. In the ventilation scan, the patient inhales radioactive gas, which follows the same pathway as air in normal breathing. In pathological conditions, the diminished areas of ventilation are visible on the scan. In the perfusion scan, a radioisotope is injected intravenously, enabling visualization of the blood supply to the lungs. When a pulmonary embolus is present, the blood supply beyond the embolus is restricted, revealing poor or no visualization of the affected area.

Ventilation–perfusion scans are often not useful in patients dependent on mechanical ventilation because the ventilation component of the scan is difficult to perform. Ventilation–perfusion mismatches may make interpretation of ventilation–perfusion scans difficult in patients with lung diseases, such as pneumonia. Because of these limitations, pulmonary angiography may be appropriate in the critically ill patient, especially if a pulmonary embolus is suspected.[11]

Pulmonary Angiography

Pulmonary angiography involves the rapid injection of a radiopaque substance for radiographic studies of the pulmonary vasculature. Suspected pulmonary embolus is the most common indication for pulmonary angiography. A radiopaque substance is injected into one or both arms, the femoral vein, or into a catheter that has been placed in the pulmonary artery. A positive test result is indicated by the impaired flow of the radiopaque substance through a narrowed vessel or by the abrupt cessation of flow of the substance in a vessel.

Bronchoscopy

Bronchoscopy involves the direct visualization of the larynx, trachea, and bronchi through a flexible fiberoptic bronchoscope. Bronchoscopy is used diagnostically to examine tissues, collect secretions, determine the extent and location of pathologic process, and obtain a biopsy. In addition, bronchoscopy is used therapeutically as a means to remove foreign bodies or secretions from the tracheobronchial tree, treat postoperative atelectasis, and excise lesions.

In preparation for a bronchoscopy, a history and physical examination should be performed. A chest radiograph, clotting studies, and ABGs also are obtained. The patient often receives intravenous sedation or analgesia before the procedure. If the purpose of the bronchoscopy is therapeutic, medications that suppress a cough or diminish secretions are avoided (e.g., intratracheal topical anesthetics, atropine, and codeine).

Careful monitoring of the patient is indicated after a bronchoscopy. The nurse assesses for any evidence of complications, which may include laryngospasm, fever, hemodynamic changes, cardiac dysrhythmias, pneumothorax, hemorrhage, or cardiopulmonary arrest.

Thoracentesis

In thoracentesis, a needle is inserted into the pleural space to remove air, fluid, or both; obtain specimens for diagnostic evaluation; or instill medications. A chest radiograph, coagulation studies, and patient education are essential before a thoracentesis. Some patients may require medication to reduce anxiety. Unlike bronchoscopy, thoracentesis requires the cooperation of the patient; therefore, a local anesthetic, rather than moderate sedation, is used to minimize the pain and discomfort that accompanies the procedure. During the procedure, the patient is placed either in a chair or on the edge of the bed in an upright position with arms and shoulders raised so that the ribs lift and separate, allowing easier needle insertion. If a patient is unable to lift his or her arms, sitting on the bed with the arms placed above the head on a table is an alternative position.

During thoracentesis, the nurse's primary function is to provide comfort for the patient, perform ongoing assessment of the patient's respiratory system, dress the wound with sterile dressings on completion of the procedure, and send labeled laboratory specimens as ordered. Post-thoracentesis nursing care includes assessment for complications, including pneumothorax, pain, hypotension, and pulmonary edema.

Sputum Culture

Sputum specimens are often part of the respiratory assessment. Because healthy patients do not produce sputum, obtaining a specimen requires the patient to cough to bring up sputum from the lungs. It is essential that the nurse distinguish sputum from saliva before sending the specimen to the laboratory.

In most cases, sputum specimens are obtained to examine for culture and sensitivity. The specimen is examined for specific microorganisms and their corresponding drug sensitivities. In addition, sputum specimens are also required for studies of cytology and acid-fast bacilli. Culture of acid-fast bacilli requires serial collection (usually over 3 days) and is used to identify the presence of tuberculosis and mycobacteria.

Pulmonary Function Tests

The flow of air in and out of the lungs provides tangible measures of lung volumes. Although these volumes are referred to as measures of "pulmonary function," in reality they are measures of *pulmonary anatomy*. In the evaluation of ventilation, structure or anatomy often determines function. Ventilatory or pulmonary function tests measure the ability of the chest and lungs to move air into and out of the alveoli.

Pulmonary function tests include volume measurements, capacity measurements, and dynamic measurements. These measurements are influenced by exercise and disease. Age, sex, body size, and posture are other variables that are taken into consideration when the test results are interpreted. Figure 23-13 in Chapter 23 illustrates pulmonary function tests showing normal lung volumes and capacity.

VOLUME MEASUREMENTS

Volume measurements show the amount of air contained in the lungs during various parts of the respiratory cycle. Measures of lung volume include tidal volume (VT), inspiratory reserve volume (IRV), expiratory reserve volume (ERV), and residual volume (RV; see Chapter 23, Table 23-1).

CAPACITY MEASUREMENTS

Capacity measurements quantify part of the pulmonary cycle. They are a combination of the previous volumes, and include inspiratory capacity (IC), functional residual capacity (FRC), vital capacity (VC), and total lung capacity (TLC; see Chapter 23, Table 23-1).

DYNAMIC MEASUREMENTS

The following measurements, called *dynamic measurements*, provide data about airway resistance and the energy expended in breathing (work of breathing).

- *Respiratory rate or frequency* is the number of breaths per minute. At rest, the respiratory rate is about 15 breaths/minute.
- *Minute volume*, sometimes called *minute ventilation*, is the volume of air inhaled and exhaled per minute. It is calculated by multiplying tidal volume by respiratory rate. At rest, the minute volume is approximately 7,500 mL/minute.
- *Dead space* is the part of the tidal volume that does not participate in alveolar gas exchange. The dead space (measured in milliliters) is the air contained in the airways (anatomical dead space) plus the volume of alveolar air that is not involved in gas exchange (physiological dead space; e.g., air in an unperfused alveolus due to pulmonary embolism or, more commonly, air in underperfused alveoli). Adult anatomical dead space is usually equal to the body weight in pounds (e.g., 140 mL in a 140-lb person). In a healthy person, dead space is composed only of anatomical dead space. Physiological dead space occurs in certain disease states. Dead space is calculated by subtracting the partial pressure of arterial carbon dioxide ($PaCO_2$) from the partial pressure of alveolar carbon dioxide ($PACO_2$). The normal value of dead space in healthy adults is typically less than 40% of the tidal volume. The dead space–tidal volume ratio is used to follow the effectiveness of mechanical ventilation.
- *Alveolar ventilation*, the complement of dead space, is expressed as the *volume of tidal air that is involved in alveolar gas exchange*. This volume is represented as volume per minute by the symbol $\dot{V}A$. $\dot{V}A$ is a measure of ventilatory effectiveness. It is more relevant to the blood gas values than either the dead space or tidal volume because these last two measures include physiological dead space. $\dot{V}A$ is calculated by subtracting the dead space (VD) from the tidal volume (VT) and multiplying the result by the respiratory rate (f):

$$\dot{V}_A = (V_T - V_D) \times f$$

About 2,300 mL of air (functional residual capacity [FRC]) remains in the lung at the end of expiration. Each new breath introduces about 350 mL of air into the alveoli. The ratio of new alveoli air to total volume of air remaining in the lungs is:

$$\frac{350 \text{ mL}}{2300 \text{ mL}}$$

Therefore, new air is only about one seventh of the total volume contained in the lungs. The normal is 5,250 mL/minute (350 mL/breath × 15 breaths/minute = 5,250 mL/minute). A normal breath (tidal volume) can replace 7,500 mL of air per minute (500 mL/breath × 15 breaths/minute = 7,500 mL/minute), requiring 0.008 second/mL:

$$\frac{1 \text{ minute}}{7{,}500 \text{ mL}} \times \frac{60 \text{ seconds}}{1 \text{ minute}} = 0.008 \text{ second/mL}$$

Therefore, the FRC of the lungs can be completely replaced in 18.4 seconds (2,300 mL × 0.008 second/mL = 18.4 seconds) if air diffusion is uniform. This slow turnover rate prevents rapid fluctuations of gas concentrations in the alveoli with each breath.

clinical applicability challenges

Self-Challenge: Critical Thinking

Mrs. J, an 84-year-old woman, has been admitted to the intensive care unit (ICU) with a diagnosis of pneumonia. She has a history of dementia, which makes it difficult to obtain reliable information during the health history. Her family tells you that she has been short of breath and is having difficulty breathing. On physical examination, her respiratory rate is 26 breaths/minute, and she uses accessory muscles for breathing. Her mucous membranes are pale. When auscultating her lungs, you hear coarse crackles in the bases. Arterial blood gases (ABGs) are PaO_2, 65 mm Hg; $PaCO_2$, 33 mm Hg; HCO_3, 23 mEq/L; pH 7.46.

1. *Describe some of the differences in the respiratory assessment of the older patient.*
2. *Interpret the patient's ABGs.*
3. *Explain why coarse crackles were heard when auscultating the patient's lungs.*
4. *Discuss what findings you anticipate on the patient's chest radiograph.*
5. *What additional assessment data should you obtain?*

Study Questions

1. *Normal breath sounds that are heard over the periphery of the lung are called*
   a. *bronchial breath sounds.*
   b. *bronchovesicular breath sounds.*
   c. *vesicular breath sounds.*
   d. *loud crackles.*
2. *Mixed venous blood has an oxygen saturation that is*
   a. *60% to 80%, which is lower than arterial blood.*
   b. *80% to 90%, which is lower than arterial blood.*
   c. *30% to 40%, which is lower than arterial blood.*
   d. *95% or greater, which is the same as arterial blood.*
3. *Consider the following arterial blood gas (ABG) analysis: $Pa{O_2}$, 86 mm Hg; pH, 7.31; $Pa{CO_2}$, 52 mm Hg; HCO_3, 24 mEq/L. Which condition is indicated by these values?*
   a. *Respiratory alkalosis*
   b. *Metabolic alkalosis*
   c. *Metabolic acidosis*
   d. *Respiratory acidosis*
4. *The primary abnormality in respiratory alkalosis is*
   a. *decreased $Pa{CO_2}$.*
   b. *increased $Pa{CO_2}$.*
   c. *decreased HCO_3.*
   d. *increased HCO_3.*
5. *A high $S\bar{v}O_2$ level may be the result of*
   a. *pain and anxiety.*
   b. *anemia.*
   c. *hypothermia.*
   d. *hyperthermia.*
6. *The measurement of end-tidal carbon dioxide ($ETCO_2$) occurs*
   a. *at the end of the alveolar plateau.*
   b. *at the beginning of the expiratory upstroke phase.*
   c. *at the end of the inspiratory downstroke phase.*
   d. *at the end of the expiratory upstroke phase.*
7. *Which of the following are routine procedures to carry out before a thoracentesis?*
   a. *Coagulation studies, chest radiograph, sputum culture, arterial blood gases (ABGs)*
   b. *Patient education, chest radiograph, coagulation studies*
   c. *Sputum culture, patient education, coagulation studies*
   d. *Patient education, coagulation studies, ABGs*
8. *The correct order in which one performs an assessment of the respiratory system is*
   a. *inspection, auscultation, percussion, palpation.*
   b. *auscultation, percussion, inspection, palpation.*
   c. *inspection, palpation, percussion, auscultation.*
   d. *auscultation, palpation, inspection, percussion.*
9. *Serial sputum cultures are typically required for which of the following?*
   a. *To test for acid-fast bacillus and mycobacteria*
   b. *Postoperative productive cough*
   c. *Preoperative productive cough*
   d. *To test for methicillin-resistant* Staphylococcus aureus
10. *When comparing end-tidal carbon dioxide ($ETCO_2$) values with $Pa{CO_2}$ values in the healthy adult*
    a. *the $ETCO_2$ is usually 2 to 5 mm Hg more than $Pa{CO_2}$.*
    b. *the $Pa{CO_2}$ is usually 2 to 5 mm Hg more than the $ETCO_2$.*
    c. *the $Pa{CO_2}$ and $ETCO_2$ are the same.*
    d. *the $Pa{CO_2}$ and the $ETCO_2$ should not be compared.*
11. *A potential mechanical cause of a prolonged expiratory upstroke when assessing a patient's end-tidal carbon dioxide ($ETCO_2$) is*
    a. *a disconnection between the endotracheal tube and the ventilator tubing.*
    b. *a hole in the ventilator tubing.*
    c. *a kink in the ventilator tubing.*
    d. *a filled water reservoir (trap).*

REFERENCES

1. Bickley LS: Bates' Guide to Physical Examination and History Taking (8th Ed). Philadelphia, Lippincott Williams & Wilkins, 2003
2. Lee WW, Mayberry K, Crapo R, et al: The accuracy of pulse oximetry in the emergency department. Am J Emerg Med 18(4):427–431, 2000
3. Grap MJ: Pulse oximetry. Crit Care Nurse 18(1):94–99, 1998
4. Barker SJ, Tremper KK, Hyatt J: Effects of methemoglobinemia on pulse oximetry and mixed venous oximetry. Anesthesiology 70(1): 112–117, 1989
5. Anderson ST, Hajduczek J, Barker SJ: Benzocaine-induced methemoglobinemia in an adult: Accuracy of pulse oximetry with methemoglobinemia. Anesth Analg 67(11):1099–1101, 1988
6. Eisenkraft JB: Pulse oximeter desaturation due to methemoglobinemia. Anesthesiology 68(2):279–282, 1988
7. Varon AJ: Methemoglobinemia and pulse oximetry. Crit Care Med 20(9):1363–1364, 1992
8. Christensen MA, Bloom J, Sutton KR: Comparing arterial and end-tidal carbon dioxide values in hyperventilated neurosurgical patients. Am J Crit Care 4:116–121, 1995
9. Velmahos GC, Chan LS, Tatevossian R, et al: High-frequency percussive ventilation improves oxygenation in patients with ARDS. Chest 116(2):440–446, 1999
10. Cortiella J, Mlcak R, Herndon D: High-frequency percussive ventilation in pediatric patients with inhalation injury. J Burn Care Rehabil 20(3):232–235, 1999
11. Dettenmeier PA: Radiographic Assessment for Nurses. St. Louis, Mosby, 1995
12. Kelley WN: Textbook of Internal Medicine (3rd Ed). Philadelphia, Lippincott-Raven, 1997
13. Fischbach FT: A Manual of Laboratory and Diagnostic Tests (7th Ed). Philadelphia, Lippincott Williams & Wilkins, 2004

OTHER SELECTED READING

Ahrens T, Sona C: Capnography applications in acute and critical care. AACN Clin Issues 14(2):123–132, 2003

Ahrens T, Schallom L, Bettorf K, et al: End-tidal carbon dioxide measurements as a prognostic indicator of outcome in cardiac arrest. Am J Crit Care 10(6):391–398, 2001

Attin M, Cardin S, Doering L, et al: An educational project to improve knowledge related to pulse oximetry. Am J Crit Care 11(6):529–534, 2002

Berry BE, Pinard AE: Assessing tissue oxygenation. Crit Care Nurse 22(3):22–42, 2002

Connolly M: Black, white, and shades of gray: Common abnormalities in chest radiographs. AACN Clin Issues 12(2):259–269, 2001

Frakes MA: Measuring end-tidal carbon dioxide: Clinical applications and usefulness. Crit Care Nurse 21(5): 23–37, 2001

Kirksey KM, Holt-Ashley M, Goodroad B: An easy method for interpreting the results of arterial blood gas analysis. Crit Care Nurse 21(5):49–54, 2001

Ruffolo DC, Headley JM: Regional carbon dioxide monitoring: A different look at tissue perfusion. AACN Clin Issues, 14(2): 168–175, 2003

Schallom L, Ahrens T: Hemodynamic applications of capnography. J Cardiovasc Nurs, 15(2): 56–70, 2001

St. John RE. End-tidal carbon dioxide monitoring. Crit Care Nurse, 23(4): 83–88, 2003

chapter 25

Patient Management: Respiratory System

DONNA L. CHARLEBOIS ■ SIDENIA S. EARVEN ■
CHARLES A. FISHER ■ ROSE LEWIS ■ PAUL K. MERREL

objectives

Based on the content in this chapter, the reader should be able to:

- Identify the two opposing forces that cause the negative pressure during respiration.
- Summarize the desired outcomes of the various bronchial hygiene techniques.
- Compare and contrast situations in which chest physiotherapy (including postural drainage) is useful and those in which it is contraindicated.
- Discuss two goals of oxygen delivery.
- Describe the nursing assessment of patients on oxygen therapy.
- List three complications of oxygen therapy.
- Compare and contrast indications for, and complications of, orotracheal intubation and nasotracheal intubation.
- Summarize procedures commonly performed in the intensive care unit that can precipitate pneumothorax.
- Compare and contrast the principles governing chest tube drainage systems.
- Discuss nursing interventions necessary to prevent complications in a patient with a chest tube drainage system.
- Discuss the pharmacology for the treatment of bronchospasm.
- Explain causes of agitation in critically ill patients.
- Analyze the process by which each of the following conditions can cause respiratory failure: benzodiazepine overdose, asthma, and pulmonary embolus.
- Differentiate between the principles of negative-pressure ventilation and positive-pressure ventilation. In positive-pressure ventilation, differentiate between pressure-cycled and volume-cycled ventilators.
- Compare and contrast intermittent mandatory, assist-control, pressure-support, and pressure-controlled ventilation.
- Summarize strategies to maximize oxygen delivery with the goal of achieving a nontoxic FIO_2 setting.

- Summarize adverse effects of positive end-expiratory pressure, how they are identified, and the appropriate treatment for each.
- Compare and contrast the advantages and disadvantages of tracheostomy versus endotracheal intubation.
- Name four nursing interventions for the ventilated patient, and explain the impact of each on decreasing the length of mechanical ventilation.
- Access one Internet resource and identify two points applicable to ventilators or ventilated patient care.

Respiration is necessary to sustaining life, and the nurse plays an important role in helping the critically ill patient breathe. The nurse must be knowledgeable and skilled in assessing patient needs, providing quick and efficient care, evaluating results of intervention, and supporting, teaching, and preparing the patient and family. Techniques, equipment, and procedures vary according to the patient's respiratory status. Bronchial hygiene, artificial airways, chest tubes, pharmacological agents, and various types of ventilatory support are discussed in this chapter.

BRONCHIAL HYGIENE

Bronchial hygiene is helpful in preventing and treating pulmonary complications. The primary phases of lung function that most bronchial hygiene aims to improve are ventilation and diffusion (Fig. 25-1). These are accomplished through the therapeutic goals of mobilization and removal of secretions and improved gas exchange.

Specific bronchial hygiene depends on existing pulmonary dysfunction. The normal airway has a functioning mucociliary "escalator" with a cough reflex and normal mucus production. In contrast, the hospitalized patient may have pneumonia or atelectasis, or may not be able to deep breathe, cough, or clear mucus effectively owing to weakness, sedation, or pain.

Assessment of the need for and the effectiveness of various methods of bronchial hygiene is based on physical assessment, chest radiography, measurement of arterial blood gases (ABGs), and additional sources of information as indicated. Any one or a combination of the following measures may be used: coughing and deep breathing maneuvers, chest physiotherapy (CPT), and bronchodilator aerosol therapy (discussed later in the chapter).

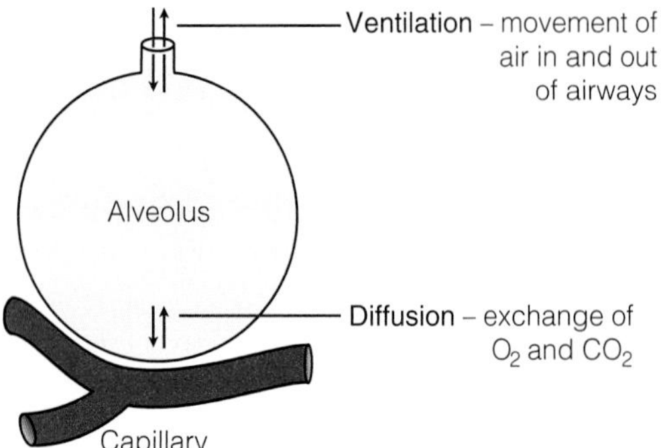

figure 25-1 Primary lung functions: ventilation and diffusion.

Methods of Bronchial Hygiene

COUGHING AND DEEP BREATHING

Effective coughing is necessary for the patient to clear secretions. The objectives of deep breathing and coughing are to promote lung expansion, mobilize secretions, and prevent the side effects of retained secretions (atelectasis and pneumonia). The efficacy of these techniques is limited to patients who are able to cooperate.

Ideally, the patient is positioned upright on the edge of the bed or chair with the feet supported. He or she is instructed to take a slow, deep breath, hold it for at least 2 to 3 seconds, and exhale slowly. If secretions are auscultated, then a cough is initiated after a maximum inspiration. Even if secretions are not auscultated, the patient should be instructed and encouraged to cough and deep breathe as a prophylactic measure. Incentive spirometers (IS) are available to encourage and quantify deep breathing by giving immediate visual feedback to the patient. Ideally, the patient uses the IS hourly while awake, completing 10 breaths each session, and increases the volume of breaths progressively. The nurse should coach the patient in this process and then document the use and progress of IS volumes.

CHEST PHYSIOTHERAPY

Postural drainage, positioning, and chest percussion and vibration are methods of CPT used to augment the patient's efforts and improve pulmonary function. These may be used in sequence in different lung drainage positions and should be preceded by bronchodilator therapy (if ordered) and followed by deep breathing and coughing. Changing the patient's position from supine to upright affects gas exchange. Positioning the patient in the lateral position may also improve gas exchange, especially in unilateral lung disease. By placing the "good" lung down, improved oxygenation results.[1] This improvement occurs because shunting is decreased when the "good" lung is in the dependent position.

Postural Drainage

Postural drainage positions facilitate gravitational drainage of pulmonary secretions into the main bronchi and trachea based on anatomy of the lung segments (Fig. 25-2). The focus of the postural drainage should be on the lobes affected by atelectasis and on increasing mucus removal

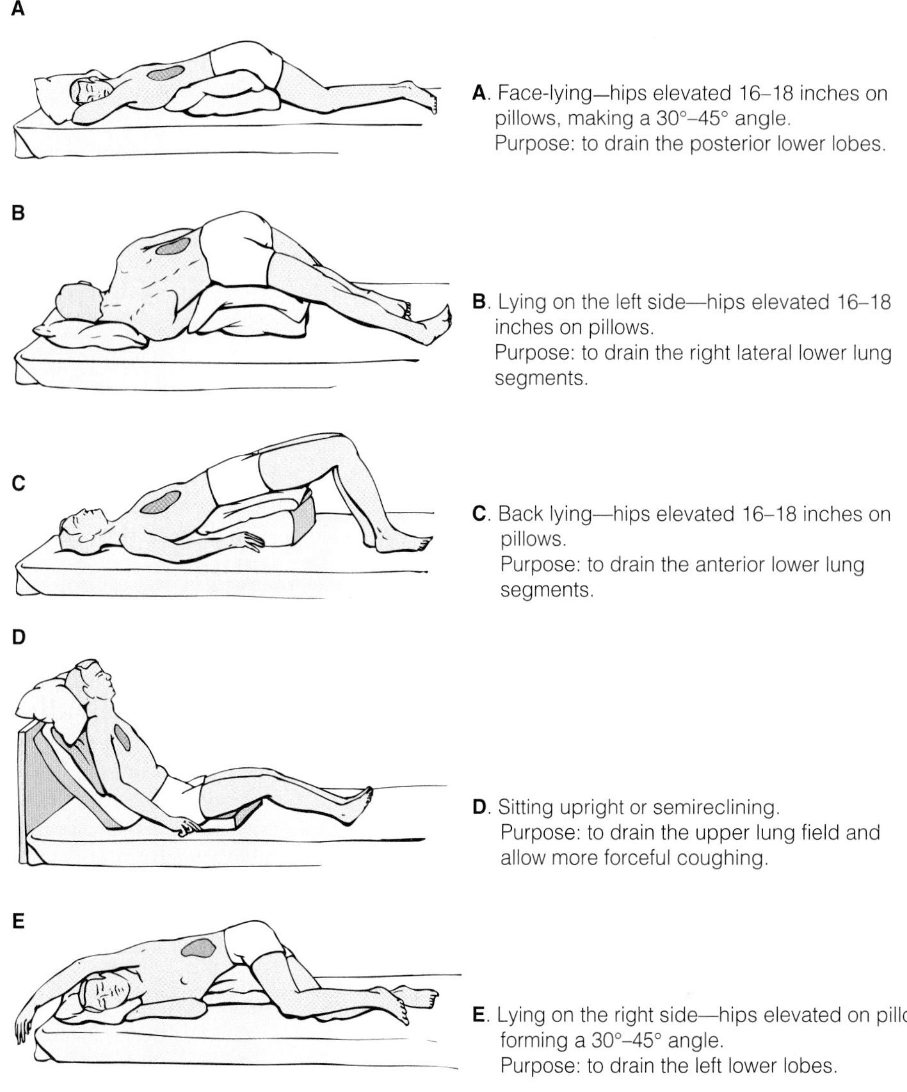

A
A. Face-lying—hips elevated 16–18 inches on pillows, making a 30°–45° angle.
Purpose: to drain the posterior lower lobes.
B
B. Lying on the left side—hips elevated 16–18 inches on pillows.
Purpose: to drain the right lateral lower lung segments.
C
C. Back lying—hips elevated 16–18 inches on pillows.
Purpose: to drain the anterior lower lung segments.
D
D. Sitting upright or semireclining.
Purpose: to drain the upper lung field and allow more forceful coughing.
E
E. Lying on the right side—hips elevated on pillows forming a 30°–45° angle.
Purpose: to drain the left lower lobes.

figure 25-2 Positions used in lung drainage.

with suctioning or by cough effort. Postural drainage is not indicated in all positions for all critically ill patients. Contraindications are listed in Box 25-1. The nurse must closely monitor the patient who is in a head-down position for aspiration, respiratory distress, and dysrhythmias. Altered techniques may include gentle percussion and using a mechanical percussor to stimulate mucus movement while avoiding surgical areas.

Chest Percussion and Vibration

Chest percussion and vibration, performed by a trained health care professional, are used to dislodge secretions. Percussion involves striking the chest wall with the hands formed into a cupped shape by flexing the fingers and placing the thumb tightly against the index finger. The patient's position depends on the segment of lung to be percussed. A towel or pillowcase is draped over the area to be percussed, and percussion is performed for 3 to 5 minutes per position. Percussion is never performed over the spine, over the sternum, or below the thoracic cage. Percussion and vibration are performed only on the rib cage. If performed correctly, percussion does not hurt the patient or redden the skin. A clapping sound (as opposed to slapping) indicates correct hand position. Mechanical percussors are also available.

Vibration is done during a prolonged pursed-lip exhalation. Vibration increases the velocity and turbulence of exhaled air to loosen secretions. This technique is accomplished by placing the hands side by side with fingers extended and applying the flat of the palm over the affected chest area. The patient inhales deeply, and then slowly exhales. While the patient exhales, the nurse vibrates the patient's chest by quickly contracting and relaxing arm and shoulder muscles. Vibration is used instead of percussion if the chest wall is extremely painful.

Contraindications and Adaptations

Modern critical care beds may have a percussion module built in, allowing for more frequent CPT. No single method has been shown to be superior, and there are many contraindications to using these techniques (see Box 25-1). Recent studies have questioned the efficacy of CPT, except in segmental atelectasis caused by mucus obstruction and in diseases that result in increased sputum production (at least 30 mL/day), such as cystic fibrosis and bronchiectasis.[2]

box 25-1 *Contraindications to Chest Physiotherapy*

Contraindications to Postural Drainage

- Increased intracranial pressure
- After meals/during tube feeding
- Inability to cough
- Hypoxia/respiratory instability
- Hemodynamic instability
- Decreased mental status
- Recent eye surgery
- Hiatal hernia
- Obesity

Contraindications to Percussion/Vibration

- Fractured ribs/osteoporosis
- Chest/abdominal trauma or surgery
- Pulmonary hemorrhage or embolus
- Chest malignancy/mastectomy
- Pneumothorax/subcutaneous emphysema
- Cervical cord trauma
- Tuberculosis
- Pleural effusions/empyema
- Asthma

Bronchoscopy is an alternative treatment used to remove mucus plugs that result in atelectasis. CPT may produce bronchospasm in asthmatic patients and may spread infected material to uninfected lung tissue in patients with unilateral pneumonia.

The inclusion of CPT in the plan of care should be individualized and evaluated in terms of derived benefit versus potential risks, and should be discontinued when it fails to promote treatment goals. In patients who cannot tolerate CPT, turning the patient laterally every 2 hours aids in draining the lungs and prevents stagnation of secretions. Progressive mobility from sitting up in a chair, to weight bearing, to ambulation is used in all ventilated patients as part of pulmonary hygiene as well as to increase patient strength and endurance. Patients with an artificial airway or an ineffective cough may require suctioning after CPT.

To be effective, CPT must be accompanied by the postural drainage position specific to the affected area of the lung. Patients with unilateral disease are positioned with the healthy lung down for better ventilation and perfusion.[3] Positioning the patient with the diseased lung down is likely to cause hypoxemia with ventilation–perfusion mismatching and shunting. Positioning, however, is changed if the patient has a lung abscess. In such cases, the preferred position is with the diseased lung down because the abscessed lung in a gravity-dependent position can drain its purulent contents into the opposite lung. The abscessed lung would then contaminate the healthy lung, and gas exchange would most likely be affected.

Recent studies have demonstrated improved oxygenation in patients with acute respiratory failure who were placed in the prone position (although this maneuver may not ultimately improve survival).[4] Prone positioning is an advanced technique used with critically ill patients who have acute lung injury (ALI) or acute respiratory distress syndrome (ARDS). The resulting enhanced oxygenation is attributed to recruitment of collapsed lung areas.[5] Patients who are ventilated benefit from having the head of the bed elevated 30 degrees at all times.[6] The rationale is to promote lung expansion and prevent aspiration that can occur in the recumbent position in intubated patients.

OXYGEN THERAPY

The administration of oxygen therapy to a patient is designed to correct hypoxemia (low blood oxygen levels). When tissue oxygen availability is decreased, it is referred to as *hypoxia*. If external or internal respiration is impaired, supplemental oxygen is vital to maintain the patient's cellular function. Oxygen therapy corrects hypoxemia, decreases the work of breathing, and decreases myocardial work. Any disease process that alters gas exchange can cause hypoxemia.

Asthma, bronchitis, pneumonia, ALI and ARDS, chronic obstructive pulmonary disease (COPD), and emphysema are disease processes that alter oxygen supply. Traumatic events that lead to pneumothorax or hemothorax, as well as surgical events such as pneumonectomy and lobectomy, or events causing large pleural effusions can significantly alter gas exchange. Oxygen delivery by nasal cannula may provide sufficient additional oxygen to reduce air hunger and shortness of breath. A patient with COPD may also have a need for continuous oxygen because of permanent alterations in the lungs, which result in lowered oxygen delivery, especially with stress, illness, infection, and exercise. Patients with COPD or emphysema should be monitored closely for carbon dioxide retention and narcosis associated with the delivery of too high a concentration of oxygen. These patients normally tolerate higher levels of carbon dioxide because their chemoreceptors no longer respond to the normally accepted partial pressure of carbon dioxide (Pco_2) levels and serum pH. These patients' primary drive to breathe comes from their oxygen, rather than carbon dioxide, levels. The desired goals for all patients on oxygen therapy is a stable arterial oxygen saturation (Sao_2) level, eupneic respirations, and a decrease in anxiety and shortness of breath. These goals should be accomplished through delivery of the least amount of supplemental oxygen needed, so the nurse continuously monitors the patient on oxygen for the desired result and complications (Box 25-2). Appropriate physician or advanced practice nurse orders are necessary to initiate this therapy.

Patient Assessment

Assessment of the patient's oxygen need is based on the disease process and the severity of the hypoxemia. The nursing assessment considers the patient's level of consciousness, vital signs (including the rate and depth of breathing), nailbed color, airway patency or presence of an artificial airway, Sao_2, and ABGs. The use of accessory muscles or abdominal breathing may indicate severe distress, and the inability to speak (or the tendency to respond using only one-syllable words) is ominous. A patient with

box 25-2 ***Complications of Oxygen Therapy***

- Respiratory arrest
- Discomfort with skin breakdown from straps and masks
- Dry mucous membranes, epistaxis, or infection in the nares
- Oxygen toxicity (prolonged high levels seen in acute lung injury [ALI] or acute respiratory distress syndrome [ARDS])
- Absorptive atelectasis
- Carbon dioxide narcosis (manifested by altered mental status, confusion, headache, somnolence)

asthma who comes in with bilateral wheezes but who can communicate in full sentences is less likely to have increased dyspnea and require intubation than the patient with asthma who sits bolt upright, only nods the head to questions, and is using the shoulder and neck accessory muscles to breathe. Laboratory data, including hemoglobin, hematocrit, ABGs, and chest radiographs, may be obtained to assist in correcting electrolyte and pH imbalances. A full assessment, which may include collection of an ABG, takes time, whereas assessment of the person's vital signs, SaO_2, and respiratory effort and symptoms can be done quickly and repeatedly. To establish baseline activity tolerance and respiratory function, it may be necessary to involve the family if the patient is not able to communicate in full sentences. The usual symptoms exhibited by a patient with asthma or COPD need to be compared with the presenting symptoms to establish the severity of the patient's illness. Oxygen therapy should be initiated for distress and hypoxemia. After a thorough assessment, including laboratory data, the oxygen delivery method is adjusted to best meet the therapeutic goal.

The patient's acuity and underlying disease process dictate the level of oxygen delivery required. The choice of oxygen delivery method is based on the assessment and presentation of the patient, the SaO_2 on room air, and the desired outcome. The desired oxygen level for a patient with COPD may be much lower than that for a patient with pneumonia who does not have COPD. The patient with pneumonia tolerates higher levels of oxygenation for longer periods than the patient with COPD, who is susceptible to carbon dioxide narcosis.

The patient is reassessed after oxygen is applied. Signs of improvement include reduction of respiratory rate, a more comfortable breathing pattern, an increased SaO_2, and the patient's own subjective statement of improved breathing with decreased anxiety or distress. Altered mental status may indicate hypoxemia, but may also be due to pH, electrolyte, or carbon dioxide changes. The nurse assesses the patient's respiratory status as often as needed until the desired results are achieved. ABGs guide therapy, especially in patients known to have carbon dioxide retention or continued lethargy or sedation, and in those unable to clear secretions. Ultimately, the ABGs indicate success or failure of efforts to correct the underlying hypoxemia.

Oxygen Delivery Systems

There are several methods of oxygen delivery available for patients. The choice of a delivery method depends on the patient's condition. Oxygen delivery systems are traditionally divided into high-flow and low-flow systems (Box 25-3).

Low-flow oxygen devices work by supplying oxygen at flow rates less than the patient's inspiratory volume. The rest of the volume is pulled from room air (entrained). Because of this oxygen and room air mixing (entrainment), the actual fraction of inspired oxygen (FIO_2) delivered to the patient is difficult to specify. Low-flow oxygen devices are suitable for patients with normal respiratory patterns, rates, and ventilation volumes. High-flow oxygen devices supply flow rates high enough to accommodate two to three times the patient's inspiratory volume. These devices are suitable for patients with high inspiratory and cellular metabolic requirements.

Oxygen delivery devices all deliver different levels of oxygen. Selection of the device is based on the desired FIO_2.[7] For example, a patient admitted with pneumonia who has an SaO_2 of 88% might improve to the desired level with a nasal cannula at 2 L/minute. In contrast, a patient who has an SaO_2 of 88% but who also has a partial pressure of arterial oxygen (PaO_2) of 52 mm Hg, and is using accessory muscles, may require a higher flow or a non-rebreather oxygen mask. Both patients are monitored for improved SaO_2 and respiratory rate and pattern. If increased distress, desaturation, or both are noted, more extreme interventions (such as intubation) may be necessary.

If lower concentrations of oxygen are needed, the system selected is usually nasal cannula. The cannula can be used even with mouth breathers because oxygen fills the nasopharynx and is entrained with inspiration. The exact concentration of oxygen depends on the patient's inspired tidal volume (V_T). If the patient hypoventilates, the oxygen concentration increases in the upper airway. In contrast, if hyperventilation occurs, the concentration of oxygen decreases owing to large amounts of room air diluting the oxygen delivered. A simple calculation for nasal cannula delivery is to add another 4% for each liter FIO_2 delivered to the room air value of 21% (see Box 25-3). Each of the other oxygen delivery devices delivers a variable FIO_2, based on breathing pattern and what device is used, as well as the oxygen flow in liters per minute.

If the oxygen concentration must be constant, as is the case for patients with COPD, Venturi systems (e.g., the Venturi mask) are used. The Venturi mask delivers an exact percentage of oxygen regardless of the patient's tidal volume. Patients with COPD may require oxygen delivery by the Venturi system. These patients are "sensitive" to oxygen, and a small increase in the percentage of FIO_2 delivered may result in an elevated $PaCO_2$ and respiratory depression. The patient with COPD may have a respiratory drive based on his or her PaO_2, and with this disease process, ventilation decreases with an increased FIO_2, resulting in hypercapnia. The carbon dioxide level can be detected through serial ABG monitoring, which may reveal large increases in $PaCO_2$ with small increases in oxygen flow.

As higher concentrations of oxygen are needed, the nasal cannula is replaced by a mask system. A simple mask delivers the lowest concentrations of oxygen, and a high-

box 25-3
Oxygen Delivery Methods With Delivered Fraction of Inspired Oxygen (FIO_2)

Nasal Cannula

FLOW (L/min)	FIO_2
1	21%–25%
2	25%–28%
3	28%–32%
4	32%–36%
5	36%–40%
6	40%–44%

Face Mask

FLOW (L/min)	FIO_2
5–6	40%
6–7	50%
7–10	60%

Face Tent
Variable oxygen delivery of 21% to 50%; depends on patient breathing (21% delivered with compressed air and up to 50% delivered with 10 L/min oxygen flow attached). Air is mixed with the oxygen flow in the mask, resulting in variable delivery with humidification. Often used for humidification as well as oxygen delivery in patients who do not like the claustrophobic feeling associated with more traditional masks.

Venturi Mask

OXYGEN FLOW (MINIMAL RATE)	FIO_2 SETTING*
4 L/min	25%
4 L/min	28%
6 L/min	31%
8 L/min	35%
8 L/min	40%
10 L/min	50%

*FIO_2 setting is based on Venturi setting/adapter used and oxygen flow.

Non-rebreather Mask
The non-rebreather mask is used in severe hypoxia to deliver the highest oxygen concentration. The one-way valve on one side allows for the exhalation of carbon dioxide. The mask delivers 80% to 95% FIO_2 at a flow rate of 10 L/min depending on the patient's rate and depth of breathing, with some room air entrained through the open port on the mask. However, the mask should fit snugly to prevent additional entrainment of room air.

Tracheostomy Collar and T-piece
The T-piece is a T-shaped adapter used to provide oxygen to either an endotracheal or tracheostomy tube. The flow rate should be at least 10 L/min with humidification. Flow can also be provided by a ventilator. The tracheostomy collar may also be used and is usually the preferred method because it is more comfortable than the T-piece. The strap on the tracheostomy collar is adjusted to keep the collar on top of the tracheostomy. With both the T-piece and tracheostomy collar, the goal is to provide a high enough flow rate to ensure that there is a minimum amount of entrained room air.

flow non-rebreather mask, the highest concentration. If a patient's PaO_2 and SaO_2 cannot be maintained using the non-rebreather mask, respiratory failure, with the need for intubation and mechanical ventilation, is imminent.

Complications of Oxygen Delivery

The delivery of oxygen can cause patients discomfort, skin breakdown, and other complications. Long-term oxygen by nasal cannula, even with humidification, can cause dry mucous membranes, epistaxis, or infection in the nares. Nasal cannula tubing, face masks (including the straps), and tracheostomy collars can cause skin breakdown along the face, bridge of the nose, back of the neck, or behind the ears. Oxygen delivery can fail if the tubing is disconnected from the wall, leading to hypoxia with dysrhythmias or increased dyspnea. The edematous or malnourished patient is at higher risk for alteration in skin integrity, and contaminated oxygen delivery devices should be replaced. Contamination can occur with copious secretions coughed onto a tracheostomy collar or with mucus on any other device used. A "no smoking" rule must be enforced for all patients while on oxygen therapy to prevent fires.

The nurse routinely inspects the skin and mucous membranes of the mouth and nares for signs of breakdown. Should skin injury occur, further breakdown could be prevented by providing skin barriers or cushions, and possibly changing to another type of device. For example, if the bridge of the nose is irritated by a face mask, switching to a nasal cannula may relieve the discomfort to the nose, as long as the patient receives the same oxygen level. The mask may cause some patients anxiety with the feeling of suffocation, and, as with all devices, the nurse should ensure the patient's comfort. Finally, disposable humidification systems need to be changed according to manufacturer specifications to prevent infections from the systems. Oxygen humidification sets for any device are routinely changed at least every 72 hours. The key to preventing any complication, including hypoxemia, is accurate and timely assessment of oxygenation parameters and monitoring for complications of the therapies by the nurse.

Oxygen toxicity starts to occur in patients breathing a concentration of more than 50% for longer than 25 hours. Patients who are ventilated with high oxygen concentrations for prolonged periods are at risk for oxygen toxicity. To prevent the pathological cellular changes of oxygen toxicity, the patient's FIO_2 should be decreased as tolerated to the lowest possible setting as long as the PaO_2 remains greater than 60 mm Hg. The pathophysiological changes with oxygen toxicity occur at the alveolar level and may progress from capillary leakage to pulmonary edema and possibly to ALI if the high FIO_2 continues for several days. Once the oxygen concentration is decreased to safer levels, the pathophysiological cellular changes may reverse, but if high FIO_2 levels continue, there may be permanent cellular changes and pulmonary function impairment.

Carbon dioxide narcosis is a risk in patients with COPD who are "sensitive" to oxygen, and an increased FIO_2 may result in an elevated $PaCO_2$, hypoventilation, and respiratory depression or respiratory arrest. Oxygen must therefore be administered with caution to patients with COPD and often at low levels to prevent respiratory depression. Absorptive atelectasis may develop in patients on high FIO_2. Absorptive atelectasis is a result of less nitrogen in the delivered gas mixture. Because nitrogen is not absorbed, it normally exerts a pressure in the alveoli, keeping the alveoli open. When nitrogen is "washed out," the oxygen replacing it is absorbed, resulting in alveolar collapse (atelectasis).

Respiratory arrest is a complication that can occur even in patients on oxygen therapy. Nurses prevent this complication by monitoring the patient's overall respiratory status, neurologic assessment, vital signs with SaO_2, and ABGs to evaluate for signs of impending respiratory failure. Respiratory arrest can also occur for reasons such as mucus plugging in the tracheobronchial airways, or plugging of a tracheostomy or endotracheal tube. Respiratory failure from fatigue due to increased work of breathing can occur quickly in a patient with pulmonary compromise, such as a patient with COPD and new-onset pneumonia. Aspiration of food or gastric contents can also lead to respiratory arrest and occurs regularly in hospitalized patients with dysphagia (e.g., from a stroke or secondary to prolonged intubation with vocal cord paralysis). The nurse must monitor the vulnerable patient more frequently when there is a clear comorbidity that may result in respiratory failure or arrest.

ARTIFICIAL AIRWAYS

Rigorous bronchial hygiene and carefully monitored oxygen therapy may eliminate the need for an artificial airway or ventilatory support. An artificial airway and ventilatory support become mandatory if these measures fail to provide adequate oxygenation and removal of carbon dioxide. Artificial airways have a fourfold purpose:

- Establishment of an airway
- Protection of the airway, with the cuff inflated
- Provision of continuous ventilatory assistance
- Facilitation of airway clearance

Knowledgeable, aggressive nursing care is required to maintain airway patency, maximize therapeutic effects, and minimize damage to the patient's natural airway.

The selection of the appropriate artificial airway is important. Because all artificial airways increase airway resistance, it is essential that the largest tube possible be used for intubation. The cuff on the endotracheal or tracheostomy tube must be very compliant (soft) so that trauma to the trachea, vocal cords, and subglottic area is minimized. The competency of the cuff must be established before intubation. Approximately 10 mL of air is injected into the cuff before use, and the clinician checks for leaks.

Nasopharyngeal and Oropharyngeal Airways

If a patient is sedated and lying supine or becomes unconscious, tongue and airway muscle tone is decreased, causing the tongue to occlude the airway. Although an oropharyngeal or nasopharyngeal airway maintains the air passage, it does not eliminate the potential for aspiration. Figure 25-3 illustrates some frequently used artificial airways. The nasopharyngeal airway (nasal trumpet) is a flexible tube that is inserted nasally past the base of the tongue to maintain airway patency. This airway may be better tolerated than the oropharyngeal airway in patients with an intact gag reflex.

OROPHARYNGEAL AIRWAY

An oropharyngeal airway is never placed in a conscious patient, because it stimulates the gag reflex and can cause vomiting and aspiration. Before placing an artificial airway, the nurse makes sure any possible obstruction is cleared. Insertion of an oropharyngeal airway follows three steps:

1. Gently open the patient's mouth using a crossed finger technique or a modified jaw thrust.

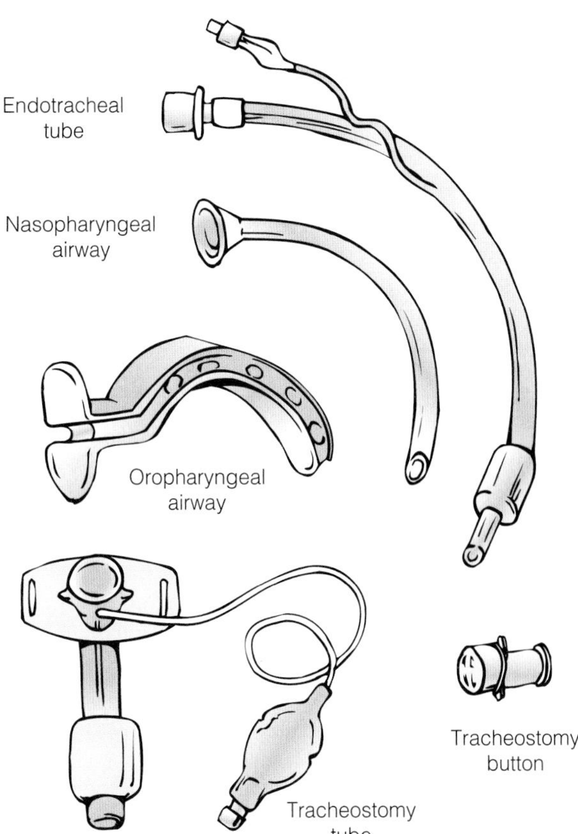

figure 25-3 Five frequently used artificial airways.

2. Hold down the tongue with a depressor and guide the airway over the back of the tongue. (An optional method is to position the tip of the airway toward the roof of the mouth [curved end towards the roof] and gently advance the airway by rotating it 180 degrees.)
3. Monitor the patient frequently for airway patency by listening to breath sounds. Provide oropharyngeal suction as needed for emesis or oral secretions.

Oral suctioning is important to maintain oral hygiene when the patient is intubated because the patient's ability to swallow can be limited. Oral suctioning is done as needed for copious oral secretions, and after suctioning the endotracheal or tracheostomy tubes to maintain oral hygiene and comfort. Oral care is a routine nursing function that includes removal of posterior oropharyngeal secretions to minimize the buildup of oral secretions on top of the endotracheal tube cuff.

Oral suctioning is performed using a Yankauer device (tonsil-tip suction apparatus). The larger openings on the Yankauer tip allow for suctioning of thick or copious secretions better than other suction catheters designed for suctioning through endotracheal or nasotracheal tubes, which are smaller in diameter. In addition, the smaller suction catheters are flexible, which may cause them to kink. The Yankauer device is angled to allow it to follow the contour of the oral cavity along the palate. This facilitates suctioning in the posterior oropharynx and the buccal pouches, where secretions may collect. After suctioning, the nurse rinses the tubing with tap water to clear it of thick secretions and ensure that the suction will continue to function in the future.

To remove an oropharyngeal airway, the oropharynx is suctioned and the airway is gently removed.

NASOPHARYNGEAL AIRWAY

The insertion of a nasopharyngeal airway involves the following steps:

1. Determine and select the correct tube length by measuring from the tip of the nose to the earlobe. Use a tube with the largest outer diameter that will fit the patient's nostril.
2. Lubricate the tube with water, water-soluble jelly, or lidocaine jelly, which will alleviate discomfort.
3. Reassure the patient and familiarize him or her with the procedure.
4. Insert the airway into the nostril up to the end of the nasal trumpet.
5. Have the patient exhale with the mouth closed. (If the tube is in the correct position, air can be felt exiting from the tube opening.)
6. Open the patient's mouth, depress the tongue, and look for the tube's tip just behind the uvula.

In patients who require frequent nasotracheal suctioning, nasopharyngeal airways are frequently used to prevent patient discomfort and airway trauma from repeated suction catheter introduction through the nares. Nasotracheal suctioning is best done using a red rubber suction catheter, which is more flexible and better tolerated than standard plastic catheters. Nasotracheal suctioning is done as a sterile procedure. The catheter is lubricated with water-soluble jelly and passed to the back of the nasopharynx initially. Supplemental oxygen is given before suctioning and in between each suction attempt. The oxygen can be given using a manual resuscitation bag (MRB) with mask and gently bagging with each inspiration to provide a high FIO_2. Other high-flow devices, such as a Venturi mask, may also be used. The nurse or respiratory therapist then asks the patient to cough, which opens the epiglottis and allows the catheter to be advanced. A change in the sound of the cough and the return of sputum with suctioning indicates passage into the tracheal tree. The technique of nasotracheal suctioning is difficult and should be attempted only by experienced practitioners. The novice intensive care unit (ICU) nurse should seek the help of experienced clinicians to learn this skill.

The nasopharyngeal airway may have to be gently rotated to withdraw it from the nares. Be prepared for the potential for epistaxis with nasopharyngeal airway removal.

Endotracheal Tubes

An endotracheal tube is inserted if the patient needs ventilation or protection of the airway from aspiration. Equipment listed in Box 25-4 is assembled before intubation. The endotracheal tube can be inserted nasally or orally. The advantages and disadvantages of each placement are listed in Table 25-1.

To reduce the incidence of complications, personnel with rigorous credentials must perform tracheal intubation. The nurse explains the procedure to the patient and family. The patient is positioned on his or her back with a small blanket under the shoulder blades to hyperextend the neck and open the airway. Air is injected into the endotracheal cuff before insertion to ensure an intact cuff, and then the cuff is deflated. The stylet is a malleable thick wire with a blunt end that is used to stiffen the flexible endotracheal tube for insertion. The end of the stylet must be kept at least 1 inch from the end of the endotracheal tube to prevent perforation of the trachea. The stylet is inserted to the correct position and the remaining stylet is

box 25-4
Equipment for Endotracheal Intubation

- Laryngoscope with blades and intact bulb
- Suction setup with Yankauer suction
- Correct size endotracheal tube with stylet*
- 10-mL syringe for cuff inflation
- Adhesive tape, twill tape, or Velcro endotracheal tube holder
- Magill forceps (may be used with nasal intubation)
- Pulse oximetry
- Oxygen source
- Manual resuscitation bag with mask
- End-tidal CO_2 monitor or disposable detector
- Sedation and paralytic medication

*In adults, tube size is usually 8.0 initially unless the procedure is difficult, the patient is small, or a difficult intubation is anticipated, in which case smaller sizes are used. An endotracheal tube larger than 7.0 mm facilitates bronchoscopy.

table 25-1 Airway Placement

Type	Advantages	Disadvantages
Nasal endotracheal	Patient comfort Prevents tube obstruction from biting Easily anchored and reduced risk of extubation Oral hygiene more effective Used in patients with maxillofacial trauma or cervical spine injuries	Can kink and obstruct airway Predisposes to acute sinusitis, which may result in bacteremia Epistaxis a frequent complication Pressure necrosis of the nares Tube and cuff can cause tracheoesophageal fistula, erosion, and vocal chord paralysis High risk for shearing off nasal polyps in patients with asthma
Oral endotracheal	Less trauma during intubation than nasal route Permits use of a larger endotracheal tube* Avoids nasal/sinus complications	Predisposes to mouth sores Uncomfortable for patient Pressure sores develop on lips, gums, and tongue Easily obstructed by biting, necessitates a bite block Tube and cuff can cause tracheal damage, tracheo-esophageal fistula, and vocal chord paralysis Tube, bite block, and tube-securing tape complicate oral hygiene Self-extubation easier (from patient pushing on endotracheal tube with tongue) Difficult to secure (beards, failure of tape to adhere to skin) Makes communication difficult

*Facilitates work of breathing because the larger endotracheal tube allows improved flow, and bronchoscopy is done only with an endotracheal tube of at least 7.5 mm.

bent over the distal end of the endotracheal tube to maintain endotracheal tube stiffness. The physician or other qualified health care professional shapes the endotracheal tube with the stylet to facilitate placement through the vocal cords before insertion.

Before the procedure, the nurse confirms that the suction is working properly. Using an MRB and mask, the nurse preoxygenates the patient. The physician may use topical anesthetics, sedatives, or a short-acting neuromuscular blocking agent to facilitate rapid and nontraumatic intubation. Newer, short-acting intravenous anesthetics facilitate rapid intubation, and a lidocaine bolus reduces the reflex to cough.

The nurse assists during intubation by providing suction as necessary and monitoring the patient's SaO_2 by pulse oximetry, as well as the patient's heart rate and blood pressure. Intubation attempts should be held and the patient oxygenated with the MRB if the SaO_2 falls below 90%. Hypoxemia during intubation may cause bradycardia, hypotension, dysrhythmias, and other complications.

After placement of the endotracheal tube, the cuff is inflated. The chest is auscultated bilaterally for equal breath sounds, and the abdomen is auscultated for evidence of esophageal intubation. Waterproof tape is used to secure the endotracheal tube, and the centimeter mark is noted at the lips, teeth, or nares for the nasotracheal tube. The level of the endotracheal tube must be noted to prevent changing of position, which could result either in right mainstem bronchus placement with left lung collapse or self-extubation. A portable chest x-ray is obtained immediately after the insertion to confirm proper tube placement, which is about 2 to 3 cm above the carina (but below the clavicular heads, as appropriate).

Complications of endotracheal tube placement are noted in Box 25-5. Initially during intubation, complications of hypoxemia, gastric intubation, mainstem intubation, and oral or tracheal tissue damage can occur. Vomiting during the procedure can lead to aspiration with resultant lung injury. If the patient has prolonged hypoxemia and hypercapnia (as might result with a difficult intubation), dysrhythmias such as bradycardia or tachycardia can occur, possibly leading to hypotension or hypertension.

Once the patient is intubated, potential complications include disconnection, failure of the ventilator, tube obstruction, sinusitis, and tracheoesophageal fistula. Vocal chord paralysis or laryngeal or tracheal stenosis may present after extubation. Accidental extubation in a critically ill patient is a preventable complication. The most challenging cases involve confused patients who attempt to self-extubate. Orienting the patient to the need for the endotracheal tube and offering assurances that you will help make him or her more comfortable are the first

box 25-5 *Complications of Intubation*

- Laryngospasm/bronchospasm
- Hypoxemia/hypercapnia during intubation
- Laryngeal edema resulting in stridor with extubation
- Trauma/bleeding to nasal, oral, esophageal, tracheal, or laryngeal sites
- Fractured teeth
- Nosocomial infection (pneumonia, sinusitis, abscess)
- Displacement of tube (right mainstem intubation, gastric intubation)
- Aspiration of oral or gastric contents
- Tracheal stenosis/tracheomalacia
- Laryngeal damage, paralysis, and necrosis
- Dysrhythmias, hypertension, hypotension

interventions. Occasionally, physical or pharmacological restraints are necessary.

Many of the complications can be avoided by ensuring adequate fixation of the endotracheal tube, securing ventilator tubing properly, suctioning only as needed, and following other care maintenance protocols. These include oral care to remove secretions and maintaining the head of the bed at 30 degrees to help prevent aspiration. Following aseptic policies decreases nosocomial infections, and maintaining proper cuff pressure helps to prevent tracheal erosion. Ultimately, the patient on long-term ventilation may require a tracheostomy to continue ventilatory support and weaning.

SUCTIONING

The presence of an artificial tube prevents glottic closure. As a result, the patient is unable to use the normal clearing mechanism (i.e., effective coughing). In addition, the foreign object increases production of secretions. Suctioning, therefore, becomes paramount for removing secretions and maintaining airway patency. Suctioning is not without risks and should be done only when needed.[8] Complications of suctioning are listed in Box 25-6. Indications for suctioning include visual observation of secretions in the airway, determination of the presence of secretions or mucus plugs by chest auscultation, coughing, an increase in peak airway pressure, a decrease in tidal volume during pressure ventilation, or deterioration of the patient's oxygenation as noted by decreased Sao_2.

The procedure for suctioning is given in Box 25-7. The nurse performs suctioning as a sterile procedure, using practices recommended by the Centers for Disease Control and Prevention. In-line suction catheters are available for use in patients on high levels of positive end-expiratory pressure (PEEP) who do not tolerate disconnection of the ventilator tubing for suctioning. In addition, in-line suction catheters are used for patients with copious secretions requiring frequent suctioning, or those with grossly bloody secretions. Patients who are identified as having the potential for long-term mechanical ventilation and patients who have been reintubated after a failed extubation are candidates for the use of the continuous aspiration of subglottic secretions (CASS) endotracheal tube. This device is used to prevent the subglottic accumulation of secretions that may lead to aspiration, and is discussed later in the section on ventilator-associated pneumonia (VAP).[9]

box 25-6 *Complications of Suctioning*

- Hypoxemia
- Dysrhythmias
- Vagal stimulation (bradycardia, hypotension)
- Bronchospasm
- Elevated intracranial pressure (ICP)
- Atelectasis
- Tracheal mucosal trauma
- Bleeding
- Nosocomial infection

box 25-7 *Procedure for Suctioning*

Equipment

Sterile suction catheter
Sterile gloves
Sterile normal saline for irrigation, when indicated
Sterile disposable container

Technique

1. Perform routine procedures before suctioning: Administer medication, assemble equipment, explain the procedure to the patient, adjust bed to comfortable working position, prepare suction pressure, wash hands, and don gloves.
2. Hyperoxygenate the patient with 100% oxygen, using a manual resuscitation bag (MRB) or the ventilator. If the ventilator method is used, preoxygenation must last at least 2 minutes. Return to the previous oxygen setting after suctioning is completed. (Clinical research shows that the use of the patient's ventilator for preoxygenation delivers higher oxygen concentrations and lower peak pressures than those generated with an MRB).[5] In patients who do not tolerate suctioning with hyperoxygenation, a positive end-expiratory pressure (PEEP) attachment should be on the MRB at the appropriate setting, or in-line suctioning should be used to avoid loss of PEEP and desaturation.
3. Quickly but gently insert the catheter as far as possible into the artificial airway without application of suction.
4. Withdraw the catheter 1 to 2 cm, and apply intermittent suction while rotating and removing the catheter. Limit suction pressure to –80 to –120 mm Hg. Aspiration should not exceed 10 to 15 seconds. (Prolonged aspiration can lead to severe hypoxia, hemodynamic instability, and, ultimately, cardiac arrest.)
5. Hyperoxygenate the patient before and after each subsequent pass of the catheter for at least 30 seconds, and before reconnection to the ventilator.
6. Monitor heart rate and rhythm and pulse oximetry during and after suctioning.
7. Discontinue the procedure if the patient does not tolerate it, as evidenced by dysrhythmias, bradycardia, or a drop in Sao_2.
8. Remove equipment.
9. Perform oral hygiene. Clean suction tubing.
10. Wash your hands.
11. Document procedure.

HYPEROXYGENATION AND SALINATION

The patient must be hyperoxygenated using the ventilator set to 100% if an in-line system is used. Patients not on ventilators also need to be hyperoxygenated before suctioning. The patient should be instructed to take deep breaths while connected to a 100% oxygen source. Patients incapable of taking a deep breath should be assisted using an MRB with mask, timing a squeeze on the MRB with the patient's own breath.[10] The presence of epiglottitis or croup is an absolute contraindication to any kind of suctioning of patients without an artificial airway. The routine instillation of normal saline has become increasingly questionable. In a test tube, saline and sputum act like oil and water, and they do not form a mixture. Therefore, it is unlikely that saline instillation liquefies or increases the amount of sputum obtained during suction. In addition, saline instillation causes oxygenation to decrease and may predispose patients to nosocomial infection by transporting bacteria to lower airways.[11–13]

Endotracheal tube care and cuff pressure monitoring are discussed in more detail later in this chapter, in the section on assessment and management of the ventilated patient. Once the patient is intubated, the patient loses the ability to communicate easily. This inability to communicate can become a major stressor during the ventilated period.

CHEST TUBES

The chest tube is a drain. Its purposes are to remove air, fluid, or blood from the pleural space; restore negative pressure to the pleural space; re-expand a collapsed or partially collapsed lung; and prevent reflux of drainage back into the chest.

Physiological Principles

A short review of chest anatomy and pleural pressures is provided for an understanding of chest tubes and drainage systems.

CHEST ANATOMY

The chest is composed of three compartments: the mediastinum, a right pleural cavity, and a left pleural cavity. Each pleural cavity is lined with a thin, slippery membrane called the *parietal pleura.* A similar membrane covers the lung and is called the *visceral pleura.* A thin layer of fluid with a total volume of 5 to 15 mL acts as a lubricant between the visceral and parietal pleurae, allowing them to slide smoothly over each other during breathing.

Pleural fluid is secreted by capillaries of the parietal pleura and removed by the lymphatics of the parietal pleura. Pleural fluid can come from interstitial spaces of the lung through the visceral pleura, or leak from the peritoneal cavity through holes in the diaphragm. Lymphatics can remove approximately 20 times the amount normally secreted.[14] Because the two pleurae lie in contact with each other, the pleural space is a "potential" space only. If the area between these membranes becomes an actual space, the lung collapses.

PLEURAL PRESSURES

The lung is kept expanded within the chest cavity by intrapleural negative pressure. Two opposing forces create the negative pressure. The first is the tendency of the chest wall to spring upward and outward. The second is the tendency of the elastic alveolar tissue to contract. An analogy for these forces is two microscope slides held together by a drop of water placed between them. One is not able to pull the slides apart because of the surface tension of the fluid. Compare the lung to the two slides: one slide is the visceral pleura and the other is the parietal pleura, and the drop of water is pleural fluid. As in the analogy of the slides, the opposing forces attempt to pull the pleurae in different directions. A negative pressure is generated that holds the lung tightly to the chest wall, preventing lung collapse. During inspiration, the intrapleural pressures become more negative, favoring the flow of gas into the lungs. On expiration, the pressures become less negative (increasing toward atmospheric pressure), and gas flows out of the lungs (Table 25-2).

table 25-2 The Effect of Breathing on Intrapleural Pressure

Ventilation Cycle	Intrapleural Pressures
At rest	–5 cm H_2O
Inspiration	–6 to –12 cm H_2O
Expiration	–4 to –8 cm H_2O

All gases move from an area of higher pressure to an area of lower pressure. During inspiration, the chest cavity enlarges through diaphragmatic contraction. This increases lung space and causes intrapleural pressure to fall below atmospheric pressure (760 mm Hg at sea level). Air flows down a pressure gradient, from the relatively high atmospheric pressure into the area of low pressure in the lungs. During expiration, this process is reversed. The diaphragm recoils, decreasing the space in the chest cavity and compressing the lungs. Intrapleural pressure is now higher than atmospheric pressure, causing air to move out of the lungs. After the respiratory muscles relax, the pressure between the outside air and the lungs is equalized, and there is no air movement between breaths.

Equipment

Equipment needed for chest tube insertion is listed in Box 25-8.

box 25-8
Equipment for Chest Tube Insertion

- Chest tube tray or thoracotomy tray (with scalpel)
- Chest tube
- 1% Lidocaine
- Antiseptic (povidone–iodine)
- Sterile gloves
- Large hemostats
- Suture material (0-0 or 2-0 silk) on a cutting needle
- Bacteriostatic ointment or petroleum gauze
- Sterile gauze with a slit
- Tape—both wide and narrow, or an occlusive dressing
- Chest tube drainage system and suction
- Sterile water for water-seal systems
- Medication for pain and sedation

CHEST TUBE

Most chest tubes are multifenestrated, transparent tubes with distance and radiopaque markers. This enables the physician or other qualified health care professional to visualize the tube on chest x-ray and position it correctly in the pleural space. All openings in the tube must be placed within the rib cage to ensure that air leaks do not develop either in subcutaneous tissue or outside the chest wall. Chest tubes are categorized as pleural or mediastinal, depending on the location of the tube's tip. Patients can have more than one tube in different locations, depending on the purposes of the tubes.

Larger tubes (20 to 36 French) are used to drain blood or thick pleural secretions. Smaller tubes (16 to 20 French) are used to remove air.

DRAINAGE SYSTEM

To reestablish intrapleural negative pressure, a seal for the chest tube that prevents outside air from entering the system is required. The simplest way to accomplish this is to use an underwater system of drainage. A review of multichamber systems can provide a basis for understanding all of the commonly used disposable drainage units. Knowledge of these systems enables the nurse to safely manage the most complex chest tube drainage setup. Modern chest drainage systems are composed of disposable materials and may be configured in either two- or three-chamber systems. The two-chamber system has a water seal and a collection chamber, whereas the three-chamber system adds a suction control chamber.

Two-Chamber System

In a two-chamber system, the first chamber is the collection receptacle and the second chamber is the water seal. In a disposable system that requires water, sterile water is added to the second chamber to the 2-cm level to achieve the seal. This level represents the negative pressure that is exerted on the pleural space as the water closes the chest drain to outside air, acting as a one-way valve. The water seal allows air to escape, while preventing outside air from entering the pleural space. A fluid level higher than 2 cm of water exerts a greater negative pressure on the pleural space and may prevent resolution of the air leak. In addition, a higher column of water in the water seal chamber can make breathing more difficult because the patient has a longer column fluid to move during respiration. Figure 25-4 depicts disposable chest drainage systems.

The patient's chest tube is connected to a 6-foot length of latex tubing that is attached to an outlet on the top of the drainage collection chamber. The second chamber (the water seal) has a vent that remains open, allowing air from the pleural space to escape as it bubbles through the water seal to the atmosphere. Except for the vented cap, the drainage system from the chest tube insertion site to the bottle is airtight.

The fluid level in the water seal fluctuates ("tidals") during respiration. During inspiration, pleural pressures become more negative, causing the fluid level in the water seal chamber to rise. During expiration, pleural pressures become more positive, causing the fluid level to descend. If the patient is being mechanically ventilated, this process is reversed. Bubbling should be seen in the underwater seal chamber only during expiration (or during inspiration with positive-pressure ventilation) as air and fluid drain from the pleural cavity. Constant bubbling indicates either an air leak in the system or a bronchopleural fistula, as discussed later in the section on Assessment and Management.

Three-Chamber System

In the three-chamber system, a suction control chamber is added to the two-chamber system. This is the safest way to regulate the amount of suction. The third bottle is configured similarly to the underwater seal chamber. In a disposable system that requires water, suction is achieved by adding water to the prescribed level in the suction chamber, usually –20 cm.

In this system, it is the height of the water column in the third chamber, and not the amount of wall suction, that determines the amount of suction applied to the chest tube, most commonly –20 cm H_2O. Once the wall suction exceeds the force necessary to "lift" this column of fluid, any additional suction simply pulls air from a vented cap atop the chamber up through the water. The amount of wall suction applied to the third chamber should be sufficient to create a "gently rolling" bubble in the suction control chamber. Vigorous bubbling results in water loss, changing suction pressure and increasing the noise level in the patient's room. It is important to assess for water loss and to add sterile water as necessary to maintain the prescribed level of suction. The bubbling should be assessed for gentle action, and the water level (–20 cm H_2O) assessed every 8 hours and when the patient's clinical picture changes.

SUCTION

Dry suction (waterless) systems use a spring mechanism to control the suction level and can provide higher levels of suction with easier setup.[15] The dry suction systems can be easily adjusted for any setting between –10 and –40 cm H_2O, and allow for safer use if the device is accidentally tipped over. If this happens, the drainage can be returned to the correct collection chamber without replacing the unit, resulting in cost savings. Dry suction systems that can deliver higher levels of suction may be necessary in patients with large bronchopleural fistulas, hemorrhage, or obesity.

The Emerson Pleural Suction Pump may be used instead of wall suction. It can be set up using a two- or three-bottle system, as well as disposable chest drainage systems. In contrast to the wall unit, the pressure control knob on the front of the pump controls the suction generated. The amount of pressure is registered on the suction dial.

Heimlich valves are reserved for the treatment of pneumothoraces (usually spontaneous or traumatic) on an outpatient basis or in the field by paramedics. The valve is composed of a small-bore chest tube attached to a one-way valve, which is enclosed in a plastic case. The one-way valve allows air to escape, but not re-enter, the pleural space. The Heimlich valve is not appropriate for fluid removal.[16]

Chest Tube Placement

If injury, surgery, or any disruption in the integrity of the lungs and chest cavity occurs, placement of a chest tube is warranted. In addition, iatrogenic pneumothorax can

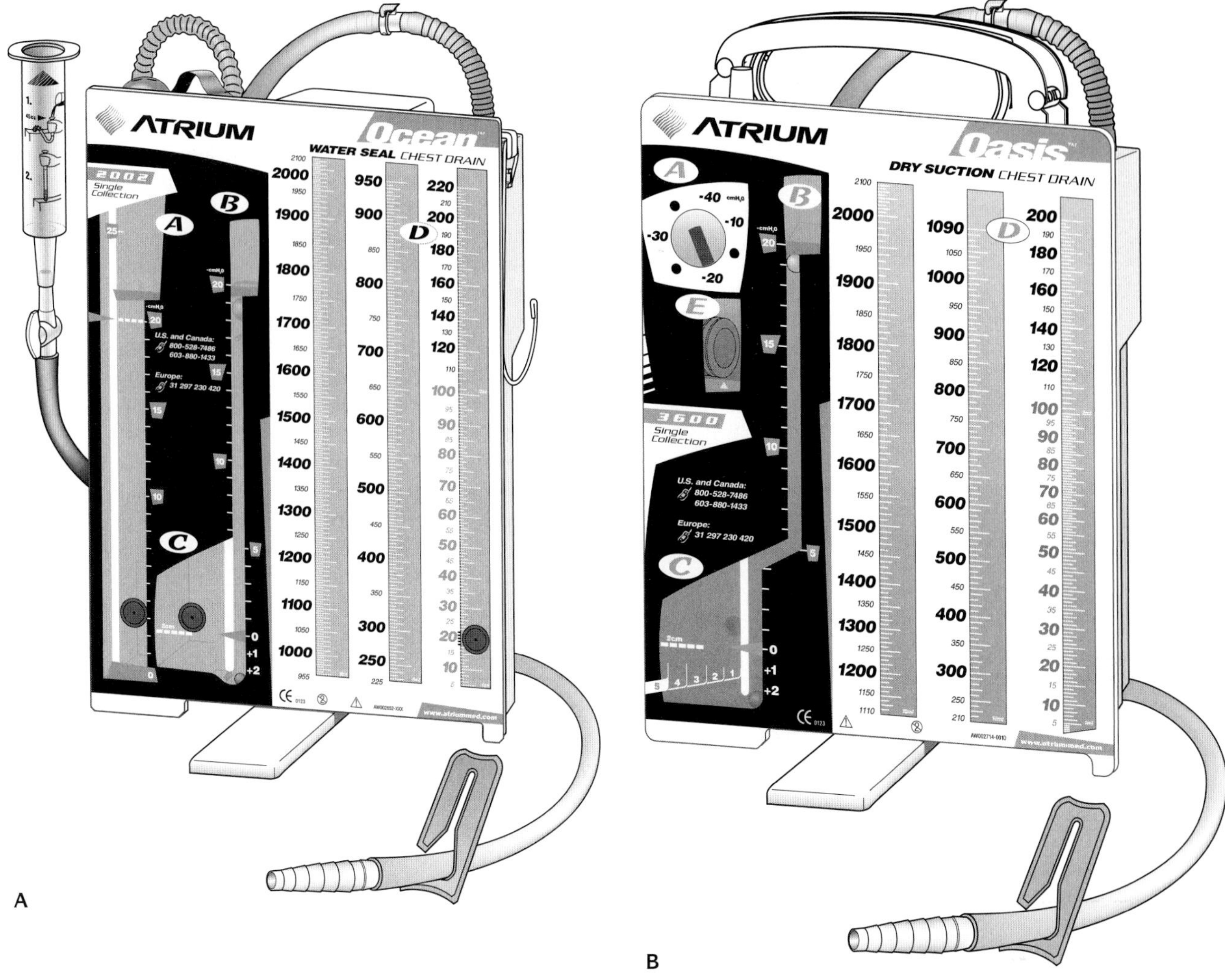

figure 25-4 Chest tube drainage systems. (**A**) The Atrium Ocean™ is an example of a water seal chest drain system composed of a drainage chamber and water seal chamber. The suction control is determined by the height of the water column in that chamber (usually 20 cm). (*A*, suction control chamber; *B*, water seal chamber; *C*, air leak zone; and *D*, collection chamber). (**B**) The Atrium Oasis™ is an example of a dry suction water seal system that uses a mechanical regulator for vacuum control, a water seal chamber, and a drainage chamber. (*A*, dry suction regulator; *B*, water seal chamber; *C*, air leak monitor; D, collection chamber; and *E*, suction monitor bellows.) Courtesy of Atrium Medical Corporation, Hudson, New Hampshire.

occur in the ICU during thoracic central line placement, thoracentesis, or cardiopulmonary resuscitation (CPR), or after transbronchial lung biopsy. Indications for chest tube placement are listed in Table 25-3.

Chest tube insertion can be accomplished in the operating room, in the emergency department, or at the bedside. Placement is based on the principle that because of their different densities and weights, air rises and liquid sinks. The insertion site for air removal is near the second intercostal space along the mid-clavicular line. The insertion site for liquid drainage is near the fifth or sixth intercostal space on the mid-axillary line. Fluid may occasionally become loculated (walled off), requiring ultrasonography or computed tomography (CT) guidance for drainage tube placement. After heart surgery, placement can be in the mediastinum to drain blood from around the heart.

The nurse prepares the patient and family for the procedure, answering any questions they may have. The nurse also prepares the patient physically. Because parietal pleurae are innervated from the intercostal and phrenic nerves, this is a painful procedure, and administration of analgesics is indicated. The patient is positioned in a Fowler's or semi-Fowler's position. After the skin has been cleaned and anesthetized, the physician or other qualified health care professional makes a small skin incision. A hemostat is used to penetrate the pleural space (Fig. 25-5). The tract made by the hemostat is then dilated with a finger. The proximal end of the tube is clamped with the hemostat and then inserted into the pleural space. If the placement is difficult, a metal trocar can be used to penetrate the chest wall, leaving the tube in place and removing the trocar.

After insertion, the external end of the tube is connected to a chest drainage unit. It is important to remember that the ends of both the chest tube and the drainage system tubing must remain sterile as they are connected. To prevent the tube from dislodging, the tube is sutured to the skin

table 25-3 Indications for Chest Tube Placement

Indication	Cause
Hemothorax	Chest trauma Neoplasms Pleural tears Excessive anticoagulation Post-thoracic surgery/open lung biopsy
Pneumothorax	
Spontaneous: >20%	Bleb rupture Symptomatic patient Presence of lung disease
Tension	Mechanical ventilation Penetrating puncture wound Prolonged clamping of chest tubes Lack of seal in chest tube drainage system
Bronchopleural fistula	Tissue damage Tumor Aspiration of toxic chemicals
Pleural effusion	Neoplasms Serious cardiopulmonary disease Inflammatory conditions
Chylothorax	Trauma Malignancy Congenital abnormalities

around the insertion site. The ends of the suture are wrapped around the tube and tied off. Bacteriostatic ointment or petroleum gauze can be applied to the incision site. Petroleum gauze has been preferred because it is thought to prevent air leaks; however, it also has the potential to macerate the skin and predispose the site to infection. A 4×4 gauze pad with a split is positioned over the tube and taped occlusively to the chest. All connections from the insertion site to the drainage collection system are securely taped to prevent air leaks, as well as inadvertent disconnection. The proximal tube is taped to the chest to prevent traction on the tube and sutures if the patient moves.

A postinsertion chest x-ray is always ordered to confirm proper positioning. The lungs are auscultated, and the condition of the tissue around the insertion site is evaluated for the presence of subcutaneous air. This assessment provides a baseline for determining improvement or worsening of the patient's condition. Daily chest radiographs may be necessary, or are obtained as needed to assess the clinical picture. Pain management continues to be an issue throughout the duration of chest tube use. Dressings are changed per institutional protocol, or as needed if soiled or loose.

Chest tubes are removed after drainage is minimal and 12 to 25 hours after placing the chest tube to water seal. Placement to water seal only (without suction) identifies persistent air leaks or reaccumulation of fluid with a repeat chest x-ray. Other indications for removal of the chest tube are listed in Box 25-9. When the tube is placed to water seal, disconnect the suction tube to facilitate atmospheric venting. Premature clamping or removal of the tube may cause reaccumulation of the pneumothorax.

Before removing the chest tube, the patient is placed in a Fowler's or semi-Fowler's position. Premedication is recommended to alleviate pain and discomfort. The dressing over the insertion site is removed and the area is cleaned. The suture is clipped. The tube is removed in one quick movement at peak inspiration or during expiration to prevent entraining air back into the pleural cavity through the chest tube eyelets. Immediately after tube removal, the lung fields are auscultated for any change in breath sounds, and an occlusive sterile dressing is applied over the site. A chest x-ray is usually obtained several hours later to look for the presence of residual air or fluid.

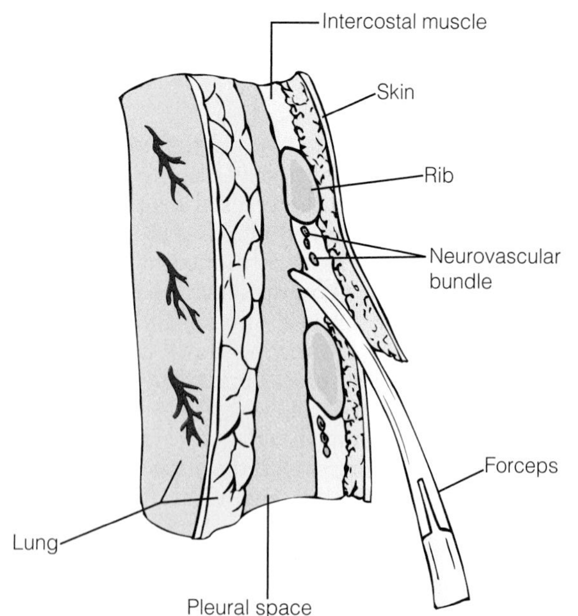

figure 25-5 Forceps penetrate the pleural space to create a track for the chest tube.

Assessment and Management

Nursing care is directed at maintaining patency and proper functioning of the chest tube drainage system. Vigilant and expert nursing care can prevent serious complications in the patient with a chest tube and drainage system. The latex tubing is frequently drained into the collection container. Coiling the latex tubing loosely on the bed prevents kinks and pooling of blood in a dependent loop hanging on the floor. The chest tube drainage system is never raised

box 25-9
Indications for Chest Tube Removal

- One day after cessation of air leak
- Drainage of less than 50–100 mL of fluid per day
- 1–3 days post cardiac surgery
- 2–6 days post thoracic surgery
- Obliteration of empyema cavity
- Serosanguineous drainage from around the chest tube insertion site

above the chest or the drainage will back up into the chest. At frequent intervals, the chest tube drainage system is checked for drainage, suction level, and water seal integrity. The system should be secured to the foot of the patient's bed or taped to the floor to avoid accidental overturning and possible reaccumulation of the pneumothorax. All tubing connections should be inspected for leaks and secured with tape to prevent accidental disconnection.

To check for chest tube patency and respiratory cycle fluctuations, the suction must be momentarily disconnected (system placed only to water seal—not clamped). Use a step-by-step system to evaluate and troubleshoot the system:

1. Assess cardiopulmonary status and vital signs every 2 hours and as needed.
2. Check and maintain tube patency every 2 hours and as needed.
3. Monitor type and amount of drainage.
4. Mark amount of drainage on collection chamber in hourly or shift increments and document in output record.
5. Prevent dependent loops from forming in tubing.
6. Refill water systems with sterile water to the water seal level and prescribed suction level (secondary to evaporation).
7. Assess for tidaling in the water seal chamber with respiration or mechanical ventilation breaths.
8. Assess for the location of air leaks (constant bubbling in the water seal chamber). Turn off the suction. Begin at the insertion site; occlude the chest tube or drainage tube (briefly) below each connection point until the drainage unit is reached.
9. Check that all tubing connections are securely sealed and taped.
10. Assess the patient for pain, intervene as needed, and reassess appropriately.
11. Assess the actual chest tube insertion site for signs of infection and subcutaneous emphysema with dressing changes.
12. Change the dressing every other day or per unit guideline, when soiled, and when ordered.[17]

DRAINAGE MONITORING

The nurse assesses and documents the color, consistency, and amount of drainage, while remaining alert to significant changes. A sudden increase indicates hemorrhage or sudden patency of a previously obstructed tube. A sudden decrease indicates chest tube obstruction or failure of the chest tube or drainage system. The following nursing actions are recommended to reestablish chest patency:

- Attempt to alleviate the obstruction by repositioning the patient.
- If the clot is visible, straighten the tubing between the chest and drainage unit and raise the tube to enhance the effect of gravity.

Studies have suggested that milking and stripping techniques may not be beneficial for maintenance of chest tube patency.[17] These techniques may excessively increase intrapleural and intrapulmonary pressures, affecting ventricular function or causing trauma from aspiration of lung tissue into chest tube eyelets. However, this procedure may be necessary in cases of active bleeding to prevent blood clotting in the tubing that could lead to cardiac or pleural tamponade.[17]

WATER SEAL MONITORING

Monitoring the water seal of the chest tube drainage system is as important as observing the drainage. Visual checks are made to ensure water seal chambers are filled to the 2-cm water line. If suction is applied, the nurse ensures the water line in the suction chamber is at the ordered level (usually −20 cm H_2O) because water evaporates over time, decreasing the amount of suction being applied. Only sterile water should be added to the system. If an Emerson Pleural Suction Pump is used, the suction gauge is checked. The air vent opening must never be occluded. Disconnect the suction tubing briefly to accurately assess the water level in the chamber.

Respiratory fluctuations are observed in the water seal chamber. The absence of fluctuations can indicate that the lung is re-expanded or that there is an obstruction in the system. Continuous vigorous bubbling in the water seal chamber, without suction, indicates continued pneumothorax, or it can indicate the tube has been displaced or disconnected, or the drainage system is damaged. The entire system has to be checked for disconnections and the chest tube inspected to see if it is displaced outside the chest. In the setting of mechanical ventilation at high volumes and pressures, bubbling in a chest tube system that persists may indicate a bronchopleural fistula when there is no pneumothorax or other known cause.

POSITIONING

The ideal position for a patient with a chest tube is semi-Fowler's. Turning the patient every 2 hours enhances air and fluid evacuation. The nurse teaches patients how to support or "splint" the chest wall near the tube insertion site using a pillow, bath blanket, or their arms. Coughing, deep breathing, and ambulation are encouraged. Administration of pain medication before these exercises decreases pain and enhances lung expansion.

Complications

The most serious complication resulting from chest tube placement is tension pneumothorax, which can develop if there is any obstruction in the chest tube drainage system. Clamping chest tubes as a routine practice predisposes patients to this complication. Clamping of chest tubes is recommended in only two situations:

- To locate the source of an air leak if bubbling occurs in the water seal chamber (*clamping is done only momentarily*).
- To replace the chest tube drainage unit (*clamping is done only momentarily*).

If the tube must be clamped, padded hemostats are used to avoid cutting the vinyl chest tube.

Occasionally, the chest tube may fall out or be accidentally pulled out. In such a circumstance, the insertion site is quickly sealed off using petroleum gauze covered with dry gauze and occlusive tape dressing to prevent air from entering the pleural cavity.

Transporting the Patient With Chest Tubes

As in any transport situation for critically ill patients, constant assessment is necessary to prevent inadvertent chest tube removal, resulting in recurrent pneumothorax. Maintain chest drainage system integrity by positioning the drainage system below the level of the chest. Secure the system to the foot of the bed, and ensure that the tubing does not become crushed or kinked. If the system requires suction to evacuate the pleural space, portable suction must be implemented. Frequent assessment of the patient and the drainage system should be done per unit guidelines, and as needed, to check for air leak, dressing integrity, water seal integrity, water level, and drainage.

PHARMACOLOGICAL AGENTS

Bronchodilator Therapy

Asthma is characterized by recurrent airway inflammation and increased hypersensitivity to a wide range of stimuli (noxious fumes and gases, air pollutants, animal dander, extreme cold, and exercise). The hypersensitivity leads to hyperreactivity of the airways with obstruction, with symptoms widely variable even in the same individual. Asthma is an episodic disease with recurrent exacerbations and periods without symptoms. The management goals include symptom control to maintain normal activities, prevention of exacerbations, and minimization of pharmacological side effects and toxicity. Pharmacological therapy is designed around multiple classes of drugs and aimed at reducing inflammation, treating acute symptoms, and maintaining a plan for the short- and long-term therapy. The agents discussed in Table 25-4 include short- and long-acting bronchodilators, corticosteroids, anti-inflammatory agents, and other agents. Bronchospasm may also be present in COPD and can be treated with the same pharmacological agents.

BRONCHODILATORS

Bronchodilators act principally to dilate the airways by relaxing bronchial smooth muscles. The goals of bronchodilator therapy are to relax the airways, mobilize secretions, and reduce mucosal edema. Bronchodilator therapy can be delivered through metered-dose inhalers, preferably with a spacer attachment, or nebulization. Regardless of the mode of delivery, assessment before, during, and after the therapy is essential.

Assessment before and after treatment includes breath sounds, pulse, and respiratory rate. The last two commonly increase during bronchodilator therapy and can remain elevated for as long as 1 to 1.5 hours after treatment. ABGs may be indicated. (In people with asthma, measurement of peak expiratory flow rate with a peak flow meter before and after a treatment measures the improvement in airway obstruction.) Objective evaluation is crucial, but subjective information is also valuable. How does the patient feel? Is breathing better than before the treatment? How long does the effectiveness of the treatments last? What, if any, are the side effects (jitteriness, palpitations, inability to concentrate, increased heart rate), and how long do these symptoms last?

Bronchodilators may be divided into three categories based on their mechanism and site of action. These are beta$_2$-adrenergic agonists, anticholinergic agents, and methylxanthines.

Beta$_2$-Adrenergic Agonists

The bronchodilator effects of beta-adrenergic agonists result from the stimulation of beta$_2$-adrenergic receptors in the bronchial smooth muscle. In addition, these agents may decrease the release of mediators from mast cells and basophils. Beta$_1$-adrenergic receptors in the heart may also be stimulated, leading to undesired cardiac effects. Newer beta agonists are more specific for the beta$_2$ receptor, although they retain some beta$_1$ activity.

Beta agonists may be administered orally or inhaled. Aerosolized or inhaled therapy is preferred. It has been shown to produce comparable bronchodilation and fewer systemic adverse effects.

Beta agonists are the bronchodilators of choice for the treatment of acute exacerbation of asthma because of their rapid onset of action. Beta agonists produce less bronchodilation in patients with COPD than in those with asthma. Albuterol (2.5 to 5 mg diluted in 3 mL normal saline) is the bronchodilator of choice in the acute setting and may be administered on an as-needed basis.[18] Until recently, all available inhaled beta agonists, such as albuterol, had short durations of action (4 to 6 hours). Salmeterol is the first long-acting beta agonist and has a duration of action of 12 hours. Salmeterol cannot be used for acute exacerbations of asthma because of its slow onset of action.

Anticholinergic Agents

Anticholinergic agents produce bronchodilation by reducing intrinsic vagal tone to the airways. They also block reflex bronchoconstriction caused by inhaled irritants.

Atropine is the prototype anticholinergic agent but is used infrequently. It is readily absorbed from the respiratory tract but produces unwanted systemic effects (e.g., blurred vision, drying of respiratory secretions, tachycardia, anxiety). Ipratropium, a quaternary amine that is not well absorbed from the respiratory tract, produces fewer systemic adverse effects and has taken the place of atropine. It is most effective in patients with COPD when used on a regular basis. It decreases submucosal gland secretion and relaxes bronchial smooth muscle. Ipratropium should not be used alone in acute exacerbations because of its slower onset of effect compared with beta agonists. It has been shown to be effective during status asthmaticus when administered through a nebulizer in combination with beta agonists.

Methylxanthines

The use of methylxanthines in the treatment of bronchospastic airway disease is controversial. The mechanism of action of these agents is poorly understood. They inhibit phosphodiesterase, an enzyme that catalyzes the breakdown of cyclic adenosine monophosphate. They may also possess some degree of anti-inflammatory activity and may augment respiratory muscle contractility.

Theophylline, the prototype methylxanthine, may be used chronically in the treatment of bronchospastic disease but is usually considered third- or fourth-line therapy.

table 25-4 Action, Dosage, and Side Effects of Pulmonary Drugs

Agent	Usual Dose	Common Adverse Effects	Comments
Albuterol (Proventil, Ventolin)	*Aerosol* 1–2 inhalations every 4–6 h *Solution for inhalation* 2.5 mg tid–qid	Palpitations, tachycardia, anxiety, irritability, tremor, GI upset, cough, dry mouth, hoarseness, flushing, headache	Shake well before using; allow 1 full minute between inhalations.
Metaproterenol (Alupent, Metaprel)	*Inhaler* 2–3 inhalations every 3–4 h Maximum dose: 12 inhalations daily *Solution for inhalation* One treatment every 4–6 h	Palpitations, tachycardia, anxiety, irritability, tremor, GI upset, cough, dry mouth, hoarseness, flushing, headache	Shake well before using; allow 1 full minute between inhalations.
Salmeterol (Serevent)	*Asthma/bronchospasm* 1–2 inhalations every 12 h Maximum dose: 4 inhalations daily	Palpitations, tachycardia, anxiety, irritability, tremor, GI upset, cough, dry mouth, hoarseness, flushing, headache	Shake well before using; allow 1 full minute between inhalations; should not be used for relief of acute asthmatic symptoms.
Terbutaline (Brethine, Bricanyl)	*Asthma/bronchospasm* *Aerosol* 1–2 inhalations every 4–6 h	Palpitations, tachycardia, anxiety, irritability, tremor, GI upset, cough, dry mouth, hoarseness, flushing, headache	Shake well before using; allow 1 full minute between inhalations.
Beclomethasone (Beclovent, Vanceril)	2 inhalations tid–qid or 4 inhalations bid Maximum dose: 20 inhalations daily	Throat irritation, hoarseness, coughing, dry mouth, oral thrush; adrenal suppression with large doses over a prolonged period; rare cases of immediate and delayed hypersensitivity reactions	Use bronchodilator therapy several minutes before using inhaled steroid therapy to enhance penetration.
Methylprednisolone (Solu-Medrol)	125 mg IV every 6 h initially; dose tapered according to patient response; may switch to oral prednisone when tapering	Hyperglycemia, impaired immune response, hypertension, fluid retention, psychosis, steroid myopathy, fragile skin	Long-term use should be avoided due to adverse effects.
Prednisone (Deltasone)	40–60 mg qid initially then taper based on patient response	Hyperglycemia, impaired immune response, hypertension, fluid retention, osteoporosis, hyperkalemia	Long-term oral therapy should be avoided if possible; inhaled therapy is preferred for chronic use if necessary.
Triamcinolone (Azmacort)	2 inhalations tid–qid Maximum dose: 16 inhalations daily	Throat irritation, hoarseness, coughing, dry mouth, oral thrush; adrenal suppression with large doses over a prolonged period	Use bronchodilator therapy several minutes before using inhaled steroid therapy to enhance penetration.
Ipratropium (Atrovent)	Initial dose: 2 inhalations qid Maximum dose: 12 inhalations daily	*Aerosol/inhalation solution* Cough, dry mouth, nervousness, agitation, dizziness, headache, GI upset, palpitations, urinary retention, constipation, worsening narrow angle glaucoma	Must be used regularly to achieve benefit in patients with COPD.
Cromolyn (Intal, Gastrocrom, Nasalcrom)	20 mg inhaled capsule or nebulizer solution or 2 sprays of aerosol qid	Lacrimation, urinary frequency, dizziness, headache, rash, cough, wheezing, nasal irritation, sneezing, epistaxis, unpleasant taste	Must be used regularly to achieve benefit.
Nedocromil (Tilade)	2 inhalations qid	Cough, pharyngitis, rhinitis, bronchospasm, dry mouth, unpleasant taste, GI upset, dizziness, headache	Must be used regularly to achieve benefit.

(continued)

table 25-4 ■ Action, Dosage, and Side Effects of Pulmonary Drugs (Continued)

Agent	Usual Dose	Common Adverse Effects	Comments
Theophylline (Aerolate, Bronkodyl, Elixophyllin, Quibron-T, Slo-bid, Slo-Phyllin, Theo-Dur, Theolair, Uniphyl)	*Asthma/bronchospasm* *Regular release preparations* Initial dose: 16 mg/kg (up to 400 mg) in three to four divided doses *Time-release preparations* Initial dose: 12 mg/kg (up to 400 mg) in two to three divided doses Maximum dose: 13 mg/kg daily	GI irritation, diarrhea, increased gastroesophageal reflux, palpitations, tachycardia, potentiation of diuresis Toxic levels—possible cardiac dysrhythmias, convulsions, and death *Theophylline therapeutic range:* 10–20 mg/L (some references list 5–15 mg/L)	Do not chew or crush enteric-coated or sustained-release capsules or tablets; take at the same time, with or without food each day; do not change from one brand to another without consulting a physician. *Drug–drug interactions:* Agents that may decrease theophylline concentrations include **phenobarbital, phenytoin, ketoconazole, rifampin,** and **smoking**. Agents that may increase theophylline concentrations include **allopurinol, cimetidine, corticosteroids, erythromycin,** and **ciprofloxacin**.
Montelukast (Singulair)	10 mg PO qd PM	Dizziness, fatigue, abdominal pain, rash, asthenia, influenza, cough, nasal congestion	*Drug–drug interactions:* Agents that may decrease montelukast concentrations include **rifampin** and **phenobarbital.**
DNase (Pulmozyme)	2.5 mg inhaled daily	Laryngitis, hoarseness, hemoptysis	Evaluate for thick, tenacious secretions.

Some patients with severe disease who are not controlled with beta agonists, anticholinergics, or anti-inflammatory agents may benefit from theophylline. Aminophylline, the intravenous form of theophylline, is rarely used in acute exacerbations because of the lack of evidence that it is beneficial in this situation.

Theophylline has a narrow therapeutic index. Depending on the clinical situation, serum drug concentration should be monitored to ensure efficacy and prevent toxicity. The accepted therapeutic range is 10 to 20 μg/mL, although some references use 5 to 15 μg/mL.[18] Theophylline interacts with a variety of other medications that may alter its serum concentration. These include erythromycin, ciprofloxacin, and cimetidine. Patients with liver disease or congestive heart failure eliminate theophylline more slowly and may be at an increased risk for development of toxicity. The level should be monitored 12 to 25 hours after the loading dose is administered, and as frequently as clinical condition, liver, and renal function dictate.

ANTI-INFLAMMATORY AGENTS

Anti-inflammatory agents interrupt the development of bronchial inflammation and have a prophylactic or preventive action. They may also reduce or terminate ongoing inflammation in the airway. Anti-inflammatory agents include corticosteroids, mast cell stabilizers, and leukotriene receptor antagonists.

Corticosteroids

Corticosteroids are the most effective anti-inflammatory agents for the treatment of reversible airflow obstruction. Corticosteroid therapy should be initiated simultaneously with bronchodilator therapy because the onset of action may take 6 to 12 hours. They may be administered parenterally, orally, or as aerosols. In acute exacerbations, high-dose parenteral steroids (intravenous methylprednisolone) are used and then tapered as the patient tolerates. Short courses of oral therapy may be used to prevent the progression of acute attacks. Long-term oral therapy is associated with systemic adverse effects and should be avoided if possible. If necessary, the chronic use of inhaled corticosteroids, such as fluticasone, is preferred because of the decreased risk of systemic adverse effects.

Mast Cell Stabilizers

The two available mast cell stabilizers are cromolyn and nedocromil. They are thought to stabilize the mucous membrane and prevent the release of mediators from mast cells. These agents are not indicated for acute exacerbations of asthma because they are used *prophylactically* to prevent acute airway narrowing after exposure to allergens (e.g., exercise, cold air). A 4- to 6-week trial may be required to determine the efficacy in individual patients. The desired end point is to reduce the frequency and severity of asthma attacks and enhance the effects of concomitantly administered bronchodilator and steroid therapy. As a result, it may be possible to decrease the dose of bronchodilators or corticosteroids in patients who respond to mast cell stabilizers.

Leukotriene Receptor Antagonists

Leukotriene receptor antagonists, such as montelukast, may be used in the management of exercise-induced bronchospasm, asthma, allergic rhinitis, and urticaria. These agents block the activity of endogenous inflammatory mediators, particularly leukotrienes. These mediators cause increased vascular permeability, mucus secretion, airway edema, bronchoconstriction, and other inflammatory cell–mediated activities. The leukotriene receptor antagonist is administered once daily and is usually well tolerated. It is not to be administered for acute conditions, but as a part of an ongoing program of therapy.[19]

CYSTIC FIBROSIS AGENT (DNase)

DNase is used in patients with cystic fibrosis to break down molecules in tenacious secretions to facilitate expectoration, as well as decrease the amount of medium for bacterial growth. This also improves gas flow through airways. It is administered as an inhalation daily.[19]

Antibiotics

Pneumonia is often treated empirically until the results of cultures and sensitivities are available. Then, the antibiotic regimen is tailored to eradicate the specific pathogenic organism (Table 25-5). Commonly, broad-spectrum antibiotics or combination therapy is used. The critically ill patient is at increased risk for development of pneumonia owing to mechanical ventilation, decreased immune responses, use of corticosteroids, debilitated general health, and cross-infection by health care workers.

Empirical therapy for community-acquired pneumonia includes therapy directed toward the most common organisms associated with this type of pneumonia. These organisms include *Streptococcus pneumoniae* and *Haemophilus influenzae*. Methicillin-resistant *Staphylococcus aureus* (MRSA) should be suspected in patients admitted to the hospital from a nursing home. *Legionella* should be suspected in patients with severe multilobar pneumonia. Patients infected with the human immunodeficiency virus (HIV) should be empirically treated for *Pneumocystis carinii* pneumonia.

Nosocomial pneumonia is often associated with gram-negative bacilli, such as *Pseudomonas aeruginosa*, or it may be polymicrobial. Aspiration is a concern in mechanically ventilated patients or patients unable to protect their airway. Aspiration pneumonia is associated with anaerobic organisms (e.g., *Actinomyces* species). Atypical organisms (*Mycoplasma pneumoniae*, *Chlamydia pneumoniae*, and *Legionella* species) should also be considered, as should viral infection.

Sedative Agents

Critically ill patients frequently require pharmacological intervention for analgesia, sedation, control of anxiety, and facilitation of mechanical ventilation. The selection of appropriate pharmacological agents is based on the cause of the agitation (Box 25-10), underlying illness, possible adverse effects, history of previous drug use, and cost. Agents most commonly used in the ICU include opiates, benzodiazepines, haloperidol, and propofol (Diprivan) (Table 25-6).

These agents can be given as bolus doses, by continuous infusion, or by using a combination of the two approaches. When administering these agents by continuous infusion, it is important to closely monitor the patient's response and adjust the dose to meet the needs of each individual. This is best done by using an objective pain or sedation rating scale for consistent assessment and documentation of the medication's efficacy. Such a protocol can help prevent the prolonged use of these agents and can lower the cumulative amount required for the control of pain or agitation. This can contribute to a decreased length of hospital stay and decreased length of mechanical ventilation.[20–23]

table 25-5 ■ Antibiotic Therapy in Pulmonary Disease

Pulmonary Infection	Empirical Therapy
Community-acquired pneumonia	Ceftriaxone 1–2 g daily or cefotaxime 2 g every 8 h; adjust dose for renal function
Methicillin-resistant *Staphylococcus aureus* (MRSA) pneumonia	Vancomycin 750–1500 mg every 12 h; adjust dose for weight and renal function
Legionella pneumonia	Erythromycin 1 g every 6 h, azithromycin 500 mg PO or IV
Pneumocystis carinii pneumonia	Trimethoprim/sulfamethoxazole (TMP/SMZ) 15 mg/kg (as TMP) every 6–8 h; adjust dose for renal function
Nosocomial pneumonia	Ceftriaxone 1–2 g daily or ceftazidime 2 g every 8 h; adjust for renal function; used if *Pseudomonas* is suspected Cefotaxime 2 g every 8 h; adjust for renal function
Aspiration pneumonia	Clindamycin 600 mg every 6 h or 900 mg every 8 h Ampicillin/sulbactam 1.5–3 g every 6 h; adjust for renal function Ticarcillin/clavulanate 3.1 g every 4–6 h; adjust for renal function
Mycoplasma pneumoniae pneumonia	Erythromycin 500 mg every 6 h
Chlamydia pneumoniae pneumonia	Doxycycline 100 mg every 12 h Erythromycin 500 mg every 6 h

box 25-10
Etiologies of Agitation in Critically Ill Patients

Pain
Mechanical ventilation
Dyspnea
Hypoxia
Metabolic disarray
Withdrawal from alcohol or drugs
Anxiety
Sleep deprivation
Immobility
Sepsis
Age
Steroid administration
Alzheimer's disease

When using a continuous infusion, if an increase in dosage is necessary, an additional small bolus dose should be given to facilitate rapid increase to the new desired blood level. Patients who have received large amounts of opiates or benzodiazepines for 2 or more weeks must have their dosage tapered gradually to prevent symptoms of withdrawal. As a rule, the dose may be decreased by 20% to 25% a day. Some protocols promote the conversion of benzodiazepine infusions to the oral route before stopping the infusion. This is done to maintain an appropriate level of sedation and to wean patients who have required prolonged sedation.

Neuromuscular Blocking Agents

If metabolic demands and work of breathing continue to compromise ventilatory or hemodynamic stability after maximization of sedation, neuromuscular blocking agents may be required. The goal of therapy with neuromuscular blocking agents is to maximize oxygenation and prevent complications, such as barotrauma (alveolar rupture that can result in death), which can be caused by high ventilatory pressures.

The use of neuromuscular blocking agents is usually required if the pressure-controlled inverse ratio mode of ventilation is used. Neuromuscular blocking agents do *not* possess analgesic or sedative properties. When neuromuscular blocking agents are used, sedation and analgesia are required, along with patient and family education. A chemically paralyzed patient should never be left unattended.

Many recent reports of prolonged paralysis after use of neuromuscular blocking agents have prompted many institutions to initiate protocols for instituting, monitoring, and withdrawing neuromuscular blocking agents. These range from the use of peripheral nerve stimulators to assess the level of neuromuscular blockade, to the routine daily discontinuation of neuromuscular blocking agents to assess neurological status and the need for continued administration.

Commonly used neuromuscular blocking agents are vecuronium (Norcuron), atracurium (Tracrium), and cisatracurium (Nimbex). Each has advantages and disadvantages related to concomitant drug effects, underlying illness, and cost.

VENTILATORY SUPPORT

When a patient is unable to maintain a patent airway, adequate gas exchange, or both, despite aggressive management with the interventions discussed previously, more invasive support with intubation and mechanical ventilation must be considered. This step carries its own risks and imposes significant physical and psychological burdens on the patient and family. Every effort should be made to avoid mechanical ventilation, but it is usually necessary at the point at which respiratory distress becomes respiratory failure.

Respiratory failure is defined as the inability to maintain adequate respiration as measured by arterial blood pH, $Paco_2$, and Pao_2. "Adequate" means a pH greater than 7.25, a $Paco_2$ less than 50 mm Hg, and a Pao_2 greater than 50 mm Hg (even with the patient on oxygen). If the ABGs deteriorate beyond these parameters, mechanical ventilatory support is often indicated. Patients are predisposed to development of acute respiratory failure if any of the systems involved in respiration are compromised or overwhelmed (Table 25-7). The degree of risk for development of respiratory failure depends on the patient's ability to move air, secretions, and oxygenated blood. Often, it

table 25-6 ■ Pharmacological Options in Critically Ill Patients

Agents	Comments	Antagonist
Opiates Morphine sulfate Fentanyl	Can cause hypotension and respiratory distress	Naloxone
Benzodiazepines		
Midazolam	Shorter acting	Flumazenil
Lorazepam	Lower cost	Flumazenil
Haloperidol (Haldol)	Monitoring for prolongation of OT interval, extrapyramidal symptoms needed	
Propofol (Diprivan)	For short-term use; may cause hypotension, bradycardia, myocardial depression; lipid-based: included in nutritional assessment to prevent overfeeding; no analgesic effects	

table 25-7 Possible Events Leading to Respiratory Failure

Body System	Event
Nervous system	Head trauma
Brainstem	Poliomyelitis
Spinal cord and nerves	Cervical (C1–C6) fractures
	Overdose
Muscular system	Myasthenia gravis
Primary—diaphragm	Guillain-Barré
Secondary—respiratory	
Skeletal system	Flail chest
Thorax	Kyphoscoliosis
Respiratory system	Obstruction
Airways	Laryngeal edema
	Bronchitis
	Asthma
Alveoli	Emphysema
	Pneumonia
	Fibrosis
Pulmonary circulation	Pulmonary embolus
Cardiovascular system	Congestive heart failure
	Fluid overload
	Cardiac surgery
	Myocardial infarction
Gastrointestinal system	Aspiration
Hematological system	Disseminated intravascular coagulation
Genitourinary system	Renal failure

is the nurse who initially recognizes the onset of acute respiratory failure. Identification of high-risk patients, serial monitoring and evaluation of respiratory status, and institution of appropriate measures may forestall or negate the need for ventilatory assistance. Before intubation and ventilation, the patient may have required increased FIO_2 to meet his or her oxygen demand.

When ventilatory assistance is required, the objective of mechanical ventilation is to support the patient through an episode of illness. Clinical goals of mechanical ventilation may include reversal of hypoxemia; reversal of acute respiratory acidosis; relief of respiratory distress; prevention or reversal of atelectasis; resting of ventilatory muscles; reduction in systemic oxygen consumption, myocardial oxygen consumption, or both; reduction in intracranial pressure (ICP); and stabilization of the chest wall. Mechanical ventilation is not curative and can actually cause complications (as discussed later in this chapter).

Physiological Principles

To understand the effects of modern mechanical ventilation, the reader is encouraged to review the physiology of normal respirations and lung compliance, as discussed in Chapter 23. The relationship between intrapulmonary pressures during inspiration and expiration is reversed during mechanical ventilation. The ventilator delivers air by pumping it into the patient; therefore, pressures during inspiration are positive. The positive pressure pumped into the lungs results in increased intrathoracic pressures and decreased venous return during inspiration. With the institution of positive end-expiratory pressure (PEEP), even greater pressures are generated during inspiration. During expiration, the pressure in the lungs decreases to the "baseline" PEEP level and continues to be positive throughout expiration. Most patients compensate for this hindrance to venous return by increasing peripheral venous tone. If conditions of decreased sympathetic response (e.g., hypovolemia, drugs, or older age) are present, hypotension may develop. In addition, a large tidal volume (>10 to 12 mL/kg) that generates pressures of 35 cm H_2O or more not only reduces cardiac output, but increases the risk of pneumothorax.

Positive pressure can result in barotrauma. Barotrauma occurs when air leaks from the alveoli into the pleural space; this is called a *pneumothorax.* Another form of lung injury is called *volutrauma* and is caused by delivery of large tidal volumes in patients with stiff, noncompliant lungs. With volutrauma, fractures develop in the alveoli that allow fluid and protein to seep into the lungs. This phenomenon is a form of noncardiogenic pulmonary edema. Lung damage from either barotrauma or volutrauma can increase mortality, especially in susceptible patients (e.g., those with asthma or ARDS). To prevent lung injury, it is important to determine lung compliance so that the ventilatory support can be appropriately adjusted to minimize airway pressures.

COMPLIANCE

Compliance refers to the ability of the lung to distend. In terms of its compliance, the lung is frequently compared with a balloon. Initially, it is hard to inflate a balloon until it is stretched (noncompliant). After repeated inflations, this elastic resistance is lost (overly compliant), and the balloon becomes very easy to blow up. In conditions that reduce the lung's elasticity, such as inflammation, fibrotic changes, or edema, the lung requires more force to inflate. A patient on a ventilator with normal lungs should have a compliance near 100 mL/cm H_2O (normal). In contrast, a patient on a ventilator with pulmonary disease that causes "stiff" lungs (e.g., ARDS, sarcoidosis) may have a compliance as low as 20 to 30 mL/cm H_2O, indicating a severely compromised lung.

As the volume of gas is delivered to a patient on a mechanical ventilator, the ventilator's pressure gauge slowly rises from zero to peak inspiratory pressure (PIP). The rise in pressure is caused by the airways' resistance (to flow), as well as by lung and chest wall compliance (Box 25-11). A graph of pressure over time, depicting inspiration, would look like the example shown in Figure 25-6. Dynamic pressures and PIP can give an indication of both airway resistance and lung compliance.

STATIC PRESSURE

One of the measurements used to obtain compliance is static pressure or plateau pressure.[24] Plateau pressure is obtained by pushing the end-inspiratory hold button on a ventilator at the end of a maximum inspiration. This holds the volume of delivered air in the patient's chest by preventing exhalation. The PIP drops to a plateau pressure with this maneuver, which reflects the pressure

box 25-11
Factors Decreasing Compliance

Airway Factors
Peak flow
Size of airways
Airway obstructions
External obstructions (kinked ventilator tubing or water in the tubing)

Lung Factors
Elasticity (stiffness) of the lung
Presence of auto-PEEP
Shunt (ARDS)

Chest Wall Factors
Chest wall deformities
Position of patient
External compression of chest wall or diaphragm (distended abdomen, obesity)

necessary to hold the lungs open. A graph depicting static pressure and PIP can been seen in Figure 25-7. Static compliance is determined by dividing the effective tidal volume by the plateau pressure minus the total PEEP:

$$V_T/(\text{plateau pressure} - \text{PEEP}) = \text{static compliance}$$

A higher compliance means that the lung is more easily distended, whereas a lower compliance means that the lung is stiffer and difficult to distend. In other words, a higher compliance is better. Low compliance may be due to stiff lungs as with ARDS, a restrictive chest wall (i.e., kyphoscoliosis), or ventilation of only a small portion of lung, such as occurs with partial lung collapse. Serial measurements of compliance can alert the nurse to sudden decreases, which may be due to pneumothorax, mucus plugging, or pulmonary edema.

Equipment

Many different ventilatory support systems are available. Manual resuscitators are typically used in emergencies, such as acute respiratory failure. Several types of mechanical ventilators are in use, and they offer a variety of modes.

MANUAL RESUSCITATORS

The nurse's first line of defense for acute respiratory failure is the MRB, sometimes referred to as an Ambu-bag or bag-valve device. During cardiopulmonary resuscitation or hyperinflation with bagging and suctioning of any mechanically ventilated patient, MRBs with reservoirs must be used and connected to an oxygen source to deliver 74% to 100% concentrations of oxygen. MRBs without reservoirs may deliver a lower FIO_2 but must also be connected to an oxygen source.

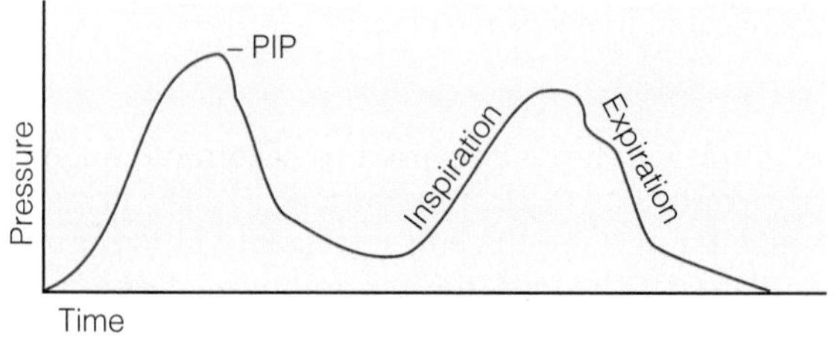

figure 25-6 Graph displaying peak respiratory pressure (PIP).

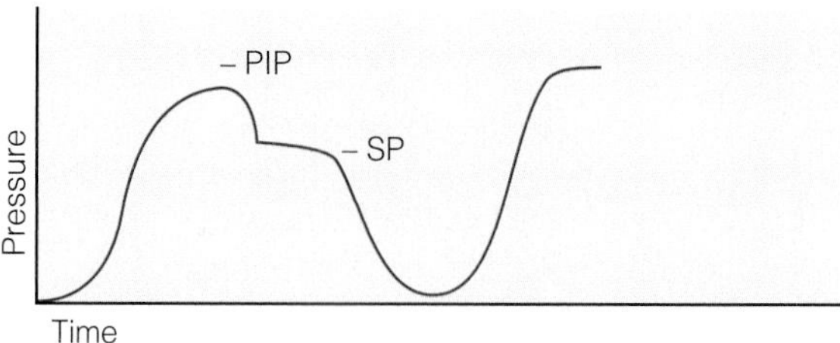

figure 25-7 Graph depicting static pressure (SP); peak inspiratory pressure (PIP).

Knowledge of the bag and skill in using it are vital. The function of this simple ventilator can be compared with that of the more sophisticated models. The following guidelines pertain to the manual resuscitator:

- The force of squeezing the bag determines the tidal volume delivered to the patient.
- The number of hand squeezes per minute determines the assisted respiratory rate.
- The force and rate that the bag is squeezed determine the peak flow.

While the bag is being used, one must carefully observe the patient's chest rise to determine whether the bag is ventilating properly and whether any gastric (abdominal) distension is developing. In addition, the amount of resistance encountered can roughly indicate lung compliance. If a patient becomes progressively harder to "bag," an increase in secretions, pneumothorax, worsening bronchospasms, or other condition that might decrease the patient's compliance must be considered. Breaths delivered to a conscious patient must be timed to coincide with spontaneous inspiratory effort or the discomfort of dyssynchronous breathing will create anxiety, and the patient will not tolerate the additional ventilation.

When delivering breaths with an MRB, the nurse allows time for complete exhalation between breaths to prevent air trapping (referred to as auto-PEEP), which can cause hypotension and barotrauma, especially in patients with obstructive airway disease.

MECHANICAL VENTILATORS

The goal of mechanical ventilation is to maintain alveolar ventilation appropriate for the patient's metabolic needs and to correct hypoxemia and maximize oxygen transport. Ventilators are classified into two categories: negative-pressure ventilators and positive-pressure ventilators. Regardless of which type or model is used, the nurse must be familiar with the ventilator's function and limitations. The following discussion of ventilators is in order of evolution of ventilator technology and subsequent use in clinical practice.

Negative-Pressure Ventilators

Early negative-pressure ventilators were known as "iron lungs." The patient's body was encased in an iron cylinder and negative pressure was generated by a large piston to enlarge the thoracic cage. This caused alveolar pressures to fall, and a pressure gradient was formed so that air flowed into the lungs. The iron lung was used most frequently during the poliomyelitis epidemics of the 1930s and 1940s,[25] but iron lungs are still occasionally used today. Intermittent short-term negative-pressure ventilation is sometimes used in patients with chronic diseases. Rarely, this method of support is chosen for patients who are not candidates for aggressive mechanical ventilation as provided through an artificial airway. These patients suffer from a wide variety of conditions such as COPD, diseases of the chest wall (kyphoscoliosis), and neuromuscular diseases (Duchenne's muscular dystrophy, amyotrophic lateral sclerosis [ALS]).

The iron lung is cumbersome to use and very large. Most negative-pressure ventilators in use today are more portable. To improve mobility and comfort, there is a device that fits like a tortoise shell, forming a seal over the chest. A hose connects the shell to a negative-pressure generator. The thoracic cage is literally pulled outward to initiate inspiration. The use of negative-pressure ventilators is restricted in clinical practice, however, because they limit positioning and movement and they lack adaptability to large or small body torsos.

Positive-Pressure Ventilators

Figure 25-8 shows a typical positive-pressure ventilator.

Volume Ventilators. The volume ventilator is commonly used in critical care settings. The basic principle of this ventilator is that a designated volume of air is delivered with each breath. The amount of pressure required to deliver the set volume depends on the patient's lung compliance and patient–ventilator resistance factors. Therefore, PIP must be monitored in volume modes because it varies from breath to breath. With this mode of ventilation, a respiratory rate, inspiratory time, and tidal volume are selected for the mechanical breaths.

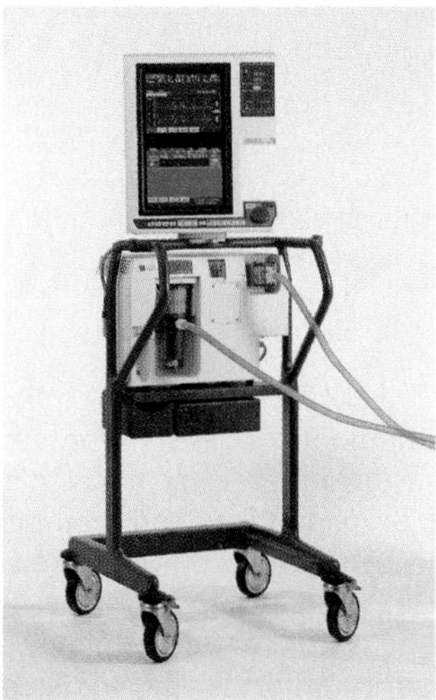

figure 25-8 The Puritan-Bennett 840™ Ventilator System is an example of a positive-pressure ventilator that has volume, pressure, and mixed modes designed for adult, pediatric, and infant ventilation. Courtesy of Tyco Healthcare/Nelicor Puritan Bennett, Pleasanton, California.

Pressure Ventilators. The use of pressure ventilators is increasing in critical care units. A typical pressure mode delivers a selected gas pressure to the patient early in inspiration, and sustains the pressure throughout the inspiratory phase. By meeting the patient's inspiratory flow demand throughout inspiration, patient effort is reduced and comfort increased. Although pressure is consistent with these modes, volume is not. With changes in resistance or compliance, volume will change. Therefore, exhaled tidal volume is the variable to monitor closely. With pressure modes, the pressure level to be delivered is selected, and with some mode options (i.e., pressure controlled [PC], described later), rate and inspiratory time are preset as well.

High-Frequency Ventilators. The high-frequency ventilator accomplishes oxygenation by the diffusion of oxygen and carbon dioxide from high to low gradients of concentration. This diffusion movement is increased if the kinetic energy of the gas molecules is increased. High-frequency ventilators use small tidal volumes (1 to 3 mL/kg) at frequencies greater than 100 breaths/minute.[26] The breathing pattern of a person on a high-frequency ventilator is somewhat analogous to the breathing pattern of a panting dog; panting entails moving small volumes of air at a very fast rate.

Theoretically, a high-frequency ventilator would be used to achieve lower peak ventilatory pressures, thereby lowering the risk of barotrauma and improving ventilation–perfusion matching because of its different flow delivery characteristics. Clinical data are lacking so far to show that use of a high-frequency ventilator improves outcomes. Potential adverse effects associated with high-frequency ventilators include gas trapping and necrotizing tracheobronchitis, when used in the absence of adequate humidification.[27]

Ventilator Modes

Several different modes of ventilatory control are available on ventilators. Figure 25-9 and Table 25-8 compare these modes. Volume modes include assist-control (A/C) mode and synchronized intermittent mandatory ventilation (SIMV) mode. Pressure modes include pressure-support ventilation (PSV) mode, pressure-controlled ventilation (PCV) mode, volume-guaranteed pressure options (VGPO) mode, continuous positive airway pressure (CPAP)/PEEP mode, and noninvasive bilevel positive airway pressure ventilation (BiPAP) mode. There is no one best mode for managing patients in respiratory failure, although each mode has its advantages and disadvantages.

VOLUME MODES

Assist-Control Mode

In A/C mode, a mandatory (or "control") rate is selected. If the patient wishes to breathe faster, he or she can trigger the ventilator and receive a full-volume breath. This mode of ventilation is often used fully to support a patient, such

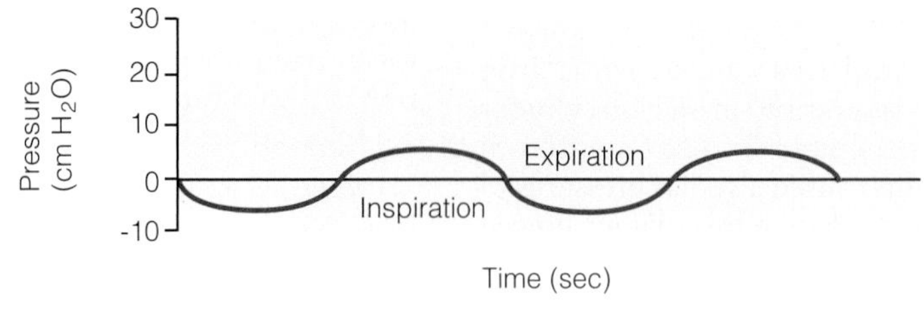

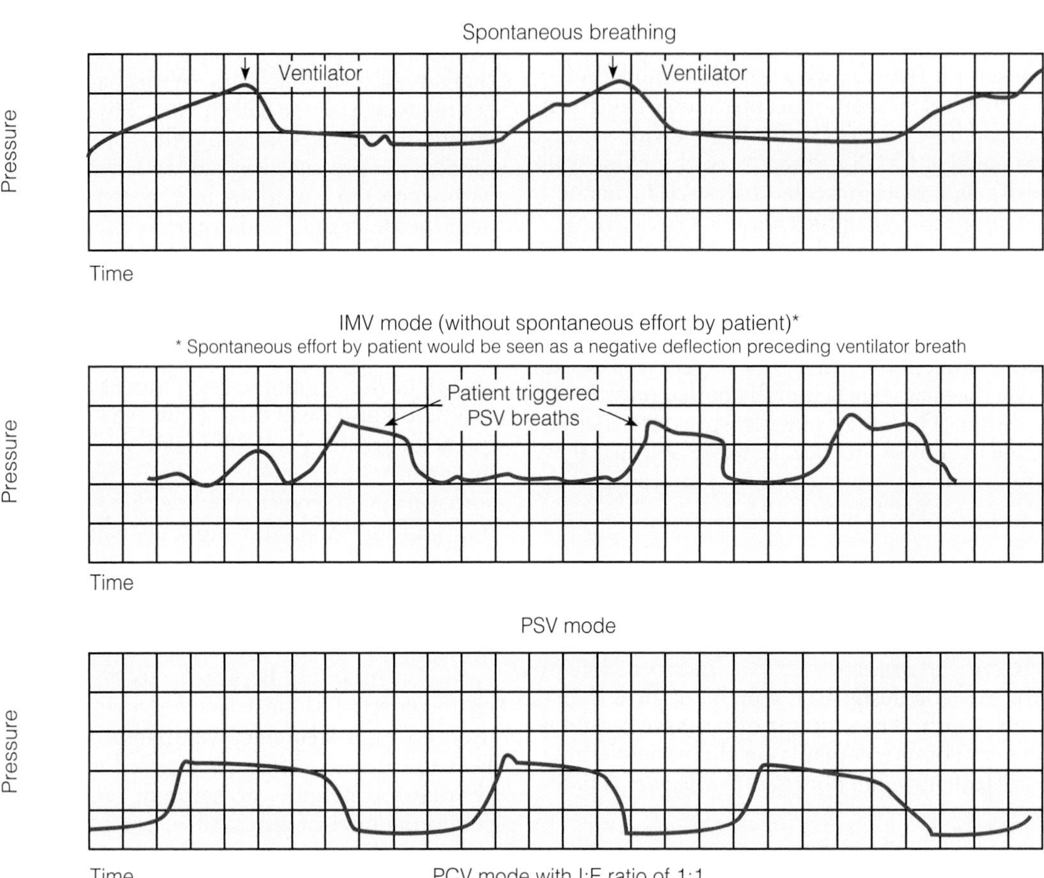

figure 25-9 Comparison of ventilatory modes using continuous airway pressure monitoring.

as when the patient is first intubated or when the patient is too weak to perform the work of breathing (e.g., when emerging from anesthesia).

Synchronized Intermittent Mandatory Ventilation Mode

In SIMV mode, the rate and tidal volume are preset. If the patient wants to breathe above this rate, he or she may. However, unlike the A/C mode, any breaths taken above the set rate are spontaneous breaths taken through the ventilator circuit. The tidal volume of these breaths can vary drastically from the tidal volume set on the ventilator, because the tidal volume is determined solely by the patient's spontaneous effort. Adding pressure support (discussed in the next section) during spontaneous breaths can minimize the risk of increased work of breathing. In the past, SIMV has been used as a popular weaning mode. To wean the patient, the mandatory breaths were gradually decreased, thereby allowing the patient to assume more and more of the work of breathing.

PRESSURE MODES

Pressure-Support Ventilation Mode

PSV mode augments or assists spontaneous breathing efforts by delivering a high flow of gas to a selected pressure level early in inspiration, and maintaining that level throughout the inspiratory phase. The patient's effort determines the rate, inspiratory flow, and tidal volume. When PSV mode is used as a stand-alone mode of ventilation, the pressure support level is adjusted to achieve the approximate targeted tidal volume and respiratory rate. At high pressure levels, PSV mode provides nearly total ventilatory support.

Specific uses of PSV are to promote patient comfort and synchrony with the ventilator, to decrease the work of breathing necessary to overcome the resistance of the

table 25-8 Comparison of Modes of Ventilation

Ventilatory Mode	Indications	Advantages/Disadvantages	Special Monitoring
A/C	Often used as initial mode of ventilation	Advantages: Ensures vent support during every breath; Each breath same tidal volume. Disadvantages: Hyperventilation, air trapping	Work of breathing may be increased if sensitivity or flow rate is too low.
SIMV	Often used as initial mode of ventilation and for weaning	Advantages: Allows spontaneous breaths (tidal volume determined by patient) between vent breaths; weaning is accomplished by gradually lowering the set rate and allowing the patient to assume more work. Disadvantages: Patient–ventilator asynchrony possible	
PSV	Intact respiratory drive in patient necessary Used as a weaning mode, and in some cases of dyssynchrony	Advantages: Decreases work of breathing, increases patient comfort. Disadvantages: Should not be used in patients with acute bronchospasm	Adjust PSV level to maintain desired respiratory rate and tidal volume. Monitor for changes in compliance, which can cause tidal volume to change. Monitor respiratory rate and tidal volume at least hourly.
PCV	Used to limit plateau pressures that can cause barotrauma Severe ARDS	Disadvantages: Patient–ventilator asynchrony possible, necessitating sedation/paralysis	Monitor tidal volume at least hourly. Monitor for barotrauma, hemodynamic instability.
IRV	Usually used in conjunction with PCV Increases ratio I:E to allow for recruitment of alveoli and improve oxygenation	Disadvantages: Almost always requires paralysis	Monitor for auto-PEEP, barotrauma, and hemodynamic instability.
VGPO	Combines advantages of pressure ventilation with guaranteed tidal volume	Advantages: Ensures a delivered tidal volume. Disadvantages: Requires sophisticated knowledge of the mode and waveform analysis	
CPAP	Constant positive airway pressure for patients who breathe spontaneously	Advantages: Used in intubated or nonintubated patients. Disadvantages: On some systems, no alarm if respiratory rate falls	Monitor for increased work of breathing.
Noninvasive (Bi-Pap)	Nocturnal hypoventilation in patients with neuromuscular disease, chest wall deformity, obstructive sleep apnea, and COPD; to prevent intubation; to prevent reintubation initially after extubation	Advantages: Decreased cost when patients can be cared for at home; no need for artificial airway. Disadvantages: Patient discomfort or claustrophobia	Monitor for gastric distension, air leaks from mouth.

endotracheal tube, and for weaning. As a weaning tool, PSV is thought to increase the endurance of the respiratory muscles by decreasing the physical work and oxygen demands during spontaneous breathing. Because the level of pressure support can be gradually decreased, endurance conditioning is enhanced.

In PSV mode, the inspired tidal volume and respiratory rate must be monitored closely to detect changes in lung compliance. In general, if compliance decreases or resistance increases, tidal volume decreases and respiratory rate increases. PSV mode should be used with caution in patients with bronchospasm or other reactive airway conditions.

Pressure-Controlled Ventilation Mode

The PCV mode is used to control plateau pressures in conditions such as ARDS where compliance is decreased and the risk of barotrauma is high. It is used when the patient has persistent oxygenation problems despite a high FIO_2 and high levels of PEEP. The inspiratory pressure level, respiratory rate, and inspiratory–expiratory (I:E) ratio must be selected. Tidal volume varies with compliance and airway resistance and must be closely monitored. Sedation and the use of neuromuscular blocking agents are frequently indicated, because any patient–ventilator asynchrony usually results in profound drops in the SaO_2. This is especially true when inverse ratios are used. The "unnatural" feeling of this mode often requires muscle relaxants to ensure patient–ventilator synchrony.

Most ventilators operate with a short inspiratory time and a long expiratory time (1:2 or 1:3 ratio). This promotes venous return and allows time for air to exit the lungs passively. Inverse ratio ventilation (IRV) mode reverses this ratio so that inspiratory time is equal to, or longer than, expiratory time (1:1 to 4:1). Inverse I:E ratios are used in conjunction with pressure control to improve oxygenation in patients with ARDS by expanding stiff alveoli by using longer distending times, thereby providing more opportunity for gas exchange and preventing alveolar collapse.

As expiratory time is decreased, one must monitor for the development of hyperinflation or auto-PEEP. Regional alveolar overdistension and barotrauma may occur owing to excessive total PEEP.[28] When the PCV mode is used, the mean airway and intrathoracic pressures rise, potentially resulting in a decrease in cardiac output and oxygen delivery. Therefore, the patient's hemodynamic status must be monitored closely.

Volume-Guaranteed Pressure Options Mode

VGPO mode ensures delivery of a prescribed tidal volume while using a decelerating flow pattern through a "pressure" breath. The options include both spontaneous and control rate parameters, and the volume guarantee is provided differently, depending on the ventilator.[29] VGPO can be used in acutely ill patients as well as more stable, weaning patients. Some examples include the volume support (VS) and pressure-regulated volume control (PRVC) options (Siemens Medical), as well as pressure augmentation (PA; Bear Medical Systems).

In the acutely ill, unstable patient, this option may provide pressure ventilation while guaranteeing tidal volume and minute ventilation at a set rate. In the spontaneously breathing patient, the option is used as a "safety" when pressure ventilation is desired. The use of a volume guarantee in the spontaneously breathing patient may be especially important at night (when respiratory rates and volumes normally decrease) and in patients for whom secretions are a problem (because secretions increase resistance and result in decreased spontaneous volumes).[21]

CONTINUOUS POSITIVE AIRWAY PRESSURE/POSITIVE END-EXPIRATORY PRESSURE MODE

CPAP is the term used when PEEP is supplied during spontaneous breathing. PEEP is the term used to describe positive end-expiratory pressure with positive-pressure (machine) breaths. CPAP assists spontaneously breathing patients to improve their oxygenation by elevating the end-expiratory pressure in the lungs throughout the respiratory cycle. CPAP can be used for intubated and nonintubated patients. It may be used as a weaning mode and for nocturnal ventilation (nasal or mask CPAP) to splint open the upper airway, preventing upper airway obstruction in patients with obstructive sleep apnea.

PEEP is positive pressure exerted at the end of exhalation. It is common practice to use low levels of PEEP (2 to 5 cm H_2O) in the intubated patient. PEEP is increased in 2- to 5-cm H_2O increments when FIO_2 levels are greater than 50% to attain an acceptable SaO_2 (<90%) or PaO_2 (>60 to 70 mm Hg). PEEP is most often necessary in patients with refractory hypoxemia (e.g., those with ARDS), where the PaO_2 deteriorates rapidly despite greater concentrations of oxygen administration.

PEEP is used to keep alveoli stented open and it may recruit alveolar units that are totally or partially collapsed. This end-expiratory pressure increases the functional residual capacity (FRC) by reinflating collapsed alveoli, maintains the alveoli in an open position, and improves lung compliance. This decreases shunt and improves oxygenation. In addition, there is some evidence that keeping the alveoli open enhances surfactant regeneration. High levels of PEEP should rarely be interrupted because it may take several hours to recruit alveoli again and restore the FRC; until this occurs, oxygenation may suffer.[21]

In the patient who does not have adequate circulating blood volume, institution of PEEP decreases venous return to the heart, decreases cardiac output, and decreases oxygen delivery to the tissues. If hypotension or decreased cardiac output results from PEEP application, restoring circulating intravascular volume with administration of intravenous fluids may correct the hypotension. Another serious complication of PEEP is barotrauma. It can occur in any mechanically ventilated patient but is most common when high levels of PEEP are used (≥10 to 20 cm H_2O) in lungs with high ventilating pressures and low compliance, and in patients with obstructive airway disease. The development of barotrauma is an emergency and usually requires placement of a chest tube.

Noninvasive Bilateral Positive Airway Pressure Ventilation Mode

BiPAP (Respironics, Inc.) is a noninvasive form of mechanical ventilation provided by means of a nasal mask, nasal prongs, or a full-face mask. It is used in the treatment of patients with chronic respiratory insufficiency to manage acute or chronic respiratory failure without intubation and conventional mechanical ventilation. It is also used as a bridge to weaning patients from mechanical ventilation, and as an alternative to conventional mechanical ventilation in patients who are ventilated in their homes.[30] The system allows the clinician to select two levels of positive-pressure support: an inspiratory pressure support level (referred to as IPAP) and an expiratory pressure called EPAP (PEEP/CPAP level).[26] Because BiPAP allows for the provision of assisted inspiration and therefore ventilation, application of this mode to those patients who hypoventilate as well as experience obstruction during sleep is possible.[21]

BiPAP is beneficial in patients with worsening hypoventilation, obstructive apneic episodes, or both. It is also useful to avoid intubation in patients with respiratory failure and hypercarbia, and to avoid reintubation after extubation in borderline cases. Use of a full-face mask may increase the risk of aspiration and of rebreathing carbon dioxide; therefore, ventilation with a full-face mask should be used cautiously. Thick or copious secretions and poor cough may be relative contraindications to BiPAP.

Use of Mechanical Ventilators

SETTING VENTILATOR CONTROLS

The nurse must know how to monitor the various ventilators, modes, and controls before giving mechanical ventilatory support to a patient. The following section discusses the various controls and settings and their implications for nursing care. In some institutions, the respiratory therapists share responsibility for managing the ventilator, but the nurse still needs to be fully aware of the implications for the patient of the mode and level of mechanical support.

Ventilator settings must be frequently evaluated against patient response. Iatrogenically induced complications include overventilation (which causes respiratory alkalosis) and underventilation (which causes respiratory acidosis or hypoxemia). ABG studies determine the effectiveness of mechanical ventilation. Patients with chronic pulmonary disease, however, should be ventilated to stay relatively close to their normal ABG values. This usually means accepting relatively high carbon dioxide levels, lower-than-average oxygenation, or both.

Fraction of Inspired Oxygen

Most ventilators allow for easy adjustment of oxygen percentage (FIO_2) by means of a dial. Oxygen analyzers, either in-circuit or external, allow the nurse to ascertain the FIO_2 that is being delivered. Initially a patient is placed on a high level of FIO_2 (60% or higher). Subsequent changes in FIO_2 are based on ABGs and the SaO_2. Usually the FIO_2 is adjusted to maintain an SaO_2 of greater than 90% (roughly equivalent to a PaO_2 >60 mm Hg). Oxygen toxicity is a concern when an FIO_2 of greater than 60% is required for more than 25 hours; therefore, most clinicians attempt to use strategies to allow for maintenance of an FIO_2 of 60% or less.

Respiratory Rate

The number of breaths per minute delivered to the patient can be directly dialed on most ventilator models. The nurse double-checks the functioning of the ventilator by observing the patient's respiratory rate. In the pressure ventilator, the inspiratory time determines the duration of inspiration by regulating the gas flow rate. The higher the flow rate, the faster peak airway pressure is reached and the shorter the inspiration; conversely, the lower the flow rate, the longer the inspiration. A very high flow rate may produce turbulence, shallow inspirations, and uneven distribution of volume.

Respiratory rate times tidal volume equals minute ventilation ($RR \times V_T = MV$). In turn, minute volume determines alveolar ventilation. These two parameters are adjusted according to the $PaCO_2$. Increasing the minute volume decreases the $PaCO_2$; conversely, decreasing the minute volume increases the $PaCO_2$. In special cases, hypoventilation or hyperventilation is desired. For example, in a patient with head injury, respiratory alkalosis may be required to promote cerebral vasoconstriction, with a resultant decrease in ICP. In this case, the tidal volume and respiratory rate are increased to achieve the desired alkalotic pH by manipulating the $PaCO_2$. In contrast, a patient with COPD whose baseline ABGs reflect an elevated $PaCO_2$ should not be hyperventilated. Instead, the goal should be restoration of the baseline $PaCO_2$. These patients usually have a large carbonic acid load, and lowering their carbon dioxide levels rapidly may result in seizures. Rate adjustments may also be necessary to enhance patient comfort or when rapid rates cause air trapping that result in auto-PEEP.

Tidal Volume

In the volume ventilator, the number of milliliters of air to be delivered with each breath is set by the clinician. Tidal volumes of 10 to 15 mL/kg of body weight were traditionally used. Research has identified a phenomenon of iatrogenic lung injury (dubbed *volutrauma*) in which forces produced in the lungs by the large tidal volumes may aggravate the damage inflicted on the lungs by the pathological process that necessitated mechanical ventilation.[31] For this reason, lower tidal volume targets (6 to 8 mL/kg) are now recommended.

Peak Flow

Peak flow is the velocity of gas flow per unit of time, and is expressed in liters per minute. On many volume ventilators, this is a separate dial. If auto-PEEP (due to inadequate expiratory time) is present, peak flow is increased to shorten inspiratory time so that the patient may exhale completely. However, increasing peak flow increases turbulence, which is reflected in increasing airway pressures.

Pressure Limit

On volume-cycled ventilators, the pressure limit dial limits the highest pressure allowed in the ventilator circuit. Once the high pressure limit is reached, inspiration is terminated. Therefore, if the pressure limit is being constantly reached, the designated tidal volume is not being delivered to the patient. The cause of this can be coughing, accumulation of secretions, kinked ventilator tubing, pneumothorax, decreasing compliance, or a pressure limit set too low.

Positive End-Expiratory Pressure

The PEEP control adjusts the pressure that is maintained in the lungs at the end of expiration. PEEP and CPAP can be visualized on the respiratory pressure gauge or display. Instead of returning to zero (atmospheric pressure) at the end of expiration, the pressure value drops to the PEEP/CPAP level. Reduction of PEEP is considered if the patient has a Pa_{O_2} of 80 to 100 mm Hg on an F_{IO_2} of 50% or less, is hemodynamically stable, and has stabilization or improvement of the underlying illness. To evaluate whether the effects of PEEP are beneficial, monitoring of ABGs, Sa_{O_2}, compliance, and hemodynamic pressures (including cardiac output and blood pressure) is necessary. Baseline values are obtained before changes in PEEP are made. PEEP is usually increased in increments of 2 to 5 cm H_2O. The patient is monitored for adverse effects, such as hypotension and dysrhythmias. If these occur, the PEEP is reduced. If higher PEEP is tolerated, the patient is stabilized on the new PEEP settings for approximately 15 minutes. The monitored parameters are then repeated.

Hemodynamic measurements (cardiac output, pulmonary artery pressure [PAP], central venous pressure [CVP], and pulmonary artery wedge pressure [PAWP]) are taken at end-expiration with the patient on PEEP. Accuracy in selecting the point of end-expiration on the waveform tracing is facilitated by using continuous airway monitoring[28] (Fig. 25-10). PEEP does not need to be discontinued before obtaining hemodynamic measurements. Hemodynamic measurements can be inaccurate (as an indicator of volume status) if a patient is on high PEEP or the position of the transducer is not leveled at the phlebostatic axis. The position of the catheter within the pulmonary circulation should also be verified on a chest x-ray.

Attempts are made to minimize removing the patient from the ventilator when using high levels of PEEP. Oxygenation can deteriorate and be slow to rebound because it takes a significant amount of time for the effects of PEEP to be reestablished. Therefore, if the patient is being oxygenated using an MRB, it must be equipped with a valve that allows levels of PEEP to be dialed in. An in-line suction apparatus may be helpful to prevent breaking the PEEP circuit to suction the patient.

Sensitivity

The sensitivity function controls the amount of patient effort needed to initiate an inspiration, as measured by negative inspiratory effort. Increasing the sensitivity (requiring less negative force) decreases the amount of work the patient must do to initiate a ventilator breath. Likewise, decreasing the sensitivity increases the amount of negative pressure that the patient needs to initiate inspiration and increases the work of breathing.

RESPONDING TO ALARMS

Mechanical ventilators are used to support life. Alarm systems are necessary to warn the nurse of developing problems. Alarm systems can be categorized according to volume and pressure (high and low). Low-pressure alarms warn of disconnection of the patient from the ventilator or circuit leaks. High-pressure alarms warn of rising pressures. Electrical failure alarms are necessary for all ventilators. A nurse or respiratory therapist must respond to every ventilator alarm. Alarms must never be ignored or disarmed. Some clinical troubleshooting guidelines are presented in Table 25-9.

Ventilator malfunction is a potentially serious problem. Nursing or respiratory therapists perform ventilator checks every 2 to 4 hours, and recurrent alarms may alert the clinician to the possibility of an equipment-related issue. When device malfunction is suspected, a second person manually ventilates the patient while the nurse or therapist looks for the cause. If a problem cannot be promptly corrected by ventilator adjustment, a different machine is procured so the ventilator in question can be taken out of service for analysis and repair by technical staff.

ENSURING HUMIDIFICATION AND THERMOREGULATION

Mechanical ventilation bypasses the upper airway, thereby negating the body's protective mechanism for humidifying and warming inspired air. These two processes must be

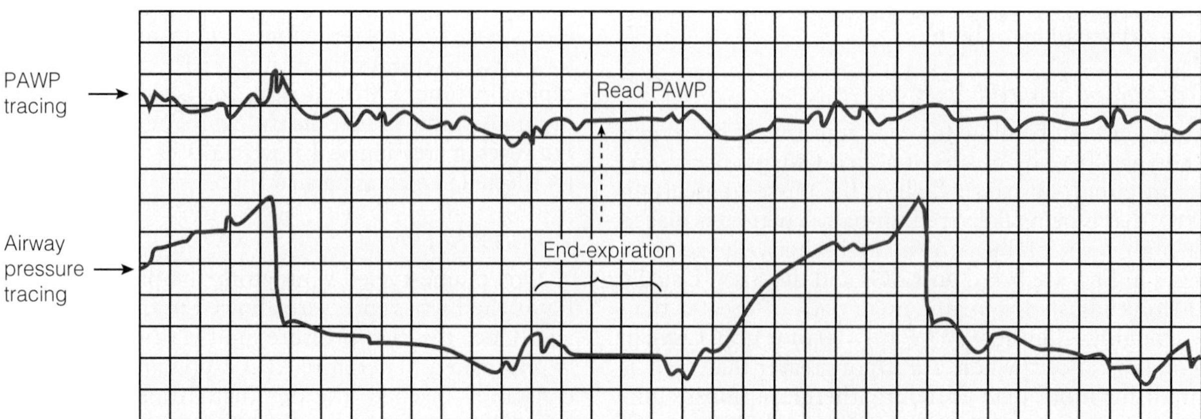

figure 25-10 Use of continuous airway pressure monitoring to assist in identifying point of end-expiration.

added to the ventilator circuit in the form of a humidifier with a temperature control. All air delivered by the ventilator passes through the water in the humidifier, where it is warmed and saturated. Because of this, insensible water loss is decreased. In most instances, the temperature of the air is about body temperature. In some rare instances (severe hypothermia), the air temperatures can be increased. Caution is advised because prolonged inhalation of gas at high temperatures can cause tracheal burns. An empty humidifier contributes to drying the airway, often with resultant mucus plugging and less ability to suction out secretions.

As air passes through the ventilator to the patient, water condenses in the corrugated tubing. This moisture is considered contaminated and must be drained into a receptacle and not back into the sterile humidifier. If the water is allowed to build up, resistance is developed in the circuit and PEEP is generated. In addition, if moisture accumulates near the endotracheal tube, the patient can aspirate the water. The nurse and respiratory therapist jointly are responsible for preventing this condensation buildup. The humidifier is an ideal medium for bacterial growth. Institutional policies should describe the frequency of ventilator circuit changes.

table 25-9 Troubleshooting the Ventilator

Problem	Possible Causes	Action
Volume or pressure alarm	*Patient related*	
	Patient disconnected from ventilator	Reconnect STAT.
	Loss of delivered V_T	Auscultate neck for possible leak around endotracheal tube (ETT) cuff.
		Review chest film for endotracheal tube placement—may be too high.
		Check for loss of V_T through chest tube.
	Decrease in patient-initiated breaths	Evaluate patient for cause: check respiratory rate, ABGs, last sedation.
	Increased compliance	May be due to clearing of secretions or relief of bronchospasms.
	Ventilator related	
	Leaks	Check all tubing for loss of connection, starting at patient and moving toward humidifier.
		Check for change in ventilator settings.
		(*Note:* If problem is not corrected STAT, MRB patient until ventilator problem is corrected.)
High-pressure or peak-pressure alarm	*Patient related*	
	Decreased compliance	
	Increased dynamic pressures	Suction patient.
		Administer inhaled β-agonists.
		If sudden, evaluate for pneumothorax.
		Evaluate chest film for ETT placement in right main stem bronchus.
		Sedate if patient is bucking the ventilator or biting the ETT.
	Increased static pressure	Evaluate ABGs for hypoxia, fluids for overload, chest film for atelectasis.
		Auscultate breath sounds.
	Ventilator related	
	Tubing kinked	Check tubing.
	Tubing filled with water	Empty water into a receptacle: Do not drain back into the humidifier.
	Patient–ventilator asynchrony	Recheck sensitivity and peak flow settings.
		Provide sedation/paralysis if indicated.
Abnormal ABGs	*Patient related*	
Hypoxia	Secretions	Suction.
	Increase in disease pathology	Evaluate patient and chest film.
	Positive fluid balance	Evaluate I & O.
Hypocapnia	Hypoxia	Evaluate ABGs and patient.
	Increased lung compliance	Evaluate for wean potential.
Hypercapnia	Sedation	Increase respiratory rate or V_T settings.
	Fatigue	
	Ventilator related	
Hypoxia	FIO_2 drift	Check ventilator with oxygen analyzer.
Hypocapnia	Settings not correct	Decrease respiratory rate, V_T, or MV.
Hypercapnia	Settings not correct	Increase respiratory rate, V_T, or MV.
Heater alarm	Adding cold water to humidifier	Wait.
	Altered setting	Reset.
	Cold air blowing on humidifier	Redirect air flow.

Complications of Mechanical Ventilation

Complications that can occur with mechanical ventilation are listed in Box 25-12. Although all of these adverse consequences will occur over time in some ventilated patients, the incidence of these complications can be minimized by good preventive care practices.

ASPIRATION

Aspiration can occur before, during, or after intubation. The potential for development of nosocomial pneumonia or ARDS is increased if aspiration occurs. The risk of aspiration after intubation can be minimized by maintaining appropriate cuff inflation, evacuating gastric distension with suction, suctioning the oropharynx (especially before cuff deflations), and elevating the head of the patient's bed 30 degrees or more at all times.[32] Elevation of the head of the bed is limited when the patient has femoral site intravenous lines; however, the bed can be raised up to 15 to 20 degrees and then placed in slight reverse Trendelenburg position to approximate 30 degrees of elevation.

box 25-12
Complications of Mechanical Ventilation

Airway
- Aspiration
- Decreased clearance of secretions
- Nosocomial or ventilator-acquired pneumonia

Endotracheal Tube
- Tube kinked or plugged
- Rupture of piriform sinus
- Tracheal stenosis or tracheomalacia
- Mainstem intubation with contralateral lung atelectasis
- Cuff failure
- Sinusitis
- Otitis media
- Laryngeal edema

Mechanical
- Hypoventilation with atelectasis
- Hyperventilation with hypocapnia and respiratory alkalosis
- Barotrauma (pneumothorax or tension pneumothorax, pneumomediastinum, subcutaneous emphysema)
- Alarm "turned off"
- Failure of alarms or ventilator
- Inadequate nebulization or humidification
- Overheated inspired air, resulting in hyperthermia

Physiological
- Fluid overload with humidified air and sodium chloride (NaCl) retention
- Depressed cardiac function and hypotension
- Stress ulcers
- Paralytic ileus
- Gastric distension
- Starvation
- Dyssynchronous breathing pattern

BAROTRAUMA

Mechanical ventilation involves "pumping" air into the chest, creating positive pressures during inspiration. If PEEP is added, the pressures are increased and continued throughout expiration. These positive pressures can rupture an alveolus or emphysematous bleb. Air then escapes into, and is trapped in, the pleural space, accumulating until it begins to collapse the lung. Eventually the collapsing lung impinges on the mediastinal structures, compressing the trachea and eventually the heart; this is called *tension pneumothorax.* Signs and symptoms of tension pneumothorax are listed in Box 25-13. Signs of pneumothorax include extreme dyspnea, hypoxia (indicated by a decrease in SaO_2), and an abrupt increase in PIP. Breath sounds may be decreased or absent on the affected side; however, this sign may not be reliable in the patient on positive-pressure ventilation. Observation of the patient may reveal a tracheal deviation (to the opposite side) or the sudden development of subcutaneous emphysema. The most ominous signs of tension pneumothorax are hypotension and bradycardia that can deteriorate into a cardiac arrest without timely medical intervention. The physician or other qualified health care professional may decompress the chest by inserting a needle to evacuate the trapped air until a chest tube can be inserted.

VENTILATOR-ASSOCIATED PNEUMONIA

Ventilator-associated pneumonia (VAP) is the second most common hospital-acquired infection and the leading cause of death from nosocomial infections.[33] Intubated patients have a 10-fold increase in the incidence of nosocomial pneumonia, and the critically ill patient who is mechanically ventilated is especially at risk for development of VAP. Factors that lead to nosocomial pneumonia are oropharyngeal colonization, gastric colonization, aspiration, and compromised lung defenses. Mechanical ventilation, reintubation, self-extubation, presence of a nasogastric tube, and supine position are a few of the associated risk factors for VAP.[32] Maintenance of the natural gastric acid barrier in the stomach plays a major role in decreasing incidence and mortality from nosocomial pneumonia. The widespread use of

box 25-13 ***Signs and Symptoms of Tension Pneumothorax***

- Tachycardia
- Tachypnea
- Agitation
- Diaphoresis
- Midline tracheal shift
- Muffled heart tones
- Absent breath sounds over affected lung
- Hyperresonance to percussion over affected lung
- Elevation in peak airway pressures in ventilated patients
- Decrease in saturation of oxygen in arterial blood (SaO_2) or arterial oxygen tension (PaO_2)
- Hypotension
- Cardiac arrest

antacids or histamine type 2 receptor (H_2) blockers can predispose the patient to nosocomial infections because they decrease gastric acidity (increase alkalinity). Used to guard against stress bleeding, these medications may increase colonization of the upper gastrointestinal tract by bacteria that thrive in a more alkaline environment.

VAP is defined as nosocomial pneumonia in a patient who has been mechanically ventilated (by endotracheal tube or tracheostomy) for at least 48 hours at the time of diagnosis. A patient should be suspected of having a diagnosis of VAP if the chest x-ray shows new or progressive and persistent infiltrates. Other signs and symptoms can include a fever higher than 100.4°F (38°C), leukocytosis, new-onset purulent sputum or cough, and worsening gas exchange.[34]

There are numerous strategies for the prevention of VAP. The first step in preventing VAP is to prevent colonization by pathogens of the oropharynx and gastrointestinal tract.[34,35] Basic nursing care principles, such as meticulous handwashing and the use of gloves when suctioning patients orally or through the endotracheal tube, are essential. Gloves should also be worn when suctioning through closed-suction devices. In addition, critically ill patients have an increased risk for colonization by the microorganisms contributed by poor oral hygiene.[36] Oral care for a mechanically ventilated patient involves brushing the patient's teeth (approximately every 2 to 4 hours), using antiseptic solutions and alcohol-free mouthwash to cleanse the mouth, applying a water-based mouth moisturizer to maintain the integrity of the oral mucosa, and thoroughly suctioning oral secretions.[35] Additional nursing studies evaluating the effectiveness of various methods of oral care in the prevention of VAP are needed in the mechanically ventilated population to establish oral care guidelines. No evidence-based protocols on oral care and prevention of VAP exist.[32,37,38]

In patients receiving enteral feedings, the head of the bed should be elevated 30 to 45 degrees (unless contraindicated) to decrease the risk of aspiration.[32] Long-term (i.e., longer than 3 days) endotracheal tubes and gastric tubes should be placed orally (unless contraindicated or not tolerated by the patient). This intervention reduces the risk of the patient contracting infectious maxillary sinusitis, which is associated with the development of VAP.[39] Last, the use of an endotracheal tube that provides a port for the continuous aspiration of subglottic secretions (CASS) appears to prevent the development of VAP in the first week of intubation, and may decrease the overall incidence of VAP.[9,40] The use of the CASS endotracheal tube is typically reserved for those patients who can be identified as potentially requiring long-term ventilation.

DECREASED CARDIAC OUTPUT

Decreased cardiac output, as reflected by hypotension, may be observed at the initiation of mechanical ventilation. Although this is often attributed to the drugs used for intubation, the most important contribution to this phenomenon is lack of sympathetic tone and decreased venous return owing to the effects of positive pressure within the chest. In addition to hypotension, other signs and symptoms can include unexplained restlessness, decreased levels of consciousness, decreased urine output, weak peripheral pulses, slow capillary refill, pallor, fatigue, and chest pain. Increasing fluids to correct the relative hypovolemia usually treats hypotension in this setting.

WATER IMBALANCE

The decreased venous return to the heart is sensed by the vagal stretch receptors located in the right atrium. This sensed hypovolemia stimulates the release of antidiuretic hormone (ADH) from the posterior pituitary. The decreased cardiac output, leading to decreased urine output, compounds the problem by stimulating the renin–angiotensin–aldosterone response. The patient who is mechanically ventilated and hemodynamically unstable and requires large amounts of fluid resuscitation can experience extensive edema, including scleral and facial edema.

COMPLICATIONS ASSOCIATED WITH IMMOBILITY

Many complications that contribute to the morbidity and mortality of mechanically ventilated patients are the result of immobility. These include muscle wasting and weakness, contractures, loss of skin integrity, pneumonia, deep venous thrombosis (DVT) that can result in pulmonary embolus, constipation, and ileus.

GASTROINTESTINAL PROBLEMS

Gastrointestinal complications associated with mechanical ventilation include distension (due to air swallowing), hypomotility and ileus (due to immobility and the use of narcotic analgesics), vomiting, and breakdown of the intestinal mucosa due to the lack of normal nutritional intake. This breakdown allows translocation of bacteria from the gut into the bloodstream, leading to increased risk of bacteremia in patients who are unable to be fed enterally. Maintenance of an adequate bowel elimination pattern is necessary to prevent abdominal distension with resulting impingement on diaphragmatic excursion.

Many mechanically ventilated patients are already malnourished because of underlying chronic disease. Research verifies that the many side effects of clinical starvation can lead to pulmonary complications and death, as listed in Box 25-14.

MUSCLE WEAKNESS

The muscles used in respiration, like other muscles, become deconditioned and may even atrophy with prolonged disuse. The ventilated patient's respiratory muscles may not

box 25-14
Side Effects of Clinical Starvation

- Atrophy of respiratory muscles
- Decreased protein
- Decreased albumin
- Decreased cell-mediated immunity
- Decreased surfactant production
- Decreased replication of respiratory epithelium
- Intracellular depletion of adenosine triphosphate (ATP)
- Impaired cellular oxygenation
- Central respiratory depression

be used (other than in passive movement) while on the ventilator, especially if muscle relaxants, heavy sedation, or both have been part of the care plan. A retraining period to exercise and strengthen the respiratory muscles may be necessary before ventilatory support can be discontinued. Especially at risk for "critical illness myopathies" are those who have been on steroids in combination with muscle relaxants.

Muscle weakness also occurs as a result of muscle fatigue. Those patients requiring mechanical ventilation typically have one or more reasons for an increase in the work of breathing. These include an increase in carbon dioxide production, physiological dead space (non–gas-exchanging air passages), or both; decreased lung compliance; and increased airway resistance, as with bronchospasm or thick secretions. When the work of breathing exceeds the capacity of weakened muscles, the patient begins to display abnormal respiratory mechanics with inefficient use of these muscles. This often occurs during a weaning trial after prolonged ventilation. The accepted intervention for fatigue in this setting is returning to muscle rest on the ventilator. This carries the risk, however, of contributing further to muscle atrophy.[41]

Assessment and Management

The patient who needs ventilatory support also needs primary nursing care. One of the greatest contributions the nurse can make to decreasing costs, length of stay, and mortality in patients with respiratory problems is to implement interventions that prevent or minimize complications. Because mechanical ventilation is supportive rather than curative, focus of care for the mechanically ventilated patient is holistic. The nurse must interact effectively with each member of the health care team to achieve desired patient outcomes. Examples of nursing diagnoses and collaborative problems for the patient who needs ventilatory support are given in Box 25-15. Box 25-16 summarizes care of the patient on a ventilator. The mechanical ventilator, the artificial airway, and the care that is required to maintain mechanical ventilation require specialized nursing knowledge and skills that are discussed in the following sections. Special considerations for the pediatric patient are given in Box 25-17.

box 25-15 ***Examples of Nursing Diagnoses and Collaborative Problems for the Patient Who Needs Ventilatory Support***

- Ineffective Coping
- High Risk for Impaired Gas Exchange
- Excess Fluid Volume
- Impaired Acid–Base Status
- Ineffective Breathing Pattern
- Ineffective Airway Clearance
- Impaired Tissue Perfusion
- Alteration in Body Image (related to intubation or tracheostomy)
- Impaired Thought Processes—Agitation or Anxiety
- Risk for Infection
- High Risk for Complications Associated with Mechanical Ventilation
- High Risk for Complications Associated with Tracheostomy

ENDOTRACHEAL TUBE CARE

To prevent tube movement, tube migration, or inadvertent extubation, endotracheal tubes must be anchored securely. Anchoring can be accomplished with adhesive tape or with specially manufactured tube immobilization appliances. Usual practice is to retape the endotracheal tube every 1 to 2 days or when soiled or insecure. In orally intubated patients, the position of the endotracheal tube should be changed from side to side to facilitate oral care and prevent areas of pressure necrosis. The disadvantage of frequent retaping is that patients with fragile skin or prolonged intubation may experience skin breakdown. Twill tape can be substituted for adhesive tape in these situations and for heavily bearded patients. Retaping by two people is desirable to prevent accidental tube displacement. Sinusitis is relatively common in nasally intubated patients and can cause bacteremia and sepsis. Signs of sinusitis (fever, purulent nasal drainage) must be reported immediately.

The final step in retaping is to compare tube placement with placement before retaping. Endotracheal tube placement is verified by radiography after initial intubation. The position in centimeters at the lips/teeth or nostril is recorded; this placement is verified every shift to detect inadvertent position changes. Tube placement is checked, after retaping, by comparing the centimeter markings at the lips/teeth or nostril with the last radiological documentation of position. Placement of an oral bite block can prevent biting on the tube, which can cause airway narrowing (the high-pressure alarm on the ventilator will sound) or tube displacement. Oral inspection and hygiene are of paramount importance when a bite block is used. The use of a swivel connector (connecting the tube to the ventilator circuit), along with anchoring a large loop of tubing to the bed, facilitates patient movement without tube movement.

Persistent coughing may suggest that the endotracheal tube has migrated to touch the carina, requiring the tube to be withdrawn to an appropriate level. The pilot cuff balloon is protected from inadvertent disruption; cuff rupture or endotracheal tube occlusion with a mucus plug usually requires reintubation. If a patient is prematurely extubated for any reason, the airway must be kept patent. Oxygenation and ventilation may be provided with an MRB and mask until reintubation can be accomplished.

TRACHEOSTOMY CARE

In patients requiring long-term mechanical ventilation, the airway is converted to a tracheostomy at some point to prevent the complications of endotracheal intubation, such as tracheal stenosis and vocal cord paralysis. The preferred method of airway management is the tracheostomy tube for long-term ventilation. A review of the literature reveals no consensus as to optimal timing for tracheostomy, although the most common time seems to be about 21 days after intubation.[42] Practice at some institutions has been for earlier tracheostomy (e.g., at 7 to 14 days on the ventilator)

(text continues on page 552)

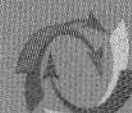

box 25-16 collaborative care guide *for the Patient on Mechanical Ventilation*

OUTCOMES	INTERVENTIONS
Oxygenation/Ventilation	
A patent airway is maintained. Lungs are clear to auscultation. Patient is without evidence of atelectasis. Peak, mean, and plateau pressures are within normal limits. Arterial blood gases (ABGs) are within normal limits.	▪ Auscultate breath sounds q2–4h and PRN. ▪ Suction as needed for rhonchi, coughing, or oxygen desaturation. ▪ Hyperoxygenate and hyperventilate before and after each suction pass. ▪ Monitor airway pressures q1–2h. ▪ Monitor airway pressures after suctioning. ▪ Administer bronchodilators and mucolytics as ordered. ▪ Perform chest physiotherapy if indicated by clinical examination or chest x-ray. ▪ Turn side to side q2h. ▪ Consider kinetic therapy or prone positioning as indicated by clinical scenario. ▪ Get patient out of bed to chair or standing position when stable. ▪ Monitor pulse oximetry and end-tidal CO_2. ▪ Monitor ABGs as indicated by changes in noninvasive parameters, patient status, or weaning protocol.
Circulation/Perfusion	
Blood pressure, heart rate, cardiac output, central venous pressure (CVP), and pulmonary artery pressure remain stable on mechanical ventilation.	▪ Assess hemodynamic effects of initiating positive-pressure ventilation (e.g., potential for decreased venous return and cardiac output). ▪ Monitor electrocardiogram (ECG) for dysrhythmias related to hypoxemia. ▪ Assess effects of ventilator setting changes (inspiratory pressures, tidal volume, positive end-expiratory pressure [PEEP], and fraction of inspired oxygen [FIO_2]) on hemodynamic and oxygenation parameters. ▪ Administer intravascular volume as ordered to maintain preload.
Fluids/Electrolytes	
Intake and output (I & O) measurements are balanced. Electrolyte values are within normal limits.	▪ Monitor hydration status in relation to clinical examination, auscultation, amount and viscosity of lung secretions. ▪ Assess patient weight, I & O totals, urine specific gravity, or serum osmolality to evaluate fluid balance. ▪ Administer electrolyte replacements (IV or enteral) per physician's order.
Mobility	
Patients will maintain/regain baseline functional status related to mobility and self-care. Joint range of motion is maintained.	▪ Collaborate with physical/occupational therapy staff to encourage patient effort/participation to increase mobility. ▪ Progress activity to sitting up in chair, standing at bedside, ambulating with assistance as soon as possible. ▪ Assist patient with active or passive range-of-motion exercises to all extremities at least every shift. ▪ Keep extremities in physiologically neutral position using pillows or appropriate splint/support devices as indicated.

(continued)

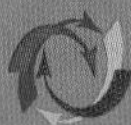

box 25-16 collaborative care guide *for the Patient on Mechanical Ventilation (Continued)*

OUTCOMES	INTERVENTIONS
Safety Endotracheal tube will remain in proper position. Proper inflation of endotracheal tube cuff is maintained. Ventilator alarm system remains activated.	■ Securely stabilize endotracheal tube in position; use respiratory therapy expertise for best method. ■ Note and record the "cm" line on endotracheal tube position at lip or teeth. ■ Use patient self-protective devices or sedation per hospital protocol. ■ Evaluate endotracheal tube position on chest x-ray (by viewing film or by report). ■ Keep emergency airway equipment and manual resuscitation bag readily available, and check each shift. ■ Inflate cuff using minimal leak technique, or pressure less than 25 mm Hg by manometer. ■ Monitor cuff inflation/leak every shift and PRN. ■ Protect pilot balloon from damage. ■ Perform ventilator setting and alarm checks q4h (minimum) or per hospital protocol.
Skin Integrity Patient is without evidence of skin breakdown.	■ Assess and document skin integrity at least every shift. ■ Turn side to side q2h; reassess bony prominences for evidence of pressure injury. ■ When patient is out of bed to chair, provide pressure relief to sitting surfaces at least q1h. ■ Remove self-protective devices from wrists, and monitor skin per hospital policy.
Nutrition Nutritional intake meets calculated metabolic need (e.g., basal energy expenditure equation). Patient will establish regular bowel elimination pattern.	■ Consult dietitian for metabolic needs assessment and recommendations. ■ Provide early nutritional support by enteral or parenteral feeding, start within 48 hours of intubation. ■ Monitor actual delivery of nutrition daily with I & O calculations. ■ Weigh patient daily. ■ Administer bowel regimen medications as ordered, along with adequate hydration.
Comfort/Pain Control Patients will indicate/exhibit adequate relief of discomfort/pain while on mechanical ventilation.	■ Document pain assessment, using numerical pain rating or similar scale when possible. ■ Provide analgesia as appropriate, document efficacy after each dose. ■ Prevent pulling and jarring of the ventilator tubing and endotracheal or tracheostomy tube. ■ Provide meticulous oral care q1–4h. ■ Administer sedation as indicated.

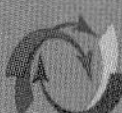

box 25-16 collaborative care guide *for the Patient on Mechanical Ventilation (Continued)*

OUTCOMES	INTERVENTIONS
Psychosocial	
Patient participates in self-care and decision making related to own activities of daily living (ADLs) (e.g., turning, bathing). Patient communicates with health care providers and visitors.	■ Encourage patient to move in bed and attempt to meet own basic comfort/hygiene needs independently. ■ Establish a daily schedule for bathing, out of bed, treatments, and so forth with patient input. ■ Provide a means for patient to write notes and use visual tools to facilitate communication. ■ Encourage visitor conversations with patient in normal tone of voice and subject matter. ■ Teach visitors to assist with range-of-motion and other simple care delivery tasks, to facilitate normal patterns of interaction.
Teaching/Discharge Planning	
Patient cooperates with and indicates understanding of need for mechanical ventilation. Potential discharge needs are assessed.	■ Provide explanations to patient/significant others regarding: Rationale for use of mechanical ventilation Procedures such as suctioning, airway care, other pulmonary toilet Plan for and progress toward weaning and extubation ■ Initiate early social work to screen for needs, resources, and support systems.

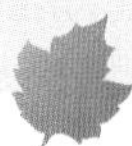

box 25-17
Considerations for the Pediatric Patient on Mechanical Ventilation

The nurse caring for a pediatric patient on ventilatory support must protect the physiological safety and stability of the patient while ensuring adequate psychosocial and emotional support for the child *and* his or her family members. These needs generate a complex set of priorities:

Maintain the Airway

- Assess endotracheal tube position every shift and PRN; reassess with any signs of respiratory distress.
- Change tape on artificial airway every other day and PRN (use two people); check integrity every shift. Mark the position of the endotracheal tube at tape with permanent marker to provide a visual "quick reference" point.
- Protect the child from self-extubation as needed with use of age-appropriate soft restraints.

Ensure Patient–Ventilator Synchrony

- Offer a developmentally appropriate explanation and encouragement to the child regarding the purpose of ventilation and the benefit of "breathing with the machine." Involve the family to reinforce these ideas.
- When clinically necessary, titrate sedation and paralytics to suppress patient effort and allow full mechanical ventilation (younger patients on ventilators should *always* receive sedation).
- Collaborate with the respiratory therapist on the care plan to maintain adequate ventilation and oxygenation. Begin systematic weaning process when the patient's condition permits.

Address Patient Comfort Issues

- Titrate ordered analgesia to age-appropriate pain scale or physiological parameters.
- Use comfort measures to calm, soothe, and reassure the child (and family) as needed.
- Administer anxiolytic/amnesic medications per order to help reduce physical and psychological stressors related to experience of acute illness and related interventions.

Provide Secure, Supportive Environment for the Child and Family

- Encourage and facilitate consistent presence of parents and other significant family members at the bedside to maintain the child's normal social and emotional ties.
- Involve the family in care plan development and hands-on interventions when appropriate.
- Facilitate communication between family members and health care team members.
- Consult the chaplain, social worker, and psychologist as needed for additional support or intervention.

to facilitate earlier weaning, particularly if the patient has multiple comorbidities and demonstrates difficulty weaning, or has trauma or neurological diagnoses associated with prolonged need for an artificial airway. Tracheostomy is also done for patient comfort and safety when mobilizing the patient, and may lead to decreased ventilator weaning time. In addition to long-term ventilation, indications for tracheostomy include upper airway obstruction, airway edema from anaphylaxis, failed intubation, multiple intubations (high risk for complications), complications of endotracheal tube intubation, absence of protective reflexes, home care, conditions where endotracheal tube intubation is not possible (e.g., facial trauma, cervical fractures), and the desire for improved patient comfort.

The advantages of tracheostomy over endotracheal intubation include faster weaning (at least in part because of decreased dead space), enhanced patient comfort, enhanced communication, and the possibility of oral feeding. The tracheostomy is inserted into the trachea, thereby avoiding the mouth, upper airway, and glottis, and this decreases problems of airway resistance and occlusion. Box 25-18 lists the equipment necessary for performing a tracheostomy.

Tracheostomy is not without disadvantages. These include hemorrhage, infection, pneumothorax, and the need for an operative procedure that is itself a risk. Complications of tracheostomy are given in Box 25-19. The most serious complication is erosion into the innominate artery, which can result in exsanguination. If bleeding occurs, the cuff can be hyperinflated in an attempt to control bleeding until emergency surgery can be initiated. Recently, the practice of bedside percutaneous tracheostomy using a progressive dilation technique has been touted to decrease the morbidity and cost incurred with an operative procedure. Less infection and bleeding have also been cited as advantages over the standard procedure.[43]

The nurse can prevent complications by assessing for them with each patient interaction, and during tracheostomy care. Proper fixation of the tracheostomy tube reduces the movement of the tube in the airway and limits friction injury to the tracheal wall or larynx. Maintaining the cuff pressure at the minimum required to prevent air leak on the ventilator reduces the risk of tissue breakdown due to excessive pressure on the trachea wall. The tracheostomy tube must be firmly secured. The ventilator tubing should have enough length to allow movement without pulling on the tracheostomy and to allow for procedures. A tracheostomy swivel connector, with or without flex tubing, reduces the tension on the tracheostomy while the patient is on the ventilator. A confused or very mobile patient can easily decannulate himself or herself; patient restraints may be needed to prevent accidental decannulation. Orienting the patient to the need for an artificial airway and providing pain control and sedation (if needed to improve patient tolerance of the tracheostomy) are measures that are taken before resorting to restraint application. If restraints are needed, a physician's order is required, with regular review of continued need. Patients must be closely monitored for potential injury, and circulatory checks with removal of restraints must be performed frequently.

Tracheostomy care includes frequent changing of tracheal ties and dressing, although initial ties are not changed until at least 25 to 48 hours after placement to allow for hemostasis of the site. The sutures from either a percutaneous or surgical tracheostomy are left in place for 48 to 72 hours or even up to a week (per hospital protocol) to prevent decannulation. As with retaping of the endotracheal tube, changing of tracheostomy ties should be a two-person procedure. The ties should be tied so that one to two fingers can be inserted between the ties and the skin, allowing minimal movement of the tracheostomy tube but maintaining comfort. It is mandatory to maintain a mid-

box 25-19 *Complications of Tracheostomy*

- Acute hemorrhage at the site
- Air embolism
- Aspiration
- Tracheal stenosis
- Erosion into the innominate artery with exsanguination
- Failure of the tracheostomy cuff
- Laryngeal nerve damage
- Obstruction of tracheostomy tube
- Pneumothorax
- Subcutaneous and mediastinal emphysema
- Swallowing dysfunction
- Tracheoesophageal fistula
- Infection
- Accidental decannulation with loss of airway

box 25-18 *Equipment for Tracheostomy*

- Percutaneous tracheostomy kit, either percutaneous or surgical*
- Surgical drapes, towels, gowns, gloves and sutures, prep equipment, and povidone–iodine (Betadine) solution
- Suction setup
- Correct size tracheostomy tube*
- 10-mL syringe for cuff inflation
- Twill tape, or Velcro tracheostomy holder†
- Pulse oximetry
- Oxygen source
- Manual resuscitation bag with mask
- End-tidal CO_2 monitor or disposable detector
- Sedation and paralytic medication
- Bronchoscopy cart (visualize correct placement for percutaneous approach)

*In adults, tube size is usually 8.0 mm initially unless the procedure is difficult. Percutaneous tracheostomy kits come with special tracheostomy tubes designed for that use. Smaller sizes can be used, and there are pediatric tracheostomy tubes.

†Initially the tracheostomy tube is sutured to the neck in both surgical and percutaneous procedures. Sutures are removed after 48 to 72 hours. Tracheostomy is secured at all times with twill tape or a Velcro tracheostomy holder, even with the sutures in place, to prevent accidental dislodgment.

line position for the tracheostomy to prevent pressure on surrounding tissue. The stoma is cleansed with half-strength hydrogen peroxide and observed for wound healing, bleeding, and signs of infection. The routine practice of inner cannula cleaning or changes may not be necessary, according to a recent study.[44] The routine care for tracheostomy is cleaning at least every 8 hours and as needed, changing the inner cannula daily (or according to facility policy), and changing soiled tracheostomy ties as needed, progressing to daily and as-needed care. This longer care interval usually occurs after 7 to 10 days or when secretion and tracheostomy drainage are minimal. The routine care of tracheostomies is always performed as a sterile procedure while in the hospital.

If decannulation occurs within the first 7 days of tracheostomy insertion, the patient may be reintubated with an endotracheal tube if emergent tracheostomy tube replacement cannot be done safely. An obturator and a new, appropriately sized tracheostomy tube is kept at the bedside. If inadvertent decannulation occurs after a tract has developed, the tube is carefully replaced using the obturator.

Tube Cuff Pressure Monitoring

Tube cuff pressures are monitored every shift to prevent overdistension and excess pressure on the tracheal wall mucosa, which can cause complications such as tracheal stenosis. If a patient is on the ventilator, the best pressure is the lowest possible pressure without incurring a loss of inspiratory volume. Physiologically, pressures of about 20 to 30 mm Hg obliterate capillary circulation to the tracheal mucosa. If a cuff leak is suspected, auscultation at the neck for the sound of air escaping above the cuff can determine whether the seal is adequate.

One method used to inflate a cuff is called the *minimal occluding volume.* Air is injected slowly during ventilator inspiration while auscultation is performed over the trachea. When the harsh "squeak" of air escaping is no longer audible, the minimal occluding volume has been reached, and the tube cuff is occluding the airway without excessive pressure on the trachea. Extra air should not be added. Best practice in ICUs is the actual measurement of cuff pressure using a manometer. This device is attached to the endotracheal tube pilot balloon to obtain a reading, which should not exceed 25 mm Hg. If a leak is still present above this level of inflation, slight repositioning of the endotracheal tube in the patient's airway may correct the problem. Changing to a larger or longer endotracheal tube may be necessary with increasing pressures to seal the airway. The cuff pressure should be assessed with the manometer every 6 to 8 hours, and when a leak is noted, to help prevent aspiration of subglottic secretions.

Discharge Planning and Patient Teaching

Discharge planning is necessary for patients who will be discharged to home with tracheostomies. Rationales for tracheostomy care include promotion of ostomy healing, prevention of infection, maintenance of a patent airway, and increased patient comfort. Before discharge, the nurse must:

- Explain the rationale and procedure for home tracheostomy care to the patient and the caregiver.[45]
- Arrange for home care supplies, oxygen, and suction equipment to be set up at the home before discharge.
- Arrange for home health care if an additional caregiver is needed to hold the tracheostomy in place while changing the tracheal ties if the patient cannot assist.
- Provide a contact number where questions about tracheostomy care can be answered 24 hours per day, 7 days per week.
- Review the tracheostomy care procedure with the caregiver and monitor the caregiver performing this care.
- Ensure that the caregiver can perform the care, following the steps completely, and is able to recite indications for calling the physician or 911.

If prepackaged tracheostomy kits are not being used, the following will be needed for home tracheostomy care:

- Bottles of hydrogen peroxide (H_2O_2), and sterile normal saline (NS; or sterile water)
- Twill tape, or pre-made Velcro tracheal ties
- Disposable sterile cotton swabs, a sterile basin, a sterile brush or pipe cleaners for inner cannula cleansing
- Scissors, procedure gloves (nonsterile)
- Suction equipment, catheters, and self-inflating resuscitation bag and mask, oxygen supply (suctioning with bagging is taught as a separate procedure for home care)
- Sterile 4 × 4 gauze pads, and sterile precut drain sponges to fit the tracheostomy
- Sterile, packaged disposable inner cannulas
- Protective eyewear and masks

Teaching the patient and family caregiver tracheostomy care allows for independence and self-care, and is an essential component for discharge teaching. Communication about the procedure and reassurance during the training process reduce anxiety and improve cooperation. The procedure in the Patient Teaching Guide in Box 25-20 is designed for the tracheostomy patient who is going home and who tolerates periods of time off the tracheostomy collar without experiencing a decrease in SaO_2.

NUTRITIONAL SUPPORT

Respiratory muscles, like all other body muscles, need energy to work. If energy needs are not met, muscle fatigue occurs, leading to discoordination of respiratory muscles and a decrease in tidal volume. Hypomagnesemia and hypophosphatemia have been implicated in muscle fatigue caused by depleted levels of adenosine triphosphate (ATP). In prolonged starvation, the body cannibalizes the intercostal and diaphragmatic muscles for energy.

Metabolic needs in critically ill patients are much higher than in normal subjects. Basic caloric requirements are usually increased by 25% for hospital activity and stress associated with treatment. Adequate nutrition is a prerequisite for weaning from mechanical ventilation; nutritional support should be instituted early. If the gastrointestinal tract is intact, enteral nutrition is preferred and can be provided through a feeding tube.

Many chronically ill patients, such as those with COPD, have long-standing protein and calorie malnutrition. Initial tube feeding is started slowly, with close monitoring of blood glucose levels. The nurse observes the patient for signs of intolerance, such as diarrhea and hyperosmolar

box 25-20

Caring for a Tracheostomy at Home

Procedure for Tracheostomy Care

ELEMENT	RATIONALE	PRECAUTIONS AND CONSIDERATIONS
1. Wash hands.	Reduces microorganisms on hands, standard precautions	Protective eyewear or face mask should be worn with copious secretions, especially in patients with forceful coughs.
2. Bag and suction trachea as needed to remove secretions.	Preoxygenates to reduce risk of hypoxemia and cough during the tracheostomy care procedure	
3. Don procedure gloves and remove soiled dressing.	Reduces microorganisms	
4. Remove soiled gloves and prepare prepackaged kit or supplies; prepare supplies and place approximately 100 mL in two bowls, one with hydrogen peroxide (H_2O_2), and the other with normal saline (NS).		
5. Don new procedure gloves.	Reduces microorganisms, standard precautions	
6. Remove tracheostomy collar and oxygen supply; remove inner cannula and place into H_2O_2 bowl. (See Precautions and Considerations for use of disposable inner cannulas and single-lumen tracheostomy tubes.)	Inner cannula can now be cleaned.	When using disposable inner cannulas omit steps 6 to 8 and 10. Remove disposable inner cannula and replace with new inner cannula. With single-lumen tracheostomy tubes, skip steps 6 to 8 and 10. (Many institutions change inner cannulas as often as every 8 to 12 hours. Periodic cleaning or changing of the inner cannula tube is thought necessary to identify narrowing of the inner cannula from encrusted or tenacious secretions. Evidence suggests that frequent inner cannula changes are not necessary.[46,47])
7. Cleanse inner cannula with small brush or pipe stem cleaners.	Removes debris and thick secretions	
8. Rinse inner cannula with NS poured over the cannula and let soak; remove and let cannula dry.	Removes H_2O_2 and debris	
9. Moisten cotton swabs and 4 × 4 gauze pads with NS, then cleanse stoma site and outer cannula and neckplate, wiping with swabs and 4 × 4 pads.	Cleanses outer stoma and cannula of secretions; use NS alone to cleanse delicate skin around stoma because H_2O_2 can lead to skin and mucous membrane irritation	
10. Insert and lock inner cannula in place.	Secures inner cannula	
11. Pat dry the skin surrounding the stoma with a dry 4 × 4 pad.	Dry skin reduces likelihood of microorganism growth and skin breakdown	

box 25-20
Caring for a Tracheostomy at Home (Continued)

Procedure for Tracheostomy Care

ELEMENT	RATIONALE	PRECAUTIONS AND CONSIDERATIONS
12. Prepare new tracheostomy ties or use premade tie; cut twill tape long enough to wrap around the neck twice.	Length appropriate for wrapping around the neck and tying on the side of the neck	Premade Velcro trach ties are available and easy to use: review manufacturer's guideline.
13. The patient or an assistant holds the neckplate securely.	Prevents accidental decannulation	
14. Remove old twill tape or premade tracheostomy tie.	Allows for clean tracheostomy tie application	Patient or assistant holds tracheostomy in place until new tie is secured; if patient unable to assist, tie the new twill tape into place first, then remove the old twill tape or have another health care worker stabilize the tracheostomy when replacing ties to prevent decannulation.
15. Apply twill tape and secure through eyes on neckplate; insert both ends into eyes, bring one end back around the neck and tie on one side of the neck; apply Velcro tracheostomy tie through both eyes, adjusting with Velcro to correct tightness.	Resecures the tracheostomy with the knot on the side of the neck; allows knot to be observed when using twill tape	Tighten tracheostomy tie to allow one finger to be inserted between tie and neck for venous flow and comfort. Twill tape loosens when wet, which may lead to an increased risk of tube dislodgement.
16. Tuck the precut drain sponge under the neckplate; change drain sponge as needed.	Absorbs stoma secretions	Use only precut tracheostomy drain gauze; cutting a 4 × 4 pad causes frayed edges that may be a possible source for infection.
17. Replace tracheostomy collar for humidification and oxygen.	Returns humidified oxygen to tracheal airway	Humidified air or oxygen prevents drying of secretions that can lead to obstruction.
18. Remove all soiled supplies and wash hands after procedure.	Reduces microorganisms and standard procedure	

Call the Physician or 911

- Indications for calling the physician at home include elevated temperature, oozing or frank bleeding, foul odor from the stoma or secretions, and a change in color or increased secretions around the tracheostomy opening.
- Reasons for calling 911 include obstruction, loss of tracheostomy from the stoma, respiratory distress from other causes, severe bleeding, severe distress from febrile condition, and other potential medical emergencies.

dehydration. If the patient tolerates feedings, the rate is gradually increased until the desired rate is achieved. If tube feedings cannot be tolerated, parenteral hyperalimentation should be considered (see Chapter 40).

Patients who require long-term mechanical ventilation typically need 2,000 to 2,500 calories per day. Overly large caloric loads increase carbon dioxide production and can precipitate respiratory failure in a compromised patient. When available, metabolic chart determinations (also called *indirect calorimetry*) are the best way to assess individual nutritional requirements. Nutritionists are invaluable in determining the caloric needs and establishing caloric goals for ICU patients.

EYE CARE

Eye care of the patient on mechanical ventilation is important. Many ICU patients are comatose, sedated, or chemically paralyzed and therefore have lost the blink reflex or ability to close their eyelids completely. This can lead to corneal dryness and ulceration.

Few studies have established the efficacy of one eye care measure compared with another. Current practices include instillation of lubricating drops or ointment, taping the eyes, applying eye shields, or applying a moisture chamber.[48] Scleral edema is common in the ventilated patient. Raising the head of the bed may reduce scleral edema.

ORAL CARE

Frequent oral care must be performed for all mechanically ventilated patients. Oral care not only increases comfort and decreases thirst, but preserves the integrity of the oropharyngeal mucosa. An intact mucosa helps prevent infection and colonization of organisms that may lead to systemic, possibly life-threatening infection. As noted in the VAP discussion, there is no evidence-based protocol or definitive critical care guideline for the oral care of ventilated patients (endotracheal or tracheostomy). Nursing skills manuals do present guidelines for oral care in patients with and without teeth, and incapacitated patients.[8] These general oral care guidelines are not suitable for patients with an endotracheal tube and do not provide evidence-based support for using or not using an antibacterial agent, such as chlorhexidine, in the mouthwash. Oncology- and gerontology-based research and guidelines for oral care do substantiate the impact of oral mucosal changes on a person's well-being.[49,50] Oral care in critical care depends on unit-variable guidelines and usually is based on the nurse's experience and knowledge as well as on product availability, with conflicting advice on the most appropriate choice of solutions and equipment.[49] Suggested guidelines for oral care in critically ill, mechanically ventilated patients may include the following (summarized from the available literature):

1. Systematic assessment of the oral mucosa is performed daily, and with each cleaning.
2. A scheduled, regular oral care regimen should be established, using products that remove plaque and cleanse the mouth without causing pain or irritation. A non–alcohol-based mouthwash should be used, and the teeth should be brushed a minimum of every 8 hours. Toothbrushes should have soft bristles and should be used with toothpaste. In patients with bleeding disorders or a low platelet count, a toothette (foam brush) is substituted for a toothbrush.
3. Oral suctioning and care to remove subglottic secretions should occur every 1 to 2 hours. Alternatively, in long-term mechanically ventilated patients who are candidates, a CASS tube may be used to remove subglottic secretions. Each oral care should include suctioning of the subglottic secretions to prevent aspiration.
4. Guidelines for use of a chlorhexidine-based mouthwash do not exist, nor do they for hydrogen peroxide or other antibacterial or antifungal mouthwashes. Mouthwash should be compatible with the patient's condition, and should not cause pain due to additives for flavor, alcohol, or strength. Using half-strength solutions diluted with water may help the patient tolerate more frequent oral care.
5. Follow unit and manufacturer's guidelines for products, and evaluate oral care needs for the individual patient. Establish a care plan that meets the patient's needs. Factors to take into account include the frequency of oral care, the products to be used, and daily assessment of oral mucosa.

PSYCHOLOGICAL CARE

The ventilated patient is often subjected to extreme physical and emotional stress in the ICU environment. Psychological distress can be caused by sleep deprivation, sensory overstimulation (as well as sensory deprivation of familiar cues), pain, fear, the inability to communicate, and commonly used pharmacological agents. Treatments can often seem dehumanizing. In many cases, the prognosis is poor and the possibility of death is ever-present.

Feelings of helplessness and lack of control can be overwhelming. The patient may attempt to gain some element of control through constant demanding or exhibition of other "inappropriate" behavior. If the patient is incapable of dealing with stress through coping mechanisms, he or she may exhibit depression, apathy, and lack of emotional involvement. These reactions may be exacerbated in patients with a history of psychiatric problems or drug or alcohol abuse.

Assisted ventilation can precipitate a psychological dependence in those with primary respiratory disorders. If for the first time in years a patient is receiving enough oxygen to meet metabolic needs and does not have to struggle for air, he or she may be reluctant to give up the ventilator. Weaning can become even more stressful for this patient.

Facilitating Communication

A number of interventions can facilitate communication with the patient who has an endotracheal or tracheostomy tube. Before assessing the patient's ability to communicate, provide the patient with his or her eyeglasses or hearing aid (if applicable). Complete explanations from staff members regarding any procedures may help decrease the patient's stress. The caregiver can use verbal and nonverbal communication skills. Nonverbal communication may include sign language, gestures, or lip reading. If the patient is unable to use these forms of nonverbal communication, helpful devices include pencil and paper, "grease" boards, and picture or alphabet boards.

Once he or she is off the ventilator and tolerating the tracheostomy collar, the tracheostomy patient can communicate by using "buttons" that occlude the tracheostomy tube. The buttons allow for the passage of air around the tracheostomy to the vocal chords. The Kirshner button mentioned later in this chapter in weaning section is one type of button. Two other buttons are the Passy-Muir valve and the Shiley speaking valve. The Passy-Muir valve is a one-way valve that allows air to enter during inspiration, then closes to allow the air to flow over the vocal chords with exhalation. The Shiley speaking valve works in the same way as the Passy-Muir valve, but has a side port for oxygen tubing to be attached, providing oxygen support without using a tracheostomy collar. Patients with copious secretions are at risk for obstruction of these valves. They must be monitored very closely. In addition, patients at high risk for aspiration, and especially patients with laryngeal or pharyngeal dysfunction, should be carefully assessed before one of these devices is used. The nurse should store these valves in a container clearly identified with the patient's name for safekeeping because each type of valve is relatively costly. The patient should be taught to remove the valve with excessive sputum during cough and call for assistance to clean the valve before reuse. The tracheostomy patient with a speaking valve is at increased risk for aspiration because the cuff must be deflated for the patient to communicate.

Caring for the Family

Family members must deal with a strange environment, a critically ill loved one, and the financial strain imposed by the illness. Nursing support is given by familiarizing the family with the physical surroundings, supplying information about visitation policies, and providing frequent progress reports on the patient's condition.

Studies show improvement in patient outcomes from increased presence of loved ones during hospitalization. Based on these findings and on increased patient and family satisfaction, many ICUs have instituted open visitation policies and increased involvement of family members in patient care. Critical care patients and especially the elderly benefit from increased visitation, and despite some conflicting results, studies support that there is no detrimental effect on the physiological status of critically ill patients when increased visitation is permitted.[51–53] Nurses increasingly recognize the importance of family visitation for the patient. The presence of family during invasive procedures or during a code has been associated with positive outcomes, and studies show family and caregivers reported the benefit of being at the bedside.[53,54]

Often nurses do not consider family needs a priority. Ideally, the nurse establishes open communication with the patient and family, proactively arranges for visits, and provides the family with information.[55] As noted in the article on visitation policies in critical care, most nurses are more liberal with critical care visitation than stated policy.[55] A system that includes liberal visitation policies and flexibility for individual patient and family needs promotes a healing environment and supports the family as partners in the care plan.

Weaning From Mechanical Ventilation

As soon as the patient is placed on mechanical ventilation, plans begin for weaning the patient from mechanical support. The process to achieve this goal includes correcting the cause of respiratory failure, preventing complications, and restoring or maintaining physiological and psychological functional status. Patients can be categorized into two groups: those requiring short-term ventilation (≤3 days) and those requiring long-term ventilation (>3 days).[56]

Each patient is evaluated daily for readiness to wean. Box 25-21 and Box 25-22 present guidelines for weaning

box 25-21
Guidelines for Weaning From Short-Term Ventilation

Patients are often intubated electively for surgical or other procedures, or more urgently owing to respiratory distress related to underlying pulmonary disease or traumatic injury. The other common reason for intubation is the need for airway protection because of airway swelling (e.g., as a result of acute inhalation injury) or significant change in mental status (e.g., as with cerebrovascular accident [CVA] or head injury). Once the procedure is completed or the patient is stabilized, the goal should be extubation as soon as the patient is able to protect the airway. The weaning process in this setting may proceed rapidly, based on individual patient response to reducing ventilatory support.

Readiness Criteria

- Hemodynamically stable, adequately resuscitated, and not requiring vasoactive support
- Sa_{O_2} >92% on Fi_{O_2} ≤40%, positive end-expiratory pressure (PEEP) ≤5 cm H_2O
- Chest x-ray reviewed for correctable factors; treated as indicated
- Metabolic indicators (serum pH, major electrolytes) within normal range
- Hematocrit >25%
- Core temperature >36°C and <39°C
- Adequate management of pain/anxiety/agitation
- No residual neuromuscular blockade
- Arterial blood gases (ABGs) normalized or at patient's baseline

Weaning Intervention

- Reduce ventilator rate, then convert to pressure-support ventilation (PSV) only.
- Wean PSV as tolerated to ≤10 cm H_2O.
- If patient meets tolerance criteria for at least 2 hours on this level of support *and* meets extubation criteria (see later), may extubate.
- If patient fails tolerance criteria, increase PSV or add ventilator rate as needed to achieve "rest" settings (consistent respiratory rate <20 breaths/minute) and review weaning criteria for correctable factors.
- Repeat wean attempt on PSV 10 cm after rest period (minimum 2 hours). If patient fails second wean trial, return to rest settings and use "long-term" ventilation weaning approach.

Tolerance Criteria

If the patient displays any of the following, the weaning trial should be stopped and the patient returned to "rest" settings.

- Sustained respiratory rate greater than 35 breaths/minute
- Sa_{O_2} <90%
- Tidal volume ≤5 mL/kg
- Sustained minute ventilation >200 mL/kg/minute
- Evidence of respiratory or hemodynamic distress:
  Labored respiratory pattern
  Increased anxiety, diaphoresis, or both
  Sustained heart rate >20% higher or lower than baseline
  Systolic blood pressure >180 mm Hg or <90 mm Hg

Extubation Criteria

- Mental status: alert and able to respond to commands
- Good cough and gag reflex, able to protect airway and clear secretions
- Able to move air around endotracheal tube with cuff deflated and end of tube occluded

Adapted from evidence-based practice guidelines used in the Surgical/Trauma Intensive Care Unit, University of Virginia Health System, Charlottesville, Virginia.

box 25-22
Guidelines for Weaning From Long-Term Ventilation

Patients on mechanical ventilation for longer than 72 hours or those having failed short-term weaning often display significant deconditioning as a result of acute or chronic complex illness, or both. These patients usually require a period of "exercising" respiratory muscles to regain the strength and endurance needed for successful return to spontaneous breathing. Goals for this process are:

- To have the patient tolerate two to three daily weaning trials of reduction in ventilatory support without exercising to the point of exhaustion
- To rest the patient between weaning trials and overnight on ventilator settings that provide diaphragmatic rest, with minimal or no work of breathing for the patient

Readiness Criteria

- Same as for short-term ventilation (see Box 25-21), with emphasis on hemodynamic stability, adequate analgesia/sedation (record scores on flow sheet), and normalizing volume status

Weaning Intervention

- Transfer to pressure-support ventilation (PSV) mode, adjust support level to maintain patient's respiratory rate at less than 35 breaths/minute.
- Observe for 30 minutes for signs of early failure (same tolerance criteria as with short-term ventilation; see Box 25-21).
- If tolerated, continue trial for 2 hours, then return patient to "rest" settings by adding ventilator breaths or increasing PSV to achieve a total respiratory rate of less than 20 breaths/minute.
- After at least 2 hours of rest, repeat trial for 2 to 4 hours at same PSV level as previous trial. If the patient exceeds the tolerance criteria (listed in Box 25-21), stop the trial and return to "rest" settings. In this case, the next trial should be performed at a higher support level than the "failed" trial.
- Record the results of each weaning episode, including specific parameters and the time frame if "failure" observed, on the bedside flow sheet.
- The goal is to increase the length of the trials and reduce the PSV level needed on an incremental basis. With each successive trial, the PSV level may be decreased by 2 to 4 cm H_2O, the time interval may be increased by 1 to 2 hours, or both, while keeping the patient within tolerance parameters. The pace of weaning is patient-specific and tolerance may vary from day to day. Review readiness criteria for correctable factors daily *and* each time the patient "fails" a weaning trial.
- Ensure nocturnal ventilation at "rest" settings (with a respiratory rate of <20 breaths/minute) for at least 6 hours each night until the patient's weaning trials demonstrate readiness to discontinue ventilatory support.

Discontinuing Mechanical Ventilation

The patient should be weaned until ventilator settings are FIO_2 ≤40%, PSV ≤10 cm H_2O, and positive end-expiratory pressure (PEEP) ≤8 cm H_2O. Once these settings are well tolerated, the patient should be placed on continuous positive airway pressure (CPAP) 5 cm H_2O or (if tracheostomy in place) on tracheostomy collar. If the patient meets tolerance criteria over the first 5 minutes, the trial should be continued for 1 to 2 hours. If clinical observation and arterial blood gases (ABGs) indicate that the patient is maintaining adequate ventilation and oxygenation on this "minimal" support, the following options should be considered:

- If the patient meets extubation criteria (see Box 25-21), this step should be attempted.
- If the patient is on tracheostomy collar, the trials should be continued two to three times per day with daily increases in time on tracheostomy collar by 1 to 2 hours per trial until total time off the ventilator reaches 18 hours per day. At this point, the patient may be ready to remain on tracheostomy collar for longer than 25 hours unless the tolerance criteria are exceeded.
- Ventilator weaning is considered successful once the patient achieves spontaneous ventilation (extubated or on tracheostomy collar) for at least 25 hours.

Adapted from evidence-based practice guidelines used in the Surgical/Trauma Intensive Care Unit, University of Virginia Health System, Charlottesville, Virginia.

from short-term ventilation and long-term ventilation, respectively. It is important to perform this assessment and address weaning impediments before initiating weaning trials. Many weaning indices have been advocated for use in predicting weaning readiness. Some look exclusively at respiratory factors such as muscle strength and endurance (e.g., negative inspiratory pressure [NIP], positive expiratory pressure [PEP], weaning index, or ratio of frequency to tidal volume). Others are integrated indices that look at a broad range of physiological factors that influence weaning readiness; these are not only predictors, but tools to assist in identifying and improving factors that influence the weaning process.[57]

In addition to controversy concerning weaning indices, there is disagreement and lack of evidence regarding which approach to weaning is best. Some clinicians maintain total ventilatory support up until the time of weaning trials; others use intermittent trials of increasing frequency and duration. The theoretical advantages of a gradual approach to weaning support include the following: (1) over time, the patient on partial rather than full ventilation is exposed to lower levels of pressure and volume, therefore reducing the risk of complications; and (2) a weaning approach that requires the patient to perform some level of work to breathe imposes an "exercise" regimen that should reduce deconditioning and atrophy of the muscles used in respiration.[41]

The performance of the diaphragm, as well as accessory muscles of respiration, depends on both the endurance and strength of the muscles. The effectiveness of diaphragmatic contraction is a function of both the resting length of muscle fibers and the speed with which they contract. Both of these factors are affected by physiological changes that change the resting position of the diaphragm. With COPD, the resting length is shorter (weakening force of contraction), and with diaphragmatic distension, ascites, or morbid obesity, the diaphragm must push down abdominal contents as it contracts. Reactive airway disease increases the resistance to air flow, with increased workload for muscles of respiration. Any of these abnormalities can lead to significant fatigue of these muscles and respiratory distress.[58]

Respiratory muscle fatigue impedes weaning. It may take as long as 25 hours of complete rest (the mechanical ventilator assumes all of the work of breathing for the patient) for recovery of fatigued respiratory muscles. Therefore, it is common practice to increase ventilatory support at night to ensure rest. This can be accomplished with any of the "resting" modes, so long as the patient's respiratory rate is less than 20 breaths/minute. The intent here is to promote and simulate the normal decrease in rate and work of breathing that occurs during each person's sleep/rest cycle.

Weaning trials are discontinued if signs of fatigue or respiratory distress develop. The weaning tolerance criteria and observations are summarized in Box 25-21 and Box 25-22. The use of sedatives and narcotics during weaning should be limited to only the level of medication clearly needed to control pain or anxiety. Special considerations for weaning an older patient from a ventilator are given in Box 25-23.

Regardless of the mode or approach, certain factors have been found to influence weaning success positively. These include the use of collaborative, multidisciplinary teams to formulate comprehensive plans of care based on assessment of individual patients, the use of standardized weaning protocols that are assigned to each patient on the basis of individual assessment, and the use of critical pathways.[59] The interplay of these strategies—all designed to promote consistency of, and rationale for, practice—truly leads to outcomes showing that the whole (process) is greater than the sum of its parts.

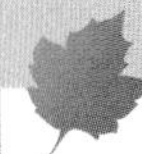

box 25-23

Overcoming Barriers to Ventilator Weaning in the Older Patient

An elderly patient on mechanical ventilation poses a unique challenge to caregivers. Successful weaning requires effective nursing interventions to address the patient's basic care needs.

- **Alteration in sleep/rest pattern:** Learn the patient's normal sleep habits, establish a restful environment, and minimize interruptions for at least 6 hours each night and 2 hours of midday rest. Consult the pharmacist or physician for sleep medication PRN at bedtime.
- **Nutrition and hydration:** Consult the dietitian and begin delivery of recommended nutrition as soon as possible. Assess patient tolerance and increase to goal rate per order. Evaluate fluid balance each shift (intake and output, weight, clinical examination) and discuss changes in intake and the possible need for diuretics with the physician.
- **Management of analgesia and sedation:** Administer analgesia per order, assessing need and effect of intervention by pain scale or physiological parameters. Carefully evaluate possible etiology of anxiety or agitation; when pharmacological intervention is indicated, titrate to achieve desired response using standardized sedation scale.
- **Alteration in bowel elimination:** Learn the patient's "usual" elimination pattern if possible; start with similar intervention and add more aggressive bowel regimen as needed to establish regular bowel movements. Evaluate factors (e.g., medications) that may alter bowel function, and ensure adequate hydration (by enteral route if possible).
- **Activity/mobility status:** Consult the physical or occupational therapist to evaluate functional capacity and initiate appropriate therapy. Begin getting patient out of bed as soon as possible, and encourage active range-of-motion exercises and participation in activities of daily living.

SHORT-TERM VENTILATION WEANING

Patients typically intubated for a short time include those who are intubated for surgical procedures, for an acute exacerbation of an underlying lung disease that can be easily reversed, and for airway protection during an acute neurological event (e.g., drug overdose). Weaning within a short time is desirable because physiological changes caused by the mechanical ventilation begin within 72 hours (see Box 25-21).

Frequently used predictive criteria for short-term weaning success are an NIP of no more than –20 cm H_2O (more negative, e.g., –30 cm H_2O), PEP of at least +30 cm H_2O (more positive, e.g., +45 cm H_2O), and spontaneous minute volume of less than 12 L/minute. NIP and PEP give an indication of respiratory muscle strength. The choice of weaning method does not seem to be important.

Weaning procedures may vary slightly from hospital to hospital, but general guidelines remain the same. For instance, weaning is usually initiated in the morning when the patient is rested. The patient is made comfortable, and the nurse elevates the head of the bed. Pharmacological agents for comfort, such as bronchodilators or sedatives, are administered as indicated. By explaining the procedure, the nurse helps the patient through some of the discomfort and apprehension. Before a weaning trial, the nurse ensures a patent airway and suctions if necessary.

Support and reassurance help the patient through the discomfort and apprehension as the nurse remains with the patient after initiation of the weaning process. The nurse also evaluates and documents the patient's response to weaning.

LONG-TERM VENTILATION WEANING

The longer a patient requires mechanical ventilation, the greater the potential for development of volume–pressure trauma, which consists of multiple alveolar fractures and leaky alveolar–capillary membranes.[60] The process of long-term weaning often takes weeks. Usually this process is

insights into clinical research

Henneman E, Dracup K, Ganz T, et al: Using a collaborative weaning plan to decrease duration of mechanical ventilation and length of stay in the intensive care units for patients receiving long term ventilation. Am J Crit Care 11(2):132–140, 2002

While intensive care units (ICUs) are faced with length-of-stay issues, weaning patients off long-term ventilation becomes more challenging. The purpose of this study was to evaluate the effectiveness of two structures that support communication and are needed to promote collaborative decision making in improving outcomes for patients receiving long-term ventilation. The structures are a weaning board and a flow sheet. "Long term" was defined as 7 days or more.

The sample consisted of all patients admitted to the medical ICU who received mechanical ventilation for 7 or more days. The intervention was termed "the collaborative weaning plan" and consisted of five parts: (1) the multidisciplinary team developed the weaning plan during morning rounds; (2) the plan of care for weaning was then documented on a weaning board; (3) data on the weaning process and the patient's response to each weaning trial were documented on the flow sheet; (4) any member of the ICU team could fill in the weaning board or the flow sheet; (5) the processes used to wean patients were not manipulated during the intervention period. Eighty-two patients were in the experimental group and 55 in the comparison group. Results showed that outcomes, such as days of ventilation, length of stay, cost, mortality, reventilation, and readmission were better in the experimental group than in the comparison group. These results, despite limitations, indicate that significant improvements in patient outcomes can be obtained by using interventions aimed at improving communication among members of the health care team.

complicated, and involves multiple delays and setbacks. During long-term weaning, the patient may fail a weaning trial and should then be rested on the ventilator before another trial is attempted. The rest period is to allow the recovery of the respiratory muscles. Patients who fail a weaning trial often exhibit rapid, shallow breathing patterns consistent with their respiratory muscle weakness. Regular reevaluation of the weaning plan by the multidisciplinary team, coupled with continuous communication with the patient and family, is necessary (see Box 25-22).

METHODS FOR VENTILATOR WEANING

Various methods have been studied for weaning from the ventilator. Controversies exist over which methods are best. Some of the most common weaning methods include T-piece or CPAP trials and a gradual PSV reduction.[61] Comprehensive assessment of the patient's needs and progress toward weaning, monitoring of the weaning parameters, and following established goals promote successful weaning. Multidisciplinary and comprehensive approaches to weaning based on a health care professional (nurse) monitoring and promoting a weaning plan with continuity have demonstrated positive outcomes.[62]

insights into clinical research

Epstein C, Mokadem N, Peerless J: Weaning older patients from long-term mechanical ventilation. Am J Crit Care 11(4):369–377, 2002

As the number of older persons in the United States increases, the number of older adults who experience traumatic injuries and undergo surgical procedures will also increase. In the United States, the percentage of older adults in the intensive care unit (ICU) ranges from 42% to 48%. With greater numbers of older adults requiring intensive care, the use of long-term mechanical ventilation has increased. This study group defined long-term mechanical ventilation as lasting 3 days or more. This pilot study looked at 10 trauma/surgical patients older than 60 years of age who required 3 or more days of mechanical ventilation. The purpose of this study was to describe the clinical course of weaning in critically ill older adults who were receiving long-term ventilation to determine whether differences exist between patients who can be weaned and those who cannot, and whether systemic factors (age) play a role in these differences.

Participants were monitored daily until they were successfully weaned for 24 hours. Available clinical data were collected every day and weaning decisions were made using these data and the Burns Weaning Assessment Program (BWAP). The BWAP is a 26-item checklist of general and respiratory factors used to assess readiness for weaning. Results of this pilot study showed that the six patients who could be weaned from ventilatory support were significantly younger (mean age, 70 years; median age, 71.5 years; range, 60–80 years) than the four patients who could not be weaned (mean age, 76 years; median age, 80 years; range, 63–82 years). Patients who could be weaned, however, were ready by day 11 of their stay in the ICU, and those who could not be weaned were not ready until day 17.

Results of this study are not surprising and lead to the same conclusions as other studies in geriatrics. Older critically ill patients must generate enormous adaptive responses to the stressors of injury to regain hemostasis. Older adults have many of the risk factors that prolong mechanical ventilation, including respiratory muscle weakness, a blunted ventilatory response to hypoxemia, increased atelectasis due to diminished production of surfactant, and a greater susceptibility to infection. The multidimensional and interactive effects of these factors on weaning from mechanical ventilation most likely are more problematic for older patients than for younger patients.

T-piece Trial

The T-piece is connected to the patient at the desired FIO_2 (usually slightly higher than the previous ventilator setting). The patient's response to and tolerance of the trial are continuously observed. The duration of T-piece trials is not standardized, and some clinicians extubate if an initial trial of 30 minutes ends with acceptable ABGs and patient response. Some use trials of increasing frequency and duration to evaluate and build the patient's endurance with periods of rest on the ventilator between trials. When the latter method is used, the patient is usually deemed ready to be extubated after 25 successive hours on a T-piece.

Synchronized Intermittent Mandatory Ventilation Method

The SIMV mode was initially heralded as the optimal weaning mode, allowing for some spontaneous breathing (to prevent respiratory muscle atrophy) while providing a backup rate. Weaning with the SIMV method entails a gradual reduction in the number of delivered breaths until a low rate is reached (usually 4 breaths/minute). The patient is then extubated if all other weaning criteria are met. However, low levels of SIMV (fewer than 4 breaths/minute) may result in a high level of work and fatigue. SIMV plus PSV may be used to decrease the work of breathing associated with spontaneous breaths. It has been suggested that using the combined modes may result in prolonged weaning duration.[63] As a result, PSV "standalone" mode is often preferred for weaning trials.

Continuous Positive Airway Pressure Method

CPAP entails breathing through the ventilator circuit with a small amount (or zero amount) of positive pressure. The use of CPAP versus the use of a T-piece for weaning is controversial. Often the decision to use one over the other is determined by observing the patient's response, or is simply based on the clinician's preference.

Pressure-Support Ventilation Method

Low levels of PSV decrease the work of breathing associated with endotracheal tubes and ventilator circuits. Weaning using the PSV mode entails a progressive decrease in pressure based on the patient maintaining an adequate tidal volume (8 to 12 mL/kg) and a respiratory rate of less than 25 breaths/minute. PSV is associated with less work of breathing than with volume modes, so longer weaning trials may be tolerated.

ADJUNCTS TO WEANING

Several adjuncts to long-term weaning are used to improve weaning tolerance and patient comfort. The fenestrated tracheostomy tube provides for communication during weaning periods, improving patient interaction. The fenestrated tracheostomy tube has an opening in the outer cannula but not the inner cannula. With the inner cannula in place and the cuff inflated, the patient is easily mechanically ventilated. During the weaning process, the inner cannula is removed, the cuff deflated, the outer cannula capped, and supplemental oxygen supplied by nasal cannula. This system permits air to pass the vocal cords, allowing verbal communication by the patient. The cuff should never be inflated while the inner cannula is capped because the patient will be unable to breathe. The Kirshner button or Shiley speaking valve provides communication during weaning periods for patients with tracheostomy tubes. These provide less resistance than the fenestrated tracheostomy tube, and with the Shiley valve, supplemental oxygen can be given through a side port. Humidified air with a tracheostomy collar may be required to keep the airway moist and prevent secretions from drying. Use of a large endotracheal tube (>7.0 mm) decreases resistance to breathing and decreases the work of breathing. A larger endotracheal tube also supports bronchoscopy to remove secretions when needed. Tracheostomy in many instances is more comfortable for patients and allows for improved oral care, improved communication, and tracheostomy collar or Kirshner button trials.

EXTUBATION CRITERIA

Whichever mode or combination of modes is used for weaning, extubation cannot occur until several criteria are met based on short-term or long-term ventilation (see Box 25-21 and Box 25-22). Before extubation, the patient must be able to maintain his or her own airway, as evidenced by an appropriate level of consciousness and the presence of cough and gag reflexes. In all patients, but especially in those with a history of difficult intubation or reactive airway disease, the "cuff leak test" should be performed before extubation. This entails deflation of the tube cuff (after suctioning of the oropharynx) and a brief period of occluding the endotracheal tube to demonstrate an air leak with patient inspiration. Absence of a leak can indicate edema, and may predict laryngeal stridor postextubation. If the cuff leak test fails, the patient may be given corticosteroids to reduce edema for 25 to 48 hours, then reassessed for cuff leak. Direct visualization of the trachea with a bronchoscope may be obtained before extubation to determine if the edema has resolved.

Extubation should never occur unless a qualified person is available to reintubate emergently if the patient does not tolerate extubation. After explaining the procedure and preparing the patient, the nurse suctions the patient's tube and posterior oropharynx. Equipment includes an MRB and mask at bedside. After the nurse loosens the endotracheal tube securing device or tape, the cuff is deflated. The endotracheal tube is removed quickly while having the patient cough. The patient's mouth is suctioned and humidified oxygen is applied immediately. The patient is evaluated for immediate signs of distress: stridor, dyspnea, and decrease in SaO_2. Treatment for stridor includes inhaled racemic epinephrine and sometimes administration of intravenous steroids (because steroids do not work immediately, they are given before extubation in those at risk). If these interventions fail, immediate reintubation may be necessary.

Home Care and Mechanical Ventilation

Certain patients requiring invasive mechanical ventilation may be candidates for home care. Conditions that may warrant home care ventilator management include:[64]

- Neurologic disorders (e.g., ALS, Guillain-Barré syndrome, multiple sclerosis, muscular dystrophy, myasthenia gravis, poliomyelitis, polymyositis, spinal cord injury)
- Restrictive disorders (e.g., interstitial pulmonary fibrosis, kyphoscoliosis, obesity, sarcoidosis)
- Obstructive disorders (e.g., bronchiectasis, bronchiolitis obliterans, bronchopulmonary dysplasia, chronic bronchitis and emphysema, cystic fibrosis, sleep apnea syndromes)

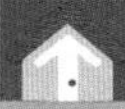

box 25-24 *Home Care for Ventilator-Assisted Patients*

- The caregivers, patient, nurse, and physician meet to discuss the patient's and caregivers' desire for home care. The team presents a realistic overview, including the need for extensive caregiver teaching before discharge, and the need for a high level of caregiver commitment owing to the extensive daily care needs of the patient.
- This initial meeting is followed by a multidisciplinary meeting with representatives from Nursing, Medicine, Social Work, Physical and Occupational Therapy, Respiratory Therapy, Speech Therapy, Nutrition, and Pharmacy, to discuss the patient's and caregivers' resources and formulate a teaching plan.
- Funding for home care management must be in place before discharge.
- Extensive assessment of the patient's physical status as well as an assessment of home and caregiver resources is imperative before initiating the process of preparing patients and caregivers for home care of a ventilator-assisted patient.

Patient's Physical Status

- Are acute diseases resolved, chronic conditions under control, all infectious processes cured or under definitive treatment?
- Does the patient have stable pulmonary function, minimal ventilator settings (low F_{IO_2} and simplest ventilatory mode), and pulmonary secretion control with adequate cough or tracheal suction?
- Does the patient have a stable metabolic and nutritional status, and simplified medication and nutrition regimen?

Caregiver Resources

- Are multiple caregivers available (minimum one more for backup)?
- Is the caregiver motivated, realistic, flexible, committed, and in good health?

Home

- Are adequate electrical circuits available for ventilator equipment?
- Is there adequate heating and cooling, a phone, a safe water supply, and storage space?
- Is there adequate room for safe patient evacuation in the case of an emergency?
- Caregiver and patient goals must be identified, and a teaching plan formulated with an approximate timeline toward discharge:
  - Ventilator, tracheostomy, suctioning teaching
  - Nutrition, hydration, medication teaching
  - Patient personal care, hygiene, percutaneous endoscopic gastrostomy (PEG) care, bowel and bladder care teaching
  - Techniques for maintenance of patient's strength and flexibility
  - Communication techniques, recreational activities for patient
  - Safe patient positioning and transferring techniques
  - Troubleshooting tracheostomy and ventilator
  - Troubleshooting signs of acute illness, exacerbation of chronic illnesses, or progression of underlying illness
  - Emergency plans, caregiver cardiopulmonary resuscitation (CPR) training
  - Conference with patient and caregivers regarding end-of-life issues and wishes, with specific scenarios reviewed
  - Conference with patient and caregivers regarding alternatives, if home care does not work out
  - Conference regarding ways to meet the psychological needs of the patient and caregivers
- The team performs ongoing evaluation of the patient's and caregivers' readiness and progress toward discharge and adjusts the teaching plan and discharge date accordingly.
- Predischarge and discharge:
  - Caregivers gradually take over the patient's total care while in the hospital, with staff supervising and assisting in troubleshooting.
  - The respiratory therapy home care coordinator assesses the home and arranges for delivery of equipment.
  - The respiratory therapy home care coordinator notifies the local electrical company, fire department, and rescue squad of patient on ventilator before discharge.
  - The respiratory therapy home care coordinator completes home ventilator management teaching.
  - A physician is identified to follow the patient on discharge.
  - A contact person is identified from the hospital unit (case manager, primary nurse).
  - A referral for home health care (e.g., Physical or Occupational Therapy, Speech, Counseling, Nursing, Social Work, Nutrition) is provided.
  - Arrangements are made for ventilation on ventilator to be used at home at least 3 days before discharge.
  - The caregiver changes the tracheostomy before discharge.
  - When the discharge date is established by the team, caregiver, and patient, Social Work arranges for transportation.
  - Equipment needed for transportation home (e.g., suction machine, ventilator) is secured and established to be in good working order.
  - Discharge orders are in place at least 2 days before discharge.
  - Discharge medications are obtained before discharge.

A discharge planning guide for a patient who is a candidate for home care management on a ventilator is given in Box 25-24.

New Frontiers and Challenges for Ventilated Patients

Ventilated patients present major challenges to nurses because they are prone to iatrogenic complications and higher mortality and morbidity rates. It is important that nurses apply current research findings to practice so that clinical and financial outcomes may improve. Research such as that focusing on surfactant, partial liquid ventilation, the use of low-volume ventilation, and appropriate fluid management in ARDS will provide new challenges for nurses responsible for implementing the changes in clinical practice. Ventilator weaning by use of weaning teams, outcomes managers, and weaning protocols shows promise for future improvement in outcomes, lowering hospital costs, and more effective weaning from ventilators.[64–66] These system approaches continue to show promise in reducing days on the ventilator and number of complications. They will continue to be popular initiatives for hospitals that are attempting to find the best outcomes in terms of high-quality and cost-effective solutions for patients.

Nurses can use current journals and the World Wide Web to search for information to learn about the most up-to-date information and research. The new nurse should seek access to a health science library database to obtain the most current research for his or her area of practice, as well as subscribe to nursing journals. Four excellent sources for the new nurse for advanced topics are (1) *AACN Procedure Manual for Critical Care*, (2) *AACN Protocols for Practice: Care of the Mechanically Ventilated Patient*, (3) *AACN Clinical Issues*, and (4) *Egan's Fundamentals of Respiratory Care* (referenced in the bibliography). These resources provide more in-depth coverage of topics related to ventilators, pathophysiology, and care of the patient. The new frontiers of nursing and health care will continue to require that nurses keep abreast of rapidly changing practice by continually updating their knowledge. The key to excellent nursing care is evidence-based practice. The challenge for new nurses is to integrate the knowledge, therapies, adverse effects, and clinical skills surrounding respiratory care into all aspects of clinical practice. The ever-changing technology and research of the 21st century will continually challenge nurses to update their clinical practice with the latest evidence-based practice and research to provide the respiratory patient with the highest-quality care.

case study ■ ASPIRATION PNEUMONIA

Mr. Jones is a 62-year-old man who presented in the emergency department (ED) with decreased mental status, nausea and vomiting, and shortness of breath. His history includes hypertension, smoking, and chronic obstructive pulmonary disease (COPD). According to his family, he became acutely short of breath after an episode of vomiting this morning. He was also more difficult to arouse over the course of the morning. On presentation to the ED, the patient was moaning; his respiratory rate was labored at 28 breaths/minute; his temperature was 101.7°F (38.7°C), and his SaO_2 was 86% on room air, but other vital signs were stable. A stat chest x-ray was done, which showed a right lower lobe infiltrate. ABGs were drawn with the following results: pH 7.30; $PaCO_2$ 62 mm Hg; PaO_2 60 mm Hg; bicarbonate 19 mEq/L; base excess −2. After discussion with the patient and family, the decision was made to intubate Mr. Jones secondary to his increased work of breathing due to suspected aspiration pneumonia. After successful intubation, the patient was suctioned. Moderate amounts of green sputum with some food particles were sent for cultures. In addition, blood and urine cultures were sent. The patient was placed on the following ventilator settings: FIO_2 0.40; synchronized intermittent mandatory ventilation (SIMV) rate 8; pressure support 10; and positive end-expiratory pressure (PEEP) 5 cm H_2O. After 72 hours of antibiotics and aggressive pulmonary toilet, the patient was successfully weaned and extubated. ■

clinical applicability challenges

Self-Challenge: Critical Thinking

1. *How would you assess Mr. Jones' readiness to wean from the ventilator?*
2. *Once weaning readiness is ensured, what sort of "weaning plan" may be incorporated for this patient?*
3. *What interventions can the nurse implement to prevent further aspiration in this patient?*
4. *What other nursing interventions should be implemented for the mechanically ventilated patient?*

Study Questions

1. *Which areas are appropriately percussed or vibrated regardless of the patient's position or the affected lobes?*
   a. *Over the clavicles, breast tissue, sternum, or shoulder blades*
   b. *Over surgical sites or fractured ribs only with mechanical percussor*
   c. *Over any area with a mechanical percussor*
   d. *Over the ribs in the areas designated for bronchial drainage*
2. *What lateral position improves ventilation and perfusion in patients with unilateral pulmonary disease, excluding an abscessed lung?*
   a. *Healthy lung up*
   b. *Healthy lung down*
   c. *Prone position*
   d. *Supine position*
3. *What oxygen delivery device delivers a constant concentration of oxygen regardless of the patient's position, tidal volume, or respiratory rate?*
   a. *Low-flow nasal cannula at 6 L/minute*
   b. *Low-flow non-rebreather mask at 10 L/minute*
   c. *High-flow aerosol mask at 6 L/minute*
   d. *High-flow Venturi mask at 10 L/minute*

4. *What bed position has been shown to improve outcomes and reduce aspiration for ventilated patients?*
   a. *Lateral position with reverse Trendelenburg*
   b. *Supine position (flat) with reverse Trendelenburg*
   c. *Head of bed elevated no more than 20 degrees*
   d. *Head of bed elevated greater than 30 degrees*
5. *The criteria that may terminate weaning from mechanical ventilation include*
   a. *respiratory rate greater than 30 breaths/minute, increased accessory muscle use, Sao_2 less than 90%, electrocardiographic changes.*
   b. *respiratory rate less than 30 breaths/minute, no accessory muscle use, Sao_2 greater than 90%, electrocardiogram normal.*
   c. *mild anxiety, tidal volume greater than 5 mL/kg, occasional increased systolic blood pressure and heart rate.*
   d. *normal $Paco_2$, stable neurological status, diaphoresis.*
6. *Which modes of ventilation are typically used for weaning? (Choose two.)*
   a. *Pressure control/inverse I:E ratio*
   b. *Assist control*
   c. *Pressure support ventilation (PSV)*
   d. *Synchronized intermittent mandatory ventilation (SIMV)*
7. *The normal amount of pleural fluid found within the pleural space is*
   a. *50 to 60 mL.*
   b. *5 to 15 mL.*
   c. *0 to 5 mL.*
   d. *75 to 100 mL.*
8. *To decrease bronchospasm, albuterol acts primarily on the*
   a. *alpha receptors.*
   b. *$beta_1$ receptors.*
   c. *delta receptors.*
   d. *$beta_2$ receptors.*
9. *DNase improves airflow in the patient with cystic fibrosis by*
   a. *relaxing bronchial smooth muscle.*
   b. *breaking down large molecules in thick secretions.*
   c. *narrowing large airways.*
   d. *stabilizing mast cell membranes.*
10. *Management and weaning of the patient on mechanical ventilation are best accomplished by which of the following?*
   a. *A comprehensive care plan including all appropriate nursing interventions*
   b. *Physician order sets to address the expected medications, laboratory studies, and interventions needed by patients on ventilatory support*
   c. *A collaborative multidisciplinary process for planning and delivering care*
   d. *Randomization of patients to different prescribed modes of ventilation*
11. *Which of the following issues is the nursing priority in weaning an elderly patient from ventilatory support?*
   a. *Adequate nutritional support and balanced intake and output (I & O)*
   b. *An effective regimen for treating pain, anxiety, or agitation*
   c. *Establishing regular sleep/rest and bowel elimination patterns*
   d. *All of the above*

REFERENCES

1. West JB: Respiratory Physiology: The Essentials (6th Ed). Philadelphia, Lippincott Williams & Wilkins, 2003
2. Bakow ED: Bronchial hygiene. In Dantzker DR, MacIntyre NR, Bakow ED (eds): Comprehensive Respiratory Care, pp 422–438. Philadelphia, WB Saunders, 1995
3. Peruzzi WT, Smith B: Bronchial hygiene therapy. Crit Care Clin 11(1):79–96, 1995
4. Gattinoni L, Tognoni G, Pesenti A, et al: Effect of prone positioning on the survival of patients with acute respiratory failure. N Engl J Med 345(8):568–573, 2001
5. Doering LV: The effect of positioning on hemodynamics and gas exchange in the critically ill: A review. Am J Crit Care 2:208–216, 1993
6. Pappert D, Rossaint R, et al: Influence of positioning on ventilation-perfusion relationships in severe adult respiratory distress syndrome. Chest 106:1511–1516, 1994
7. Malloy R, Pierce M: Oxygen therapy. In Dantzker DR, MacIntyre NR, Bakow ED (eds): Comprehensive Respiratory Care, pp 499–519. Philadelphia, WB Saunders, 1995
8. Perry AG, Potter PA: Clinical nursing skills and techniques (5th Ed). St. Louis, Mosby, 2002
9. Valles J, Artigas A, Rello J, et al: Continuous aspiration of subglottic secretions in preventing ventilator-associated pneumonia. Ann Intern Med 122:179–186, 1995
10. AARC Clinical Practice Guideline: Endotracheal suctioning of mechanically ventilated adults and children with artificial airways. Respir Care 38(5):500–504, 1993
11. Grap MJ, Glass C, et al: Endotracheal suctioning: Ventilator vs manual delivery of hyperoxygenation breaths. Am J Crit Care 5:192–197, 1996
12. Schwenker D, Ferrin M, Gift AG: A survey of endotracheal suctioning with instillation of normal saline. Am J Crit Care 7(4):255–260, 1998
13. Blackwood B: Normal saline instillation with endotracheal suctioning: Primum non nocere (first do no harm). J Adv Nurs 29(4):928–934, 1999
14. Braunwald E, Fauci AS, Kasper DL, et al. (eds): Harrison's Principles of Internal Medicine (15th Ed). New York, McGraw-Hill, 2001
15. Gross SB: Current challenges, concepts, and controversies in chest tube management. AACN Clin Issues 4(2):260–275, 1993
16. Lanken PN, Hanson CW III, Manaker S (eds): The Intensive Care Unit Manual, p 384. Philadelphia, WB Saunders, 2001
17. Lynn-McHale DJ, Carlson KK (eds): AACN Procedure Manual for Critical Care, pp 138–140. Philadelphia, WB Saunders, 2001
18. Lanken PN, Hanson CW III, Manaker S (eds): The Intensive Care Unit Manual, pp 838–840. Philadelphia, WB Saunders, 2001
19. McEvoy GK (ed): AHFS Drug Information 2001. Bethesda, MD, American Society of Health System Pharmacists, 2001
20. Argour R: Sedation and pain management in critically ill adults. Crit Care Nurse 20(5):39–58, 2000
21. Kollef MH, Levy NT, Ahrens TS, et al: The use of continuous IV sedation is associated with prolongation of mechanical ventilation. Chest 114(2):541–548, 1998
22. Covington H: Use of propofol for sedation in the ICU. Crit Care Nurse 18(4):34–39, 1998
23. Weinart CR, Chlan L, Gross C: Sedating critically ill patients: Factors affecting nurses' delivery of sedative therapy. Am J Crit Care 10(3):156–167, 2001
24. Slutsky AS: Consensus conference on mechanical ventilation: January 28–30, 1993 at Northbrook, Illinois, USA. Intensive Care Med 20:64–79, 1994
25. Levine S, Henson D: Negative pressure ventilation. In Tobin MJ (ed): Principles and Practice of Mechanical Ventilation, pp 393–411. New York, McGraw-Hill, 1994
26. Slutsky AS: Consensus conference on mechanical ventilation: January 28–30, 1993 at Northbrook, Illinois, USA. Intensive Care Med 20:150–162, 1994
27. MacIntyre NR: High-frequency ventilation. In Tobin MJ (ed): Principles and Practice of Mechanical Ventilation, pp 455–460. New York, McGraw-Hill, 1994
28. Pierce LN: Traditional and nontraditional modes of mechanical ventilation. In Chulay M, Burns S (eds): Protocols for Practice: Care

of the Mechanically Ventilated Patient Series, pp 1–33. Aliso Viejo, CA, American Association of Critical-Care Nurses, 1998
29. Burns SM: Mechanical ventilation and weaning. In Kinney MR, et al. (eds): AACN Clinical Reference for Critical Care Nursing (4th Ed), p 621. St. Louis, Mosby, 1998
30. Elliott M: Noninvasive mechanical ventilation by nasal or face mask. In Tobin MJ (ed): Principles and Practice of Mechanical Ventilation, pp 427–453. New York, McGraw-Hill, 1994
31. Bidani A, Tzouanakis AE, et al: Permissive hypercapnia in acute respiratory failure. JAMA 272(12):957–962, 1994
32. Harris JR, Miller TH: Preventing nosocomial pneumonia: Evidence-based practice. Crit Care Nurse 20(1):51–68, 2000
33. Kollef MH: Current concepts: The prevention of ventilator-associated pneumonias. N Engl J Med 340(8):627–634, 1999
34. Centers for Disease Control and Prevention: Guidelines for prevention of nosocomial pneumonia. MMWR 46(RR-1):1–79, 1997; also available at http://www.phppo.cdc.gov/cdcrecommends/AdvSearchResultsV.asp
35. Hixson S, Sole ML, King T: Nursing strategies to prevent ventilator-associated pneumonia. AACN Clin Issues 9:76–90, 1998
36. Fourrier F, et al: Colonization of dental plaque: A source of nosocomial infections in intensive care unit patients. Crit Care Med 26:301–308, 1998
37. Barnason S, Graham J, Wild MC, et al: Comparison of two endotracheal tube securement techniques on unplanned extubation, oral mucosa, and facial skin integrity. Heart Lung 27(6):409–417, 1998
38. Brooks JA: Postoperative nosocomial pneumonia: Nurse-sensitive interventions. AACN Clin Issues 12(2):305–323, 2001
39. Holzapfel L, Chastang C, Demingeon G, et al: A randomized study assessing the systematic search for maxillary sinusitis in nasotracheally mechanically ventilated patients: Influence of nosocomial maxillary sinusitis on the occurrence of ventilator-associated pneumonia. Am J Respir Crit Care Med 159(3):695–701, 1999
40. Grap MJ, Munro CL: Ventilator-associated pneumonia: Clinical significance and implications for nursing. Heart Lung 26(6):419–429, 1997
41. Dries DJ: Weaning from mechanical ventilation. J Trauma 43(2): 372–384, 1997
42. Heffner JE: Timing of tracheotomy in mechanically ventilated patients. Am Rev Respir Dis 147:768–771, 1993
43. Zavotsky KE, D'Amelio LF: Bedside percutaneous tracheostomy: Implications for critical care nurses. Crit Care Nurse 15(5):37–43, 1995
44. Fiorell M, Burns SM, et al: Are frequent tracheostomy inner cannula changes necessary? NTI Research Abstract. Am J Crit Care 5(3):235, 1996
45. Lynn-McHale DJ, Carlson KK (eds): AACN Procedure Manual for Critical Care, pp 56–63 (4th Ed). Philadelphia, WB Saunders, 2001
46. Henneman EA, Ellstrom K, St. John R: Airway management. In Chulay M, Burns S (eds): Protocols for Practice: Care of the Mechanically Ventilated Patient Series. Aliso Viejo, CA, American Association of Critical Care Nurses, pp 1–44. 1998
47. Burns SM, Spilman M, Wilmoth D, et al: Are frequent inner cannula changes necessary? A pilot study. Heart Lung 27:58–62, 1998
48. Cortese D, Capp L, McKinley S: Moisture chamber versus lubrication for the prevention of corneal epithelial breakdown. Am J Crit Care 4(6):425–428, 1995
49. Miller M, Kearney N: Oral care for patients with cancer: A review of the literature. Cancer Nurs 25(4):251–254, 2001
50. Fitzpatrick J: Oral health care needs of dependent older people: Responsibilities of nurses and care staff. J Adv Nurs 32(6):1325–1332, 2000
51. Tullman DF, Dracup K, Lindquist R, et al: Creating a healing environment for elders. AACN Clin Issues 11(1):34–50, 2000
52. Messner RL: Visiting hours: What's really best? RN 59(10):27–30, 1996
53. Fontaine DK, Briggs LP, Pope-Smith B: Designing humanistic critical care environments. Crit Care Nurs Q 25(3):21–34, 2001
54. Meyers TA, Eichhorn DJ, Guzzetta CE, et al: Family presence during invasive procedures and resuscitation: The experience of family members, nurses, and physicians. Am J Nurs 100(2):32–43, 2000
55. Simon SK, Phillips K, Badalamenti S, et al: Current practices regarding visitation policies in critical care units. Am J Crit Care 6(3):210–217, 1997
56. Burns SM, Clochesy JM, et al: Weaning from long-term mechanical ventilation. Am J Crit Care 4(1):4–22, 1995
57. Burns SM, Burns JE, Truwit JD: Comparison of five clinical weaning indices. Am J Crit Care 3(5):342–352, 1994
58. Smith-Blair N: Mechanisms of diaphragm fatigue. AACN Clin Issues 13(2):307–319, 2002
59. Henneman EA: Liberating patients from mechanical ventilation: A team approach. Crit Care Nurse 21(3):25–33, 2001
60. Burns SM: Weaning from long-term mechanical ventilation. In Chulay M, Burns S (eds): Protocols for Practice: Care of the Mechanically Ventilated Patient Series, pp 1–33. Aliso Viejo, CA, American Association of Critical Care Nurses, 1998
61. Knebel AR: Ventilator weaning protocols and techniques: Getting the job done. AACN Clin Issues 7(4):550–559, 1996
62. Burns SB, Dempsey E: Long-term ventilator management strategies: Experience of two hospitals. AACN Clin Issues 11(3):425–441, 472–474, 2000
63. Aloi A, Burns SM: Continuous airway pressure monitoring in the critical care setting. Crit Care Nurse 15(2):66–74, 1995
64. Glass CA: Home care management of ventilator-assisted patients. In Chulay M, Burns S (eds): Protocols for Practice: Care of the Mechanically Ventilated Patient Series. Aliso Viejo, CA, American Association of Critical Care Nurses, pp 1–26. 1998
65. Henneman E, Dracup K, Ganz T, et al: Effect of a collaborative weaning plan on patient outcome in the critical care setting. Crit Care Med 29(2):297–303, 2001
66. Burns SM: The long-term mechanically ventilated patient: An outcomes management approach. Crit Care Nurs Clin North Am 10(1):87–97, 1998

OTHER SELECTED READING

Baun MM, Stone KS, Rogge JA: Endotracheal suctioning: Open versus closed with and without positive end-expiratory pressure. Crit Care Nurs Q 25(2):13–26, 2002

Bezanson JL, et al: Predictors and outcomes associated with early extubation in older adults undergoing coronary artery bypass surgery. CE Online. Am J Crit Care 10(6):383–390, 2001

Cattapan SE, Fahey PJ: Weaning from mechanical ventilation. Update on latest strategies: Protocol-directed approaches may improve outcomes. J Crit Illness 18(3):117–122, 2003

Combes A, Figliolini C, Trouillet J, et al: Factors predicting ventilator-associated pneumonia recurrence. Crit Care Med 31(4):1102–1107, 2003

Douglas SL, Daly BJ: Caregivers of long-term ventilator patients: Physical and psychological outcomes. Chest 123(4):1073–1081, 2003

Kirschenbaum L, Azzi E, Sfeir T, et al: Effects of continuous lateral rotation therapy on the prevalence of ventilator-associated pneumonia in patients requiring long-term ventilatory care. Crit Care Med 30(9):1224–1230, 2002

Kress JP, Pohlman AS, O'Connor MF, et al: Daily interruption of sedative infusions in critically ill patients undergoing mechanical ventilation. N Engl J Med 342(20):1471–1477, 2000

Pierson DJ: Indications for mechanical ventilation in adults with acute respiratory failure. Proceedings of the 29th Respiratory Care Journal Conference: Invasive mechanical ventilation in adults: Implementation, management, weaning and follow-up, part I. Respir Care 47(3):249–265, 2002

Smyrnios NA, Connolly A, Wilson M, et al: Effects of a multifaceted, multidisciplinary hospital-wide quality improvement program on weaning from mechanical ventilation. Crit Care Med 30(6):1224–1230, 2002

Wolfe JA: Lung protection strategies for mechanical ventilation. Rt J Respir Care Practitioners 15(6):22, 24, 44, 2002

Zeitoun SS, DeBarros AL, Diccini S: A prospective, randomized study of ventilator-associated pneumonia in patients using a closed vs. open suction system. J Clin Nurs 12(4):484–489, 2003

chapter

26

Common Respiratory Disorders

COLONEL JANET R. HARRIS ■
LIEUTENANT COLONEL MARY E. TENHET*

objectives

Based on the content in this chapter, the reader should be able to:

- Discuss the pathophysiology of pneumonia.
- Compare and contrast the signs and symptoms of selected pulmonary disorders.
- Discuss the management of selected pulmonary disorders.
- Describe the pathophysiology of chronic obstructive lung disease (COPD) and associated signs and symptoms found on physical examination.
- Explain various laboratory and diagnostic tests performed in COPD.
- Discuss the medical, pharmacological, and surgical management of COPD.

*The views of the authors are their own and do not reflect the official policy or position of the Department of the Army, the Department of Defense, or the United States Government.

PNEUMONIA

Pneumonia is a common infection that is found in both the community and hospital. It is encountered by critical care nurses when it complicates the course of a serious illness or leads to acute respiratory distress. In the United States, pneumonia is the leading cause of death from infectious disease, the second most common nosocomial (hospital-acquired) infection, and the sixth leading cause of death.[1,2] About 4.8 million cases of pneumonia (1.8 cases per 100 persons), including 1.4 million hospital discharges with a diagnosis of pneumonia, are reported each year.[1] In 1998, 91,871 people died of pneumonia: a rate of 34 per 100,000 population.[1] Elderly patients (older than 65 years of age) died of pneumonia at a significantly higher rate: 241.2 per 100,000 population.[1]

Community-acquired pneumonia (CAP) is an acute infection of the pulmonary parenchyma in an individual who is not hospitalized or residing in a long-term care facility before the onset of symptoms. In the outpatient setting, CAP has a low mortality rate (1% to 5%). However, the mortality rate climbs to 12% in patients requiring hospitalization and 40% in those requiring admission to the intensive care unit (ICU).[3] According to guidelines developed by the American Thoracic Society (ATS),[3] patients with severe CAP require admission to the ICU. Severe CAP is defined as the presence of one of four major criteria or the presence of two of five minor criteria[3,4] (Box 26-1).

Hospital-acquired (nosocomial) pneumonia (HAP) is defined as pneumonia occurring more than 48 hours after admission, which excludes infection that is incubating at the time of admission. The ATS further classifies HAP as either early-onset or late-onset. Early-onset HAP occurs within 2 to 5 days of hospitalization, and late-onset HAP occurs after 5 days of hospitalization.[5] HAP occurs at a rate of 5 to 10 cases per 1,000 hospital admissions, and the incidence increases by 6- to 20-fold in patients receiving mechanical ventilation.[5]

The ATS HAP guidelines state that the criteria defining severe CAP can also be used to define severe HAP.[5] Severe HAP may occur in the ICU, with patients receiving mechanical ventilation being at the greatest risk, or it may precipitate admission to the ICU.[6] HAP independently contributes to mortality in critically ill patients; the attributable mortality rate is 11% to 33%.[7]

box 26-1
American Thoracic Society Criteria for Diagnosis of Severe Community-Acquired Pneumonia

Major Criteria

- Need for mechanical ventilation
- Requirement for vasopressors for >4 hours (septic shock)
- Acute renal failure (urine output <80 mL in 4 hours or serum creatinine >2 mg/dL in the absence of chronic renal failure)
- Increase in size of infiltrates by >50% in presence of clinical nonresponse to treatment or deterioration

Minor Criteria

- Respiratory rate >30 breaths/minute
- Systolic BP ≤90 mm Hg
- Diastolic BP <60 mm Hg, multilobar disease
- PaO_2/FIO_2 ratio <250

From American Thoracic Society: Guidelines for the management of adults with community-acquired pneumonia. Am J Respir Crit Care Med 163:1730–1754, 2001, with permission.

Etiology

Bacteria, viruses, mycoplasmas, other infectious agents such as fungi, and foreign material can all cause pneumonia. The specific etiology varies greatly depending on the type of pneumonia (CAP or HAP). Gram-positive organisms predominate in CAP, whereas enteric gram-negative bacilli predominate in HAP. *Streptococcus pneumoniae* (pneumococcus) is the most common cause of CAP and also the most frequent cause of mortality in CAP.[3,8] Even in the approximately 50% of cases of CAP in which the causative organism is not identified, *S. pneumoniae* is believed to predominate.[3] Drug-resistant *S. pneumoniae* is frequently seen in individuals older than 65 years of age.[3] The so-called atypical pathogens may also play a role. The term *atypical* is misleading. The ATS uses "atypical" to identify a group of pathogens, including *Mycoplasma pneumoniae*, *Chlamydia pneumoniae*, and *Legionella* species, rather than to identify an atypical clinical course.[3] The exact role "atypical" pathogens play in CAP is controversial because their frequency of detection as causal agents depends on the diagnostic test used.[3] Other pathogens that should be considered in severe CAP requiring admission to the ICU include *Haemophilus influenzae*, *Staphylococcus aureus*, *Mycobacterium tuberculosis*, respiratory viruses, and endemic fungi.[3]

The enteric gram-negative bacilli and *S. aureus* (gram-positive) are the most frequently identified organisms in HAP.[2,5,7] More than one organism may be identified in over 30% of patients with HAP, and HAP is frequently polymicrobial.[5,7] Polymicrobial HAP is particularly common (>50%) in patients receiving mechanical ventilation (ventilator-associated pneumonia). Highly resistant gram-negative organisms (e.g., *Pseudomonas aeruginosa*, *Acinetobacter* species) and methicillin-resistant *S. aureus* are frequently seen in late-onset HAP but may occur in early-onset HAP in patients with risk factors for these pathogens.[5,7] The spectrum of potential pathogens can be defined by assessment of a variety of factors, including the severity of the pneumonia, presence of comorbidities, prior therapy (including antibiotics), and length of hospitalization.[5]

Pathophysiology

Pneumonia is an inflammatory response to inhaled or aspirated foreign material or the uncontrolled multiplication of microorganisms invading the lower respiratory tract. This response results in the accumulation of neutrophils and other effector cells in the peripheral bronchi and alveolar spaces. The pathogenesis of bacterial HAP is depicted in the theoretical model postulated by the Centers for Disease Control and Prevention (CDC; Fig. 26-1). The body's defense system, which includes anatomical, mechanical, humoral, and cellular defenses, is designed to repel and remove organisms entering the respiratory tract. Many systemic diseases increase the patient's risk of pneumonia by altering the respiratory defense mechanism. Pneumonia develops when normal pulmonary defense mechanisms are either impaired or overwhelmed, allowing microorganisms to multiply rapidly.

Pathogens may enter the lower respiratory tract and cause pneumonia in four ways: aspiration, inhalation, hematogenous spread from a distant site, and translocation. The primary route of bacterial entry into the lungs is aspiration of microorganisms from the oropharynx. Aspiration occurs frequently (>45% of the time) in healthy individuals while they sleep. The risk of clinically significant aspiration is increased in patients with a depressed level of consciousness or dysphagia; in those who have endotracheal or enteral tubes; or in those receiving enteral feedings. For example, aspiration occurs more often (>70% of the time) and more extensively in patients with a depressed level of consciousness.[7] Another potential source of pneumonia-causing bacteria is inhalation of bacteria-laden aerosols from contaminated respiratory equipment. Inhalation is an effective entry mechanism for *Legionella* species, *M. tuberculosis*, certain viruses, and fungi. Hematogenous spread may be an effective mechanism; the pulmonary circulation provides a potential portal of entry for microbes. The pulmonary capillaries form a dense network in the walls of the alveoli that is ideal for gas exchange. Hematogenous microbes from distant sites of infection can migrate through this network and cause pneumonia. (Pneumonia can also cause bacteremia. Secondary bacteremia after pneumonia has been reported in 6% to 20% of pneumonia cases.) Finally, translocation of bacterial toxins from the gut lumen to the mesenteric lymph nodes and eventually to the lungs may possibly cause bacterial pneumonia. However, translocation has not yet been confirmed as a pathophysiological mechanism.

Colonization of the oropharynx and the stomach plays an important role in the pathophysiology of bacterial pneumonia.[9] (Colonization is the presence of microorganisms other than the normal flora in the absence of clinical evidence of infection.) Gram-positive bacteria and anaerobic bacteria normally live in the oropharynx, and it is hypothesized that they occupy bacterial binding sites in the oropharyngeal mucosa. When normal oropharyngeal flora are destroyed, these binding sites are susceptible to colonization by pathogenic bacteria. The gram-negative or pathogenic gram-positive organisms that have colonized the oropharynx are readily available for aspiration into the tracheobronchial tree. Risk factors associated with oropharyngeal colonization include previous antibiotic therapy, increased age, depressed level of consciousness, dental plaque, smoking, and chronic diseases, such as chronic obstructive pulmonary disease (COPD), alcoholism, diabetes mellitus, and malnutrition.

The stomach can serve as a reservoir for bacteria. This organ is normally sterile because of the bactericidal activity of hydrochloric acid. However, when gastric pH increases above normal (pH >4), microorganisms are able to multiply. Gastric colonization increases retrograde colonization of the oropharynx and increases the risk of pneumonia. Individuals at risk for gastric colonization include the elderly; those with achlorhydria, ileus, or upper gastrointestinal disease; and those receiving antacids, histamine-2 antagonists, or enteral feedings.[7]

Risk factors increase the likelihood of pneumonia through one of the many mechanisms identified in the theoretical model (see Fig. 26-1). Risk factors for HAP are grouped into three categories: host-related, treatment-related, and infection control–related risk factors (Box 26-2).

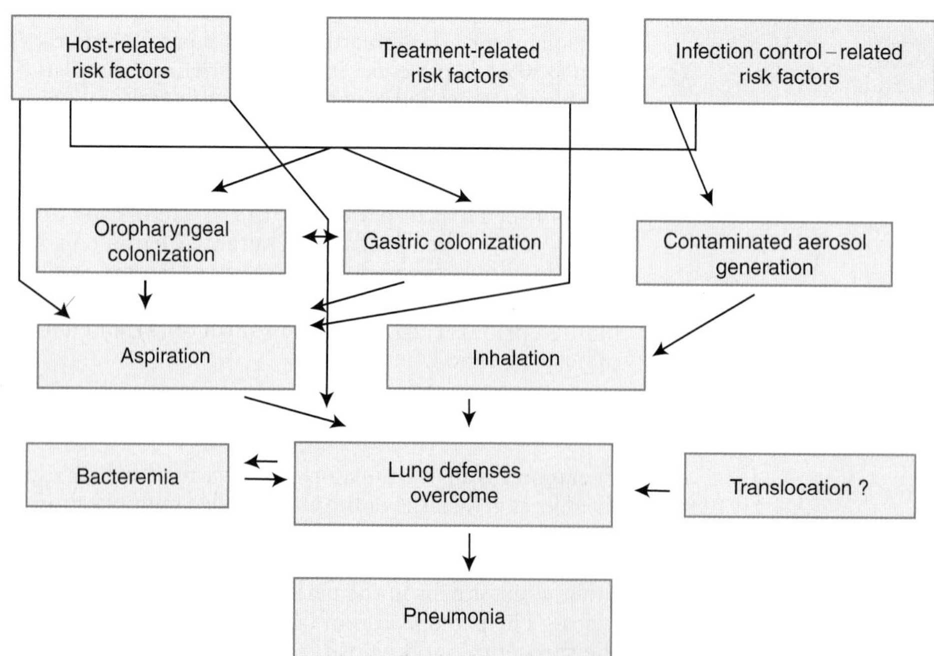

figure 26-1 Theoretical model for nosocomial pneumonia developed by the Centers for Disease Control and Prevention (CDC) Hospital Infection Control Practices Advisory Committee and modified by the author based on empiric evidence. (From Harris JR, Miller TH: Preventing nosocomial pneumonia: Evidenced-based practice. Crit Care Nurse, 20(1):51–66, 2000.)

box 26-2
Risk Factors for Hospital-Acquired and Community-Acquired Pneumonia

Community-Acquired Pneumonia
- Age <2 years or >65 years
- Smoking
- Alcohol abuse
- Comorbidities: pulmonary disease, cardiovascular disease, hepatic disease, renal disease, central nervous system disease, immunosuppression

Hospital-Acquired Pneumonia

Host-Related Risk Factors
- Increased age
- Altered level of consciousness
- Chronic obstructive pulmonary disease (COPD)
- Severe illness
- Malnutrition
- Shock
- Blunt trauma
- Severe head trauma
- Chest trauma
- Smoking
- Dental plaque

Treatment-Related Risk Factors
- Mechanical ventilation
- Reintubation or self-extubation
- Bronchoscopy
- Nasogastric tube
- Presence of intracranial pressure (ICP) monitor
- Prior antibiotic therapy
- Elevated gastric pH
- Histamine type 2 receptor blockers
- Antacid therapy
- Enteral feedings
- Head surgery
- Upper abdominal or thoracic surgery
- Supine position

Infection Control–Related Factors
- Poor handwashing
- Changing ventilator tubing less than every 48 hours

Risk factors for hospital-acquired pneumonia reprinted with permission from Harris JR, Miller TH: Preventing nosocomial pneumonia: Evidenced-based practice. Crit Care Nurse 20(1):51–66, 2000.

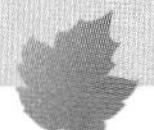

box 26-3
Pneumonia in the Older Patient

- **Presentation.** The usual symptoms (fever, chills, increased white blood count) may be absent. Confusion and tachypnea are common presenting symptoms in older patients with pneumonia. Other symptoms in the older patient include weakness, lethargy, failure to thrive, anorexia, abdominal pain, episodes of falling, incontinence, headache, delirium, and nonspecific deterioration.
- **Prevention.** People 65 years of age and older should receive both the pneumococcal vaccine (a one-time vaccination) and yearly influenza vaccines. The Health Care Financing Agency has approved the use of standing orders to give the vaccines to Medicare patients.

Assessment

HISTORY

Knowledge of risk factors and symptoms can assist in the identification of potential pathogens causing CAP and HAP. Hemoptysis implies tissue necrosis and is more common with pyogenic streptococcal pneumonia, anaerobic lung abscesses, *S. aureus*, necrotizing gram-negative organisms, and invasive *Aspergillus*.[10] Extrapulmonary symptoms may indicate specific pathogens; diarrhea and abdominal discomfort are present with *Legionella* species, and otitis media and pharyngitis are present with *Mycoplasma pneumoniae*.[10] The clinical presentation in the older adult may vary somewhat from what is "typical" in a younger person (Box 26-3).

Historical information may also be extremely helpful in diagnosis of CAP and HAP. It is necessary to include information about contact with animals, especially birds, bats, rats, and rabbits, which can assist with the diagnosis of histoplasmosis, psittacosis, tularemia, and plague.[8,10] In addition, a complete history may assist in the differential diagnosis. Diseases that may mimic pneumonia include congestive heart failure, atelectasis, pulmonary thromboembolism, drug reactions, pulmonary hemorrhage, and acute respiratory distress syndrome.

PHYSICAL FINDINGS

A comprehensive cardiovascular and pulmonary assessment should be completed, with a focus on the ATS major and minor criteria (see Box 26-1). The nurse should assess for signs of hypoxemia (duskiness or cyanosis) and dyspnea (nasal flaring). Patients present with new-onset respiratory symptoms (e.g., cough, sputum production, dyspnea) that are usually accompanied by fever and chills. Inspection of the chest includes assessing respiratory pattern and respiratory rate, observing the patient's posture and work of breathing, and inspecting for the presence of intercostal retractions. Percussion of the chest frequently reveals dullness with lobar pneumonia. Decreased breath sounds are heard on auscultation. Fine early crackles (formerly called *rales*) or bronchial breath sounds are heard over the area of consolidation.

DIAGNOSTIC STUDIES

The workup for severe pneumonia, whether CAP or HAP, is similar. Table 26-1 summarizes the current ATS recommendations. The diagnostic evaluation must be performed rapidly to prevent delays in initiation of antibiotic therapy.

All patients should have a chest radiograph (posteroanterior and lateral views) to identify both the presence and location of infiltrates. The chest radiograph is helpful in differentiating pneumonia from other conditions and identifying severe pneumonia, which is indicated by the presence of multilobular, rapidly spreading or cavitary infiltrates.

The value of examining lower respiratory secretions with Gram's stain and culturing sputum is controversial.

table 26-1 Diagnostic Studies in Patients With Severe Community-Acquired Pneumonia or Severe Hospital-Acquired Pneumonia

Study	Rationale
Chest radiograph (anterior–posterior and lateral)	Identify presence and severity of infiltrates. Assess for pleural effusions. Determine severity of pneumonia by identifying the presence of multilobar, rapidly spreading, or cavitary infiltrates.
Two sets of blood cultures from separate sites	Can isolate the etiologic pathogen in 8%–20% of cases.
Complete blood count Serum electrolytes Renal and liver function	Document the presence of multiple-organ dysfunction. Help define severity of illness.
Arterial blood gases	Define severity of illness. Determine need for supplemental oxygen and mechanical ventilation.
Thoracentesis (if pleural effusion >10 mm identified on lateral decubitus film) Pleural fluid studies, including: White blood count with differential Protein Glucose Lactate dehydrogenase (LDH) pH Gram stain and acid-fast stain Culture for bacteria, fungi, and mycobacteria	Rule out empyema.

From data in American Thoracic Society: Guidelines for the management of adults with community-acquired pneumonia. Am J Respir Crit Care Med 163:1730–1754, 2001, and American Thoracic Society: Hospital-acquired pneumonia in adults: Diagnosis, assessment of severity, initial antimicrobial therapy, and preventive strategies. Am J Respir Crit Care Med 153:1711–1725, 1996.

The ATS does not recommend routine use of Gram's stain and sputum culture and advises that results must be interpreted cautiously.[3,5] However, the Infectious Disease Society of America (IDSA) recommends routine Gram's stain and culture of deep-cough specimens.[8] Lower respiratory secretions can be easily obtained in intubated patients using endotracheal aspiration. Nonquantitative endotracheal aspiration cultures may assist in excluding certain pathogens and may be helpful in modifying initial empirical treatment.[5] Routine use of quantitative invasive diagnostic techniques (bronchoscopy with protected specimen brush [PSB] or bronchoalveolar lavage [BAL]) in severe pneumonia is not recommended by the ATS, CDC, or IDSA.[3,5,7,8] Current guidelines suggest that BAL or PSB be used only in selected circumstances, such as in nonresponse to antimicrobial therapy, immunosuppression, suspected tuberculosis in the absence of a productive cough, pneumonia with suspected neoplasm or foreign body, or conditions that require lung biopsy.[3,5,7,8,11]

Management

ANTIBIOTIC THERAPY

Antibiotic therapy is the cornerstone of treatment for both CAP and HAP. Patients should initially be treated empirically, based on the severity of disease and the likely pathogens.[3,5] Table 26-2 presents ATS guidelines for treatment of severe CAP, and Table 26-3 presents ATS guidelines for treatment of severe HAP. Initial therapy should be instituted rapidly. Data show that hospitalized patients with CAP who receive their first dose of antibiotic therapy within 8 hours of arrival at the hospital have reduced mortality at 30 days.[3,12] Initial therapy should not be changed within the first 48 to 72 hours unless progressive deterioration is evident or initial microbiological (blood or respiratory) cultures indicate a need to modify therapy.[3,5]

The optimal duration of therapy for either CAP or HAP has not yet been established. Factors to consider when determining the duration of therapy include concurrent illness, bacteremia, severity of pneumonia at the onset of antibiotic therapy, infecting pathogen(s), and rapidity of clinical response.[3,5] Recommended duration of therapy is 7 to 10 days for *S. aureus* or *H. influenzae;* 10 to 14 days for *M. pneumoniae* and *C. pneumoniae;* and 14 to 21 days for *P. aeruginosa* and *Acinetobacter*, multilobar involvement, malnutrition, or a necrotizing gram-negative bacillus.[3,5,8]

SUPPORTIVE THERAPY

Oxygen therapy is required to maintain adequate gas exchange. Mechanical ventilation to correct hypoxemia is frequently required in both severe CAP and HAP (see Acute Respiratory Failure). Humidified oxygen should be administered by mask or intubation to promote ciliary movement

table 26-2 Antibiotic Therapy for Severe Community-Acquired Pneumonia*†

Organisms	Therapy‡§
No Risk for Pseudomonas aueruginosa	
Streptococcus pneumoniae (including DRSP)	Intravenous β-lactam (cefotaxime, ceftriaxone)‖
Legionella spp	plus either
Hemophilus influenzae	Intravenous macrolide (azithromycin)
Enteric gram-negative bacilli	or
Staphylococcus aureus	Intravenous fluoroquinolone
Mycoplasma pneumoniae	
Respiratory viruses	
Miscellaneous	
Chlamydia pneumoniae	
Mycobacterium tuberculosis	
Endemic fungi	
Risk for Pseudomonas aueruginosa	
All of the above pathogens plus *P. aeruginosa*	Selected intravenous antipseudomonal β-lactam (cefepime, imipenem, meropenem, piperacillin/tazobactam)¶ plus intravenous antipseudomonal quinolone (ciprofloxacin) or Selected intravenous antipseudomonal β-lactam (cefepime, imipenem, meropenem, piperacillin/tazobactam) plus either Intravenous macrolide (azithromycin) or Intravenous nonpseudomonal fluoroquinolone

* Excludes patients at risk for HIV.
† In roughly one third to one half of the cases no etiology was identified.
‡ Combination therapy required.
§ In no particular order.
‖ Antipseudomonal agents such as cefepime, piperacillin/tazobactam, imipenem, and meropenem are generally active against drug-resistant *S. pneumoniae* (DRSP) and other likely pathogens in this population, but are not recommended for routine use unless the patient has risk factors for *P. aeruginosa*.
¶ If β-lactam allergic, replace the listed β-lactam with aztreonam and combine with an aminoglycoside and an antipneumococcal fluoroquinolone as listed.
Reprinted with permission from the American Thoracic Society: Guidelines for the management of adults with community-acquired pneumonia. Am J Respir Crit Care Med 163:1730–1754, 2001.

of mucus. Aggressive pulmonary toilet is indicated to mobilize secretions, open closed alveoli, and promote oxygenation. Adequate nutritional support is critical. In addition, a nutritional consult should be initiated with implementation of appropriate enteral or parenteral therapy.

Prevention

Pneumonia is the sixth leading cause of death in the United States; therefore, prevention of both CAP and HAP is essential. Primary measures to prevent CAP include the use of influenza and pneumococcal vaccines.[3,8] All immunocompetent patients 65 years of age or older should receive the pneumococcal vaccine.[3] In addition, individuals 64 years of age or younger should be immunized if they have chronic illnesses, such as cardiovascular disease, chronic pulmonary disease (COPD, but not asthma), diabetes mellitus, alcoholism, chronic liver disease, cerebrospinal fluid leaks, and functional or anatomic asplenia; belong to special populations, such as Alaska natives or other Native Americans; or live in special social settings, such as long-term care facilities.[3] The ATS recommends influenza vaccine for three target groups: persons at a high risk of influenza complications, persons who may transmit influenza to high-risk patients (e.g., health care workers); and any person who wishes to decrease the chance of becoming infected with influenza.[3] High-risk patients include individuals older than 65 years of age, residents of long-term care facilities, patients with chronic cardiovascular or pulmonary disease, patients who required regular medical care or hospitalization during the preceding year, and pregnant women in the second or third trimester during influenza season. Because cigarette smoking is a risk factor for both HAP and CAP pneumonia, smoking cessation, particularly in patients who have previously had pneumonia, is an important preventive strategy.[3]

A complete understanding of the pathogenesis of HAP enables the critical care nurse to develop strategies about interventions that prevent the onset of pneumonia.[13] The CDC considers education the cornerstone of an effective infection control program and the prevention of HAP.[7] The CDC has published comprehensive guidelines on the prevention of HAP.[7] World Wide Web access to the CDC guidelines is available at http://www.cdc.gov.

table 26-3 Antibiotic Therapy for Patients With Severe Hospital-Acquired Pneumonia*

Organisms	Therapy
Severe HAP Early Onset	
Core organisms	Cephalosporin
Enteric gram-negative bacilli (nonpseudomonal)	Second-generation
Enterobacter species	or nonpseudomonal third-generation
Escherichia coli	β-lactam/β-lactamase inhibitor combination
Klebsiella species	If allergic to penicillin
Proteus species	Fluoroquinolone
Serratia marcescens	
Haemophilus influenzae	
Methicillin-sensitive *Staphylococcus aureus*	
Streptococcus pneumoniae	
HAP With Risk Factors (Pseudomonas), Early Onset or Severe HAP Late Onset	
Core organisms plus	Aminoglycoside or ciprofloxacin
Pseudomonas aeruginosa	plus one of the following:
Acinetobacter species	Antipseudomonal penicillin
Methicillin-resistant *S. aureus*	β-lactam/β-lactamase inhibitor
	Ceftazidime or cefoperazone
	Imipenem
	Aztreonam[†]
	± Vancomycin

* Excludes patients with immunosuppression

[†] Aztreonam efficacy is limited to enteric gram-negative bacilli and should not be used in combination with an aminoglycoside if gram-positive or *Haemophilus influenzae* infection is of concern.

Reprinted with permission from the American Thoracic Society: Hospital-acquired pneumonia in adults: Diagnosis, assessment of severity, initial antimicrobial therapy, and preventive strategies. Am J Respir Crit Care Med 153:1711–1725, 1996.

PLEURAL EFFUSION

The pleural space is a potential space between the visceral and parietal pleurae that lines the lungs and interior chest wall. There is a continuous flow of fluid from the parietal pleura of the chest wall to the visceral pleura, and the fluid is eventually absorbed by the pulmonary lymphatics.

Pathophysiology

Pleural effusion is the accumulation of pleural fluid due to an increased rate of fluid formation, a decreased rate of fluid removal, or both.[14] This is caused by at least one of the five following mechanisms:

- Increased pressure in subpleural capillaries or lymphatics
- Increased capillary permeability
- Decreased colloid osmotic pressure of the blood
- Increased intrapleural negative pressure
- Impaired lymphatic drainage of the pleural space

TRANSUDATES

Transudative pleural effusions are an ultrafiltrate of plasma, indicating that the pleural membranes are not diseased.[14] The fluid accumulation is caused by systemic factors that affect the formation and absorption of pleural fluid. The most common cause of transudative pleural effusions and the most common cause of pleural effusions in the ICU is congestive heart failure.[14,15] In congestive heart failure, an increase in pulmonary venous pressure contributes to the formation of pleural effusions. Treatment focuses on decreasing venous hypertension and improving cardiac output.[14,15] Another cause of transudative pleural effusions is atelectasis, which may cause pleural fluid to accumulate because of a decrease in pleural pressure. The fluid continues to accumulate until the pleural–parietal pleural interstitial pressure gradient returns to normal.[14] Other causes of transudative pleural effusions include cirrhosis, nephrotic syndrome, and peritoneal dialysis.

EXUDATES

Exudative pleural effusions result from leakage of fluid across an injured capillary bed into the pleural or adjacent lung.[14] Fluid with a high protein content leaks across the disrupted capillary bed. Exudative pleural effusions may also result from infected fluid accumulating in the mediastinum, retroperitoneum, or peritoneum, and they can move into the low-pressure space of the pleural cavity.[14] Exudative pleural effusions satisfy any one of the following criteria[14]:

- Pleural fluid-to-serum protein ratio greater than 0.5
- Pleural fluid-to-serum lactate dehydrogenase (LDH) ratio greater than 0.6
- Pleural fluid LDH that is two thirds of the upper normal limit for serum LDH

Pneumonia is the most common cause of exudative pleural effusions, although the incidence varies with the infective agent. Exudative pleural effusions are frequently seen in pneumonia caused by *S. pneumoniae* and are less commonly associated with pneumonia produced by *S. aureus* and gram-negative bacilli.[14] Empyema, a cause of exudative pleural effusions, refers to gross pus in the pleural cavity and requires drainage with a chest tube.[14] The second most common cause of exudative pleural effusions is metastatic disease (e.g., lung, breast, gastric, or ovarian cancer).[14] Approximately one third of exudative pleural effusions caused by malignancies are bloody. If a massive effusion opacifies an entire hemithorax, metastatic disease should be suspected.[14]

Exudative pleural effusions occur in approximately 50% of patients with pulmonary embolism.[14,15] The presence of a pleural effusion on chest radiology in a patient with chest pain and dyspnea is suggestive of pulmonary effusion. Mechanisms that produce these effusions include ischemia-induced increased pleural capillary permeability, imbalance in vascular and pleural space hydrostatic pressures, and pleuropulmonary hemorrhage.[15]

A hemothorax is a bloody exudative pleural effusion and is diagnosed by a pleural fluid-to-blood hematocrit ratio greater than 50%.[14,15] Trauma is the most common cause of a hemothorax (see Chapter 55). Hemothorax can result from invasive procedures (placement of central venous catheter, thoracentesis), pulmonary infarction, malignancies, or a ruptured aortic aneurysm. Hemothorax is a rare complication of anticoagulation therapy.[15]

Assessment

HISTORY AND PHYSICAL FINDINGS

Subjective findings include shortness of breath and pleuritic chest pain, depending on the amount of fluid accumulation. Objective findings include tachypnea and hypoxemia if ventilation is impaired, dullness to percussion, and decreased breath sounds over the involved area.

DIAGNOSTIC STUDIES

A lateral decubitus chest radiograph is the best demonstration of free pleural fluid. When a pleural effusion is suspected on the basis of physical examination and is confirmed radiologically, it is necessary to obtain a sample of pleural fluid for diagnosis by diagnostic thoracentesis (aspiration of fluid from the pleural space). The laboratory tests performed on the pleural fluid obtained by thoracentesis are listed in Table 26-4. Evaluation of the pleural fluid is necessary to distinguish transudative from exudative effusions. When the distance between the pleural fluid line to the inside of the chest wall on lateral decubitus view is less than 1 cm, the pleural effusion is difficult to obtain by thoracentesis and not likely to be clinically significant.[14,15] In addition, the associated risk of pneumothorax outweighs the benefit of the thoracentesis.[15]

table 26-4 Assessment of Pleural Fluid

Test	Comment
Red blood cell count >100,000/mm³	Trauma, malignancy, pulmonary embolism
Hematocrit >50% of peripheral blood	Hemothorax
White blood cell count (WBC)	
>50,000–100,000/mm³	Grossly visible pus, otherwise total WBC less useful than WBC differential
>50% Neutrophils	Acute inflammation or infection
>50% Lymphocytes	Tuberculosis, malignancy
>10% Eosinophils	Most common: hemothorax, pneumothorax; also benign
>5% Mesothelial cells	Asbestos effusions, drug reaction, paragonimiasis; tuberculosis *less likely*
Glucose <60 mg/dL	Infection, malignancy, tuberculosis, rheumatoid
Amylase >200 units/dL	Pleuritis, esophageal perforation, pancreatic disease, malignancy, ruptured ectopic pregnancy Isoenzyme profile: salivary–esophageal disease, malignancy (especially lung) Isoenzyme profile: pancreatic–pancreatic disease
pH <7.2	Infection (complicated parapneumonic effusion and empyema), malignancy, esophageal rupture, rheumatoid or lupus pleuritis, tuberculosis, systemic acidosis, urinothorax
Triglyceride >110 mg/dL	Chylothorax
Microbiological studies	Etiology of infection
Cytology	Diagnostic of malignancy

Adapted from Sahn SA: State of the art: The pleura. Am Rev Respir Dis 138:184–234, 1988; From Zimmerman LH: Pleural effusions. In Goldstein RH, et al (eds): A Practical Approach to Pulmonary Medicine, p 199. Philadelphia, Lippincott-Raven, 1997.

Management

Treatment of the underlying cause is necessary. Removal of the pleural effusion by thoracentesis or chest tube placement may be indicated depending on the etiology and size of effusion. The primary indication for therapeutic thoracentesis is relief of dyspnea.

PNEUMOTHORAX

A pneumothorax occurs if air enters the pleural space between the visceral and parietal pleurae, producing partial or complete lung collapse.

Pathophysiology

During spontaneous breathing, two opposing forces generate negative pleural pressures. Pressure in the airways is positive during expiration (+3 mm Hg) and negative during inspiration (–2 mm Hg).[15] However, pleural pressure remains subatmospheric on both inspiration (average, –9 mm Hg) and expiration (average, –5 mm Hg).[15] Therefore, airway pressure remains higher than pleural pressure throughout the respiratory cycle. Sudden communication of the pleural space with either alveolar or external air allows gas to enter (Fig. 26-2). When the pleural pressure rises, the elasticity of the lung causes it to collapse. The lung continues to collapse until either the pressure gradient no longer exists or the pleural defect closes.[15,16] Lung collapse produces a decrease in vital capacity, an increase in the alveolar–arterial partial pressure of oxygen ($P_{AO_2} - Pa_{O_2}$) gradient, a ventilation–perfusion mismatch, and an intrapulmonary shunt resulting in hypoxemia.[15,16] In the patient without underlying lung disease, hypercapnia does not occur because the uninvolved lung functions to maintain adequate alveolar ventilation. In the patient with underlying pulmonary disease (COPD), hypercapnia is common because the abnormal gas exchange produced by the pneumothorax is superimposed on preexisting abnormal gas exchange.[15]

There are two types of pneumothorax: spontaneous and traumatic. Spontaneous pneumothorax is any pneumothorax that results from the rupture of air into the pleural space without obvious cause. Primary spontaneous pneumothorax occurs in the absence of underlying lung disease, and secondary spontaneous pneumothorax occurs as a complication of underlying lung disease.[15,17] Primary spontaneous pneumothorax occurs primarily in young (adolescence to 30 years of age), tall men. Family history and cigarette smoking are important risk factors.[17,18] Secondary spontaneous pneumothorax largely occurs in patients who have COPD.[17] Other causes of secondary spontaneous pneumothorax include asthma, cystic fibrosis, *Pneumocystis carinii* pneumonia, sarcoidosis, necrotizing pneumonia, and histiocytosis X.[15,17]

The most common causes of a traumatic pneumothorax in critically ill patients are invasive procedures and barotrauma.[15] (See Chapter 55 for a discussion of blunt and penetrating trauma as causes of pneumothorax.) Accidental entry of air into the pleural space during an invasive procedure causes iatrogenic pneumothorax. Central line catheter insertions cause approximately 36,000 pneumothoraces per year, which affect 1% of the patients receiving central line catheters.[15] Pulmonary barotrauma occurs in approximately 10% of patients receiving mechanical ventilation.[15] Barotrauma includes parenchymal interstitial gas, pneumomediastinum, subcutaneous emphysema, pneumoperitoneum, and pneumothorax.[15] Pulmonary interstitial gas or emphysema is the initial radiographic indication of barotrauma. The mechanically ventilated patient is at risk for development of a tension pneumothorax. A tension pneumothorax occurs when the pressure of air in the pleural space exceeds atmospheric pressure. As pressures in the thorax increase, the mediastinum shifts to the contralateral side, placing torsion on the inferior vena cava and decreasing venous return to the right side of the heart[17] (see Fig. 26-2).

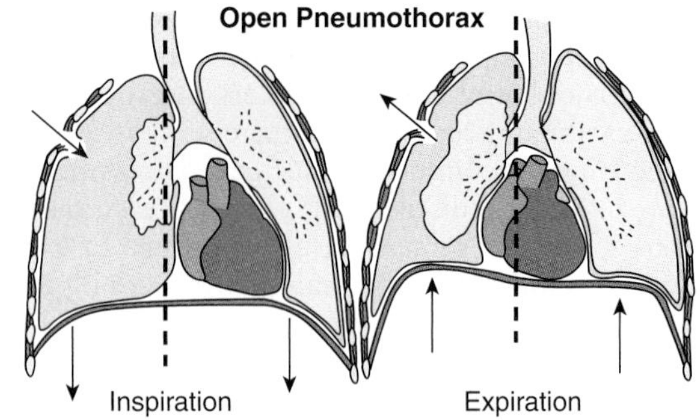

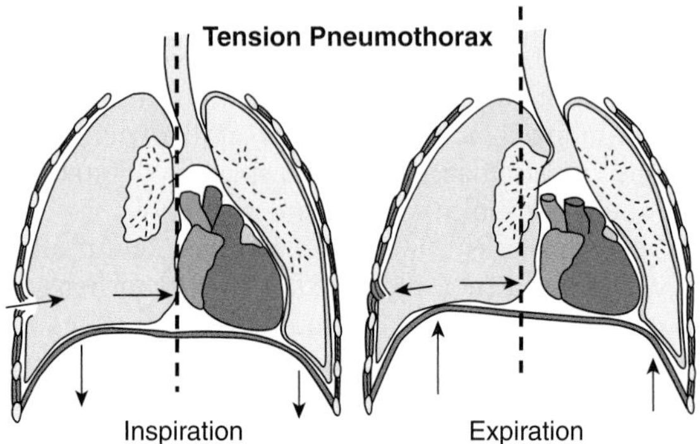

figure 26-2 Open or communicating pneumothorax (*top*) and tension pneumothorax (*bottom*). In an open pneumothorax, air enters the chest during inspiration and exits during expiration. There may be slight inflation of the affected lung due to a decrease in pressure as air moves out of the chest. In tension pneumothorax, air can enter but not leave the chest. As the pressure in the chest increases, the heart and great vessels are compressed and the mediastinal structures are shifted toward the opposite side of the chest. The trachea is pushed from its normal midline position toward the opposite side of the chest and the unaffected lung is compressed. (From Porth C: Pathophysiology: Concepts of Altered Health States [6th Ed], p 636. Philadelphia, Lippincott Williams & Wilkins, 2002.)

Assessment

HISTORY AND PHYSICAL FINDINGS

The patient complains of sudden onset of acute pleuritic chest pain localized to the affected lung. The pleuritic chest pain is usually accompanied by shortness of breath, increased work of breathing, and dyspnea. Chest wall movement may be uneven because the affected side does not expand as much of the healthy side. Breath sounds are distant or absent. Chest percussion produces a hyperresonant sound. Tachycardia occurs frequently in all types of pneumothorax. Tension pneumothorax is a life-threatening condition manifested by respiratory distress (Box 26-4).

DIAGNOSTIC STUDIES

To assess for the presence of a pneumothorax, a chest radiograph should be obtained with the patient in the upright or decubitus position. The chest film shows contralateral mediastinal shift, ipsilateral diaphragmatic depression, and ipsilateral chest wall expansion in the patient with tension pneumothorax.[15] When clinical symptoms of tension pneumothorax are present in a patient on mechanical ventilation, treatment should not be delayed to obtain radiographic confirmation. Arterial blood gases (ABGs) are used to assess for hypoxemia and hypercapnia.

Management

Supplemental oxygen should be administered to all patients with pneumothorax because oxygen accelerates the rate of air resorption from the pleural space.[16] A chest tube is placed in the apical and anterior aspect of the pleural space to assist air removal. Connecting the chest tube to underwater seal drainage alone is usually adequate to resolve the pneumothorax. Initially placing the chest tube to suction risks reexpansion pulmonary edema due to rapid reinflation of the collapsed lung.[16] If the pneumothorax persists after 12 to 24 hours of underwater seal drainage, 15 to 20 cm H_2O suction should be applied to facilitate closure.[16] In approximately one third of patients with COPD, persistent air leaks require multiple chest tubes to evacuate the pneumothorax.[16]

A tension pneumothorax is a life-threatening condition requiring immediate treatment; if untreated, it leads to cardiovascular collapse. If a chest tube is not immediately available, a large-bore (16- or 18-gauge) needle should be placed into the anterior second intercostal space. After needle insertion, a chest tube is placed and connected to underwater seal drainage. When the tension pneumothorax is relieved, the effect is rapid and occurs as an improvement in oxygenation, a decrease in heart rate, and an increase in blood pressure.

box 26-4 ***Symptoms of Tension Pneumothorax***

- Hypoxemia (early sign)
- Apprehension
- Respiratory distress (severe tachypnea)
- Increasing peak and mean airway pressures, decreasing compliance, and auto–positive end-expiratory pressure (auto-PEEP) in patients receiving mechanical ventilation
- Cardiovascular collapse (heart rate >140 beats/minute with any of the following: peripheral cyanosis, hypotension, pulseless electrical activity)

PULMONARY EMBOLISM

Pulmonary embolism and deep venous thrombosis (DVT) are both part of the spectrum of disease known as venous thromboembolism. Pulmonary embolism is obstruction of a pulmonary artery with a thrombosis that has broken free from its site of origin and migrated to the pulmonary vasculature (Fig. 26-3); pulmonary embolism results from DVT, which is clot formation inside a vein. At least 5 million episodes of venous thromboembolism occur annually, and approximately 10% of these episodes lead to pulmonary embolism.[19] At least 10% of patients with pulmonary embolism (50,000) die each year.[19] The incidence of venous thromboembolism varies. The risk of venous thromboembolism is greatest in surgical patients; approximately 50% of patients undergoing elective hip replacement and 70% undergoing elective knee replacement have venous thromboembolism.[19] Marik and associates[20] reported a 12% incidence of venous thrombosis in medical and surgical ICU patients, 92% of whom had received prophylaxis. Risk factors increasing the incidence of venous thromboembolism are listed in Box 26-5.

Pathophysiology

Pulmonary embolism and DVT are part of a common disease entity, venous thromboembolism. Virchow's triad (venous stasis, hypercoagulability, vein wall damage) has long been acknowledged in the pathophysiology of venous thromboembolism. Venous stasis is an important factor in the formation of DVT and permits red blood cells, platelets, white blood cells, and fibrin to adhere, primarily to a venous valve, producing a thrombus.[21] Hypercoagulability may occur as a result of trauma or surgery. Damage to the vessel wall causes adherence of blood platelets and activation of clotting factors.

Thrombus formation is frequently bilateral and often asymptomatic. Although most thrombi form in the calf, most pulmonary emboli (80% to 90%) arise from venous thrombi that extend into the proximal veins (popliteal and iliofemoral) of the lower extremities.[19,21] Proximal venous thrombi pose an approximate 50% risk of embolism.[19]

Occlusion of a pulmonary artery by an embolus produces both pulmonary and hemodynamic changes. Alveoli are ventilated but not perfused, producing areas of mismatched ventilation and perfusion. As a result, well-ventilated alveoli are underperfused and gas exchange is compromised (increased respiratory dead space). Pulmonary vascular constriction resulting from a lack of carbon dioxide, which is normally present in pulmonary arterial blood, shifts ventilation from the underperfused alveoli. Accompanying physiological changes include increased minute ventilation, decreased vital capacity, increased airway resistance, and decreased diffusing capacity.[21]

The severity of hemodynamic change in pulmonary embolism depends on the size of the embolus and degree of pulmonary vascular obstruction, as well as on the preexisting status of the cardiopulmonary system. In patients with no previous cardiopulmonary disease, there is a relationship between the degree of pulmonary artery obstruction and the pulmonary artery pressure. Increased right ventricular afterload results from obstruction of the pul-

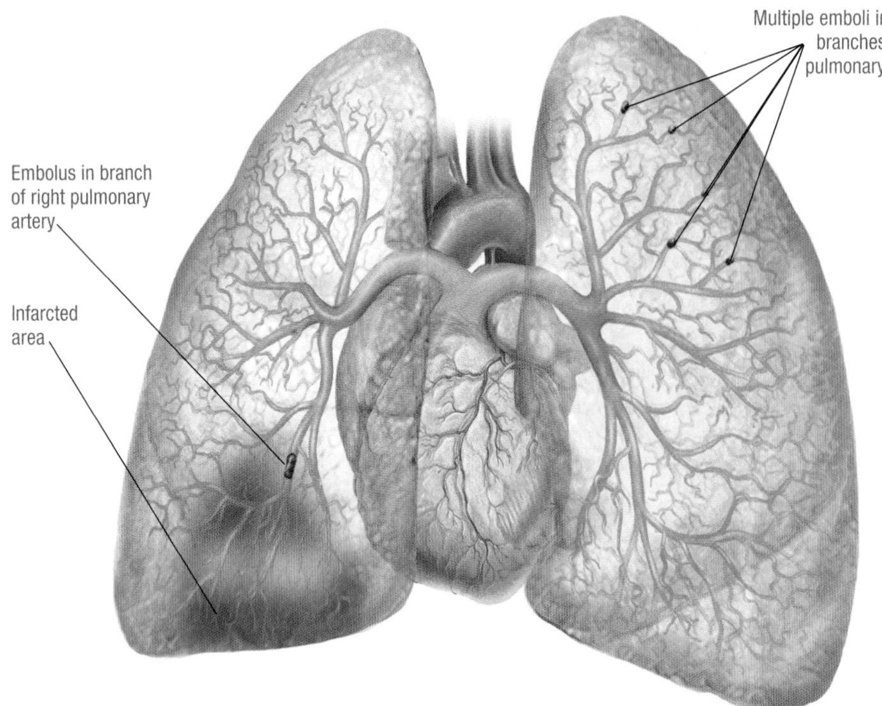

figure 26-3 Sites of pulmonary emboli. (From Anatomical Chart Company: Atlas of Pathophysiology. Springhouse, PA, Springhouse, 2002.)

monary vascular bed by embolism. In patients with no preexisting cardiopulmonary disease, obstruction of less than 20% of the pulmonary vascular bed produces compensatory events that minimize adverse hemodynamic consequences.[19] Cardiac output is maintained by increases in both right ventricular stroke volume and heart rate, and recruitment and distension of pulmonary vessels occur, producing normal or near-normal pulmonary artery pressure and pulmonary vascular resistance.[19] When the degree of pulmonary vascular obstruction exceeds 30% to 40%, increases in pulmonary artery pressure occur, followed by modest increases in right atrial pressure.[19] As the degree of pulmonary artery obstruction exceeds 50% to 60%, compensatory mechanisms are overcome, producing a decrease in cardiac output and dramatic increases in right atrial pressure.[19] Patients with preexisting cardiopulmonary disease have degrees of pulmonary hypertension that are disproportionate to the degree of embolic obstruction.[19] Severe pulmonary hypertension may develop from a relatively small reduction of pulmonary blood flow.

Assessment

Both pulmonary embolism and DVT are frequently clinically unsuspected, causing significant diagnostic and therapeutic delays and substantial morbidity and mortality. Patients with lower extremity DVT frequently do not exhibit erythema, pain, swelling, or tenderness.[22] Clinical evaluation may indicate a need for further studies but is not reliable for confirmation or exclusion of the diagnosis of DVT.[22] Similarly, clinical manifestations associated with pulmonary embolism are not adequately sensitive or specific for diagnosis or exclusion of pulmonary embolism. Signs and symptoms of pulmonary embolism are listed in Box 26-6. Dyspnea is the most frequent symptom in patients with angiographically confirmed pulmonary embolism. Other signs and symptoms (in order of frequency) are pleuritic chest pain, cough, apprehension, leg swelling, and pain.[23] A diagnostic algorithm for suspected pulmonary embolism is presented in Figure 26-4.

Management

Heparin and thrombolytic agents are used to treat pulmonary embolism. However, anticoagulation with heparin is the mainstay for treatment. Guidelines developed by the American College of Chest Physicians (ACCP) for the treatment of venous thromboembolism are shown in Table 26-5.[24]

Patients with DVT or pulmonary embolism should be treated with unfractionated intravenous heparin or adjusted-dose subcutaneous heparin. (For subcutaneous treatment with unfractionated heparin, give 250 U/kg every 12 hours to obtain an activated partial thromboplastin time [aPTT] with therapeutic range at 6 to 8 hours.) The heparin dosage should prolong the aPTT to a range that corresponds to a plasma heparin level of 0.2 to 0.4 U/mL by protamine sulfate, or 0.3 to 0.6 U/mL by an amidolytic anti-factor Xa assay (grade A1).[24]

Low-molecular-weight heparin (LMWH) can be substituted for unfractionated heparin in patients with DVT and in stable patients with pulmonary embolism. Treatment with heparin or LMWH should continue for at least 5 days, overlapped with oral anticoagulation for at least 4 to 5 days (grade A1).[24]

The recommended length of anticoagulation therapy varies, depending on the patient's age, comorbidities, and the likelihood of recurrence of pulmonary embolism or

box 26-5
Risk Factors for Thromboembolism

Hereditary Thrombophilias

- Protein C deficiency
- Protein S deficiency
- Antithrombin III deficiency
- Factor V Leiden mutation
- Prothrombin 20210 G–A variation
- Hyperhomocysteinemia

Acquired Medical Predisposition

- Prior venous thromboembolism
- Age >40 years
- Malignant neoplasia
- Congestive heart failure
- Cerebrovascular accident
- Nephrotic syndrome
- Estrogen therapy
- Pregnancy and the postpartum period
- Obesity
- Prolonged immobilization
- Antiphospholipid antibody syndrome
- Lupus anticoagulant
- Inflammatory bowel disease

Acquired Surgical Predisposition

- Major thoracic or abdominal surgery requiring general anesthesia and lasting >30 minutes
- Hip arthroplasty
- Knee arthroplasty
- Knee arthroscopy
- Hip fracture
- Major trauma
- Open prostatectomy
- Spinal cord injury
- Neurosurgical procedures

Reprinted with permission from Fedullo PF: Pulmonary embolism and deep vein thrombosis. In Shoemaker W, Grenvik A, Ayres S, et al (eds): Textbook of Critical Care (4th Ed), p 1494. Philadelphia, Saunders/Harcourt Health Sciences, 2000.

box 26-6 ***Signs and Symptoms of Pulmonary Embolism***

Small to Moderate Embolus

- Dyspnea
- Tachypnea
- Tachycardia
- Chest pain
- Mild fever
- Hypoxemia
- Apprehension
- Cough
- Diaphoresis
- Decreased breath sounds over affected area
- Rales
- Wheezing

Massive Embolus

A more pronounced manifestation of the above signs and symptoms, plus the following:

- Cyanosis
- Restlessness
- Anxiety
- Confusion
- Hypotension
- Cool, clammy skin
- Decreased urinary output
- Pleuritic chest pain: associated with pulmonary infarction
- Hemoptysis: associated with pulmonary infarction

Signs of Pulmonary Embolism in Intensive Care Patients

- Worsening hypoxemia or hypocapnia in a patient on spontaneous ventilation
- Worsening hypoxemia and hypercapnia in a sedate patient on controlled mechanical ventilation
- Worsening dyspnea, hypoxemia, and a reduction in $Paco_2$ in a patient with chronic lung disease and known carbon dioxide retention
- Unexplained fever
- Sudden elevation in pulmonary artery pressure or central venous pressure in a hemodynamically monitored patient

DVT. In most patients, anticoagulation therapy with warfarin should be continued for 3 to 6 months.[24] The first episode of idiopathic DVT should be treated for at least 6 months.[24] Patients with new-onset DVT and a risk factor (cancer, inhibitor deficiency state) or recurrent venous thrombosis should be treated indefinitely.[24] Patients with massive pulmonary embolism or severe iliofemoral thrombosis may require a longer period of heparin therapy.[24] Anticoagulation using full-dose subcutaneous heparin for several months is effective in patients who have contraindications to warfarin (e.g., pregnant women) but who can safely take heparin.[24]

Thrombolytic therapy is only recommended for patients with acute massive pulmonary embolism who are hemodynamically unstable and not prone to bleeding.[24] All thrombolytic agents act systemically and have the potential to lyse a fresh platelet-fibrin clot anywhere and cause bleeding at that site.[24] Intracranial disease, recent surgery, trauma, and hemorrhagic disease are contraindications to thrombolytic therapy. Urokinase, streptokinase, and recombinant tissue plasminogen activator (tPA) are the thrombolytic agents approved for treating pulmonary embolism and venous thromboembolism. Heparin therapy is not administered concurrently with thrombolytics; however, thrombolytic therapy is followed by administration of heparin then warfarin.

An inferior vena cava filter is recommended to prevent pulmonary embolism in patients with contraindications to heparin therapy (risk of major bleed or drug sensitivity).[24] Placement of an inferior vena cava filter is also recommended in patients with recurring thromboembolism despite adequate anticoagulation, chronic recurrent embolism and pulmonary hypertension, and concurrent

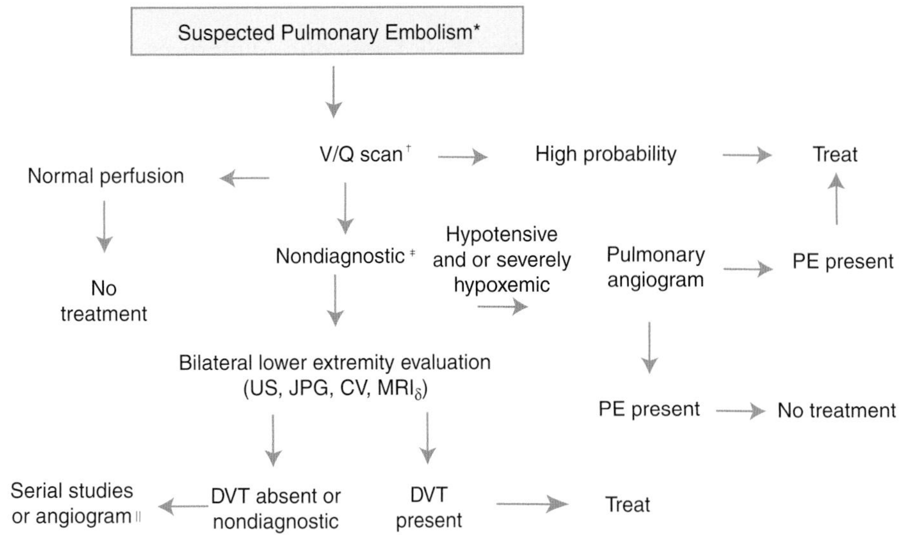

* The history, physical exam, ancillary testing and recognition of risk factors leading to suspicion of pulmonary embolism (PE) are discussed in the text. When PE is suspected and the risk of bleeding deemed low, it is appropriate to begin anticoagulation while diagnostic testing is underway.

† A perfusion scan alone may suffice. Diagnostic alternatives to the ventilation-perfusion (V/Q) scan include spiral computed tomography (CT) and magnetic imaging (MRI). These are being used increasingly, and also require institutional and reader expertise and further validation in well designed trials.

‡Patients with low probability V/Q scans and low clinical suspicion are unlikely to have PE. Others require further evaluation. There are several options when the V/Q scan (or spiral CT or lung MRI) is nondiagnostic. Pulmonary angiography is the appropriate approach if the patient is unstable. Otherwise, leg studies can be performed. If spiral CT or lung MRI is performed, a negative result should be interpreted together with the level of clinical suspicion. Although these techniques appear to be sensitive, additional studies (pulmonary angiography or leg studies) should be performed as deemed appropriate.

δ A positive test is useful. The sensitivity for compression ultrasound (US) and impendance plethysmography (IPC) is low in asymptomatic patients, and negative or nondiagnostic studies require additional data. MRI appears sensitive in this setting, but no level 1 data exists. The role of D-dimer testing in clinical algorithms is not clearly established, but recent data from a few centers suggest that the sensitivity of certain assays may help exclude VTE when combined with other diagnostic test results. General recommendations that can be extrapolated to all centers cannot be made at present.

‖Negative serial IPC in this setting has been associated with excellent outcome without anticoagulation at certain centers.

figure 26-4 Diagnostic algorithm for patients with symptoms suggestive of acute pulmonary embolism. The recommended diagnostic approach allows for some flexibility depending upon the resources at a particular institution. *CV*, cardiovascular; *PE*, pulmonary embolism; *US*, ultrasound; *DVT*, deep vein thrombosis; *MRI*, magnetic resonance imaging; *V/Q*, ventilation–perfusion. (American Thoracic Society: The diagnostic approach to acute venous thromboembolism. American J Respiratory and Critical Care Medicine 160:1043–1066, 1999.)

surgical pulmonary embolectomy or pulmonary endarterectomy procedures.[24]

Prevention

Prevention of venous thromboembolism is essential to decreasing the morbidity and mortality associated with pulmonary embolism. Prophylactic measures are based on the patient's specific risk factors. Preventive measures recommended by the ACCP are listed in Table 26-6.

CHRONIC OBSTRUCTIVE PULMONARY DISEASE

Chronic obstructive pulmonary disease (COPD) is a disease state characterized by airflow limitation that is not fully reversible. The airflow limitation is usually both progressive and associated with an abnormal inflammatory response of the lungs to noxious particles or gases or an inherited deficiency of α_1-antitrypsin.[25,26] The term COPD is applied to several disease entities, including emphysema and chronic bronchitis.[27]

COPD is a major cause of chronic morbidity and mortality throughout the world. The World Health Organization (WHO) estimates that COPD shares fourth and fifth place with human immunodeficiency virus (HIV)/acquired immunodeficiency syndrome (AIDS) as a single cause of death (behind heart disease, cerebrovascular disease, and acute respiratory infection), causing 2.74 million deaths in 2000.[25] The WHO estimates that COPD was the 12th highest cause of morbidity and mortality in 1990 and that it will be 5th by 2020.[25]

Pathophysiology

As COPD progresses, pathophysiological changes usually occur in the following order: mucus hypersecretion, ciliary dysfunction, airflow limitation, pulmonary hyperinflation, gas exchange abnormalities, pulmonary hypertension, and cor pulmonale.[25] The peripheral airways become the major site of obstruction in patients with COPD. The structural changes in the airway wall are the most important cause of the increase in peripheral airway resistance. Inflammatory changes such as airway edema and mucus hypersecretion also contribute to narrowing of the peripheral airways.[25]

table 26-5 American College of Chest Physicians Recommendations for Treatment of Venous Thromboembolism

Anticoagulation Guidelines for	Recommended Therapy
Unfractionated Heparin	
Suspected VTE	• Obtain baseline aPTT, PT, CBC. • Check for contraindications to heparin therapy. • Give heparin 5,000 U IV. • Order imaging study.
Confirmed VTE	• Re-bolus with heparin 80 U/kg IV, and start maintenance infusion at 18 U/kg/h. • Check aPTT at 6 h; maintain a range corresponding to a therapeutic heparin level. • Start warfarin therapy on day 1 at 5 mg; adjust subsequent daily dose according to INR. • Stop heparin after 4 to 5 days of combined therapy, when INR is >2.0 (2.0–3.0). • Anticoagulate with warfarin for at least 3 mo (target INR 2.5; 2.0–3.0).
LMW Heparin	
Suspected VTE	• Obtain baseline aPTT, PT, CBC. • Check for contraindication to heparin therapy. • Give unfractionated heparin, 5,000 U IV. • Order imaging study.
Confirmed VTE	• Give LMWH (enoxaparin), 1 mg/kg subcutaneously q12h. • Start warfarin therapy on day 1 at 5 mg; adjust subsequent daily dose according to the INR. • Consider checking platelet count between days 3 and 5. • Stop LMWH after at least 4–5 days of combined therapy, when INR is >2.0 on 2 consecutive days. • Anticoagulate with warfarin for at least 3 mo (goal INR 2.5; 2.0–3.0).

VTE, venous thromboembolism; *aPTT,* activated partial thromboplastin time; *PT,* prothrombin time; *INR,* international normalized ratio; *CBC,* complete blood count; *LMWH,* low-molecular-weight heparin.

From American College of Chest Physicians: Fifth ACCP consensus conference on antithrombotic therapy. Chest 114(5 Suppl):565S, 567S, 1998, with permission.

Mucus hypersecretion is caused by the stimulation of the enlarged mucus-secreting glands and the increased number of goblet cells by inflammatory mediators such as leukotrienes, proteinases, and neuropeptides.[25] Ciliated epithelial cells undergo squamous metaplasia, leading to impaired mucociliary clearance,[25] which is usually the first physiological abnormality to occur in COPD. This abnormality may be evident for many years before any other abnormalities develop.[25] Expiratory airflow limitation is an essential finding in COPD. As the disease process progresses, forced expiratory volume in 1 second (FEV_1) and forced vital capacity (FVC) decrease; this is related to the increased thickness of the airway wall, loss of alveolar attachments, and loss of lung elastic recoil. Frequently, the first sign of developing airflow limitation is a decrease in the FEV_1/FVC ratio.[25] According to the 2001 Global Initiative for Chronic Obstructive Lung Disease (GOLD), the presence of a postbronchodilator FEV_1 less than 80% of the predicted value in combination with an FEV_1/FVC ratio less than 70% confirms the presence of airflow limitation that is not fully reversible (Table 26-7). In severe COPD, air is trapped in the lungs during forced expiration, leading to an abnormally high functional residual capacity (FRC). As FRC increases, this leads to pulmonary hyperinflation.[25]

In advanced COPD, peripheral airway obstruction, parenchymal destruction, and pulmonary vascular irregularities reduce the lung's capacity for gas exchange, resulting in hypoxemia (low blood oxygen) and hypercapnia (high blood carbon dioxide).[25] A ventilation–perfusion ratio mismatch is the driving force behind hypoxemia in patients with COPD, regardless of the stage of the disease.[28] Chronic hypercapnia usually indicates inspiratory muscle dysfunction and alveolar hypoventilation.[25] As hypoxemia and hypercapnia progress late in COPD, pulmonary hypertension often develops, which causes hypertrophy of the right ventricle, better known as cor pulmonale.[25] Right-sided heart failure leads to further venous stasis and thrombosis that may potentially result in pulmonary embolism and further compromise the pulmonary circulation.[25] Last, COPD is associated with systemic inflammation and skeletal muscle dysfunction that may result in limitation of exercise capacity and decline of health status.[25]

Assessment

HISTORY

A detailed medical history of a new patient with known or suspected COPD should assess the following:

table 26-6 American College of Chest Physicians Recommendations for Prevention of Venous Thromboembolism (VTE)

Patient Population	Recommended Therapy	Grade*
Low-risk general surgery	Early ambulation	C1
Moderate-risk general surgery	LDUH, LMWH, intermittent pneumatic compression, or elastic stockings	A1
Higher-risk general surgery	LDUH, or higher-dose LMWH	A1
Very–high-risk general surgery with multiple risk factors	LDUH, or LMWH combined with intermittent pneumatic compression	B1
Total hip replacement surgery	LMWH, started 12–24 h after surgery Warfarin, started before or immediately after surgery, *or* Adjusted-dose heparin, started before surgery; Adjuvant use of elastic stockings or intermittent pneumatic compression	A1
Total knee replacement surgery	LMWH, warfarin, or intermittent pneumatic compression	A1
Acute spinal cord injury	LMWH Elastic stockings and intermittent pneumatic compression may have benefit when used with LMWH; however, they appear ineffective when used alone	B1 C1
Trauma patients with identifiable risk factor for thromboembolism	LMWH, as soon as safe Intermittent pneumatic compression if LMWH will be delayed or is contraindicated For high-risk patients with suboptimal prophylaxis, consider screening with duplex ultrasonography or filter placement in the inferior vena cava	A1 C1 C2
Myocardial infarction	LDUH or full-dose anticoagulation Intermittent pneumatic compression or elastic stockings when heparin is contraindicated	A1 C1
Ischemic stroke and lower extremity paralysis	LDUH or LMWH Intermittent pneumatic compression with elastic stockings	A1 B1
Medical patients with risk factors for VTE (including congestive heart failure and chest infections)	LDUH or LMWH	A1
Patients with long-term indwelling central vein catheters	Warfarin (1 mg/day), or LMWH qd, to prevent axillary–subclavian venous thrombosis	A1
Patients receiving a spinal puncture or epidural catheter placement	LMWH should be used with caution	C1

LDUH, low-dose unfractionated heparin; LMWH, low-molecular-weight heparin.

*A1: Methods strong, results consistent—randomized clinical trials (RCTs), no heterogeneity, effect clear that benefits do (or do not) outweigh risks.

A2: Methods strong, results consistent—RCTs, no heterogeneity, effect equivocal—uncertain whether benefits outweigh risks.

B1: Methods strong, results inconsistent—RCTs, heterogeneity present, effect clear that benefits do (or do not) outweigh risks.

B2: Methods strong, results inconsistent—RCTs, heterogeneity present, effect equivocal—uncertain whether benefits outweigh risks.

C1: Methods weak—observational studies, effect clear that benefits do (or do not) outweigh risks.

C2: Methods weak—observational studies, effect equivocal—uncertain whether benefits outweigh risks.

From American College of Chest Physicians: Fifth ACCP consensus conference on antithrombotic therapy. Chest 114(5 Suppl):439S–769S, 1998, with permission.

- *Exposure to risk factors*, such as smoking, and occupational or environmental exposures.
- *Past medical history*, including asthma, allergy, sinusitis or nasal polyps, respiratory infections in childhood, and other respiratory diseases.
- *Family history of COPD or other chronic respiratory disease.*
- *Pattern of symptom development.* COPD typically develops in adults, and most patients are aware of the occurrence of increased breathlessness, increased frequency of winter "colds," and some social restriction for a number of years before seeking medical attention.
- *History of exacerbations or previous hospitalizations for respiratory disorder*. Patients may be conscious of periodic worsening of symptoms even if these episodes have not been identified as acute exacerbations of COPD. Common conditions that trigger exacerbations of COPD are listed in Box 26-7.
- *Comorbidities* such as heart disease and rheumatic disease, which may also contribute to restriction of activity.
- *Appropriateness of current medical treatments*, such as beta blockers commonly prescribed for heart disease. Beta blockers are usually contraindicated in COPD.

table 26-7 Stages of Chronic Obstructive Pulmonary Disease (COPD) and Their Treatment

Stage	Characteristics	Recommended Treatment
ALL		• Avoidance of risk factor(s) • Influenza vaccination
0: At Risk	• Chronic symptoms (cough, sputum) • Exposure to risk factor(s) • Normal spirometry	
I: Mild COPD	• FEV_1/FVC <70% • FEV_1 ≥80% predicted • With or without symptoms	• Short-acting bronchodilator when needed
II: Moderate COPD	IIA: • FEV_1/FVC <70% • 50% ≤ FEV_1 <80% predicted • With or without symptoms	• Regular treatment with one or more bronchodilators • Rehabilitation • Inhaled glucocorticosteroids if significant symptoms and lung function response
	IIB: • FEV_1/FVC <70% • 30% ≤ FEV_1 <50% predicted • With or without symptoms	• Regular treatment with one or more bronchodilators • Rehabilitation • Inhaled glucocorticosteroids if significant symptoms and lung function response or if repeated exacerbations
III: Severe COPD	• FEV_1/FVC <70% • FEV_1 <30% predicted or presence of respiratory failure or right heart failure	• Regular treatment with one or more bronchodilators • Inhaled glucocorticosteroids if significant symptoms and lung function response or if repeated exacerbations • Treatment of complications • Rehabilitation • Long-term oxygen therapy if respiratory failure • Consider surgical treatments

FEV_1, forced expiratory volume in 1 second; *FVC*, forced vital capacity.

Patients must be taught how and when to use their treatment, and treatments being prescribed for other conditions should be reviewed. Beta-blocking agents (including eye drop formulations) should be avoided.

From Pauwels RA, et al: Global Strategy for the Diagnosis, Management, and Prevention of Chronic Obstructive Pulmonary Disease: National Heart, Lung, and Blood Institute and World Health Organization Global Initiative for Chronic Obstructive Lung Disease (GOLD). Respir Care 46:810, 2001, with permission.

- *Impact of disease on patient's life*, including limitation of activity, missed work and economic consequences, effect on family routines, or feelings of depression or anxiety.
- *Social and family support.*
- *Possibilities for reducing risk factors, especially smoking cessation.*[25]

PHYSICAL FINDINGS

A physical examination is rarely diagnostic in COPD, although it remains an important aspect of patient care.[25] The physical examination should include:

Inspection

- *Central cyanosis* or bluish discoloration of the mucosal membranes. This feature may be present but is difficult to detect in artificial light and in many racial groups.
- *Common chest wall abnormalities*, which reflect the pulmonary hyperinflation seen in COPD, including relatively horizontal ribs, "barrel-shaped" chest, and protruding abdomen.
- *Flattening of the hemidiaphragms*, which may be associated with paradoxical indrawing of the lower rib

box 26-7 *Conditions That Trigger Exacerbations of Chronic Obstructive Pulmonary Disease*

- Infections: bacterial or bacterial superinfection of a primary viral process (acute tracheobronchitis)
- Left ventricular failure
- Cardiac dysrhythmias
- Pneumothorax
- Pulmonary thromboembolism
- Upper airway obstruction
- Aspiration
- Rhinitis or sinusitis
- Asthma
- Gastroesophageal reflux

From Honig EG, Ingram RH: Chronic bronchitis, emphysema, and airways obstruction. In Braunwald E, et al (eds): Harrison's Principles of Internal Medicine, pp 1494–1497. New York, McGraw-Hill, 2001, with permission.

cage on inspiration, reduced cardiac dullness, and widening xiphisternal angle.
- *Resting respiratory rate*, which is often increased to more than 20 breaths per minute, and breathing may be shallow.
- *Pursed-lip breathing*, which may serve to slow expiratory flow and permit more efficient lung emptying.
- *Resting muscle activation*, which may be indicative of respiratory distress. While lying supine, patients with COPD often use the scalene and sternocleidomastoid muscles.
- *Ankle or lower leg edema*, which may be an indication of right heart failure.

Palpation and Percussion

- *Palpation and percussion*, which are often unhelpful in COPD.
- *Heart apex beat*, which may be difficult to detect due to pulmonary hyperinflation.
- *Pulmonary hyperinflation*, which also leads to downward displacement of the liver and an increase in the ability to palpate this organ without its actually being enlarged.

Auscultation

- *Reduced breath sounds*. Patients with COPD often have reduced breath sounds.
- *Wheezing*. Occurrence during quiet breathing is a useful indicator of airflow limitation. However, wheezing heard only after forced expiration is of no diagnostic significance.
- *Inspiratory crackles*, which occur in some COPD patients but are of little assistance diagnostically.
- *Heart sounds*, which are best heard over the xiphoid area.

Symptoms of COPD include cough, sputum production, and shortness of breath on exertion. Characteristic features of an acute exacerbation of COPD are listed in Box 26-8.[29]

box 26-8 ***Signs and Symptoms of Acute Exacerbations of Chronic Obstructive Pulmonary Disease***

- Worsening of previously stable disease
- Increased dyspnea
- Increased wheeze
- Increased cough
- Increased sputum volume
- Increased sputum tenacity and purulence
- Variable degrees of water retention
- Worsening gas exchange and ventilation–perfusion relationships
- Increased hyperventilation
- Increased work of breathing
- Chest tightness

From Honig EG, Ingram RH: Chronic bronchitis, emphysema, and airways obstruction. In Braunwald E, et al (eds): Harrison's Principles of Internal Medicine, New York, McGraw-Hill, 2001, with permission.

DIAGNOSTIC STUDIES

Laboratory and diagnostic tests in COPD are summarized in Table 26-8.

Spirometry

Expiratory airflow limitation is the hallmark diagnostic sign of COPD. Because spirometry is the most reproducible and objective measure of airflow limitation, it remains the gold standard for diagnosing COPD and monitoring its progression.[25] Spirometry is performed in patients with chronic cough and sputum production even without dyspnea. Spirometry measures the maximal volume of air forcibly exhaled from the point of maximal inspiration (FVC) and the volume of air exhaled during the first second of this exercise (FEV_1). The ratio of these two measurements (FEV_1:FVC) is then calculated.[26] Spirometry measurements are evaluated by comparison of the results with appropriate reference values based on age, height, sex, and race.

Figure 26-5 demonstrates a normal spirogram and a spirogram characteristic of a patient with COPD with mild to moderate airflow limitation. Patients with COPD have decreased FEV_1 and FVC, and the degree of spirometric abnormality generally reflects the severity of the disease[25] (see Table 26-8). By itself, the FEV_1:FVC ratio is the most sensitive measure of airflow limitation, and an FEV_1:FVC ratio less than 70% is considered an early sign of airflow limitation in patients whose FEV_1 remains normal (at least 80% of the predicted value).

Arterial Blood Gases

ABG measurements should be performed in all patients with an FEV_1 less than 40% predicted or when clinical signs of respiratory failure or right-sided heart failure are present (i.e., central cyanosis, ankle swelling, increase in the jugular venous pressure).[25] Respiratory failure is indicated by a partial pressure of arterial oxygen (PaO_2) of 60 mm Hg with or without a partial pressure of arterial carbon dioxide ($PaCO_2$) of 45 mm Hg while breathing air at sea level.[25] Several precautions must be taken to ensure accurate results. First, it should be noted if the patient is currently receiving an oxygen source and the amount of oxygen delivered to the patient during the blood gas sample time. Second, if the fraction of inspired oxygen (FIO_2) has been changed, a period of 20 to 30 minutes should elapse before gas tensions are rechecked.[25]

Management

Several different management techniques, ranging from exercise training, nutrition counseling, and education, to drug therapy, oxygen use, and surgery, may be effective in the treatment of COPD. See Table 26-7 for therapeutic guidelines for the various stages of COPD. Box 26-9 provides a collaborative care guide for the patient with COPD.

table 26-8 ■ Laboratory and Diagnostic Tests for Patients With Chronic Obstructive Pulmonary Disease (COPD)

Test	Rationale
Spirometry	Measures FVC and FEV_1
Bronchodilator reversibility	Performed once during diagnosis stage and useful for the following reasons: • To rule out an asthma diagnosis (If FEV_1 returns to predicted normal range after administration of bronchodilator, airflow limitation is likely due to asthma.) • To establish a patient's best attainable lung function at that point in time • To gauge a patient's prognosis (Postbronchodilator FEV_1 is a more reliable prognostic indicator than prebronchodilator FEV_1.) • To assess potential response to treatment (An increase in FEV_1 >200 mL and 12% above prebronchodilator FEV_1 is considered significant.)
Glucocorticosteroid reversibility	Measures significant FEV_1 response (i.e., FEV_1 increase of 200 mL and 15% above baseline)
Chest radiography	Bullous disease may be evident Radiological changes seen include: • Flattened diaphragm on lateral chest film • Increased volume of retrosternal air space (signs of hyperinflation) • Hyperlucency of the lungs • Rapid tapering of vascular markings
Computed tomography and ventilation–perfusion scanning	Assessment of surgical patient to visualize airway and parenchymal disease May assist with differential diagnosis
Arterial blood gases	Performed if FEV_1 <40% predicted or if signs of respiratory failure or right heart failure are present
α_1-Antitrypsin deficiency screening	Indicated for patients in whom COPD develops at <45 years of age or who have a strong family predisposition (α_1-antitrypsin serum level below 15%–20% of normal value is highly suggestive of homozygous α_1-antitrypsin deficiency)
Hematocrit	Smokers can develop polycythemia in the presence of arterial hypoxemia. (Hematocrit >55% is defined as polycythemia.)

FEV_1, forced expiratory volume in 1 second; FVC, forced vital capacity.

From Pauwels RA, et al: Global Strategies for the Diagnosis, Management, and Prevention of Chronic Obstructive Pulmonary Disease: National Heart, Lung, and Blood Institute and World Health Organization Global Initiative for Chronic Obstructive Lung Disease (GOLD). Respir Care 46:798–825, 2001, with permission.

NONPHARMACOLOGICAL THERAPY

The main goals of pulmonary rehabilitation are to decrease symptoms, improve quality of life, and increase physical and emotional participation in day-to-day activities.[25] The 2001 GOLD guidelines for the diagnosis, management, and prevention of COPD recommend a comprehensive pulmonary rehabilitation program.

Exercise Training

An exercise training program for COPD may consist of bicycle ergometry, treadmill exercise, or timed walking, and may range in frequency from daily to weekly, in duration from 10 to 45 minutes per session, and in intensity from 50% peak oxygen consumption to maximum tolerated.[25] Many physicians advise patients to exercise on their own (i.e., walking 20 minutes daily) if they are unable to participate in a structured exercise program. The benefits of pulmonary rehabilitation in COPD patients include the following:

- Improved exercise capacity
- Reduced (perceived) intensity of breathlessness
- Improved health-related quality of life
- Reduced number of hospitalizations and days in the hospital

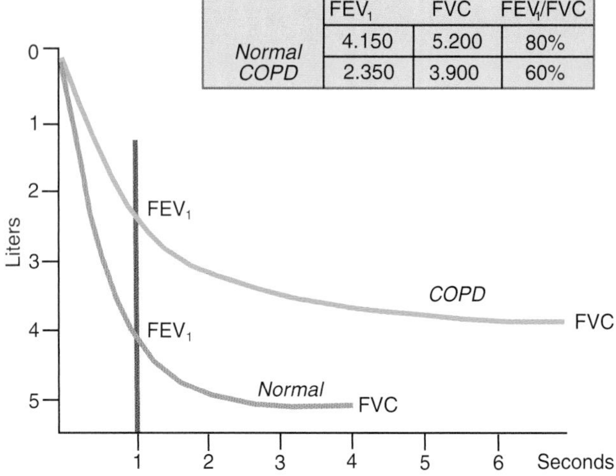

figure 26-5 Normal spirogram and spirogram typical of patients with mild to moderate chronic obstructive pulmonary disease (COPD). *FVC*, forced vital capacity; *FEV*$_1$, forced expiratory volume in 1 second. (National Heart, Lung and Blood Institute, World Health Organization: Global Initiative for Chronic Obstructive Lung Disease: Global Strategy for the Diagnosis, Management, and Prevention of Chronic Obstructive Pulmonary Disease: NHLBI/WHO Workshop, 2001.)

- Reduced COPD-associated anxiety and depression
- Improved arm function due to strength and endurance training of the upper limbs
- Benefits that extend well beyond the immediate period of training
- Improved survival[25]

Nutritional Counseling

Malnutrition is a common problem in patients with COPD and is present in over 50% of patients with COPD admitted to the hospital. The incidence of malnutrition varies with the degree of gas exchange abnormality. Malnutrition results in wasting of respiratory muscles and further respiratory muscle weakness. A complete nutritional assessment should be conducted to identify strategies to maximize the patient's nutritional status. Preventive measures may include providing small, frequent meals for those patients who become breathless while eating; correcting poor dentition; and managing comorbidities (i.e., pulmonary sepsis, lung tumors) appropriately.[25] Improving the nutritional state of weight-losing patients with COPD can lead to increased respiratory muscle strength.[25]

Education

Smoking cessation is the single most effective method of reducing the risk for development of COPD and slowing its progression.[25] In addition, it is the most cost-effective method. A brief (3-minute) counseling session to encourage a smoker to quit results in smoking cessation rates of 5% to 10%. Every smoker should have such a counseling session at every visit to a health care provider.[30] Numerous effective pharmacotherapies (i.e., nicotine replacement products) exist today for smoking cessation, and their use is advised if counseling is unsuccessful in helping a patient quit smoking.[25] It is necessary to stress the importance of elimination or reduction of exposures to various noxious substances in the workplace. Secondary prevention achieved through surveillance and early detection is also very important.[25] Finally, measures should be implemented to reduce or avoid indoor air pollution from biomass fuel, which is burned for cooking and heating in poorly ventilated dwellings. Patients should be advised to check public announcements of air quality, and, depending on the severity of their disease, they should avoid vigorous exercise outdoors or stay indoors if possible during days when pollution levels are high.[25]

PHARMACOLOGICAL THERAPY

According to the 2001 GOLD guidelines, pharmacological treatment for stable patients with COPD mainly includes bronchodilators and glucocorticosteroids. Other pharmacological treatments are sometimes used.

Bronchodilators

Bronchodilators are the cornerstone of symptom management in patients with COPD and are prescribed on an as-needed or a regular basis to prevent or reduce symptoms. Bronchodilators improve emptying of the lungs, reduce hyperinflation at rest and during exercise, and improve exercise performance.[25] They increase the FEV_1 by widening the smooth muscle tone of the airways rather than by altering the elastic recoil properties of the lung.[25] Long-acting bronchodilators are the most convenient. Inhalation is the preferred route of administration. The major bronchodilator agents are beta$_2$-adrenergic agonists, anticholinergics, and theophylline; a combination of these drugs may be effective.[25] The choice of the particular form of bronchodilator therapy depends on availability and the patient's response in terms of symptom relief and side effects. Combination therapy, rather than an increased dose of a single agent, may lead to improved efficacy and a decreased risk of side effects. Table 26-9 summarizes information about the most commonly used bronchodilators.

Glucocorticoids

Regular treatment with inhaled glucocorticosteroids for COPD is appropriate only for patients with symptomatic disease and a documented spirometric response to glucocorticosteroids, or in patients with an FEV_1 less than 50% predicted and repeated exacerbations requiring treatment with antibiotics or oral glucocorticosteroids.[26] Extended treatment with inhaled glucocorticosteroids may alleviate symptoms but does not alter the long-term decline in FEV_1 typically seen in patients with COPD. The dose–response relationships and long-term safety of inhaled glucocorticosteroids in COPD are not fully known, and long-term treatment with oral glucocorticosteroids is not recommended.[25]

Other Pharmacological Agents

Several other drugs may be useful but are not universally recommended. Antibiotics should not be used in COPD except for treatment of infectious exacerbations and other bacterial infections.[25] Mucolytic agents have

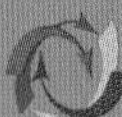

box 26-9 collaborative care guide *for the Patient With Chronic Obstructive Pulmonary Disease*

OUTCOMES	INTERVENTIONS
Oxygenation/Ventilation	
Patient has arterial blood gases within normal limits and pulse oximeter value >90%.	■ Assess respiratory rate, effort, and breath sounds q2–4h. ■ Obtain arterial blood gases per order or signs of respiratory distress. ■ Monitor arterial saturation by pulse oximeter. ■ Provide supplemental oxygen by nasal cannula or face mask using lowest possible FIO_2 and flow rate. ■ Provide humidification with oxygen. ■ Provide intubation and mechanical ventilation as necessary (refer to Collaborative Care Guide for the Patient on Mechanical Ventilation, Chapter 25).
Patient maintains normal rate and depth of respiration.	■ Monitor respiratory rate, pattern, and effort (e.g., use of accessory muscles). ■ Assess respirations during sleep; note sleep apnea or Cheyne-Stokes patterns.
Patient has clear chest x-ray.	■ Obtain chest x-ray qd.
Patient has clear breath sounds.	■ Monitor breath sounds for crackles, wheezes, or rhonchi q2–4h. ■ Administer diuretics per order. ■ Administer bronchodilators and mucolytics as indicated.
There is no evidence of atelectasis or pneumonia.	■ Encourage nonintubated patients to use incentive spirometer, cough, and deep breathe q2–4h and PRN. ■ Assess quantity, color, and consistency of secretions. ■ Turn side to side q2h. ■ Mobilize out of bed to chair.
Circulation/Perfusion	
Blood pressure, heart rate, and hemodynamic parameters are within normal limits.	■ Monitor vital signs q1–2h. ■ Monitor pulmonary artery pressures and right atrial pressure q1h and cardiac output, systemic venous resistance, and peripheral venous resistance q6–12h if pulmonary artery catheter is in place. ■ Assess for signs of right ventricular dysfunction (e.g., increased central venous pressure, neck vein distension, peripheral edema).
Patient is free of dysrhythmias.	■ Maintain patent IV access. ■ Monitor for atrial dysrhythmias due to right atrial dilation and ventricular dysrhythmias due to hypoxemia and hypoxia.
Serum lactate will be within normal limits.	■ Monitor lactate qd until it is within normal limits. ■ Administer red blood cells, positive inotropic agents, colloid infusion as ordered to increase oxygen delivery.
Fluids/Electrolytes Renal function is maintained as evidenced by urine output >30 mL/h, normal laboratory values.	■ Monitor intake and output q1–2h. ■ Monitor blood urea nitrogen, creatinine, electrolytes, Mg, PO_4. ■ Replace potassium, magnesium, and phosphorus per order or protocol. ■ Take daily weights.
Patient is euvolemic.	■ Administer fluid volume and diuretics based on vital signs, physical assessment, secretion viscosity, as ordered.
Mobility/Safety	
There is no evidence of loss of muscle tone or strength.	■ Promote standing at bedside, sitting up in chair, ambulating with assistance as soon as possible. ■ Establish activity program. ■ Monitor response to activity.

(continued)

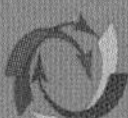

box 26-9 collaborative care guide ***for the Patient With Chronic Obstructive Pulmonary Disease (Continued)***

OUTCOMES	INTERVENTIONS
Patient maintains joint flexibility.	■ Consult with physical therapist. ■ Use passive and active range of motion q4h while awake.
There is no evidence of infection. White blood cells (WBCs) are within normal limits.	■ Monitor systemic inflammatory response syndrome criteria: increased WBC count, increased temperature, tachypnea, tachycardia. ■ Use strict aseptic technique during procedures and monitor others. ■ Maintain invasive catheter tube sterility. ■ Per hospital protocol, change invasive catheters, culture blood, line tips, or fluids.
There is no evidence of DVT.	■ Initiate DVT prophylaxis within 24 hours of admission. ■ Monitor for leg pain, redness, or swelling.
Skin Integrity	
There is no evidence of skin breakdown.	■ Turn side to side q2h. ■ Remove self-protective devices from wrists, and monitor skin per hospital policy. ■ Assess risk of skin breakdown using objective tool (e.g., Braden Scale). Consider pressure relief/reduction mattress.
Nutrition	
Caloric and nutrient intake meet metabolic requirements per calculation (e.g., Basal Energy Expenditure).	■ Provide parenteral, enteral, or oral nutrition within 48 hours. ■ Consult dietitian or nutritional support service. ■ Avoid high-carbohydrate load if patient retains CO_2. ■ Monitor albumin, prealbumin, transferrin, cholesterol, triglycerides, glucose.
Comfort/Pain Control	
Patient is comfortable and evaluates pain as <4 on the pain scale.	■ Assess pain/comfort q4h. ■ Administer analgesics and sedatives cautiously, closely monitoring respiratory rate, depth, and pattern. ■ Differentiate between agitation caused by discomfort or caused by hypoxia before medication administration. ■ Elevate head of bed to improve breathing comfort.
Psychosocial	
Patient demonstrates decreased anxiety.	■ Assess vital signs during treatments, discussions, and so forth. ■ Cautiously administer sedatives. ■ Consult social services, clergy as appropriate. ■ Provide for adequate rest and sleep. ■ Provide support during periods of dyspnea.
Teaching/Discharge Planning	
Patient/significant others understand procedures and tests needed for treatment.	■ Prepare patient/significant others for procedures such as chest physical therapy, bronchoscopy, pulmonary artery catheter insertion, or laboratory studies.
Significant others understand the severity of the illness, ask appropriate questions, anticipate potential complications.	■ Explain the causes and effects of COPD and the potential for complications, such as pneumonia or cardiac dysfunction. ■ Encourage significant others to ask questions related to the ventilator, pathophysiology, monitoring, treatments, and so forth.
In preparation for discharge to home, patient understands activity levels, dietary restrictions, medication regimen, metered inhaler.	■ Make appropriate referrals and consults early during hospitalization. ■ Initiate family education regarding proper use of metered inhaler, signs and symptoms of respiratory failure, and appropriate actions.

table 26-9 ■ Commonly Used Bronchodilator Drugs

Drug*	Metered-Dose Inhaler (μg)†	Nebulizer (mg)†	Oral (mg)†	Duration of Action (h)
β_2 agonists				
Fenoterol	100–200	0.5–2.0	—	4–6
Salbutamol (albuterol‡)	100–200	2.5–5.0	4	4–6
Terbutaline	250–500	5–10	5	4–6
Formoterol	12–24	—	—	12+
Salmeterol	50–100	—	—	12+
Anticholinergics				
Ipratropium bromide	40–80	0.25–0.5	—	6–8
Oxitropium bromide	200	—	—	7–9
Methylxanthines§				
Aminophylline (SR)	—	—	225–450	Variable, up to 24
Theophylline (SR)	—	—	100–400	Variable, up to 24

*Not all products are available in all countries.
† Doses: β-agonists refer to average dose given up to four times daily for short-acting and two times daily for long-acting preparations; anticholinergics are usually given three to four times daily.
‡ Albuterol is a North American generic term.
§ Methylxanthines require dose titration depending on adverse effects and plasma theophylline levels.
From Pauwels RA, et al: Global Strategies for the Diagnosis, Management, and Prevention of Chronic Obstructive Pulmonary Disease: National Heart, Lung, and Blood Institute and World Health Organization Global Initiative for Chronic Obstructive Lung Disease (GOLD). Respir Care 46:798–825, 2001, with permission.

minimal overall benefits, and their widespread use is not recommended based on current research. However, patients with viscous sputum may benefit from mucolytics.[25] α_1-Antitrypsin augmentation therapy may be useful in young patients with severe hereditary α_1-antitrypsin deficiency and confirmed emphysema. However, α_1-antitrypsin augmentation therapy is very expensive, and it may not be available in most countries.[25] *N*-acetylcysteine, an antioxidant, has been shown to reduce the frequency of COPD exacerbations and could play a role in the treatment of patients with recurrent exacerbations. This drug is not currently available for routine use; results of ongoing trials must first be thoroughly evaluated.[25] Immunostimulators have been shown to decrease the severity but not the frequency of exacerbations of COPD. The regular use of immunostimulators cannot be recommended based on limited evidence.[25] Antitussives, when used regularly, are contraindicated in patients whose COPD is stable. The coughing mechanism plays a significant protective role in patients with COPD.[25] Inhaled nitric oxide, a vasodilator, has been evaluated in patients with COPD and hypoxemia caused primarily by ventilation–perfusion mismatching, and gas exchange worsens related to altered hypoxic regulation of ventilation–perfusion balance.[25] Therefore, nitric oxide is contraindicated in patients whose COPD is stable. Finally, almitrine bismesylate, a respiratory stimulant that increases ventilation at any level of carbon dioxide under hypoxemic conditions, has been studied in both stable respiratory failure and acute exacerbations. However, it is not recommended for regular use.[25]

OXYGEN THERAPY

Oxygen therapy is one of the principal nonpharmacological treatments for patients with severe COPD (Box 26-10). Oxygen therapy can be administered as long-term continuous therapy, during exercise, and in the relief of acute dyspnea. The goal of such long-term oxygen therapy is to increase the baseline PaO_2 at rest to at least 60 mm Hg at sea level or produce an oxygen saturation in arterial blood (SaO_2) of at least 90%; this preserves vital organ function by ensuring an adequate delivery of oxygen.[25] Oxygen therapy is initiated for patients with severe COPD (stage III) if:

- PaO_2 is at or below 55 mm Hg or SaO_2 is at or below 88%, with or without hypercapnia
- PaO_2 is between 55 mm Hg and 60 mm Hg or SaO_2 is below 90%, if there is evidence of pulmonary hypertension, congestive heart failure, or polycythemia[25]

The long-term administration of oxygen (more than 15 hours per day) to patients with chronic respiratory failure has been shown to increase survival.[25] However, caution should be exercised in administration of supplemental oxy-

box 26-10 *Oxygen Use*

Many patients with chronic respiratory diseases will receive oxygen on a continual or intermittent basis. When these patients are admitted or visits made to their home, the nurse reviews oxygen safety. The nurse also verifies the patient's knowledge of the oxygen dose and checks his or her ability to read the reserve volume in the tank or oximizor. The patient is taught (if the patient can do this) to check a pulse oximetry reading at rest and with exercise. Nutritional counseling is necessary for patients too short of breath to eat solid foods.

gen in this select group of patients. A rapid increase in PaO_2 causes an increase in $PaCO_2$, which can put patients at risk for respiratory arrest. The properties involved with carbon dioxide retention include an increased carbon dioxide production or an increase in the alveolar dead space ventilation, which promotes rapid, shallow breathing and a decrease in the hypoxic drive to breathe.[31] Therefore, supplemental oxygen is titrated upward very cautiously, using oxygen administered through low-flow nasal cannulas or a Venturi mask. If successful oxygenation (SaO_2 of 90% or greater) is not obtained without a progression of respiratory acidosis, intubation and mechanical ventilation is usually performed.[31]

SURGICAL THERAPY

Lung Volume Reduction Surgery

Lung volume reduction surgery (LVRS) is a surgical procedure in which parts of the lung are resected to reduce hyperinflation, thereby improving the mechanical efficiency of the respiratory muscles, increasing the elastic recoil pressure of the lung, and ultimately improving expiratory flow rate.[25] Currently, LVRS, or pneumectomy, is designed to relieve dyspnea and improve lung function (FEV_1, FVC, ABGs, and exercise capacity) in severely disabled patients with stage III emphysema who have exhausted medical alternatives.[32–34] For patients awaiting eventual lung transplantation, LVRS provides a means to obtain immediate symptomatic improvement (significant increase in oxygenation and decreased arterial carbon dioxide).[34]

Specifically, LVRS resects severely emphysematous lung tissue, resulting in improved elastic recoil in the remaining pulmonary parenchyma, which decreases hyperinflation and improves diaphragmatic function.[32] The goal of stapler resection is to reduce the overall volume of each lung by 25% to 30%.[34] Some studies have documented improvements in FEV_1 and FVC in the range of 50% to 100% and a decrease in total lung capacity from 15% to 20% after LVRS.[33,35] Usually, a subsequent 25% to 50% improvement of airflow and exercise capacity occurs.[32] The etiology of this physiological improvement is unclear, but it may be related to increases in elastic recoil properties of the remaining lung.[33] Recent studies have indicated the pulmonary effects last more than 1 year after LVRS.[35–37]

Attempts to standardize LVRS have met with much difficulty because of the tremendous inherent subjectivity in selection of patients and the selection of lung areas to be resected.[38] Little consensus exists regarding exact guidelines for selection of ideal and suboptimal candidates for surgery. Reports have shown that patients with bilateral upper lobe–dominant disease do somewhat better after LVRS than other patients.[38] Patients who meet the following criteria may be considered for LVRS:

- Age younger than 75 years
- FEV_1 at least 25% predicted
- $PaCO_2$ less than 45 mm Hg
- Predominant upper lobe emphysema on computed tomography (CT) scan
- Residual volume greater than 200%
- Demonstration of severe dyspnea despite optimal medical therapy
- Excellent cardiac performance, with left ventricular ejection fraction greater than 45%
- No other comorbidities
- Demonstrable preoperative motivation to have the surgery with agreement to participate in 4 to 6 weeks of pulmonary rehabilitation[25,32,33]

Contraindications to LVRS include active smoking, marked obesity or cachexia, and inability to undertake pulmonary rehabilitation successfully.[32]

Depending on the volume of tissue to be removed, LVRS is performed through a median sternotomy or thoracotomy, or using video-assisted thoracoscopic surgery. The target for LVRS, as predetermined by CT and ventilation–perfusion scanning, is the hyperinflated portion of the diseased lung with well-demarcated areas of trapped air or dead space.[36] Usually, tissue from the upper lobe or the least functional lung is removed first.[33,34]

Early, uncontrolled studies show hospital mortality rates of 5% to 18% for LVRS; average hospital stays of 9 to 18 days, with frequent significant air leaks; and costs of $33,000 to $70,000 per case.[32] Because of the large number of potential candidates, the high costs associated with the procedure, and unanswered questions about the benefits of LVRS, the use of LVRS in the United States has been restricted to a multicenter, randomized, controlled trial—the National Emphysema Treatment Trial (NETT). NETT is designed to compare LVRS with the best available medical therapy,[32] and the results indicate the following:

- Physiological benefits from LVRS may begin to dissipate as early as 1 year after surgery.
- Accelerated declines of FEV_1 averaging 100 mL per year may occur and are particularly marked in those patients with the greatest postoperative gains in airflow.
- Improvements in dyspnea and exercise tolerance may be sustained for as long as 3 years, but may then begin to decline.[32]

Morbidity in LVRS is related to persistent postoperative air leaks, difficulty with postoperative weaning from the ventilator, and postoperative nosocomial pulmonary infections.[33] In addition, a recent study confirmed that older patients and those undergoing cardiac surgery in combination with LVRS are at increased risk for postoperative respiratory failure.[39] Until the results of this and similar controlled studies are known and the risk–benefit ratio is satisfactorily resolved, LVRS will remain an experimental palliative surgical procedure.[25,32]

Other Surgical Procedures

Patients with severe COPD (stage III) may also consider bullectomy and lung transplantation.[25] Bullectomy is a surgical procedure for bullous emphysema, which is effective in alleviating dyspnea and improving overall lung function.[25] Patients with very advanced COPD are candidates for lung transplantation. Lung transplantation has been shown to improve quality of life and functional capacity.[25]

Prevention

Influenza vaccines reduce serious illness and death by about 50% in patients with COPD.[25] Vaccines containing killed or live, inactivated viruses are recommended, because they are more efficacious in elderly patients with COPD. Vaccines are administered either once (autumn) or twice (autumn and winter) each year. There is currently no evidence for recommending the general use of pneumococcal vaccine for COPD.[25] However, some experts do recommend pneumococcal vaccine administration once each year for patients with COPD and chronic bronchitis and every other year for asplenic patients or patients at risk for decreased antibody levels (e.g., in transplantation or in chronic renal failure).[3,5,40]

Chronic Bronchitis

Chronic bronchitis is defined as the presence of a productive cough of more than 250 mL of sputum per day for at least 3 months per year over 2 consecutive years, in the absence of other medical causes.[40] Chronic bronchitis without airflow obstruction is referred to as *simple bronchitis*, whereas chronic bronchitis with airflow obstruction is referred to as *chronic obstructive bronchitis*.[26]

PATHOPHYSIOLOGY

Airway obstruction is caused by inflammation of the major and small airways in chronic bronchitis (Fig. 26-6). Subsequently, edema and hyperplasia of submucosal glands and excess mucus excretion into the bronchial tree occur, resulting in a chronic productive cough.[26] Cigarette smoking is the major causal factor in the development of chronic bronchitis.[40] Other causes of chronic airway irritation include air pollutants and occupational exposure to nitrogen, sulfur oxides, or endotoxin.[40] Nonspecific pathological changes in the lung, including infiltration of airway mucosa and submucosa with neutrophils and mononuclear cells, smooth muscle hypertrophy, and enlargement of the submucosal secretory glands, may also contribute to the development of chronic bronchitis.[40]

Once the airway lumen is occluded by secretions and narrowed by a thickened wall, patients develop airflow obstruction and COPD. Acute bacterial or viral infection in patients with existing chronic bronchitis can increase airway and parenchymal damage, impair mucociliary clearance, obstruct bronchioles, and contribute to chronic epithelial damage and bacterial colonization that further exacerbate symptoms and airway obstruction.[40] Common bacteria isolated from the secretions of patients with chronic bronchitis include *H. influenzae*, *Haemophilus parainfluenzae*, *S. pneumoniae*, *Moraxella catarrhalis*, *Klebsiella pneumoniae*, and *Chlamydia trachomatis*.[40] Even in nonsmoking patients, acute viral infection may lead to the chronic airway inflammation and chronic sputum production characteristic of chronic bronchitis.[40] In contrast to emphysema, chronic bronchitis may have a reversible component if the source of chronic infection or irritation is treated. These patients normally do not have hyperinflation or abnormal diffusion test results.

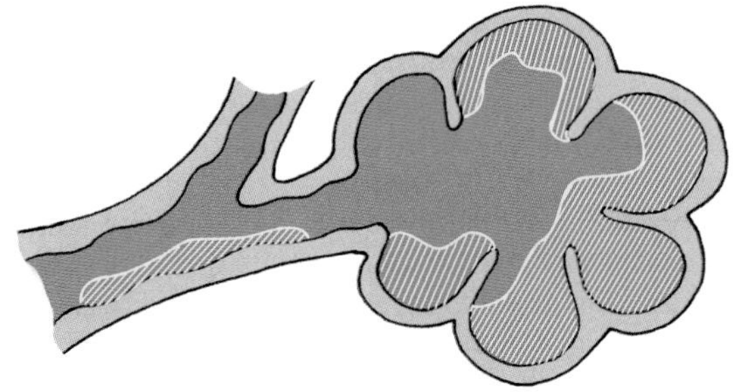

figure 26-6 Bronchitis inflammation and thickening produce narrowing of airways. Lined areas indicate secretions.

ASSESSMENT

Excessive bronchial secretions and subsequent airway obstruction and vasoconstriction lead to ventilation–perfusion mismatching. Patients do not compensate by increasing their ventilation and, therefore, develop hypoxemia, cyanosis, and eventually cor pulmonale with peripheral edema.[26] Hence, these patients are termed "blue bloaters."[26] Common physical signs and symptoms may include:

- Copious sputum expectoration arising from sleep
- Sputum that is usually mucoid, often with brownish discoloration
- Increased sputum volume or changes in color from whitish to yellow or green (signs of a endobronchial infection)
- Hemoptysis occurring during acute exacerbations
- Decreased breath sounds, wheezes or rhonchi
- Resting respiratory rate greater than 16 breaths per minute
- Prolonged forced expiratory time (greater than the normal 4 seconds)[40]

Table 26-10 lists common patterns of disease in advanced COPD in terms of history, physical examination, chest radiograph, and laboratory and diagnostic tests. These patterns may become increasingly apparent as the disease progresses.[27] Manifestations of severe chronic bronchitis exacerbations are listed in Box 26-11.

MANAGEMENT

Patients with chronic bronchitis without airflow obstruction require no specific pharmacological treatment.[40] An essential prophylactic measure involves rigorous bronchial hygiene to promote the clearance of secretions, which provide an ideal medium for bacterial growth in peripheral airways. It is important to prevent the development of an acute inflammatory process to avoid exacerbations. Other preventive measures include smoking cessation, immunization against influenza virus and *S. pneumoniae*, and prompt antibiotic treatment for acute exacerbations caused by bacterial tracheobronchitis.[40]

Chronic bronchitis with airflow obstruction does require pharmacological treatment. The major goals of drug therapy in chronic bronchitis with COPD are to reverse or slow the progression of airway obstruction and mucosal edema, decrease secretion volume, alleviate bronchial smooth muscle spasm, and decrease airway inflammation.[40] Primary agents include inhaled bronchodilators (beta$_2$-adrenergic agents, anticholinergic agents, corticosteroids) and theophylline.[40] Clinicians must be aware of the frequent adverse effects of beta agonists and theophylline, such as tachycardia, atrial dysrhythmias, and restlessness.[40] In addition to drug therapy, the previously described surgical treatment of COPD applies to patients with chronic bronchitis.

table 26-10 Patterns of Disease in Advanced Chronic Obstructive Pulmonary Disease

	Type A: "Pink Puffer" (Emphysema Predominant)	Type B: "Blue Bloater" (Bronchitis Predominant)
History and physical examination	Major complaint is dyspnea, often severe, usually presenting after age 50 y. Cough is rare, with scant clear, mucoid sputum. Patients are thin, with recent weight loss common. They appear uncomfortable, with evident use of accessory muscles of respiration. Chest is very quiet without adventitious sounds. No peripheral edema.	Major complaint is chronic cough, productive of mucopurulent sputum, with frequent exacerbations due to chest infections. Often presents in late 30s and 40s. Dyspnea usually mild, though patients may note limitations to exercise. Patients frequently overweight and cyanotic but seem comfortable at rest. Peripheral edema is common. Chest is noisy, with rhonchi invariably present; wheezes are common.
Laboratory and imaging studies	Hemoglobin usually normal (12–15 g/dL). Pa_{O_2} normal to slightly reduced (65–75 mm Hg) but Sa_{O_2} normal at rest. Pa_{CO_2} normal to slightly reduced (35–40 mm Hg). Chest radiograph shows hyperinflation with flattened diaphragms. Vascular markings are diminished, particularly at the apices.	Hemoglobin usually elevated (15–18 g/dL). Pa_{O_2} reduced (45–60 mm Hg) and Pa_{CO_2} slightly to markedly elevated (50–60 mm Hg). Chest radiograph shows increased interstitial markings ("dirty lungs"), especially at bases. Diaphragms are not flattened.
Pulmonary function tests	Airflow obstruction ubiquitous. Total lung capacity increased, sometimes markedly so. DLCO reduced. Static lung compliance increased.	Airflow obstruction ubiquitous. Total lung capacity generally normal but may be slightly increased. DLCO normal. Static lung compliance normal.
Special evaluations		
Ventilation–perfusion ($\dot{V}/\dot{Q}$) matching	Increased ventilation to high $\dot{V}/\dot{Q}$ areas (i.e., high dead space ventilation).	Increased perfusion to low $\dot{V}/\dot{Q}$ areas.
Hemodynamics	Cardiac output normal to slightly low. Pulmonary artery pressures mildly elevated and increase with exercise.	Cardiac output normal. Pulmonary artery pressures elevated, sometimes markedly so, and worsen with exercise.
Nocturnal ventilation	Mild to moderate degree of oxyhemoglobin desaturation not usually associated with obstructive sleep apnea.	Severe oxyhemoglobin desaturation, frequently associated with obstructive sleep apnea.
Exercise ventilation	Increased minute ventilation for level of oxygen consumption. Pa_{O_2} tends to fall; Pa_{CO_2} slightly.	Decreased minute ventilation for level of oxygen consumption. Pa_{O_2} may rise; Pa_{CO_2} may rise significantly.

DLCO, diffusing capacity of lung for carbon monoxide.
From Tierney L, et al: Chronic obstructive pulmonary disease (COPD). In Tierney L, et al (eds): Current Medical Diagnosis & Treatment (40th Ed), pp 283–288. New York, McGraw-Hill, 2001, with permission.

Emphysema

The ATS[41] defines emphysema as a loss of lung elasticity and abnormal, permanent enlargement of the air spaces distal to the terminal bronchioles with destruction of the alveolar walls and capillary beds without obvious fibrosis (Fig. 26-7). Most patients with COPD have a combination of chronic bronchitis (mucus hypersecretion) and emphysema rather than "pure" bronchitis or emphysema[27] (see Table 26-10).

There are three types of emphysema: centrilobular emphysema, panacinar emphysema, and paraseptal emphysema (Fig. 26-8). Centrilobular emphysema is most common in smokers and often localizes in the upper lung zones. Panacinar emphysema is most frequently found in patients with α_1-protease inhibitor deficiency and is often localized in the lower lobes. Paraseptal emphysema is also most common in smokers and is localized peripherally, with possible formation of large bullae.[33]

PATHOPHYSIOLOGY

The enlargement of the air spaces in emphysema results in hyperinflation of the lungs and increased total lung capacity.[27] Emphysema is believed to result from the breakdown of elastin by enzymes, called *proteases*, which digest proteins. These proteases, especially elastase, are released from neutrophils, alveolar macrophages, and other inflammatory cells.[26] Two recognized conditions that cause emphysema are smoking and inherited α_1-antitrypsin deficiency. Smoking contributes to increased inflammatory cells in the alveoli, enhanced release of elastase from neutrophils, increased elastase activity in macrophages, and activation of mast cells that release mast cell elastases.[26] α_1-Antitrypsin usually protects the lung from the destructive inflammatory cells; however, the elastic tissue destructive process continues unabated in patients with an inherited α_1-antitrypsin deficiency.[26]

Almost all individuals who develop emphysema before 40 years of age have an α_1-antitrypsin deficiency. Evidence has shown that cigarette smoking decreases levels of α_1-antitrypsin and increases the number of macrophages in the alveolar walls. This vicious cycle promotes increased numbers of neutrophils. A hereditary deficiency in α_1-antitrypsin is responsible for about 1% of all cases of COPD.[26] Smoking and repeated respiratory tract infections

box 26-11 ***Manifestations of Severe Exacerbations of Chronic Bronchitis***

Constitutional Signs

Temperature frequently subnormal

White blood cell count varies—may be slightly ↑, normal, or ↓

Central Nervous System Disturbances

Headache

Confusion

Hallucinations

Depression

Drowsiness

Somnolence

Coma

Papilledema

Cardiovascular Signs

Diaphoresis

Tachycardia

Blood pressure varies: normal, ↑, or ↓

Vasoconstriction initially followed by vasodilation

Neuromuscular Signs

Fine tremors

Asterixis

Flaccidity

Convulsions

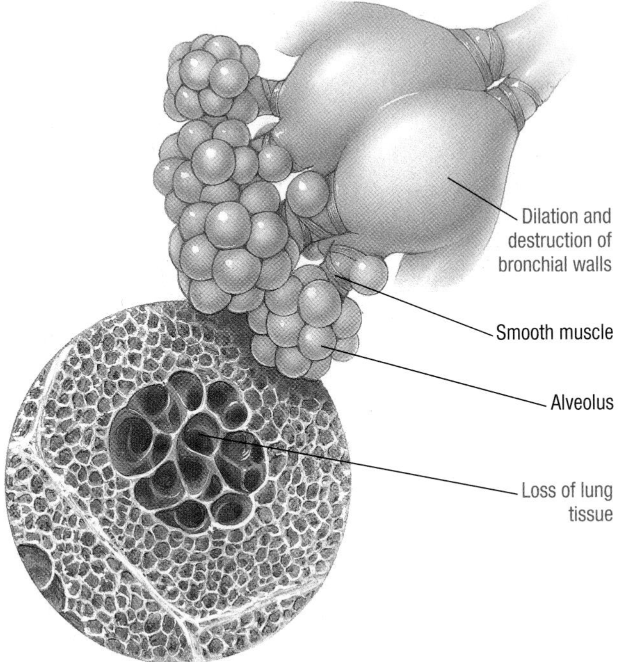

figure 26-7 Lung changes in emphysema. Air spaces are enlarged in the emphysematous lung. (From Anatomical Chart Company: Atlas of Pathophysiology, p 89. Springhouse, PA: Springhouse, 2002.)

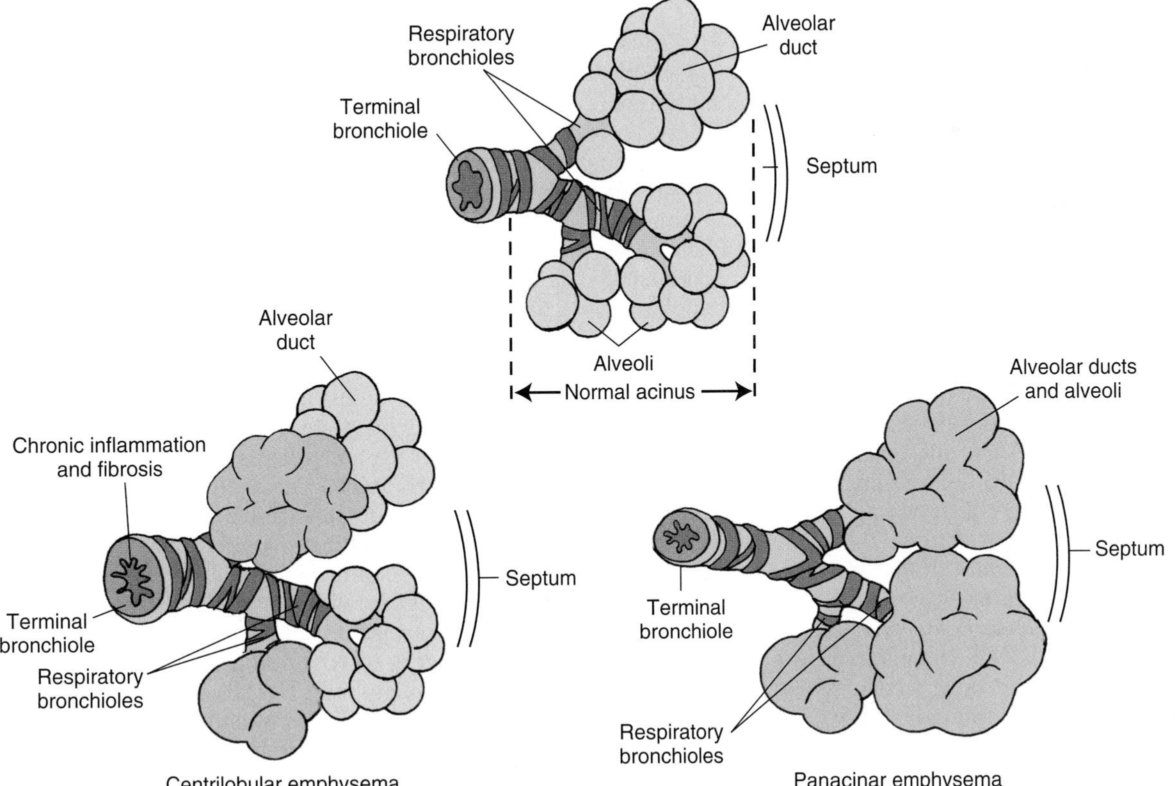

figure 26-8 Types of emphysema. The acinus, the gas-exchanging structure of the lung distal to the terminal bronchiole, consists of the terminal bronchiole, respiratory bronchioles, alveolar ducts, alveolar sacs, and alveoli. In centrilobular (proximal acinar) emphysema, the respiratory bronchioles are mainly involved. In paraseptal (distal acinar) emphysema, the alveolar ducts are mainly affected. In panacinar (panlobular) emphysema, the acinus is uniformly damaged. (From Porth CM: Pathophysiology: Concepts of Altered States [5th Ed], p 541. Philadelphia, Lippincott-Raven, 1998. Courtesy of Dmitri Kavetnikov, artist.)

further decrease α_1-antitrypsin levels, adding to the risk of emphysema in individuals with low α_1-antitrypsin levels.[26]

A common phenomenon in emphysema is spontaneous pneumothorax related to rupture of thinned parenchyma.[33] Patients may experience acute severe dyspnea and respiratory failure depending on the amount of pulmonary reserve (see the discussion of barotrauma in section on Pneumothorax).

ASSESSMENT

Patients with pulmonary emphysema are referred to as "pink puffers" because their oxygen levels are usually satisfactory and their skin remains pink.[26] There is a proportionate loss of ventilation and perfusion area in the lung. In severe COPD, air is trapped in the lungs during forced expiration, leading to abnormally high residual volume.[26] These patients develop a "puffing style" of breathing. Table 26-10 lists common findings of emphysema in terms of history, physical examination, chest radiography, and laboratory and diagnostic tests. Common physical examination findings include increased basal respiratory rate; barrel-shaped chest; decreased breath sounds; soft, dry rales in lung bases; right-sided S_3 gallop auscultated substernally; supraclavicular wasting and nasal flaring; and evidence of pulmonary hypertension, including an increased second heart sound, jugular venous distension, and right ventricular heave.[33] Cyanosis may be present in advanced cases of emphysema.

MANAGEMENT

The medical and surgical therapies described for COPD also pertain to patients with emphysema (see COPD, Management). Preventive measures include an annual influenza vaccine and a pneumococcal vaccine every 5 to 10 years.[33] Medical therapy involves smoking cessation, pulmonary rehabilitation, and oxygen therapy in all patients who are hypoxemic (Pa_{O_2} less than 55 mm Hg or oxygen saturation Sa_{O_2} less than 88%).[33] Pharmacological therapy includes bronchodilators (beta$_2$ agonists, anticholinergics, and theophylline), possibly mucolytics, and α_1-protease inhibitor replacement in young patients with homozygous disease. In addition, adequate nutrition is important. Patients with advanced emphysema (FEV_1 less than 750 mL) may experience significant weight loss related to a variety of reasons, including increased energy expended during breathing secondary to the use of accessory muscles; performing activities of daily living; and reduced caloric intake.[33] Patients who are overweight and hypercapnic should strive to lose weight to diminish the respiratory workload.[33]

Two surgical treatments available for patients with emphysema are LVRS and lung transplantation. Currently, LVRS is the only recognized therapy that can increase respiratory function (FEV_1, FVC, ABGs, and exercise capacity) in moderate to severe emphysema.[33] Some studies have documented an improvement in FEV_1 and FVC in the range of 50% to 100% after LVRS.[33] For end-stage emphysema, the only definitive surgical treatment is single-lung transplantation. Because of the short supply of donor lungs, lung transplantation is usually reserved for younger patients (younger than 60 years of age) with α_1-protease inhibitor deficiency.[33] Studies have indicated improvements in exercise performance and ABGs after lung transplantation.

ACUTE ASTHMA

Asthma is defined as a chronic inflammatory disease of the airways[42] characterized by airway hyperresponsiveness to a variety of stimuli. It is manifested as variable airway obstruction that resolves either spontaneously or after bronchodilator administration.[43] Based on symptoms and lung function, the National Asthma Education and Prevention Program (NAEPP) has classified asthma as mild intermittent, mild persistent, moderate persistent, or severe persistent (Table 26-11).

According to the CDC, asthma is a worldwide epidemic. In the United States in 1998, as many as 17.3 million people had asthma, which represents a threefold increase since 1980.[44] In the United States during the past decade, prevalence rates have increased by 29%, hospital admissions have increased by 300%, and the asthma death rate has increased by 31%.[44] More than 5,000 people die of asthma annually in the United States, and most cases are believed to be preventable.[44]

Pathophysiology

Inflammation may be present throughout the bronchial tree, from large airways to the alveoli. This inflammation is characterized by mast cell activation, inflammatory cell infiltration, edema, denudation and disruption of the bronchial epithelium, collagen deposition beneath the basement membrane, goblet cell hyperplasia (which contributes to mucus hypersecretion), and smooth muscle thickening (Fig. 26-9). This inflammatory process contributes to airway hyperresponsiveness, airflow limitation, pathological damage, and associated respiratory symptoms (i.e., wheezing, shortness of breath, and chest tightness).[45]

Factors contributing to the airflow limitation in asthma include acute bronchoconstriction, airway mucosal edema, chronic formation of mucus plugs, and airway remodeling.[46]

The T lymphocytes (helper T [Th] cells) are believed to play a crucial role in the inflammation process.[47] Th1 cells serve a protective role against airway inflammation, and Th2 cells promote development of chronic airway inflammation. Recent studies suggest that possible early childhood viral and bacterial infections may contribute to Th2 cell stimulation and result in asthma pathogenesis.[47]

The etiology and pathogenesis of asthma are not fully understood.[48] Asthma is familial but does not occur in a pattern consistent with a single major gene.[49] Asthma is frequently associated with clinical manifestations of atopy (familial allergy to common aeroallergens) and elevated serum immunoglobulin E (IgE) concentration, but some evidence suggests that allergy and asthma may be inherited separately.[48] Passive exposure to environmental tobacco smoke appears to be a risk factor for the development of childhood asthma.[48] The most common precipitant of an acute asthmatic exacerbation is an upper respiratory tract viral infection.[43] Other potential infectious causal factors include infection with *C. pneumoniae*, tracheobronchitis related to herpes simplex, and exposure to aspirin or other nonsteroidal anti-inflammatory cyclooxygenase-1

table 26-11 Classification of Asthma Severity

	Symptoms	Nighttime Symptoms	Lung Function
Mild intermittent	Symptoms ≤2 times a week Asymptomatic and normal PEF between exacerbations Exacerbations brief (few hours to few days); intensity may vary	≤2 times a month	FEV_1 or PEF ≥80% predicted PEF variability ≤20%.
Mild persistent	Symptoms >2 times a week but <1 time a day Exacerbations may affect activity	>2 times a month	FEV_1 or PEF >80% predicted PEF variability 20%–30%
Moderate persistent	Daily symptoms Daily use of inhaled short-acting beta$_2$-agonist Exacerbations affect activity Exacerbations ≥2 times a week; may last days	>1 time a week	FEV_1 or PEF >60% to <80% predicted PEF variability >30%
Severe persistent	Continual symptoms Limited physical activity Frequent exacerbations	Frequent	FEV_1 or PEF ≤60% predicted PEF variability >30%

FEV_1, forced expiratory volume in 1 second; PEF, peak expiratory flow.
Adapted from National Asthma Education and Prevention Program, Expert Panel Report 2: Guidelines for the Diagnosis and Management of Asthma. National Institutes of Health publication no. 97-4051. Bethesda, MD, National Institutes of Health, 1997.

inhibitors, which can lead to life-threatening asthmatic reactions in selected patients.[43] Common triggers of asthma exacerbations are given in Box 26-12.[50,51]

Assessment

HISTORY AND PHYSICAL FINDINGS

The medical history should address the following areas:

- Symptoms and symptom patterns
- Precipitating and aggravating factors
- Development of disease
- Current treatment
- Effect of symptoms on activities of daily living
- Impact of asthma on the patient and family
- Perceptions of the disease by the patient and family (parent, if appropriate)[46]

The physical examination should focus on the following areas:

- Vital signs
- Height/weight and a comparison of normal values for age
- Inspection of skin for evidence of atopic dermatitis or eczema
- Mouth breathing
- Dark discoloration beneath the lower eyelids ("allergic shiners")
- Edematous or pale nasal mucosa
- Clear nasal discharge
- Hypertrophy of tonsils and adenoids
- Presence of tearing and periorbital edema
- Lung auscultation for wheezing
- Hyperexpansion of the thorax
- Use of accessory muscles
- Presence of tachypnea[52]

Signs and symptoms vary with the degree of bronchospasm. Patients may complain of shortness of breath associated with wheezing, especially during the late night and early morning hours, along with disruption of sleep.[48] Additional findings, including tachycardia, retractions, restlessness, anxiety, inspiratory/expiratory wheezing, hypoxemia, hypercapnia, cough, sputum production, expiratory prolongation, cyanosis, and an elevated pulsus paradoxus (systolic blood pressure in expiration exceeding that in inspiration by more than 10 mm Hg), may be observed in patients who have severe attacks.[48] Table 26-12 presents the signs and symptoms of airway dysfunction as they relate to asthma severity.

DIAGNOSTIC STUDIES

Objective measures in the diagnosis and measurement of asthma severity consist of spirometry and pulmonary function testing.[52] Allergy testing may be performed to ascertain precipitating allergens.[46] Spirometry measurements of the FVC, FEV_1, and FEV_1:FVC ratio are performed before and after the patient inhales a short-acting bronchodilator, which determines whether airflow obstruction is present and whether it is reversible.[47] An increase of at least 12% and 200 mL in FEV_1 after inhaling a short-acting bronchodilator indicates significant reversibility and

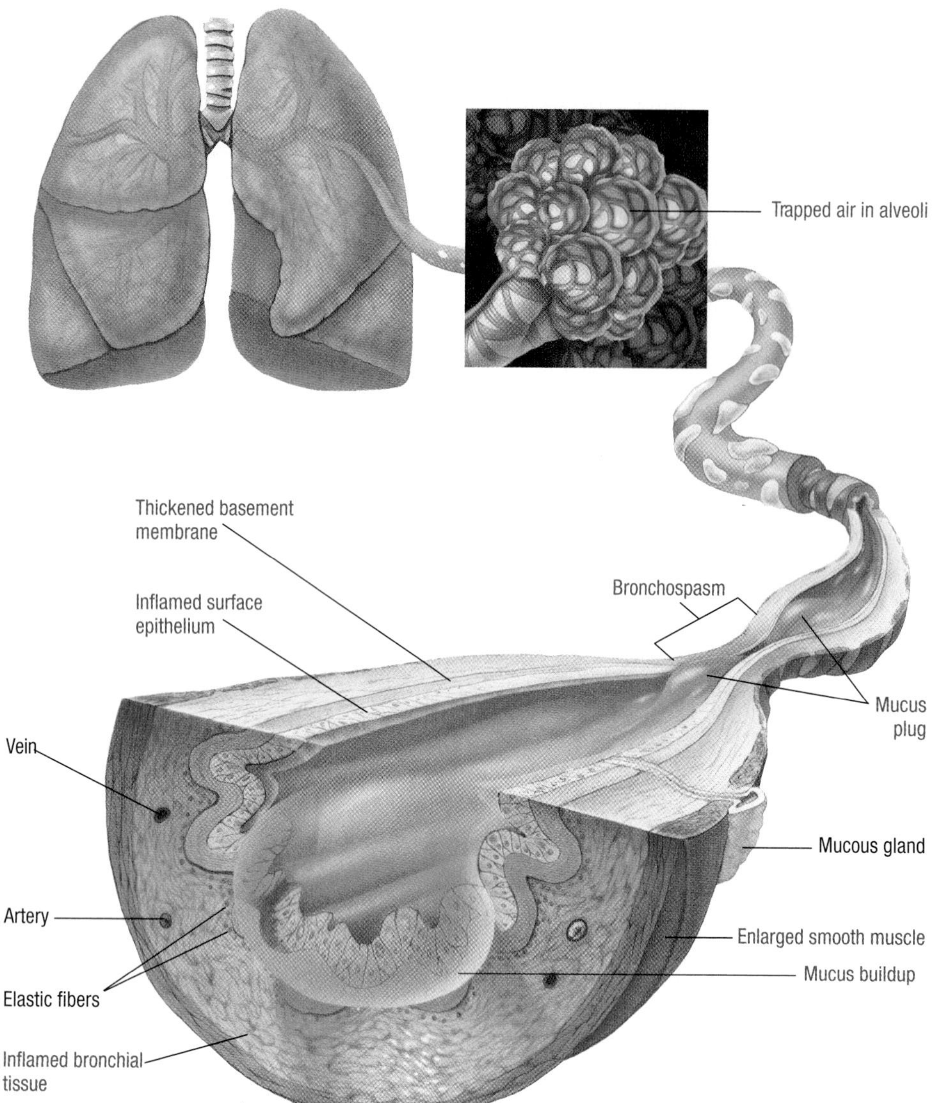

figure 26-9 Asthmatic bronchus. (From Anatomical Chart Company: Atlas of Pathophysiology, p 83. Springhouse, PA: Springhouse, 2002.)

box 26-12 ***Common Triggers of Asthma***

- Viral respiratory infections
- Environmental allergens (domestic dust mite, tobacco smoke, animals with fur, cockroach, outdoor and indoor pollens and mold, perfume, wood-burning stoves)
- Exercise, temperature, humidity
- Occupational and recreational allergens or irritants
- Medications (aspirin, nonsteroidal anti-inflammatory drugs, and beta blockers)
- Food (sulfites)
- Emotions

From National Heart, Lung, and Blood Institute, National Institutes of Health: Global Initiative for Asthma, p 249. Bethesda, MD, National Heart, Lung, and Blood Institute, 2003. Also available at: www.ICSI.org.

confirms the presence of asthma.[51] The FVC_1:FEV ratio is less than 75% predicted. Airway resistance is increased, so FEV is reduced out of proportion to FVC reduction.[53] Portable peak flow meters are used to monitor ongoing lung function. Patients are instructed how to measure peak expiratory flow, an indicator of the degree of airflow obstruction in the large airways, by using the peak flow meter on a regular basis.[47]

Management

The level of treatment is based on the child's or adult's level of asthma severity, which changes with time, age, and compliance with treatment.[52] Frequent reassessments of the level of severity are necessary to provide adequate therapy. The overall goals of therapy are to prevent chronic and troublesome symptoms; prevent exacerbations of symptoms; maintain normal activity levels; maintain normal pulmonary function; optimize pharmacotherapy and minimize side effects; and satisfy the patient's and the family's

table 26-12 Classification of Severity of Asthma Exacerbations

	Mild	Moderate	Severe	Impending Respiratory Failure
Symptoms				
Breathlessness	With activity	With talking	At rest	At rest
Speech	Sentences	Phrases	Words	Mute
Signs				
Body position	Able to recline	Prefers sitting	Unable to recline	Unable to recline
Respiratory rate	Increased	Increased	Often >30/min	>30/min
Use of accessory respiratory muscles	Usually not	Commonly	Usually	Paradoxical thoracoabdominal movement
Breath sounds	Moderate wheezing at mid- to end-expiration	Loud wheezes throughout expiration	Loud inspiratory and expiratory wheezes	Little air movement without wheezes
Heart rate (beats/min)	<100	100–120	>120	Relative bradycardia
Pulsus paradoxus (mm Hg)	<10	10–25	Often >25	Often absent
Mental status	May be agitated	Usually agitated	Usually agitated	Confused or drowsy
Functional Assessment				
PEF (% predicted or personal best)	>80	50–80	<50 or response to therapy lasts <2 hours	<50
Sao_2 (%, room air)	>95	91–95	<91	<91
Pao_2 (mm Hg, room air)	Normal	>60	<60	<60
$Paco_2$ (mm Hg)	<42	<42	≥42	≥42

Adapted from National Asthma Education and Prevention Program, Expert Panel Report 2: Guidelines for the Diagnosis and Management of Asthma. National Institutes of Health publication no. 97-4051. Bethesda, MD, National Institutes of Health, 1997.

expectations and goals for asthma care.[46] A stepwise pharmacological approach is recommended in treating patients with asthma. The main goal is to gain control quickly and to "step down" to the lowest medication level required to maintain asthma control.[46] A list of quick-relief asthma medications is presented in Table 26-13. A flow chart outlining the stepwise approach is shown in Figure 26-10.

Asthma education and self-management training are critical to helping the asthmatic patient control airway inflammation. The 1997 NAEPP guidelines describe the critical components of asthmatic patient education. An important aspect of asthmatic patient education programs is training in the necessary management skills. These skills include proper medication administration, understanding the need for maintenance medications, knowing the early warning signs of an asthma attack, making decisions on the basis of self-monitoring of symptoms and peak flow results, and maintaining control of environmental asthma triggers (i.e., dust mites, fur-bearing animals).[54] Recent studies have confirmed that appropriate therapy, coupled with structured asthma education, significantly improve short-term compliance with therapy and decreases asthma morbidity.[47] Long-term asthma management requires regular follow-up care with a clinician experienced in long-term asthma to maintain optimal asthma control and avoid preventable complications.[48]

Status Asthmaticus

Status asthmaticus is a medical emergency. It is an acute refractory asthma attack that has not responded to rigorous therapy with beta$_2$-adrenergic compounds or intravenous theophylline. Patients present with a dramatic picture of acute anxiety, markedly labored breathing, tachycardia, and diaphoresis. Deterioration of pulmonary function results in alveolar hypoventilation with subsequent hypoxemia, hypercapnia, and acidemia. A rising $Paco_2$ in a patient with an acute asthmatic attack is often the first objective indication of status asthmaticus.

The treatment of status asthmaticus involves the institution of multiple therapeutic modalities. All patients with status asthmaticus demonstrate hypoxemia and require oxygen therapy. Patients are also usually dehydrated and require fluid resuscitation. Pharmacological agents include methylxanthines, sympathomimetic amines, and corticosteroids. If pulmonary function cannot be improved and respiratory failure ensues, patients may require intubation and assisted ventilation (see Chapter 25). A spontaneous pneumothorax may occur during severe acute asthmatic attacks, as well as during positive-pressure mechanical ventilation[48] (see section on Pneumothorax, Management).

table 26-13 Quick-Relief Medications for Asthma*

Drug	Important Formulations	Usual Adult Dosage	Cost†	Comments
Short-Acting Inhaled Beta₂-Agonists				
Albuterol (Proventil, Ventolin)	MDI: 90 μg/puff, 200 puffs/canister	Two puffs 5 min before exercise Two puffs q4–6h as needed	$21.70/17 g	Preferred formulation in most cases. Chlorofluorocarbon propellant.
	Nebulizer solutions: 5 mg/mL (0.5%)	1.25–5 mg (0.25–1 mL) in 2–3 mL of normal saline q4–8h as needed	$14.99/20 mL	Administer with powered nebulizer. More frequent dosing is acceptable for acute or severe exacerbations. May mix with cromolyn or ipratropium nebulizer solutions.
	Unit dose: 0.083%, 3 mL	One dose q4–8h as needed	$1.24/unit	
	Dry powder (Ventolin Rotocaps): 200 μg/capsule	One or two capsules q4–6h as needed	$32.15/100 200-μg capsules	Rotohaler required for inhalation.
	Tablets: 2 mg, 4 mg	2–4 mg orally q6–8h	$31.14/100 2-mg tablets	Extended-release 4-mg tablet (Proventil Repetab) available for use q12h.
Albuterol HFA (Proventil HFA)	MDI: 90 μg/puff, 200 puffs/canister	Two puffs 5 min before exercise Two puffs q4–6h as needed	$29.41/6.7 g	Nonchlorofluorocarbon propellant.
Bitolterol (Tornalate)	MDI: 370 μg/puff, 300 puffs/canister	Two or three puffs q6–8h as needed	$43.68/15 mL	Chlorofluorocarbon propellant.
	Nebulizer solution, 2 mg/mL (0.2%)	0.5–2 mg (0.25–1 mL) in 2–3 mL of normal saline q4–8h as needed	$15.75/30 mL	Administer with powered nebulizer. May not mix with other nebulizer solutions.
Pirbuterol				
(Maxair)	MDI: 200 μg/puff, 300 puffs/canister	Two puffs q4–6h as needed	$42.96/25 g	Chlorofluorocarbon propellant.
(Maxaire Autoinhaler)	MDI: 200 μg/puff, 400 puffs/canister	Two puffs q4–6h as needed	$47.76/14 g	Breath-activated MDI system. Chlorofluorocarbon propellant.
Terbutaline				
(Brethaire)	MDI: 200 μg/puff, 300 puffs/canister	Two puffs q4–6h as needed	$26.27/7.5 g	Chlorofluorocarbon propellant.
(Brethine, Bricanyl)	Tablets: 2.5 mg, 5 mg	2.5–5 mg orally three times a day	$46.25/100 5-mg tablets	Tremor, nervousness, palpitations common; therefore not recommended.
	Injection solution, 1 mg/mL	0.25 mg (0.25 mL) subcutaneously; may be repeated once in 30 min	$1.87/1 mg per mL	Onset of action 30 min. Not limited to beta₂-agonist effects.
Anticholinergics				
Ipratropium bromide	MDI: 18 μg/puff, 200 puffs/canister	Two to four puffs q6h	$38.87/14 g	Chlorofluorocarbon propellant.
	Unit dose nebulizer solution, 0.2 mg/mL (0.02%), 2.5 mL (0.5 mg)	0.25–0.5 mg (1–2 mL) q6h	$2.54/unit	

(continued)

table 26-13 Quick-Relief Medications for Asthma* (Continued)

Drug	Important Formulations	Usual Adult Dosage	Cost†	Comments
Systemic Corticosteroids				
Methylprednisolone (many)	Tablets: 4 mg	40–60 mg/day as single dose or in two divided doses for 3–10 days	$11.00/4-mg Dose-Pack	
Methylprednisolone sodium succinate (many)	Intravenous injection solution vials: 40, 125, 500 mg	0.5–1 mg/kg q6h	$5.64/125-mg vial	
Prednisolone (many)	Tablets: 5 mg Syrup: 15 mg/5 mL	40–60 mg/day as single dose or in two divided doses for 3–10 days	$0.05/5-mg tablet $67.39/240-mL syrup	
Prednisone (many)	Tablets: 1, 2.5, 5, 10, 20, 50 mg	40–60 mg/day as single dose or in two divided doses for 3–10 days	$0.04/5 mg	

*Only drugs available in the United States are listed.

†Cost to pharmacist (average wholesale price, generic when possible) for quantity listed. Source: Drug Topics Red Book 19(3), March 2000.

From Tierney L, et al: Acute respiratory failure. In Tierney L, et al (eds): Current Medical Diagnosis & Treatment (40th Ed). New York, McGraw-Hill, 2001, with permission.

ACUTE RESPIRATORY FAILURE

Acute respiratory failure is a sudden and life-threatening deterioration in pulmonary gas exchange, resulting in carbon dioxide retention and inadequate oxygenation.[31] Acute respiratory failure remains a major cause of morbidity and mortality in the intensive care setting, despite the technological advances in diagnosis, monitoring, and management that have been made in the past four decades.[55] Recently, a study of over 1,400 patients found that 44% of patients diagnosed with acute respiratory failure who required admission to the ICU died in the hospital; in the past 20 years, this statistic that has not changed significantly.[56] Acute respiratory failure may be responsible for as much as 10% to 15% of admissions to medical ICUs and for as much as 50% to 75% of those patients who require ICU hospital stays longer than 7 days.[55]

Pathophysiology

Acute respiratory failure is defined as a PaO_2 of 50 mm Hg or less, a $PaCO_2$ greater than 50 mm Hg, and an arterial pH less than 7.35.[26,31] This definition is valid only in cases in which baseline ABGs are assumed to be normal.[57] In patients with established chronic hypoxemia or hypercapnia, acute respiratory failure is indicated by the acute deterioration of blood gases relative to their previous levels rather than their absolute values.[57] In patients with chronic lung disease, ABGs associated with classic acute respiratory failure may not be present because these patients have adapted to blood gas levels outside this range, consistent with their disease process.[26]

Acute respiratory failure may be caused by a variety of pulmonary and nonpulmonary diseases (Box 26-13). Respiratory failure may result from malfunction of the respiratory center, abnormal respiratory neuromuscular system, chest wall diseases, airway obstruction, or parenchymal lung disorders.[57] Many factors may precipitate or exacerbate acute respiratory failure (Box 26-14).

A vicious positive feedback mechanism characterizes the deleterious effects of continued hypoxemia and hypercapnia. Hypoxemia affects every organ and tissue and hypercapnia impairs cellular functions.[57] Hypoxemia in respiratory failure may be caused by any of these conditions, separately or in various combinations: Table 26-14 lists the causes of hypoxemia.[57,58] Hypercapnia results from alveolar hypoventilation and ventilation–perfusion mismatching when there is no compensation by increased ventilation of well-perfused regions.[57] In acute hypercapnia, arterial blood pH is decreased, indicating acute respiratory acidosis. Patients with advanced COPD and chronic hypercapnia may exhibit an acute rise of $PaCO_2$ to a high level, a decrease of blood pH, and a significant increase in serum bicarbonate during the onset of acute respiratory failure.[57]

Hypoxemia and hypercapnia may have precipitous effects, which include the following:

- Increased pulmonary vascular resistance
- Cor pulmonale

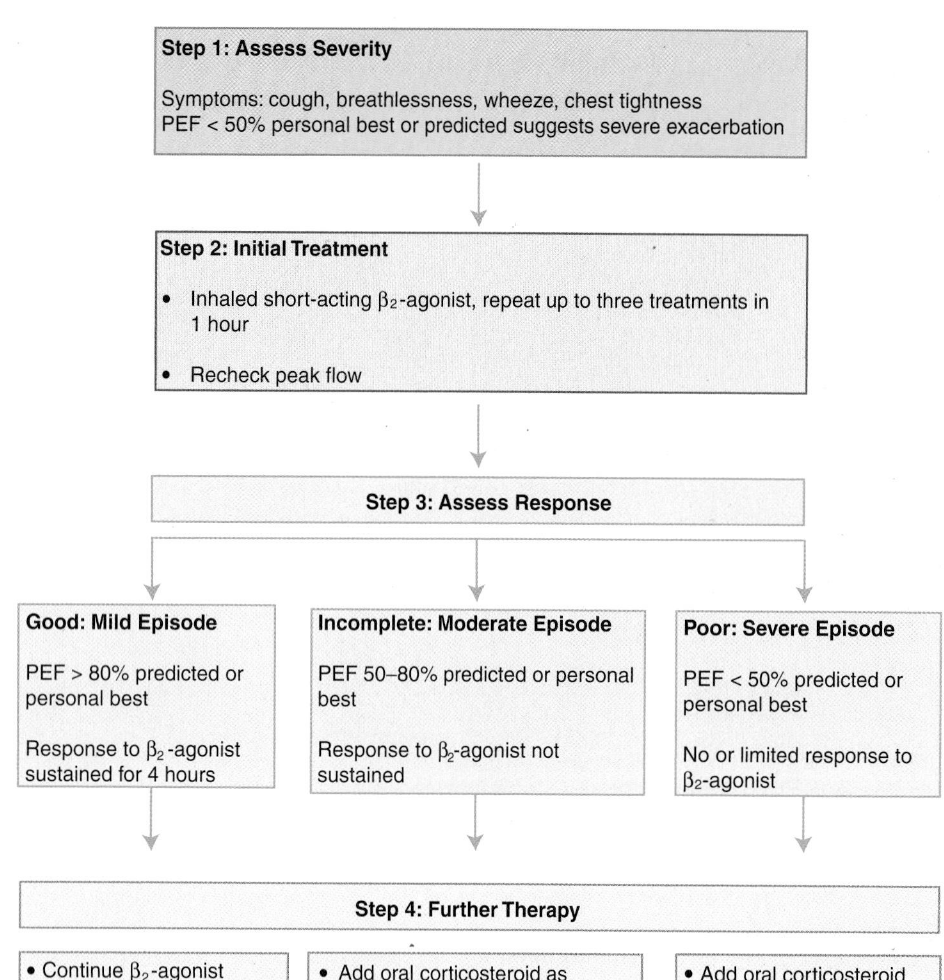
Step 1: Assess Severity
Symptoms: cough, breathlessness, wheeze, chest tightness
PEF < 50% personal best or predicted suggests severe exacerbation
Step 2: Initial Treatment
• Inhaled short-acting β2-agonist, repeat up to three treatments in 1 hour
• Recheck peak flow
Step 3: Assess Response
Good: Mild Episode
PEF > 80% predicted or personal best
Response to β2-agonist sustained for 4 hours
Incomplete: Moderate Episode
PEF 50–80% predicted or personal best
Response to β2-agonist not sustained
Poor: Severe Episode
PEF < 50% predicted or personal best
No or limited response to β2-agonist
Step 4: Further Therapy
• Continue β2-agonist every 3 – 4 hours as needed for 24 – 48 hours
• Double usual dose of inhaled corticosteroid for 7 – 10 days
• Contact clinician for follow-up within 3 days
• Add oral corticosteroid as previously prescribed by clinician
• Continue β2-agonist every 3–4 hours as needed
• Consult clinician urgently (this day) for instructions
• Add oral corticosteroid
• Repeat β2-agonist immediately
• Immediate transport to hospital emergency room, consider ambulance

figure 26-10 Peak expiratory flow rate–based plan for management of asthma exacerbations. *PEF,* peak expiratory flow. (Modified from National Asthma Education Program: Expert Panel Report II. Guidelines for the diagnosis and management of asthma. Washington, DC: U.S. Department of Health and Human Services, 1997. NIH publication 97-4051. From Givelber RJ, O'Connor GT: Asthma. In Goldstein RH, et al [eds]: A Practical Approach to Pulmonary Medicine, pp 68–84. Philadelphia, Lippincott-Raven, 1997.)

- Right-sided heart failure
- Impaired left ventricular function
- Reduced cardiac output
- Cardiogenic pulmonary edema
- Diaphragmatic fatigue from increased workload of respiratory muscles[57]

Classification

Acute respiratory failure is classified as *acute hypoxemic respiratory failure* (type I), *acute hypercapnic respiratory failure* (type II), or *combined hypoxemic and hypercapnic respiratory failure* (type I and type II).[55] Type I failure is a direct defect in oxygenation. Type II failure is a direct defect in ventilation. However, in many instances, the distinction is not clear; many patients exhibit signs and symptoms of a combined type I and type II respiratory failure.[55]

ACUTE HYPOXEMIC RESPIRATORY FAILURE (TYPE I)

Type I acute respiratory failure is the result of abnormal oxygen transport secondary to pulmonary parenchymal disease, with increased alveolar ventilation resulting in a low $Pa{CO_2}$.[57] The principal problem in type I acute respiratory failure is the inability to achieve adequate oxygenation, as evidenced by a $Pa{O_2}$ of 50 mm Hg or less and a $Pa{CO_2}$ of 40 mm Hg or less.[55] The most common cause of hypoxemia is ventilation–perfusion mismatch.[59] However, right-to-left shunt and alveolar hypoventilation are the most clinically significant causes of type I failure.[55] The major causes of type I respiratory failure are listed in Table 26-15.

ACUTE HYPERCAPNIC RESPIRATORY FAILURE (TYPE II)

Type II acute respiratory failure, or ventilatory failure, is the result of inadequate alveolar ventilation[57] and is charac-

box 26-13
Causes of Acute Respiratory Failure

Intrinsic Lung/Airway Diseases

Large Airway Obstruction

- Congenital deformities
- Acute laryngitis, epiglottitis
- Foreign bodies
- Intrinsic tumors
- Extrinsic pressure
- Traumatic injury
- Enlarged tonsils and adenoids
- Obstructive sleep apnea

Bronchial Diseases

- Chronic bronchitis
- Asthma
- Acute bronchiolitis

Parenchymal Diseases

- Pulmonary emphysema
- Pulmonary fibrosis and other chronic diffuse infiltrative diseases
- Severe pneumonia
- Acute lung injury from various causes (acute respiratory distress syndrome)

Cardiovascular Disease

- Cardiac pulmonary edema
- Massive or recurrent pulmonary embolism
- Pulmonary vasculitis

Extrapulmonary Disorders

Diseases of the Pleura and the Chest Wall

- Pneumothorax
- Pleural effusion
- Fibrothorax
- Thoracic wall deformity
- Traumatic injury to the chest wall: flail chest
- Obesity

Disorders of the Respiratory Muscles and the Neuromuscular Junction

- Myasthenia gravis and myasthenia-like disorders
- Muscular dystrophies
- Polymyositis
- Botulism
- Muscle-paralyzing drugs
- Severe hypokalemia and hypophosphatemia

Disorders of the Peripheral Nerves and Spinal Cord

- Poliomyelitis
- Guillain-Barré syndrome
- Spinal cord trauma (quadriplegia)
- Amyotrophic lateral sclerosis
- Tetanus
- Multiple sclerosis

Disorders of the Central Nervous System

- Sedative and narcotic drug overdose
- Head trauma
- Cerebral hypoxia
- Cerebrovascular accident
- Central nervous system infection
- Epileptic seizure: status epilepticus
- Metabolic and endocrine disorders
- Bulbar poliomyelitis
- Primary alveolar hypoventilation
- Sleep apnea syndrome

box 26-14 ***Precipitating Factors Leading to Acute Respiratory Failure***

- Changes of tracheobronchial secretions
- Infection: viral or bacterial
- Disturbance of tracheobronchial clearance
- Drugs: sedatives, narcotics, anesthesia, oxygen
- Inhalation or aspiration of irritants, vomitus, foreign body
- Cardiovascular disorders: heart failure, pulmonary embolism, shock
- Mechanical factors: pneumothorax, pleural effusion, abdominal distension
- Trauma, including surgery
- Neuromuscular abnormalities
- Allergic disorders: bronchospasm
- Increased oxygen demand: fever, infection
- Inspiratory muscle fatigue

From Farzan S: Respiratory failure. In Farzan S (ed): A Concise Handbook of Respiratory Diseases (4th Ed), pp 371–386. Stamford, CT, Appleton & Lange, 1997, with permission.

terized by marked elevation of carbon dioxide with relative preservation of oxygenation.[55] Hypoxemia results from reduced alveolar pressure of oxygen (PAO_2) and is proportionate to hypercapnia.[57] Three factors contribute to type II failure: decreased ventilatory drive, respiratory muscle fatigue or failure, and increased work of breathing.[59] Various factors may influence a decreased ventilatory drive, such as medications/drugs (narcotics, benzodiazepines, barbiturates, alcohol), brainstem lesions, hypothyroidism, morbid obesity, and sleep apnea.[55,59] Respiratory muscle fatigue or failure is caused by neuromuscular dysfunction due to the following diseases: amyotrophic lateral sclerosis, Guillain-Barré syndrome, myasthenia gravis, muscular dystrophy, and polymyositis.[59] Increased work of breathing most commonly occurs in COPD (increased dead space) or asthma (elevated airway resistance), and it may also result from thoracic abnormalities (restriction on lungs) such as pneumothorax, rib fractures, or pleural effusions.[59] Extensive burns may produce increased carbon dioxide production from the hypermetabolic state, requiring increased minute ventilation.[59] The major causes of type II respiratory failure are listed in Table 26-15, including hypercapnic respiratory failure.[31]

table 26-14 Causes of Hypoxemia in Acute Respiratory Failure

Mechanism	Effect
Inhalation of a hypoxic gas mixture or severe reduction of barometric pressure—occurs in toxic fume inhalation, in fires that consume oxygen in combustion, and at high altitudes because of reduced barometric pressure.	Decrease in the partial pressure of inhaled oxygen
Alveolar hypoventilation—commonly seen in ventilatory failure hypoxemic patients.	Increased alveolar PCO_2 Decreased alveolar PO_2 Arterial hypoxemia
Impairment of diffusion—prevents complete equilibration of alveolar gas with pulmonary capillary blood.	Usually small effect and easily compensated by a small increase in inspired oxygen (FIO_2); present in emphysema and diffuse lung injury
Ventilation–perfusion mismatching—uneven ventilation of various lung regions and units whose perfusion frequently fails to match the changes in ventilation.	Most common cause of oxygen desaturation High ventilation–perfusion units contribute to dead space Supplemental oxygen reverses hypoxemia
Right-to-left shunt—the result of continuous perfusion of nonventilated lung regions.	Indicates closure of air passages, especially the distal airways and alveoli. Classic sign—changes in FIO_2 have little effect on PaO_2 when the true shunt fraction exceeds 30%.
Reduced oxygen in mixed venous blood—may occur from abnormal pulmonary gas exchange, too high or too low cardiac output, or high metabolic rate (fever).	Increased oxygen extraction from arterial blood results in decreased PaO_2.

From Farzan S: Respiratory failure. In Farzan S, (ed): A Concise Handbook of Respiratory Diseases (4th Ed), pp 371–386. Stamford, CT, Appleton & Lange, 1997, with permission.

COMBINED HYPOXEMIC AND HYPERCAPNIC RESPIRATORY FAILURE (TYPE I AND TYPE II)

The combined type of acute respiratory failure develops as a consequence of a combined inadequate alveolar ventilation and abnormal gas transport.[57] This condition is commonly seen in asthmatic exacerbations, emphysema complicated by a lower respiratory tract infection, severe pneumonia, pulmonary edema, and pulmonary embolism.[55] Any potential cause of type I failure may lead to combined failure, especially if increased work of breathing and hypercapnia are involved. Situations producing respiratory muscle fatigue or neuromuscular weakness may be compounded by pneumothorax or pleural effusion, which would result in hypoxemia superimposed on the primary hypercapnia.[55]

Assessment

HISTORY

A complete medical and social history should be obtained from the patient or a family member to determine the patient's baseline respiratory status on admission. The ATS has provided specific standards for assessment of adult patients with actual or potential pulmonary dysfunction, which address process and outcome variables.[60] Box 26-15 presents the nursing assessment guide based on these standards. These comprehensive standards are used in assessment, goal setting, intervention, and evaluation to ensure that patients receive high-quality health care.[61] Self-management categories address the patient's capacity for self-care (physical, cognitive, psychosocial, socioeconomic, and environmental). The health care professional will find this a valuable tool in the continual assessment process of patients with pulmonary disorders.

PHYSICAL FINDINGS

Presentation of acute respiratory failure may vary, depending on the underlying disease, precipitating factor(s), and the degree of hypoxemia, hypercapnia, or acidosis.[57] It is essential to determine whether intubation and positive-pressure ventilation are required as emergency measures; this is the most critical assessment objective.[55] Typically, intubation and ventilation are necessary in patients with depressed mental status or coma, severe respiratory distress, extremely low or agonal respiratory rate, obvious respiratory muscle fatigue, peripheral cyanosis, or impending cardiopulmonary arrest.[55] Patients with altered mental status are at risk for aspiration of gastric contents. In any of these situations, immediate intervention is vital and should not be postponed pending the results of ABG studies or chest radiography.[55]

The classic symptom of hypoxemia is dyspnea,[62] although this may be completely absent in ventilatory failure resulting from depression of the respiratory center.[57] Other presenting symptoms of hypoxemia include cyanosis, restlessness, confusion, anxiety, delirium, tachypnea, tachycardia, hypertension, cardiac dysrhythmias, and tremor.[62] Peripheral cyanosis of the skin, lips, or nail beds suggests

table 26-15 Evaluation and Management of Common Causes of Acute Respiratory Failure

Etiology	Key Clinical Findings	Key Diagnostic Tests	Specific Therapy
Normal Alveolar–Arterial Gradient: Acute Hypercapnic Respiratory Failure			
Reduced FIO_2	Geographic location (altitude)	Ambient FIO_2	Change location
CNS depression	History of drug overdose, head trauma, or anoxic encephalopathy Comatose	Response to naloxone Toxicology screen Electrolytes (glucose, calcium, sodium) CT head, EEG	Naloxone, charcoal Correct electrolytes Neurological evaluation
Neuromuscular dysfunction	Neck trauma or neuromuscular disease Received paralytic medications (2)	Cervical spine films Review medications CXR: elevated hemidiaphragms Upright/supine PFTs (reduced VC, NIF, PEF in supine position)	Stabilize cervical spine Discontinue paralytics Noninvasive ventilation
Increased Alveolar–Arterial Gradient: Acute Hypoxemic Respiratory Failure			
Alveoli/interstitium			
Cardiogenic pulmonary edema	Rales, diaphoresis	CXR: pulmonary edema PA line: elevated PCWP, ECG, echocardiogram	Diuresis Reduce LVEDP
Adult respiratory distress syndrome	Rales PaO_2 <55 mm Hg with FIO_2 >60%	CXR: pulmonary edema PA line: normal or low PCWP	Treat underlying cause
Pneumonia	Fever Lung sounds: rales and/or egophony	CXR: diffuse or lobar infiltrate CBC: leukocytosis Sputum Gram's stain, blood culture	Antibiotics: empirical therapy tailored to likely pathogens
Pleural effusion	Lung sounds: egophony	CXR: pleural effusion; contralateral mediastinal shift Thoracentesis	Drainage Treat underlying cause Consider pleurodesis
Atelectasis	Diminished breath sounds Postoperative	CXR: volume loss, ipsilateral mediastinal shift	Reduce sedation Pulmonary toilet Consider bronchoscopy
Pneumothorax	Diminished breath sounds Chest wall asymmetry Tracheal deviation	CXR: pneumothorax; contralateral mediastinal shift	Decompression: chest tube
Alveolar hemorrhage	Hemoptysis	CXR: localized or diffuse infiltrate; air bronchograms Sputum: hemosiderin-laden macrophages ANCA, antiGBM, sputum AFB, cytology, Gram's stain, urinalysis	Protect uninvolved lung Identify bleeding site and etiology If localized, consider resection, embolization
Pulmonary infarct	Tachypnea, tachycardia Pleuritic CP, hemoptysis Risk for DVT; hypercoagulable	CXR: wedge-shaped peripheral infiltrate Abnormal $\dot{V}/\dot{Q}$scan or PA gram	Heparin anticoagulation Consider thrombolysis and IVC filter
Airways			
Asthma	Wheezing (may be absent if severe airflow obstruction)	Reduced PEF	Beta-agonists Corticosteroid Theophylline Consider HELIOX
Chronic obstructive pulmonary disease	Wheezing: infrequent		Titrate oxygen carefully to SaO_2 >89% Beta-agonists Ipratropium bromide Corticosteroid Theophylline Antibiotics: if clinical evidence of infection

(continued)

table 26-15 Evaluation and Management of Common Causes of Acute Respiratory Failure (Continued)

Etiology	Key Clinical Findings	Key Diagnostic Tests	Specific Therapy
Acute airway obstruction			
Foreign body	Witnessed aspiration	CXR	Localize and remove foreign body using bronchoscope
Epiglottitis	Odynophagia, drooling	Lateral neck films	Racemic epinephrine, antibiotics, HELIOX
Vascular disease			
Pulmonary embolus	See pulmonary infarct	CXR: nonspecific Abnormal $\dot{V}/\dot{Q}$scan or PA gram	Heparin anticoagulation Consider thrombolysis and IVC filter
Lymphatic disease			
Lymphangitic carcinomatosis	History of neoplasm	CXR: reticular infiltrates Cytology from PA line	Treat underlying disease

AFB, acid fast bacilli; ANCA, anti-neutrophilic cytoplasmic antibody; antiGBM, anti-glomerular basement membrane antibody; CBC, complete blood cell count; CNS, central nervous system; CP, chest pain; CT, computed tomography; CXR, chest x-ray; DVT, deep venous thrombosis; ECG, electrocardiogram; EEG, electroencephalogram; HELIOX, helium and oxygen mixture; IVC, inferior vena cava; LVEDP, left ventricular end-diastolic pressure; NIF, negative inspiratory force; PA, pulmonary artery; PA gram, pulmonary arteriogram; PCWP, pulmonary capillary wedge pressure; PEF, peak expiratory flow; PEFR, peak expiratory flow rate; PFTs, pulmonary function tests; VC, vital capacity; $\dot{V}/\dot{Q}$, ventilation–perfusion.

From Powell CA, Joyce-Brady MF: Acute and chronic respiratory failure. In Goldstein RH, et al (eds): A Practical Approach to Pulmonary Medicine, pp 300–302. Philadelphia, Lippincott-Raven, 1997, with permission.

the presence of profound arterial hypoxemia, usually with a PaO_2 less than 50 mm Hg.[55]

The cardinal symptoms of hypercapnia are dyspnea and headache.[62] Other clinical manifestations of hypercapnia include peripheral and conjunctival hyperemia, hypertension, tachycardia, tachypnea, impaired consciousness, papilledema, and asterixis.[62] Uncorrected carbon dioxide narcosis leads to diminished alertness, disorientation, increased intracranial pressure, and ultimately unconsciousness.[55] Other physical findings on examination may include use of accessory muscles of respiration, intercostal or supraclavicular retraction, and paradoxical abdominal movement if diaphragmatic weakness or fatigue is present.[57] See Table 26-15 for more details concerning clinical findings.

DIAGNOSTIC STUDIES

Because the signs and symptoms of acute respiratory failure are nonspecific and insensitive, the physician must request an ABG analysis[62] to determine the exact level of PaO_2, $PaCO_2$, and blood pH in cases of suspected acute respiratory failure. Only determination of the blood gases and pH can confirm the diagnosis.[57] Other diagnostic tests necessary to determine the etiology of acute hypoxemic respiratory failure include chest radiography, sputum examination, pulmonary function testing, angiography, ventilation–perfusion scanning, CT, toxicology screen, complete blood count, serum electrolytes, cytology, urinalysis, bronchogram, bronchoscopy, electrocardiography, echocardiography, and thoracentesis.[31] See Table 26-15 for more details about the use of these diagnostic tests in acute respiratory failure.

Management

Treatment of acute respiratory failure warrants immediate intervention to correct or compensate for the gas exchange abnormality and identify the cause.[31] Therapy is directed toward correcting the cause and alleviating the hypoxia and hypercapnia.[26] Although the recommended therapeutic intervention may vary according to the specific disease's pathological process, general management principles are applicable to every patient with acute respiratory failure (Table 26-16). See Table 26-15 for specific therapies for the management of common causes of acute respiratory failure.[31]

If alveolar ventilation is inadequate to maintain PaO_2 or $PaCO_2$ levels related to respiratory or neurological failure, endotracheal intubation and mechanical ventilation may be lifesaving.[26] The initial assessment and the decision to initiate mechanical ventilation should be performed rapidly to minimize the life-threatening complications associated with extended hypoxemia (e.g., cardiac dysrhythmias, anoxic encephalopathy).[31] Controlled oxygen therapy and mechanical ventilation are used to increase PaO_2 by increasing FIO_2 and to normalize pH by increasing minute ventilation.[31] See Chapter 25 for further information on airway management and care of the patient on a ventilator.

Patients with acute hypoxemic respiratory failure should receive immediate treatment with rapidly increased FIO_2 and continuous pulse oximetry monitoring until an SaO_2 of 90% or higher is obtained.[55] Correction of hypoxemia in the acute setting takes precedence over possible attenuation of hypoxic respiratory drive.[55] Therefore, once hypoxemia is reversed, oxygen is titrated to the minimum level necessary for correction of hypoxemia and prevention of significant carbon dioxide retention.[55]

Patients with acute hypercapnic respiratory failure should be immediately assessed for either an impaired central respiratory drive associated with sedative or narcotic therapy or for underlying bronchospasm secondary to an asthma exacerbation or COPD.[55] Reversal agents (opiate antagonists, e.g., naloxone) are used in the case of impaired central respiratory drive, and inhaled bronchodilators and systemic corticosteroids are used in the case of underlying bronchospasm.[55]

box 26-15
Nursing Assessment Guide for Adult Patients With Pulmonary Dysfunction

History and Symptoms Profile

Pulmonary Symptoms*

- Dyspnea
- Cough
- Sputum
- Hemoptysis
- Wheeze
- Chest pain (e.g., pleuritic)

Extrapulmonary Symptoms*

- Night sweats
- Headaches on awakening
- Weight changes
- Fluid retention
- Nasal stuffiness, discharge
- Fatigue
- Orthopnea, paroxysmal nocturnal apnea
- Snoring, sleep disturbances, daytime drowsiness
- Sinus problems

Pulmonary Risk Factors

- Smoking history: type (cigarettes, cigar, pipe); amount per day; duration (years)
- Childhood respiratory diseases/symptoms
- Family history of respiratory disease
- Alcohol and chemical substance abuse (e.g., heroin, marijuana, cocaine)
- Environmental exposures: location (e.g., home, work, region); type (e.g., asbestos, silica, gases, aerosols); duration
- Obesity or nutritional depletion
- Compromised immune system function (e.g., IgG deficiency, HIV infection, α_1-antitrypsin deficiency)

Previous History

- Pulmonary problems
- Treatments
- Number of hospitalizations
- Medical diagnosis(es)
- Immunizations

Self-Management Capacity

Physical Ability (0 to 4 scale, 0 = independent, 4 = dependent)

- Lower extremity (e.g., walking, stair climbing)
- Upper extremity (e.g., shampooing, meal preparation)
- Activities of daily living: toileting, hygiene, feeding, dressing
- Activity pattern during a typical day
- Patient statement re: management of problems
- Sensory-perceptual factors (e.g., vision, hearing)

Cognitive Ability

- Mental age
- Memory
- Knowledge about diagnosis and treatment of pulmonary problems, or risk factors of pulmonary disease
- Judgment

Psychosocial-Cultural Factors

- Self-concept: self-esteem, body image, role(s), changes
- Value system (e.g., spiritual and health beliefs)
- Coping mechanisms
  - Displaced anger
  - Anxiety
  - Hostility
  - Dependency
  - Withdrawal
  - Isolation
  - Avoidance
  - Denial
  - Noncompliance
  - Acceptance

Socioeconomic Factors

- Social support system
  - Family
  - Significant others
  - Friends
  - Community resources
  - Government resources
- Financial situation/health insurance
- Employment/disability

Environmental Factors

- Home
- Community
- Worksite
- Health care setting (e.g., hospital, nursing home)

---

*Consider onset, duration, character, and precipitating, aggravating, and relieving factors of symptoms.

Modified from American Thoracic Society Medical Section of the American Lung Association: Standards of nursing care for adult patients with pulmonary dysfunction, Am Rev Respir Dis 144:231, 1991. From Kríder SJ: Interview and respiratory history. In Wilkins RL, et al (eds): Clinical Assessment in Respiratory Care (4th Ed), p 26. St. Louis, Mosby, 2000, with permission.

table 26-16 Management in Respiratory Failure

Management Principle	Therapeutic Intervention
Establishment and maintenance of an adequate airway	• Use oropharyngeal or nasopharyngeal tubes for upper airway obstruction during transient loss of consciousness. • Tracheal intubation may be necessary to prevent aspiration, maintain airway patency, and provide effective suctioning. • Strictly adhere to adequate tracheobronchial toilet (i.e., deep breathing, coughing, tracheobronchial suctioning).
Oxygenation	• Increase the inspired oxygen (FIO_2) concentration by administration of oxygen via a Venturi mask or nasal cannula. • Improve cardiac output, correct anemia, and reduce metabolic rates (fever) to improve tissue oxygenation. • Consider continuous positive airway pressure or expiratory positive airway pressure via a nasal or facial mask for alert and cooperative patients. • Mechanical ventilatory support may be needed in more severe cases with refractory and progressive hypoxemia.
Correction of acid–base disturbance	• Correct pH disturbances: In acute hypercapnia with acidosis, improve alveolar ventilation by providing mechanical ventilatory support, establishing and maintaining an adequate airway, treating bronchospasm, and controlling heart failure, fever, and sepsis. • Consider bicarbonate administration in acute respiratory acidosis or metabolic acidosis.
Restoration of fluid and electrolyte balance	• Prevent excessive intravenous fluid administration and, conversely, poor fluid intake. • Monitor fluid intake and output closely. • Perform daily body weight measurement. • Prevent and treat promptly hypokalemia and hypophosphatemia.
Optimization of cardiac function	• Maintain adequate cardiac output. • Consider use of pulmonary artery catheter for accurate hemodynamic monitoring.
Identification and treatment of underlying correctable conditions and precipitating causes	• Prevent or treat respiratory tract infections (viral, bacterial, or fungal). • Prevent potential airway obstruction by maintenance of proper tracheobronchial hygiene, recognize increased tracheobronchial secretions, changes in their characteristics, or difficulty in their elimination due to various factors. • Identify and treat congestive heart failure appropriately. • Recognize and treat bronchospasm with bronchodilators and corticosteroids. • Assess for organic or metabolic disorder affecting the central nervous system or neuromuscular function. • Assess tolerance to sedative, hypnotic, and narcotic drugs in patients with chronic ventilatory insufficiency. In case of a narcotic drug overdose, a proper antidote may be administered. • Avoid indiscriminate use of oxygen; it may potentiate carbon dioxide retention or result in carbon dioxide narcosis. • Remove air or fluid in the pleural cavity. • Prevent and treat abdominal distension by insertion of a nasogastric tube. • For trauma and surgical patients, assess limitation of the thoracic wall movement, ineffective cough, immobility, and lack of deep breathing. • Control fever and other causes of increased metabolism. • Assess diaphragmatic fatigue; if present, mechanical ventilatory support is indicated to rest these muscles and restore their contractility. • Promptly identify and adequately treat hypophosphatemia, hypokalemia, and hypocalcemia.
Prevention and early detection of potential complications	• Most of these complications occur in mechanically ventilated patients (see Chapter 25).
Nutritional support	• Enteral alimentation is preferred over parenteral feeding because bowel wall integrity is maintained. • Recommend high-lipid formulas over high carbohydrates to limit carbon dioxide production.
Periodic assessment of the course, progress, and response to therapy	• Perform frequent arterial blood gas measurements. • Monitor arterial oxygen saturation by pulse oximetry.
Determination of a need for mechanical ventilatory support	• Continuously assess the patient's respiratory status and need for ventilator support (see Chapter 25).

From Farzan S: Respiratory failure. In Farzan S (ed): A Concise Handbook of Respiratory Diseases (4th Ed), pp 371–386. Stamford, CT, Appleton & Lange, 1997, with permission.

clinical applicability challenges

Self-Challenge: Critical Thinking

A 65-year-old man with a 10-year history of COPD seeks medical attention because he feels increasingly short of breath since contracting a "heavy chest cold." His typical chronic productive daily cough has "turned yellow"; his usual dyspnea (after climbing two flight of stairs) has become more severe; and he becomes short of breath even when walking one city block on level ground. He denies fever, chills, or chest pain. He takes oral theophylline and aerosolized albuterol daily but continues to smoke 10 cigarettes per day.

The patient is afebrile. His vital signs are respirations 24 breaths/minute; pulse rate 96 beats/minute and regular; blood pressure 138/74 mm Hg lying, right arm, and 134/74 mm Hg sitting, right arm. He appears chronically ill but is in no acute distress. He is able to speak without apparent dyspnea. Physical examination shows increased lateral chest diameter (barrel chest), use of accessory muscles of respiration, low diaphragms, and distant breath sounds throughout both lung fields. Rhonchi are heard over mainstem bronchi, followed by several nonproductive coughs, which clear the rhonchi. A chest radiograph is negative.

1. *What other subjective data about this patient would you want to obtain?*
2. *What potential infectious organisms would you consider?*
3. *What would you include in your differential diagnosis?*
4. *What is the appropriate treatment for this patient?*
5. *What would be your educational plan for this patient?*
6. *What are the indications for hospitalization in similar patients?*

Study Questions

1. *A 65-year-old woman presents with increased shortness of breath over the past week and a previous diagnosis of emphysema. Pulmonary function studies would most likely demonstrate*
   a. *decreased forced expiratory volume, increased total lung capacity, increased residual volume.*
   b. *increased forced expiratory volume, decreased total lung capacity, increased residual volume.*
   c. *decreased forced expiratory volume, decreased total lung capacity, decreased residual volume.*
   d. *increased forced expiratory volume, increased total lung capacity, decreased residual volume.*
2. *Understanding the importance of avoiding respiratory irritants is a teaching concern for the patient described in question 1. Select the single most important cause of respiratory irritation.*
   a. *Inhaling dust or fumes*
   b. *Breathing cold air*
   c. *Cigarette smoke*
   d. *Allergens*
3. *When treating chronic bronchitis with airflow obstruction, you would be least likely to order*
   a. *antibiotics.*
   b. *corticosteroids.*
   c. *bronchodilators.*
   d. *theophylline.*
4. *All of the following signs and symptoms are associated with emphysema except*
   a. *purse-lipped breathing.*
   b. *barrel-shaped chest.*
   c. *usually thin appearance.*
   d. *continuous cough with copious sputum.*
5. *In pneumonia, which of the following is the primary route by which organisms enter into the lower respiratory tract?*
   a. *Inhalation*
   b. *Aspiration*
   c. *Translocation*
   d. *Hematogenous spread from a distant site*
6. *The most common cause of a pleural effusion in critically ill patients is*
   a. *cirrhosis.*
   b. *pneumonia.*
   c. *congestive heart failure.*
   d. *hemothorax.*
7. *The primary treatment for a transudate pleural effusion is*
   a. *treatment of the underlying cause.*
   b. *thoracentesis.*
   c. *antibiotics.*
   d. *oxygen therapy.*
8. *The most common cause of a pneumothorax in critically ill patients is*
   a. *trauma.*
   b. *COPD.*
   c. *invasive procedures and barotrauma.*
   d. Pneumocystis carinii *pneumonia.*
9. *Signs and symptoms of pulmonary embolism in intensive care patients include all of the following except*
   a. *unexplained fever.*
   b. *sudden decrease in pulmonary artery pressure or central venous pressure.*
   c. *worsening hypoxemia or hypocapnia in a spontaneously ventilated patient.*
   d. *worsening hypoxemia and hypercapnia in a sedate patient on controlled mechanical ventilation.*

REFERENCES

1. Centers for Disease Control and Prevention: Fast stats. Natl Vital Stat Rep 48(11):1–5, 2001
2. Centers for Disease Control and Prevention: National Nosocomial Infections Surveillance (NNIS) system report, data summary from January 1990–May 1999. Am J Infect Control 27:520–532, 1999
3. American Thoracic Society: Guidelines for the management of adults with community-acquired pneumonia. Am J Respir Crit Care Med 163:1730–1754, 2001
4. Ewig S, et al: Severity of community-acquired pneumonia. Am J Respir Crit Care Med 158:1102–1108, 1998
5. American Thoracic Society: Hospital-acquired pneumonia in adults: Diagnosis, assessment of severity, initial antimicrobial therapy, and preventive strategies. Am J Respir Crit Care Med 153:1711–1725, 1996
6. Harris JR, et al: Risk factor for nosocomial pneumonia in critically ill trauma patients. AACN Clin Issues 11(2):198–231, 2000
7. Centers for Disease Control and Prevention: Guidelines for prevention of nosocomial pneumonia. Morb Mortal Wkly Rep 46(RR-1):1–80, 1997 (CDC guidelines also available at: http://www.cdc.gov)

8. Bartlett JG, et al: Practice guidelines for the management of community-acquired pneumonia in adults. Clin Infect Dis 31:347–382, 2000
9. Johanson WG Jr, Dever LL: Microbial flora and colonization of the respiratory tract. In Fishman AP (ed): Fishman's Pulmonary Diseases and Disorders, pp 1883–1890. New York, McGraw-Hill, 1998
10. Niederman MS: Acute infectious pneumonia. In Irwin RS, et al (eds): Intensive Care Medicine (3rd Ed), pp 879–899. Philadelphia, Lippincott Williams & Wilkins, 1999
11. Mandell LA, Campbell J, Douglas G: Nosocomial pneumonia guidelines. Chest 113:118S–193S, 1998
12. Meeham RP, et al: Quality of care, process, and outcomes in elderly patients with pneumonia. JAMA 278:2080–2084, 1997
13. Harris JR, Miller TH: Preventing nosocomial pneumonia: Evidenced-based practice. Crit Care Nurse 20(1):51–66, 2000
14. Zimmerman LH: Pleural effusions. In Goldstein RH, et al (eds): A Practical Approach to Pulmonary Medicine, pp 195–205. Philadelphia, Lippincott-Raven, 1997
15. Sahn SA: Pleural disease in the intensive care unit. In Grenvik A, et al (eds): Textbook of Critical Care (4th Ed), pp 1548–1560. Philadelphia, WB Saunders, 2000
16. Berk JL: Pneumothorax. In Goldstein RH, et al (eds): A Practical Approach to Pulmonary Medicine, pp 206–223. Philadelphia, Lippincott-Raven, 1997
17. Strange C: Pleural diseases. In Scanlan CL, et al (eds): Egan's Fundamentals of Respiratory Care (7th Ed), pp 475–490. St. Louis, Mosby, 1999
18. Tierney L, et al (eds): Current Medical Diagnosis & Treatment (40th Ed). New York, McGraw-Hill, 2001
19. Fedullo PF: Pulmonary embolism and deep venous thrombosis. In Grenvik A, et al (eds): Textbook of Critical Care (4th Ed), pp 1493–1507. Philadelphia, WB Saunders, 2000
20. Marik PE, et al: The incidence of deep venous thrombosis in ICU patients. Chest 111:661–664, 1997
21. Weg JG: Venous thromboembolism–pulmonary embolism and deep vein thrombosis. In Irwin RS, et al (eds): Intensive Care Medicine (3rd Ed), pp 650–673. Philadelphia, Lippincott Williams & Wilkins, 1999
22. American Thoracic Society: The diagnostic approach to acute venous thromboembolism. Am J Respir Crit Care Med 160: 1043–1066, 1999
23. Arroliga AC: Pulmonary vascular disease. In Scanlan CL, et al (eds): Egan's Fundamentals of Respiratory Care (7th Ed), pp 491–505. St. Louis, Mosby, 1999
24. American College of Chest Physicians: Fifth ACCP consensus conference on antithrombotic therapy. Chest 114(5 Suppl):439S–769S, 1998
25. National Heart, Lung and Blood Institute and World Health Organization: Global initiative for chronic obstructive lung disease: Global strategy for the diagnosis, management, and prevention of chronic obstructive pulmonary disease: NHLBI/WHO workshop. Respir Care 46:798–825, 2001
26. Porth C: Pathophysiology: Concepts of Altered Health States (5th Ed), pp 529–564. Philadelphia, Lippincott Williams & Wilkins, 1998
27. Tierney L, et al: Chronic obstructive pulmonary disease (COPD). In Tierney L, et al (eds): Current Medical Diagnosis & Treatment (40th Ed), pp 283–288. New York, McGraw-Hill, 2001
28. Rodriguez-Roisin R, MacNee W: Pathophysiology of chronic obstructive pulmonary disease. Eur Respir Monogr 3:107–126, 1998
29. British Thoracic Society: British Thoracic Society COPD guidelines summary. Thorax 52(Suppl 5):S1–S32, 1997
30. Britton J, Knox A: Helping people to stop smoking: The new smoking cessation guidelines. Thorax 54:1–2, 1999
31. Powell CA, Joyce-Brady MF: Acute and chronic respiratory failure. In Goldstein R, et al (eds): A Practical Approach to Pulmonary Medicine, pp 296–308. Philadelphia, Lippincott-Raven, 1997
32. Honig EG, Ingram RH: Chronic bronchitis, emphysema, and airways obstruction. In Braunwald E, et al (eds): Harrison's Principles of Internal Medicine (15th Ed), pp 1494–1497. New York, McGraw-Hill, 2001
33. Karlinsky J: Emphysema. In Goldstein R, et al (eds): A Practical Approach to Pulmonary Medicine, pp 224–239. Philadelphia, Lippincott-Raven, 1997
34. Nunley DR, et al: Critical care aspects of lung transplantation. In Grenvik A, et al (eds): Textbook of Critical Care (4th Ed), pp 1972–1981. Philadelphia, WB Saunders, 2000
35. Brenner M, et al: Rate of FEV_1 change following lung volume reduction surgery. Chest 113:652–659, 1998
36. Russi E, et al: Lung volume reduction surgery for emphysema. Eur Respir J 10:208–218, 1997
37. Gelb A, et al: Lung function 4 years after lung volume reduction surgery for emphysema. Chest 116:1608–1615, 1999
38. Daniel TM: Present status of lung volume reduction surgery in Virginia. Virginia Pulm J 6(1):1–8, 2000
39. Chatila W, et al: Acute respiratory failure after lung volume reduction surgery. Am J Respir Crit Care Med 162(4):1292–1296, 2000
40. Wu DMH, Center DM: Chronic bronchitis and bronchiectasis. In Goldstein R, et al (eds): A Practical Approach to Pulmonary Medicine, pp 240–246. Philadelphia, Lippincott-Raven, 1997
41. American Thoracic Society: Standards for the diagnosis and care of patients with chronic obstructive pulmonary disease. Am J Respir Crit Care Med 152:S77–S120, 1995
42. McFadden E: Diseases of the respiratory system: Asthma. In Braunwald E, et al (eds): Harrison's Principles of Internal Medicine (15th Ed), pp 1456–1463. New York, McGraw-Hill, 2001
43. O'Donnell WJ, Drazen JM: Life-threatening asthma. In Grenvik A, et al (eds): Textbook of Critical Care (4th Ed), pp 1451–1459. Philadelphia, WB Saunders Company, 2000
44. Centers for Disease Control and Prevention: Surveillance for asthma: United States, 1960–1995. Morb Mortal Wkly Rep 47(Suppl):1–27, 1998
45. National Heart, Lung and Blood Institute, National Institutes of Health: Practical Guide for the Diagnosis and Management of Asthma. Publication no. 97-4053. Bethesda, MD, National Institutes of Health, 1997
46. American Academy of Allergy, Asthma, and Immunology: Pediatric Asthma Promoting Best Practice: Guide for Managing Asthma in Children. Rochester, NY, University of Rochester, 1999
47. Janson S: Biologic markers of airway inflammation in asthma. AACN Clin Issues 11:232–240, 2000
48. Givelber RJ, O'Connor GT: Asthma. In Goldstein R, et al (eds): A Practical Approach to Pulmonary Medicine, pp 68–84. Philadelphia, Lippincott-Raven, 1997
49. Drazen JM, Turino GM: Progress at the interface of inflammation and asthma: Report of an ATS-sponsored workshop, November 1993. Am J Respir Crit Care Med 152:386–387, 1995
50. National Heart Lung and Blood Institute, National Institutes of Health: Global Initiative for Asthma. Bethesda, MD, National Heart, Lung, and Blood Institute, 1998
51. Institute for Clinical Systems Improvement: Diagnosis and Management of Asthma, p 35. Bloomington, IN, Institute for Clinical Systems Improvement, 2000 (also available at: www.ICSI.org)
52. Velsor-Friedrich B, Foley M: School-based management of the child with an acute asthma episode. AACN Clin Issues 12:282–292, 2001
53. Al-Asad K, Karlinsky JB: Pulmonary function tests. In Goldstein R, et al (eds): A Practical Approach to Pulmonary Medicine, p 27. Philadelphia, Lippincott-Raven, 1997
54. National Heart Lung and Blood Institute, National Institutes of Health: National Asthma Education and Prevention Program. Expert Panel Report 2: Guidelines for the Diagnosis and Management of Asthma, p 146. Bethesda, MD, National Institutes of Health, 1997
55. Van Hoozen B, Albertson TE: Acute respiratory failure. In Burton GG, et al (eds): Respiratory Care: A Guide to Clinical Practice (4th Ed), pp 1107–1132. Philadelphia, JB Lippincott, 1997
56. Vasileyev S, et al: Hospital survival rates of patients with acute respiratory failure in modern respiratory intensive care units. Chest 107(4):1083–1088, 1995
57. Farzan S: Respiratory failure. In Farzan S (ed): A Concise Handbook of Respiratory Diseases (4th Ed), pp 371–386. Stamford, CT, Appleton & Lange, 1997
58. Marini JJ, Wright LA: Acute respiratory failure. In Baum GL, et al (eds): Textbook of Pulmonary Diseases (6th Ed), pp 919–939. Philadelphia, Lippincott-Raven, 1998
59. Christie HA, Goldstein LS, Respiratory failure and the need for ventilatory support. In Scanlan CL, et al (eds): Egan's Fundamentals of Respiratory Care (7th Ed), pp 819–831. St. Louis, Mosby, 1999
60. American Thoracic Society: Standards of nursing care for adult patients with pulmonary dysfunction. Am Rev Respir Dis 144:231, 1991
61. Krider SJ: Interview and respiratory history. In Wilkins RL, et al (eds): Clinical Assessment in Respiratory Care (4th Ed), pp 11–50. St. Louis, Mosby, 2000

62. Tierney L, et al: Acute respiratory failure. In Tierney L, et al (eds): Current Medical Diagnosis & Treatment (40th Ed), pp 346–351. New York, McGraw-Hill, 2001

OTHER SELECTED READING

American College of Radiology: ACR appropriateness criteria for suspected lower extremity deep vein thrombosis. Radiology 215(Suppl): 49–53, 2000.

Behnia M, Cummings O: Desquamative interstitial pneumonia masquerading as acute life-threatening pulmonary embolism. Am J Crit Care 13(3); 199–201, 2004

Caroci A, Lareau S: Descriptors of dyspnea by patients with chronic obstructive pulmonary disease versus congestive heart failure. Heart Lung 33(2):102–110, 2004

Cicutto L, Downey G: Biological markers in diagnosing, monitoring, and treating asthma: A focus on non-invasive measurements. AACN Clin Issues 15(1):97–111, 2004

El-Masri M, Williamson K, Fox-Wasylyshyn S: Severe acute respiratory syndrome: Another challenge for critical care nurses. AACN Clin Issues 15(1):150–159, 2004

Gelinas C, Fortier M, Viens C, et al: Pain assessment and management in critically ill intubated patients: A retrospective study. Am J Crit Care 13(2):126–135, 2004

Holcomb S: Asthma update. Dimens Crit Care Nurs 23(3):101–110, 2004

Jeng C, Chang W, Wai P, et al: Comparison of oxygen consumption in performing daily activities between patients with chronic obstructive pulmonary disease and a health population. Heart Lung 32(2): 121–130, 2003

Kanervisto M, Paavilainen E, Astedt-Kurki P: Impact of chronic obstructive pulmonary disease on family functioning. Heart Lung 32(6):360–367, 2003

Koschel M: Pulmonary embolism. AJN 104(6):46–50, 2004

Meek P, Lareau S, Hu J: Are self-reports of breathing effort and breathing distress stable and valid measures among persons with asthma, persons with COPD, and healthy persons? Heart Lung 32(5): 335–346, 2003

chapter

27

Acute Respiratory Distress Syndrome

MARY VAN SOEREN

objectives

Based on the content in this chapter, the reader should be able to:

- Compare and contrast the causes, definition, assessment findings, and outcomes between acute lung injury (ALI) and acute respiratory distress syndrome (ARDS).
- Relate the assessment and diagnostic findings of ARDS to the pathophysiological processes.
- Describe mechanical ventilation strategies used to prevent ventilator-associated lung injury (VALI).
- Explain the management of patients with ARDS and rationales for the interventions.
- Discuss potential complications of ARDS and the related interventions.

Acute respiratory distress syndrome (ARDS) represents a complex clinical syndrome (rather than a single disease process) and carries a high risk of mortality. The severity of the clinical course, the uncertainty of the outcome, and the reliance on the full spectrum of critical care resources for treatment means that the entire health care team is challenged. For nearly 30 years, researchers and clinicians have investigated the nature of the pathological process and explored treatment options with the goal of improving outcome. Through this application of research to practice we know that some previous strategies have been ineffective, and new innovations in mechanical ventilation, sedation, nutrition, and pharmacological intervention are now important research initiatives. A key role for the critical care nurse is early detection and prevention of ARDS. Therefore, with respect to ARDS, it is essential for critical care nurses to be knowledgeable of risk factors, assessment tools and protocols, and preventive strategies.

DIAGNOSTIC CRITERIA AND INCIDENCE

ARDS was first described in 1967 and was termed adult (rather than acute) respiratory distress syndrome because of a misconception that the syndrome occurred only in adults. Recognition of the prevalence of this syndrome in younger patients led to the current terminology. Diagnostic criteria for ARDS have been hard to define because ARDS is at the extreme end of a continuum of acute, hypoxic lung injury resulting in acute respiratory failure. In 1994, the American-European Consensus Conference members proposed diagnostic criteria for acute lung injury (ALI) and ARDS, with ALI as the less severe form of this syndrome manifested by hypoxia and noncardiogenic lung edema[1] (Table 27-1).

The causes of ARDS are many and diverse.[2] The syndrome may be precipitated by either direct or indirect pulmonary injury, possibly in previously healthy people who

table 27-1 Comparison of Acute Lung Injury (ALI) and Acute Respiratory Distress Syndrome (ARDS)

Criterion	ALI	ARDS
Pao_2:Fio_2 ratio, regardless of PEEP level	Less than 300	Less than 200
Chest x-ray	Bilateral infiltrates	Bilateral infiltrates
Pulmonary artery wedge pressure	Less than 18 mm Hg or no indication of left atrial hypertension	Less than 18 mm Hg or no indication of left atrial hypertension

PEEP, positive end-expiratory pressure; *Pao_2:Fio_2 ratio,* ratio of arterial oxygen to inspired oxygen.
Adapted from Bernard GR, Artigas A, Brigham KL, et al: The American-European Consensus conference on ARDS: Definitions, mechanisms, relevant outcomes, and clinical trials co-ordination. Am J Respir Crit Care Med 149:818–824, 1994.

are exposed to an insult (Box 27-1). Symptoms may not manifest for up to 72 hours after the initial insult, making association with the cause sometimes difficult. For example, direct injury occurs through aspiration, pulmonary infection (bacterial, fungal, viral, or mycobacterial), near-drowning, thoracic trauma, and toxic inhalation. Indirect injury that results in ARDS includes sepsis syndrome, burns, trauma, multiple blood transfusions, cardiopulmonary bypass, pancreatitis, and fat emboli. The question of whether these causes result in the same pathological changes in the lung is under investigation, but the clinical presentation and treatment are similar.[3] Most patients with ARDS require a period of mechanical ventilation support.

Current research findings indicate that the incidence of ARDS has been difficult to determine because of the variation in diagnostic criteria.[4] It is estimated that 150,000 cases per year occur in the United States with an associated mortality rate of 30% to 70%.[2] This statistic represents a decrease from the 90% mortality rate over the last decades. The patients most at risk for development of ARDS are elderly (older than 65 years), with a severe acute illness on presentation to critical care (e.g., sepsis) or with additional risk factors such as a preexisting chronic disorder.[2,5] However, any individual with one of the potential precipitating causes of ARDS is susceptible, and nurses need to be vigilant for early warning signs—even, for example, in a young trauma patient. ARDS has developed in approximately one third of patients with sepsis (regardless of the bacterial source) or severe trauma.[6] Critical care techniques to provide life support for individuals with ARDS have reached a point where death results from complications such as ventilator-acquired pneumonia, sepsis, or multiorgan dysfunction, rather than from respiratory failure.[7]

box 27-1 ***Risk Factors for Acute Respiratory Distress Syndrome (ARDS)***

Indirect Pulmonary Injury

- Shock of any etiology
- Sepsis
- Hypothermia
- Hyperthermia
- Drug overdose
- Disseminated intravascular coagulation (DIC)
- Multiple transfusions
- Cardiopulmonary bypass
- Eclampsia
- Burns
- Pancreatitis
- Severe nonthoracic trauma

Direct Pulmonary Injury

- Pulmonary infections
- Toxic inhalation
- Aspiration (gastric fluids, near-drowning)
- Pneumonitis

Systemic Inflammatory Response Syndrome (SIRS) Criteria

SIRS is manifested by two or more of the following:

- Temperature greater than 100.4°F (38°C) or less than 96.8°F (36°C)
- Heart rate greater than 90 beats/minute
- Respiratory rate greater than 20 breaths/minute or an arterial carbon dioxide tension ($Paco_2$) less than 32 mm Hg
- White blood cell count greater than 12,000 cells/mm^3 or less than 4,000 cells/mm^3 OR more than 10% immature (band) forms

PATHOPHYSIOLOGY

In 1967, Ashbaugh and others described ARDS in case reports of 12 patients presenting with acute tachypnea, decreased lung compliance, diffuse pulmonary infiltrates on chest x-ray, and hypoxemia. Later researchers used histological examination of lungs of patients with ARDS to show lung fibrosis that was unlike other diseases. This led to new understanding that the pathological process was not limited to the lung endothelium, but was a result of alterations of lung epithelium and vascular tissue, and the development of hyaline membranes. Pathological changes in lung vascular tissue, increased lung edema, and impaired gas exchange are hallmarks of the pathophysiology. The pathological pulmonary alterations of ARDS are directly related to a cascade of events resulting from release of cellular and biochemical mediators. The activation, interactions, and multisystem actions of biological mediators are extremely complex.

Systemic Inflammatory Response Syndrome

Systemic inflammatory response syndrome (SIRS) describes the inflammatory response occurring throughout the body as a result of some systemic insult. Most patients with ARDS manifest the symptoms that define SIRS (see Box 27-1), and the respiratory system may be the earliest and most common organ system to be involved in the systemic response. Thus, an understanding of the pathophysiology of SIRS and knowledge of the interventions used for SIRS are important in relation to ARDS. Often, patients with SIRS develop multisystem organ dysfunction (MODS), primarily in the liver and kidney. As endothelial damage progresses and tissue hypoxia ensues from the severely impaired gas exchange, the inflammatory response is perpetuated and the SIRS cascade intensifies (upregulates) with the release of more mediators. ARDS and MODS are therefore part of a vicious cycle and the continuum of SIRS.[3] Determination of the triggers for SIRS and ARDS that are present in some individuals but not others and investigation of how to stop the cascade pathways are the subjects of ongoing research.

Pathological Changes in Acute Respiratory Distress Syndrome

Mediators released as a result of either direct or indirect injury can precipitate ARDS, including lipopolysaccharide (LPS) in gram-negative bacterial sepsis. There is a relationship between clinical presentation (severe acute hypoxia resistant to improvement with supplemental oxygen, tachypnea, and dyspnea), mediator release (interleukins, tumor necrosis factor-α [TNF-α], and platelet-activating factor [PAF]), and pathological changes (microvascular permeability, pulmonary hypertension, and pulmonary endothelial damage). Some primary mediators responsible for lung damage in ARDS and their major actions as they relate to ARDS are listed in Table 27-2.[2]

Adequate pulmonary gas exchange depends on open, air-filled alveoli; intact alveolar–capillary membranes; and normal blood flow through the pulmonary vasculature. In ARDS, diffuse alveolar–capillary membrane damage occurs and increases membrane permeability. Alterations in alveolar–capillary membrane integrity allow fluids to move from the vascular space into the interstitial and alveolar space. The resultant interstitial and alveolar edema and eventual alveolar collapse impair both oxygenation and ventilation. The pathogenesis of ARDS is illustrated in Figure 27-1. Inflammatory mediators cause the pulmonary vascular bed to vasoconstrict. Pulmonary hypertension and reduced blood flow to portions of the lung result. Because of the reduction in blood flow and decreased hemoglobin in capillaries, there is a decrease in oxygen available for diffusion and transport, further impairing oxygenation.

The pathological changes affect pulmonary blood vessels, gas exchange, and lung and bronchial mechanics (Fig. 27-2). The overall picture of ARDS is one of impaired diffusion of oxygen and elimination of carbon dioxide into pulmonary capillary blood. Ventilation is impaired because of a decrease in lung compliance and an increase in airway resistance. Increased membrane permeability, fluid-filled and collapsed alveoli, and dysfunctional surfactant, a substance that normally decreases the surface tension of alveoli and prevents their collapse, cause decreased lung compliance. Mediator-induced bronchoconstriction causes airway narrowing and increased airway resistance, restricting the flow of air into the lungs.

There is progression in the pathological changes associated with ARDS, starting with increasing pulmonary edema in the early stages and progressing to inflammation, fibrosis, and impaired healing in the later stages. Recognizing the dynamic nature of the morphological changes involved with ARDS enables the nurse to understand the changes in physical assessment, mechanical ventilation strategies, treatment, and management that occur throughout the patient's critical care stay.

Stages of Acute Respiratory Distress Syndrome

There are distinct stages in the progression of ARDS[2] (Table 27-3). In stage 1, diagnosis is difficult because the signs of impending ARDS are subtle. Clinically, the patient exhibits increased dyspnea and tachypnea, but there are few radiographic changes. At this point, neutrophils are sequestering; however, there is no evidence of cellular damage. Within 24 hours (a critical time for early treatment), the

table 27-2 Examples of Pathological Responses to Biological Mediators

Response	Biological Mediators
Persistent inflammatory response	Cytokines: interleukins (IL-1, IL-6), interferon-γ (INF-γ), tumor necrosis factor-α (TNF-α) complement, thromboxane
Endothelial membrane disruption	Complement, thromboxane, kinins, TNF-α, toxic oxygen metabolites, leukotrienes, prostaglandins (PGE_1 and PGE_2)
Selective vasoconstriction	Thromboxane, TNF-α, platelet-activating factor (PAF), toxic oxygen metabolites
Systemic vasodilation	Complement, prostaglandins, TNF-α, IL-1, IL-6
Myocardial depression	Complement, leukotrienes, TNF-α, myocardial depressant factor
Bronchoconstriction	Complement, thromboxane, leukotrienes, PAF

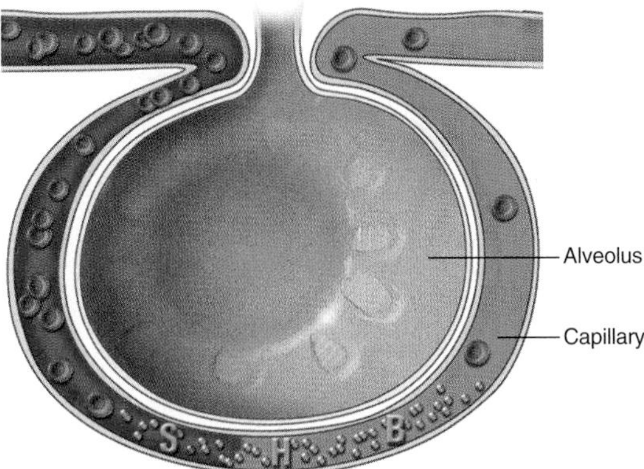

Phase 1. Injury reduces normal blood flow to the lungs. Platelets aggregate and release histamine (H), serotonin (S), and bradykinin (B).

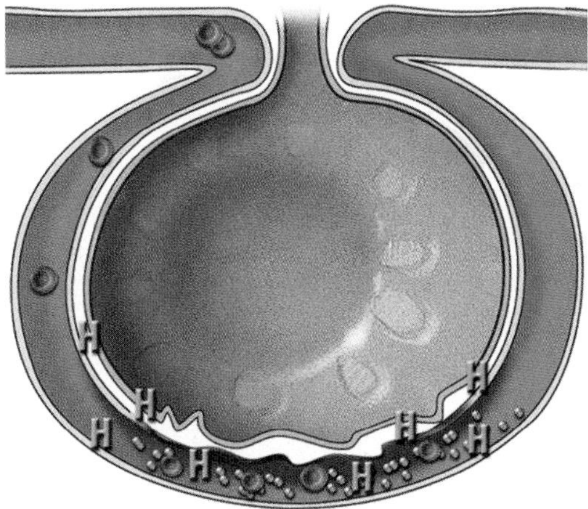

Phase 2. Those substances, especially histamine, inflame and damage the alveolar–capillary membrane, increasing capillary permeability. Fluids then shift into the interstitial space.

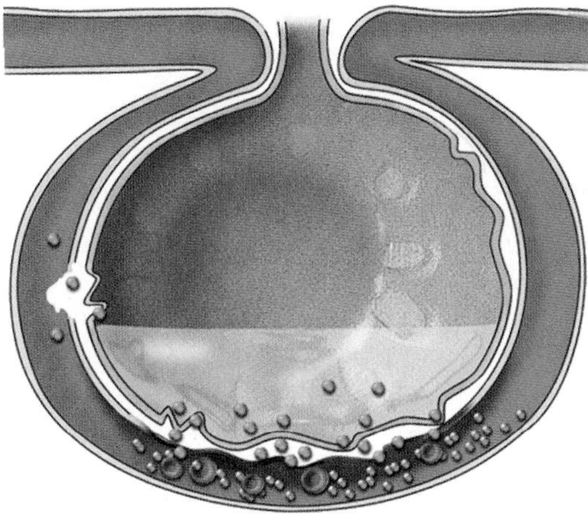

Phase 3. As capillary permeability increases, proteins and fluids leak out, increasing interstitial osmotic pressure and causing pulmonary edema.

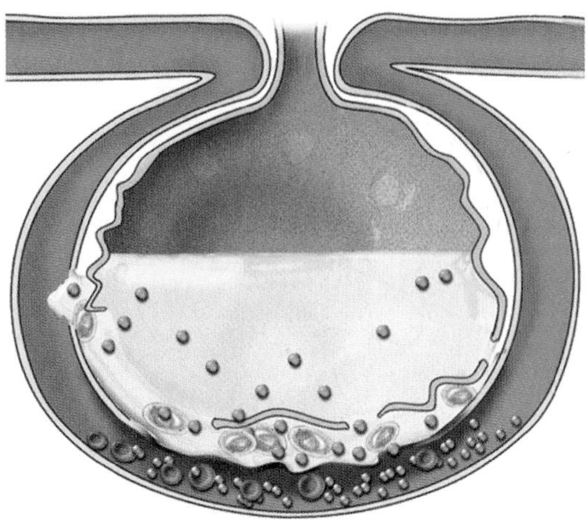

Phase 4. Decreased blood flow and fluids in the alveoli damage surfactant and impair the cell's ability to produce more. As a result, alveoli collapse, impeding gas exchange and decreasing lung compliance.

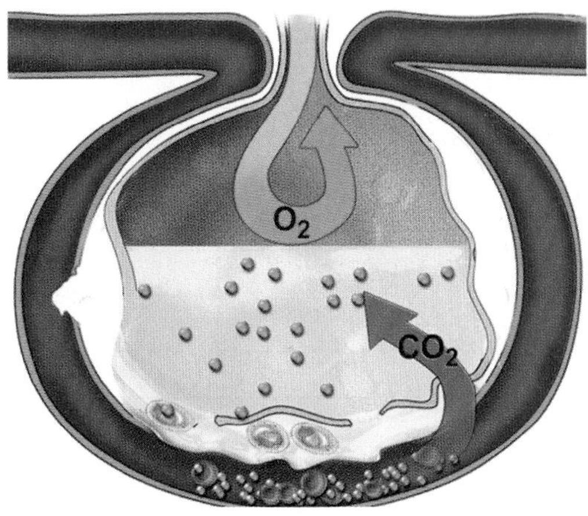

Phase 5. Sufficient oxygen cannot cross the alveolar–capillary membrane, but carbon dioxide (CO_2) can and is lost with every exhalation. Oxygen (O_2) and CO_2 levels decrease in the blood.

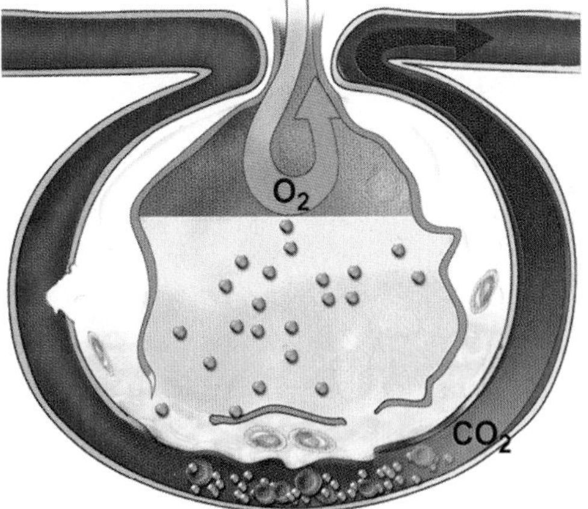

Phase 6. Pulmonary edema worsens, inflammation leads to fibrosis, and gas exchange is further impeded.

figure 27-1 Pathogenesis of acute respiratory distress syndrome (ARDS). Changes in lung epithelium and vascular endothelium result in fluid and protein movement, changes in lung compliance, and disruption of the alveoli with accompanying hypoxia. (Source: Anatomical Chart Company: Atlas of Pathophysiology, pp 79, 81. Springhouse, PA, Springhouse, 2001.)

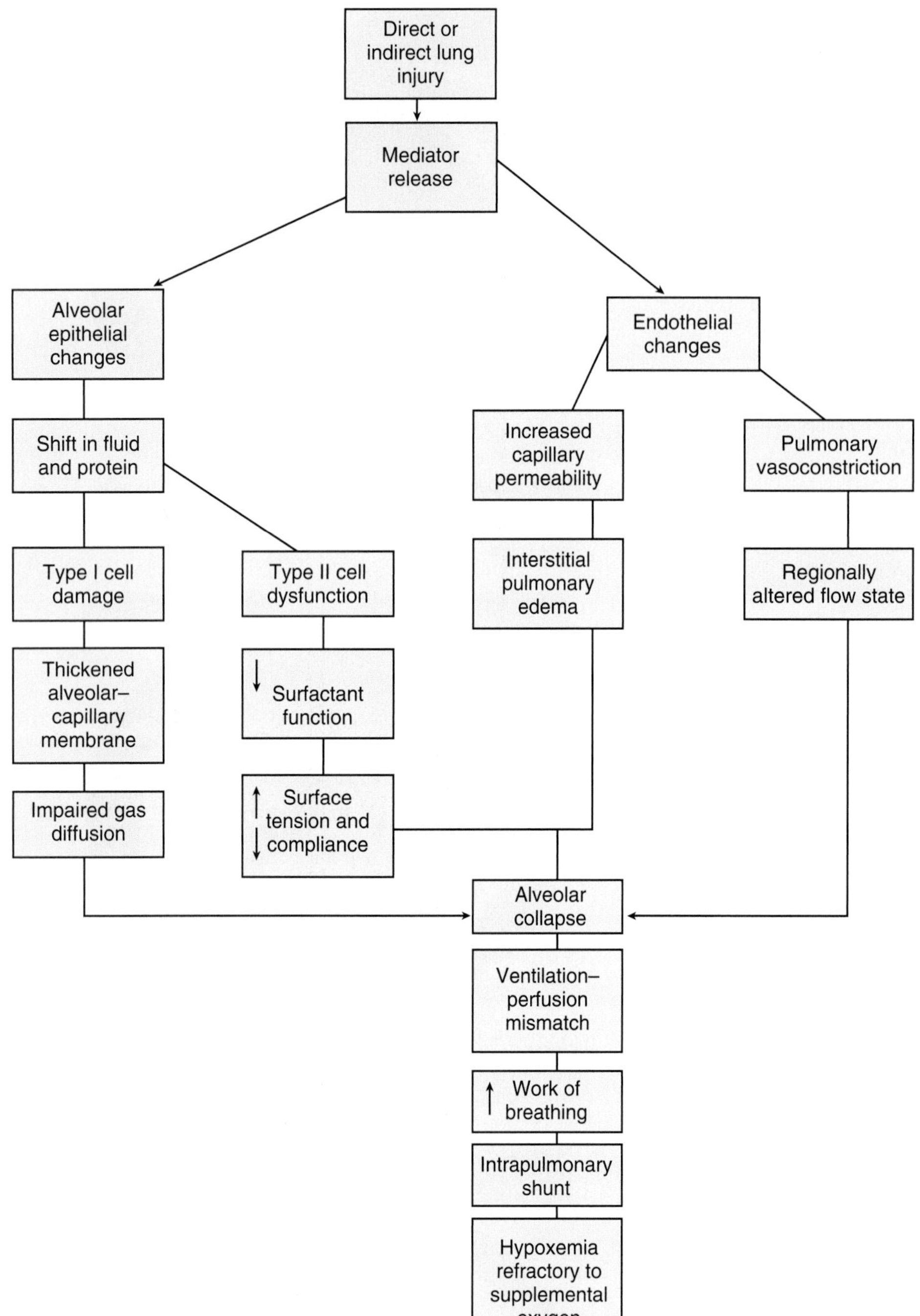

figure 27-2 Pathophysiological cascade is initiated by injury resulting in mediator release. The multiple effects result in changes to the alveoli, vascular tissue, and bronchi. The ultimate effect is ventilation–perfusion mismatching and refractory hypoxemia.

symptoms of respiratory distress increase in severity, with cyanosis, coarse bilateral crackles on auscultation, and radiographic changes consistent with patchy infiltrates. It is at this point (stage 2) that the mediator-induced disruption of the vascular bed results in increased interstitial and alveolar edema. The endothelial and epithelial beds are increasingly permeable to proteins. The hypoxia is resistant to supplemental oxygen administration, and mechanical ventilation will most likely be commenced in response to a worsening ratio of arterial oxygen to inspired oxygen (PaO_2/FIO_2 ratio).

From the 2nd to the 10th day after injury (stage 3), evidence of SIRS is present, with hemodynamic instability, generalized edema, the possible onset of nosocomial infections, increasing hypoxemia, and lung involvement. Air bronchograms may be evident on chest radiography as well as decreased lung volumes and diffuse interstitial markings.

Stage 4, which develops after 10 days, is typified by few additional radiographic changes. There is increasing multiorgan involvement, SIRS, and increases in the arterial carbon dioxide tension ($PaCO_2$) as progressive lung fibrosis and emphysematous changes result in increased dead space. Fibrotic lung changes result in ventilation management difficulties, with increased airway pressure and development of pneumothoraces.

table 27-3 Clinical Presentation and Pathological Changes During Acute Respiratory Distress Syndrome (ARDS)

Radiographic Change	Clinical Presentation	Pathological Change
Stage 1 (first 12 hr): Normal chest x-ray	Dyspnea, tachypnea	Neutrophil sequestration, no evidence of cellular damage
Stage 2 (24 hr): Patchy alveolar infiltrate, primarily in dependent lung areas; normal heart size	Dyspnea, tachypnea, cyanosis, tachycardia, coarse crackles	Neutrophil infiltration, vascular congestion, fibrin strands, increased interstitial and alveolar edema
Stage 3 (2–10 days): Diffuse alveolar infiltrates, possibly air bronchograms, decreased lung volume, normal heart size	Hyperdynamic hemodynamic parameters, systemic inflammatory response syndrome (SIRS) presentation	Type II cell proliferation, microemboli formation, increased interstitial and alveolar inflammatory exudate
Stage 4 (>10 days): Persistent infiltrates, new pneumonic infiltrates, recurrent pneumothorax	Multiple organ involvement, difficulty maintaining adequate oxygenation, sepsis, pneumonia	Type II cell hyperplasia, thickening of interstitial wall with fibrosis, macrophages, fibroblasts, remodeling of arterioles

From van Soeren MH, Diehl-Jones WL, Maykut RJ, et al: Pathophysiology and implications for treatment of acute respiratory distress syndrome. AACN Clin Issues 11(2):179–197, 2000.

ASSESSMENT

History

The need for a complete and accurate history for the patient presenting with ARDS is important. The history may provide information that allows for removal of the precipitating cause, interrupting the ensuing mediator response. A thorough history may be difficult to obtain because the cause may occur before admission. This is a syndrome of uncertain outcome and, often, a long critical care admission; therefore, the health care team plays a large role in providing support to both the patient and the family. Developing a relationship early (e.g., by taking the time to obtain a thorough history) may assist with care throughout the course of admission.

All health care team members contribute information to the history. Information about past relevant incidents, the use of medical and complementary therapies, and social factors may be helpful for the person's care. Items of importance include assessment of risk factors for the development of ARDS (see Box 27-1), a social history to assess risk behaviors (e.g., human immunodeficiency virus status, smoking, substance abuse), medications (including over-the-counter [OTC] medications), and complementary therapies (all exogenous substances, including inhalations). This information is obtained in addition to the history of the present illness and presenting signs and symptoms.

Physical Examination

Acute respiratory failure initially may present within a few hours to several days, depending on the initial insult, and does not always progress to ARDS.[8] Monitoring patients who meet the SIRS criteria (see Box 27-1) may aid identification of those who are at risk for development of ARDS. No unexplained change in respiratory rate should be taken lightly because there are few reliable early indicators of impending ALI or ARDS. Vital signs throughout the progression of ARDS vary, but the general trend is hypotension, tachycardia, and hyperthermia or hypothermia. Respiration, initially rapid and labored, varies once mechanical ventilation is instituted.

Early signs and symptoms of respiratory failure include tachypnea, dyspnea, and tachycardia. Breath sounds often are clear in this phase. Patients with acute respiratory failure may exhibit neurological changes, such as restlessness and agitation associated with impaired oxygenation and decreased perfusion to the brain. Use of accessory respiratory muscles is evident. The cardiovascular response is tachycardia to improve cardiac output as compensation for poor tissue oxygenation. These attempts to reduce hypoxia represent an adaptive sympathetic nervous system response. In both ALI and ARDS, these attempts to reduce hypoxia will likely be ineffective because mediators are already circulating and triggering a cascade of systemic responses.

As the pathological changes progress, lung auscultation may reveal crackles secondary to an increase in secretions and narrowed airways; however, the bubbling crackles of cardiogenic pulmonary edema may be minimal. Assessment must be considered in the context of the presenting or initiating disease. For example, pneumonia, one risk factor for ARDS, may confound the ability to diagnose early-stage lung sound changes. The patient may be increasingly restless and confused secondary to hypoxia. Decreases in arterial oxygen saturation (SaO_2) are early signs of impending decompensation.

The ability to compensate decreases with increasing pathological changes to the lung, pulmonary vasculature, and bronchi. Dependent lung fields have decreased breath sounds as fluid accumulation and alveoli collapse occur. Agitation may give way to lethargy, an ominous sign in which interventions to support ventilation and oxygenation are required quickly. Other later stages of progression result from tissue hypoxia and include dysrhythmias, chest pain, decreased renal function, and decreased bowel sounds. These are indications of multisystem involvement as highly perfused organ systems respond to decreased oxygen delivery with diminished function.

In the later stages of ARDS, mechanical ventilation support is required. Consolidation of the lungs with fluid reduces breath sounds. Lung compliance is decreased and increasing difficulties maintaining ventilation in the face of increasing resistance ensue. Unexplained changes in ventilation (such as a decreased PaO_2 or increased peak inspiratory pressure) cannot be minimized because development of spontaneous pneumothoraces is a frequent complication of ARDS in the later stages. Transmitted sounds, poor air entry throughout all lung fields, and diffuse crackles coupled with ventilation make breath sounds difficult to assess. A further complicating event is myocardial depression, a mediated response. Therefore, in spite of persistent tachycardia, cardiac output decreases and hypotension results.

Diagnostic Studies

Throughout the stages of ARDS, the reliance on diagnostic tests is important (Table 27-4). In the early stages, the need to establish cause may require specific tests, such as blood cultures, bronchoalveolar lavage cultures, and computed tomography (CT) examinations for abscess (e.g., abdominal abscesses). In later stages, further vigilance is required to intervene for early management of any nosocomial infections. Ongoing monitoring of routine blood chemistry and hematology is done to ensure stability in metabolic parameters and optimization of existing function.

Recent research has focused on the use of plasma and bronchoalveolar lavage samples for detection of mediators, particularly elevated amounts of interleukin-1 (IL-1) and tumor necrosis factor-α (TNF-α), as early markers for diagnosis of ARDS.[9] This is currently experimental but will likely provide further information within the next 5 years. Of particular interest and importance are the following tests in the management of ARDS.

BLOOD GAS ANALYSIS

Deterioration of arterial blood gases (ABGs), despite interventions, is a hallmark of ARDS. Initially, hypoxemia (an arterial oxygen tension, or PaO_2, of <60 mm Hg) may improve with supplemental oxygen; however, refractory hypoxemia (no improvement of PaO_2 with supplemental oxygen) and a persistently low SaO_2 eventually develop. Early in acute respiratory failure, dyspnea and tachypnea

table 27-4 Integrated Assessment of the Patient With Acute Respiratory Distress Syndrome (ARDS)

Stage	Physical Examination	Diagnostic Test Results
Stage 1 (first 12 hr)	• Restlessness, dyspnea, tachypnea • Moderate to extensive use of accessory respiratory muscles	• *ABG:* Respiratory alkalosis • *CXR:* No radiographic changes • *Chemistry:* Blood results may vary depending on precipitating cause (e.g., elevated white blood cell count, changes in hemoglobin) • *Hemodynamics:* Elevated PAP, normal or low PAWP
Stage 2 (24 hr)	• Severe dyspnea, tachypnea, cyanosis, tachycardia • Coarse bilateral crackles • Decreased air entry to dependent lung fields • Increased agitation and restlessness	• *ABG:* Decreased SaO_2 despite supplemental oxygen administration • *CXR:* Patchy bilateral infiltrates • *Chemistry:* Increasing acidosis (metabolic) depending on severity of onset • *Hemodynamics:* Increasingly elevated PAP, normal or low PAWP
Stage 3 (2–10 days)	• Decreased air entry bilaterally • Impaired responsiveness (may be related to sedation necessary to maintain mechanical ventilation) • Decreased gut motility • Generalized edema • Poor skin integrity and breakdown	• *ABG:* Worsening hypoxemia • *CXR:* Air bronchograms, decreased lung volumes • *Chemistry:* Signs of other organ involvement: decreased platelets and hemoglobin, increased white blood cell count, abnormal clotting factors • *Hemodynamics:* Unchanged or becoming increasingly worse
Stage 4 (>10 days)	• Symptoms of MODS, including decreased urine output, poor gastric motility, symptoms of impaired coagulation **OR** • Single-system involvement of the respiratory system with gradual improvement over time	• *ABG:* Worsening hypoxemia and hypercapnia • *CXR:* Air bronchograms, pneumonthoraces • *Chemistry:* Persistent signs of other organ involvement: decreased platelets and hemoglobin, increased white blood cell count, abnormal clotting factors • *Hemodynamics:* Unchanged or becoming increasingly worse

ABG, arterial blood gas; *CXR,* chest radiograph; *MODS,* multisystem organ dysfunction syndrome; *PAP,* pulmonary artery pressure; *PAWP,* pulmonary artery wedge pressure.

are associated with a decreased $PaCO_2$. Hypercarbia develops as gas exchange and ventilation become increasingly impaired. Arterial pH in the early phase may be high (>7.45), a finding that is consistent with respiratory alkalosis secondary to rapid respirations and a low $PaCO_2$. The arterial pH measurements in ARDS are typically lower because of respiratory and ventilatory failure and tissue hypoxia, anaerobic metabolism, and subsequent metabolic acidosis. Base excess and deficit follow a similar trend, depending on the degree of tissue and organ hypoxia.

Measurement of arterial lactate is commonly ordered as an indication of tissue hypoxia and anaerobic metabolism. An elevated blood lactate concentration is common in early ARDS and resolves as oxygenation improves. Lactate measurement is not done routinely once adequate, although perhaps not optimal, oxygenation has been achieved.

RADIOGRAPHIC STUDIES

In the early phase of ARDS, the chest radiographic changes are usually negligible. Within a few days, the chest x-ray findings show patchy bilateral alveolar infiltrates, usually in the dependent lung fields. This may be mistaken for cardiogenic pulmonary edema. Over time, these patchy infiltrates progress to diffuse infiltrates, consolidation, and air bronchograms. CT of the chest also shows areas of infiltrates and consolidation of lung tissue. Daily chest x-rays are important in the continuing evaluation of the progression and resolution of ARDS and for ongoing assessment of potential complications, especially pneumothoraces.

INTRAPULMONARY SHUNT MEASUREMENT

An intrapulmonary shunt is a type of ventilation–perfusion mismatch. It may be defined as the percentage of cardiac output that is not oxygenated owing to pulmonary blood flowing past collapsed or fluid-filled and nonventilated alveoli (a physiological shunt), absence of blood flow to ventilated alveoli (alveolar dead space), or a combination of both of these conditions (silent unit; see Chapter 23, Fig. 23-16). Normally, an intrapulmonary shunt of 3% to 5% is present in all people. Advanced respiratory failure and ARDS are associated with a shunt of 15% or more because of the pathological changes in blood flow, endothelial disruption, and alveolar collapse. As the intrapulmonary shunt increases to 15% and greater, more aggressive interventions, including mechanical ventilation, are required because this level of shunt is associated with profound hypoxemia and may be life-threatening.

The intrapulmonary shunt fraction (Qs/Qt) is calculated using the arterial oxygen content (CaO_2), the mixed venous oxygen content ($C\bar{v}O_2$), and the capillary oxygen content (CcO_2):

$$Qs/Qt = (CcO_2 - CaO_2) \div (CcO_2 - C\bar{v}O_2)$$

Oxygen content is determined by hemoglobin (Hgb), oxygen saturation (SO_2), and partial pressure of oxygen (PO_2), measured by calculating the oxygen content in the pulmonary capillary bed, in the systemic arterial system, and in the mixed venous blood from the pulmonary artery. The formulas to calculate oxygen content are:

$$CcO_2 = (Hgb \times 1.36 \times SaO_2) + (100 \times 0.0031)$$

$$CaO_2 = (Hgb \times 1.36 \times SaO_2) + (PaO_2 \times 0.0031)$$

$$C\bar{v}O_2 = (Hgb \times 1.36 \times S\bar{v}O_2) + (P\bar{v}O_2 \times 0.0031)$$

The intrapulmonary shunt fraction may be estimated using a simple calculation, the ratio of arterial oxygen to inspired oxygen (i.e., the PaO_2/FIO_2 ratio). In general, a PaO_2/FIO_2 ratio greater than 300 is normal, a value of 200 is associated with an intrapulmonary shunt of 15% to 20%, and a value of 100 is associated with an intrapulmonary shunt of more than 20%.

LUNG COMPLIANCE, AIRWAY RESISTANCE, AND PRESSURES

Lung mechanics are altered in ARDS, resulting in reduced alveolar ventilation and pulmonary gas exchange. Lung compliance, or distensibility, is decreased as the alveoli become fluid-filled or collapsed. More effort and greater pressure are required to move air into the lungs as they become increasingly "stiff." In addition, the resistance to airflow into and out of the lungs increases with the accumulation of secretions and mediator-induced bronchoconstriction. Because the patient with ARDS requires mechanical ventilation to support oxygenation and ventilation, lung compliance and airway resistance can be evaluated by assessing ventilator pressures and tidal volume changes.

Precise measurement of airway resistance involves measurement of airflow velocity and airway diameter; however, airway resistance may be estimated by comparing the ventilator peak inspiratory pressure to the plateau (static) pressure at end inspiration. A difference between these two pressures of 10 cm H_2O or less would suggest a normal airway resistance, whereas a difference greater than 10 cm H_2O would suggest increased resistance. Although evaluating the airway resistance by calculating the difference between the peak inspiratory pressure and the plateau pressure does not provide an exact measurement, this method is useful for trending changes and evaluating the effectiveness of interventions that are directed toward reducing airway resistance.

Lung compliance likewise may be estimated and trended. The static lung compliance calculation uses the plateau pressure and requires use of a specific constant associated with different types of mechanical ventilators. Dynamic lung compliance is less precise because its calculation uses the peak inspiratory pressure, which does not eliminate resistance factors; however, it is simpler and may be useful to trend through the course of ARDS.

$$Cdyn = V_T \div (PIP - PEEP)$$

where Cdyn = dynamic lung compliance; V_T = tidal volume; PIP = peak inspiratory pressure; and PEEP = positive end-expiratory pressure. The normal dynamic lung compliance is approximately 100 mL/cm H_2O.

Close monitoring of airway pressures, including the mean airway pressure, the peak inspiratory pressure, and the plateau pressure, is an important component of patient assessment in ARDS. Increases in these pressures as tidal volumes are maintained to achieve a normal $PaCO_2$ indicate reduced compliance and increased resistance to airflow. As airway pressures rise, the lung epithelium is traumatized, resulting in further lung tissue damage. Volutrauma (lung epithelial damage) or barotrauma from persistently elevated airway pressures thus has additional deleterious effects on ventilation and oxygenation.[10]

Possible nursing diagnoses for a patient with ARDS are given in Box 27-2.

MANAGEMENT

Therapeutic modalities for the treatment of ARDS have remained elusive. Treatment is supportive; that is, while contributing factors are corrected or reversed and the lungs heal, care is taken that treatment does no further damage. Figure 27-3 describes the current status of the management of ARDS.[2,8,10,11]

Oxygenation and Ventilation

OXYGEN DELIVERY

One of the hallmarks of ARDS is refractory hypoxemia; therefore, attention to improving oxygen delivery is paramount. Strategies include optimizing normal oxygen delivery parameters, including hemoglobin, cardiac output, and oxygen saturation. Oxygen delivery is the amount of oxygen delivered to the tissues and organs every minute and depends on the flow of oxygenated blood through the tissue beds. Oxygen delivery is determined by hemoglobin, arterial oxygenation, and cardiac output:

$$DaO_2 = CO \times (Hgb \times SaO_2 \times 1.38) + (PaO_2 \times 0.0031)$$

where DaO_2 = oxygen delivery; CO = cardiac output; Hgb = hemoglobin; SaO_2 = arterial oxygen saturation; and PaO_2 = arterial oxygen tension.

Adequate oxygen delivery, defined as a DaO_2 of greater than 800 mL O_2/minute, is essential to meet tissue requirements for oxygen, thereby preventing anaerobic metabolism and hypoxia, which can trigger and perpetuate SIRS. Critically ill patients with ARDS have high demands for oxygen to maintain organ function.

Hemoglobin combines with oxygen to form oxyhemoglobin; therefore, sufficient amounts of hemoglobin are necessary to carry oxygen to the cells. There is little research to support the intuitive concept that normal or increased hemoglobin is required to promote oxygen delivery in patients with SIRS or ARDS. Recent studies on transfusion requirements indicate that values of approximately 8.0 g/dL are sufficient for critically ill patients, except for those with cardiac disease. Therefore, transfusion to maintain normal hemoglobin is no longer accepted therapy and should be discouraged.[12]

Cardiac output is typically altered in ARDS because of the SIRS response, the effect of hypoxemia on the myocardium, and the decrease in venous return induced by mechanical ventilation. Evaluation of the cardiac output is important to assess oxygen delivery and initiate appropriate interventions. Therapies to optimize cardiac output are directed toward enhancing preload and contractility and normalizing afterload. Use of a thermodilution pulmonary artery catheter to assess oxygen delivery and consumption is routine for patients with ARDS to ensure that the appropriate interventions are instituted.

Fluid administration to ensure adequate intravascular volume and optimize preload is important before other interventions are initiated. Controversy exists regarding the administration of crystalloids or colloids in patients with ARDS because of the increased permeability of capillaries and the risks of worsening pulmonary function.[8] In general, the pulmonary artery wedge pressure (PAWP) should be maintained at greater than 12 mm Hg and breath sounds and ABGs closely monitored during fluid administration.

Positive inotropic agents, such as dopamine or dobutamine, are used to enhance contractility and increase cardiac output.[8,13] Vasoconstrictors, such as norepinephrine, may be added to the therapies to counteract the SIRS-induced vasodilation. Vasoconstricting agents, however, must be administered cautiously because many vascular beds, especially in the lungs, are constricted, also as a result of SIRS mediators and hypoxia. Patients receiving inotropic or vasoactive drugs require regular evaluation of cardiac output, systemic vascular resistance, and PAWP, in addition to continuous arterial blood pressure monitoring.

MECHANICAL VENTILATION

The goal of therapy is to improve tissue oxygenation and ventilation. Methods to deliver appropriate levels of oxygen and allow for removal of carbon dioxide include types of mechanical ventilation and positioning. Techniques to limit ventilator-associated (or induced) lung injury (VALI), including the use of low tidal volumes (<6 mL/kg predicted body weight), the use of adequate PEEP (to reduce the risk of using a high fraction of inspired oxygen and precipitating oxygen toxicity), and limiting plateau pressures to 30 cm H_2O or less are under study, as are novel therapies such as extracorporeal lung-assist technology, partial liquid ventilation, and high-frequency oscillation ventilation

box 27-2 *Examples of Nursing Diagnoses and Collaborative Problems for the Patient With Acute Respiratory Distress Syndrome*

- Impaired Gas Exchange related to refractory hypoxemia and pulmonary interstitial/alveolar leaks found in alveolar capillary injury states
- Ineffective Airway Clearance related to increased secretion production and decreased ciliary motion
- Ineffective Breathing Patterns related to inadequate gas exchange, increased secretions, decreased ability to oxygenate adequately, fear, or exhaustion
- Anxiety related to critical illness, fear of death, role changes, or permanent disability
- Risk for Infection related to invasive monitoring devices and endotracheal tube

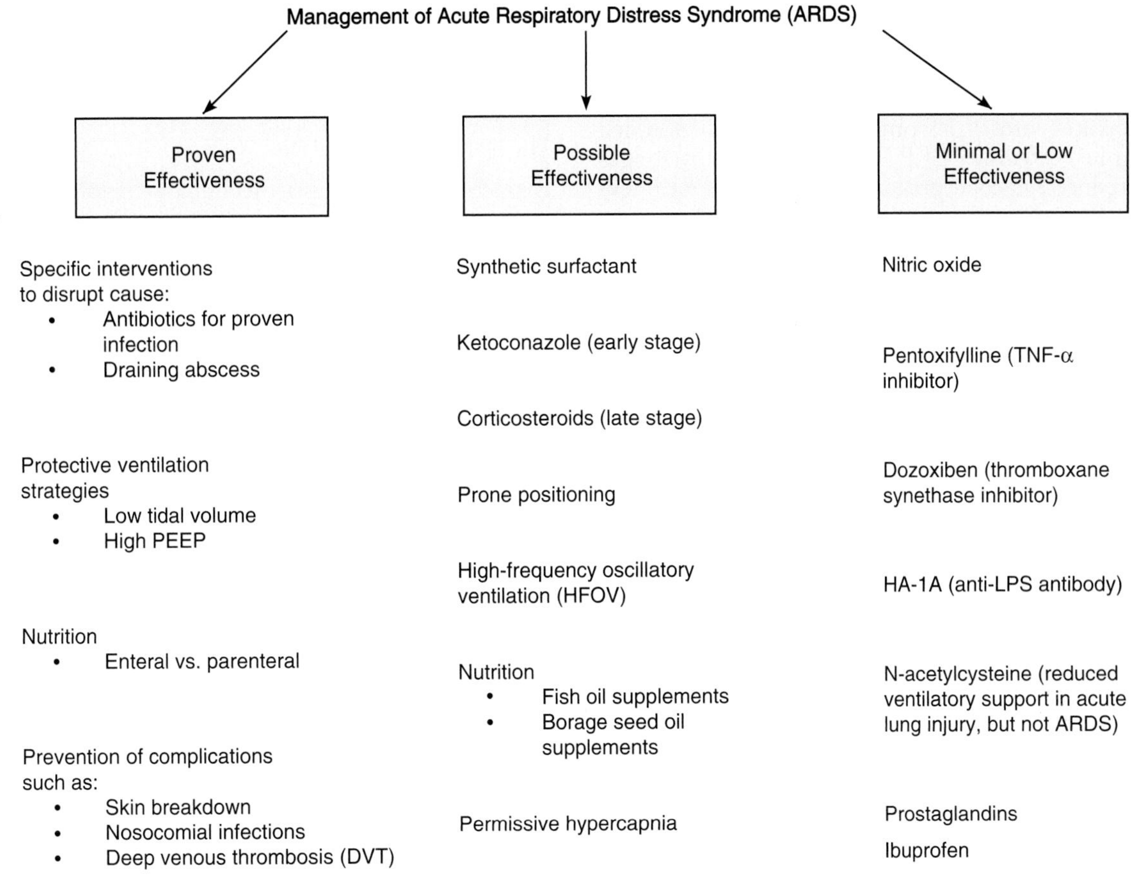

figure 27-3 Management of acute respiratory distress syndrome (ARDS). Treatment involves interventions of proven, possible, or minimal to low effectiveness. Therapies supported by multicentered trials are included in the proven list. No item in this list, except specific interventions to disrupt cause, have been shown to treat ARDS; rather, they provide adjunct therapy to reduce complications or length of ventilator days. Items that appear in the possible effectiveness category have support through limited individual studies with promising results. One of the primary issues in obtaining proof of efficacy includes a lack of randomized controlled trials for many treatments currently in use. *PEEP,* positive end-expiratory pressure; *TNF-α,* tumor necrosis factor-α.

(HFOV).[2,11,14] Kinetic bed therapy and prone positioning have been implicated in improvements in oxygenation in patients with ARDS, but there remains no conclusive evidence that mortality is decreased.[15]

Multiple modes of mechanical ventilation are available to support the patient with respiratory failure. In general, the principle of "do no harm" includes use of the lowest fraction of inspired oxygen (FIO_2) to achieve adequate oxygenation and use of small tidal volumes (<6 mL/kg) to minimize airway pressures, thus preventing or reducing lung damage (barotrauma and volutrauma) while maintaining the $PaCO_2$ within a relatively normal range. PEEP prevents collapse and opens alveolar sacs, allowing diffusion of gases across the alveolar–capillary membrane. Recommended values for PEEP are 10 to 15 cm H_2O, but values in excess of 20 cm H_2O are acceptable to reduce inspired oxygen requirements or maintain adequate oxygenation.

Several modes of mechanical ventilation are directed toward minimizing airway pressures and iatrogenic lung injury, associated with conventional volume-controlled mechanical ventilation.[12,14] Pressure-controlled ventilation limits the peak inspiratory pressure to a set level (as opposed to volume-controlled ventilation, which delivers a set tidal volume despite the pressure required to move the set volume into the lungs). Pressure-controlled ventilation also uses a decelerating inspiratory airflow pattern to minimize the peak pressure while delivering the necessary tidal volume. Patients on pressure-controlled ventilation mode typically require significant amounts of sedation and pharmacological paralysis to prevent attempts at breathing and dyssynchrony with the ventilator. Airway pressure release ventilation is similar to pressure-controlled ventilation but with the advantage of allowing the patient to initiate breaths; therefore, these patients do not require the same level of sedation or paralysis to achieve pressure-limited ventilation.[16]

Inverse ratio ventilation is another strategy thought to improve alveolar recruitment.[2] Reversal of the normal inspiratory:expiratory ratio (I:E ratio) to 2:1 or 3:1 prolongs inspiration time, preventing complete exhalation. An inverse I:E ratio is achieved through manipulation of the mechanical ventilator. This increased end-expiratory volume creates auto-PEEP (intrinsic PEEP) that is added to the applied extrinsic PEEP. The theoretical advantages include reduced alveolar pressures and overall PEEP levels. This therapy requires patients to be sedated or given paralytics to improve tolerance.

Permissive hypercapnia is a strategy that allows the $Pa{CO_2}$ to rise slowly above normal through reduction of tidal volume, therefore limiting the plateau and peak airway pressures. A $Pa{CO_2}$ between 55 and 60 mm Hg and a pH of 7.25 to 7.35 are tolerated when achieved in a gradual fashion.[2]

HFOV uses very low tidal volumes delivered at rates between 60 and 100 breaths/minute, resulting in lower airway pressures and reduced barotrauma. Deleterious effects of HFOV include increased trapping of air in the alveoli (auto-PEEP) and increased mean airway pressures to high levels in some patients. Research is ongoing as to the possible effectiveness of this mode of ventilation.[11]

Regardless of the recent interest in ventilation strategies, no method has been shown to be superior in the treatment of ARDS, and ventilation management and choice remains a complex decision based on the application of multiple methods for individual cases. Larger randomized, controlled trials are needed before a full understanding of which strategy provides the optimal patient support is achieved.

EXTRACORPOREAL LUNG-ASSIST TECHNOLOGY

Extracorporeal lung-assist technology involves the use of large vascular cannulas to remove blood from the patient. A pumping device and circuit circulate the blood, and one or two "artificial lungs" remove carbon dioxide and oxygenate the blood.[2,11] Extracorporeal membrane oxygenation (ECMO) and extracorporeal carbon dioxide removal ($ECCO_2R$) may potentially be effective in the management of ARDS, but at present their use is controversial. These highly invasive, high-risk technologies allow the lungs to "rest" because near-apneic ventilation or ventilation with small tidal volumes and slow respiratory rates greatly reduces airway pressures while gas exchange takes place in the artificial membrane lungs. The need for intensive resources and personnel with a high degree of expertise, coupled with the potential for devastating complications (particularly intracranial hemorrhage) and a lack of conclusive benefits for patients with ARDS, make extracorporeal lung-assist technology of limited use. In the pediatric population, the use of ECMO has demonstrated benefit with improved survival rates[17] (Table 27-5).

insights into clinical research

Rocker G, MacKenzie M-G, Williams B, et al: Noninvasive positive pressure ventilation: Successful outcome in patients with acute lung injury/ARDS. Chest 115(1):173–177, 1999

There is increasing support for the use of noninvasive positive-pressure ventilation (NPPV) in the treatment of acute respiratory failure secondary to exacerbation of chronic obstructive pulmonary disease (COPD), particularly in patients presenting with hypercarbic respiratory failure. However, there are few reports on the use of NPPV in patients with ALI/ARDS. With the recognition of the importance of avoiding the potential complications and adverse effects of intubation and mechanical ventilation, application of this technique may be beneficial for some patients with ALI/ARDS.

In this pilot study, Rocker and colleagues reported the outcome of treating ten patients (3 men, 7 women, mean age 47 years) who met the American–European diagnostic criteria for ARDS, with NPPV. The method used for NPPV was a full facemask connected to a ventilator with continuous positive airway pressure adjusted to maintain the fraction of inspired oxygen ($F{IO_2}$) at less than 60% with an arterial oxyhemoglobin saturation of more than 90%. Success was defined as the withdrawal of facemask ventilation without the need for further assisted ventilation for an additional 72 hours. Failure was defined as the need for conventional intubation or further provision of NPPV within a 72-hour period from the end of a previous NPPV trial. Use of NPPV was assessed 108 times, with the technique implemented 12 times. Results showed that the overall survival rate was 70% (7 of 10), with 3 intensive care unit (ICU) deaths occurring 5, 8, and 16 days after ICU admission. The overall success rate for the NPPV trials was 6 of 12 (50%). The average duration of successful NPPV was 64.5 hours (range, 23.5 to 80.5 hours), with ICU discharge in the next 24 to 48 hours for three of six patients. Unsuccessful episodes lasted an average of 7.3 hours (range, 0.1 hour to 116 hours), followed by the need for conventional ventilation for an additional 5 days. The length of ICU stay was reduced with successful NPPV (3.7 days) versus 7 days when the treatment failed and conventional ventilation was used. No patients experienced complications related to NPPV, such as skin necrosis, gastric distension, nosocomial pneumonia, or evidence of barotrauma. The average APACHE II (Acute Physiology and Chronic Health Evaluation) scores of greater than 20 and only one patient with multiple organ failure suggest a group of less severely ill patients that may indicate limitations for use of NPPV, but further study is required.

In this report, intubation and mechanical ventilation was avoided 50% of the time. NPPV may be a useful strategy to limit ventilator-associated lung injury such as barotrauma or volutrauma and nosocomial pneumonia. In patients with ARDS, NPPV reduces the work of breathing and preserves a tidal volume compatible with adequate alveolar ventilation. The use of NPPV may be limited to less severely ill patients with ALI/ARDS; however, those who respond should benefit from improvements in respiratory rate, respiratory muscle activity, and gas exchange as well as reduction in complications associated with treatment and decreased length of stay.

table 27-5 Additional Treatment Options and Their Implications for Neonates and Children

Treatment	Use in Pediatric Patients	Potential Complications
Extracorporeal membrane oxygenation (ECMO)	Used as cardiac support pretransplantation and as salvage therapy in severe lung injury. 18,000 cases in Extracorporeal Life Support Organization database. Survival rates of more than 80% in neonates and 40%–50% in older children.[17]	Use of exogenous anticoagulation may lead to cellular damage and bleeding; intracranial hemorrhage; neurological damage; sepsis; multisystem organ dysfunction (MODS).
Nitric oxide	Used in management of pulmonary hypertension in children and neonates.	With high levels (>60%) of nitric oxide, formation of methemoglobin and resultant methemoglobinemia leads to decreased hemoglobin oxygen binding capacity, causing seizures, coma, cardiac dysrhythmias, and death. Nitrogen dioxide toxicity and rebound pulmonary hypertension and dyspnea can result if nitric oxide is suddenly discontinued.
Surfactant	Accepted therapy in neonates because of outcome studies demonstrating improved oxygenation, earlier extubation, and fewer intensive care unit days. Some promising evidence with children as well.[17]	No major adverse effects.

PARTIAL LIQUID VENTILATION

Phase II clinical trials are underway using perfluorocarbons in the prevention of lung injury and infection for patients with ALI and ARDS.[11] The use of liquid breathing with perfluorocarbons as the medium for gas exchange is thought to provide decreased surface tension, assist with distension of collapsed alveoli, and remove inflammatory debris. In the pediatric setting, partial liquid ventilation has gained wider acceptance; however, promising results indicate further use in the future in the adult population. Similar to ECMO, the requirement of resources not readily available in nonacademic centers may limit any proliferation of use for some time even if efficacy is established, but this therapy may be a focus of innovative treatment in the next decade.

POSITIONING

Frequent position change is well established as a means to prevent and reverse atelectasis and facilitate removal of secretions from the airways. Although not a treatment for ARDS, turning a patient side to side, having the patient sit upright, and using the Trendelenburg position for postural drainage are necessary interventions to prevent worsening of respiratory failure due to atelectasis and pneumonia. Continuous lateral rotation using a kinetic therapy bed turns patients slowly 60 degrees to each side over 11 minutes and is useful to enhance secretion removal.[15]

Prone positioning, in the patient's bed or using a Stryker frame, improves pulmonary gas exchange, facilitates pulmonary drainage in the dorsal lung regions, and aids resolution of consolidated dependent alveoli (in the supine position), particularly in the dorsal lung regions. The evidence for the effectiveness of prone positioning, now a common intervention with ARDS, is variable. Randomized, controlled trials are under way and these results will be necessary before support for prone positioning becomes clear.[11,14] There are alternative explanations for the improved oxygenation associated with prone positioning, and the question of whether the improvement in oxygenation persists beyond 4 hours remains controversial.[16] The risks associated with this technique include loss of airway control through accidental extubation, loss of vascular access, facial edema and development of pressure areas, and difficulties with cardiopulmonary resuscitation (CPR). Recommendations from the University of Pennsylvania on the steps involved in prone positioning appear in Balas[10] (Box 27-3).

Pharmacological Therapy

TREATMENT

Most of the pharmacological agents used in the ARDS population are supportive. Many agents have been developed as treatments directed toward specific mediators to disrupt or interfere with the development of SIRS. Most of these promising pharmacological interventions have ultimately proven to be ineffective in humans, notably anti-TNF drugs, most anti-inflammatory mediators, and inhaled gases such as nitric oxide.[2,14] Of the treatments now available, the most promising are surfactant, corticosteroids (used in late-stage ARDS), and ketoconazole (used for prevention and in the very early stages).

Antibiotic therapy is appropriate in the presence of a known microorganism but should not be used prophylactically.[18] The signs of SIRS are similar to those of infection (i.e., tachycardia, fever, increased white blood cell count), thus creating the temptation to treat the patient with SIRS with antimicrobial therapy. It is essential to identify a source of infection (isolation of specific bacteria through blood, wound, pulmonary, and other cultures) before ini-

box 27-3
Summary of Key Steps to Consider for Prone Positioning

1. Recruit an interdisciplinary team to evaluate the patient's condition and determine if a trial of prone positioning is warranted.
2. Organize the team to ensure familiarity with the procedure and patient care while prone.
   - Use your hospital's evidence-based procedure
   - Equipment on site
   - Assign and clarify team roles during proning
3. Prepare the patient for the procedure.
   - Provide explanation to patient and family
   - Consider insertion of feeding tube, nasogastric tube, or both as necessary
4. Assess and document the patient's pre-proning status.
   - Hemodynamic and ventilatory parameters, skin or wound condition, and so forth.
5. Protect and maintain the patient's airway.
   - Secure endotracheal tube
   - Apply in-line suction if not already in place
6. Use safety precautions to ensure body position will be maintained during the proning procedure.
7. Administer adequate sedation, analgesic, and anxiolytic medication.
8. Complete the procedure as per protocol. Note: Risks of inadvertent extubation or line displacement are high during the procedure.
9. Assess, evaluate, and monitor the patient's condition.
10. Continue preventive care for pressure areas, eyes, and skin.

tiation of antibiotics. Prophylactic antibiotic therapy has not been shown to improve outcome. Emphasis is on prevention of infection, especially nosocomial infection related to the use of invasive vascular catheters and ventilators (e.g., ventilator-associated pneumonia [VAP]).

Bronchodilators and mucolytics are useful in ARDS to assist in maintaining airway patency and reducing the inflammatory reaction and accumulation of secretions in the airways. The response to therapy is evaluated by monitoring airway resistance and pressures and lung compliance.

Exogenous surfactant replacement therapy has been used for several years in neonates with hyaline membrane disease to decrease alveolar surface tension and facilitate the maintenance of open alveoli[17] (see Table 27-5). Administration of surfactant to adults with ARDS has shown some usefulness, but requires further investigation. A phase II trial is underway using synthetic surfactant with novel inhalation techniques to improve drug delivery.[19]

The use of corticosteroids to decrease the inflammatory response in late stages of ARDS is regaining popularity with recent case studies and one randomized, controlled trial supporting low doses in the 7- to 10-day range of ARDS.[2,8] Further research is underway to determine whether these results remain consistent in larger studies.

Newer pharmacological agents directed toward blocking mediators and the SIRS inflammatory cascade are under investigation, but none has proven effective in treating ARDS. Nitric oxide is an inhaled gas that causes selective pulmonary vasodilation and therefore reduces the deleterious effects of pulmonary hypertension. In spite of widespread use, to date, nitric oxide has not been shown to improve mortality or oxygenation beyond the first 24 hours of therapy,[20] although there is some evidence of effectiveness for children and neonates[17] (see Table 27-5). Other agents that have demonstrated no positive effects on the outcomes of ARDS are[2]:

- Antioxidants, such as *N*-acetylcysteine. *N*-acetylcysteine, a glutathione analog, replenishes glutathione, a natural antioxidant, possibly decreasing endothelial damage caused by oxygen radicals and reducing the ventilatory time in patients with mild to moderate ALI, but not ARDS.
- Antilipid mediators, such as prostacyclin (prostaglandin I_2 [PGI_2]), and nonsteroidal anti-inflammatory drugs (NSAIDs), such as ibuprofen or indomethacin. These agents theoretically interact with the arachidonic acid cascade metabolites, which produce lung endothelial injury and inflammation.
- Monoclonal antibodies. These agents were developed to interfere with specific mediators that increase white blood cell (neutrophil) adhesion and activation, contribute to the inflammatory response, and cause endothelial injury.
- Pentoxifylline. This drug was thought to be an effective anticytokine agent.

SEDATION

Effective use of sedation to promote comfort and reduce respiratory effort, thus decreasing oxygen demand, is an important consideration for nurses dealing with patients with ARDS. Neuromuscular blocking agents and general anesthetics such as propofol are all used to decrease the work of breathing and facilitate ventilation for patients with ARDS. These have long- and short-term side effects. The risks include polyneuropathy of critical illness, overfeeding with lipids, and prolongation of days requiring ventilation.[21] Recent studies have focused on distinguishing between pain, anxiety, and delirium, all possible reasons for patients in critical care to require pharmacological interventions. It is vital for all people administering these agents to realize why each is being given, what the goals of therapy are, and what the long-term implications of overuse can be. These considerations are balanced with the need to decrease oxygen demand and provide comfort for patients requiring intensive ventilation management and undergoing potentially uncomfortable procedures.

Nutritional Support

Early initiation of nutritional support is essential for patients with ARDS because we now realize that nutrition plays an active therapeutic role in recovery from critical illness.[22] There are two major theoretical reasons to use early enteral feeding as a therapeutic intervention in SIRS and ARDS. Mediators (TNF-α and IL-1 in particular) stimulate release of proteolytic enzymes that stimulate protein catabolism from skeletal muscle. Persistent protein loss is compounded by interstitial loss through capillary leak and downregulation of messenger RNA (mRNA) production of intravascular proteins such as albumin. Earlier in this chapter, reference was made to changes in circulatory patterns due to hypoxic sympathetic nervous system reactions. In this way, there is decreased perfusion to the gut. After resuscitation, increases in neutrophil release further damage the injured, reperfused colon through increased vascular endothelial permeability, thus releasing normal gut bacteria into the systemic circulation and leading to increases in the incidence of peritonitis, pneumonia, and sepsis. The mechanism through which enteral feeding improves outcome remains unproven, but the reduction in mortality in the critically ill who are enterally fed indicates that this practice is of general benefit.

A balanced caloric, protein, carbohydrate, and fat intake is calculated based on metabolic needs, with particular attention paid to specific amino acids, lipid, and carbohydrate intake. Patients with SIRS or ARDS usually require 35 to 45 kcal/kg/day. High-carbohydrate solutions are avoided to prevent excess carbon dioxide production. Intralipids are judiciously administered to prevent further upregulation of the lipid mediators of SIRS, which contribute to inflammation and lung injury.

The problem that faces the practitioner is the ability to deliver enteral nutrition in the face of decreased gut motility. Insertion of small bowel feeding tubes may be considered. The role of total parenteral nutrition is controversial and some clinicians rarely use it, either alone or in combination with enteral nutrition.[23] The risk of aspiration associated with enteral feeding needs to be appreciated, and careful monitoring of absorption and gut function is essential.

A collaborative care guide for the patient with ARDS is given in Box 27-4.

PREVENTION OF COMPLICATIONS

Complications of ARDS are primarily related to SIRS, VALI, and immobility imposed by critical illness. The most serious of these is the development of MODS due to hypoxemia, hypoxia, and the persistent inflammatory response. The mortality rate of ARDS continues to be more than 60% when associated with MODS.[2]

Mechanical ventilation with high levels of PEEP, high tidal volumes, and volume-controlled modes predisposes the patient with ARDS to volutrauma and barotrauma, as previously described. Barotrauma may present as a pneumothorax, pneumomediastinum, or subcutaneous or interstitial emphysema. Prompt chest tube insertion is required for the presence of a pneumothorax. Prevention of volutrauma and barotrauma by maintaining the lowest possible airway pressures, PEEP, and tidal volumes may be achieved through the use of pressure-limiting modes of mechanical ventilation.

Immobility due to bed rest, sedation, or pharmacological paralysis has multisystem effects. Nosocomial pneumonia not infrequently is acquired from accumulation of secretions in the airways and atelectasis secondary to immobilization, with bacterial access through the endotracheal tube. As discussed, frequent repositioning and prone positioning accompanied by chest physiotherapy help to reduce stasis of secretions and facilitate removal. Endotracheal suctioning using the endotracheal tube to remove secretions is necessary but poses risks related to disconnecting the ventilator and introducing microorganisms. The use of in-line suction catheters reduces incidence of nosocomial pneumonia related to suctioning. Suctioning only when indicated (to avoid inducing a reduction in the $Sa{O_2}$), using sterile technique, and avoiding use of saline instillation reduce the transmission of bacteria into the lungs.

Deep venous thrombosis (DVT) and subsequent pulmonary embolus may be life-threatening complications of immobility. Initiation of DVT prophylaxis within 48 hours of admission minimizes the risk for development of DVT. Low-dose heparin, graded elastic stockings, external pneumatic compression devices, frequent mobilization, and ambulation have shown utility in reducing DVT formation.

The physiological aging process compounds the severity of the metabolic insults and complications of ARDS (Box 27-5).

case study ■ ACUTE RESPIRATORY DISTRESS SYNDROME

Mr. Jenkins, a 25-year-old man, presented to the emergency department (ED) after a 3-week history of cough and respiratory symptoms. He had seen his family physician 5 days before admission and had been put on oral antibiotics for community-acquired pneumonia. His sister had brought him into the ED 2 days ago because his symptoms had not improved. He was afebrile at that time. His oxygen saturation was 95% on room air and his physical examination and chest x-ray were consistent with a right lower lobe community-acquired pneumonia. The man was sent home to complete the course of antibiotics, with instructions to call the family physician if there was no improvement.

Today he has returned to the ED. At the time of admission, his oxygen saturation was 88% on 100% oxygen by facemask. His vital signs were: temperature 104°F (40°C); respirations 36 breaths/minute; pulse rate 115 beats/minute; and blood pressure 100/50 mm Hg. The patient was orally intubated and mechanically ventilated using lung-protective strategies. After intubation, his blood pressure fell to 60/30 mm Hg and he was started on dopamine infusion after volume resuscitation with normal saline. Arterial blood gases (ABGs) on admission were as follows: pH 7.16; $Pa{O_2}$ 73 mm Hg; $Pa{CO_2}$ 47 mm Hg; bicarbonate 16 mEq/L; and $Sa{O_2}$ 90% on an $FI{O_2}$ of 80% using assist-control ventilation with tidal volumes initially at 8 mL/kg and then reduced to 6 mL/kg. Sedation was started with morphine and midazolam infusions. Early enteral feeding was started within 12 hours of intubation; however, decreased gastric motility secondary to sepsis limited achieving a goal rate until 5 days. At the time of admission, the patient's chest x-ray indicated diffuse bilateral patchy infiltrates. His pulmonary artery wedge pressure (PAWP) was 14 mm Hg. He was admitted to the intensive care unit with a diagnosis of sepsis/ARDS as a result of pneumonia.

(text continues on page 625)

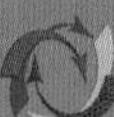

box 27-4 collaborative care guide *for the Patient With Acute Respiratory Distress Syndrome (ARDS)*

OUTCOMES	INTERVENTIONS
Oxygenation/Ventilation	
Patent airway will be maintained. A PaO_2:FIO_2 ratio of 200 to 300 or more will be maintained, if possible.	■ Auscultate breath sounds every 2 to 4 hours and as required. ■ Intubate to maintain oxygenation and ventilation and decrease work of breathing. ■ Suction endotracheal airway when appropriate (see Chapter 25, Box 25-16, Collaborative Care Guide for the Patient on Mechanical Ventilation). ■ Hyperoxygenate and hyperventilate before and after each suction pass.
Lung-protective ventilation strategies will be used. Maintain a low tidal volume (<6 mL/kg), a plateau pressure less than or equal to 30 cm H_2O, and PEEP levels titrated to pressure–volume curve.	■ Monitor airway pressures every 1 to 2 hours. ■ Monitor airway pressures after suctioning. ■ Administer bronchodilators and mucolytics. ■ Obtain a PEEP study to determine optimal oxygen delivery. ■ Consider a change in ventilator mode to prevent barotrauma and volutrauma.
The risk of atelectasis, ventilator-associated pneumonia (VAP), and barotrauma will be reduced and oxygenation will be improved.	■ Turn side-to-side every 2 hours. ■ Perform chest physiotherapy every 4 hours, if tolerated. ■ Consider kinetic therapy or prone positioning. ■ Take chest x-ray daily.
Oxygenation will be maximized (a PaO_2 of 55 to 80 mm Hg or an SaO_2 of 88% to 95%).	■ Monitor pulse oximetry and end-tidal carbon dioxide. ■ Monitor arterial blood gases as indicated by changes in noninvasive parameters. ■ Monitor intrapulmonary shunt (Qs/Qt and PaO_2:FIO_2 ratio). ■ Increase PEEP and FIO_2 to decrease intrapulmonary shunting, using lowest possible FIO_2. ■ Consider permissive hypercapnea to maximize oxygenation. ■ Monitor for signs of barotrauma, especially pneumothorax. ■ Consider risk of prolonged hyperoxia and decrease FIO_2 to less than 65% as soon as able.
Circulation/Perfusion	
Blood pressure, cardiac output, central venous pressure (CVP), and pulmonary artery pressures remain stable related to mechanical ventilation.	■ Assess hemodynamic effects of initiation of mechanical ventilation (e.g., decreased venous return and cardiac output). ■ Monitor electrocardiogram (ECG) for dysrhythmias related to hypoxemia. ■ Assess hemodynamic effects of changes in inspiratory pressure settings, tidal volume, PEEP, and ventilatory modes. ■ Assess effects of ventilator setting changes on cardiac output and oxygen delivery. ■ Administer intravascular volume to maintain preload.
Blood pressure, heart rate, and hemodynamic parameters are optimized to therapeutic goals (e.g., DaO_2 greater than 600 mL O_2/m^2).	■ Monitor vital signs every 1 to 2 hours. ■ Monitor pulmonary artery pressures and right atrial pressure every hour and cardiac output, systemic vascular resistance, peripheral vascular resistance, DaO_2, and oxygen consumption ($\dot{V}O_2$) every 6 to 12 hours, if pulmonary artery catheter is in place. ■ Administer intravascular volume as indicated by real or relative hypovolemia, and evaluate response. ■ Consider monitoring gastric mucosal pH as a guide to systemic perfusion.

(continued)

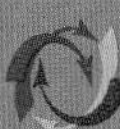

box 27-4 collaborative care guide
for the Patient With Acute Respiratory Distress Syndrome (ARDS) (Continued)

OUTCOMES	INTERVENTIONS
Serum lactate will be within normal limits.	■ Monitor lactate as required until it is within normal limits. ■ Administer red blood cells, positive inotropic agents, and colloid infusion as ordered to increase oxygen delivery.
Fluids/Electrolytes	
Patient is euvolemic.	■ Monitor hydration status to reduce viscosity of lung secretions.
Urine output is greater than 30 mL/hr (or >0.5 mL/kg/hr).	■ Monitor intake and output. ■ Avoid use of nephrotoxic substances and overuse of diuretics. ■ Administer fluids and diuretics to maintain intravascular volume and renal function.
There is no evidence of electrolyte imbalance or renal dysfunction.	■ Replace electrolytes as ordered. ■ Monitor blood urea nitrogen (BUN), creatinine, serum osmolarity, and urine electrolytes as required.
Mobility/Safety	
There is no evidence of complications related to bed rest and immobility.	■ Initiate deep venous thrombosis (DVT) prophylaxis. ■ Reposition frequently. ■ Mobilize to chair when acute phase is past, hemodynamic stability and hemostasis achieved. ■ Consult physiotherapist. ■ Conduct range-of-motion and strengthening exercises when able.
Physiological changes are detected and treated without delay.	■ Monitor mechanical ventilator alarms and settings and patient parameters (e.g., tidal volume) every 1 to 2 hours. ■ Ensure appropriate settings and narrow limits for hemodynamic, heart rate, and pulse oximetry alarms.
There is no evidence of infection; white blood cell count is within normal limits.	■ Monitor for systemic inflammatory response syndrome (SIRS) criteria (increased white blood cell count, increased temperature, tachypnea, tachycardia). ■ Use strict aseptic technique during procedures, and monitor others. ■ Maintain sterility of invasive catheters and tubes. ■ Change chest tube and other dressings and invasive catheters. ■ Culture blood and other fluids and line tips when they are changed.
Skin Integrity	
Skin will remain intact.	■ Assess skin every 4 hours and each time patient is repositioned. ■ Turn every 2 hours. ■ Consider pressure relief/reduction mattress, kinetic therapy bed, or prone positioning. ■ Use Braden Scale to assess risk of skin breakdown.
Nutrition	
Caloric and nutrient intake will meet metabolic requirements per calculation (e.g., basal energy expenditure).	■ Provide enteral nutrition within 24 hours. ■ Consult dietician or nutritional support service. ■ Consider small bowel feeding tube if gastrointestinal motility is an issue for enteral feeding. ■ Monitor lipid intake. ■ Monitor albumin, prealbumin, transferrin, cholesterol, triglycerides, and glucose.

(continued)

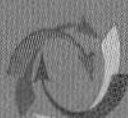

box 27-4 collaborative care guide *for the Patient With Acute Respiratory Distress Syndrome (ARDS) (Continued)*

OUTCOMES	INTERVENTIONS
Comfort/Pain Control	

Patient will be as comfortable as possible as evidenced by stable vital signs or cooperation with treatments or procedures.	■ Objectively assess comfort/pain using a pain scale.
	■ Provide analgesia and sedation as indicated by assessment.
	■ Monitor patient cardiopulmonary and pain response to medication.
	■ If patient is receiving neuromuscular blockade for ventilatory control:
	  ■ Use peripheral nerve stimulator to assess pharmacological paralysis.
	  ■ Provide continuous or routine (every 1 to 2 hours) intravenous sedation and analgesia.

Psychosocial	
Patient demonstrates decreased anxiety.	■ Assess vital signs during treatments, discussions, and the like. ■ Cautiously administer sedatives. ■ Consult social services, clergy, as appropriate. ■ Provide for adequate rest and sleep.
Teaching/Discharge Planning	
Patient/significant others understand procedures and tests needed for treatment.	■ Prepare patient/significant others for procedures, such as bronchoscopy, pulmonary artery catheter insertion, or laboratory studies. ■ Explain the causes and effects of ARDS and the potential for complications, such as sepsis, barotrauma, or renal failure.
Significant others understand the severity of the illness, ask appropriate questions, and anticipate potential complications.	■ Encourage significant others to ask questions related to the ventilator, the pathophysiology of ARDS, monitoring, and treatments.

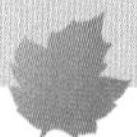

box 27-5
Considerations for the Older Patient With Acute Respiratory Distress Syndrome (ARDS)

- People who are 65 years of age or older are at increased risk for multisystem organ involvement with less chance of recovering from ARDS; therefore, the mortality rate is increased in this population.
- Because of increased immunosuppression with aging, the elderly are at greater risk for infection; therefore, nosocomial infections, such as urinary tract infections and ventilator-associated pneumonia (VAP), are more common.
- Hemodynamic instability adds metabolic insults to already-decreased renal function, thus predisposing this group to renal failure.
- Decreased stroke volume; possible coronary artery disease (CAD), atherosclerosis, or both, and increased systolic blood pressure and peripheral vascular resistance alter hemodynamic recovery.
- Decreased maximal oxygen uptake associated with decreased lung volumes puts elderly patients at greater risk for ventilator-associated lung injury (VALI).
- Decreased muscle mass associated with aging makes recovery from prolonged immobility more difficult. Therefore, an elderly person with ARDS may require prolonged rehabilitation.
- Generalized peripheral edema, multiple invasive tests, and prolonged bed rest, combined with the decreased skin integrity associated with old age, increase the elderly patient's potential for development of pressure ulcers and skin tears.
- Elderly patients with ARDS are at risk for not receiving the same quality and quantity of treatment and care as younger patients, due to the effects of ageism. The patient's age is one factor to consider in outcome and prognosis, but not the only one.
- The incidence of comorbid conditions, especially non–insulin-dependent diabetes mellitus and CAD, increases with age. Research findings indicate that the presence of comorbidity increases the risk of death for patients with ARDS.
- The patient and family may request no initiation of, or early removal from, life support based on previously expressed wishes. A person's life experience or vision of risk related to prolonged illness with high possibility of mortality may influence this decision, and these wishes should be respected.

Sputum specimens were sent after bronchoscopy and broad-spectrum antibiotics were started. An infectious diseases consult was requested. The diagnosis was penicillin-resistant *Streptococcus pneumoniae* pneumonia, explaining why the choice of antibiotic, normally very effective in a healthy young person in this area, was ineffective.

The patient remained on assist-control mechanical ventilation and dopamine infusion. He was chemically paralyzed with morphine and benzodiazepine infusions. During the next 48 hours, the nurses obtained cardiac outputs and ABGs every 6 hours; conducted hourly assessments of respiratory parameters, vital signs, breath sounds, mental status, and urine output; and performed frequent side-to-side turning with chest physiotherapy every 4 hours. Drugs and fluids were collaboratively titrated based on the assessment parameters. The ventilator settings were adjusted to decrease the FIO_2 and minimize airway pressures. The peak plateau pressures were reduced to 30 cm H_2O, and the blood gases stabilized, although they were still abnormal. Multiple combinations of ventilation strategies were used to improve oxygenation, including permissive hypercapnia and inverse ratio ventilation.

Over a 35-day course, the patient experienced worsening hypoxemia and was placed on high-frequency oscillation ventilation (HFOV) with nitric oxide. His complications remained largely respiratory, with development of nosocomial pneumonia and multiple pneumothoraces. In spite of aggressive interventions, all efforts by the health care team failed, and multisystem organ failure developed. The final decision to withdraw active treatment was made by the health care team and family when thrombocytopenia developed in the patient in the face of worsening hypoxemia (FIO_2 100% with an SaO_2 of 66%). Ventilation was withdrawn and the patient died. ■

clinical applicability challenges

Self-Challenge: Critical Thinking

1. *Discuss risk factors for ARDS that may have been present for the patient in the case study.*
2. *Explain the rationale for the ventilator settings that were used for the patient in the case study.*
3. *Role-play an interaction that you would have with the patient's family during the course of his illness and at the time of his death.*

Study Questions

1. *In late-stage ARDS, difficulty maintaining oxygenation and ventilation is a result of*
   a. *interstitial pulmonary edema.*
   b. *fibroproliferative changes to the lung.*
   c. *neutrophil infiltration of the vascular system.*
   d. *decreased pulmonary artery wedge pressure (PAWP).*
2. *Pressure-limited mechanical ventilation is appropriate for patients with ARDS because it*
   a. *helps to reduce volutrauma and barotrauma.*
   b. *increases airway pressures.*
   c. *limits pulmonary artery pressures.*
   d. *limits lung compliance.*
3. *Changes in positive end-expiratory pressure (PEEP) are often necessary to decrease the risk associated with*
   a. *pulmonary embolus associated with immobility.*
   b. *high levels of oxygen administered to the patient.*
   c. *high levels of carbon dioxide associated with respiratory distress.*
   d. *the release of inflammatory mediators.*
4. *Complications associated with ARDS include all of the following except*
   a. *deep venous thrombosis (DVT).*
   b. *multiorgan failure.*
   c. *pneumothorax.*
   d. *intracranial hemorrhage.*
5. *The most effective treatment for ARDS is*
   a. *lung-protective ventilation.*
   b. *prone positioning.*
   c. *removal of the inciting cause.*
   d. *use of multiple ventilation strategies.*

REFERENCES

1. Bernard GR, Artigas A, Brigham KL, et al: The American-European Consensus Conference on ARDS: Definitions, mechanisms, relevant outcomes, and clinical trials coordination. Am J Respir Crit Care Med 149:818–824, 1994
2. van Soeren MH, Diehl-Jones WL, Maykut RJ, et al: Pathophysiology and implications for treatment of acute respiratory distress syndrome. AACN Clin Issues 11(2):179–197, 2000
3. Domenighetti G, Stricker H, Waldispuehl B: Nebulized prostacyclin (PGI_2) in acute respiratory distress syndrome: Impact of primary (pulmonary injury) and secondary (extrapulmonary injury) disease on gas exchange. Crit Care Med 29(1):57–62, 2001
4. Meade MO, Guyatt GH, Cook RJ, et al: Agreement between alternative classifications of acute respiratory distress syndrome. Am J Respir Crit Care 163:490–493, 2001
5. Luhr OR, Karlsson M, Thorsteinsson A, et al: The impact of respiratory variables on mortality in non-ARDS and ARDS patients requiring mechanical ventilation. Intensive Care Med 26:508–517, 2000
6. Navarrete-Navarro P, Ruiz-Bailen M, Rivera-Fernandez R, et al: Acute respiratory distress syndrome in trauma patients: ICU mortality and prediction factors. Intensive Care Med 26:1624–1629, 2000
7. Luce JM: Acute lung injury and the acute respiratory distress syndrome. Crit Care Med 26:369–376, 1998
8. Phillips JK: Management of patients with acute respiratory distress syndrome. Crit Care Nurs Clinics North Am 11(2):233–247, 1999
9. Pittet JF, Mackersie RC, Martin TR, et al: Biological markers of acute lung injury: Prognostic and pathogenic significance. Am J Respir Crit Care Med 155:1187–1205, 1997
10. Balas MC: Prone positioning of patients with acute respiratory distress syndrome: Applying research to practice. Crit Care Nurse 20(1):24–36, 2000
11. Wilmoth D. New strategies for mechanical ventilation: lung protective ventilation. Crit Care Nurs Clin North Am 11(4):447–454, 1999
12. Hebert PC, Wells G, Blanjchman MA, et al: A multi-center, randomised, controlled clinical trial of transfusion requirements in critical care. N Engl J Med 340:409–417, 1999
13. Vieillard-Baron A, Girou E, Valente E, et al: Predictors of mortality in acute respiratory distress syndrome: Focus on the role of right heart catheterization. Am J Respir Crit Care Med 161(5):1597–1601, 2000
14. Meade MO, Herridge MS: An evidence-based approach to acute respiratory distress syndrome. Respir Care 46:1368–1379, 2001
15. Staudinger T, Kofler J, Mullner M, et al: Comparison between prone positioning and continuous rotation of patients with adult respiratory distress syndrome: Results of a pilot study. Crit Care Med 29(1): 51–56, 2001
16. Amato M, Barbas C, Medeiros D, et al: Effect of a protective ventilation strategy on mortality in the acute respiratory distress syndrome. N Engl J Med 338:347–354, 1998
17. Moloney-Harmon PA: When the lung fails: Acute respiratory distress syndrome in children. Crit Care Clin North Am 11(4):519–528, 1999
18. Kollef MH, Sherman G, Ward S, et al: Inadequate antimicrobial treatment of infections. Chest 115:462–474, 1999

19. Spragg RG, Lewis JF: Pathology of the surfactant system of the mature lung. Am J Respir Crit Care 163:280–282, 2001
20. Matthay MA, Pittet JF, Jayr C: Just say NO to inhaled nitric oxide for the acute respiratory distress syndrome. Crit Care Med 26:1–2, 1998
21. Kress PJ, Pohlman RN, O'Connor MF, et al: Daily interruption of sedative infusions in critically ill patients undergoing mechanical ventilation. N Engl J Med 342:1471–1477, 2000
22. Cheever KH: Early enteral feeding of patients with multiple trauma. Crit Care Nurse 19(6):40–51, 1999
23. Heyland DK: Parenteral nutrition in the critically-ill patient: More harm than good? Proc Nutr Soc 59(3):457–466, 2000

OTHER SELECTED READING

American Thoracic Society: International Consensus Conferences in Intensive Care Medicine: Ventilator-associated lung injury in ARDS. Am J Respir Crit Care Med 160:2118–2124, 1999

Arnold JH: Partial liquid breathing: Are we headed in the right direction? Crit Care Med 28:1675–1676, 2000

Artigas A, Bernard GR, Carlet J, et al: The American-European Consensus Conference on ARDS, Part 2: Ventilatory, pharmacologic, supportive therapy, study design strategies and issues related to recovery and remodeling. Am J Respir Crit Care Med 157:1332–1347, 1998

Brook AD, Ahrens TS, Scaiff R, et al: Effect of nursing implemented sedation protocols on the duration of mechanical ventilation. Crit Care Med 27:2609–2615, 1999

Curley MAQ: Prone positioning of patients with acute respiratory distress syndrome: A systematic review. Am J Crit Care 8(6):397–405, 1999

Gadel JE, DeMichele SJ, Karlstad, MD, et al: Effect of enteral feeding with eicosapentaenoic acid, γ-linolenic acid, and antioxidants in patients with acute respiratory distress syndrome. Crit Care Med 27(8):1409–1420, 1999

Gattinoni L, Tognoni G, Pesenti A, et al: Effect of prone positioning on the survival of patients with acute respiratory failure. N Engl J Med 345(8):568–573, 2001

Howard AE, Courtney-Shapiro C, Kelso L, et al: Comparison of three methods of detecting acute respiratory distress syndrome: Clinical screening, chart review, and diagnostic coding. Am J of Crit Care 13(1):59–64, 2004

Heyland DK, Drover J: Does immunonutrition make an impact? It depends on the analysis. Crit Care Med 28(3):906–907, 2000

Hynes-Gay P, Chu N, Murray C, et al: The use of high-frequency oscillatory ventilation in adult ARDS patients. CACCN J 12(1):12–16, 2001

Karima R, Matsumoto S, Higashi H, et al: The molecular pathogenesis of endotoxic shock and organ failure. Molec Med Today 5(3):123–132, 1999

Knight JA: Free radicals: Their history and current status in ageing and disease. Ann Clin Lab Sci 28:331–346, 1998

Murray TA, Patterson LA: Prone positioning of trauma patients with acute respiratory distress syndrome and open abdominal incisions. Crit Care Nurse 22(3):52–56, 2002

Osterman M, Keenan SP, Seiferling RA, et al: Sedation in the intensive care unit: A systematic review. JAMA 283:1451–1459, 2000

Pugin J, Verghese G, Widmer MC, et al: The alveolar space is the site of intense inflammatory and profibrotic reactions in the early phase of acute respiratory distress syndrome. Crit Care Med 27:304–312, 1999

Ranieri VM, Suter PM, Tortorella C, et al: Effects of mechanical ventilation of inflammatory mediators in patients with acute respiratory distress syndrome: A randomized controlled trial. JAMA 282(1):54–61, 1999

Shibata K, Cregg N, Englebert D, et al: Hypercapnic acidosis may attenuate acute lung injury by inhibition of endogenous xanthine oxidase. Am J Respir Crit Care Med 158:1578–1584, 1998

Stewart TE, Meade MO, Cook DJ, et al: Evaluation of a ventilation strategy to prevent barotrauma in patients at high risk for acute respiratory distress syndrome. N Engl J Med 338:355–361, 1998

Zilberberg MD, Epstein SK: Acute lung injury in the medical ICU: Comorbid conditions, age, etiology and hospital outcome. Am J Respir Crit Care Med 157:1159–1164, 1998

PART

six

Renal System

INTERNET RESOURCES

Topic	Web Page Address
American Association of Kidney Patients	www.aakp.org
American Nephrology Nurses Association	www.annanurse.org
American Society for Artificial Internal Organs	www.asaio.com
American Society of Nephrology	www.asn-online.org
American Society of Pediatric Nephrology	www.aspneph.com
Atlas of Diseases of the Kidney	www.kidneyatlas.org
Continuous Renal Replacement Therapies	www.crrt.com
European Renal Association	www.era-edta.org
Forum of End Stage Renal Disease Networks	www.esrdnetworks.org
International Society for Peritoneal Dialysis	www.ispd.org
International Society of Nephrology	www.isn-online.org
Kidney & Urologic Foundation of America, Inc.	www.kidneyurology.org/homepage.htm
The Kidney Foundation of Canada	www.kidney.ca
National Institute of Diabetes, Digestive, and Kidney Diseases	www.niddk.nih.gov
National Kidney and Urologic Diseases Information Clearinghouse	www.kidney.niddk.nih.gov
National Kidney Foundation	www.kidney.org
Nephron Information Center	www.nephron.com
NephroWorld	www.nephroworld.com
Polycystic Kidney Disease Foundation	www.pkdcure.org/home.htm
Renalnet	www.renalnet.org
Renalworld	www.renalworld.com
TransWeb (Information about Transplantation and Donation)	www.transweb.org
U.S. Renal Data Systems	www.usrds.org
United Network for Organ Sharing	www.unos.org
World Foundation for Renal Care	www.worldrenal.org

chapter

28

Anatomy and Physiology of the Renal System

KARA L. ADAMS

objectives

Based on the content in this chapter, the reader should be able to:

- Identify the structures comprising the nephron: glomerulus, proximal tubule, loop of Henle, and distal and collecting tubules.
- Describe the impact of afferent and efferent blood supply on renal function.
- Differentiate the functions of the nephron, including glomerular filtration, passive and active transport, tubular secretion, and clearance.
- Compare normal fluid pressures in the nephron and how they affect glomerular filtration rate (GFR).
- Explain the relationship of antidiuretic hormone (ADH), renin, and aldosterone to fluid regulation by the kidneys.
- Explain the mechanisms used by the kidneys to help maintain homeostasis.
- Describe the physiological roles for the predominant electrolytes.

With each contraction of the heart, the kidneys receive 20% to 25% of the cardiac output. This means that approximately 1.2 L of blood pass through the kidneys each minute, and the body's entire blood volume is filtered through the kidneys 340 times per day. With this large volume of blood, the kidneys have a dominant role in filtration and a minor role in metabolism. Therefore, the kidneys have a large requirement for pressure and a relatively smaller requirement for oxygen. The regulation and maintenance of the concentration of solutes in the extracellular fluid (ECF) of the body are the primary functions of the kidney. The kidneys remove metabolic waste products and excess concentrations of constituents and conserve substances present in normal or low quantities.

MACROSCOPIC ANATOMY OF THE RENAL SYSTEM

The kidneys are bean-shaped organs that lie in a retroperitoneal position in the abdomen, one on each side of the vertebral column (Fig. 28-1). The kidneys are partially protected by the last pair of ribs, with the right kidney slightly lower than the left because of the location of the liver. A tough, fibrous coat, known as the renal capsule, surrounds each kidney. The adrenal glands, which are discussed in more detail in Chapter 42, cap the kidneys.

The adult kidneys are approximately 12 cm long, 6 cm wide, and 2.5 cm thick. The weight of the kidneys ranges between 125 and 170 g in men and 115 and 155 g in

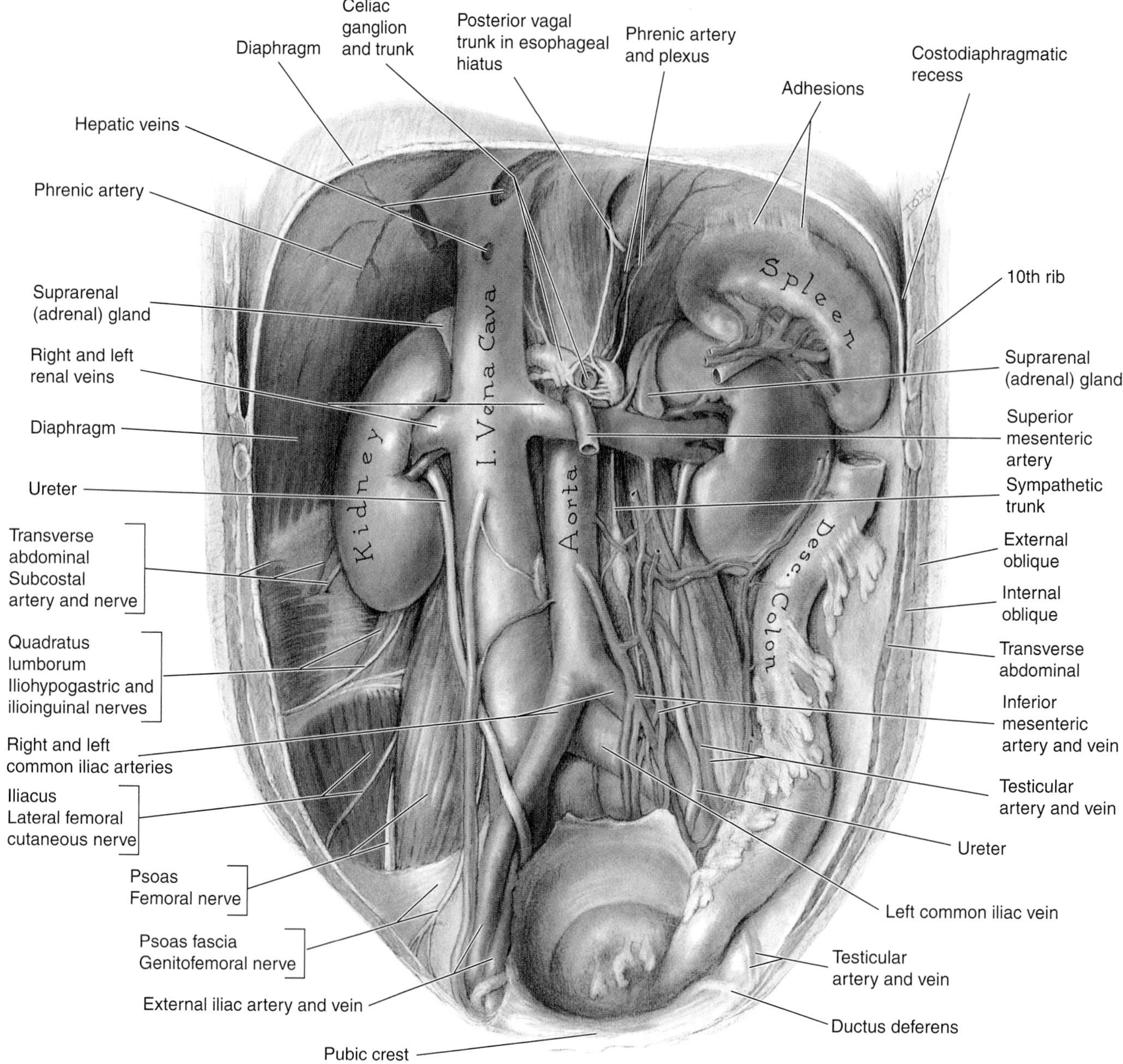

figure 28-1 Anatomy of the kidneys and urinary system. (Used with permission from Moore KL, Dalley AF: Clinically Oriented Anatomy [4th Ed.], p 281. Philadelphia, Lippincott Williams & Wilkins, 1999.)

women. The size and weight of the kidneys are clinically valuable indicators in ultrasound-guided differential diagnosis of renal failure (see Chapter 29).

There are two distinct layers of the kidney: the renal cortex and the renal medulla (Fig. 28-2). The renal cortex is the outer portion of the kidney and has two regions: the cortical region and the juxtamedullary ("next to the medulla") region. The cortex contains the glomeruli, the proximal tubules, the cortical loops of Henle, the distal tubules, and the cortical collecting ducts. The inner layer, the medulla, in addition to the cortical structures, contains the renal pyramids. The pyramids contain the medullary loops of Henle and the medullary portions of the collecting ducts, which join together to form a minor calyx. Minor calyces come together to form a major calyx. The renal calyces further join to become the conduit for directing the flow of urine into the ureter.

Urine exits the kidney at an oblique angle through the fibromuscular structure, the ureter. Peristalsis helps maintain the flow of urine through the ureter. The ureter enters the bladder in the trigone region. The trigone region of the bladder is so called for the three structures that form the shape of a triangle: the two ureters and the urethra. The peristaltic actions in the ureter and the angle of entry at the bladder help to prevent the reflux of urine. Urine exits the bladder through the urethral orifice via the urethra. The male urethra is about 20 cm long; the female urethra is about 3 to 5 cm long.

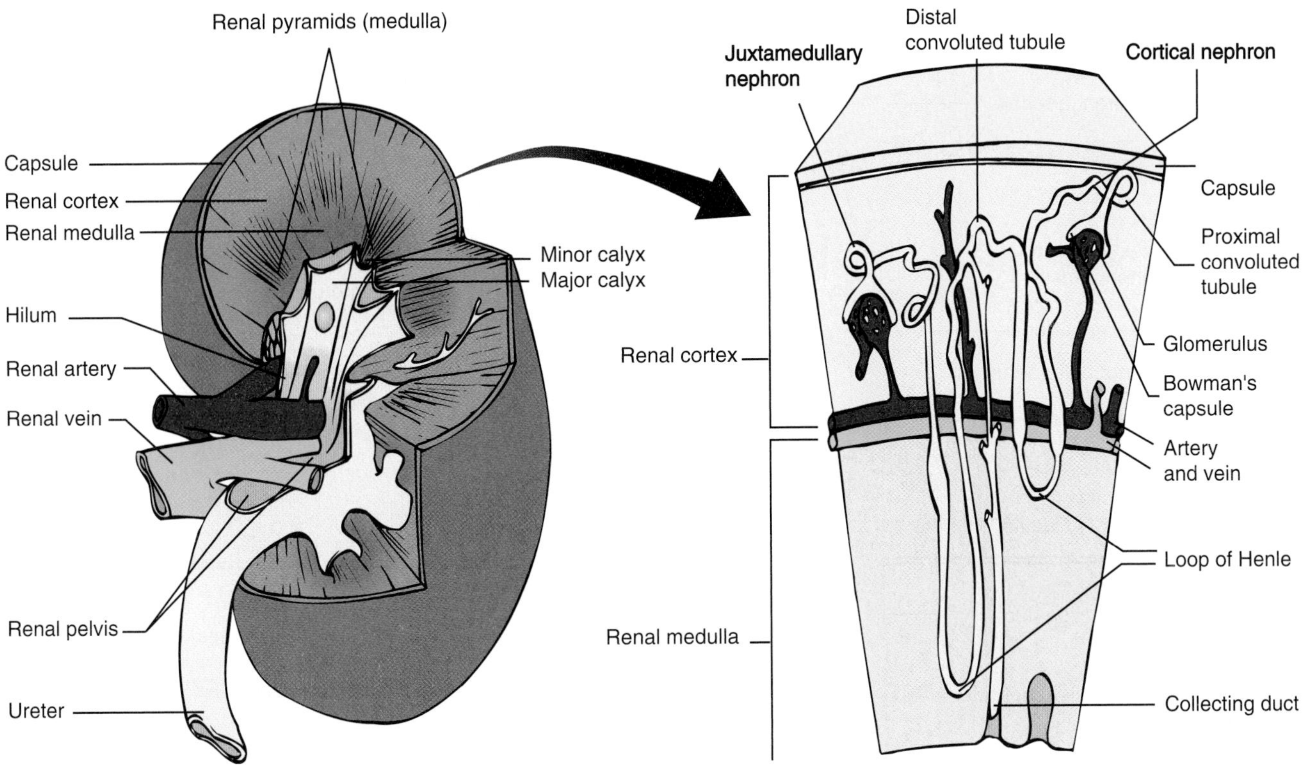

figure 28-2 Macroscopic anatomy of the kidney.

On the medial aspect of each kidney there is an indentation known as the hilum. It is through this indentation that the renal arteries and nerves enter and the renal veins, lymphatics, and ureters exit (see Fig. 28-2).

The kidneys receive their blood supply from the renal artery, a branch of the descending aorta. The renal artery divides into several smaller branches known as the interlobar arteries (Fig. 28-3). Further branching produces numerous afferent arterioles. Each afferent arteriole forms a tuft of capillaries, known as the glomerulus, where blood is filtered. Leaving the glomerulus is the efferent arteriole. The efferent arteriole branches to form a second capillary bed, known as the peritubular capillaries (see Fig. 28-3). The peritubular capillaries surround the loop of Henle to reabsorb more water and solutes as needed for homeostasis. Reconnecting, this vast network of vessels eventually returns to the central circulation through the renal veins.

The kidneys were once thought to function in the normal homeostasis of systemic blood pressure because of the effect of hydrostatic pressure on filtration. It is now known that the glomerular filtration rate (GFR) is relatively stable over a wide range of arterial blood pressures. The reason for this stability is that the afferent arterioles adjust their diameter in response to the pressure of blood coming to them. If the blood pressure decreases, the smooth muscles of the afferent arterioles relax. This causes dilation of these arterioles, which increases the perfusion of the glomeruli and maintains the GFR at its normal rate. Conversely, with an increase in blood pressure, these vessels constrict. There is a limit, however, to this autoregulatory mechanism. Below a mean arterial pressure of 90 mm Hg and above a mean of 250 mm Hg, the GFR is proportional to perfusion pressure. For example, if the systemic blood pressure falls greatly, such as in shock, the GFR will fall to near zero, thereby producing near anuria.

MICROSCOPIC ANATOMY OF THE RENAL SYSTEM AND NORMAL RENAL PHYSIOLOGY

Urine, the end product of kidney function, is formed from the blood by the smallest unit of the kidney, the nephron (see Fig. 28-3). Each human kidney consists of about 1 million nephrons, all of which function identically; therefore, kidney function can be explained by describing the function of one nephron (Table 28-1). A nephron is composed of a glomerulus, a proximal tubule, a loop of Henle, and a distal tubule. Several distal tubules drain into a collecting duct.

Approximately 80% of the filtrate is returned to the bloodstream by reabsorption in the proximal tubule. In a healthy person, all the filtered glucose and amino acids; much sodium, chloride, hydrogen, and other electrolytes; and uric acid and urea are reabsorbed here. The proximal tubule cells also secrete substances (e.g., some drugs, organic acids, and organic bases) into the filtrate.

In the loop of Henle, the filtrate (urine) becomes highly concentrated. This part of the nephron is composed of a

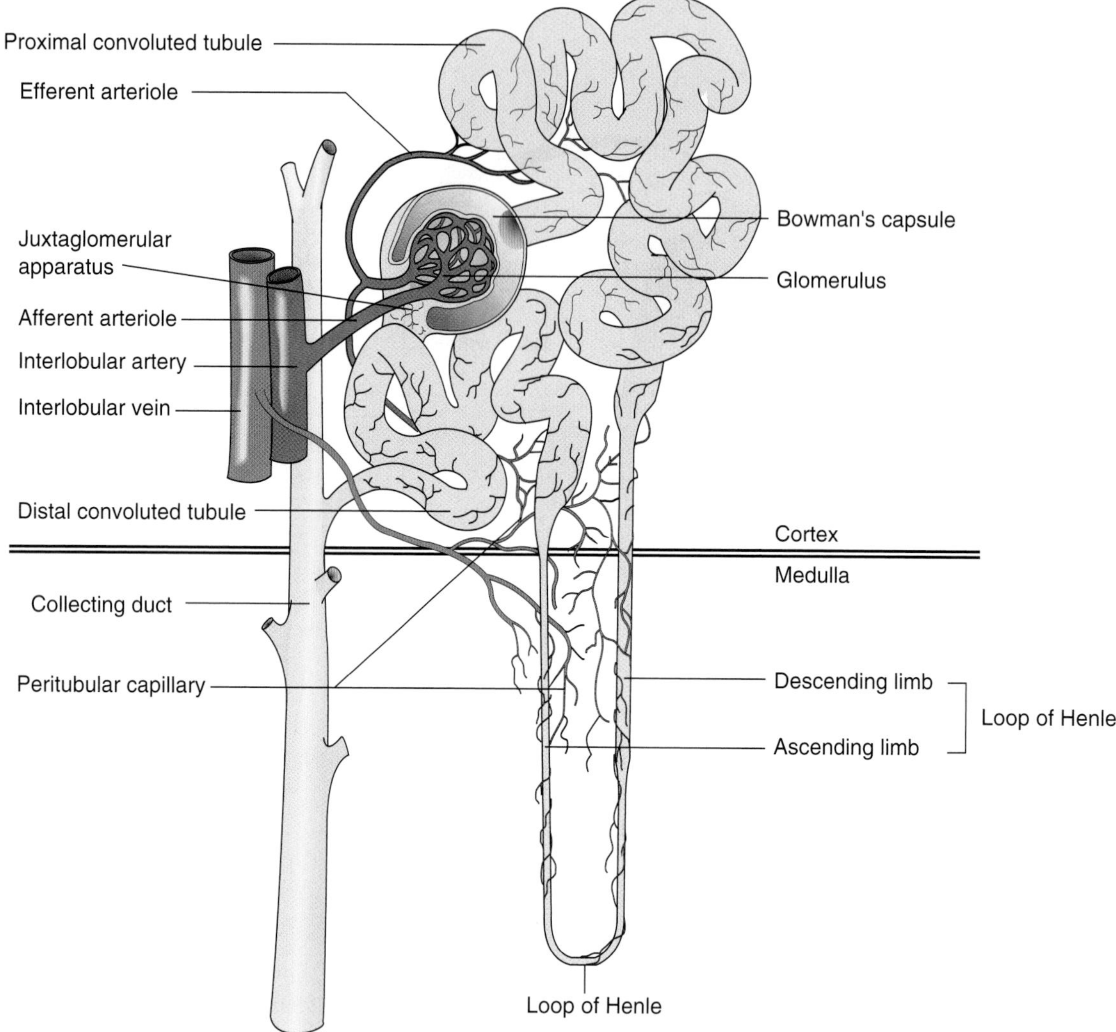

figure 28-3 Renal blood supply. The afferent arteriole feeds the glomerulus. Exiting the glomerulus is the efferent arteriole, which divides into a second capillary network, the peritubular capillaries. (Used with permission from Porth CM: Pathophysiology: Concepts of Altered Health States [6th Ed.], p 675. Philadelphia, Lippincott Williams & Wilkins, 2002.)

thin-walled descending portion and a thick-walled ascending portion. Loops of Henle belonging to juxtamedullary nephrons dip into the medulla of the kidney, which contains a highly concentrated interstitial fluid. (The thin walls of the descending portion are quite permeable.) This permeability, together with the high concentration of the interstitial fluid at this point, causes water to move by osmosis from the filtrate into the interstitial fluid. This makes the filtrate quite concentrated by the time it reaches the ascending limb of the loop.

The thicker-walled ascending limb is relatively impermeable to water, but it contains ion carriers that actively transport chloride ions out of the filtrate. This creates an electrochemical gradient that "pulls" the positively charged sodium ions out of the filtrate as well. This exit of electrolytes without water now makes the filtrate more dilute than before.

In the distal tubule, sodium again is reabsorbed by active transport, and hydrogen, potassium, and uric acid can be added to the urine by tubular secretion.

The collecting ducts receive the contents from many distal tubules. There is no further electrolyte reabsorption or secretion, and, in the well-hydrated person, no further water reabsorption as well. Water reabsorption without electrolyte reabsorption can occur in the collecting ducts under the stimulus of antidiuretic hormone (ADH).

Juxtaglomerular Apparatus

The nephron is arranged so that the initial portion of the distal tubule lies at the juncture of the afferent and efferent arterioles, which is very near the glomerulus. Here, macula densa cells of the distal tubule lie in approximation to the juxtaglomerular cells of the wall of the afferent arteriole.

table 28-1 Nephron Functions

Nephron Structure	Function	Concentration of Filtrate Along the Nephron
Glomerulus	Free filtration of blood through Bowman's capsule to produce filtrate Hydrostatic and osmotic pressure forces create net filtration pressure	Isosmotic
Proximal convoluted tubule	Reabsorbs sodium, potassium, calcium, glucose, ketone bodies, and amino acids by active transport Reabsorbs chloride and bicarbonate by electromechanical gradient Reabsorbs water by osmosis Reabsorbs urea by diffusion	Isosmotic
Loop of Henle		
Thin descending limb	Reabsorbs sodium by active transport Further reabsorption of chloride by electromechanical gradient Reabsorbs water by osmosis Reabsorbs urea by diffusion	Isosmotic
Thick ascending limb	Reabsorbs sodium and chloride by active transport Blocks water reabsorption at thick ascending limb Reabsorbs bicarbonate by electromechanical gradient	Hypo-osmotic
Distal tubule	Reabsorbs sodium by active transport and aldosterone Reabsorbs water by osmosis Reabsorbs phosphorus, chloride, and bicarbonate by electromechanical gradient	Hypo-osmotic
Collecting tubule	Antidiuretic hormone (ADH) promotes selective water reabsorption Secretes or reabsorbs bicarbonate and hydrogen ions to maintain pH Secretes potassium and hydrogen ions depending on body requirements or effects of drugs Secretes some creatinine Actively reabsorbs potassium	Depends on body requirements for fluid

Both these cell types (juxtaglomerular and macula densa cells) plus some connective tissue cells constitute the juxtaglomerular apparatus (Fig. 28-4). A major function of the juxtaglomerular cells is to secrete renin, which thereby initiates the renin–angiotensin–aldosterone system. Research suggests that the macula densa cells may have a role in autoregulation by altering blood flow rates in the nephron. When a decrease in sodium chloride concentration is sensed, the macula densa cells initiate two signals: one signal to reduce afferent arteriole tone (increasing afferent arteriole hydrostatic pressure) and a second to increase renin release from the juxtaglomerular cells. In this manner, the juxtaglomerular apparatus helps maintain and promote glomerular filtration.

Glomerulus

The glomerulus consists of a tuft of capillaries fed by the afferent arteriole, drained by the efferent arteriole. The glomerulus is surrounded by Bowman's capsule. High hydrostatic pressure in the afferent arteriole causes rapid filtration. Fluid that is filtered from the capillaries into this capsule then flows into the tubular system, which is divided into four sections: the proximal tubule, the loop of Henle, the distal tubule, and the collecting duct (see Fig. 28-3). Lower hydrostatic pressure in the efferent circulation allows reabsorption. Most of the water and electrolytes are reabsorbed into the blood in the peritubular capillaries that surround the tubular structures. The end products of metabolism remaining in the tubules pass into the urine.

Glomerular filtration is determined by net filtration pressure. Hydrostatic pressure and osmotic pressure forces are major factors. Hydrostatic pressure is driving or "pushing" pressure. Osmotic pressure is defined as the pressure exerted by water (or any solvent) on a semipermeable membrane as it attempts to cross the membrane into an area containing more molecules that cannot cross the semipermeable membrane. The pores in the glomerular capillary make it a semipermeable membrane that permits smaller molecules and water to cross, but prevents larger molecules (e.g., plasma proteins) from crossing. Protein concentrations are the greatest factors in determining an osmotic pressure, and therefore osmotic pressure is often referred to as *colloid osmotic pressure.*

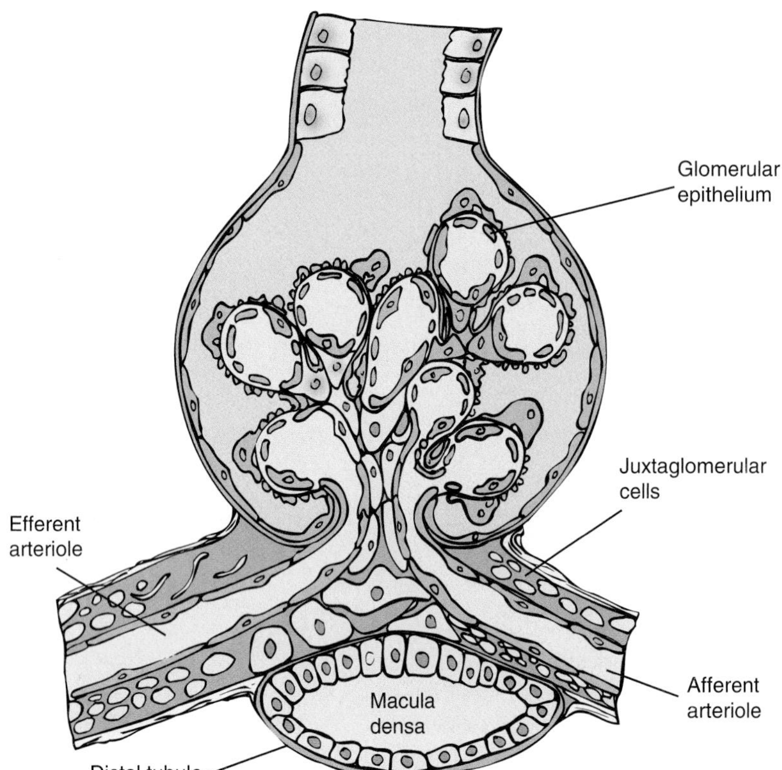

figure 28-4 The juxtaglomerular apparatus. The macula dense cells lie in close proximity to the afferent and efferent arterioles, which help to regulate nephron functions.

Four forces are considered when determining net filtration of fluid. These forces are:

1. Glomerular hydrostatic pressure, which promotes filtration
2. Bowman's capsule hydrostatic pressure, which opposes filtration
3. Glomerular colloid osmotic pressure, which opposes filtration
4. Bowman's capsule colloid osmotic pressure, which promotes filtration

Under normal conditions, the concentration of proteins in Bowman's capsule is thought to be negligible, and therefore is not considered as part of the net filtration pressure equation (Fig. 28-5). Glomerular hydrostatic pressure is about 60 mm Hg and is autoregulated under most circumstances. Filtrate hydrostatic pressure in Bow-

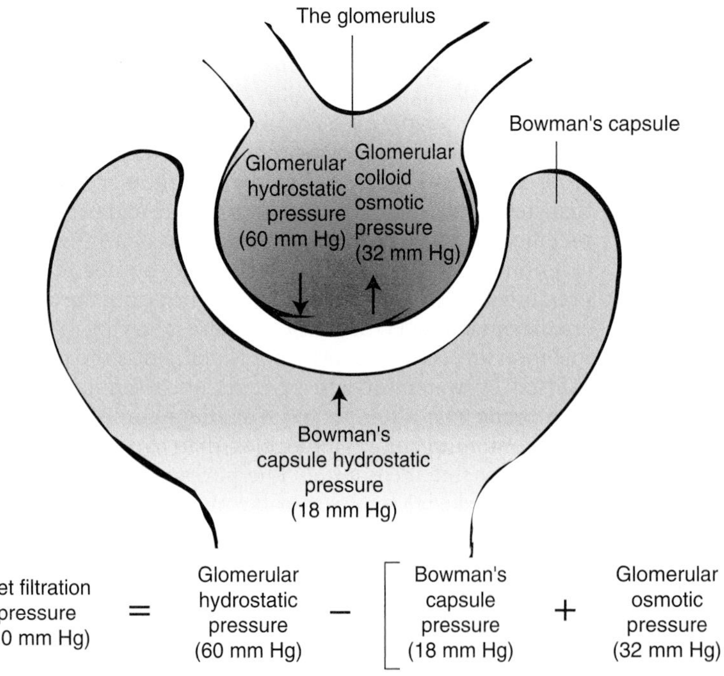

figure 28-5 Interaction of hydrostatic and osmotic forces for glomerular filtration.

man's capsule, about 18 mm Hg, results from the presence of filtrate in the capsule and opposes blood hydrostatic pressure. Glomerular osmotic pressure, derived from protein concentrations in the blood, is about 32 mm Hg. As mentioned, the filtrate also exerts a negligible osmotic pressure. The sum of these pressures is the net gradient that favors movement of filtrate from the bloodstream into Bowman's capsule.

The rate at which the filtrate is formed is termed the *glomerular filtration rate* (GFR). In the typical healthy person, this amounts to the formation of 125 mL of filtrate per minute. Major clinical factors that influence the GFR are the blood hydrostatic pressure and the filtrate osmotic pressure. Hypoproteinemia, as in starvation, lowers filtrate osmotic pressure and increases the GFR. The GFR decreases with severe hypotension because of a drop in blood hydrostatic pressure, when autoregulatory control may be lost. Other factors that decrease the hydrostatic pressure (and therefore the GFR) are afferent arteriole constriction and renal artery stenosis.

From the 20% to 25% of the cardiac output that goes to the kidneys in a resting adult, about 125 mL of filtrate is produced each minute. This totals 180 L/day and is about 4.5 times the total amount of fluid in the body. Obviously, not all this filtrate could be excreted as urine. As this filtrate passes from Bowman's capsule through the remainder of the nephrons, all but about 1.5 L/day is returned to the bloodstream. Similarly, at plasma glucose levels of less than 200 mg/dL, none of the filtered glucose is found in the urine when it enters the collecting tubules. The volume and content of the urine are the result of tubular reabsorption and tubular secretion.

Tubules

TUBULAR REABSORPTION

Reabsorption is accomplished by active transport, osmosis, and diffusion. It occurs in all parts of the nephron as substances moving from the lumen into the peritubular capillaries.

Active Transport

Active transport involves the binding of a molecule of a substance to a carrier, which then moves the molecule from one side of the membrane to the other against the concentration gradient of that substance. Because it helps molecules to move in a direction opposite the one they would move by simple diffusion, the carrier acts like a pump. Many processes for active transport use the sodium–potassium pump. Therefore, the small oxygen requirements of the kidneys are closely linked to the active transport processes that occur in the nephron.

In tubular cells, the carrier is located in the cell membrane nearest the peritubular capillaries, and it transports material out of the tubular cell into the peritubular fluid. This lowers the intracellular concentration of the type of molecule being transported. The decreased concentration enables more of those molecules to diffuse from the urine (filtrate) into the tubule cell. These molecules, in turn, exit the cell and enter the peritubular fluid by active transport. The movement of molecules increases the peritubular fluid concentration of the molecule, and this increase stimulates the diffusion of the molecule into the peritubular capillaries. In the nephrons, reabsorption by active transport removes molecules from the filtrate (urine) back to the bloodstream.

Because active transport involves carrier molecules and energy exchanges, there is an upper limit to the number of molecules of a substance that can be transported at one time. This maximum limit for reabsorption rates is called T_{max}. Glucose is an example of a molecule that appears in the same concentrations that it appears in the blood. As serum glucose rises, filtrate glucose also rises. The renal tubules reabsorb the filtered glucose at faster and faster rates, until all of this molecule's active transport mechanisms are being used. At this T_{max}, more glucose is appearing in the filtrate than can be reabsorbed, and glucose is excreted in the urine. This "spilling" of glucose into the urine indicates serum levels higher than T_{max}.

Osmosis

The active transport of sodium is responsible for the osmotic reabsorption of water from the filtrate in the proximal (and later, in the distal) tubule. As sodium ions are actively transported out of the cell and into the peritubular fluid, they make the osmotic pressure of this peritubular fluid higher than that of the cellular or tubular fluid. Water is thereby osmotically "pulled out" of the tubular fluid. Both water and sodium then diffuse into peritubular capillaries and are returned to the bloodstream. This movement of positively charged sodium ions also creates an electrochemical gradient that draws negatively charged ions (especially chloride) out of the tubular fluid and back into the bloodstream.

Diffusion

Urea is an example of a molecule that is reabsorbed by diffusion. Under the high pressures in the glomerular capillaries, urea is filtered. In the tubules, as water is reabsorbed into the bloodstream, urea follows by simple diffusion. No selective permeability prevents its return to the bloodstream, and no transport mechanism is required. The reabsorption rates of urea range from 40% to 60% of what is filtered and depend entirely on water reabsorption rates.

TUBULAR SECRETION

Secretion involves active transport and is performed only by distal tubule cells. Substances move from the peritubular capillaries through tubule cells into the filtrate. Many substances that are secreted do not occur naturally in the body (e.g., penicillin). Naturally occurring bodily substances that are secreted include uric acid, potassium, and hydrogen ions.

In the distal tubule, the active transport of sodium uses a carrier system that is also involved in the tubular secretion of hydrogen and potassium ions (Fig. 28-6). In this relationship, every time the carrier transports sodium out of the tubular fluid, it carries either a hydrogen or a potassium ion into the tubular fluid on its "return trip." Thus, for every sodium ion reabsorbed, a hydrogen or potassium ion must be secreted, and vice versa. The choice of cation to be secreted depends on the ECF concentration of these ions (hydrogen and potassium).

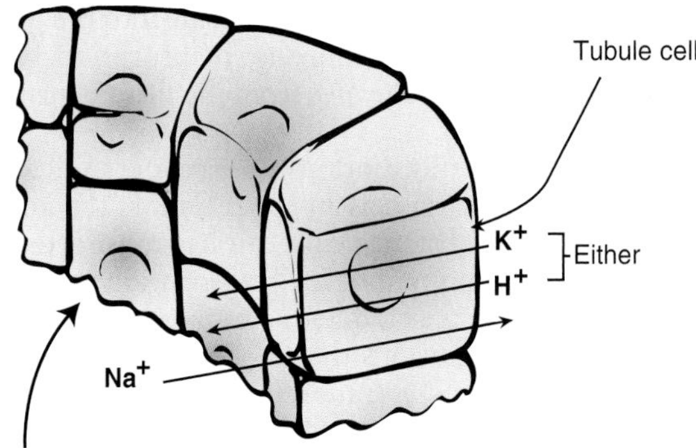

figure 28-6 Cation exchange in the distal tubule.

Knowledge of this cation exchange system in the distal tubule helps to explain some of the relationships that these electrolytes have with one another. For example, it is clear why an aldosterone blocker may cause hyperkalemia. The aldosterone blocker reduces sodium reabsorption. Such reduced reabsorption of sodium also reduces the tubular secretion of either hydrogen or potassium. The hydrogen excess can be buffered, but the potassium simply rises to above-normal levels, leading to hyperkalemia. Similarly, the cation exchange system helps to explain why there can be an initial fall in plasma potassium as severe acidosis is corrected therapeutically. In severe acidosis, the nephrons attempt to compensate by increasing hydrogen ion secretion. As acidosis is therapeutically corrected (e.g., by sodium bicarbonate administration), potassium ions are secreted. Another concern is a shift of potassium into cells. As hydrogen ions no longer need to be secreted, potassium ions become the sole exchange for sodium ions, leading, it is thought, to a reduction in plasma potassium.

HORMONAL INFLUENCES

Through the reabsorption of sodium and the passive "following" of water and chloride, it is possible to make urine of the same osmolality as blood. Under conditions of dehydration, however, urine is very concentrated, whereas if a great deal of water is consumed, urine is more dilute than blood. This final regulation of urine (and, therefore, serum osmolality and volume) is under the influence of three hormones: ADH, renin, and aldosterone.

Antidiuretic Hormone

Osmoreceptors in the hypothalamus are sensitive to serum osmolality. During dehydration, when serum osmolality rises, osmoreceptors in the hypothalamus respond by stimulating the hypothalamus to secrete ADH, which increases the permeability of collecting tubule cells to water. This permits the reabsorption of water alone (without electrolytes), which in turn decreases the concentration of the ECF. Negative feedback loops regulate ADH secretion. This means that as the concentration of the ECF returns to normal, the stimulus for ADH secretion disappears, and ADH secretion is stopped.

Renin

Another hormone that influences urine concentration is renin. When the GFR falls because of dehydration or blood loss, the juxtaglomerular apparatus secretes renin. Subnormal sodium levels in the filtrate also stimulate renin secretion. Renin converts angiotensin, which is secreted by the liver, into angiotensin I. Pulmonary capillary cells in turn convert angiotensin I into angiotensin II (see Chapter 42, Fig. 42-9).

Aldosterone

Angiotensin II constricts the smooth muscle surrounding the arterioles. This increases blood pressure, which increases the GFR. Angiotensin II also triggers the secretion of aldosterone by the adrenal cortex (see Chapter 42, Fig. 42-9). Aldosterone is the third hormone that influences urine osmolality. By increasing sodium reabsorption in distal tubule cells, aldosterone causes an increase in renal water reabsorption. This increases blood pressure and decreases serum osmolality. Simultaneously, potassium is excreted in the urine in exchange for the sodium reabsorption. Therefore, aldosterone also is secreted in response to subnormal serum sodium and elevated potassium levels.

FUNCTIONS OF THE RENAL SYSTEM

Renal Clearance

From the previous discussion, an important concept in renal function emerges: *clearance*. As the filtrate moves along the nephron, it contains a large proportion of metabolic end products. These products are removed (cleared) from the blood and exit the body in the urine. Indeed, of each 125 mL of glomerular filtrate formed per minute, about one half, or 60 mL, returns to the blood without urea, and about one half is excreted with urea. Stated another way, 60 mL of plasma is "cleared" of urea each minute in normally functioning kidneys. In the same way, 125 mL of plasma is cleared of creatinine, 12 mL of uric acid, 12 mL of potassium, 25 mL of sulfate, 25 mL of phosphate, and so forth each minute.

It is possible to calculate renal clearance by simultaneously sampling urine and plasma. By dividing the quantity of substance found in each milliliter of plasma into the quantity found in the urine, the milliliters cleared per minute can be calculated. This method is used as one means of testing kidney function.

Other methods of assessing renal function involve chemicals that are known to be filtered only, or both filtered and secreted. Insulin, for example, is filtered only and neither absorbed nor secreted. Therefore, the clearance of insulin provides a measure of glomerular filtration. Mannitol can be used similarly. Para-aminohippurate sodium (PAH) or iodopyracet (Diodrast) are drugs that are secreted in addition to being filtered. As such, their clearance provides an index of plasma flow through the kidneys. They also can be used together with a filtered-only drug in assessing tubular secretion and therefore the health of tubular cells.

The sodium concentration in the urine can also serve as an index of tubular health in certain situations. For example, in acute renal failure, an increased clearance of sodium can indicate acute tubular necrosis (ATN). Accordingly, supernormal blood levels of filtered substances (creatinine and other nitrogenous wastes) indicate a fall in glomerular filtration and therefore in nephron health.

Regulation

In addition to excreting nitrogenous wastes as urea and other byproducts of metabolism, the kidneys help to regulate the electrolyte concentration and the pH of the ECF (i.e., the blood and interstitial fluid of the body).

ELECTROLYTE CONCENTRATION

Electrolytes are substances that, when in water, disassociate and become charged. When charged, the solution is capable of carrying an electrical current. Positively charged electrolytes are cations; negatively charged electrolytes are anions. Most electrolytes are dissolved in body fluids, although some are bound to proteins or deposited as solids to form bones and teeth.

Despite the complex physiology associated with electrolytes, electrolytes have four main functions in homeostasis:

1. Cell metabolism and contribution to body structures
2. Facilitation of water movement between body compartments
3. Help in the maintenance of acid–base balance
4. Maintenance and production of membrane potentials in nerve and muscle cells

The functions of individual electrolytes are given in Table 28-2. For normal functions to occur, the concentration of electrolytes must be carefully maintained. Energy, usually in the form of adenosine triphosphate (ATP), is often required to maintain this balance. As described earlier in this chapter, the kidneys play a crucial role in electrolyte balance. In addition to being lost in the urine, electrolytes

table 28-2 Electrolyte Functions

Electrolyte	Normal Range	Functions
Sodium (Na^+)	135–145 mEq/L	Exerts an extracellular osmolality, thereby regulating movement of body fluids Facilitates nerve impulses through active transport and the sodium–potassium pump
Potassium (K^+)	3.5–5 mEq/L	Maintains nervous impulse conduction in the heart Promotes skeletal muscle function Plays small role in osmotic regulation Assists with acid–base regulation
Chloride (Cl^-)	100–110 mEq/L	Maintains electroneutrality by passively following the positively charged ions Helps regulate osmotic pressure differences between intracellular and extracellular fluid compartments Regulates body water balance with sodium Combines with H^+ in gastric mucosal cells to make hydrochloric acid
Calcium (Ca^{2+})	8.5–10.0 mg/dL (total) 4.4–5.4 mg/dL (ionized)	Major structural component of bones and teeth Plays role in blood coagulation Promotes muscle contraction and nervous impulse transmission Decreases neuromuscular irritability
Phosphorus (PO_4^-)	2.5–4.5 mg/dL	A structural component of bones and teeth Helps maintain acid–base balance Energy production (ATP) Delivery of oxygen to tissues as a component of 2,3-DPG
Magnesium (Mg^{2+})	1.8–2.5 mEq/L	Ensures the cross-membrane transport of sodium and potassium in the sodium–potassium pump Promotes neuromuscular excitability Plays role in heart contraction Facilitates transmission of central nervous system impulses Part of many enzymatic reactions for carbohydrate and protein metabolism

are lost from the gastrointestinal tract in the stool and through the skin in sweat.

Sodium

The sodium content of a normal adult is approximately 142 mEq/L of ECF. As the most abundant extracellular electrolyte, sodium exerts an extracellular osmolality, thereby regulating movement of body fluids. Sodium plays a role in nerve impulses through active transport and the sodium–potassium pump. The balance of sodium is carefully regulated by the kidneys, with hormonal influences of aldosterone and ADH. Regulation occurs primarily through reabsorption (or excretion) in the proximal tubule under the influence of aldosterone.

Potassium

In contrast to sodium, potassium is the most abundant intracellular electrolyte, with an approximate plasma concentration of only 4.5 mEq/L. Potassium, among other substances and factors, is critical in the maintenance of nervous and impulse conduction in the heart. Because of the small plasma concentration, potassium plays little role in osmotic regulation. Although some potassium may be lost in sweat and feces, the kidneys excrete approximately 80% to 90% of the potassium lost by the body. In cases of hyperkalemia, aldosterone release facilitates increased potassium excretion. Potassium also assists with acid–base regulation through the cellular exchange with hydrogen ions.

Chloride

Chloride is the most abundant extracellular anion. Negatively charged, chloride passively follows the positively charged sodium to maintain electroneutrality. All positive charges and negative charges must be in equilibrium. Therefore, chloride passively follows the secretion or reabsorption of the predominant cations, sodium and potassium. A large amount of chloride is also found in the gastric mucosal cells in the form of hydrochloric acid.

Calcium

Calcium has both structural and functional roles in homeostasis. In the form of calcium phosphate, it is the major structural component of bones and teeth. In the free, plasma form, calcium has a function in clotting, muscle contraction, and nervous impulse transmission. In the ionized form, about half is bound to plasma proteins, such as albumin.

Unlike the other electrolytes, calcium is absorbed from the small intestine under the influence of vitamin D, with the remaining ingested calcium lost in the feces. Excretion also occurs in the proximal convoluted tubule of the kidneys.

Parathyroid hormone (PTH) is produced and released by the parathyroid glands. A low calcium concentration stimulates its release. PTH facilitates the shift of calcium in its solid form (calcium phosphate, found in the bones) to its ionized form. PTH also increases the calcium absorbed from the intestine by signaling the kidneys to activate vitamin D. Reabsorption of calcium at the renal tubules is also increased under the influence of PTH. Calcitonin, secreted by the thyroid gland, is another hormone that plays a comparatively small role in calcium regulation. Calcitonin acts in opposition to PTH in an effort to reduce plasma calcium levels.

Phosphorus

Like calcium, phosphorus has both structural and functional roles. Approximately 85% is found in the organic form in bones and teeth. The remaining phosphorus is in the inorganic, ionized forms, HPO_4^{2-} and $H_2PO_4^-$. Carried in two forms, phosphate is able to accept or donate an ion, thereby assisting with acid–base balance. The intracellular ionized form plays a role in many critical metabolic processes, with its primary function being the formation of ATP. Phosphorus is required for the delivery of oxygen to tissues because it is the primary substrate for 2,3-diphosphoglycerate (2,3-DPG).

PTH regulates phosphorus, with effects directly opposite those of calcium. PTH causes an increase in calcium plasma concentration and promotes excretion of phosphorus. PTH also causes release of phosphorus in the bones and shifts it to the ECF. Presumably, this would cause an increase in phosphorus; however, PTH also decreases the transport of phosphate ions by the kidney tubules, so more phosphate ions are lost in the urine.

Magnesium

Magnesium is a predominantly intracellular ion. Magnesium ensures the cross-membrane transport of sodium and potassium in the sodium–potassium pump. In addition, magnesium functions in the maintenance of neuromuscular excitability and in the transmission of central nervous system (CNS) impulses. It also plays a role in enzymatic reactions for carbohydrate and protein metabolism. Often, reactions requiring calcium require magnesium as well.

pH

If buffers and the respiratory mechanism for pH homeostasis are insufficient, the kidneys then take part, although much more slowly than the respiratory system. Although respiratory control of carbon dioxide, and therefore hydrogen ion levels, can take only seconds to achieve, 48 to 72 hours may pass before the renal system can change the serum acid–base balance significantly.

Alkalosis occurs as a result of too few hydrogen ions or too many bicarbonate ions. To compensate, the body must conserve hydrogen ions. In renal compensation for alkalosis, tubular reabsorption of hydrogen ions is increased and secretion is decreased. This increases the hydrogen ion concentration of the ECF and thereby decreases the alkalosis.

Acidosis occurs as a result of too many hydrogen ions and too few bicarbonate ions. To compensate, the body must secrete hydrogen ions. Renal compensation for acidosis involves an increase in the hydrogen ion secretion of the tubule cells, especially in the distal tubule cells. In this case, bicarbonate and sodium ions are continually being filtered from the glomerulus. Also, hydrogen ion secretion by distal tubule cells causes an increase in sodium reabsorption. Such sodium reabsorption can increase bicarbonate reabsorption electrochemically. Therefore, as hydrogen ions are being eliminated from the ECF, sodium and bicarbonate ions are being added to it. Both serve to decrease the acidosis (Fig. 28-7).

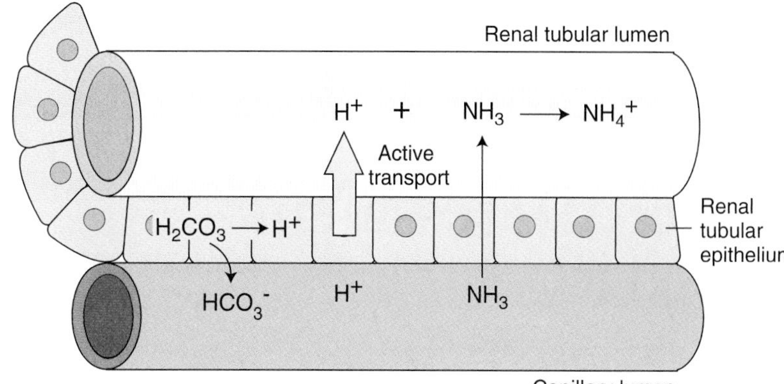

figure 28-7 Renal compensation for acidosis. Hydrogen (H^+) is moved from blood into the filtrate by active transport and exits in the urine as ammonium (NH_4^+). HCO_3^-, bicarbonate; NH_3, ammonia.

Urine can be acidified (by hydrogen ion secretion) only to a pH level of 4.0 to 4.5. If the tubular secretion of hydrogen ions was the only mechanism operating, only a few hydrogen ions could be secreted before the critical shut-off level of 4.0 was reached. This would occur because hydrogen would combine with urinary chloride to make hydrochloric acid. Not many of these strong hydrochloric acid molecules are needed to make the urine pH 4.0. The formation of hydrochloric acid would then stop tubular hydrogen ion secretion before sufficient compensation for acidosis could be obtained. This does not occur because tubule cells deaminate certain amino acids and secrete the nitrogenous component as ammonia. This ammonia combines with hydrogen in the urine to form ammonium. Because tubule membranes are not permeable to ammonium, much of it is secreted in this form. Some ammonia combines with chloride to form ammonium chloride.

Other Renal Functions

Renal interstitial (not nephron) cells manufacture and secrete two hormones, calcitriol and erythropoietin, the actions of which are unrelated to urine formation. Calcitriol is a hormone that increases plasma calcium concentration by increasing intestinal absorption of calcium, promoting bone resorption, and stimulating the renal tubular reabsorption of calcium. Erythropoietin is a glycoprotein hormone that stimulates the bone marrow to produce red blood cells. Any process that decreases the oxygen content in the blood, such as bleeding or hypoxemia, is sensed by the kidney and initiates the release of erythropoietin. This increases the arterial oxygen content required to maintain cell integrity.

The kidneys also activate vitamin D.

clinical applicability challenges

Self-Challenge: Critical Thinking

1. *Your postoperative patient is experiencing severe hypotension and increased blood urea nitrogen (BUN) levels. Explain the effect of hypotension on glomerular filtration rate (GFR), renin secretion, and the kidney's attempt to maintain homeostasis.*

Study Questions

1. *In the glomerulus, urine is formed by*
   a. *secretion.*
   b. *filtration.*
   c. *reabsorption.*
   d. *b and c.*
2. *Aldosterone stimulates increased sodium reabsorption by distal tubule cells. One consequence of elevated plasma aldosterone levels would be*
   a. *metabolic acidosis.*
   b. *hypokalemia.*
   c. *metabolic alkalosis.*
   d. *supernormal urine sodium levels.*
3. *Hyperglycemia increases the osmotic pressure of the filtered urine in the nephron. This would cause*
   a. *increased sodium and water reabsorption, leading to oliguria.*
   b. *decreased sodium and water reabsorption, leading to diuresis.*
   c. *decreased glomerular filtration, leading to prerenal azotemia.*
   d. *increased glomerular secretion of proteins into the filtrate.*
4. *What does parathyroid hormone (PTH) cause?*
   a. *An increase in calcium concentration*
   b. *A decrease in phosphorus concentration*
   c. *Potassium secretion*
   d. *a and b*

OTHER SELECTED READING

Guyton AC, Hall JE: Textbook of Medical Physiology (10th Ed). Philadelphia, WB Saunders, 2000

Huether SE, McCance KL: Pathophysiology: The Biologic Basis for Disease in Adults and Children (4th Ed). St. Louis, Mosby, 2001

Koeppen BM, Stanton BA: Renal Physiology (3rd Ed). St Louis, Mosby, 2001

Porth CM: Essentials of Pathophysiology: Concepts of Altered Health States (6th Ed). Philadelphia, Lippincott Williams & Wilkins, 2002

Rose BD, Rennke HG: Renal Pathophysiology: The Essentials. Baltimore, Williams & Wilkins, 1994

Seeley RR, Stephens TD, Tate P, et al: Anatomy and Physiology (6th Ed). New York, McGraw-Hill, 2002

Sherwood L: Human Physiology: From Cells to Systems (5th Ed). Los Angeles, Brooks-Cole, 2004

Valtin H, Schafer JA: Renal Function (3rd Ed). Boston, Little, Brown, 1995

chapter

29

Patient Assessment: Renal System

KARA ADAMS

objectives

Based on the content in this chapter, the reader should be able to:

- Analyze the relationship between the physiological function of the kidneys and the signs and symptoms that indicate renal dysfunction.
- Formulate a plan for collecting assessment data for patients with renal disorders and fluid and electrolyte imbalance.
- Explain the components of the urinalysis.
- Describe diagnostic and laboratory blood tests used to evaluate renal status.
- Discuss methods to evaluate fluid balance.

Assessment of the renal system involves determining how well the kidneys perform their many functions. It also includes gathering information about other systems. The nurse plays a vital role in assessing renal function and fluid and electrolyte balance. A careful assessment of the history and physical findings, along with interpretation of laboratory results, can provide early clues to the diagnosis of disorders of water and volume imbalance and other complications of renal dysfunction in the critically ill patient.

HISTORY

The patient history provides important information that helps determine the cause, severity, treatment, and management of renal dysfunction. It involves gathering information about the present illness, current signs and symptoms (system review), and significant past health history. A format for renal assessment is summarized in Box 29-1.

To begin, the patient is asked about his or her perception of the chief complaint. The description should include the onset, duration, and frequency of the complaint; the setting in which it developed; and factors that lessen or aggravate the problem. The complaint's significance to the patient and its impact on the patient's life should be ascertained. The patient is asked if this is the first time that this has occurred.

Once the patient has described the presenting problem, the nurse inquires about past medical history and family history. This information may offer clues to the underlying cause of the problem. A history of polycystic kidney disease, renal calculi, or hereditary nephritis is common in patients with kidney disease. Certain systemic diseases, such as the following, also may contribute to the development of renal failure:

- Diabetes mellitus
- Systemic lupus erythematosus
- Hypertension
- Sickle cell anemia
- Wegener's granulomatosis
- Goodpasture's syndrome

box 29-1
Factors in Renal Assessment

History

- Chief complaint (description of signs and symptoms, treatments, and response to treatments)
- Medical history
- Family history
- Medication history

Physical Examination

- Skin (turgor, temperature, dryness/moisture, scratches, lesions)
- Mucous membranes
- Presence of edema, ascites
- Respiratory rate, lung sounds
- Blood pressure, heart rate, rhythm, sounds
- Behavioral changes, mental status
- Test for tetany (Chvostek's sign, Trousseau's sign)
- Paresthesias, numbness, weakness, tremors of extremities

The patient is asked if there is history of heart disease because chronic congestive heart failure can affect renal function. Have there been problems with the liver, such as hepatitis or cirrhosis? The patient should also identify any recent illnesses, including infections, surgeries, or severe injuries, because endotoxins, severe hypotension, and skeletal muscle destruction can result in kidney damage. Some cellular contents that can be nephrotoxic at high levels include myoglobin, potassium, organic acids, and phosphorus. Because another common cause of kidney disease can be exposure to nephrotoxic agents, the nurse should ascertain whether the patient has been exposed to such agents as aminoglycosides, furosemide, radiographic dyes, or other drugs and chemical agents. Is there possible exposure to environmental agents at home or work, such as cleaning products, pesticides, lead (such as paint or gas fumes), and mercury? Does the patient have serious allergic reactions?

When the patient has end-stage renal disease (ESRD) and is receiving dialysis, the nurse asks about the following:

- Cause(s) of ESRD
- Date dialysis began
- Type of dialysis (hemodialysis or peritoneal dialysis)
- History of transplantation
- Date, time, and place of last dialysis
- Common problems, complications, and management associated with treatments

When the patient is receiving hemodialysis, the nurse asks if there have been problems with the arteriovenous fistula or graft, such as scar tissue, aneurysms, redness, or infection.

The nurse also needs to know all current medications, including over-the-counter and home remedy drugs. This may also be the time to ask about alcohol intake and the use of illicit drugs.

Next, the nurse conducts a review of signs and symptoms to determine further the patient's health status. How has the person's health been in general? Have there been any changes in hearing or vision? Have activity levels changed? Is there fatigue, muscle weakness, or problems with walking? How has the person been sleeping? The gastrointestinal system review can include questions about diet, changes in appetite, bowel elimination, and abdominal tenderness or fullness.

The patient is questioned about fluid intake, thirst, and urination:

- Have you ever had any dysuria, nocturia, polyuria, or incontinence?
- Have you ever experienced any flank pain or hematuria? Can you describe it?
- Have you noticed a change in the amount, color, smell, or pattern of voiding?
- Have you had a recent change in weight? When and with what was it associated?
- Have you noticed any swelling? Does the swelling dissipate with extremity elevation?
- Have you ever passed a renal stone?
- Have you ever had difficulty with starting urination (hesitancy), urgency, dribbling at end of urination, or stopping the stream?
- Have you ever experienced burning during urination?
- Do you have any history of urinary tract infections; if so, how were they treated?

The nurse explores factors such as shortness of breath, number of pillows used for sleep, and unusual tightness of shoes, waistband, or rings. Has there been puffiness around the eyes? The patient is asked to describe any skin problems, such as dryness, itching, bruising, rashes, or bumps. Has there been poor healing of cuts and scratches?

The patient's neurological status is addressed, including a history of fainting, seizures, localized weakness, numbness, tingling or burning sensations, asterixis (involuntary jerking commonly seen in the hands, tongue, or feet), tremors, paralysis, foot-drop, and restless leg syndrome. Has the patient or family noticed any memory loss, decreased interest in the environment, lethargy, or difficulty with usual activities?

PHYSICAL EXAMINATION

The physical examination provides objective data that are used to substantiate and clarify the history. The history guides the physical examination and helps determine areas of the examination that require more depth. If time permits, the nurse reviews the chart, including laboratory results, before beginning the physical examination. This can help identify data that require follow-up during the physical examination.

The nurse begins the physical examination by observing the patient's overall appearance, including facial expression, height and weight, position in bed, grooming, personal hygiene, and signs of distress. The nurse observes the patient's level of responsiveness, cognition, and interaction with people, including positive, negative, or unusual responses.

Because patients with renal problems usually have significant problems with fluid and electrolyte balance, the nurse evaluates the patient's volume status throughout the examination. The nurse may begin by taking the blood pressure (noting pulse pressure and a positive pulse paradoxus) and temperature. Patients with ESRD tend to have low temperatures because they are usually immunosuppressed.

Throughout the physical examination, the nurse inspects the skin on the extremities and trunk for color and evidence of excoriation, bruising, or bleeding; palpates for moistness, dryness, temperature (using the back of the fingers), and edema; and checks mobility and turgor by lifting a fold of skin and noting the ease (mobility) and speed with which it returns into place (turgor). To assess hydration further, the nurse inspects the tongue and mucous membranes in the mouth and looks for a saliva pool under the tongue.

When examining the neck, the nurse observes for jugular vein distension and determines the need to measure jugular venous pressure. Distension of the jugular veins may indicate that the patient is in a state of fluid overload.

The anterior and posterior chest is inspected for respiratory rate, rhythm, depth, and effort. Deformities of the thorax, shape of chest, or bulging of interspaces during expiration are noted. The precordial area is observed and palpated for heaves, pulsations, and thrills. The nurse listens for heart rate and rhythm, extra heart sounds, murmurs, clicks, and pericardial friction rub. Fluid overload often results in the presence of a third or fourth heart sound.

Anterior and posterior lung fields are auscultated. The nurse notes the quality of vesicular breath sounds and the presence of adventitious breath sounds (crackles, wheezes, rubs).

After auscultating the posterior chest, the nurse can assess kidney tenderness. To do this, the nurse places one hand over the posterior costovertebral angle (CVA). Then, using the fist of the second hand, he or she gently percusses the CVA and notes whether the patient has discomfort (Fig. 29-1).

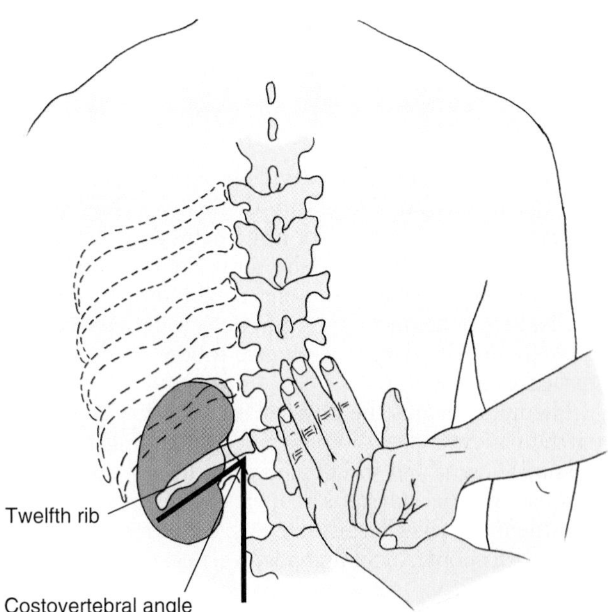

figure 29-1 Assessment of costovertebral angles (CVA).

The nurse inspects the abdomen and then listens for bowel sounds. In addition to auscultating bowel sounds, the nurse auscultates the renal arteries for the presence of bruits by placing the stethoscope above and to the left and right of the umbilicus. A bruit is an abnormal sound that resembles a blowing or swishing noise, similar to the sound of a cardiac murmur. The presence of a renal bruit often indicates renal stenosis, which means there may be diminished blood flow to the kidney. This diminished blood flow may result in acute or chronic renal dysfunction (Fig. 29-2).

Next, the nurse percusses and palpates the abdomen, and then palpates the liver border to determine enlargement. If ascites is suspected, the nurse measures abdominal girth and may check for a fluid wave or shifting dullness.

If the patient is at risk for excess vascular volume, the nurse looks for hypertension; pulmonary edema; rales; engorged, elevated neck veins; liver congestion and enlargement; congestive heart failure; and shortness of breath. Signs and symptoms related to excess extravascular volume include pitting edema of feet, ankles, hands, and fingers; periorbital edema; sacral edema; and ascites.

While examining the extremities, the nurse can check the quality of the peripheral pulses; observe for tremors; test for paresthesia, numbness, and weakness; and palpate fingernails and toenails, checking for color, shape, and capillary refill time.

If the patient has an arteriovenous graft or fistula for dialysis, the nurse assesses it for patency and for adequate circulation to the extremity distal to the access. Palpating

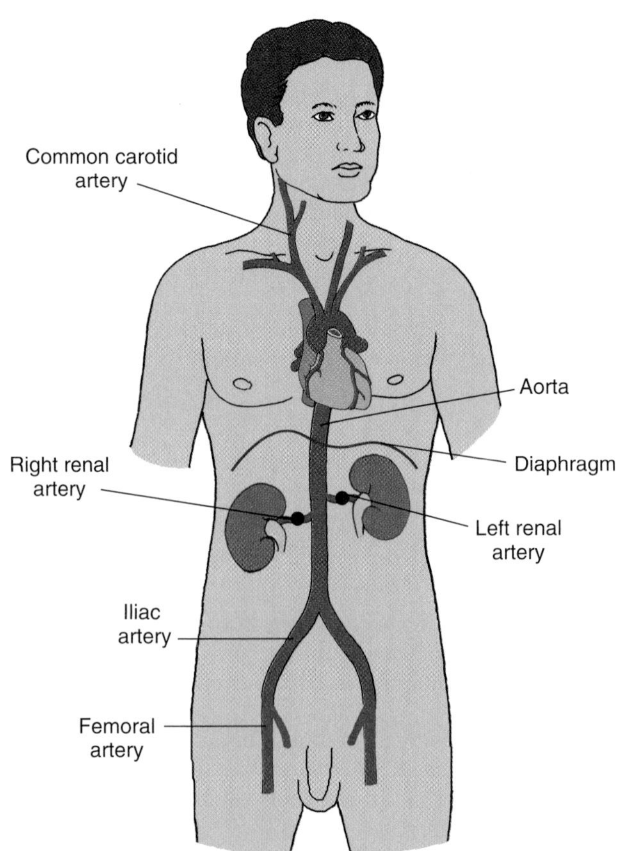

figure 29-2 Sites for auscultation of renal bruits.

for a thrill and auscultating for the presence of a bruit help to assess patency of the graft. If assessment reveals a change, the physician or practitioner must be notified urgently because the graft may be saved through radiological or surgical intervention. If the patient has temporary dialysis access, the exit site is inspected for signs of inflammation or infection. Often the lumens of the temporary access have high doses of heparin to maintain patency, so flushing or use of the device is clarified with the physician or practitioner beforehand.

Patients with renal impairment may be at risk for hypocalcemia, hypomagnesemia, or both. Physical assessment of these electrolyte changes can be achieved by checking for Chvostek's or Trousseau's signs. Chvostek's sign occurs when there is facial irritability after tapping the facial nerve in front of the auditory meatus with the finger. Trousseau's sign occurs then there is spasm of the hands and feet (carpopedal spasm) in response to arm compression (for example, as with a blood pressure cuff).

During the history and examination, the nurse has observed the patient's level of consciousness and mental status. If more data are needed, the nurse may use tools such as the Glasgow Coma Scale and Folstein Mini Mental Examination.

ASSESSMENT OF RENAL FUNCTION

Laboratory Studies

URINE STUDIES

Urinalysis

The nurse inspects the urine for color, clarity, and odor. Normally, the urine is clear and yellow to straw-colored, and smells of ammonia. Changes in the characteristics of the urine can indicate kidney damage, infection, excretion of drugs, or the kidney's compensation for systemic homeostatic imbalance. Cloudy urine may indicate infection, whereas very clear and colorless urine may be a sign of diuresis, either induced pharmacologically or by diabetes insipidus. Blood in the urine may actually appear bright red or dark brown. If hematuria is present in a man older than 50 years, additional radiological evaluation (such as cystoscopy) is considered to rule out a malignancy.[1] Urinalysis is used to identify more specifically the components of the urine.

Urine Volume

The difference between the glomerular filtration rate (GFR) and the amount of water reabsorbed determines the urine volume. A normal patient must reabsorb 179 L/day when the GFR is 180 L. This is the equivalent of roughly more than 99% of filtered volume. Patients with renal disease and impairment may actually excrete an appropriate amount of urine. For example, a patient with severe renal disease may have a GFR of 10 L but still excrete 1 L, or 90% reabsorption. Thus, urine volume is of little diagnostic importance in this setting. One exception to this is in the setting of acute anuria. In acute anuria, a patient may be making normal volume and experience an abrupt change in pattern. Causes of acute anuria include:

- Complete bilateral obstruction (i.e., abdominal compartment syndrome)
- Glomerulonephritis
- Bilateral vascular occlusion

Trends in urine production, however, can provide important clues to the body's recruitment of important compensatory responses, as in hypovolemia. The body initiates the renin–angiotensin–aldosterone system to maintain the crucial water balance (see Chapter 28).

Urine pH

Normal urinary pH is acidic, with a range between 5.0 and 6.5, depending primarily on dietary intake. The kidneys play a tremendous role in acid–base balance (see Chapter 28). The urine will become increasingly acidic (lower pH) when the body is attempting to conserve sodium. Clinically, urinary pH is important in two settings. First, an alkaline urinary pH (above 7.5) suggests the presence of a urinary tract infection. Second, a low, or acidic pH, indicates the kidney may be compensating for a serum acidosis. Physiologically, in this state, the kidneys reabsorb more bicarbonate and excrete more hydrogen ions to buffer the serum acidosis.

Urine Protein

Most proteins are large molecules and under normal conditions should not penetrate Bowman's capsule. Normal urinary protein levels, therefore, are zero to trace. Proteinuria usually indicates damage to the capillary structures, as in the case of glomerular diseases (glomerulonephritis) and intrarenal acute renal failure. For diagnostic purposes, a 24-hour sample of urine is used to assess for proteinuria. Single dipstick measurements are not as sensitive and may lead to false-positive values.

Urine Glucose and Ketones

Glucose, like most proteins, is not present in the urine under normal conditions. Unlike proteins, glucose is freely filtered but reabsorbed in the proximal tubule. Glucose becomes detectable if the serum glucose is elevated (greater than 200 mg/dL) as the filtered load exceeds the kidney's reabsorptive abilities.

Ketone bodies are byproducts of fat metabolism and are formed in states of insulin deficiency. Three ketone bodies are formed: β-hydroxybutyric acid (the primary ketone formed), acetoacetic acid, and acetone. The latter two ketone bodies are detected in the urine. Acetone may be measured in the serum.

Urinary Sediment

Sediment is particulate matter that, when examined, can reveal certain physiological conditions in the renal system. Sediment in general refers to casts, red cells, white cells, epithelial cells, and crystals. Casts are the breakdown products of cellular material formed in the collecting tubules. Urinary stasis, as in prerenal disease, may promote cast formation. Casts can be made up of different types of cells and thus, the shape, composition, and size of the casts can help in the identification of the presence and etiology of a disease.

Red Blood Cells. Red blood cells may be microscopic or grossly visible. The most common type of bleeding in adults is extrarenal. Red blood cells enter the urine anywhere along the urinary tract. Any injury or damage to the structures making up the urinary tract can cause hematuria. Kidney stones, trauma, and prostatic disease are examples of extrarenal causes of hematuria.

Microscopic bleeding can be present in glomerular diseases, such as glomerulonephritis. When assessing the results of the urinalysis, take note of the presence of red blood cell casts and the red blood cell morphology. Glomerular bleeding is often associated with some type of fragmentation of the red blood cell, whereas extrarenal bleeding often leaves the cell intact. The presence of red blood cell casts is virtually diagnostic of glomerulonephritis.

Myoglobin makes the urine appear red; however, when the urine is inspected under the microscope, there is no evidence of red blood cells. Myoglobin is a component of skeletal muscle breakdown, or rhabdomyolysis. Crush injuries or protracted down times are the greatest predictors of this disease. When muscle begins to break down, it releases the myoglobin, which is similar in chemical structure to hemoglobin. Because of its large molecular size, myoglobin blocks the renal tubules, placing patients at very high risk for intrarenal failure.

White Blood Cells. White blood cells in the urine (pyuria) usually indicate infection anywhere along the urinary tract. Leukocyte esterase is an enzyme that can be detected in the urine. This enzyme is present along the urinary tract as a component of the local immune response. High levels of this enzyme can indicate infection. The presence of nitrates may also aid in the diagnosis of a bacterial infection along the urinary tract.

Specific Gravity and Osmolality

The specific gravity of the urine tests the kidneys' ability to concentrate and dilute the urine. The specific gravity measures the buoyancy of a solution compared with water and depends on the number of particles in the solution and their size and weight. There are three methods used to obtain this measurement in clinical practice: a multiple-test *dipstick* that has a reagent area for specific gravity, the *urinometer*, and the *refractometer* (TS meter). The urinometer has been in clinical use for many years and requires enough urine to float the urinometer. Its results are questionable. The refractometer gives highly reproducible results and requires only one drop of urine for the measurement. In addition, this instrument can be used to measure the total solids in plasma (hence the name, *TS* meter), which is a good indicator of the plasma protein concentration and can be a useful indicator of a patient's fluid balance (especially if serial determinations are done).

The normal kidney has the capacity to dilute the urine to a specific gravity of 1.001 and to concentrate the urine to at least 1.022. For reference, the specific gravity of water is 1.000. Normally, a person's water balance determines whether the urine is concentrated or dilute; dilute urine is an indicator of water excess, and concentrated urine indicates water deficit. In many renal diseases, the ability of the kidneys to form concentrated urine is lost, and the specific gravity can become "fixed" at 1.010. This finding is often seen in acute tubular necrosis, acute nephritis, and chronic renal disease. A falsely high specific gravity can be seen when high–molecular-weight substances, such as protein, glucose, mannitol, and radiographic contrast material, are present in the urine. Therefore, a greater degree of accuracy can be obtained by checking the urine osmolality in these cases.

Osmolality measures only the number of solute particles present in a solution. Recall that the main determinants of osmolality are the sodium, urea, and glucose. In states of volume depletion or excess, several neuroendocrine responses interact to maintain homeostasis, thereby affecting the urinary osmolality. Because of this dynamic interaction, particularly in critical illness, single measurements of the osmolality are of little diagnostic importance. The urinary osmolality is often followed for the evaluation of patients with hyponatremia.

Normal urine osmolality ranges from 300 to 900 mOsm/kg/24 hours. Because of this wide range, more information about renal function is obtained when simultaneous serum and urine samples are collected and interpreted. In renal disease, one of the first functions to be lost is the ability to concentrate urine. This can result in the urine osmolality becoming fixed within 150 mOsm of the simultaneously determined serum osmolality.

Urinary Sodium Concentration

The urinary sodium excretion is used as an indicator of renal function in differentiating the oliguria associated with acute renal failure from other prerenal causes. States of poor kidney perfusion are usually associated with a decrease in urinary sodium concentration (usually less than 10 mEq/L). This is a compensatory reaction generated by the activation of the renin–angiotensin–aldosterone system. Activation of this neuroendocrine response allows for increased reabsorption of sodium (reduced excretion) with a subsequent increase in water reabsorption. The root cause of kidney hypoperfusion can be anything that causes a reduction in effective circulating volume: Volume depletion and heart failure are two examples. If hypoperfusion persists, acute renal failure may ensue. In acute renal failure (because of damage to the tubular transport mechanisms), urine sodium concentration usually is greater than 30 to 40 mEq/L despite oliguria. However, when the urine pH is alkaline, urine sodium concentration does not reflect sodium balance accurately, and the chloride concentration becomes a better indicator of volume status.

Fractional Excretion of Sodium Test

The fractional excretion of sodium (FE_{Na}) test gives a more precise estimation of the amount of filtered sodium that remains in the urine and is more accurate in predicting tubular injury than the urinary sodium concentration.[2] One benefit of the FE_{Na} compared with the urinary sodium is that it removes the confounding effect of water. It can be calculated by using the following formula:

$$\left[(U/P)\,Na/(U/P)\,Cr\right] \times 100$$

in which *U* and *P* are the urinary and plasma concentrations of sodium and creatinine, respectively. (Although volume measurements are necessary to derive the absolute urinary excretion of both sodium and creatinine, these cancel out in deriving the formula.)

The test requires the determination of both serum and urinary sodium and creatinine concentrations on simultaneously obtained samples. Values less than 1% indicate prerenal azotemia, or underperfusion. Values greater than 1% (and frequently greater than 3%) are indicative of acute renal failure.

BLOOD STUDIES

Creatinine and Creatinine Clearance

Creatinine is a byproduct of normal muscle metabolism and is excreted in the urine primarily as the result of glomerular filtration, with a small percentage secreted into the urine by the kidney tubules. Therefore, creatinine is the most important indicator of GFR. The amount of creatinine excreted in the urine is directly related to muscle mass and normally remains constant unless significant muscle wasting (a catabolic state) occurs. Normal serum values for creatinine are 0.6 to 1.2 mg/dL.

The creatinine clearance can be defined as the amount of blood that is cleared of creatinine in 1 minute and is an excellent clinical indicator of renal function. As renal function diminishes, creatinine clearance decreases. To obtain an accurate creatinine clearance, the nurse collects all urine made in a 24-hour period and obtains a blood specimen at some point during the urine collection. Thus, it is essential for the nurse to communicate to other team members that a 24-hour collection is in progress. For consistency, the blood sample is usually collected at the midpoint of the urine collection. It is important to note the exact beginning and ending time of the urine collection.

The actual creatinine clearance is calculated by the following formula:

$$\text{Creatinine clearance} = \frac{\text{UV}}{\text{PC}}$$

where *U* is the urine creatinine concentration; *V*, the urine volume; and *PC*, the plasma creatinine concentration.

The expression *UV* tells how much creatinine appears in the urine during the period of collection. This can be converted readily to milligrams per minute, which is the standard reference point. Dividing this value by the plasma creatinine concentration (which must be converted from milligrams per 100 mL to milligrams per milliliter) tells the minimum number of milliliters of plasma that must have been filtered by the glomeruli to produce the measured amount of creatinine in the urine. The final result is usually expressed in milliliters per minute. The normal range varies between 80 and 120 mL/minute, depending on the person's size, age, and sex. The results can be adjusted to a standard body size of 1.73 m^2 (body surface area [BSA]), which can be derived from standard tables if the patient's height and weight are known; it averages between 120 and 125 mL/minute/1.73 m^2 BSA. After age 40 years, normal creatinine clearance values generally decrease 6.5 mL/minute per decade because of a decline in GFR.

There are also formulas that estimate creatinine clearance based on a single serum creatinine level. An estimate may be done when there is difficulty collecting a 24-hour urine sample or when spot-checking the creatinine clearance will assist prompt treatment (as in the case of drug nephrotoxicity). The estimate may be accurate only in patients with chronic renal failure with stable renal function who are not edematous or extremely overweight.

$$\text{Creatinine clearance (estimated)} = \frac{(140 - \text{age}) \times \text{weight in kg}}{(\text{PCr in mg/dL}) \times 72}$$

where PCr is plasma creatinine; note that for women, the final result is multiplied by 0.85.

When the kidneys are damaged by a disease process, the creatinine clearance decreases and the serum creatinine concentration rises. The urine creatinine excretion decreases initially until the blood level rises to a point at which the amount of creatinine appearing in the urine is equal to the amount being produced by the body. For example, a healthy person with a serum creatinine concentration of 1 mg/dL and a creatinine excretion of 1 mg/minute has a creatinine clearance of 100 mL/minute. When the person experiences a 50% loss of renal function, the serum creatinine rises to 2 mg/dL, and the person will continue to excrete 1 mg/minute of creatinine in the urine when balance is restored. When the person has rapidly changing renal function and oliguria (e.g., acute renal failure), the creatinine clearance is less reliable. Until renal function stabilizes, serum creatinine levels provide a better indication of the rate and direction of change. In patients with rhabdomyolysis, the serum creatinine is elevated out of proportion to the reduction of GFR as the result of chemical conversion of muscle creatine to creatinine. In this situation, the serum creatinine is less reliable as an indicator of renal function.

Blood Urea Nitrogen

The blood urea nitrogen (BUN) level has been used for many years as an indicator of kidney function, but unlike the serum creatinine, the BUN level can be influenced by many factors. At low urine flow rates, more sodium and water, and consequently more urea, are reabsorbed. Therefore, when the patient is volume depleted, the BUN tends to rise out of proportion to any change in renal function. A normal value for the BUN is considered to be 8 to 20 mg/dL.

Increased urea production can result from increased protein intake (tube feedings and some forms of hyperalimentation) or increased tissue breakdown, as with crush injuries, febrile illnesses, steroid or tetracycline administration, and reabsorption of blood from the intestine in a patient with intestinal hemorrhage. The BUN also may be elevated in the dehydrated patient because the lack of fluid volume causes a concentrated value. The patient in shock and the patient with congestive heart failure may have an elevated BUN secondary to decreased renal perfusion. The opposite is true for patients with decreased protein intake or liver disease (both of which reduce urea production) and for patients with large urine volumes secondary to excessive fluid intake.

The BUN can be of significant value, however, when used as a comparison with the serum creatinine concentration. Normally, there is a ratio of 10:1 (urea:creatinine). Discrepancies in this ratio might suggest a potentially correctable situation, as noted in Box 29-2.

box 29-2
Factors Affecting the Serum Urea:Creatinine Ratio

Decreased Urea:Creatinine Ratio (<10:1)
- Liver disease
- Protein restriction
- Excessive fluid intake

Increased Urea:Creatinine Ratio (>10:1)
- Volume depletion
- Decreased "effective" blood volume
- Catabolic states
- Excessive protein intake

Osmolality

The *osmolality* of a solution is an expression of the total number (concentration) of particles in the solution and is independent of the size, molecular weight, and electrical charge of the molecules. All substances in solution contribute to the osmolality. For example, 1 mol (gram molecular weight) of sodium chloride dissociates incompletely into Na and Cl ions and produces 1.86 osm when dissolved in 1 kg of solvent (such as plasma). A mole of nonionic solute (e.g., glucose or urea) produces only 1 osm when dissolved in 1 kg of solvent. The total concentration of particles in a solution equals the osmolality and is normally reported in units of osmoles per kilogram of solvent. In the clinical setting (because of much smaller concentrations), the osmolality is reported in milliosmoles (thousandth of an osmole, abbreviated mOsm) per kilogram of solvent (plasma or serum).

The normal *serum osmolality* consists primarily of sodium and its accompanying anions, with urea and glucose contributing about 5 mOsm each. Therefore, when the serum sodium, urea, and glucose concentrations are known, the osmolality of plasma can be calculated by the following formula:

$$\text{Osmolality} = 2\text{Na} + \text{BUN}/2.6 + \text{glucose}/18$$

The calculated osmolality normally is within 10 mOsm of the measured osmolality. The normal adult average osmolality is 280 to 290 mOsm/kg and remains quite constant. Because water can move freely between the blood, interstitial fluid, and tissues, any change in the osmolality of one body compartment produces a shift in body fluids. Therefore, the osmolality of the plasma is the same as that of other body compartments except in rapidly changing conditions, when a slight lag may occur.

A decrease in the serum osmolality can occur only when the serum sodium is decreased. An increase in the serum osmolality can occur whenever the serum sodium, urea, or glucose is elevated or when abnormal compounds are present in the blood, such as drugs, poisons, or metabolic waste products, such as lactic acid. Symptoms usually do not occur until the osmolality is greater than 350 mOsm/kg. Coma can occur when the osmolality is 400 mOsm/kg or greater.

Nonspecific Studies

Hematocrit and Hemoglobin. The normal hemoglobin for men is 13.5 to 17.5 g/dL and 12 to 16 g/dL for women. The normal hematocrit should be 40% to 52% for adult men and 37% to 48% for adult women. False elevations of hematocrit can be seen with dehydration or after dialysis. Low hematocrits may be a dilutional value due to hypervolemia. The kidney is the primary site for the production of erythropoietin. It stimulates the bone marrow to release mature red blood cells. Many patients with ESRD produce insufficient amounts of erythropoietin, which can result in chronic anemia. These patients can also have bleeding problems due to impaired platelet function and immunological abnormalities.

Uric Acid. The normal uric acid serum level is between 2 and 8.5 mg/dL. It is excreted primarily by the kidneys, with some in the stool. Uric acid may be elevated because of excessive production from cell breakdown or because it is not adequately excreted by the kidney.

Diagnostic Studies

RADIOLOGICAL STUDIES

Radiological studies of the kidneys that may be useful in evaluating renal abnormalities include roentgenography, ultrasonography, and radionuclide studies. These studies and their purposes are summarized in Table 29-1.

RENAL BIOPSY

Renal biopsy is the most invasive but most definitive diagnostic tool used in the comprehensive renal evaluation. It is used to define the histological counterpart of the clinical picture, provide etiological clues for diagnosis, assess prognosis, and guide therapy. It is also used as an assessment tool for insurability, employment, or disability. Contraindications to biopsy include serious bleeding disorders, excessive obesity, and severe hypertension (Table 29-2).

Renal biopsies are usually performed percutaneously with a biopsy needle, but an open renal biopsy under general anesthesia still is performed. Preparation for a renal biopsy includes obtaining informed consent, prebiopsy clotting studies, preoperative blood typing, and sedation (usually diazepam, 5 to 10 mg) and establishing intravenous access to prevent or treat complications. After the biopsy, the patient's vital signs are checked every 15 minutes for the first 2 hours, hourly for 4 hours, and then every 4 hours for the first 24 hours. The patient's urine is examined for blood. The major complication is bleeding, which can occur either retroperitoneally or into the urinary tract. Other complications that can occur are biopsy of other abdominal viscera, such as bowel, pancreas, liver, spleen, or vessels, and tears in the diaphragm or pleura.

RENAL ANGIOGRAPHY

Assessment of the renal vasculature may be accomplished by ultrasonography. When precise measurements are required, evaluation of renal blood flow may be used. This procedure may be performed in conjunction with cardiac catheterization. Access is obtained by percutaneous technique: An introducer, or sheath, is inserted into the femoral artery and a small catheter is passed to the bifurcation of the renal arteries. Contrast medium is injected to provide radiological visualization of blood flow. Preparation for a renal angiogram is similar to that for renal biopsy, and includes obtaining informed consent, preprocedure clotting studies,

table 29-1 Radiological Study of Kidneys

Diagnostic Test	Purpose
Roentgenography	
• Radiograph of kidney–ureter–bladder (KUB)	Detect abnormal calcifications, renal size
• Tomography	Determine renal outlines and abnormalities
• Intravenous pyelography (IVP)	Detect anatomical abnormalities of the kidneys and ureters
• Retrograde pyelography	Assess renal size, evaluate ureteral obstruction, localize and diagnose tumors, obstructions
• Antegrade pyelography	Distinguish cysts from hydronephrosis
• Renal arteriography and venography	Evaluate possible renal arterial stenosis, renal mass lesions, renal vein thrombosis, and venous extension of renal cell carcinoma
• Digital subtraction angiography	Visualize major arterial vessels
Ultrasonography	Delineate renal outlines Measure longitudinal and transverse dimensions of the kidneys Evaluate mass lesions Examine perinephric area Detect and grade hydronephrosis
Radionuclide scintillation imaging (renal scan)	
• Static imaging	Evaluate location, size, and contour of functional renal tissue; may reveal areas of inhomogeneity or filling defects
• Dynamic imaging	Monitor the passage of a radiopharmaceutical agent through the vascular, renal parenchymal, and urinary tract compartments
Magnetic resonance imaging	Determine anatomical abnormalities

table 29-2 Indications for Renal Biopsy

Clinical Condition	Biopsy Indicated	Expected Gain
Orthostatic proteinuria	No	—
Isolated hematuria and/or proteinuria	No*	—
Hematuria and/or proteinuria with ↓ GFR	Yes	D,P,T
Nephrotic syndrome	Yes	D,P,T
Systemic disease with renal abnormalities	Yes†	D,P,T
Classic ARF	No	—
ARF with		
1. azotemia >3 wk	Yes	D,P
2. moderate proteinuria	Yes	D,T
3. anuria	Yes	D,T
4. eosinophilia or eosinophiluria	Yes	D,T
Post-transplant ↓ in GFR	Yes	D,P,T

GFR, glomerular filtration rate; D, diagnosis; P, prognosis; T, therapy; ARF, acute renal failure

* Biopsy may be indicated for insurance, administrative reasons, and so forth.

† Biopsy may or may not be indicated, depending on clinical picture.

preoperative blood typing, and sedation (usually midazolam, 1 to 2 mg, or diazepam, 5 to 10 mg), and establishing intravenous access to prevent or treat complications. After the angiogram, the patient's vital signs are checked every 15 minutes for the first 2 hours, hourly for 4 hours, and then every 4 hours for the first 24 hours. Pressure is applied locally when the arterial access is removed. Because the artery is accessed, life-threatening bleeding can ensue. Therefore, the access site is assessed for bleeding with the same frequency as the vital signs are assessed. Diligence in application of pressure to the site and conducting site assessment is imperative. Watch for development of bradycardia because pressure applied to the groin area may stimulate the vagus nerve.

ASSESSMENT OF ELECTROLYTES AND ACID–BASE BALANCE

The role of the kidney is central in maintaining fluid volume and ionic composition of body fluids. When the kidneys properly regulate the excretion of water and ions, homeostasis is achieved. When they fail to adapt adequately, imbalances occur. Electrolyte values and signs and symptoms of imbalance are summarized in Table 29-3. All of the electrolytes need to be monitored closely by the critical care nurse because minor shifts can be lethal.

table 29-3 Disorders of Electrolyte Balance

Electrolyte Imbalance	Signs and Symptoms	Diagnostic Test Results
Hyponatremia	• Muscle twitching and weakness • Lethargy, confusion, seizures, and coma • Hypotension and tachycardia • Nausea, vomiting, and abdominal cramps • Oliguria or anuria	• Serum sodium <135 mEq/L • Decreased urine specific gravity • Decreased serum osmolality • Urine sodium >100 mEq/24 h • Increased red blood cell count
Hypernatremia	• Agitation, restlessness, fever, and decreased level of consciousness • Hypertension, tachycardia, pitting edema, and excessive weight gain • Thirst, increased viscosity of saliva, rough tongue • Dyspnea, respiratory arrest, and death	• Serum sodium >145 mEq/L • Urine sodium <40 mEq/24 h • High serum osmolality
Hypokalemia	• Dizziness, hypotension, dysrhythmias, electrocardiogram (ECG) changes, and cardiac arrest • Nausea, vomiting, anorexia, diarrhea, decreased peristalsis, and abdominal distention • Muscle weakness, fatigue, and leg cramps	• Serum potassium <3.5 mEq/L • Coexisting low serum calcium and magnesium levels not responsive to treatment for hypokalemia usually suggest hypomagnesemia • Metabolic alkalosis • ECG changes, including flattened T waves, elevated U waves, depressed ST segment
Hyperkalemia	• Tachycardia changing to bradycardia, ECG changes, and cardiac arrest • Nausea, diarrhea, and abdominal cramps • Muscle weakness and flaccid paralysis	• Serum potassium >5 mEq/L • Metabolic acidosis • ECG changes, including tented and elevated T waves, widened QRS complex, prolonged PR interval, flattened or absent P waves, depressed ST segment
Hypochloremia	• Muscle hypertonicity and tetany • Shallow, depressed breathing • Usually associated with hyponatremia and its characteristic symptoms, such as muscle weakness and twitching	• Serum chloride <98 mEq/L • Serum pH >7.45 (supportive value) • Serum CO_2 >32 mEq/L (supportive value)
Hyperchloremia	• Deep, rapid breathing • Weakness • Diminished cognitive ability, possibly leading to coma	• Serum chloride >108 mEq/L • Serum pH <7.35, serum CO_2 <22 mEq/L (supportive values)
Hypocalcemia	• Anxiety, irritability, twitching around the mouth, laryngospasm, seizures, positive Chvostek's and Trousseau's signs • Hypotension and dysrhythmias due to decreased calcium influx	• Serum calcium <8.5 mg/dL • Low platelet count • ECG changes: lengthened QT interval, prolonged ST segment, arrhythmias • Possible changes in serum protein levels
Hypercalcemia	• Drowsiness, lethargy, headaches, irritability, confusion, depression, or apathy • Weakness and muscle flaccidity • Bone pain and pathological fractures • Heart block • Anorexia, nausea, vomiting, constipation, and dehydration • Flank pain	• Serum calcium >10.5 mg/dL • ECG changes: signs of heart block and shortened QT interval • Azotemia • Decreased parathyroid hormone level • Sulkowitch urine test results: increased calcium precipitation
Hypomagnesemia	• Nearly always coexists with hypokalemia and hypocalcemia • Hyperirritability, tetany, leg and foot cramps, positive Chvostek's and Trousseau's signs, confusion, delusions, and seizures • Dysrhythmias, vasodilation, and hypotension	• Serum magnesium <1.5 mEq/L • Coexisting low serum potassium and calcium levels

(continued)

table 29-3 Disorders of Electrolyte Balance (Continued)

Electrolyte Imbalance	Signs and Symptoms	Diagnostic Test Results
Hypermagnesemia	• Uncommon, caused by decreased renal excretion (renal failure) or increased intake of magnesium • Diminished reflexes, muscle weakness to flaccid paralysis • Respiratory distress • Heart block, bradycardia • Hypotension	• Serum magnesium >2.5 mEq/L • Coexisting elevated potassium and calcium levels
Hypophosphatemia	• Muscle weakness, tremor, and paresthesia • Peripheral hypoxia	• Serum phosphate <2.5 mg/dL • Urine phosphate >1.3 g/24 hours
Hyperphosphatemia	• Usually asymptomatic unless leading to hypocalcemia, then evidenced by tetany and seizures	• Serum phosphate >4.5 mg/dL • Serum calcium <9 mg/dL • Urine phosphorus <0.9 g/24 hours

From Anatomical Chart Company: Atlas of Pathophysiology, pp 30–31. Springhouse, PA, Springhouse, 2002.

Sodium Balance

Serum sodium concentration is normally 135 to 145 mEq/L. It is regulated by the kidneys and depends on the sodium concentration in the extracellular fluid. When the concentration rises, the kidneys retain water in response to antidiuretic hormone (ADH). When the concentration falls, aldosterone promotes sodium retention by the kidneys (see Chapter 42, Fig. 42-9). When the kidneys malfunction, this balance is not maintained. A low serum sodium usually indicates water intake in excess of sodium and is characterized by an increase in body weight. A high serum sodium usually indicates water loss in excess of sodium and is reflected in weight loss. Sodium is essential for maintaining the osmolality of extracellular fluids, neuromuscular function, acid–base balance, and various other cellular chemical reactions.

Hyponatremia is important because it can produce a wide range of neurological symptoms, including death. The severity of symptoms depends on the degree of hyponatremia and the rate at which it has developed. Usually, symptoms do not occur until the serum sodium is below 120 mEq/L.[2] For patients with hyponatremia, the severity of symptoms encountered depends on how rapidly the sodium concentration was lowered, as well as the value. Hyponatremia requires further evaluation. Figure 29-3 illustrates the etiologies and evaluation for hyponatremia.

Symptoms of hypernatremia generally are the same as those of hyperosmolality and result from central nervous system dehydration. Mental confusion, stupor, seizures, coma, and death may occur, in addition to other signs of dehydration, such as fatigue, muscle weakness and cramps, and anorexia. The serum osmolality usually is above 350 mOsm/L before significant symptoms are noted. This corresponds to a serum sodium level of 165 to 170 mEq/L.

Potassium Balance

Potassium is essential for regulating nerve impulse conduction and muscle contraction and is involved in numerous other body functions, including intracellular osmolality and acid–base balance. The normal serum potassium concentration is 3.5 to 5 mEq/L. Potassium balance is maintained by dietary intake and renal excretion. Ninety-eight percent of potassium is located in the skeletal muscle; therefore, the balance of this electrolyte also is strongly tied to the exchanges between the intracellular and extracellular compartments in the body.

Hypokalemia can result from inadequate potassium intake, excessive potassium loss through the kidneys, gastrointestinal loss, and extracellular-to-intracellular potassium shifts. Also, diuretic therapy can contribute to potassium excretion, further compounding the problem.

Hyperkalemia may be caused by a decrease in the renal excretion of potassium or transcellular shifts of potassium. This is seen most often in acidosis, cell injury or destruction, and hyperglycemia.

Calcium and Phosphate Balance

Calcium and phosphate are regulated reciprocally in the body by vitamin D, parathyroid hormone, and calcitonin. The calcium and phosphate salts are normally deposited in bone. When calcium levels are high, phosphate levels are low. Because in renal failure the kidneys are unable to eliminate phosphate, patients with renal failure often have high phosphate and low calcium levels.

Calcium's primary function is maintenance of bone and tooth strength. It also plays an important role in myocardial and skeletal contractility. Calcium also maintains cellular permeability and assists in blood coagulation. The normal serum concentration of calcium is 8.5 to 10.5 mg/dL. Serum calcium consists of ultrafiltrable calcium and the calcium that is bound to protein, primarily albumin. Ultrafiltrable calcium includes ionized calcium and the calcium that is in a complex with bicarbonate, citrate, and phosphate.[3]

Phosphate is essential for the formation of adenosine triphosphate (ATP). Phosphate also assists in the maintenance of cell membrane structure, oxygen delivery, and cellular immunity. The normal phosphate level is 3 to 4.5 mg/dL.

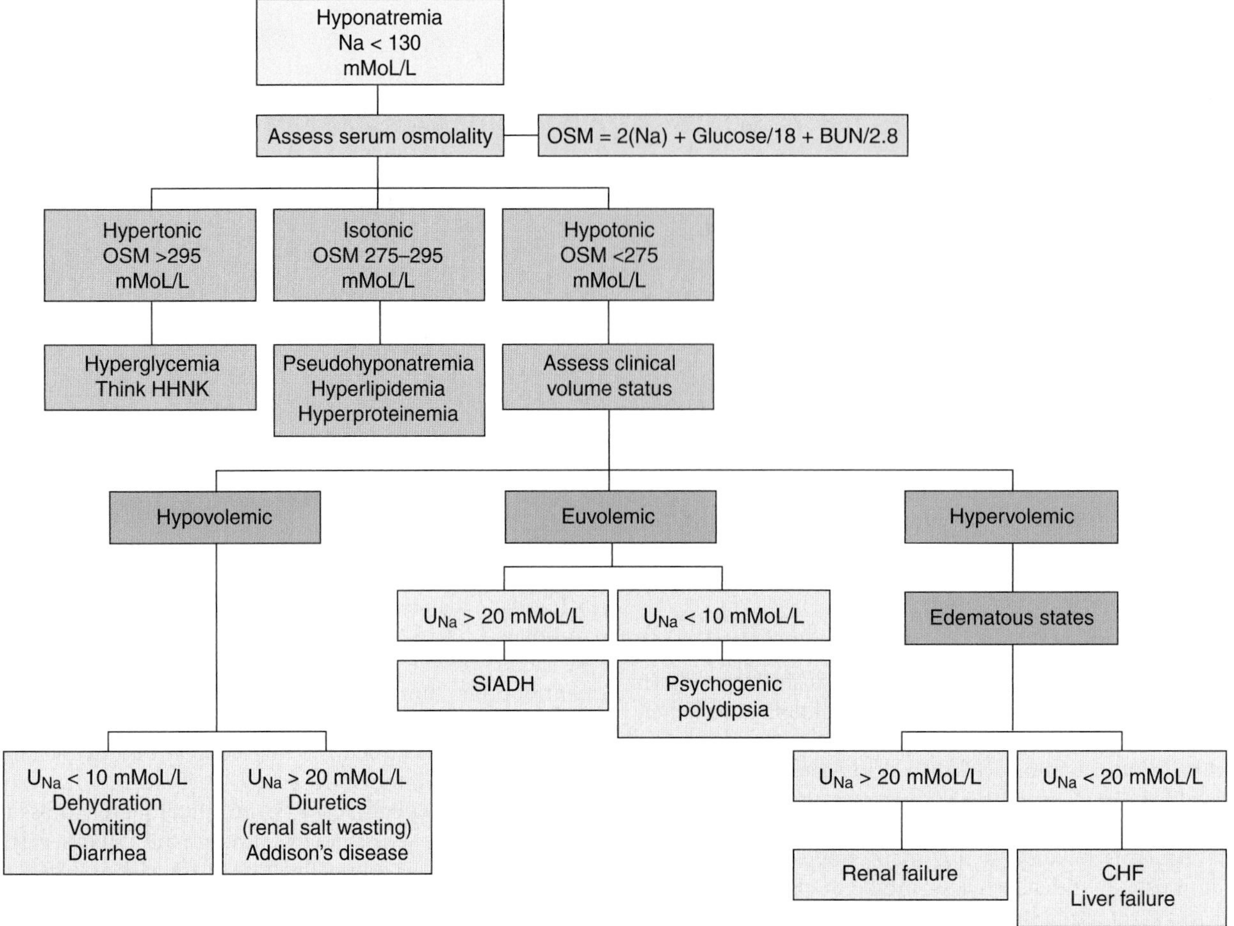

figure 29-3 Assessing hyponatremia. *Na,* sodium; *OSM,* osmolality; *BUN,* blood urea nitrogen; *HHNK,* hyperglycemic hyperosmolar nonketotic (coma); U_{Na}, urine sodium; *SIADH,* syndrome of inappropriate antidiuretic hormone secretion; *CHF,* congestive heart failure.

Magnesium Balance

The magnesium ion is the second major intracellular ion. The normal serum concentration is 1.4 to 2.1 mEq/L. Magnesium balance is necessary for the functional integrity of the neuromuscular system. The parathyroid glands regulate both magnesium and calcium. Sodium is necessary for magnesium reabsorption. Magnesium can accumulate in the serum, bone, and muscle in renal failure, causing numerous problems.

Acid–Base Balance

A normal acidity or alkalinity (pH of 7.35 to 7.45) of the body fluid is essential for life. The body maintains acid–base balance by the buffer system, the respiratory system, and the renal system. The buffer and respiratory systems are able to react quickly to changes in body pH. However, the kidneys take more time to adjust to changes in body pH.

Five major processes are associated with the regulation of acid–base balance by the renal system: hydrogen ion excretion; sodium ion reabsorption; bicarbonate ion generation and reabsorption; phosphate salt and titratable acid excretion; and ammonia synthesis and ammonium excretion.[3] Acid–base imbalances may result when the kidneys are unable to perform those processes adequately. Acid–base balances are summarized in Table 29-4.

THE ANION GAP

To maintain chemical neutrality, the total concentration of cations and anions in the blood (and other body fluids) must be equivalent in terms of milliequivalents per liter. However, because there are a number of anions and cations present in blood that are not routinely measured, a "gap" exists between the total concentration of cations and anions and the concentration normally measured in the plasma:

$$Na^+ + K^+ \text{ versus } Cl^- + HCO_3^-$$

The anion gap is composed primarily of an excess of unmeasured anions, including plasma proteins, inorganic phosphates and sulfates, and organic acids. The unmeasured cations that exist in smaller concentrations are primarily calcium and magnesium.

The anion gap usually is calculated by using the following formula:

$$Na^+ + \left(Cl^- + HCO_3^-\right)$$

and has a normal mean of approximately 12 mEq/L (range, 8 to 16 mEq/L). Potassium is usually, but not always, omitted from the formula because of its relatively low concentration and narrow range of fluctuation. However, departures from this "normal" anion gap may have impor-

table 29-4 Disorders of Acid–Base Balance

Disorder/Causes	Pathophysiology	Signs/Symptoms	Diagnosis
Respiratory Acidosis • Airway obstruction or parenchymal lung disease • Mechanical ventilation • Chronic metabolic alkalosis as respiratory compensatory mechanisms try to normalize pH • Chronic bronchitis • Extensive pneumonia • Large pneumothorax • Pulmonary edema • Asthma • Chronic obstructive pulmonary disorder (COPD) • Drugs • Cardiac arrest • Central nervous system (CNS) trauma • Neuromuscular diseases • Sleep apnea	When pulmonary ventilation decreases, partial pressure of carbon dioxide in arterial blood ($Paco_2$) increases and CO_2 level rises. Retained CO_2 combines with water (H_2O) to form carbonic acid (H_2CO_3), which dissociates to release free hydrogen (H^+) and bicarbonate (HCO_3^-) ions. Increased $Paco_2$ and free H^+ ions stimulate the medulla to increase respiratory drive and expel CO_2. As pH falls, 2,3-diphosphoglycerate (2,3-DPG) accumulates in red blood cells, where it alters hemoglobin (hgb) to release oxygen. The hgb picks up H^+ ions and CO_2 and removes them from the serum. As respiratory mechanisms fail, rising $Paco_2$ stimulates kidneys to retain HCO_3^- and sodium (Na^+) ions and excrete H^+ ions. As the H^+ ion concentration overwhelms compensatory mechanisms, H^+ ions move into cells and potassium (K^+) ions move out. Without enough oxygen, anaerobic metabolism produces lactic acid.	• Restlessness • Confusion • Apprehension • Somnolence • Asterixis • Headaches • Dyspnea and tachypnea • Papilledema • Depressed reflexes • Hypoxemia • Tachycardia • Hypertension/hypotension • Atrial and ventricular dysrhythmias • Coma	• Arterial blood gas (ABG) analysis: $Paco_2$ >45 mm Hg; pH <7.35 to 7.45; and normal HCO_3^- in the acute stage and elevated HCO_3^- in the chronic stage
Respiratory Alkalosis • Acute hypoxemia, pneumonia, interstitial lung disease, pulmonary vascular disease, or acute asthma • Anxiety • Hypermetabolic states such as fever and sepsis • Excessive mechanical ventilation • Salicylate toxicity • Metabolic acidosis • Hepatic failure • Pregnancy	As pulmonary ventilation increases, excessive CO_2 is exhaled. Resulting hypocapnia leads to reduction of H_2CO_3, excretion of H^+ and HCO_3^- ions, and rising serum pH. Against rising pH, the hydrogen–potassium buffer system pulls H^+ ions out of cells and into blood in exchange for K^+ ions. H^+ ions entering blood combine with HCO_3^- ions to form H_2CO_3, and pH falls. Hypocapnia causes an increase in heart rate, cerebral vasoconstriction, and decreased cerebral blood flow. After 6 hours, kidneys secrete more HCO_3^- and less H^+. Continued low $Paco_2$ and vasoconstriction increases cerebral and peripheral hypoxia. Severe alkalosis inhibits calcium (Ca^{2+}) ionization; increasing nerve/muscle excitability.	• Deep, rapid breathing • Lightheadedness or dizziness • Agitation • Circumoral and peripheral paresthesias • Carpopedal spasms, twitching, and muscle weakness	ABG analysis showing $Paco_2$ <35 mm Hg; elevated pH in proportion to decrease in $Paco_2$ in the acute stage but decreasing toward normal in the chronic stage; normal HCO_3^- in the acute stage but less than normal in the chronic stage

(continued)

table 29-4 Disorders of Acid–Base Balance (Continued)

Disorder/Causes	Pathophysiology	Signs/Symptoms	Diagnosis
Metabolic Acidosis			
• Excessive acid accumulation • Deficient HCO_3^- stores • Decreased acid excretion by the kidneys • Diabetic ketoacidosis • Chronic alcoholism • Malnutrition or a low-carbohydrate, high-fat diet • Anaerobic carbohydrate metabolism • Underexcretion of metabolized acids or inability to conserve base • Diarrhea, intestinal malabsorption, or loss of sodium bicarbonate from the intestines • Salicylate intoxication, exogenous poisoning, or, less frequently, Addison's disease • Inhibited secretion of acid	As H^+ ions begin accumulating in the body, chemical buffers (plasma HCO_3^- and proteins) in cells and extracellular fluid (ECF) bind them. Excess H^+ ions decrease blood pH and stimulate chemoreceptors in the medulla to increase respiration. Consequent fall of partial pressure of $Paco_2$ frees H^+ ions to bind with HCO_3^- ions. Respiratory compensation occurs but is not sufficient to correct acidosis. Healthy kidneys compensate, excreting excess H^+ ions, buffered by phosphate or ammonia. For each H^+ ion excreted, renal tubules reabsorb and return to blood one Na^+ ion and one HCO_3^- ion. Excess H^+ ions in ECF passively diffuse into cells. To maintain balance of charge across cell membrane, cells release K^+ ions. Excess H^+ ions change the normal balance of K^+, Na^+, and Ca^{2+} ions, impairing neural excitability.	• Headache and lethargy progressing to drowsiness, CNS depression, Kussmaul's respirations, hypotension, stupor, and coma and death • Associated gastrointestinal (GI) distress leading to anorexia, nausea, vomiting, diarrhea, and possibly dehydration • Warm, flushed skin • Fruity-smelling breath	• Arterial pH <7.35; $Paco_2$ normal or <34 mm Hg as respiratory compensatory mechanisms take hold; HCO_3^- may be <22 mEq/L • Urine pH <4.5 in the absence of renal disease • Elevated plasma lactic acid in lactic acidosis • Anion gap >14 mEq/L in high–anion gap metabolic acidosis, lactic acidosis, ketoacidosis, aspirin overdose, alcohol poisoning, renal failure, or other disorder characterized by accumulation of organic acids, sulfates, or phosphates • Anion gap 12 mEq/L or less in normal anion gap metabolic acidosis from HCO_3^- loss, GI or renal loss, increased acid load, rapid intravenous (IV) saline administration, or other disorders characterized by HCO_3^- loss
Metabolic Alkalosis			
• Chronic vomiting • Nasogastric tube drainage or lavage without adequate electrolyte replacement • Fistulas • Use of steroids and certain diuretics (furosemide [Lasix], thiazides, and ethacrynic acid [Edecrin]) • Massive blood transfusions • Cushing's disease, primary hyperaldosteronism, and Bartter's syndrome • Excessive intake of bicarbonate of soda, other antacids, or absorbable alkali • Excessive amounts of IV fluids, high serum concentrations of bicarbonate or lactate • Respiratory insufficiency • Low serum chloride • Low serum potassium	Chemical buffers in ECF and intracellular fluid bind HCO_3^- in the body. Excess unbound HCO_3^- raises blood pH, depressing chemoreceptors in the medulla, inhibiting respiration and raising $Paco_2$. CO_2 combines with H_2O to form H_2CO_3. Low oxygen limits respiratory compensation. When blood HCO_3^- rises to 28 mEq/L, the amount filtered by renal glomeruli exceeds reabsorptive capacity of the renal tubules. Excess HCO_3^- is excreted in urine, and H^+ ions are retained. To maintain electrochemical balance, Na^+ ions and water are excreted with HCO_3^- ions. When H^+ ion levels in ECF are low, H^+ ions diffuse passively out of cells and extracellular K^+ ions move into cells. As intracellular H^+ ion levels fall, calcium ionization decreases, and nerve cells become permeable to Na^+ ions. Na^+ ions moving into cells trigger neural impulses in peripheral nervous system and in CNS.	• Irritability, picking at bedclothes (carphology), twitching, and confusion • Nausea, vomiting, and diarrhea • Cardiovascular abnormalities due to hypokalemia • Respiratory disturbances (such as cyanosis and apnea) and slow, shallow respirations • Possible carpopedal spasm in the hand, due to diminished peripheral blood flow during repeated blood pressure checks	• Blood pH >7.45; HCO_3^- >29 mEq/L • Low potassium (<3.5 mEq/L), calcium (<8.9 mg/dL), and chloride (<98 mEq/L)

From Anatomical Chart Company: Atlas of Pathophysiology, pp 32–33. Springhouse, PA, Springhouse, 2002.

table 29-5 Causes of an Altered Anion Gap

Increased Anion Gap	Decreased Anion Gap
Increased unmeasured anions • Endogenous metabolic acidosis Lactic acidosis Ketoacidosis Uremic acidosis • Exogenous anion ingestion Ethylene glycol Methanol Paraldehyde Salicylates Penicillin Carbenicillin • Increased plasma proteins Hyperalbuminemia	Increased unmeasured cations • Normal cations Hypercalcemia Hyperkalemia Hypermagnesemia • Abnormal cations Increased globulins (e.g., myeloma) Lithium
Decreased unmeasured cations • Hypokalemia • Hypocalcemia • Hypomagnesemia	Decreased unmeasured anions • Hypoalbuminemia

tant diagnostic significance in acid–base disorders, especially metabolic acidoses.

The most common abnormality of the anion gap is an increase that is associated with increased concentrations of lactate, ketone bodies, or inorganic phosphate and sulfate that are found in lactic acidosis, ketoacidosis, and uremia, respectively. Other forms of acidosis associated with ingestion of toxins, such as ethylene glycol, methanol, paraldehyde, and salicylates, also may produce significant increases in the anion gap.

Decreases in the anion gap are less common but equally important. They can occur because of increases in unmeasured cations or because of decreases in unmeasured anions. Table 29-5 lists the causes of altered anion gap.

ASSESSMENT OF FLUID BALANCE

The nurse's role in the assessment of problems of fluid balance includes accurate measurement of intake and output, weight, and vital signs. The most sensitive indices of changes in body water content are serial weights and intake and output patterns.[2] Although vital signs can provide supporting data, they may not be abnormal until significant volume or water deficits occur. Assessment of fluid imbalance needs to be based on keen observation and recognition of pertinent symptoms.

Weight

Weight is one of the single most important tests for critically ill patients. The admission weight is compared with that obtained in the history. Of note is whether the weight has changed significantly over the past 1 to 2 weeks. Weights should be carefully measured at the same time, with the same scale, and with the same linens daily. Variations in the procedure should be noted and made known to the physician. One liter of fluid equals 1 kg of body weight, equivalent to 2.2 pounds. A kilogram scale provides for greater accuracy because drug, fluid, and diet measurements can be calculated easily using the metric system.

Rapid daily gains and losses of weight usually are associated with changes in fluid volume and not nutritional factors. Critically ill patients often experience unmeasured insensible losses, such as ventilation and wound losses. Fever can increase the amount of fluid lost through the skin and lungs by as much as 75 mL/1°F above baseline. Serial weights often are more reliable, and weight changes usually pick up imbalances before any symptoms are apparent. In addition to the fluid balance perspective, weights are also used to calculate drug dosages and, for the patient receiving dialysis, determine the amount of fluid to be removed during therapy.

Intake and Output

An accurate intake and output record provides valuable data for evaluating and treating fluid and electrolyte imbalances. It is important that the nurse teach the patient or visitors to assist in this assessment. Intake and output is measured and recorded as it occurs and totaled at the end of every shift. In the presence of excessive losses or deterioration of cardiac, hepatic, renal, or respiratory function, more detailed recording of every source of fluid intake and output is necessary, and calculations may be required every 1 to 4 hours.

In the critically ill patient, intake and output are monitored every 1 to 2 hours. The intake and output values are summed to provide an overall balance at the end of a 24-hour period. A net balance is calculated by subtracting the output from the intake:

$$\text{24-hour fluid balance} = \text{total intake} - \text{total output}$$

Depending on the patient's condition, daily therapeutic goals, and response to interventions, the net balance may be neutral, positive, or negative. The 24-hour balance is compared with the daily weight to assess overall balance. If the net daily balance is positive, but the daily weight reflects a loss over the last 24 hours, insensible losses may be the cause of the discrepancy.

Intake should include all liquids, such as water, juices, or soup, and any foods that are high in water content (e.g., oranges, grapefruit, gelatin, and ice cream). It is useful to keep a list of equivalents for fruits, ice cubes and chips, and other sources of fluid. Output should include urinary and intestinal losses and estimates of respiratory and cutaneous losses when the patient's temperature or the ambient temperature is high. Also recorded are other sources of fluid loss that are present, such as ileostomy or other enteric drainage, wound drainage, or thoracic drainage. See Box 29-3 for pediatric considerations.

In severe electrolyte and fluid imbalances, the time and type of fluid intake and the time and amount of each voiding must be recorded. In the event that renal function decreases, this information may aid immeasurably in the diagnosis and possible prevention of prerenal azotemia or acute renal failure. Risk factors for excessive fluid loss are given in Box 29-4.

Hypovolemia and Hypervolemia

The critical care nurse must be continually on the alert to detect early changes in the patient's volume status. Seldom is the diagnosis made on the basis of one parameter. The first clue may be the patient's general appearance; after observing this, the nurse seeks and notes more specific parameters.

Symptoms vary with the degree of imbalance; some are seen early in imbalance states, and others are not evident until severe imbalances are present. Table 29-6 lists the signs and symptoms of hypovolemia and hypervolemia.

In volume depletion, the patient may complain of orthostatic lightheadedness when assuming the sitting or standing position (this also can occur from inactivity and autonomic dysfunction). Development of tachycardia on assuming the upright position and a decrease in blood pressure (orthostatic hypotension), as opposed to the normal rise, are frequent early findings. Later, the pulse may become rapid, weak, and thready. There may be early dryness of the skin, with loss of elasticity, sunken eyes, loss of axillary sweating, and a dry, coated tongue. When severe volume depletion occurs, thirst, decreased urine volume, and weight loss may be noted; however, weight loss and orthostatic blood pressure and pulse changes may be the only findings.[4]

Laboratory studies, such as a high urine osmolality and low urinary sodium, may facilitate the diagnosis. Other guidelines, such as elevated hematocrit, decreased central venous pressure, and decreased pulmonary wedge pressure, may corroborate the diagnosis.

In fluid overload, the patient, if alert, may complain of puffiness or stiffness in the hands and feet. Later, periorbital edema or puffiness, followed by pitting edema of the dependent parts (feet and ankles if upright; sacral area and poste-

box 29-4 *Risk Factors for Excessive Fluid Loss*

- **Fever:** A patient with a fever of 40°C (104°F) and a respiratory rate of 40 breaths/minute can lose as much as 2,500 mL of fluid in a 24-hour period from the respiratory tract and from the skin.
- **Environment:** Hot, dry climates can increase evaporative sweat losses to 1,500 mL/hour to maintain body evaporative heat loss. This can increase to between 2 and 2.5 L/hour for short times in acclimatized people exercising in hot climates.
- **Hyperventilation:** Hyperventilation can increase respiratory water losses as a result of either disease or use of nonhumidified respirators or oxygen delivery systems.
- **Gastrointestinal tract:** Vomiting, nasogastric suction, diarrhea, and enterocutaneous drainage or fistulas can increase gastrointestinal losses.
- **Third-spacing:** Formation of pleural or peritoneal effusions and edema from liver, renal, or hepatic disease or from the diffuse capillary leak syndrome can result in a loss of effective intravascular volume. Drainage of peritoneal or pleural fluid, when formation of these third spaces still is occurring, can result in further effective intravascular losses because of continued fluid shifts from the vascular compartment to the third space.
- **Burns:** Fluid loss into burned tissues can result in a significant decrease in effective intravascular volume. Because both evaporative and transudative losses through the burned skin can result in very large losses of fluid daily, the burned patient requires special attention to maintain fluid and electrolyte balance. Formulas for determining burn area and fluid resuscitation are discussed in Chapter 53.
- **Renal losses:** Inappropriate solute and fluid loss from the kidneys can occur because of renal salt wasting. This is seen in the diuretic phase of acute tubular necrosis, in some rare patients with true renal salt wasting, and as a result of excessive diuretic administration. It also may occur as a result of solute diuresis from high-protein or high-saline enteral and parenteral alimentation and from administration of osmotic agents, such as mannitol and radiocontrast agents. Finally, fluid can be lost during the generation phase of metabolic alkalosis, in which compensatory urinary bicarbonate excretion obligates renal sodium excretion. This frequently results in volume depletion.

box 29-3 *Considerations for the Pediatric Patient*

Catheterization is often avoided in pediatric patients. Careful weight of diapers is used to achieve accurate measurement of output. A scale is zeroed with the child's dry diaper and again after each void. Weight is converted to volume using the formula where 1 kg = 1 L.

Oliguria in the critically ill child is defined as urine output less than 0.5 to 1 mL/kg/hour.

table 29-6 ■ Signs and Symptoms of Hypovolemia and Hypervolemia

Parameters	Hypovolemia	Hypervolemia
Skin and subcutaneous tissues	Dry, less elastic	Warm, moist, pitting edema over bony prominences; wrinkled skin from pressure of clothing
Face	Sunken eyes (late symptom)	Periorbital edema
Tongue	Dry, coated (early symptom); fissured (late symptom)	Moist
Saliva	Thick, scanty	Excessive, frothy
Thirst	Present	May not be significant
Temperature	May be elevated	May not be significant
Pulse	Rapid, weak, thready	Rapid
Respirations	Rapid, shallow	Rapid dyspnea, moist rales, cough
Blood pressure	Low, orthostatic hypotension; small pulse pressure	Normal to high
Weight	Loss	Gain

rior thighs if supine) will occur, followed by dyspnea or ascites, depending on etiology (i.e., cardiac decompensation and systemic fluid overload versus hepatic disease). Urine volume and urine sodium may be normal, increased, or decreased, depending on the etiology. In most diseases with fluid retention, except for the syndrome of inappropriate ADH secretion, urine sodium is reduced. The hematocrit is decreased, reflecting hemodilution.

The pulse may be rapid and auscultation of the heart may reveal the presence of a third heart sound (S_3), fourth heart sound (S_4), or a murmur secondary to volume overload. Respirations may be increased because of pulmonary congestion, and auscultation of the chest may reveal rales. A chest film may reveal pulmonary vascular congestion, increased alveolar lung markings, cardiac dilation, frank pulmonary congestion, and pleural effusions.

All data should be evaluated in the light of other evidence. Trends usually are more significant than isolated values. For example, when a decrease in urine output is noted, a systematic assessment should be done to determine why this is happening and what nursing interventions are most appropriate. Depending on the stability of the patient, the health care team may use advanced physiological monitoring (e.g., pulmonary artery catheter) to guide assessment and management. Factors affecting water balance are listed in Table 29-7.

Hemodynamic Monitoring

Hemodynamic monitoring offers the clinician an improved assessment of the patient's overall status. For a detailed discussion, refer to Chapter 17. Although physical assessment may provide insight into the volume status, changes in physical assessment are reflected later than changes in hemodynamic assessment parameters, such as central venous pressure. Through improved monitoring, interventions are guided by information on a real-time basis. Table 29-8 provides an overview of the causes of altered parameters for the assessment of preload.

Based on data from the history, physical examination, and laboratory and diagnostic tests, nursing diagnoses are developed for the patient with renal problems. Box 29-5 lists possible nursing diagnoses.

case study ■ ACUTE RENAL INSUFFICIENCY

Mrs. Russell is a 75-year-old woman who presented to the emergency department, complaining of shortness of breath, chills, and malaise for 4 days. Initially, she attributed her symptoms to the flu and treated it with ibuprofen and rest. She has a history of mild congestive heart failure (ejection fraction of 35%) and diabetes, which she states is controlled through diet. Additional medications include metoprolol 25 mg twice daily, furosemide 10 mg/day, and lisinopril 10 mg/day. During physical examination, the patient's vital signs are as follows: temperature 38°C, heart rate 75 beats/minute, respiratory rate 24 breaths/minute, and blood pressure 102/68 mm Hg. Oxygen saturation is 93% on oxygen at 2 L/minute by nasal cannula. A chest radiograph is obtained, which reveals a right lower lobe infiltrate. The patient is admitted to the unit with a diagnosis of community-acquired pneumonia and is placed on IV antibiotics.

Initial blood work obtained on arrival to the unit reveals the following: sodium 135 mEq/L; chloride 99 mEq/L; potassium 3.4 mEq/L; carbon dioxide 27 mEq/L; glucose 182 mg/dL; BUN 32 mg/dL; creatinine 1.5 mg/dL. Urinalysis reveals the following: specific gravity 1.014; pH 6.8; urine osmolality (U_{osm}) 750 mOsm/kg; urinary sodium (U_{Na}) 22 mEq/L; urinary chloride (U_{Cl}) 6 mEq/L. The patient is experiencing acute renal insufficiency, as evidenced by a rising BUN and creatinine. This renal insufficiency is primarily due to volume depletion secondary to increased insensible losses from her persistent fever. The patient's heart failure and diabetes also place her at increased risk for acute renal insufficiency. Heart failure causes decreased blood flow to the kidneys, initiating the counterproductive compensatory mechanism of water retention. The patient's

table 29-7 Factors Affecting Water Balance

	Water Excess	Water Deficiency
Intake		

Thirst	Decreased thirst threshold
	Increased osmolality
	Potassium depletion
	Hypercalcemia
	Fever
	Dry mucous membranes
	  Poor oral hygiene
	  Unmisted O_2 administration
	Hypotension
	Psychiatric disorders
		Increased thirst threshold
		Decreased osmolality
		Lack of access
		Psychiatric disorders

Parenteral fluids	Excessive D_5W	Deficient replacement
		Osmotic loads
		  Hyperalimentation
		  Hyperglycemia
		  Mannitol
		  Radiographic contrast agents

Output		
Sweating		High ambient temperature High altitude Fever

Renal excretion	Inappropriate ADH release
	Appropriate ADH release
	  Congestive failure
	  Decompensated cirrhosis
	  Volume depletion
	    Adrenal insufficiency
	    Renal salt wasting
	    Hemorrhage
	    Diuretics
	  Burns
	  Hypothyroidism
	Renal disease
	  ARF
	  Chronic renal failure
	  Nephrotic syndrome
	  Acute glomerulonephritis
	Nonsteroidal anti-inflammatory agents
		Excess excretion
		  Central
		  Nephrogenic
		    Potassium depletion
		    Hypercalcemia
		    Lithium administration
		    Demeclocycline (Declomycin)
		    Methoxyflurane (Penthrane)

D_5W, Dextrose 5% in water; *ADH*, antidiuretic hormone; *ARF*, acute renal failure

sodium level is 135 mEq/L, which is relatively low for a patient who is volume depleted. Diabetic nephropathy will also cause decreased microvascular blood flow. Mrs. Russell's urine sodium is low in light of volume depletion. Furosemide administration causes sodium loss to promote water excretion.

To improve the patient's blood flow, the nurse administers normal saline at a rate of 125 mL/hour, monitoring carefully for volume overload. Ongoing nursing assessment includes assessment and reassessment of lung sounds, observation for the development of jugular venous distension, and accurate output measurement. The patient's metoprolol and lisinopril are continued (to promote cardiac performance), but the ibuprofen is discontinued due to its nephrotoxic effects. On day 5, the patient is discharged and instructed to use another pain reliever and antipyretic, such as acetaminophen. ■

clinical applicability challenges

Self-Challenge: Critical Thinking

1. *Explain why Mrs. Russell is experiencing renal insufficiency. Describe the influence of Mrs. Russell's past medical history on her renal function.*
2. *What interventions may be required to improve Mrs. Russell's renal function?*
3. *Explain the findings of Mrs. Russell's urinary sodium.*

table 29-8 Etiologies of Altered Preload

Hemodynamic Parameter	Increased	Decreased
Preload	Renal failure Volume or blood administration Vasopressors Cardiogenic shock Bradycardia Cardiac tamponade Constrictive pericarditis	Hemorrhage Diuresis Diaphoresis Vomiting Diarrhea Poor intake Third spacing Vasodilators Septic shock Neurogenic shock Anaphylactic shock Tachycardia Loss of atrial kick
Right-sided preload	Right ventricular failure Tricuspid/pulmonic valve disease Ventricular septal defect Right ventricular papillary muscle dysfunction	
Left-sided preload	Left ventricular failure Mitral/aortic valve disease Left ventricular papillary muscle dysfunction	

Study Questions

1. *Which laboratory value is most useful in assessing renal function?*
   a. *Potassium*
   b. *Blood urea nitrogen (BUN)*
   c. *Creatinine*
   d. *Uric acid*
2. *Which of the following diagnostic tests assesses renal blood flow?*
   a. *Renal angiography*
   b. *Computed tomography*
   c. *Ultrasonography*
   d. *a and c*
3. *Which of the following findings would you expect to see in a patient who is volume depleted?*
   a. *Fractional excretion of sodium (FE_{Na}) less than 1%*
   b. *Decreased urinary sodium*
   c. *Increased urinary sodium*
   d. *a and b*
4. *Hypokalemia can be caused by all of the following except*
   a. *nasogastric tube drainage.*
   b. *administration of loop diuretics.*
   c. *acidosis.*
   d. *diarrhea.*
5. *Signs and symptoms of hypocalcemia include*
   a. *edema, dry skin, bradycardia.*
   b. *thirst, high urine specific gravity, hypotension.*
   c. *muscle weakness, bone pain, hypertension.*
   d. *cramps, tetany, positive Chvostek's and Trousseau's signs.*

box 29-5 *Examples of Nursing Diagnoses and Collaborative Problems for the Patient With Renal Problems*

- Pain related to urinary retention
- Acute Pain: Dysuria related to infection
- Acute Pain: Dysuria related to urinary obstruction
- Urinary Retention related to urinary tract obstruction
- Impaired Urinary Elimination related to catheterization
- Self-Concept Disturbance related to loss of bladder control
- Alteration in Electrolyte Balance related to impaired kidney function
- Excess Fluid Volume related to impaired kidney function
- Impaired Urinary Elimination related to impaired kidney function

REFERENCES

1. Bickley L: Bates' Guide to Physical Examination and History Taking (8th Ed). Philadelphia, JB Lippincott, 2003
2. Toto KH: Fluid balance assessment: The total perspective. Crit Care Nurs Clin 19(4):383–400, 1998
3. Metheny NM: Fluid and Electrolyte Balance: Nursing Considerations. Philadelphia, Lippincott Williams & Wilkins, 2000
4. Woodrow P: Assessing fluid balance in older people: Fluid replacement. Nurs Older People 14(10):29–30, 2003

OTHER SELECTED READING

Gould KA, Stark J: Quick resource for electrolyte imbalance. Crit Care Nurs Clin 10(4):477–490, 1998

Henke K, Eigsti J: Renal physiology: Review and practical application in the critically ill patient. Dim Crit Care Nurs 22(3):125–132, 2003

Suhayda R, Walton JC: Preventing and managing dehydration. MEDSURG Nurs 11(6):267–79, 2002

Weber J, Kelley J: Health Assessment in Nursing (2nd Ed). Philadelphia, Lippincott Williams & Wilkins, 2003

chapter 30

Patient Management: Renal System

KARA ADAMS

objectives

Based on the content in this chapter, the reader should be able to:

- Explore the physiological principles involved in renal replacement therapy: hemodialysis, continuous renal replacement therapies, and peritoneal dialysis.
- Analyze the differences in equipment and procedures used in renal replacement therapy.
- Explain the types of vascular access used in hemodialysis and continuous renal replacement therapies.
- Compare and contrast the indications, assessment and management, and complications for each renal replacement therapy.
- Explore the psychosocial and teaching needs surrounding renal replacement therapy for patients and their families.
- Analyze the specific fluid therapies chosen based on physiological alterations.
- Describe the nursing assessments and interventions for patients receiving fluid therapy.
- Explain the nursing management of selected electrolyte disorders.

Renal function may be replaced by a process called *dialysis*, which is a life-maintaining therapy used in acute and chronic renal failure. Critical care nurses may encounter patients suffering from the effects of acute renal failure or patients already on some form of chronic dialysis who subsequently become critically ill. Critical care nurses must be familiar with various dialysis therapies to help care for patients with complex illnesses. This chapter discusses the three most common forms of renal replacement therapy (hemodialysis, continuous renal replacement therapies [CRRTs], and peritoneal dialysis) as well as common fluid and electrolyte imbalances experienced by critically ill patients.

PHYSIOLOGY

All forms of dialysis make use of the principles of osmosis and diffusion to remove waste products and excess fluid from the blood. A semipermeable membrane is placed between the blood and a specially formulated solution called *dialysate*. Dissolved substances, such as urea and creatinine, diffuse across the membrane from an area of greater concentration (blood) to an area of lesser concentration (dialysate). Water molecules move across the membrane by osmosis to the solution that contains fewer water molecules. Dialysate is formulated with varying concentrations of dextrose or sodium to produce an osmotic gradient, thereby pulling excess water from the circulatory system. This process of fluid moving across a semipermeable membrane in relation to forces created by osmotic and hydrostatic pressures is called *ultrafiltration*. These basic principles are the foundation of any dialysis therapy. The manner in which they are accomplished varies depending on the therapy.

EXTRACORPOREAL THERAPIES

Hemodialysis and the CRRTs use an extracorporeal (outside the body) circuit. Therefore, they require access to the patient's circulation and anticoagulation of the circuit.

Access to Circulation

The three most common methods used to access a patient's circulation are through a vascular catheter, an arteriovenous fistula, or a synthetic vascular graft. Patients who suddenly need hemodialysis or CRRT have a venous catheter, whereas patients already receiving chronic hemodialysis probably have either an arteriovenous fistula or a synthetic vascular graft. Box 30-1 lists nursing interventions for the patient with dialysis vascular access.

VENOUS CATHETERS

Dual-lumen catheters inserted into large veins are used for acutely ill patients who need hemodialysis, continuous venovenous hemofiltration (CVVH), or continuous venovenous hemofiltration with dialysis (CVVH/D). Venous catheters are also used for hemodialysis when there is no other means of access to the circulation. Veins commonly used are the femoral, internal jugular, or subclavian. The site chosen depends on the patient's anatomy and vein accessibility and the physician's experience and preference.

Dual-lumen venous catheters also are used temporarily for patients on acute dialysis who are critically ill or patients on chronic dialysis who are waiting for a more permanent access to mature. Tunneled dual-lumen central venous catheters are often used as a permanent means of access in patients in whom all other means of entry into the circulatory system have been exhausted. The tunneled catheter has an implantable Dacron cuff around which tissue grows and acts as a barrier against infection. If possible, the catheter should be placed in the right or left internal jugular vein because catheters placed in the subclavian vein can cause stenosis. The stenosis can cause increased venous pressure and edema that may thwart future efforts to create an arteriovenous fistula or place a graft.

Whenever venous catheters are used, care must be taken to avoid accidental slippage and dislodgement during hemodialysis. Femoral catheters are usually secured with sutures as well as with tape to the leg, whereas central venous catheters in the upper body are sutured to the skin. The length of time catheters are left in place depends on catheter function and institution policy. In general, central venous catheters may be used for up to 3 to 4 weeks. More permanent internal jugular vein catheters often function for many months before problems force their removal. Catheters left in place between dialysis treatments usually are filled with a concentrated heparin–saline solution after dialysis and plugged to prevent clotting. These catheters

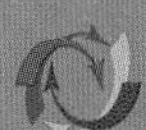

box 30-1 nursing interventions for the Patient With Dialysis Vascular Access

Dual-Lumen Venous Catheter

- Verify central line catheter placement radiographically before use.
- Do not inject IV fluids or medication into the catheter. Both lumens of the catheter usually are filled with concentrated heparin.
- Do not unclamp the catheter unless preparing for dialysis therapy. This can cause blood to fill the lumen and clot.
- Maintain sterile technique in handling vascular access.
- Observe catheter exit site for signs of inflammation or catheter kinking.

Arteriovenous Fistula or Graft

- Do not take blood pressure or draw blood from the access limb.
- Listen for bruit, and palpate for thrill q8h.
- Make sure there is no tight clothing or restraints on the access limb.
- Check access patency more frequently when patients are hypotensive. Hypotension can predispose to clotting.
- In the event of postdialysis bleeding from the needle site, apply just enough pressure to stop the flow of blood and hold until bleeding stops. Do not occlude the vessel.

should *never* be used for any purpose other than hemodialysis without first checking with dialysis unit personnel. Cleansing and dressing of the insertion site are the same as with other central lines.

If the catheters are removed at the end of dialysis, pressure is applied to the puncture sites until complete clotting occurs. The site is checked for several hours thereafter so that any recurrent bleeding can be detected. Removal of the more permanent tunneled catheter requires use of local anesthetic at the exit site and careful dissection around the Dacron cuff to free it from the attached subcutaneous tissue.

Catheter patency must be maintained. Thrombolytics may be used to dissolve clots in venous catheters. Thrombolytics are enzymes derived from streptococcal bacteria that are capable of activating the fibrinolytic system and dissolving intravascular thrombi. These agents can help preserve vascular access and reduce the need for surgery or catheter reinsertion. However, their use is associated with inherent risks and side effects, including local pain, bleeding, and an allergic response.

In the early days of dialysis, vascular access was created at every treatment by cannulating an artery to remove blood from the body and a vein to return dialyzed blood to the patient. The lines carrying blood to the dialyzer were called *arterial lines*, and the lines returning blood to the body were called *venous lines*. The two lumens of the venous catheter used in dialysis are still designated as arterial and venous. The arterial lumen is longer than the venous lumen so it can catch blood flowing by and allow it to be pumped out of the body. Blood is returned upstream from the arterial lumen to avoid pulling out the blood that has just been dialyzed and returned to the body. The lumens are distinguished by the presence of colored clamps: red on the arterial lumen and blue on the venous lumen.

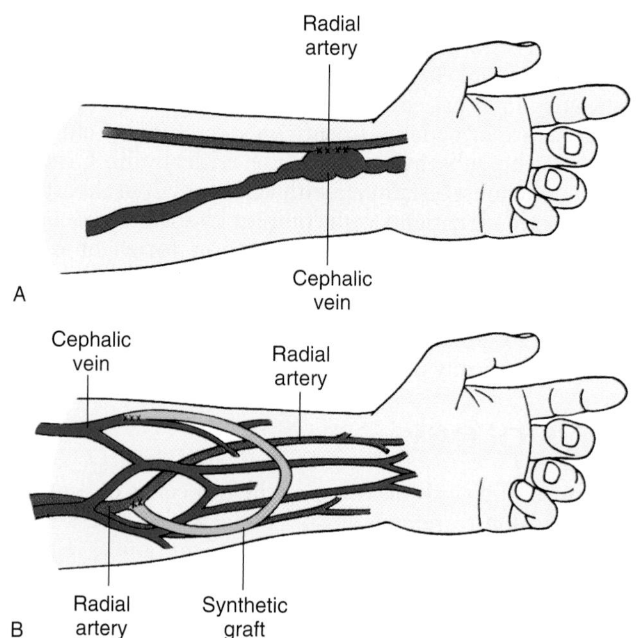

figure 30-1 Methods of vascular access for hemodialysis. (**A**) Arteriovenous fistula. (**B**) Synthetic graft.

ARTERIOVENOUS FISTULAS

The arteriovenous fistula technique was developed in 1966 in an effort to provide long-term access for hemodialysis. To create the arteriovenous fistula, a surgeon anastomoses an artery and a vein, creating a fistula or artificial opening between them (Fig. 30-1A). Arterial blood flowing into the venous system results in a marked dilation of the vein, which can then be punctured easily with a 15- or 16-gauge dialysis fistula needle. Two venipunctures are made at the time of dialysis: one for blood outflow and one for blood return.

After the arteriovenous fistula incision has healed, the site is cleansed by normal bathing or showering. To avoid scar formation, excessive bleeding, or hematoma of the arteriovenous fistula, care is taken to avoid traumatic venipuncture, excessive manipulation of the needles, and repeated use of the same site for venipuncture. Adequate pressure must be put on the puncture sites after the needles are removed. In addition, blood pressure measurements and venipunctures should *not* be performed on the arm with the fistula.

Most arteriovenous fistulas are developed and ready to use 1 to 3 months after surgery. After initial healing has occurred, patients are taught to exercise the arm to assist in vessel maturation. They also are encouraged to become familiar with the quality of the "thrill" felt at the site of anastomosis so that they can report any change in its presence or strength. A loud, swishing sound termed a *bruit* indicates a functioning fistula. Box 30-2 presents a patient teaching guide for the care of arteriovenous fistulas.

Although arteriovenous fistulas usually have a long life, complications may occur. These include thrombosis, aneurysm or pseudoaneurysm, or arterial insufficiency causing a "steal syndrome." This syndrome occurs when

box 30-2
Caring for an Arteriovenous Fistula

- Wash the fistula site with antibacterial soap each day and always before dialysis.
- Refrain from picking the scab that forms after completion of dialysis therapy.
- Check for redness, feeling of excess warmth, or the beginning of a pimple on any area of access.
- Ask the dialysis care team to rotate needles at the time of dialysis treatment.
- Check blood flow several times each day by feeling for a pulse or thrill. If this is not felt, or if there is a change, call your health care provider or dialysis center.
- Refrain from wearing tight clothes or jewelry on the access arm. Also avoid carrying anything heavy or doing anything that will put pressure on the access site.
- Avoid sleeping with your head on the arm where the access site is located.
- Remind caregivers and staff not to use a blood pressure cuff on, or draw blood from, the arm where the access site is located.
- Apply only gentle pressure to the access site after the needle is removed. Too much pressure stops flow of blood to the access site.

shunting of blood from the artery to the vein produces ischemia of the hand, causing pain or coldness in the hand. Surgical intervention can remedy all of these problems and restore adequate fistula flow.

SYNTHETIC GRAFTS

The synthetic graft is made from polytetrafluoroethylene (PTFE), a material manufactured from an expanded, highly porous form of Teflon. The graft is anastomosed between an artery and a vein and is used in the same manner as an arteriovenous fistula (see Fig. 30-1B).

For many patients whose own vessels are not adequate for fistula formation, PTFE grafts are extremely valuable. PTFE segments are also used to patch areas of arteriovenous grafts or fistulas that have stenosed or developed areas of aneurysm. It is best to avoid venipuncture in new PTFE grafts for 2 to 4 weeks while the patient's tissue grows into the graft. When tissue growth progresses satisfactorily, the graft has an endothelium and wall composition similar to the patient's own vessels.

The procedures for preventing complications in grafts are the same as those used for arteriovenous fistulas. However, certain complications are seen more frequently with grafts than with fistulas, including thrombosis, infection, aneurysm formation, and stenosis at the site of anastomosis.

Anticoagulation

Blood in the extracorporeal system, such as the dialyzer and blood lines, clots rapidly unless some method of anticoagulation is used. Heparin is the drug of choice because it is simple to administer, increases clotting time rapidly, is monitored easily, and may be reversed with protamine. Trisodium citrate 4% may also be used for CRRT. This agent chelates calcium, thereby inactivating the clotting cascade.

Specific heparinization procedures vary, but the primary goal of all methods is to prevent clotting in the dialyzer with the least amount of anticoagulation. Two methods commonly used are intermittent and constant infusion.

SYSTEMIC ANTICOAGULATION

Typically, the circuit is initially primed with a dose of heparin, followed by smaller intermittent doses of anticoagulation or heparin administered at a constant rate by an infusion pump. This results in systemic anticoagulation, in which the clotting times of the patient and the dialyzer essentially are the same.

Definitive guidelines are difficult to provide because methods and dialyzer requirements vary. The normal clotting time of 6 to 10 minutes may be increased to 30 to 60 minutes. The effect of heparin usually is monitored by the activated clotting time, prothrombin time (PT), or partial thromboplastin time (PTT).

The patient's need for heparinization and an appropriate beginning heparin dose should be assessed routinely before dialysis, especially in the critically ill patient who may be actively bleeding or at risk for bleeding. The patient's platelet count, serum calcium level, and results of coagulation studies are valuable in assessing current function of the clotting process. Often, little or no heparin can be used when the patient has serious alterations in one or more factors needed for effective clotting.

REGIONAL ANTICOAGULATION

Systemic heparinization does not usually present a risk unless the patient has overt bleeding (e.g., gastrointestinal bleeding, epistaxis, or hemoptysis), is 3 to 7 days postsurgery, or has uremic pericarditis. In these situations, other methods to prevent clotting of the extracorporeal system can be used. One method is regional heparinization, in which the patient's clotting time is kept normal while the clotting time of the dialyzer is increased. This is accomplished by infusing heparin at a constant rate into the dialyzer and simultaneously neutralizing its effects with protamine sulfate before the blood returns to the patient.

Like systemic heparinization, regional heparinization has no associated standard heparin–protamine ratio. Frequent monitoring of the clotting times is the best way to achieve effective regional heparinization. Because of the rebound phenomenon that has occurred after regional heparinization, low-dose heparinization may be used, even in the presence of overt bleeding. With this method, minimal heparin doses are used throughout dialysis. Although some clotting may take place in the dialyzer, the small blood loss is preferable to the risk of profound bleeding.

Bleeding problems occasionally occur because of accidental heparin overdose. This may be caused by infusion pump malfunction or an error in setting the delivery rate. Because of the hazards, heparin delivery must be monitored carefully and frequently.

Another way to prevent dialyzer clotting and reduce the risk of bleeding due to heparin is to infuse a small initial heparin dose (e.g., 250 U) and use frequent normal saline flushes of the extracorporeal system, or use saline flushes alone.

Some dialysis centers perform regional citrate anticoagulation in which citrate is infused into the system before the dialyzer binds calcium, obstructing the normal clotting pathway. The citrate–calcium complex is then cleared from the blood by the dialyzer, and the anticoagulant effect is reversed by infusing calcium chloride before the blood returns to the patient. The patient's sodium levels may rise because the citrate is administered in the form of sodium citrate.[1] Citrate has a higher pH, and therefore patients may also become metabolically alkalotic.

INTERMITTENT HEMODIALYSIS

In hemodialysis, water and excess waste products are removed from the blood as it is pumped by the dialysis machine (Fig. 30-2) through an extracorporeal circuit (Fig. 30-3) into a device called a *dialyzer*, or *artificial kidney*. The blood is in one compartment, and the dialysate is in another compartment. There, the blood flows through a semipermeable membrane. The semipermeable membrane is a thin, porous sheet made of cellulose or a synthetic material. The pore size of the membrane permits diffusion of low–molecular-weight substances such as urea, creatinine, and uric acid. In addition, water mol-

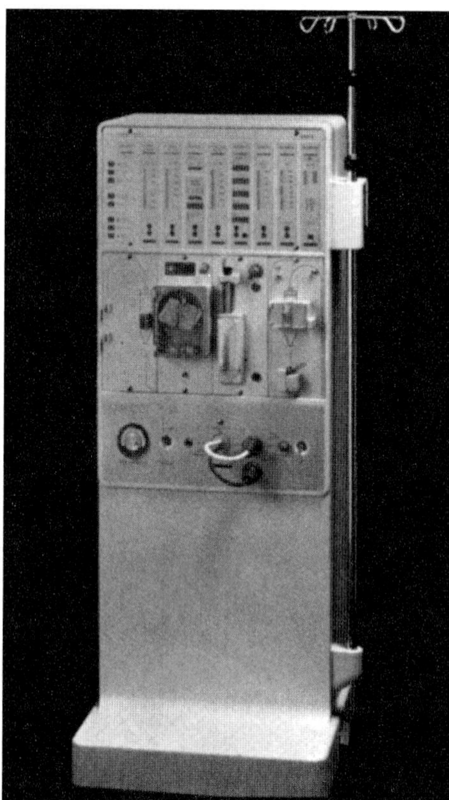

figure 30-2 Hemodialysis delivery unit, which includes an automatic blood pressure cuff, heparin infusion pump, and blood pump. This machine displays a continuous readout of ultrafiltration goal, rate, and total fluid removed and monitors dialysate temperature and conductivity. It can vary the sodium concentration of the dialysate. (Fresenius 2008, Fresenius VSA, Inc., Concord, CA.)

ecules are small and move freely through the membrane, but most plasma proteins, bacteria, and blood cells are too large to pass through the pores of the membrane. The difference in the concentration of the substances in the two compartments is called the *concentration gradient.*

The blood, which contains waste products such as urea and creatinine, flows into the blood compartment of the dialyzer, where it comes into contact with the dialysate, which contains no urea or creatinine. A maximum gradient is established so that these substances move from the blood to the dialysate. These waste products fall to more normal levels as the blood passes through the dialyzer repeatedly at a rate ranging from 200 to 400 mL/minute over 2 to 4 hours.

Excess water is removed by a pressure differential created between the blood and fluid compartments. This pressure differential is aided by the action of the dialyzer pump and usually consists of positive pressure in the blood path and negative pressure in the dialysate compartment. This is the process of *ultrafiltration.* Hemodialysis:

- Removes byproducts of protein metabolism, such as urea, creatinine, and uric acid
- Removes excess water
- Maintains or restores the body buffer system
- Maintains or restores the level of electrolytes in the body

Indications for Hemodialysis

Hemodialysis is indicated in chronic renal failure and for complications of acute renal failure. These include uremia, fluid overload, acidosis, hyperkalemia, and drug overdose. Table 30-1 compares hemodialysis, CRRT, and peritoneal dialysis.

Contraindications to Hemodialysis

Hemodialysis may be contraindicated in patients with coagulopathies because the extracorporeal circuit needs to be heparinized. Hemodialysis may also be difficult to perform in patients who have extremely low cardiac output or who are sensitive to abrupt changes in volume status. For these critically ill patients, CRRT may be the optimal choice. In addition, intermittent hemodialysis may not keep up with the metabolic needs of a highly catabolic patient. In this case, CRRT would probably be chosen. Patients treated chronically for renal failure may be given the choice to undergo hemodialysis or peritoneal dialysis.

Equipment

DIALYZERS

Dialyzers are designed to provide a parallel path through which blood and dialysate flow and to have a maximal membrane surface area between the two. Dialyzers vary in size, physical structure, and type of membrane used to construct the blood compartment. All these factors determine the potential efficiency of the dialyzer, which refers to its ability to remove water (ultrafiltration) and waste products (clearance).

The hollow-fiber dialyzer is the most commonly used configuration. In this design, the blood path flows through hollow fibers composed of semipermeable membrane, and the dialysate path is encased in a rigid plastic tube. Dialysate surrounds each hollow fiber. This provides a large surface area to cleanse the blood. Blood and dialysate flow in opposite directions from each other (countercurrent flow); as blood travels through the dialyzer, it is constantly exposed to a fresh flow of dialysate. This countercurrent flow maintains the concentration gradient between the two compartments and provides the most efficient dialysis.

Synthetic membranes are used most commonly because they are highly biocompatible. They remove waste products efficiently, and there is little reaction between the blood and the membrane material. Because the synthetic membranes are highly permeable to water, they should be used only with a machine that controls the amount of ultrafiltration.

The size, efficiency, and metabolic needs of the patient are considered when choosing a dialyzer. A patient with a larger body surface area who has greater metabolic needs benefits from use of a larger and more efficient dialyzer, whereas a patient with a smaller body surface area and lower metabolic needs benefits from a smaller, less permeable dialyzer.

DIALYSATE

The dialysate, or "bath," is a solution composed of water and the major electrolytes of normal serum. It is made in a clean system with filtered tap water and chemicals. It is

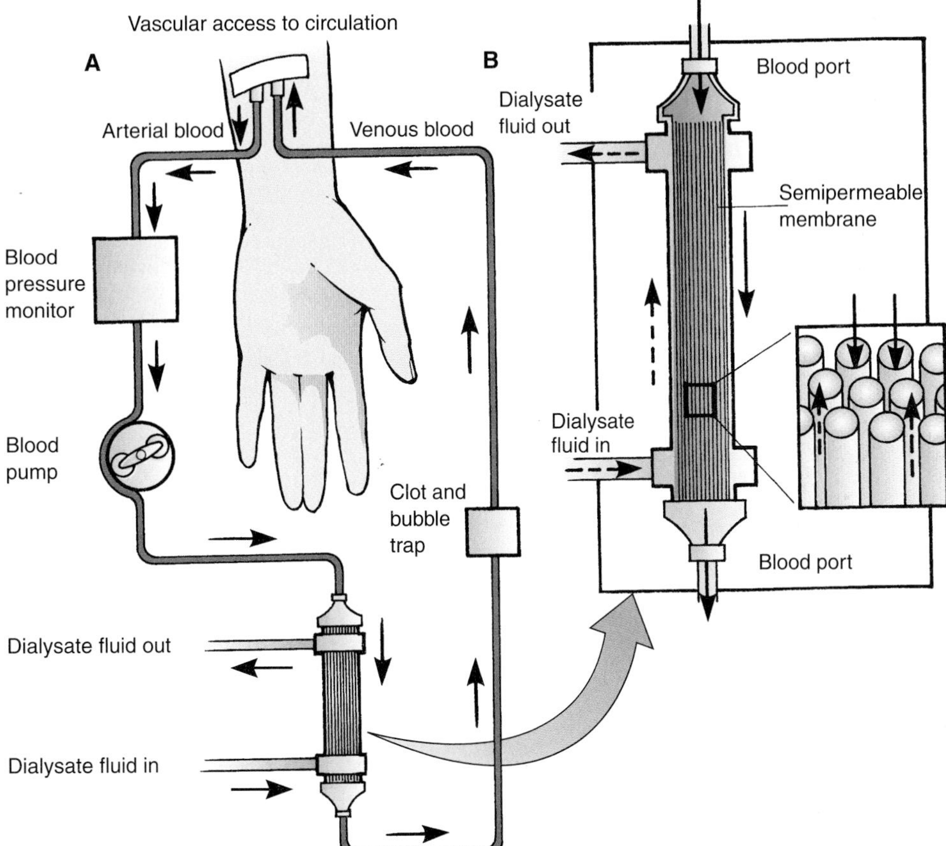

figure 30-3 Hemodialysis system. (**A**) Blood from an artery is pumped into (**B**) a dialyzer, where it flows through the cellophane tubes, which act as the semipermeable membrane (*inset*). The dialysate, which has the same chemical composition as the blood except for urea and waste products, flows in around the tubules. The waste products in the blood diffuse through the semipermeable membrane into the dialysate. (Used with permission from Smeltzer SC, Bare BG: Brunner & Suddarth's Textbook of Medical–Surgical Nursing [10th Ed], p 1286. Philadelphia, Lippincott Williams & Wilkins, 2004.)

not a sterile system; bacteria are too large to pass through the membrane, and the potential for infection of the patient is minimal. However, because bacterial byproducts can cause pyrogenic reactions, especially in highly permeable membranes, water used to make dialysate must be bacteriologically safe. Dialysate concentrates usually are provided by commercial manufacturers. A standard bath usually is used for patients receiving chronic dialysis, but variations may be made to meet specific patient needs.

DIALYSATE DELIVERY SYSTEM

A single delivery unit provides dialysate for one patient, whereas a multiple delivery system may provide dialysate for as many as 20 patient units. In either system, an automatic proportioning device and metering and monitoring devices ensure precise control of the water–concentrate ratio.

The single delivery unit is usually used in patients on acute dialysis. It is a mobile unit, and dialysate requirements are easily tailored to meet individual patient needs.

ACCESSORY EQUIPMENT

Hardware used in most dialysis systems includes a blood pump, infusion pumps for heparin delivery, and monitoring devices for detection of unsafe temperatures, dialysate concentration, pressure changes, air, and blood leaks. All dialysis delivery systems consist of a single compact unit that includes the dialysate delivery equipment and blood monitoring components (see Fig. 30-2). Disposable items used in addition to the artificial kidney include dialysis tubing for transport of blood between the dialyzer and patient, pressure transducers for protection of monitoring devices from blood exposure, and a normal saline bag and tubing for priming the system before use.

HUMAN COMPONENT

Expertise in the use of highly technical equipment is gained through theoretical and practical training in the clinical setting. However, the operation and monitoring of various kinds of dialysis equipment differ. Reference to the manufacturer's instruction manuals gives the nurse guidelines for the safe operation of equipment. The technical aspects of hemodialysis may seem overwhelming at first, but they can be learned fairly rapidly. A more important aspect, the critical thinking and synthesis of patient assessment data that the nurse uses when caring for a patient during dialysis, takes longer to learn.

Assessment and Management

The degree and complexity of problems arising during hemodialysis vary among patients and depend on many factors. Important variables are the patient's diagnosis, stage of illness, age, other medical problems, fluid and electrolyte balance, prior experience with hemodialysis, and emotional state. Because an increasing number of older adults are receiving dialysis, it also is important to consider the normal decreases in cardiac function and other system changes due to the aging process (Table 30-2).

table 30-1 Comparison of Hemodialysis, Continuous Renal Replacement Therapy (CRRT), and Peritoneal Dialysis

	Hemodialysis	CRRT	Peritoneal Dialysis
Access	Arteriovenous fistula or graft; dual-lumen venous catheter	Arteriovenous fistula or graft; dual-lumen venous catheter	Temporary or permanent peritoneal catheter
Anticoagulation requirements	Systemic heparinization or frequent saline flushes	Systemic anticoagulation with heparin or trisodium citrate may be indicated depending on patient's coagulation studies before starting therapy	May only need heparin intraperitoneally Not absorbed systemically
Length of treatment	3–4 h, three to five times per week, depending on patient acuity	Continuous through day; may last as many days as needed	Continuous (cycled) or intermittent exchanges; time between exchanges = 1–6 h
Advantages	Quick, efficient removal of metabolic wastes and excess fluid Useful for drug overdoses and poisonings	Best choice for patient who is hemodynamically unstable because less blood is outside body than with hemodialysis and blood flow rates are slower; amount of fluid removed can still be achieved but over a much longer period of time Good for hypercatabolic patients who receive large amounts of intravenous fluids	Continuous removal of wastes and fluid Better hemodynamic stability Fewer dietary restrictions
Disadvantages	May require frequent vascular access procedures Places strain on a compromised cardiovascular system Potential blood loss from bleeding or clotted lines Requires specially trained staff to perform therapy	Requires vascular access procedures; potential blood loss from clotting or equipment leaks; uses an extra piece of equipment Requires specially trained staff to perform therapy	Contraindicated after abdominal surgery or in presence of many scars Waste products may be removed too slowly in a catabolic patient Danger of peritonitis

PREPROCEDURE

A predialysis assessment is the first step in managing the patient having hemodialysis. It consists of a review of the patient's history and clinical findings, response to previous dialysis treatment, laboratory results (such as electrolytes), consultation with other caregivers, and the nurse's direct assessment of the patient.

The nurse evaluates fluid balance before dialysis so that corrective measures may be initiated at the beginning of the procedure. Blood pressure, pulse, weight, intake and output, tissue turgor, and other symptoms assist the nurse in estimating fluid overload or depletion. Monitoring tools, such as pulmonary artery pressure, also help determine cardiovascular fluid load.

The term *dry weight* or *ideal weight* is used to express the weight at which fluid volume is in a normal range for a patient who is free of the symptoms of fluid imbalance. It provides a guideline for fluid removal or replacement. The figure is not absolute. It requires frequent review and revision, especially in patients receiving dialysis in whom frequent weight changes occur.

After reviewing the data and while consulting with the physician, the dialysis nurse establishes objectives regarding fluid removal and restoration of electrolyte balance for the dialysis treatment. The objectives vary from one dialysis to the next in the patient whose condition may change rapidly. For example, fluid removal may take precedence over correction of an electrolyte imbalance, or vice versa.

Anxiety and apprehension, especially during the first dialysis, may contribute to change in blood pressure, restlessness, and gastrointestinal upset. The presence of a competent and caring nurse during dialysis may increase the patient's sense of security enough to avoid the need for an antianxiety drug that might precipitate changes in vital signs.

A basic explanation of the procedure and its place in the total care plan for the patient also may allay some of the anxiety experienced by the patient and family. They must understand that dialysis is being used to support normal body function rather than to "cure" the kidney problem.

PROCEDURE

The nurse begins the procedure by checking the equipment (Box 30-3). After predialysis preparation and a safety check of equipment, the nurse is ready to begin hemodialysis. Access to the circulatory system is gained by one of several options: a dual-lumen catheter, an arteriovenous fistula, or graft. The dual-lumen catheter is opened under aseptic conditions according to institutional policy. Two large-gauge (15- or 16-gauge) needles are needed to cannulate a graft or fistula.

table 30-2 Normal Aging Changes That Affect Fluid Balance

Physiological Component	Normal Changes With Increasing Age	Nursing Implications
Total body water	About 6% reduction in total body water Decrease in ratio of intracellular fluid	Increased risk of fluid volume deficit
Renal function	Reduction in renal weight by 50 g between 40 and 80 y of age Loss of 30%–50% of glomeruli by 70 y of age Thickening of glomerular and tubular basement membranes from 20 to 90 y of age Decrease in GFR from 20 to 90 y of age Decrease in ability to concentrate urine (maximum ability to concentrate urine is urine specific gravity of 1.022–1.026)	Greater difficulty in eliminating heavy solute loads (drugs, glucose, protein, electrolytes) Slower conservation of fluids in response to fluid restriction
Regulatory functions	Decrease in secretion of aldosterone from adrenal cortex Decreased response of zona glomerulosa Decreased response of distal tubule to vasopressin Decreased ability to form and excrete ammonia Decreased glucose tolerance Decreased sensation of thirst	Diminished ability to conserve sodium and excrete potassium Reduced ability to correct acid–base imbalance Increased risk of hyperglycemia and osmotic diuresis Decreased ability to recognize fluid deficit
Skin changes	Decreased skin elasticity Atrophy of sweat glands Diminished capillary bed	Skin turgor is poor indicator of state of hydration Skin is less effective in cooling body temperature
Cardiovascular function	Decreased baroreceptor sensitivity Decreased cardiac output (1%/y from 20 to 80 y of age) Decreased stroke volume (0.7%/y from 20 to 80 y of age) Decrease in renal plasma flow from 600 mL/min in second decade to 300 mL/min by eighth decade Decreased elasticity of arteries Increased vascular rigidity, causing increased peripheral resistance	Diminished ability to manage hypotension associated with shock Increased frequency of peripheral edema Increased risk of orthostatic hypotension, dizziness, falls
Respiratory function	Decreased compliance of chest wall Decreased elasticity of lung tissue Decreased number of alveoli Decreased strength of expiratory muscles Decreased normal partial pressure of oxygen	Increased difficulty in regulating pH associated with major illness, surgery, burns, or trauma
Gastrointestinal function	Decreased volume of saliva Decreased volume of gastric juice Decreased calcium absorption	Mouth may be drier Increased risk of hyponatremia and hypokalemia during vomiting and gastric suction Increased need for dietary calcium and vitamin D

GFR, glomerular filtration rate.
Adapted from Metheny NM: Fluid and Electrolyte Balance: Nursing Considerations, p 413. Philadelphia, Lippincott Williams & Wilkins, 2000, with permission.

box 30-3 nursing interventions for *Checking Hemodialysis and Continuous Venovenous Hemofiltration With Dialysis (CVVH/D) Equipment*

- Prime lines and dialyzer or filter to expel all air before starting treatment.
- Test all alarms before connecting the patient to the circuit.
- Respond to all alarms immediately.
- Replace wet pressure transducers if they interfere with transmission of pressure reading.
- Inspect and tighten all connections before initiating treatment.

Figure 30-3 illustrates the hemodialysis circuit. After vascular access is established, blood begins to flow, assisted by the blood pump. The part of the disposable circuit before the dialyzer is designated the arterial line, both to distinguish the blood in it as blood that has not yet reached the dialyzer and in reference to needle placement. The arterial needle is placed closest to the arteriovenous anastomosis in a graft or fistula to maximize blood flow. A clamped saline bag always is attached to the circuit just before the blood pump. In episodes of hypotension, blood flow from the patient can be clamped while the saline is opened and allowed to infuse rapidly to correct blood pressure. Blood transfusions and plasma expanders also can be attached to the circuit at this point and allowed to drip in, assisted by the blood pump. Heparin infusions may be located either before or after the blood pump, depending on the equipment in use.

The dialyzer is the next important component of the circuit. Blood flows into the blood compartment of the dialyzer, where exchange of fluid and waste products takes place. Blood leaving the dialyzer passes through an air detector that shuts down the blood pump if any air is detected. At this point in the pathway, any medications that can be given during dialysis are infused through a medication port. However, unless otherwise ordered, most medications are withheld until after dialysis.

Blood that has passed through the dialyzer returns to the patient through the venous, or postdialyzer line. After the prescribed treatment time, dialysis is terminated by clamping off blood from the patient, opening the saline line, and rinsing the circuit to return the patient's blood.

A dialysis nurse is in constant attendance during acute hemodialysis. Blood pressure and pulse are recorded at least every half hour when the patient's condition is stable. All machine pressures and flow rates are checked and recorded on a regular basis. The nurse assesses the patient's responses to fluid and solute removal and the condition and function of the patient's vascular access. Standard Precautions, one tier of the Centers for Disease Control and Prevention Isolation Guidelines, are followed. A protective face shield and gloves are worn by the nurse performing hemodialysis because of the risk of exposure to blood. The dialysis nurse and critical care nurse work together to care for the patient, and they must coordinate their specific patient care responsibilities.

POSTPROCEDURE

The results of a dialysis treatment can be determined by assessing the amount of fluid removed (as assessed by postdialysis weight) and the degree to which electrolyte and acid–base imbalances have been corrected. Blood drawn immediately postdialysis may show falsely low levels of electrolytes, urea nitrogen, and creatinine. The process of equilibration is thought to continue for some time after dialysis because these substances move from inside the cell to the plasma.

Complications

DIALYSIS DYSEQUILIBRIUM

Uremia must be corrected slowly to prevent dysequilibrium syndrome, which is a set of signs and symptoms ranging from headache, nausea, restlessness, and mild mental impairment to vomiting, confusion, agitation, and seizures. This is thought to occur as the plasma concentration of solutes, such as urea nitrogen, is lowered. Blood urea and nitrogen play a role in calculating the serum osmolarity. Because of the blood–brain barrier, solutes are removed much more slowly from brain cells. Therefore, plasma becomes hypotonic in relation to the brain cells. This results in a shift of water from plasma to the brain cells and causes cerebral edema and symptoms of dysequilibrium syndrome. This syndrome can be avoided by dialyzing patients for short periods, such as 1 to 2 hours on 3 or 4 consecutive days.

HYPOVOLEMIA

Fluid overload is treated during dialysis by removing excess water. Because this removal depends on shifting fluid from other body compartments to the vascular space, care must taken to avoid removing fluid so rapidly during dialysis that it leads to volume depletion. Excessive fluid removal may lead to hypotension, and little is gained if intravenous (IV) fluids are given to correct the problem. Therefore, it is better to reduce the volume overload over two or three dialyses, unless pulmonary congestion is life-threatening.

HYPOTENSION

Normal saline in bolus amounts of 100 to 200 mL is used to correct hypotension. Dialysis machines now aid in preventing hypotension because the amount of ultrafiltration is controlled at the push of a button. It is also possible to vary the sodium concentration of dialysate. A higher sodium level in the dialysate means that less sodium is removed from the blood. A higher serum sodium assists the body as it shifts fluid from the interstitial to the intravascular compartment. Blood volume expanders, such as albumin, are sometimes used in patients with a low serum protein.

The use of antihypertensive drugs in patients who undergo dialysis may precipitate hypotension during dialysis. To avoid this, standard practice in many dialysis units is to omit antihypertensive drugs 4 to 6 hours before dialysis. Restriction of fluids and sodium before and during the dialysis phases is a more desirable method for control of hypertension. Sedatives and tranquilizers also may cause hypotension and should be avoided, if possible.

HYPERTENSION

Fluid overload, dysequilibrium syndrome, renin response to ultrafiltration, and anxiety are the most frequent causes of hypertension during dialysis. Hypertension during dialysis is usually caused by sodium and water excess. This can be confirmed by comparing the patient's present weight to his or her ideal or dry weight. If fluid overload is the cause of hypertension, ultrafiltration usually brings about a reduction in the blood pressure.

Some patients who may be normotensive before dialysis become hypertensive during dialysis. The rise may occur either gradually or abruptly. The cause is not well understood, but it may be the result of renin production in response to ultrafiltration and an increase in renal ischemia. Patients must be carefully monitored because the vasoconstriction caused by the renin response is limited. Once a decrease in blood volume surpasses the ability to maintain blood pressure through vasoconstriction, hypotension can occur precipitously.

MUSCLE CRAMPS

Muscle cramps may occur during dialysis as a result of excess fluid removal, which results in diminished intravascular volume and reduced muscle perfusion. Cramps are treated by lowering the rate of ultrafiltration, giving a saline bolus of 100 to 200 mL, and either administering 10 mL of 23.4% saline or increasing the sodium content of the dialysate.[2]

DYSRHYTHMIAS AND ANGINA

Dysrhythmias and angina may occur in patients with underlying cardiac disease in response to fluid removal. Decreasing the rate of fluid removal may help. Medication may be needed to control cardiac rhythm.

CONTINUOUS RENAL REPLACEMENT THERAPIES

In CRRT, blood circulates outside the body through a highly porous filter similar to that used with hemodialysis. The process is similar to hemodialysis in that water, electrolytes, and small to medium-sized molecules are removed by ultrafiltration. CRRT is accompanied by a simultaneous reinfusion of a physiological solution, and it occurs continuously for an extended period. A pump, slightly different from that used in hemodialysis, is used and often incorporates a weighing system so fluids can be intricately balanced hour to hour (Fig. 30-4).

CRRTs include continuous arteriovenous hemofiltration, continuous arteriovenous hemofiltration with dialysis, continuous venovenous hemofiltration (CVVH), and CVVH with dialysis (CVVH/D; Table 30-3). This discussion focuses primarily on CVVH and CVVH/D because these therapies are replacing the arteriovenous procedures. Access to the circulation for CVVH and CVVH/D is the same as that used for short-term hemodialysis. The extracorporeal circuit is similar to the hemodialysis circuit (Fig. 30-5). A pump is added to assist blood flow. The rate of blood flow is typically much slower than in hemodialysis. The ultrafiltration rate is titrated to reach an hourly goal and is based on the patient's cardiac and pulmonary status.

When CVVH is used, a replacement fluid is ordered and is connected either before or after the filter, depending on patient characteristics and institutional practice. When dialysis is added to the CVVH process, it is called CVVH/D. Adding the dialysate increases the ability to remove wastes. Therefore, it is used when uremia must be aggressively managed, such as with the highly catabolic patient. CVVH and CVVH/D can be performed and managed by the critical care nurse. Typically, competency assessment and validation are performed before the nurse cares for patients with CRRT.

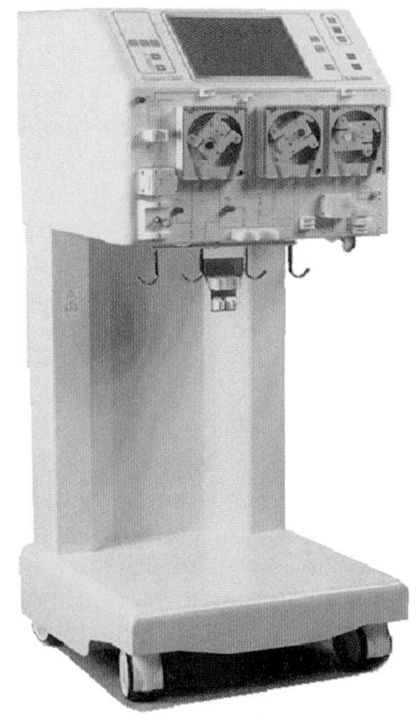

A

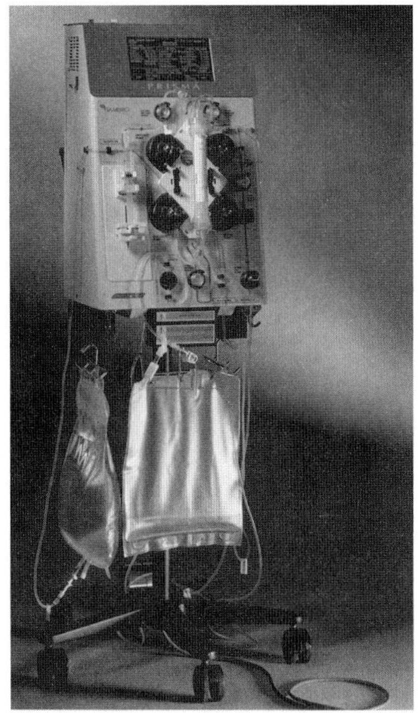

B

figure 30-4 Devices for administering continuous renal replacement therapy (CRRT) offer an integrated fluid warmer for the heating of infusion and dialysate fluids, a weighing system to reduce the possibility of error in assessing fluid balance, and a battery backup that allows treatments to continue when the patient is moved. (**A**) Diapact pump, B-Braun McGraw Corporation. (**B**) PRISMA, Gambro Corporation.

table 30-3 Continuous Renal Replacement Therapies

Type of Therapy	Mechanism of Action	Indications
Continuous venovenous hemodialysis	Blood is driven through low-permeability dialyzer, and countercurrent flow of dialysis solution is delivered on dialysate compartment. Ultrafiltrate produced during membrane transit corresponds to the patient's weight loss; solute clearance is mainly achieved by diffusion; replacement solution is not needed. Efficiency of clearance is limited to small molecules.	Fluid and solute clearance
Continuous venovenous hemofiltration (CVVH)	Blood is driven through highly permeable filter via extracorporeal circuit in venovenous mode. Ultrafiltrate produced during membrane transit is replaced partially or completely to achieve blood purification and volume control; ultrafiltration is in excess of patient weight loss; replacement solution is needed.	Fluid and solute clearance
Slow continuous hemofiltration	Blood is driven through highly permeable filter via extracorporeal circuit in venovenous mode. Ultrafiltrate produced during membrane transit is not replaced and corresponds exactly to patient weight loss.	Only for fluid control in overhydration status
Continuous venovenous hemofiltration with dialysis (CVVH/D)	Blood is driven through highly permeable dialyzer, and countercurrent flow of dialysis solution is delivered on the dialysate compartment. Ultrafiltrate produced during membrane transit is in excess of the patient's weight loss; solute clearance is obtained both by diffusion and convection; replacement solution is needed to obtain fluid balance (sometimes referred to as "push-pull" dialysis).	For combined convection and diffusion clearance

Adapted from Bellomo R, Ronco C: Continuous renal replacement therapy in the intensive care unit. Intensive Care Med 25:781–789, 1999, with permission.

Indications for Continuous Renal Replacement Therapy

CRRT is indicated in the following circumstances: in patients with a high risk of hemodynamic instability who do not tolerate the rapid fluid shifts that occur with hemodialysis, in those who require large amounts of hourly IV fluids or parenteral nutrition, and in those who need more than the usual 3- to 4-hour hemodialysis treatment to correct the metabolic imbalances of acute renal failure. Table 30-4 presents criteria for initiating CRRT. CVVH is used when patients primarily need excess fluid removed, whereas CVVH/D is used when patients also need waste products removed due to uremia. For a comparison of CRRT with hemodialysis and peritoneal dialysis, see Table 30-1.

Contraindications to Continuous Renal Replacement Therapy

CRRT is contraindicated once patients become hemodynamically stable or no longer require continuous therapy, and intermittent hemodialysis should be used. It may be difficult to achieve access to circulation in some patients with coagulopathies, which may prolong initiation of therapy. Patient and family discussion is imperative before initiation of therapy; patients may not wish to receive CRRT, and it is essential that patient wishes be considered.

Equipment

A typical CVVH/D setup is shown in Figure 30-5. Blood exits the body through the arterial limb of the vascular access. The first infusion line shown is for the anticoagulation. Located just before the blood pump is a line that measures pressure in the prefilter portion of the circuit, known as the arterial pressure. The blood pump, which propels blood into the filter, is next. An infusion port just after the blood pump is usually connected to normal saline for flushing the circuit or for attaching the replacement fluid. A bag of dialysate is shown flowing through the filter and surrounding the hollow fibers in which the blood travels. As the dialysate exits the filter, it passes through a sensor that detects microscopic amounts of blood, thereby warning of filter rupture. The dialysate and excess fluid removed from the patient are collected in a graduated collection device for easy measurement. Meanwhile, the blood exits the filter and passes into a drip chamber, where air and foam are trapped instead of entering the patient's circulation. The drip chamber also contains a line to which a syringe can be attached to raise and lower the blood level and another line that measures pressure in the postfilter section of the circuit, known as venous pressure. A clamp is located after the drip chamber and automatically engages if air tries to pass through it. The arterial and venous pressure transducers are protected by a disposable filter. As blood returns to the body, replacement fluid is infused. In some systems, the line for replacement fluid is placed before the blood pump

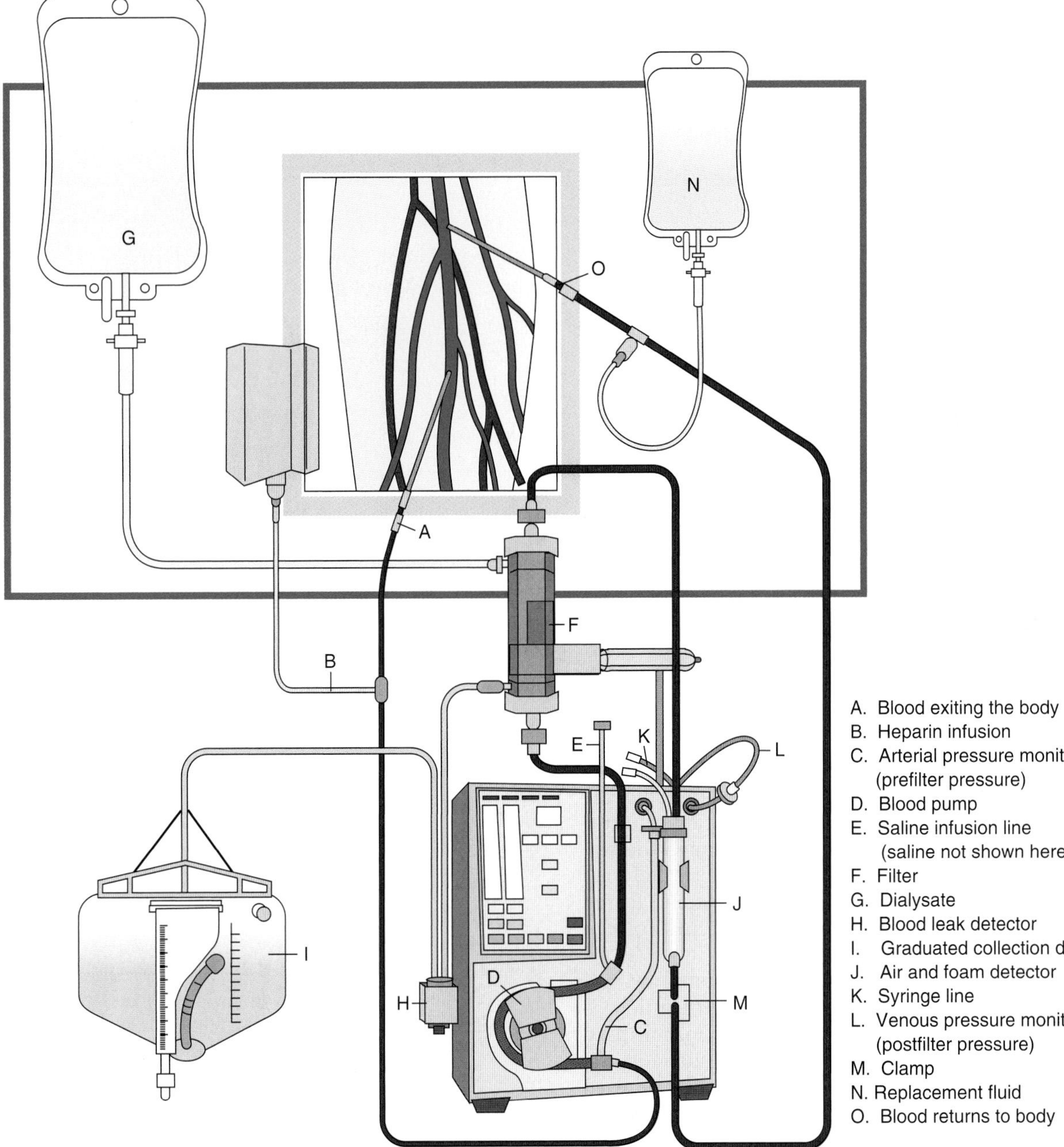

figure 30-5 Continuous venovenous hemofiltration with dialysis (CVVH/D). (Baxter Health Care Corporation, Renal Division, McGaw Park, IL)

so it can be infused before the blood reaches the filter. The total amount of blood in the circuit is about 150 mL.

Assessment and Management

PREPROCEDURE

Baseline hemodynamics, vital signs, and weight are obtained before initiation of therapy. The filters used in the continuous therapies are much more porous than those used in hemodialysis, and the circuit does not contain a mechanism to control the amount of fluid removed. Thus, the potential exists for uncontrolled losses of a large amount of fluid. Because of this, an hourly fluid balance goal is set by the physician. Fluid is replaced each hour in varying amounts to achieve the goal (Box 30-4).

PROCEDURE

Before therapy is initiated, the equipment is checked (see Box 30-3). The lines and filter are primed to expel air from the circuit. Arterial and venous lines are connected to the corresponding port of the access catheter, and the blood pump is turned on. Blood starts to flow through the tubing. Ultrafiltration begins to produce plasma water (ultrafiltrate) that starts to flow into the

table 30-4 Conditions That Warrant Continuous Renal Replacement Therapy (CRRT)*

Clinical Condition	Assessment Findings
Oliguria	Urine output <200 mL/12 h
Anuria	Urine output <50 mL/12 h
Severe acidemia due to metabolic acidosis	pH <7.1
Azotemia (urea)	>30 mmol/L
Hyperkalemia or rapidly rising serum potassium levels	Serum potassium >6.5 mEq/L
Suspected uremia organ involvement	Pericarditis, encephalopathy, neuropathy, myopathy
Severe alterations in serum sodium levels	Serum sodium >160 mmol/L or <115 mmol/L
Clinically significant organ edema	Pulmonary edema
Drug overdose with dialyzable toxin	Aspirin overdose
Coagulopathy requiring large amounts of blood products in patient at risk of pulmonary edema or acute respiratory distress syndrome (ARDS)	Disseminated intravascular coagulation (DIC)

*One of these conditions is sufficient grounds for the initiation of CRRT. Two of these conditions make CRRT essentially mandatory. Combined derangements suggest the initiation of CRRT even before some of these conditions have been reached.

Adapted from Bellomo R, Ronco C: Continuous renal replacement therapy in the intensive care unit. Intensive Care Med 25:781–789, 1999, with permission.

collection device. Most experts recommend controlling the amount of ultrafiltrate by raising or lowering the collection device until the desired hourly rate of ultrafiltration is achieved. Blood flow rates through the circuit average 100 mL/hour, and the standard dialysate flow rate is 1 L/hour. Substances are adequately cleared when ultrafiltration produces 500 to 600 mL/hour of ultrafiltrate.

Anticoagulation, if indicated, is administered as therapy begins. Low-dose heparin is the standard anticoagulant used in patients at risk of bleeding. It may be used along with saline flushes to prevent circuit clotting. Saline flushes without low-dose heparin may be used when the patient has a low platelet count. A typical protocol is to flush 100 mL through the circuit every half hour. Another method of anticoagulation is to infuse 4% trisodium citrate before the filter. This anticoagulates only the extracorporeal part of the circuit. It chelates calcium, which is then replaced through infusion in a central line. For this process to be effective, the dialysate solution must be calcium free. The patient needs to be closely monitored to prevent hypercalcemia or hypocalcemia.[3]

Hourly maintenance of the CVVH/D system includes measuring blood and dialysate flows, calculating net ultrafiltration and replacement fluid, titrating anticoagulants, assessing the integrity of the vascular access, and monitoring hemodynamic parameters and blood circuit pressures. The nephrologist sets a goal for hourly fluid balance, and the critical care nurse is responsible to see that it is met. Box 30-5 lists interventions in monitoring fluid and electrolyte balance. By comparing total intake and output, the hourly net fluid balance is calculated.

box 30-4
Example Showing Hourly Fluid Goal With Intake and Output in Fluid Replacement in CVVH/D

1. The patient needs to have 200 mL of fluid removed per hour.
2. The patient receives 500 mL/h of intravenous fluid (e.g., blood transfusions and parenteral nutrition).
3. The patient has 400 mL of nasogastric drainage and 100 mL of wound drainage in 1 hour.
4. Peritoneal dialysate is added at the rate of 1,000 mL/h to increase clearance.
5. The total amount of fluid in the collecting bag at the end of one hour is 2,500 mL. (Remember, 1,000 mL is peritoneal dialysate, so 1,500 mL has been filtered from the patient's plasma.)

To calculate the amount of replacement fluid, add the input fluid of 500 mL of IV fluid and 1,000 mL of peritoneal dialysate. Output is the 1,500 mL that has been filtered from the patient's plasma, 400 mL of nasogastric drainage, and the 100 mL of wound drainage. Total output is 2,000 mL, and the total input is 1,500 mL. The difference is 500 mL. The hourly fluid removal goal of 200 mL is subtracted, indicating 300 mL has been removed in excess of the goal and needs to be replaced this hour.

The amount of replacement fluid is determined by the difference between desired and net fluid balance. Fluid balance and replacement should be recorded on a bedside flow sheet.[3]

In CVVH, replacement fluid may be infused prefilter or postfilter. Both techniques have advantages and disadvantages. When fluid is given prefilter, it decreases blood viscosity and increases blood flow through the filter. This enhances ultrafiltrate (plasma fluid) production and solute removal and decreases the frequency of clotting. The disadvantage is the increased need for fluid replacement. If replacement fluid is given postfilter, there is less total fluid loss and less need for replacement fluid. However, there is an increased incidence of filter clotting and decreased filter life. The method chosen depends on the system used and institutional preference.[3]

Electrolytes, urea nitrogen, creatinine, and glucose levels are drawn before the procedure is started and then at least twice daily. Electrolyte imbalances can be corrected by altering the composition of the replacement fluid or by custom-mixing the dialysate.[3] Anticoagulation is monitored by checking activated clotting times or PT and PTT. Although frequency is determined by each institution, it is not unusual to check clotting times every 1 or 2 hours to prevent clotting of the filter and blood lines.[3]

No one policy delineates the optimal time to change the circuit. Many institutions put a 24- to 48-hour limit on circuit life, although there are reports of filters lasting an average of 4 days. System performance is monitored by checking the amount of urea nitrogen in the filtrate compared with the amount of urea nitrogen prefilter. A decreasing ratio indicates inadequate performance. A decreasing rate of ultrafiltration and increases in the venous pressure indicate clotting in the filter.[3]

Treatment may be interrupted to transport the patient for a diagnostic test or procedure to fix a mechanical problem with the circuit or vascular access. Treatment may be terminated if the patient shows signs of recovering renal function. When it is determined that continuous therapy can be terminated, the blood is returned to the patient. First, the ultrafiltrate outlet is clamped, and the dialysate is turned off. Then, anticoagulation is turned off, and the blood is returned to the patient through a saline flush. Once the lines are clear, they are disconnected from the vascular access. Then the vascular access is heparinized per unit policy. Documentation includes fluid balance, condition of the access, and the patient's response to treatment. The tubing and filter are disposable. When working with the circuit and ultrafiltrate, the nurse uses Standard Precautions. Box 30-6 lists some nursing diagnoses and collaborative problems associated with hemodialysis and CRRT.

box 30-5 nursing interventions for *Monitoring Fluid and Electrolyte Balance During CVVH/D*

- Draw electrolytes, blood urea nitrogen, and creatinine before initiating treatment and then at least twice daily.
- Assess vital signs, central pressure readings (if available), breath sounds, heart sounds, weight, intake, and output before initiating treatment and at least every half hour during treatment.
- Collaborate with nephrologist to determine hourly fluid balance.
- Record all intake and output when calculating replacement fluid for the next hour.
- Administer replacement fluid tailored to the patient's electrolytes, or obtain custom mixed dialysate from the pharmacy.
- If hypotension occurs, administer saline boluses (100–200 mL), reduce ultrafiltration by raising the collecting device, and, if necessary, obtain an order for 5% albumin.
- Observe patient for signs of electrolyte imbalances (i.e., electrocardiographic changes and muscle weakness, as with hypokalemia).

Technical Complications in Continuous Venovenous Hemofiltration With Dialysis

ACCESS PROBLEMS

Blood flows used in CVVH/D are much lower than for hemodialysis, making it more likely that a catheter will provide adequate flow. However, a poorly functioning access jeopardizes the entire CVVH/D procedure. Often, the position of the patient's extremity affects blood flow. If the access is in a limb, the limb should be gently immobilized. An obstruction, such as a clot or kink in the arterial lumen of the catheter, results in less blood being delivered to the circuit and manifests as lowered arterial and venous pressures. Clots or kinks in the venous lumen of the catheter raise venous pressures as blood tries to return against an obstruction. The treatment may be temporarily halted while the nurse manually flushes each lumen to determine patency. If blood flow still cannot be established, the nephrologist is notified immediately to replace the catheter.

box 30-6 *Examples of Nursing Diagnoses for the Patient Undergoing Hemodialysis or Continuous Renal Replacement Therapy (CRRT)*

- Excess Fluid Volume related to renal impairment
- Deficient Fluid Volume related to renal replacement therapy of fluid removal
- Ineffective Tissue Perfusion related to decreased renal perfusion
- Risk for Infection risk factors: invasive devices, malnutrition

CLOTTING

An early sign of filter clotting is a reduced rate of ultrafiltration, which cannot be corrected by increasing blood flow or by lowering the collection device. As clotting progresses, venous pressure rises, arterial pressure drops, and the blood lines appear dark. Clotting times are low. A saline bolus may help determine the location and extent of clotting. It may be possible to return some of the patient's blood before changing the circuit, but if clotting is extensive this should not be attempted. Box 30-7 lists some nursing interventions for maintaining blood flow through a CVVH/D circuit.

AIR IN THE CIRCUIT

If the connections are loose, or a prefilter infusion line runs dry, air disrupts the system by collecting in the drip chamber and setting off the air detector alarm and triggering the clamp on the venous line to close. The nurse assesses the circuit's integrity to detect the source of air. Before resetting the line clamp, the nurse makes sure all bubbles have been tapped out of the drip chamber, all connections are tight, and there is no danger of air getting into the patient's bloodstream.[3]

BLOOD LEAKS

Blood appears in the ultrafiltrate if there is any rupture inside the filter. The blood leak alarm sounds and the blood pump stops. Testing the ultrafiltrate with a dipstick can verify a microscopic leak. Blood can be safely returned to the patient as long as there is no gross blood in the ultrafiltrate. Then the circuit should be changed. A gross leak is readily identifiable. Blood should not be returned to the patient, and the patient's hematocrit should be checked to determine the need for transfusion.

Physiological Complications in Continuous Venovenous Hemofiltration With Dialysis

HYPOTENSION

If blood pressure and intravascular filling pressures fall below optimal, the nurse can increase the infusion rate of replacement fluid or give a normal saline bolus of 100 to 200 mL. At the same time, the ultrafiltrate collection device is raised to decrease ultrafiltration until pressures stabilize. An infusion of 5% albumin may also help stabilize blood pressure. If this situation persists, the physician is consulted to adjust the net ultrafiltration goal.

HYPOTHERMIA

Some patients experience chills and lowered body temperature while their blood is circulating outside the body. If this happens, it may be advisable to use a blood warmer to warm either the dialysate or the replacement fluid. Advancements in the technologies used to perform CRRT have improved the precision of fluid balance and reduced the hypothermia that can develop with any extracorporeal therapy. The primary development therapy has been the automatic fluid weighing system, which automates all intake and output fluid calculations.

Psychological Aspects of Renal Replacement Therapies

The psychological impact of short-term renal replacement therapy is different from that of lifelong therapy. Although the patient depends on a machine in both situations, in short-term therapy there is usually hope that the patient may recover renal function. Therefore, concerns usually focus on the discomfort associated with insertion of the temporary vascular access and the dialysis treatment. Once these situations are handled, the patient and family then must cope with the uncertainty of how long renal failure will last and how long dialysis will be necessary.

Patients who develop chronic renal failure must deal with the fact that renal replacement therapy will be necessary for the rest of their lives. At first, patients usually deny a great deal of what is happening to them. This may continue for some time and prevent some patients from accepting necessary aspects of their treatment regimen. Other patients who feel considerably better after starting dialysis may enter a "honeymoon phase" and appear quite euphoric for a while. Patients should progress through the normal grieving stages and develop healthy coping mechanisms to deal with their long-term treatment.

Hemodialysis Applied to Other Therapies

The technical equipment and knowledge needed to perform hemodialysis are often applied to other therapies that involve an extracorporeal blood process, such as hemoperfusion and therapeutic apheresis. *Hemoperfusion* is used primarily for the treatment of drug overdose. Blood is pumped from the body and perfused through a

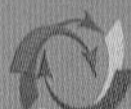

box 30-7 nursing interventions for *Maintaining Blood Flow Through A Continuous Venovenous Hemofiltration With Dialysis (CVVHID) Circuit*

- Check clotting times at initiation and at the prescribed intervals throughout treatment.
- Flush system as often as needed with saline to assess appearance of filter and circuit.
- Monitor ultrafiltration rates, venous and arterial pressure, and color of blood in circuit.
- If system is clotting, return as much blood as possible to the patient before changing the system.

column of charcoal or other absorbent materials that bind the drug. This leads to a rapid reduction in serum levels and avoids potential tissue damage caused by an abnormally high drug level. This therapy is particularly useful for drugs that are fat bound or whose molecular structure is too large to be removed by hemodialysis. A hemodialysis blood pump and air detector often are used with hemoperfusion cartridges and tubing.

Therapeutic plasma exchange, or *apheresis*, is another therapy that may be performed using standard hemodialysis equipment in conjunction with a plasma separator cell and replacement fluids. Apheresis is used to treat diseases caused or complicated by circulating immune complexes or their abnormal proteins. During the procedure, the patient's whole blood is separated into its major components, and the offending components are removed.

PERITONEAL DIALYSIS

Peritoneal dialysis and hemodialysis accomplish the same objective and operate on the same principle of diffusion. However, in peritoneal dialysis, the peritoneum is the semipermeable membrane, and osmosis is used to remove fluid, rather than the pressure differentials used in hemodialysis. To access the peritoneal cavity, a Tenckhoff (peritoneal) catheter is inserted (Fig. 30-6). Intermittent peritoneal dialysis is an effective alternative method of treating acute renal failure when hemodialysis is not available or when access to the bloodstream is not possible. It sometimes is used as an initial treatment for renal failure while the patient is being evaluated for a hemodialysis program. For a comparison of peritoneal dialysis with hemodialysis and CRRT, see Table 30-1.

Peritoneal dialysis has the following advantages over hemodialysis:

- The required technical equipment and supplies are less complicated and more readily available.
- There is less need for highly skilled personnel.
- The adverse effects associated with the more efficient hemodialysis are minimized. This may be important for patients with severe cardiac disease, who cannot tolerate rapid hemodynamic changes.

Peritoneal dialysis also has a few disadvantages.

- It requires more time to remove metabolic wastes adequately and to restore electrolyte and fluid balance.
- Repeated treatments may lead to peritonitis.
- Long periods of immobility may result in complications, such as pulmonary congestion and venous stasis.

Because fluid is introduced into the peritoneal cavity, peritoneal dialysis is contraindicated in patients who have existing peritonitis, in those who have undergone recent or extensive abdominal surgery, and in those who have abdominal adhesions. In the event of a cardiac arrest, the patient's abdomen is drained immediately to maximize the efficiency of chest compressions.

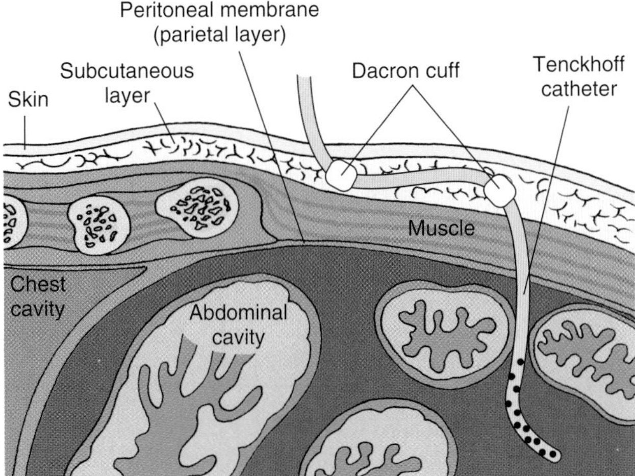

figure 30-6 A Tenckhoff (peritoneal) catheter is used to access the peritoneal cavity. A Dacron cuff wrapped around the catheter helps to reduce complications related to infection.

Equipment

SOLUTIONS

As in hemodialysis, peritoneal dialysis solutions contain "ideal" concentrations of electrolytes but lack urea, creatinine, and other substances that are to be removed. Unlike dialysate used in hemodialysis, solutions must be sterile. Dextrose concentrations of the solutions vary; a 1.5%, 2.5%, or 4.25% dextrose solution can be used. Use of 2.5% or 4.25% solutions usually is reserved for more fluid removal and occasionally for better solute clearance. If peritoneal dialysate does not contain potassium, a small amount of potassium chloride may have to be added to the dialysate to prevent hypokalemia. The patient's serum potassium must be monitored closely to regulate the amount of potassium to be added.

AUTOMATED PERITONEAL DIALYSIS SYSTEMS

Automated peritoneal dialysis systems have built-in monitors and a system of automatic timing devices that cycle the infusion and removal of peritoneal fluid. For this reason, they are called *cyclers*, and they may be used in the intensive care setting. They are convenient because they eliminate the need to change solution bags constantly. Most cyclers also have a log that retains cycle-by-cycle information on ultrafiltration. Setting up the cycler requires attaching the appropriate strength of large-volume (5 L) solution bags to the cycler tubing, using aseptic technique. The cycler is programmed to deliver a set amount of dialysate per exchange for a certain length of time. When the time is up, the patient is automatically drained and then refilled. Cyclers are usually used when patients have a permanent peritoneal access device.

Assessment and Management

PREPROCEDURE

Before peritoneal dialysis begins, the nurse must perform the following interventions:

1. Prepare the patient for catheter insertion and the dialysis procedure by giving a thorough explana-

tion of the procedure. A consent form may be signed according to hospital policy.
2. Ask the patient to empty the bladder just before the procedure to avoid accidental puncture with the trocar.
3. Give a preoperative medication, as ordered, to enhance relaxation during the procedure.
4. Warm the dialyzing fluid to body temperature or slightly warmer, using a device manufactured solely for this purpose. It is not recommended that peritoneal dialysate be warmed in microwave ovens due to uneven heating of the fluid and inconsistency from one microwave to another.
5. Take and record baseline vital signs, such as temperature, pulse, respirations, and weight. An in-bed scale is ideal for frequent monitoring of the patient's weight.
6. Take the patient's history, identifying abdominal surgery or trauma.
7. Examine the abdomen before the catheter is inserted.
8. Follow specific orders, obtained before the procedure, regarding fluid removal, replacement, and drug administration.

PROCEDURE

The following items are needed for the procedure:

- Peritoneal dialysis administration set
- Peritoneal dialysis catheter set, which includes the catheter, a connecting tube for connecting the catheter to the administration set, and a metal stylet
- Trocar set of the physician's choice
- Ancillary drugs: local anesthetic solution (2% lidocaine), aqueous heparin (1,000 U/mL), potassium chloride, broad-spectrum antibiotics

The physician makes a small midline incision just below the umbilicus under sterile conditions. A trocar is inserted through the incision into the peritoneal cavity. The obturator is removed, and the catheter is inserted and secured.

The dialysis solution flows into the abdominal cavity by gravity as rapidly as possible (5 to 10 minutes; Fig. 30-7). If it flows in too slowly, the catheter may need to be repositioned. When the solution is infused, the tubing is clamped, and the solution remains in the abdominal cavity for 30 to 45 minutes. Next, the solution bottles or bags are placed below the abdominal cavity, and the fluid is drained out of the peritoneal cavity by gravity. If the system is patent and the catheter well placed, the fluid drains in a steady, forceful stream. Drainage should take no more than 20 minutes.

This cycle is repeated continuously for the prescribed time, which varies from 12 to 36 hours, depending on the purpose of the treatment, the patient's condition, and the proper functioning of the system. Dialysis effluent is considered a contaminated fluid, and gloves are worn while handling it.

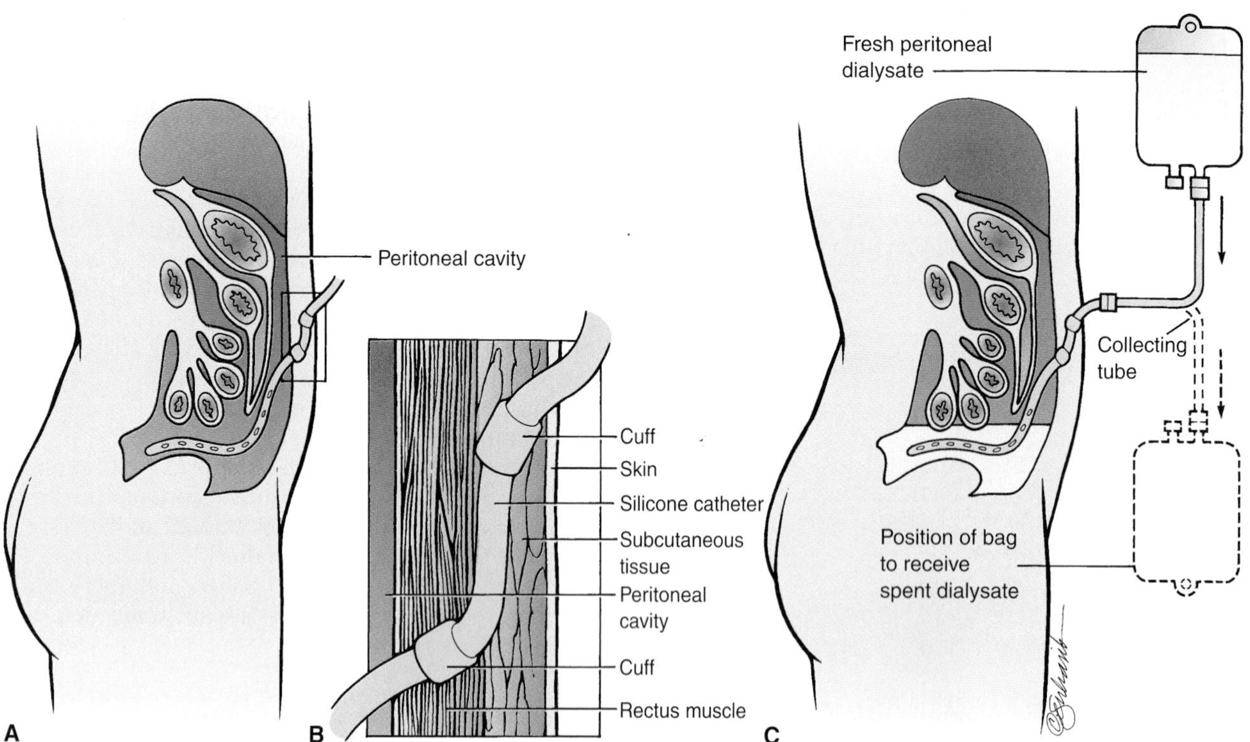

figure 30-7 Continuous ambulatory peritoneal dialysis. (**A**) The peritoneal catheter is implanted through the abdominal wall. (**B**) Dacron cuffs and a subcutaneous tunnel provide protection against bacterial infection. (**C**) Dialysate flows by gravity into the peritoneal catheter and then into the peritoneal cavity until the next drainage period. Dialysis thus continues on a 24-hour-a-day basis during which the patient is free to move around and engage in his or her usual activities. (Used with permission from Smeltzer SC, Bare BG: Brunner & Suddarth's Textbook of Medical–Surgical Nursing [10th Ed], p 1293. Philadelphia, Lippincott Williams & Wilkins, 2004.)

POSTPROCEDURE

After the procedure, the nurse must perform the following interventions:

1. Maintain accurate records of intake and output and weights obtained from the same scale for assessment of volume depletion or overload.
2. Monitor blood pressure and pulse frequently. Orthostatic blood pressure changes and increased pulse rate are valuable clues that help the nurse evaluate the patient's volume status.
3. Detect signs and symptoms of peritonitis early. Low-grade fever, abdominal pain, and cloudy peritoneal fluid all are possible signs of infection.
4. Maintain sterility of the peritoneal system. Masks and sterile gloves must be worn while the abdominal dressing is being changed. Solution bags or bottles are changed in as controlled a physical environment as possible to avoid contamination (e.g., avoiding areas of high traffic and high air flow).
5. Detect and correct technical difficulties early before they result in physiological problems. Slow outflow of the peritoneal fluid may indicate early problems with the patency of the peritoneal catheter.
6. Prevent complications of bed rest and provide an environment that helps the patient in accepting bed rest for prolonged periods.
7. Prevent constipation. Difficult or infrequent defecation decreases the clearance of waste products and cause the patient more discomfort and distension.

Technical Complications

INCOMPLETE RECOVERY OF FLUID

The fluid that is removed should equal or exceed the amount inserted. Commercially prepared dialysate contains approximately 1,000 to 2,000 mL of fluid. If, after several exchanges, the volume drained is less (by 500 mL or more) than the amount inserted, an evaluation must be made. Signs of fluid retention include abdominal distension or complaints of fullness. The most accurate indication of the amount of unrecovered fluid is weight.

If the fluid drains slowly, the catheter tip may be buried in the omentum or clogged with fibrin. Turning the patient from side to side, elevating the head of the bed, and gently massaging the abdomen may facilitate drainage.

If fibrin or blood exists in the outflow drainage, heparin needs to be added to the dialysate. The specific dose, which is ordered by the physician, is 500 to 1,000 U/L.

LEAKAGE AROUND THE CATHETER

Superficial leakage after surgery may be controlled with extra sutures and a decrease in the amount of dialysate instilled into the peritoneum. Increases in intra-abdominal pressure may also cause dialysate leaks. Therefore, continued vomiting, coughing, and jarring movements should be avoided during the initial postoperative period. The abdominal dressing must be checked frequently to detect leakage. Dialysate leaks can be distinguished from other clear fluids by checking with a dextrose test strip. Dialysate tests positive because of its dextrose content. A leaking catheter must be corrected because it acts as a pathway for bacteria to enter the peritoneum.

BLOOD-TINGED PERITONEAL FLUID

Blood-tinged peritoneal fluid is expected in the initial outflow but should clear after a few exchanges. Gross bleeding at any time is an indication of a more serious problem and must be investigated immediately.

Physiological Complications

PERITONITIS

Peritonitis is a serious, but manageable, complication of peritoneal dialysis. Signs of peritonitis include low-grade fever, abdominal pain when fluid is being inserted, and cloudy peritoneal drainage fluid. Early detection and treatment reduces the patient's discomfort and prevents more serious complications.

Treatment begins as soon as a sample of peritoneal fluid is obtained for culture and sensitivity. The patient is started on a broad-spectrum antibiotic, which is usually added to the dialysate solution, although it also can be given intravenously. Depending on the severity of the infection, the patient's condition should improve dramatically after 8 hours of antibiotic therapy.

CATHETER INFECTION

During the daily dressing change, the nurse examines the exit site closely for signs of infection, such as tenderness, redness, and drainage around the catheter. In the absence of peritonitis, a catheter infection usually is treated with an oral, broad-spectrum antibiotic. Box 30-8 lists nursing

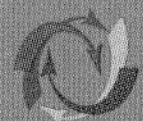

box 30-8 nursing interventions for *Preventing Infection During Peritoneal Dialysis*

- Maintain aseptic technique throughout dialysis procedure.
- Use sealed plastic dialysate bags.
- Change dialysis tubing regularly per protocol.
- Swab or soak tubing connections and injection ports with bactericidal solution before adding medications or breaking closed system.
- Assess patient continuously for signs and symptoms of peritonitis (pain, cloudy effluent, fever).
- Change exit site dressing daily using aseptic technique until healing occurs. Assess daily for increase in inflammation or drainage.
- If infection is suspected, obtain appropriate culture, and begin antibiotic according to protocol or physician's order.

interventions for preventing infections during peritoneal dialysis.

HYPOTENSION

Hypotension may occur if excessive fluid is removed. Vital signs are monitored frequently, especially if a hypertonic solution is used. Lying and sitting blood pressure readings are especially useful for evaluating fluid status. Progressive drops in blood pressure and weight are signs of fluid deficit.

HYPERTENSION AND FLUID OVERLOAD

If all the dialysate solution is not removed in each cycle, hypertension and fluid overload may occur. If there is hypertension and a weight increase, the nurse assesses catheter patency and notes the exact amount of fluid in the dialysate bottle. Some manufacturers add 50 mL to a 1,000-mL bottle. Over a period of hours, this can make a considerable difference.

The nurse also observes the patient for signs of respiratory distress and pulmonary congestion. In the absence of other symptoms of fluid overload, hypertension may be the result of anxiety and apprehension. Nonpharmacological measures to reduce anxiety are preferable to administering sedatives and tranquilizers.

HIGH BLOOD UREA NITROGEN AND CREATININE

Blood urea nitrogen and creatinine levels are closely monitored because they help evaluate the effectiveness of the dialysis. When levels remain high, it indicates inadequate clearance of these waste products.

HYPOKALEMIA

The serum potassium is monitored closely because hypokalemia is a common complication of peritoneal dialysis. When the serum potassium level is low, potassium chloride is added to the dialysate.

HYPERGLYCEMIA

Supplemental insulin can be added to the dialysate to control hyperglycemia. Blood glucose levels should be monitored closely in patients with diabetes mellitus and hepatic disease.

PAIN

Patients may experience mild abdominal discomfort at any time during the procedure. It is probably related to the constant distension or chemical irritation of the peritoneum. If a mild analgesic does not provide relief, inserting 5 mL of 2% lidocaine directly into the catheter may help. The patient may be more comfortable if nourishment is given in small amounts, when the fluid is draining out rather than when the abdominal cavity is distended.

Severe pain may indicate more serious problems of infection or paralytic ileus. Infection is not likely in the first 24 hours. Aseptic technique and prophylactic antibiotics minimize the risk of infection. Periodic cultures of the outflowing fluid help in the early detection of pathogenic organisms.

IMMOBILITY

Immobility may lead to hypostatic pneumonia, especially in the debilitated or older patient. Deep breathing, turning, and coughing should be encouraged during the procedure. Leg exercises and the use of elastic stockings may prevent the development of venous thrombi and emboli.

DISCOMFORT

Peritoneal dialysis results in slower clearance of waste products than hemodialysis; therefore, it is rarely associated with the dysequilibrium seen with hemodialysis. However, boredom is a frequent problem because the treatment is longer. Nursing measures are directed toward making the patient as comfortable as possible. Diversions such as reading, watching television, and visitors should be encouraged. Educating the patient about peritoneal dialysis and involving the patient in the care may reduce some of the anxiety and discomfort.

Peritoneal Dialysis as a Chronic Treatment

Intermittent peritoneal dialysis (IPD) has been used for chronic therapy for some time, but it requires the patient to remain stationary for 10 to 14 hours, three times per week. Because of this inconvenience to the patient and increased staff time needed if this therapy is performed in-center, IPD seldom is used and is not available in many dialysis centers.

Peritoneal dialysis has gained popularity as a chronic form of dialysis therapy, especially since continuous ambulatory peritoneal dialysis (CAPD) has become available. CAPD is easily taught to patients and does not limit ambulation between dialysate fluid exchanges. It uses the dialysis fluid that is continuously present in the peritoneal cavity 24 hours a day, 7 days a week. Dialysis fluid is drained by the patient and replaced with fresh solution three to five times per day. The number of solution exchanges needed per day depends on the patient's individual needs. Although the patient is required to perform dialysis techniques every day, CAPD is attractive to many patients with end-stage renal disease (ESRD) because they can accomplish it easily and independently. CAPD may also be preferred in patients who benefit from a slow, continuous removal of sodium and water, such as in those with refractory congestive heart failure.

Continuous cyclic peritoneal dialysis (CCPD) is another variation of chronic peritoneal dialysis therapy. Patients who choose this form of therapy perform IPD at night during sleep using a cycling machine and in the morning instill dialysis fluid, which remains in the abdomen during the whole day. This is most convenient for patients who require the help of working family members to perform their exchanges.

As with acute peritoneal dialysis, peritonitis is the greatest potential problem with chronic forms of dialysis. Peritoneal catheters are permanent and inserted in the operating room. Such catheters have one or two Dacron cuffs that the surgeon sutures to the abdominal wall or subcutaneous tissue or both to anchor the catheter and provide a permanent seal against invading bacteria. Patients are taught how to recognize any potential problem associated with the catheter or treatment and to seek help from the CAPD team when needed.

Patients who perform IPD, CAPD, or CCPD at home usually visit the dialysis unit every 4 to 8 weeks. At this time, a nursing assessment is performed, techniques are reviewed, and required blood studies are obtained. All health team members, including the physician, nurse, dietitian, and social worker, work together with the patient and family to ensure successful adaptation to the chosen mode of treatment. A discharge planning guide for the patient undergoing chronic peritoneal dialysis is given in Box 30-9.

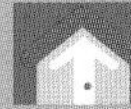

box 30-9 *Peritoneal Dialysis*

- Discuss basic information about normal kidney function.
- Discuss basic information about the disease process.
- Discuss the basic principles of peritoneal dialysis.
- Demonstrate catheter and exit site care.
- Demonstrate measurement of vital signs and weight measurement.
- Discuss monitoring and management of fluid balance.
- Discuss basic principles of aseptic technique.
- Demonstrate the CAPD exchange procedure using aseptic technique (CCPD patients should also demonstrate exchange procedure in case of failure or unavailability of cycling machine).
- Demonstrate cycler set up procedure and maintenance if on CCPD.
- Discuss complications of peritoneal dialysis; prevention, recognition, and management of complications.
- Demonstrate procedure for adding medications to the dialysis solution.
- Demonstrate procedure for obtaining sterile dialysis fluid samples.
- Discuss routine laboratory work needed and implications of results.
- Discuss dietary restrictions and importance of maintaining normal weight.
- Discuss medications: name of medications, their actions, potential side effects, and when to contact the physician.
- Discuss ordering, storage, and inventory of dialysis supplies.
- Describe plan for follow-up continuing care.
- Demonstrate maintenance of home dialysis records, including daily weights.
- Describe actions in case of emergency.

Used with permission from Smeltzer SC, Bare BG: Brunner & Suddarth's Textbook of Medical–Surgical Nursing (10th Ed), p. 1296. Philadelphia, Lippincott Williams & Wilkins, 2004.

PHARMACOLOGICAL MANAGEMENT OF RENAL DYSFUNCTION

When the kidneys fail, treatment such as dialysis may be used to achieve fluid and electrolyte balance. Pharmacological treatment may be initiated to enhance an already functional kidney, attempt to recover renal function, or optimize fluid balance.

Diuretics

Diuretics are drugs that promote fluid removal through increased urine production. There are three major classes of diuretics: loop, thiazide, and potassium-sparing. Table 30-5 presents information about the various diuretics. In addition, acetazolamide and mannitol may be used to promote fluid removal. The ultimate goal of diuretic therapy is to improve cardiopulmonary status. It may be necessary to use combination therapy to achieve the desired therapeutic end point. Drugs from different classes are chosen to maximize urine production in combination therapy.

Diuretics may be administered orally or intravenously. The effect is more immediate with IV therapy. The patient is monitored for breath sounds, pulmonary pressure, and peripheral edema to determine his or her response to therapy. Careful laboratory assessment of the blood urea nitrogen and creatinine level is required to monitor for development or worsening of acute renal failure. Ideally, the patient's pulmonary status and fluid balance improve while the glomerular filtration rate remains normal.

Diuretics have both desirable and undesirable effects (see Table 30-5). Overdiuresis is the most common side effect. The nurse must monitor for fluid volume depletion, especially when diuretic regimens are altered or initiated. Signs of volume depletion are discussed in Chapter 29. Other side effects include hyponatremia, hypokalemia, hyperkalemia, hypocalcemia, hypercalcemia, hypomagnesemia, and acid–base disturbances. A reduction in volume from vomiting, third-spacing of fluid, diuretic therapy, or other conditions may have the same consequences. A reduction in the effective circulatory volume can lead to acute renal failure, put increased work on the heart, and result in many metabolic derangements. The most effective management strategy is to replace only that volume required to achieve adequate perfusion. In cases where a delicate balance exists between diuresis and overdiuresis, a pulmonary artery catheter may be inserted to guide therapy. Box 30-10 lists nursing diagnoses for patients taking diuretics.

Hypokalemia is another common side effect of diuretics, particularly the loop and thiazide diuretics. In general, hypokalemia is a benign condition that can be managed effectively with potassium supplementation. If left untreated, patients may experience harmful, sometimes life-threatening, cardiac dysrhythmias.

Vasoactive Drugs

Sometimes the cause of decreased effective circulatory volume is reduced cardiac contractility. This compensation can put an increased burden on the failing heart. In such a case, an inotropic agent (such as dobutamine or milrinone) may be added to the plan of care to improve the forward flow of the heart, thereby improving the effective circulatory volume and stopping the cascade of counterproductive compensatory mechanisms. A failing heart, such as in congestive heart failure, can cause reduced blood flow to the

table 30-5 Diuretic Agents

Drug	Mechanism	Complication(s)	Management and Prevention
Loop diuretics Examples: furosemide (Lasix), ethacrynic acid (Edecrin), bumetanide (Bumex)	Powerful diuretics that act primarily in the thick segment of the medullary and cortical ascending limbs of loop of Henle Cause loss of sodium, chloride, and potassium Increase calcium excretion	Volume depletion	Monitor daily weights, intake and output, signs and symptoms of volume depletion.
		Hypokalemia	Potassium supplements or extra-dietary potassium may be necessary when loop diuretics are used routinely.
		Hyponatremia	
		Hypocalcemia	Monitor calcium levels and administer supplemental calcium as indicated.
		Hypomagnesemia	Usually no intervention is required because body stores of magnesium are quite high.
Thiazides Examples: chlorothiazide (Diuril), hydrochlorothiazide (HCTZ)	Act by inhibiting sodium reabsorption in distal tubule and, to a lesser extent, inner medullary collecting duct Cause loss of sodium, chloride, and potassium Decrease urinary calcium excretion	Hypercalcemia	Monitor calcium levels; loop diuretic may be indicated if calcium levels are persistently elevated.
		Hypokalemia	Potassium supplements or extra-dietary potassium may be necessary when these agents are used routinely.
		Hypomagnesemia	Usually no intervention is required because body stores of magnesium are quite high.
Potassium-sparing diuretics Examples: spironolactone (Aldactone), triamterene (Dyrenium), amiloride (Midamor)	Conserve potassium Spironolactone inhibits action of aldosterone, thereby reducing sodium reabsorption while increasing potassium reabsorption Triamterene acts on distal renal tubule to depress exchange of sodium Effects of amiloride are apparently due to inhibition of sodium entry into cell from luminal fluid	Hyperkalemia	Potassium supplements are contraindicated, as are salt substitutes containing potassium. Often combined with thiazides for effective diuresis; hypokalemic tendency of thiazides may offset hyperkalemic tendency of triamterene and spironolactone.
Carbonic anhydrase inhibitors Example: acetazolamide (Diamox)	Decrease proximal tubular sodium reabsorption Not very effective when administered alone Facilitate excretion of bicarbonate	Metabolic acidosis	Monitor pH and bicarbonate.
Osmotic diuretics Example: Mannitol	Nonreabsorbable polysaccharide that pulls water into vascular space, thereby increasing glomerular flow	Hyperosmolarity	Monitor serum osmolarity. Withhold mannitol therapy if serum osmolarity is >300–305 mMol/L.

Adapted from Metheny NM: Fluid and Electrolyte Balance: Nursing Considerations, p 53. Philadelphia, Lippincott Williams & Wilkins, 2000, with permission.

kidney and potentiate acute renal failure. The same compensatory mechanisms used in volume depletion operate in an attempt to restore renal function. Namely, the renin–angiotensin–aldosterone system is activated to increase sodium and water retention and achieve renal and peripheral vasoconstriction. Other common inotropic agents are described in detail in Chapter 18.

Dopamine is a vasoactive drug at higher doses but can stimulate dopamine receptors in the kidneys when infused at lower doses. Stimulation of dopamine receptors causes renal vasodilation and increase renal blood flow. Although this practice is commonly used to prevent or treat acute renal failure in some settings, several studies[2] have found that there is no improvement in clinical outcome and a lack of sufficient clinical evidence to support its routine use.

DISORDERS OF FLUID VOLUME

Critically ill patients often have imbalances in fluid homeostasis related to their primary underlying disease. Fluid imbalance occurs when there is an excess or deficit of fluid

box 30-10 *Examples of Nursing Diagnoses for the Patient Undergoing Diuretic Therapy*

- Impaired Gas Exchange related to increased pulmonary hydrostatic pressure secondary to congestive heart failure
- Potential for Deficient Fluid Volume related to effect of diuretic therapy
- Risk for Electrolyte Imbalance
- Risk for Cognitive Impairment related to electrolyte imbalance

and may be either absolute or relative. Medications, such as diuretics, put patients at increased risk of fluid imbalance. Infection increases metabolic demand and insensible loss, and fluid volume deficits may develop. Regardless of patient diagnosis, assessment of fluid balance (see Chapter 28) and careful management are mainstays of patient care in the critical care setting.

Fluid Volume Deficit

When fluid loss exceeds intake, a fluid volume deficit exists. A fluid volume deficit is a physiological situation in which fluids are lost in an isotonic fashion (both fluid and electrolytes are lost together). Dehydration is the loss of water alone, resulting in a hyperosmolar state. Although the critically ill patient typically can have both a fluid volume deficit and dehydration states simultaneously, this discussion is limited strictly to disorders of fluid volume deficit.

Several patient populations are particularly vulnerable to development of fluid volume deficits. Young children at prespeech developmental levels cannot communicate thirst; therefore, during times when fluid requirements increase, they do not increase their fluid intake of their own accord. Debilitated patients, such as patients after stroke, may not be able to communicate their needs or have swallowing disturbances and cannot manage their own intake of fluid. Elderly patients are at particular risk of a fluid volume deficit because of the multisystem changes associated with aging. For a review of the changes associated with aging and nursing implications for fluid volume assessment and management, see Table 30-2.

CAUSES

Gastrointestinal Loss

Physiologically, the body produces approximately 5 L of gastrointestinal fluid. In the gastrointestinal tract, fluids help to act as a carrier of important enzymes and buffers to aid in digestion. In the distal small intestine and large intestine, fluid is reabsorbed, leaving only approximately 150 mL lost through the stool daily.

Excess loss from any site from which fluids are ordinarily lost may cause a fluid imbalance. Conditions such as vomiting and diarrhea may cause an increase beyond the typical 150 mL and result in a fluid volume deficit. In addition, surgically placed drainage tubes and nasogastric tubes used for suction may cause such a deficit.

Infection

Infection causes fluid deficits in several ways:

1. Infection can increase metabolic demand, increasing insensible water loss. When patients are not critically ill, they often mitigate this imbalance by increasing fluid intake. When they have widespread infections or a self-care deficit, which may occur in the elderly, fluid intake may not be sufficient to restore fluid balance.
2. Mediators are released as part of the immune response. These mediators cause a loosening of the capillary tight junctions, resulting in the third-spacing of fluids.
3. Carbon dioxide production increases due to increased metabolism. To maintain pH balance, tachypnea may develop. Although only a very small amount of fluid is lost daily through the respiratory tract, water loss may become clinically significant when the respiratory rate is greater than 35 breaths per minute.

Renal Loss

The kidneys filter approximately 180 L per day. However, urine output is only 1% to 2% of total blood volume filtered (see Chapter 28). Reabsorption of fluid is influenced by a complex regulatory system that includes the actions of aldosterone, angiotensin, and antidiuretic hormone (ADH). A defect in any one of the regulatory functions can cause a disruption in renal fluid balance.

Several endocrine disorders may disrupt the renal regulatory system. Adrenal insufficiency, the absence of glucocorticoids and aldosterone, can cause a reduction in the absorption of sodium, thereby promoting water loss. Diabetes insipidus is a profound reduction in ADH, which reduces the amount of fluid reabsorbed at the distal convoluted tubule. Water loss predominates in diabetes insipidus, and therefore volume imbalance is related to dehydration.

Serum osmolarity is predicted by sodium, glucose, and blood urea nitrogen. Normally, glucose does not influence the overall osmolarity. However, in profound hyperglycemia, the influence of glucose increases greatly. Serum osmolarity increases and is sensed by the osmoreceptors, thereby pulling fluids into the vascular space and initiating an osmotic diuresis. Two conditions that pathologically increase glucose are diabetic ketoacidosis (DKA) and hyperglycemic, hyperosmolar, and nonketotic (HHNK) coma. Both of these disorders are discussed in more detail in Chapter 44.

Diuretic therapy is intended to treat fluid volume excess. However, overadministration of diuretics may result in a fluid volume deficit. It is important to recognize the immediate onset that diuretics can have when administered intravenously, initiated for the first time, or adjusted in dosage (see Table 30-5 for more information).

Third-Spacing of Fluid

Third-spacing of fluid is the movement of fluid from the vascular space to the interstitial space. To create a movement of fluid between body compartments, there is an alteration in capillary permeability because of inflammation, ischemia, or injury. Causes of third-spacing of fluids are numerous and include infection; systemic inflammatory response syndrome (SIRS), such as in pancreatitis; hypoalbuminemia, such as in liver failure; burns; intestinal obstruction; and surgery. The amount of fluid lost depends on the degree of the pathophysiological alteration. Regardless of cause, the fluid lost is not functioning to maintain vascular volume, and therefore a fluid volume deficit exists. When fluid leaks out of the vascular space, daily weights can increase, paradoxically, despite intravascular volume depletion.

MANAGEMENT: FLUID VOLUME REPLACEMENT

To correct a fluid volume deficit, it is necessary to treat the underlying cause and replace the lost fluid. The main purposes of fluid administration include replacement of lost fluid, maintenance of fluid balance, and replacement of lost electrolytes. Several types of fluids, which have different physiological effects, are available. Administration of fluids may occur using the gastrointestinal tract or an IV route. When chronic replacement is required, such as in patients with long-term tube feeding, the gastrointestinal approach is used. Enteral access is required when patients are unable to take fluids by mouth. When rapid restoration of fluid balance is required, the IV route is preferred. Occasionally, both routes are used.

Maintenance Fluids

Under normal conditions, the average healthy adult requires about 2.5 L/day. This volume replaces fluids lost through the feces, the respiratory tract, sweating, and the urine. Patients who are unable to consume their usual intake of fluid are often prescribed IV maintenance fluids of 2 to 3 L/day. When determining the rate of administration of maintenance fluid, factors such as medical history (renal failure), age (young or old), confounding water excesses (congestive heart failure), and ongoing assessment parameters (edema formation) must be considered.

Replacement Fluids

Critically ill patients are often unable to consume the additional fluid required to replace the lost fluid. In this case, IV administration beyond baseline maintenance fluids is required for homeostasis. This is achieved by either administering a bolus of fluid or increasing the total daily fluid intake. When fluid loss occurs acutely, the loss must be replaced immediately to maintain tissue perfusion. The type of fluid given depends on the type of fluid lost. When whole blood is lost, such as in trauma or surgery, blood may be administered. When intravascular volume is depleted, such as in diarrhea, isotonic solutions may be administered. The rate of administration depends on the patient's medical history and amount of volume lost.

Crystalloids. Crystalloid solutions are prepared with a specified balance of water and electrolytes. Box 30-11 provides a description of commonly used crystalloid solutions. These fluids are described separately, but they are most commonly used in combination. Fluids are classified as hypotonic (osmolarity <250 mEq/L), isotonic (osmolarity approximately 310 mEq/L), or hypertonic (osmolarity >376 mEq/L).

Dextrose solutions are given to provide free water and some calories to prevent protein catabolism. The 5% solution contains 50 g of dextrose for every liter of fluid and

box 30-11
Common Crystalloid Solutions

5% Dextrose in water (D_5W): no electrolytes, 50 g dextrose
- Supplies about 170 cal/L and free water to aid in renal excretion of solutes
- Should not be used in excessive volumes in patients with increased antidiuretic hormone (ADH) activity or to replace fluids in hypovolemic patients

0.9% NaCl (isotonic saline): Na^+ 154 mEq/L, Cl^- 154 mEq/L
- Isotonic fluid commonly used to expand the extracellular fluid in presence of hypovolemia
- Because of relatively high chloride content, it can be used to treat mild metabolic alkalosis

0.45% NaCl (1/2 strength saline): Na^+ 77 mEq/L, Cl^- 77 mEq/L
- A hypotonic solution that provides sodium, chloride, and free water (sodium and chloride provided in fluid allow kidneys to select and retain needed amounts)
- Free water desirable as aid to kidneys in elimination of solutes

0.33% NaCl (1/3 strength saline): Na^+ 56 mEq/L, Cl^- 56 mEq/L
- A hypotonic solution that provides sodium, chloride, and free water
- Often used to treat hypernatremia (because this solution contains a small amount of sodium, it dilutes the plasma sodium while not allowing the level to drop too rapidly)

3% Saline
- Grossly hypertonic solution used only to treat severe hyponatremia
- Use this solution only in settings where the patient can be closely monitored

Lactated Ringer's solution: Na^+ 130 mEq/L, K^+ 4 mEq/L, Ca^{2+} 3 mEq/L, Cl^- 109 mEq/L, lactate (metabolized to bicarbonate) 28 mEq/L
- Approximately isotonic solution that contains multiple electrolytes in about same concentrations as found in plasma (note that this solution is lacking magnesium and phosphate)
- Used in the treatment of hypovolemia, burns, and fluid lost as bile or diarrhea
- Useful in treating mild metabolic acidosis

Adapted from Metheny NM: Fluid and Electrolyte Balance: Nursing Considerations, p 181. Philadelphia, Lippincott Williams & Wilkins, 2000, with permission.

provides approximately 170 calories per liter. When pure dextrose solutions such as 5% dextrose in water (D_5W) are administered, the dextrose is metabolized, resulting in the administration of free water. When given intravenously, free water decreases the plasma osmolarity, thereby promoting the movement of water evenly into all body compartments. Free water does not stay in the vascular space; therefore, pure dextrose solutions should not be used when intravascular replacement of fluids is required.

Saline solutions are commonly used and are available in different strengths, such as 0.9% and 0.45%. Normal saline, or 0.9% saline, is an isotonic solution. Approximately one fourth of the fluid administered remains in the vascular space, and the remaining fluid moves into the extracellular space 1 hour after administration. During critical illness, the amount that exits into the extracellular space can increase due to increased capillary permeability.

Half-strength saline, in comparison, is a hypotonic solution. Additional free water is administered with this solution, making it an ideal maintenance fluid. Occasionally, half-strength saline is administered to replace fluids lost when there is concurrent hypernatremia.

Saline solutions, such as 3% saline, are hypertonic and may be given for the treatment of symptomatic hyponatremia. The hypertonicity pulls fluid from the extravascular space to the vascular space. Hypertonic solutions should be administered only where patients may be closely monitored because fluid volume excess can develop rapidly. Some studies have shown that hypertonic saline solutions, such as 3% or 7.5% saline, may be beneficial during resuscitation.

Colloids. Colloids are high–molecular-weight substances and therefore do not cross the capillary membrane under normal conditions. Table 30-6 describes commonly prepared colloid solutions.

Albumin is the most abundant circulating protein in the body and accounts for 80% of the colloid oncotic pressure. For therapeutic uses, albumin is prepared from donor plasma. With albumin, there is no risk of bloodborne diseases, such as hepatitis or human immunodeficiency virus (HIV) infection. Albumin is available in two concentrations, 5% and 25%, and both preparations contain some sodium. The 5% solution is similar in osmolarity to plasma. In contrast, the 25% solution is hypertonic, thereby pulling extravascular water into the vascular space. Both preparations of albumin can cause the intravascular volume to expand beyond the volume of albumin infused because of the increased oncotic pressure generated. Care must be taken when administering albumin to patients at high risk of volume overload. Use of albumin should also be limited in patients with profound capillary leak syndrome (e.g., in

table 30-6 **Common Colloid Solutions**

Solution	Contents	Indications	Comments
Albumin	Available in two concentrations: 5%: oncotically similar to plasma 25%: hypertonic Both 5% and 25% solutions contain about 130–160 mEq/L of sodium	Used as volume expander in treatment of shock May be useful in treating burns and third-spacing shifts	Cost is approximately 25–30 times more than for crystalloid solutions. Increased interstitial oncotic pressure in disease states in which there is increased capillary leaking (e.g., burns, sepsis) may occur; this may result in increased vascular space loss of fluid. Use caution with rapid administration; watch for volume overload.
Hetastarch	Synthetic colloid made from starch (6%) and added to sodium chloride solution	May be used to expand plasma volume when volume is lost from hemorrhage, trauma, burns, and sepsis	Plasma volume expansion effects decrease over 24–36 h. Starch is eliminated by kidneys and liver; therefore, use caution in patients with liver and kidney impairment. Mild, transient coagulopathies may occur. Transient rise in serum amylase may occur.
Dextran	Glucose polysaccharide substance, available as low–molecular-weight dextran (dextran 40) or high–molecular-weight dextran (dextran 70) No electrolyte content	May be used to expand plasma volume when volume is lost from hemorrhage, trauma, burns, and sepsis	Has been associated with greater risk of allergic reaction than albumin or hetastarch. Interference with blood cross-matching may occur. May cause coagulopathy; has more profound effect on coagulation than hetastarch.

sepsis, acute respiratory distress syndrome, and pancreatitis[3]). Although albumin is a protein, it is inefficient and expensive when used for malnutrition.

The starches dextran and hetastarch, which differ from each other only slightly, have an oncotic pressure similar to albumin. Both substances are used to expand plasma volume by exerting an oncotic pressure and thereby pulling water from the extravascular space to the vascular space. Hetastarch is metabolized by both the kidneys and liver. The diuresis that may occur with hetastarch is an osmotic diuresis and does not reflect an increase in effective renal circulatory volume. Both dextran and hetastarch may cause coagulopathies; however, dextran has a more profound effect on coagulation.

Fluid Volume Excess

Fluid volume excess occurs when there is the retention of sodium, resulting in the reabsorption of water. Electrolytes typically remain unchanged when there is an increase in total body water and electrolytes increase in parallel. Many critically ill patients may have mixed disturbances with manifestations of the confounding compensatory mechanisms. Causes of fluid volume excess include overadministration of fluids, edematous disorder (e.g., congestive heart failure, kidney or liver failure), excessive sodium intake, and medications (e.g., steroids, desmopressin acetate).

When the kidneys are functioning normally and regulating fluid balance, the body typically rids itself of excess fluid and fluid overload is not manifested clinically. When the kidneys sense a decrease in effective circulatory volume, the compensatory mechanisms prevent the excretion of excess water, such as in congestive heart failure.

Management of fluid volume excess is directed toward correction of the underlying disorder. If this is not feasible, efforts are geared to prevention of pulmonary compromise by attempting to rid the body of the excess sodium and water. In cases of volume overload, there is an increase in pulmonary hydrostatic pressure, which promotes movement of water into the alveoli, thereby impeding gas exchange. Sodium restriction reduces the amount of water reabsorption but does contribute to acute correction of volume overload. Diuretics are the mainstay of treatment for acute resolution of fluid volume excess (see Table 30-5).

MANAGEMENT OF ELECTROLYTE IMBALANCES

Electrolyte disorders commonly occur in critically ill patients, typically in combination with other conditions. Management of the underlying problem ensures long-term restoration of balance. However, acute management of electrolyte disorders is often required to maintain cellular integrity.

Sodium

Sodium is the major extracellular cation. It is a major predictor of serum osmolarity and controls movement of water. Disorders of sodium are typically associated with water disorders (Table 30-7).

Hyponatremia may be associated with volume excess, such as in edematous disorders (e.g., heart, kidney, or liver failure), or with volume deficit, such as when volume loss is exceeded by sodium loss (e.g., in gastrointestinal fluid, diuretic overuse, or adrenal insufficiency). Low sodium with euvolemia is manifested as the syndrome of inappropriate ADH secretion (SIADH; see Chapter 44). Pseudohyponatremia may occur in association with hyperlipidemia and hypoproteinemia; the total body sodium remains unchanged, but the actual sodium measurement is altered.

Management of hyponatremia is aimed at correcting the underlying cause (see Table 30-7). When the hyponatremia is associated with hypervolemia, diuretics may be beneficial. When the disorder is associated with euvolemia, such as in SIADH, water restriction may be useful. In conditions in which there is both sodium loss and water loss, administration of hypertonic saline at slow rates may help improve clinically significant hyponatremia.

Hypernatremia may occur as an isolated condition when there is a loss of free water, which raises the sodium level. Increased insensible loss of fluid, such as occurs in sweating, hyperventilation, or fever, is the most common cause of this type of hypernatremia. The fluid volume deficit associated with the hypernatremia depends almost entirely on the degree of insensible loss. Endocrine disorders, such as hyperaldosteronism, or Cushing's disease, can result in hypernatremia and are associated with total body water excess. Administration of hypertonic fluids, such as sodium bicarbonate, 3% saline, or albumin, may also cause hypernatremia.

Management of hypernatremia is primarily aimed at restoring fluid balance (see Table 30-7). Correcting the underlying cause of the increased sodium is also important.

Potassium

Potassium is the major intracellular ion. Potassium plays a key role in neuromuscular functioning, and high or low levels may result in alterations in the cardiac rhythm. Because of the narrow range of extracellular potassium balance, renal function is essential to regulation of potassium. In critically ill patients, disorders of potassium are common and have numerous causes (see Table 30-7).

Hypokalemia is most commonly caused by an absolute deficiency in potassium. Losses of potassium occur through the kidneys, gastrointestinal tract, sweat, and intracellular shifting. Although relative deficiencies may occur, such as in metabolic alkalosis, they are rare compared with the absolute deficits. Management of hypokalemia involves replacement of depleted potassium to restore potassium balance. It may be necessary to check the magnesium level in patients who do not respond to potassium replacement. Box 30-12 presents nursing considerations in potassium replacement.

Hyperkalemia is caused by reduced renal excretion, excessive administration of potassium replacements, transcellular shifts, and measurement error. Patients with renal failure are at particular risk. Dialysis is typically used to manage hyperkalemia in patients with ESRD. Noncompliance with dialysis can certainly cause hyperkalemia and is a frequent reason for hospital admission. Potassium replacement therapy, although performed frequently in

table 30-7 Management of Electrolyte Disorders

Electrolyte	Selected Medical Conditions Associated With Disturbance	Collaborative Interventions
Sodium		
Hyponatremia	Congestive heart failure Liver failure Kidney failure Hyperlipidemia Hypoproteinemia SIADH GI Loss Adrenal insufficiency Thiazide diuretics Drugs: NSAIDs, tricyclic antidepressants, SSRIs, chlorpropamide, omeprazole Tumors associated with ectopic excessive ADH production: oat cell carcinoma, leukemia, lymphoma Pulmonary disorders: pneumonia, acute asthma AIDS	Review medication profile and patient history. Monitor for sites of fluid losses or gains. Monitor fluid balances and for signs and symptoms of electrolyte disturbance. Attempt to manage underlying cause. Correction of electrolyte may require sodium replacement (3% saline) or water restriction, depending on etiology of disorder.
Hypernatremia	Profound dehydration usually in patients not able to ask for water (i.e., debilitated elderly or children), in those with impaired thirst regulation (i.e., elderly), or in those with heatstroke Hypertonic tube feedings without water supplementation	Assess in patients at particular risk of hypernatremia, including debilitated or elderly patients, acutely or critically ill children, and patients receiving tube feedings.
	Increased insensible water loss (i.e., excessive sweating, second- and third-degree burns, hyperventilation) Excessive administration of sodium-containing fluids (3% saline, sodium bicarbonate)	Monitor laboratory values closely in patients with insensible fluid losses and in those receiving parenteral administration of sodium-containing fluids.
	Diabetes insipidus	For comprehensive review of management of diabetes insipidus, see Chapter 44. Administer therapeutic medications, including vasopressin, DDAVP. Administer hypotonic fluids (½ saline to free water, D_5W).
Potassium		
Hypokalemia	GI loss: diarrhea, laxatives, gastric suction Renal loss: potassium-losing diuretics, hyperaldosteronism, osmotic diuresis, steroids, some antibiotics Intracellular shifts: alkalosis, excessive secretion or administration of insulin, hyperalimentation Poor intake: anorexia nervosa, alcoholism, debilitation	Monitor laboratory values closely in patients at particular risk of hypokalemia. Pay particular attention to potassium level in patients receiving digoxin. Administer potassium either PO or IV (see Box 30-12). Monitor magnesium levels in patients who are refractory to potassium replacement.
Hyperkalemia	Pseudohyperkalemia: prolonged tight application of tourniquet; fist clenching and unclenching immediately before or during blood draws, hemolysis of blood sample Decreased potassium excretion: oliguric renal failure, potassium-sparing diuretics, hypoaldosteronism High potassium intake: improper use of oral potassium supplements; rapid IV potassium administration Extracellular shifts: acidosis, crush injuries, tumor cell lysis after chemotherapy	Ensure that minimal negative pressure is used to obtain all laboratory samples, particularly when drawn through small-gauge needles. Restrict potassium-sparing diuretics. Promote excretion: sodium polystyrene sulfonate PO or per rectum, dialysis, potassium-losing diuretics (e.g., furosemide) Emergency management measures: calcium IV, sodium bicarbonate, IV insulin with glucose, $beta_2$-adrenergic agonists
Calcium		
Hypocalcemia	Surgical hypoparathyroidism Primary hypoparathyroidism Malabsorption (alcoholism) Acute pancreatitis	Monitor for signs and symptoms associated with low calcium, especially for seizures, and stridor. Administer calcium IV for acute replacement (See Box 30-12).

(continued)

table 30-7 Management of Electrolyte Disorders (Continued)

Electrolyte	Selected Medical Conditions Associated With Disturbance	Collaborative Interventions
	Excessive administration of citrated blood Alkalotic states Drugs (loop diuretics, mithramycin, calcitonin) Hyperphosphatemia Sepsis Hypomagnesemia Medullary carcinoma of thyroid Hypoalbuminemia	Ensure adequate dietary intake for patients at particular risk.
Hypercalcemia	Hyperparathyroidism Malignant neoplastic disease Drugs (thiazide diuretics, lithium, theophylline) Prolonged immobilization Dehydration	Administer bisphosphonates, such as etidronate or mithramycin, especially when disorder is related to malignancy. Administer diuretics, such as loop diuretics, to promote renal excretion. Provide fluid replacement with 0.9% saline.
Magnesium		
Hypomagnesemia	Inadequate intake: starvation, total parenteral nutrition without adequate Mg^{2+} supplementation, chronic alcoholism Increased GI loss: diarrhea, laxatives, fistulas, nasogastric tube suction, vomiting Increased renal loss: drugs (loop and thiazide diuretics, mannitol, amphotericin B), diuresis (uncontrolled diabetes mellitus, hypoaldosteronism) Changes in magnesium distribution: pancreatitis, burns, insulin, blood products	Monitor for hypokalemia in patients with low magnesium because kidneys are not able to conserve potassium when magnesium level is low. Administer magnesium IV for acute replacement (see Box 30-12). Administer PO preparations for long-term replacement.
Hypermagnesemia	Renal failure Excessive intake of magnesium-containing compounds (e.g., antacids, mineral supplements, laxatives)	Avoid administration of magnesium-containing compounds to patients in renal failure. In extreme cases, dialysis may be indicated.
Phosphorus		
Hypophosphatemia	Refeeding syndrome Alcoholism Phosphate-binding antacids Respiratory alkalosis Administration of exogenous insulin IV Burns	Ensure nutritional intake. Monitor phosphorus for the few days after initiation of enteral or parenteral nutrition. Administer by oral supplementation (Neutra-Phos capsules) or IV (see Box 30-12).
Hyperphosphatemia	Renal failure Chemotherapy Excessive administration of phosphate compounds	Prevention is mainstay of therapy; avoid administration of phosphorus to patients in renal failure. Administer calcium acetate. Administer IV fluids to promote renal excretion. In severe cases, administration of high levels of glucose with insulin may help shift phosphorus intracellularly.

AIDS, acquired immunodeficiency syndrome; DDAVP, desmopressin acetate; GI, gastrointestinal; NSAID, nonsteroidal anti-inflammatory drug; SSRI, selective serotonin reuptake inhibitor.

critical care settings, must be performed carefully; particular attention should be paid to cardiac signs and laboratory reassessments. Acidosis of any cause can potentiate hyperkalemia; therefore, patients who are acidotic must be carefully monitored for potassium shifts.

The primary goal of management is resolution of the acidosis. However, clinically significant hyperkalemia must be resolved using the measures described in Table 30-7. Temporizing measures for hyperkalemia center on stabilization of cell membrane (calcium) and shifting potassium from the extracellular to the intracellular spaces (bicarbonate, insulin). These measures resolve the potassium imbalance temporarily and give clinicians time to address the underlying problem. If it is anticipated that correction of this problem will take some time, the excretion of potassium is facilitated by administering sodium polystyrene, dialysis, and diuretics. Drawing laboratory samples can cause hemolysis of cells, which causes

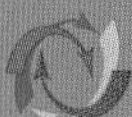

box 30-12 nursing interventions for *Intravenous Electrolyte Replacement*

Potassium

Dilution

- Do not administer undiluted potassium directly IV.
- Keep all vials of undiluted potassium away from patient care area.
- Dilution of potassium depends on the amount of fluid the patient can tolerate. Highly concentrated potassium solutions can cause irritation, pain, and sclerosing of vein.
- Typical concentrations of potassium are 10–40 mEq/100 mL. Premixed bags are available.

Peripheral IV Administration

- In collaboration with prescribing provider, consider the addition of small volume of lidocaine to minimize pain.
- Administer in central vein if available.
- For mild to moderate hypokalemia, rates of 10–20 mEq/h are recommended.
- Rates >40 mEq/h are not recommended.
- Use infusion pump to administer replacement.

Monitoring

- Monitor urinary output, blood urea nitrogen, and creatinine in patients receiving potassium replacement. Patients with impaired renal function or oliguric renal failure may experience transient hyperkalemia. Consider smaller replacement dosages and periodic reevaluation.
- When rate of administration exceeds 10 mEq/h, monitoring of cardiac rhythm is recommended.
- Assess magnesium level because correction of potassium may be refractory to potassium replacement with concurrent hypomagnesemia.

Calcium

Dilution

- Calcium can be delivered as calcium gluconate (4.5 mEq of elemental Ca^{2+}) or calcium chloride (13.5 mEq of elemental Ca^{2+}).
- Calcium can be irritating to veins. If peripheral administration is required, calcium gluconate is recommended because damage can occur to surrounding soft tissues.

Administration

- Administer by slow IV push through central vein or administer by mixing with compatible IV fluids.
- Administer slowly (over 1–2 h) for patients receiving digoxin.

Magnesium

Administration

- Administer with caution to patients with renal failure because magnesium is primarily excreted by the kidneys.
- During emergencies, such as torsades de pointes, magnesium may be injected directly.
- In mild to moderate hypomagnesemia, a rate of infusion of 1–2 g over 1 h is advisable.

Monitoring

- Monitor for hypotension or flushing during administration.
- Monitor deep tendon reflexes periodically during administration.

Phosphorus

- Phosphorus IV replacement is available as sodium or potassium phosphate. Note that phosphorus is dosed in millimoles, whereas sodium and potassium are dosed in milliequivalents.
- Administer sodium phosphate for patients with renal failure.
- Do not administer with calcium.
- Administer over several hours, typically 15–30 mmol phosphorus over 4–6 h.

liberation of the abundant intracellular potassium. Evaluating trends and assessing the overall clinical picture prevents unnecessary treatment and therefore prevents hypokalemia.

Calcium

Almost all of the calcium in the body is contained in the bone, and the remaining 1% is either bound to albumin (50% plasma calcium) or in an ionized form. The primary function of calcium is promotion of the neuromuscular impulse. Several clotting factors also depend on calcium.

Hypocalcemia has numerous causes (see Table 30-7). Most hypocalcemia is a relative deficiency; causes include intracellular shifting, decreased circulating protein, and binding with fatty acids (pancreatitis). The relative hypocalcemia that occurs with a massive transfusion of blood is common in the critical care setting. The blood is mixed with citrate to prevent coagulation; when the blood is infused, the citrate binds to calcium, causing a relative calcium deficiency. Trisodium citrate used for anticoagulation in CRRT also results in hypocalcemia.[1] Other causes of hypocalcemia include increased renal excretion (loop diuretics) or decreased absorption (malabsorption syndromes).

Calcium is transported in its ionized form, provides some of the structural components in bone, and is also bound to albumin. A low albumin level can therefore be one cause of a low calcium level. The calcium level should be corrected for the low albumin before consideration of calcium replacement. Replacement of calcium is required to prevent complications of bleeding and decreased impulse transmission. For a review of nursing considerations in calcium replacement, see Box 30-12.

Hypercalcemia, which is less common in the critical care setting, is most often caused by malignancy. Treatment is supportive and involves administration of diuretics and IV fluids, sometimes simultaneously.

Magnesium

About two thirds of the magnesium in the body is in the skeletal system, and the remaining one third is in the intracellular space. About 1% circulates in the extracellular space. Magnesium is a catalyst for hundreds of enzymatic reactions and plays a role in neurotransmission and cardiac contraction. Magnesium is primarily excreted by the kidneys.

Hypomagnesemia is caused by loss of magnesium through the gastrointestinal tract or (less commonly) the kidneys. Alcoholism is a significant cause. The etiological mechanism is not completely understood, but it is thought that decreased dietary intake due to malnutrition, decreased absorption, and increased gastrointestinal losses (due to periodic emesis) all play a role. Several drugs may also cause hypomagnesemia, including loop diuretics, aminoglycosides, amphotericin B, *cis*-platinum, cyclosporine, and citrate. For a review of the causes of hypomagnesemia, see Table 30-7.

Magnesium is available in a variety of preparations, including 50%, 20%, or 10% solutions. It is important to pay particular attention to how the replacement preparation is ordered; the replacement solution should be "dosed" in grams instead of milliliters. For a review of nursing considerations in magnesium replacement, see Box 30-12.

Phosphorus

Phosphorus is the major intracellular anion. The source of adenosine triphosphate (ATP), phosphorus is implicated in many life-sustaining processes, such as muscle contraction, neuromuscular impulse conduction, and the regulation of several intracellular and extracellular electrolyte balances.

Hypophosphatemia may be caused by several metabolic disorders, including refeeding syndrome and alcoholism, intracellular shifting due to respiratory alkalosis, binding by medications, such as phosphate-binding magnesium-containing antacids, and excessive excretion of phosphate, such as in diabetic ketoacidosis (see Table 30-7). Refeeding syndrome occurs when the patient is fed, either enterally or parenterally, after some time of starvation. During starvation, protein catabolism occurs, depleting all of the intracellular phosphorus. When a large glucose load is administered, as occurs with refeeding, it is thought that the insulin response shifts the phosphorus intracellularly.

Management of hypophosphatemia may be problematic, particularly for patients on a mechanical ventilator. Contraction of all muscles, including the diaphragm, depends on ATP. Replacement of phosphorus is indicated in critically ill patients to achieve adequate pulmonary function. Once the critical illness abates, the hypophosphatemia typically resolves as well. However, replacement with either sodium or potassium phosphate is indicated in the meantime. For a review of nursing considerations in phosphorus replacement, see Box 30-12.

Hyperphosphatemia is commonly associated with renal failure due to reduced elimination of phosphorus. Because of the inverse relationship with calcium, the high phosphorus may also be associated with hypocalcemia. Administration of phosphate binders and calcium supplementation are indicated.

clinical applicability challenges

Self-Challenge: Critical Thinking

1. *Keeping track of fluid balance during a continuous venovenous hemofiltration with dialysis (CVVH/D) treatment is difficult unless you can organize the data so they are easily accessible. Start with an hourly fluid loss goal. Remember that you must account for hourly intake (including dialysate, any intravenous lines, any flushes, oral intake, blood products, and replacement fluid) and hourly output (including ultrafiltrate and dialysate, any urine output, gastric drainage) to calculate the next hour's replacement fluid. Devise a flow sheet that lets you keep track of fluid balance at a glance.*
2. *You are caring for a male patient, and his renal function is not recovering. He must continue dialysis after discharge from the hospital. He has diabetes mellitus but has good eyesight and dexterity, and he has a supportive family. There are plenty of outpatient dialysis units in the area. Develop a teaching plan that explores the different forms of chronic dialysis to help your patient decide which one is best for him.*
3. *Your hospital is setting up a program to perform continuous venovenous hemofiltration with dialysis (CVVH/D). You are asked to help develop a protocol in collaboration with the acute care dialysis nurses. To prepare for the meeting, outline responsibilities for equipment setup and patient teaching.*
4. *D.F. is a 65-year-old man with a history of diabetes and hypertension. A year ago he began experiencing some shortness of breath and was found to have congestive heart failure. He has been treated with the following medications: furosemide 20 mg orally (PO) once a day; KCl 20 mEq PO once a day; metformin 500 mg PO twice daily; enalapril 10 mg PO once a day; and metoprolol 25 mg PO twice daily. His shortness of breath has worsened over the last two days. He was seen in the clinic and was admitted for evaluation. Admission data are as follows: temperature 36.3°C; pulse 120 beats/minute; blood pressure 87/50 mm Hg; respiratory rate 18 breaths/minute; oxygen saturation by pulse oximetry (Spo_2): 94% (on 50% fraction of inspired oxygen [Fio_2]). Laboratory test results include: Na^+: 130 mEq/L; K^+: 3.5 mEq/L; Cl^-: 100 mEq/L; carbon dioxide: 18 mMol/L; blood urea nitrogen: 45 mg/dL; creatinine: 2.3 mg/dL; glucose: 162 mg/dL. Explain the pathophysiological basis of D.F.'s symptoms.*
   - *What are D.F.'s risk factors for developing renal insufficiency?*
   - *What additional laboratory tests might you anticipate to be ordered to evaluate D.F.'s renal function?*
   - *What are some of the nursing care priorities for this patient? What treatments could you anticipate for this patient?*

   D.F. is recommended to undergo a cardiac catheterization to rule out an ischemic component to his heart failure.

   - *Describe additional risk factors D.F. has for undergoing a cardiac catheterization.*
   - *What medications may interfere with the cardiac catheterization?*

- *What are some interventions that may be initiated to reduce the risk factors?*

Study Questions

1. *Which statement about hemodialysis is not true?*
   a. *Hemodialysis rapidly removes metabolic wastes and excess fluid.*
   b. *Heparin is always needed to keep the blood from clotting in the system.*
   c. *Hemodialysis removes excess body water by effecting a pressure differential between the blood and fluid compartments.*
   d. *Hemodialysis can restore a physiological level of electrolytes.*
2. *When a continuous venovenous hemofiltration with dialysis (CVVH/D) filter and lines begin to turn dark, ultrafiltration diminishes, and venous pressure rises, what does the nurse do?*
   a. *Calls the dialysis nurse immediately to change the circuit.*
   b. *Checks the patient's blood pressure and oxygen saturation.*
   c. *Administers a saline bolus to inspect the circuit for clotting.*
   d. *Immediately gives the patient more heparin because he is probably clotting.*
3. *You are performing a peritoneal dialysis exchange and notice that the drained fluid is cloudy. What do you do?*
   a. *Obtain a sample of the drained fluid, send it to the laboratory for culture and sensitivity and cell count, and obtain an order for an antibiotic.*
   b. *Wait until the next exchange to see if it clears up.*
   c. *Send a sample of the drained fluid for urea nitrogen, creatinine, and electrolytes.*
   d. *Do nothing because the fluid usually becomes clear spontaneously.*
4. *Which of the following formulas most accurately calculates hourly fluid balance for patients on continuous renal replacement therapy (CRRT)?*
   a. *Fluid balance = total negative balance + total positive balance + replacement fluid*
   b. *Fluid replacement = total planned daily balance divided by 24 (hours)*
   c. *Fluid replacement = insensible losses – total fluid balance + 100 (mL)*
   d. *Fluid Replacement = total fluid out – total fluid in ± desired hourly balance*
5. *Which of the following fluid therapies is the best choice for restoration of fluid balance for a patient with pancreatitis?*
   a. D_5 *1/2 NS*
   b. *3% NaCl*
   c. D_5 *NS*
   d. *5% Albumin*
6. *Administration of hetastarch may cause all of the following except*
   a. *coagulopathies.*
   b. *difficulties with future blood cross-matching.*
   c. *volume overload.*
   d. *an increase in amylose.*
7. *Initial intervention for the management of hyperkalemic emergencies includes*
   a. *sodium polystyrene.*
   b. *intravenous calcium.*
   c. *intravenous fluid bolus.*
   d. *12-lead electrocardiogram.*
8. *Correction of the potassium for hypokalemia is closely related to balance of which one of the following electrolytes?*
   a. *Sodium*
   b. *Magnesium*
   c. *Calcium*
   d. *Albumin*

REFERENCES

1. Barbour C, Devenish L, Locke J, et al: Regional anticoagulation using anticoagulant citrate dextrose solution in conjunction with commercially prepared dialysate solutions containing calcium in continuous venovenous hemodiafiltration. Blood Purif 17:19–49, 1999
2. Kellum JA, Decker JM: Use of dopamine in acute renal failure: A meta-analysis. Crit Care Med 29(8):1526–1531, 2001
3. Cook D, Guyatt G: Colloid use for fluid resuscitation: Evidence and spin. Ann Intern Med 135:205–208, 2001

OTHER SELECTED READING

Bellomo R, Baldwin I, Ronco C, et al (eds): Atlas of Hemofiltration. Philadelphia, WB Saunders, 2001

Daugirdis J: Acute hemodialysis prescription. In Daugirdis J, Ing T (eds): Handbook of Dialysis (3rd Ed). Boston, Little, Brown, 2000

Gokal R, Nolf K, Fredief RT, et al (eds): The Textbook of Peritoneal Dialysis. Boston, Kluwer Academic Publishers, 2000

Gray RJ, Sands JJ (eds): Dialysis Access: A Multidisciplinary Approach. Philadelphia, Lippincott Williams & Wilkins, 2002

Gutch L, Stoner M, Corea A (eds): Review of Hemodialysis for Nurses and Dialysis Personnel (6th Ed). St. Louis, Mosby-Year Book, 1999

Metheny N (ed): Fluid and Electrolyte Balance: Nursing Considerations (4th Ed). Philadelphia, Lippincott Williams & Wilkins, 2000

Pestans C: Fluids and Electrolytes in the Surgical Patient (5th Ed). Philadelphia, Lippincott Williams & Wilkins, 2000

Schrier RW: Renal and Electrolyte Disorders (6th Ed). Philadelphia, Lippincott Williams & Wilkins, 2003

chapter 31

Renal Failure

DORENE HOLCOMBE ■ NANCY KERN FEELEY

objectives

Based on the content in this chapter, the reader should be able to:

- Explain the causes of acute renal failure.
- Describe urine production during the nonoliguric, oliguric, and diuretic phases of acute tubular necrosis (ATN).
- Differentiate between the three types of acute renal failure based on history and physical examination, laboratory values, and diagnostic tests.
- Identify the main etiologies and clinical stages of chronic renal failure.
- Identify factors that can contribute to the progression of chronic renal failure.
- Discuss the clinical manifestations and management of renal failure.
- Develop a collaborative care plan for managing acute renal failure resulting from cardiogenic shock.

ACUTE RENAL FAILURE

Acute renal failure occurs in 5% of hospitalized patients and accounts for as much as 20% of the patients treated in intensive care units (ICUs).[1,2] In hospitalized patients with acute renal failure, the mortality rate exceeds 40% to 50%; in ICU patients who have multisystem organ failure and require dialysis, the mortality rate increases to 70% to 80%.[1,3] These discouraging mortality rates have not changed in the last three decades despite advances in technology and dialysis. However, the demographics of patients have changed over the last few decades, with patients in general being older and having an increased number of comorbid conditions.[2,3] On a more optimistic note, the ability to recover normal renal function in patients who survive acute renal failure is in excess of 45%.[1,4]

Acute renal failure is a clinical syndrome in which there is a sudden loss of renal function (i.e., occurring over hours to a few days) that results in derangements in fluid and electrolyte balance, acid–base homeostasis, calcium/phosphate metabolism, blood pressure regulation, and erythropoiesis. The hallmark of acute renal failure is a decreased glomerular filtration rate (GFR), reflected by an accumulation of blood urea nitrogen (BUN) and serum creatinine—a condition termed *azotemia.* Serum creatinine is the better marker because increases in serum creatinine are relatively unaffected by nonrenal mechanisms. Changes in serum creatinine levels that suggest acute renal failure include:

- An increase of 0.5 mg/dL or a doubling of creatinine from baseline in patients with a baseline creatinine level of less than 2 mg/dL
- An increase of 1 mg/dL in patients with a baseline creatinine level greater than 2 mg/dL
- A decrease in measured creatinine clearance of more than 25%[1]

Urine output patterns in acute renal failure can manifest as oliguria (<400 mL/day), nonoliguria (>400 mL/day), or anuria (<50 mL/day). Categorization of acute renal failure as oliguric or nonoliguric is diagnostically significant because the oliguric form is associated with higher morbidity and mortality rates. Anuria is rare and suggests obstructive uropathy, a vascular catastrophe resulting in a cessation of renal perfusion, or acute cortical necrosis.[1] Any sudden and complete cessation of urinary flow in a patient with a Foley catheter should alert the nurse to inspect, flush, or change the urinary catheter.

Causes of Acute Renal Failure

There are over 50 identified pathophysiological pathways that lead to the syndrome of acute renal failure.[1] To aid in the establishment of a diagnostic and management plan, acute renal failure is organized into three general categories according to precipitating factors and the symptoms manifested (Box 31-1).

PRERENAL ACUTE RENAL FAILURE

Prerenal acute renal failure accounts for 60% to 70% of cases.[3] It is characterized by any physiological event that results in renal hypoperfusion. Most commonly, precipitating events include hypovolemia and cardiovascular failure; however, any other event that leads to an acute decrease in "effective renal perfusion" can fall into this category (see Box 31-1). For example, in sepsis, a systemic inflammatory response triggers a cascade of events that results in a vasodilated hypotensive state despite no net loss in body fluids.

INTRARENAL ACUTE RENAL FAILURE

The intrarenal category of acute renal failure is characterized by actual damage to the renal parenchyma and accounts for 25% to 40% of cases.[3] Intrarenal acute renal failure has many possible causes. One way to help categorize these causes is by anatomical compartment: glomerular, vascular, interstitial, and tubular. The glomerular etiologies, which result in acute glomerulonephritis, include immune complex–mediated causes (e.g., as seen with poststreptococcal glomerulonephritis), and include diseases that cause vasculitis, such as Wegener's granulomatosis and antiglomerular basement membrane disease. Interstitial causes include acute allergic interstitial nephritis, usually caused by pharmacological agents, and infectious causes like pyelonephritis. Vascular etiologies include acute renal artery or vein occlusion, malignant hypertension, and microangiopathic processes like atheroembolic disease or hemolytic–uremic syndrome (HUS) and thrombotic thrombocytopenic purpura (TTP). Finally, the tubules of the kidney can be primarily affected because of obstruction or acute tubular necrosis (ATN). Obstructive causes include multiple myeloma and heme pigments (e.g., myoglobin in rhabdomyolysis and hemoglobin in massive hemolysis).

By far the most common cause of intrarenal hospital-acquired acute renal failure is ATN.[1] ATN is caused by either a prolonged prerenal condition (ischemic ATN) or by the effects of toxins on the tubules (toxic ATN). Examples of potential toxins to the tubules include pharmacological agents, such as aminoglycosides, amphotericin B, and chemotherapeutic agents; heavy metals; organic solvents; and radiocontrast dye (Box 31-2).

POSTRENAL ACUTE RENAL FAILURE

Postrenal acute renal failure accounts for 5% to 10% of the cases of ARF.[3] Any obstruction in the flow of urine from the collecting ducts in the kidney to the external urethral orifice can result in postrenal acute renal failure. Postrenal obstruction can result from ureteral blockage (as with bilateral renal stones), urethral blockage (as from stricture and benign prostatic hypertrophy), or from an extrinsic source such as a retroperitoneal tumor or fibrosis. Another source of postrenal acute renal failure is a dysfunctional bladder (e.g., as might be caused by ganglionic blocking agents that interrupt autonomic supply to the urinary system). Elderly men and the young are the groups most commonly affected with postrenal acute renal failure.[1] Children are at risk secondary to congenital anomalies and elderly men are at risk because of the high prevalence of benign or malignant prostatic hypertrophy.

Pathophysiology of Acute Renal Failure

PRERENAL ACUTE RENAL FAILURE

The pathophysiology of prerenal acute renal failure is centered on the kidneys' response to inadequate perfusion. A decrease in renal perfusion results in the release

box 31-1
Precipitating Causes of Acute Renal Failure

Prerenal

Decreased intravascular volume
- Dehydration
- Hemorrhage
- Hypovolemic shock
- Hypovolemia (gastrointestinal losses, diuretics, diabetes insipidus)
- Third-spacing (burns, peritonitis)

Cardiovascular failure
- Heart failure
- Myocardial infarction
- Cardiogenic shock
- Valvular heart disease

Renal artery stenosis or thrombosis

Drugs
- Angiotensin-converting enzyme (ACE) inhibitors
- Nonsteroidal anti-inflammatory drugs (NSAIDs)—inhibit prostaglandin-mediated afferent arteriolar vasodilation
- Calcineurin inhibitors (e.g., tacrolimus, cyclosporine)—cause preglomerular vasoconstriction

Decreased "effective renal perfusion"
- Sepsis
- Cirrhosis
- Neurogenic shock

Intrarenal

Acute glomerulonephritis
- Immune complex–mediated (postinfectious, lupus nephritis, cryoglobulinemia, immunoglobulin A [IgA] nephropathy)
- With vasculitis (Wegener's granulomatosis, antiglomerular basement membrane disease, polyarteritis nodosa)

Vascular disease
- Malignant hypertension
- Microangiopathic hemolytic–uremic syndrome (HUS)
- Thrombotic thrombocytopenic purpura (TTP)
- Scleroderma
- Eclampsia
- Atheroembolic disease
- Acute cortical necrosis

Acute interstitial disease
- Allergic interstitial nephritis
- Acute pyelonephritis

Tubular obstruction
- Multiple myeloma
- Heme pigments (rhabdomyolysis, massive hemolysis)
- Acute urate nephropathy
- Ethylene glycol or methanol toxicity

Acute tubular necrosis (ATN)
- Ischemia
- Nephrotoxins
- Kidney transplant rejection

Postrenal

Ureteral obstruction
- Intrinsic (stones, transitional cell carcinoma of the ureter, blood clots, stricture)
- Extrinsic (ovarian cancer; lymphoma; metastatic cancer of the prostate, cervix, or colon; retroperitoneal fibrosis)

Bladder problems
- Tumors
- Blood clots
- Neurogenic bladder (spinal cord injury, diabetes mellitus, ischemia, drugs)
- Stones

Urethral obstruction
- Prostate cancer or benign prostatic hypertrophy
- Stones
- Stricture
- Blood clots

of the enzyme renin from juxtaglomerular cells in the walls of the afferent arterioles. This activates the renin–angiotensin–aldosterone cascade, the end result being the production of angiotensin II and the release of aldosterone from the adrenal cortex. Angiotensin II causes profound systemic vasoconstriction, and aldosterone induces sodium and water retention. These effects help the body preserve circulatory volume so as to maintain adequate blood flow to essential organs like the heart and brain. In the kidneys, angiotensin II also helps maintain the GFR by increasing efferent arteriolar resistance and by stimulating intrarenal vasodilator prostaglandins (which dilate the afferent arteriole), increasing hydrostatic pressure in the glomeruli.[2] In this way, the kidneys can preserve the GFR over a wide range of mean arterial pressures. However, when renal perfusion is severely compromised, the capacity for autoregulation is overwhelmed and the GFR falls.

It is of clinical importance that even with moderate hypovolemia or congestive heart failure, certain drugs, like angiotensin-converting enzyme (ACE) inhibitors and nonsteroidal anti-inflammatory drugs (NSAIDs), can overwhelm the kidney's ability to autoregulate. This is because these drugs disrupt some of the autoregulatory mechanisms like prostaglandin-mediated afferent arterial vasodilation, in the case of NSAIDs, and increased efferent arteriolar resistance, in the case of ACE inhibitors. Predisposing factors for NSAID- and ACE inhibitor–induced prerenal failure are hypovolemia, baseline renal insufficiency, liver disease, heart failure, and diseases of the renal arteries.[1]

In prerenal acute renal failure, once autoregulatory capacity is overwhelmed and the GFR decreases, changes in urinary composition and volume occur in a predictable pattern. When the GFR decreases, the amount of tubular fluid is reduced, and the fluid travels through the tubule more slowly. This results in increased sodium and water reabsorption. Because of the reduced renal circulation, the solutes reabsorbed from the tubular fluid are removed more slowly than normal from the interstitium of the renal medulla. This results in increased medullary tonicity, further augmenting water reabsorption from the distal

box 31-2
Common Causes of Acute Tubular Necrosis (ATN)

Ischemic

Hemorrhagic hypotension
Severe volume depletion
Surgical aortic cross-clamping
Cardiac surgery
Defective cardiac output
Septic shock
Pancreatitis
Immunosuppression (cyclosporine, tacrolimus)
Nonsteroidal anti-inflammatory drugs (NSAIDs)

Nephrotoxic

Drugs, including antimicrobials (aminoglycosides, amphotericin), cyclosporine, anesthetics, chemotherapeutic agents
Heavy metals (mercury, lead, *cis*-platinum, uranium, cadmium, bismuth, arsenic)
Radiological contrast agents
Organic solvents (carbon tetrachloride)
Fungicides and pesticides
Plant and animal substances (mushrooms, snake venom)

tubular fluid. As a result of these events, the urinary volume is reduced to less than 400 mL/day (17 mL/hour), the urine specific gravity is increased, and the urine sodium concentration is low (usually <5 mEq/L; Fig. 31-1). Because of these characteristic changes associated with renal underperfusion, measurement of urinary volume, urinary sodium, and specific gravity is a simple method of determining the effect of management on renal perfusion.

An increase in systemic blood pressure does not necessarily imply improvement in renal perfusion. This may be especially evident when drugs such as norepinephrine are used to correct the hypotension associated with states of volume depletion. These drugs may be associated with further reduction in renal blood flow as a consequence of constriction of the renal arteries. This is manifested by a further fall in urinary volume and rise in specific gravity.

In turn, if the hypoperfusion state is more appropriately and specifically treated by replacement of volume, improvement of cardiac output, correction of dysrhythmias, or a combination of these approaches, the improved renal perfusion will be manifested as an increased urinary volume and urine sodium concentration, and as a decreased specific gravity of the urine. This ability to reverse prerenal acute renal failure is the key to its diagnosis.

INTRARENAL ACUTE RENAL FAILURE

Just as there are many causes of intrarenal acute renal failure, there are also many pathophysiological pathways that lead to it (Fig. 31-2). Because ATN is the most common hospital-acquired form of intrarenal acute renal failure, this discussion focuses on the pathophysiology of ATN. The pathophysiology of ATN is complex, but because of intense and ongoing research, there is an increased understanding of the factors contributing to this condition. Ischemia and nephrotoxicity are two major underlying causes of ATN (Fig. 31-3).

Ischemic Acute Tubular Necrosis

Ischemic ATN results from prolonged hypoperfusion. Thus, prerenal acute renal failure and ischemic ATN are actually a continuum, a fact that underscores the importance of prompt recognition and treatment of the prerenal state. When renal hypoperfusion persists for a sufficient time (the exact duration of which is unpredictable and varies with clinical circumstances), renal tubular epithelia become hypoxic and sustain damage to the point that restoration of renal perfusion no longer effects an improvement in glomerular filtration. Ischemia results in decreased adenosine triphosphate (ATP) production in renal cell mitochondria, which robs the cells of a needed energy supply. Part of this energy is used to keep the proper concentration of electrolytes in the cell through electrolyte exchange channels. Some of the cellular electrolyte disturbances from ischemia are decreased intracellular potassium, magnesium, and phosphate, and increased intracellular sodium, chloride, and calcium. Increased intracellular calcium specifically has been shown to predispose the cells to injury and dysfunction.[5]

Cellular insults also occur during reperfusion from the formation of oxygen free radicals. Eventually, these cellular insults cause the tubular cells to swell and become necrotic. The necrotic cells then slough off and obstruct the tubular lumen. These sloughed cells also allow backleak of tubular fluid because of altered function of their basement membrane, contributing to the decreased GFR seen in this disorder.

A final contributor to the pathophysiology of ischemic ATN is profound renal vasoconstriction, which reduces renal blood flow by as much as 50%.[2] These hemodynamic disturbances further compromise renal oxygen delivery and add to the ischemic damage. Vasoconstrictors involved include norepinephrine from sympathetic nervous system activation, angiotensin II, and possibly endothelin, a powerful vasoconstrictor released by damaged vascular endothelial cells of the kidney.

Toxic Acute Tubular Necrosis

The pathophysiology of toxic ATN begins with a concentration of a nephrotoxin in the renal tubular cells, which causes necrosis. These necrotic cells then slough off into the tubular lumen, causing obstruction and impairing glomerular filtration in a manner similar to that of ischemic ATN. Significant differences between toxic ATN and ischemic ATN, however, include the fact that in toxic ATN, the basement membrane of the renal cells usually remains intact and the injured necrotic areas are more localized. In addition, nonoliguria occurs more often with toxic ATN and the healing process is often more rapid.

Although the potential nephrotoxins in toxic ATN are many (see Box 31-2), aminoglycoside antibiotics and radiocontrast dye deserve special mention because of frequency with which they are seen as causes in hospitalized patients. Aminoglycoside nephrotoxicity occurs in 5% to 15% of patients treated with these drugs.[2] The onset of acute renal failure secondary to aminoglycosides is usually delayed,

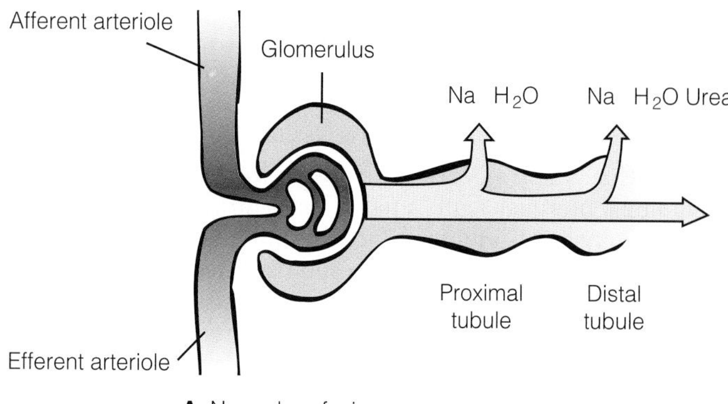

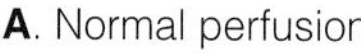

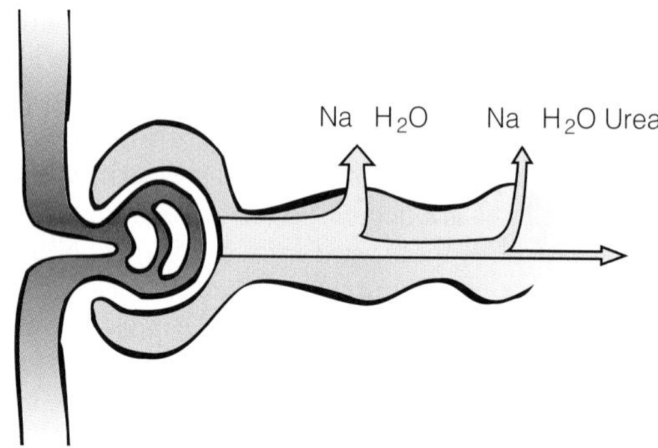

figure 31-1 (**A**) Normal perfusion of the kidney compared with (**B**) underperfusion, as seen in prerenal acute renal failure. Underperfusion of the kidney results in decreased renal blood flow and glomerular filtration, an increase in the fraction of filtrate reabsorbed in the proximal tubule, and low urine flow with low sodium (*Na*) content and increased concentration. *H_2O*, water; *OSM,* osmolarity.

often beginning 7 to 10 days after the onset of therapy. The toxicity of these agents is dose dependent and, because these agents are primarily eliminated by the kidneys, dosage must be adjusted in patients with preexisting renal impairment. To be sure the correct therapeutic range is being achieved, peak and trough blood levels are drawn frequently. Offending agents (listed in decreasing order of the severity with which they produce dose-dependent proximal tubule damage) are neomycin, tobramycin, gentamicin, amikacin, and streptomycin. Several studies have suggested that a single daily dose of gentamicin may result in less nephrotoxicity than dosing the same total amount of medication in three daily doses.[2] Besides dosage, increased risk factors for aminoglycoside toxicity are volume depletion, advanced age, and cardiac surgery.[2]

Radiocontrast-associated nephropathy usually begins within 48 hours of intravenous (IV) radiocontrast administration, peaks in 3 to 5 days, and returns to baseline in 7 to 10 days. Patients at greatest risk for contrast nephropathy are those with diabetes, especially those with diabetes and underlying renal failure. Other patients at risk are the elderly, those with intravascular volume depletion or multiple myeloma, and those who receive a large contrast load.[2]

An important way to reduce the risk of this type of acute renal failure is by aggressive hydration with IV saline before and after contrast dye administration. A novel but largely unsubstantiated approach to preventing radiocontrast-associated nephropathy in patients with underlying renal impairment is the administration of acetylcysteine (Mucomyst, 600 mg twice daily) along with hydration. This approach is based primarily on one prospective, randomized, placebo-controlled study in patients with moderate renal insufficiency (mean serum creatinine 2.4 mg/dL ±1.3 standard deviation) who were given a nonionic, low-osmolality radiocontrast agent.[6] Acetylcysteine may offer protection to these patients through its antioxidant properties (radiocontrast nephropathy may in part be mediated

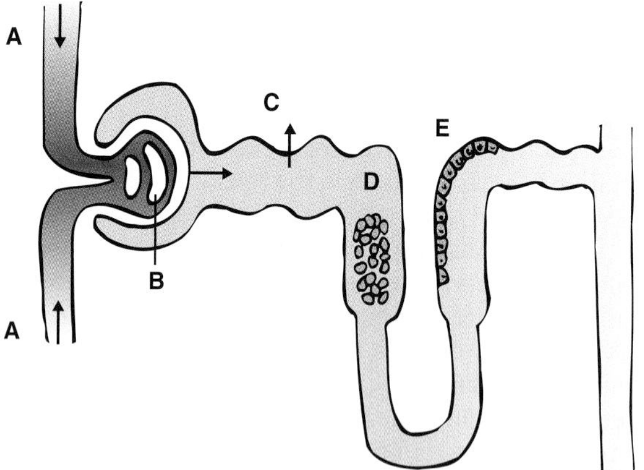

figure 31-2 Potential mechanisms of intrarenal acute renal failure include (**A**) decreased filtration pressure because of constriction in the renal arterioles, (**B**) decreased glomerular capillary permeability, (**C**) increased permeability of the proximal tubules with backleak of filtrate, (**D**) obstruction of urine flow by necrotic tubular cells, and (**E**) increased sodium delivery to the macula densa, which causes an increase in renin–angiotensin production and vasoconstriction at the glomerular level.

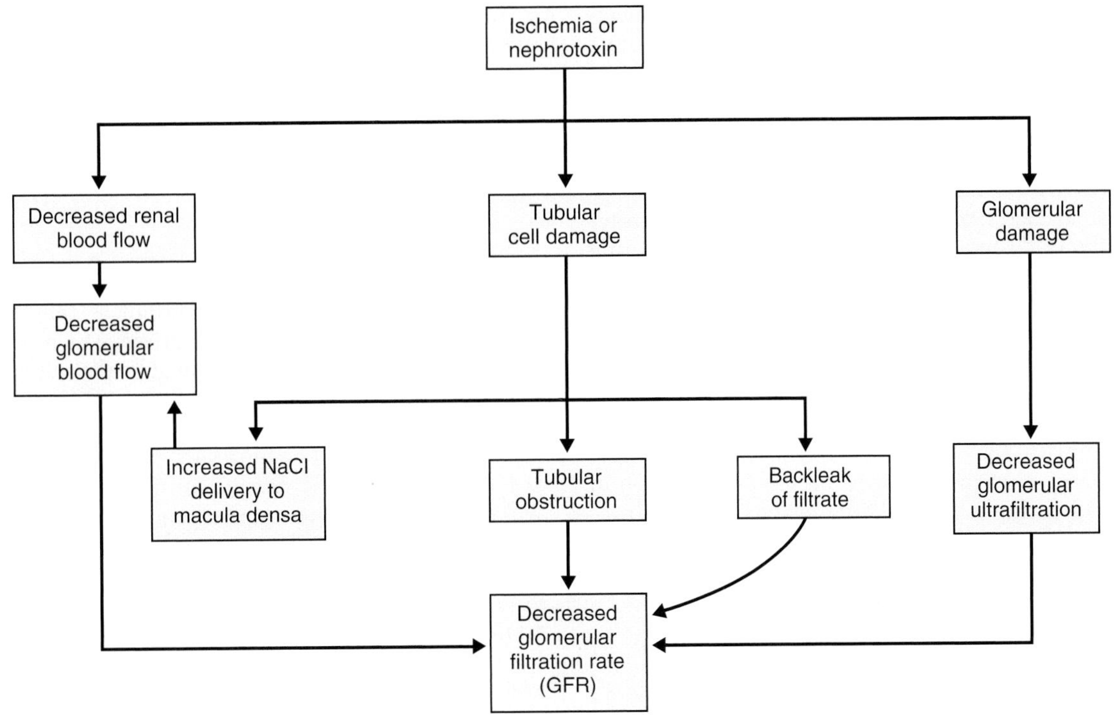

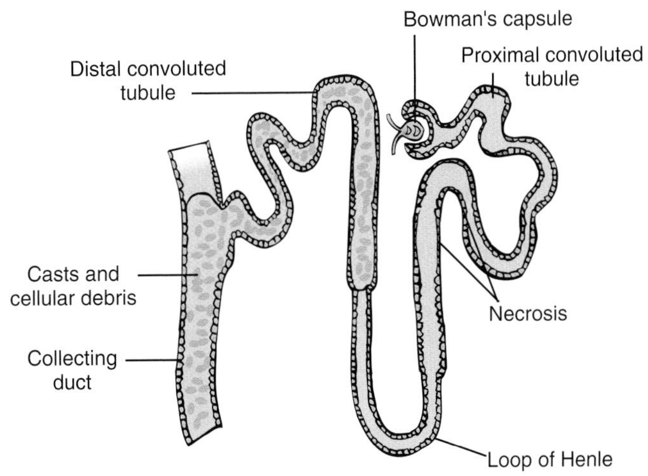

Acute tubular necrosis

figure 31-3 Ischemic ATN results from prolonged hypoperfusion. A sequence of pathophysiological processes results in the sloughing off of necrotic cells that block the tubular lumen. Toxic ATN occurs when a nephrotoxin becomes concentrated in the renal tubular cells that cause necrosis. The necrotic cells slough off and obstruct the tubular lumen, similar to ischemic ATN. In toxic ATN, the basement membrane of the renal cells usually remains intact, and the necrotic areas are more localized.

by the generation of reactive oxygen species that cause direct toxic damage to renal cells and ischemia). Although these results are promising, more rigorous studies need to be conducted before the use of acetylcysteine can be considered a standard of care. When contrast nephropathy does occur, it is usually mild, nonoliguric, and reversible. There are cases, however, when dialysis is needed to bridge the gap before renal function is restored.

POSTRENAL ACUTE RENAL FAILURE

Obstruction can occur at any point in the urinary tract. When urine cannot get around the obstruction, resulting congestion causes retrograde pressure through the collecting system and nephrons. This slows the rate of tubular fluid flow and lowers the GFR. As a result, the reabsorption of sodium, water, and urea is increased, leading to a lowered urine sodium concentration and increased urine osmolality and BUN. Serum creatinine levels also increase. With prolonged pressure from urinary obstruction, the entire collecting system dilates, compressing and damaging nephrons. This results in dysfunction of the concentrating/diluting mechanism, and the urine osmolality and urine sodium concentration become similar to those of plasma. This circumstance can be avoided by prompt removal of the obstruction.

Because a single well-functioning kidney is adequate to maintain homeostasis, the development of acute renal failure from obstruction requires blockage of both kidneys (i.e., urethral or bladder neck obstruction or bilateral ureteral obstruction) or unilateral ureteral obstruction in patients with a single kidney. After relief of the obstruction, there is often a profound diuresis that may be as great as 1 L/hour.[2] If electrolytes and water are not replenished as needed, this diuresis can be very dangerous.

Clinical Course of Acute Tubular Necrosis

The course of ATN can be divided into four clinical phases: onset phase, oliguric or nonoliguric phase, diuretic phase, and recovery phase.

ONSET PHASE

The onset (initiating) phase begins with an initial insult and lasts until cell injury occurs. During this phase, injury is evolving and the health care team members need to attempt to prevent disease progression. The onset phase lasts from hours to days, depending on the cause, and is heralded by the appearance of signs of renal failure (e.g., decreased urine output, increased serum creatinine). The major goal during this phase is to determine the cause of the ATN and initiate treatment to prevent irreversible tubular damage.

OLIGURIC OR NONOLIGURIC PHASE

The second phase of ATN is characterized as either oliguric or nonoliguric. Patients who present with oliguric ATN more frequently require renal replacement therapy, are less likely to recover renal function, and have a higher associated mortality rate.[7–9] This presentation of ATN is most commonly the result of ischemic insult. Oliguric ATN is marked by fluid overload, azotemia, electrolyte abnormalities (i.e., hyperkalemia, hyperphosphatemia, and hypocalcemia), metabolic acidosis, and symptoms of uremia. The main goal during this period is to support renal function and keep the patient alive until renal injury heals. Major causes of death during this period are from hyperkalemia, gastrointestinal bleeding, and infection. Oliguric ATN lasts approximately 12 days, although it may last only a few days or as long as 30 days.[10]

The nonoliguric presentation of ATN, seen in 50% of patients, is most commonly associated with toxic injury (e.g., from aminoglycoside antibiotics).[9] Because of the higher volume of urine output with this presentation, fluid complications are minimized. The higher volume of urine output and the fact that nonoliguric kidneys tend to retain the ability to concentrate urine to some degree results in a decreased need for dialysis in these patients. However, because potassium excretion parallels that seen in oliguria, hyperkalemia remains a major risk. The duration of nonoliguric ATN is typically short, lasting an average of 5 to 8 days.

DIURETIC PHASE

The diuretic phase lasts 1 to 2 weeks and is characterized by a gradual increase in urine output as renal function starts to return. The degree of diuresis, which can exceed 4 to 5 L/day, is primarily determined by the state of hydration at the time the patient enters this stage. Thus, patients who are receiving hemodialysis or who are nonoliguric tend to diurese less. The diuresis is thought to result from the osmotic pull of retained substances (i.e., urea and sodium), which act as osmotic agents. Although the urine output may be normal or elevated, renal concentrating ability is still impaired. This puts patients at risk for fluid volume deficits and electrolyte abnormalities like hyponatremia and hypokalemia. Primary goals during this stage are to maintain hydration, prevent electrolyte depletion, and continue to support renal function.

RECOVERY PHASE

The recovery phase of ATN lasts from several months to a year. It is the time it takes for renal function to return to normal or near-normal levels. If significant renal cell damage has occurred, especially damage to the basement membrane (which cannot regenerate), residual renal impairment may result. Of patients who survive ATN, about 45% recover normal renal function, but at least 5% require long-term dialysis.[2,4] Major health care team goals in this phase revolve around patient education. To foster and maintain the return of renal function, it is critical that patients and family members understand what precipitated the acute renal failure episode, and what follow-up care and preventive measures are necessary to prevent a recurrence in the future.

Diagnosis of Acute Renal Failure

Diagnosis of acute renal failure begins with a determination of whether the acute renal failure is prerenal, intrarenal, or postrenal. The assessment tools used to make this determination include the history and physical examination, laboratory tests, and diagnostic studies. Special considerations for assessing renal function in older patients are given in Box 31-3.

HISTORY AND PHYSICAL EXAMINATION

Essential to any assessment, including that of acute renal failure, is the history and physical examination. By taking a detailed history, clues to the categorization and exact cause of the acute renal failure can be obtained. Important indications in the history that would suggest prerenal acute renal failure include any event or condition that may have contributed to decreased renal perfusion (e.g., acute myocardial infarction, cardiovascular surgery, cardiac arrest, high fever, any shock state, and the use of certain drugs, such as NSAIDs). Also, a history of atherosclerotic

box 31-3

Assessing Renal Function in the Older Adult

As the body ages, physiological systemic and kidney-specific changes occur that are important to take into consideration when evaluating renal function. For example:

- After the age of 30 years, arteriosclerosis starts to develop, including in the renal arteries, which can result in significant damage.
- Changes in the musculoskeletal system in older people results in a decreased muscle mass and body weight. These changes must be kept in mind when assessing renal function because of the possibility of a consequent decreased baseline serum creatinine value. A minimal increase in the serum creatinine level that would be considered within normal limits for a young adult may actually signify major renal impairment in an older adult.
- Kidney-specific changes that occur with aging include a decrease in the total number of functioning glomeruli, a decrease in renal blood flow (by 10% per decade from age 30 years), and a decrease in glomerular filtration rate (GFR) of about 7 to 10 mL/minute per decade after age 40 years.[11-13]

In view of these systemic and kidney-specific changes, an accurate assessment of GFR using a 24-hour urine study or an isotopic study is essential. The Cockroft-Gault formula below, which takes into account sex, age, and weight, although perhaps less precise, could also be used. Once the true GFR is identified, therapy (especially drug therapy) can be guided more safely.

$$\text{Creatinine clearance for men} = \frac{(140 - \text{age}) \times \text{weight in kg}}{72 \times \text{serum creatinine}}$$

$$\text{Creatinine clearance for women} = 0.85 \times \text{creatinine clearance for men}$$

disease may be a clue to renal artery stenosis, another precipitant of prerenal acute renal failure. Clues to an intrarenal cause provided by the history include any prolonged prerenal event or condition as well as exposure to nephrotoxins, especially aminoglycoside antibiotics and radiocontrast dye. It is also important to collect information regarding systemic diseases, like lupus or a vasculitis, recent streptococcal infections, and causes for tubular obstruction like rhabdomyolysis (a history of trauma or a patient found unconscious for an unknown amount of time). Finally, a history of cardiac catheterization, anticoagulation, and thrombolytic therapy increases the possibility of atheroembolic intrarenal diseases. Findings that may point to postrenal acute renal failure include any history of abdominal tumors or calculi, and especially a history of benign prostatic hypertrophy in elderly men. A family history of urolithiasis or benign prostatic hypertrophy may be contributory.

The physical examination, particularly fluid status, is critical to the diagnosis of acute renal failure. In prerenal acute renal failure, a state of decreased renal perfusion related to dehydration or hypovolemia is heralded by poor skin turgor, dry mucous membranes, weight loss, and reduced jugular venous distension. In contrast, when decreased perfusion is related to vasodilation, third-spacing, cardiovascular disease (e.g., heart failure), or a combination of these factors, findings of increased extracellular fluid (ECF) may be manifested. These findings include edema, ascites, and weight gain. For critical care patients, hemodynamic monitoring values help determine intravascular fluid status as well as cardiac functioning. Surveillance values include central venous pressure (CVP), pulmonary artery wedge pressure (PAWP), and cardiac output (cardiac index). By correlating physical examination findings with the history, hemodynamic values, and laboratory tests, potential prerenal etiologies can be narrowed down further.

Although no specific physical examination finding prompts consideration of intrarenal acute renal failure, many examination findings are helpful clues to potential causes of intrarenal acute renal failure. For example, signs of a streptococcal throat infection, lupus (e.g., a butterfly mask rash), or embolic phenomena (e.g., discolored toes and livido reticularis, a semipermanent bluish mottling of the skin in the extremities) may all suggest an intrarenal cause. Again, correlation with the history and laboratory studies helps narrow the list of potential causes.

Findings on physical examination that may suggest a postrenal cause include a distended bladder, an abdominal mass, an enlarged or nodular prostate gland, and, most obviously, a kinked or obstructed Foley catheter.

LABORATORY STUDIES

Laboratory assessment, critical to the diagnosis and categorization of acute renal failure, includes both serum and urinary values. For a basic comparison of laboratory values in prerenal acute renal failure, postrenal acute renal failure, and ATN, see Table 31-1. In addition to helping to differentiate between prerenal, intrarenal, and postrenal acute renal failure, blood and urine tests are also helpful for distinguishing ATN from other types of intrarenal acute renal failure. In some circumstances, the diagnosis may be difficult, such as with rapidly progressive glomerulonephritis. In rapidly progressive glomerulonephritis, significant urine sediment abnormalities are not seen and the urine chemistries look more like those seen in prerenal azotemia than those observed in ATN. Often this in itself is a clue to the diagnosis. There are, however, many specific urine and blood tests that aid in the diagnosis of acute renal failure, particularly intrarenal acute renal failure, and they should be considered carefully (Box 31-4).

Urinary Values

Obtaining a urine specimen for diagnostic chemistries and indices is invaluable in establishing the diagnosis and determining the type of acute renal failure. The urine specimen should be obtained *before* a diagnostic challenge of diuretics is administered because these agents may alter the urine's chemical composition. The urine sodium concentration, osmolality, and specific gravity are especially helpful in distinguishing between prerenal acute renal failure and ATN because these values reflect the concentrating ability of the kidney. In prerenal failure, the hypoperfused kidney actively reabsorbs sodium and water in an attempt to increase circulatory volume. Consequently, the urine sodium level and the fractional excretion of sodium (FE_{Na})

table 31-1 Acute Renal Failure: Comparison of Laboratory Findings in Prerenal Failure, Postrenal Failure, and Acute Tubular Necrosis (ATN)

Value	Prerenal	Postrenal	ATN
Urine volume	Oliguria	May alternate between anuria and polyuria	Anuria, oliguria, or nonoliguria
Urine osmolality	Increased (>500 mOsm/kg H_2O)	Varies, increased or equal to serum	250–300 mOsm/kg H_2O
Urine specific gravity	Increased (>1.020)	Varies	Approximately 1.010
Urine sodium	<20 mEq/L	Varies	>40 mEq/L
Urine sediment	Normal, few casts	Normal, may be crystals	Granular casts, tubular epithelial cells
Fe_{Na}	<1%	>1%	>1% (often >3%)
BUN:Cr	>20:1	10:1 to 15:1	10:1 to 15:1

FE_{Na}, fractional excretion of sodium; *BUN:Cr*, blood urea nitrogen–creatinine ratio.

are low (<20 mEq/L and <1%, respectively), whereas the urine osmolality and concentration of nonreabsorbable solutes are high. In contrast, in ATN where there is parenchymal damage to the kidney, the tubular cells can no longer effectively reabsorb sodium or concentrate the urine. As a result, the urine sodium concentration is often greater than 40 mEq/L, the FE_{Na} is greater than 1%, and the urine osmolality is close to that of plasma (isosthenuria). Unfortunately, there is a limit to the usefulness of these indices because of overlap in these values for prerenal acute renal failure and ATN (i.e., urine sodium concentration values in the 20- to 40-mEq/L range). Values at the extremes thus are most useful.

The sediment in a urinalysis is also very helpful in diagnosing and distinguishing the types of acute renal failure. In prerenal acute renal failure, the urinary sediment is normal with only a few hyaline casts, whereas in ATN, coarse, muddy-brown granular casts and tubular epithelial cells are typically found. In postrenal acute renal failure, the sediment is often normal but can be helpful in diagnosing stones.

Blood Urea Nitrogen and Creatinine Levels

Serum tests for BUN and creatinine are essential not only for diagnosing acute renal failure, but for helping distinguish between prerenal acute renal failure and ATN or postrenal acute renal failure. In prerenal acute renal failure, the BUN–creatinine ratio is increased from the normal ratio of 10:1 to more than 20:1. This finding is caused by a state of dehydration, by the fact that as the tubules become more permeable to water in prerenal acute renal failure, urea is also reabsorbed, or by both of these factors. In ATN and postrenal acute renal failure, when the concentrating ability of the kidneys is impaired, both the BUN and creatinine increase proportionally, maintaining the normal 10:1 ratio.

DIAGNOSTIC STUDIES

One important diagnostic test in the evaluation of acute renal failure is renal ultrasonography. This test is especially useful in ruling out a high obstruction and has the advantage of being noninvasive. With a high obstruction, dilation of the urinary collecting system is detectable on ultrasonography within 1 to 2 days of the onset of the obstruction.[2] Ultrasonography may also reveal proximal renal calculi as a cause of postrenal obstruction. Last, it can be used to estimate renal size, which is helpful in distinguishing between acute and chronic renal failure. In chronic renal insufficiency, the kidneys are often small (<9 cm) and echogenic.

Other studies that may be useful in diagnosing acute renal failure are computed tomography (CT) and magnetic resonance imaging (MRI) to evaluate for masses, vascular disorders, and filling defects in the collecting system, and a renal arteriogram to evaluate for renal artery stenosis. It is important to keep in mind with selected studies that contrast dye used in the studies is allergenic and nephrotoxic, and thus benefits of the study must be weighed against potential risks. Finally, a renal biopsy may be helpful in patients thought to have intrarenal acute renal failure that is not ATN, especially if significant proteinuria or unexplained hematuria is revealed on urinalysis.[2] In addition to having diagnostic value, the results of a biopsy may help determine prognosis and therapy.

CHRONIC RENAL FAILURE

Chronic renal failure is a slow, progressive, irreversible deterioration in renal function that results in the kidney's inability to eliminate waste products and maintain fluid and electrolyte balance. Ultimately, it leads to end-stage renal disease (ESRD) and the need for renal replacement therapy or renal transplantation to sustain life.

Currently there are more than 300,000 dialysis and renal transplant recipients in the United States, and in 1999 alone, more than 80,000 patients were newly diagnosed. Among patients receiving dialysis, incidence rates are 43% higher in men than in women, and are higher with increasing age. The incidence rates in patients on

box 31-4
Diagnostic Clues in Acute Renal Failure

Urine
- Urate crystals: tumor lysis, especially lymphoma (urate nephropathy)
- Oxalate crystals: ethylene glycol nephrotoxicity, methoxyflurane nephrotoxicity
- Eosinophils: allergic interstitial nephritis, especially methicillin
- Positive benzidine without red blood cells: hemoglobinuria or myoglobinuria
- Pigmented casts: hemoglobinuria or myoglobinuria
- Massive proteinuria: acute interstitial nephritis, thiazide diuretics, hemorrhagic fevers (i.e., Korean, Scandinavian)
- Abnormal urine protein electrophoresis: multiple myeloma
- Anuria: renal cortical necrosis, bilateral obstruction, renal vascular catastrophe

Plasma
- Marked hyperkalemia: rhabdomyolysis, tissue necrosis, hemolysis
- Marked hypocalcemia: rhabdomyolysis
- Hypercalcemia: hypercalcemic nephropathy
- Hyperuricemia: tumor lysis, rhabdomyolysis, toxin ingestion
- Marked acidosis: ethylene glycol, methyl alcohol
- Elevated creatine kinase or myoglobin levels: rhabdomyolysis
- Low complement levels: systemic lupus erythematosus (SLE), postinfectious glomerulonephritis, subacute bacterial endocarditis
- Abnormal serum protein electrophoresis: multiple myeloma
- Positive antibody to glomerular basement membrane: Goodpasture's syndrome
- Positive antineutrophilic cytoplasmic antibody: small vessel vasculitis (Wegener's granulomatosis or polyarteritis nodosa)
- Positive antinuclear antibody (ANA) or antibody to double-stranded DNA: SLE
- Positive antibodies to streptolysin O: poststreptococcal glomerulonephritis
- Elevated lactate dehydrogenase (LDH) level, elevated serum bilirubin level, or decreased haptoglobin level: hemolytic–uremic syndrome (HUS) or thrombotic thrombocytopenic purpura (TTP)

dialysis are 311% higher in the African-American population than in the white population. Hispanics and Native Americans also have higher incidence rates than whites, but the difference in rates is not as dramatic.[14] These differences in incidence rates are important to keep in mind when considering patient risk factors and populations to which increased health education regarding prevention should be targeted.

The causes of chronic renal failure are numerous (Box 31-5), but diabetes mellitus and hypertension are by far the two most common, accounting for more than 30% and 20% of cases of ESRD, respectively.[14] Other causes include glomerulonephritis (both primary and secondary to systemic diseases), interstitial nephritis, congenital malformations, genetic disorders, neoplasms, hepatorenal syndrome, obstructive uropathy, and microangiopathic etiologies such as scleroderma and atheroembolic disease.

box 31-5
Causes of Chronic Renal Failure

- Diabetes mellitus
- Hypertension
- Glomerulonephritis
  - Primary (IgA nephropathy, postinfectious glomerulonephritis)
  - Secondary (HIV nephropathy, lupus, cryoglobulinemia, Wegener's granulomatosis, Goodpasture's syndrome, polyarteritis nodosa, amyloidosis)
- Interstitial nephritis (allergic interstitial nephritis, pyelonephritis)
- Microangiopathic vascular disease (atheroembolic disease, scleroderma)
- Congenital disease
- Genetic disease (polycystic kidney disease, medullary cystic kidney disease)
- Obstructive uropathy
- Neoplasms or tumors
- Transplant rejection
- Hepatorenal syndrome

Pathophysiology of Chronic Renal Failure

In discussing the general pathophysiology involved in the progression of chronic renal failure, it is important to have an understanding of the *intact nephron theory*. Because each of the over one million nephrons in each kidney is an independent functioning unit, as renal disease progresses, nephrons can lose function at different times. When an individual nephron becomes diseased, nephrons in close proximity increase their individual filtration rates by increasing the rate of blood flow and hydrostatic pressure in their glomerular capillaries. This hyperfiltration response in the nondiseased nephrons enables the kidneys to maintain excretory and homeostatic functions, even when up to 70% of the nephrons are damaged. Eventually, however, the intact nephrons reach a point of maximal filtration and any additional loss of glomerular mass is accompanied by an incremental loss in GFR and subsequent accumulation of filterable toxins.

The mechanisms involved in the progressive destruction of nephrons vary depending on the primary cause of the renal failure. However, specific identifiable secondary insults can rapidly accelerate the process of nephron loss. Such secondary insults include an alteration in renal perfusion, as observed in congestive heart failure or intravascular volume depletion; the administration of nephrotoxic agents; urinary obstruction; and urinary infections.[15] In addition to the primary and potential secondary insults, nephron loss can be accelerated by the hyperfiltration mechanism itself. This is why many interventions to slow down the progression of renal failure involve measures that reduce glomerular hydrostatic pressure. One such example is the use of ACE inhibitors, which prevent angiotensin II–mediated efferent arteriolar vasoconstriction and subsequent nephron hyperfiltration. Finally, recent studies have suggested a variety of other mechanisms may also contribute to renal scarring independent of the primary insult. These include alterations in circulating lipids, electrolytes like calcium and phosphate, and hormones.[2] Therapies aimed at these mechanisms may offer promise for management of chronic renal failure in the future.

DIABETIC NEPHROPATHY

Because of the extremely high prevalence of diabetes and hypertension as causes of chronic renal failure, an understanding of the renal pathophysiology specific to these entities and knowledge of interventions designed to slow down or even prevent progression to ESRD is imperative. Renal failure is a major complication of diabetes, with an incidence of 40% in patients with type 1 diabetes mellitus and 40% to 63% in patients with type 2 diabetes mellitus.[10] In diabetes, the microvasculature in the organ systems of the body, including the kidneys, is damaged. In the kidneys, primarily the afferent and efferent arterioles and the glomerular capillaries are affected. Glomerular changes include thickening of the basement membrane, deposits of immunoglobulin G (IgG) and albumin, and diffuse glomerulosclerosis. Late in diabetic nephropathy, tubular atrophy and interstitial fibrosis also occur.[10] The exact physiological mechanism for these structural alterations is unclear, but hyperglycemia is a major contributor. In the classic Diabetes Control and Complications Trial (DCCT)—a prospective, randomized, multicenter trial done to assess the effectiveness of tight blood glucose control on the complications of type 1 diabetes—strict blood glucose control was found to delay and possibly even prevent the progression of diabetic nephropathy.[16]

At the onset of diabetic nephropathy, patients may have an increased GFR (as high as 140 mL/minute) because of hyperfiltration, slightly enlarged kidneys, and microalbuminuria (30 to 300 mg/day of albumin in the urine). Over the course of approximately 10 to 20 years, hypertension and overt proteinuria develop, with consequent hypoalbuminemia and edema, as well as mild azotemia. In 50% of these patients, ESRD develops within 7 to 10 years.[10]

HYPERTENSIVE NEPHROSCLEROSIS

The effect of systemic hypertension on the kidneys results in a condition known as *nephrosclerosis.* Hypertensive nephrosclerosis involves the development of sclerotic lesions in the renal arterioles and glomerular capillaries that cause them to become thickened and narrowed, and eventually necrotic. Hypertensive nephrosclerosis can be benign or malignant. In benign nephrosclerosis, associated with chronic mild or moderate hypertension, renal impairment occurs over many years. Malignant nephrosclerosis, associated with malignant hypertension, can lead to permanent renal failure rapidly if blood pressure is not immediately reduced. Often symptoms like blurred vision and a severe headache accompany this crisis situation.

Because hypertensive nephrosclerosis is directly caused by hypertension, its incidence is greater in populations with a higher incidence of primary hypertension (e.g., elderly people, African-American people). Among African Americans, the incidence of patients with ESRD receiving dialysis due to hypertension is over 30%.[14] The signs of hypertensive nephrosclerosis vary depending on the severity of the renal damage and the acuteness of the hypertension. Some signs that may be present include proteinuria, azotemia, and hematuria with red blood cell casts. Unfortunately, like hypertension itself, patients often remain asymptomatic until extensive damage is done. To prevent or delay the progression of hypertensive nephropathy, blood pressure control is essential. This is an area where patient education can have a great impact in decreasing the incidence of ESRD. Educating patients about the complications of uncontrolled hypertension is particularly important and may foster the patient's active involvement in controlling his or her blood pressure.

Preventing the Progression of Chronic Renal Failure

An important characteristic of chronic renal failure is continuous progression. Slowing the rate of progression to ESRD once chronic renal failure develops is a focus of extensive and ongoing research. Because secondary insults to the kidney, as previously mentioned, accelerate progression of the renal failure, monitoring for and avoiding these insults is paramount. This includes avoiding fluid volume deficits, urinary obstructions, and urinary tract infections (and aggressively treating these conditions if they occur). It also involves avoiding nephrotoxins like aminoglycoside antibiotics and IV radiocontrast dye. If such agents are deemed necessary, they must be used judiciously. Even one exposure to IV contrast agents in a patient with renal insufficiency may result in ESRD. As in the case with acute renal failure, adequate hydration before and after dye administration may help prevent further renal damage.

Strict control of blood glucose levels, with the goal of keeping glycosylated hemoglobin (HbA_{1c}) within the normal range, is critical to preventing and retarding the progression of renal failure in people with diabetes. Blood pressure control is also essential for preventing the progression of renal failure from almost any primary etiology, not just hypertension or diabetes.[15] Control of hypertension entails lifestyle changes (e.g., exercise, salt restriction, and avoidance of excessive alcohol) as well as pharmacological therapy if necessary. Regarding pharmacological therapy, ACE inhibitors have been shown to offer a selective advantage in slowing the progression of diabetic nephropathy.[15,16] This is presumably because of their ability to decrease intraglomerular pressure by blocking the effect of angiotensin II on the afferent and efferent arterioles. Recently it has been demonstrated that angiotensin receptor blockers (ARBs), which also block the effect of angiotensin II, slow the progression of diabetic nephropathy as well.[17,18] Certainly, for patients who cannot tolerate ACE inhibitors (currently the mainstay of antihypertensive therapy in diabetic patients), ARBs may be a good alternative.

A protein-restricted diet as a means to slow the progression of renal failure is controversial, but the evidence seems to support the view that moderate protein restriction (0.8 g/kg/day) in patients may help. However, caution with protein restriction, especially in critically ill patients who are in a catabolic state, is important to prevent malnutrition. Malnutrition itself is a major determinant of morbidity and mortality in patients with renal failure.[15] Ways to avoid malnutrition include providing protein with high biological value, ensuring that adequate caloric requirements are met, and closely monitoring nutritional assessment parameters (i.e., body weight, serum albumin and prealbumin levels, and total protein levels). Because of the complexity of nutritional requirements in critically ill patients, collaboration with a dietitian is essential.

A final means by which the progression of renal failure may be slowed is by controlling serum lipids. Hyperlipidemia is commonly seen with chronic renal failure, especially in the settings of diabetes and nephrotic syndrome, and is hypothesized to contribute to renal failure. Although as of yet no controlled long-term human studies have assessed the efficacy of lipid reduction in renal disease, multiple animal and human studies have demonstrated a correlation between hyperlipidemia and progressive renal failure.[15] The means by which lipids may contribute to renal failure is unclear, but lipid droplets in the glomerular capillaries may accelerate the formation of sclerotic lesions, cause direct cell injury when metabolized, or effect injury through both of these mechanisms. Because the use of lipid-lowering agents is safe in diverse renal diseases, their use may be prudent, especially because lowering lipids decreases the risk of cardiovascular events (the primary cause of mortality in patients with ESRD).

Clinical Course of Chronic Renal Failure

The progression of chronic renal failure is commonly classified into three stages: decreased renal reserve, renal insufficiency, and ESRD. These stages occur along a continuum.

DECREASED RENAL RESERVE

Decreased renal reserve is characterized by a 40% to 50% loss of renal function. During this stage, the kidneys are still able to maintain excretory and regulatory functions and patients are typically asymptomatic. The early signs of renal failure, like slightly increased BUN and serum creatinine levels, are evident only after 50% to 60% of renal function is lost. If a patient is diagnosed during the decreased renal reserve stage, it usually is inadvertent or because of high suspicion based on comorbidity (e.g., diabetes).

RENAL INSUFFICIENCY

In renal insufficiency, residual renal function is only 20% to 40% of normal. By this time, solute clearance, the ability to concentrate urine, and hormone secretion are compromised. Consequently, signs of renal failure (including azotemia, electrolyte imbalances, and anemia) begin to manifest. Common symptoms during this stage include fatigue, polyuria, and nocturia.

END-STAGE RENAL DISEASE

The final stage of chronic renal failure is ESRD. It is characterized by a residual renal function of less than 15% of normal. At this point, all the normal regulatory, excretory, and hormonal functions of the kidney are severely impaired. ESRD is evidenced by marked elevations in BUN and serum creatinine levels, anemia, electrolyte imbalances (i.e., hypocalcemia, hyperkalemia, hyperphosphatemia), and fluid overload. Usually the patient is oliguric, with urine osmolality similar to plasma osmolality. Uremic symptoms are manifested and include nausea, vomiting, anorexia, altered sensorium, weakness, and fatigue. If treatment with dialysis or transplantation is not initiated, the patient will die. Considerations for the pediatric patient with ESRD are given in Box 31-6.

MANAGEMENT OF RENAL FAILURE

Although some distinct differences exist between the way acute renal failure and chronic renal failure is managed, many of the clinical manifestations and complications encountered are the same. Thus, the general management of renal failure is addressed here, noting any differences between acute and chronic renal failure as necessary. In either type of renal failure, management begins with treating the primary insult. Common nursing diagnoses and collaborative problems for patients with acute renal failure are given in Box 31-7. An overview of the management of patients with acute renal failure is provided in the accompanying Collaborative Care Guide (Box 31-8).

Managing Fluid Balance Alterations

Clinical management of fluid balance is of primary importance in patients with renal failure and is the area where differences in the management of acute and chronic renal failure are perhaps most dramatic.

box 31-6

Considerations for the Pediatric Patient With End-Stage Renal Disease

Children with end-stage renal disease (ESRD) often experience growth failure. In fact, 50% of these children are 2 standard deviations below normal in regard to height compared with age-matched children from the general population.[19] Investigational therapies directed at this problem that should be considered when managing a child with ESRD include nutritional supplementation, correction of acidosis, and the administration of recombinant human growth hormone (rhGH). Peritoneal dialysis, because it is associated with fewer dietary restrictions than hemodialysis and because it causes fewer interruptions in the daily routine (including schooling), is the preferred mode of dialytic treatment in the pediatric population. Early transplantation, the optimal solution to ESRD in children, can prevent growth retardation and should be sought aggressively.

box 31-7 *Nursing Diagnoses and Collaborative Problems for the Patient With Acute Renal Failure*

- Fluid Volume Excess related to decreased kidney function
- Alteration in Cardiac Output: Decreased related to fluid volume excess, disturbances in renin–angiotensin system
- Altered Nutrition: Less than Body Requirements related to anorexia, nausea and vomiting, dietary restrictions, and altered oral mucous membranes
- Impairment of Skin Integrity related to poor nutritional status, immobility, and edema
- Anxiety related to unexpected serious illness and uncertain prognosis, unfamiliar environment, and current symptoms
- Activity Intolerance related to fatigue, anemia, retention of waste products, and dialysis procedure
- Sleep Pattern Disturbance related to fragmented sleep
- Potential for Infection related to decreased functioning of immune system
- Knowledge Deficit: pathophysiology and etiology of acute episode, dietary restrictions, medications, complications, prognosis, and need for follow-up care

ACUTE RENAL FAILURE

In prerenal acute renal failure and the early stages of ischemic ATN, the cause of the renal failure is inadequate renal perfusion, often due to intravascular volume deficits. After using laboratory, physical assessment, and hemodynamic clues to make a rapid diagnosis of intravascular volume depletion, therapy involves prompt administration of replacement fluids, such as blood and crystalloids. The replacement solutions used should reflect the type of losses (e.g., for a patient with a hemorrhagic condition, blood would be the replacement fluid of choice). Often in acute renal failure, even if signs and symptoms of intravascular volume deficits are not present, large boluses of IV fluid challenges are given. Reversal of acute renal failure after such a bolus is therapeutic as well as diagnostic of prerenal acute renal failure.

Fluid administration in acute renal failure is also indicated in the diuretic phase of ATN, when extensive diuresis may occur, and for the prevention or alleviation of tubular obstruction seen in obstructive causes of acute renal failure, including ATN and many postrenal etiologies. In any oliguric state, however, caution must be taken to prevent fluid overload. In a sustained oliguric state, like the oliguric stage of ATN, fluid is restricted to the previous day's urine output amount plus 500 to 800 mL to account for insensible losses.

Diuretics are often used in acute renal failure to increase urinary flow to prevent or reverse oliguria, to help alleviate conditions of fluid overload, to prevent tubular obstruction, or to achieve a combination of these goals. Furosemide, a loop diuretic, and mannitol, an osmotic diuretic, are of proven benefit in preventing tubular obstruction in certain obstructive causes of acute renal failure, such as heme pigment obstruction and tumor lysis syndrome. In states of fluid overload, like pulmonary edema and heart failure, diuretics are also useful. Often in these situations, furosemide is administered every 6 hours, with the initial dose ranging between 20 and 100 mg depending on whether the patient has taken furosemide regularly. If within an hour the response is inadequate, the dose may then be doubled. This process may be repeated until adequate urine output is achieved. Sometimes even a continuous furosemide drip is required.[3] In addition, a thiazide diuretic, like hydrochlorothiazide, may be administered with furosemide because of the synergistic action of these diuretics in promoting urinary excretion.

With the use of diuretics, caution must be taken to avoid complications of dehydration, electrolyte imbalances, and side effects. Tinnitus and hearing impairment (reversible and irreversible) have been reported after IV furosemide administration. Ototoxicity is associated with rapid injection, excessively high doses, or concomitant therapy with other ototoxic drugs. The manufacturer recommends controlled IV infusion (not to exceed 4 mg/minute) for high-dose parenteral furosemide therapy.

The use of diuretics to convert oliguria to nonoliguria, unlike the aforementioned uses of diuretics, has not been substantiated consistently in medical research. Nevertheless, diuretics often are administered with this purpose in mind. In this situation, high-dose loop diuretics (often combined with a thiazide diuretic) or mannitol may be tried. If the patient has an inadequate response, the diuretics should not be continued for risk of side effects. With mannitol administration, extreme caution must be used because of its dramatic effect of increasing circulatory volume. Such a dramatic increase in circulatory volume may not be tolerated by the patient's cardiovascular system and may exacerbate conditions like heart failure and ultimately worsen the acute renal failure.

Dopamine is another agent that has been traditionally used in acute renal failure because of its ability to cause renal vasodilation at "renal doses" (1 to 3 μg/kg/minute), thereby increasing renal perfusion. The efficacy of this agent to affect the course of acute renal failure, however, has not been substantiated despite many clinical trials, and some studies have even shown deleterious effects.[1,4] Nevertheless, some clinicians may institute a trial of dopamine, particularly in a combination with fluid resuscitation, in patients with prerenal acute renal failure.

If fluid complications arise and cannot be controlled by fluid restrictions and pharmacological agents, dialysis (discussed in detail in Chapter 30) or isolated ultrafiltration may be necessary. This is often the case in oliguric patients who are receiving large amounts of IV fluids hourly owing to medications and nutritional supplements. People in whom acute renal failure develops secondary to hypoperfusion or tubular injury may have a delayed recovery time, necessitating maintenance dialysis until the tissue repairs itself and normal function returns. For these patients, discharge planning should take into consideration the need for outpatient dialysis therapy (which may last for several weeks to months), the need to modify the person's diet and consumption of fluids, and the psychosocial implications of these measures for the patient and his or her family members.

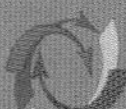

box 31-8 **collaborative care guide** *for the Patient With Acute Renal Failure (ARF)*

OUTCOMES	INTERVENTIONS
Coordination of Care All appropriate team members and disciplines will be involved in the plan of care.	■ Develop the plan of care with the patient, family, primary physician, nephrologist, pulmonologist, cardiologist, registered nurse, advanced practice nurse, social worker, respiratory therapist, physical therapist, occupational therapist, dietitian, chaplain, and dialysis staff.
Oxygenation/Ventilation Patient will have adequate gas exchange as evidenced by: ■ Arterial blood gases (ABGs) within normal limits ■ Functional oxygen saturation (Spo_2) greater than 92% ■ Clear breath sounds ■ Normal respiratory rate and depth ■ Normal chest x-ray	■ Monitor ABGs and continuous pulse oximetry. ■ Monitor acid–base status. ■ Monitor for signs and symptoms of pulmonary distress from fluid overload. ■ Provide routine pulmonary toilet, including the following: ■ Airway suctioning ■ Chest percussion ■ Incentive spirometer ■ Frequent turning ■ Mobilize out of bed to chair. ■ Support patient with oxygen therapy, mechanical ventilation, or both as indicated. Involve respiratory therapist.
Circulation/Perfusion Patient's blood pressure, heart rate, and hemodynamic parameters will be within normal limits. Patient will have adequate tissue perfusion as evidenced by: ■ Adequate hemoglobin levels ■ Euvolemic status ■ Optimal urine output depending on phase of acute renal failure ■ Appropriate level of consciousness	■ Monitor vital signs every 1 to 2 hours. ■ Monitor pulmonary artery pressure and right atrial pressure every hour and cardiac output, systemic vascular resistance, and peripheral vascular resistance every 6 to 12 hours if pulmonary artery catheter is in place. ■ Assess vital signs continuously or every 15 minutes during dialysis. ■ Monitor hemoglobin and hematocrit levels daily. ■ Assess evidence of tissue perfusion (pain, pulses, color, temperature, and signs of decreased organ perfusion such as an altered level of consciousness, ileus, and decreasing urine output). ■ Administer intravascular crystalloids or blood products as indicated.
Fluids/Electrolytes Patient will be euvolemic. Patient will achieve normal electrolyte balance. Patient will achieve optimal renal function.	■ Monitor fluid status, including input and output (fluid restriction), daily weight, urine output trends, vital signs, central venous pressure (CVP), and pulmonary artery wedge pressure (PAWP). ■ Monitor for signs and symptoms of hypervolemia (hypertension, pulmonary edema, peripheral edema, jugular venous distension, and increased CVP). ■ Monitor serum electrolytes daily. ■ Monitor renal parameters, including urine output, blood urea nitrogen (BUN), serum creatinine, acid–base status, urine electrolytes, urine osmolality, and urine specific gravity. ■ Administer fluids and diuretics to maintain intravascular volume and renal function, per order. ■ Replace electrolytes as ordered.

(continued)

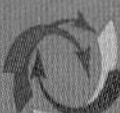

box 31-8 collaborative care guide *for the Patient With Acute Renal Failure (ARF) (Continued)*

OUTCOMES	INTERVENTIONS
	■ Treat patient with, and monitor response to, dialysis therapies if indicated. ■ Monitor and maintain dialysis access for chosen intermittent or continuous dialysis method: ***Continuous Veno–Veno Dialysis*** ■ Monitor and regulate ultrafiltration rate hourly based on patient's response and fluid status. ■ Provide fluid replacements as ordered. ■ Assess and troubleshoot hemofilter and blood tubing hourly. ■ Protect vascular access from dislodgement. ■ Change filter and tubing per protocol. ■ Monitor vascular access for infection. ***Peritoneal Dialysis*** ■ Slowly infuse warmed dialysate. ■ Drain after appropriate dwell time. ■ Assess drainage for volume and appearance. ■ Send cultures daily. ■ Assess access site for infection. ***Intermittent Hemodialysis*** ■ Assess shunt for thrill and buzzing sound (bruit) every 12 hours. ■ Avoid constrictions (i.e., blood pressures), phlebotomy, and intravenous fluid administration in arm with shunt. ■ Assess for infection. ■ Monitor perfusion of related extremity.
Mobility Patient will remain free of complications related to bed rest and immobility.	■ Initiate deep venous thrombosis prophylaxis. ■ Reposition frequently. ■ Mobilize to chair when possible. ■ Consult physical therapist. ■ Conduct range-of-motion and strengthening exercises.
Protection/Safety Patient will be protected from possible harm.	■ Assess need for wrist restraints if patient is intubated, has a decreased level of consciousness, is unable to follow commands, or is acutely agitated, or for affected extremity during hemodialysis. Explain need for restraints to patient and family members. If restrained, assess response to restraints and check every 1 to 2 hours for skin integrity and impairment in tissue perfusion. Follow hospital protocol for use of restraints. ■ Use siderails on bed and safety belts on chairs as appropriate. ■ Follow seizure precautions.
Skin Integrity Patient will have intact skin.	■ Assess skin integrity and all bony prominences every 4 hours. ■ Turn every 2 hours. ■ Consider a pressure relief/reduction mattress. Use Braden Scale to assess risk of skin breakdown. ■ Use superfatted or lanolin-based soap for bathing and apply emollients for pruritus. ■ Treat pressure ulcers according to hospital protocol. Involve enterostomal nurse in care.

(continued)

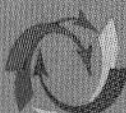

box 31-8 collaborative care guide ***for the Patient With Acute Renal Failure (ARF) (Continued)***

OUTCOMES	INTERVENTIONS
Nutrition Patient will be adequately nourished as evidenced by: ■ Stable weight not less than 10% below, or greater than 20% above, ideal body weight ■ An albumin level of 3.5 to 4.0 g/dL ■ A total protein level of 6 to 8 g/dL ■ A total lymphocyte count of 1,000 to 3,000 × 10^6/L	■ Consult dietitian to direct and coordinate nutritional support. ■ Observe sodium, potassium, protein, and fluid restriction as indicated. ■ Provide small, frequent feedings. ■ Provide parenteral or enteral feeding as ordered. ■ Monitor albumin, prealbumin, total protein, hematocrit, hemoglobin, and white blood cell counts, and monitor daily weights to assess effectiveness of nutritional therapy.
Comfort/Pain Control Patient will be as comfortable and as pain free as possible as evidenced by: ■ No complaints of discomfort ■ No objective indicators of discomfort	■ Monitor for signs and symptoms of respiratory distress related to fluid overload and support oxygenation as needed. Keep head of bed elevated and teach breathing techniques to minimize oxygen distress, such as pursed-lip breathing. ■ Plan fluid restrictions over 24 hours, allowing for periodic sips of water and ice chips to minimize thirst. ■ Provide frequent mouth and skin care. ■ Assess quantity and quality of discomfort. ■ Provide a quiet environment and frequent reassurance. ■ Observe for complications that may cause discomfort, such as infection of vascular access device, peritonitis or inadequate draining during peritoneal dialysis, and gastrointestinal disturbances (nausea, vomiting, diarrhea, constipation). ■ Administer analgesics, antiemetics, antidiarrheals, laxatives (non-magnesium and non-phosphate containing), stool softeners, antihistamines, sedatives, or anxiolytics as needed and monitor response.
Psychosocial Patient will demonstrate a decrease in anxiety as evidenced by: ■ Vital signs within normal limits ■ Level of consciousness within normal limits ■ Subjective reports of decreased anxiety levels ■ Objective assessment of decreased anxiety level	■ Assess vital signs. ■ Explore patient and family concerns. ■ If the patient is intubated, develop interventions for effective communication. ■ Arrange for flexible visitation to meet needs of the patient and family. ■ Provide for adequate rest and sleep. ■ Provide frequent information and updates on condition and treatment, and explain equipment. Answer all questions. ■ Consult social services and clergy as appropriate. ■ Administer sedatives and antidepressants as appropriate and monitor response.

(continued)

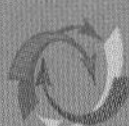

box 31-8 collaborative care guide *for the Patient With Acute Renal Failure (ARF) (Continued)*

OUTCOMES	INTERVENTIONS
Teaching/Discharge Planning	
Patient and family members will understand procedures and tests needed for treatment during the acute phase and maintenance of a patient with chronic disease. Patient and family members understand the severity of the illness, ask appropriate questions, and anticipate potential complications. In preparation for discharge to home, the patient and family members will demonstrate an understanding of renal replacement therapy, fluid and dietary restrictions, and the medication regimen.	■ Prepare the patient and his or her family members for procedures, such as insertion of dialysis access, dialysis therapy, or laboratory studies. ■ Explain the causes and effects of renal failure and the potential for complications, such as hypertension and fluid overload. ■ Encourage family members to ask questions related to the pathophysiology of renal failure, dialysis, and dietary or fluid restrictions. ■ Make appropriate referrals and consults early during hospitalization. ■ Initiate family education regarding home care of the patient on dialysis, what to expect, maintenance of renal function, and when to seek medical attention.

CHRONIC RENAL FAILURE

In chronic renal failure, fluid and salt restriction is a mainstay of therapy to prevent fluid overload. Diuretics are also used to delay the need for dialysis. Patients usually are able to respond to diuretics until they reach ESRD, at which point extensive renal damage prevents an adequate response. By the time chronic renal failure progresses to ESRD, oliguria is typically manifested and signs and symptoms of fluid overload like edema, hypertension, pulmonary edema, heart failure, and jugular vein distension occur unless dialytic therapy is instituted. In these patients, an ongoing assessment of fluid status, including obtaining accurate intake and output measurements with daily weights and monitoring for fluid complications, is imperative.

Managing Acid–Base Alterations

Acute and chronic kidney failure typically results in metabolic acidosis because of the nephrons' inability to secrete and excrete hydrogen ions and reabsorb bicarbonate ions as renal failure progresses. In critically ill patients, this acid–base disturbance may be intensified because such patients are in a high catabolic state, which increases the release of intracellular acids into the circulation. Clinical manifestations of metabolic acidosis include deep, rapid respirations (Kussmaul respirations), an altered mental status, hyperkalemia, and tachycardia. In severe metabolic acidosis, bradycardia and hypotension may manifest because of myocardial depression and vasodilation. There is also a dramatic depression of the patient's level of consciousness, often resulting in a stuporous or comatose state. A long-term consequence of metabolic acidosis, seen in patients with chronic renal failure, is bone demineralization as bone phosphate and carbonate are used as buffers against excess hydrogen ion.

Laboratory assessments of acid–base status using ABGs and venous carbon dioxide content guide therapy. Patients with a plasma bicarbonate level less than 15 mEq/L or a blood pH less than 7.3 are treated. Therapy involves the administration of alkaline medications (e.g., Shohl's solution, Bicitra, sodium bicarbonate tablets), dialysis, or both. When using citrate-containing medications, such as Bicitra or Shohl's solution, it is important that these medications not be given with aluminum-containing phosphate binders. Using these agents together would put the patient at risk for aluminum toxicity because citrate significantly increases aluminum absorption from the gastrointestinal tract.

The use of IV sodium bicarbonate is reserved for severe acidosis (evidenced by a blood pH <7.2 or a plasma bicarbonate level <12 to 14 mEq/L) because of potential complications of extracellular volume excess, metabolic alkalosis, and hypokalemia. Intractable acidosis is an indication for dialysis, which removes excess hydrogen ions and adds a buffer to the body. In hemodialysis, the buffer is bicarbonate; in peritoneal dialysis, it is lactate, which is metabolized to bicarbonate. An important caveat to keep in mind when correcting metabolic acidosis is that rapid correction can lead to acute hypocalcemia and tetany. This is because the amount of ionized calcium decreases in an alkalotic state owing to increased binding of calcium with albumin and inorganic substances such as phosphate. Throughout any kind of acid–base therapy, serum bicarbonate, pH, and calcium and potassium levels must be closely monitored.

Managing Cardiovascular Alterations

Alterations in the cardiovascular system can cause or accelerate acute and chronic renal failure. In addition, cardiovascular complications can arise as a result of renal failure. Common cardiovascular complications in acute and chronic renal failure include hypertension and hyperkalemia. Pericarditis, another cardiovascular complication of renal disease, is primarily seen with chronic renal failure.

HYPERTENSION

Hypertension as a complication of renal failure results from excess retention of water and sodium, overactivation of the sympathetic nervous system, and stimulation of the renin–angiotensin–aldosterone system. Because controlling blood pressure is essential to prevent end-organ damage and reduce the risk of life-threatening cardiovascular events, adequate treatment is essential. Management may include fluid and sodium restrictions, diuretic administration, antihypertensive therapy, and dialysis to remove excess fluid. Extensive patient teaching regarding nonpharmacological and pharmacological treatment and the potential complications of uncontrolled hypertension is an integral part of management.

HYPERKALEMIA

Hyperkalemia is a life-threatening condition seen in patients with acute and chronic renal failure. As the GFR decreases, the ability of the kidneys to excrete excess potassium diminishes. In critically ill patients, this renal impairment is frequently compounded by states of increased catabolism, acidosis, cellular injury, the administration of potassium-based medications, and blood transfusions, all of which can raise serum potassium levels. If not recognized and treated, hyperkalemia leads to fatal arrhythmias.

Assessment of hyperkalemia involves close monitoring of serum potassium levels as well as monitoring the effects of potassium on the electrical conduction system of the heart. Characteristic electrocardiogram (ECG) changes occur as potassium levels rise (Fig. 31-4). The first ECG changes that occur, usually when serum potassium is in the range of 6 to 7 mEq/L, are the appearance of tall, tented T waves and a prolonged PR interval. Next, there is a loss of the P wave and a slight widening of the QRS complex. At this point, the serum potassium is usually in the range of 8 to 9 mEq/L. From here, the QRS complex continues to widen until a sine wave (wavy line) pattern develops. This ominous sign is closely followed by ventricular fibrillation or standstill.

In evaluating hyperkalemia, it should be noted that patients with long-standing elevations in serum potassium are more refractory to its effects on the heart than patients in whom hyperkalemia develops suddenly. Thus, potassium and ECG changes must be evaluated together to determine the acuteness of the situation. Other effects of hyperkalemia that are monitored include paresthesias, hyporeflexia, and muscle weakness (which typically begins in the lower extremities and ascends to the trunk and upper extremities).

Mild hyperkalemia (a serum potassium level <6 mEq/L without ECG changes) may be treated with dietary potassium restriction, diuretics, and potassium-binding resins (e.g., sodium polystyrene sulfate). Sodium polystyrene is given orally (25 to 50 g mixed with 100 mL of 20% sorbitol) or as an enema (50 g in 50 mL of 70% sorbitol and 150 mL tap water). This drug must be used with caution in critically ill and hemodynamically unstable patients because of its association with colonic necrosis in this population.[1] Sodium polystyrene should not be used in any patient with gastrointestinal obstruction.

Treatment of life-threatening hyperkalemia entails taking steps to antagonize the effects of potassium on the heart, promote intracellular shifting of potassium, and remove potassium from the body. Antagonizing the effects of potassium on the heart is achieved with IV calcium gluconate or chloride and is the first priority for patients with substantial ECG changes. Intracellular shifting of potassium is done next to bridge the gap until potassium removal from the body can be executed. Means to shift potassium into the cell include IV insulin and dextrose administration and IV bicarbonate administration. β-Agonist therapy can also effect transcellular potassium shifting, but is impractical owing to the need to use 10 to 20 times the dose used for reactive airway disease. Removal of potassium from the body entails, as previously mentioned, diuretic administration and the use of potassium exchange resins. If these measures do not control hyperkalemia, dialysis must be initiated. Obviously, in a patient with ESRD, who is likely already receiving dialysis therapy, dialysis is initiated immediately along with other emergent therapy in life-threatening hyperkalemia.

PERICARDITIS

Pericarditis due to uremia (uremic pericarditis) is a complication seen primarily in ESRD. This type of pericarditis is characterized by aseptic inflammation of the pericardial

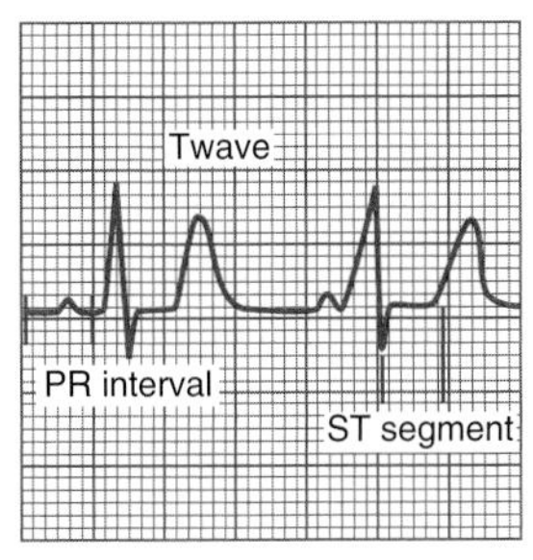

A. Peaked T waves, prolonged PR interval, depressed ST segment

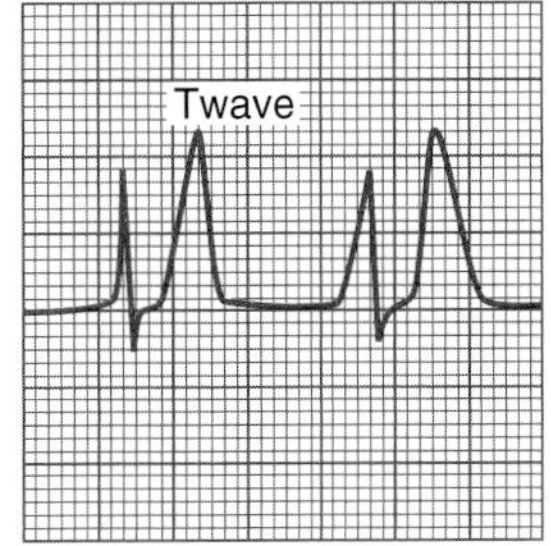

B. Lost P wave

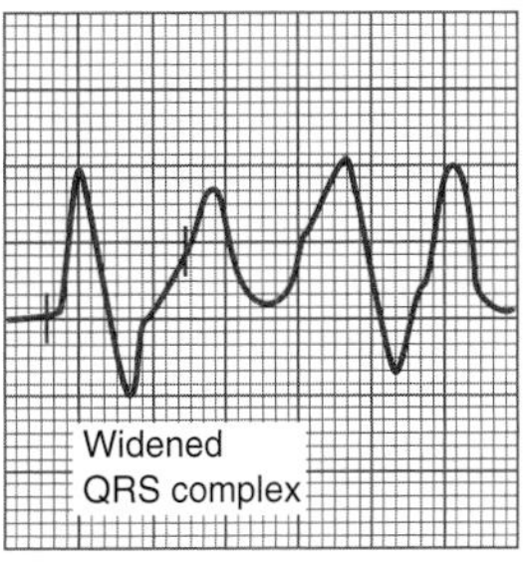

C. Widened QRS complex

figure 31-4 Typical electrocardiogram (ECG) findings indicative of various degrees of hyperkalemia. (**A**) When the serum potassium (K^+) level is about 6–7 mEq/L, the T waves become peaked, the PR interval is prolonged, and the ST segment is depressed. (**B**) At about 8–9 mEq/L, the P wave is lost. (**C**) At about 10–11 mEq/L, the QRS complex widens.

membrane, which causes the pericardial capillaries to become permeable to fluid, red blood cells, fibrinogen, and albumin. The consequent serous or serosanguineous exudate in the pericardial cavity (pericardial effusion) can increase the intrapericardial pressure and compromise ventricular contractility, stroke volume, and cardiac output. Pericardial tamponade, which results when the accumulation of exudate is so large adequate cardiac output cannot be maintained, is a life-threatening emergency. The exact etiology of uremic pericarditis is unknown, but it is associated with prolonged inadequate dialysis therapy, uremic toxins, infectious agents, and heparin administration.

Chest pain, fever, and a pericardial friction rub are the classic triad of findings associated with pericarditis. The chest pain is characteristically sharp and steady and is relieved by sitting forward and intensified by breathing deeply. A pericardial fiction rub is auscultated in 90% of symptomatic patients and is pathognomonic of acute pericarditis.[10] In addition to these findings, there are typical ECG changes in pericarditis. The most notable are widespread ST elevations with an upward concavity (versus the upward convexity typical in an acute myocardial infarction). In a large pericardial effusion, signs and symptoms are more dramatic and include dyspnea, tachycardia, mental confusion, weakness, increased jugular venous distension, peripheral edema, and a paradoxical pulse greater than 10 mm Hg during inspiration. At this point, a friction rub may or may not be heard. Tamponade, which can develop rapidly (e.g., from a major bleed into the pericardial cavity) or slowly, results in very distended neck veins, tachypnea, a narrowed pulse pressure, an increased PAWP, muffled heart sounds, diminished peripheral pulses, and a decreased level of consciousness.

Therapy for uremic pericarditis includes aggressive dialysis therapy, usually daily, until symptoms disappear. Also, because anticoagulation during dialysis may precipitate or enhance bleeding into the pericardial space, low-dose, regional, or no heparin may be prescribed. Systemic steroids and NSAIDs may also be used, but have variable results. Cardiac tamponade is an emergency that requires urgent pericardiocentesis to relieve the pressure on the heart. For the patient in whom recurrent pericarditis develops or the pericardium becomes constrictive, surgical creation of a pericardial window or pericardiectomy may be necessary.

CARDIOVASCULAR DISEASE IN CHRONIC RENAL FAILURE

Cardiac diseases are two to five times more prevalent among the ESRD population; they are the major cause of death in this population. In fact, in patients on dialysis, cardiovascular mortality is 10- to 20-fold higher than among the general population, and for patients younger than 45 years, mortality is over 100 times greater than among the general population.[14] The predominant cardiac disorders in ESRD are left ventricular hypertrophy (LVH, found in 75% of patients on dialysis), coronary artery disease (CAD), cardiomyopathy, congestive heart failure, and valvular dysfunction.

Because these disorders develop over a period of at least a few years, they usually present early in chronic renal failure and continue to progress as renal function declines. This association between renal failure and cardiovascular disease may occur because cardiovascular disease causes renal dysfunction (i.e., heart failure) or because renal failure causes an increased risk of cardiovascular disease, or because another factor (hypertension or diabetes mellitus) causes both renal dysfunction and cardiovascular disease. In any case, monitoring for cardiovascular disease, reducing modifiable risk factors, and treating specific cardiovascular conditions when present are essential to decrease ESRD mortality.

Diagnostic tests useful in assessing for cardiovascular disease in these high-risk patients include routine ECGs, echocardiography, and cardiac stress testing. Pharmacological rather than exercise stress testing is the stress test of choice because patients with chronic renal failure are often unable to attain the level of exercise needed to make exercise stress tests useful. More invasive tests for symptomatic patients include a thallium scan and coronary angiography.

Modifiable risk factors that can contribute to cardiovascular disease and that should be a central focus of management in patients with chronic renal failure include blood pressure, hypervolemia, anemia, smoking, hyperglycemia, calcium and phosphate imbalances, and metabolic acidosis. As with the general population, disease-specific treatment (e.g., antiplatelet therapy and β blocker administration for coronary artery disease) must be instituted as appropriate.

Managing Pulmonary Alterations

A frequent complication in patients with oliguric acute renal failure or ESRD is the development of pulmonary edema. This complication results from fluid overload, heart failure, or both. Clinical manifestations include dyspnea; the presence of crackles on auscultation; the production of pink, frothy sputum; tachypnea; tachycardia; decreased arterial oxygen saturation (SaO_2); and evidence of fluid overload on chest x-ray. Management involves fluid and sodium restriction, treating underlying cardiac disease, and possibly the use of diuretics if the patient's kidneys can respond to them. Frequently, pulmonary edema becomes life-threatening, necessitating intubation, emergent dialysis, or both to improve arterial oxygenation and restore fluid balance.

Other pulmonary complications in renal failure include pleural effusions, pleuritic inflammation and pain, uremic pneumonitis, and pulmonary infections. Pleuritic inflammation and uremic pneumonitis are seen more frequently with ESRD and are due to the effect of uremic toxins on the lungs and inadequate dialysis. Pulmonary infections, on the other hand, are common in both acute and chronic renal failure, especially in critically ill patients. Factors associated with renal failure that contribute to pulmonary infections include decreased pulmonary macrophage activity, a generalized immunocompromised state, tenacious sputum, and a depressed cough reflex. Collaborative management includes culturing sputum, administering broad-spectrum antibiotics until organism-specific sensitivities are available, and teaching and encouraging pulmonary toilet measures (i.e., coughing and deep breathing).

Managing Gastrointestinal Alterations

A potentially life-threatening gastrointestinal complication in both acute and chronic renal failure is gastrointestinal bleeding. Proposed etiologies for gastrointestinal bleeding as it relates to renal failure include platelet and blood-clotting abnormalities; anticoagulation use associated with dialysis, access patency, or both; ingestion of irritating drugs (e.g., NSAIDs, aspirin); and increased ammonia production in the gastrointestinal tract from urea breakdown. Ammonia is known to be irritating to mucosal surfaces. Physiological stress, especially in critically ill patients, is another proposed contributor. Assessment parameters include examining all vomitus and stool for gross and occult blood, monitoring iron, hemoglobin, hematocrit, and red blood cell indices, and paying close attention to signs of intravascular volume depletion. If gastrointestinal bleeding is suspected, radiographic and endoscopic examinations are often required to diagnose and treat specific lesions. Management depends on the specific lesion, but often includes volume restoration with crystalloids and blood products as well as the administration of histamine type 2 receptor (H_2) blockers, proton pump inhibitors, or both.

Other gastrointestinal complications associated with renal failure primarily occur in chronic renal failure and include anorexia, nausea, vomiting, diarrhea, constipation, and oral cavity alterations such as stomatitis, a metallic taste in the mouth, and fetor uremicus (the smell of urine and ammonia on the breath). Oral alterations and symptoms of anorexia, nausea, and vomiting are partially attributable to high levels of uremic toxins, which affect the intestinal mucosa and stimulate vomiting centers in the brain. Collaborative management involves initiating (or providing) adequate dialysis and administering antiemetics. Good oral hygiene is also essential.

The complication of constipation is seen frequently in patients with renal failure owing to decreased bulk and fluid in the diet and the administration of oral iron supplements and calcium-based phosphate binders. Diarrhea may also occur as a result of intestinal irritation from uremia. Collaborative management includes increasing dietary bulk; administering bulk-forming laxatives, stool softeners, or both; administering antidiarrheal agents; or a combination of these therapies. For patients with ESRD, magnesium-containing medications, including cathartics like magnesium citrate, should be avoided because of the risk of hypermagnesemia in these patients. In addition, Fleet enemas, which contain large amounts of phosphate that could be absorbed systemically, should not be used.

Managing Neuromuscular Alterations

Neuromuscular alterations include sleep disturbances, cognitive process disturbances, lethargy, muscle irritability, and peripheral neuropathies, including *restless leg syndrome* and *burning feet syndrome*. Restless leg syndrome is characterized by a discomfort in the legs, especially at night, which is sometimes relieved by continuous movement of the extremities. Burning feet syndrome consists of paresthesias and numbness in the soles of the feet and lower parts of the legs. These neuromuscular complications are associated primarily with ESRD and are thought to be the result of electrolyte imbalances, metabolic acidosis, and the effect of uremic toxins on motor and sensory nerves. Cognitive process disturbances, like a difficulty in concentrating and impaired short-term memory, are linked to elevations of BUN in the cerebral vasculature, which can result in cerebral edema. Extensive cerebral edema can result in seizures, projectile vomiting, and even coma or death.

Frequent assessments for cognitive disturbances, seizure activity, and other neuromuscular alterations are important. In addition to thorough neuromuscular examinations, nerve conduction studies and diagnostic tests, including electroencephalograms (EEGs) and head CT, may be used. Collaborative management involves implementing emergency treatment, as in the case of sustained seizure activity; maintaining electrolyte balance; correcting metabolic acidosis; using regular dialysis; and providing extensive patient teaching. Specific points that need to be included during patient teaching are the importance of preventing injury to the extremities by heat or trauma when paresthesias are present and that alterations in neuromuscular function often improve with regular dialysis or transplantation. This is qualified, however, by the fact that if components of the patient's neuropathies are due to other comorbid conditions, like diabetes, the problem may respond only minimally to dialysis or renal transplantation.

Cognitive alterations encountered are important to remember during any patient teaching. Because of difficulties in concentrating and impairments in short-term memory, teaching should be provided in short, frequent sessions with reinforcement of material and should include the family as much as possible. These points are especially true for critically ill patients who are, by definition, in a crisis situation.

Managing Hematological Alterations

Hematological system alterations are major complications in acute and chronic renal failure. These alterations include an increased bleeding tendency, an impaired immune system, and anemia.

INCREASED BLEEDING TENDENCY

The increased bleeding tendency in renal failure is attributable to a decrease in clotting factors, impaired platelet aggregation and adhesion, and prothrombin consumption. These alterations are thought to be due to uremia, but their exact pathophysiological mechanisms are unknown. Assessment involves the monitoring of platelet counts and bleeding times, coagulation studies, and assessing for bleeding, especially gastrointestinal bleeding. Collaborative management includes administering blood products as needed, protecting the patient from injury, and avoiding medications that alter platelet function, like NSAIDs and aspirin. Often heparin (for dialysis) and aspirin (for myocardial infarction prevention) are indicated in patients with renal failure. In such cases, the effects of these medications on platelets must be closely monitored. One potential and serious complication of heparin is heparin-induced thrombocytopenia; the development of this complication mandates discontinuation of the drug.

IMPAIRMENTS IN THE IMMUNE SYSTEM

Patients with renal failure are in an immunocompromised state, which sets the stage for infections (a major cause of mortality in acute and chronic renal failure). The impairments in the immune system are thought to be due to malnutrition and the effects of uremia on white blood cells. These effects include, among others, depressed T-cell– and antibody-mediated immunity, impaired phagocytosis, decreased chemotaxis of white blood cells, decreased complement proteins, and decreased bacterial opsonization.[10]

Assessing the patient for infection and monitoring laboratory indicators of infection must be done continuously. Regarding temperature as a gauge of infection, the baseline body temperature in uremic patients is decreased and thus any increase in temperature above baseline is significant. Collaborative management includes frequent handwashing, removing invasive catheters as soon as possible (or avoiding their use altogether), and obtaining cultures of blood and other body fluids that may be infected to identify specific organisms and determine appropriate antimicrobial therapy.

ANEMIA

Anemia associated with renal failure is attributable to three main mechanisms: erythropoietin deficiency, decreased red blood cell survival time, and blood loss due to an increased bleeding tendency. Of these three mechanisms, erythropoietin deficiency has the most dramatic effect.

More than 90% of the hormone erythropoietin is produced in the kidneys. It is a glycoprotein that stimulates red blood cell production in response to hypoxia and is essential to maintaining normal red blood cell counts. As kidney disease progresses and nephrons are damaged, this hormone is inadequately synthesized and a hypoproliferative anemia, resulting in normocytic normochromic red blood cells, results. Before the production of erythropoietin by human recombinant techniques, this hormone deficiency caused most patients with chronic renal failure to be in a severely anemic state, requiring frequent blood transfusions.

Decreased red blood cell survival time in renal failure occurs in the form of a mild hemolysis. The exact mechanism for this hemolysis is unclear, but it may be related to dialysis therapy or the effect of uremia on red blood cells. The average survival of red blood cells in uremia is only 70 days, which contrasts with the normal 120-day life span of a red blood cell in the general population.

In addition to the three aforementioned mechanisms of anemia, other factors can contribute to anemia in patients with renal failure, particularly those who are critically ill. Examples are malnutrition, frequent laboratory blood sampling, dialyzer malfunction and sequestration of blood in the dialyzer, and infectious states. Treating anemia in patients with renal failure is extremely important for many different reasons, including increasing the oxygen-carrying capacity of the blood, increasing intravascular volume, and preventing the negative consequences of anemia on the cardiovascular system. Concerning the cardiovascular system, anemia exacerbates myocardial, cerebral, and peripheral ischemia and increases the risk for development (or acceleration) of LVH. Correcting anemia has also been shown to have a positive impact on quality-of-life issues in patients with renal failure, including increases in appetite, energy, and work capacity.

Diagnosis of anemia entails diagnostic studies and a thorough history and physical examination. Diagnostic metabolic parameters that should be monitored include hemoglobin, hematocrit, red blood cell indices, and reticulocyte counts. In addition, the stool or vomitus should be tested for occult blood. Iron studies also need to be obtained because iron deficiency itself can cause anemia and because adequate iron stores are needed for erythropoietin to be effective. Specific iron indices that should be obtained include total serum iron, total iron-binding capacity, and serum ferritin levels. Finally, nutritional parameters and levels of folic acid, pyridoxine, and vitamin B_{12}, all of which affect red blood cell production, need to be monitored.

A thorough history and physical examination involves questioning patients about potential sites of bleeding (e.g., by asking about stool color), assessing for signs and symptoms of anemia (i.e., angina, tachycardia, skin and mucous membrane pallor, appetite suppression, weight loss, decreased energy levels, fatigue), assessing for sources of blood loss, assessing for inflammation or infection, and assessing for other diseases that can cause anemia (e.g., lupus, sickle cell anemia).

Collaborative management of anemia includes minimizing blood loss, administering oral or IV iron supplements, providing vitamin supplementation, aggressively treating infections, ensuring adequate nutrition, and administering erythropoietin, blood products, or both. Goals for iron therapy and erythropoietin administration in the ESRD population are a transferrin saturation greater than 20%, serum ferritin levels greater than 100 mg/mL, and a hemoglobin level of 11 to 12 mg/dL. These goals and guidelines to achieve them are detailed in the National Kidney Foundation Dialysis Outcomes Quality Initiative (NKF-DOQI) guidelines on anemia.[20]

Certain points regarding erythropoietin and the management of anemia deserve special mention. One is that the full effect of erythropoietin takes weeks to materialize, and hence in patients with profound anemia, blood administration is indicated. In addition, erythropoietin administration may result in an elevation of blood pressure. In some cases modification of antihypertensive therapy may be needed. When there is an inadequate response to erythropoietin despite increased dosages, reasons for erythropoietin resistance need to be explored. These include occult infections, inflammatory states, hyperparathyroidism, aluminum toxicity, malnutrition, iron deficiency, and bone marrow malignancy.

Important caveats regarding iron preparations exist as well. One is that oral iron is poorly absorbed if taken with phosphate binders, antacids, H_2-blockers, or proton pump inhibitors, all of which are commonly prescribed to patients with renal failure. On the other hand, IV iron has much better bioavailability but carries the risk of an allergic, sometimes life-threatening, reaction.

Extensive patient teaching about anemia is crucial. It should at minimum include information about medication therapy, timing of iron supplements, potential causes and signs and symptoms of worsening anemia, and information on energy conservation techniques. Information on measures to decrease bleeding, such as the use of a soft toothbrush and the avoidance of NSAIDs, is also helpful.

Managing Alterations in Drug Elimination

Because many pharmacological agents, their metabolites, or both are excreted by the kidneys, extreme caution must be used when administering medication to patients with renal failure. Depending on the patient's GFR, adjustments may need to be made in drug dosage, the interval between drug dosages, or both. Important to consider, especially in acute renal failure, is that the GRF is often unstable, and thus the GFR must be monitored frequently to dose medications accurately. As in patients without renal failure, monitoring serum levels of certain medications to be sure they are within the therapeutic range is essential. For patients receiving dialysis, the health care team must be cognizant of which drugs are dialyzed out during therapy to ensure appropriate timing of drug administration. For a listing of frequently encountered antimicrobial agents in critical care that are affected by renal failure, hemodialysis, or both, see Table 31-2.

Managing Skeletal Alterations

In renal failure, alterations in calcium and phosphate balance occur early and set the precedent for hyperparathyroidism and bone disease (renal osteodystrophy). As the GFR decreases, glomerular filtration of phosphate also decreases and serum phosphate levels begin to rise. This results in decreased serum ionized calcium levels because of binding of the calcium with the phosphate. Calcium levels also decrease owing to the failing kidneys' inability to convert vitamin D to its active form (dihydroxycholecalciferol or vitamin D_3), which is needed for adequate intestinal absorption of calcium. In response to decreased ionized calcium levels, the parathyroid glands secrete parathyroid hormone (PTH), which causes the reabsorption of calcium and phosphate salts from bones. This increases the serum calcium level but does so at the expense of bone density and mass. PTH also causes calcium reabsorption and phosphate excretion in the kidneys; however, as renal failure progresses, this effect of PTH is not realized. Eventually, as calcium and phosphate continue to be reabsorbed from bones, both levels rise in the serum concomitantly. This results in an elevation in the normal calcium–phosphate product (serum calcium multiplied by serum phosphate) of 40 mg/dL. When the product exceeds 70 mg/dL, calcium phosphate crystals can form and precipitate in various parts of the body (a condition known as *metastatic calcifications*), including the brain, eyes, gums, valves of the heart, myocardium, lungs, joints, blood vessels, and skin. Other insults to bones that can occur in renal disease include bone demineralization in response to metabolic acidosis and osteomalacia, a condition of low bone turnover. Osteomalacia is believed to be caused by aluminum deposits in the bone. The events related to bone disease in renal failure are summarized in Figure 31-5.

Complications resulting from renal bone disease include bone pain, fractures, pseudogout from deposits of calcium oxalate in synovial fluid, periarthritis from calcifications of the joints, and pruritus. Metastatic calcifications can result in calcified blood vessels and valves, skin lesions, red-eye syndrome from crystal deposition in the conjunctiva, and, most seriously, ischemic ulcers. Laboratory data, including levels of calcium, phosphate, aluminum, alkaline phosphatase (AP), intact PTH, and vitamin D_3, help make the diagnosis. Radiographic findings and bone biopsies also may be helpful.

Management involves phosphate regulation, calcium and active vitamin D (calcitriol) supplementation, prevention of aluminum toxicity, and controlling metabolic acidosis. Measures to control phosphate levels include dietary restrictions and phosphate-binding medications. Commonly used phosphate binders are calcium acetate (Phos-lo), calcium carbonate (Tums), and sevelamer hydrochloride (Renagel). Sevelamer is unique in that it is a calcium-free phosphate binder. In patients with high calcium levels it is preferred over calcium-based binders because it lessens the risk of hypercalcemia and further elevations in the calcium–phosphate product. Aluminum hydroxide binders, once a mainstay of therapy, are now infrequently used because of the effects of aluminum toxicity on the bones as well as the nervous system. Aluminum toxicity causes erythropoietin resistance as well.

Active vitamin D supplements are administered to increase serum calcium levels in hypocalcemic patients as well as to decrease PTH secretion. Besides causing a decrease in PTH indirectly through the elevation of serum calcium, active vitamin D also directly inhibits PTH secretion by binding to vitamin D receptors on the parathyroid gland. Active vitamin D may be given orally (calcitriol) or intravenously (Calcijex). In either case, caution must be exercised with the administration of these agents to avoid hypercalcemia and elevations in the calcium–phosphate product. In general, active vitamin D should be given only when the calcium–phosphate product is less than 65 mg/dL. A synthetic analog of active vitamin D that can also be used is paricalcitol (Zemplar). This drug has the advantage of causing less dramatic increases in serum calcium and phosphate levels while still causing PTH suppression. Rarely, a parathyroidectomy is indicated to treat hyperparathyroidism unresponsive to other therapies.

Patient teaching concerning bone disease and its management is complex and needs to be continually reinforced. Particular areas that should be included are the purpose and timing of medications (e.g., phosphate binders must be given with meals to be effective), dietary modifications, and the complications of untreated bone disease.

Managing Integumentary Alterations

Alterations in the integumentary system in renal failure include xerosis (dryness), pruritus, ecchymoses and purpura, and a pale bronze skin discoloration. Contributing factors to these alterations are anemia, decreased activity of sweat and sebaceous glands, retained skin pigments, abnormal blood clotting and capillary fragility, deposition of calcium phosphate crystals into the skin, hyperparathyroidism, hyperphosphatemia, and possibly increased mast cell activity and histamine secretion. Uremic frost, a white, powdery substance composed of urates on the skin, is due to crystallization of urea. It is usually seen only in severely uremic patients for whom needed dialytic therapy is being withheld. A concerning complication that can occur from these skin alterations, particularly pruritus and xerosis, is localized infection from excoriation. In addition, substantial patient discomfort and psychological disturbances from skin disfigurement may occur.

table 31-2 ■ Impact of Renal Failure and Hemodialysis on Commonly Used Antimicrobials in Critical Care

Drug	Percentage of Drug Renally Excreted	Adjustment for Renal Failure		Effect of Hemodialysis
		GFR 10–50 mL/min	*GFR <10 mL/min*	
Aminoglycosides*				
Amikacin†	95%	100% of normal dose every 24–48 hr	100% of normal dose every 48–72 hr	Dialyzed
Gentamicin†	95%	100% of normal dose every 24–48 hr	100% of normal dose every 48–72 hr	Dialyzed
Tobramycin†	95%	100% of normal dose every 24–48 hr	100% of normal dose every 48–72 hr	Dialyzed
Cephalosporins				
Cefazolin†	75%–95%	100% of normal dose every 12 hr	100% of normal dose every 24–48 hr	Dialyzed
Cefepime†	85%	100% of normal dose every 16–24 hr	100% of normal dose every 24–48 hr	Dialyzed
Cefotaxime (active metabolite in end-stage renal disease)	60%	100% of normal dose every 8–12 hr	100% of normal dose every 24 hr	Dialyzed
Cefotetan	75%	50% of normal dose	25% of normal dose	Dialyzed
Ceftazidime	60%–85%	100% of normal dose every 24–48 hr	100% of normal dose every 48 hr	Dialyzed
Ceftriaxone	30%–65%	Normal dose	Normal dose	Dialyzed
Penicillins				
Amoxicillin	50%–70%	100% of normal dose every 8–12 hr	100% of normal dose every 24 hr	Dialyzed
Ampicillin	30%–90%	100% of normal dose every 6–12 hr	100% of normal dose every 12–24 hr	Dialyzed
Mezlocillin	65%	100% of normal dose every 6–8 hr	100% of normal dose every 8 hr	Not dialyzed
Nafcillin	35%	Normal dose	Normal dose	Not dialyzed
Penicillin G	60%–85%	75% of normal dose	20%–50% of normal dose	Dialyzed
Piperacillin	75%–90%	100% of normal dose every 6–8 hr	100% of normal dose every 8 hr	Dialyzed
Ticarcillin†	85%	1–2 g every 8 hr	1–2 g every 12 hr	Dialyzed
Quinolones				
Ciprofloxacin	50%–70%	50%–75% of normal dose	50% of normal dose	Slightly dialyzed
Levofloxacin	67%–87%	250 mg every 24–48 hr (500-mg initial dose)	250 mg every 48 hr (500-mg initial dose)	No data
Tetracyclines				
Doxycycline	35%–45%	Normal dose	Normal dose	Not dialyzed
Tetracycline†	48%–60%	100% of normal dose every 12–24 hr	100% of normal dose every 24 hr	Not dialyzed
Miscellaneous Antibacterials				
Azithromycin	6%–12%	Normal dose	Normal dose	Not dialyzed
Aztreonam	75%	50%–75% of normal dose	25% of normal dose	Moderately dialyzed
Clarithromycin	15%–25%	75% of normal dose	50%–75% of normal dose	No data; give after dialysis

(continued)

table 31-2 ■ Impact of Renal Failure and Hemodialysis on Commonly Used Antimicrobials in Critical Care (Continued)

Drug	Percentage of Drug Renally Excreted	Adjustment for Renal Failure		Effect of Hemodialysis
		GFR 10–50 mL/min	*GFR <10 mL/min*	
Erythromycin	15%	Normal dose	50%–75% of normal dose	Not dialyzed
Imipenem	20%–70%	50% of normal dose	25% of normal dose	Dialyzed
Metronidazole	20%	Normal dose	50% of normal dose	Dialyzed
Sulfamethoxazole	70%	100% of normal dose every 18 hr	100% of normal dose every 24 hr	Dialyzed
Trimethoprim	40%–70%	100% of normal dose every 18 hr	100% of normal dose every 24 hr	Dialyzed
Vancomycin[†]	90%–100%	1.0 g every 24–96 hr	1.0 g every 4–7 days	Not dialyzed
Antifungals				
Amphotericin B	5%–10%	Normal dose	100% of normal dose every 24–36 hr	Not dialyzed
Fluconazole	70%	Normal dose	Normal dose	Dialyzed
Ketoconazole	13%	Normal dose	Normal dose	Not dialyzed
Antivirals				
Acyclovir	40%–75%	100% of normal dose every 12–24 hr	50% of normal dose every 24 hr	Dialyzed
Ganciclovir	90%–100%	100% of normal dose every 24–48 hr	100% of normal dose every 48–96 hr	Dialyzed
Antituberculars				
Amantadine[†]	90%	100% of normal dose every 48–72 hr	100% of normal dose every 7 days	Not dialyzed
Ethambutol	75%–90%	100% of normal dose every 24–36 hr	100% of normal dose every 48 hr	Dialyzed
Isoniazid	5%–30%	Normal dose	Normal dose	Dialyzed
Rifampin	15%–30%	50%–100% of normal dose	50%–100% of normal dose	Not dialyzed

GFR, glomerular filtration rate.
*Aminoglycosides are nephrotoxic and ototoxic and have a narrow therapeutic window. Serum levels must be monitored frequently for efficacy and toxicity.
[†]These drugs require adjustment in dose, frequency, or both when a patient's GFR is more than 50 mL/min as well.
Modified from Aronoff G, Berns J, Brier M, et al: Drug Prescribing in Renal Failure (4th Ed). Philadelphia, American College of Physicians, 1999.

Collaborative management for skin alterations includes phosphate regulation, active vitamin D administration, correction of anemia, antihistamine medications, and meticulous skin care and turning to prevent skin breakdown. Dialysis therapy helps as well by removing metabolic waste products. However, because of potential allergies to the dialysis system components, dialysis therapy can also aggravate some conditions like pruritus. Patient education should include information on factors contributing to skin alterations, the importance of keeping the skin clean and well moisturized, and ways to avoid excoriation (such as keeping the fingernails trimmed).

Managing Alterations in Dietary Intake

The goals of nutritional therapy in renal failure are to minimize uremic symptoms; reduce the incidence of fluid, electrolyte, and acid–base imbalances; minimize symptoms of anemia; decrease the patient's vulnerability to infections; and limit catabolism. Dietary restrictions related to managing comorbid conditions and reducing cardiovascular risk also need to be considered. Because of the complexity of achieving a nutritional therapy plan that meets these goals, a collaborative health care team approach, including the ongoing participation of a dietitian, is essential. This is particularly the case in critical care, where patients usually are in a catabolic state and are at risk for substantial malnutrition.

Renal diet prescriptions include restrictions in fluid, sodium, potassium, and phosphate intake and may include supplementations of iron, vitamins, and calcium. Calorically, critically ill patients with renal disease need a high-calorie diet with a total of 30 to 44 kcal/kg/day, most of which should come from a combination of carbohydrates and lipids. In addition, amino acids, both essential and nonessential, must be administered to minimize catabolism. Protein restriction to decrease symptoms of uremia and slow the progression of renal failure is controversial (refer to the section on preventing the progression of chronic renal failure), but may be beneficial. Protein restriction should never, however, compromise meeting anabolic goals, which would expose the patient to the risk of malnutrition. Usually, moderate protein restriction of 0.8 g/kg/day in patients not receiving dialysis and up to 1.5 g/kg/day in patients on dialysis is prescribed. In crit-

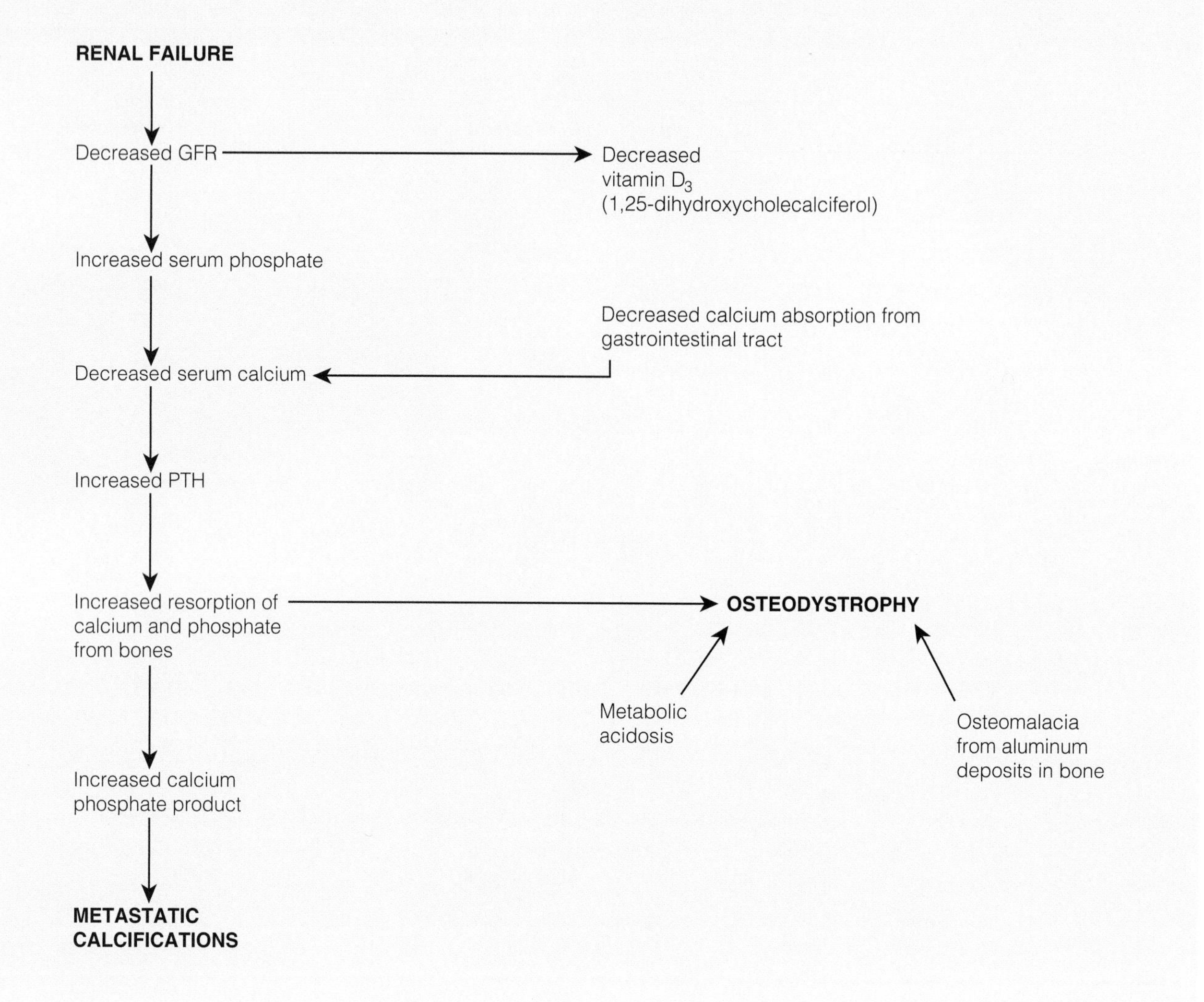

figure 31-5 Effects of renal failure on the skeletal system.

ically ill patients, parenteral nutrition may need to be instituted because of impaired bowel function or severe malnutrition. In oliguric patients, the high hourly volume requirements needed for parenteral nutrition often must be offset by dialysis or isolated hemofiltration.

To determine the effectiveness of nutritional therapy, continual laboratory monitoring of serum protein, albumin and prealbumin, electrolytes, hemoglobin, hematocrit, and urea levels is essential. Patient weight, volume status, and energy levels are additional monitoring parameters. Nutritional education, including information on dietary restrictions, the use and timing of phosphate binders, vitamin and mineral supplements, and measures of nutritional status should be provided.

Managing Alterations in Psychosocial Functioning

Patients in acute and chronic renal failure often experience feelings of fear, anxiety, and powerlessness. In addition, patients frequently have an alteration in self-concept as well as body image disturbances because of both physical and functional changes that occur in renal failure. Patients and their families may have difficulty coping owing to stress, limited resources or support, inadequate or ineffective coping mechanisms, interruptions in usual family roles, or a combination of these factors. It is important that the health care team attend to these and other psychosocial complications of renal failure to treat the patient and family holistically. Specific interventions include thorough patient and family teaching, active involvement of the patient and his or her family members in the management of the condition, provision of adequate rest and sleep to the patient, exploring the patient's and family's feelings and concerns, providing support, and obtaining the active involvement of social services and clergy as appropriate. Considerations for discharge planning are given in Box 31-9.

case study ■ ACUTE RENAL FAILURE

Mr. Burns, a 66-year-old African-American man with known heart failure, presented to the emergency department (ED) with severe dyspnea and mild chest discomfort.

box 31-9 *Acute Renal Failure*

- Explain the pathophysiology of acute renal failure in understandable terms. Use appropriate teaching aids (e.g., pictures, kidney models).
- Explain the etiology of acute renal failure and ways to decrease risk of further or future kidney damage, including control of hypertension, strict control of blood glucose levels (in patients with diabetes), the maintenance of normal serum lipid levels, and the avoidance of nephrotoxins.
- Explain the level of renal function the patient can expect to have after the acute phase is over.
- Explain and provide written guidelines on diet and fluid restrictions. Teach the patient how to reduce thirst (e.g., by sucking on sour, hard candy) and stress that any substance that is liquid at room temperature counts as fluid intake.
- Demonstrate how to check blood pressure, pulse, respirations, and weight. Teach the patient about the importance of weighing himself or herself at the same time, on the same scale, and with similar amounts of clothing to monitor weight accurately.
- Provide instruction on how to monitor for and avoid infections. Instruct the patient to report any occurrence of an infection to a health care professional.
- Describe the purpose, action, and adverse effects of medications. Point out when medications need to be taken (e.g., phosphate binders are taken with meals) and what medications should not be taken together.
- Explain the importance of rest during the recovery phase; assist the patient in planning for exercise as tolerated.
- Teach the patient ways to minimize the risk of bleeding.
- Explain the purpose of dialysis and the importance of regular treatments.
- Explain the need for ongoing follow-up with health care professionals.

An initial physical examination was significant for extra heart sounds (S_3 and S_4); bilateral crackles in the lower half of his lung fields; labored, tachypneic breathing; and a functional oxygen saturation (SpO_2) of 89% on room air. The patient's skin was cool and dry, and he had +2 lower extremity edema. His ECG showed normal sinus rhythm with ST depressions in V_1 to V_4. Laboratory data revealed normal cardiac enzyme values and the following serum chemistries: sodium 136 mEq/L; chloride 91 mEq/L; carbon dioxide 21 mEq/L; creatinine 1.2 mg/dL; BUN 15 mg/dL. A Foley catheter was inserted, and 40 mL of dark amber urine was obtained and sent for urinalysis, which came back negative.

After being placed on 4 L oxygen by nasal cannula and given IV furosemide, the patient was admitted to the cardiovascular intensive care unit (CVICU). During his first day in the CVICU, the patient became increasingly dyspneic and hypoxemic and eventually required oral intubation to stabilize his arterial oxygen saturation (SaO_2). A pulmonary artery catheter was placed and the following initial readings were recorded: central venous pressure (CVP) 15 mm Hg (normal = 0 to 8 mm Hg); pulmonary artery wedge pressure (PAWP) 29 mm Hg (normal = 8 to 12 mm Hg); and cardiac output 2.5 L/minute (normal = 2.5 to 4.5 L/minute). The patient's PAWP remained high throughout the day despite frequent administration of IV furosemide (in response to which he put out only 800 mL of urine throughout the day) and being placed on a dobutamine drip. His total fluid intake that day was 2400 mL. That night, his temperature rose to 101.3°F (38.5°C). A pan-culture was ordered, and the patient was started on gentamicin and cefotaxime.

On the patient's second day in the CVICU, he went into ventricular fibrillation, which converted to normal sinus rhythm with a systolic blood pressure of 60 mm Hg after three consecutive defibrillations. He subsequently needed both dobutamine and norepinephrine (Levophed) to maintain a mean arterial pressure of 65 mm Hg. He continued to receive IV furosemide to maintain a urine output of 40 mL/hour. By day 3, the patient had gained 3 kg since admission and had course crackles throughout his lung fields. His PAWP was 22 mm Hg and his urine output was 20 mL/hour. Furosemide administration was discontinued owing to lack of response. Bloodwork revealed the following: sodium 130 mEq/L; potassium 5.0 mEq/L; chloride 90 mEq/L; carbon dioxide 21 mEq/L; creatinine 5.4 mg/dL; BUN 58 mg/dL; calcium 7.8 mg/dL; phosphate 6.0 mg/dL. The results of urinalysis were as follows: sodium 63 mEq/L; osmolality 372 mOsm/kg H_2O; specific gravity 1.008; FE_{Na} 5.2%; granular sediment with tubular epithelial cells.

In light of these laboratory findings, the patient's worsening fluid overload, and his hemodynamic instability, Mr. Burns was started on continuous renal replacement therapy (CRRT). In addition, adjustments were made in the dosing of his prescribed pharmacological agents based on his GFR. On CRRT, he was able to remove 2 L of fluid in 24 hours and his PAWP decreased to 14 mm Hg. By day 4, his oxygenation had improved and he no longer needed norepinephrine to maintain an adequate blood pressure. Unfortunately, on day 5, ventricular fibrillation developed once again, and Mr. Burns was pronounced dead after 45 minutes of cardiac life support. ■

CASE ANALYSIS

Mr. Burns' acute renal failure, as evidenced by his more-than-doubling serum creatinine value from admission, was the result of inadequate renal perfusion due to cardiogenic shock. Inadequate renal perfusion is a cause of prerenal acute renal failure, but if sustained long enough, can lead to ATN. The high urine sodium concentration and FE_{Na} indicate that Mr. Burns' kidneys are no longer able to reabsorb sodium and water appropriately given his hypoperfused state. The inability of his kidneys to reabsorb water appropriately is also shown by his urine osmolality and specific gravity. If his kidneys were able to reabsorb water and concentrate his urine, these values would be much higher. Finally, renal tubular damage is indicated by his urinary sediment findings. All these laboratory tests show the inadequate perfusion to his kidneys was sustained long enough for ATN to develop.

clinical applicability challenges

Self-Challenge: Critical Thinking

1. *Develop a collaborative care plan that could have been used for Mr. Burns.*
2. *Role-play an interaction with Mr. Burns' spouse, who wants to know "why his kidneys stopped working."*
3. *Suppose that Mr. Burns had lived, but needed ongoing renal replacement therapy to sustain his life (i.e., he was in ESRD). Develop a teaching plan for him regarding his fluid restrictions.*

Study Questions

1. *Two major causes of intrarenal acute renal failure are*
   a. *dehydration and increased cardiac output.*
   b. *calculi in the ureters and hypovolemic shock.*
   c. *aminoglycoside antibiotics and radiocontrast dye administration.*
   d. *an obstructed Foley catheter and benign prostatic hypertrophy.*
2. *During which phase of acute tubular necrosis (ATN) are hyperkalemia, gastrointestinal bleeding, infection, and vascular volume overload major potential problems?*
   a. *Onset phase*
   b. *Oliguric phase*
   c. *Diuretic phase*
   d. *Recovery phase*
3. *A laboratory finding indicative of prerenal acute renal failure is*
   a. *a fractional excretion of sodium (FE_{Na}) less than 1%.*
   b. *a blood urea nitrogen:serum creatinine ratio (BUN:Cr) greater than 20:1.*
   c. *normal urinary sediment.*
   d. *all of the above.*
4. *Which of the following statements is true about chronic renal failure?*
   a. *Sometimes it is reversible.*
   b. *Hypertension is the most common cause.*
   c. *Ultimately, it leads to end-stage renal disease (ESRD).*
   d. *It has a sudden onset.*
5. *The causes of metabolic acidosis in renal failure include*
   a. *increased renal secretion and excretion of hydrogen ions.*
   b. *decreased reabsorption of bicarbonate.*
   c. *increased exhalation of carbon dioxide.*
   d. *a decrease in catabolism.*
6. *The purpose of administering hypertonic glucose and insulin when treating hyperkalemia is to*
   a. *promote diuresis and renal clearance of potassium.*
   b. *antagonize the effects of excess potassium ions on the electrical conduction system of the heart.*
   c. *promote the shift of potassium from the extracellular fluid to the intracellular fluid.*
   d. *exchange sodium for potassium ions in the intestine.*
7. *Decreased erythropoietin production in renal failure results in*
   a. *decreased red blood cell survival.*
   b. *impaired white blood cell function.*
   c. *decreased red blood cell production.*
   d. *an inability of platelets to function properly.*

REFERENCES

1. Albright R: Acute renal failure: A practical update. Mayo Clin Proc 76(1):67–74, 2001
2. Mindell J, Chertow G: A practical approach to acute renal failure. Med Clin North Am 81(3):731–748, 1997
3. Agrawal M, Swartz R: Acute renal failure. Am Fam Physician 61(7):2077–2088, 2000
4. DuBose T, Warnock D, Mehta R, et al: Acute renal failure in the 21st century: Recommendations for management and outcomes assessment. Am J Kidney Dis 29(5):793–799, 1997
5. Edelstein C, Ling H, Wangsiripaisan A, et al: Emerging therapies for acute renal failure. Am J Kidney Dis 30(5):S89–S95, 1997
6. Tepel M, van der Giet M, Schwarzfeld C, et al: Prevention of radiographic-contrast-agent-induced reductions in renal function by acetylcysteine. N Engl J Med 343(3):180–184, 2000
7. Barretti P, Soares V: Acute renal failure: Clinical outcome and causes of death. Ren Fail 19(2):253–257, 1997
8. Parker R, Himmelfarb J, Tolkoff-Rubin N, et al: Prognosis of patients with acute renal failure requiring dialysis: Results of a multicenter study. Am J Kidney Dis 32(3):432–443, 1998
9. Johnson J, Johnston J, Flick R, et al: Acute renal failure in recipients of organ transplantation and nontransplantation patients: Comparison of characteristics and mortality. Ren Fail 19(3):461–473, 1997
10. Lancaster L (ed): Core Curriculum for Nephrology Nursing (4th Ed). Pitman, NJ, AJ Jannetti, 2001
11. Davison A: Renal disease in the elderly. Nephron 80:6–16, 1998
12. Bevan M: The older person with renal failure. Nurs Standard 14(33):48–54, 2000
13. Brown W, Schmitz P: Acute and chronic kidney disease. Clin Geriatr Med 14(2):211–236, 1998
14. United States Renal Data System: USRDS 2001 Annual Data Report. Bethesda, MD, National Institutes of Health, National Institute of Diabetes and Digestive and Kidney Diseases, 2001
15. Malhotra D, Tzamaloukas A: Nondialysis management of chronic renal failure. Med Clin North Am 81(3):749–766, 1997
16. The Diabetes Control and Complications Trial Research Group: The effect of intensive treatment of diabetes on the development and progression of long-term complications in insulin-dependent diabetes mellitus. N Engl J Med 329(14):977–986, 1993
17. Parving H, Lehnert H, Brochner-Mortensen J, et al: The effect of irbesartan on the development of diabetic nephropathy in patients with type 2 diabetes. N Engl J Med 345(12):870–878, 2001
18. Lewis E, Hunsicker L, Clarke W, et al: Renoprotective effect of the angiotensin-receptor antagonist irbesartan in patients with nephropathy due to type 2 diabetes. N Engl J Med 345(12):851–860, 2001
19. Balinsky W: Pediatric end-stage renal disease: Incidence, management and prevention. J Pediatr Health Care 14(6):304–308, 2000
20. National Kidney Foundation: NKF-DOQI clinical practice guidelines for the treatment of anemia of chronic renal failure. Am J Kidney Dis 30(Suppl 3):S192–S240, 1997

OTHER SELECTED READING

Baer C: Care of the critically ill chronic renal failure patient: Crises, challenges, and choices. Crit Care Nurs Clin North Am 10(4):433–448, 1998

Baigent C, Burbury K, Wheeler D: Premature cardiovascular disease in chronic renal failure. Lancet 356:147–152, 2000

Biddle G, Firanek C, Brouwer D, et al: Highlights for nephrology nurses from the updated NKF-K/DOQI guidelines. Nephrol Nurs J 28(1):45–50, 2001

Daugirdas J, Blake P, Ing T: Handbook of Dialysis (3rd Ed). Boston, Little, Brown, 2001

Haney S: Drug use in renal failure. Crit Care Nurs Clin North Am 14(1):77–80, 2002

Kohli H, Bhaskaran M, Muthukumar T, et al: Treatment-related acute renal failure in the elderly: A hospital-based prospective study. Nephrol Dial Transplant 15(2):212–217, 2000

Lancaster L (ed): Core Curriculum for Nephrology Nursing (4th Ed). Pitman, NJ, AJ Jannetti, 2001

Zakynthinos E, Theodorakopoulou M, Konstaninidis K, Zakynthinos S: Hemorrhagic cardiac tamponade in critically ill patients with acute renal failure. Heart Lung, 33(1):55–60, 2004

PART
one
two
three
four
five
six
seven
eight
nine
ten
eleven
twelve

Nervous System

INTERNET RESOURCES

Topic	Web Page Address
American Academy of Physical Medicine and Rehabilitation	www.aapmr.org
American Association of Neuroscience Nurses	www.aann.org
American Association of Spinal Cord Injury Nurses	www.aascin.org
American Spinal Injury Association	www.asia-spinalinjury.org
Brain Injury Association of America	www.biausa.org
Brain Injury Resource Center	www.headinjury.com
Brain Trauma Foundation	www.braintrauma.org
British Trauma Society	www.trauma.org
The Center for Neuro Skills: Traumatic Brain Injury Resource Guide	www.neuroskills.com
Center for Paralysis Research	www.vet.purdue.edu/cpr
Guillain-Barré Syndrome Foundation International	www.guillain-barre.com
The International Brain Injury Association	www.internationalbrain.org
International Spinal Development & Research Foundation	www.spine-research.org
Miami Project to Cure Paralysis	www.miamiproject.med.miami.edu
Myasthenia Gravis Foundation of America	www.myasthenia.org
National Institute of Neurological Disorders and Stroke	www.ninds.nih.gov
National Spinal Cord Injury Association	www.spinalcord.org
National Stroke Association	www.stroke.org
NeuroLand	www.NeuroLand.com
Paralyzed Veterans of America	www.pva.org
The Perspectives Network	www.tbi.org
Society of Trauma Nurses	www.traumanursesoc.org
Spinal Cord Injury Network	www.spinalcordinjury.net
The Spinal Cord Injury Resource Center	www.spinalinjury.net
Spinal Cord Society	http://members.aol.com/scsweb

chapter

32

Anatomy and Physiology of the Nervous System

MARY CIECHANOWSKI ■ DONNA MOWER-WADE ■
SANDRA W. MCLESKEY ■ LOUIS STOUT

objectives

Based on the content in this chapter, the reader should be able to:

- Describe the cellular units of the nervous system.
- Briefly explain the physiology of a nerve impulse.
- Discuss two functions of cerebrospinal fluid.
- Explain the functions of the thalamus.
- Define the reticular activating system.
- Briefly define the sensory system and the motor system.
- List three spinal cord reflexes and explain the baroreceptor reflex.
- Explain the anatomy and physiology of pain and the gate theory of pain regulation.
- Explain the concept of homeostasis.
- Explain the acute stress response.
- Explain why the stress response could be helpful or harmful, depending on the situation

We now know that the brain is a central organ that coordinates activity of most, if not all, body systems through its influence on the endocrine and immune systems as well as its more generally appreciated influence on skeletal muscle and autonomic function. Its influence is modulated by sensory perceptions that convey a picture of the external and internal environments, and also by internal circuits having to do with emotional state and levels of arousal. Therefore, the brain can be thought of as the integrative organ that drives our responses to environmental influence. Moreover, separation of the brain and spinal cord from the periphery is more anatomical than conceptual, and modern nurses must always keep in mind that the brain has a profound influence on almost everything that happens in the periphery, and vice versa.

Traditionally, the nervous system is discussed with reference to both anatomical and functional divisions. Anatomical components are the central nervous system (CNS), comprising the brain and spinal cord, and the peripheral nervous system (PNS), comprising the cranial and spinal nerves. The nervous system is functionally separated into the sensory, integrative, and motor (somatic and autonomic) divisions. Content in this chapter is ordered according to both divisions. First, however, cell anatomy and physiology are discussed.

CELLS OF THE NERVOUS SYSTEM

The cellular units are the *neuron*—the basic functional unit—and its attendant cells, the *neuroglia*.

Neuroglia

Neuroglia constitute the supportive tissue associated with the neurons. In the CNS, there are three types of neuroglia: microglia, astrocytes, and oligodendroglia. The oligodendroglia produce the myelin that covers nerve fibers in the CNS. In the PNS, the counterpart of the myelin-producing oligodendroglial cell is the Schwann cell.

Under most circumstances, neurons lose their ability to undergo mitosis early in the life of the individual. However, neuroglia retain mitotic abilities throughout a person's life span. Because of this, malignant or benign proliferative lesions originating in the CNS involve neuroglia rather than neurons. As the neuroglial tumor enlarges, however, it adversely affects adjacent neurons—early by exerting pressure, and later by promoting an inflammatory reaction along with the pressure.

Neurons

The basic functional unit of the nervous system is the neuron (or *nerve cell*), and all information and activity, whether sensory, motor, or both, is accomplished by neurons. The neuron consists of a nerve cell body or *soma* that contains nuclear and cytoplasmic material and processes, either axons or dendrites, that arise from the soma (Fig. 32-1). *Axons* normally carry nerve impulses away from the cell body, whereas *dendrites* conduct impulses toward the cell body. Axons and dendrites may be merely microscopic knobs or areas on the cell body surface, or they may be cylindrical processes that can extend to over 1 m (3¼ ft) in length. A specialized structure at the end of the axon is called the *axon terminal*. This is a bulbous ending (sometimes called a *bouton*) that forms a synapse with another neuron. The axon terminal contains vesicles of neurotransmitter that are released into the synapse, diffuse across to the postsynaptic neuron, and bind to specific receptors on the membrane of the postsynaptic cell. Binding of a particular neurotransmitter to its specific receptor on the postsynaptic neuron either depolarizes or hyperpolarizes the postsynaptic neuron in the area of the synapse. Axons and dendrites are referred to collectively as *nerve fibers*. A bundle of nerve fibers together with their coverings is called a *tract* in the CNS and a *nerve* in the periphery.

Some nerve fibers are covered with a lipid–protein sheath termed the *myelin sheath*, which appears to be formed in the CNS by the oligodendrocytes. Other fibers remain unmyelinated. All nerve fibers in the PNS are covered by a *neurilemma*. This is a sheath formed by the Schwann cells, which wrap themselves around the fiber. Some Schwann cells around particular fibers secrete myelin; others do not (see Fig. 32-1). The neurilemma of a myelinated fiber comes in contact with the axon at periodic intervals. These periodic constrictions of the neurilemmal sheath are termed the *nodes of Ranvier*. The nodes of Ranvier produce faster nerve impulse conduction by allowing the impulse to jump from one node to the next (saltatory conduction).

Neurons are very diverse, with many specialized anatomical features that are important to their function. Some neurons are extremely large or may give rise to extremely long nerve fibers. Transmission velocities in long, myelinated fibers may be as high as 100 m/second, whereas unmyelinated neurons with very short, unmyelinated processes demonstrate velocities of 1 m/second. Some neurons connect to many different neurons, perhaps thousands of other neurons, in a "network," whereas others have relatively few connections to other cells of the nervous system.

It has been estimated that there are 12 billion neurons in the human CNS. Three-fourths of these neurons are located in the cerebral cortex, where conscious thought and feeling reside, as well integrative processing and smoothing of planned motor movements. This processing includes not only the determination of appropriate and effective responses, but the storage of memory and the development of associative motor and thought patterns.

CHARACTERISTICS OF NEURONS

Resting Membrane Potential

As is true of all cells, the neuronal cell membrane contains sodium–potassium pumps that keep the inside of the neuron more negatively charged than the outside interstitial fluid. The cytoplasm of all cells contains anions (negatively charged ions) that are too large to leave the cell. Many ions, including sodium, potassium, and chloride, are small enough to diffuse through tiny pores in the cell membrane. If it were not for the sodium–potassium pump, the concentrations of these ions would be equal on the inside of the cell compared with the outside. However, the sodium–potassium pump in the cell membrane pumps sodium ions out of the cell almost as fast as they enter. For every two sodium ions that are pumped out, one potassium ion is pumped into the cell. Because of this, there is a net positive charge leaving the cell and the large anions cannot be counterbalanced. Thus, under resting conditions when no impulse is being conducted, the inside of the neuron is negative with respect to the outside as long as the sodium–potassium pumps are operating. This internal relative negativity is the *resting membrane potential* of the neuron and typically measures about −85 mV.

In addition, as a result of activity of the sodium–potassium pump, sodium ion concentration inside the cell is much lower than outside, and potassium ion concentration is much higher inside the cell than outside. These

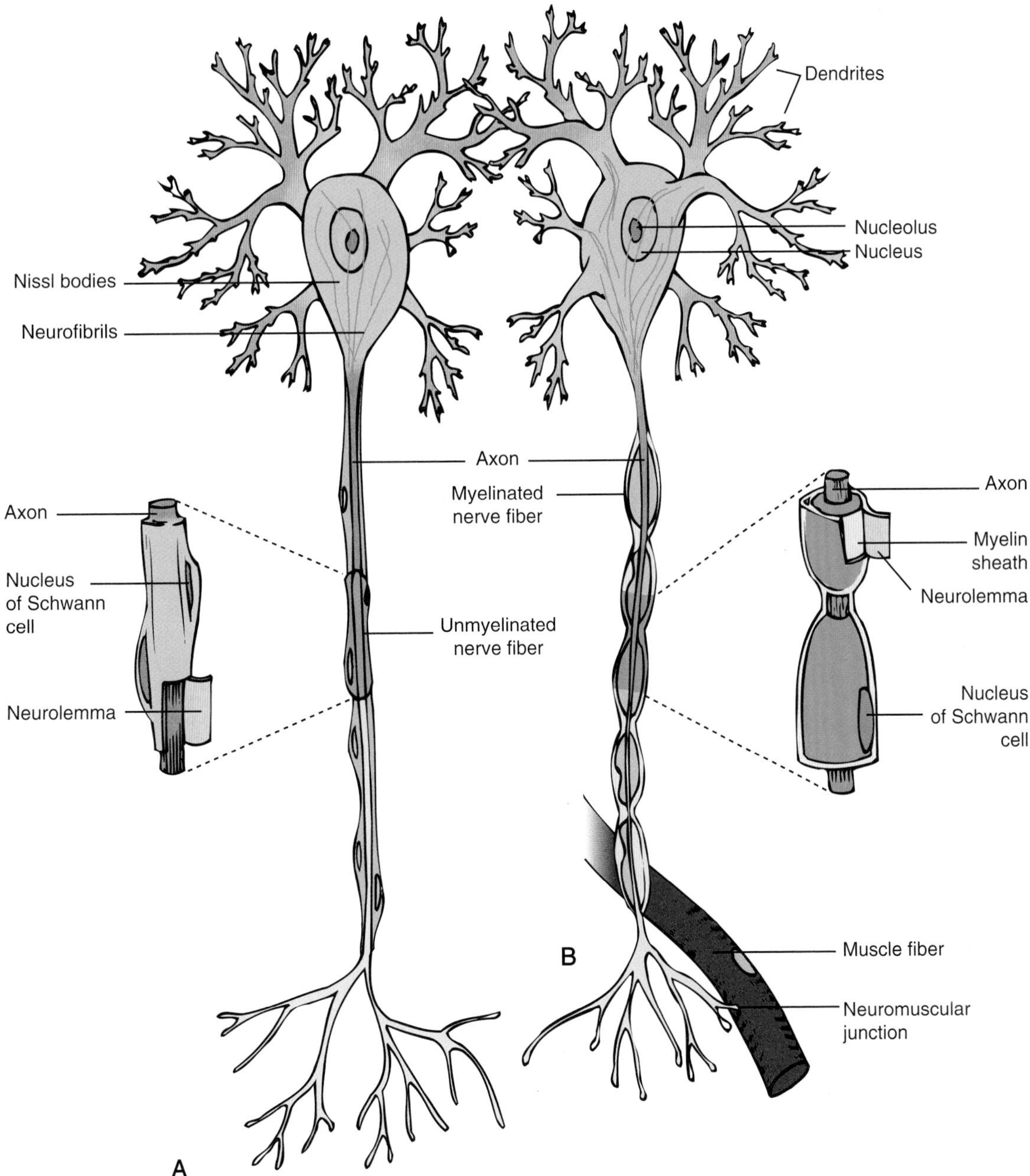

figure 32-1 Typical efferent neurons. (**A**) Unmyelinated fiber. (**B**) Myelinated fiber.

concentration gradients are important for depolarization produced by synaptic transmission and also for conduction of the action potential down the axon (Fig. 32-2).

Synaptic Transmission

Submicroscopic spaces between the axon (or axons) of one neuron and the dendrite (or dendrites) or soma of another are called *synapses*. Axons or dendrites may branch, enabling the axon of one neuron to synapse with dendrites or somas of several neurons. Typically, axons from many neurons synapse with the dendrite(s) or soma of a single neuron. A synapse consists of a presynaptic axon terminal, a postsynaptic neuron, and the small (150 to 1000 Å) space between elements called a *synaptic cleft* (Fig. 32-3A). When an action potential is conducted down the presynaptic axon and depolarizes the axon terminal, vesicles of neurotransmitter are released into the synaptic cleft, diffuse across the cleft, and bind to specific receptors on the postsynaptic cell membrane. The binding of neurotransmitter to its receptor causes a change in the membrane potential of the postsynaptic cell, either a depolarization or a hyperpolarization.

In an extremely short time (millionths of a second), the neurotransmitter detaches from the receptor site. It may then reattach or be inactivated. Inactivation occurs in two basic ways, depending on the neurotransmitter. For example, the catecholamine neurotransmitters and serotonin are taken back into the axon terminal by specific reuptake

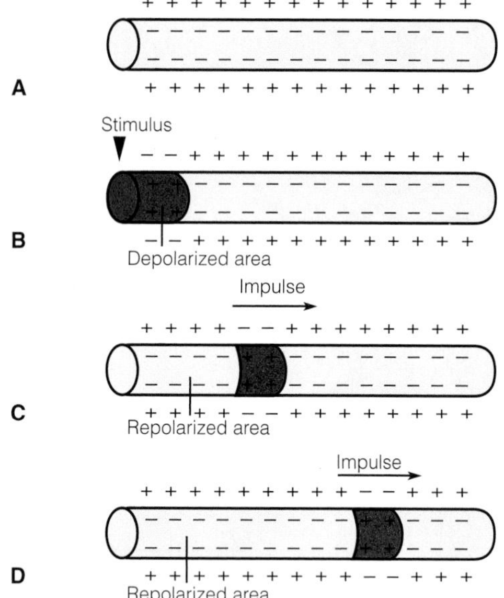

figure 32-2 Propagation of impulses. (**A**) Resting membrane. (**B**) Action potential, first stage: stimulation of fiber results in depolarization. (**C**) Action potential, second stage: repolarization occurs as the resting potential is restored. (**D**) Propagation of impulses continues in direction of arrow.

pumps, and repackaged in vesicles to be reused. In contrast, acetylcholine is destroyed by an enzyme, acetylcholinesterase, present in the synaptic cleft. In either case, the neurotransmitter is available to bind to its receptors on the postsynaptic membrane only for a very short time. For activity of the neural pathway to continue, rapid, repetitive, discrete stimulation of neurons is necessary. In this way, neural pathways can be stimulated over prolonged periods by repeated depolarizations of presynaptic neurons, or activity of a specific pathway can be turned on or off almost instantaneously.

From the preceding discussion, it can be seen that synaptic transmission is a one-way street—from the axon across the synaptic cleft to the dendrite or soma of the next neuron. It cannot proceed in the opposite direction. It also can be seen that decreased destruction or decreased reuptake of a transmitter can increase the effect of this transmitter on the postsynaptic membrane. Similarly, increased destruction or increased reuptake of a transmitter reduces its postsynaptic effects. Several classes of pharmacological agents take advantage of these facts. For instance, acetylcholinesterase inhibitors such as neostigmine are used to increase the amount of acetylcholine remaining in the synapse of the neuromuscular junction to counteract the effects of paralytic drugs given during anesthesia. Serotonin

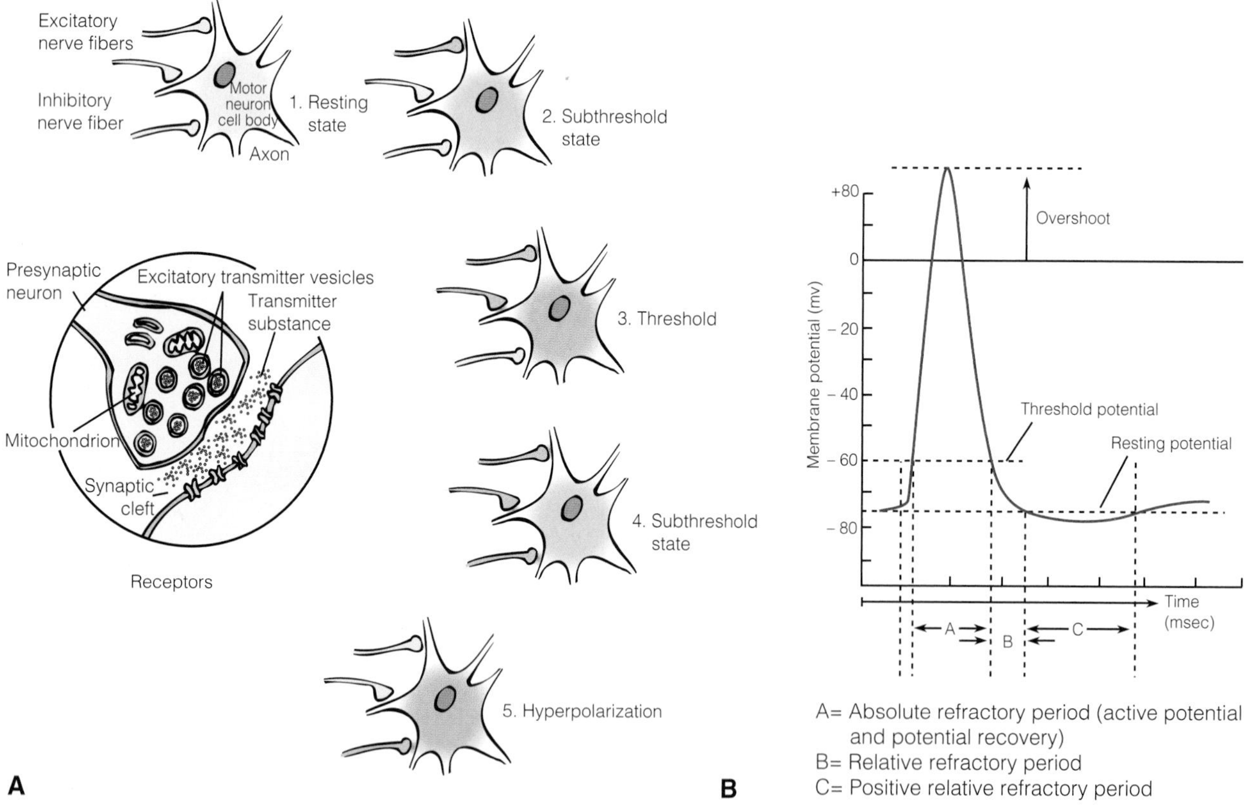

figure 32-3 Conduction at synapses. (**A**) A neuron may be excited or inhibited by transmitter substances liberated by presynaptic nerve fiber endings. Two excitatory and one inhibitory fiber are shown. (*1*) During the resting state, no impulses are received. (*2*) During the subthreshold state, impulses from only one excitatory fiber cannot cause the postsynaptic neuron to mount an action potential. (*3*) The threshold is reached by the addition of impulses from a second excitatory fiber. This enables the postsynaptic neuron to mount an action potential. (*4*) The subthreshold state is restored by impulses from an inhibitory fiber. (*5*) When the inhibitory fiber alone is carrying impulses, the postsynaptic neuron is in a state of hyperpolarization and is unable to fire. (**B**) The time course of a neural action potential.

or norepinephrine reuptake pump inhibitors increase the amount of serotonin or norepinephrine in the synapse and have therapeutic effects in depressed patients.

Each neuron synthesizes and stores only one major neurotransmitter in its axon terminal. Major neurotransmitters include serotonin, acetylcholine, gamma-aminobutyric acid (GABA), glycine, glutamate, and the catecholamines, dopamine, norepinephrine, and epinephrine. It was not known until the 1970s that peptides could act as neurotransmitters. Examples of these neuropeptides are the endogenous opioids (endorphins and enkephalins) and substance P, all of which appear to be involved in pain sensation. The endorphins and enkephalins, often described as the body's own morphine, contribute to a decrease in pain sensation. Substance P excites sensory neurons that respond to painful stimuli, so it is thought to be involved in transmission of pain information from the periphery to the CNS.

Each major neurotransmitter has multiple receptors. For instance, epinephrine can bind to $alpha_1$, $alpha_2$, $beta_1$, and $beta_2$ receptors, and acetylcholine can bind to neuronal nicotinic, skeletal muscle nicotinic, or muscarinic receptors, which are further subdivided into m_1, m_2, and m_3. The postsynaptic membrane of each synapse contains only one receptor type for the particular neurotransmitter synthesized by the presynaptic neuron. The receptor subtype dictates the effects of a neurotransmitter in a particular synapse on the postsynaptic cell (hyperpolarization or depolarization). Therefore, the same neurotransmitter might be either hyperpolarizing or depolarizing to a given postsynaptic neuron, depending on the receptor subtype present on the postsynaptic cell. However, GABA receptors are always hyperpolarizing, and GABA is the most important inhibitory neurotransmitter in the nervous system. Likewise, glutamate and glycine are always depolarizing (excitatory) neurotransmitters.

Neuronal Thresholds and the Action Potential

A depolarizing impulse that reaches a neuron's dendrites or soma through action of a neurotransmitter binding to its receptors causes the membrane to depolarize locally. This is accomplished through action of the receptor. The local depolarization produced by the receptor causes voltage-sensitive sodium channels locally in the membrane to open and sodium ions are transmitted down their concentration gradient from outside the neuron to inside. This causes further local depolarization. If enough sodium channels open locally, the resulting depolarization is large enough to open sodium channels in adjacent areas, depolarizing a larger area of the membrane. As mentioned, for a given nerve cell there typically are many other neurons that synapse with its soma or dendrites. Some of these synapsing neurons release neurotransmitter that interacts with the nerve cell's receptors to depolarize the postsynaptic neuron. These synapsing neurons would be excitatory because their influence is to depolarize the postsynaptic neuron and bring it closer to achieving a propagating action potential. Other synapsing neurons release other neurotransmitters that interact with their receptors to hyperpolarize the postsynaptic neuron. These synapsing neurons would be inhibitory because hyperpolarization of the postsynaptic neuron prevents a propagating action potential. The nerve cell body algebraically sums the depolarizing and hyperpolarizing influences. If the depolarizing influences outweigh the hyperpolarizing influences, the membrane potential of the nerve cell body may reach a certain value called *threshold.* At that point, an action potential is generated at the point where the axon leaves the soma. The action potential is propagated down the length of the axon by the process of sodium channel openings in the area of the advancing action potential, followed by complete depolarization of that area. After a time, sodium channels close and the membrane in that area can repolarize through activity of the sodium–potassium pump and through opening of voltage-sensitive potassium channels. As potassium accumulates within the cell, either by entry through the voltage-sensitive potassium channels or the sodium–potassium pump, the membrane potential is reestablished. The action potential is thus propagated down the entire length of the axon to the axon terminal. At that point, depolarization of the axon terminal causes neurotransmitter to be released, which diffuses across the synapse and binds to specific receptors, causing a depolarizing or hyperpolarizing change in the postsynaptic neuron.

Neuronal thresholds can also be influenced by hormones. For example, *thyroxine* lowers thresholds of certain neurons, and one sign of hyperthyroidism is the presence of exaggerated spinal reflexes, such as the knee jerk and ankle jerk.

Figure 32-3B depicts the time course of a neuronal action potential as monitored by electrodes inserted into an axon. Compared with cardiac action potentials, neuronal action potentials are quite short, with durations of approximately 5 to 15 milliseconds. Like the cardiac action potential, there are absolute and relative refractory periods during which the neuron cannot easily be reexcited. However, these refractory periods are very short because repeated impulse conduction is necessary to maintain tonic activity of particular neural pathways. For instance, the motor pathways that supply muscles of posture must be tonically active to maintain a steady contraction in these muscles that keep us erect. Other pathways that have tonic activity include the autonomic motor pathways (sympathetic and parasympathetic), as discussed later in this chapter.

The electrical activity of the action potential can be monitored in certain clinical situations. For example, the electroencephalogram depicts multiple action potentials from surface neurons of the brain. Nerve conduction studies can be done on peripheral nerves to diagnose areas of compression or entrapment, which slow action potentials.

NERVE REGENERATION

If a nerve fiber is severed, the portion distal to the cut will die. The part still attached to the cell body will regenerate. In peripheral neurons, the neurilemma itself provides a channel that can be followed by a regenerating fiber so that it may become reattached to its original anatomical connection (Fig. 32-4). Regeneration also occurs in the absence of a neurilemma, as in the case of CNS neurons. Because there is no channel to ensure correct anatomical

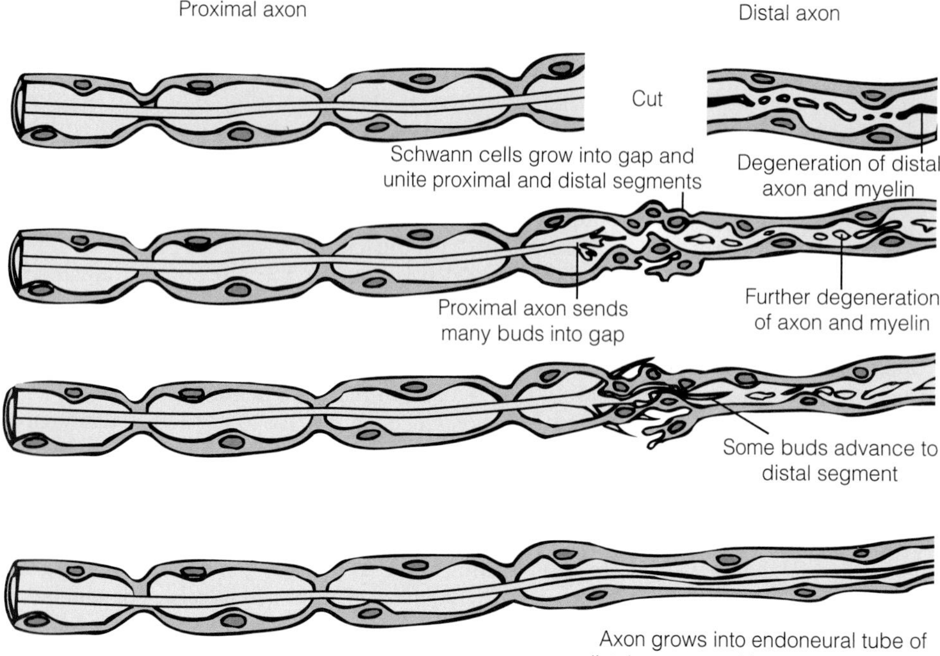
Proximal axon
Distal axon
Cut
Schwann cells grow into gap and unite proximal and distal segments
Degeneration of distal axon and myelin
Proximal axon sends many buds into gap
Further degeneration of axon and myelin
Some buds advance to distal segment
Axon grows into endoneural tube of distal segments. New myelin is formed.

figure 32-4 Diagram of changes that occur in a nerve fiber that has been cut and then regenerates.

reconnection, though, most such regenerations do not produce recovered function. The regrowing stump may wind aimlessly among other structures or curl into a useless tangle. A bigger hindrance to functional regeneration in the CNS has been discovered, however—an overgrowth of neuroglial cells that occurs in response to injury. This produces a neuroglial thicket that acts as a barrier to the reconnection of severed neuronal networks.

It is important to note that the preceding paragraph deals with nerve processes, axons, or dendrites that are cut by an injury. If the soma is damaged by injury or the nerve cell is killed by lack of oxygen or a neurotoxin, there will be no regeneration. Moreover, under ordinary circumstances, a neuron that dies cannot be replaced because neurons do not normally undergo mitosis in people older than 2 years of age.

CENTRAL NERVOUS SYSTEM

The CNS comprises the brain and spinal cord. It receives sensory input through sensory neurons whose dendrites run within spinal and cranial nerves, and it sends out motor impulses through axons of motor neurons that run in these same nerves. The CNS also contains large numbers of neurons that are entirely contained within it. These neurons are termed *internuncial neurons*, or *interneurons*, and may exist inside the brain and spinal cord or connect one with the other.

The CNS, including the spinal cord, is covered by three layers of tissue collectively called the *meninges* and consisting of the pia mater, the arachnoid layer, and the dura mater (Fig. 32-5). The *pia mater* is the layer that lies next to the CNS. Next is the *arachnoid layer*, which contains a substantial vascular supply. Last is the *dura mater*, the thickest layer of all, lying next to the bones surrounding the CNS.

The CNS is richly supplied with blood vessels that bring oxygen and nutrients to the cells there. However, many substances cannot easily be exchanged between blood and brain because the endothelial cells of the vessels and the astrocytes of the CNS form extremely tight junctions collectively referred to as the *blood–brain barrier*. In particular, polar molecules and large molecules such as proteins do not cross the blood–brain barrier, but lipid-soluble molecules cross with ease. Many drugs penetrate the brain poorly because they do not have sufficient lipid solubility to cross the blood–brain barrier.

The space between the arachnoid layer and the pia mater, termed the *subarachnoid space*, contains cerebrospinal fluid (CSF). CSF is another means for supplying nutrients (but not oxygen) to the CNS. It also serves a protective function by cushioning the brain and spinal cord.

Cerebrospinal Fluid

CSF is a clear, colorless fluid that flows in the ventricles of the brain and the subarachnoid space of the brain and spinal cord. As mentioned, CSF functions as a fluid shock absorber, keeping the delicate CNS tissues from being mechanically injured by surrounding bony structures. It also plays a role in the exchange of nutrients between the plasma and cellular compartments. CSF is actually a plasma filtrate that is exuded by the capillaries in the roofs of each of the four ventricles of the brain. As such, it is similar to plasma without the large plasma proteins, which stay behind in the bloodstream. Red blood cells, which contain the hemoglobin that is responsible for most oxygen transport in blood, are not present in CSF. Therefore, the CSF is a poor source of oxygen, although it contains glucose, amino acids, and other nutrients that might be needed by the cells of the CNS. Most of the CSF is made in the lateral ventricles, which are located in each cerebral hemisphere. It moves from there through

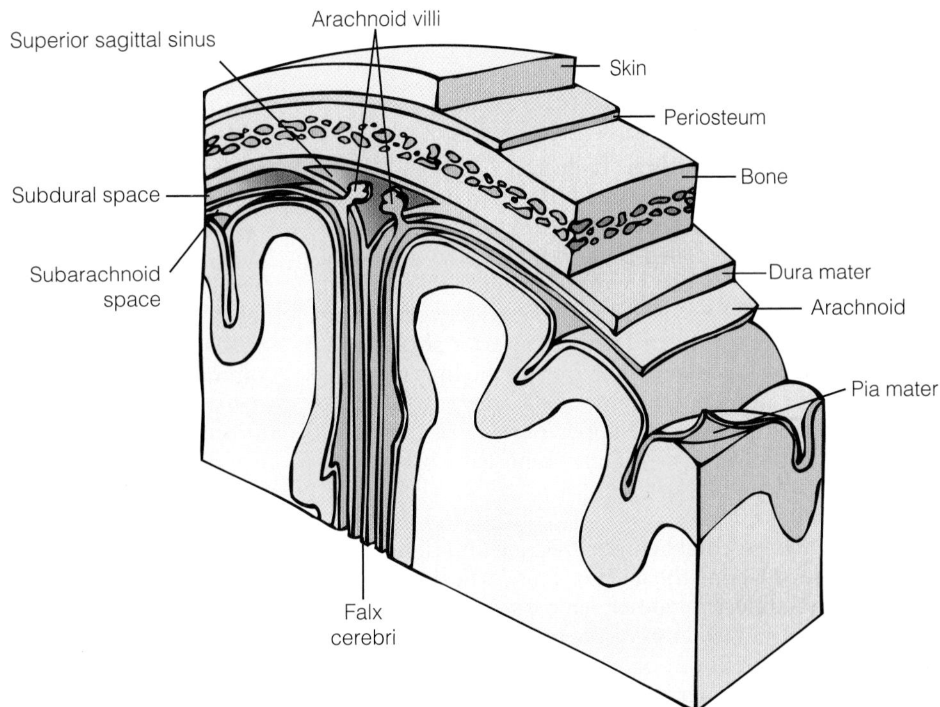

figure 32-5 The cranial meninges. The arachnoid villi shown within the superior sagittal sinus are one site of passage of cerebrospinal fluid (CSF) into the blood.

the ducts into the third ventricle of the diencephalon (Fig. 32-6). From there it travels through the aqueduct of Sylvius of the midbrain and enters the fourth ventricle in the medulla oblongata. Most of it then passes through holes (foramina) in the roof of this ventricle and enters the subarachnoid space. A small amount diffuses down into the spinal canal. In the subarachnoid space, the CSF is reabsorbed into the bloodstream at certain points called the *arachnoid villi.*

The formation and reabsorption of CSF is governed by the same hydrostatic and colloid osmotic forces that regulate the movements of fluid and small molecules between the plasma and interstitial fluid compartments. Briefly reviewed, the action of these forces is as follows. Two opposing push–pull forces influence the movement of water and small molecules through the semipermeable capillary membranes. One force is composed of plasma oncotic pressure and CSF hydrostatic pressure. It favors movement of water and small molecules from the CSF compartment into the plasma. The movement of water and small molecules in the opposite direction is influenced by the force of plasma hydrostatic pressure and CSF oncotic pressure. These two opposing forces are exerted simultaneously and continually. In the ventricles, the flow of CSF out of the ventricles reduces CSF hydrostatic pressure. This tips the influence in favor of the movement of water and small molecules from plasma to ventricles. The low plasma hydrostatic pressure of blood in the venous sinuses next to the arachnoid villi tips the scales in favor of the movement of water and solute from the CSF compartment back into the bloodstream. Death of cells lining the CSF compartment releases proteins into the CSF. This elevates CSF oncotic pressure and retards reabsorption (while also hastening CSF formation if the damage is in ventricle walls). Increased CSF proteins from this or other causes can provoke or exacerbate a condition of excess CSF called *hydrocephalus.*

Because the CSF is formed in the ventricles and must travel to the arachnoid to be reabsorbed, any impediment to its flow impairs its absorption. The aqueduct of Sylvius or the foramina in the roof of the fourth ventricle may become clogged by adhesions from an infection (meningitis), clots from a subarachnoid hemorrhage, a tumor, or

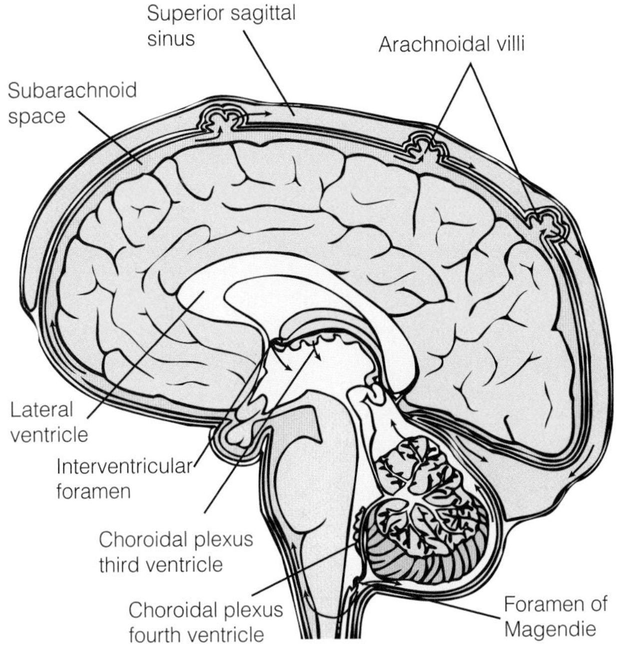

figure 32-6 Diagram of the flow of cerebrospinal fluid (CSF) from the time of its formation from blood in the choroid plexuses until its return to the blood in the superior sagittal sinus. (From Hickey JV: The Clinical Practice of Neurological and Neurosurgical Nursing [5th Ed]. Philadelphia, Lippincott Williams & Wilkins, 2003.)

a congenital abnormality. This produces a hydrocephalus with increased pressure in the CSF.

Brain

The basic anatomy of the brain is illustrated in Figure 32-7. The parts of the brain, in descending order, are the cerebral hemispheres (the cerebrum), diencephalon, midbrain, pons varolii (usually called the *pons*), medulla oblongata (usually called the *medulla*), and cerebellum. The general appearance of the brain can be viewed as a stem extending upward from the spinal cord with an inferior small flowering overgrowth (cerebellum) covering the lower part of the stem and a large superior flowering overgrowth (cerebrum) covering most of the upper portion of the stem. The medulla, pons, and midbrain compose the brainstem.

CEREBRUM

Each of the two cerebral hemispheres (left and right) has a layer of cortex covering the surface. This cortical layer consists of several different types of neurons with accompanying neuroglia arranged in six distinctive layers according to cell type and function. Some of these neurons project myelinated axons deeper into the cortex with ultimate destinations lower in the CNS or in the opposite cortex. Because myelin is white, these areas of myelinated axons appear as so-called white matter. Deep within each hemisphere are several collections of nerve cell bodies, termed the *basal ganglia*, and a lateral ventricle containing CSF. The left and right hemispheres are connected and communicate with each other by a transverse band of white matter termed the *corpus callosum*, formed by myelinated axons traveling between each side of the cortex. Each hemisphere has four lobes named for and generally underlying each of the following skull bones: frontal, parietal, temporal, and occipital. For the most part, each hemisphere serves the contralateral side of the body (fibers cross over in the CNS). One notable exception, however, is Broca's speech area. This area of the cortex subserves all motor speech functions and is located in a posterolateral area of the left frontal lobe for all right-handed and many left-handed people. Damage to this area in an adult produces motor dysphasia.

Many areas of the cerebrum operate together to produce coordinated human function. The process of communication provides a good example of this coordination. *Verbal communication* depends on the ability to interpret speech and translate thought into speech. Ideas usually are communicated between people by either the spoken or the written word. With the spoken word, the input of sensory information occurs through the primary auditory cortex. In auditory association areas, the sounds are interpreted as words and the words as sentences. These sentences are then interpreted by a common integrative area of the cortex as thoughts.

The common integrative area also develops thoughts to be communicated. Letters seen by the eyes are associated with words and sentences in the visual association areas and then integrated into thought in the common integrative area. Operating in conjunction with facial regions of the somesthetic sensory area, the common integrative area initiates a series of impulses, each representing a syllable or word, and transmits them to the secondary motor area controlling the larynx and mouth. The speech center, in addition to controlling motor activity of the larynx and mouth, sends impulses to the respiratory center of the secondary motor cortex to provide appropriate breath patterns for the speech process.

Cortex

As mentioned, the cortex is the most superficial layer of the cerebrum. It is responsible for all higher mental func-

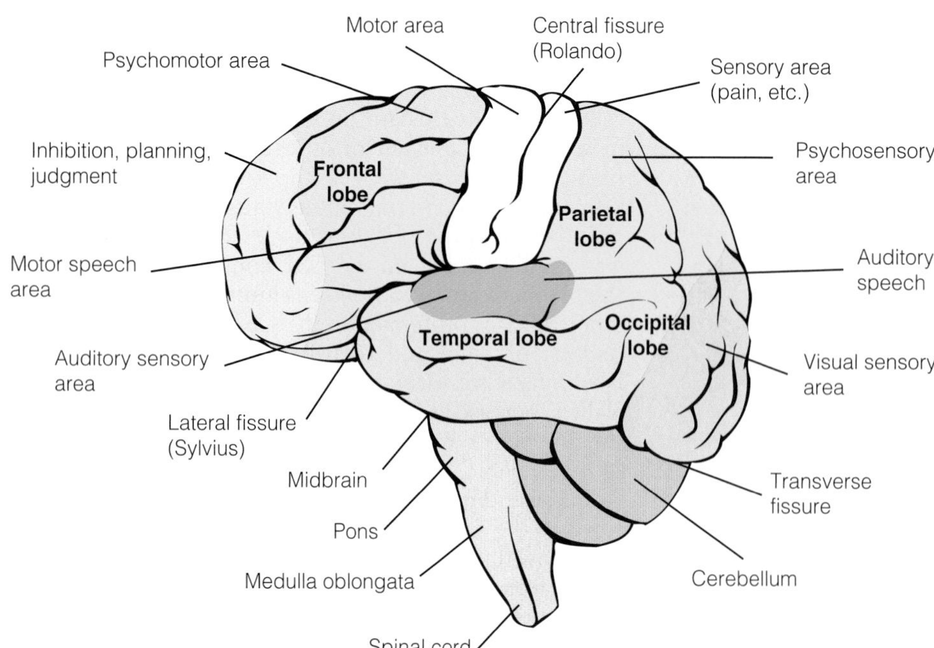

figure 32-7 The human brain, showing the lobes and fissures of the cerebrum. Major functional areas are also indicated.

tions, such as judgment, language, memory, creativity, and abstract thinking. It also functions in the perception, localization, and interpretation of all sensations and governs all voluntary motor activities (see Fig. 32-7). Various areas of the cortex have been identified as having different motor and sensory functions, but some of these areas are being implicated in other functions as well. For example, the occipital area, which usually takes sensory impulses from the eyes and integrates them into visual images, is now known to function in some learning processes of blind people.

Basal Ganglia

The basal ganglia function in cooperation with other lower brain parts in providing circuitry for basic and subconscious bodily movements. They provide the necessary background muscle tone for discrete voluntary movements, smoothness and coordination in functions of muscle antagonists, and the basic automatic subconscious rhythmic movements involved in walking and balance. Lesions of the basal ganglia produce various clinical abnormalities, such as chorea, hemiballismus, and Parkinson's disease.

DIENCEPHALON

The diencephalon, a major division of the cerebrum, lies below the cerebral hemispheres. The diencephalon is a paired structure on each side of the third ventricle, directly above the brainstem. The most important areas of the diencephalon are the thalamus and the hypothalamus, described in the following sections. The subthalamus is the ventral portion of the thalamus, and the epithalamus is an area that contains the pineal gland, thought to play an important role in diurnal rhythms (Fig. 32-8).

Thalamus

The *thalamus* (see Fig. 32-8) functions as a sensory and motor relay center. That is, its neurons receive sensory impulses from synapsing neurons that originate at lower levels in the spinal cord or brainstem and relay sensory input, including sight, sound, and touch, to the sensory cortex. The thalamus also functions in the gross awareness of certain sensations, most notably pain. Discrete localization and the finer perceptual details of sensations are cortical functions, but awareness occurs at the thalamic and even midbrain areas. Finally, the thalamus is involved in the reticular activating systems (RAS), the neural system that promotes wakefulness and consciousness and possibly some aspects of attention.

Hypothalamus

The *hypothalamus* is the seat of neuroendocrine interaction. It controls visceral, autonomic, endocrine, and emotional function. It is connected to the reticular formation of the brainstem as well as the diencephalon, the cortex, and the pituitary gland. This area of the brain also contains some of the centers for coordinated parasympathetic and sympathetic stimulation, as well as those for temperature regulation, appetite regulation, regulation of water balance by antidiuretic hormone (ADH), and regulation of certain rhythmic psychobiological activities (e.g., sleep).

BRAINSTEM

A major subdivision of the brain, the brainstem consists of the midbrain, pons, and medulla and contains respiratory and autonomic control centers, as well as many tracts of myelinated motor axons that are passing through on their way down to the spinal cord, or sensory axons passing through on their way up to the thalamus. In addition, areas of the brainstem are important in coordinating activity of the cerebellum with the rest of the brain. Also, 10 of the 12 cranial nerves originate from this area (Fig. 32-9).

Midbrain

The midbrain lies between the diencephalon and the pons. It contains the aqueduct of Sylvius, many ascending and descending nerve fiber tracts (white matter), and cen-

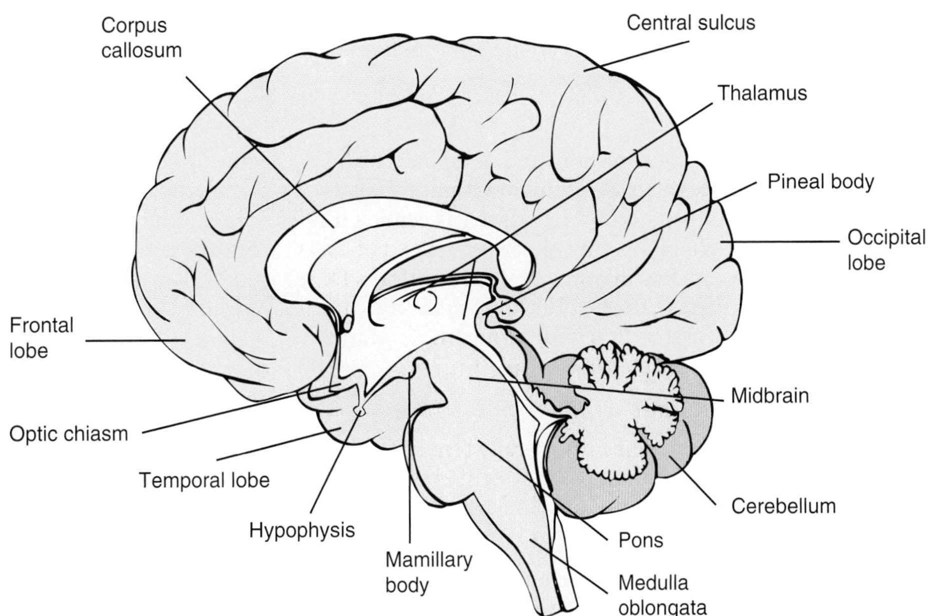

figure 32-8 Lateral view of the human brain, showing the parts of the brainstem, the cerebellum, and other major landmarks. (From Cohen H: Neuroscience for Rehabilitation [2nd Ed]. Philadelphia, Lippincott Williams & Wilkins, 1999.)

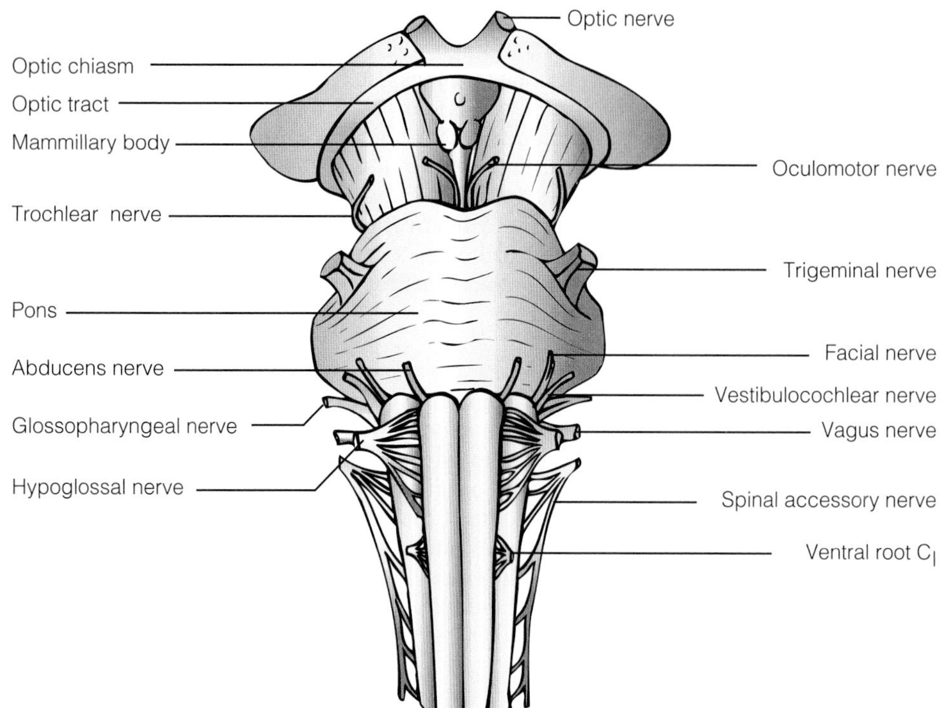

figure 32-9 Anterior surface of the brainstem, showing the emergence and entrance of most of the cranial nerves. (From Parent A: Carpenter's Human Neuroanatomy [9th Ed]. Baltimore, Williams & Wilkins, 1996.)

ters for auditory and visually stimulated nerve impulses. The *Edinger-Westphal nucleus* in the midbrain contains the autonomic reflex centers for pupillary accommodations to light. It receives sensory fibers from the retina by cranial nerve II and sends motor impulses by way of sympathetic and parasympathetic fibers (cranial nerve III) to the smooth muscles of the iris. Impaired pupillary accommodation means that at least one of these inputs or outputs is damaged or that the midbrain is suffering insult (often from tentorial herniation or stroke). Cranial nerve IV also originates in the midbrain.

Pons

The *pons* lies between the midbrain and the medulla and has cell bodies of fibers contained in cranial nerves V, VI, VII, and VIII. It contains pneumotaxic and apneustic respiratory centers and fiber tracts connecting higher and lower centers, including the cerebellum.

Medulla Oblongata

The *medulla* lies between the pons and the spinal cord. It contains centers that regulate vital functions such as breathing, cardiac rate, and vasomotor tone, as well as centers for vomiting, gagging, coughing, and sneezing reflex behaviors. It also contains the fourth ventricle. Cranial nerves IX, X, XI, and XII originate in the medulla. Impairment of any of the vital functions or reflexes involving these cranial nerves suggests medullary damage.

Functionally Integrated Brainstem Systems

Four networks of neurons in the brainstem should be mentioned. They are the integrated systems responsible for posture and equilibrium, consciousness, emotional reactions, and sleep.

Bulboreticular Formation. The bulboreticular formation is a network of neurons in the brainstem that helps maintain balance and erect posture. This area receives sensory information from a variety of sources, including the peripheral sensory receptors that are relayed from the spinal cord, the cerebellum, the inner ear vestibular apparatus, the motor cortex, and the basal ganglia. Therefore, the bulboreticular formation is an integrative network for sensory information and motor information that has to do with body posture and balance. Output from the bulboreticular formation travels down descending fibers to internuncial neurons in the spinal cord, which synapse with motor neurons. This output alters the tonus of muscles maintaining balance and erect posture and positions of major body parts (trunk, appendages) necessary for the performance of discrete actions (e.g., writing at a table, walking).

Reticular Activating System. The RAS is an ascending nerve fiber system originating in the midbrain and thalamus. The RAS is stimulated by sensory impulses from various sources. These include input from the optic and acoustic cranial nerves, somesthetic impulses from the dorsal column and spinothalamic pathways, and fibers from the cortex. Therefore, the RAS is an integrative system that receives sensory information concerning light, sound, and touch that may indicate a need for alertness. Excitatory output of the RAS extends to a variety of higher centers, including the cortex. In this way, the RAS can stimulate these centers to maintain alertness. The stimulation of the cortex by the RAS seems to be the major physiological basis for consciousness, alertness, and attention to various environmental stimuli. Decreased activity of the RAS produces decreased alertness or levels of consciousness, including stupor and coma. Inactivation of the RAS can result from anything that interrupts the entry of a critical amount of sensory input or from any damage that prevents the RAS fibers from sending impulses to the cortex.

Limbic System. The hypothalamus, the cingulate gyrus of the cortex, the amygdala and hippocampus in the temporal lobes, and the septum and interconnecting nerve fiber tracts among these areas comprise a functional unit of the brain called the limbic system. This system provides a neural substrate for emotions (e.g., terror, intense pleasure, eroticism). This region of the brain is involved in emotional experience and in the control of emotion-related behavior. Also, it is here that neural pathways provide a connection between higher brain functioning and endocrine or autonomic activities.

Sleep Centers. The release of stored serotonin from axon terminals in the diencephalon, medulla, thalamus, and a small forebrain area, collectively called DMTF, results in inactivation of the RAS and activation of the DMTF. DMTF activity results in the four stages of sleep. During sleep stages III and IV, parasympathetic activity (with decreased heart rate, respiratory rate, and so forth) predominates and sleepwalking, sleep talking, and nocturnal enuresis occur.

Rhythmic discharges (about four to eight times per night, from 10 to 20 minutes per episode) from the pontine nuclei during sleep result in rapid eye movement (REM) sleep, during which approximately 80% of all dreaming occurs and sympathetic nervous system activity predominates. Based on circadian rhythmicity and decreasing cerebral serotonin levels, the RAS is reactivated in the morning, after 6 to 8 hours of sleep.

CEREBELLUM

The cerebellum (see Fig. 32-8) is located just superior and posterior to the medulla. It receives "samples" of all ascending somesthetic sensory input and all descending motor impulses. Use of these connections enables the cerebellum to match intended motor stimuli (before they reach the muscles) with actual sensory data. This ensures an optimal match for voluntary motor "intention" with actual motor action, with time to alter the motor message in case of error. It sends its own messages to the basal ganglia and cortex and to parts of the brainstem.

The cerebellum functions to produce smooth, steady, harmonious, and coordinated skeletal muscle actions; maintain equilibrium; and control posture without any jerky or uncompensated movements or swaying. The cerebellum is also involved in motor learning and is responsible for reflexive activities that occur when motor learning is complete, such as correcting one's balance when riding a bike. Cerebellar disease can produce typical symptoms, the most prominent of which are disturbances of gait, equilibrium ataxia (overstability or understability of the walk), inability to perform rapid repetitive movements, and characteristic intention tremors.

Spinal Cord

The spinal cord lies within the neural canal of the vertebral column, extending down and filling the neural canal to the level of about the second lumbar vertebra. A pair of spinal nerves exits between adjacent vertebrae the entire length of the vertebral column. Each spinal nerve exits the spinal column at its respective level (e.g., C5, T11, L1, S1). However, because the cord is shorter than the spinal column, the level of the cord that gives rise to a particular pair of spinal nerves is above the vertebra of that level. For instance, the two spinal nerves that leave the spinal column between the L4 and L5 vertebrae have to travel down the spinal canal from the cord level L4, which is actually up at about vertebral level T11. Below the point at which the cord terminates, the neural canal is filled with descending spinal nerves collectively known as the *cauda equina* (horse's tail), which exit the spinal canal at the vertebra that corresponds to the cord level from which they arose (Fig. 32-10). Because neurons occupy less space in the canal at lower lumbar levels, it is here that spinal taps may be performed safely. This anatomical fact also explains why injuries to lumbar and lower thoracic vertebrae can produce impairment at disproportionately lower body levels.

Within the cord lie ascending sensory fibers and descending motor fibers, many of which are myelinated and appear as white matter. Interneurons, and the nerve cell bodies and dendrites of the second-order somatic (voluntary) and first-order autonomic motor neurons, are not myelinated and appear as gray matter. The central area of the cord contains nerve cell bodies and internuncial neurons (i.e., nerve cells contained entirely within the cord) and also appears as gray matter. The gray matter has left and right dorsal and ventral projections, giving it an "H"-shaped appearance (Fig. 32-11). Nerve cell bodies of motor neurons supplying skeletal muscles lie in the ventral horns. Left and right lateral projections or horns of gray matter referred to as the *intermediolateral cell column* exist in the thoracic and upper lumbar cord. Within these lie the nerve cell bodies of the sympathetic preganglionic neurons.

It is important to realize that the spinal cord is really an extension of the brain and contains many integrative and processive functions. For instance, the substantia gelatinosa contains nerve terminals of descending neurons, and also interneurons, that function to moderate ascending pain impulses (see later).

PERIPHERAL NERVOUS SYSTEM

The PNS consists of 12 pairs of cranial nerves and 31 pairs of spinal nerves and includes all neural structures lying outside the pia mater of the spinal cord and brainstem. The parts of the PNS inside the spinal canal and attached to the ventral and dorsal surfaces of the cord are called the spinal nerve roots. Those attached to the ventrolateral surface of the brainstem are the cranial nerve roots.

Functionally, the PNS is separated into sensory and motor divisions. The sensory division includes sensory neurons that innervate the skin, muscles, joints, and viscera and provide sensory information about the environment outside and inside the body to the CNS. The motor division includes motor neurons that innervate skeletal muscles and the autonomic nervous system (ANS) that innervates smooth and cardiac muscle and the glands. The ANS is responsible for regulating the ongoing functions of many organ systems, such as blood pressure, heart rate, and gastrointestinal activity.

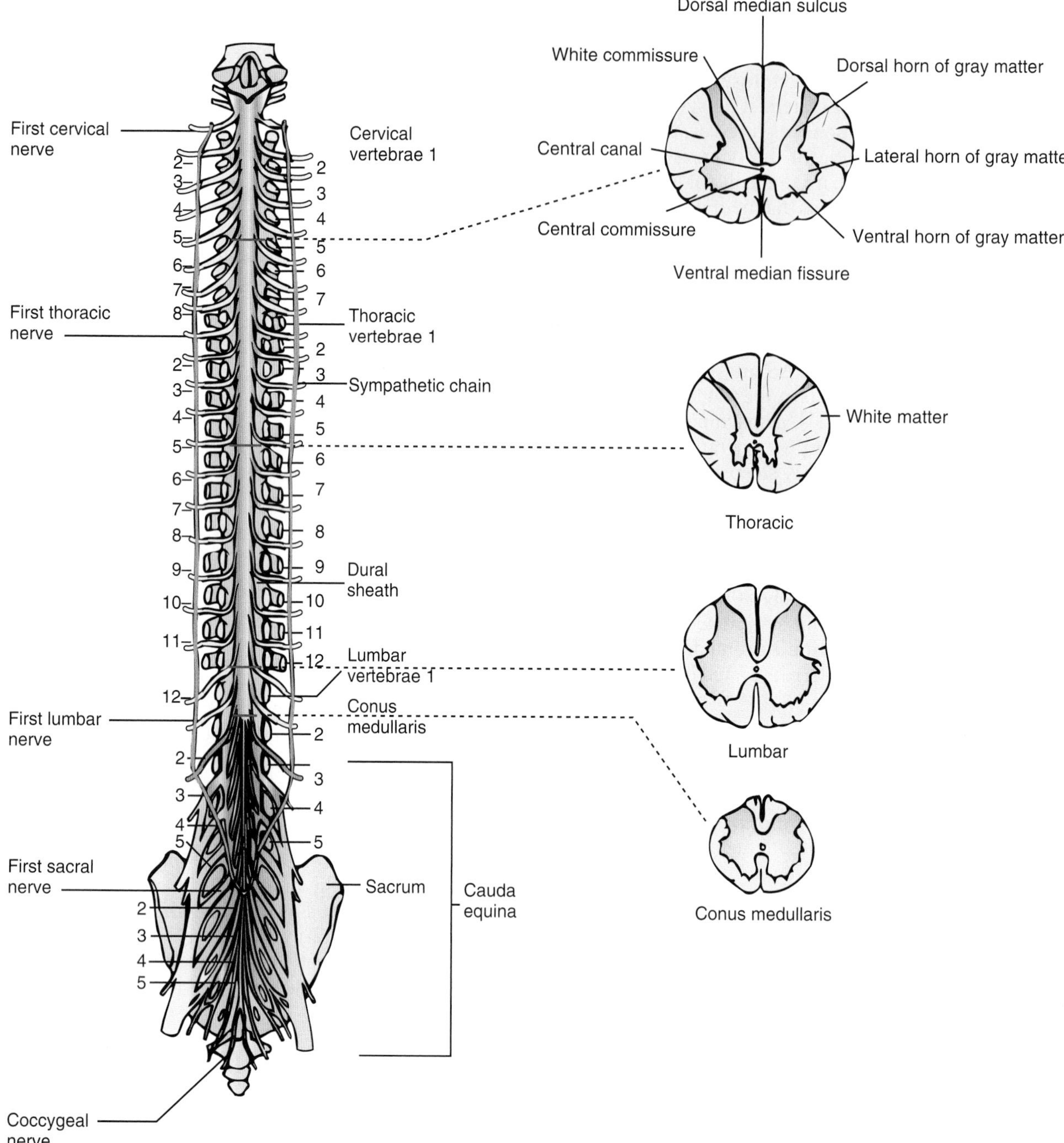

figure 32-10 The spinal cord within the vertebral canal. The spinal canal and meninges have been opened. The spinal nerves and vertebrae are numbered on the left. Cross (transverse) sections with regional variations in gray matter and increasing proportions of white matter as the cord is ascended appear on the right.

Cranial Nerves

The 12 pairs of cranial nerves supply motor and sensory fibers mostly to the structures of the head, neck, and upper back, although cranial nerve X, the vagus nerve, supplies the viscera to about the level of the waist (Table 32-1). Most cranial nerves originate in the brainstem (see Fig. 32-9), except cranial nerves I and II, which originate in the diencephalon. Cranial nerves are classified as either sensory, motor, or mixed (carrying both sensory and motor signals). They bring input from the special senses (vision, hearing, smell) and somatic sensory input from the face and head into the brain. They also send motor commands out to the muscles and glands of the head and neck to control facial expression, eye movements, movements of the structures in the mouth and throat, movements of the head and neck, and autonomic functions of the eyes, salivary glands, and viscera in the chest and upper abdomen. Most cranial nerves contain fibers of more than one functional type; thus, most cranial nerves

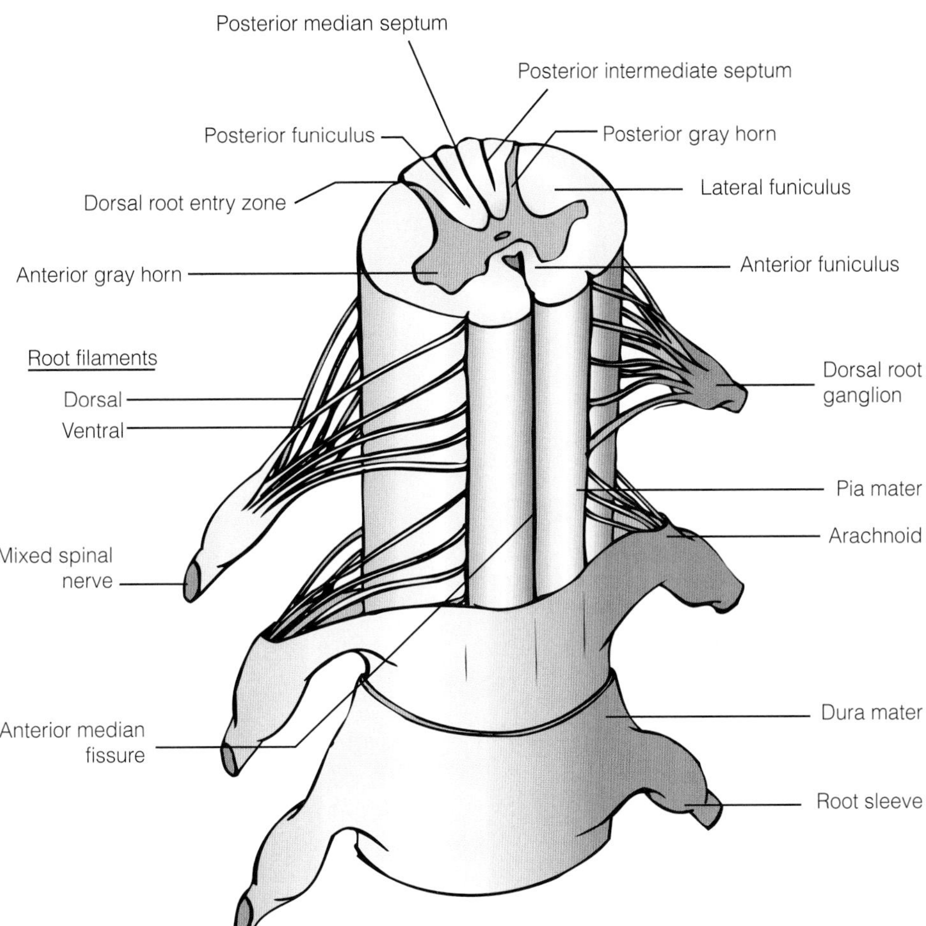

figure 32-11 Spinal cord, nerve roots, and meninges. (From Parent A: Carpenter's Human Neuroanatomy [9th Ed]. Baltimore, Williams & Wilkins, 1996.)

are associated with more than one nucleus in the brainstem (see Table 32-1).

Spinal Nerves

Spinal nerves are attached to the spinal cord in pairs; there are 8 cervical, 12 thoracic, 5 lumbar, 5 sacral, and 1 coccygeal pair of spinal nerves (see Fig. 32-10). Spinal nerves contain both sensory and motor fibers. Each spinal nerve attaches to the cord by a dorsal and a ventral root. The dorsal root houses the nerve cell bodies of sensory neurons. Motor axons, whose nerve cell bodies lie in the gray matter of the ventral horn of the cord, traverse the ventral root. Thus, damage to the dorsal root may impair sensory function without impairing motor function, and vice versa. However, a spinal nerve injury distal to the roots could damage both sensory and motor functioning. A dermatome is the area of skin innervated by sensory fibers from a particular spinal nerve emanating from a particular segment of the spinal cord.

Sensory Division

The sensory division of the nervous system is composed of sensory receptors, sensory neurons, sensory pathways, and perceptive areas of the brain.

SENSATIONS AND SENSORY RECEPTORS

Sensations often are divided into the special senses (e.g., vision, hearing, and smell) and those termed *somesthetic sensations* (e.g., pain, touch, and stretch). In this section, only somesthetic sensations are discussed. Such sensations provide information about, for example, body position and conditions of the external and internal environment. These are called proprioceptive, exteroceptive, and visceral sensations, respectively.

Proprioceptive sensations describe the physical position state of the body, such as muscle tension, joint flexion or extension, tendon tension, and deep pressure in dependent parts, such as the feet while one is standing or the buttocks while one is sitting. *Exteroceptive sensations* monitor conditions on the body surface, such as temperature and pain. *Visceral sensations* are similar to exteroceptive sensations, except that they originate from within the body and monitor pain, pressure, and fullness from internal organs.

The sensory receptors for somesthetic sensations are basically dendrites, which can have the form of free nerve endings or specialized receptors. Free nerve endings are nothing more than small, filamentous branches of dendrites. They detect crude sensations of touch, pain, heat, and cold. The precision is crude because different neurons have overlapping distributions of their dendrites. These nerve endings are the most widely distributed and most numerous of sensory receptors, and perform the general

table 32-1 The Cranial Nerves

Cranial Nerve	Tract(s)	Function	Location of Origin
I. Olfactory	Sensory	Sense of smell	Diencephalon
II. Optic	Sensory	Vision	Diencephalon
III. Oculomotor	Parasympathetic Motor	Pupillary constriction Elevation of upper eyelid and four of six extraocular movements	Midbrain
IV. Trochlear	Motor	Downward, inward movement of the eye (superior oblique)	Midbrain
VI. Abducens	Motor	Lateral deviation of eye (lateral rectus)	Pons
V. Trigeminal	Motor Sensory	Muscles of mastication and opening jaw Tactile sensation to the cornea, nasal and oral mucosa, and facial skin	Pons
VII. Facial	Parasympathetic Motor Sensory	Secretory for salivation and tears Movement of the forehead, eyelids, cheeks, lips, ears, nose, and neck to produce facial expression and close eyes Tactile sensation to parts of the external ear, auditory canal, and external tympanic membrane Taste sensation to the anterior two-thirds of the tongue	Pons

(continued)

table 32-1 The Cranial Nerves (Continued)

Cranial Nerve	Tract(s)	Function	Location of Origin
VIII. Vestibulocochlear (also known as acoustic or cochlear)	Sensory	*Vestibular branch:* Equilibrium *Cochlear branch:* Hearing	Pons
IX. Glossopharyngeal	Parasympathetic Motor Sensory	Salivation Voluntary muscles for swallowing and phonation Sensation to pharynx, soft palate, and posterior one-third of tongue Stimulation elicits gag reflex	Medulla
X. Vagus	Parasympathetic Motor Sensory	Autonomic activity of viscera of thorax and abdomen Voluntary swallowing and phonation Involuntary activity of visceral muscles of the heart, lungs, and digestive tract Sensation to the auditory canal and viscera of the thorax and abdomen	Medulla
XI. Spinal accessory	Motor	Sternocleidomastoid and trapezius muscle movements	Medulla
XII. Hypoglossal	Motor	Tongue movements	Medulla

Artwork from Evans MJ: Neurologic Neurosurgical Nursing (2nd Ed), pp 7–8. Springhouse, PA, Springhouse, 1995.

discriminatory functions. The more specialized sensory receptors discriminate between very slight differences in degrees of touch, pain, heat, and cold. Indeed, the special exteroceptive end organs for detecting light touch, warmth, and cold differ structurally from one another and are specific in their function. The physiological basis for this specific function has not been determined, but is presumed to be based on some specific physical effect on the receptor itself.

Sensation from the viscera may come from specialized sensory receptors, such as baroreceptors and chemoreceptors that reside in arterial walls, or stretch receptors in sphincters. In contrast, visceral pain is the result of stimulation of unmyelinated, raw sensory nerve endings, usually by stretch, as might happen during swelling or distension, or by pressure on the organ as might happen from compression by a tumor. For both specialized or unspecialized visceral receptors, the sensory fibers run within the autonomic nerves (sympathetic or parasympathetic) back to CNS centers that are closely associated with autonomic motor responses. For this reason, these sensory fibers are sometimes referred to as *autonomic afferent fibers.* This is a somewhat misleading name because the autonomic nervous system is purely a motor system (see later), and the name refers only to the anatomic location of sensory fibers within the nerves that also carry autonomic motor fibers.

Stimulation of a sensory receptor initiates an electrical charge (generator potential) that depolarizes the sensory dendrite, causing a series of nerve impulses to travel along the sensory dendrite to the cell body. As mentioned, the sensory neuron cell body is contained in the dorsal root ganglion just outside the spinal cord. The sensory neuron sends axons into the spinal cord (or brain in the case of cranial nerves), where it synapses with projection neurons in either brain or spinal cord that carry impulses to the appropriate centers in the brain, including the thalamus, where the sensation finally may be perceived consciously. As mentioned previously, the projection neuron may synapse in the thalamus with another neuron, which relays the sensory impulse to the sensory cortex.

When the sensation first stimulates the sensory receptor in the periphery, there is a burst of impulses; if the stimulus persists, the frequency of impulses transmitted begins to decrease. All sensory receptors show this phenomenon of *adaptation* to varying degrees and at different rates. Adaptations to light touch and pressure occur in a few seconds, whereas pain and proprioceptive sensations adapt very little, if at all, and at a very slow rate. This adaptation results in our being unaware of the touch of our clothing to our skin, or the pressure on our buttocks while we are seated. Determination of the intensity of the sensation is made on a relative rather than an absolute basis.

Although there are structurally different receptors for detecting each type of sensation, the area of the brain to which the information is transmitted determines the *modality*, or type of sensation, a person feels. The thalamus and sensory cortex operate together to attribute various sensory qualities and intensities to nerve impulse information they receive.

SENSORY PATHWAYS

As mentioned, sensory neurons that enter the cord synapse with projection neurons that carry the sensory information up the spinal cord. There are a number of pathways by which sensory information is transmitted up the cord by axons of the projection neurons. Depending on the type of somesthetic receptor involved, fibers of sensory neurons may, on entering the cord, do one of three things. First, they may send axons up the cord to the medulla on the same side of the body as the sensory receptor. This tract of myelinated axons (white matter) is called the *dorsal column.* In the medulla, the sensory neurons synapse with projection neurons that cross over to the opposite side of the brain and travel to the thalamus. This tract is called the *medial lemniscus* (Fig. 32-12). It is used for the conduction of impulses originating from stimulation of joint, muscle, and tendon

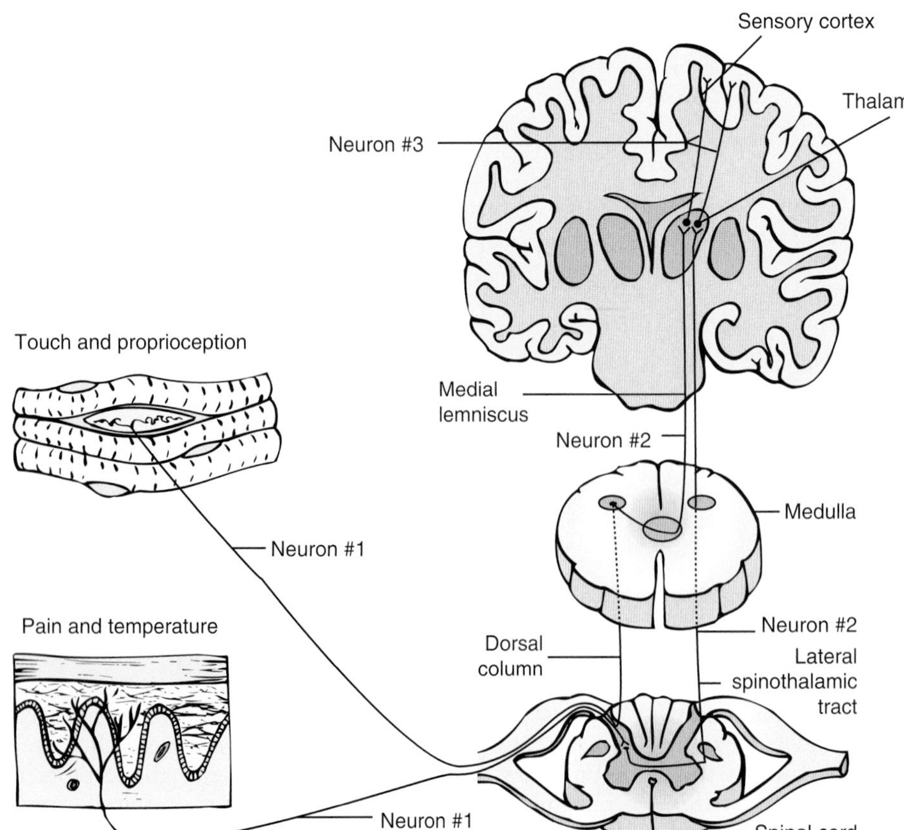

figure 32-12 Pathways of ascending tracts. Sensory neurons enter the cord at the dorsal horn. Axons of sensory neurons for touch and proprioception ascend in the dorsal columns to the medulla, where they synapse with second-order projection neurons that cross (decussate) to the opposite side before ascending to the thalamus in the tract called the medial lemniscus. First-order neurons for pain and temperature enter the dorsal gray matter of the cord, where they synapse with second-order projection neurons that cross to the opposite side and ascend in the lateral spinothalamic tract to the thalamus. Third-order neurons connect both pathways from thalamus to the sensory cortex.

proprioceptors; vibration-sensitive receptors; and receptors in the skin involved in precise localization of touch.

Second, the sensory neurons may synapse immediately on entering the cord with projection neurons that immediately cross over to the opposite side of the cord. Fibers from these projection neurons then travel up the white matter of the cord to the thalamus. This is called the *spinothalamic pathway* (see Fig. 32-12). It conducts impulses concerned with pain, temperature, poorly localized touch, and sex organ sensations. Both the dorsal column/medial lemniscus pathway and the spinothalamic pathway involve crossing of the sensory information from each side of the body to the opposite side of the CNS. Therefore, sensations on each side of the body are perceived by the thalamus and sensory cortex on the opposite side. In the thalamus, neurons of both the dorsal column pathway and the spinothalamic pathway synapse with other neurons that transmit impulses to the appropriate area of the sensory cortex. Because of their final destination in the cortex, impulses from either pathway give rise to consciously perceived sensations.

Third, certain sensory neurons may synapse with a projection neuron belonging to the *spinocerebellar pathway.* Spinocerebellar neurons do not cross over. They carry impulses only as far as the cerebellum (and possibly lower brainstem). This pathway carries impulses originating from stimulation of joint, muscle, and tendon proprioceptors. Because this pathway ends at the cerebellum, it transmits sensory information that never is perceived consciously. Instead, these data are used in reflex postural adjustments.

Motor Division

The motor division comprises the areas of the brain, descending fiber tracts, and motor neurons involved in producing or altering movement or adjusting tonus of skeletal, cardiac, and smooth muscles and in regulating the secretions of the various exocrine and certain endocrine gland cells. Muscle and glandular tissues are referred to as the *effector organs* of this system.

The motor division can be divided on the basis of motor neurons and effector organs into *somatic* and *autonomic* subdivisions (Fig. 32-13). The former involves skeletal muscles and the motor neurons innervating them. The latter is composed of smooth muscle, cardiac muscle, and gland cells plus the sympathetic and parasympathetic fibers innervating them.

SOMATIC MOTOR DIVISION

Figure 32-14 depicts the major descending fiber tracts from motor areas of the cortex. The most prominent of these tracts is the corticospinal tract, often called the *pyramidal tract* because it originates from pyramid-shaped nerve cell bodies in the cortex. The corticospinal tract is heavily myelinated and appears as white matter in the brain and spinal cord. The fibers cross to the opposite side in an area of the medulla referred to as the *decussation* (crossing over) of the pyramids. There are several other motor tracts that originate in the cortex or in the cerebellum. These tracts may cross over in the brain or in cord centers. Motor fibers from the brain ultimately stimulate somatic motor neurons, the nerve cell bodies of which lie in the anterior (ventral) horn of the gray matter in the cord. The axons of these motor neurons travel within spinal nerves and terminate adjacent to the membranes of skeletal muscle cells. The space between the somatic motor neuron axon and the muscle cell is termed the *neuromuscular junction.* When stimulated by signals arriving at their level in the cord, somatic motor neurons conduct impulses to the ends of their axons. As the impulse arrives there, it triggers the release of acetylcholine molecules that are stored in vesicles in the axon terminal. The acetylcholine diffuses across the neuromuscular junction and binds with nicotinic

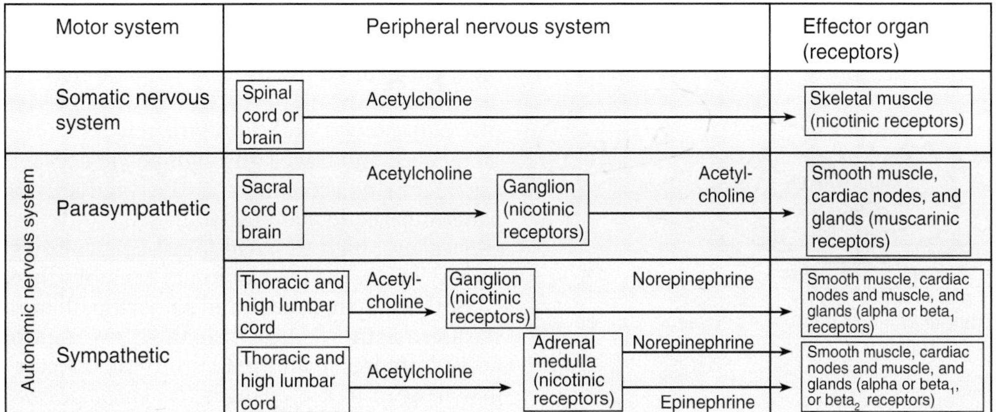

figure 32-13 A comparison between the divisions of the motor systems. The somatic nervous system (*pink*) sends cholinergic motor axons from the spinal cord or brain to the skeletal muscles. Acetylcholine released from these axon terminals binds to nicotinic receptors on skeletal muscles to cause contraction. The autonomic nervous system is composed of parasympathetic (*blue*) and sympathetic (*green*) divisions. For both directions, preganglionic cholinergic neurons originate in the brain or spinal cord and send their axons to ganglia in the periphery, where they synapse with postganglionic neurons having ganglionic nicotinic receptors. Postganglionic neurons of the parasympathetic division are cholinergic and synapse with muscarinic receptors on end organs. Postganglionic neurons of the sympathetic division are noradrenergic and synapse with alpha or beta$_1$ receptors on end organs. The adrenal medulla is innervated by preganglionic sympathetic neurons. Acetylcholine released by these neurons binds to ganglionic nicotinic receptors on cells of the adrenal medulla, causing them to release norepinephrine and epinephrine into the bloodstream.

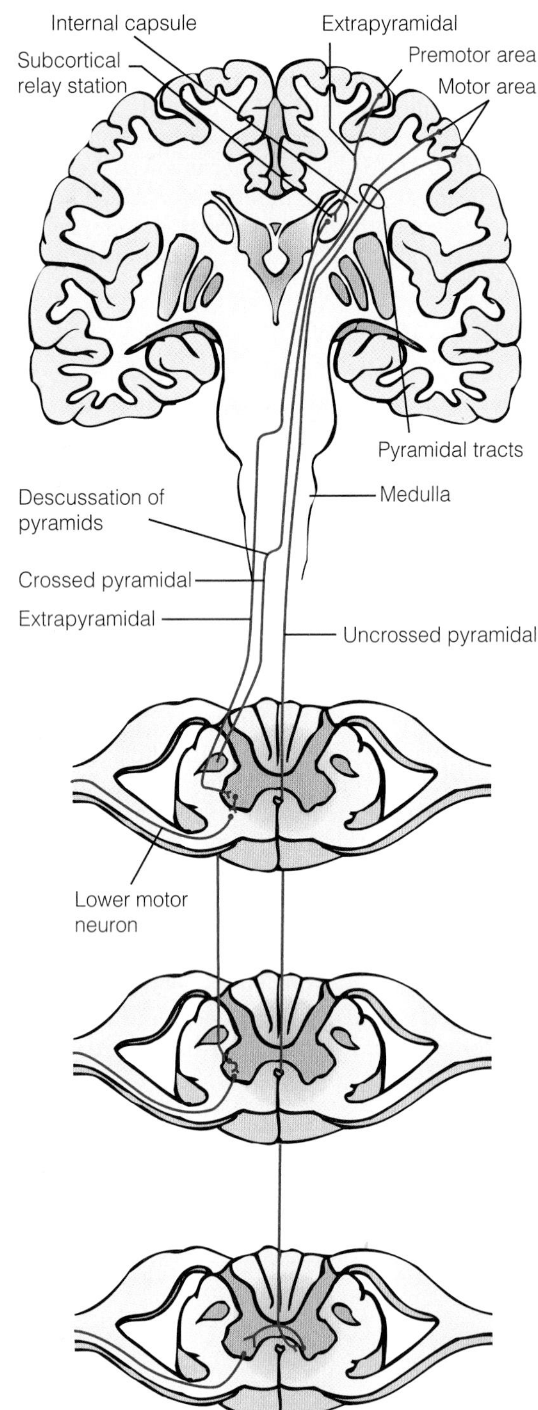

figure 32-14 Diagram of motor pathways between the cerebral cortex, one of the subcortical relay centers, and lower motor neurons in the spinal cord. Decussation (crossing) of fibers means that each side of the brain controls skeletal muscles on the opposite side of the body.

receptor sites on a skeletal muscle cell membrane. This triggers a chain of events leading to muscle contraction. Thus, willed intentional motor movements whose impetus arose in the cortex are enacted by the effects of acetylcholine on nicotinic skeletal muscle receptors.

Not shown in Figure 32-14 are descending fiber tracts that stimulate motor neurons responsible for the movement of skeletal muscles of the head (e.g., tongue, face, jaw). The general pattern and myoneural transmitter are the same, except the somatic motor neuron nerve cell bodies lie in certain areas of the brain and exit through cranial nerves. These fibers must also cross over from the opposite side before synapsing with the motor neurons.

Also not shown in Figure 32-14 are several extrapyramidal (not part of the pyramidal [i.e., corticospinal] tracts) tracts arising from the brainstem centers (e.g., bulboreticular formation, midbrain). Some of these cross over; others do not. Fibers in these tracts descend the cord and ultimately stimulate either somatic motor neurons, which stimulate skeletal muscle cells, or other motor neurons (gamma efferent) that alter the tensions of stretch receptor organelles (muscle spindles) in the skeletal muscles. Alteration of spindle tension provokes a spinal reflex arc that efficiently alters skeletal muscle tonus. These extrapyramidal pathways conduct impulses that produce the automatic coordinated alterations in skeletal muscle tonus and movement that are necessary for gross motor movements (e.g., walking) and for appropriate posture for conduction of finer movements (e.g., sitting at a desk with arm flexed in preparation for writing).

AUTONOMIC MOTOR DIVISION

The autonomic division contains both *sympathetic* and *parasympathetic motor fibers.* They are responsible for contraction and relaxation of smooth muscle, rate and strength of contraction of cardiac tissue, secretion of exocrine glands, and secretion of the adrenal medulla. They also influence the secretion of the islets of Langerhans in the pancreas.

The sympathetic and parasympathetic sections differ on the basis of the anatomical distribution of nerve fibers, the secretion of two different neurotransmitters by the postganglionic fibers of the two divisions, and the antagonistic effects of the two divisions on some of the organs they innervate (Table 32-2). Figure 32-15 shows the anatomy of the sympathetic and parasympathetic nervous systems. The CNS center immediately responsible for sympathetic outflow resides in the intermediolateral column of the thoracic cord. In contrast, 80% of parasympathetic activity originates in the brain and travels through cranial nerve X (the vagus nerve), and approximately 20% originates in the sacral cord and travels through pelvic nerves. Unopposed vagal activity accounts for the bradycardia and other parasympathetic manifestations seen in the early weeks of cervical and high thoracic spinal cord injuries, when cord activity below the level of injury temporarily ceases.

Both the sympathetic and parasympathetic motor pathways are composed of a chain of two neurons carrying nerve impulses from the CNS to the effector organ. The first neuron in the chain is the *preganglionic neuron;* the second is the *postganglionic neuron.* (A *ganglion* is a group of cell bodies.) Nerve cell bodies of preganglionic sympathetic neurons lie in the lateral horns of the gray matter of the thoracic and high lumbar segments of the cord (the intermediolateral cell columns); their axons exit the cord in the spinal nerve roots. The nerve cell bodies of preganglionic parasympathetic neurons lie either in certain areas of the brain and send their axons down cranial nerve X (the vagus nerve), or in the lateral horns of gray matter in the sacral cord and send their axons down the pelvic nerves.

table 32-2 Responses of Effector Organs to Autonomic Nerve Impulses and Circulating Catecholamines

		Adrenergic & Noradrenergic Responses	
Effector Organs	**Muscarinic Response**	***Receptor Type***	***Response****
Eye			
Radial muscle of iris	—	α	Contraction (mydriasis)
Sphincter muscle of iris	Contraction (miosis)		
Ciliary muscle	Contraction for near vision	β	Relaxation for far vision
Heart			
Sinoatrial node	Decrease in heart rate; vagal arrest	β_1	Increase in heart rate
Atria	Decrease in contractility	β_1	Increase in contractility and conduction velocity
AV node and conduction system	Decrease in conduction velocity; atrioventricular block	β_1	Increase in conduction velocity
Ventricles	—	β_1	Increase in contractility and conduction velocity
Arterioles			
Coronary, skeletal muscle, pulmonary, abdominal viscera, renal	—	α β_2	Constriction Dilation
Skin and mucosa, cerebral, salivary glands	—	α	Constriction
Systemic Veins	—	α β_2	Constriction Dilation
Lung			
Bronchial muscle	Contraction	β_2	Relaxation
Bronchial glands	Stimulation	?	Inhibition (?)
Stomach			
Motility and tone	Increase	α, β_2	Decrease (usually)
Sphincters	Relaxation (usually)	α	Contraction (usually)
Secretion	Stimulation		Inhibition (?)
Intestine			
Motility and tone	Increase	α, β_2	Decrease
Sphincters	Relaxation (usually)	α	Contraction (usually)
Secretion	Stimulation		Inhibition (?)
Gallbladder and Ducts	Contraction		Relaxation
Urinary Bladder			
Detrusor	Contraction	β	Relaxation (usually)
Trigone and sphincter	Relaxation	α	Contraction
Ureter			
Motility and tone	Increase (?)	α	Increase (usually)
Uterus	Variable[†]	α, β_2	Variable[†]
Male Sex Organs	Erection	α	Ejaculation
Skin			
Pilomotor muscles	—	α	Contraction
Sweat glands	Generalized secretion	α	Slight, localized secretion[‡]
Spleen Capsule	—	α β_2	Contraction Relaxation
Adrenal Medulla	—		—
Liver	—	α, β_2	Glycogenolysis
Pancreas			
Acini	Secretion	α	Decreased secretion

(continued)

table 32-2 Responses of Effector Organs to Autonomic Nerve Impulses and Circulating Catecholamines (Continued)

		Adrenergic & Noradrenergic Responses	
Effector Organs	**Muscarinic Response**	***Receptor Type***	***Response****
Islets	Insulin and glucagon secretion	α	Inhibition of insulin and glucagon secretion
		β_2	Insulin and glucagon secretion
Salivary Glands	Profuse, watery secretion	α	Thick, viscous secretion
		β_2	Amylase secretion
Lacrimal Glands	Secretion		—
Nasopharyngeal Glands	Secretion		—
Adipose Tissue	—	β_1	Lipolysis
Juxtaglomerular Cells	—	$\beta(\beta_1?)$	Renin secretion
Pineal Gland	—	β	Melatonin synthesis and secretion

*α and β_1—norepinephrine and epinephrine; β_2—epinephrine only.
† Depends on stage of menstrual cycle, amount of circulating estrogen and progesterone, pregnancy, and other factors.
‡ On palms of hands and in some other locations ("adrenergic sweating").
From Ganong WF: Review of Medical Physiology: Los Altos, CA, Lange Medical Publications, 2003

As mentioned, axons of preganglionic sympathetic neurons exit the cord and enter the ventral roots of spinal nerves. They then leave the spinal nerve to enter a nearby sympathetic ganglion (by a connecting pathway termed a *ramus*). In a sympathetic ganglion, the preganglionic neuron synapses with a postganglionic one. The postganglionic sympathetic neuron then may reenter the spinal nerve or exit the ganglion by a special sympathetic nerve and travel to the effector organ. Preganglionic sympathetic neurons may also send axons up or down the sympathetic ganglion chain, where they synapse with postganglionic sympathetic neurons at different levels. In this way, the sympathetic nervous system maintains communication between its different levels up and down the cord. This anatomy makes possible unitary activation of the sympathetic system so that all sympathetic end organs are stimulated maximally during the same time. This type of activation is important for the total sympathetic response involved in flight or fight. In contrast, the parasympathetic system is more diffuse, with more indirect communication between vagal parasympathetic centers in the brain and sacral parasympathetic centers, and relative independence of activity.

Axons of preganglionic parasympathetic neurons leave the CNS by certain cranial or spinal nerves and travel to the effector organ. At or near the effector organ, they synapse with the postganglionic neuron, which innervates the effector organ.

Acetylcholine is the neurotransmitter synthesized by *all* preganglionic autonomic neurons—both sympathetic and parasympathetic (see Fig. 32-13). Neurons that use acetylcholine as their neurotransmitter are called *cholinergic neurons*. When an action potential is conducted down the axon of a preganglionic autonomic neuron, acetylcholine is released into the synapse between the axon terminal and the membrane of the postganglionic neuron. It diffuses across the synapse and binds to nicotinic receptors on the membrane of the postganglionic neuron, depolarizing that membrane and, depending on the strength of the depolarization, it may cause the postganglionic neuron to develop an action potential. The nicotinic acetylcholine receptors on the postganglionic neuron at its synapse with the preganglionic neuron are similar to, but slightly different from, the nicotinic acetylcholine receptors on the skeletal muscle membrane at the neuromuscular junction. This is why drugs such as vecuronium and tubocurarine are able to block the skeletal muscle nicotinic receptors without affecting ganglionic nicotinic receptors at normal doses.

Acetylcholine also is the neurotransmitter synthesized by the axons of postganglionic parasympathetic neurons (see Fig. 32-13). An action potential conducted down the axon of a postganglionic parasympathetic neuron (as the result of a strong depolarizing influence received from the preganglionic neuron) causes acetylcholine to be released from the axon terminal into the synapse. The acetylcholine diffuses across the synapse and binds to *muscarinic* acetylcholine receptors on the parasympathetic end organ. These receptors cause changes in the end organ cell that result in smooth muscle contraction, glandular secretion, or hyperpolarization of the sinoatrial node of the heart (causing a decrease in heart rate) or slowing in the speed of conduction in the atrioventricular node of the heart. Table 32-2 shows the effects of acetylcholine on the muscarinic receptors in the various effector organs of the parasympathetic nervous system. As noted previously, the activity of the acetylcholine is terminated by acetylcholinesterase, an enzyme in the synapse. Because muscarinic receptors are structurally different from nicotinic receptors, although both can bind acetylcholine, drugs have been developed that affect only muscarinic receptors and not nicotinic receptors. An example of such a drug is atropine, which blocks muscarinic receptors and prevents the binding of acetylcholine. This and similar drugs are called *mus-*

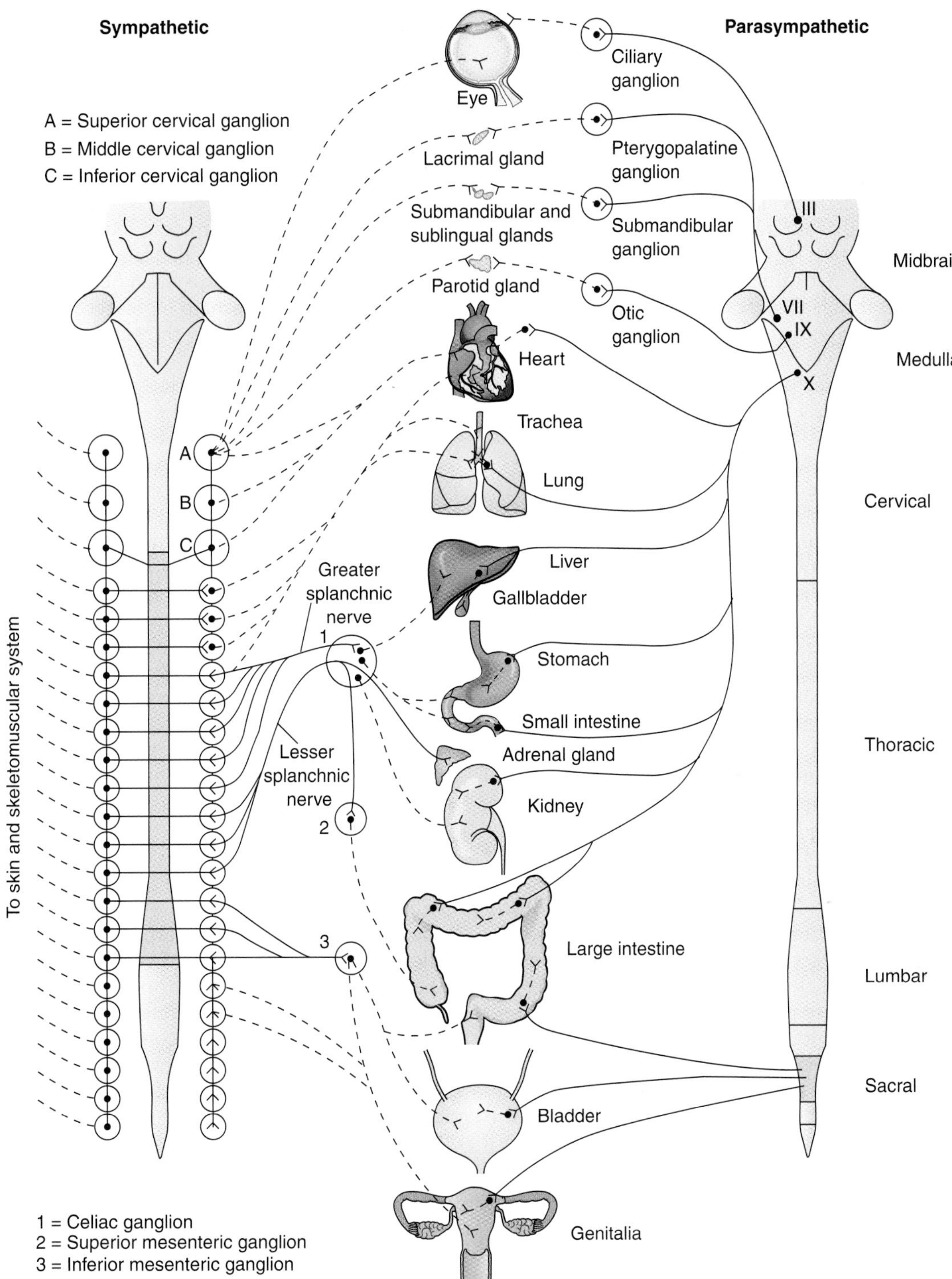

figure 32-15 The autonomic nervous system and the organs it affects. The left side illustrates the actions of the sympathetic nervous system. The right side illustrates the parasympathetic nervous system. (Porth CM: Pathophysiology: Concepts of Altered Health States [6th Ed]. Philadelphia, Lippincott Williams & Wilkins, 2002.)

carinic antagonists (also known as *anticholinergics*), and their effects are opposite to those of acetylcholine at muscarinic receptors.

Postganglionic sympathetic neurons synthesize norepinephrine, also called noradrenaline. For this reason, they and other neurons that use norepinephrine as their neurotransmitter are called *noradrenergic neurons.* When an action potential is conducted down a postganglionic sympathetic neuron (because of a strong depolarizing influence received from the preganglionic neuron), norepinephrine is released from the axon terminal into the synapse. It diffuses across the synapse and binds to receptors on the cell membrane of the effector organ. These receptors may be alpha or beta receptors. Alpha receptors may be alpha$_1$ or alpha$_2$ receptors, and beta receptors may be beta$_1$ or beta$_2$ receptors. The heart has mostly beta$_1$ receptors, and the smooth muscle of the arteries and veins has mostly alpha$_1$ and alpha$_2$ receptors. The sympathetic nervous system innervates organs with alpha$_1$, alpha$_2$, and beta$_1$ receptors and norepinephrine activates these receptors to cause changes in the effector organs that have them. For instance, activation of beta$_1$ receptors in the sinoatrial node by norepinephrine released from sympathetic axon terminals results in depolarization of the sinoatrial node and an increase in heart rate. Activation of alpha$_1$ or alpha$_2$ receptors in the arteries results in increased contraction by arteriolar smooth muscle and an increase in blood pressure. Table 32-2 shows effects of activation of alpha and beta receptors on various effector organs.

The adrenal medulla is innervated by the sympathetic nervous system through preganglionic (cholinergic) sympathetic neurons. When an action potential is conducted down their axons, these neurons release acetylcholine from their axon terminals into their synapses. The acetylcholine diffuses across the synapse and binds to nicotinic receptors on the cell membranes of the adrenal medullary cells, triggering the release of some norepinephrine but mostly epinephrine from the adrenal cells into the bloodstream. Circulating norepinephrine and epinephrine can both bind to alpha and beta receptors on sympathetic effector organs, similar to synaptic norepinephrine that is released from sympathetic nerve terminals. However, there is one important difference between norepinephrine and epinephrine. As mentioned, beta$_2$ receptors are not innervated by the sympathetic nervous system, and norepinephrine does not bind or activate beta$_2$ receptors to any degree. However, epinephrine is a powerful stimulator of beta$_2$ receptors, which it reaches through the bloodstream after being secreted by the adrenal medulla. Thus, dilation of bronchiolar smooth muscle or dilation of blood vessels in skeletal muscles are important effects of beta$_2$ receptors that are mediated by circulating epinephrine rather than by norepinephrine released from sympathetic nerve terminals or the adrenal medulla.

Although the sympathetic nerves originate in the thoracic and high lumbar cord, and parasympathetic nerves originate with nuclei that send axons down various cranial nerves or sacral spinal nerves, inputs into the patterns of autonomic function can be regulated or triggered by centers in the hypothalamus, medulla, and bulboreticular formations. These centers in the CNS send impulses along descending fibers to the appropriate preganglionic autonomic neuron. In the cord, such fibers travel by special descending tracts in the white matter until they reach the appropriate level of the cord. Thus, any interruption of these descending fibers (e.g., transection of cervical tracts) impedes or prevents stimulation of preganglionic autonomic neurons in the thoracic, lumbar, and sacral regions of the cord.

Inputs into the centers in the brainstem and hypothalamus that regulate sympathetic or parasympathetic outflow come from diffuse areas throughout the brain, including visual or auditory centers and areas of the brain associated with conscious thought or planning. Therefore, when we see an alarming sight, such as a car bearing down on us, or hear a frightening noise, sympathetic centers are stimulated and sympathetic outflow increases. Conversely, if we smell food, parasympathetic outflow might increase to prepare the digestive glands for secretion.

In many organ systems, the sympathetic and parasympathetic systems are antagonistic. For instance, the sympathetic system increases the rate of firing of the sinoatrial node and increases the speed of conduction in the atrioventricular node of the heart, whereas the parasympathetic system does the opposite. The parasympathetic system activates the gastrointestinal tract, whereas the sympathetic system inhibits it. Although this is a recurring theme, it is not an absolute rule. Thus, sympathetic stimulation constricts blood vessels (through alpha receptors), but blood vessels are not innervated by the parasympathetic system, so an opposite effect is not produced by the parasympathetic system. The sympathetic system stimulates cardiac ventricular contractility (through beta$_1$ receptors), but the ventricles are not innervated by the parasympathetic system, so contractility is not affected by it. The two systems actually work together in the male genitalia, where the parasympathetic system mediates erection while the sympathetic system mediates ejaculation.

It is important to realize that both the sympathetic and parasympathetic systems are tonically active most of the time. One or the other may be more active at a given time, but it is rare that either of them is completely silent. Therefore, a person's heart rate at any given time is an algebraic summation of the positive effects of the sympathetic system and the negative effects of the parasympathetic system. At rest, parasympathetic influence is strongest and the heart rate is slow. With exertion or strong emotion, sympathetic activation increases and the heart rate speeds up.

REFLEXES

Basically, a reflex is a motor response to a sensory input. Reflexes have three components. There is a sensory component, which may consist of only one sensory input or multiple inputs. There is an integrative CNS component that processes the sensory component and "decides" whether it is strong enough to warrant a motor response. Finally, the motor component executes the response. The motor component can consist of one motor nerve and one muscle, or several motor nerves and several muscles. The three components together constitute a "reflex arc" (Fig. 32-16). Reflexes are mediated by lower areas of the brain or by the spinal cord, so that they happen without conscious thought. We become aware of the sensory input and the motor response when they are communicated to our cortex, but by then, the reflex is over. However, if we know that a reflexive action is likely, such as when we see someone about to strike our knee with a reflex hammer, we can often suppress a reflex by willing ourselves not to perform the motor action. This capability illustrates that the cortex has input into the integrative component of the reflex. If higher centers are damaged, the reflex will still occur. For example, people with spinal cord transections still have reflexes in areas supplied by spinal nerves below the transection. Of course, they are unaware that these reflexes are taking place because they cannot receive sensory input to their cortex from below the level of the transection.

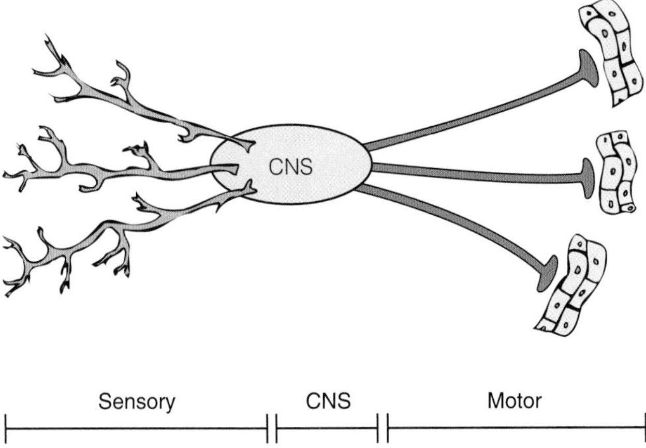

figure 32-16 Schematic representation of a reflex arc. *CNS*, central nervous system.

Brain Reflexes

Brain reflexes include those involving the *cardioregulatory* and *vasomotor centers* of the medulla, plus the pupillary adjustment center, which involves the midbrain. Additional reflexes mediated by brain centers include the gag reflex, blink reflex, vomiting, and swallowing.

Because of its importance to critical care, the baroreceptor reflex will be used as an illustration of a brain reflex. The sensory components of the baroreceptor reflex are stretch receptors in various arteries, the most important of which are in the carotid sinuses and the aortic arch. These stretch receptors are really specialized dendrites of sensory nerves that sense the stretch in the arterial wall that is produced by the pulse. If the blood pressure is high, the stretch receptors are highly stimulated, whereas if the blood pressure is low, the stretch receptors are not stimulated very much. The stretch receptors send nerve impulses down their dendrites to sensory ganglia near the brain in their respective nerves (cranial nerve IX—the glossopharyngeal nerve—in the case of the carotid sinuses, and cranial nerve X—the vagus nerve—in the case of the aortic arch) that are proportional to the degree of stretch. This information is communicated by sensory axons to autonomic centers in the medulla that process the information and compare it with a "set point" that represents the degree of stimulation they should receive if blood pressure were normal. If the medullary centers receive too little stimulation from the baroreceptors, they send impulses to sympathetic centers to increase sympathetic outflow. This stimulates sympathetic nerves supplying the heart to increase their release of norepinephrine, which binds to beta$_1$ receptors in the sinoatrial node to increase heart rate and beta$_1$ receptors in the ventricles to increase contractility. Sympathetic nerves supplying the veins release norepinephrine, which binds to alpha receptors, causing constriction of the veins, which increases venous return to the heart. Sympathetic nerves supplying the arteries release norepinephrine, which binds to alpha receptors, causing constriction of the arteries, which raises the blood pressure. The combination of increased venous return to the heart, increased heart rate, and increased contractility raises the cardiac output, which also increases the blood pressure. Finally, sympathetic nerves supplying the juxtaglomerular apparatus in the kidney release norepinephrine, which binds to beta$_1$ receptors there, stimulating renin release. Through a series of events, renin stimulates the formation of angiotensin II, which is a potent arterial constrictor, increasing blood pressure directly; it also acts on the kidney (through aldosterone) to cause sodium and water retention. Increased retention of sodium and water further increases venous return to the heart, causing additional increased cardiac output and blood pressure. Therefore, activation of the sympathetic nervous system in response to decreased stimulation of the baroreceptors produces many consequences at the effector organs, all of which separately and together cause a rise in blood pressure. If the stretch on the baroreceptors is too high (according to the normal set point), the sympathetic nervous system is inhibited, sympathetic outflow decreases, and consequences at the effector organs are diminished.

Spinal Cord Reflexes

In one type of cord reflex, the sensory component of the reflex is the sensory neurons that send their axons to the cord through one of the spinal nerves, the CNS integrative component is the spinal cord, and the motor component is the motor neurons that supply skeletal muscles. Deep tendon reflexes belong in this classification, as does the *withdrawal reflex* (Fig. 32-17A). These reflexes are present at each level of the spinal cord, bilaterally.

The sensory component of the withdrawal reflex is pain that originates in nociceptors, specialized dendrites of sensory neurons. Impulses are conducted through dendrites of the sensory neurons to the dorsal horn of the spinal cord and from there along sensory axons into the cord. These impulses stimulate cord interneurons, which, if the sensory input is strong enough, stimulate motor neurons whose axons innervate skeletal muscles, causing contraction. When contracted, the skeletal muscles produce withdrawal of the body part from the painful stimulus. The withdrawal reflex depends on the appropriate anatomical connections between sensory neurons, interneurons, and motor neurons in the cord. If these become nonfunctional (e.g., spinal shock or physical trauma), this and other spinal reflexes do not occur.

The withdrawal reflex of one foot is associated with another reflex, the *crossed extensor reflex* (see Fig. 32-17B). This reflex involves stimulation of various extensor muscles in the opposite leg so that a person's weight is fully supported by the other leg while one lower extremity is withdrawn from a painful stimulus. Such a reflex is complex and involves many levels of the cord. Any imbalance, however slight, during the operation of this reflex in a normal person triggers the occurrence of additional reflexes involving the bulboreticular formation, cerebellum, and various muscles of arms and trunk to maintain balance and posture.

Another cord reflex is the *stretch reflex* or *deep tendon reflex*, most commonly illustrated by the clinical test of the knee jerk reflex (see Fig. 32-17C). In the deep tendon reflex, the sensory component is a specialized sense organ, the muscle spindle, which sends its signals along a spinal nerve

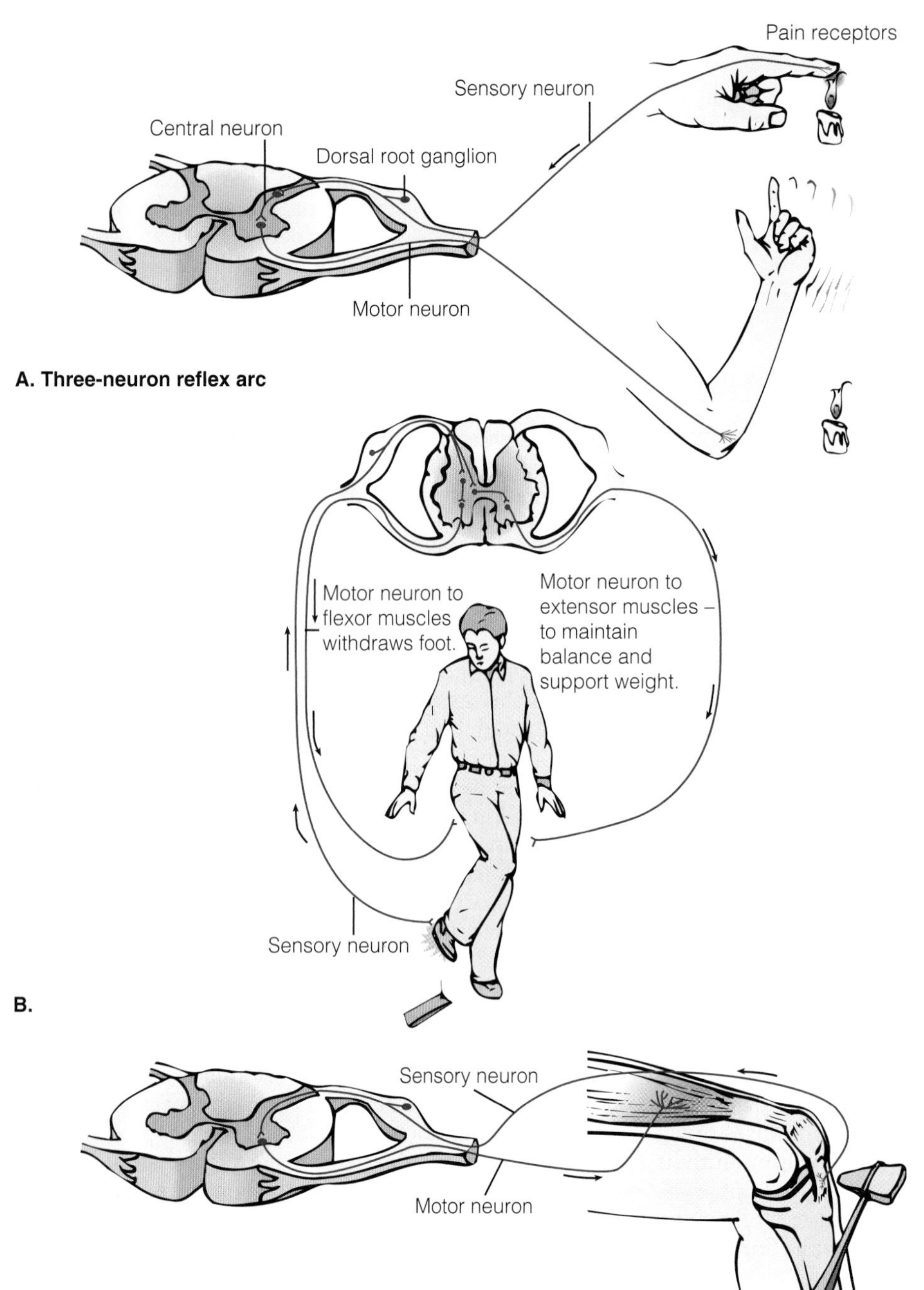

figure 32-17 Reflex arcs showing pathways of impulses in response to a stimulus. (**A**) The withdrawal reflex involves a three-neuron reflex arc: sensory, central, and motor neurons. (**B**) The flexor and crossed extensor reflexes. (**C**) Example of a stretch reflex, involving only a two-neuron reflex arc: sensory and motor neurons.

to the dorsal horn of the spinal cord. The CNS component is a single synapse of the sensory axon terminal with the motor nerve cell body. The motor component is the motor axon supplying the skeletal muscle. In the knee jerk test, a reflex hammer blow stretches the quadriceps tendon, which stretches the muscle spindle, which sends impulses through the dendrite and axon of its nerve cell to release neurotransmitter from the axon terminal. This causes the motor neuron cell body in the spinal cord to depolarize. If the depolarization is strong enough, an action potential is conducted down the axon of the motor neuron to depolarize the muscle through release of acetylcholine into the synapse at the neuromuscular junction, as discussed previously. This causes contraction of the quadriceps, which causes the lower leg to kick forward. Other deep tendon reflexes of clinical importance are the ankle jerk and the biceps and triceps reflexes. All work similarly to the knee jerk.

We can use the example of deep tendon reflexes in the extremities to illustrate the principle of neuronal threshold and the soma's summation of inhibitory and excitatory influences, as explained previously (see Fig. 32-3). Certain descending nerve fibers from the brainstem deliver low-level inhibition to motor neurons in the cord that supply muscles in the extremities. These inhibitory influences on the motor neuron are not enough to prevent development of an action potential when a strong stimulus is received from the sensory neuron that supplies the muscle spindle that is stretched when a tendon is tapped. The action potential in the motor neuron depolarizes the axon supplying the neuromuscular junction, causing a muscle contraction in the stretched muscle. However, this contraction stretches the muscle spindle again, which is communicated to the cord and might therefore cause an additional reflexive action potential to develop in the motor neuron, which would produce a second contraction of the muscle. However, this normally does not happen because the inhibitory influences arriving from the brain are strong enough to prevent the second action potential. When the spinal cord is severed, the descending inhibitory axons are also severed and the inhibitory input does not reach the motor neuron. Consequently, a tap on a tendon produces multiple jerks, called *clonus*, because the motor neuron is no longer hyperpolarized by the inhibitory input. Therefore, when the spindle is stretched by the first contraction, impulses communicated to its axon are able to reexcite the motor neuron more easily and cause a second, or even a third or fourth contraction.

An important feature of all cord reflexes involving skeletal muscles is *reciprocal inhibition*, which occurs in the antagonist muscle of the one stimulated. For example, when a flexor reflex stimulates the biceps, it also inhibits its antagonist, the triceps, and provides for more efficient performance of motor activities in the upper arm.

Spinal cord activities also include autonomic reflex circuits, which aid in the control of visceral functions of the body. Sensory input arises from visceral sensory receptors and is transmitted to the spinal cord, where reflex patterns appropriate to the sensory input are determined. The signals are then transmitted to autonomic motor neurons in the gray matter of the spinal cord, which send impulses to the sympathetic nerves innervating visceral motor end organs.

A most important autonomic reflex is the *peritoneal reflex*. Tissue damage in any portion of the peritoneum results in the activation of this reflex, which slows or stops all motor activity in nearby viscera, such as the intestine. Other autonomic cord reflexes are capable of modifying local blood flow in response to cold, pain, and heat. This vascular control by autonomic reflexes in the spinal cord can operate as a backup mechanism for the usual brainstem control patterns in patients with transectional injuries at the brainstem. Alternatively, because the autonomic reflexes arising lower in the cord of a patient with a cervical transectional injury are not modulated by brainstem centers as they are in patients without a transection, sensory input to autonomic centers in the cord can cause extreme motor responses, similar to the development of clonus with unmodulated deep tendon reflexes. However, these motor reflexes are sympathetic, and their out-of-control state in spinally injured patients is called *autonomic hyperreflexia*.

Also included in the autonomic reflexes of the spinal cord are those causing the emptying of the urinary bladder and the rectum. These reflexes are mediated by the sacral parasympathetic system. When the bladder or bowel becomes distended, sensory signals from stretch receptors in the bladder or bowel wall are transmitted by sensory neurons to the internuncial neurons of the upper sacral and lower lumbar segments of the cord. These neurons in turn stimulate parasympathetic motor neurons innervating the smooth muscle in the wall of the bladder or bowel, and their respective internal smooth muscle sphincters also are reflexively inhibited by the internuncials. The result is a reflex contraction of bladder or bowel and an opening of the respective smooth muscle sphincter, thereby permitting defecation or micturition.

In addition to their smooth muscle sphincters, both the bladder and bowel have skeletal muscle sphincters that are controlled by motor neurons. Descending motor fibers from the cortex synapse with the motor neurons, and in toilet-trained individuals, keep the skeletal muscle sphincters in a state of contraction, inhibiting the reflex emptying of bladder or bowel at times or places deemed inappropriate by the individual. When an appropriate time and place is reached, the individual can consciously relax the skeletal muscle sphincter and either void or defecate reflexively. Toilet training of infants must await the functional maturation of these descending motor fibers. Cord transection or other damage above the level of the cord housing the neurons for the bladder or bowel evacuation reflexes interrupts some or all of these descending fibers. This produces a condition in which the patient cannot consciously control (prevent) the emptying of the bladder or bowel, or both. As long as the sacral cord and associated spinal nerves are functioning, voiding or defecation proceeds reflexively in such a patient. Damage to or interrupted function of the level of the cord housing the anatomical neuronal connections for these reflexes (as in, for example, spina bifida, spinal shock, or severe injuries to the lower sacral or lumbar cord) or damage to the spinal nerves supplying the bladder or rectum prevents reflex evacuation of bladder or bowel, or both. Such a patient may exhibit retention with overflow, but does not possess any effective mechanism for emptying the bladder or bowel.

PAIN

The sensation of pain warrants special consideration because it plays such an important protective role. Whenever there is tissue damage, pain receptors, called *nociceptors*, are stimulated and send impulses back to the spinal cord. These impulses are transmitted up to the brain, where they are perceived, as previously explained. Pain is usually felt while tissue is undergoing damage and ceases when the damage ends. Stimulation of the nociceptors is caused by the release of substances from damaged tissue and from activation of the inflammatory response. Damaged cells release potassium and hydrogen ion, both of which can stimulate nociceptors. However, the inflammatory response that is evoked in response to tissue damage is responsible for much of the stimulation of nociceptors. For instance, histamine can stimulate nociceptors and prostaglandins and leukotrienes can sensitize nociceptors to other stimuli. All of these substances are released by inflammatory cells (macrophages, neutrophils, and other white blood cells) that are attracted to the area of tissue injury. In addition, activated platelets participating in clot formation in response to tearing of blood vessels release serotonin, which also stimulates nociceptors. Finally, the nociceptor itself may release substance P when it is stimulated, which sensitizes it to other activating substances.

Pain Pathways and Their Modulation

The sensation of pain is transmitted to the spinal cord and up to the brain in the same manner as previously described for sensations in general. To review, the nociceptor is really a specialized dendrite of a sensory neuron, whose cell body is in the dorsal root ganglion of the spinal nerve. When the nociceptor is stimulated enough to mount an action potential, the impulse travels to the dorsal horn, and then down the sensory nerve's axon into the dorsal horn, where it synapses with one or more projection neurons. The projection neurons carry the pain message to the thalamus where pain is first perceived. The projection neurons synapse in the thalamus with neurons that carry the message to the sensory cortex, where the pain is perceived as a localized sensation.

There is an important difference, however, in how pain messages are transmitted to the thalamus and cortex compared with other sensations. This difference is in the way the pain impulse can be modulated by spinal influences before it ascends the cord. In brief, gating mechanisms exist in an area in the gray matter called the *substantia gelatinosa* at all levels of the dorsal cord. These mechanisms, which are described in the following, are capable of regulating the number of pain impulses that can enter the ascending tracts and travel to the brain.

To regulate ascending pain impulses, an area of the brainstem called the *periaqueductal gray* sends axons to the nucleus raphe magnus in the medulla. These axons synapse with neurons that send axons from the nucleus raphe magnus to all levels of the cord in the substantia gelatinosa. These neurons regulate the ability of pain-stimulated sensory neurons to stimulate projection neurons of the spinothalamic tract. Thus, the descending fibers control the entry of pain impulses into the spinal pain conduction system at the level of the cord where the particular sensory neuron enters (Fig. 32-18). What cannot be conducted at least to the thalamus cannot be perceived.

How do the descending fibers modulate stimulation of the projection neurons by the sensory neurons? When researchers answered this question, we also obtained the answer to another perplexing question: How do the opioid drugs relieve pain? The neurons that descend from the nucleus raphe magnus in the medulla as well as the modulating internuncial neurons use previously undiscovered small protein neurotransmitters collectively referred to as the *endogenous opioid peptides:*

- Leucine-enkephalin
- Methionine-enkephalin
- Beta-endorphin
- Dynorphin
- Alpha-neoendorphin

When the endogenous opioid peptides are released into a synapse and bind to their receptors on the postsynaptic cell, they produce hyperpolarization of the postsynaptic cell. As explained previously, that makes the postsynaptic cell less likely to be able to conduct an action potential along its axon. Therefore, the descending fibers that synapse with the projection neurons can produce hyperpolarization in the projection neurons, lessening or perhaps even eliminating the pain messages that would otherwise be conducted upward by the projection neurons. Therefore, the endogenous opioid neurotransmitters, by binding to their receptors on the projection neurons, lessen the perception of pain in the thalamus and cortex. Under extreme circumstances, these descending pathways may be so inhibitory to projection neurons as to eliminate all ascending pain messages, producing complete analgesia to pain. This phenomenon is sometimes seen in victims of automobile crashes or wounded soldiers, who continue to function, oblivious to their wounds.

What stimulates areas of the periaqueductal gray and nucleus raphe magnus to send these descending inhibitory messages to the substantia gelatinosa, resulting in the release of opioid neurotransmitters and diminution of ascending pain signals? Unfortunately, we know very little about this, but it is possible that acupuncture and electrical stimulation devices for pain control are stimulating these pathways, causing inhibition of the projection neurons by the descending neurons' release of opioid neurotransmitters.

We now know that the opioid drugs work in the same way as the endogenous opioid neurotransmitters. They bind to opioid receptors on the projection or internuncial neuron, producing hyperpolarization and a decrease in the amount of pain stimulus reaching the thalamus and the cortex. There are neurons that use the endogenous opioids as neurotransmitters in the brain as well, and opioid drugs also bind to the receptors that these neurons supply. These effects may increase the analgesic effects of the drug, or they may be responsible for other effects, such as the somnolence or dizziness that opioid drugs produce. In addition, there are opioid receptors in the intestinal tract that are stimulated by endogenous opioids and by opioid drugs. These receptors inhibit peristalsis in the intestinal tract, and this effect is responsible for the constipation and nausea often seen with opioid drugs.

Pain is a complex sensation. There is great variation in pain thresholds among different people and within the same person at different times. These variations can partly be explained by the modulation of pain pathways by endogenous opioid neurotransmitters. In addition, the amount of tissue injury and presence of chemical mediators can increase the pain experience qualitatively, quantitatively, temporally, and spatially. However, pain perception is also influenced by expectations and by cultural influences. It is helpful to remember that pain is a *perception* and that we have to take a person's word in describing that perception to us. It is impossible to judge a patient's pain by their appearance, their actions, or physical or laboratory signs. The complexity of the pain pathways can make the clinical management of pain difficult, but every patient's description of his or her pain should be taken seriously. Opioid addiction is practically unknown in patients without a history of drug abuse who receive opioids for pain relief. Pain medication should be administered to most patients based on their own self-report of their pain.

Referred Pain

Referred pain is pain perceived as arising from a site that is different from its true point of origin. The "true point of origin" for this type of pain usually is some visceral organ or deep somatic structure, and the "point of refer-

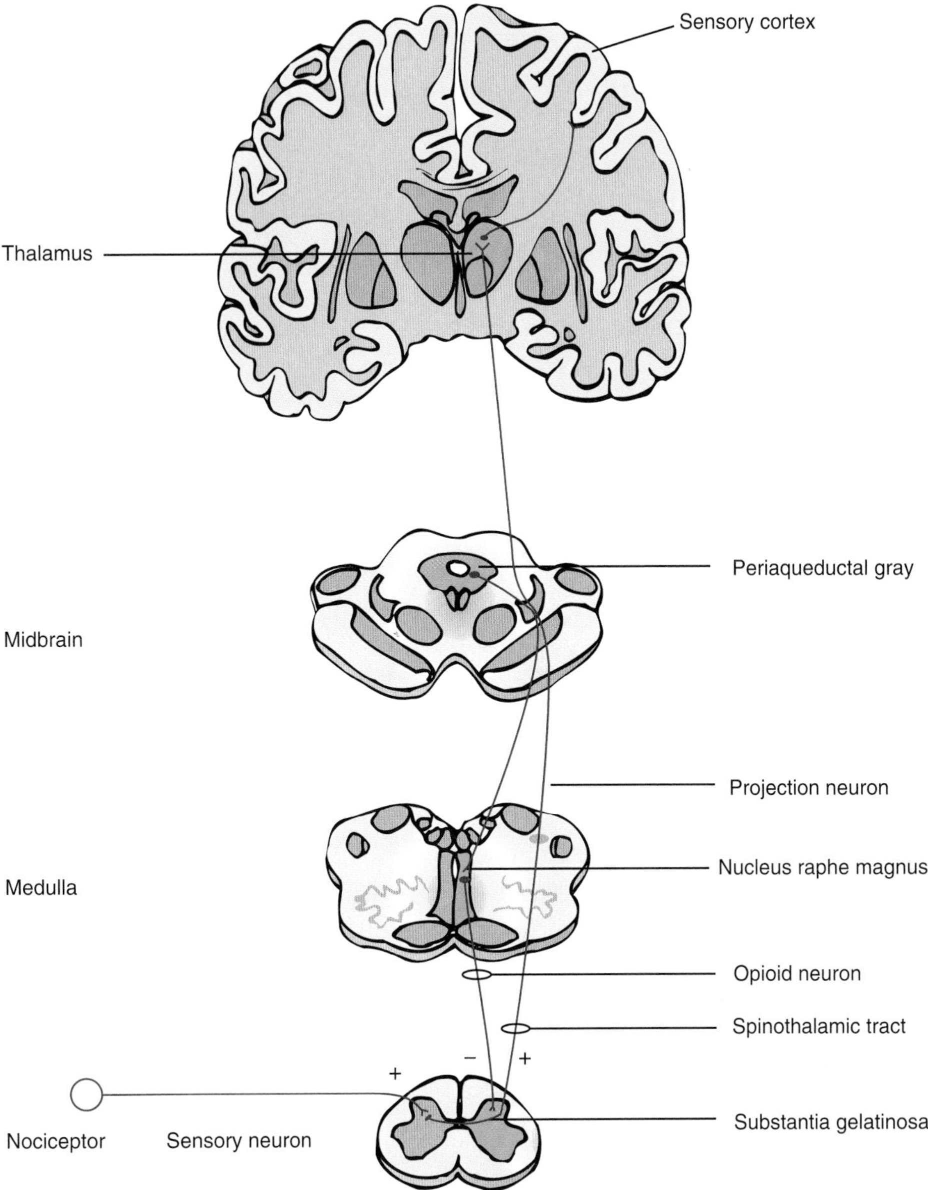

figure 32-18 Modulation of ascending pain impulses by descending opioid neurons with origins in the nucleus raphe magnus with input from the periaqueductal gray. The sensory neuron's influence on the projection neuron is stimulatory (depolarizing), designated by the plus sign, but the influence of the opioid neuron is inhibitory (hyperpolarizing), designated by the minus sign. Therefore, if the strength of impulses descending in the opioid neuron is high, the projection neuron will experience fewer action potentials and send fewer pain impulses up to the thalamus.

ence" is some area of the body surface. Well-known examples include the referring of pain from severe cardiac ischemia to the left arm or the referring of diaphragmatic pain to the neck and shoulder.

The most generally accepted theory for referred pain is that the two sensory neurons, one from the region of the true point of origin and one from the point of reference, enter the same segment of the spinal cord and synapse with the same projection neuron. There is no way for the cortex to know whether a given projection neuron was originally stimulated by pain from the true point of origin or from the referred area. In localizing the source of the pain stimulus, the cortex relies on prior experience regarding the person's geographical knowledge of his or her own body. Because surface areas are more familiar to a person than the locations of the visceral or deep somatic structures, the referred locale is used preferentially over the more unfamiliar but true point of origin (Fig. 32-19).

THE NEUROHORMONAL STRESS RESPONSE

Homeostasis

In the middle of the 19th century, the French physiologist, Claude Bernard (1813–1878), coined the term *milieu intérieur* to mean the internal environment to which body cells are exposed. He stated that to maintain proper cell functioning, the *milieu intérieur* must be constant and proper.[1,2]

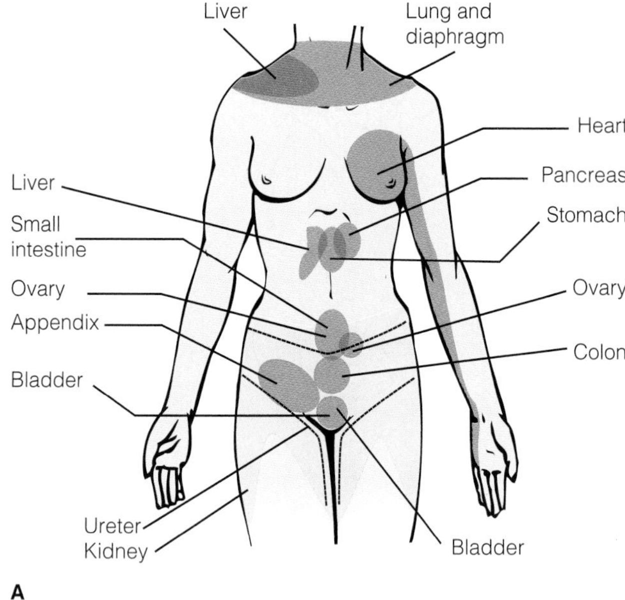

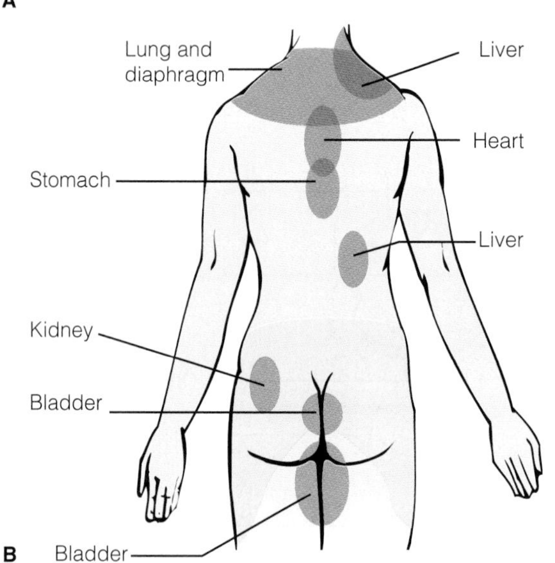

figure 32-19 Areas of referred pain. (**A**) Anterior view. (**B**) Posterior view.

> The living body, though it has need of the surrounding environment, is nevertheless relatively independent of it. This independence which the organism has of its external environment, derives from the fact that in the living being, the tissues are in fact withdrawn from direct external influences and are protected by a veritable internal environment which is constituted, in particular, by the fluids circulating in the body.*

Although Bernard thought the blood constituted the *milieu intérieur*, we now realize that each tissue and cell type probably has its own environment that may be different from that of other tissues or cell types. However, the idea of a constant and appropriate internal environment remains valid to this day. Bernard was the first to advance the concept that bodily processes are constantly responding to the external environment with mechanisms that maintain constancy of the *milieu intérieur*: "The constancy of the internal environment requires such a perfection in the organism that external variations are instantly compensated for and balanced."[1] The concept of a constant internal environment was expanded by Walter Canon in the early 20th century to include all bodily process and structures, and was termed *homeostasis.*

Homeostasis is defined as the situation in which attributes of the body such as blood pressure, level of alertness, and muscle tone remain constant or change appropriately for different situations. The constant nature of these attributes is due to the right balance between stimulatory and inhibitory neuronal and hormonal influences. In addition, structural components, such as the composition of blood, composition of extracellular fluid (ECF), and bones, tendons, muscles, and internal organs, remain essentially constant even though their components are being constantly degraded and resynthesized. Again, this structural constancy is maintained through a combination of neural and hormonal mechanisms. Homeostasis is a dynamic equilibrium—dynamic because of the constant degradation and renewal, or stimulation and inhibition, and an equilibrium because there is a balance between these opposing processes such that conditions remain constantly the same. When stressors disturb the dynamic equilibrium, compensatory mechanisms return it to its previous steady state (Fig. 32-20).

Disruption of Homeostasis

Although each of us is continually exposed to psychological and physiological stressors, we are usually able to maintain a state of emotional and physical health through compensatory mechanisms that maintain homeostasis. In fact, it has been shown that some level of stress is beneficial to health. However, in the event of stress that overwhelms compensatory mechanisms, we can become ill (Fig. 32-21). Overwhelming stressors may become so because of their large magnitude over time, or because of their sudden onset. Individuals who present as patients in critical care settings have usually experienced recent, severe

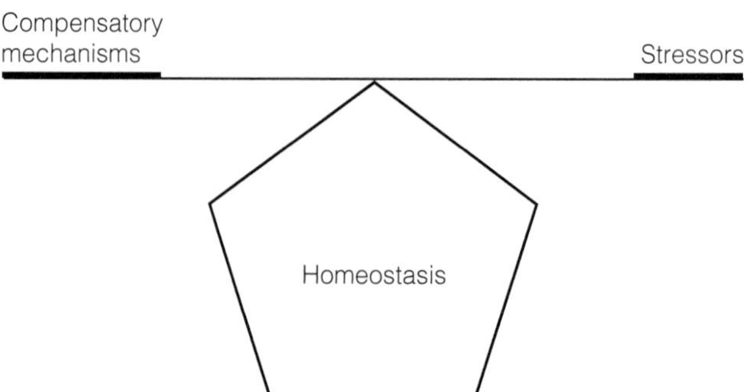

figure 32-20 Homeostasis is maintained when compensatory mechanisms are strong enough to overcome the imbalance induced by increased stress.

*Opening lecture in general physiology given to the *College de France*, as quoted in Schultz SG: The internal environment. In Johnson LR (ed): Essential Medical Physiology (2nd Ed). New York, Raven Press, 1998.

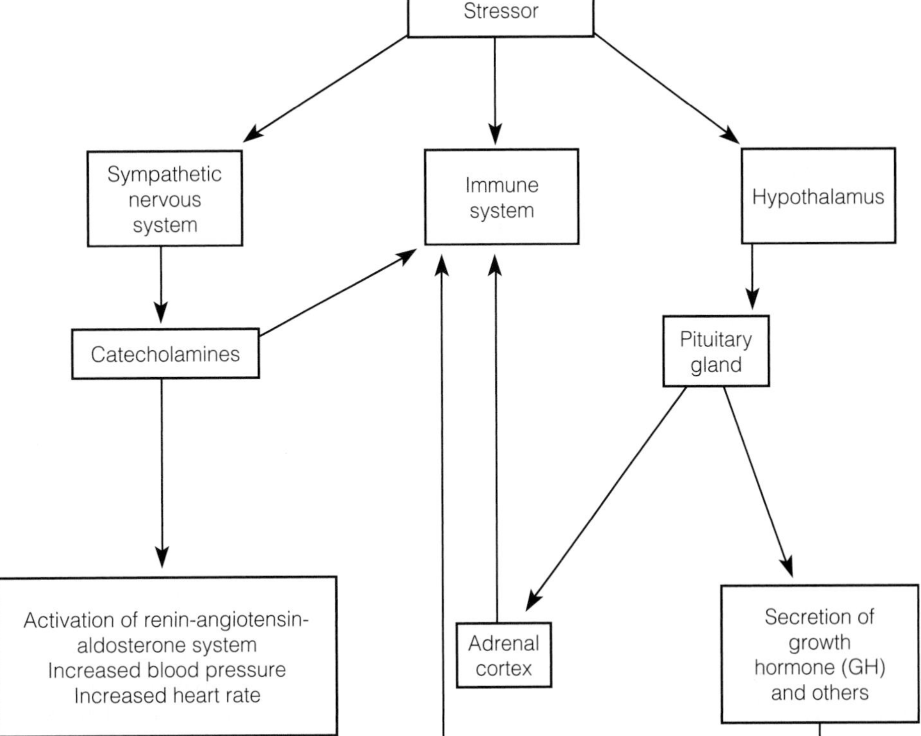

figure 32-21 The stress response induces increased activity in the sympathetic nervous system, including the adrenal medulla, which activates the renin–angiotensin–aldosterone system and increases the blood pressure and heart rate, among other things. The stress response also activates the pituitary gland, which secretes increased growth hormone; the adrenal cortex, which secretes increased cortisol; and the immune system.

physiological stressors, but these are superimposed on their level of chronic physiological and psychological stress. In addition, the patient is exposed to continuous stressors that are byproducts of the critical care setting, such as monitoring devices, invasive procedures, and the continual presence of devices for intravenous access, endotracheal intubation, and others.

Although others, especially Walter Cannon (who also coined the term *homeostasis*), presented some of these theories earlier, Dr. Hans Selye was the most prolific researcher and author on the topic of stress.[3,4] *Stress* is any external or internal factor that affects the normal state of dynamic equilibrium in an individual. These factors, or *stressors*, can be either physical or psychological. Regardless of whether the person consciously perceives a threat, the body responds with certain intrinsic reactions. When the effects are realized by the conscious mind, the individual perceives a *stressful experience*. The *stress response* is how a person reacts to the stressors that he or she encounters (i.e., the person's physiological adaptation or psychological coping mechanisms). One person may have compensatory mechanisms with a large capacity to handle stressors, whereas another person may not. Therefore, exposure to a given stressor does not elicit the same response in all individuals. This difference may be based on internal conditioning factors such as age, sex, and genetics, and external factors such as culture, previous life events, exposure to this or similar stressors, diet and nutrition, and medications.

Stressors may be either psychological or physiological in origin. Psychological stressors are additive in nature (e.g., life events such as a job change, divorce, marriage) and have a physiological impact. Physiological stressors, such as injury or infection, disrupt homeostasis, eliciting the stress response in an attempt to restore it. If homeostasis is not restored quickly, illness will result.

GENERAL ADAPTATION SYNDROME

Selye and his collaborators noted commonalities in responses to different stressors in different individuals. They termed these commonalities the *general adaptation syndrome*. Although this term has fallen from favor, and the changes they noted are probably not as general as they thought, the concept of a generalized response to stress remains. They also defined the three basic stages to the stress syndrome as the *alarm reaction*, *stage of resistance*, and *stage of exhaustion*.

- *Alarm reaction*. During this initial stage, the threat is perceived, either consciously or subconsciously, and body processes are modified to counteract it. The sympathetic nervous system is stimulated by the stressor and there is a subsequent response through the release of norepinephrine, epinephrine, adrenocorticotropic hormone (ACTH), and ADH. Stimulation of the sympathetic nervous system raises heart rate and blood pressure and stimulates the renin–angiotensin–aldosterone system, which results in sodium and water retention, increasing the blood pressure further. and release cortisol, which has multiple, far-reaching effects on nearly every organ. ADH raises blood pressure by causing intense vasoconstriction and also causes the kidney to retain water, further raising blood pressure. These effects are additive to those elicited by the sympathetic nervous system and the renin–angiotensin–aldosterone system.

- *Stage of resistance.* During the second stage, the stress is being compensated for by increased activity of the stress responses evoked during the alarm phase. Cortisol secretion, the sympathetic nervous system, and other mechanisms triggered in the alarm reaction may continue to be activated at a lower, more constant level. This phase may continue for a long time, even years, if the increased levels of stress response mechanisms are maintained. However, the increased levels of stress response mechanisms come at a price—the use of additional resources of energy and nutrients. It is during this stage that symptoms of disease may become chronic if the compensatory responses are not adequate to control them.
- *Stage of exhaustion.* The ability to mount a stress response has limits. Therefore, the stress response can be activated only for a finite time or to a finite degree. If the stressor is not removed or adaptation does not occur, the individual will no longer be able to resist the stressor. At this point, homeostasis is no longer achievable. A shock state may occur (see Chapter 54), and, without appropriate intervention, organ failure and death may rapidly ensue.

THE STRESS RESPONSE

Acute Stress

Consider a prehistoric man walking on the African veldt. Suddenly, a lion springs from behind some vegetation. The man's eyes capture an image of the lion, which is communicated to the visual areas in his occipital cortex. From there, the image is sent to and processed by his prefrontal and frontal cortex and perceived as a threat. This information of threat is communicated to many centers in his brain, including those supplying the autonomic nervous system. Immediately, sympathetic outflow is greatly increased by activation of brainstem sympathetic centers and through unitary activation of the sympathetic nervous system (remember the autonomic ganglia that communicate with each other at all levels of the spinal cord), increasing the rate of firing of his sympathetic nerves, releasing norepinephrine into sympathetic synapses. At the same time, parasympathetic outflow is greatly inhibited, decreasing activity of the gastrointestinal system and the need of those organs for blood. The man's heart rate and cardiac contractility (beta$_1$ receptors) are greatly increased, both of which increase his cardiac output, and his resistance arterioles constrict (alpha receptors). Increased cardiac output and increased arteriolar resistance raises his blood pressure. At the same time, veins also constrict (alpha receptors), increasing venous return to his heart and increasing cardiac output still more. The adrenal medulla is stimulated by sympathetic outflow (neuronal nicotinic receptors) to secrete some norepinephrine, but mostly epinephrine, into the bloodstream. The epinephrine stimulates alpha and beta$_1$ receptors all over the man's body, causing the same effects as norepinephrine does at those receptors. It also stimulates beta$_2$ receptors on his bronchiolar smooth muscle, causing relaxation and dilation of the bronchioles, enabling him to inspire and expire greater volumes of air. In addition, it stimulates beta$_2$ receptors on arterioles in his skeletal muscle beds, causing profound dilation, increasing the capacity of these beds for blood flow. Because arterioles to digestive and other internal organs are constricted by virtue of alpha receptor activation, the greatly increased cardiac output is directed to skeletal muscle beds, supplying the muscle cells with increased amounts of oxygen and glucose to sustain increased contraction. Blood flow to the brain is also greatly increased by the increased cardiac output because arterioles supplying the brain have few alpha receptors, so they remain fully dilated. Stimulation of beta$_1$ receptors in the juxtaglomerular apparatus of the kidney by norepinephrine (from sympathetic nervous system nerve terminals and the adrenal medulla) and epinephrine (from the adrenal medulla) causes the release of renin, which activates the renin–angiotensin–aldosterone system. Angiotensin II, synthesized in response to activation of the renin–angiotensin–aldosterone system, causes additional arteriolar constriction, increasing blood pressure still further. It also causes the release of aldosterone, which causes the kidney to retain sodium and water. Sodium and water retention increases the preload to the heart, increasing cardiac output still further.

In addition, communication of the threatening sight to the hypothalamus activates many neurohormonal mechanisms controlled by the pituitary. We consider only three of these. First, the hypothalamus increases its synthesis and release of ADH from the posterior pituitary. ADH causes the kidney to retain water, further increasing the preload and cardiac output. It is also a potent arteriolar vasoconstrictor, increasing blood pressure still further. Second, the hypothalamus increases its secretion and release of corticotropin-releasing hormone (CRH), which causes the anterior pituitary to secrete additional ACTH, which in turn causes the adrenal cortex to release increased quantities of cortisol. Cortisol has far-reaching effects on many organs that increase their ability to respond to stress. Third, through increased synthesis and release of growth hormone–releasing hormone (GHRH) by the hypothalamus, growth hormone (GH) synthesis and release by the anterior pituitary is increased. Like cortisol, GH has many far-reaching effects on many organs, but its overall effect is to increase the activity of tissue repair mechanisms and utilization of nutrients.

Finally, the man's immune system is activated by the stress response. This activation is achieved by multiple influences, only a few of which are mentioned here. First, GH increases the ability of many cells of the immune system, such as neutrophils and T and B lymphocytes, to carry out their functions, including phagocytosis, antigen presentation, and antibody production. In addition, the physiologically high levels of cortisol affect the immune system's ability to respond to foreign antigens. (Levels produced by pharmacological doses of corticosteroids are much higher than those produced by stress and are immunosuppressive.) The effects of physiologically elevated levels of cortisol in response to stress on immune function are complex and may involve effects on the ability of immune cells to exit the circulation and go to sites of tissue injury, or their ability to respond to antigen presentation. Finally, catecholamines also affect the immune system's ability to respond to tissue injury or foreign antigens. The net response of the immune system to acute influences of the stress response is generally considered to be an increased ability to mount an inflammatory response and respond to a foreign antigen. Figure 32-21 summarizes the effects on various body systems.

Returning to our prehistoric man threatened by a lion, the changes produced in his body by the threatening sight of a lion all have the effect of increasing the ability of his muscles to help him run faster or fight harder to escape the lion, and increasing his ability to respond to tissue injury that might result from his encounter with the lion. These changes constitute the alarm reaction characterized by Selye. The lion threat represents an acute stressor that would end very quickly, either because the man escaped or was killed. If the man was successful in escaping the lion, the stress response would extinguish itself and his physiological state would gradually return to normal.

The question that arises for modern humans is "How are the changes of the alarm reaction beneficial for stresses encountered in modern times?" If one is running to get away from a dangerous situation or to catch a bus, is injured in an automobile crash, or contracts an acute illness, the acute stress response is very likely still beneficial. However, if one undergoes an acute emotional stress, such as an intense argument or the death of a loved one, the alarm reaction is invoked, the same as it would be for a more physiologically oriented stress. In such circumstances, we do not need increased ability to fight or run away, decreased activity of our gastrointestinal system, or increased ability for tissue repair. Therefore, in these circumstances, the acute stress response is at best superfluous, and at worst consumes resources and unnecessarily creates wear and tear on body systems.

Chronic Stress

Selye's "stage of resistance" describes our ability to handle chronic stress. Chronic stressors that affected prehistoric humans included starvation or extreme heat or cold. Responses to these stressors included some of the same mechanisms as outlined earlier for acute stress, but at diminished levels that are more sustainable over a long period. However, responses to these stressors also included additional mechanisms that conserve body stores of nutrients and energy. These responses include cortisol, but also insulin, glucagon, and GH. The chronic stress response in prehistoric times probably did not include response to diseases. Because disease processes could not be treated, affected individuals quickly died during the acute stress response. The mechanisms that evolved prehistorically to handle chronic stress may or may not be appropriate to handle modern stressors such as chronic disease or the chronic emotional stress associated with constant deadlines or commuting in heavy traffic. Moreover, with modern medical care, we now have the ability to maintain individuals with extremely high levels of chronic stress due to disease, their emotional state, and the stress induced by our interventions. In intensive care units we measure many aspects of homeostasis, such as electrolyte levels, blood cell counts, cardiac functioning, and hormonal levels and adjust our care to preserve homeostasis (a proper *milieu intérieur*).

In many such situations, the chronic stress responses as they have been handed down to us from prehistoric times may actually be counterproductive and decrease our ability to maintain homeostasis. In addition, increased activity of stress responses may increase the likelihood of degenerative diseases of the circulatory system, such as atherosclerosis, leading to vascular events in the heart, periphery, or brain; disorders of glucose metabolism that lead to type 2 diabetes; or, perhaps, disorders of the immune system that lead to inflammatory diseases. These types of diseases are all the result of a complex interplay between a person's genetic makeup, his or her life experiences (including exposure to antigens and infectious diseases), and level of both physiological and psychological stress.

CONCLUSION

As we have seen, the brain coordinates activities of many body systems directly or through its influence on the endocrine system and the immune system. This control is modulated at every level by sensory input that informs the brain about our interactions with the environment, including our internal environment (*milieu intérieur*). Cortical and subcortical processing of sensory information enables us to form purposeful movements to carry out our activities and respond to threats to homeostasis. Special considerations are made for older and pediatric patients when applying principles of neurological anatomy and physiology to clinical practice. These considerations are outlined in Boxes 32-1 and 32-2.

clinical applicability challenges

Self-Challenge: Critical Thinking

1. *Describe how voluntary movement is achieved by discussing the motor pathways in the somatic motor division, beginning with the cortex and ending with muscle contraction.*
2. *Describe the pathway of pain as it travels from the nociceptor to the sensory cortex.*

Study Questions

1. *Which of the following regarding an action potential is false?*
   a. *Sodium–potassium pumps maintain membrane potential of the cell.*
   b. *Action potentials of neurons inside the brain can be monitored by an electroencephalogram (EEG).*
   c. *The inside of the cell is more positively charged than the outside.*
   d. *The action potential has self-propagated conduction.*
2. *Which structure is part of the brainstem?*
   a. *Cerebral cortex*
   b. *Thalamus*
   c. *Basal ganglia*
   d. *Pons*
3. *What is the function of the limbic system?*
   a. *Sleep–wake cycle*
   b. *Voluntary and subconscious bodily movements*
   c. *Control of emotion-related behavior*
   d. *Production of cerebrospinal fluid (CSF)*

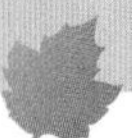

box 32-1

Considerations for the Older Patient

With increasing age:

- Cerebral atrophy results in a decrease in total brain weight and volume, especially in the frontal and temporal lobes, enlargement of the ventricles, and a loss of gray matter.
- Cerebral atrophy causes the dura mater and bridging veins to become tightly adherent to the skull; thus, they are easily torn with significant movement of the cranial contents leading to subdural hematoma formation.
- Cerebral atrophy creates more space for intracranial blood to be concealed, so the older patient may manifest only subtle symptoms, which may lead to a delay in diagnosis.
- Axonal loss or decreases in myelination result in a loss of white matter.
- There is atrophy of the hippocampus, which correlates with a decline in learning and memory and cognitive impairments.
- A decreased number of neuronal cells and degeneration of dendrites and dendritic spines in cortical pyramidal cells leads to declining synaptic transmission and slowed impulse conduction.
- There is decreased production, release, and metabolism of neurotransmitters.
- Altered circulation in the inner ear and fewer functional cochlear cells lead to reduced hearing.
- A decreased number of olfactory cells in nasal mucosa leads to a reduced sense of smell.
- There is an increase in wakefulness and arousal from sleep, and a decrease in slow-wave sleep leading to changes in sleep patterns.
- The odontoid process in the cervical spine is most commonly fractured because of osteoporosis and degenerative joint disease.
- Central cord syndrome occurs more frequently because of spinal stenosis.
- The patient is more prone to severe brain injury and may have less reserve to survive a severe injury.
- The incidence of dementia somewhat increases. Those who develop dementia have a decline in cognitive and emotional abilities, which can affect memory, language, visuospatial skills, complex cognition, emotion, and personality.

Impairment of sensation, proprioception, gait, vision, hearing, and delayed response time are a few factors that predispose older individuals to injury. Because of the age-related changes in the brain, older people are at higher risk for injury and have less chance for survival after a severe injury.

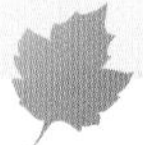

box 32-2

Considerations for the Pediatric Patient

- All brain cells are present at birth and rapidly change in organization and chemical composition. Development of brain cells is complete by 5 years of age.
- Collateral circulation is abundant to provide perfusion to the brain when there is pathology.
- Small children have thin skulls that can be easily penetrated.
- Because of an infant's immature, flexible skull, a great deal of force is needed to cause a skull fracture.
- An infant's brain is quite compressible, which permits fluid accumulation that leads to extracerebral collections as a result of trauma.
- After a traumatic brain injury, there is a higher incidence of early seizures (within first 7 days) in children younger than 5 years of age.
- In infancy the head accounts for one-fourth of the body length and one-third of the body weight; thus, infants and young children are prone to brain injury because of the head's disproportion to the rest of the body.
- Global cerebral blood flow is higher in children than in adults. Increases to age 5 are followed by a gradual decline to adult levels by age 19 years.
- Cranial sutures do not fuse until 16 to 18 months of age. As a result, if there is a gradual increase in intracranial volume during infancy, head circumference may increase. The areas in which the major sutures intersect in the anterior and posterior portions of the skull are known as *fontanels*. Increased intracranial pressure produces a bulging, full anterior fontanel.
- The spine is very flexible and bends easily, which means spinal cord injuries are less common after pediatric trauma compared with adult trauma.
- Pediatric spinal ligaments are relatively lax, the neck and paraspinous and paravertebral muscles are incompletely developed, and the vertebral facets are more shallow than those of the adult. This laxity of the spine can protect the child during minor trauma but may result in subluxation and spinal cord injury if major acceleration–deceleration forces are applied to the head, neck, or vertebral column.
- Pediatric vertebrae are softer and more cartilaginous than adult vertebrae and thus less likely to fracture. As a result, when the child does sustain a spinal cord injury, it is often present without radiographic abnormality (spinal cord injury without radiographic abnormality, or SCIWORA).
- Cervical spine injuries in infants and young children tend to be at cervical spine levels C1–5 compared with those in adults (C5–7).

Young children are highly active, curious, and spontaneous. They lack knowledge and judgment skills. All of these factors place them at risk for injury. Seventy-five percent of children hospitalized for trauma have a brain injury. Although most pediatric brain injuries are mild, CNS injuries are the most common cause of pediatric traumatic death. Unlike adults, whose recovery after trauma tends to plateau within 6 months to 1 year, children often continue to show recovery of motor, speech, and intellectual function for several years after injury.

4. *Which is not a function of cranial nerve III (oculomotor)?*
   a. *Upper eyelid elevation*
   b. *Extraocular movements*
   c. *Sight*
   d. *Pupillary response*
5. *Which of the following areas of referred pain is not associated with the corresponding organ?*
   a. *Cardiac: left arm*
   b. *Diaphragm: shoulder*
   c. *Stomach: epigastrium*
   d. *Appendix: left lower abdominal quadrant*

REFERENCES

1. Conti F: Claude Bernard: Primer of the second biomedical revolution. Nat Mol Cell Biol 2:703–708, 2001
2. Conti F: Claude Bernard's Des Fonctions du Cerveau: An ante litteram manifesto of the neurosciences? Nat Neurosci 3:979–985, 2002
3. Selye H: The general adaptation syndrome and the diseases of adaptation. J Clin Endocrinol 6:117, 1946
4. Selye H: Stress Without Distress. Philadelphia, JB Lippincott, 1974

OTHER SELECTED READING

Ashburn MA, Rice LJ: The Management of Pain. Philadelphia, Churchill Livingstone, 1998

Burton H: Visual cortex activity in early and late blind people. J Neurosci 23(10):4005–4011, 2003

Cohen H: Neuroscience for Rehabilitation (2nd Ed). Philadelphia, Lippincott Williams & Wilkins, 1999

Dellasega C: Assessment of cognition in the elderly. Nurs Clin North Am 33(3):395–405, 1998

Fisher MD: Pediatric traumatic brain injury. Crit Care Nurse Q 20(1):36–51, 1997

Hickey JV: The Clinical Practice of Neurological and Neurosurgical Nursing (5th Ed.) Philadelphia, Lippincott Williams & Wilkins, 2003

Horner A, VanDemark M, Jensen GA: The challenge of assessing a patient with dementia and head injury. AACN Clin Issues 13(1):73–83, 2002

Kandel E, Schwartz JH, Jessell TM: Principles of Neural Science (4th Ed). New York, McGraw-Hill, 2000

Levin DL, Morriss FC: Essentials of Pediatric Intensive Care (2nd Ed). New York, Churchill Livingstone, 1997

McHugh JM, McHugh WB: Pain: Neuroanatomy, chemical mediators, and clinical implications. AACN Clin Issues 11(2):168–178, 2000

McLone DG: Pediatric Neurosurgery: Surgery of the Developing Nervous System (4th Ed). Philadelphia, WB Saunders, 2001

Minton MS, Hickey JV: A primer of neuroanatomy and neurophysiology. Nurs Clin North Am 34(3):555–572, 1999

Olmstead JMD, Olmsted EH: Claude Bernard and the Experimental Method in Medicine. New York, Henry Schuman, 1952

Parent A: Carpenter's Human Neuroanatomy (9th Ed). Baltimore, Williams & Wilkins, 1996

Pudelek B: Geriatric trauma: Special needs for a special population. AACN Clin Issues 13(1):61–72, 2002

Victor M, Ropper AH: Adams and Victor's Principles of Neurology (7th Ed). New York, McGraw-Hill, 2001

chapter

33

Patient Assessment: Nervous System

GENELL HILTON

objectives

Based on the content in this chapter, the reader should be able to:

- Gather neurological data in an orderly and objective manner.
- Correlate such data over time.
- Recognize patterns of assessment findings that imply a significant change in neurological condition for the patient.
- Evaluate the effect of neurological dysfunction on the patient's living patterns.
- Relate the procedures of selected neurodiagnostic tests to nursing implications for patient care.

Assessment and care of a patient with a neurological problem constitute one of the biggest challenges for many critical care nurses. In basic nursing education and even in many critical care courses, assessment of the nervous system is frequently covered last. In addition, the curriculum may not address the nervous system to the depth or complexity of other body systems. It is not uncommon, then, for even the experienced caregiver to feel uncertain when gathering data about the nervous system.

There are four major objectives in the nursing assessment of a patient with a real or potential neurological problem. The first objective is to gather data about the functioning of the nervous system in an objective and orderly manner, avoiding inconsistencies in data collection or inadequate data collection. It is essential that examination results be recorded clearly so changes in findings can be easily identified. A standard neurological check sheet should be used by all the nursing staff, with clearly defined grading scales or terms listed.

The second objective of neurological assessment is to correlate and trend the data over time. For such a correlation to be of value, the results of history, physical assessment, and diagnostic tests must be interrelated. Use of a patterned format helps establish medical and nursing diagnoses and guides the nurse in choosing and evaluating therapy.

The third objective of neurological assessment is to analyze the data to develop a list of potential or actual diagnoses. Minor changes in neurological status may be the first indication that the patient's physical condition is worsening. It is the responsibility of the nurse providing care to the patient to recognize these changes, correlate these findings to the pathophysiological process, and intervene appropriately.

The fourth objective of the neurological nursing assessment is to determine the effect of dysfunction on the patient's daily living and ability to care for himself or herself. Up to this point, the goals of physicians and nurses in the care of a patient with a neurological problem have been similar. Each discipline uses many of the same questions and techniques to determine normal and abnormal nervous system functioning. The focus of nursing is to help patients cope with real or potential changes in daily living and self-care.

These objectives of neuroassessment are the same for all patients. However, when the patient is a child, all aspects of this process can be difficult (Box 33-1). In older patients, it is necessary to take the normal changes of aging into account when assessing for neurological problems, and to remember that older adults are at increased risk for certain medical conditions that predispose them to neurological problems (or could be confused with a neurological problem). Special considerations for older adults are given in Box 33-2.

HISTORY

Neurological assessment begins with the nurse's first encounter with the patient. Conversation with the patient and family is a vital source of data needed to evaluate overall functioning.

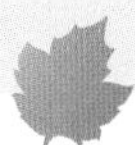

box 33-1

Neuroassessment of the Pediatric Patient

- History may be difficult to obtain.
- Language skills may be limited so that the degree of confusion is difficult to assess.
- If the nurse is unfamiliar with normal children's behavior, deviation from the norm may not be apparent.
- Variations in physical capability and limitations in motor, social, and language skills can add to the difficulty of assessing the injured pediatric patient.
- When a child's level of consciousness is assessed, special attention should be given to the comments of the caregiver. A child may seem calm to the nurse, but if the caregiver insists the child is "not acting right," further evaluation is warranted.
- Children who allow the nurse to examine them or perform painful diagnostic tests without protest are cause for special concern.
- Pupil checks can most easily be accomplished by permitting the child, if his or her condition allows, to play with the flashlight; changes in pupils can be noted with the change in level of light.
- A modified Glasgow Coma Scale can be used for assessing infants and toddlers.

Modified Glasgow Coma Scale for Infants, Toddlers, and Children

Best Eye-Opening Response	**Score**
Spontaneous	4
To verbal stimulus	3
To pain stimulus	2
None	1
Best Motor Response	
Normal spontaneous movement	6
Localizes pain	5
Withdraws to pain	4
Abnormal flexion	3
Abnormal extension	2
None	1
Best Verbal Response	
Smiles, interacts	5
Consolable	4
Cries to pain	3
Moans to pain	2
None	1

A total score of 3 to 8 suggests severe impairment, 9 to 12 suggests moderate impairment, and 13 to 15 suggests mild impairment.

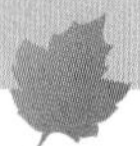

box 33-2

Neuroassessment of the Older Patient

When assessing an older adult, it is necessary to ascertain the person's previous level of functioning to adequately assess the person's status. The following should be taken into consideration when the nurse assesses an older adult's neurological function.

- Motor function may be affected by decreased strength, alterations in gait, changes in posture, and increased tremors.
- Vision may be decreased, pupils may be less reactive, color discrimination may be decreased, gaze may be impaired, and night vision may be diminished.
- Hearing may be diminished and changes in Rinne test findings may be noted. The nurse should bear in mind that an undetected hearing impairment can lead to the erroneous assumption that a person has more neurological deficits than he or she actually has.
- Changes in sensory function may include decreased reflexes, decreased vibratory and position sense, and decreased two-point discrimination.
- Older adults are at increased risk for depression, nutritional abnormalities, stroke, transient ischemic attacks (TIAs), and dementia.
- Older adults may have impaired sleep patterns.

Analysis of the Current Problem

Analysis of the current problem (i.e., the problem bringing the person to the health care facility) entails eliciting a chief complaint from the patient and obtaining a history of the present illness. The chief complaint is a one- or two-sentence description, in the words of the patient, highlighting his or her reason for seeking care. This description may or may not have anything to do with the reality of the person's situation, but it does give the nurse insight into the patient's view of the condition. In some situations, it may be necessary to have a family member or friend present who can confirm and clarify the patient's responses.

Obtaining a history of the present illness allows the nurse to delve into the details of the chief complaint. The history should include a description of any precipitating events; a description of the characteristics of the symptoms; the severity, timing, and duration of the symptoms; and a description of factors that aggravate or alleviate the symptoms (Box 33-3).

Review of Systems

The review of systems is done to gain an overview of systemic conditions or symptoms, information that may help the nurse uncover the patient's problems. Questions are organized from head to toe and are aimed at identifying neurological problems. Potential findings of the review of systems that may indicate neurological disease are given in Box 33-3.

box 33-3

Neurological Assessment: Components of the Patient History

History of Present Illness

P Precipitating events (e.g., travel, a fall, infection, prodromal symptoms, drug ingestion)
Q Quality of symptoms (a complete description of presenting symptoms)
R Relief of symptoms (aggravating or alleviating factors)
S Severity of symptoms (a description of how incapacitating the symptoms are and how they affect the person's lifestyle)
T Timing (the duration of the symptoms, including the initial onset and frequency)

Review of Systems

HEENT Dizziness, headaches, vision changes, sensitivity to light, auditory changes, tinnitus, sinus infections, difficulty swallowing, hoarseness, slurred speech, sinusitis, infection
Cardiovascular Palpitations, history of coronary artery disease, vascular problems
Respiratory History of chronic pulmonary disease, episodes of shortness of breath, recurrent infections
Gastrointestinal Nausea, vomiting, diarrhea or constipation, weight loss, history of gastrointestinal problems
Genitourinary Incontinence, impotence
Musculoskeletal Weakness or paralysis, decreased range of motion, muscle stiffness or pain, spinal problems
Neurological Syncope, confusion, difficulty with concentration, speech problems, paresthesias, tremors, gait disturbances
Psychiatric History of psychiatric problems, mood swings, delusions or hallucinations

Pertinent Medical History

Family history Stroke, diabetes mellitus, hypertension, seizures, headaches, cancer
Medical history Stroke, diabetes mellitus, hypertension, vascular disease, cancer, seizures, infections, renal or hepatic disease, psychiatric or neurological disease, trauma
Surgical history Neurological or HEENT surgery
Social history Use of alcohol, cigarettes, or drugs; exposure to toxins
Medications Antiepileptics, psychotropics, antihypertensives, anticoagulants, sedatives, oral contraceptives

HEENT, head, eyes, ears, nose, throat.

Pertinent Medical History

Significant past medical and surgical history should be ascertained because certain conditions may predispose the patient to neurological problems (see Box 33-3). In addition, the family history, particularly a history of stroke, hypertension, or seizures, is important to obtain. A review of medications can shed light on the patient's symptomatology because certain medications, such as sedatives and psychotropics, play a role in the onset of neurological symptoms or can mask or exacerbate symptoms.

PHYSICAL EXAMINATION

Mental Status

The mental status examination includes tests to evaluate level of consciousness and arousal, orientation to the environment, and thought content.

The quality of a patient's level of consciousness is the most basic and most critical parameter requiring assessment. It is an assessment that demonstrates the functioning of the cerebral hemispheres as well as that of the reticular activating system, which is responsible for arousal. The level of a patient's awareness of, response to, and interaction with the environment is also the most sensitive indicator of nervous system dysfunction. Several systems are used for grading alterations in arousal and awareness. Terms such as *lethargic*, *stuporous*, and *semicomatose* are in common use in many areas (Box 33-4).

Orientation to the environment involves assessing not only the patient's ability to respond, but the content of his or her response. This is assessed by asking the patient questions such as, "What is your name? Where are you right now? What is the month/year/date/time?" An increase in the number of wrong answers might indicate increasing confusion and deterioration in neurological status. Likewise, an increase in the number of correct answers may indicate neurological improvement.

In instances where brain injury is suspected, the Glasgow Coma Scale (GCS) has proven to be a reliable tool for assessing arousal and level of consciousness (Box 33-5). The GCS allows the examiner to record objectively the patient's response to the environment in three major areas: eye opening, movement, and verbalization. In each category, the best response is scored. The GCS uses two responses, best eye-opening response and best verbal response, to assess arousal and level of consciousness. Best eye-opening response is scored from 1 to 4, with 1 as no response and 4 as spontaneous eye opening. Best verbal response addresses orientation and ranges from 1 to 5, with 1 again indicating no response and 5 indicating an oriented patient. The intubated patient is usually noted to have a verbal score of 1T, which should be added into the total score. In this way, recognition is given to the patient's inability to speak secondary to the presence of the endotracheal tube.

The maximum total score for a fully awake and alert person is 15. A minimum score of 3 indicates a completely unresponsive patient. An overall score of 8 or below is associated with coma; if maintained over time, it may be one predictor of a poor functional recovery. This scoring system was designed as a guide for rapid evaluation of the acutely ill or severely injured patient whose status may change quickly. It is not useful as a guide for evaluation of patients in long-standing comas or during prolonged recovery from severe brain injury.

An alternative to grading scales, such as the GCS and the stimulus–reaction level scale in Box 33-6, is to describe what stimulus is used and what the patient's response is. A suggested order of stimuli follows:

1. Call the patient by name.
2. Call his or her name louder.
3. Combine calling the patient's name with light touch.
4. Combine calling the patient's name with vigorous touch ("shake and shout").
5. Create pain by applying noxious stimuli.

When noxious stimuli are needed to evoke a response, the nurse should pay careful attention to where the painful stimulus is applied. A misplaced examiner's hand can cause serious skin or tissue injury. Areas to avoid include the skin

box 33-4
Clinical Terminology for Grading Responsiveness

Alert (full consciousness): normal
Awake: may sleep more than usual or be somewhat confused on first awakening, but fully oriented when aroused
Lethargic: drowsy but follows simple commands when stimulated
Obtunded: arousable with stimulation; responds verbally with a word or two; follows simple commands; otherwise drowsy
Stuporous: very hard to arouse; inconsistently may follow simple commands or speak single words or short phrases; limited spontaneous movement
Semicomatose: movements are purposeful when stimulated; does not follow commands or speak coherently
Comatose: may respond with reflexive posturing when stimulated or may have no response to any stimulus

box 33-5
The Glasgow Coma Scale

Best Eye-Opening Response	**Score**
Spontaneously	4
To speech	3
To pain	2
No response	1
Best Motor Response	**Score**
Obeys commands	6
Localizes stimuli	5
Withdrawal from stimulus	4
Abnormal flexion (decorticate)	3
Abnormal extension (decerebrate)	2
No response	1
Best Verbal Response	**Score**
Oriented	5
Confused conversation	4
Inappropriate words	3
Garbled sounds	2
No response	1

A total score of 3 to 8 suggests severe impairment, 9 to 12 suggests moderate impairment, and 13 to 15 suggests mild impairment.

box 33-6
A Stimulus–Reaction Level Scale

Level	Description
1	Alert; no delay in response
2	Drowsy but responsive to gentle stimulation; confused about either name, place, or time
3	Very drowsy; responds to strong stimulation with orienting eye movements, obeying commands or localizing, and actively attempting to remove stimulus
4	Unconscious; localizes but not successful in removing stimulus
5	Unconscious; withdrawal movements to any stimulation
6	Unconscious; stereotypical flexion movements to pain
7	Unconscious; stereotypical extension movements to pain
8	Unconscious; no response to pain stimulation

of the nipples and genital area. Instead, one should apply pain to the big toenail, the knuckles or nails of the fingers, the sternum, or the supraorbital ridge; all provide sufficient data to elicit a patient's response to pain. When stimulating the supraorbital ridge, one should take care not to damage the eye itself.

More complex information about nervous system functioning can be obtained by gathering data about the patient's ability to integrate attention, memory, and thought processes (Box 33-7). Such a mental status examination also may uncover clues about the presence of additional problems affecting the patient's lifestyle. The Mini-Mental State Examination (MMSE) is a widely used cognitive assessment tool that is easy and rapid to administer and has good interrater reliability. It is frequently used to monitor disease progression in patients with dementia or other progressive disease states. The MMSE is composed of questions related to orientation, registration, attention and calculation, recall, and language. Points are assigned for correct answers, with a maximum of 30 points. Scores of less than 20 many indicate neurological disease.

When gathering such a wealth of data, assessment of the patient's ability to communicate becomes paramount. Use of language requires comprehension of verbal and nonverbal symbols and the ability to use those symbols to communicate with others. Evaluation of the patient's understanding normally is accomplished through the spoken word. However, speech dysfunctions can make such evaluations exceedingly difficult (Table 33-1).

box 33-7
Format for Mental Status Examination

Attention
Digit span forward and backward

Remembering
Short-term: recall of three items after 5 minutes
Long-term: recall of mother's maiden name, recall of breakfast menu, events of previous day, etc.

Feeling (Affective)
Facial, body expression of mood
Verbal description of affect
Congruence of verbal, body indicators of mood

Language
Content and quantity of spontaneous speech
Naming common objects, parts of objects
Repetition of phrases
Ability to read and explain short passage in newspaper, magazine
Ability to write to dictation, spontaneously

Thinking
Fund of information (e.g., current president, preceding three)
Knowledge of current events
Orientation to person, place, time (tested as part of arousal, see consciousness)
Calculation: add two numbers, subtract 7 from 100
Problem-solving: What would you do if you found a stamped envelope on the street? What would you do if you smelled smoke in a theater?

Spatial Perception
Copy drawings: square, cross, three-dimensional cube
Draw clock face, map of room
Point out right and left side of self
Demonstrate: putting on a coat, blowing out match, using a toothbrush

Motor Function

Evaluation of motor function consists of two components—motor response to stimuli and motor strength and coordination. Assessment of motor response involves evaluating the type of stimuli necessary to elicit a motor response. This gives the health care team information regarding the level of awareness necessary to obtain a motor response as well as the patient's ability to follow commands. Evaluation of motor strength and coordination gives an indication of potential problems with motor neuron pathways or the cerebellum.

MOTOR RESPONSE TO STIMULI

The nurse first attempts to elicit a motor response by asking the patient to move an extremity. If no response is forthcoming, the patient is unable to carry out verbal commands; therefore, noxious stimuli should be used to elicit a motor response. Localization to painful stimuli is characterized by an organized attempt to remove the stimulus, which entails movement of the extremity across midline. This contrasts to withdrawal, in which the patient simply pulls away from the noxious stimulus, rather than attempting to remove it (Fig. 33-1). Appropriate responses, such as localization or withdrawal, mean that the sensory and corticospinal pathways are functioning (see Fig. 33-1A, B). There may be monoplegia or hemiplegia, indicating that the corticospinal pathways are interrupted on one side.

table 33-1 Patterns of Speech Deficits

Type	Deficit Location	Speech Patterns
Fluent dysphasia	Left parietal–temporal lobes (Wernicke's area)	• Fluent speech that lacks coherent content • Impaired understanding of spoken word in spite of normal hearing • May have normal-sounding speech rhythm but no intelligible words • May use invented, meaningless words (neologism), word substitution (paraphasia), or repetition of words (perseveration, echolalia)
Nonfluent dysphasia	Left frontal area (Broca's area)	• Slow speech with poor articulation • Inability to initiate sounds • Comprehension usually intact • Usually associated with impaired writing skills
Global dysphasia	Diffuse involvement of frontal, parietal, and occipital areas	• Nonfluent speech • Inability to understand spoken or written words
Dysarthria	Corticobulbar tracts; cerebellum	• Loss of articulation, phonation • Loss of control of muscles of lips, tongue, palate • Slurred, jerky, or irregular speech but with appropriate content

Inappropriate responses include decorticate rigidity and decerebrate rigidity. Flexion of the arms, wrists, and fingers; adduction of the upper extremities; and extension, internal rotation, and plantar flexion of the lower extremities characterize *decorticate rigidity* (see Fig. 33-1C). Such rigidity results from lesions of the internal capsule, basal ganglia, thalamus, or cerebral hemisphere that interrupt corticospinal pathways.

Decerebrate rigidity consists of extension, adduction, and hyperpronation of the upper extremities and extension of the lower extremities, with plantar flexion of the feet (see Fig. 33-1D). Many times, the person also has clenched teeth. Injury to the midbrain and pons results in decerebration. At times, the inappropriate responses of decortication and decerebration may switch back and forth. If there is no response to noxious stimuli or only very weak flexor responses (i.e., flaccidity), the patient probably has extensive brainstem dysfunction (see Fig. 33-1E).

Abnormal motor responses in a comatose patient include *tonic contraction*, which is consistent muscular contraction, and *clonus*, which is alternating muscle spasticity and relaxation.

MOTOR STRENGTH AND COORDINATION

The second component of the motor assessment addresses strength and coordination. Muscle weakness is a cardinal sign of dysfunction in many neurological disorders. The nurse can test extremity strength by offering resistance to various muscle groups, using the nurse's own muscles or gravity. As a quick test to detect weakness of the upper extremities, the nurse can have the patient hold the arms straight out with palms upward and eyes closed and observe for any downward drift or pronation of the forearms. This is referred to as *pronator drift*. A similar test for the lower extremities involves having the patient raise the legs, one leg at a time, straight off the bed against the examiner's resistance. Weakness noted in any of these tests can indicate damage to the motor neuron pathways of the pyramidal system, which transmits commands for voluntary movement. Motor function for each extremity is reported as a fraction, with 5 as the denominator:

0/5 = No muscle contraction
1/5 = Flicker or trace of contraction
2/5 = Moves but cannot overcome gravity
3/5 = Moves against gravity but cannot overcome resistance of examiner's muscles
4/5 = Moves with some weakness against resistance of examiner's muscles
5/5 = Normal power and strength

Muscle groups should be assessed individually, initially without resistance and then against resistance, to obtain a thorough evaluation. Upper extremity muscle strength should be evaluated by asking the patient to shrug the shoulders (trapezius and levator scapulae muscles), raise the arms (deltoid muscle), flex the elbow (biceps muscle), extend the arm (triceps muscle), and extend the wrist (extensor carpi radialis longus muscle). Lower extremity muscle strength should be evaluated by asking the patient to raise the leg (iliopsoas muscle), extend the knee (quadriceps muscle), dorsiflex and plantar flex the foot (anterior tibialis and gastrocnemius muscles, respectively), and, last, flex the knee (hamstring muscle).

Assessment of movement and strength in a patient who cannot follow commands or is unresponsive can be difficult because participating in muscle strength testing

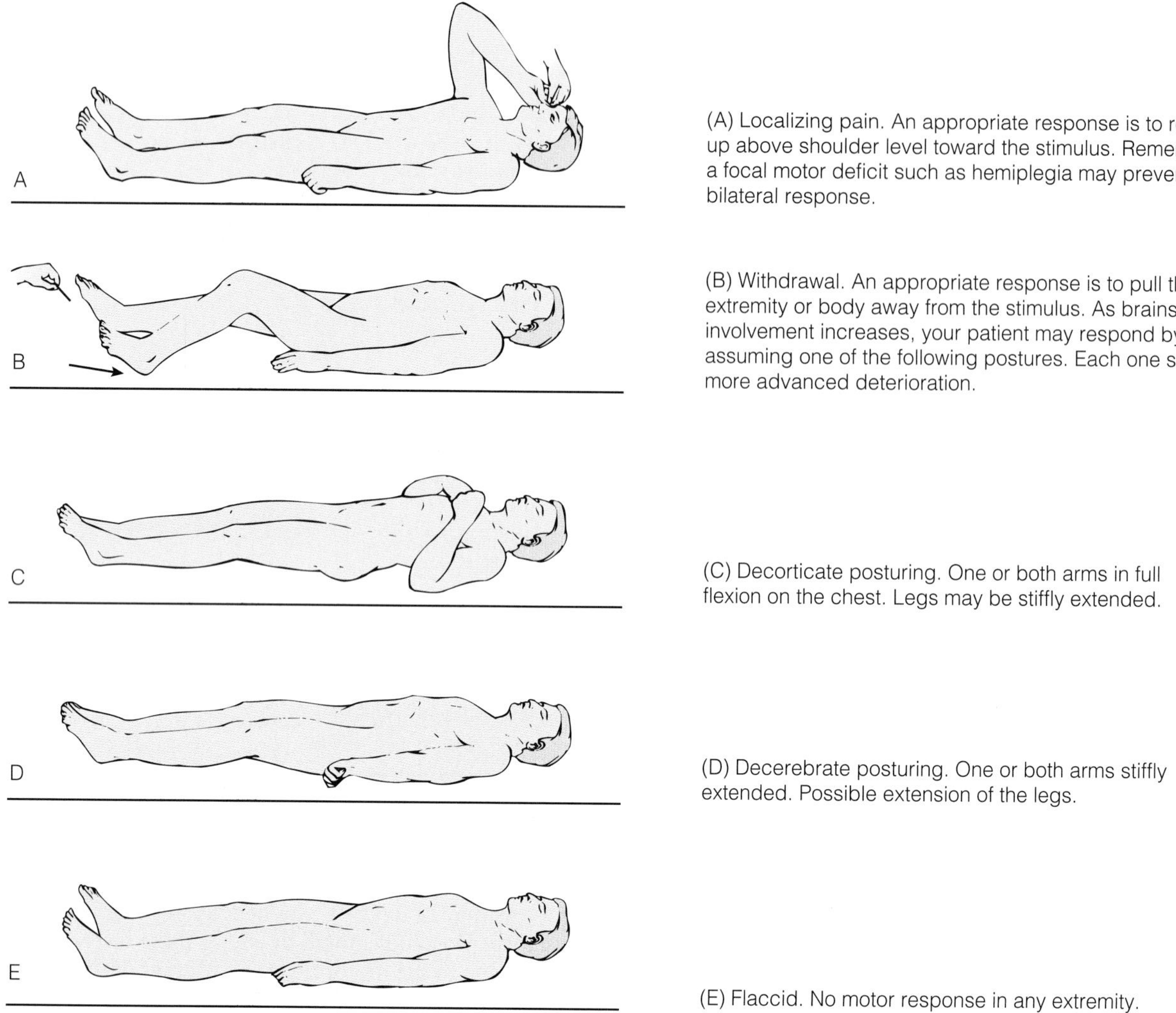

A
(A) Localizing pain. An appropriate response is to reach up above shoulder level toward the stimulus. Remember, a focal motor deficit such as hemiplegia may prevent a bilateral response.
B
(B) Withdrawal. An appropriate response is to pull the extremity or body away from the stimulus. As brainstem involvement increases, your patient may respond by assuming one of the following postures. Each one shows more advanced deterioration.
C
(C) Decorticate posturing. One or both arms in full flexion on the chest. Legs may be stiffly extended.
D
(D) Decerebrate posturing. One or both arms stiffly extended. Possible extension of the legs.
E
(E) Flaccid. No motor response in any extremity.

figure 33-1 Motor responses to pain. When a painful stimulus is applied to an unconscious patient's supra-orbital notch, the patient will respond in one of these ways.

against gravity requires the patient's understanding and cooperation. Unless the patient is able to mount a motor response secondary to painful stimuli, the nurse may not have the opportunity to test for muscle strength in any sort of reliable manner. Therefore, for comatose patients, it is important to note what, if any, stimuli initiate a response and to describe or grade the type of response obtained.

The nurse also assesses each extremity for size, muscle tone, and smoothness of passive movement. Dysfunctions noted here can indicate problems in the basal ganglia (also called the *extrapyramidal system*). These pathways normally suppress involuntary movements through controlled inhibition. Assessment findings may include the "clasp-knife" phenomenon, in which initially strong resistance to passive movement suddenly decreases. Alternatively, "lead-pipe" rigidity may be present, which is steady, continuous resistance to passive movement and is characteristic of diffuse hemispheric damage. "Cogwheel" rigidity, which is a series of small, regular, jerky movements felt on passive movement, is characteristic of Parkinson's disease. The nurse also should be alert to involuntary movements, from mild fasciculation (muscle twitching) to violent, flailing movement of an extremity. Descriptive terms for involuntary movements are given in Box 33-8.

Hemiparesis (weakness) and hemiplegia (paralysis) are unilateral dysfunctions resulting from a lesion contralateral to the corticospinal tract. Paraplegia may result from thoracic or lumbar spinal cord or peripheral nerve dysfunctions. Quadriplegia is associated with high cervical spinal cord lesions, brainstem dysfunction, and large bilateral lesions in the cerebrum.

The cerebellum is responsible for smooth synchronization, balance, and ordering of movements. It does *not* initiate any movements, so a patient with cerebellar dysfunction is not paralyzed. Instead, ataxia, dysmetria, and lack of synchronization of movement are common manifestations. Some of the more common tests for cerebellar synchronization of movement with balance include the following:

- **Romberg test.** This test is performed by having the patient stand with his or her feet together, first with the eyes open, then with the eyes closed. The nurse looks for sway or direction of falling, and is prepared to catch the patient if necessary.
- **Finger-to-nose test.** This test is performed by having the patient touch one finger to the examiner's

box 33-8
Types of Involuntary Movements

Tremor	Purposeless movement
Resting	Lesion in basal ganglia
Intention	Lesion in cerebellum
Asterixis	Metabolic derangement
Physiological	Due to fatigue or stress
Fasciculation	Twitching of resting muscles due to peripheral nerve or spinal cord lesion or to metabolic influences such as cold or anesthetic agents
Clonus	Repetitive movement; elicited with stretch reflex and implies lesion of the corticospinal tracts
Myoclonus	Nonrhythmic movement; single jerk-like movements; symmetrical; unknown etiology
Hemiballismus	Flailing movement of extremity; violent movement; not present during sleep; lesion in subthalamic nuclei of basal ganglia
Chorea	Irregular movements; involves limbs and facial muscles; asymmetrical movements at rest; involuntary movements may increase when purposeful movement is attempted
Athetosis	Slow, writhing movements

finger, then touch his or her own nose. Overshooting or past-pointing the mark is called *dysmetria.* Both sides are tested individually.

- **Rapidly alternating movement (RAM) test.** The patient's ability to perform RAMs is checked on each side by having the patient oppose each finger and thumb in rapid succession or by performing rapid pronation and supination of the hand on the leg. Inability to perform RAMs is termed *adiadochokinesia;* performing RAMs poorly or clumsily is termed *dysdiadochokinesia.*
- **Heel-to-shin test.** This test is performed by having the patient extend the heel of one foot down the anterior aspect of the shin, moving from the knee to the ankle.

Pupillary Changes

Assessment of pupillary response is an important component of the neurological examination. Pupils are examined for size (best specified in millimeters) and shape (Fig. 33-2). The patient focuses on a distant point in the room. To isolate the eye being examined, the examiner places the edge of one hand along the patient's nose. A bright light is directed into one eye, and the briskness of pupillary constriction (direct response) is noted. The other pupil also should constrict (consensual response). The procedure is

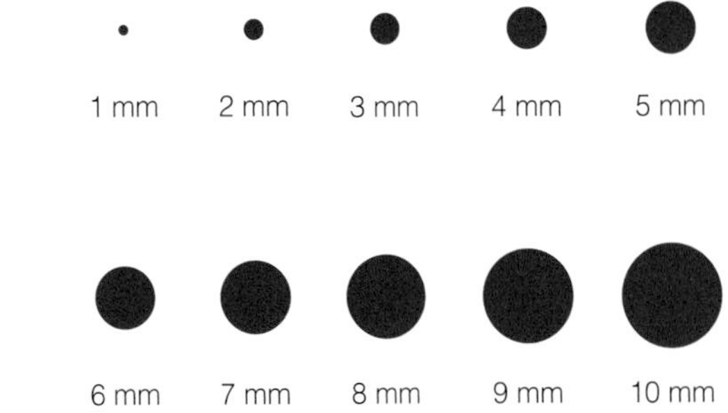

figure 33-2 Pupil size chart.

then repeated with the other eye. *Anisocoria* (unequal pupils) is normal in a small percentage of the population, but can also indicate neural dysfunction. If it is a normal variant, the difference in pupil size should be less than 1 mm.

Pupil reactivity is also assessed with respect to *accommodation.* To test accommodation, an object is held 8 to 12 inches in front of the patient's face. The patient focuses on the object as the examiner moves it toward the patient's nose. The pupils should constrict as the object gets closer, and the eyes turn inward to maintain a clear image. The normal response to testing is documented as PERRLA, or Pupils Equal, Round, Reactive to Light and Accommodation.

Some important pupillary abnormalities are shown in Figure 33-3. Causes of small, reactive pupils include metabolic abnormalities and bilateral dysfunction in the diencephalon. Large, fixed pupils (5 to 6 mm) that may show slight rhythmic constriction and dilation when stimulated may indicate midbrain damage. Midposition-fixed pupils (4 to 5 mm) also may indicate midbrain dysfunction, with sympathetic and parasympathetic pathways interrupted. Pinpoint, nonreactive pupils are seen after damage to the pons area of the brainstem (thus the phrase "pontine pupils are pinpoint"), with selected eye medications, and with opiate administration. A unilaterally dilated, nonreactive ("blown") pupil is seen with third cranial (oculomotor) nerve damage when the uncal portion of the temporal lobe herniates through the small opening in the tentorium. When structures are compressed around the opening in the tentorium or fold of dura that separates the cerebrum from the cerebellum and brainstem, loss of functioning of the parasympathetic nerves to the pupil on that side results in ipsilaterally dilated pupils. A quick guide to changes in pupil size is given in Box 33-9.

The assessment of pupillary response for comatose patients is the same as for conscious patients. Pupil reactivity to light, by direct and consensual response, is easily obtained. It may be impossible to ascertain reactivity to accommodation, however, because the patient may be unable to cooperate.

Vital Signs

Vital sign assessment is crucial to the neurological examination. Changes in temperature, heart rate, and blood pressure are considered late findings in neurological deterioration. Changes in respiratory rate, on the other hand, can indicate progression of neurological impairment and are frequently seen early in neurological deterioration.

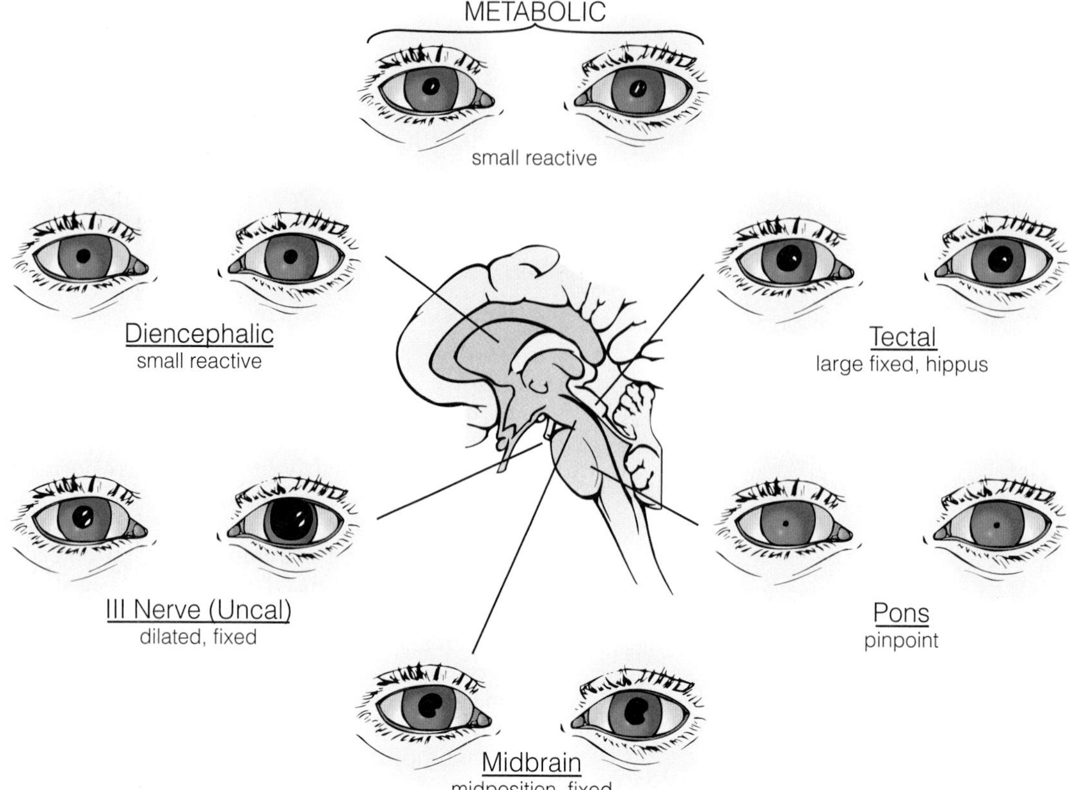

figure 33-3 Abnormal pupils. (Adapted from Plum F, Poser J: The Diagnosis of Stupor and Coma [3rd Ed]. Philadelphia, FA Davis.)

RESPIRATIONS

Variations in respiratory pattern are commonly associated with neurological injury. Shallow, rapid respirations can indicate a problem with maintenance of a patent airway or the need for suctioning. Snoring respirations or stridor can also indicate a partially obstructed airway. The inability to maintain an effective airway may be associated with a high cervical spinal cord lesion or progressive diaphragmatic paralysis (seen with neurodegenerative diseases), or it may be associated with a decreasing level of consciousness.

Changes in respiratory pattern can also be a direct indication of increasing intracranial pressure (ICP) (see Chapter 36, Fig. 36-6). Cheyne-Stokes respirations (crescendo–decrescendo respirations alternating with periods of apnea) are frequently noted in neurological disease.

Hypoventilation after cerebral trauma can lead to respiratory acidosis. As the blood carbon dioxide increases and blood oxygen decreases, cerebral hypoxia and edema can result in secondary brain injury, thereby extending the amount of damage. *Hyperventilation* after cerebral trauma produces respiratory alkalosis with decreased blood carbon dioxide levels. This causes vasoconstriction of cerebral vessels, contributing to decreased cerebral blood flow.

TEMPERATURE

Normal regulation of temperature occurs in the hypothalamus. Diffuse cerebral damage can result in alterations in temperature. Central nervous system (CNS) fevers may be very high and differentiate themselves from other causes of fever by their resistance to antipyretic therapy. Hypothermia occurs with metabolic causes, pituitary damage, and spinal cord injuries.

PULSE

Variations in heart rate and rhythm may also be associated with neurological injury. An increase in ICP may lead to episodes of tachycardia and can predispose the patient to alterations in electrocardiogram (ECG) pattern, such as ventricular or atrial arrhythmias. As pressure rises, bradycardia results and may be considered a terminal event.

BLOOD PRESSURE

Blood pressure is controlled at the level of the medulla. Therefore, specific damage to this area or encroaching

box 33-9
Quick Guide to Causes of Pupil Size Changes

Pinpoint pupils
- Drugs: opiates
- Drops: medications for glaucoma
- "Nearly dead": damage in the pons area of the brainstem

Dilated pupils
- Fear: panic attack, extreme anxiety
- "Fits": seizures
- "Fast living": cocaine, crack, phencyclidine (PCP)

edema secondary to injury in other areas results in alterations in blood pressure. Hypotension is not normally associated with neurological injury except in instances of impending cerebral herniation. On the other hand, hypotension must be avoided in the postinjury stage because it can lead to decreased cerebral perfusion, hypoxia, and extension of the initial injury.

Hypertension is much more commonly seen. In the intact brain, the mechanism of cerebral autoregulation, on which cerebral perfusion depends, maintains blood flow to the brain at a constant, despite wide variations in systemic pressure. After injury, however, autoregulatory mechanisms fail and cerebral blood flow varies dramatically with variations in systemic pressure. As blood pressure rises, cerebral blood flow and, consequently, volume increase, resulting in an increase in ICP. Likewise, as blood pressure drops, cerebral blood flow drops, resulting in ischemia.

Cranial Nerve Function

Cranial nerve assessment varies depending on whether the patient is conscious or unconscious. Assessment of the cranial nerves in the unconscious patient is important because it provides data regarding brainstem function. Many components must be eliminated, but a significant number of the cranial nerves can still be assessed. For specific physiological information about the cranial nerves, see Chapter 32.

CRANIAL NERVE I (OLFACTORY NERVE)

The first cranial nerve contains sensory fibers for the sense of smell. This test usually is deferred unless the patient complains of an inability to smell. The nurse tests the nerve, with the patient's eyes closed, by placing aromatic substances near the nose for identification. Fragrances that have a distinct smell (e.g., soap, coffee, or cinnamon) should be used. Ammonia should not be used because the patient will respond to irritation of the nasal mucosa rather than to the odor. Each nostril is checked separately. Loss of smell may be caused by a fracture of the cribriform plate or a fracture in the ethmoid area. The patient also may have anosmia (loss of sense of smell) from a shearing injury to the olfactory bulb after a basilar skull fracture or from cerebrospinal fluid (CSF) leak.

CRANIAL NERVE II (OPTIC NERVE)

Assessment of cranial nerve II involves evaluation of visual acuity and visual fields. Gross visual acuity is checked by having the patient read ordinary newsprint, noting the patient's preinjury need for glasses. Visual fields are tested by having the patient look straight ahead with one eye covered. The examiner moves a finger from the periphery of each quadrant of vision toward the patient's center of vision. The patient should indicate when the examiner's finger is seen. This is done for both eyes, and the results are compared with the examiner's visual fields, which are assumed to be normal (Fig. 33-4). Damage to the retina produces a blind spot. An optic nerve lesion produces partial or complete blindness on the same side. Damage to the optic chiasm results in *bitemporal hemianopsia*, blindness in both lateral visual fields (Table 33-2). Pressure on the optic tract can cause *homonymous hemianopsia*, half-blindness on the opposite side of the lesion in both eyes.

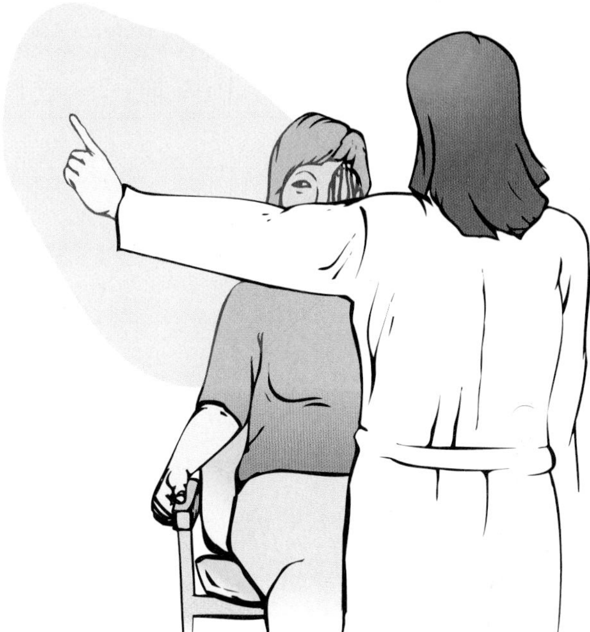

figure 33-4 Confrontational method of testing visual fields.

A lesion in the parietal or temporal lobe may produce contralateral blindness in the upper or lower quadrant of vision, respectively, in both eyes (*quadrant deficit*). Damage in the occipital lobe can cause homonymous hemianopsia with central vision sparing.

CRANIAL NERVES III (OCULOMOTOR NERVE), IV (TROCHLEAR NERVE), AND VI (ABDUCENS NERVE)

Cranial nerves III, IV, and VI are checked together because they all innervate extraocular muscles. The parasympathetic fibers of the oculomotor nerve are responsible for lens accommodation and pupil size through control of the ciliary muscles. This is the nerve tested when a nurse elicits pupillary response. The motor fibers of the oculomotor nerve innervate the muscles that elevate the eyelid and those that move the eyes up, down, and medially. These include the superior rectus, inferior oblique, inferior rectus, and medial rectus muscles. The trochlear nerve innervates the superior oblique muscle to move the eyes down and in. The lateral rectus muscle moves the eyes laterally and is innervated by the abducens nerve. Diplopia, nystagmus, conjugate deviation, and ptosis may indicate dysfunction of these cranial nerves. In the conscious patient, these nerves are tested by having the patient follow the examiner's finger as he or she moves it in all directions of gaze (Fig. 33-5).

Ocular position and movement are among the most useful guides to the site of brain dysfunction in the comatose person. When observing the eyes at rest, it is not uncommon to note a slight divergence of gaze. If both eyes are conjugately deviated to one side, there is possible dysfunction either in the frontal lobe on that side or in the contralateral pontine area of the brainstem. Downward deviation suggests a dysfunction in the midbrain.

Although the unconscious patient cannot participate in the examination by voluntarily moving the eyes through

table 33-2 Visual Field Defects Associated With Defects of the Visual System

VISUAL FIELD DEFECT	Left	Right	DESCRIPTION
Anopsia	○	●	Blindness in one eye; due to complete lesion of the right optic nerve, as in trauma.
Bitemporal hemianopsia (central vision)	◐	◑	Blindness in both lateral visual fields; due to lesions around the optic chiasm such as pituitary tumors or aneurysms of the anterior communicating artery. Affected fibers originate in the nasal half of each retina.
Homonymous hemianopsia	◐	◐	Half-blindness involving both eyes with loss of visual field on the same side of each eye; due to lesion of temporal or occipital lobe with damage to the optic tract or optic radiations (blindness occurs on the side opposite the lesion; here, the lesion occurred in the right side of the brain, resulting in loss of vision in the left visual field of both eyes)
Quadrant deficit	◔	◔	Blindness in the upper or lower quadrant of vision in both eyes, resulting from a lesion in the parietal or temporal lobe

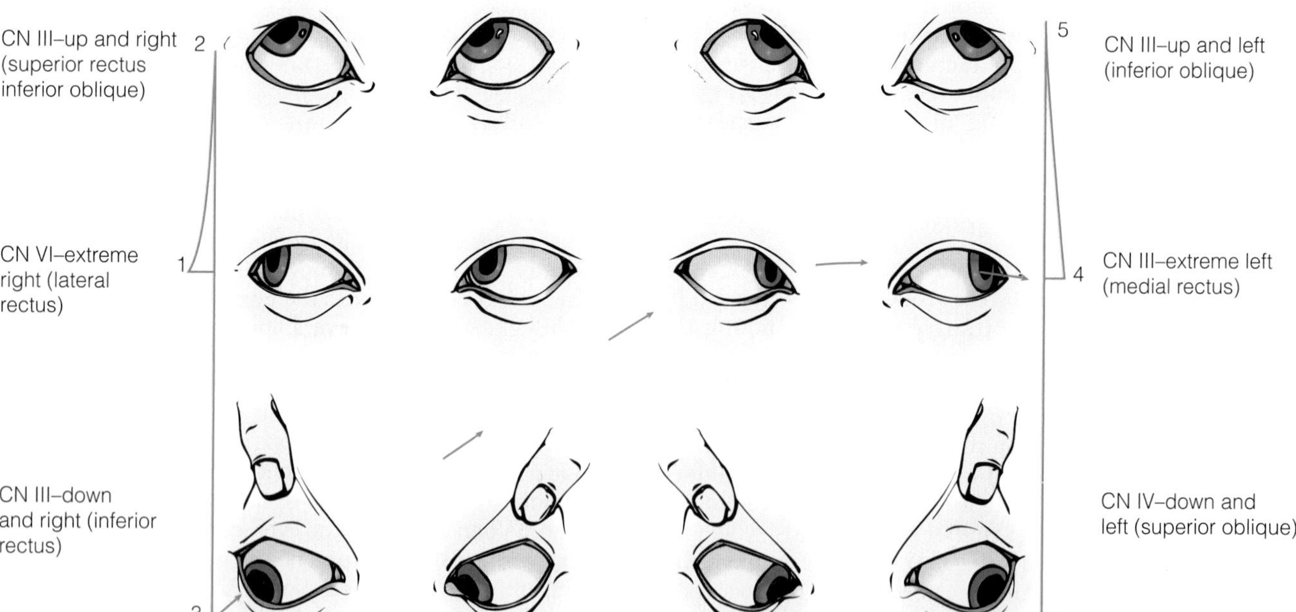

figure 33-5 Muscles used in conjugate eye movements in the six cardinal directions of gaze. Lead the patient's gaze in the sequence numbered 1 through 6. *CN III,* oculomotor nerve; *CN IV,* trochlear nerve; *CN VI,* abducens nerve.

fields of gaze, the examiner still can test the range of ocular movement by assessing the oculocephalic ("doll's eyes" test) and oculovestibular (caloric ice-water test) reflexes. The oculocephalic reflex can be assessed by quickly rotating the patient's head to one side and observing the position of the eyes (Fig. 33-6). This maneuver must *never* be performed in a person with possible cervical spine injury. A normal response consists of initial conjugate deviation of the eyes in the opposite direction, then, within a few seconds, smooth and simultaneous movement of both eyes back to midline position. This response indicates an intact brainstem. An abnormal reflex response occurs when one eye does not follow the normal response pattern. Absence of any ocular movement when the head is rotated briskly to either side or up and down indicates an absent reflex and portends severe brainstem dysfunction.

The examiner tests the oculovestibular reflex by elevating the patient's head 30 degrees and irrigating each ear separately with 30 to 50 mL of ice water (Fig. 33-7). This test should never be performed in a patient who does not have an intact eardrum or who has blood or fluid collected behind the eardrum. Also, the external ear canal should be unobstructed by cerumen or debris. In an unconscious patient with an intact brainstem, the eyes exhibit horizontal nystagmus with slow, conjugate movement toward the irrigated ear followed by rapid movement away from the stimulus. When the reflex is absent, both eyes remain fixed in midline position, indicating midbrain and pons dysfunction. The oculovestibular reflex can usually be elicited later than the oculocephalic reflex.

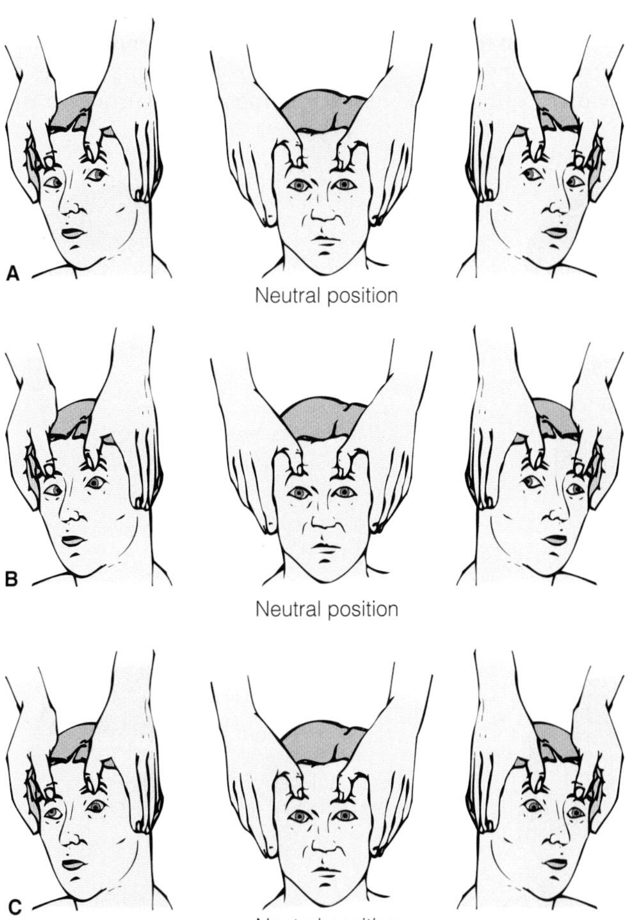

figure 33-6 Test for oculocephalic reflex response (doll's eyes phenomenon). (**A**) Normal response—when the head is rotated, the eyes turn together to the side opposite to the head movement. (**B**) Abnormal response—when the head is rotated, the eyes do not turn in a conjugate manner. (**C**) Absent response—as head position is changed, eyes do not move in the sockets.

CRANIAL NERVE V (TRIGEMINAL NERVE)

Cranial nerve V has three divisions: ophthalmic, maxillary, and mandibular. The sensory portion of this nerve controls sensation to the cornea and face. The motor portion controls the muscles of mastication. This nerve is partially tested by checking the corneal reflex; if it is intact, the patient will blink when the cornea is stroked with a wisp of cotton or a drop of normal saline is placed in the eye. Care must be taken not to stroke the eyelash because that can cause the eye to blink regardless of the presence of a corneal reflex. Facial sensation can be tested by comparing light touch and pinprick on symmetrical sides of the face. The ability to chew or clench the jaw also should be observed.

CRANIAL NERVE VII (FACIAL NERVE)

The sensory portion of cranial nerve VII is concerned with taste on the anterior two thirds of the tongue. The motor portion controls muscles of facial expression (Fig. 33-8). With a central (supranuclear) lesion, there is muscle paralysis of the lower half of the face on the side opposite the lesion. The muscles around the eyes and forehead are unaffected. With a peripheral (nuclear or infranuclear) lesion, there is complete paralysis of facial muscles on the same side as the lesion.

The most common type of peripheral facial paralysis is Bell's palsy, which consists of ipsilateral facial paralysis. There is drooping of the upper lid with the lower lid slightly everted. Facial lines on the same side are obliterated with the mouth drawn toward the normal side.

In the comatose patient, motor function of the facial muscles and jaw can be ascertained by observing spontaneous muscle activity such as yawning, grimacing, or chewing. Symmetry of movement may be assessed, and facial droops may be observed.

CRANIAL NERVE VIII (ACOUSTIC NERVE)

Cranial nerve VIII is divided into the cochlear and vestibular branches, which control hearing and equilibrium, respectively. The cochlear nerve is tested by air and bone conduction. A vibrating tuning fork is placed on the mastoid process; after the patient can no longer hear the fork, he or she should be able to hear it for a few seconds longer when it is placed in front of the ear (Rinne test). The patient may complain of tinnitus or decreased hearing if this nerve is damaged. The vestibular nerve may not be evaluated routinely. The nurse should be alert, however, to complaints of dizziness or vertigo from the patient.

CRANIAL NERVES IX (GLOSSOPHARYNGEAL NERVE) AND X (VAGUS NERVE)

Cranial nerves IX and X usually are tested together. The glossopharyngeal nerve supplies sensory fibers to the posterior third of the tongue and the uvula and soft palate. The

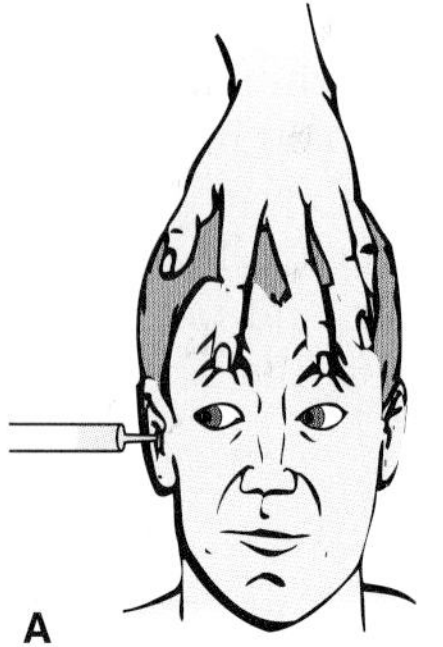

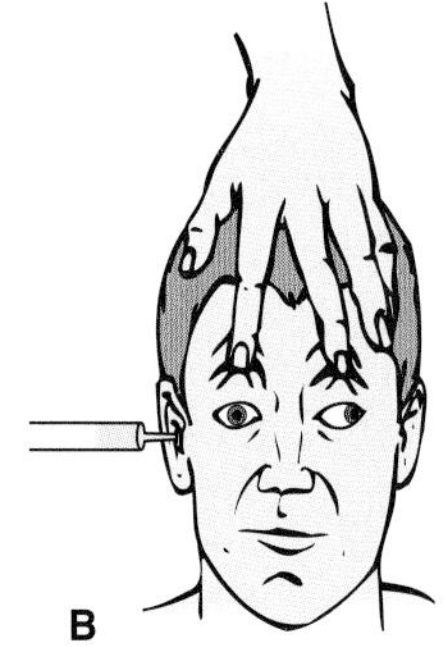

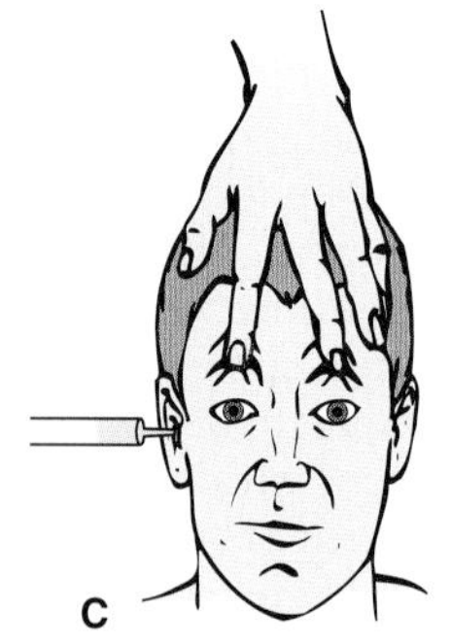

figure 33-7 Test for oculovestibular reflex response (caloric ice-water test). (**A**) Normal response—ice water infusion in the ear produces conjugate eye movements. (**B**) Abnormal response—infusion produces dysconjugate or asymmetrical eye movements. (**C**) Absent response—infusion produces no eye movements.

vagus nerve innervates the larynx, pharynx, and soft palate and conveys autonomic responses to the heart, stomach, lungs, and small intestines. Autonomic vagal functions usually are not tested because they are checked during the general physical examination. These nerves can be tested by eliciting a gag reflex, observing the uvula for symmetrical movement when the patient says "ah," or observing midline elevation of the uvula when both sides are stroked. Inability to cough forcefully, difficulty with swallowing, and hoarseness may be signs of dysfunction.

CRANIAL NERVE XI (SPINAL ACCESSORY NERVE)

Cranial nerve XI controls the trapezius and sternocleidomastoid muscles. The examiner tests this nerve by having the patient shrug the shoulders or turn the head from side to side against resistance.

CRANIAL NERVE XII (HYPOGLOSSAL NERVE)

Cranial nerve XII controls tongue movement. This nerve can be checked by having the patient protrude his or her tongue. The examiner checks for deviation from midline, tremor, and atrophy. If deviation is noted secondary to nerve damage, it will be to the side of the cerebral lesion.

Testing cranial nerve function completely is time consuming and exacting. A partial and quicker screening assessment may be performed, focusing on nerves in which dysfunction may indicate serious problems or interfere with activities of daily living (Table 33-3). The cranial nerves of primary importance in a screening examination are the

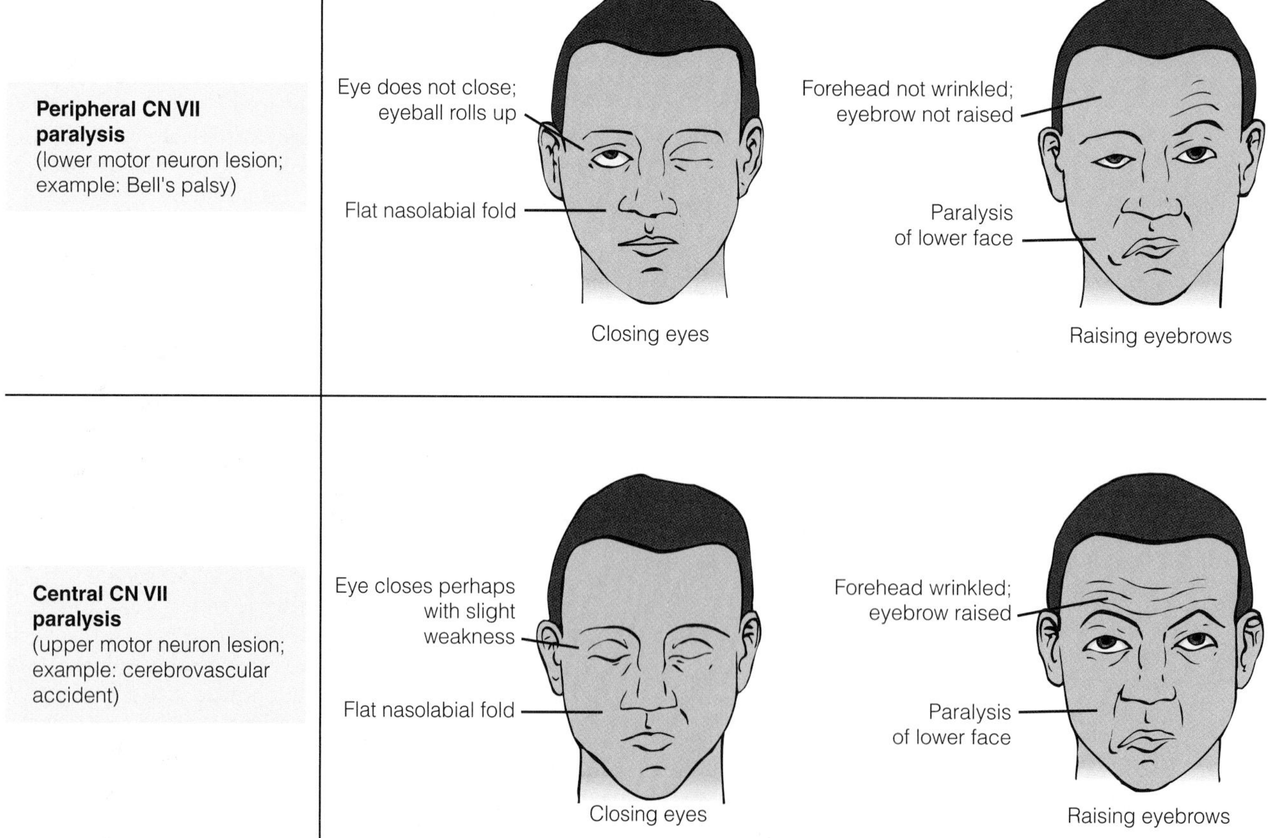

figure 33-8 Facial movements with upper and lower motor neuron facial paralysis. *CN VII,* facial nerve.

table 33-3 A Quick Screening Test for Cranial Nerve Function

	Nerve	Reflex	Procedure
II III	Optic Oculomotor	Pupil constriction (protection of the retina)	Shine a light into each eye and note if the pupil on that side constricts (direct response). Next, shine a light into each eye and note if the opposite pupil constricts (consensual response).
V VII	Trigeminal Facial	Corneal reflex (protection of the cornea)	Approaching the eye from the side and avoiding the eyelashes, touch the cornea with a wisp of cotton. Alternatively, a drop of sterile water or normal saline may be used. A blink response should be present.
IX X	Glossopharyngeal Vagus	Airway protection	Touch the back of the throat with a tongue depressor. A gag or cough response should be present.

optic, oculomotor, trigeminal, facial, glossopharyngeal, and vagus nerves.

Reflexes

A reflex occurs when a sensory stimulus evokes a motor response. Cerebral control and consciousness are not required for a reflex to occur. Superficial and deep reflexes are tested on symmetrical sides of the body and compared by noting the strength of contraction elicited on each side.

Cutaneous, or superficial, reflexes occur when certain areas of skin are lightly stroked or tapped, causing contraction of the muscle groups beneath. Such reflexes are graded simply as normal, abnormal (pathological), or absent. An example is the plantar reflex. A sensory stimulus is applied by briskly stroking the outer edge of the sole and across the ball of the foot with a dull object, such as a tongue blade or key. The normal motor response is downward or plantar flexion of the toes. An abnormal response (Babinski's sign) is upward or dorsiflexion of the big toe, with or without fanning of the other toes. A positive Babinski's sign can indicate a lesion in the pyramidal tract.

Muscle stretch reflexes, also called deep tendon reflexes, are elicited by a brisk tap with a reflex hammer. The target for this sensory stimulus is a stretched tendon of a muscle group. The desired motor response is contraction of the stimulated muscle group. Deep tendon reflexes are commonly graded on a scale of 0 to 4:

4+: A very brisk response; evidence of disease, electrolyte imbalance, or both; associated with clonic contractions
3+: A brisk response; possibly indicative of disease
2+: A normal response
1+: A response in the low-normal range
0: No response; possibly evidence of disease or electrolyte imbalance

Hyperreflexia is associated with upper motor neuron disease, whereas areflexia is associated with lower motor neuron dysfunction, such as spinal cord lesions. Reflexes can be tested on the comatose patient. It is anticipated that, depending on the severity and location of the neuronal damage, either hyperreflexia or areflexia will be present.

Sensation

The last component of the neurological examination involves a sensory assessment. Normal sensory findings depend on an intact spinal cord, sensory pathways, and peripheral nervous system. The primary forms of sensation are tested first. These include perception of touch (cotton wisp), pain (pinprick), temperature (hot, cold), proprioception (limb position), and vibration. With the patient's eyes closed, multiple and symmetrical areas of the body are tested, including the trunk and extremities.

The nurse assesses the perception of touch by asking the patient to close the eyes and identify when and where he or she feels a cotton wisp or cotton swab on the skin. Pain is assessed with the use of a pin or the sharp edge of a cotton swab, moving in a head-to-toe direction on both sides of the body. Temperature, if tested, uses glass tubes of hot and cold water and proceeds in the manner described previously. Two-point discrimination may also be tested and refers to the patient's ability to distinguish between two closely located points. Discrimination of sharp versus dull is also a commonly used test.

Proprioception is tested by asking the patient, again with the eyes closed, to identify the direction of movement (e.g., moving a finger upward and then asking the patient if the finger is up or down). The same test is performed on the other hand, as well as both lower extremities. The nurse assesses vibration using a tuning fork placed over a bony prominence. The patient is asked to identify when vibration is felt.

The patient's ability to perceive the sensation should be noted, with distal areas compared with proximal areas and right and left sides compared at corresponding points. The nurse should also determine whether sensory change involves one entire side of the body. Abnormal results may indicate damage somewhere along the pathways of the receptors in the skin, muscles, joints and tendons, spinothalamic tracts, or sensory area of the cortex (Table 33-4).

table 33-4 Testing Superficial and Deep Sensations

Sensation	Stimuli	Dysfunction
Spinothalamic Tracts Carry Impulses for		
Pain	Alternate sharp and dull ends of a pin, asking patient to discriminate between the two (superficial pain). Squeeze nail beds; apply pressure on the orbital rim; rub sternum (deep pain).	• Ipsilateral sensory loss implies a peripheral nerve lesion. • Contralateral sensory loss is seen with lesions of the spinothalamic tract or in the thalamus.
Light touch	Use a wisp of cotton on skin and ask patient to identify when it touches.	• Bilateral sensory loss may indicate a spinal cord lesion. • Paresthesia is an abnormal sensation, such as itching or tingling.
Temperature	Use test tubes filled with hot and cold water or use small metal plates of varying temperatures. (Test only if pain and light touch sensations are abnormal.)	• Causalgia is a burning sensation that can be caused by peripheral nerve irritation.
Posterior Columns Carry Impulses for		
Vibration	Apply a vibrating tuning fork on bony prominences, and note patient's ability to sense and locate vibrations bilaterally.	• Ipsilateral sensory loss may be due to spinal cord injury or to peripheral neuropathy.
Proprioception	Move the patient's finger or toe up and down and ask patient to identify final resting position.	• Contralateral loss may occur from lesions of the thalamus or of the parietal lobes.

Cortical forms of sensation also should be tested. When primary sensation is intact, but interpretation of the sensory input is altered, then damage to the parietal lobe may be anticipated. Problems with discriminative sensation include those involving stereognosis, graphesthesia, and point localization.

The ability to recognize and identify objects by touch is called *stereognosis* and is a function of the parietal lobe. The inability to recognize objects by touch, sight, or sound is termed *agnosia*. This may be tested by placing an object in a patient's hand and asking him or her, with the eyes closed, to identify the object solely based on touch. Identification of an object by the sense of sight is a function of the parieto-occipital junction. The temporal lobe is responsible for identification of objects by sound. Each of these senses should be tested separately. For example, a patient may not be able to identify a whistle by its sound but may recognize it immediately if he or she holds it or looks at it.

Graphesthesia is the ability to recognize numbers or letters traced lightly on the skin. Bilateral sides are compared. *Point localization* refers to the ability to locate the precise spot on the body touched by the examiner. One version of dysfunction in this area is called *extinction phenomenon*, the inability to recognize bilateral sensations when the examiner simultaneously touches two symmetrical areas on opposite sides of the body.

In a comatose patient, it is impossible to perform a complete test for sensation because patient cooperativity is required. However, use of painful stimuli to elicit a response gives a gross indication that some degree of sensory function remains intact. More detailed data would be unavailable, though.

Signs of Trauma or Infection

Signs of trauma or infection may be evident on examination:

- **Battle's sign** (bruising over the mastoid areas) suggests a basal skull fracture.
- **Raccoon's eye** (periorbital edema and bruising) suggests a frontobasilar fracture.
- **Rhinorrhea** (drainage of CSF from the nose) suggests fracture of the cribriform plate with herniation of a fragment of the dura and arachnoid through the fracture.
- **Otorrhea** (drainage of CSF from the ear) usually is associated with fracture of the petrous portion of the temporal bone.
- **Signs of meningeal irritation** include nuchal rigidity (i.e., pain and resistance to neck flexion), fever, headache, and photophobia. A positive Kernig's sign (i.e., pain in the neck when the thigh is flexed on the abdomen and the leg is extended at the knee) also may be present. Brudzinski's sign (involuntary flexion of the hips when the neck is flexed toward the chest) is another indication of meningeal inflammation. Kernig's sign and Brudzinski's sign are shown in Figure 33-9.

Signs of Increased Intracranial Pressure

The prevention of increased ICP, or intracranial hypertension, is of key importance to the nurse's role when caring for a patient with a neurological injury. It is first essential for the nurse to establish a baseline neurological assessment on the patient, on which further deterioration can be based.

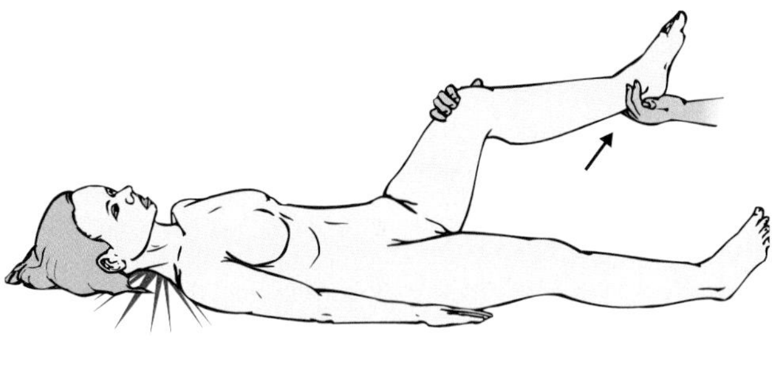

A. Kernig's sign

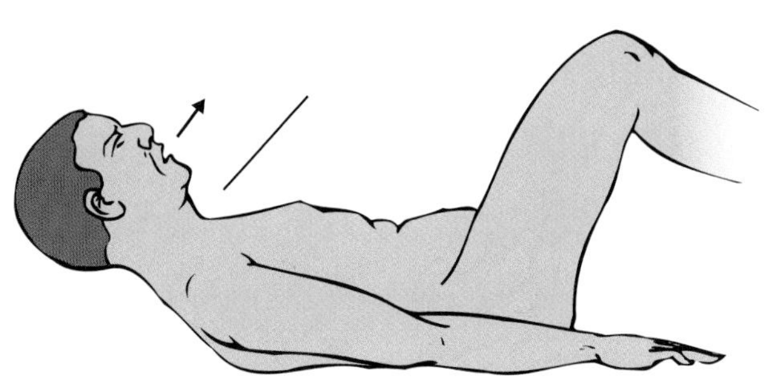

B. Brudzinksi's sign

figure 33-9 Two signs of meningeal irritation.

In general terms, increased ICP is manifested by deterioration in all aspects of neurological functioning.

Level of consciousness decreases as ICP rises. Initially, the patient may evidence restlessness, confusion, and combativeness. This then decompensates into lower levels of consciousness, ranging from lethargy to obtundation to coma. Pupillary reactions begin to diminish, with sluggishly reactive pupils and eventually fixed, dilated pupils. Frequently, because of the potential for injury to be ipsilateral, one pupil dilates before the other one does, resulting in unequal pupils.

Motor function also declines and the patient will begin to show abnormal motor activity. For example, the patient who initially may have localized to painful stimuli now shows either abnormal flexion or extension. Late findings are changes in vital signs. Variations in respiratory patterns are evidenced, eventually resulting in complete apnea. Cushing's triad (characterized by a rising systolic pressure, dropping diastolic pressure, and bradycardia) is considered a sign of impending herniation (see Chapter 36).

Evaluation of Dysfunction in the Patient's Living Patterns

Neurological nursing assessment would be incomplete if the process consisted solely of gathering data and identifying abnormal functions. Nursing expertise should expand the scope to include an evaluation of the impact of dysfunction on the patient's living patterns and ability to care for self. For example, diplopia (double vision) is an abnormal finding and may be an indicator of problems with the ocular muscles or with the nervous system; however, it also may be a clue suggesting difficulty in carrying out daily activities.

NEURODIAGNOSTIC STUDIES

Many diagnostic tests are available to help diagnose neurological and neurosurgical problems. Such neurodiagnostic testing is performed in conjunction with a thorough neurological examination. The availability and diagnostic accuracy of current technology benefit the patient in an acute setting by shortening the time required to arrive at a diagnosis and institute therapy. The choice of which investigative test to perform should be based on the examiner's ability to integrate the findings with neurological assessment and locate the cause of the abnormality.

The nurse's role in neurodiagnostic testing involves patient and family preparation and monitoring the critically ill patient for potential complications during and after the procedure. Although there has been a definite increase in the number of tests that can be performed at the bedside, many still require the patient to be transported to the imaging department or even out of the institution, further expanding the role of the critical care nurse. Table 33-5 summarizes some of the diagnostic tests and outlines nursing implications.

Neuroradiological Techniques

Conventional radiographs of the skull and spine are used to identify fractures, dislocations, and other bony anomalies, especially in the setting of acute trauma. In addition, radiographs may be diagnostic when displacement of the calcified pineal gland is visible, which is an immediate clue to the presence of a space-occupying lesion. Air inside the skull also suggests an open skull fracture, such as a frontal or basilar skull fracture, that may not be readily apparent externally. However, the use of plain films has decreased in recent years as computed tomography (CT) and magnetic resonance imaging (MRI) have proven to be better diagnostic tools.

Spinal films are still used as an initial screening in suspected vertebral or spinal cord trauma. They allow for visualization of the spine to evaluate complaints of pain or noted motor and sensory impairment. In the suspected spinal cord injured–patient, visualization of the cervical spine through C7 is indicated to rule out a cervical spine injury. Frequently, however, it is difficult to visualize through C7; therefore, it is sometimes necessary for another individual to pull down on the patient's arms to drop the shoulders low enough for the film to be taken. In addition, visualization of C1-2 is indicated, which may be obtained by an odontoid or Waters' view. This film is taken through the open mouth of the patient and necessitates patient cooperation. In instances where complete clearance is impossible, CT must be used to rule out cervical spinal injury.

The procedure for plain films of the skull and spine requires careful patient positioning and is relatively painless. The nurse's role involves monitoring the patient and attendant equipment during the procedure and being alert for complications related to patient position and the length of the procedure. In the spinal cord injured–patient, care should be taken to ensure stabilization of the neck by a hard cervical collar and logrolling during testing.

table 33-5 Neurodiagnostic Tests

Diagnostic Test	Description	Information Obtained	Nursing Considerations and Interventions
Computed tomography, or CT scan (invasive and noninvasive)	A scanner takes a series of radiographic images all around the same axial plane. A computer then creates a composite picture of various tissue densities visualized. The images may be enhanced with the use of IV contrast dye.	CT scans give detailed outlines of bone, tissue, and fluid structures of the body. They can indicate shift of structures due to tumors, hematomas, or hydrocephalus. A CT scan is limited in that it gives information only about structure of tissues, not about functional status.	Instruct the patient to lie flat on a table with the machine surrounding, but not touching, the area to be scanned. Patient also must remain as immobile as possible; sedation may be required. The scan may not be of the best quality if the patient moves during the test or if the x-ray beams were deflected by any metal object (i.e., traction tongs, ICP monitoring devices).
Magnetic resonance imaging (MRI)	A selected area of the patient's body is placed inside a powerful magnetic field. The hydrogen atoms inside the patient are temporarily "excited" and caused to oscillate by a sequence of radiofrequency pulsations. The sensitive scanner measures these minute oscillations, and a computer-enhanced image is created.	An MRI scan creates a graphic image of bone, fluid, and soft-tissue structures. It gives a more defined image of anatomical details and may help one diagnose small tumors or early infarction syndromes.	Risk factors for this technique are not well identified. This test is contraindicated in patients with previous surgeries where hemostatic or aneurysm clips were implanted. The powerful magnetic field can cause such clips to move out of position, placing the patient at risk for bleeding or hemorrhage. Other contraindications include cardiac pacemakers, prosthesic valves, bullet fragments, and orthopedic pins. Inform patient that the procedure is very noisy. Use caution if patient is claustrophobic. The patient (and caregivers) must remove all metal objects with magnetic characteristics (e.g., scissors, stethoscope).
Positron emission tomography (PET); single-photon emission computed tomography (SPECT)	The patient either inhales or receives by injection radioactively tagged substances, such as oxygen or glucose. A gamma scanner measures the radioactive uptake of these substances, and a computer produces a composite image, indicating where the radioactive material is located, corresponding to areas of cellular metabolism.	These diagnostic tests are the only ones to measure physiological and biochemical processes in the nervous system. Specific areas can be identified as to functioning and nonfunctioning. Cerebral metabolism and cerebral blood flow can be measured regionally. PET and SPECT scans help diagnose abnormalities (tumors, vascular disease) and behavioral disturbances, such as dementia and schizophrenia, that may have a physiological basis.	The patient receives only minimal radiation exposure because the half-life of the radionuclides used is from a few minutes to 2 h. Testing may take a few hours. The patient must remain very still and immobile. Procedure is very expensive.

(continued)

table 33-5 Neurodiagnostic Tests (Continued)

Diagnostic Test	Description	Information Obtained	Nursing Considerations and Interventions
Cerebral angiography (invasive)	This is a radiographic contrast study in which radiopaque dye is injected by a catheter into the patient's cerebral arterial circulation. The contrast medium is directed into each common carotid artery and each vertebral artery, and serial radiographs are then taken.	The contrast dye illuminates the structure of the cerebral circulation. The vessel pathways are examined for patency, narrowing, and occlusion, as well as structural abnormalities (aneurysms), vessel displacement (tumors, edema), and alterations in blood flow (tumors, arteriovenous malformations).	In preparation for this test, inform the patient as to the location of the catheter insertion (femoral artery is a common site) and that a local anesthetic will be used. Also warn that a warm, flushed feeling will occur when the dye is injected. After this procedure, assess the puncture site for swelling, redness, and bleeding. Also check the skin color, temperature, and peripheral pulses of the extremity distal to the site for signs of arterial insufficiency due to vasospasm or clotting. A large amount of contrast medium may be needed during this test, with resulting increased osmotic diuresis and risk of dehydration and renal tubular occlusion. Other complications include temporary or permanent neurological deficit, anaphylaxis, bleeding or hematoma at insertion site, and impaired circulation to the extremity used for injection.
Digital subtraction angiography (invasive)	In this test, a plain radiograph is taken of the patient's cranium. Then, radiopaque dye is injected into a large vein, and serial radiographs are taken. A computer converts the images into digital form and "subtracts" the plain radiograph from the ones with the dye. The result is an enhanced radiographic image of contrast medium in the arterial vessels.	Extracranial circulation (arterial, capillary, and venous) can be examined. Vessel size, patency, narrowing, and degree of stenosis or displacement can be determined.	There is less risk to the patient for bleeding or vascular insufficiency because the injection of dye is intravenous rather than intraarterial. The patient must remain absolutely motionless during the examination (even swallowing will interfere with the results).
Radioisotope brain scan (noninvasive)	In this test, radioactive isotope is usually injected intravenously. The scanning device produces films of areas of concentration of the isotope within the patient's head.	Because damaged brain tissue absorbs more isotope, the presence of an intracranial lesion can be diagnosed, as well as cerebral infarction or contusion. Lack of uptake of the isotope may indicate cerebral brain death.	Minimal patient preparation is required. The isotope may not be readily available within the institution. Movement will make the test difficult to interpret. This test is less commonly used than CT scan or MRI.

(continued)

table 33-5 Neurodiagnostic Tests (Continued)

Diagnostic Test	Description	Information Obtained	Nursing Considerations and Interventions
Myelography (invasive)	A myelogram is a radiographic study in which a contrast substance (either air or dye) is injected into the lumbar subarachnoid space. Fluoroscopy, conventional radiographs, or CT scans are used to visualize selected areas.	The spinal subarachnoid space is examined for partial or complete obstructions due to bone displacements, spinal cord compression, or herniated intervertebral disks.	Instruct the patient as for a lumbar puncture. In addition, advise that a special table will tilt up or down during the procedure. Postprocedure care is determined by the type of contrast material used. Oil-based contrast dye: • flat in bed for 24 h • force fluids • observe for headache, fever, back spasms, nausea, and vomiting Water-based contrast dye: • head of bed elevated for 8 h • keep patient quiet for first few hours • do not administer phenothiazines • observe for headache, fever, back spasms, nausea, vomiting, and seizures
Electroencephalogram, or EEG (noninvasive)	An EEG is a recording of electrical impulses generated by the brain cortex that are sensed by electrodes on the surface of the scalp.	Analysis of the resulting tracings helps detect and localize abnormal electrical activity occurring in the cerebral cortex. It aids in seizure focus detection, localization of a source of irritation such as a tumor or abscess, and diagnosis of metabolic disturbances and sleep disorders.	Reassure the patient that he or she will not feel an electrical shock or pain during this test. The nurse also may need to clarify for the patient that the machine cannot "read minds" or indicate the presence of mental illness. The patient's scalp and hair should be free of oil, dirt, creams, and sprays because they can cause electrical interference and thus an inaccurate recording. Inform the EEG technician of electrical devices around the patient that may cause interference during the procedure (e.g., cardiac monitor, ventilator).
Cortical evoked potentials (noninvasive) Somatosensory evoked potentials (SSEPs) Brainstem auditory-evoked response (BAER) Visual evoked potentials (VEPs)	In this test, a specialized device senses central or cortical cerebral electrical activity by skin electrodes in response to peripheral stimulation of specific sensory receptors. The sensory receptors stimulated can be those for vision, hearing, or tactile sensation. The signals are graphically displayed by a computer, and characteristic peaks, and the intervals between them, are measured.	Cortical evoked potentials provide a detailed assessment of neuron transmission along particular pathways. It has value in determining the integrity of visual auditory and tactile pathways in patients with multiple sclerosis and spinal cord injury. This test also may be used in the assessment of a sensory pathway before, during, and after surgery.	This test may be used in conscious as well as unconscious patients and can be performed at the bedside. The patient must be as motionless as possible during some phases of this test to minimize musculoskeletal interference. Depending on the sensory pathway being tested, the patient may be instructed to watch a series of geometric designs or listen to a series of clicking noises.

(continued)

table 33-5 Neurodiagnostic Tests (Continued)

Diagnostic Test	Description	Information Obtained	Nursing Considerations and Interventions
Transcranial Doppler sonography (TCD)	This is a test in which high-frequency ultrasonic waves are directed from a probe toward specific cerebral vessels. The ultrasonic energy is aimed through cranial "windows," areas in the skull where the bony table is thin (temporal zygoma) or where there are small gaps in the bone (orbit or foramen magnum). The reflected sound waves are analyzed for shifts in frequency, indicating flow velocity.	The speed or velocity at which blood travels through cerebral vessels is an indicator of the size of the vascular channel and the resistance to blood flow. An approximation of cerebral blood flow may be determined. Cerebral autoregulation can be monitored by observing the response of intracranial vessels to changes in arterial carbon dioxide and to the partial occlusion of the proximal vessels, as may occur in vasospasm.	The test is noninvasive and may be performed at the bedside by the physician or ultrasound technician in 30–60 min. There are no known adverse effects, and the procedure may be repeated as often as necessary. The testing is accomplished with the patient initially supine, and later on his or her side, with the head flexed forward.
Lumbar puncture (invasive)	A hollow needle is positioned in the subarachnoid space at L3–4 or L4–5 level, and CSF is sampled. The pressure of the CSF also is measured. Normal pressure varies with age from 45 mm H_2O in full-term newborns to 120 mm H_2O in adults.	The CSF is examined for blood and for alterations in appearance, cell count, protein, and glucose. The opening pressure is roughly equivalent to the ICP for most patients, if done recumbent and no block is present.	This test is contraindicated in patients with suspected increased ICP because a sudden reduction in pressure from below may cause brain structures to herniate, leading to death. In preparation for this test, position the patient on side with knees and head flexed. Explain to the patient that some pressure may be felt as the needle is inserted and not to move suddenly or cough. After this procedure, keep the patient flat for 8 to 10 hours to prevent headache. Encourage liberal fluid intake.

Computed Tomography

Computed tomography (CT) scanning has been in use in the United States since 1973. CT scanning uses intersecting x-ray beams through the brain and skull to measure the density of tissues through which the x-ray beams pass. The denser the material (i.e., skull), the whiter it appears on the film (Fig. 33-10). The less dense the material (i.e., air), the darker it appears on the film. With mathematical reconstruction, multiple views or slices of the brain can be seen, which allows for a very precise, detailed picture of the brain and its contents.

The CT scan permits more refined measurement of the density of tissues, blood, and bone in the body compared with that afforded by conventional radiographs. For example, cerebral edema appears less dense and therefore is of a lighter color than normal tissue. The value of this technique is illustrated best in the trauma setting, where the ability to image rapidly and accurately the intracranial contents and position of vertebrae and spinal cord has dramatically changed the treatment of neurological patients.

CT scans are recommended in the initial workup of seizures, headache, and loss of consciousness, and for the diagnosis of suspected hemorrhage, tumors, and other lesions. CT scanning can reliably detect conditions such as skull fractures, tissue swelling, hematomas, tumors, and abscesses. However, it has been noted that some vascular lesions are not as reliably documented using CT scan as they are with MRI. Therefore, MRI is indicated if these lesions are suspected.

Use of a contrast medium can enhance a CT scan. Using radiographic contrast material allows better visualization of vascular areas and enhances lesions previously seen on noncontrast films. Serial CTs may allow the health care team to follow neurological progression and therefore to intervene in a rapid manner. Care should be taken in the patient with renal failure or renal insufficiency because contrast clearance may be impaired.

Sometimes two technologies are used in combination, such as myelography with CT scanning, to provide a more refined image of anatomical structures of the spinal cord and vertebral column. With current technology, a routine

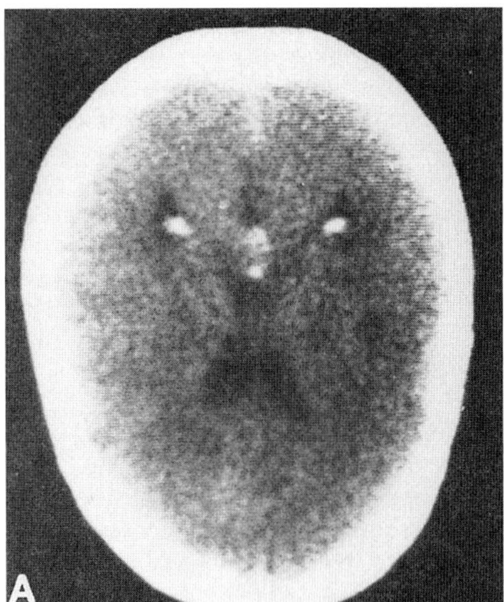

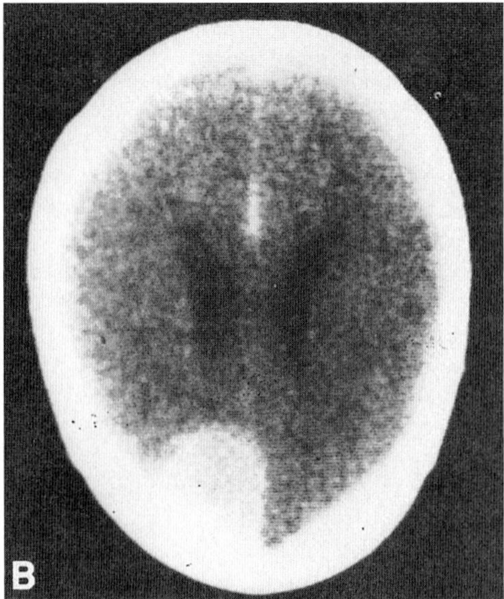

figure 33-10 Computed tomography (CT) scan of the brain. (**A**) Normal scan. (**B**) Scan showing a large mass in the left frontal lobe. (Reprinted with permission from Hickey J: The Clinical Practice of Neurological and Neuroscience Nursing [5th Ed], p 97. Philadelphia, Lippincott Williams & Wilkins, 2003.)

scan now takes less than 5 minutes to survey the patient, analyze the data, and display a finished image.

Nursing management is focused on patient education to obviate any potential complications, such as poor patient tolerance. The patient should be aware that he or she must lie very still during the procedure and that he or she may experience feelings of claustrophobia. In addition, the nurse should ascertain whether the patient has any pre-existing allergies, particularly if contrast is to be used. The nurse may need to remain with the patient during the procedure to continue to monitor neurological status and vital signs.

Magnetic Resonance Imaging

Magnetic resonance imaging (MRI), known in the past as nuclear magnetic resonance imaging, has become widely available in medium and large medical centers. This modality uses nonionizing forms of radiation to produce computerized cross-sectional images in much the same fashion as a CT scan. It provides much more finely detailed images, however, that look remarkably like anatomical slices of the body. An MRI is superior to a CT scan in the early diagnosis of cerebral infarction and the detection of demyelinating disorders, such as multiple sclerosis. It is also helpful in diagnosing small lesions, such as tumors and hemorrhages, which might not appear on a CT scan. However, traditional CT scanning is superior for scanning for bony abnormalities, which are visualized poorly on an MRI.

Although superior in many ways to CT scanning, MRI has its limitations. Its powerful magnetic fields interfere with the functioning of devices such as cardiac pacemakers. Patients with surgical clips and prosthetic implants made of ferrous metal cannot be scanned. It is also difficult to study patients on life-support equipment because most ventilators and monitors are constructed in part of ferrous metal. If emergency therapy is needed, the patient must be removed from the scanning chamber and the imaging suite before resuscitation can begin.

Positron Emission Tomography and Single-Photon Emission Computed Tomography

Positron emission tomography (PET) is a process in which molecules labeled with radioactive isotopes are located in the brain and recorded by radiation-sensitive detectors outside the head. PET has the capacity to measure cerebral blood flow and cerebral metabolism as the isotope-labeled glucose or oxygen is used in the body. It is superior to previous technologies that could image structure only, not function. It currently assists in the diagnosis of Alzheimer's disease, which shows a characteristic pattern of glucose consumption, as well as in Parkinson's disease, Huntington's disease, and Tourette's syndrome. However, the complexity of the testing, the comparatively high cost per scan, and the need to have a cyclotron nearby to produce the short-lived radioactive isotopes make this modality impractical and unwieldy in the clinical setting.

Single-photon emission computed tomography (SPECT) combines the imaging ability of conventional nuclear medicine scanners with the technology of transaxial CT scanning to overcome some limitations. Using more stable radioisotopes, SPECT scanning has been able to detect diminished perfusion in an area of stroke before there is conventional CT evidence of infarction, as well as alterations in regional blood flow in patients with Alzheimer's disease.

Angiography and Digital Subtraction Angiography

Cerebral angiography remains the study of choice for evaluating cerebrovascular problems (Fig. 33-11). It is the only test that can reveal large and small aneurysms and arteriovenous malformations and their relationship to adjacent structures and vessels. It involves the passage of a radiographic catheter through a large artery (usually femoral)

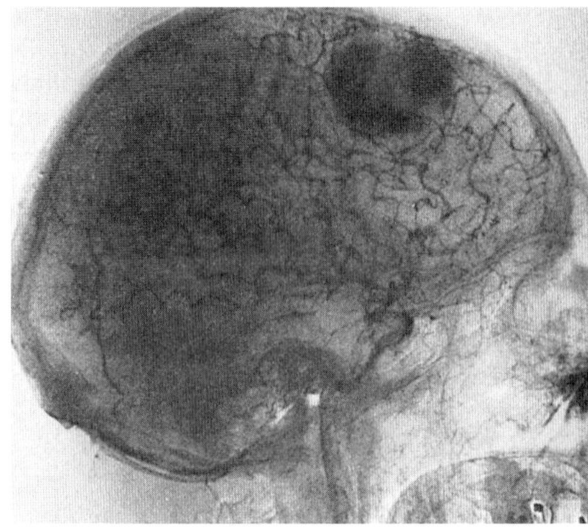

figure 33-11 Cerebral angiogram showing an abnormal, large, space-occupying lesion at one o'clock. (Reprinted with permission from Hickey J: The Clinical Practice of Neurological and Neuroscience Nursing [5th Ed], p 108. Philadelphia, Lippincott Williams & Wilkins, 2003.)

to each of the arterial vessels bringing blood to the brain and spinal cord. Radiopaque contrast dye is then injected into each vessel. A rapid sequence of films is taken after the dye has passed through small arterial branches and capillaries and into the venous circulation. In this way, the vessel lumen and size and the presence of any occlusions can be visualized. Cerebral angiography has been used before surgery to help decide the appropriateness of medical versus surgical management. It has also been combined with balloon angioplasty in instances of vascular occlusion or coiling in the treatment of aneurysms.

Digital subtraction angiography makes use of radiographic contrast to illuminate the cerebral circulation, but in considerably smaller quantities than required for conventional angiography. The dye may be injected into the arterial or the venous systems. Films are taken before and after the dye injection and converted into digital information in the accompanying computer. The images are "subtracted" from each other, removing all images in common. The resultant image displays only the enhanced circulatory system, free of other anatomical distortion.

The major complications associated with angiography include stroke, vasospasm, or renal failure secondary to the contrast load. Contraindications to angiography include identified allergies to contrast, anticoagulant therapy, and kidney and liver disease.

Cerebral Blood Flow Studies

In the diagnostic setting, cerebral blood flow is evaluated most commonly by a radioisotope brain scan. A radioactive isotope, such as technetium-99m, is injected intravenously. In unusual circumstances, the isotope can also be administered orally or intra-arterially. The brain is then scanned to determine which areas show an accumulation of the radioactive substance. If there is blood flow to the brain, damaged areas absorb more of the isotope than areas without damage. Cerebral blood flow studies are indicated in the detection of either increased or decreased blood flow during operative procedures or to assess for vasospasm. They may also be used after carotid endarterectomy. The test may be used to determine brain death, which is evidenced if there is no flow to the cerebral hemispheres. In certain disorders, such as carbon monoxide poisoning, there may be increased blood flow to the brain, yet anoxic brain death may still occur.

Normal cerebral blood flow is 50 to 55 mL per 100 g of cerebral tissue per minute. Flow in gray matter is four times higher than flow in white matter. The measurement of cerebral flow assists with decision making regarding treatment and in the identification of complications.

Myelography

Myelography is a contrast study of the spinal cord and surrounding structures. It involves the introduction of water-soluble material (metrizamide) into the CSF through a lumbar or cisternal puncture, performed under fluoroscopy, after approximately 10 mL of CSF has been removed. Myelography is indicated in the evaluation of herniated intervertebral disks, spinal cord tumors, and congenital problems, and in the assessment of spinal cord trauma. Because metrizamide is lighter than CSF, it allows for better visualization of nerve roots and surrounding structures. However, because of its rapid dispersal into the subarachnoid space, the patient's position cannot be adjusted. At times, a heavier, oil-based preparation is used (iophendylate [Pantopaque]), which must be removed at the end of the procedure. Because metrizamide does not require removal, the patient should be kept well hydrated to facilitate dye excretion. It is also potentially toxic to cerebral tissue, as evidenced by grand mal seizures, so the patient must remain with the head up at least 30 to 45 degrees, and phenothiazine medications, which increase the toxic symptoms, must be avoided.

Ultrasonography and Noninvasive Cerebrovascular Studies

B-mode imaging (brightness modulated) involves visualization of the structure of vessel walls and the presence of atherosclerotic plaques. It does so by recording the reflection of ultrasonic waves. A two-dimensional image is produced of the pulsating vessel, allowing for analysis of minor plaques.

Transcranial Doppler ultrasonographic studies provide a noninvasive means for monitoring intracranial hemodynamics at the bedside. The examination is performed through cranial "windows," areas in the skull where the bone is relatively thin, such as the temporal area, or where there are small spaces between bones, such as the orbit. The ultrasonic probe transmits sound waves at certain frequencies to a specified depth. The resultant reflected signal from blood traveling through cerebral vessels is interpreted for speed or velocity. As resistance or vascular size changes, it is reflected as a change in blood flow velocities. The data may be used to monitor therapy, aid in determining prognosis, and provide early recognition of cerebral vasospasm in patients after subarachnoid hemorrhage or severe head injury. Serial Doppler studies in patients with an aneurysm provide data regarding postoperative vasospasm and alleviate the need for repeat angiograms.

Carotid and vertebral artery duplex scans provide anatomical imaging of blood vessels combined with hemodynamic information. Doppler studies at the cranial window provide information about direction of flow, pulsatile rhythmicity, and resistance to flow of the cerebral vasculature. The nurse should be aware of whether the patient has any history of arrhythmias or cardiac disease because these may alter the hemodynamic profile and findings of the test.

Electrophysiological Studies

ELECTROENCEPHALOGRAPHY

Using electroencephalography (EEG), a record is made of the brain's electrical activity. Small plate electrodes are placed in specific locations on the patient's scalp, and 16 to 21 channels transcribe the electrical potentials generated by the brain. Waveforms are classified in terms of voltage and amplitude. An EEG is most valuable in the diagnosis and treatment of patients with seizures. In addition, it may help localize structural abnormalities, such as tumors and abscesses, and aid in the differentiation of structural and metabolic abnormalities. It also may provide confirmatory criteria in the diagnosis of brain death. In recent years, a modified form of EEG has been used at the bedside in critical care to monitor the effects of pharmacological agents that reduce cerebral blood flow and hence reduce electrical activity. This is termed *continuous EEG monitoring* and is rapidly becoming a standard of care in many facilities. It is intended to detect subclinical or nonconvulsive seizure activity in patients who are taking medications that suppress electrical activity.

A computerized technique that dramatically compresses standard EEG data and converts them into a more easily interpreted and colorized form is *compressed spectral array*. This technique is also seen at the bedside in neurological intensive care units to monitor patients with severe head injuries.

EVOKED POTENTIALS

An evoked potential is an electrical manifestation of the brain's response to an external stimulus: auditory, visual, somatic, or a combination of these. The measurement of such a response provides an assessment of the function of neuropathways from the periphery through the spinal cord and brainstem and finally to cortical structures (Fig. 33-12). This technique has been most helpful in the diagnosis of

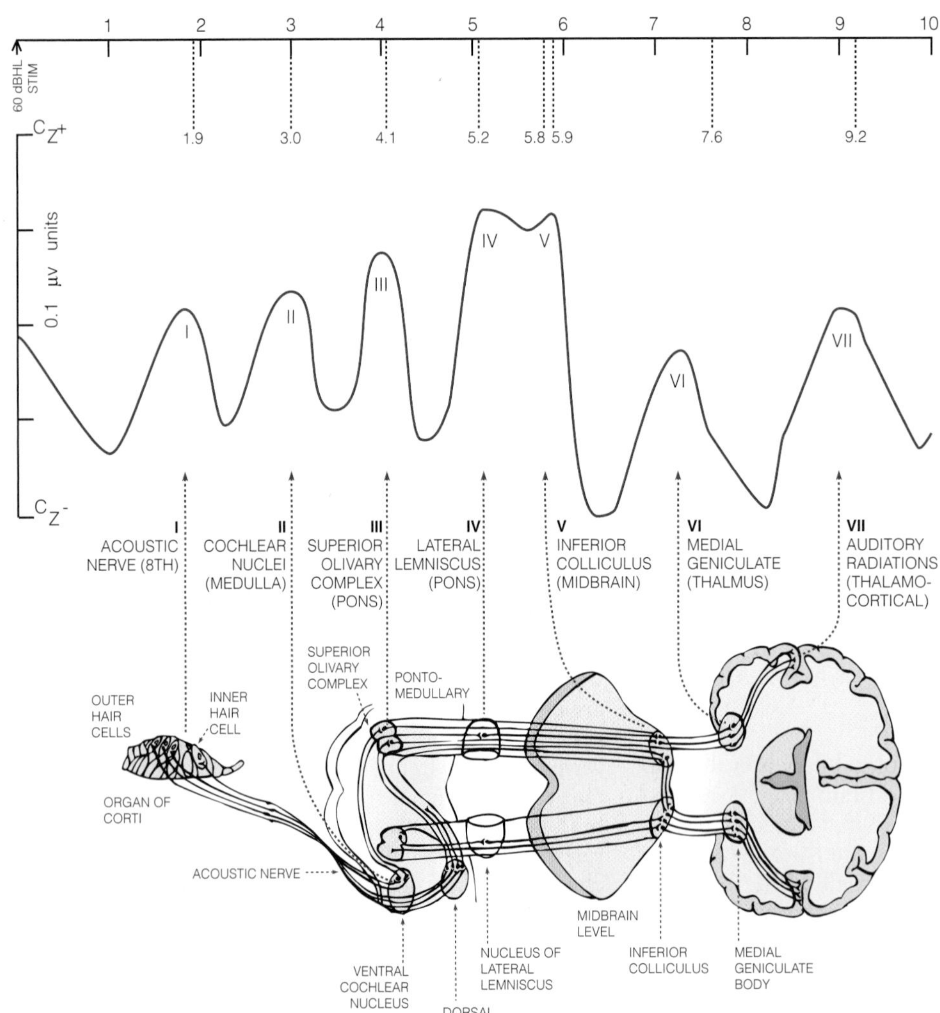

figure 33-12 The waveform of a normal brainstem auditory evoked response. (Courtesy of Grass-Telefactor, an Astro-Med, Inc. Product Group, West Warwick, RI.)

table 33-6 Normal and Abnormal Values for Cerebrospinal Fluid

Characteristic	Normal	Abnormal
Color	Clear, colorless	Cloudy often due to presence of WBC or bacteria Xanthochromic due to presence of RBC
WBC	0–5/mm^3, all mononuclear	Elevated count accompanies many conditions (tumor, meningitis, subarachnoid hemorrhage, infarct, abscess)
RBC	None	Presence may be due to traumatic tap or subarachnoid hemorrhage
Chloride	120–130 mEq/L	Low concentration associated with meningeal infection and tuberculous meningitis Elevated level not neurologically significant
Glucose	50–75 mg/100 mL	Decreased level associated with presence of bacteria in CSF Elevated level not neurologically significant
Pressure	70–180 mm H_2O	Low pressure associated with inaccurate placement of needle, dehydration, or block along subarachnoid space or at foramen magnum Elevated pressure associated with benign intracranial hypertension; cerebral edema; CNS tumor, abscess, or cyst; hydrocephalus; muscle tension or abdominal compression; subdural hematoma
Protein	14–45 mg/100 mL	Decreased level not neurologically significant Increased level associated with demyelinating or degenerative disease, Guillain-Barré syndrome, hemorrhage, infection, spinal block, tumor

(From Cammermeyer M, Appeldorn C [eds]: Core Curriculum for Neuroscience Nursing. [4th ed.] Chicago, American Association of Neuroscience Nurses, 1996)

multiple sclerosis and Guillain-Barré syndrome and in determining the prognosis for reversibility of coma in the brainstem-injured patient. It also may be used during surgery to monitor potential injury during manipulations of spinal nerves and structures.

The three most frequently used techniques in head trauma evaluation are somatosensory evoked potentials (SSEPs), which use electrical shock as a stimulus; brainstem auditory evoked response (BAER), which uses click or sound stimulus; and visual evoked potentials, which use light stimulus. SSEPs assess neurological function in specific neural pathways postinjury and detect further CNS insults from secondary processes, such as hypoxia and hypertension.

Lumbar Puncture for Cerebrospinal Fluid Examination

A lumbar puncture for CSF analysis may be performed to help diagnose autoimmune disorders or infections. Occasionally, it is performed to verify subarachnoid hemorrhage, although a CT scan is the procedure of choice and is safer for such a patient. CSF is obtained by the insertion of an 18- to 22-gauge needle between the vertebrae at the L3-4 or L4-5 levels. The fluid is sent for content analysis and for culture, sensitivity, and other serological tests (Table 33-6). Pressure readings may also be obtained for diagnostic use.

If a lumbar puncture is done in a patient with elevated ICP, herniation can be a life-threatening complication. Complications that can result from a CSF leak include a postprocedure headache, nuchal rigidity, fever, and difficulty voiding. Treatment involves the injection of blood into the dura, called a *blood patch*, to stop the leak.

clinical applicability challenges

Self-Challenge: Critical Thinking

1. *You have just been assigned to the care of a newly admitted patient diagnosed with a right cerebral cerebrovascular accident (CVA). Outline how you would perform an initial assessment, in particular detailing the neuroassessment of the comatose patient.*
2. *Discuss the indications and limitations of the diagnostic tests appropriate for the patient with a cerebral aneurysm.*

Study Questions

1. *A trauma patient is admitted with a Glasgow Coma Scale (GCS) score of 11. He is hemodynamically stabilized and has been intubated. He opens his eyes to painful stimuli and withdraws from the stimuli. His current GCS score is*
   a. *7T*
   b. *10T*
   c. *9*
   d. *7*
2. *Slow, writhing movements are called*
   a. *fasciculations.*
   b. *myoclonus.*
   c. *chorea.*
   d. *athetosis.*
3. *An upper motor neuron lesion (i.e., a stroke) may cause dysfunction in which cranial nerves?*
   a. *Peripheral cranial nerve VII (facial nerve)*
   b. *Central cranial nerve VII (facial nerve)*
   c. *Cranial nerve I (olfactory nerve)*
   d. *Cranial nerve VIII (acoustic nerve)*

4. *Drainage of cerebrospinal fluid (CSF) from the nose suggests fracture of the cribriform plate and is called*
   a. *otorrhea.*
   b. *Battle's sign.*
   c. *rhinorrhea.*
   d. *Kernig's sign.*
5. *A diagnostic test that might be of particular interest in the diagnosis of multiple sclerosis and Guillain-Barré syndrome is*
   a. *electroencephalography (EEG).*
   b. *evoked potentials.*
   c. *myelography.*
   d. *digital subtraction angiography.*

OTHER SELECTED READING

Arbour R: Using bispectral index monitoring to detect potential breakthrough awareness and limit duration of neuromuscular blockade. Am J Crit Care 13(1):66–73, 2004

Arbour R: Continuous nervous system monitoring, EEG, the bispectral index, and neuromuscular transmission. AACN Clin Issues 14(2):185–207, 2003

Bader MK, Littlejohns LR, March K: Brain tissue oxygen monitoring in severe brain injury, II: Implications for critical care teams and case study. Crit Care Nurse 23(4):29–40, 2003

Bickley BS: Bates' Guide to Physical Examination and History Taking (8th Ed). Philadelphia, Lippincott Williams & Wilkins, 2002

Fischbach FT: A Manual of Laboratory and Diagnostic Tests (7th Ed). Philadelphia, Lippincott Williams & Wilkins, 2003

Hickey JV: The Clinical Practice of Neurological and Neurosurgical Nursing (5th Ed). Philadelphia, Lippincott Williams & Wilkins, 2002

Jones S: An algorithm for train-of-four monitoring in patients receiving continuous neuromuscular blocking agents. Dim Crit Care Nurs 22(2):50–59, 2003

Littlejohns LR, Bader MK, March K: Brain tissue oxygen monitoring in severe brain injury, I: Research and usefulness in critical care. Crit Care Nurse 23(4):17–25, 2003

McQuillan KA, Von Rueden KT, Hartsock R, et al. (eds): Trauma Nursing from Resuscitation to Rehabilitation (3rd Ed). St. Louis, WB Saunders, 2001

Olson D, Chioffi S, Macy G, et al: Potential benefits of bispectral index monitoring in critical care: A case study. Crit Care Nurse 23(4): 45–52, 2003

Olson D, Cheek D, Morgenlander J: The impact of bispectral index monitoring on rates of propofol administration. AACN Clin Issues 15(1):63–73, 2004

Stewart-Amidei C, Kunkel J: AANN's Neuroscience Nursing: Human Responses to Neurologic Dysfunction (2nd Ed). Philadelphia, WB Saunders, 2001

chapter 34

Patient Management: Nervous System

MONA N. BAHOUTH ■ KAREN L. YARBROUGH

objectives

Based on the content in this chapter, the reader should be able to:

- Define intracranial pressure and intracranial hypertension.
- Discuss several physiological principles affecting intracranial pressure, including the Monro-Kellie model, compliance, autoregulation, and cerebral perfusion.
- List indications for intracranial pressure monitoring.
- Describe currently available methods of monitoring intracranial pressure.
- List three possible complications associated with intracranial pressure monitoring, and troubleshooting strategies.
- Identify various strategies to manage increased intracranial pressure.
- Describe the pharmacological agents used for patients experiencing a neurological emergency.

Intracranial pressure (ICP) is defined as the pressure in the cranial vault relative to atmospheric pressure. Understanding general principles regarding the concepts of ICP provides the critical care nurse with a framework that he or she can then apply to multiple neurological conditions. In addition, a working knowledge of the pharmacological agents used in neurological emergencies, such as steroids, antihypertensive agents, diuretics, analgesics, sedatives, barbiturates, and anticonvulsants (for the brain-injured patient), better prepares the nurse to handle these situations.

PHYSIOLOGICAL PRINCIPLES

Intracranial Dynamics

Concepts of ICP management and intervention strategies are based on the principle that the skull is a rigid box, a nonexpansile, noncontractile space. Its contents are divided into three intracranial sections: blood maintained in the blood vessels, cerebrospinal fluid (CSF), and brain parenchyma. The brain's ability to self-regulate is based on the Monro-Kellie doctrine of fixed intracranial volume. This doctrine states that the volume of the intracranium is equal to the volume of the cerebral blood (3% to 10%); plus the volume of the CSF (8% to 12%); plus the volume of brain tissue, which consists of more than 80% water. As long as the total intracranial volume remains the same, ICP remains constant. To maintain this equilibrium, there cannot be any increase in volume of one of these components without a compensatory decrease in the other two. Any alterations in the volume of any of these three components within the cranial vault, without a response from the other two components, may lead to a change in ICP. A normal ICP measurement varies between 0 and 15 mm Hg. By most standards, an ICP measurement greater than 15 mm Hg is considered intracranial hypertension, or increased ICP.

Basic physiological responses to illness in any of the three components in the intracranial vault can cause increased ICP (Table 34-1).

CEREBRAL BLOOD FLOW

Autoregulation is defined as the ability of an organ to maintain consistent blood flow despite marked changes in arterial circulatory and perfusion pressures. The normal brain has the ability to autoregulate *cerebral blood flow* (CBF). Normally, autoregulation ensures a constant blood flow through the cerebral vessels over a range of perfusion pressures by changing the diameter of vessels in response to changes in arterial pressures. This mechanism is the brain's protective device against the constantly fluctuating changes of blood pressure. When autoregulation is impaired, the CBF is dictated by and fluctuates in correlation with the systemic blood pressure. In patients with impaired autoregulation, any activity that causes an increase in blood pressure, such as coughing, suctioning, or restlessness, can cause an increase in CBF that could also increase ICP.

The first of three components that may undergo changes as the body attempts to maintain a consistent intracranial volume is the CBF. Normal CBF is provided by a cerebral perfusion pressure (CPP) in the range of 60 to 100 mm Hg. The brain receives approximately 750 mL/minute of arterial blood (15% to 20% of total cardiac output when at rest).[1] For autoregulation to be functional, carbon dioxide levels must be in an acceptable range and hemodynamic pressures must be within the following ranges: CPP over 60 mm Hg, mean arterial pressure (MAP) under 160 mm Hg, systolic pressure between 60 and 140 mm Hg, and ICP under 30 mm Hg. Factors that alter the ability of the cerebral vessels to constrict or dilate, such as hypoxia, hypercapnia, and brain trauma, also interfere with autoregulation. Carbon dioxide is the most potent vasodilator of cerebral vessels, causing increased CBF and increased volume, leading to increased ICP.

CEREBROSPINAL FLUID CIRCULATION

CSF also contributes to fluctuations in intracranial hemodynamics. CSF is a clear fluid produced predominantly in the choroid plexus in the lateral, third, and fourth ventricles. It fills the ventricles and subarachnoid space and protects the brain and spinal cord from injury. Circulation of CSF occurs in a closed system; it is predominantly reabsorbed by the arachnoid villi located in the subarachnoid space and dispersed into the venous system through the superior sagittal sinus (see Chapter 32, Fig. 32-6). Along the entire CSF cycle, potential disturbances in production, circulation, and absorption can contribute to changes in ICP. For instance, overproduction of CSF in the choroid plexus overwhelms the circulatory system. Obstruction of CSF circulation through the ventricles leads to dilation of the ventricular system. Marked slowing of absorption in the arachnoid villi because of blood or infectious debris interferes with the reabsorption of CSF, thereby leading to systemic overload. These processes summarize the basic etiologies of obstructive or communicating hydrocephalus (dilation of the ventricles).

PARENCHYMA

The third and most difficult intracranial component to manipulate without surgical intervention is the brain parenchyma. However, the brain tissue does respond to increased ICP and changes within the other two intracranial components. The brain can accommodate or compensate for minimal changes in volume by partial collapse of the cisterns, ventricles, and vascular systems, in turn decreasing production and increasing reabsorption of CSF.

The following is a summary of compensatory mechanisms to maintain normal ICP:

- Shunting of CSF into the spinal subarachnoid space
- Increased CSF absorption
- Decreased CSF production
- Shunting of venous blood out of the skull

table 34-1 Potential Causes of Increased Intracranial Pressure

Contributing Physiology	Intracranial Component Involved	Potential Cause	Potential Treatment
Overproduction of CSF	CSF space	Choroid plexus papilloma	Surgical removal, diuretics
Inadequate CSF reabsorption (communicating hydrocephalus)	CSF space	Subarachnoid hemorrhage, infection	Drainage of CSF from lumbar intrathecal site, shunt placement
Blockage of CSF circulation (obstructive hydrocephalus)	CSF space	Posterior fossa tumor, head injury, birth defects (spina bifida)	Ventricular drainage, surgical removal of obstruction
Edema (vasogenic, cytotoxic)	Brain tissue	Tumor, infection, infarction, hypoxia, arteriovenous malformation	Drainage of CSF, removal of lesion, adequate oxygenation
Expansile mass	Brain tissue	Tumor, abscess, intracerebral hemorrhage	Surgical removal, steroids
Vasospasm	Intracranial circulation	Subarachnoid hemorrhage	Hypervolemia, hypertensive therapy, calcium channel antagonists
Vasodilation	Intracranial circulation	Elevated $Paco_2$, systemic vasodilators (alpha-adrenergic agents)	Hyperventilation, removal of offending agent

During the compensatory period, ICP remains fairly constant. When these compensatory mechanisms have been exhausted, however, pressure increases rapidly until shifting of brain tissue toward open spaces in the skull occurs and the blood supply to the medulla is cut off. The ability of the intracranial content to compensate depends on the location of the lesion, the rate of expansion, and the compliance or volume-buffering capacity of the system.

Volume–Pressure Curve

The intracranial volume–pressure curve, also called a *pressure–volume index*, demonstrates the relationship between changes in intracranial volume and changes in ICP. The rate at which ICP rises in response to a change in intracranial volume depends on the compliance of the brain. The term *compliance* is defined as a change in volume resulting from a change in pressure. The term *elastance* refers to a change in pressure resulting from a change in volume. Elastance is often described as compliance and the two terms become interchangeable. When the intracranial compartment has low compliance (stiffness), a small volume change causes a large increase in ICP. In Figure 34-1, the curve illustrates compliance, as the compensatory mechanisms maintain ICP in the normal range during increases in intracranial volume. Little change occurs in ICP during the initial increase in volume because the volume added to the cranium is compensated for by volume displacement. As the compensatory mechanisms become exhausted, the volume added becomes greater than the volume displaced,

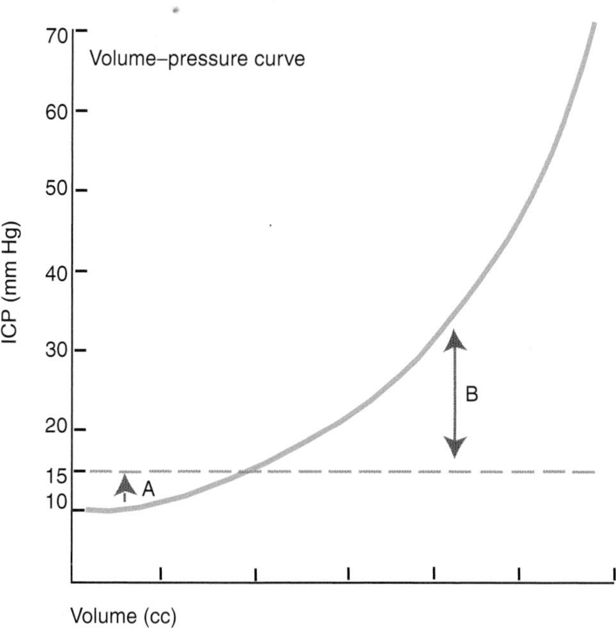

figure 34-1 Volume–pressure curve. Volume–pressure response (VPR), also referred to as the pressure–volume index (PVI), provides a method of estimating the compensatory capacity of the intracranial cavity. Note that the intracranial pressure (ICP) remains within the normal limit of 0–15 mm Hg as long as compliance is normal and fluid can be displaced by the additional volume (**A**). Once the compensatory system is exhausted, a small additional volume causes a greater increase in pressure (**B**). Acute changes can cause serious and sometimes fatal neurological deterioration.

and there is a larger increase in ICP with any incremental volume increase. The cranial contents become stiffer, and free communication of CSF between the lateral ventricles and infratentorium is lost.

Knowledge of the patient's position on the volume–pressure curve is useful in monitoring and selecting appropriate interventions. Estimating a patient's location on this curve can be accomplished by temporarily increasing the intraventricular volume. This is performed with the injection of approximately 1 mL of normal saline into the ventricle through an intraventricular device, under sterile conditions, and noting changes in the pressure response.

Many factors contribute to increased ICP along the volume–pressure curve. Drastic increases in ICP may result from hypercarbia, hypoxia, rapid eye movement sleep, pyrexia, or the administration of certain anesthetics. A major reason for controlling and decreasing ICP is the maintenance of cerebral oxygenation by adequate CBF, which is estimated clinically by the measurement of CPP.

Cerebral Perfusion Pressure

Cerebral perfusion pressure is the blood pressure gradient across the brain. CPP is calculated by subtracting the mean ICP from the mean systemic arterial pressure (MAP): CPP = MAP – ICP. When the CPP is greater than 100 mm Hg, there is a potential for hyperperfusion and increased ICP. When the CPP is less than 60 mm Hg, blood supply to the brain is inadequate, and neuronal hypoxia and cell death may occur. If MAPs and ICPs are equal, CPP is zero, indicating no CBF. CBF may also cease totally at pressures somewhat above zero. Patients with hypotension, such as postcardiac resuscitation or trauma patients, with normal ICPs (0 to 15 mm Hg) may have impaired CPP.

The autoregulation system for maintenance of constant blood flow does not function at pressures less than 40 mm Hg. Because an acutely injured brain requires a higher CPP than a normal brain, a minimum CPP of 70 mm Hg is required for maintenance of adequate cerebral perfusion and potentially improved outcomes in head-injured patients.[2] When CPP decreases, the cardiovascular response is a rise in systemic pressure.

When brain damage is severe, as with widespread brain edema or when blood flow has been arrested in the brain, CBF may be reduced at relatively normal levels of CPP.[3] This is caused by an impedance to the flow of blood across the cerebrovascular bed. If autoregulation is impaired, CBF may not increase despite increases in CPP. Increased ICP leads to ischemia, brain stiffness, and possible herniation.

CAUSES OF INCREASED INTRACRANIAL PRESSURE

Cushing's Syndrome

Cushing's syndrome is the classic syndrome of increased ICP and includes increased pulse pressure, decreased pulse, and decreased respirations with pupillary changes. This syndrome usually occurs only in association with posterior fossa lesions and seldom with the more commonly observed supratentorial mass lesions, such as subdural hematomas. When these classic Kocher-Cushing signs do accompany a supratentorial lesion, they are associated with a sudden pressure increase and usually herald a state of decompensation. Brain damage usually is irreversible if prolonged, and death is imminent without emergent intervention.

Cerebral Edema

Cerebral edema leading to increased ICP is a process common to multiple neurological illnesses. Its presence leads to secondary complications related to the expansion of brain tissue within the closed space of the cranium. Independently, cerebral edema can cause marked increases in ICP and must be treated aggressively. In general, once edema begins, its progression is rapid and difficult to control.

Treatment of cerebral edema includes the use of corticosteroids as well as osmotic diuretics directed at the reduction of ICP. These agents work by increasing plasma osmolarity, which draws fluid out of the brain tissue and into the bloodstream. The goal of therapy is to maintain plasma osmolarity up to 320 mOsm/L. See Chapter 36 for further information about cerebral edema.

VASOGENIC EDEMA

The most common type of cerebral edema is vasogenic edema, which is characterized by a disruption in the blood–brain barrier and the inability of the cell walls to control movement of water in and out of the cells. Capillary permeability is affected and fluid and protein are allowed to leak from the plasma into the extracellular space, resulting in increased extracellular fluid volume predominantly in the white matter. Common processes leading to vasogenic edema include brain tumors, cerebral abscess, and both ischemic and hemorrhagic stroke.

CYTOTOXIC EDEMA

Cytotoxic edema is characterized by swelling of the individual neurons and endothelial cells, which increases fluid in the intracellular space and reduces available extracellular space, affecting the gray matter. Eventually the cell membrane cannot maintain an effective barrier and both water and sodium enter the cell, causing swelling and loss of function. Cytotoxic edema occurs after injuries such as anoxia or hypoxic injury.

Herniation

Herniation is defined as the displacement of tissue through rigid openings. Shifting of brain tissue through rigid openings in the skull leads to displacement of midline brain structures and compression of elegant structures in the central nervous system (CNS), causing traditional clinical herniation syndromes. See Chapter 36 for more information about herniation syndromes.

INTRACRANIAL PRESSURE MONITORING

Monitoring ICP provides information that facilitates interventions to prevent secondary cerebral ischemia and brainstem distortion. For ICP monitoring to be safe, effective, and within cost-containment guidelines, the indications for monitoring, methods of monitoring, and ethical considerations for patient care and nursing practice must be taken into account for each patient. In addition to diagnosis, factors that affect patient selection include the patient's prognosis, potential benefit from invasive ICP monitoring and therapy, and the availability of medical and nursing personnel. ICP monitoring helps improve patient outcome by providing information on the likelihood of cerebral herniation and facilitating calculation of CPP. It is also helpful in guiding the use of potentially harmful treatments, such as hyperventilation, mannitol, and barbiturates.

Intracranial Pressure Monitoring Devices

Various devices, such as intraventricular catheters, fiberoptic devices, and epidural monitors, are used to monitor ICP. A chosen ICP device should have pressure range capability of 0 to 100 mm Hg, accuracy within the ICP range of 0 to 20 mm Hg ±2 mm Hg, and a maximum error of 10% in the range of 20 to 100 mm Hg of ICP.[4] The type of monitor used depends on several clinical factors, type of neurological process, and the patient's symptoms on presentation (Fig. 34-2). A variety of advantages and disadvantages exist with each of the devices; therefore, an awareness of potential complications is essential in the bedside management of the patient undergoing such monitoring (Table 34-2). Recent guidelines provided by the Brain Trauma Foundation consortium rank available devices by consensus preference (Box 34-1).

Intraventricular catheters (IVCs) remain the most widely used ICP monitoring device. The catheter is a tubular instrument that is placed inside fluid-filled cavities in the ventricles. CSF is synthesized in these cavities and flows out to circulate over the surface of the brain. IVCs can be inserted under sterile conditions at the bedside in the

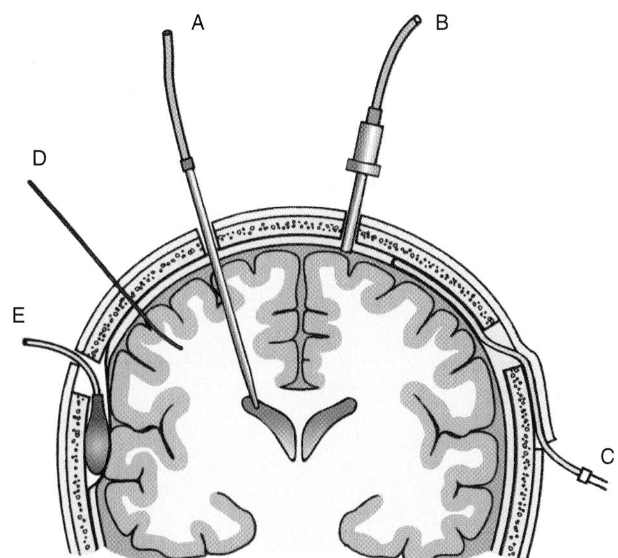

figure 34-2 Intracranial pressure (ICP) monitoring systems. (**A**) intraventricular; (**B**) subarachnoid; (**C**) subdural; (**D**) parenchymal; (**E**) epidural.

table 34-2 Advantages and Disadvantages of Intracranial Pressure Monitoring Devices

Monitoring Site	Advantages	Disadvantages
Intraventricular (ventriculostomy)	• Very accurate • True central direct measure of ICP • Can withdraw CSF to decrease ICP or measure compliance • Ease of CSF sampling	• Need transducer repositioned with every change in head position • High risk of serious infection • Difficult insertion in patients with small or displaced ventricles • Risk for intracerebral bleeding or edema along the cannula track
Intraventricular (fiberoptic catheter)	• Versatile; may be placed in ventricle or subarachnoid space • No adjustment of transducer with head movement	• Separate monitoring system required • Fragile catheter • Unable to recalibrate once device is placed
Intraparenchymal	• Ease of insertion • True brain pressures	• Infections rare, but serious
Lumbar/subarachnoid	• Simple to do single readings • No penetration of the brain parenchyma • Decreased risk for infection • Can sample CSF • Direct pressure management	• Contraindicated with evidence of increased ICP • Requires intact skull • Transducer repositioned with head movement
Subdural	• Ease of insertion	• Risk for serious infection
Epidural	• Low risk of infections • No transducer adjustment with head movement	• Imperfect correlation with intradural pressure (sensing through dura) • Operating room for placement • Unable to recalibrate once device is placed • Unable to drain CSF

intensive care unit (ICU) or in the operating room during surgical cases. They are considered the most accurate, low-cost, and reliable device used to measure ICP. IVCs are also unique in that they allow for simultaneous monitoring and treatment of ICP by intermittently draining CSF. Figure 34-3 depicts an IVC system in use.

Fiberoptic monitors use fiberoptic technologies to measure ICP. The tip of the fiberoptic probe has a transducer, which is inserted into brain parenchyma, the ventricles it surrounds, or the subdural space. Fiberoptic monitors are easily inserted and their use is increasing. Fiberoptic ventricular catheters provide similar benefits to IVCs, but at a higher cost. Of similar precision are parenchymal ICP monitors with fiberoptic or strain gauge catheter tip transduction; however, these devices are subject to potential measurement drift (especially after 5 days of monitoring).

Subarachnoid, subdural, and epidural monitors are less accurate and less frequently used than the other types of monitors. Epidural monitors are placed into the epidural space between the inner surface of the skull and the dura mater to monitor ICP.

box 34-1
Brain Trauma Foundation Device Ranking

1. IVC devices (most frequently used and most reliable)—fluid-coupled catheter with external strain gauge or catheter tip pressure transducer
2. Parenchymal catheter tip pressure transducer device
3. Subdural devices—catheter tip pressure transducer or fluid-coupled catheter with an external strain gauge
4. Subarachnoid fluid-coupled device with an external strain gauge
5. Epidural devices

COMPLICATIONS OF INTRACRANIAL PRESSURE MONITORING DEVICES

Each type of monitoring system has potential complications. To ensure accurate measurements and reduce morbidity, it is necessary to be alert to problems associated with ICP monitoring systems that could cause incorrect ICP measurements and complications. When the monitor indicates a change in ICP, the nurse must first determine whether the reading is accurate. If the reading is accurate, an attempt is then made to determine the reason for the pressure change. Table 34-3 provides a guide to troubleshooting ICP lines.

As with any invasive procedure, complications may occur. In critically ill patients with neurological problems, the risk–benefit ratio for any therapy must be considered before the implementation of that therapy. For instance,

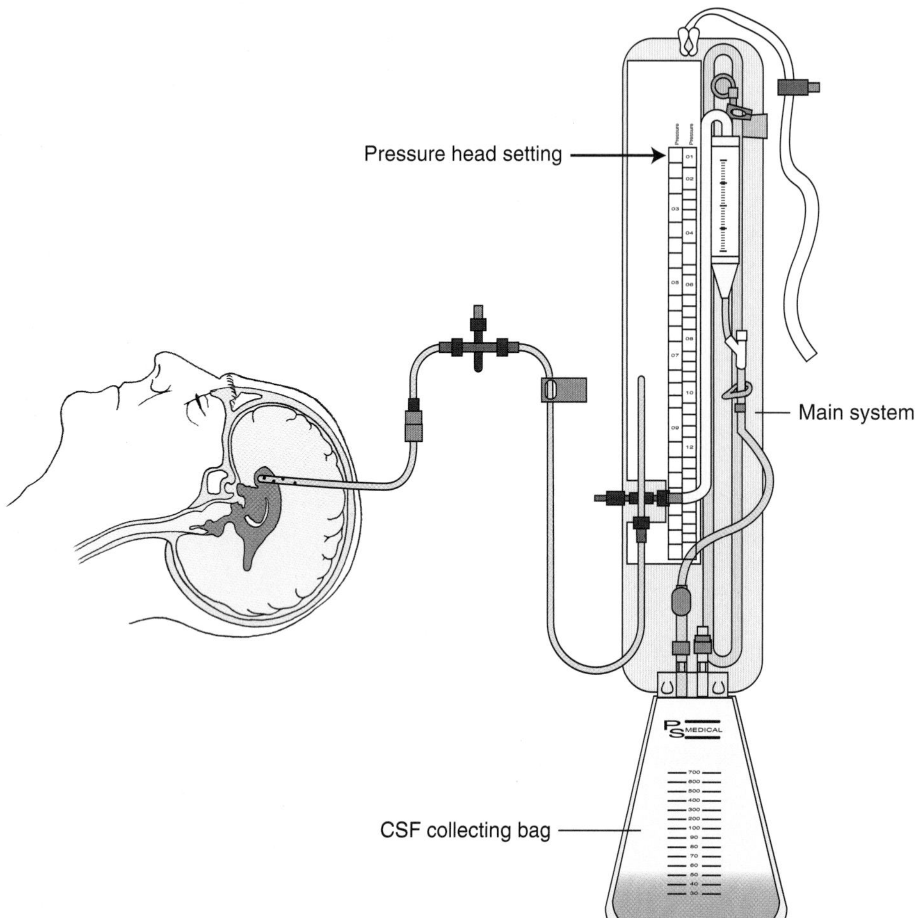

figure 34-3 Intraventricular catheter system. (Courtesy of Medtronic Neurologic Technologies, Goleta, California.)

IVCs carry the potential risks of catheter misplacement, obstruction, infection, and hemorrhage.

Because drainage holes responsible for the collection of excessive CSF are very small, it is easy for the catheter to become obstructed; the nurse must monitor for this complication. Malfunction or obstruction occurs at a rate of 6% to 10% in patients with an IVC and is significantly higher in patients with parenchymal or ventricular fiberoptic catheter tip devices, at a rate of 9% to 40%.[5] Higher rates of obstruction have been correlated with malignant elevations of ICP greater than 50 mm Hg. A reduction in catheter infections has been reported with recent changes in insertion techniques, antibiotic prophylaxis, and improved CSF sampling methods.[5] Hemorrhage associated with IVC placement is poorly described in the literature, prompting the reporting of a 1.1% to 2.8% risk of hematoma formation. The hemorrhage rate is highly dependent on the choice of device.

Results of Intracranial Pressure Monitoring

Normal measurements of ICP range between 0 and 10 mm Hg, with an upper limit of 15 mm Hg. During coughing or straining, a normal ICP may increase to 100 mm Hg. In acute situations, patients often become symptomatic at pressures ranging from 20 to 25 mm Hg.

A patient's tolerance of a change in ICP varies with the acuteness of its onset. Patients with a slower buildup of ICP, as with the example of expanding brain tumors, are more tolerant of elevations in ICP than are patients whose ICP increases rapidly, such as those with acute subdural hematoma. Uncontrolled ICP between 20 and 25 mm Hg is considered extremely dangerous for the head-injured patient. Sustained ICP greater than 60 mm Hg usually is fatal.

ICP may rise to the level of the MAP. The greater the variations in the mean ICP, the more nearly exhausted are the compensatory mechanisms for intracranial volume increases.

Although protocols vary, measures to reduce ICP are usually initiated if the patient shows neurological deterioration, such as a score of 7 or less on the Glasgow Coma Scale (GCS) or an ICP of 15 mm Hg or greater. Both systolic and diastolic blood pressures should be noted, although ICP is monitored and trended routinely as a mean pressure. Because there is a linear relationship between pulse pressure and ICP, pulse pressure may be used to estimate intracranial elastance, particularly in the patient with cerebral vasoparalysis.

INTRACRANIAL PRESSURE WAVEFORMS

Waveforms of ICP provide an index of ICP dynamics, such as changes in intracerebral compliance. The appearance of ICP waveforms varies according to the measurement technique being used, the patient's pathological status and activities, interventions, or environmental changes. Hemo-

table 34-3 Troubleshooting Intracranial Pressure Lines

Problem	Cause	Nursing Considerations and Interventions
No ICP waveform	Air between the transducer diaphragm and pressure source	Eliminate air bubbles with sterile saline.
	Occlusion of intracranial measurement device with blood or debris	Flush intracranial catheter or screw as directed by physician: 0.25 mL sterile saline is often used.
	Transducer connected incorrectly	Check connection, and be sure the appropriate connector for amplifier is in use.
	Fiberoptic catheter bent, broken	Replace fiberoptic catheter.
	Incorrect gain setting for pressure or patient having plateau waves	Adjust gain setting for higher pressure range.
	Trace turned off	Turn power on to trace.
False high-pressure reading	Transducer too low	Place the venting port of the transducer at the level of the foramen of Monro. For every 2.54 cm (1 in) the transducer is below the pressure source, there is an error of approximately 2 mm Hg.
	Transducer incorrectly balanced	With transducer correctly positioned, rebalance. Transducer should be balanced every 2 to 4 h and before the initiation of treatment based on a pressure change.
	Monitoring system incorrectly calibrated	Repeat calibration procedures.
	Air in system: air may attenuate or amplify pressure signal	Remove air from monitoring line.
High-pressure reading	Airway not patent: an increase in intrathoracic pressure may increase $Paco_2$	Suction patient. Position. Initiate chest physiotherapy.
	Ventilator setting incorrect	Check ventilator settings.
	Positive end-expiratory pressure (PEEP)	Draw arterial blood gases because hypoxia and hypercarbia cause increases in ICP.
	Posture	Head should be elevated 15–30 degrees unless contraindicated by other problems, such as fractures.
	Head and neck	The head should be positioned to facilitate venous drainage.
	Legs	Limit knee flexion.
	Excessive muscle activity during decerebrate posturing in patients with upper brainstem injury may increase ICP.	Muscle relaxants or paralyzing agents sometimes are indicated.
	Hyperthermia Excessive muscle activity Increased susceptibility to infection	Initiate measures to control muscle movement, infection, and pyrexia.
	Fluid and electrolyte imbalance secondary to fluid restrictions and diuretics	Draw blood for serum electrolytes, serum osmolality. Note pulmonary artery pressure. Evaluate input and output with specific gravity.
	Blood pressure: vasopressor responses occur in some patients with elevating ICP.	Use measures to maintain adequate CPP.
	Low blood pressure associated with hypovolemia, shock, and barbiturate coma may increase cerebral ischemia.	
False low-pressure reading	Air bubbles between transducer and CSF	Eliminate air bubbles with sterile saline.
	Transducer level too high	Place the venting port of the transducer at the level of the foramen of Monro. For every 2.54 cm (1 in) the transducer is above the level of the pressure source, there will be an error of approximately 2 mm Hg.

(continued)

table 34-3 Troubleshooting Intracranial Pressure Lines (Continued)

Problem	Cause	Nursing Considerations and Interventions
False low-pressure reading	Zero or calibration incorrect	Rezero and calibrate monitoring system.
	Collapse of ventricles around catheter	If ventriculostomy is being used, there may be inadequate positive pressure. Check to make sure a positive pressure of 15 to 20 mm Hg exists. Drain CSF slowly.
	Otorrhea or rhinorrhea	These conditions cause a false low-pressure reading secondary to decompression. Document the correlation between drainage and pressure changes.
	Leakage of fluid from connections	Eliminate all fluid leakage.
	Dislodgement of catheter from ventricle into brain	Contact physician regarding appropriate diagnostic studies and intervention. Use soft catheter designed for intraventricular measurement.
	Occlusion of the end of a subarachnoid screw by the necrotic brain	In most cases, remove screw.

dynamic and respiratory oscillations can be observed in ICP traces.

Sometimes the waveforms closely resemble arterial pressure waveforms; at other times they resemble central venous pressure waveforms. To varying degrees, oscillations corresponding to intracranial arterial pulsations with retrograde venous pulsations are seen with each heartbeat (Fig. 34-4). In patients with ICP less than 20 mm Hg, a slower waveform, synchronous with respiration and caused by changes in intrathoracic pressure, can be seen (see Fig. 34-4, middle). Alterations in arterial driving force, disturbance of venous outflow, and cerebral vasodilation correlate with changes in waveform appearances. At times, a small "a" wave is superimposed on diastole, reflecting right arterial pressure.

Some patients exhibit waveform variation, most commonly A, B, and C waves. *A waves*, also known as *plateau waves*, are spontaneous, rapid increases of pressure ranging from 50 to 200 mm Hg, occurring at variable intervals (see Fig. 34-4, bottom). They tend to occur in patients with moderate elevations of ICP, last 5 to 20 minutes, and fall spontaneously. Plateau waves usually are accompanied by a temporary increase in neurological deficit.

Although the mechanism of A waves has not been established firmly, it is thought that they indicate decreased intracranial compliance; therefore, these waveforms should be identified and treated quickly. They may result from an increase in blood volume with a simultaneous decrease in blood flow. The sudden reversal of high pressure may be caused by increased CSF absorption. Falls in CPP with intact autoregulation and low intracranial compliance have been correlated with the initiation of plateau waves. Plateau waves may also be set off by a vasodilating stimulus or by nonspecific stimuli, such as hypoventilation or hyperventilation, pain, and aroused mental activities.

B waves are small, sharp, rhythmic waves with ICPs up to 50 mm Hg, occurring at a frequency of 0.5 to 2 per minute. They correspond to changes in respiration, providing clues to periodic respiration related to poor cerebral compliance or pulmonary dysfunction. B waves often are seen with

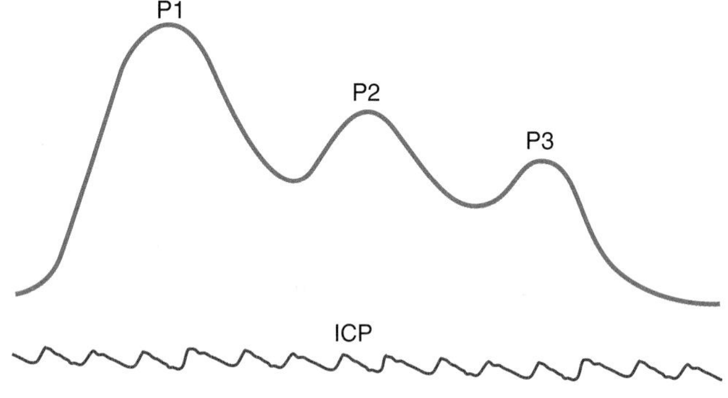

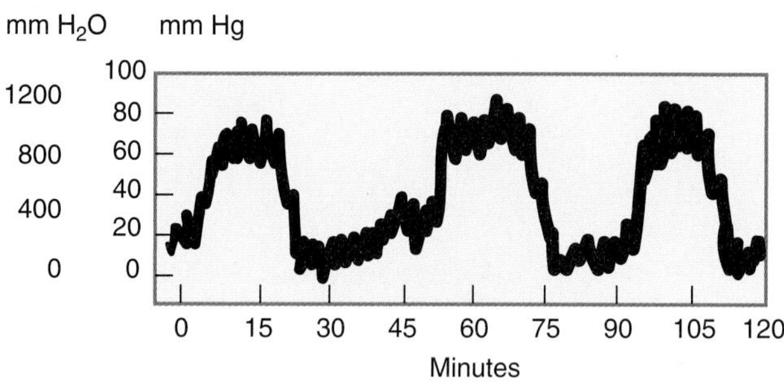

figure 34-4 Intracranial pressure (ICP) waveforms. *Top,* A normal ICP pulse waveform may demonstrate three or more descending peaks. P1, the pressure wave, originates from choroid plexus pulsations. P2, the tidal wave, is more variable in shape and amplitude and ends on the dicrotic notch. P3, the dicrotic wave, follows the dicrotic notch and tapers down to the diastolic position unless retrograde venous pulsations cause a few more peaks. The P2 portion of the waveform most directly reflects the state of intracerebral compliance. As mean ICP rises, P2 progressively elevates, causing the pulse wave to appear more rounded. When a state of decreased compliance exists, the P2 component is equal to or higher than P1. *Middle,* An ICP waveform demonstrating hemodynamic and respiratory oscillations. Note the vascular pressure-type notches in the waveforms and the baseline variations that reflect respirations. *Bottom,* "A," or plateau waves, associated with decreased intracranial compliance, may be secondary to an increase in blood volume with a simultaneous decrease in blood flow.

Cheyne-Stokes respirations (see Chapter 36). They may precede A waves and increase as compliance decreases. At times, they occur in patients with normal ICP and no papilledema. They may be secondary to oscillations of cerebral blood volume.

C waves are small, rhythmic waves with ICPs up to 20 mm Hg, occurring at a rate of approximately six per minute. They are related to blood pressure. Like A waves, they indicate severe intracranial compression, with limited remaining volume residual in the intracranial space.

Computerized systems are being developed to analyze waveforms and integrate ICP, CPP, and other relevant parameters.

Indications for Intracranial Pressure Monitoring

ICP monitoring is primarily a means for therapy guidance. There remains insufficient scientific evidence to support any treatment standards in regard to ICP devices. However, general guidelines exist to provide direction in therapy for patients at risk for and with increased ICP. Diagnostic conditions that may be indications for ICP measurement include head injury, stroke, brain tumors, cardiac arrest, and surgery. The decision to use ICP monitoring should be based on clinical and radiographic evaluation and computed tomography (CT) scan diagnosis.

Currently, ICP monitoring is not indicated for patients with mild to moderate head injury, defined as a GCS score of 9 to 15. ICP monitoring may, however, be appropriate for comatose patients or patients suffering severe head injury with or without abnormalities on a head CT scan. Severe head injury is defined as a GCS score of 3 to 8 after cardiopulmonary resuscitation. Abnormal CT scan findings are defined as the presence of hematoma, contusion, edema, or compressed basal cisterns. ICP monitoring is also appropriate for patients suffering head trauma with a negative CT scan who have two or more of the following criteria: age greater than 40 years, any motor posturing, or systolic blood pressure less than 90 mm Hg.

The upper limit of normal ICP is defined by most centers as 15 mm Hg. Although no prospective, randomized trial has been completed, a summary of the literature suggests that ICP monitors are beneficial in:

- Providing earlier detection of intracranial mass lesion
- Limiting indiscriminate use of therapies with potentially harmful consequences
- Reducing ICP through CSF drainage, thereby improving CPP
- Assisting in determining prognosis
- Possibly improving outcomes[4]

Nontraumatic neurological disorders that may benefit from ICP monitoring are subarachnoid hemorrhage, intracerebral hemorrhage, ischemic infarction, infection, hydrocephalus, and, rarely, brain tumors with associated edema or with significant lesion volume.

Coagulopathy, systemic infection, CNS infection, or infection at the site of device insertion are relative contraindications to the placement of ICP monitors.

MANAGEMENT OF INCREASED INTRACRANIAL PRESSURE

In the stage between the onset of increased ICP and herniation, many treatments are available to reduce ICP and maintain adequate cerebral perfusion. No single management routine is appropriate for all patients. In addition to clinical pathways and nursing care protocols, algorithms for the incremental application and weaning of ICP management have been developed. Figure 34-5 provides an algorithm for first-tier (conventional) and second-tier (refractory) treatments of increased ICP. First-tier therapy includes ventricular CSF drainage (as discussed previously), mannitol administration, respiratory support, and sedation and analgesia. Second-tier therapy includes hypothermia, barbiturate coma, optimized hyperventilation, hypertensive CPP therapy, and decompressive craniectomy.

Most management techniques for increased ICP are oriented toward control of cerebral blood volume and CSF circulation, the two major mechanisms responsible for the regulation of ICP. Although protocols vary, measures to reduce ICP are usually initiated when the patient's ICP increases to approximately 15 mm Hg.

Although no one therapeutic regimen has been accepted universally, the goals of treatment for the patient with increased ICP are as follows: reduce ICP, optimize CPP, and avoid brain shift.

First-Tier Therapy

MANNITOL ADMINISTRATION

Mannitol, a hypertonic crystalloid solution that decreases cerebral edema, is also used as first-tier therapy for reducing ICP after brain injury. It is typically administered as a bolus intravenous (IV) infusion over 10 to 30 minutes in doses ranging from 0.25 to 2 g/kg body weight. Studies have demonstrated mannitol's effect on ICP, CPP, CBF, and brain metabolism and have also shown a beneficial effect on long-term neurological outcome. More recently, hypertonic saline has also been shown effective.[6–8] The immediate plasma-expanding effect of mannitol, which reduces blood viscosity, increases CBF and cerebral oxygen metabolism, permitting cerebral arterioles to decrease in diameter. This lowers cerebral blood volume and ICP, while maintaining constant CBF. Ideally, to reduce potential side effects and optimize the risk–benefit ratio, mannitol administration should be based directly on ICP measurements. However, mannitol may be safely administered when it is not possible to measure ICP.

Mannitol is excreted in the urine. If it is administered in large doses and serum osmolarity is greater than 320 mOsm, there is a significant risk for development of acute tubular necrosis (ATN). Therefore, it is customary to measure serum osmolarity every 6 to 8 hours to a target of less than 320 mOsm.

A Foley catheter must be inserted when mannitol is administered. When mannitol is used during the early resuscitation phase of hypovolemic head-injured patients, crystalloid solutions are infused simultaneously to correct hypovolemia. Adjunct crystalloid fluid administration facilitates rapid renal excretion of mannitol, preventing renal

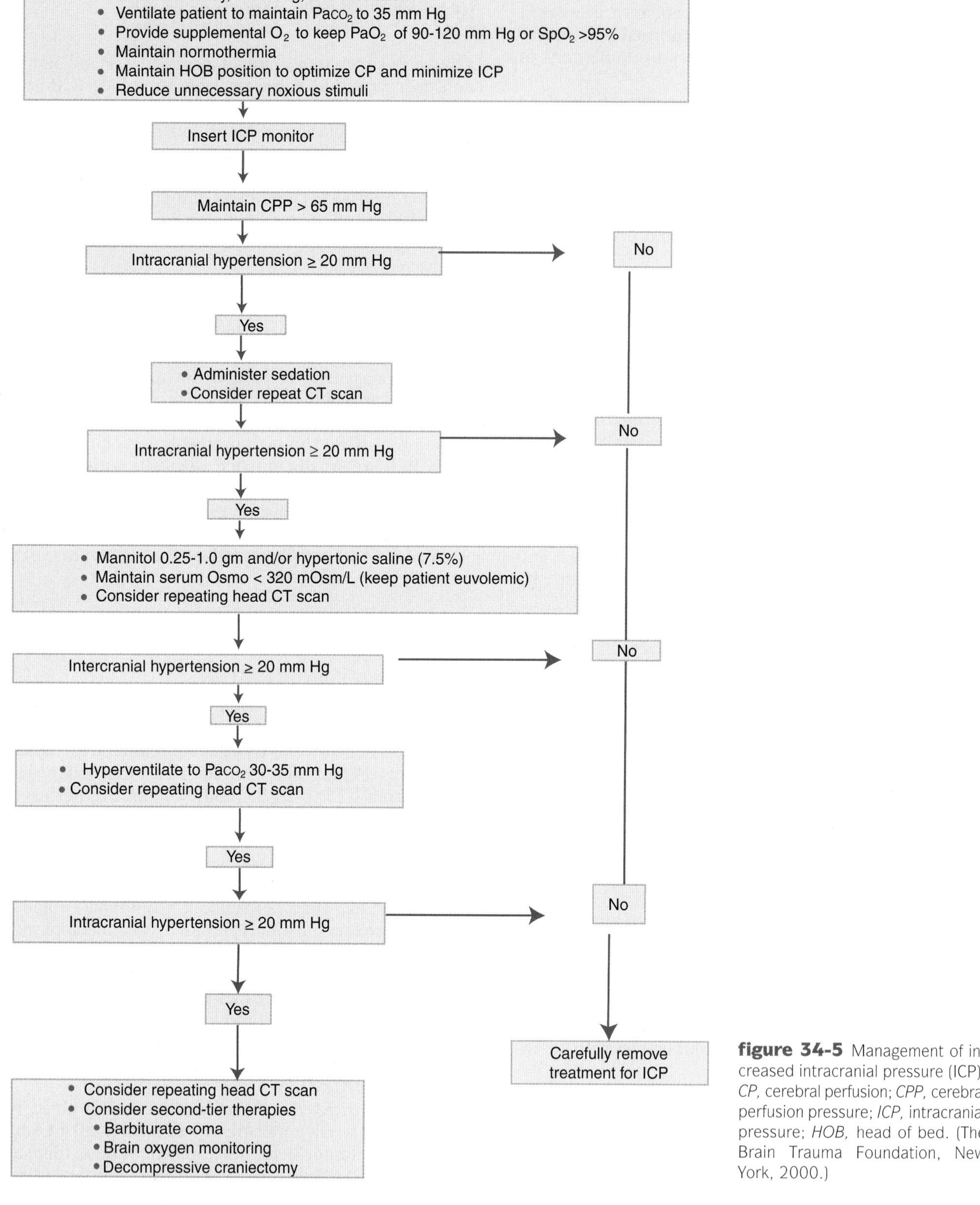

figure 34-5 Management of increased intracranial pressure (ICP). *CP,* cerebral perfusion; *CPP,* cerebral perfusion pressure; *ICP,* intracranial pressure; *HOB,* head of bed. (The Brain Trauma Foundation, New York, 2000.)

failure. In the early phases of acute brain injury, mannitol is recommended as monotherapy because of the risk for massive diuresis, causing depletion of intravascular volume and electrolytes, when mannitol is combined with furosemide.

Furosemide is a loop diuretic that is frequently used for the critically ill patient experiencing congestive heart failure. It is also used in patients who are experiencing fluid retention due to poorly functioning kidneys. A critically ill patient who is hypovolemic or has poor blood flow to the kidneys experiences renal dysfunction and low urinary output. Furosemide increases reabsorption of sodium in the loop of Henle, and the result is increased urinary output. Furosemide is indicated in adults, infants, and children for the treatment of edema associated with congestive heart failure, cirrhosis of the liver, and renal disease, including nephritic syndrome.

Furosemide is particularly useful when an agent with greater diuretic potential is desired. Excessive diuresis may cause dehydration and blood volume reduction with circulatory collapse and possible vascular thrombosis and embolism, particularly in older patients. As with any effective diuretic, electrolyte depletion may occur during furosemide therapy, especially in patients receiving higher doses and a restricted salt intake. Symptoms of electrolyte imbalance include dryness of mouth, thirst, weakness, lethargy, drowsiness, restlessness, muscle pains or cramps, muscular fatigue, hypotension, oliguria, tachycardia, dysrhythmias, or gastrointestinal disturbances such as nausea and vomiting.

RESPIRATORY SUPPORT

Mean airway pressure is the leading factor affecting ICP in the patient who is ventilated. Positive airway pressure is transmitted to the intracranial cavity through the mediastinum. Therefore, any condition decreasing pulmonary compliance or use of positive end-expiratory pressure increases the mean airway pressure and decreases the MAP and CPP.

Hyperventilation remains controversial in the management of increased ICP. Inducing hypocarbia is an effective way to reduce CBF because of its strong vasoconstrictive effect on the cerebral arteries. The arterial carbon dioxide tension ($Paco_2$) should be lowered gradually to avoid a rebound effect of vasodilation from overcorrection. When hyperventilation is discontinued, ventilation rates should be gradually returned to normal. Severe, prolonged hyperventilation has been conclusively shown to worsen the outcome of patients with a severe head injury. Severe hyperventilation is defined as a $Paco_2$ of less than 25 mm Hg by jugular venous oxygen saturation monitor. Extreme hyperventilation is believed to cause secondary ischemia by constricting cerebral vasculature.[4]

In the absence of a malignant increase in ICP, chronic prolonged hyperventilation therapy (a $Paco_2$ less than 25 mm Hg) should be avoided after a traumatic brain injury. Also, the use of prophylactic hyperventilation therapy (a $Paco_2$ less than 35 mm Hg) during the first 24 hours after a traumatic brain injury should be avoided because it can compromise cerebral perfusion during a time of critically reduced CBF. CBF after trauma is 30 mL/100 g/minute during the first 8 hours after injury and 20 mL/100 g/minute during the first hour.[9] Hyperventilation may become necessary for brief periods when there is acute neurological deterioration, or if increased ICP is refractory to sedation, paralysis, CSF drainage, and osmotic diuretics. Therefore, the literature suggests avoiding hyperventilation during the first 5 days after a traumatic injury and most directly during the first 24 hours after trauma.[4]

Suctioning should be approached thoughtfully to avoid hypoxemia as well as increased intrathoracic pressures. Limiting the duration of passes of the suction catheter to no more than 10 seconds, to be repeated no more than once or twice, avoids overstimulation of the cough reflex and decreases the incidence of increased intrathoracic pressure and ICP.

ANALGESIA AND SEDATION

Before starting patients on analgesics or sedatives, every effort should be made to implement nonpharmacological management techniques for pain, agitation, anxiety, and confusion. However, patients with impaired neurological function may require analgesia and sedation to decrease anxiety and diminish awareness of noxious stimuli. Also, the treatment of pain lowers energy expenditures, thereby facilitating healing. Further, analgesics and sedatives may potentiate each other, allowing patients to be calm and comfortable at lower doses.[10]

In patients with a severe head injury (GCS score of less than 8), pain medications and sedatives are used to:

- Reduce agitation, discomfort, and pain
- Facilitate mechanical ventilation by suppressing coughing
- Limit responses to stimuli, such as suctioning, which may increase ICP

A patient with a neurological emergency must be treated for pain and provided sedation. The patient with a brain injury does require frequent neurological assessments that may be affected by pain medications; however, the patient has a right to adequate pain relief. A neurologist should be consulted early in the patient's hospital course to assist in the proper dosing of medications so that frequent neurological assessments can be performed.

Analgesics

Opiate narcotics primarily affect the CNS. Fentanyl and morphine are two of the most frequently used opiate narcotics that:

- Limit pain caused by injuries and nursing interventions
- Facilitate mechanical ventilation
- Potentiate the effect of sedatives[10]

Potentially life-threatening adverse effects of narcotics include respiratory depression, depression of the cough reflex, mood changes, nausea, and vomiting. As a result, a patient may experience hypoxia; therefore, intubation equipment must be readily available at all times when a patient is receiving narcotics. Naloxone reverses CNS depression, which can occur with the administration of fentanyl and morphine, and therefore must also be readily available whenever narcotics are administered. Vital signs, including pulse oximetry, must be monitored diligently when a patient receives IV pain medication. With proper dosing and diligent nursing observation, narcotics can be used effectively in the critically ill patient.

The basic principles of narcotic administration are adequate pain relief and safe administration. The infusion should begin with the lowest possible dose and be titrated until pain relief is obtained. When a patient with a brain injury also has severe pain caused by multiple traumatic injuries, a continuous infusion of fentanyl or morphine is indicated. A typical pain management regimen may include a continuous morphine infusion starting at 1 to 2 mg/hour, or fentanyl 50 to 100 µg/hour and titrated every 15 to 30 minutes until the patient appears comfortable. For a patient with moderate pain, a 24-hour regimen of opiate narcotic administration has been proven to provide increased pain relief versus a PRN schedule of opiate dosing.

For the patient who can communicate, a verbal pain scale is used to assess pain. Standardized rating scales, such as a 1 to 10 pain scale, should be used to quantify and evaluate pain status and response to therapy. In addition to location, quality, and duration of pain, the nurse must document the effectiveness of analgesics every hour for 4 hours with initial administration, and then every 4 hours.[10]

When the patient is unable to communicate, physiological parameters are used to determine the effectiveness of pain management. The nurse should assess heart rate, respiratory rate, use of accessory muscles for breathing, and blood pressure. Adequate pain management leads to less patient movement, such as thrashing, which increases metabolic activity. The following clues can be used to determine if adequate pain relief has been obtained for the patient who cannot communicate:

- Ease of breathing
- The mechanically ventilated patient breathing in concert with ventilator
- Possible decrease in heart rate
- Less agitation as indicated by restful sleep state
- Cooperation with nursing interventions without excessive combative behavior

Narcotics can be safely administered to the older patient. However, the older critically ill patient may be especially susceptible to respiratory depression and therefore require lower dosages. Also, narcotics decrease gastric motility and may cause constipation. For the older patient confined to bed, prophylactic administration of a stool softener is normal practice. (For all patients receiving narcotics, documentation of the number of bowel movements is essential.) Older individuals may also be susceptible to nausea and vomiting with the administration of narcotics. Protection of the airway is especially important in the older patient with a neurological diagnosis. Finally, insertion of an orogastric tube to decompress the stomach may be used in older patients.

Sedatives

The most commonly used sedatives in the ICU are benzodiazepines, which potentiate the effects of analgesic agents. Midazolam, diazepam, and lorazepam are used frequently for sedation before ICU procedures and as needed to treat anxiety. Lorazepam is frequently used for alcohol withdrawal as well as for anticonvulsant therapy. Midazolam is most often used for sedation before procedures to produce amnesia of immediate events. Benzodiazepines cause little change in CBF, ICP, and cerebral metabolic rate. Side effects of sedatives include respiratory depression, hypotension, and somnolence. It is mandatory that resuscitation equipment be available at all times when a patient is provided IV benzodiazepines. Benzodiazepines should be administered at the lowest possible dose that produces effective sedation, without causing somnolence. As with analgesic agents, frequent vital signs must be obtained with the administration of sedatives. Recommended minimal documentation of vital signs should be every hour for 4 hours, then every 4 hours, and 15 minutes after every dosage change.

Various scales may be used to document the patient's response to sedation. Target sedation levels for most patients are commensurate with ease of arousal. For the patient who cannot communicate (as discussed earlier with analgesic use), the assessment of physiological parameters can be used to determine the patient's response to sedation. A patient must be assessed to eliminate all reasons for severe anxiety, which may interfere with recovery from a critical illness. Pharmacological management of sedation is only one strategy to treat anxiety. Nursing measures to provide comfort must be offered in addition to medications.

Anesthetics

Propofol (Diprivan) is a fat-soluble anesthetic that is administered as a continuous infusion to decrease agitation in the critically ill patient. Studies have shown that propofol may decrease CBF, ICP, CPP, and cerebral metabolic function.[11] Propofol is easily titrated based on patient response. It also has a short half-life and can be discontinued for frequent neurological assessments. Propofol can cause a decreased level of consciousness in 2 minutes. Common side effects include hypotension; therefore, frequent blood pressure monitoring must be performed, especially if the patient has increased ICP. Also, diligent airway protection must be provided for the patient receiving propofol. He or she must be intubated and mechanically ventilated when propofol is administered to prevent respiratory depression. For these reasons, the patient who is provided a continuous infusion of propofol must be cared for in the ICU, with constant critical care nurse surveillance.

Other cautions with propofol are related to the handling of the drug. Propofol is manufactured by using a fat emulsion, making it a powerful medium for bacterial growth. Propofol must be handled meticulously to prevent the risk of bacterial or fungal infection associated with its use. Propofol IV lines should be changed frequently, usually every 12 hours. In addition, the ICU team calculates the number of fat calories provided by propofol and includes these in the total number of calories required by the patient.

Second-Tier Therapy

HYPOTHERMIA

Induced therapeutic hypothermia is the intentional lowering of a patient's body temperature, usually by heat exchange through a heart-lung machine or by surface cooling. Hypothermia continues to be used in the management of patients with severe traumatic brain injury, despite the lack of unequivocal evidence supporting its use.[12] It is a well-described method of preventing post-ischemic brain damage after total circulatory arrest for cardiothoracic surgery.

BARBITURATE COMA

Induced barbiturate coma has been used in severe cases of refractory elevated ICP. Criteria for the use of barbiturates in the head-injured patient include a GCS score of less than 7; ICP greater than 25 mm Hg for 10 minutes when the patient is at rest; and maximum use of CSF drainage, mannitol, analgesia, and sedation. Usually either pentobarbital or thiopental is used to induce a barbiturate coma; the usual length of the coma is 72 hours.

Barbiturates suppress seizure activity and reduce cerebral metabolic activity and cerebral oxygen demand. Barbiturates affect CBF, metabolic demand, electroencephalographic (EEG) activity, and systemic hemodynamics. CBF may decrease by 50%. The barbiturate appears to have a direct restrictive effect on cerebral vasculature by diverting small amounts of blood from well-perfused areas to ischemic areas, thereby improving cerebral pressure. Vascular spasms are reduced by improving CBF. Barbiturate administration decreases the systemic blood pressure, which may prevent the disruption of the blood–brain barrier. The effects of noxious stimuli such as ICU noise, positioning, and suctioning are blunted. The total muscle relaxation and immobilization reduces cerebral venous pressure. Both blood pressure and ICP become less labile.

Before the administration of barbiturates, the following must be provided for the patient: a secure airway with mechanical ventilation; ICP, blood pressure, cardiac, and pulmonary artery monitoring; and continuous EEG monitoring. An EEG is obtained before administration of a barbiturate so that spontaneous electrocortical activity is documented. The EEG pattern of burst suppression is the most common method to establish barbiturate dosing. The loading dose of phenobarbital is 5 to 10 mg/kg over 30 minutes followed by a maintenance dose of 1 mg/kg/hour until EEG burst suppression is achieved. The initial dose may be supplemented with 200 mg IV for burst suppression. Barbiturates are metabolized in the liver and excreted in the kidneys; therefore, liver or kidney function affects serum barbiturate levels. Barbiturate serum levels alone are poor guides to measure therapeutic efficacy and systemic toxicity.

The patient in a barbiturate coma is totally dependent on the critical care nurse to maintain his or her safety. Clinical neurological evaluation is impossible, making extensive accurate monitoring of physiological responses to therapy mandatory. The critical care team must manage artificial ventilation; all vital functions must be provided for the patient. Hypotension secondary to vasodilation is frequently experienced, and a reduction in cardiac output may occur. Vasopressor agents such as dopamine or norepinephrine (Levophed) should be available when barbiturates are administered. Potential complications include deep venous thrombosis (DVT), pulmonary emboli, pneumonia, and infections.

Barbiturates should be discontinued with any of the following clinical findings:

- ICP less than 15 mm Hg for 24 to 72 hours
- Systolic blood pressure less than 90 mm Hg despite the use of vasopressors
- Progressive neurological impairment, as evidenced by deterioration of brainstem auditory evoked responses
- Cardiac arrest

At the time of discontinuation, the barbiturate is tapered gradually over 24 to 72 hours. Arousal is gradual and prolonged, even after blood levels have been zero for several days. The patient must be weaned slowly and carefully from mechanical ventilation, monitoring for residual muscle weakness that occurs with barbiturate therapy. Patients may experience facial weakness for several days after the barbiturate has been discontinued. Occasionally the patient may experience dysarthria, related to weakness of the muscles of speech. During the first 24 hours of barbiturate withdrawal, slow, abnormal muscle movements may be observed.

ANTIHYPERTENSIVE THERAPY

The regulation of blood pressure is an important aspect of managing the patient with increased ICP. Pharmacological management of increased ICP includes the aggressive administration of antihypertensives to manipulate systolic and mean arterial blood pressures to maintain adequate CPP.

Blood pressure is directly related to cerebral blood volume, perfusion pressure, ischemia, and compliance. The brain determines blood flow based on its metabolic needs at rest and in stress states. Under stress, the caloric needs of the injured brain may increase more than 100%, and CBF must increase to match its metabolic demand, or cerebral tissue death occurs. Because autoregulation is often impaired in the injured brain, the patient with ischemic or traumatic injury may require antihypertensive therapy to treat life-threatening hypertension and protect the brain from secondary injury.

For brain-injured patients, the preservation of CPP and maintenance of systemic oxygen availability are two important goals. Most head-injured patients have increased metabolic oxygen consumption, mild hypertension, and increased cardiac indices. Brain-injured patients are at risk for secondary injury caused by hypotension and hypoxia. Invasive blood pressure monitoring is routinely used to provide continuous and accurate blood pressure measurements during the acute management phase of a head-injured patient. MAP is calculated and helpful both for evaluating CPP and measuring the efficacy of antihypertensive therapy.

The brain-injured patient must also be monitored continuously for any adverse effect from drug therapies. In addition to the MAP, the cardiac output is monitored in the acute management of a head-injured patient. Cardiac output is one of the most important parameters that must be measured in a critically ill patient. Drug therapies to manage blood pressure may cause a precipitous increase or decrease in cardiac output. A low cardiac output places the head-injured patient in jeopardy of further ischemic injury. When the cardiac output is too high, excess myocardial work may lead to myocardial injury. The cardiac output is individualized to a patient's weight, creating the cardiac index. Cardiac index is usually maintained at 3 L/minute/m^2 because the brain-injured patient frequently has increased metabolic needs. The systemic vascular resistance (SVR) is used clinically to assess arterial perfusion. An increased SVR may indicate profound arterial vasoconstriction, which may impede blood flow through arterial vessels. A low SVR may indicate vasodilation, leading to stasis of the blood. In this case, low blood flow may occur to vital organs. Several classes of cardiac medications affect the SVR. In head-injured patients, pulmonary artery capillary wedge pressure is usually maintained at 12 to 15 mm Hg. In addition, noninvasive continuous pulse oximetry and arterial blood gas measurement are used to determine arterial oxygen content.

Different classes of antihypertensive medications can be used to treat systemic hypertension in the critically ill patient.[13] An agent that will not cause acute hypotension must be carefully chosen. A patient with a head injury may also experience myocardial ischemia and be at risk for developing a myocardial infarction and rapid supraventricular dysrhythmias. The danger exists that if a dysrhythmia is not managed aggressively, hypotension may develop. Antidysrhythmics can be safely used in head-injured patients. As with any medication, the patient must be assessed for the development of adverse effects associated with cardiovascular medications, including bradycardia, hypotension, myocardial ischemia, tachycardia, and decreased cardiac output.

Angiotensin-converting enzyme (ACE) inhibitors and beta blockers are often used to treat hypertension in the head-injured patient with systemic hypertension. Beta blockers are most often used because of their safe side effect profile, although they may cause bradycardia. Calcium channel blockers are usually avoided in head-injured patients because of their potential to exacerbate cerebral edema. Table 34-4 lists major classes of pharmacological agents used to treat neurological emergencies.

Acute hypertension is defined as a systolic blood pressure greater than 185 mm Hg and a diastolic blood pressure greater then 110 mm Hg. The blood pressure must be gently decreased to avoid problems with cerebral autoregulation dysfunction. In the emergency department or ICU, hydralazine and labetalol are frequently used to treat acute hypertension. Both agents must be administered slowly to avoid hypotension. If the patient remains hypertensive after hydralazine or labetalol administration, nitroprusside may be used. Nitroprusside is a potent vasodilator and can lower the blood pressure quickly. It is administered as a continuous infusion, is easily titrated, and has a relatively short half-life. Nitroprusside must be used in the ICU or emergency department, where continuous blood pressure monitoring can be provided. Hypotension may occur if the infusion is increased too quickly.

DECOMPRESSIVE CRANIECTOMY

Another strategy under investigation for the management of refractory intracranial hypertension is decompressive craniotomy. This therapy is based on the concept that ICP can be reduced through surgical release of the rigid skull. Although promising, studies of adult and pediatric patients are equivocal at this time in terms of patient outcome. Further studies are in progress to evaluate the risks and benefits of craniectomy for patients with head injury and large-territory cortical infarction. Evaluation of long-term morbidity and mortality as well as the best timing of this procedure continues.[14–16]

Nursing Management

Nursing care activity can compound primary and secondary intracranial insults, contributing to rapid deterioration in the unstable patient who has lost intracranial compliance, autoregulation, and vasomotor tone.[17] Patient positioning, emotional state, pain status, hemodynamic as well as respiratory status, and seizure activity can all contribute to a patient's ICP. The following sections describe a few patient management strategies for the reduction of ICP (Table 34-5).

POSITIONING

Primary positioning strategies for the patient with impending or increased ICP include placement of the head and neck in a neutral position. Extreme neck flexion, extension, or rotation restricts venous drainage from the head through the internal jugular venous system and the vertebral venous plexus, increasing the total intracranial content. Decerebrate or decorticate posturing may also increase ICP.

Head of bed elevation has been shown to promote venous drainage and decrease ICP. The head is elevated 15 to 30 degrees, unless contraindicated by spine or limb fractures.

Tracheostomy ties and cervical collars should be frequently checked for proper fit. Flexion of the hips greater than 90 degrees should be avoided because it contributes to both intra-abdominal and thoracic pressures (also impairing venous outflow).

ENVIRONMENTAL CONSIDERATIONS

Environmental stimuli contributing to pain, stress, or anxiety can increase cerebral metabolic rates and blood flow, confounding the management of increased ICP. Pain control and sedation are essential to reduce environmental overload, with consideration for the need for serial neurological assessments in the critically ill patient. ICU anxiety and discomfort cannot be underestimated and should be considered in the patient who is neurologically impaired. Periods of uninterrupted sleep and rest should be provided between activities. Only essential interventions should be performed during times of poor intracranial compliance, and activities should be spaced to avoid a cumulative effect. Also, avoiding unnecessary painful procedures, such as frequent blood draws, is helpful. Methods for decreasing restless movements for the anxious patient should also be incorporated.

NEUROMUSCULAR BLOCKADE

Neuromuscular blockading (NMB) agents are used to induce muscle paralysis to treat severe acute lung injury in the brain-injured patient. An NMB agent blocks the transmission of acetylcholine at the motor end plate, producing skeletal muscle paralysis. Reversal of NMB agents is provided by acetylcholinesterase inhibitors such as neostigmine, edrophonium, and pyridostigmine. The use of an NMB agent requires mechanical ventilation with full support. Resuscitation equipment must be present at all times when a patient is treated with an NMB agent. For a conscious patient, the inability to move and communicate is frightening; therefore, concurrent administration of analgesia and sedation is mandatory.[18] Analgesia and sedation provide the added benefit of producing amnesia.

Complications common with most NMB agents are tachycardia, hypotension, and dysrhythmias. Cardiac medications such as antidysrhythmics, diuretics, and calcium channel and beta blockers can potentiate the action of NMB drugs. Certain antibiotics such as aminoglycosides and clindamycin can potentiate the action of paralytic agents. Alterations in body temperature or acid–base balance and electrolyte disturbances also alter the action of NMB agents.

A troubling complication of paralytic therapy is prolonged polymyopathy. Weakness of skeletal muscles can

(text continues on page 792)

table 34-4 Major Classes of Pharmacological Agents Used to Treat Neurological Emergencies

Class	Medication	Mechanism of Action	Comments
Direct vasodilators	Sodium nitroprusside Nitroglycerin Hydralazine	Directly dilate the peripheral vasculature and lower vascular resistance Sodium nitroprusside: start at 0.3 μg/kg/min, maximum continuous IV infusion 10 μg/kg/min Nitroglycerin: start at 5 μg/min, then titrate as needed upward q 5 min (max 100 μg/min) Hydralazine: 10–20 mg IV, may be repeated as needed	• Dilate the cerebral vasculature • Increase cerebral blood volume and ICP, decrease MAP and CPP • Sodium nitroprusside: at high doses may cause cyanide toxicity, check thiocyanate levels, protect infusion from light • Nitroglycerin: venous dilation, caution with high doses; may cause hypotension • Hydralazine: used in hypertensive emergency, may cause hypotension and headache
Beta-adrenergic antagonists	Metoprolol Esmolol	Beta-adrenergic receptor antagonist Metoprolol: 5 mg IV q 3–5 min × 3 doses, followed by PO administration 25–50 mg PO bid and may increase to 50–100 mg PO bid Esmolol: for hypertensive emergency, bolus dose 500 μg/kg over 1 min, then 50–200 μg/kg/min	• Do not affect CBF • Use with caution with Cushing's response, can potentiate bradycardia
Mixed alpha- and beta-adrenergic antagonists	Labetalol	Selective alpha- and nonselective beta-adrenergic receptor antagonist Labetalol: for hypertensive emergency, start 20 mg IV over 3–5 min, followed by 40–80 mg IV every 10 min PRN up to 300 mg, or IV infusion 0.5–2 mg/min	• Reduce SVR • Improve CPP and do not increase ICP • May slow heart rate
Calcium channel antagonists	Verapamil Diltiazem	Prevent transport of calcium ions in vascular smooth muscle, resulting in vasodilation, decreased myocardial contractility, decreased heart rate Verapamil: for supraventricular tachycardia, 5–10 mg IV over 2 min, followed by 40–80 mg tid–qid Diltiazem: 20 mg over 2 min, continuous infusion 5–15 mg/h	• Use with caution, may cause cerebral vasodilation with increased ICP • Contraindicated in patients with tumors and cerebral edema
Angiotensin-converting enzyme (ACE) inhibitors	Lisinopril	Shift the upper and lower limits of blood brain autoregulation by inhibiting angiotensin II–mediated vascular tone in large cerebral arteries, while small vessels vasoconstrict Lisinopril: start 10 mg/d, titrate to 80 mg/d PRN	• Preserve CBF after single dose • Increase CBF with chronic treatment • Have the potential to increase ICP in patients with intracranial hypertension by increasing CBF
Osmotic diuretic	Mannitol	Indicated for intracranial hypertension Mannitol: 0.25–2 g/kg IV over 30–60 min	• If infused too quickly, may contribute to renal insufficiency
Loop diuretic	Furosemide	Indicated for pulmonary edema and adjunct therapy for hypertension Furosemide: 20–80 mg IV, increase dose 20–40 mg IV q6–8h until desired effect	• May cause potassium loss; check electrolytes q8–12h with initial therapy
Nondepolarizing muscle blockading agents	Pancuronium	Skeletal muscle paralysis Bolus 0.04–0.1 mg/kg Continuous infusion	• May cause tachycardia and dysrhythmias • Patient must be mechanically ventilated
	Atracurium	Skeletal muscle paralysis Bolus 0.4–0.5 mg/kg IV Continuous infusion 4–12 μg/kg/min IV	• Rare occurrence of prolonged weakness after discontinuation of drug infusion • Patient must be mechanically ventilated • Use in patients with hepatic and renal impairment

(continued)

table 34-4 Major Classes of Pharmacological Agents Used to Treat Neurological Emergencies (Continued)

Class	Medication	Mechanism of Action	Comments
	Cisatracurium	Skeletal muscle paralysis Bolus 0.1–0.2 mg/kg Continuous infusion 2.5–3 μg/kg/min IV	• Rare incidence of prolonged weakness after continuous IV infusion • Patient must be mechanically ventilated • Use in patients with hepatic and renal impairment
Sedatives	Diazepam Lorazepam Midazolam	Benzodiazepines are sedatives and hypnotics that induce anterograde amnesia Diazepam and lorazepam are also used to stop seizure activity Diazepam: 10–20 mg IV no faster than 2 mg/min, then repeat q4h Lorazepam: 0.05–0.2 mg/kg/dose, up to 8 mg, may repeat every 15 min, continuous infusion 1 mg/hr and titrate to goal, not to exceed 8 mg/h Midazolam: 0.1–0.3 mg/kg bolus, no faster than 4 mg/min, continuous infusion 0.05 mg/kg/h up to 1.0 mg/kg/h	• May cause somnolence, hypotension, delirium, hallucinations, respiratory depression • Titrate to goal using sedation scale • Lorazepam/midazolam: use with caution in patients with hepatic/renal failure, contraindicated in patients with acute narrow-angle glaucoma or in shock, and in older patients
Anticonvulsants	Phenytoin Carbamazepine	Indicated for tonic-clonic seizures and partial seizures Phenytoin: loading dose 15–20 mg/kg for status epilepticus, no faster than 50 mg/kg; maintenance dose 200–500 mg qd or in divided doses tid Carbamazepine: 200 mg bid, maintenance 200–400 tid	• May cause ataxia, lethargy, movement disorders, rash, coarse facies, lymphadenopathy • May decrease theophylline, oral contraceptive, and warfarin levels • Phenytoin levels may increase with methsuximide and alcohol • Phenytoin levels may decrease when used with valproic acid and tegretol • Contraindicated with alcohol ingestion, sinus bradycardia, heart block
Analgesics	Morphine Fentanyl Hydromorphone	Opiate analgesics blunt the pain response by interfering with central and peripheral pain pathways Morphine: bolus 1–4 mg Continuous infusion 0.07–0.5 mg/kg/h Fentanyl: bolus 50–100 μg over 1–2 min, continuous infusion 0.7–10 μg/kg/h Hydromorphone: continuous infusion 7–15 μg/kg/h	• May cause respiratory depression; must have naloxone readily available • Have resuscitation equipment nearby at all times • Use the lowest dose that provides adequate pain relief • Use a 1–10 pain scale to assess effectiveness of pain relief • For severe pain, around-the-clock administration or a continuous infusion of pain medication provides more efficient pain relief than PRN dosing • Use lower doses in older patients • Use nonpharmacological approaches to pain management • Side effects: decrease gastric motility, nausea/vomiting, tremulousness
Anesthetic	Propofol	Propofol is an intravenous general anesthetic agent that can be used to treat agitation in the ICU Propofol: bolus not necessary, continuous infusion 5–50 μg/kg/min	• Patient must be mechanically ventilated • Must have dedicated IV line • Must use aseptic technique • May cause hypotension • Must provide analgesics and sedation • Use for the shortest period possible
Barbiturates	Phenobarbital Pentobarbital	Used to produce CNS depression and reduce the spread of an epileptic focus Phenobarbital: loading dose 6–8 mg/kg IV; maintenance dose 1–3 mg/kg/24 h IV Pentobarbital: loading dose 3–10 mg/kg over 30 min; maintenance dose 0.5–3.0 mg/kg/h	• May cause respiratory depression and cardiac depression • Patient must be mechanically ventilated • Continuous EEG monitoring for barbiturate-induced coma

table 34-5 Nursing Considerations for Patients at Risk for Increased Intracranial Pressure

Problem	Nursing Action	Rationale
Adequate ventilation	• Assess respiratory patterns and rate	• Indicates neurological changes, pain status, and patency of airway
	• Suctioning: Preoxygenate with 100% O_2, one or two catheter passes, no more than 10 sec per catheter insertion	• Prevents increased CO_2 (vasodilator that increases ICP); decreases coughing stimulation and increased intrathoracic pressure
	• Monitor continuous pulse oximetry and blood gases	• Alerts nurse to airway problems; good indicator of hemodynamics of respiration
Neurological assessment	• Evaluate patient baseline neurological status at beginning of shift (preferably with previous shift RN)—mental status, pupil shape, size, and response, motor function	• Subtle changes from baseline indicate deterioration and the need for early intervention
	• Assess vital signs—note trends (review ordered parameters for notification of physician)	• Mean arterial pressure directly correlates with ICP in patient with loss of autoregulation
	• Review nursing actions and emergency algorithm for neurologic deterioration (available medications—mannitol, hyperventilation, etc)	• Ensures optimal benefit to patient and decreases secondary injury from prolonged ICP
Positioning	• Place head of bed flat or at 30 degrees elevation per orders	• Promotes cerebral perfusion or facilitates venous drainage; orders based on physiological process
	• Maintain head in neutral position	• Promotes jugular outflow
	• Avoid hip flexion	• Decreases intrathoracic pressure
	• Assess agitation in restrained patients	• Increases ICP
	• Turn patient q2h, instructing patient to exhale with turn	• Prevents skin breakdown and avoids Valsalva maneuver during repositioning
	• Carry out passive range-of-motion exercises	• Prevents contractures while avoiding Valsalva-inducing isometric contractions
	• Avoid clustering of patient activities (e.g., turning, bathing, suctioning)	• Produces prolonged ICP spikes
	• Use therapeutic interventions for emotional upset—speak with soft voice, use caution with unpleasant conversations, decrease noxious stimuli (noise), use therapeutic touch	• Causes elevations in ICP; comatose patients still respond to unpleasant environmental stimuli
Transport of patient with invasive ICP monitor	• Confirm time of test or possibility of completing as portable study	• Avoids excessive delays in uncontrolled and potentially overstimulating environment
	• Prepare respiratory therapy and other assistants during transport	• Adequate oxygenation remains a priority; multiple lines necessitate additional manpower
	• Gather transport supplies (sedation if ordered, transport monitor, antihypertensives)	• Prepare for intervention with any adverse patient response during travel specific to contributors of increased ICP
	• Assist with transfer of patient to diagnostic table with RN at head of bed monitoring device	• Ensures patient protection and provides for monitor equipment recalibration for accuracy of monitoring
	• Monitor and record hemodynamics and ICP dynamics during study	• Monitors patient response to procedure
Temperature control	• Frequent temperature checks (oral or rectal preferred if no contraindications)	• Cerebral metabolic rate increases with elevated body temperature
	• Confirm orders for early treatment of fever and aggressively treat	• Increased CBF increases ICP
	• Provide gradual cooling with cooling blanket, closely monitored	• Shivering increases ICP
Glycemic control	• Monitor serum glucose and fingersticks as ordered (q4–6h)—adhere closely to sliding scale protocols in nondiabetic patients	• Alterations in glucose can produce neurological changes (i.e., changes in metabolic rate)
	• Maintain euvolemia with normal saline	• Hypotonic glucose intravenous solutions should be avoided

(continued)

table 34-5 Nursing Considerations for Patients at Risk for Increased Intracranial Pressure

Problem	Nursing Action	Rationale
Bowel and bladder regimens	• Administer daily stool softeners as ordered	• Reduces risk for straining and increased intra-abdominal pressure, which increases ICP
	• Avoid enemas	• Prevents Valsalva maneuver
	• Assess patency of Foley catheters	• Important to monitor amount of diuresis, especially in patients treated with osmotic diuretics
	• Document strict intake and output	• Important to maintain euvolemia
Seizure precautions	• Seizure precautions per hospital protocol (padding, etc.)	• Prevents injury in high-risk patients
	• Monitor serum anticonvulsant drug levels	• Maintains therapeutic levels

occur with prolonged NMB. A condition known as acute quadriplegic myopathy syndrome (AQMS), or postparalytic quadriparesis, is one of the most devastating complications caused by prolonged use of an NMB agent.[18] This condition is manifested by prolonged weakness of the upper and lower extremities. The extraocular motor muscles are usually spared in this condition, so patients with AQMS can move their eyes. A patient may also experience painful muscle fibrillations. For this reason, the smallest dosage of an NMB agent should be used to obtain adequate respiratory support.

Clinical research has not provided sufficient information to recommend a standard NMB agent. A consensus of critical care experts has produced several recommendations, though.[18] For patients requiring skeletal paralysis to facilitate adequate mechanical ventilation, pancuronium is recommended. Pancuronium can induce adequate paralysis in 2 to 3 minutes. However, another NMB agent should be chosen for patients with a cardiovascular history because tachycardia is a side effect of pancuronium. For patients with hepatic or renal disease, cisatracurium or atracurium is recommended. Cisatracurium and atracurium have a lower threshold for causing cardiovascular side effects. Atracurium is recommended for use in a critically ill patient with multiple organ dysfunction syndrome and brain injury.[18]

Peripheral nerve stimulation monitoring is mandatory with NMB therapy.[18] A peripheral nerve stimulator is a small hand-held device used in the ICU to monitor the depth of NMB in the patient receiving prolonged paralytic therapy. This device delivers a small jolt of energy to the ulnar surface of the wrist, causing the thumb to twitch. The train-of-four method is used to measure the efficacy and depth of NMB. The peripheral nerve stimulator delivers four 2-Hz stimuli of 0.2 millisecond delivered at intervals of 0.5 second to the ulnar nerve at the wrist. Normally, the thumb twitches four times when the peripheral nerve stimulator is activated. The nurse observes thumb movements after peripheral nerve stimulation. If the thumb twitches two or three times, NMB dosing is usually sufficient. If four thumb twitches occur, paralysis is ineffective. If no twitches occur, paralysis is excessive and the dose of the NMB agent must be reduced. The use of peripheral nerve stimulation monitoring every 4 hours, with a dosage change as necessary, may help prevent complications associated with NMB therapy.

Excellent nursing care also can help prevent some of the complications caused by NMB agents. A rigid turning schedule must be maintained to prevent the development of pressure ulcers. Aspiration precautions must be maintained at all times. Also, DVT prophylaxis must be implemented before induction of paralysis.

Seizure Prophylaxis

Seizure activity markedly elevates the cerebral metabolic rate and CBF. It can lead to hypoxia and hypercapnia. In a patient with increased ICP, seizure prophylaxis should be considered to prevent additional neurological injury.

Anticonvulsant therapy may be used to prevent early post-traumatic seizure, especially in patients at risk for seizure (Box 34-2). Phenytoin and carbamazepine are good options for prevention of early (less than 7 days) post-traumatic seizure.

The treatment of choice for acute-onset seizures (such as tonic-clonic seizures) in the critically ill patient is diazepam. Initially, the nurse may administer diazepam 5 to 10 mg IV over 2 to 3 minutes and repeat 5 mg IV every 5 minutes for a total of four doses. The patient should be placed on his or her side and an oxygen mask applied. When seizure activity has subsided, the nurse should obtain a serum glucose to determine if hypoglycemia is a contributing cause. An EEG may also be ordered to determine if the patient is continuing to experience subclinical seizure and to determine seizure focus.

box 34-2 ***Patients at Increased Risk for a Post-Traumatic Seizure***

Patients with:

- GCS score <10
- Subdural hematoma
- Cortical contusion
- Epidural hematoma
- Depressed skull fracture
- Intracerebral hematoma
- Penetrating head wounds
- Seizure within 24 hours of injury

case study ■ ACUTE HEAD TRAUMA

Mr. Jenkins, a 28-year-old man, was involved in a motor vehicle accident (MVA). The patient was in good health when his car sustained a driver-side impact and rolled over into a ditch. Air bags were deployed. The emergency medical team needed 15 minutes to extricate Mr. Jenkins from his car. A preliminary examination at the scene showed loss of consciousness, a GCS score of 10, and a respiratory rate of 8 breaths/minute, with a pulse oximetry reading of 89%. Cervical traction was applied. The patient was intubated and required full airway support. The patient was immediately stabilized using Advanced Cardiac Life Support (ACLS) principles and transported by helicopter to a trauma center. Rapid CT scans of the patient's head, chest, and abdomen were obtained. Laboratory specimens and blood were sent for type and cross-match.

A history was obtained from the patient's wife:

- Current medications: None.
- Medical history: Unremarkable.
- Surgical history: Appendectomy, age 21 years.
- Social history: Lives with wife, no children. Employed full time as a computer analyst. Denies smoking, alcohol, and recreational drug use history. Has not traveled outside the United States in the last 12 months.
- Family history: Mother age 60 years with hypertension, father age 62 years with diabetes, one brother and two sisters, all healthy.
- Admission diagnostics: Head CT scan negative: no hemorrhage, no early ischemic changes, no signs of midline shift or mass effect. Chest and abdomen CT scans: unremarkable.
- Laboratory values: Following laboratory values within normal limits: comprehensive metabolic panel including electrolyte panel and liver function tests; coagulation parameters: prothrombin time (PT), partial thromboplastin time (PTT), international normalized ratio (INR); white blood cell (WBC) count and platelets. Complete blood count (CBC) reveals hemoglobin 8.0 g/100 mL (normal 13 to 18 g/100 mL) and hematocrit 28% (normal, 42% to 52%).
- Review of systems: Patient unable to respond and unremarkable.
- Physical examination:

General: Well-nourished male, eyes closed. Vital signs: blood pressure 188/66 mm Hg; heart rate 45 beats/minute; respiratory rate supported by mechanical ventilation at 16 breaths/minute; pulse oximetry 93%.

Head, eyes, ears, nose, throat (HEENT): Head with multiple lacerations, right temporal contusion, orbits edematous with raccoon's eyes, no obvious skull depression, no obvious neck injuries, cervical collar in place.

Lungs: Bilateral chest expansion, coarse rhonchi throughout.

Cardiovascular: Heart sounds S_1 and S_2, no murmurs or palpitations, +1 thready peripheral pulses, no peripheral edema or jugular venous congestion.

Gastrointestinal: No bowel sounds, abdomen distended.

Genitourinary: Nondistended.

Skin: Diaphoretic, ecchymosis throughout body, multiple lacerations.

Musculoskeletal: Obvious right femur fracture.

Neurological examination: Patient obtunded, no response to commands, no verbal output, no spontaneous motor output.

Cranial nerves: Pupils symmetric and responsive to light, fixed oculomotor movements, facial symmetry, tongue appears midline, no gag or cough.

Motor examination: Moves all extremities only with profound noxious stimuli.

Sensory/coordination/gait examinations: Unable to assess.

Clinical impression: Patient is 28-year-old male, status post MVA with multiple fractures and acute head injury. The patient's femur fracture required immediate surgical repair. The patient was admitted to the ICU for critical care management.

- Problem list: Traumatic brain injury, acute lung injury, femur fracture.

The patient was admitted to the ICU immediately after surgical repair of his femur. Every hour, the ICU nurse checked his vital signs and performed a neurological assessment, including level of consciousness, motor activity, and pupillary status. He received two units of packed red blood cells during surgery for low hemoglobin and hematocrit. The patient remained mechanically intubated, and a chest x-ray revealed minimal interstitial markings indicating aspiration pneumonia. His pain was managed with a continuous infusion of morphine 2 mg/hour.

On day 2, the patient started to respond to verbal stimuli and followed simple commands to show two fingers bilaterally. He still required mechanical ventilation because of heavy sedation; respirations were synchronous with the ventilator. Lorazepam 1 mg/hour was started. A sedation score was used to assess the patient's response to sedation; he appeared to be sleeping and comfortable but easily arousable.

On day 3, during a routine neurological assessment, the nurse discovered that the patient's left pupil was fixed and dilated; there was no spontaneous motor movement, and no response to central or peripheral noxious stimuli. The nurse immediately contacted the house officer and prepared the patient for transport for a stat brain CT scan. The CT scan revealed a left temporal hemorrhage with 4-mm midline shift and mild edema. A neurosurgical consultation was immediately obtained. An intraventricular device was inserted to monitor ICP, and the patient was taken to the operating room for immediate decompressive surgery. Initial mean ICP was 43 mm Hg.

During surgery, the patient received several therapies to reduce ICP, including mannitol infusion and mild hyperventilation. In the recovery area, the nurse titrated mannitol administration based on serial serum osmolarities (every 6 hours). The patient's ICP on return to the unit was 12 mm Hg. Postsurgical orders included monitoring of MAP, CPP, and ICP hourly, head of bed at 30 degrees, and strict intake and output (I/O) monitoring. Nitroprusside, which was started in the operating room for refractory hypertension, was continued with orders to keep the systolic blood pressure less than 160 mm Hg.

On day 4, the patient continued to experience transient episodes of increased ICP that responded to conservative measures, including:

- Maintaining his neck in a neutral position
- Providing adequate pain relief
- Spacing nursing interventions to avoid agitation
- Minimizing loud conversation and informing the patient before any uncomfortable procedures
- Minimizing cough

His blood pressure remained 140/70 mm Hg and the nitroprusside infusion was discontinued. The patient required IV hydralazine as needed to maintain a systolic blood pressure of less than 160 mm Hg and a diastolic blood pressure of less than 90 mm Hg.

During the evening shift on day 4, the patient experienced a 2-minute episode of tonic-clonic seizure activity. He responded to urgent dosing of diazepam 5 mg. A repeat dose of 5 mg was needed after 5 minutes when the patient continued to show generalized seizure activity. After a second dosing of diazepam, seizure activity stopped. The patient was given a loading dose of phenytoin with an order written for phenytoin 250 mg twice daily. An EEG was obtained, which revealed no subclinical seizure activity. The patient remained agitated in the postictal state. A repeat head CT scan was obtained, which showed no new hemorrhage or shift. ICP was 35 mm Hg and persisted, despite aggressive management with mannitol, drainage of CSF, analgesics, and sedation. Propofol infusion was initiated and mechanical ventilation continued. Mannitol infusion was titrated to serum osmolarity every 8 hours. His ICP gradually decreased to 12 mm Hg. Mannitol was gradually weaned.

On day 5, the patient continued with an elevated ICP of 25 mm Hg. An arterial blood gas (ABG) test showed severe hypoxia and hypercarbia attributed to severe acute lung injury. A nondepolarizing NMB agent was used to assist ventilatory synchronization. The patient was started on a continuous infusion of cisatracurium. Lorazepam and fentanyl infusions were initiated simultaneously for continued sedation and analgesia. Propofol was discontinued. The nurse tested the train-of-four every 4 hours and with every dose change, targeting one of four twitches as indicating the dose of cisatracurium required to prevent complications of prolonged NMB.

On day 6, the patient's ICP was continuously 10 mm Hg and below. Mannitol was no longer indicated. Acute lung injury was improving, as evidenced by chest x-ray and ABGs. The NMB agent was titrated to off. After discontinuation, there was no evidence of prolonged generalized weakness or polymyopathy. The patient still required sedation and analgesia, but was responsive to noxious stimuli.

On day 7, the patient's ICP remained below 10 mm Hg. A CT scan of his brain revealed no further hemorrhage or mass effect. The IVC device was removed.

The patient slowly regained alertness and function after multisystem trauma and secondary brain injury, including intracranial hemorrhage and hypoxia. The patient required prolonged ventilation due to lung injury, but was successfully weaned from the ventilator. As the patient recovered, his need for sedation and analgesia decreased. The patient remained on anticonvulsant therapy throughout the rehabilitation phase. He required acute and long-term rehabilitation, including speech, occupational, and physical therapy. The patient will require vocational retraining to determine and optimize his abilities. ■

clinical applicability challenges

Self-Challenge: Critical Thinking

1. *Identify three pathophysiological problems leading to increased ICP.*
2. *Discuss the pharmacological and nonpharmacological interventions for the management of increased ICP.*

Study Questions

1. *Monitoring of ICP may be indicated for which of the following conditions?*
   a. *Abnormal brain CT scan*
   b. *Inability to obey commands or utter recognizable words despite cardiopulmonary stabilization*
   c. *A Glasgow Coma Scale score of less than 8*
   d. *All of the above*
2. *Interventions to decrease increased ICP include all of the following except*
   a. *mannitol.*
   b. *hypoventilation.*
   c. *morphine as needed.*
   d. *maintaining the head in a neutral neck position.*
3. *Nondepolarizing neuromuscular blockading (NMB) agents are used as last-effort therapy for managing mechanical ventilation and increased ICP. Which one of the following statements regarding the use of NMB agents is not true?*
   a. *The patient must be mechanically ventilated.*
   b. *The patient requires adjunctive analgesia therapy.*
   c. *The patient should not receive sedation with NMB agents.*
   d. *Depth of neuromuscular blockade is measured using a peripheral nerve stimulator.*
4. *Principles of opiate administration for pain management for the patient who experiences a neurological emergency include all of the following except*
   a. *opiate analgesics cannot be administered to a head-injured patient because frequent neurological examinations will not be possible.*
   b. *a visual or verbal pain score should be used to assess pain.*
   c. *as-needed dosing of an opiate analgesic provides more effective pain relief than a continuous infusion of an analgesic agent.*
   d. *the lowest dose possible of an opiate analgesic should be administered to provide adequate pain relief.*

REFERENCES

1. March K: Intracranial pressure monitoring and assessing intracranial compliance in brain injury. Crit Care Nurs Clin North Am 12(4):429–436, 2000
2. Ter Minassian A, Dube L, Guilleux AM, et al: Changes in intracranial pressure and cerebral autoregulation in patients with severe traumatic brain injury. Crit Care Med 30(7):1616–1622, 2002

3. Ghajar J: Intracranial pressure monitoring techniques. New Horiz 3(3):395–399, 1995
4. Brain Trauma Foundation, American Association of Neurological Surgeons, Joint Section on Neurotrauma and Critical Care: Guidelines for the management of severe traumatic brain injury. J Neurotrauma 17(6/7):449–554, 2000
5. Kapadia F, Rodriguez C, Jha AN: A simple technique to limit ICP catheter infection. Br J Neurosurg 11:335–336, 1997
6. Adelson PD, Bratton S, Carney N, et al: Guidelines for the acute medical management of severe traumatic brain injury in infants, children, and adolescents: Use of hyperosmolar therapy in the management of severe pediatric traumatic brain injury. Pediatr Crit Care Med 4:S40–S44, 2003
7. Roberts I, Schierhout G, Wakai A: Mannitol for acute traumatic brain injury. Cochrane Database 2:CD001049, 2003
8. Vialet R, Albanese J, Thomachot L, et al: Isovolume hypertonic solutes in the treatment of refractory posttraumatic intracranial hypertension. Crit Care Med 31(6):1683–1687, 2003
9. Cruz J: Low clinical ischemic threshold for cerebral blood flow in severe acute brain trauma. J Neurosurg 80:143–147, 1994
10. Jacobi J, Fraser G, Coursin D: Clinical practice guidelines for the sustained use of sedatives and analgesics in the critically ill adult. Crit Care Med 30(1):119–141, 2002
11. Wagner BK, O'Hara DA: Pharmacokinetics and pharmacodynamics of sedatives and analgesics in the treatment of agitated critically ill patients. Clin Pharmacokinet 33(6):426–453, 1977
12. Harris OA, Colford JM, Good MC, et al: The role of hypothermia in the management of severe brain injury: A meta-analysis. Arch Neurol 59(7):1077–1083, 2002
13. Joint National Committee on Prevention, Detection, and Evaluation and Treatment of High Blood Pressure: The Sixth Report of the Joint National Committee on Prevention, Detection, and Evaluation and Treatment of High Blood Pressure. Arch Intern Med 157(21):2413–2446, 1997
14. Albanese J, Leone M, Alliez J, et al: Decompressive craniectomy for severe traumatic brain injury: Evaluation of the effects at one year. Crit Care Med 31(10):2535–2538, 2003
15. Figaji A, Fieggen A, Peter J: Early decompressive craniotomy in children with severe traumatic brain injury. Childs Nerv Syst 19(9):666–673, 2003
16. Jaeger M, Soehle M, Meixensberger J: Effects of decompressive craniectomy in brain tissue oxygen in patients with intracranial hypertension. J Neurol Neurosurg Psychiatry 74(4):513–515, 2003
17. Wong F: Prevention of secondary brain injury. Crit Care Nurse 20:18–27, 2000
18. Murray M, Cowen J, DeBlock H, et al, for the Society of Critical Care Medicine: Clinical practice guidelines for sustained neuromuscular blockade in the adult critically ill patient. Crit Care Med 30(1):142–156, 2002

OTHER SELECTED READING

Arbour R: Aggressive management of intracranial dynamics. Crit Care Nurse 18(3):30–40, 1998

Caplan L: Caplan's Stroke: A Clinical Approach. Boston, Butterworth Heinemann, 2000

Cruz J, Minoja G, Okuchi K: Major clinical and physiological benefits of early high doses of mannitol for intraparenchymal temporal lobe hemorrhages with abnormal papillary widening: A randomized trial. Neurosurgery 51(3):628–637, 2002

Deray M, Resnick T, Alvarez L: Complete Pocket Reference for the Treatment of Epilepsy. Miami, C.P.R. Educational Services, 2001

Dunn LT: Raised intracranial pressure. J Neurol Neurosurg Psychiatry 73:23–27, 2002

Haltiner AM, Newell DW, Temkin NR: Side effects and mortality associated with use of phenytoin for early post-traumatic seizure prophylaxis. J Neurosurg 91:588–592, 1999

Jones PA, Andrews PJ, Midgley S: Measuring the burden of secondary insults in head injured patients during intensive care. J Neurosurg Anesthesiol 6:4–14, 1994

Kidd KC, Criddle L: Using jugular venous catheters in patients with traumatic brain injury. Crit Care Nurse 21(6):17–22, 2001

Kolb S, Litt B: Management of epilepsy and co-morbid disorders in the emergency room and intensive care unit. In Ettinger A, Devinsky O (eds): Managing Epilepsy and Co-Existing Disorders, pp 515–533. Woburn, MA, Butterworth-Heinemann, 2002

Krauss JJ, Metzler MD, Coplin WM: Critical care issues in stroke and subarachnoid hemorrhage. Neurol Res 24:S47–S57, 2002

Mokri B: The Monro-Kellie hypothesis: Applications in CSF volume depletion. Neurology 56:1746–1748, 2001

Robertson CS, Cormio M: Cerebral metabolic management. New Horiz 3(3):410–422, 1995

Sahjpaul R, Girotti M: Intracranial pressure monitoring in severe traumatic brain injury. Can J Neurol Sci 27:143–147, 2000

Schwab S, Steiner T, Aschoff A, et al: Early hemicraniectomy in patients with complete middle cerebral artery infarction. Stroke 29:1888–1893, 1998

Segal S, Gallagher AC, Shefler AG, et al: Survey of the use of intracranial pressure monitoring in children in the United Kingdom. Intensive Care Med 27:236–239, 2001

VanderSchaaf IC, Ruigrok YM, Rinkel GJ, et al: Study design and outcome measures in studies on aneurismal subarachnoid hemorrhage. Stroke 33(8):2043–2046, 2002

Wong F: Prevention of secondary brain injury. Crit Care Nurse 20:18–27, 2000

chapter

35

Common Neurosurgical and Neurological Disorders

BARBARA FITZSIMMONS ■ EILEEN BOHAN*

objectives

Based on the content in this chapter, the reader should be able to:

- Describe a classification system for brain tumors.
- Discuss the surgical management of brain tumors.
- Name the medical and surgical options for the patient with a cerebral aneurysm or arteriovenous malformation.
- Differentiate between partial and generalized seizures.
- Review the current antiepileptic drugs used to manage epilepsy.
- Describe the classification of stroke.
- Discuss the nursing management of a patient who has experienced an acute ischemic stroke.
- Identify the pathophysiological basis of Guillain-Barré syndrome
- Explain the pharmacological management of myasthenia gravis.

During the course of their illness, many patients with neurological diseases require critical care management. Routine neurosurgical procedures usually involve a short intensive care unit (ICU) admission. In addition, complications of the tumor or treatments may necessitate readmission. ICU admission follows the use of thrombolytic therapy for stroke and may be required to treat the patient with stroke and increased intracranial pressure (ICP). Patients with myasthenia gravis or Guillain-Barré syndrome may require an ICU stay for respiratory sequelae of their disease. The nurse clinician is better prepared to manage the acute and chronic needs of this patient population if she or he understands the course of the disease, as well as the medical and surgical tools available for these disorders. This chapter provides an overview of the etiology, signs and symptoms, diagnostic workup, and current management of the neurosurgical and neurological disorders most often encountered in the ICU environment.

*We would like to thank the following people for their advice and support: Drs. Henry Brem, Richard Clatterbuck, Ira Garonzik, Gregory Krauss, Frederick Lenz, Rafael Tamargo, and Robert Wityk, and Pamela Sanders, RN.

NEUROANATOMY

The following discussion is not intended to be a complete overview of neuroanatomy (see Chapter 32 for a complete discussion). Instead, it provides a basic review to understand better the topics presented in this chapter.

Cerebrum

The cerebrum is divided into two hemispheres. The area controlling speech is referred to as the *dominant* hemisphere. The left hemisphere is the control center for speech in right-handed people and more than 75% of left-handed individuals. A band of fibers known as the *corpus callosum* unites the two hemispheres. Each cerebral hemisphere is composed of four lobes: the frontal, parietal, temporal, and occipital. Cerebral lesions usually cause symptoms on the opposite side of the body (contralateral). Table 35-1 summarizes the specific functions of each lobe.[1,2]

Cerebellum

Situated in the posterior fossa of the skull, the cerebellum sits below the occipital lobe and behind the brainstem. It is separated from the brainstem by the fourth ventricle, at the level of the pons. The cerebellum is made up of two hemispheres, separated by the vermis. It contains three peduncles, which connect it to the cerebrum, the brainstem, and the spinal cord.

Lesions in the cerebellum may result in ataxia, causing gait unsteadiness toward the side of the abnormality; difficulty with equilibrium and uncoordinated movements; difficulty with fine voluntary movements; intention tremor; nystagmus; and decreased muscle tone. Lesions of the cerebellar hemispheres produce symptoms to the side of the lesion (ipsilateral). Signs of increased ICP may occur, given the relationship of the cerebellum to the fourth ventricle.

Brainstem

Communication between the brain and the spinal cord takes place in the brainstem. It is composed of the midbrain, pons, and medulla oblongata. Cranial nerves III through XII originate from these structures. In addition to cranial nerve deficits, lesions in the brainstem may cause vomiting and may affect respiratory rate, breathing patterns, and sensory/motor functions.

Ventricles

The ventricular system is composed of two lateral ventricles, surrounded by the cerebral hemispheres; the third ventricle in the diencephalon; and the fourth ventricle, surrounded by the cerebellum, pons, and medulla oblongata. The choroid plexus in the lateral ventricles produces cerebrospinal fluid (CSF), which flows into the third and fourth ventricles, and then into the subarachnoid space. If there is an obstruction of the ventricular system, CSF is unable to circulate, and hydrocephalus develops. Patients with hydrocephalus usually present with urinary incontinence, balance difficulties, and cognitive impairment.[3] Figure 35-1 demonstrates hydrocephalus caused by an intraventricular brain tumor.

Brain Vasculature

Two major sets of vessels supply the brain with blood: the carotid or anterior circulation and the vertebral or posterior circulation. Each system comes off the aortic arch as a pair of vessels: the left and right common carotid arteries and the left and right vertebral arteries. Each carotid bifurcates to form the internal and external carotid artery. The vertebral arteries arise from the subclavian arteries. The vertebrals join to form the basilar artery, which in turn divides to form the two posterior cerebral arteries, which supply the medial and inferior surfaces of the brain and the lateral portions of the temporal and occipital lobes.

The circle of Willis (Fig. 35-2) is the area in which the branches of the basilar and internal carotid arteries unite. The circle of Willis is composed of the two anterior cerebral arteries, the anterior communicating artery, the two posterior cerebral arteries, and the two posterior communicating arteries. This circular network permits blood to circulate from one hemisphere to the other and from the anterior to the posterior areas of the brain. This system allows for collateral circulation if one vessel is occluded. It is not unusual, however, for some vessel in the circle of Willis to be atrophic or even absent. This accounts for different clinical presentations among patients with the same lesion. For example, a person with an occluded carotid artery and a fully patent circle of Willis may be totally asymptomatic, but a patient in whom the circle of Willis is incomplete may demonstrate a massive cerebral infarction.[4]

Neuromuscular Junction

Later in this chapter, myasthenia gravis is discussed. To understand the basis for this disease, it is necessary to have some basic knowledge about the neuromuscular junction. Chapter 32 provides a complete review of neu-

table 35-1 Cerebrum: Function By Location

Lobe	Function	Dominant Hemisphere
Frontal	Contralateral motor skills; personality; behavior; intellect; emotions; urinary/fecal continence; smell	Motor (Broca's area) speech; language-dependent memory
Parietal	Contralateral sensation: position, vibration, touch, temperature; contralateral lower visual fields	Receptive speech and language comprehension; numbers and calculations; left/right discrimination
Temporal	Hearing sounds, music; new memory; behavior; smell; contralateral upper visual fields	Hearing language; receptive (Wernicke's area) speech
Occipital	Perception of vision; contralateral visual fields	—

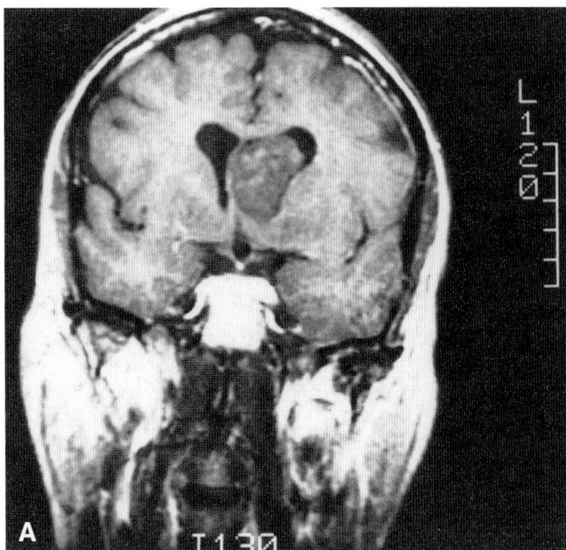

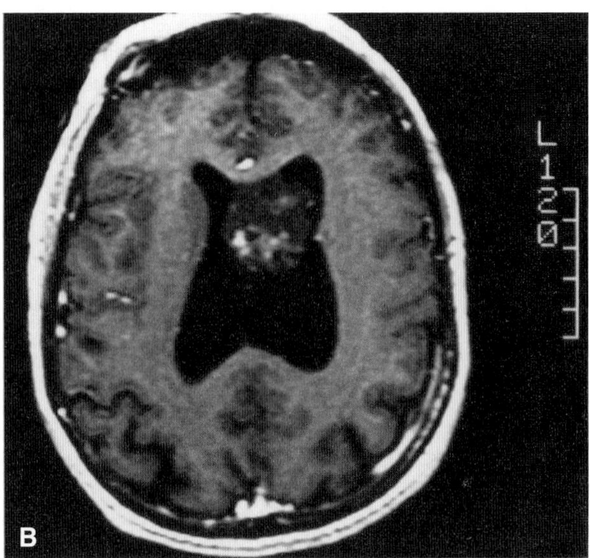

figure 35-1 (**A**) Coronal magnetic resonance imaging (MRI) view of intraventricular subependymoma. (**B**) Axial MRI view of hydrocephalus associated with intraventricular tumor. (Courtesy of Henry Brem, MD, Johns Hopkins University, Baltimore, MD.)

rons, axons, dendrites, and synapses, and the functions all of these perform.

NEUROLOGICAL SURGERY

Surgery is indicated for several neurological disorders. Neurological surgery is a common and integral part of the management of patients with brain tumors, arteriovenous malformations, and aneurysms. Craniotomy is the most common procedure performed for these problems. The following section reviews the etiology and pathophysiology of these conditions, and describes surgical approaches used for the management of these patients.

Brain Tumors

A brain tumor is broadly described as any neoplasm arising within the cranium. Tumors may originate in the brain (primary) or seed in the brain from other organs (metastatic). Pathological examination of a tumor is used to classify the tumor by cell type. Tumors are further graded based on the degree of malignancy. Classification and grade are used to predict patient outcome (Table 35-2 outlines the most common brain tumors designated by the World Health Organization [WHO] system).[5–8] Other predictors include patient age and general health, early detection, and tumor location.[9]

Although many brain tumors are low grade or "benign," their location may impede surgical removal and cause brain edema as well as shifting of the surrounding structures. This causes increased ICP. Untreated increased ICP can lead to brain herniation and can be fatal. Early diagnosis and symptom management, in addition to histological diagnosis, are important prognostic factors.

ETIOLOGY

The cause of most brain tumors is still unknown. As research improves in the area of genetics, there has been increased interest in identifying chromosomal abnormalities in many types of cancer, including brain tumors. Cytogenetic studies of glioblastoma multiforme, the most common primary brain tumor, have shown multiple chromosomal changes, with both gain and loss of certain chromosomes. It is hypothesized that this information will, at the very least, aid in the development of individualized therapies for patients with primary brain tumors. Some hereditary diseases, such as neurofibromatosis and polyposis, are associated with the development of certain types of brain tumors.[10]

Data from a familial brain tumor registry of primary brain tumors have been collected in the United States and Canada. These data showed a number of cases of first-degree relatives with gliomas. More than 50% of these cases involved high-grade gliomas. One noticeable difference from common familial tumors, such as colon and breast cancer, was that the gliomas were reported for two generations only, unlike multigenerational reporting in the other cancers. Of note, the incidence of husband-and-wife gliomas suggests that environmental factors may play a role in the development of these tumors.[11]

Other environmental factors currently being studied are electric and magnetic fields, foods (particularly those that are broken down in the stomach or bladder to form N-nitroso compounds), occupational exposure, and chemical exposure.

Ionizing radiation has been shown to increase the occurrence of some brain tumors (nerve sheath tumors, meningiomas, and gliomas) when given in high doses. Low-dose radiation exposure is a topic of discussion and controversy.[12]

To evaluate further these and other possible causes of brain tumors, large, multi-institutional collaborative studies are needed.

EPIDEMIOLOGY

Recent statistics indicate that there are approximately 35,000 new cases of primary brain tumors diagnosed in the United States each year, with an estimated 3,000

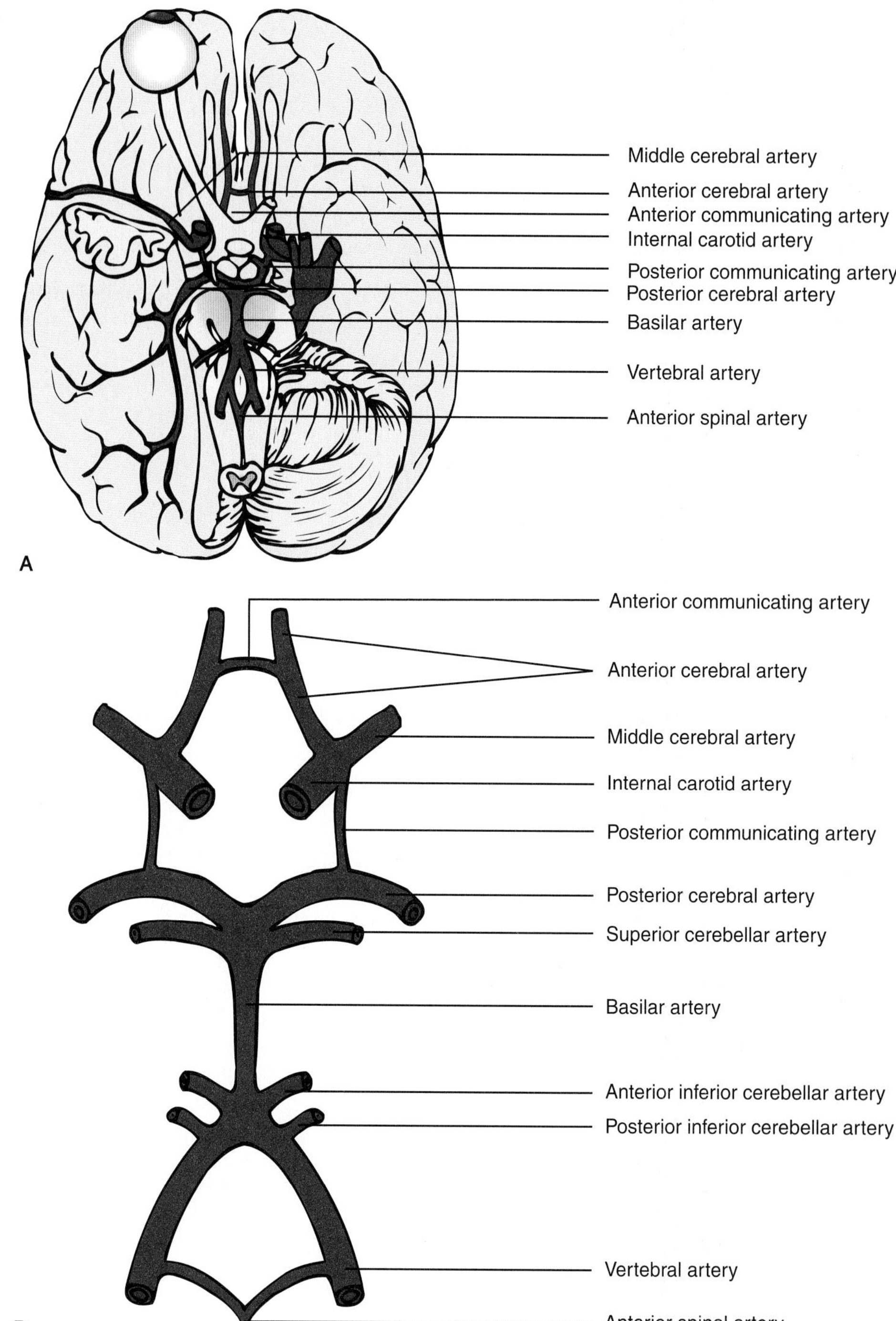

figure 35-2 Circle of Willis (arterial blood supply to the brain). (**A**) The circle of Willis seen from below the brain. (**B**) Schematic of the circle of Willis.

pediatric brain tumors. There are approximately 100,000 new cases of metastatic brain tumors in the United States yearly.[13]

Epidemiological studies have confirmed certain patterns of brain tumor incidence. There has been a significant increase in the incidence of brain tumors in developed countries over the past several decades. Some of this increase can be attributed to improved diagnostic techniques, access to medical care, and an increasing elderly population. It is suspected, however, that some of these increases are also attributable to environmental and lifestyle factors, as previously outlined.[14]

Other patterns of incidence have been documented by age, ethnicity, and sex. For example, the average age of onset for glioblastomas and meningiomas is approximately 60 years. Gliomas are diagnosed more often in the white population and in men. African Americans and women have higher rates of meningiomas.[15]

PATHOPHYSIOLOGY

The brain has its own distinct protective mechanism in the form of the blood–brain barrier. Studies undertaken in the mid-19th century showed that dyes injected intravenously (IV) were not observed in brain tissue as they were in other

table 35-2 Classification and Grading of Brain Tumors (Most Common Intracranial Tumors)

Classification/Grade	Description	Symptoms	Treatment Prognosis*
Neuroepithelial Tumors *Gliomas*	• Approximately 50% of primary brain tumors		
Astrocytic			
WHO Grade I—Pilocytic astrocytoma	• Pediatric; 85% cerebellar; slow growing; well circumscribed; cystic; benign	• Increased ICP • Focal neurological signs	• Curable with surgery (craniotomy for tumor removal)
WHO Grade II—Astrocytoma	• Infiltrative; slow growing	• Seizures • Acute or subtle onset of symptoms	• Radiation therapy (RT) for residual tumor; may hold RT after gross total resection • Young age is good prognostic factor
WHO Grade III—Anaplastic astrocytoma	• Hypercellular; anaplasia	• May have acute onset of symptoms	• RT with or without chemotherapy • High recurrence rate • Age and overall health affect prognosis
WHO Grade IV—Glioblastoma multiforme	• Poorly differentiated, with high mitotic rate; highly malignant • Most common glioma	• Rapid onset of symptoms • Increased ICP or focal signs	• Infiltrative nature: unable to accomplish complete removal of all cells • RT with or without chemotherapy • Experimental protocols • Recurrence in virtually all cases • Median survival: 12–18 mo
Oligodendroglioma	• Well differentiated; calcified; infiltrative; slow growing • Some tumors are malignant (anaplastic)	• Seizures • Headaches • Subtle onset of symptoms	• RT for residual tumor; may hold after gross total resection • RT with or without chemotherapy for anaplastic oligodendroglioma
Mixed glioma (oligoastrocytoma)	• May behave more or less aggressively, depending on features	• Dependent on location and degree of malignancy	• Variable outcome
Ependymoma	• Affects pediatric and young adult patients; originates from lining of the ventricles; frequently in posterior fossa; usually benign	• May present with hydrocephalus; symptoms related to location	• RT for residual or recurrent disease; craniospinal RT for evidence of spinal disease only • Good prognosis
Embryonal (PNET) Medulloblastoma, most common	• Pediatric; malignant; occurs mainly in posterior fossa; CSF metastasis in one-third of patients	• Symptoms by location • Hydrocephalus common	• Craniospinal RT • Poor prognosis, particularly with CSF dissemination
Peripheral Nerve Tumors	• Approximately 7% of primary brain tumors		
Vestibular schwannoma (acoustic neuroma)	• Cerebellopontine angle; benign; encapsulated • Seen in association with neurofibromatosis, type 2	• Decreased hearing • Tinnitus • Balance problems • May have other cranial nerve deficits	• Curable with surgery • Excellent prognosis • Cranial nerve deficits may be permanent or temporary; affect quality of life
Meningeal Tumors	• Approximately 27% of primary brain tumors		

(continued)

table 35-2 Classification and Grading of Brain Tumors (Most Common Intracranial Tumors) (Continued)

Classification/Grade	Description	Symptoms	Treatment Prognosis*
Meningioma	• Composed of arachnoid cells; attached to dura; usually benign; well circumscribed; may be vascular • Common locations: falx, olfactory groove, sphenoid ridge, parasellar, optic nerve	• Headaches may occur from dural stretching • Seizures and focal neurological signs	• Degree of resection (and recurrence) associated with location • Excellent prognosis with gross total resection • Atypical and malignant meningiomas have more aggressive features and less favorable outcomes
Lymphomas and Hematopoietic Tumors	• Approximately 3% of primary brain tumors		
Malignant central nervous system lymphoma	• Arise in CNS without systemic lymphoma; commonly suprasellar; diffuse brain infiltration; may be periventricular and may involve leptomeninges • Solitary or multiple	• Neurological or neuropsychiatric symptoms	• Diagnosis commonly by stereotactic biopsy or CSF cytology • Steroids may decrease or temporarily obliterate lesion on CT/MRI • RT with or without chemotherapy • High-dose methotrexate used as single agent; some studies defer RT • Increasing incidence in immunocompetent patients; decreasing in patients with AIDS • Possible improved survival with newer treatments
Germ Cell Tumors	• Approximately 1% of primary brain tumors • Developmental tumors—from gonads and extragonadal sites; germinoma (solid, enhancing on MRI) and teratoma (cystic, with fat and calcification) most common	• Symptoms are location dependent • Germinomas are often suprasellar—diabetes insipidus	• RT for germinomas; curable • Teratoma, less favorable prognosis; gross total resection equals improved survival • Chemotherapy in some cases
Sellar Tumors	• Approximately 7% of primary brain tumors		
Craniopharyngioma	• Benign; calcified, cystic tumors	• Endocrine abnormalities • Visual impairment • Cognitive/personality changes • May have increased ICP	• Gross total resection affects prognosis • RT for residual tumor
Pituitary adenoma	• 6.3% of sellar tumors • Benign; originates from adenohypophysis; classification by hormonal content • Microadenoma less than 1 cm • Macroadenoma greater than 1 cm	• Hypersecretion 70% 1. Prolactin: amenorrhea, galactorrhea 2. Growth hormone: acromegaly 3. Adrenocorticotropic hormone (ACTH): Cushing's syndrome 4. Thyroid-stimulating hormone (TSH): hyperthyroid (rare)	• Surgical: transsphenoidal for approximately 95% of surgical cases • Medical: appropriate in some cases of prolactin- and growth hormone–secreting tumors • Radiation for recurrence or for hypersecretory tumors, when medical management has failed

(continued)

table 35-2 Classification and Grading of Brain Tumors (Most Common Intracranial Tumors) (Continued)

Classification/Grade	Description	Symptoms	Treatment Prognosis*
		• Hyposecretion caused by compression of the pituitary gland • Visual field deficits (bitemporal hemianopia) • Headache • Pituitary apoplexy: acute hemorrhage or infarct of gland—emergency treatment indicated	
Metastatic Tumors	• Approximately 100,000 new cases yearly; occur in 20%–40% of patients with cancer • Originate from primary systemic tumors • Discrete, round, ring enhancing • 50% are solitary • Lung and breast are most common primary sites	• Symptoms are location dependent	• Prognosis dependent on number of tumors, tumor location, systemic disease, and patient age • Improved prognosis with gross total resection and RT

*Note: For all tumors, biopsy or craniotomy for tumor removal is necessary to establish a definitive diagnosis.

body organs. However, when injected directly into the CSF, they were absorbed into the brain but not disseminated through the brain's vascular system to the rest of the body. These studies confirmed the restricted permeability between the blood and the brain and between the blood and the CSF, but not between the brain and CSF. Tumors are able to cause disruption of this blood–brain barrier, as evidenced by computed tomography (CT) and magnetic resonance imaging (MRI) scans, which show contrast uptake at the site of many tumors. Studies by Long and others confirmed that a tumor's capillary system becomes increasingly abnormal, and permeable, with increasing malignancy, therefore causing blood–brain barrier disruption.[16–18]

Vasogenic edema, caused by increased capillary permeability and commonly seen in association with brain tumors and other brain lesions, is the direct result of blood–brain barrier disruption. As outlined in the Monro-Kellie doctrine, the contents of the cranial vault—brain, CSF, and blood—have a fixed volume. Any addition to this volume must be balanced by reduction in one of the other components. When this compensatory mechanism is no longer able to function, edema develops and ICP increases. In Figure 35-3, an MRI scan shows brain edema and mass effect caused by a glioblastoma multiforme. Some slow-growing tumors, such as meningiomas, can become quite large as a result of this compensatory mechanism and the brain's plasticity. This plasticity allows the brain to accommodate to slow tumor growth over a long period of time[18] (Fig. 35-4).

CLINICAL MANIFESTATIONS

The patient with a brain neoplasm may present with one or more signs of tumor growth. The signs may be general or focal. The most common *general* signs of brain tumors are headaches, seizures, or mental status changes. These are related to increasing ICP.

The triad of symptoms associated with increased ICP includes headache, nausea with or without vomiting, and papilledema (swelling of the optic discs). Symptoms are typically treated with corticosteroids, which are discussed later in this chapter. Clinical evidence of herniation (shift-

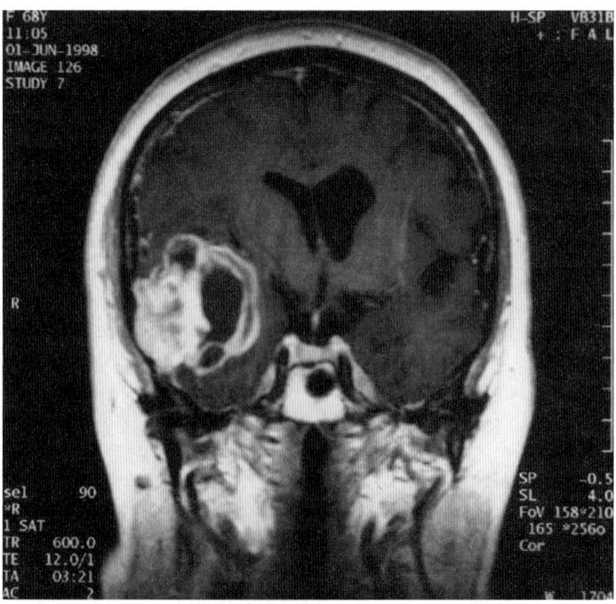

figure 35-3 Coronal MRI view of ring-enhancing glioblastoma multiforme with evidence of mass effect. (Courtesy of Henry Brem, MD, Johns Hopkins University, Baltimore, MD.)

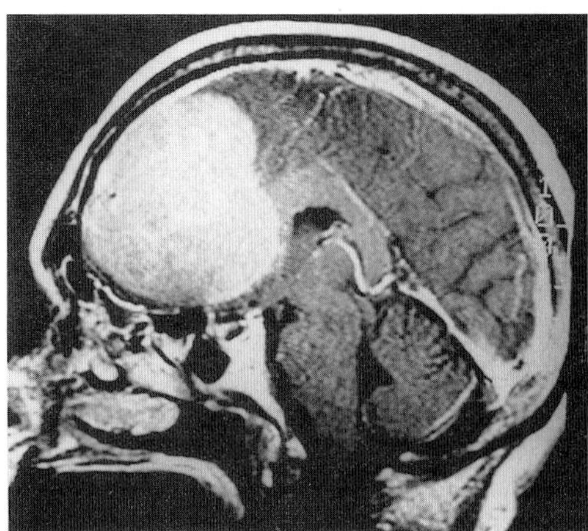

figure 35-4 Sagittal view of meningioma. (Courtesy of Henry Brem, MD, Johns Hopkins University, Baltimore, MD.)

ing of brain tissue by masses, increased ICP, or both) often requires critical care management using fluid restriction, hyperventilation, osmotic agents, and diuretics. Some situations necessitate the use of CSF drainage through an intraventricular catheter (see Chapter 34).[19–21]

The frequency of seizures depends on tumor location as well as tumor histology. Thirty-five to 50% of patients experience seizures over the course of their disease. Seizure activity is more common in patients with low-grade tumors. Tumors in the cerebral hemispheres are much more likely to cause seizure activity than posterior fossa tumors. Seizures may be focal or generalized, as discussed later in this chapter.[21,22]

Mental status changes occur as the result of mass effect on the brain caused by increased ICP or hydrocephalus. Patients may become drowsy and mentally slower as ICP increases. Cognitive changes occur in the form of problems concentrating, memory difficulties, personality changes, confusion, or disorientation. Although mental status changes are associated with frontal lobe tumors, they are also the result of increased ICP.

Focal neurological deficits may be the temporary result of tumor compression, or may be permanent, as a result of tumor destruction. These deficits are directly related to tumor location, as outlined in the Neuroanatomy section of this chapter. Figure 35-5 outlines site-specific signs and symptoms of brain tumors.

DIAGNOSIS

History taking is a key element in the process of diagnosing a brain neoplasm. The duration, frequency, and severity of symptoms should be ascertained. It is important to assess if there is a particular time of day or series of activities that initiate symptoms. Are they intermittent or continuous? Do they resolve with pharmacological management? Morning headaches and headaches that increase with Valsalva maneuver or are associated with nausea and vomiting are seen in patients with tumor-induced increased ICP.[23] The physical examination aids in further localizing the lesion. Patients may minimize or are often unaware of subtle neurological deficits. Family involvement in this discussion is useful.

Imaging studies such as CT scans and MRI are typically ordered to localize the lesion and assess the amount of edema and mass effect on surrounding structures. CT scans are often obtained to establish a differential diagnosis when a patient is seen in the emergency department. Because MRI images tumors in three dimensions (axial, coronal, and sagittal), it is the preferred diagnostic tool.[5,19] An electroencephalogram (EEG) is used to confirm the presence of seizure discharges, which may be useful in determining if anticonvulsants are needed. Magnetic resonance angiography (MRA) images the vascular anatomy and vessels that feed certain tumors. It can be a noninvasive alternative to the angiogram, which is an invasive study used to identify and perform embolization of feeding vessels to the tumor with the use of glue preparations. In some cases, angiography and embolization are performed within 24 to 48 hours of surgery for large tumors such as meningiomas.[24,25] Functional MRI (fMRI) is a type of imaging used for tumors in the dominant hemisphere or motor strip. It is believed that increased cerebral blood flow is recognized as an increased signal on the fMRI. The patient performs a particular task, and the fMRI indicates which part of the brain is activated. This is a noninvasive procedure currently used in some centers as part of the preoperative assessment of language, motor and sensory function, and tumor location.[26–29] Positron emission tomography (PET) uses radionuclides to measure cerebral blood flow and brain metabolism. It is used to differentiate low-grade from high-grade (and more metabolically active) tumors. It is also used to differentiate radiation necrosis from high-grade tumors in previously treated patients. Magnetic resonance spectroscopy (MRS) is another noninvasive radiographic technique that measures metabolite levels in brain tumors. Biological compounds such as choline can be quantitated in brain tumors. Because MRS is obtained at the same time as MRI, the anatomic and metabolic characteristics of the tumor are obtained with little additional inconvenience to the patient.[30]

CLINICAL MANAGEMENT

Once the differential diagnosis of brain tumor is obtained through history, physical examination, and imaging studies, decisions are made regarding appropriate treatment modalities. A medical and surgical plan of care is discussed with the patient and family members.

Pharmacological Management

Tumors and tumor treatments are known to cause increased ICP and are treated with corticosteroids. Corticosteroids such as dexamethasone reduce brain edema by reducing the permeability of tumor capillaries and possibly by shifting some of the fluid into the ventricular system.[23] A dose of 16 mg daily is standard in the perioperative period. It is usually given in two to four divided doses, spaced over the course of the day. Resolution of symptoms can be quite rapid. Steroids also increase the safety of the surgical procedure. They are, however, associated with significant side effects, as outlined in Table 35-3.[23]

Type 2 histamine receptor (H_2) blockers are usually prescribed for the patient taking steroids. They are used to prevent gastrointestinal symptoms that can be associated with prolonged steroid use, including ulcers and gastrointestinal bleeding. Although taking the medication

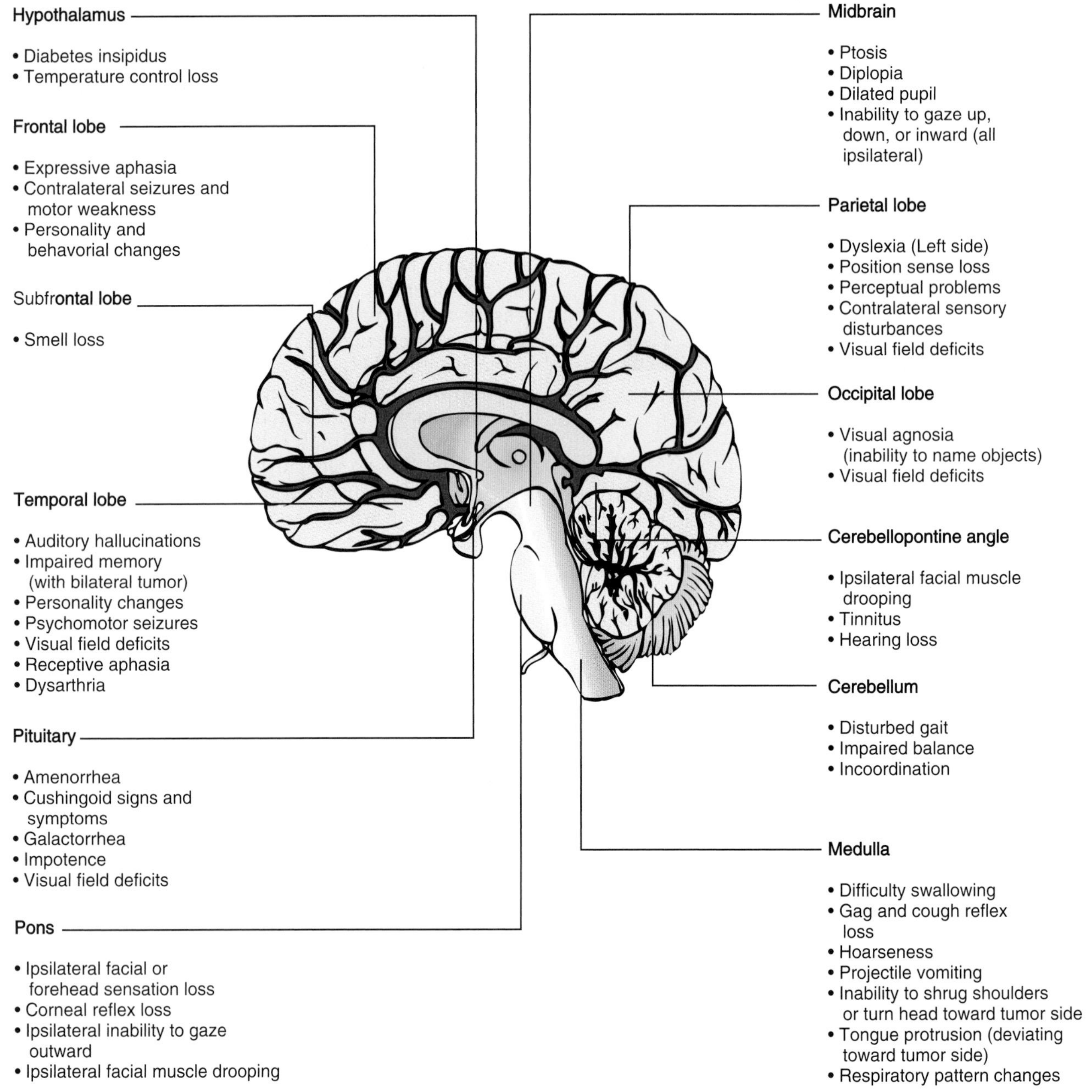

figure 35-5 Site-specific signs and symptoms of brain tumors. (Reprinted with permission from Anatomical Chart Company: Atlas of Pathophysiology, p123. Springhouse, PA, Springhouse, 2002.)

with food may be sufficient to prevent these symptoms, H_2 blockers are routinely used.[23]

Anticonvulsant therapy is initiated when the patient presents with a seizure. Many surgeons also use anticonvulsants during the perioperative period. Because some studies have shown little difference in postoperative seizures in patients receiving anticonvulsants compared with control groups without such drugs, many physicians are limiting the use of postoperative and prophylactic anticonvulsant therapy.[31] However, other studies suggest that anticonvulsant therapy may be warranted after surgery, even in patients who have not presented with seizures, specifically in the case of glioblastoma multiforme.[32] Seizures are extensively discussed later in this chapter.

Surgical Management

Clinical and radiographic evaluations are useful in obtaining a differential diagnosis. Pathologic examination of tumor tissue, however, produces the definitive diagnosis. There are two distinct surgical approaches to diagnosing and treating brain tumors. Stereotactic biopsy is used to obtain small samples of tumor tissue under CT or MRI guidance. Craniotomy is performed when tumor removal is feasible, and provides not only a pathological diagnosis, but surgical resection of the lesion. These approaches are discussed in the Surgical Approaches section of this chapter.

Over the last several decades, improvements in anesthesia, microsurgical equipment, intraoperative monitoring techniques, and pharmacological management have

table 35-3 Complications of Corticosteroid Therapy

Neurological	*Common:* Behavioral changes, insomnia, myopathy, hallucinations, hiccups, tremor, reduced taste and smell, cerebral atrophy *Uncommon:* Psychosis, dementia, seizures, dependence, paraparesis (epidural lipomatosis)
Dermatological	Thin, fragile skin; purpura; ecchymoses; striae; acne; inhibition of wound healing; Kaposi's sarcoma
Rheumatological	Osteoporosis, avascular necrosis, growth retardation, tendinous rupture
Gastrointestinal	Increased appetite, abdominal bloating, gastrointestinal bleeding and perforation, pancreatitis, liver hypertrophy
Ophthalmological	Visual blurring, cataract, glaucoma, exophthalmos, uveitis
Cardiovascular	Hypertension, atherosclerosis, arrhythmia (with IV push)
Endocrine/metabolic	Hyperglycemia, hypokalemia, hypophosphatemia, hypernatremia, hyperlipidemia, redistribution of body fat (e.g., centripetal obesity, buffalo hump), amenorrhea
Urogenital	Polyuria, genital burning (with IV push)
Miscellaneous	Opportunistic infections (including candidiasis, *Pneumocystis carinii* pneumonitis), hypersensitivity reactions, neutrophilia, lymphopenia, night sweats
Steroid withdrawal	Pseudorheumatism (very common), headache, lethargy, low-grade fever, adrenal insufficiency, pseudotumor cerebri

Used with permission from Wen PY, Black PM: Clinical presentation, evaluation and preoperative preparation of the patient. In Berger MS, Wilson CB (eds): The Gliomas, pp 328–336. Philadelphia, WB Saunders, 1999.

significantly improved intraoperative mortality rates. Postoperative morbidity has also significantly decreased. The perioperative management of the patient with a brain tumor involves a multidisciplinary team approach, as outlined in Table 35-4.[19]

Despite substantial improvements in the surgical management of the patient with a brain tumor, perioperative complications may be severe and require critical care monitoring and management (Table 35-5). The most common complications include brain edema, infection, hyponatremia or other changes in electrolytes, hemorrhage, thromboembolism, and seizures.[33,34]

Radiation Therapy

Many brain tumors are treated with adjuvant therapies, either because they are not able to be surgically resected or because of their aggressive nature. For most brain tumors, radiation therapy is the first-line treatment after biopsy or craniotomy. *External beam radiation* is usually used to treat those tumor cells that are not surgically resectable. The energy produced by radiation damages tumor DNA at the time of cell division. Because neurons do not divide, they are spared. There is, however, a maximum dose that the normal brain is able to tolerate. A standard dose of up to 6000 centigrays (cGy; also referred to as *radiation absorbed dose*, or *rad*) is administered to primary brain tumors over a period of 6 weeks. Multiple metastatic tumors receive a dose of approximately 3000 cGy divided over 10 treatments. A solitary metastasis may be treated with higher radiation doses and with a boost of focused radiation.

Only one course of external beam radiation is usually given. There are, however, other approaches to applying radiation. *Intensity-modulated radiation therapy* (IMRT) modifies the radiation beam so that a more focused dose can be given, without exposing surrounding brain tissue. *Stereotactic radiosurgery* (e.g., gamma knife and linear accelerator) is applied under MRI guidance. A three-dimensional image is obtained and radiation is given in one large dose to residual tumor, sparing normal brain tissue. *Brachytherapy* uses radioactive isotopes in seeds or liquid inserted into residual tumor. *Radiosensitizers* are agents given in addition to radiation therapy. It is postulated that some substances increase oxygen delivery to hypoxic tumors. The oxygen enhances the effects of radiation. *Hyperthermia* is also being applied with the same goal of increasing oxygen to tumors to maximize the effects of radiation.[35–40]

Chemotherapy

Malignant brain tumors require multiple treatment modalities. Chemotherapy is given in conjunction with radiation or at the time of tumor recurrence. Drugs may be administered orally or IV, but can cause systemic toxicities and have difficulty crossing the blood–brain barrier in sufficient amounts to provide benefit. Other approaches have been explored as alternatives or adjuncts to conventional chemotherapy. These include combination chemotherapy, continuous infusion chemotherapy, chemical blood–brain barrier disruption, high-dose chemotherapy and bone marrow transplantation, intra-arterial chemotherapy, and chemotherapy before radiation. All of these approaches are currently being evaluated.[41–43]

A recent advance in the treatment of malignant gliomas was formulated on the hypothesis that these tumors overwhelmingly recur within 2 cm of the site of origin and are uniformly fatal. A biodegradable polymer was developed

table 35-4 Multidisciplinary Management Guide for the Patient With a Brain Tumor

Stage	Management Team	Interventions	Nursing Considerations
Preoperative			
• History and physical	• Neurosurgeon, nurse practitioner, RN	• Baseline history and physical examination; neurological evaluation: mental status, cranial nerves, motor and sensory function, coordination, reflexes	• Preoperative teaching to begin • Involve family as much as possible
• Medications	• Physician, pharmacist, nurse practitioner, RN	• Steroids; histamine type 2 receptor (H_2) blockers, as needed; anticonvulsants for supratentorial lesions • Prescribe new medications; medication review; discuss interactions or contraindications	• Anticoagulants, nonsteroidal anti-inflammatory drugs (NSAIDs) to be discontinued (with consent of prescribing physician)
• Diagnostic testing	• Neuroradiologist	• Baseline MRI or CT scan • ECG, chest x-ray • Other diagnostic studies as indicated	• Most preoperative testing performed within 1 week of surgery
• Preoperative teaching	• By speciality: RN, neurosurgeon, neuroanesthesiologist	• Informed consent • Obtain all test results before admission day	• A written teaching pamphlet is recommended for patient and family use
• Hospital admission	• Admitting office, OR staff	• Obtain/confirm demographics	• Most patients are admitted the day of surgery
Intraoperative			
• Stereotactic biopsy	• OR team, surgeon, anesthesiologist, radiologist, pathologist	• Stereotactic frame placed; samples taken through catheter inserted under MRI/CT guidance • Histological evaluation	• May be performed in radiology suite or OR • Teaching regarding stereotactic frame • May also be done as a frameless procedure
• Craniotomy	• OR team, surgeon, anesthesiologist, pathologist	• Tumor tissue obtained for biopsy; tumor resected • Histological evaluation	• Teaching regarding general anesthesia
Postoperative			
• Critical care unit	• Critical care staff, neurosurgeon	• Hemodynamic monitoring; frequent neurological evaluations	• If possible, it is useful for patient and family to see the unit before surgery
• Nursing unit	• Floor nurses, surgeon, consulting physicians, rehabilitation medicine, pharmacist, clergy, nutritionist	• Postoperative care to include vital signs, neurological exam, wound care, cough, and deep breathing; increase activity as tolerated; advance diet as tolerated • Rehabilitation medicine consult • Evaluate for deficits and complications and provide consultations, as indicated	• More family participation in care when possible • Patients are usually out of bed within 24 hours of surgery • Recently, short hospital stays cause increased family involvement and responsibility; begin teaching while patient is on the nursing unit
Discharge Planning	• Social worker, nursing staff, consulting physicians, radiation oncologist, medical oncologist (when indicated)	• Inpatient/outpatient rehabilitation as needed (occupational therapy, physical therapy, speech, cognitive) • Outpatient therapies as needed (e.g., radiation, chemotherapy) • Hospice care (inpatient or home hospice) may be indicated, particularly in cases of recurrent malignant gliomas, refractory to conventional treatments	• Ideally, planning begins as soon as the patient arrives on the nursing unit • Family takes on greater role because patient is often discharged from the hospital 2–3 days postoperatively, particularly in cases of highly malignant tumors where home hospice is indicated

Adapted from Bohan E: Neurosurgical management of patients with central nervous system malignancies. Semin Oncol Nurs 14:8–17, 1998.

table 35-5 Critical Care Management of Brain Tumor Complications

Diagnosis	Management
Increased ICP	• Corticosteroids and antacids or histamine type 2 receptor (H_2) blockers • IV fluids: Avoid hypotonic solutions • Elevate head of bed and maintain adequate body alignment • Avoid hypotension and control hypertension; arterial line useful; if ICP monitor is available, titrate B/P to maintain a CPP of 70–80 mm Hg • Keep well oxygenated; may need to intubate • Judicious use of osmotic therapy: mannitol to expand plasma volume and draw fluid out of the brain; may be used in conjunction with furosemide • Sedation to reduce activity and decrease hypertension • Intraventricular catheter may be necessary to monitor ICP and drain CSF • Cautious use of hyperventilation for short periods only to reduce arterial carbon dioxide pressure (Pco_2) (6–24 h) • May require surgical intervention for hematoma
Wound infection, intracranial abscess, or bone flap infection	• Blood work, including complete blood count (CBC) and blood cultures • CT scan, MRI, and in some cases MR spectroscopy to identify abscess • Surgical removal of abscess or bone flap, when feasible • Appropriate wound cultures, when possible • Antibiotic therapy • Infectious disease consultation for appropriate drug, dose, and duration
Hyponatremia or hypernatremia	• Possible diabetes insipidus (DI), salt-wasting syndrome, or syndrome of inappropriate antidiuretic hormone secretion (SIADH) • For hyponatremia: fluid restriction, hypertonic saline • For hypernatremia: fluids, vasopressin
Intracranial hemorrhage	• Immediate CT scan to evaluate for early signs of a bleed • Monitor blood pressure • Check laboratory values: prothrombin time (PT), partial thromboplastin time (PTT), platelets • Management of increased ICP, as described above • May need to intubate and ventilate • Surgery may be necessary to remove blood clot
Thromboembolism: deep venous thrombosis (DVT) and pulmonary embolus (PE)	• Diagnosed through transcranial Doppler study or ventilation-perfusion scan ($\dot{V}/\dot{Q}$scan) • Heparinization *only after* CT scan has ruled out intracranial blood • Alternatively, vena cava filter (Greenfield filter) may be used • Large PEs require ICU care for further medical treatment
Seizures	• Potential for status epilepticus • Protect patient from injury • Titrate antiepileptics to therapeutic levels

Courtesy of Michael Torbey.

that delivers a continuous infusion of carmustine (BCNU) chemotherapy over a period of several weeks. The chemotherapy wafers are implanted directly into the resection cavity during surgical removal of the tumor, bypassing the blood–brain barrier and eliminating systemic toxicities.[44] The U.S. Food and Drug Administration (FDA) has approved the wafers for the treatment of malignant gliomas. Studies are underway using higher doses of this drug-impregnated wafer formulation for metastatic tumors to the brain.

Research Initiatives

Radiation and chemotherapy are targeted at damaging cell DNA, thereby killing the cell or preventing it from dividing. Other approaches have been used in an effort to address different aspects of tumor growth:

- Glioma cells are deficient in a protein that suppresses tumor growth (–p53). *Gene therapy* is being explored using adenoviruses, for example, which are engineered to replicate in and inactivate these cells. They are designed not to replicate in normal (+p53) cells.[45,46]
- *Antiangiogenic factors* are used to prevent tumors from forming their own blood supply, crucial to tumor growth.[47–49]
- *Immunotherapy* is designed to stimulate the immune system to eliminate tumors. Targeted toxins are injected into and infiltrate tumor cells. Cytokines, such as interferon and interleukin, are proteins produced by the body to stimulate an immune response. They are being combined with inactivated tumor cells as the basis for tumor vaccines.[50,51]
- Cancer cells have enzymes that resist chemotherapy. Certain drugs called *resistance modifiers* are being used to inhibit these enzymes and to increase the effectiveness of chemotherapy.[52]

Nursing Management

Some tumors are cured with surgery, while others follow a protracted course involving adjuvant therapies and treatment for recurrent disease. As part of the multidisciplinary team, the nurse plays a central role in patient care and family support throughout the course of the patient's disease. The nurse participates in the diagnosis, treatment, and follow-up care of the patient with a brain tumor.

Careful history taking and symptom evaluation contributes to the accurate diagnosis of a brain tumor. Once medications are prescribed, patient education includes discussion of dose, side effects, and contraindications. The results of tests leading to a differential diagnosis are reviewed with the patient and family. When a decision has been made to proceed with surgery, extensive teaching is required in the perioperative period. Table 35-4 outlines the nurse's role in the plan of care for this patient population. Patient teaching is better retained if it is both verbal and written. Teaching sheets are useful and can be referred to at different times during the treatment period.

Although surgery and follow-up therapies are disruptive to patient and family activities, it is important to encourage a return to normality as soon as feasible. Continuing with activities of daily living that encourage a positive and motivated attitude contributes to recovery.

Hospice

Multiple surgical procedures and adjuvant therapies are often successful in containing malignant gliomas for a period. Inevitably, these tumors recur and become resistant to all treatment modalities. In addition, patient quality of life may be so compromised that further therapy is not feasible. Home and inpatient hospice are available in most communities, and provide dedicated and supportive end-of-life care.

Aneurysms

An aneurysm is a round, saccular dilation of the arterial wall that develops as a result of weakness of the wall. Aneurysms may be congenital or degenerative arterial lesions. Concern arises if the outpouching of the vessel wall ruptures or becomes large enough to exert pressure on surrounding brain structures.

Approximately 20% to 40% of patients die from the initial bleed of their aneurysm before reaching medical care. Rebleeding is the leading cause of death in patients with a history of ruptured aneurysm. Of those who survive the initial bleeding, 35% to 40% bleed again if left untreated, with a mortality rate of about 42%. Some recent data suggest that the mortality rate from initial hemorrhage is as high as 60%. Rebleeding most often occurs around the seventh day after the original bleed. Predictors of good recovery by 1 month after the bleed include a high score on the admission Glasgow Coma Scale (GCS) and an absence of blood on the first CT scan.[53,54]

ETIOLOGY

The etiology of aneurysms is unclear, but is probably a combination of congenital and degenerative factors. Carmichael described the combination hypothesis of aneurysm formation. He found that congenital focal defects of the tunica media (the middle layer of the blood vessels made up of transverse elastic and muscle fibers) are common, but degenerative changes are necessary for the formation of aneurysms. Histological investigation of the normal vessel wall into the aneurysmal sac shows that the tunica media usually ends at the neck of the aneurysm and the internal elastic lamina becomes fragmented as it enters the sac. Consistent with this hypothesis, aneurysms are rare in children, but common into late adulthood.[53]

Although the exact cause of intracranial aneurysm is not understood, there is evidence to support that acquired and genetic factors contribute to the development of aneurysms. Genetic factors include heredity and genetically transmitted diseases. Acquired factors encompass traumatic brain injury, sepsis, cigarette smoking, and hypertension.[53]

EPIDEMIOLOGY

Aneurysms are present in 2% of the population. In the United States there are approximately 30,000 new cases of subarachnoid hemorrhage (SAH) each year that are attributed to aneurysmal rupture. The incidence of SAH is 6.0 to 7.5 cases per 100,000 individuals. They occur more often in women than in men and, as noted earlier, can be linked to cigarette smoking.[53] Aneurysm can also be associated with other pathological processes, such as polycystic kidney disease.[55,56] The incidence of aneurysms increases with age.

Seasonal variability is another epidemiological feature. Clinicians observed that there may be a seasonal variability, with increases occurring in spring and fall.

The Cooperative Study of Intracranial Aneurysms and Subarachnoid Hemorrhage reported that in 32% of cases, the hemorrhage occurred during physical activity. The study also reported that a similar proportion occurred during sleep. In summary, the incidence of SAH can be roughly divided into thirds: sleeping, active, and at rest.

PATHOPHYSIOLOGY

Arterial vessels are composed of three layers: endothelial lining, smooth muscle, and connective tissue. A defect in the smooth muscle layer, or tunica media, allows the endothelial lining to bulge through, creating an aneurysm. The two types of aneurysms are saccular (also known as "berry" because of its well-defined stem and berry-like outpouching of the medial layer of the arterial wall) and fusiform. Berry aneurysms are usually located on major cerebral arteries at the apex of branch points, which is where maximum hemodynamic stress occurs in the vessel. Fusiform aneurysms occur more commonly in the vertebrobasilar system.[56]

Most aneurysms arise from larger arteries around the anterior section of the circle of Willis. The most frequent sites of occurrence in the anterior circulation are the anterior communicating artery, the posterior communicating artery, the middle cerebral artery bifurcation, and the internal carotid artery bifurcation. In the posterior circulation, the most common locations are the basilar artery apex and the posterior inferior cerebellar artery.[53]

Hemorrhage from an aneurysm usually occurs in the subarachnoid space because aneurysm-forming vessels usually lie in the space between the arachnoid layer of the meninges and the brain. The force of the rupturing vessel can be so great that it can push blood through the pia mater and into the brain substance, causing an intracerebral hemorrhage. It can also push through the arachnoid into the subdural space, causing a subdural hemorrhage.

CLINICAL MANIFESTATIONS

Many aneurysms are silent and never cause a problem, but may be discovered on postmortem examination. If an aneurysm causes problems, it typically occurs between the ages of 35 and 60 years. Aneurysmal SAHs are graded according to their severity on the Hunt and Hess scale. In this grading system, Grade 0 is the unruptured aneurysm and Grade V is a hemorrhage with severe neurological sequelae (Table 35-6).[55] However, the Hunt and Hess scale is not the only grading system that has been developed for SAH. The World Federation of Neurological Surgeons grading scale is also used for SAH.

Approximately half of patients have some warning signs before an aneurysm ruptures. These signs may include headaches, lethargy, neck pain, a "noise in the head," and optic, oculomotor, or trigeminal cranial nerve dysfunction.

After an aneurysm has bled or ruptured, the patient usually complains of a horrific headache. The classic description is, "the worst headache of my life." There may be a decrease in the level of consciousness, cranial nerve dysfunction, visual disturbances, perhaps hemiparesis or hemiplegia, and often vomiting. All these signs are related to an increase in ICP. With an SAH, there are signs of meningeal irritation, such as a stiff and painful neck, photophobia, blurred vision, irritability, fever, positive Kernig's sign, and positive Brudzinski's sign. Exactly which deficits are present depends on the location of the aneurysm, the subsequent hemorrhage, and the severity of the bleeding.

Bleeding stops because ICP in the subarachnoid space reaches mean arterial pressure (MAP) quickly, stopping the bleeding long enough for the rupture to seal. If this does not occur, the patient dies.

When there is blood in the subarachnoid space, it irritates the brainstem, causing abnormal activity in the autonomic nervous system, often with cardiac arrhythmias and hypertension. Hypertension can also result from elevated ICP. Another complication of blood in the subarachnoid space is hydrocephalus. Blood in the subarachnoid space impedes reabsorption of CSF by the arachnoid villi. Hydrocephalus results in enlargement of the lateral and third ventricles.

DIAGNOSIS

The diagnosis of a cerebral aneurysm usually is made on the basis of history, physical examination, CT scan, lumbar puncture, and cerebral angiogram. When the nurse takes the patient's history, he or she identifies risk factors such as genetic predisposition, hypertension, and cigarette smoking. Patients with an SAH may present with a headache, neck discomfort, or both without any neurological signs. The headache may range in severity from mild to severe. A CT scan reveals hemorrhage in 92% of cases when it is obtained within 24 hours of the hemorrhage. There is a steady decline over ensuing days, with only 57% of scans being positive 5 days after an SAH occurs.[57]

If the results of a CT scan are negative and the patient is suspected of having an SAH, a lumbar puncture should be done. After a positive lumbar puncture, the gold standard is to perform a cerebral angiogram because other procedures such as MRA and CT angiography (CT-A) can yield false-negative results, leading to a misdiagnosis.[53] Transcranial Doppler ultrasonography (TCD) can also be used to diagnose and treat vasospasm, a common complication of an SAH.

Examples of nursing diagnoses and collaborative problems for the patient with a cerebral aneurysm or arteriovenous malformations (which are discussed after aneurysms) are presented in Box 35-1.

CLINICAL MANAGEMENT

The management of a patient with a ruptured or leaking aneurysm before surgical repair focuses on minimal stimulation of the patient. Some institutions initiate "aneurysm precautions," measures such as a quiet environment, bowel regimen, and limited visitors. Sedation may also be used.

table 35-6 Hunt and Hess Grading Scale for Aneurysms

Grade	Description
Grade 0	Unruptured aneurysm
Grade I	Asymptomatic Minimal headache Slight nuchal rigidity (neck stiffness)
Grade II	Moderate to severe headache Nuchal rigidity Cranial nerve deficits
Grade III	Lethargy Mental confusion Mild focal neurological deficit
Grade IV	Stupor Moderate to severe motor deficit Possible posturing
Grade V	Deep coma Posturing Declining appearance

Adapted from Mower-Wade D, Cavanaugh MC, Bush C: Protecting a patient with ruptured cerebral aneurysm. Nursing 2001 31(2):52–58, 2001.

box 35-1 ***Examples of Nursing Diagnoses and Collaborative Problems for the Patient With Cerebral Aneurysm or Arteriovenous Malformations***

- Altered Cerebral Tissue Perfusion related to interruption in cerebral blood flow or intracranial hypertension
- Pain related to meningeal irritation
- Risk for Sensory/Perceptual Alterations (visual, auditory, kinesthetic, and tactile) related to altered level of consciousness, disorientation, impaired communication skills, restricted or unfamiliar environment, photophobia
- Risk for Fluid Volume Excess related to hypervolemia used to treat vasospasm
- Risk for Fluid Volume Deficit related to fluid restriction and use of osmotics to control intracranial hypertension

Plasma volume should not be allowed to fall. Hyponatremia, which may result from cerebral salt wasting, must be anticipated.

Stool softeners are used in the management of patients with an aneurysm to prevent straining. Mild analgesics can be used to relieve headaches; acetaminophen or codeine can be used without masking neurological signs.

Blood in the subarachnoid space causes an elevated temperature. An antipyretic, usually acetaminophen, and hypothermia blankets can be used to manage fever. Dexamethasone, a steroid, is also used.

Surgical Management

Clipping. Surgical excision or clipping may be considered if the aneurysm is in an accessible area. Aneurysms of the vertebrobasilar system often present the problem of surgical inaccessibility. The accepted surgical treatment is the placement of a clip across the neck of the aneurysm. Some aneurysms may be wrapped in a gauzelike material or coated with an acrylic substance that gives the aneurysm support. Although wrapping or coating should not be the goal of surgery, there may be conditions, as with a fusiform aneurysm, in which there is no other option.[56]

In the past several years, there has been controversy over when surgical intervention should occur. The current philosophy is that surgery should occur sooner rather than later. Thus, surgery is usually performed 48 hours after the bleed occurs (Fig. 35-6).

After aneurysm clipping, the patient is maintained in a critical care environment. Maintenance of an adequate airway is vital. If the patient is intubated and suctioning is needed, it is important that the suction catheter be passed and removed quickly to prevent desaturation.

Signs of vasospasm, such as hemiparesis, visual disturbance, seizures, or a decreasing level of consciousness, should be noted and reported so that medical interventions can be rapidly implemented. Control of ICP is a collaborative effort. Nurses should keep the head of the patient's bed elevated without neck flexion or severe rotation. Also, nursing care activities should be spaced to avoid causing a sharp rise in ICP.

Coiling. One of the most valuable recent developments in the management of aneurysms has been the technique of endovascular thrombosis of aneurysms with Guglielmi detachable coils (GDCs). These are thrombogenic platinum alloy microcoils. They are soft to allow the coil to conform to the shape of the aneurysm. Coils are available in various lengths and diameters to provide maximal occlusion.[58]

The procedure used to introduce the coil into the aneurysm is similar to that used for a cerebral angiogram, using the femoral artery and fluoroscopic equipment. In this procedure, a microcatheter is passed through the aorta, around the aortic arch, and then into the vessel specific to the aneurysm. Once the catheter is in position, the coil system is advanced through the catheter into the aneurysm sac. The coil is then in position, and if placement is satisfactory, a low-voltage current is applied. The current causes the coil to detach. If the coil is successfully placed, it occludes the aneurysm and separates it from the cerebral circulation. The number of coils placed is individualized to the patient. Through this coiling procedure, the risk of hemorrhage or rehemorrhage is decreased.

A complication of this treatment is stroke. It can occur because the parent artery feeding the aneurysm becomes occluded. Stroke may also occur from the introduction of

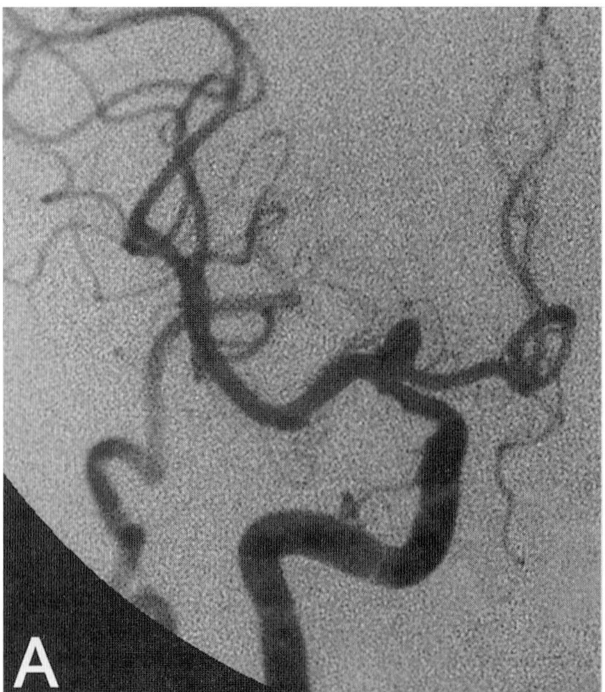

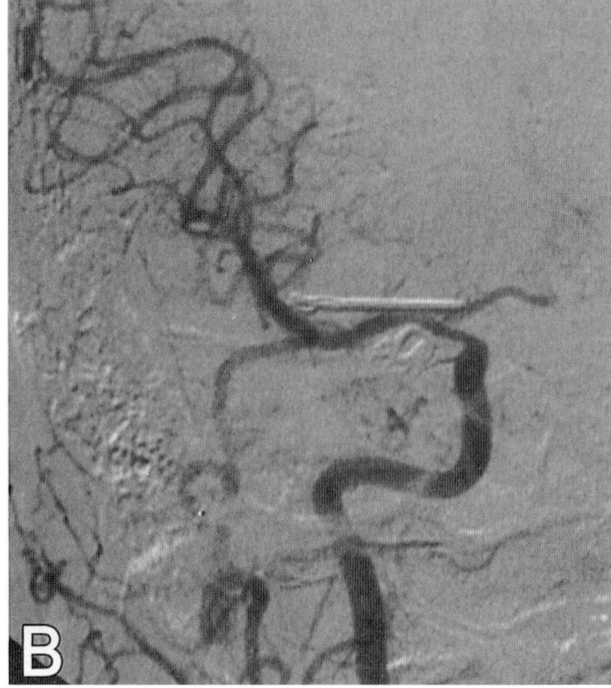

figure 35-6 Preoperative (**A**) and postoperative (**B**) angiography: clipping of right internal carotid artery termination aneurysm. (Courtesy of Rafael Tamargo, MD, and Richard Clatterbuck, MD, Johns Hopkins University, Baltimore, MD.)

air or particles into the catheter system. Additional complications of this technique are perforation or rupture of the aneurysm, vasospasm, damage to the femoral artery, and infection.

Although clipping is the preferred treatment of most aneurysms, GDC coiling is an option for patients who are considered to be surgically high risk owing to medical instability, or those who would otherwise be treated conservatively.[58]

Medical Management of Complications

As previously noted, vasospasm can occur after, as well as before, surgery in the patient with an aneurysm. Angiographic vasospasm is seen early. The peak of chronic vasospasm may not be seen until 7 to 10 days postbleed. Although the aneurysm may have been clipped successfully, vasospasm can cause the development of a large area of ischemia or infarcted brain, with severe deficits.

Vasospasm usually occurs 3 to 12 days after an SAH. The peak incidence is between days 7 and 10. Vasospasm is of clinical significance because it decreases cerebral blood flow, depriving brain tissue of oxygen and promoting accumulation of metabolic waste products, such as lactic acid.

The exact etiology of vasospasm is not clear. There appears to be a positive correlation between the size of the hemorrhage seen on CT scan and the subsequent development of spasm. Lysed red blood cells release calcium ions, which are believed to be mediators for spasm. There has been some success in using nimodipine, a calcium antagonist, after an SAH to improve patient outcomes. Nimodipine blocks the slow channel of calcium influx, which reduces the contraction of smooth and cardiac muscles without affecting skeletal muscles. The theory is that calcium channel blockers may alleviate the abnormal contraction of vascular smooth muscle that may contribute to vasospasm.[56]

"Triple H" therapy is the standard for the prevention and treatment of vasospasm. It consists of hypervolemic expansion, hemodilution, and induced hypertension in postoperative patients. Nimodipine is used with this therapy. These measures reduce smooth muscle spasm and maximize perfusion when spasm does occur.

Hypervolemia is accomplished by volume expansion, using both IV colloid and crystalloid solutions. They are given to increase intravascular volume and decrease blood viscosity. Through hypervolemia, the cerebral vessels dilate and the MAP increases, thereby improving cerebral perfusion pressure (CPP). During this therapy, the patient should be monitored for pulmonary edema and heart failure. A pulmonary artery catheter helps monitor the patient's hemodynamic status.[55]

Hemodilution through the administration of IV fluids decreases blood viscosity, increases regional cerebral blood flow, and may decrease infarction size and increase oxygen transport. The goal for hemodilution is to reduce the hematocrit by 15%. The patient's hematocrit level should be maintained between 30% and 33%, which helps improve cerebral blood flow without causing hypoxia.

Vasopressors are used to induce hypertension. The objective is to maintain systolic blood pressure at greater than 20 mm Hg over normal. Vasopressors raise the patient's blood pressure to the point where neurological deficit improves.[55]

When conventional medical therapy is not effective, acute arterial vasospasm secondary to an SAH can be managed by balloon angioplasty in centers where this technology is available. Recent advances in microballoon technology now allow access to the cerebral vasculature with soft, flexible angioplasty balloons, which mechanically dilate and improve cerebral blood flow through the major arterial segments affected by vasospasm.

Another complication after an aneurysm rupture is hydrocephalus. Hydrocephalus indicates an imbalance between the production and absorption of CSF. It may occur in patients who have experienced an SAH. When there is blood in the subarachnoid space, the red blood cells can occlude the very small channels leading from one ventricle to another. If this occurs, an obstructive hydrocephalus develops. In this case, there is an obstruction of the normal flow of CSF, often between the third and fourth ventricles, or at the exits from the fourth ventricle. There is also the potential for a reabsorption problem, whereby red blood cells occlude the arachnoid villi, impeding reabsorption and resulting in a communicating hydrocephalus. The patient may require a shunt. With a ventriculoperitoneal (VP) shunt, the proximal tip of the catheter is placed in a lateral ventricle and the distal tip is placed in the peritoneum. The shunt drains into the peritoneal cavity to treat the hydrocephalus.

Seizures may occur from blood in the subarachnoid space acting as an irritant. Typically, patients are placed on an anticonvulsant to minimize seizure risk.

Rebleeding is another complication in patients with an SAH if the aneurysm is not repaired. At least 10% of all patients with an SAH have another bleed within hours of the initial hemorrhage. Without intervention, the risk of rebleeding in the remaining patients is at least 30% during the subsequent 3 weeks. The immediate mortality rate of rebleeding is about 60%.[54]

Nursing Management

Assessment. One of the nurse's primary responsibilities is to obtain a baseline neurological assessment and perform subsequent assessments to monitor for changes. After surgery, the nurse must be alert to the development of new deficits or a worsening of preoperative deficits. The severity and duration of any postoperative disability depend largely on the location and extent of the vascular lesion and resultant ischemia. The patient must also be carefully monitored for the development of cerebral edema.

Plan. Before surgery, the nurse implements aneurysm precautions by providing a quiet environment with limited stimulation. The nurse does a bowel assessment and implements individualized interventions.

A patent airway is required. Management of the patient's fluid and electrolytes includes careful monitoring for hyponatremia, which can cause an increase in cerebral edema. Accurate intake and output measurements are imperative.

The nurse also monitors vital signs to avoid any significant change, especially in blood pressure. Hypotension must be treated immediately to prevent a drop in cerebral perfusion. Cardiac arrhythmias may be present, especially if there was bleeding into the subarachnoid space. Arrhythmias require prompt management because they may precipitate a drop in cardiac output and a consequent drop in cerebral perfusion.

A patent IV site is maintained for hydration. Continuous fluids are a part of the management of vasospasm. The IV site is monitored frequently and fluids are not interrupted for any reason. In the event of an infiltrate, the nurse restarts the line immediately.

Measures also need to be taken to manage increased ICP if it develops. Measures such as hyperventilation and osmotic diuretics are valuable tools in managing cerebral edema.

Emotional support is also a crucial part of the overall nursing care of the patient with a ruptured aneurysm. Because of an aneurysm's abrupt onset, the hospital admission cannot be planned. Often the rupture suddenly interrupts the patient's daily life and perhaps leaves the patient with neurological impairment. The patient's support system needs to be organized to tend to daily activities and responsibilities in the patient's absence. A social worker can be instrumental in helping to organize the support of friends and family.

PATIENT EDUCATION AND DISCHARGE PLANNING

Smoking and hypertension are both preventable risk factors associated with intracranial aneurysm and SAH. Patients can be instructed that cessation of smoking and control of hypertension can reduce the incidence of aneurysm formation and rupture.[54]

Patients who have undergone clipping of cerebral aneurysms should be carefully screened before MRI. Titanium clips used after 1996 are "MRI-friendly." It is necessary to ascertain the composition of the clip before MRI.

If a patient has experienced a seizure and is being maintained on anticonvulsant therapy, instructions should be given about medication monitoring and the need for compliance. In addition, the patient should be instructed about seizure safety.

Rehabilitation for specific deficits should begin early. Also, family participation in the rehabilitation plan should be encouraged. Members of the health care team, such as physical, occupational, and speech therapists, can help restore independence.[55] Services can be coordinated either for inpatient or outpatient settings, depending on the extent of impairment and insurance coverage.

case study ■ CEREBRAL ANEURYSM

Ms. A is a 32-year-old woman who collapsed while participating in a step-aerobics class. She clutched her head and fell to the floor. The Emergency Medical Services System was initiated, and she was taken to the local university hospital. Her admitting complaint was "the worst headache of my life" and photophobia. A CT scan revealed blood in the subarachnoid space. An angiogram confirmed the diagnosis of aneurysm.

She was admitted to the ICU, where her only deficit was mild right hemiparesis. She was started on nimodipine and taken to surgery 48 hours after admission. Twenty-four hours after surgery, she was transferred to an inpatient unit. During the night shift, the nurse noted that the patient's hemiparesis was increasing and she could not raise her right arm off the bed. The physician was notified, the patient was examined, and a stat CT scan was obtained to rule out a rebleed or hydrocephalus. TCD revealed vasospasm.

On admission to the ICU, triple H therapy was initiated in conjunction with nimodipine. By the next day, Ms. A's hemiparesis returned to baseline and she was transferred to the inpatient unit. After a 3-week hospitalization, she was transferred to an inpatient rehabilitation unit. ■

Arteriovenous Malformations

Arteriovenous malformations are congenital lesions consisting of dilated arteries and veins without a capillary system. Arterial blood flows directly into the venous system. Arteriovenous malformations are usually described as a "tangle" of blood vessels with a well-defined nidus that does not involve brain parenchyma. They typically enlarge with age. Although they are found throughout the CNS, approximately 90% of arteriovenous malformations are located in the cerebrum. Of these, the most common locations are the frontal and temporal lobes, most often supplied by the middle cerebral artery.[59]

EPIDEMIOLOGY

Arteriovenous malformations are relatively uncommon brain lesions. Population-based studies have estimated an occurrence rate of 1 per 100,000 persons. Autopsy studies, however, report a 1% to 4% occurrence rate.[60] There is not a statistically significant predisposition by sex, but they may occur slightly more frequently in men. The average age at diagnosis is 33 years, with 64% of arteriovenous malformations being detected in people younger than 40 years. In cases in which the patient has both an arteriovenous malformation and an aneurysm (7%), the symptomatic lesion is treated initially. In some instances, both can be surgically treated at the same time. Of the two, aneurysms are more likely to be the cause of hemorrhage.[61]

PATHOPHYSIOLOGY

Arteriovenous malformations develop as an atypical preservation of embryonic connections between arteries and veins, most likely between the fourth and eighth weeks of embryo development. This is the period in which cells begin to differentiate and capillary components to the brain develop. Arteriovenous malformations are most likely to arise at this time because of the failure of the primitive vasculature to develop an adequate capillary system. Because blood is shunted directly from the arterial to the venous circulation without benefit of a capillary bed, there is less resistance, and arteriovenous malformations receive significant blood flow. Arteries and veins enlarge to carry this increased flow, and their walls are characteristically quite thin. Arteries providing blood to the arteriovenous malformation and draining veins also become enlarged with increased flow volume in the lesion.[62]

CLINICAL MANIFESTATIONS

Hemorrhage occurs in 50% to 60% of patients with arteriovenous malformations. These hemorrhages may be subdural, intracerebral, or subarachnoid. There are differing opinions regarding whether the size of the lesion affects the likelihood of a bleed, but small size may be associated with an increased risk of hemorrhage, which may be caused by higher flow and pressure from the feeding vessels. The location of the arteriovenous malformation also affects the risk of a bleed. Periventricular, intraventricular, and posterior fossa lesions have a higher risk of a bleed.

There is an approximate 20% morbidity rate and 10% mortality rate after a bleed. The risk of a rebleed is higher in the first 2 years after the initial hemorrhage, and declines after 10 years.[60,61] Cerebral arteriovenous malformations cause approximately 4% to 5% of SAHs. An SAH caused by an arteriovenous malformation is less lethal than one caused by an aneurysm rupture, but is associated with significant neurological morbidity.[63]

Seizures are another common presenting sign of an arteriovenous malformation. The risk for a seizure increases with the size of the lesion. Patients are treated with antiepileptic drugs after presentation with a seizure, but antiepileptic drugs are not usually used prophylactically for arteriovenous malformations. Seizures are more likely to occur in patients who have large and more superficial arteriovenous malformations.

Other presenting signs include headache, increased ICP, neurological deficits referable to the location of the lesion, bruit, and visual symptoms. Cognitive decline is seen particularly in older patients with large arteriovenous malformations. This may be related to cerebral steal, which can cause ischemic changes by diverting arterial blood away from normal brain tissue to the arteriovenous malformation.[64]

Arteriovenous malformations may be graded based on features, location, and venous drainage. The Spetzler-Martin grading system assigns 1 point for lesions less than 3 cm, 2 points for 3- to 6-cm lesions, and 3 points for lesions greater than 6 cm. If the arteriovenous malformation is located in an eloquent area of the brain, it is given 1 point. No points are given for noneloquent areas. Deep venous drainage associated with the arteriovenous malformation is allotted 1 point, with no points for superficial venous drainage. A low score is associated with better outcomes and a higher score with increased morbidity from surgery.[65]

DIAGNOSIS

CT scanning and MRI are used to evaluate the presence of an arteriovenous malformation. The lesion is differentiated from tumors and other brain lesions by the presence of a hemosiderin ring around the lesion. Three-dimensional imaging is useful in establishing the malformation in relation to the surrounding anatomy. MRA is a noninvasive method of evaluating feeding and draining vessels in relation to the arteriovenous malformation nidus. Although it provides useful information, it is not consistently able to replace the more invasive angiography that is also used to evaluate feeding arteries and draining veins. Rarely, the arteriovenous malformation is not angiographically evident. This may be true of lesions that have bled, have small feeding and draining vessels, or low flow. TCD, single-photon emission computed tomography (SPECT), and PET are also used to image blood flow changes.[66]

CLINICAL MANAGEMENT

Arteriovenous malformations can be managed in a number of ways. Management decisions are based on the patient's age and medical condition, flow associated with the arteriovenous malformation, history of hemorrhage, other symptoms, and the location of the malformation.

Surgical Management

Surgery is the preferred treatment for most arteriovenous malformations. Surgery can reduce the risk of both hemorrhage and seizure. Stereotactic radiosurgery is used for relatively small lesions. Embolization with particles, liquids, balloons, or coils to the arteriovenous malformation nidus may be used to facilitate other therapies. Table 35-7 outlines procedures, indications, outcomes, and possible complications.[61,67,68]

Nursing Management

The nursing management of the patient with an arteriovenous malformation is similar to that described for a patient with a cerebral aneurysm. Baseline and follow-up neurological assessments are necessary to monitor for subtle changes or evidence of hemorrhage. Careful evaluation of focal neurological signs or evidence of cerebral edema minimizes significant postoperative morbidity.

PATIENT EDUCATION AND DISCHARGE PLANNING

Patients who have experienced a hemorrhage or seizures secondary to an arteriovenous malformation are managed in much the same way as patients with aneurysms. Safeguards and family teaching include a discussion of signs of increased ICP; seizure control, anticonvulsant therapy, and seizure safety; postoperative complications; and side effects of radiation, when appropriate.

Surgical Approaches

Neurological surgery may be performed in a number of situations:

1. To obtain tissue for pathological diagnosis
2. To remove an abnormal mass or space-occupying lesion and, consequently, to reduce mass effect (tumor, cyst, hemorrhage)
3. To repair an abnormality (e.g., aneurysm)
4. To place a device (e.g., shunt, reservoir)

A number of factors are considered when making the appropriate surgical decision. Diagnostic studies are first performed to establish a differential diagnosis. Patient age, neurological status, and concurrent medical conditions are factors in the decision to proceed with surgery and the decision regarding the appropriate approach. The most commonly used surgical procedures are briefly described in the following sections.

STEREOTACTIC BIOPSY

A stereotactic biopsy is used to obtain tissue for definitive pathological diagnosis. It is often used when a tumor is suspected but the lesion is too small or deep for surgical removal. It is usually used for tumors in eloquent areas of the brain, lesions crossing the corpus callosum, and multiple lesions that are not resectable. A stereotactic biopsy also

table 35-7 Management of Arteriovenous Malformations

Procedure	Indication	Outcome	Comments
Surgery	• Surgically accessible arteriovenous malformation (AVM)	• Removal of lesion • Decreased risk of bleed • Improved seizure control • Preoperative propranolol believed to minimize postoperative bleeding and edema • Labetalol used to keep mean arterial pressure (MAP) at 70–80 mm Hg perioperatively	• Inability to remove lesion • Risks of surgery: cerebral edema, hemorrhage, neurological deficits • Inpatient hospital stay
Radiation			
Stereotactic radiosurgery (SRS) (external beam radiation effective in only a small percentage of cases; gamma knife, proton beam, or linear accelerator is used)	• When surgery is not indicated	• Reduction in size of lesion • Noninvasive • Outpatient, no recovery period	• Lesion not removed • May take years for complete obliteration • May require multiple treatments • Continued risk of bleeding • Used for small AVMs only
Embolization	• Injection of substance to occlude the feeder vessels	• Facilitates other therapies (surgery, radiation) by reducing AVM • Useful for larger AVMs • Short hospital stay	• Does not typically cure AVM • May need more than one procedure • Need to wait days or weeks before surgery or SRS • Risk of stroke or hemorrhage

may be used to confirm the diagnosis of previously treated tumors—for example, when a malignant glioma has been treated with multiple therapies, tissue is obtained and analyzed to differentiate active tumor from treatment effect (i.e., necrosis). Also, some patients may have multiple medical problems and be too ill to proceed with a craniotomy. Others may opt to have the less invasive biopsy.

Before the biopsy, a rigid head frame is applied. Next, a contrast-enhanced CT scan or MRI is obtained by using the localizing frame. An axial image of the tumor is displayed, with a number of coordinates to indicate entry points. After the imaging is completed, the procedure can be performed in the radiology suite, or the patient may be taken to the operating room. The biopsy can be done under general or local anesthesia. After the skin is shaved and prepared, a small hole (twist drill or burr hole) is made, a needle is passed to the lesion, and one or more biopsies are obtained and immediately evaluated by a pathologist. Once sufficient tissue or cyst fluid is obtained for diagnostic purposes, the procedure is complete. Because of the possibility of sampling error, it is not unusual for the neurosurgeon to take multiple specimens from various areas of the tumor, when feasible.[69]

CRANIOTOMY

A craniotomy is performed to remove a space-occupying abnormality such as a tumor, cyst, or vascular malformation. This procedure may also be needed on an emergency basis to evacuate a hematoma or reverse a herniation syndrome. When appropriate, a craniotomy is also used to coil or clip an aneurysm.

In this procedure, a skin incision is made, the bone flap is elevated, dura is opened, and the tumor is subjected to biopsy or resection. The neurosurgical patient has quite distinct intraoperative pharmacological needs. The neuroanesthesiologist administers agents that provide the needed anesthetic effect while minimizing risks of increasing ICP or lowering seizure threshold. Rapid reversibility is also particularly important in patients receiving a craniotomy because their postoperative neurological status needs to be assessed quickly.

In addition to the equipment used during surgery to maximize safety and efficiency, there are specific tools for intraoperative monitoring that may enhance the outcome for these patients. Over the past 10 to 15 years, significant advances have taken place. Ultrasonography has been a standard of neurosurgical monitoring for some years because it can distinguish abnormal lesions from normal brain tissue and edema. Residual abnormal tissue may also be identified before closing.[70] Frameless stereotaxy is an intraoperative navigational system used to generate a three-dimensional tumor image. A CT scan or MRI is taken before surgery and markers (fiducials) are placed on the scalp. A computer image is then generated in the operating room from the imaging data. It is thought that this procedure enhances surgical safety and effectiveness by reducing craniotomy size, minimizing brain manipulation, and maximizing tumor resection.[71] Cortical mapping is used for masses in eloquent areas of the brain. Somatosensory evoked potentials (SSEPs) are recorded during surgery under general anesthesia to assess the relationship between the motor strip and the lesion to be resected. Direct cortical stimulation provides for localization of the sensory-motor cortex and is also used to minimize neurological deficits and maximize tumor removal. In some cases, greater seizure control is also accomplished with these procedures. Direct cortical stimulation requires local anesthesia and the patient to be conscious during much of the procedure.[72]

Craniotomies have been enhanced by the use of microscopes, operating loupes, self-retaining retractors, high-speed drills, ultrasonic aspirators (using sound waves), and laser (using light beams). Bipolar coagulation is used to minimize bleeding.[73] Endoscopic techniques are also used, particularly for colloid cysts and intraventricular and periventricular tumors, allowing for minimally invasive cyst and tumor removal. In these procedures, a burr hole is made and the dura opened. The endoscope is introduced to provide visualization of the lesion, and a port allows for aspiration or biopsy. In selected endoscopic cases, frameless stereotaxy is used to increase accuracy and minimize brain trauma.[74]

Postoperative management of the patient who has undergone a craniotomy or stereotactic biopsy for a brain tumor focuses on assessment of and intervention for a number of potential complications. In the immediate postoperative period, patients may be slow to respond because of the effects of general anesthesia. Temporary changes in mental status or new focal neurological signs should resolve rather quickly in this situation. If there is a significant change from the baseline examination, radiographic documentation of hemorrhage or cerebral edema is performed. A CT scan or MRI is obtained to rule out postoperative complications. Edema is expected, and can often be treated with corticosteroids. If significantly increased ICP occurs, the patient is medically managed in an intensive care environment under close observation. Occasionally, surgical intervention is required for acute postoperative hemorrhage.

TRANSSPHENOIDAL SURGERY

Transsphenoidal surgery is being used in many centers to remove pituitary tumors and cysts. The transnasal, transsphenoidal approach is replacing transcranial surgery, when appropriate. An estimated 75% to 95% of cases are performed in this manner.[75] The patient is positioned on the operating table under general anesthesia. The sphenoid sinus is opened, the sella is opened, and the tumor is removed using the surgical microscope. If there is evidence of CSF leak at the time of surgery, the sellar cavity is packed with fat tissue, typically taken from the patient's abdomen. The mucosal incision is closed with reabsorbable sutures. Nasal septal splints are applied.

This procedure is usually well tolerated. Postoperative care is aimed at increasing mobility, monitoring respiration, evaluating fluid and electrolyte balance, and observing for evidence of CSF leak. The major risks of intracranial surgery—cerebral edema and intracerebral hemorrhage—are avoided. Nasal splints are removed 2 to 4 days after surgery.[75]

NEUROLOGICAL DISORDERS

Cerebrovascular Disease

Cerebrovascular disease is the most frequent neurological disorder of adults. It is the third leading cause of morbidity and mortality in the United States after heart disease and cancer.[76] It includes any pathological process that involves the blood vessels of the brain. Most cerebrovascular disease is caused by thrombosis, embolism, or hemorrhage. The mechanism of each of these etiologies is different, but the ultimate result is damage to a focal area of the brain.

Stroke

Over the last several years, advances have been made in the treatment of stroke. Early recognition and prompt entry into the emergency medical system are essential to reduce death and disability from stroke. Media campaigns have been launched to increase public awareness about the signs and symptoms of stroke so that care may be sought promptly.

A stroke is now referred to as a "brain attack" to encourage health care professionals and the public to think about stroke with the same urgency as a "heart attack." A "brain attack" must be viewed as a medical emergency. To reverse cerebral ischemia, patients must be evaluated promptly. Ischemic brain injury occurs when arterial occlusion lasts longer than 2 to 3 hours. Delay in seeking medical care may eliminate the potential for tissue-saving therapy with thrombolytic agents.

According to the National Stroke Association, stroke is one of the leading causes of permanent disability in adults. Of long-term stroke survivors, 15% require institutional care, 30% are dependent in activities of daily living, and 60% have decreased socialization outside the home. The American Heart Association estimates that 15 to 20 billion dollars are spent annually on stroke and stroke-related disorders.[76]

A stroke may be defined as a neurological deficit that has a sudden onset, lasts more than 24 hours, and results from cerebrovascular disease. A stroke occurs when there is a disruption of blood flow to a region of the brain. Blood flow is disrupted because of an obstruction of a vessel, on account of a thrombus or embolus, or the rupture of a vessel. The clinical features seen depend on the location of the event and region of the brain the vessel perfused.[76]

ETIOLOGY

Approximately three-fourths of strokes are due to vascular obstruction (thrombi or emboli), resulting in ischemia and infarction. About one-fourth of strokes are hemorrhagic, resulting from hypertensive vascular disease (which causes an intracerebral hemorrhage), a ruptured aneurysm, or an arteriovenous malformation. Figure 35-7 outlines stroke classification.

EPIDEMIOLOGY

Approximately 750,000 strokes occur every year in the United States.[3] The incidence in men is greater than in women. It is estimated that there are 3 million stroke survivors and that stroke is a leading cause of disability and a leading diagnosis for long-term care.[76] Risk factors for stroke include smoking, hypertension, obesity, cardiac disease, hypercholesterolemia, diabetes, and use of birth control pills. Prevention efforts focus on lifestyle changes that can modify risk factors. In addition, the appropriate use of warfarin or aspirin in patients at risk for cardiac sources of emboli (e.g., atrial fibrillation) constitutes primary prevention.

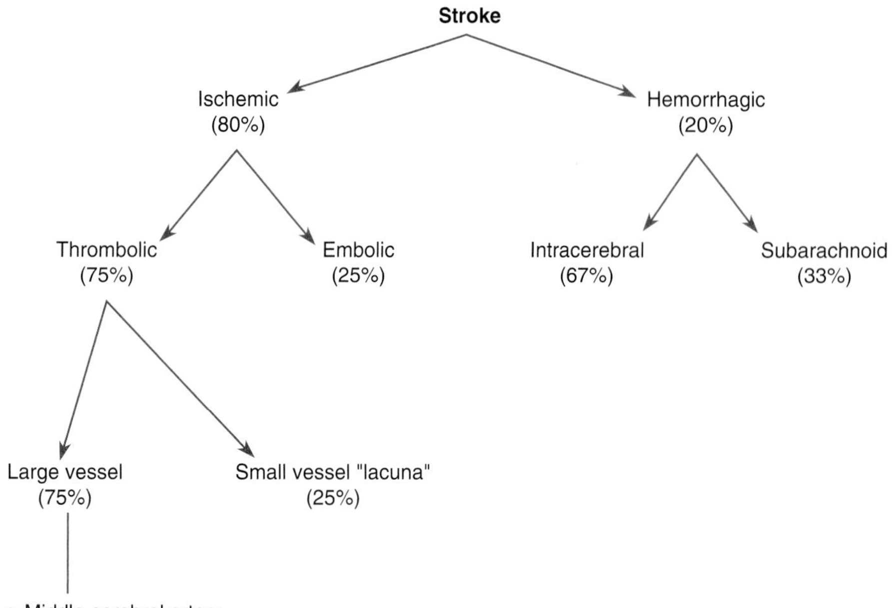

figure 35-7 Classification of stroke. (Courtesy of Eric Aldrich, MD, PhD, Johns Hopkins University, Baltimore, MD.)

PATHOPHYSIOLOGY

When blood flow to any part of the brain is impeded as a result of a thrombus or embolus, oxygen deprivation of the cerebral tissue begins. Deprivation for 1 minute can lead to reversible symptoms, such as loss of consciousness. Oxygen deprivation for longer periods can produce microscopic necrosis of the neurons. The necrotic area is then said to be *infarcted.*

The initial oxygen deprivation may be caused by general ischemia (from cardiac arrest or hypotension) or hypoxia from an anemic process or high altitude. If the neurons are ischemic only and have not yet necrosed, there is a chance to save them. This situation is analogous to the focal injury caused by a myocardial infarction. An occluded coronary artery can produce an area of infarcted (dead) tissue. Surrounding the infarcted zone is an area of ischemic tissue, which has been marginally deprived of oxygen. This ischemic tissue, as in the brain, may either be salvaged with appropriate treatment or killed by secondary events.

Cerebral ischemia is a complex process that depends on the severity and duration of the decline in cerebral blood flow. The ischemic cascade begins within seconds to minutes after perfusion failure, creating a zone of irreversible infarction and surrounding area of potentially salvageable "ischemic penumbra." The goal of acute stroke management is to salvage the ischemic penumbra, or the territory at risk. Without prompt intervention, the entire ischemic penumbra can eventually become an infarcted region.

A stroke caused by an embolus may be a result of blood clots, fragments of atheromatous plaques, lipids, or air. Emboli to the brain most often have a cardiac source, secondary to myocardial infarction or atrial fibrillation. If hemorrhage is the etiology of a stroke, hypertension often is a precipitating factor. Vascular abnormalities, such as arteriovenous malformations and cerebral aneurysms, are more prone to rupture and cause hemorrhage in the presence of hypertension.

The most frequent neurovascular syndrome seen in thrombotic and embolic strokes is due to involvement of the middle cerebral artery. This artery mainly supplies the lateral aspects of the cerebral hemisphere. Infarction to that area of the brain can cause contralateral motor and sensory deficits. If the infarcted hemisphere is dominant, speech problems result, and dysphasia may be present.

It is difficult to predict the amount of brain ischemia and infarction resulting from a thrombotic or embolic stroke. There is a possibility that the stroke will extend after the initial insult. There can be massive cerebral edema and an increase in ICP to the point of herniation and death after a huge thrombotic stroke. The area of the brain involved and the extent of the insult influence the prognosis. Because thrombotic strokes often are caused by atherosclerosis, there is risk of a future stroke in a patient who already has had one. With embolic strokes, patients also may have subsequent episodes of stroke if the underlying cause is not treated. If the extent of brain tissue destroyed from a hemorrhagic stroke is not excessive and is in a nonvital area, the patient may recover with minimal deficits. If the hemorrhage is large or in a vital area of the brain, the patient may not recover; however, if the intracerebral hemorrhage is less massive, survival is possible. For the purposes of this discussion, the focus is on the diagnosis and management of ischemic stroke.

CLINICAL MANIFESTATIONS

A stroke is usually characterized by the sudden onset of focal neurological impairment. The patient may experience signs such as weakness, numbness, visual changes, dysarthria, dysphagia, or aphasia. The manifestations of a stroke depend on the anatomical location of the lesion. Table 35-8 presents the correlation of blood supply to symptomatology in a brain attack.[77]

If symptoms resolve in less than 24 hours, the event is classified as a transient ischemic attack (TIA). Most TIAs last for only minutes to less than an hour, which further clouds recognition and prompt treatment. Furthermore, the differential diagnosis of stroke includes ruling out intracerebral hemorrhage, SAH, subdural or epidural hematoma, neoplasm, seizure, or migraine headache.[78]

DIAGNOSIS

Rapid diagnosis of a stroke is essential so that appropriate patients can receive thrombolytic therapy, the goal of which is to save damaged brain tissue and minimize permanent deficits. The patient should be taken to an emer-

table 35-8 Anterior and Posterior Blood Supply

Artery	Brain Structure	Signs/Symptoms of Occlusion
Anterior Blood Supply		
Anterior choroidal	Globus pallidus, lateral geniculate body, posterior limb of internal capsule, medial temporal lobe	Contralateral hemiplegia Hemihypesthesia Homonymous hemianopia
Ophthalmic	Orbit and optic nerve	Transient mononuclear blindness or complete unilateral blindness
Anterior cerebral	Anterior three-fourths of medial surface of cerebral hemispheres caudate nucleus, globus pallidus, and the internal capsule	Contralateral sensory and motor deficits greater in leg than arm Incontinence Deviation of the eyes and head toward the lesion Contralateral grasp reflex Abulic symptoms Arm apraxia Expressive aphasia (in dominant hemisphere occlusion) Motor or sensory aphasia (distal occlusion)
Middle cerebral	Cortical surfaces of the parietal, temporal, and frontal lobes Basal ganglia and internal capsule	Complete: Spatial neglect and homonymous hemianopia Global aphasia (left lesion) Superior trunk: Contralateral hemiplegia and hemianesthesia in face and arm Ipsilateral deviation of eyes and head Broca's aphasia (usually left-sided) Inferior trunk: Contralateral hemianopsia or upper quadrantanopia Wernicke's aphasia (left lesion) Left visual neglect (right lesion)
Posterior Blood Supply		
Vertebral	Anterolateral parts of the medulla	Contralateral impairment of pain and temperature sensation
Posterior cerebral	Occipital lobe, medial and inferior surface of temporal lobe, the midbrain, third and lateral ventricles	Contralateral hemiplegia, sensory loss, and ipsilateral visual field deficits
Posterior inferior cerebellar	Medulla and cerebellum	Medial branch: Vertigo, nystagmus, ataxia, persistent dizziness Lateral branch: Unilateral clumsiness with gait and limb ataxia Inability to stand Sudden falling Vertigo, dysarthria, oculomotor signs
Anterior inferior cerebellar	Cerebellum and pons	Horner's syndrome and contralateral loss of pain and temperature sense of the arm, trunk, and leg
Superior cerebellar	Upper part of cerebellum, midbrain	Slurred speech and contralateral loss of pain and thermal sensation
Basilar	Pons and midbrain	Limb paralysis, bulbar or pseudobulbar paralysis of cranial nerve motor nuclei, nystagmus, coma, or locked-in syndrome

Used with permission from Testani-Dufour L, Morrison CAM: Brain attack: Correlative anatomy. J Neurosci Nurs 29(1):213–224, 1997.

gency department where a neurologist can perform an initial screening and obtain appropriate neuroimaging studies. The time of symptom onset to administration of thrombolytic therapy (or "time to needle") should be within a 3-hour window. Emergency departments need to have services streamlined so that testing may be performed and treatment initiated promptly.

The patient's history helps determine what has happened to the individual. It is important to obtain a description of the neurological event; how long it lasted; and whether the symptoms are resolving, completely gone, or the same as at the time of onset. Identifying the type of symptoms can help determine and locate a possible vascular etiology. Determination of risk factors for stroke, such as hypertension, chronic atrial fibrillation, elevated serum cholesterol, smoking, oral contraceptive use, or a familial history of stroke, also aids in diagnosis.

In the emergency department, some of the tests that are frequently used to evaluate the patient with acute ischemic stroke are a CT scan of the brain without contrast, blood studies, neurological examination, and a screen performed using the National Institutes of Health Stroke Scale (NIHSS). This tool allows a score to be given for the severity of the stroke. Table 35-9 summarizes the NIHSS.[79]

table 35-9 National Institutes of Health Stroke Scale

1.a.	Level of consciousness (LOC)	Alert	0
		Drowsy	1
		Stuporous	2
		Coma	3
1.b.	LOC questions	Answers both correctly	0
		Answers one correctly	1
		Answers neither correctly	2
1.c.	LOC commands	Performs both correctly	0
		Performs one correctly	1
		Performs neither correctly	2
2.	Best gaze	Normal	0
		Partial gaze palsy	1
		Forced deviation	2
3.	Visual	No visual loss	0
		Partial hemianopia	1
		Complete hemianopia	2
		Bilateral hemianopia	3
4.	Facial palsy	Normal	0
		Minor paralysis	1
		Partial paralysis	2
		Complete paralysis	3
5.	Motor arm	No drift	0
		Drift	1
		Some effort against gravity	2
		No effort against gravity	3
		No movement	4
		Amputation, joint fusion explain:	9
6.	Motor leg	No drift	0
		Drift	1
		Some effort against gravity	2
		No effort against gravity	3
		No movement	4
		Amputation, joint fusion explain:	9
7.	Limb ataxia	Absent	0
		Present in one limb	1
		Present in two limbs	2
8.	Sensory	Normal	0
		Mild to moderate loss	1
		Severe to total loss	2
9.	Best language	No aphasia	0
		Mild to moderate	1
		Severe	2
		Mute	3

There is no definitive laboratory study that will determine if a patient has experienced a stroke. Rather, the studies are viewed in conjunction with the history, neurological examination, and results of neuroimaging studies. Laboratory studies, including complete blood cell count, electrolytes, glucose, and coagulation parameters, are obtained.[78]

An emergent CT scan should be performed to rule out intracerebral hemorrhage. Ideally, the CT scan is obtained within 60 minutes of arrival in the emergency department so that treatment decisions can be made. A CT scan can be useful in differentiating between cerebrovascular and nonvascular lesions. For example, a subdural hemorrhage, brain abscess, tumor, SAH, or intracerebral hemorrhage is visible on the CT scan. However, an area of infarction may not show on the CT scan for 48 hours.

Newer neuroimaging techniques also provide valuable information. T1- and T2-weighted, fluid-attenuated inversion recovery (FLAIR), diffusion-weighted, and perfusion-weighted MRI techniques have become widely available and are better at detecting infarction than a CT scan. The earliest changes normally appear within the first 24 hours. Using FLAIR, images can be manipulated so that only abnormal areas are hyperintense.

Another study that may be performed, based on availability of the technology, is diffusion-weighted imaging (DWI) and perfusion-weighted imaging (PWI). This technique helps identify the infarct core and penumbra, which is important because the presence of viable tissue directs interventions such as reperfusion. The ischemic penumbra surrounds the infarcted tissue. It is the marginally perfused area of the brain that has been damaged by the insult but is potentially salvageable. DWI detects acute infarction as early as a few hours after the onset of symptoms. It can reveal changes in infarcted tissue hours before a CT scan or MRI can detect any abnormality. It also discriminates acute from chronic ischemic changes. PWI looks at the region of cerebral blood flow. The difference between the diffusion defect and the perfusion defect represents the ischemic penumbra, or the "territory at risk." DWI-PWI identifies patients who are ideal candidates for thrombolytic therapy.[78,80]

Cerebral angiography has been the gold standard for evaluating cerebral vasculature. There is an estimated 1.5% to 2% associated risk of morbidity or mortality with this procedure. It can, however, demonstrate an arterial occlusion or embolus. Because of the time that it takes to perform cerebral angiography, the window of opportunity to treat a patient with thrombolytics may be missed. The vasculature can be evaluated noninvasively by the use of TCD, ultrasonography, MRA, or CT-A.

Also, an electrocardiogram (ECG) should be obtained to assess for evidence of arrhythmia or cardiac ischemia. The ECG helps determine if an arrhythmia is present, which may have caused the stroke. Atrial fibrillation is an arrhythmia in which clots form in the heart and may travel to the brain (hence a cardioembolic etiology). Other changes that might be found on an ECG are an inverted T wave, ST depression, and QT elevation and prolongation. Additional tests that can be done are transesophageal echocardiography (TEE) and Holter monitoring.

In summary, prompt performance and interpretation of a CT scan is crucial to acute stroke management. Head CT and TCD provide vital information and allow the physician to make the decision to use thrombolytic therapy. An alternate approach is urgent MRI with PWI and DWI.[80]

CLINICAL MANAGEMENT

The management of an ischemic stroke comprises four primary goals: restoration of cerebral blood flow (reperfusion), prevention of recurrent thrombosis, neuroprotection, and supportive care. The timing of each element of clinical management needs to be implemented in a decisive manner.

Optimally, patients are initially evaluated at a center that has a stroke program. Decisions in the emergency department determine the patient's treatment plan. Emergency departments may have emergi-paths, critical pathways, or protocols that have been developed by a multidisciplinary team to guide care.[81]

The focus of initial treatment should be to save as much of the ischemic area as possible. Three ingredients necessary to this area are oxygen, glucose, and adequate blood flow. The oxygen level can be monitored through arterial blood gases (ABGs), and oxygen can be given to the patient if indicated. Hypoglycemia can be evaluated with serial checks of blood glucose. Reperfusion may be accomplished by the use of IV tissue plasminogen activator (t-PA).

Cerebral perfusion pressure is a reflection of the systemic blood pressure, ICP, functioning autoregulation in the brain, and heart rate and rhythm. The parameters most easily controlled externally are the blood pressure and cardiac rate and rhythm. Arrhythmias usually can be corrected.

If the patient is a candidate for thrombolytic therapy, treatment with t-PA begins in the emergency department, and he or she is then moved to the ICU for further monitoring. If the individual is not a candidate for thrombolytic therapy, the complexity of the patient's problems determines his or her placement in the ICU, medical unit, or stroke specialty unit.

Pharmacological Management

Thrombolytic agents are exogenous drugs that dissolve clots. The U.S. Food and Drug Administration currently approves t-PA for stroke. Dissolving the clot permits reperfusion of the brain tissue. IV thrombolytic therapy should be initiated within 3 hours or less of the onset of neurological symptoms. The clock begins for the patient from the time he or she was last seen well. For example, a patient retires to bed at 11:00 P.M. and awakens at 5:00 A.M. to go to the bathroom. As he attempts to rise from the bed, he feels weak and has difficulty standing up. As he calls out for his wife's help, his speech is garbled. The last time he was awake and functioning normally was 11:00 P.M. Even if his symptoms started only a few minutes ago, the time he was last seen well was 6 hours ago. Therefore, he is already outside of the treatment window for IV t-PA.

Candidate selection for t-PA must be done carefully. The neurological examination, NIHSS score, and results of neuroimaging studies assist the physician with the decision to offer thrombolytic therapy. Box 35-2 outlines eligibility criteria for this treatment.[79] The standards for the administration of IV t-PA to treat stroke are a result of the National Institute of Neurologic Disorders and Stroke (NINDS)

box 35-2
Eligibility Criteria for Thrombolytic Therapy

Inclusion Criteria
1. Symptom onset of less than 3 hours
2. Clinical diagnosis of ischemic stroke with measurable deficit on the National Institutes of Health Stroke Scale (NIHSS)
3. Older than 38 years
4. Computed tomography (CT) criteria: absence of high-density lesion consistent with intracerebral hemorrhage; absence of significant mass effect or midline shift; absence of parenchymal hypodensity; or effacement of cerebral sulci in more than 33% of the middle cerebral artery territory

Exclusion Criteria
1. Stroke or serious head trauma within past 3 months
2. Systolic blood pressure (BP) more than 185 mm Hg or diastolic BP more than 110 mm Hg, or BP readings that require aggressive treatment
3. Conditions that could precipitate or suggest parenchymal bleeding (subarachnoid and intracerebral hemorrhage; recent-onset myocardial infarction; seizures at onset; major surgery within past 14 days; gastrointestinal or urinary tract hemorrhage within previous 21 days; and arterial puncture of a noncompressible site or lumbar puncture within previous 7 days)
4. Glucose less than 50 mg/dL or more than 400 mg/dL; international normalized ratio (INR) more than 1.7; platelet count less than 100,000/mm^3
5. Rapidly improving or deteriorating neurological signs or minor symptoms
6. Recent myocardial infarction
7. Recent treatment with IV or subcutaneous heparin within past 48 hours and elevated partial thromboplastin time (PTT)
8. Women of childbearing age who have a positive pregnancy test result

Used with permission from Hock NH: Brain attack: The stroke continuum. Nurs Clin North Am 34(3):718, 1999.

t-PA Stroke Study. A dose of IV t-PA, 0.9 mg/kg (maximum dose, 90 mg), is administered as 10% of the total dose as a bolus over 1 to 2 minutes, with the remainder infused over 60 minutes. The t-PA activates plasminogen, a naturally occurring enzyme present in the intravascular endothelium that protects against excessive clotting. Activating plasminogen initiates the process of dissolving the clot through fibrinolysis. No other antithrombotic therapy should be given for the next 24 hours. A major risk of this therapy is intracerebral hemorrhage. However, it is encouraging that this agent may prove effective in reversing neurological deficit and improving quality of life after a stroke.

The direct administration of a thrombolytic into a vessel is an alternative to IV t-PA. Such administration is effective in acute ischemic stroke and can be given up to 6 hours after the onset of symptoms. A limiting factor is that the patient must be admitted to a specialty center in which localized intra-arterial infusion of thrombolytic agents is possible. Through this approach, an occluded cerebral artery can be reopened. For intra-arterial therapy, a femoral arterial sheath is usually inserted, through which a microcatheter can be threaded, under fluoroscopy. The catheter tip is positioned into the clot and advanced as the clot dissolves. The femoral sheath usually remains in place for 24 hours in case of recurrent vessel occlusion. The advantage of this approach is that the medication can be delivered directly to its target.[78]

Aside from thrombolytic therapy, secondary treatment options for stroke include anticoagulation with antithrombotic and antiplatelet agents. If a patient experiences atrial fibrillation, anticoagulation with warfarin (Coumadin) may be warranted. The patient needs instruction about bleeding precautions, however. Education also includes the purpose of the medication, information about moderate consumption of leafy green vegetables containing vitamin K, and the importance of having blood drawn regularly to monitor prothrombin time (PT) and the international normalized ratio (INR). In addition, for safety, patients should be instructed to obtain Medic Alert cards and bracelets so they can be identified as taking an anticoagulant in the event of a medical emergency.

Antiplatelet drugs include dipyridamole-ER, ticlopidine, clopidogrel, and aspirin. These agents deter platelets from adhering to the wall of an injured blood vessel or other platelets and are given to prevent a future thrombotic or embolic event. The modified-release formula of dipyridamole increases the effect of specific factors that act as antiaggregates to reduce platelet aggregation. Ticlopidine inhibits platelet function by suppressing adenosine diphosphate–induced platelet aggregation and aggregation due to other factors. The recommended dose for ticlopidine is 250 mg twice a day. Neutropenia and thrombocytopenia are known side effects. Clopidogrel also inhibits the activity of adenosine diphosphate, but is not associated with an increased risk of neutropenia. Aspirin limits platelet adhesion and aggregation. The suggested dose of aspirin is 81 to 325 mg per day.[79] The administration of these agents plays a role in stroke prevention by decreasing the risk of future strokes.

Control of Hypertension and Increased Intracranial Pressure

The control of hypertension, ICP, and CPP may take the efforts of both the nurse and the physician. The nurse must assess for these problems, recognize them and their significance, and ensure that medical interventions are initiated.

Patients with moderate hypertension usually are not treated acutely. If their blood pressure decreases after the brain becomes accustomed to the hypertension needed for adequate perfusion, the brain's perfusion pressure will fall along with the blood pressure. If the diastolic blood pressure is above approximately 105 mm Hg, it may need to be lowered gradually. This may be accomplished effectively with labetalol.

If ICP is elevated in a patient who has had a stroke, it usually occurs after the first day. Although this is a natural response of the brain to some cerebrovascular lesions, it is destructive to the brain. The destructive response, such as edema or arterial vasospasm, can sometimes be treated or prevented. The usual methods of controlling increased ICP can be instituted: hyperventilation; fluid restriction; head elevation; avoidance of neck flexion or severe head rotation that would impede venous outflow from the head; and the use of osmotic diuretics (mannitol) to decrease cerebral edema (see Chapter 34 for more information).

Surgical Management

In patients with carotid stenosis, carotid endarterectomy may be performed to prevent a stroke. Carotid endarterectomy is a surgical procedure in which atherosclerotic plaque that has accumulated inside the carotid artery is surgically removed. Once the plaque is removed, blood flow is restored. This surgery has fallen in and out of favor during the last decade. The North American Symptomatic Carotid Endarterectomy Trial (NASCET) and the European Carotid Surgery Trial (ECST) were designed to examine the benefit of surgery for patients with symptomatic carotid stenosis. These studies determined that carotid endarterectomy is justifiable in patients with high-grade stenosis (≥70%) if the operation is performed by a skilled surgeon. The benefit of surgery increases for male patients with a prior history of stroke. Patients with less than 50% stenosis do not benefit from surgery.[82]

Nursing Management

Assessment. A thorough neurological assessment is essential to identify deficits the patient is experiencing. As previously discussed, the NIHSS is a valuable tool that can be used in the emergency department to rate severity of the stroke and determine if the individual is a candidate for t-PA (see Table 35-9). The brevity and reliability of the tool make it ideal for use in the emergency department. The NIHSS is also helpful for making subsequent assessments and should be performed in conjunction with the neurological examination.[8]

As a member of a large multidisciplinary team, the nurse must be prepared to assume a critical role to assist with the administration of thrombolytic therapy, optimize acute patient care, and move the patient to rehabilitation quickly to maximize the patient's outcome.[83] The patient needs to be carefully monitored for infection, changes in temperature, and changes in glucose level, all of which have potentially deleterious effects in patients who have had a stroke. The nurse is in the unique position to identify problems and collaborate with the physician to initiate appropriate referrals to rehabilitation medicine specialists, social workers, speech–language pathologists, or dietitians. Because of the nature of the patient's problems, the multidisciplinary approach provides comprehensive care by addressing all needs.

Plan. The nurse plays a significant role in preventing complications associated with immobility, hemiparesis, or any neurological deficit produced by a stroke. Preventive measures are particularly important in the areas of urinary tract infections, aspiration, pressure ulcers, contractures, and thrombophlebitis. Effective interventions for the treatment of acute stroke help lower the death rate and reduce the morbidity of patients who have had a stroke. The Collaborative Care Guide (Box 35-3) delineates the specific outcomes and interventions for the patient who has had a stroke.[79,84]

Emotional and Behavioral Modification. Patients who have experienced a stroke may display emotional problems, and their behavior may be different from baseline. Emotions may be labile; for example, the patient may cry one moment and laugh the next, without explanation or control. Tolerance to stress may also be reduced. A minor stressor in the prestroke state may be perceived as a major problem after the stroke. Families may not understand the behavior. Patients may show frustration or agitation with the nursing staff or their family members.

It is the nurse's role to help the family understand these behavioral changes. Also, the nurse can help modify the patient's behavior by controlling stimuli in the environment, providing rest periods throughout the day to prevent the patient from becoming overtired, giving positive feedback, and providing repetition when the patient is trying to relearn a skill.

Communication. Patients can demonstrate much frustration with their deficits. Probably no deficit produces more frustration for the patient and those trying to communicate with him or her than the one involving the production and understanding of language. Dysphasia can involve motor abilities, sensory function, or both. If the area of brain injury is in or near the left Broca's area, the memory of motor patterns of speech is affected. This results in an expressive dysphasia, in which the patient understands language but is unable to use it appropriately.

Receptive dysphasia usually is a result of injury to the left Wernicke's area, which is the control center for recognition of spoken language. The patient therefore is unable to understand the significance of the spoken word. The presence of both expressive and receptive dysphasia is referred to as *global dysphasia.* Box 35-4 summarizes differences between expressive and receptive problems.

It is important for the nursing staff to inform families that having dysphasia does not mean that a person is intellectually impaired. Communication at some level should be attempted, whether it is by writing, using picture boards, or gestures.

PATIENT EDUCATION AND DISCHARGE PLANNING

Education must provide information to patients about modifying risk factors and teach individuals to recognize the signs and symptoms of a stroke. Information can be presented regarding medication and other lifestyle modifications to manage blood pressure. Patients can be referred to smoking cessation programs. Education can also be provided about weight management and exercise programs. Compliance with medication regimens should also be stressed.

Hospitals need to organize community outreach programs regarding stroke prevention, the recognition of signs and symptoms of a stroke, its emergent nature, and the need to contact 911 at the onset of symptoms. There must be public awareness about the signs and symptoms, such as sudden onset of numbness or weakness of the face, arm, or leg; confusion; trouble speaking or understanding; vision problems; dizziness; loss of balance; or severe

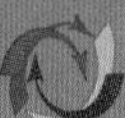

box 35-3 collaborative care guide *for the Patient Who Has Had a Stroke*

OUTCOMES	INTERVENTIONS
Neurological	
Patient will maintain adequate cerebral perfusion pressure.	■ Obtain vital signs and perform a neurological assessment to establish a baseline and to monitor for the development of additional deficits. ■ Use NIHSS for detection of early changes suggesting edema or extension of stroke. ■ Position head of bed at 30 degrees to promote venous return. ■ Implement DVT precautions to include TEDs and sequential compression devices.
Patient will not develop complications of immobility.	■ Assess for neglect. ■ Provide active or passive range of motion to all extremities every shift. ■ Establish splinting routine to affected extremities. ■ Monitor daily blood glucose. ■ Instruct in mobility aids; instruct in strategies of fall prevention.
Patient will establish an effective method of communication.	■ Assess ability to speak and to follow simple commands. ■ Arrange for consultation with speech language pathologist to differentiate language disturbances. ■ Use communication aids such as picture cards and pantomine to enhance communication. ■ Provide a calm, unrushed environment. Listen attentively to the patient. Speak in a normal tone.
Respiratory	
Patient will maintain adequate airway. Patient will maintain oxygen saturation (Spo_2) within normal limits. Atelectasis will be prevented.	■ Monitor breath sounds every shift. ■ Check oxygen saturation every shift. ■ Instruct to cough and deep breathe and incentive spirometry every 2 hours while awake. ■ Assist with removal of airway secretions as needed. Be certain to preoxygenate before suctioning.
Gastrointestinal	
Patient will receive adequate caloric intake and will not experience decrease in weight from baseline. Patient will be free from aspiration.	■ Obtain admission weight. ■ Perform cranial nerve assessment (including ability to swallow) to identify deficits. ■ Obtain consultation from speech–language pathologist to see if patient is safe to eat orally. ■ Provide proper diet and assist with feeding as needed. ■ Monitor caloric intake; implement calorie count if necessary. ■ Obtain dietary consultation to obtain recommendation for supplements.

(continued)

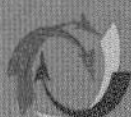

box 35-3 collaborative care guide
for the Patient Who Has Had a Stroke (Continued)

OUTCOMES	INTERVENTIONS
Genitourinary The patient will achieve urinary continence.	■ Perform assessment of usual patterns and habits. ■ Establish a toileting schedule using a bedpan, urinal, or bedside commode. ■ Monitor for the development of urinary retention or urinary tract infection. ■ Use bladder scanner to evaluate contents of bladder. ■ Avoid use of indwelling catheter to prevent infection.
Cardiovascular Patient will not experience any arrhythmias	■ Monitor vital signs closely. ■ Manage blood pressure carefully; avoid sharp drops in blood pressure that could result in hypotension and cause an ischemic event secondary to hypotension. ■ During cardiac monitoring phase, identify arrhythmias. ■ Treat arrhythmias to maintain adequate cerebral perfusion pressure and reduce chance of neurological impairment.

headache. The urgency of immediate attention must be stressed. Emergency medical personnel need to be able to identify the symptoms of a stroke and mobilize the patient to the nearest hospital with a full complement of stroke services from diagnosis to discharge.[81]

In addition, a stroke is often a life-changing experience for the patient and family. Depending on the outcome, family members may require education about how to provide care for the patient at home. Instruction about mobility, nutrition, safety, sleep, and eliminative care must occur, along with referrals for home care, if appropriate. With support, the patient will be able to achieve maximum quality of life and reintegrate into the community.

Seizures

A seizure is an episode of abnormal and excessive discharge of cerebral neurons. It can result in sensory, motor, or behavioral activities, and can be associated with changes in the level of consciousness. The specific symptoms depend on the location of the discharge in the brain. The most common sites of seizure origin are the frontal and temporal lobes and the hippocampus. Some seizures are so mild that only the patient is aware of them. Others are quite severe. The actual period of the seizure (ictal) may be followed by a postictal phase of lethargy and disorientation.

Epilepsy is a condition in which seizures are recurrent. Status epilepticus is defined as a condition of either contin-

box 35-4
Comparison of Expressive and Receptive Dysphasia

Expressive Dysphasia	Receptive Dysphasia
Hemiparesis is present because motor cortex is near Broca's area.	Hemiparesis is mild or absent because lesion is not near motor cortex. Hemianopsia or quadrantanopsia may be present.
Speech is slow, nonfluent; articulation is poor; speaking requires much effort. Total speech is reduced in quantity. Patient may use telegraphic speech, omitting small words.	Speech is fluent; articulation and rhythm are normal. Content of speech is impaired; wrong words are used.
Patient understands written and verbal speech.	Patient does not understand written and verbal speech.
Patient writes dysphasically.	Content of writing is abnormal. Penmanship may be good.
Patient may be able to repeat single words with effort. Phrase repetition is poor.	Repetition is poor.
Object naming is often poor, but it may be better than attempts to use spontaneous speech.	Object naming is poor.
Patient is aware of deficit, often experiencing frustration and depression.	Patient is often unaware of deficit.
Curses or other ejaculatory speech may be well articulated and automatic. Patient may be able to hum normally.	Patient may use wrong words and sounds.

ued seizure activity or repetitive seizures without interictal recovery, over a period of greater than 30 minutes. The symptoms may be associated with tonic-clonic, complex-partial, or absence seizures. It is a neurological emergency and requires immediate treatment.[85–87]

Pseudoseizures are nonepileptic events that may involve either motor activity or physical collapse. They can often be differentiated from epilepsy because they may involve asymmetrical motor activity, side-to-side head movements, and purposeful activity. They also may be gradual in onset. The motor activity may last for many minutes, unlike epilepsy. There is usually a brief or no "postictal" phase. Patients are likely to have either emotional or psychological disorders, and may require antidepressants, counseling, and psychiatric intervention. Pseudoseizures are more often seen in women and in adolescents and young adults. In some cases, the patient also suffers from true epilepsy. Childhood abuse is not uncommon in these patients.[88]

ETIOLOGY

Seizures may be idiopathic (primary), having no specific underlying cause, or symptomatic (secondary), having a known etiology.

Idiopathic seizures are common, accounting for more than 60% of all epilepsy. They occur most often in children younger than 10 years. Congenital and genetic causes of epilepsy are seen in approximately 10% of the population. Although inherited epilepsy is more often idiopathic, it is also associated with other conditions.

Symptomatic seizures have numerous etiologies, including vascular disease, alcohol, cerebral tumors, trauma, infection or fever, anoxia, and degenerative diseases.

A number of other variables affect seizure frequency and intensity. Fatigue and sleep deprivation may lower one's seizure threshold. Emotional and physical stress correlate with seizure onset, but are difficult to quantify. Many women who keep records of seizure activity discover that they are cyclic, occurring more frequently or increasing in severity during menstruation. Alcohol and drug abuse as well as electrolyte disturbances cause seizures, as well as intensifying already present epilepsy. Many medications have the effect of lowering seizure threshold.[89]

Status epilepticus is typically associated with drug withdrawal, metabolic disturbances, or concurrent illness in patients with known epilepsy. Common causes of new-onset status epilepticus are cerebrovascular disease, brain tumors, intracranial infections, fevers, head trauma, and metabolic disorders.[85–87]

EPIDEMIOLOGY

Three to 5% of the population experiences epilepsy. Infants and young children are most likely to experience seizures, followed in frequency by the elderly. Populations in undeveloped countries are at greater risk for development of seizures or epilepsy. This is likely because of compromised hygiene, poor nutrition, increased risk of infection, and the high percentage of children. Single seizures are much less common than epilepsy (20 per 100,000 and 50 per 100,000, respectively). Partial seizures that generalize are quite common (60%), followed by generalized seizures alone (20%), and partial seizures alone (10%). Medical treatment is effective in approximately 80% of cases.[89]

PATHOPHYSIOLOGY

Nerve cells (neurons) in the brain possess an electrical charge that reflects a balance between intracellular and extracellular components. The electrical activity of the neuronal membrane is determined by the flow of ions between these spaces. Ions such as sodium (Na^+), potassium (K^+), calcium (Ca^{2+}), and chloride (Cl^-) flow across the membrane in relationship to large, negatively charged molecules (anions) that remain inside the cell. If the permeability of these cells is altered, their excitability can change, making the neuron more likely to discharge. Hyperexcitability can result in increased random firing. When this is combined with a certain pattern of neuronal firing (synchronization), epileptogenic properties in the neuron exist.

Although it is not known exactly how the mechanisms of abnormal neuronal excitation and synchronization lead to epileptiform activity, continued exploration of cell membrane activity, environmental variables, and pharmacological responses have led to increased understanding and management of epilepsy.[90]

CLINICAL MANIFESTATIONS

The features of epilepsy are based on the location of the epileptiform discharge and the type of event. Box 35-5

box 35-5
Classification of Seizures

Generalized

Involve both hemispheres; loss of consciousness; no local onset in the cerebrum

- Tonic-clonic (grand mal)—loss of consciousness; stiffening; forced expiration (cry); rhythmic jerking
- Clonic—symmetrical, bilateral semirhythmic jerking
- Tonic—sudden increased tone and forced expiration
- Myoclonic—sudden, brief body jerks
- Atonic ("drop attacks")—sudden loss of tone; falls
- Absence (petit mal)—brief staring, usually without motor involvement

Partial

Focal; involve one hemisphere

Simple partial—no change in level of consciousness

- Motor (Jacksonian)
- Sensory (special sensory or somatosensory, e.g., visual, auditory, olfactory, epigastric)
- Autonomic (e.g., respiratory changes, flushing, tachycardia)
- Psychic (e.g., déjà vu, fear)

Complex partial—altered level of consciousness; with or without automatisms: lip-smacking, swallowing, aimless walking, verbalizations

- Simple partial followed by change in level of consciousness
- Starts with change in consciousness

Partial with secondary generalization

- Simple partial → generalization
- Complex partial → generalization
- Simple partial → complex partial → generalization

Unclassified Epileptic Seizures

provides a description of specific seizures and resulting clinical characteristics.[91]

DIAGNOSIS

The patient who presents with a seizure is initially evaluated to ascertain the cause of the seizure and establish a diagnosis of epilepsy. History taking begins with a description of the event by the patient or witnesses. This description should include:

- What the patient was doing at the time of the seizure
- Duration of the episode
- Unusual symptoms or behaviors before the seizure
- Specific features, including movements, sensations, sounds, tastes, smells, and incontinence
- Level of consciousness during and after the event
- Duration and description of symptoms after the seizure
- Reporting of any similar previous episodes and age of onset

Inquiry should be made of:

- Sleep patterns
- Alcohol or drug abuse
- History of illnesses or injuries
- Family seizure history
- Other possible variables: menstrual cycle, stress, fevers, metabolic disorders
- If other seizures have occurred, similarities in symptoms, duration, frequency, and time of day

After the first seizure occurrence, a CT scan or MRI is taken to assess for a structural lesion. An EEG is obtained to measure cerebral excitability. Scalp electrodes are placed to measure neuronal membrane activity in the underlying cerebral cortex. Rhythms may be obtained when the patient is both awake and asleep. The EEG localizes the region from which the patient's seizure arises at one time point. If additional information is needed regarding seizure patterns and characteristics, an inpatient hospital stay may be recommended in an epilepsy monitoring unit, as discussed in the following section.

Other diagnostic studies that may be obtained include PET to evaluate hypometabolic states that correlate with the epileptogenic area; SPECT to identify cerebral blood flow and perfusion differences during and after a seizure[92]; bilateral carotid amobarbital (Amytal) testing to assess speech dominance and memory; fMRI to localize seizure focus and identify its relationship to a structural lesion; and neurocognitive testing to obtain a baseline evaluation.[93]

Epilepsy Monitoring Unit

Patients who require more detailed EEG monitoring are admitted to an appropriate unit where scalp electrodes are placed. Monitoring is continuous and involves audiovisual observations. Monitoring takes place while the patient is awake and asleep. Medications may be tapered or withdrawn during these observations. Because video EEG monitoring captures ictal, postictal, and interictal data, seizures are localized, seizure activity is documented, and the patient's clinical symptoms are observed.

In situations in which localization is not obtained or is questionable, a more invasive approach may be necessary. Three different types of electrodes can be surgically implanted for intracranial recording.

Depth electrodes are typically placed bilaterally, in the hippocampus. Multiple electrodes are placed under local or general anesthesia through twist drill or burr holes for simultaneous recording. The patient is awake for the actual electrode placement, so that neurological status is constantly observed. The electrodes are attached to the scalp or bone for continuous monitoring over the next few days in the epilepsy monitoring unit. Hemorrhage, headache, and infection are possible complications. This procedure is most often used to confirm, rather than localize, seizure focus.

Subdural and epidural electrodes are typically placed unilaterally, under general anesthesia. Strips are placed through burr holes. Grids require a craniotomy, and allow for a larger region to be monitored (Fig. 35-8). They are secured to the dura, and the electrode leads exit through an incision for continuous monitoring. Infection, hemorrhage, and mass effect from cerebral edema are possible risks. Bone flap may be replaced at the end of the procedure or after the strips or grids are removed. Intracranial monitoring may be initiated before seizure surgery.[94]

CLINICAL MANAGEMENT

Pharmacological Management

In most cases, the patient with epilepsy can be medically treated. Some medications are known to be more appropriate for specific classes of seizures. Certain drugs are found most useful in the pediatric patient population. Some antiepileptic drugs are preferred as monotherapy, and others are more appropriate as adjunctive therapy with other drugs. Table 35-10 describes current antiepileptic drugs with general indications, doses, common side effects, and nursing considerations.[95]

Status epilepticus is an emergency situation and requires rapid pharmacological management. Parenteral drugs are given to provide fast drug absorption. Drugs are given IV,

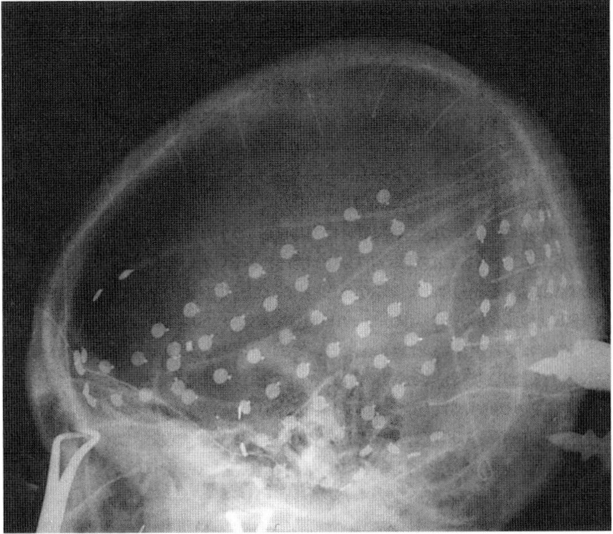

figure 35-8 Radiograph of a grid for seizure monitoring. (Courtesy of Frederick Lenz, MD, and Ira Garonzik, MD, Johns Hopkins University, Baltimore, MD.)

table 35-10 ■ Current Antiepileptic Drugs

Agent	Indications	Usual Dose	Common Adverse Effects	Comments
Carbamazepine (Tegretol)	Mono/adjunctive therapy Partial and generalized seizures	400–2000 mg	Drowsiness, fatigue, dizziness, blurred vision, rash, hyponatremia, bone marrow dyscrasia	Interactions with other AEDs; rare aplastic anemia, hepatic failure; obtain blood levels
Clobazam (Frisium)	Adjunctive therapy Partial and generalized seizures	10–30 mg	Drowsiness, fatigue, dizziness, blurred vision	Benzodiazepine; used as second-line therapy for resistance to other AEDs
Clonazepam (Klonopin)	Adjunctive therapy Partial and generalized seizures	0.5–4 mg	Sedation, cognitive, ataxia, behavior changes, leukopenia	Helpful in children with severe epilepsy
Ethosuximide (Zarontin)	Mono/adjunctive therapy Absence seizures	500–1500 mg	Nausea, somnolence	Levels affected by other AEDs
Felbamate (Felbatol)	Mono/adjunctive therapy Partial or secondary generalized seizures	1200–3600 mg	Nausea, anorexia, headache, insomnia	Effective in severe, resistant epilepsy; affects other AEDs; aplastic anemia (FDA alert); liver failure
Gabapentine (Neurontin)	Adjunctive therapy Partial and secondary generalized seizures	900–3600 mg	Sedation, dizziness, weight gain	No significant drug interactions; minimal side effects
Lamotrigine (Lamictal)	Mono/adjunctive therapy Partial and generalized seizures	200–700 mg	Rash	Affected by other AEDs
Levetiracetam (Keppra)	Adjunctive therapy for partial seizures	Begin with 250–500 mg bid Increase to 2000 mg, then 3000 mg	Somnolence, asthenia, irritability, dizziness, infection	
Oxcarbazepine (Trileptal)	Mono/adjunctive therapy Partial and secondary generalized seizures	1200–2400 mg	Cognitive, headaches, somnolence, dizziness, rash, hyponatremia	Increase dose over several weeks
Phenobarbital	Mono/adjunctive therapy Partial or generalized seizures (myoclonus/absence)	100 mg	Sedation, depression, ataxia, rash, impotence, hyperactivity	Potential CNS toxicity, especially in children; taper slowly
Phenytoin (Dilantin)	Mono/adjunctive therapy Partial and generalized seizures (not absence/myoclonus)	200–600 mg	Ataxia, dizziness, sedation, rash, gum hyperplasia	Interactions with multiple other drugs; dose guided by blood levels; less expensive
Primidone (Mysoline)	Adjunctive therapy Partial and secondary generalized seizures	500–1500 mg	Dizziness, nausea, those seen with phenobarbital	Converted to phenobarbital in the body
Tiagabine (Gabitril)	Adjunctive therapy Partial seizures	32–56 mg	Fatigue, somnolence, dizziness, incoordination	Promising for refractory partial seizures
Topiramate (Topomax)	Adjunctive therapy Partial and generalized seizures	400 mg	Cognitive, somnolence, dizziness, tremor, anorexia, paresthesias, kidney stones	Highly effective; titrate up very slowly; daily dose divided
Valproate (Depakote)	Mono/adjunctive therapy Generalized seizures; childhood epilepsy; febrile convulsions	750–4000 mg	Nausea, weight gain, endocrine, thrombocytopenia, hair loss	Interactions with other AEDs

(continued)

table 35-10 ■ Current Antiepileptic Drugs (Continued)

Agent	Indications	Usual Dose	Common Adverse Effects	Comments
Vigabatrin (Sabril)	Adjunctive therapy Partial and secondary generalized seizures	1000–3000 mg	Somnolence, dizziness, headache, mood changes, visual field changes, weight gain	Effective; use limited by neuropsychiatric and visual symptoms
Zonisamide (Zonegran)	Adjunctive therapy Partial seizures; myoclonic epilepsy	400–600 mg	Cognitive, psychiatric, somnolence, fatigue, kidney stones, rash	Does not affect other AEDs

AEDs, antiepileptic drugs.

intramuscularly, or rectally. Many fast-acting drugs are lipid soluble and have a tendency to redistribute from the plasma to the fat and muscle, thereby leading to an initial drop in blood and brain concentrations. This may lead to recurrence of seizures. The administration of repeat boluses or a continuous infusion must be done judiciously because the drugs saturate fat, and muscle and plasma levels will increase. This may result in prolonged decreased mental status, obtundation, and even death. Emergency management of status epilepticus is summarized in Box 35-6[86,87] and Figure 35-9.[85]

Surgical Management

There are situations in which antiepileptic drugs are unable to control epilepsy. Attempts at monotherapy and adjunctive therapy have been exhausted and multiple drug regimens have failed; seizure activity has compromised a patient's quality of life. In these cases, seizures are considered intractable. Surgery to obtain seizure control is considered in these situations. It may also be considered in situations in which the side effects of therapy are so debilitating that the patient is unable to function at an acceptable capacity.

In many cases, the patient is monitored before surgery in an epilepsy monitoring unit using a video EEG. Grid or strip placement to localize seizure focus and identify functional areas is often used. After surgery, the nurse performs regular, intermittent neurological examinations and has the patient attempt to perform certain tasks. Language deficits and motor weakness are observed. The goals of this procedure are to localize epileptiform discharges in relation to speech, memory, and sensory and motor function. It is also useful in identifying the relationship between seizure discharges and a focal lesion, such as a tumor, when present. This enhances the safety and accuracy of tumor surgery.

The decision to proceed with surgery depends on a thorough discussion among the multidisciplinary team members. The neurologist, neurosurgeon, patient, and family review the medical treatment used to date and establish that therapy has been maximized. They evaluate the likelihood of seizure control with surgery. Preoperative neuropsychological testing is obtained. The appropriate testing is established and discussed. Some or all of the diagnostic studies previously outlined may be indicated.

The goal of seizure surgery is to remove or disrupt the seizure focus. Table 35-11 summarizes the most commonly performed surgical procedures, along with expected outcomes, possible complications, and nursing considerations.[85,96–100]

Nursing Management

Careful history taking is a central component to the accurate diagnosis and management of epilepsy. Family history, age at onset, frequency, and a description of symptoms and their duration all aid in the development of a plan of care tailored to the patient's particular situation. Antiepileptic drugs are prescribed based on all of these data.

box 35-6
Emergency Management of Status Epilepticus

- **Blood tests:** Anticonvulsant levels; blood gases; electrolytes; complete blood count; renal and liver functions; coagulation studies. Correct severe hypoglycemia, hyperkalemia, hyponatremia
- **Electroencephalogram (EEG)**
- **Appropriate intravenous fluids**
- **Neurological evaluations**
- **Vital signs**
- **Parenteral drug treatment:** Should begin as early as possible; if patient is at home, emergency personnel should administer before hospital transfer. There is considerable variation in emergency drug treatment regimens. Figure 35-9 outlines one example.
- **Metabolic abnormalities:** May require bicarbonate for acidosis; use cautiously to prevent cerebral or pulmonary edema
- **Hypotension:** Electrocardiogram (ECG) and medical management
- **Respiratory compromise:** May require intubation and ventilatory support
- **Rhabdomyolysis:** Muscle breakdown, particularly with motor seizures, can lead to myoglobinuria, renal failure, and hyperkalemia; correct electrolyte disturbances; monitor urine output and color; may need to use mannitol and dopamine
- **Hepatic failure:** May be caused by reactions to antiepileptic therapy
- **Establish and treat cause of status:** May need to obtain brain computed tomography (CT) scan or lumbar puncture
- **Intensive care and seizure monitoring:** EEG; intra-arterial blood pressure monitoring; oximetry; central venous pressure (CVP) monitoring; monitoring of elevated intracranial pressure (ICP)

Premonitory stage
Diazepam 10 mg IV (given over 2–5 min) or rectally, repeated once 15 min later if status continues to threaten
or
Lorazepam 4 mg IV bolus
↓
If seizures continue or status develops

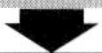

Stage of early status
Lorazepam 4 mg IV bolus (if not given earlier)
↓
If status continues after 30 min

Stage of established status
Phenobarbital IV infusion of 10 mg/kg at a rate of 100 mg/min (i.e., about 700 mg in an average adult over 7 min)
or
Phenytoin IV infusion of 15 mg/kg at a rate of 50 mg/min (i.e., about 1000 mg in an average adult over 20 min)
or
Fosphenytoin IV infusion of 15 mg PE/kg at a rate of 100 mg PE/min (i.e., about 1000 mg PE in an average adult over 10 min)
↓
If status continues after 30–60 min

Stage of refractory status
General anesthesia with either:
Propofol 2 mg/kg IV bolus, repeated if necessary, and then followed by a continuous infusion of 5–10 mg/kg/h initially, reducing to 1–3 mg/kg/h. When seizures have been controlled for 12 h, the drug dosages should be slowly tapered over 12 h
or
Thiopental: 100–250 mg IV bolus given over 20 s, with further 50 mg boluses every 2–3 min until seizures are controlled, followed by a continuous IV infusion to maintain a burst suppression pattern on the EEG (usually 3–5 mg/kg/h).
Thiopental should be slowly withdrawn 12 h after the last seizure

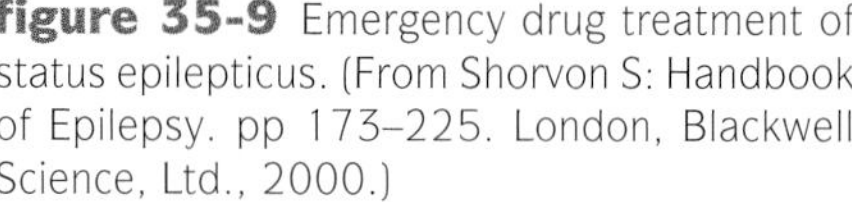

figure 35-9 Emergency drug treatment of status epilepticus. (From Shorvon S: Handbook of Epilepsy. pp 173–225. London, Blackwell Science, Ltd., 2000.)

Changes in severity or frequency of symptoms require modification of the treatment regimen. Drug therapy may last indefinitely; therefore, treatment should address both efficacy and tolerability. Side effects can compromise quality of life, necessitating the use of different, and possibly less effective, medications or multiple antiepileptic drugs.

Inpatient nursing care includes monitoring the patient during the seizure (the patient is never left alone) and providing support and protection without attempting to restrain the individual. Turning the patient to his or her side during a generalized seizure, if possible, helps maintain a patent airway.

PATIENT EDUCATION AND DISCHARGE PLANNING

Patient education should provide instructions for independent functioning. The following patient education points are critical parts of discharge planning:

- Make the home environment safe, particularly in the case of tonic-clonic epilepsy.
- Assess for injury after each seizure.
- Keep a log to record a description of the seizure and postictal period, duration, time of day, severity, and any new characteristics.
- Know the specifics of a ketogenic (high-fat, low-carbohydrate) diet, when appropriate, for children with intractable seizures.
- Be aware of state laws on driving restrictions related to epilepsy.
- Wear a Medic Alert bracelet.
- Monitor serum antiepileptic drug levels when appropriate.
- Be aware of circumstances when emergency treatment is required.
- Consult seizure experts for intractable epilepsy.

Guillain-Barré Syndrome

Guillain-Barré syndrome is thought to be an inflammatory peripheral neuropathy in which lymphocytes and macrophages strip myelin from axons. The diffuse inflammatory reaction may be seen in the peripheral nervous

table 35-11 Indications for and Outcomes of Seizure Surgery

Procedure	Indications	Expected Outcomes	Possible Complications	Nursing Considerations
Temporal lobectomy: Removal of 6 cm of temporal lobe in the nondominant hemisphere and 4–5 cm in the dominant hemisphere	• Intractable seizures • Greater than 5 years' duration • Significant quality of life compromise	• 60%–70% seizure free • 20% greatly improved seizure control	• Visual (superior quadrantanopsia) field defects • Dysphasia (usually temporary) • Mild memory problems • Depression • Transient psychiatric disturbance • Infection or bleeding	• At 1 year after surgery, it is expected that seizure status will not change • Medication management continues for 2–3 years after surgery
Hemispherectomy: Surgical removal (or disconnection) of a hemisphere in children and adolescents	• Severe seizures • Often multiple seizure types and daily seizures	• 90%–95% improvement in seizure activity • 70%–85% resolution of seizures	• Chronic bleeding into surgical cavity; neurological disability and death; late hydrocephalus	• Careful patient selection required • May see improved behavior and social development
Corpus callosectomy: Transection of the corpus callosum	• Cases of severe secondary generalized epilepsy; drop attacks	• Reduces number of generalized seizures • Seizure-free periods usually temporary and occur in only 5%–10% of patients	• Hemiparesis • Transient syndrome of mutism, urinary incontinence, and bilateral leg weakness	• Used when other options have failed • Many patients have learning disabilities
Vagal nerve stimulation: Implanted programmable signal generator in the chest with stimulating electrodes to the left vagus nerve	• Medically refractory, often partial seizures	• Reduction in seizure frequency: high stimulation, 25%; low stimulation, 15%	• Changes in voice • Dyspnea • Tingling in neck during stimulation • Rare cases of bradycardia or asystole	• Does not usually resolve seizures • Used when resective surgery is not an option

system, cranial nerves, and spinal nerve roots. It is referred to as a syndrome, as opposed to a disease, because of the combination of signs and symptoms seen in the patient.

ETIOLOGY

The etiology of Guillain-Barré syndrome is unclear, but an autoimmune response is strongly suspected. There is a preceding event or trigger that is often an infection.[101] Occasionally, vaccinations have been known to trigger Guillain-Barré syndrome.

Approximately half of the people who develop Guillain-Barré syndrome have a mild febrile illness 2 to 3 weeks before the onset of symptoms. The febrile infection is usually respiratory or gastrointestinal. Significant interest has developed in such infections and the development of autoantibodies. Some studies show a relationship between clinical findings and *Campylobacter jejuni* infection, as well as between clinical findings and cytomegalovirus infections. In the first group, patients tended to have a pure motor Guillain-Barré syndrome with predominantly distal motor involvement and a rapid onset of weakness. In the second group, there was greater involvement of the sensory system. Cranial nerves were more often involved, as were proximal muscles.[102]

Approximately 25% of patients with this disease have antibodies to either cytomegalovirus or Epstein-Barr virus. It has been suggested that an altered immune response to peripheral nerve antigens may contribute to the development of the disorder.[102]

EPIDEMIOLOGY

Guillain-Barré syndrome occurs with equal frequency in both sexes and all races. It can develop at any age. The annual incidence is approximately 2 cases per 100,000 population.[102]

PATHOPHYSIOLOGY

In Guillain-Barré syndrome, the myelin sheath surrounding the axon is lost. The myelin sheath is quite susceptible to injury by many agents and conditions, including physical trauma, hypoxemia, toxic chemicals, vascular insufficiency, and immunological reactions. Demyelination is a common response of neural tissue to any of these adverse conditions.

Myelinated axons conduct nerve impulses more rapidly than nonmyelinated axons. Along the course of a myelinated fiber are interruptions in the sheath called *nodes of Ranvier*, where there is direct contact between the cell membrane of the axon and the extracellular fluid. The membrane is highly permeable at these nodes, resulting in especially good conduction. The movement of ions into and out of the axon can occur rapidly only at the nodes of Ranvier; therefore, a nerve impulse along a myelinated fiber may jump from node to node (known as *saltatory conduction*) quite rapidly. Loss of the myelin sheath in Guillain-Barré syndrome makes saltatory conduction impossible, and nerve impulse transmission is aborted.

A current theory regarding the disease process of Guillain-Barré syndrome speculates that a primary lymphocytic T-cell mechanism is the cause of the inflammation. Cells migrate through the vessel walls to the peripheral nerve. The result is edema and perivascular inflammation. Macrophages then break down the myelin.

Another theory of causation is that the process of demyelination is initiated by an antibody attack on the myelin early in the course of the disease. Demyelination causes axon atrophy, which results in slowed or blocked nerve conduction.

CLINICAL MANIFESTATIONS

The syndrome may develop rapidly over the course of hours or days, or may take up to 3 to 4 weeks to develop. Most patients demonstrate the greatest weakness in the first weeks of the disorder. Patients are at their weakest point by the third week of the illness.

In the beginning, a flaccid, ascending paralysis develops quickly. The patient is most commonly affected in a symmetrical pattern. The patient may first notice weakness in the lower extremities that may quickly extend to include weakness and abnormal sensations in the arms. Deep tendon reflexes are usually lost, even in the earliest stages. The trunk and cranial nerves may become involved. Respiratory muscles can become affected, resulting in respiratory compromise.

Autonomic disturbances such as urinary retention and orthostatic hypotension may also occur. Superficial and deep tendon reflexes may be lost. Some patients experience tenderness and pain on deep pressure or movement of some muscles.

Sensory symptoms of paresthesias, including numbness and tingling, may occur. Pain is a complaint in a large number of patients. It is aching in nature and often compared with the feeling of muscles that have been overexerted. If there is cranial nerve involvement, cranial nerve VII, the facial nerve, is most often affected. Guillain-Barré syndrome does not affect level of consciousness, pupillary function, or cerebral function.

Symptoms may progress for several weeks. The level of paralysis may stop at any point. Motor function returns in a descending fashion. Demyelination occurs rapidly, but the rate of remyelination is approximately 1 to 2 mm per day.

DIAGNOSIS

The diagnosis of Guillain-Barré syndrome depends greatly on the patient's history and clinical progression of symptoms. As noted, onset is usually sudden and the history often reveals an upper respiratory or gastrointestinal disorder occurring 1 to 4 weeks before onset of the neurological manifestations. The history of the onset of symptoms can be revealing because symptoms of Guillain-Barré syndrome usually begin with weakness or paresthesias of the lower extremities and ascend in a symmetrical pattern.

A lumbar puncture may be performed and reveal increased protein. Also, nerve conduction studies record impulse transmission along the nerve fiber. In the patient with Guillain-Barré syndrome, the velocity of conduction is reduced.

Pulmonary function tests are done when Guillain-Barré syndrome is suspected to establish a baseline for comparison as the disease progresses. Declining pulmonary function capacity may indicate the need for mechanical ventilation and management in an ICU.

CLINICAL MANAGEMENT

Because of the risks associated with respiratory failure, bulbar symptoms, and autonomic dysfunction, all patients, except those with mild Guillain-Barré syndrome, should be admitted to a hospital that has specialized ICUs. Furthermore, patients who are older, have rapid progression or prior gastrointestinal infection, or are ventilator dependent tend to have a poor prognosis and need to be monitored closely.[103]

Certain strategies can lessen the severity of the illness and hasten recovery. A useful clinical sign of respiratory compromise is the strength of the neck flexor muscles. When the head cannot be lifted against gravity, the phrenic nerves are also affected, causing diaphragm paralysis and reduction of the forced vital capacity (FVC), the amount of air a patient can forcefully exhale after maximal inhalation. Under these circumstances, the airway cannot be successfully managed without intubation.

In addition, preventive measures need to be established so that deep venous thrombosis (DVT) and subsequent pulmonary embolism do not develop. Heparin 5000 units subcutaneously may be given along with antiembolism stockings and sequential compression devices. The autonomic nervous system fluctuations need to be monitored in terms of blood pressure changes and cardiac arrhythmias.

The first therapy proven to benefit patients with Guillain-Barré syndrome is plasmapheresis. This procedure mechanically removes humoral factors. Current recommendations are that patients with the motor-dominant form of Guillain-Barré syndrome receive plasmapheresis.[101] A dual-lumen central vascular access device and a specially trained team are needed to perform the plasmapheresis treatments. The physician may order plasmapheresis when the patient is worsening in an attempt to lessen the severity of the disease.

Intravenous immunoglobulin (IVIG) is also useful in managing Guillain-Barré syndrome. IVIG is a blood product that contains pooled plasma from many people. The major component is immunoglobulin G, with a trace amount of immunoglobulin A. Initial research indicates that immunoglobulins have a specific effect in certain subgroups, such as patients with *C. jejuni* infection.[102]

Immunoglobulins can be infused easily, even in the home setting, without expensive equipment. The optimal dosages and frequency of administration are individualized. Immunoglobulin, which binds to receptors on T cells or receptors on nerves, induces only a temporary improvement because of the turnover of T cells or the loss of antibodies from the receptors. Daily treatments with IVIG may be helpful in acute Guillain-Barré syndrome when the patient is rapidly deteriorating.

Neurologists who use IVIG for Guillain-Barré syndrome are familiar with the side effects, which include low-grade fever, chills, myalgia, diaphoresis, fluid overload, hypertension, nausea, vomiting, rash, headaches, aseptic meningitis, and neutropenia. The most serious adverse effect is acute tubular necrosis (ATN), which happens with any concomitant disease that compromises renal glomerular filtration.

Currently there are no efficacy data that favor managing Guillain-Barré syndrome with IVIG rather than plasmapheresis. The individual patient's circumstances, such as availability of resources to perform plasmapheresis, may dictate the treatment. IVIG is an attractive treatment because it can be easily administered in the critical care setting.[101]

Nursing Management

Assessment. For the patient with Guillain-Barré syndrome, careful assessment and the resultant plan help minimize the complications of immobility and move the patient toward rehabilitation without deficits. Although patients with Guillain-Barré syndrome are critically ill, their chances of returning to a productive life are good if they survive the acute stages.[102] Once Guillain-Barré syndrome is suspected, the patient is hospitalized so that frequent assessments can be performed to monitor the patient for deterioration. Because of the progressive nature of the disease, assessment should focus on the neurological examination, that is, cranial nerve involvement, motor weakness, and sensory changes. Cranial nerve deficits identify if the patient is at risk for aspiration. The patient's level of numbness, tingling, and pain should be addressed.

Cardiovascular assessment is done to monitor blood pressure and heart rate. The patient's respiratory status should also be monitored and FVC assessed at least every shift. Gastrointestinal and urinary function should come under surveillance as well. The patient is at risk for development of constipation and urinary tract infections. Other complications of immobility are the potential for pressure ulcers and DVT.

Plan. When caring for a patient with Guillain-Barré syndrome, the major goals are to prevent infections and complications of immobility, provide functional maintenance of the body systems, treat life-threatening crises promptly, and provide psychological support for the patient and family. In terms of the patient's neurological status, weakness will result in impaired mobility. Range-of-motion activities should be performed at least once per shift to minimize the patient's risk for development of contractures. Also, steps should be taken to maintain body alignment. Measures such as splint placement are implemented to prevent wrist hyperflexion and footdrop. Physical therapy should be initiated early in the course of hospitalization and continued throughout the recovery period.

Cranial nerve involvement places the patient at risk for aspiration. Adequate nutrition must be maintained. If the patient is unable to take oral feedings, tube feedings may be initiated. In addition, because of intubation or impaired verbal communication, alternate communication should be developed using communication boards, gestures, and simple signals such as eye blinking.

Respiratory failure is the most severe complication of GBS. Weakened respiratory muscles put the patient at great risk for hypoventilation and repeated pulmonary infections. Fifty percent of patients with GBS have some respiratory compromise, resulting in reduced tidal volume and vital capacity or perhaps complete respiratory arrest. A tracheostomy may be indicated if the patient requires long-term mechanical ventilation.

If there is autonomic nervous system involvement, drastic changes in blood pressure (hypotension or hypertension), heart rate, or both can occur. Cardiac monitoring allows quick identification and treatment of arrhythmias. Valsalva maneuver, coughing, and suctioning may trigger an autonomic nervous system disturbance. The patient should be monitored closely.

Comfort measures are used. For instance, frequent position changes may be helpful. When remyelination occurs, it is often uncomfortable and the patient may complain of numbness and pain. This can be an encouraging sign to the patient because the disease process is reversing.

Although the patient is incapacitated physically, he or she is fully aware of the surroundings. It is essential to provide emotional support and encouragement along each phase of the hospital course. The patient may experience a sense of helplessness and hopelessness. Frequent explanations of the interventions and of progress are useful. The patient should be allowed to participate in care as much as functionally possible.[104]

PATIENT EDUCATION AND DISCHARGE PLANNING

Education is provided about the disease process, course, and recovery. Patients need to know that the disease may progress to the point at which mechanical ventilation is required. The patient also can be informed about the Guillain-Barré Syndrome International Foundation, which provides information and resources. He or she may be discharged to a rehabilitation facility where recovery can continue. Patients may continue to show improvement for up to 2 years.

Myasthenia Gravis

Myasthenia gravis is a neuromuscular transmission disorder that is caused by an autoimmune response. *Myasthenia* is derived from the Greek words for "muscle" and "weakness," whereas *gravis* means "grave" in Latin. Therefore, the name means "grave muscle weakness," which is its primary clinical feature, along with abnormal fatigability.

ETIOLOGY

Myasthenia gravis is an autoimmune disorder. The factors that trigger the autoimmune process are not known, but the thymus gland is involved. The thymus lies behind the sternum and may extend down to the diaphragm or up to the neck. This gland plays a role in the responsiveness of T cells to foreign antigens. The thymus gland is large in children and small in adults. By adulthood, the gland has shrunken and has nearly been replaced by fat. Abnormalities in the thymus gland frequently occur in patients with myasthenia gravis. Eighty percent of patients with myasthenia gravis have thymal hyperplasia, whereas 10% have thymoma.

EPIDEMIOLOGY

Myasthenia gravis is seen more often in women than in men at a ratio of 3:2. It is primarily a disease of young women and older men. Symptoms most commonly appear in the third decade of life, although any age group may be affected. There are approximately 5 cases per 100,000 population, or 25,000 individuals with myasthenia gravis in the United States. It is not hereditary. Women with myasthenia gravis who give birth may transmit a transient type of neonatal myasthenia to the infant, yet it resolves within days after birth.[105]

PATHOPHYSIOLOGY

Myasthenia gravis is a result of circulating antibodies directed toward the skeletal muscle acetylcholine receptors. The acetylcholine receptor is a protein composed of five subunits situated in a specialized surface of the muscle membrane termed the *end plate*. When acetylcholine is released from the nerve after depolarization, it binds to the acetylcholine receptor and causes the ion channel to open. This passage of ions moving through the channel leads to depolarization of the end plate, action potential generation, and subsequent muscle fiber contraction. With this process, the depolarization of the end plate is significantly greater than what is required for action potential generation and, therefore, fluctuations in end plate depolarization do not affect action potential generation or the overall strength of muscle contraction.

The acetylcholine receptor antibodies in myasthenia gravis lead to the loss of acetylcholine receptors by increased internalization of the receptor and complement-based lysis of the muscle membrane. They may compromise ion flow through the acetylcholine receptor. The acetylcholine receptor function leads to a decrease in end plate depolarization, which may be insufficient to generate an action potential. This results in a failure of the muscle to contract. If acetylcholine receptor loss is mild, action potentials will occur. If neuromuscular transmission is stressed by repetitive nerve stimulation, which occurs with repetitive movements, the action potential is lost, and the muscle weakness occurs.[106] In summary, antibodies attack the acetylcholine receptors of the neuromuscular junction, thereby blocking the transmission of nerve impulses to muscle.

CLINICAL MANIFESTATIONS

Myasthenia gravis can be characterized as ocular myasthenia or generalized myasthenia, depending on the clinical signs and symptoms. In ocular myasthenia, patients may present with problems such as ptosis and diplopia. Approximately 6 months after onset of eye signs, half of the patients develop generalized myasthenia gravis.

In generalized myasthenia gravis, the patient may demonstrate ocular manifestations as well as difficulty with chewing, dysphagia, and dysarthria. The patient's voice may have a nasal quality. Difficulty with speech and swallowing are considered to result from bulbar involvement of the disease. Motor weakness is also apparent in this disorder. The patient often demonstrates more proximal than distal weakness. Muscle weakness can vary among patients. The patient often reports increased weakness with sustained activity and improvement with rest. Patients may also demonstrate respiratory compromise due to weakness of the respiratory muscles. This weakness can lead to respiratory failure and result in death.

DIAGNOSIS

Similar to other neurological disorders, the patient's history along with other diagnostic tests aids in an accurate diagnosis. Patients may present with complaints of double vision or drooping eyelids. Also, myasthenia gravis causes weakness of the shoulder girdle muscles. Therefore, the patient may complain of the inability to perform a variety of self-care activities, such as drying the hair with a blow dryer.

The neurological examination is also valuable in making the diagnosis. The cranial nerve examination may reveal ptosis and diplopia as well as other cranial nerve involvement. Motor weakness may be exhibited.

In addition to the neurological examination, laboratory studies are obtained. Blood is drawn for acetylcholine receptor antibodies, which are present in up to 80% of patients.

Electromyography (EMG) is helpful in the diagnosis of myasthenia gravis. In this diagnostic study, a needle electrode is inserted into a skeletal muscle and a recording of the electrical activity at rest, during voluntary activity, and with electrical stimulation is displayed on an oscilloscope. The patient should be informed that the needle causes some discomfort.[107] A decrease of the muscle action potential can be identified in approximately 74% of people with myasthenia gravis. In the patient with myasthenia gravis, this repetitive stimulation produces a rapid decline in muscle action potential because of the deficient numbers of acetylcholine receptors.

The Tensilon, or edrophonium, test is a classic diagnostic tool for confirming a diagnosis of myasthenia gravis. A positive test result lends strong support for the diagnosis of myasthenia gravis. In this test, 10 mg of IV Tensilon, a short-acting anticholinesterase agent, is given over an approximately 5-minute period. When injected, it transiently inhibits the breakdown of acetylcholine at the neuromuscular junction. A response is anticipated within 5 minutes. The test is most useful if there is improvement of ptosis or strength of the extraocular muscles. Limb strength or improved bulbar function may be difficult to interpret. When Tensilon is administered, atropine should be readily available in the event the patient develops bradycardia.[106]

A CT scan or MRI of the chest may also be done to rule out thymoma or thymal hyperplasia.

CLINICAL MANAGEMENT

The clinical management of myasthenia gravis includes the following strategies: use of medications to enhance neuromuscular transmission; long-term immunosuppression with corticosteroids, azathioprine (Imuran), cyclophosphamide (Cytoxan), or cyclosporine; short-term immunomodulation with plasmapheresis or IVIG; or thymectomy.

Pharmacological Management

Pharmacological management includes the use of anticholinesterases, steroids, or other immunosuppressive agents. Pyridostigmine (Mestinon) is available as a 60-mg tablet or a 180-mg time-span formula. The time-span tablet should not be crushed. If the patient is unable to swallow the tablet or has a nasogastric tube or percutaneous endoscopic gastrostomy, the 60-mg tablet may be crushed or the liquid form of pyridostigmine may be used. The drug inactivates cholinesterase so acetylcholine is not immediately destroyed. Through this action, more acetylcholine is available at the neuromuscular junction and the patient has improved muscle strength. Medication onset is 30 minutes after administration and peaks in 2 hours.

Pyridostigmine lasts approximately 3 to 4 hours, and the patient is dosed several times throughout the day. It should be given before meals so that the patient receives maximal benefit of the medication at mealtime. Side effects include muscarinic effects on smooth muscle and glands as well nicotinic effects. Diarrhea, abdominal cramping, increased salivation, blurred vision, bradycardia, and increased perspiration are possible muscarinic effects; muscle twitching, weakness, and fatigue are potential nicotinic side effects.[105]

If the patient cannot take oral pyridostigmine because of NPO status or intubation, IV neostigmine is comparable with the oral agent. Neostigmine bromide 1 mg is equivalent to pyridostigmine 60 mg.

Prednisone, a corticosteroid, reduces the amount of antibodies produced through the immune response, blocks the immune mechanism, and restores the chemical reaction at the neuromuscular junction. Patients may experience a temporary increase in motor weakness when steroids are initiated, thereby resulting in the need for inpatient admission. The patient needs to be educated about, and monitored for, side effects such as steroid-induced diabetes, osteoporosis, weight gain, fluid retention, cosmetic changes such as hirsutism and moon facies, mood changes, insomnia, gastric ulcers, and increased susceptibility to infection.

Other immunosuppressive agents that may be used include azathioprine and cyclophosphamide. Azathioprine slowly reduces the level of circulating acetylcholine receptor antibodies. Onset of immunosuppression is usually at 3 to 12 months, with maximum improvement in 12 to 36 months.[106] When these agents are given, the patient must be instructed about the potential hazards of these drugs. Women of childbearing age need to take precautions against pregnancy. Also, the nurse must practice the principles of safe handling of hazardous drugs. With cyclophosphamide, as with other chemotherapeutic agents, standards need to be in place so that the patient receives an accurate dose of the medication. The patient may experience hair loss and needs to be monitored for side effects such as hemorrhagic cystitis and bone marrow suppression. In addition, hospital guidelines for the safe administration of chemotherapeutic drugs must be followed.

Cyclosporine may be used for patients who are refractory to treatment or cannot tolerate the side effects of steroids. Cyclosporine has traditionally been used to achieve immunosuppression after organ transplantation. It has been shown to suppress T-cell function, resulting in a decrease of circulating acetylcholine receptor antibodies. It is usually given in divided dosages of 5 mg/kg after the morning and evening meals. The patient should be monitored for hypertension and nephrotoxicity. The onset of action is more rapid than azathioprine at 2 to 12 weeks, yet it is more costly.

There are some medications the patient should not receive. For example, D-penicillamine is contraindicated in patients with myasthenia gravis. There are other agents that can cause an increase in myasthenic weakness (Table 35-12).[106] Among these medications are some antibiotics. Both patients and health care professionals need to be cognizant of these medications. Although physicians and nurses working in the neuroscience arena are often familiar with these agents, patients may face potential difficulties in settings such as the emergency department or surgery, where the health care professional does not encounter patients with myasthenia gravis on a regular basis and may not be familiar with these medications.

Plasmapheresis

Plasmapheresis or plasma exchange may be indicated for patients in crisis or who are otherwise refractory to treatment. Plasmapheresis is initiated to remove circulating anti–acetylcholine receptor antibodies from the plasma, which results in clinical improvement.[105] This procedure is performed through a dual-lumen central vascular access device, which is similar to a dialysis catheter. A specialized team of nurses, trained in plasmapheresis, performs the treatment, usually three times a week, while the patient is an inpatient. Treatments may continue on an outpatient basis. The patient's circulating blood volume is removed through one of the lumens, filtered, and then returned through the second lumen. The patient's plasma is removed and albumin is returned, along with the solid components of the patient's blood. The procedure takes several hours, and the patient needs to be monitored for hypotension. Electrolytes and clotting factors need to be evaluated after each treatment.

The catheters must be managed appropriately because they are a potential source of infection. They can pose a

table 35-12 Medications to Avoid in Myasthenia Gravis

Category	Drug
Antibiotics	Aminoglycosides "Mycins" Tetracycline Polymixin B and E Colistin
Antiepileptic drugs	Phenytoin Mephenytoin Trimethadione
Cardiovascular medications	Quinidine Procainamide Beta blockers
Psychotropics	Lithium carbonate Phenothiazines
Muscle relaxants	Curare Succinylcholine
Others	Magnesium preparations Quinine D-Penicillamine Chloroquine

Adapted from Kernich C, Kaminski H: Myasthenia gravis: Pathophysiology, diagnosis and collaborative care. J Neurosci Nurs 27(4):207–215, 1995.

special challenge because the patient with myasthenia gravis may be receiving steroids or other immunosuppressive therapy. The nurse must also be aware that plasmapheresis removes medications, including pyridostigmine, that the patient has taken. The nurse must obtain an order from the physician to hold the medication.

Intravenous Immunoglobulin

Another treatment that may be used is IVIG. It is used either for acute disease management or as a long-term treatment for patients with myasthenia gravis who do not respond to other types of treatments. The patient's dose is individualized. Patients may exhibit clinical improvement in 2 to 4 days, and it may last for weeks or months.[105] The action of IVIG is unknown. The patient needs to be monitored for fever and chills, leukopenia, headache, fluid overload, and renal failure. Approximately 70% of patients receiving IVIG have been shown to improve rapidly in 4 to 5 days.

Thymectomy

Thymectomy is a surgical approach performed for the management of myasthenia gravis. This thoracic procedure promotes sustained remission and improvement. The fall in antibody titers after surgery further supports the use of thymectomy.[108] Patients must be aware that this procedure is performed for its long-term benefit so that they do not expect a dramatic improvement immediately after surgery. A complete remission may occur from 6 months to 10 years after thymectomy. Patients may demonstrate improvement to the point at which their medications may be reduced, thereby reducing adverse side effects.

Post-thymectomy care involves a short stay in the ICU. Pain after this procedure is managed with epidural analgesia. The patient is usually extubated immediately after the surgery. Intermittent positive-pressure breathing (IPPB) may be used to minimize postoperative respiratory complications. After the critical care stay, patients are transferred to an inpatient setting, where they are monitored for complications.

Management of Myasthenic Versus Cholinergic Crisis

Factors such as stress, respiratory infection, too rapid a steroid taper, or medication affecting the neuromuscular junction may predispose the patient to a crisis. A myasthenic crisis needs to be differentiated from a cholinergic crisis because the management of each is different.

A myasthenic crisis is characterized by a sudden exacerbation of weakness in the patient with generalized myasthenia gravis. It is usually caused by lack of medication or lack of responsiveness at the neuromuscular junction to cholinergic treatment, as well as a worsening of the disease process. The patient is unresponsive to an increase in anticholinesterase medications and can experience severe weakness, dysphagia, and respiratory compromise.

The hallmarks of cholinergic crisis are muscarinic or nicotinic side effects, namely, increased perspiration, abdominal cramping, and diarrhea. Cholinergic crisis results from too much medication that causes neuromuscular blockage (which prevents muscle depolarization because of excess acetylcholine). The patient may also experience respiratory failure. Indeed, respiratory failure may be seen in both types of crises.

In the past, the Tensilon test was used to determine if the patient was in a myasthenic or cholinergic crisis. If there was an improvement in muscle strength when Tensilon was administered, it indicated a myasthenic crisis. If there was no improvement or further deterioration of muscle strength, the patient was most likely experiencing a cholinergic crisis.[109] This test is no longer required because the withdrawal of cholinesterase drugs is necessary for improvement in both crises.[108] Respiratory and nutritional support is provided in both situations.

Nursing Management

Assessment. The nurse must focus the neurological assessment on cranial nerve involvement, motor strength, and the extent of respiratory involvement. One valuable tool in monitoring respiratory function is the use of a handheld spirometer to measure FVC. The nurse must be vigilant in monitoring the patient's respiratory status because the patient's diaphragm and intercostal muscles may become weak. In myasthenia gravis, if the patient's FVC falls below 1 L, it usually indicates respiratory failure, and intubation and mechanical ventilation are necessary.

Plan. The patient with myasthenia gravis may need assistance with activities of daily living. Adaptive equipment can help him or her perform self-care activities. Short rest periods should be planned into the day, so the patient does not fatigue easily.

Nutrition also needs to be addressed. Meals should be planned when pyridostigmine is at its peak. Aspiration precautions should be established. Thin liquids should be given only if the patient can tolerate them well. Nutrition may need to be offered through the enteral route.

Skin care also needs to be planned into the care routine, and measures should be taken to avoid pressure ulcers. Pressure relief devices can be used in bed or on chairs.

An effective method of communication should also be developed. It may be difficult to understand the patient because of the nasal quality of the voice. A communication board may be helpful as an alternate communication device.

PATIENT EDUCATION AND DISCHARGE PLANNING

Support and education about myasthenia gravis are crucial for the successful management of the disease. The patient needs to learn about the purpose of medications, medication schedules, and side effects. Patients should be instructed to adhere to their medication schedules and to contact the physician for modification if needed. Doses of medication should be kept at home and work so that they are readily available. During travel, the patient should always carry his or her medication, for example in a purse or camera case, so that it does not become lost with luggage.

It is also helpful for the patient to obtain a Medic Alert bracelet and card so that rapid identification can occur in the event of a medical emergency. If the patient is unable to communicate, successful management may hinge on health care professionals knowing that the individual has myasthenia gravis.

The patient and family should be taught to recognize signs and symptoms of a crisis. In addition, the importance of avoiding potential triggers for a crisis, such as respiratory infection or undue stress, should be emphasized. During the winter months when colds and flu occur, patients should be instructed to stay away from places where large groups of people gather, such as movies or concerts.

The patient should also be educated about community support groups. The Myasthenia Gravis Foundation can provide valuable resources to the patient. Box 35-7 lists patient teaching guidelines for myasthenia gravis.

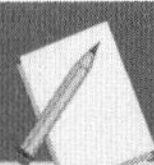

box 35-7
Living With Myasthenia Gravis

Safety

- Obtain a Medic Alert bracelet and wear it at all times. Always carry personal identification in your wallet or purse.
- Avoid respiratory infections. Stay away from concert halls and movie theaters in the winter.
- Avoid stress and stressful situations.
- Consider grinding or pureeing foods to make them easier to eat. Choose calorie-rich, nutritious snacks. Request a consultation with a dietitian if you have difficulty maintaining your weight.

Activity

- Plan frequent rest periods during the day.
- Conserve energy as much as possible.
- Avoid shopping at peak times or substitute "on-line" shopping so items can be delivered directly to your door.

Medications

- Mestinon should be taken as directed by your physician. Adjustments should be made only under the direction of your physician. Remember not to crush Mestinon Timespan.
- Mestinon should be stored at home and at work. Do not store medication in your car where it could be exposed to extreme heat and cold. When traveling, keep medication with you; do not store it in your luggage.
- Avoid medications (certain antibiotics such as aminoglycosides, anticonvulsants, and muscle relaxants) that could exacerbate myasthenia gravis.
- Do not take any over-the-counter preparations or complementary medications without first contacting your physician.
- If you are taking Imuran or cyclophosphamide, you need to follow precautions about hazardous drugs. Be certain to discuss family planning issues with your physician.

When to Call the Physician

- Call your physician if you are experiencing increased weakness, swallowing problems, or respiratory difficulties.
- Contact your physician immediately if you are hospitalized for any reason.

The Myasthenia Gravis Foundation of America is a valuable resource. Contact them for additional information and to find local support groups.

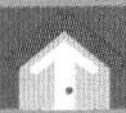

35-8 ***Neurological Dysfunction***

- Arrange for a safety assessment of the home environment to identify potential hazards to ambulation.
- Review the patient's medication profile to reinforce compliance and to ensure therapeutic monitoring.
- If the patient cannot care for himself or herself or if the family cannot provide care, consider the services of a home health agency.
- Provide resources to take home, such as written materials about neurological dysfunction, information about medications, and the name of the person to contact with questions. The home care nurse will be able to reinforce patient teaching and answer questions.
- Arrange for resources such as speech therapy, occupational therapy, and physical therapy.

Home care for the patient with neurological dysfunction is discussed in Box 35-8. Special considerations for older patients with neurological dysfunction are outlined in Box 35-9.

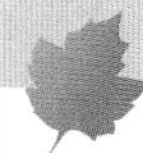

box 35-9

Neurological Dysfunction in the Older Patient

Given current improvements in health care and the overall interest of the population in nutrition and exercise, Americans are living longer, more productive lives. Consequently, people are faced with the increased risk of developing acute and chronic illnesses in later years. Although medical and surgical interventions have improved tremendously over the past several decades, the risk of complications increases significantly in the older population. Immobility is a major cause of pneumonia, deep venous thrombosis (DVT), pressure ulcers, and cognitive impairment. Strategies for preventing or minimizing these complications should be anticipated and planned for at the time of diagnosis. Pharmacological and surgical treatments need to be designed for the particular needs of the older patient. The ICU environment is particularly stressful for this patient population. The combination of a fragile neurological status and increased sensory input may lead to confusion and disorientation. Patients who are normally quite independent may find even a short ICU stay extremely demoralizing.

The resources of the multidisciplinary team should be maximally used for these patients. During the hospitalization, the nurse clinician is responsible for assessing the specific needs of the patient and instituting measures to reduce complications. In the ICU environment, a thorough neurological examination is performed at regular intervals to evaluate for subtle changes. Treatments are coordinated to provide for adequate rest. Rehabilitation therapy is used as soon as the patient is hemodynamically stable and can tolerate increases in activity. Sequential compression devices (SCDs) and active and passive range-of-

(continued)

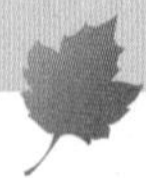

box 35-9

Neurological Dysfunction in the Older Patient (Continued)

motion exercises are used to prevent venous thrombosis. Pulmonary toilet, when appropriate, minimizes the risk of pneumonia and other pulmonary sequelae of immobility. Physicians and pharmacists modify the medication regimen to the particular needs of the older patient. Many medication combinations affect cognition, behavior, and orientation. Social work support is used to plan for transfer to the nursing unit and to anticipate the long-term home care or institutional needs of the patient. Communication with family members, who may need to take on increasing responsibility for decision making and supportive care, is necessary on a frequent and regular basis. Nutrition consultations provide for adequate oral or enteral requirements and take into account concurrent medical problems that may affect nutritional requirements. Spiritual support is often overlooked during aggressive medical therapy, a time when it is most important and when the patient may not be able to express his or her spiritual needs. A discussion of the patient's advance directives should be included in the plan of care.

clinical applicability challenges

Self-Challenge: Critical Thinking

1. *Mr. S. has recently undergone a craniotomy and has been diagnosed with glioblastoma multiforme. He is in otherwise excellent health. He is trying to decide whether to enter a protocol using a combination of radiation and experimental chemotherapy or to proceed with conventional radiation therapy. What issues should he and his family consider in making this decision?*
2. *Mr. J. is 67 years old. He has a history of uncontrolled hypertension, cigarette smoking, and type 2 diabetes. At noon, while eating lunch with his wife, his speech becomes garbled during the conversation. As his wife assists him to the bedroom to rest, he has difficulty walking because of right-sided weakness. His wife recently attended a health fair at the local senior center and she recognizes the symptoms of stroke. She immediately calls 911 and her husband is transported to the local university hospital. What factors will determine if Mr. J. is a candidate for thrombolytic therapy?*
3. *A 45-year-old woman presents to the emergency department having lost consciousness and having had jerking movements of the arms and legs, witnessed by her husband. She is now awake, but has slurring of speech, arm weakness, and lethargy. Describe the history and physical examination, diagnostic studies, and laboratory tests that will be performed in the emergency department.*
4. *Mrs. P. is a 48-year-old woman with myasthenia gravis who has had the flu for 2 days. She presents to her local emergency department complaining of increasing weakness, fatigue, and difficulty swallowing. After her initial assessment, her FVC is 0.8 L, and she is transferred to the ICU. What are the priority nursing interventions for Mrs. P.?*

Study Questions

1. *What is the most common primary brain tumor?*
   a. *Meningioma*
   b. *Acoustic neuroma*
   c. *Glioblastoma multiforme*
   d. *Pituitary tumor*
2. *A definitive diagnosis of brain tumor is obtained through:*
   a. *magnetic resonance imaging (MRI) scan.*
   b. *positron emission tomography (PET) scan.*
   c. *physical examination.*
   d. *pathological examination of tumor tissue.*
3. *The condition of recurrent abnormal and excessive discharges of cerebral neurons is*
   a. *seizure.*
   b. *epilepsy.*
   c. *postictal.*
   d. *status epilepticus.*
4. *The most common type of stroke is*
   a. *hemorrhagic.*
   b. *ischemic.*
   c. *thalamic.*
   d. *subarachnoid.*
5. *Which of the following is a contraindication to receiving tissue plasminogen activator (t-PA)?*
   a. *Recent history of surgery*
   b. *Blood glucose level of 75 mg/dL*
   c. *Score of 23 on the National Institutes of Health Stroke Scale (NIHSS)*
   d. *Blood pressure of 160/100 mm Hg*
6. *Which of the following treatment modalities is used to prevent vasospasm?*
   a. *Coiling*
   b. *Intravenous colloid solutions*
   c. *Cerebral angiography*
   d. *Drug-induced hypotension*
7. *What is the typical presentation of symptoms in a person with Guillain-Barré syndrome?*
   a. *Rapid ascending paralysis*
   b. *Deficits of cranial nerves IX and X*
   c. *Respiratory arrest*
   d. *Distal tingling of fingertips*
8. *The defect at the neuromuscular junction in myasthenia gravis is caused by*
   a. *antibody attack on acetylcholine receptor sites.*
   b. *hypokalemia resulting from impaired neuronal transmission.*
   c. *misfiring of neurons.*
   d. *overstimulation of the parasympathetic nervous system.*

REFERENCES

1. Lindsay KW, Bone I, Callander R: Neurology and Neurosurgery Illustrated. New York, Churchill Livingstone, 1986
2. Goldberg S: Clinical Neuroanatomy Made Ridiculously Simple (2nd Ed). Miami, MedMaster, 2000
3. Barker E (ed): Neuroscience Nursing: A Spectrum of Care (2nd Ed). St. Louis, Mosby, 2002
4. Minton MS, Hickey JV: A primer of neuroanatomy and neurophysiology. Nurs Clin North Am (34)3:555–572, 1999
5. Burger PC, Scheithauer BW: Tumors of the Central Nervous System. Atlas of Tumor Pathology. Washington, DC, Armed Forces Institute of Pathology, 1994

6. Chandler WF: Pituitary tumors. In Bernstein M, Berger MS (eds): Neuro-Oncology: The Essentials, pp 399–408. New York, Thieme, 2000
7. Divisions of Neuropathology at Brigham and Women's Hospital and Children's Hospital, Boston, MA: Neuropathology of central nervous system tumors. In Black PM, Loeffler JS (eds): Cancer of the Nervous System, pp 25–53. Cambridge, MA, Blackwell Science, 1997
8. World Health Organization: Classification of tumours. In Kleihues P, Cavenee WK (eds): Pathology and Genetics of Tumours of the Nervous System. Lyon, France, IARC Press, 2000
9. Louis DN, Stemmer-Rachamimov AO: Pathology and classification. In Bernstein M, Berger MS (eds): Neuro-Oncology: The Essentials, pp 18–29. New York, Thieme, 2000
10. James CD: Genetic aspects. In Bernstein M, Berger MS (eds): Neuro-Oncology: The Essentials, pp 42–48. New York, Thieme, 2000
11. Grossman S: Familial gliomas. In Berger MS, Wilson CB (eds): The Gliomas, pp 12–14. Philadelphia, WB Saunders, 1999
12. Preston-Martin S: Epidemiology. In Berger MS, Wilson CB (eds): The Gliomas, pp 2–11. Philadelphia, WB Saunders, 1999
13. Central Brain Tumor Registry of the United States, 2002–2003: Statistical report: Primary brain tumors in the United States, 1995–1999. Chicago, Central Brain Tumor Registry of the United States
14. Bohnen NI, Radhakrishnan K, et al: Descriptive and analytic epidemiology of brain tumors. In Black PM, Loeffler JS (eds): Cancer of the Nervous System, pp 3–24. Cambridge, MA, Blackwell Science, 1997
15. Wrensch MR, Minn Y, Bondy ML: Epidemiology. In Bernstein M, Berger MS (eds): Neuro-Oncology: The Essentials, pp 2–17. New York, Thieme, 2000
16. Engelhard HH: Brain tumors and the blood-brain barrier. In Bernstein M, Berger MS (eds): Neuro-Oncology: The Essentials, pp 49–53. New York, Thieme, 2000
17. Long D: Capillary ultrastructure and the blood-brain barrier in human malignant brain tumors. J Neurosurg 32:127–144, 1970
18. Thapar K, Rutka JT, Laws ER Jr.: Brain edema, increased intracranial pressure, vascular effects, and other epiphenomena of human brain tumors. In Kaye AH, Laws ER Jr (eds): Brain Tumors: An Encyclopedic Approach, pp 163–189. New York, Churchill Livingstone, 1995
19. Bohan E: Neurosurgical management of patients with central nervous system malignancies. Semin Oncol Nurs 14:8–17, 1998
20. Frank J: Management of intracranial hypertension, Med Clin North Am 77:61–75, 1993
21. Wen PY: Diagnosis and management of brain tumors. In Black PM, Loeffler JS (eds): Cancer of the Nervous System, pp 106–127. Cambridge, MA, Blackwell Science, 1997
22. Keles GE, Berger M: Functional mapping: Functional magnetic resonance imaging. In Bernstein M, Berger MS (eds): Neuro-Oncology: The Essentials, pp 130–134. New York, Thieme, 2000
23. Wen PY, Black PM: Clinical presentation, evaluation and preoperative preparation of the patient. In Berger MS, Wilson CB (eds): The Gliomas, pp 328–336. Philadelphia, WB Saunders, 1999
24. Sawaya R, Hammoud MA, et al: Intraoperative localization of tumor and margins. In Berger MS, Wilson CB (eds): The Gliomas, pp 361–375. Philadelphia, WB Saunders, 1999
25. Yamada K, Sorensen AG: Diagnostic imaging. In Bernstein M, Berger MS (eds): Neuro-Oncology: The Essentials, pp 56–77. New York, Thieme, 2000
26. Haynor DR, Maravilla K: The role of functional imaging in the surgical management of brain neoplasms. In Berger MS, Wilson CB (eds): The Gliomas, pp 337–341. Philadelphia, WB Saunders, 1999
27. Kiriakopoulos ET, Mikulis DJ: Functional magnetic resonance imaging. In Bernstein M, Berger MS (eds): Neuro-Oncology: The Essentials, pp 94–98. New York, Thieme, 2000
28. Ruge MI, Victor M, et al: Concordance between functional magnetic resonance imaging and intraoperative language mapping. Stereotact Funct Neurosurg 72:95–102, 1999
29. Schulder M, Holodny A, et al: Functional magnetic resonance image-guided surgery of tumors in or near the primary visual cortex. Stereotact Funct Neurosurg 73: 31–36, 1999
30. Vigneron DB, Nelson SJ: Magnetic resonance spectroscopy. In Bernstein M, Berger MS (eds): Neuro-Oncology: The Essentials, pp 99–114. New York, Thieme, 2000
31. Foy PM, Chadwick DW, et al: Do prophylactic anticonvulsant drugs alter the pattern of seizures after craniotomy? J Neurol Neurosurg Psychiatry 55:753–757, 1992
32. Telfeian AE, Philips MF, Crino PB, et al: Postoperative epilepsy in patients undergoing craniotomy for glioblastoma multiforme. J Exp Clin Cancer Res 20:5–10, 2001
33. Sawaya RE, Rambo W, et al: Basic principles of brain tumor surgery in adults. In Black PM, Loeffler JS (eds): Cancer of the Nervous System, pp 128–139. Cambridge, MA, Blackwell Science, 1997
34. Greenberg MS: Handbook of Neurosurgery, pp 640–655 (5th Ed). New York, Thieme, 2001
35. Dunne-Daly CF: Principles of radiotherapy and radiobiology. Semin Oncol Nurs 15:250–259, 1999
36. Grant W, Cain RB: Intensity modulated conformal therapy for intracranial lesions. Med Dosim 23:237–241, 1998
37. Kleinberg L, Grossman SA, et al: Phase I trial to determine the safety, pharmacodynamics and pharmacokinetics of RSR13, a novel radioenhancer, in newly diagnosed glioblastoma multiforme. J Clin Oncol 17:2593–2603, 1999
38. Kondziolka D, Flickinger JC, Lunsford LD: Stereotactic radiosurgery and radiation therapy. In Bernstein M, Berger MS (eds): Neuro-Oncology: The Essentials, pp 183–197. New York, Thieme, 2000
39. Nicolaou N: Radiation therapy treatment planning and delivery. Semin Oncol Nurs 15:260–269, 1999
40. Tatter S, Shaw E, et al: An inflatable balloon catheter and liquid 125I radiation source (Glia Site Radiation Therapy System) for treatment of recurrent malignant glioma: Multicenter safety and feasibility trial. J Neurosurg 99:297–303, 2003
41. Armstrong TS, Gilbert MR: Chemotherapy of astrocytomas: An overview. Semin Oncol Nurs 14:18–25, 1998
42. Grossman SA, Wharam M, et al: Phase II study of continuous infusion carmustine and cisplatin followed by cranial irradiation in adults with newly diagnosed high-grade astrocytoma. J Clin Oncol 15:2596–2603, 1997
43. Gilbert M, O'Neill A, et al: A phase II study of preradiation chemotherapy followed by external beam radiotherapy for the treatment of patients with newly diagnosed glioblastoma multiforme: An Eastern Cooperative Oncology Group study. J Neurooncol 47:145–152, 2000
44. Brem H, Langer R: Polymer-based drug delivery to the brain. Sci Med 3:2–11, 1996
45. Trask TW, Trask RP, et al: Phase I study of adenoviral delivery of the HSV-tk gene and ganciclovir administration in patients with recurrent malignant brain tumors. Mol Ther 1:195–203, 2000
46. Ram Z, Oldfield EH: Gene therapy for malignant brain tumors. In Berger MS, Wilson CB (eds): The Gliomas, pp 157–163. Philadelphia, WB Saunders, 1999
47. Fine HA, Figg WD, et al: Phase II trial of the antiangiogenic agent thalidomide in patients with recurrent high-grade gliomas. J Clin Oncol 18:708–715, 2000
48. Folkman J: Tumor angiogenesis: Therapeutic implications. N Engl J Med 285:1182–1186,1971
49. Sills AK, Sipos EP, et al: Angiogenesis inhibition in the treatment of central nervous system tumors. Adv Neurooncol 2:81–96, 1997
50. Hall WA: Targeted toxin therapy for malignant astrocytoma. Neurosurgery 46:544–551, 2000
51. Merchant RE, Young HF: Intracavitary immunotherapy. In Berger MS, Wilson CB (eds): The Gliomas, pp 599–608. Philadelphia, WB Saunders, 1999
52. Friedman HS, Pluda J, et al: Phase I trial of carmustine plus 06-benzylguanine for patients with recurrent or progressive malignant glioma. J Clin Oncol 18:3522–3528, 2000
53. Tamargo RJ, Walter KA, Oshiro EM: Aneurysmal subarachnoid hemorrhage: Prognostic features and outcomes. New Horizon 5:364–375, 1997
54. Wiebers DO and International Study of Unruptured Intracranial Aneurysms Investigators: Unruptured intracranial aneurysms: Natural history, clinical outcome, and risks of surgical and endovascular treatment. Lancet 362:103–110, 2003
55. Mower-Wade D, Cavanaugh MC, Bush C: Protecting a patient with ruptured cerebral aneurysm. Nursing 2001 31(2):52–58, 2001
56. Greenberg MS: Handbook of Neurosurgery, pp 770–803 (5th Ed). New York, Thieme, 2001
57. Kassell NF, Torner JC, Clark HJ, et al: The international cooperative study on the timing of aneurysm surgery: Part I. Overall management results. J Neurosurg 73:18–36, 1990
58. Morrison SR: Guglielmi detachable coils: An alternative therapy for surgically high-risk aneurysms. J Neurosci Nurs 29(4):232–327, 1997
59. Vale F, Hadley MN: Pathology of intracranial aneurysms and vascular malformations. In Batjer HH, et al (eds): Cerebrovascular Disease, pp 65–78. Philadelphia, Lippincott-Raven, 1997

60. Brown RD Jr: Intracranial saccular aneurysms and arteriovenous malformations. In Johnson RT, Griffin JW, McArthur JC (eds): Current Therapy in Neurologic Disease, pp 219–225. St. Louis, Mosby, 2002
61. Greenberg MS: Handbook of Neurosurgery, pp 804–814 (5th Ed). New York, Thieme, 2001
62. Garretson HD: Vascular malformations and fistulas. In Wilkins RH, Rengachary SS (eds): Neurosurgery, pp 1448–1458. New York, McGraw-Hill, 1991
63. Hillman J: Population-based analysis of arteriovenous malformation treatment. J Neurosurg 95:633–637, 2001
64. Fisher WS III: Intracranial vascular malformations: Clinical presentations. In Batjer HH, et al (eds): Cerebrovascular Disease, pp 657–667. Philadelphia, Lippincott-Raven, 1997
65. Spetzler RF, Martin NA: A proposed system for grading of arteriovenous malformations. J Neurosurg 65:476–483, 1986
66. Selman WR, Tarr RW, Ratcheson RA: Intracranial arteriovenous malformations: patient evaluation and considerations for treatment. In Batjer HH, et al (eds): Cerebrovascular Disease, pp 679–689. Philadelphia, Lippincott-Raven, 1997
67. Vinuela F, Duckwiler G, Guglielmi G: Principles of interventional neuroradiology. In Batjer HH, et al (eds): Cerebrovascular Disease, pp 691–706. Philadelphia, Lippincott-Raven, 1997
68. Latchaw RE, Madison MT, Larsen DW, et al: Intracranial arteriovenous malformations: Endovascular strategies and methods. In Batjer HH, et al (eds): Cerebrovascular Disease, pp 707–726. Philadelphia, Lippincott-Raven, 1997
69. Chen TC, Apuzzo MLJ: Principles of stereotactic neurosurgery. In Black PM, Loeffler JS (eds): Cancer of the Nervous System, p 177. Cambridge, MA, Blackwell Science, 1997
70. Sawaya R, Hammoud MA, Ligon BL, et al: Intraoperative localization of tumor and margins. In Berger MS, Wilson CB (eds): The Gliomas, pp 361–375. Philadelphia, WB Saunders, 1999
71. Kiya N, Dureza C, Fukushima T, et al: Computer navigational microscope for minimally invasive neurosurgery. Minim Invasive Neurosurg 40:110–115, 1997
72. Stapleton SR, Kiriakopoulos E, Mikulis D, et al: Combined utility of functional MRI, cortical mapping, and frameless stereotaxy in the resection of lesions in eloquent areas of brain in children. Pediatr Neurosurg 26:68–82, 1997
73. Sawaya RE, Rambo W, Ligon BL, et al: Basic principles of brain tumor surgery in adults. In Black PM, Loeffler JS (eds): Cancer of the Nervous System, pp 128–139. Cambridge, MA, Blackwell Science, 1997
74. Schroeder HWS, Wagner W, Tschiltschke W, et al: Frameless neuronavigation in intracranial endoscopic neurosurgery, J Neurosurg 94:72–79, 2001
75. Landolt AM, Schiller Z: Surgical technique: transsphenoidal approach. In Landolt AM, Vance ML, Reilly PL (eds): Pituitary Adenomas, pp 307–314. New York, Churchill Livingstone, 1996
76. Littrell KA: Brain attack emergent care of the patient with acute ischemic stroke. Adv Nurses 2(1):10–13, 2000
77. Testani-Dufour L, Morrison CAM: Brain attack: correlative anatomy. J Neurosci Nurs 29(1):213–224, 1997
78. Kasner SE: Management of acute ischemic stroke. In Stern MB, Brown MJ, Galetta SL, et al (eds): Penn Neurology 2000, pp 21–33. New York, AlphaMedica Press, 2000
79. Hock NH: Brain attack the stroke continuum. Nurs Clin North Am 34(3):689–723, 1999
80. Wityk RJ, Beauchamp NJ: Diagnostic evaluation of stroke. Neurol Clin 19:357–378, 2000
81. Bonnono C, Criddle LM, Lutsep H, et al: Emergi-paths and stroke teams: An emergency department approach to acute ischemic stroke. J Neurosci Nurs 32(6):298–305, 2000
82. Wein TH, Bornstein NM: Stroke prevention: cardiac and carotid-related stroke. Neurol Clin 19:321–341, 2000
83. Hock N: Neuroprotective and thrombolytic agents: Advances in stroke treatment. J Neurosci Nurs 30(3):175–184, 1999
84. Ulrich SP, Canale SW: Nursing Care Planning Guides, pp 241–260, Philadelphia, WB Saunders, 2001
85. Shorvon S: Handbook of Epilepsy, pp 173–225. London, Blackwell Science, 2000
86. Claassen J, Hirsch LJ, et al: Continuous EEG monitoring and midazolam infusion for refractory nonconvulsive status epilepticus. Neurology 57:1036–1042, 2001
87. Alldredge BK, Gelb AM, et al: A comparison of lorazepam, diazepam, and placebo for the treatment of out-of-hospital status epilepticus. N Engl J Med 345:631–637, 2001
88. Scott CA, Fish TR, Allen PJ: Design of an intensive epilepsy monitoring unit. Epilepsia 41(Suppl 5):S3–S8, 2000
89. Shorvon S: Handbook of Epilepsy, pp 1–16. London, Blackwell Science, 2000
90. Engel J Jr: Seizures and Epilepsy, pp. 39–70. Philadelphia, FA Davis, 1989
91. Greenberg MS: Handbook of Neurosurgery, pp 254–284 (5th Ed). New York, Thieme, 2001
92. Gulati S, Bal CS, Kalra V: Single-photon emission computed tomography (SPECT) in childhood epilepsy. Indian J Pediatr 67(Suppl):S32–S39, 2000
93. Benbadis SR, Tatum WO 4th: Advances in the treatment of epilepsy. Am Fam Physician 64:91–98, 2001
94. Spencer SS, Spencer DD: Surgery for Epilepsy, pp 54–65. Boston, Blackwell Scientific, 1991
95. Shorvon S: Handbook of Epilepsy, pp 85–172. London, Blackwell Science, 2000
96. Carson BS Sr: Indications and outcomes for lobectomy, corpus callosotomy, and hemispherectomy in pediatric neurosurgical patients. Clin Neurosurg 47:385–399, 2000
97. Hodaie M, Musharbash A, et al: Image-guided, frameless stereotactic sectioning of the corpus callosum in children with intractable epilepsy. Pediatr Neurosurg 34:286–294, 2001
98. Iannelli A, Guzzetta F, et al: Surgical treatment of temporal tumors associated with epilepsy. Pediatr Neurosurg 32:248–254, 2000
99. Morrow JI, Bingham E, et al: Vagal nerve stimulation in patients with refractory epilepsy. Effect on seizure frequency, severity and quality of life. Seizure 9:442–445, 2000
100. Olejniczak PW, Fisch BJ, et al: The effect of vagus nerve stimulation on epileptiform activity recorded from hippocampal depth electrodes. Epilepsia 42:423–429, 2001
101. Lindenbaum Y, Kissel, JT, Mendell JR: Treatment approaches for Guillain-Barré syndrome and chronic inflammatory demyelinating polyradiculoneuropathy. Neurol Clin 19(1):187–204, 2001
102. Asbury AK: Guillain-Barré syndrome. In Stern MB, Brown MJ, Galetta SL, et al (eds): Penn Neurology 2000, pp 99–114. New York, AlphaMedica Press, 2000
103. Sheikh KA: Peripheral nerve disease: Guillain-Barré syndrome. In Johnson RT, Griffin JW, McArthur JC (eds): Current Therapy in Neurologic Disease, pp 366–370. St. Louis, Mosby, 2002
104. Worsham TL: Easing the course of Guillain-Barré syndrome. RN 63(3):46–50, 52, 2000
105. Ross AP: Neurologic degenerative disorders. Nurs Clin North Am 34(3):725–742, 1999
106. Kernich C, Kaminski H: Myasthenia gravis: Pathophysiology, diagnosis and collaborative care. J Neurosci Nurs 27(4):207–215, 1995
107. Shpritz DW: Neurodiagnostic studies. Nurs Clin North Am (34)3:593–606, 1999
108. Younger DS, Raksadawan N: Therapy in neuromuscular disease. Neurol Clin 19(1):205–215, 2001
109. Hickey J (ed): The Clinical Practice of Neurological and Neurosurgical Nursing (5th Ed). Philadelphia, Lippincott Williams & Wilkins, 2003

OTHER SELECTED READING

Batjer HH, et al (eds): Cerebrovascular Disease. Philadelphia, Lippincott-Raven, 1997
Cunning S: When the DX is myasthenia gravis. RN 63(4):26–30, 2000
Dashe JF: Acute stroke evaluation and treatment. Clin Supervis 39(1):43–53, 2000
Duncan PW, et al: Development of a comprehensive assessment toolbox for stroke. Clin Geriatr Med 15(4):885–915, 1999
Grohar-Murray ME, Becker A, Reilley S, et al: Self-care actions to manage fatigue among myasthenia gravis patients. J Neurosci Nurs 30(3):191–199, 1998
Jain RK, Carmeliet PF: Vessels of death or life. Sci Am 285(6):38–45, 2001
Semin Oncol Nurs 14:1, 1998 (entire journal)
Semin Oncol Nurs 15:4, 1998 (entire journal)
Van Gijn J, Rinkel GJE: Subarachnoid haemorrhage: Diagnosis, causes and management. Brain 1124:249–278, 2001

chapter

36

Head Injury

ELIZABETH ZINK

objectives

Based on the content in this chapter, the reader should be able to:

- Identify the importance of mechanisms of injury when assessing the patient with head trauma.
- Describe various types of head injuries and their typical characteristics.
- Explain the pathophysiological processes occurring from the onset of injury through recovery, using the concepts of primary and secondary brain injury.
- Explain the importance and process of continuous neurological assessment in the head-injured patient.
- Discuss the rationale for medical and nursing management in the care of the head-injured patient.
- State the roles of the multidisciplinary health care team in caring for the patient with a head injury.

Head injury affects as many as 1.5 million Americans each year and can have devastating effects on patients and their families.[1] Estimates from the Brain Injury Association of America suggest that a person sustains a brain injury every 21 seconds. Eighty thousand patients suffer long-term disability and 50,000 patients die. Motor vehicle crashes account for 50% of all traumatic brain injuries, with violence and falls accounting for the remainder of cases.[1] The incidence of head injury is two times greater in men than in women and peaks in adolescence, young adulthood, and those older than 75 years of age[1] (Box 36-1). Critical care nurses can have an impact on the incidence of head injury through detailed patient and family teaching as well as active participation in primary prevention (e.g., helmet safety, violence prevention, fall prevention, and drug and alcohol awareness).

A thorough understanding of the pathophysiological mechanisms in head injury enables the critical care nurse to make an optimal contribution to the care of the head-injured patient. Critical care nurses play a key role in organizing the multidisciplinary care of these complex patients and their families.

MECHANISMS OF HEAD INJURY

Understanding the mechanisms of injuries, along with diagnostic testing and physical examination, aids in the expedient diagnosis of head injury. Typical mechanisms of injury include acceleration, deceleration, acceleration–deceleration, coup–contre coup, and rotational injury (Fig. 36-1):

- *Acceleration injuries* occur when a moving object strikes the nonmoving head (e.g., a bat striking the head or a missile fired into the head).

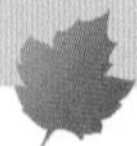

box 36-1

Risk Factors for Head Injury in the Older Patient

Elderly patients often present to the emergency department or acute care facility with a change in mental status. Head injury should not be overlooked as a cause for mental status changes. A careful history may reveal a history of falling, possibly several weeks before presentation to the health care provider. For example, in the event of a subdural hematoma, symptoms tend to manifest more slowly because cortical atrophy in older adults affords the brain more space within the cranial vault. The history may also reveal risk factors for falling, including living alone, syncope, cardiac dysrhythmias, frequent urination during the night necessitating frequent trips to the bathroom, and previous stroke. Another risk factor for head injury in the older adult is the use of anticoagulants, which can predispose the person to greater injury should a fall occur. Finally, alcohol use as a cause of falls should not be overlooked in the elderly population.

- *Deceleration injuries* occur when a moving head strikes a stationary object, such as in a fall or motor vehicle crash in which the head strikes the windshield. Acceleration–deceleration injuries often occur in motor vehicle crashes and episodes of physical violence.
- *Coup–contre coup injuries* occur when the head is struck, causing the brain to move within the cranial vault and forcibly contact the opposite pole of the skull and the region in which the initial blow was dealt. These injuries are also termed *translational injuries* because forces can be translated to opposite areas of the brain. For example, if a patient were struck with a blunt object in the back of the head, it would be necessary to assess the frontal lobes as well as the occipital lobes and cerebellum for injury.
- *Rotational injuries* occur when forces cause the brain to twist within the skull, resulting in stretching or tearing of neurons in the white matter as well as tearing of the blood vessels that tether the brain to the inside of the skull.

The possibility of cervical spine injury must also be carefully investigated and excluded before removal of immobilization devices. Head injuries can be categorized by

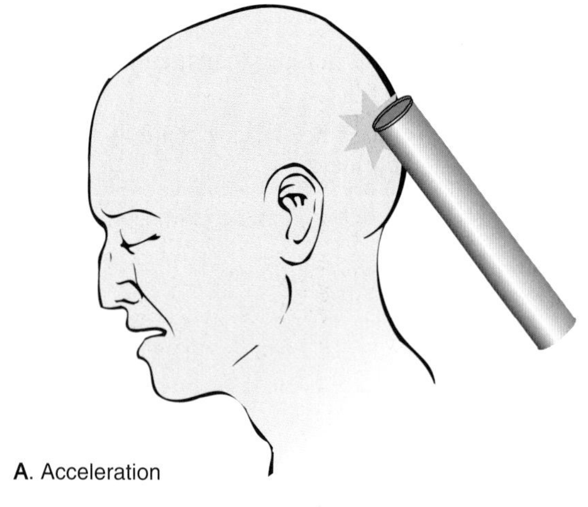

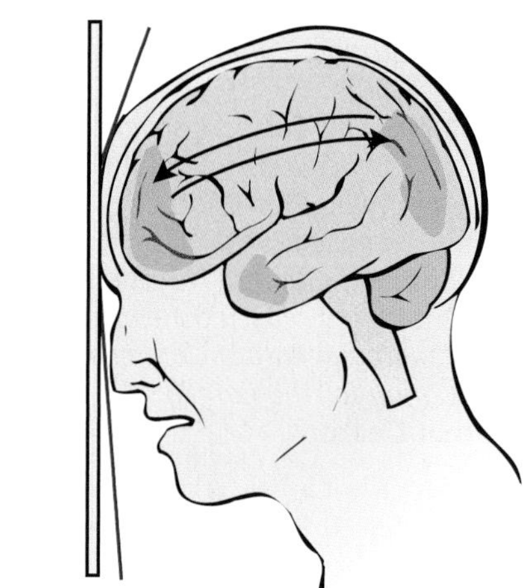

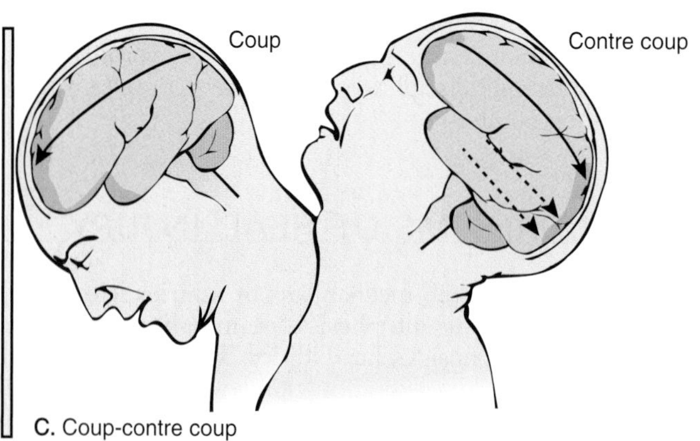

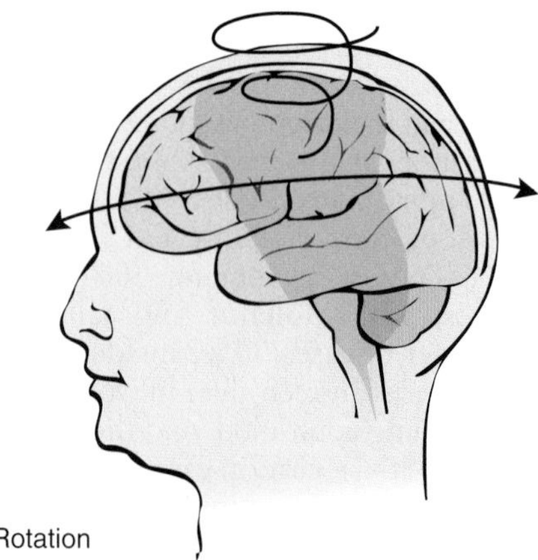

figure 36-1 Typical mechanisms of head injury. (**A**) Acceleration. (**B**) Acceleration–deceleration. (**C**) Coup-contre coup. (**D**) Rotation.

severity using the findings of diagnostic tests and the Glasgow Coma Scale (Table 36-1).

PATHOPHYSIOLOGY

Head injuries are classified as either primary or secondary. Primary injury is the result of the initial injury. The initial injury causes disruption of the electrical, chemical, and physical integrity of the cells in the area, leading to cell death. Secondary injury encompasses the physiological response to brain injury, including cerebral edema, cerebral ischemia, biochemical changes, and changes in cerebral hemodynamics. Current research and existing therapies are focused on preventing and mitigating secondary brain injury to maximize chances for a positive functional outcome.

Primary Brain Injury

SCALP LACERATION

A scalp laceration frequently causes copious amounts of bleeding due to the vascularity of the scalp, and often signifies other underlying injuries to both the skull and brain tissue. The area is carefully palpated for deformation before applying gentle pressure to stop bleeding. Skull fractures may still be present even if deformities are not palpable, so care is taken in applying pressure to scalp wounds. If underlying deformation of the skull is detected, application of dry, sterile gauze is appropriate. Scalp lacerations can be sutured at the bedside or may require surgical repair, depending on the size and extent of injury. Avulsion of areas of the scalp often require surgical reimplantation because vascular structures must also be addressed during the repair.

SKULL FRACTURE

The skull offers protection to the brain by distributing forces outward, lessening the direct impact to the brain. It is important to remember that blood vessels travel along bony grooves on the inside surface of the skull. Fractures occurring directly over these vessels can injure them, producing an epidural hematoma (discussed later in this chapter). Skull fractures may be compound (i.e., occurring with an open wound) or displaced (closed wound in which the edges of the fracture no longer meet), or they can be linear. Depressed skull fractures are fractures in which bone is pressed into the dura; this is often felt as a depression or dip on palpation. Patients with depressed skull fractures often require surgical elevation of the bone, debridement of bone fragments, and careful repair of the dura. Injury to the dura places the patient at risk for meningitis; therefore, careful monitoring for signs and symptoms is important. Studies have not shown a clear benefit to prophylactic treatment with antibiotics in preventing meningitis after basilar skull fracture and cerebrospinal fluid (CSF) leak.[2,3]

Basilar skull fractures occur at the base, or floor, of the skull, typically in the areas of the anterior fossa and middle fossa. Basilar skull fractures can be linear or compound. Careful assessment of extraocular movements is important in detecting the impingement or damage of cranial nerves that can become entrapped in a basilar skull fracture. Placement of nasogastric tubes and nasotracheal intubation should be avoided because these tubes could pass through the fractured areas of the skull and cause damage to the brain. Placement of an orogastric tube or orotracheal intubation is a better option in these patients.

Drainage of CSF from the ear or nose indicates injury to the dura. Drainage from the ear, termed *otorrhea*, typically signifies a fracture in the middle fossa. Ecchymosis (bruising) behind the ear (Battle's sign) is a delayed sign of a basilar skull fracture in the middle fossa. *Rhinorrhea*, CSF drainage from the nose, occurs with a fracture in the anterior fossa. "Raccoon eyes," a ringlike pattern of bruising around the eyes, is a late sign of this type of fracture.

Drainage from the ear or nose may be mixed with blood, making identification of CSF difficult. To assess the drainage, the nurse gently wipes a gauze pad across the area. A layering of fluids, with blood on the inside and CSF in a yellowish ring on the outside (the "halo sign"), should appear. Patients may also report a sweet or salty taste if CSF drips down the pharynx. Clear fluid can be tested for glucose to distinguish between CSF and other body fluids.

CSF leaks typically heal on their own with rest; however, in situations in which the leak persists, a lumbar catheter may be placed to drain CSF from below, reducing pressure on the site of injury. In rare cases, surgical repair and packing of the leak must be performed. A loose gauze dressing can be applied to the ear or nose to quantify the amount and character of drainage. The patient should be instructed not to blow his or her nose.

CONCUSSION

A concussion is classified as a mild traumatic brain injury and defined as any alteration in mental status resulting from trauma that may or may not involve a loss of consciousness. Often patients are unable to recall events leading up to a traumatic event, and occasionally short-term memory is affected after the event; however, not all patients experience memory disturbance. Patients with concussions may undergo observation in emergency departments or seek medical attention after the injury at a

table 36-1 Defining the Severity of Head Injury

Severity	Description
Mild	GCS score 13–15 May have lost consciousness or exhibited amnesia for 5–60 min No abnormality on CT scan and length of hospital stay <48 h
Moderate	GCS score 9–12 Loss of consciousness or amnesia for 1–24 h May have abnormality on CT scan
Severe	GCS score 3–8 Loss of consciousness or amnesia for more than 24 h May have a cerebral contusion, laceration, or intracranial hematoma

GCS, Glasgow Coma Scale.

private doctor's office because of headache or other nonspecific symptoms. However, many patients never seek medical attention. Cerebral concussions are not associated with structural abnormalities on radiographic imaging. Recovery after a concussion is usually quick and complete, but some patients may exhibit symptoms of postconcussion syndrome, which include headaches, decreased attention span, short-term memory impairment, dizziness, irritability, and emotional lability. These symptoms can last for months up to 1 year and can often be alarming to both the patient and the family. Therefore, discharge teaching must include a review of these signs and symptoms, and information regarding where to seek medical follow-up.

CONTUSION

A cerebral contusion is a focal injury that ranges in severity according to the size and extent of brain tissue injury. Contusions in the brain are the result of laceration of microvessels and usually begin on the surface of the cortex, occasionally spreading to deeper layers of the brain. The diagnosis of cerebral contusion is made using computed tomography (CT) scans. Focal neurological deficits may occur with small lesions, whereas multiple or large contusions may result in depressed level of consciousness, abnormal posturing, and coma. Mortality and morbidity associated with cerebral contusions is related to cerebral edema, which occurs in response to the brain tissue injury. When explaining this type of injury and the development of cerebral edema to a patient or family member, it is sometimes helpful to make a comparison with an injured finger that swells after the injury. Cerebral edema peaks at 24 to 72 hours after the injury, causing increased intracranial pressure (ICP) and possibly further injury to intracranial structures. These patients may progressively deteriorate over the first 72 hours and therefore require intensive anticipatory monitoring (serial neurological assessments) to prevent further brain injury. If cerebral edema is not controlled, cerebral herniation and brain death may ensue.

EPIDURAL HEMATOMA

An epidural hematoma is a collection of blood located between the dura and the inner table of the skull, usually caused by laceration of an extradural artery (Fig. 36-2). Epidural hematomas accumulate rapidly because of arterial bleeding and require prompt recognition and expeditious surgical intervention to prevent cerebral herniation. Patients with epidural hematomas may initially lose consciousness, regain consciousness, and then rapidly deteriorate to unconsciousness. Posturing and unilateral dilation of the pupil represent late signs of cerebral herniation. The only remedy for this injury is immediate surgical evacuation; *an epidural hematoma is a neurosurgical emergency.* Functional outcome depends on expedient removal of the clot and the presence of other underlying brain injury.

SUBDURAL HEMATOMA

A subdural hematoma is an accumulation of blood below the dura and above the arachnoid covering of the brain (see Fig. 36-2). Tearing of the surface veins or disruption of venous sinuses can cause a subdural hematoma. The incidence of subdural hematoma increases in the elderly and in patients with alcoholism, due to cortical atrophy, which puts tension on the bridging veins leading from the surface of the brain to the inner surface of the skull. The increased incidence of falls compounds the risk of subdural hematomas in these two subpopulations. Subdural hematomas can be separated into the following three categories based on the time from injury to the onset of symptoms: acute, subacute, and chronic.

Patients with an acute subdural hematoma manifest symptoms within 24 to 48 hours after injury because of

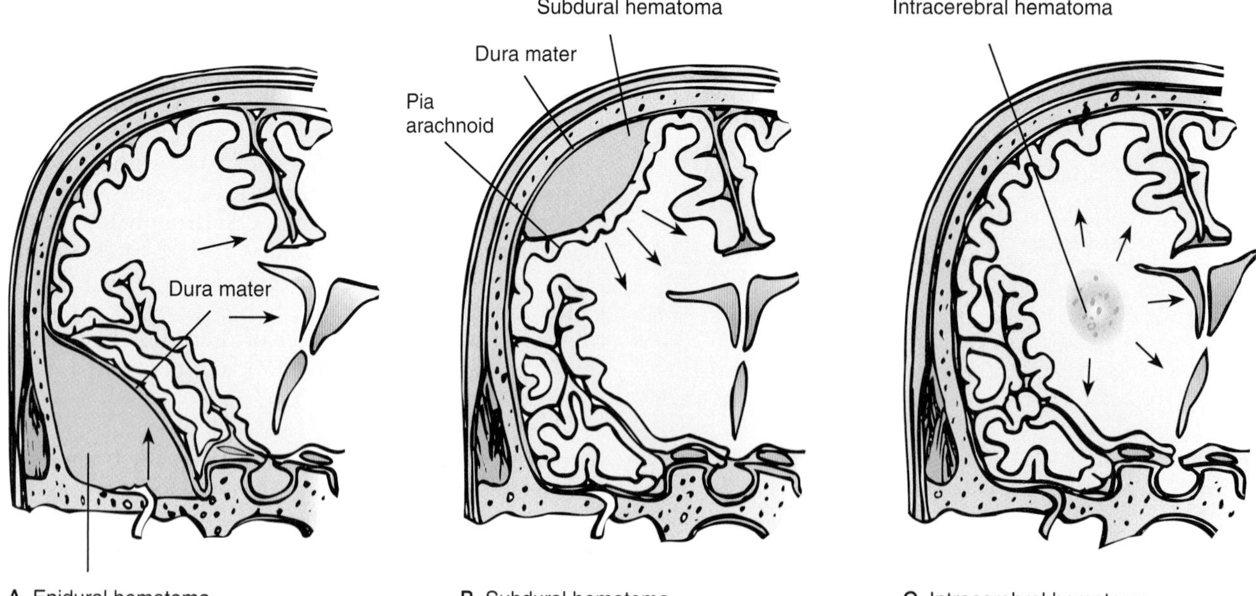

figure 36-2 Cerebral hematomas. (**A**) An epidural hematoma. (**B**) A subdural hematoma. (**C**) An intracerebral hematoma. (Used with permission from Hickey JV: The Clinical Practice of Neurological and Neuroscience Nursing [5th Ed.], p 381. Philadelphia, Lippincott Williams & Wilkins, 2002.)

slower accumulation of blood from veins. Symptoms include worsening headache, focal neurological deficit, unilateral pupillary abnormalities, and a decreasing level of consciousness. Cerebral herniation may result if increased ICP is not treated or the hematoma is not removed.

Subacute subdural hematomas are associated with an onset of symptoms 2 days to 2 weeks after injury. The onset of symptoms is slower and often more innocuous than in an acute hematoma. Surgical clot evacuation may be performed on an elective basis.

Patients with a chronic subdural hematoma may experience an initial small bleed that does not cause symptoms. However, over time, slow capillary leaking causes expansion of the mass and produces symptoms of increased ICP. A chronic subdural hematoma can be differentiated from other subtypes by a layering of blood or a thickened fibrous membrane that can sometimes be identified on CT. Chronic subdural hematomas are often seen in elderly patients with a history of falling. Cerebral atrophy affords more space for a hematoma to expand before producing symptoms. Common symptoms include headache, lethargy, confusion, and seizures. A craniotomy may be performed to remove the hematoma and drains placed to facilitate drainage of the surgical site. The head of the patient's bed may be ordered to remain flat to mitigate tension placed on bridging veins when the head is elevated. This is thought to prevent rebleeding and reaccumulation of the clot in the immediate postoperative period.

INTRACEREBRAL HEMATOMA

An intracerebral hematoma is a collection of blood within the brain tissue (see Fig. 36-2). Traumatic causes of intracerebral hematoma include depressed skull fractures, penetrating missile injuries, and sudden acceleration–deceleration. Treatment of patients with intracerebral hematoma remains controversial regarding whether surgical intervention is warranted or medical management is more appropriate. In general, surgical intervention is pursued only if the lesion continues to expand and is located close to the surface of the brain. Evacuation of a deep intracerebral hematoma may have more associated risks than benefits. Medical therapy aims to manage cerebral edema and promote adequate cerebral perfusion.

TRAUMATIC SUBARACHNOID HEMORRHAGE

Traumatic subarachnoid hemorrhage occurs with tearing or shearing of microvessels in the arachnoid layer where CSF flows around the brain. A traumatic subarachnoid hemorrhage often accompanies other severe brain injuries and appears to be associated with poor outcome and increased morbidity.[4,5] Additional complications such as hydrocephalus and cerebral vasospasm add to the complexity of the injury.

DIFFUSE AXONAL INJURY

Diffuse axonal injury (DAI) is characterized by a direct tearing or shearing of axons, which worsens during the first 12 to 24 hours as both local and diffuse edema develops. DAI prolongs or disables signal conduction from the white matter to gray matter in the brain and is thought to occur with rotational and acceleration–deceleration forces. DAI can be classified as mild, moderate, or severe based on length of coma and degree of neurological dysfunction. Mild DAI is associated with a coma lasting no longer than 24 hours; moderate DAI is characterized by a coma lasting beyond 24 hours with transient flexor or extensor posturing. Severe DAI is characterized by prolonged coma, fever, diaphoresis, and severe extensor posturing. DAI is not easily identified through radiographic imaging in the first 24 hours; however, small punctate hemorrhages may be visualized deep in the white matter, a finding that increases the clinician's suspicion for DAI. Magnetic resonance imaging (MRI) may be helpful in identifying neuronal damage after 24 hours.

CEREBROVASCULAR INJURY

Injury or dissection of the carotid and vertebral arteries due to trauma was once thought to be rare; however, current findings suggest this is not true.[6] Arterial dissection is characterized by bleeding into the blood vessel wall, causing damage to the innermost endothelial layer (i.e., the intima). Damage to the intima can result in clot formation or an intimal flap, either of which can occlude the vessel, resulting in stroke. The key to preventing stroke in these patients is early identification of the injury, exclusion of concomitant hemorrhage, and initiation of anticoagulant therapy. To detect this type of injury, magnetic resonance angiography (MRA) or cerebral angiography may be performed on patients who have sustained injury to the neck or have unexplained focal neurological deficits.

Secondary Brain Injury

Secondary brain injury encompasses all events leading to further brain damage that occur after the initiating trauma. Examples of conditions causing secondary brain injury are uncontrolled increased ICP, cerebral ischemia, systemic hypotension, and local or systemic infection. Prevention of secondary injury is crucial in preserving brain function and optimizing functional outcome.[7,8] The mechanisms by which functional neurons are endangered include inflammation, ischemia, and cerebral blood flow disturbances.[9] These secondary processes can result in cerebral infarction, coma, and herniation.[9] Prevention of hypotension, hypercarbia, hypoxemia, and seizures is extremely important in attempting to prevent further injury.[10]

Understanding intracranial dynamics and the nature of cerebral blood flow is essential to preventing and treating secondary brain injury. See Chapter 34 for a complete discussion of intracranial dynamics and the Monro-Kellie doctrine (i.e., the contents of the cranium—brain, CSF, and blood—have a fixed volume, and any addition to this volume must be balanced by reduction in one of the other components). The compliance curve (Fig. 36-3) illustrates the body's ability to compensate for additions of water, CSF, or blood into the cranial vault until a critical point is reached, at which compensation has been maximized. This critical point indicates a decrease in intracranial compliance in which a small addition of volume will cause a disproportionate increase in ICP. For example, an intubated patient with a head injury and ICP monitor is suctioned at 10 A.M., and the nurse notes an anticipated

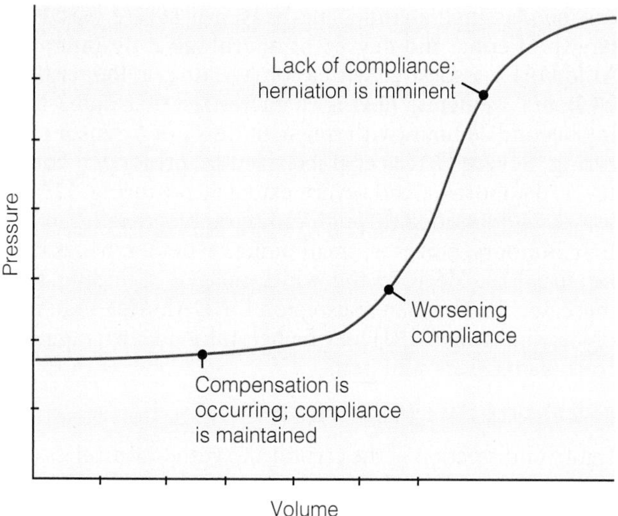

figure 36-3 The compliance curve. The body is able to compensate for the addition of water, blood, or cerebrospinal fluid (CSF) to the cranial vault until a critical point is reached where compensation has been maximized. At this point, the addition of a small amount of volume will cause a disproportionate increase in intracranial pressure (ICP).

transient increase in ICP that returns to baseline over the next 60 seconds. At 2 P.M., the patient is again suctioned, and an increase in ICP is noted. This time, however, the nurse notes that the ICP decreases very slowly and reaches a plateau at 30 mm Hg. The initial increase in ICP after suctioning occurs because of coughing and a resultant increase in intrathoracic pressure, which quickly decreases with the ICP as the patient calms. In this patient's case it appears that intracranial compliance has decreased over the 4-hour period, resulting in a prolonged elevation of ICP after suctioning. After a change in ICP is noted, the patient's neurological states should be rapidly reassessed. Possible causes for the decrease in compliance are cerebral edema (an increase in brain water), expansion of a mass lesion (i.e., hematoma), development of a new mass lesion, or hydrocephalus (an increase in CSF). A thorough understanding of intracranial dynamics and pressure–volume relationships allows the clinician to anticipate worsening patient conditions and possible treatment options.

Cerebral autoregulation is a protective mechanism that enables the brain to achieve a constant blood flow over a range of fluctuating systemic blood pressures (see Chapter 34 for a complete discussion). Several studies have shown that cerebral blood flow, which is normally 50 mL per 100 g of brain tissue per minute, can decrease up to 50% during the first 24 to 48 hours after injury.[8] Researchers have suggested that even one episode of decreased systolic blood pressure less than 90 mm Hg may lead to increased mortality in severely brain-injured adults.[11] Therefore, treatment decisions are centered around maintaining adequate cerebral perfusion pressure. (See Chapter 34 for a full discussion of cerebral perfusion pressure.)

Biochemical mechanisms may also play a role in causing secondary brain injury. Contemporary theories identify the release of excitatory amino acids, calcium ions, reactive oxygen species, and free fatty acids as well as the inflammatory cascade as major causes of (secondary) brain injury.[7,12] The excitatory amino acid glutamate has been widely implicated in cerebral ischemia because of its ability to bind to the *N*-methyl-D-aspartate (NMDA) receptor, allowing an influx of sodium and calcium into the cell and displacing potassium, a chain of events that eventually results in cellular edema. Researchers have postulated that low–blood-flow states in the brain initiate a destructive chain of events that incites the release of cytokines and other natural mechanisms of the body's defense system. The inflammatory response has been implicated as a potential cause or exacerbating factor in many disease processes, and its role in secondary brain injury warrants further investigation.

CEREBRAL EDEMA

Cerebral edema commonly occurs in patients with head injuries 24 to 48 hours after the primary insult and typically peaks at 72 hours. Cerebral edema may cause the patient's condition to worsen before it improves. Patients require increased observation during this period because of the increased risk of deterioration. It is helpful to inform families about the course of cerebral edema so that they can be aware of the potential deterioration over the first 72 hours, even if the patient appears to be progressing well. If cerebral edema is not aggressively treated, it causes herniation syndrome. The treatment of cerebral edema is discussed in Chapter 34.

Cytotoxic and vasogenic edema are discussed in this section with respect to the pathophysiology of brain injury. Cytotoxic edema occurs as the intracellular sodium–potassium pump fails, allowing an influx of sodium and water into the cell and an efflux of potassium. Vasogenic edema occurs with a disruption of the blood–brain barrier. Disruption of the blood–brain barrier can occur as a result of injury or a surgical procedure.

ISCHEMIA

Cerebral ischemia comprises a serious class of secondary injury and is a major cause of morbidity and mortality. It is unknown whether ischemia typically occurs at the time of injury or in subsequent periods.[8] Cerebral ischemia occurs whenever blood flow is either diminished or inadequate to meet metabolic demands. The end point of unresolved ischemia is infarction or tissue death, which then incites a cascade of events resulting in additional edema (see Chapter 35 for further information on cerebral ischemia and stroke).

HERNIATION SYNDROME

Herniation syndrome describes a state in which cerebral structures shift inside the cranium under high pressure. Cushing's triad describes the three late signs of herniation: increased systolic blood pressure, decreased heart rate, and an irregular respiratory pattern. Widened pulse pressure is also associated with herniation. Changes in vital signs can occur rapidly, but typically have a gradual onset as the brainstem becomes compressed. Irregular respiratory patterns vary according to the location of lesions in the brain. The examination findings of a patient with increased

table 36-2 Increased Intracranial Pressure Versus Herniation Syndrome

	Increased ICP	Herniation Syndrome
Level of arousal	Increased stimulus required	Unarousable
Motor function	Subtle motor weakness or pronator drift	Dense motor weakness, posturing or absent response
Pupillary response	Sluggish pupillary response	Unilateral dilated and fixed pupil ("blown pupil")
Vital signs	May be stable or labile	Cushing's triad (increased systolic blood pressure, decreased heart rate, irregular respiration)

Used with permission from an unpublished lecture, Lomer J, 1997.

ICP can be contrasted to those of a patient with herniation syndrome (Table 36-2).

Four common displacement syndromes include uncal herniation, tonsillar herniation, central (transtentorial) herniation, and upward cerebellar herniation. The most common syndromes in the setting of critical care and trauma are uncal and tonsillar herniation (Table 36-3).

Herniation of the medial temporal lobe through the tentorium is termed uncal herniation. Uncal herniation often produces unilateral pupillary dilation from compression of the third cranial nerve, with contralateral hemiplegia or posturing. Uncal herniation may not produce changes in vital signs until contents are further shifted downward against the brainstem, causing it to herniate through the foramen magnum. Therefore, it is important to note that changes in vital signs are often a **late sign.** Tonsillar herniation describes the downward displacement of the cerebellar tonsils through the foramen magnum, which causes compression of the cervicomedullary junction. Clinical signs include loss of consciousness early in the process, respiratory changes and arrest, flaccid paralysis, and neck pain/head tilt. Central herniation can be caused by bilateral expanding lesions or a centrally located mass lesion causing downward displacement of the cerebral hemispheres and midline structures (i.e., the basal ganglia, diencephalon, and the midbrain) through the tentorium[13] (Fig. 36-4).

Critical care nurses have the opportunity to make a significant contribution to patient outcome by performing thorough serial neurological examinations, taking into account subtle changes. Once thought to be immediately fatal, herniation syndrome has been shown to be reversible with aggressive therapy in certain circumstances.

COMA

Coma is an alteration in consciousness caused by damage to both hemispheres of the brain or the brainstem. Coma results from disruption of the reticular activating system (RAS), which is a physiological entity encompassing nuclei from the medulla through the cerebral cortex. The RAS is responsible for wakefulness, heightened arousal, and alert-

table 36-3 Herniation Syndromes

Name	Tissue Displaced	Common Causes	Clinical Signs
Central (transtentorial) herniation	Supratentorial	Compression and impaired blood flow to the brainstem Chronic increases in ICP Tumor in frontal, parietal, occipital lobes	Early altered alertness Respiratory sighs, yawns, pauses Roving eyes, small pupils Late sign: decorticate or decerebrate posturing
Uncal herniation	Supratentorial	Rapidly expanding lesions—hematoma	Early unilateral dilating pupil Once brainstem signs begin, deterioration is rapid
Upward cerebellar herniation	Infratentorial	Posterior fossa mass	Coma Cerebellar infarct if superior cerebellar arteries occluded Hydrocephalus with involvement of sylvian aqueduct
Tonsillar herniation	Infratentorial	Elevated ICP Expanding mass	Cranial nerve abnormalities Respiratory changes (apneustic/cluster breathing) Change in level of consciousness (rapid)

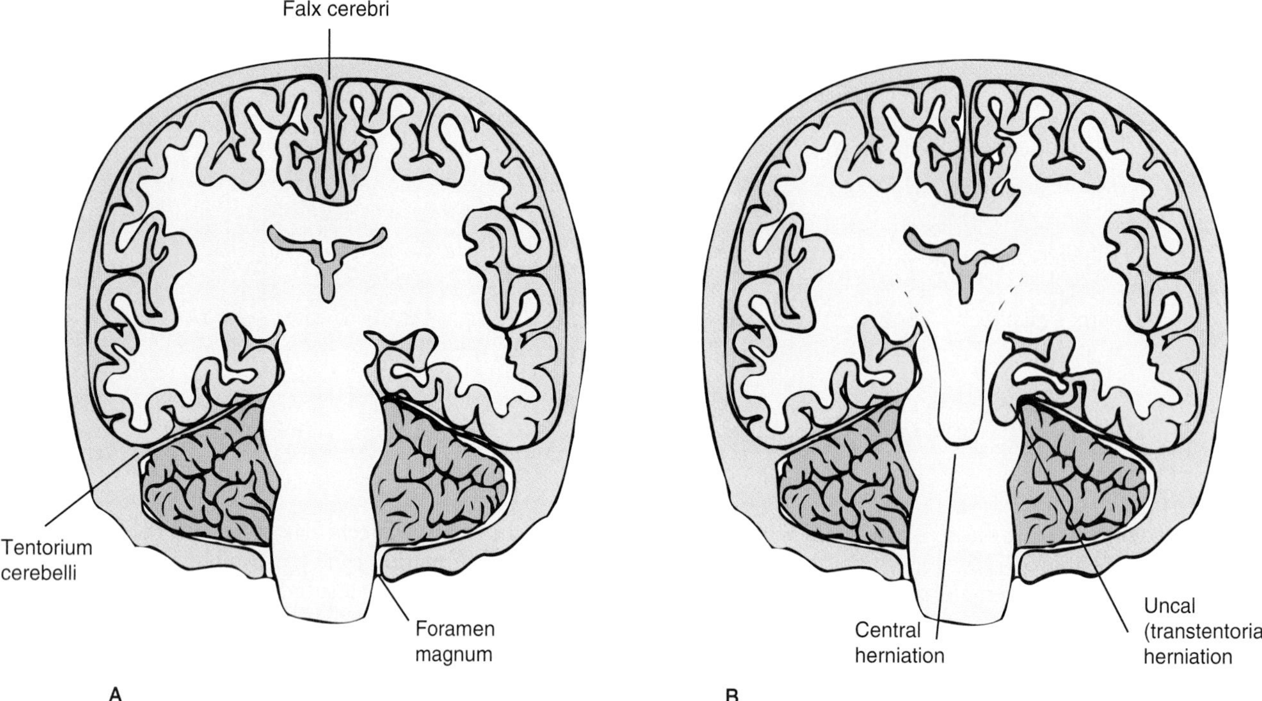

figure 36-4 (**A**) Normal brain. (**B**) Herniated brain. Herniation associated with brainstem compression is called *central herniation,* whereas herniation associated with the supratentorial structures is called *uncal (transtentorial) herniation.*

ness. Multiple causes of coma exist (Box 36-2) and must be considered in the treatment of the patient with head injury to give the patient an optimal chance of regaining consciousness. Consciousness can be placed on a continuum from full consciousness to coma, and states of coma can be subdivided into light coma, coma, and deep coma (see Chapter 33, Box 33-4).

PERSISTENT VEGETATIVE STATE

Several terms describe a persistent vegetative state, such as *irreversible coma* or *coma vigil.* A persistent vegetative state is characterized by a period of sleeplike coma followed by a return to the awake state but with a total lack of apparent cognition.[14] In a persistent vegetative state, the higher cortical functions of the cerebral hemispheres have been damaged permanently, but the lower functions of the brainstem remain intact. The patient's eyes may open spontaneously, or they may open seemingly in response to verbal stimuli. Sleep–wake cycles exist. The patient maintains normal blood pressure and respiratory control. Also seen are involuntary lip smacking, chewing, and roving eye movements.

A diagnosis of persistent vegetative state cannot be made for at least 4 weeks after onset of traumatic brain injury and coma.[14] This diagnosis elicits ethical concerns regarding quality-of-life issues. Caring for the patient in a persistent vegetative state can be a physical and emotional challenge. Dealing with alternating cycles of hope and grief on the part of family and friends can be emotionally battering. The critical care nurse should use all available resources of pastoral care, social service, and various assistance programs to work through personal thoughts and feelings. Everyone involved in the care of such patients should have a realistic understanding of the prognosis of persistent vegetative state. Supporting the family in the process of gathering information and making decisions is difficult but essential.

ASSESSMENT

Physical Examination

The two most important tenets of neurological assessment are (1) level of consciousness is the most sensitive indica-

box 36-2
Causes of Coma

- Infections of the central nervous system
- Electrolyte disturbances
- Hyperthyroidism (thyroid storm)
- Hypothyroidism (myxedema coma)
- Hypoxia
- Psychiatric conditions
  - Hysteria
  - Catatonia
- Seizures
- Structural lesions (i.c., DAI)
- Toxins
  - Drugs
  - Toxic metabolites of organ failure

tor of increased ICP, and (2) *maximum stimulus* must be applied to achieve the *maximum patient response*.

Serial neurological examinations of the patient with a head injury are paramount to the management of brain injury. The Glasgow Coma Scale (GCS; see Chapter 33, Box 33-5) is useful in assessing trends of neurological function over time; however, focal motor deficits are not taken into consideration. The advantages of the GCS are ease of use and proven consistency across evaluators.

ASSESSMENT OF COGNITIVE FUNCTION

Assessment of cognitive function and level of arousal is one of the most commonly performed assessments; however, the purpose of this section is to provide the critical care nurse with a system with which to observe subtle neurological changes. Cognitive function is usually assessed by asking three orientation questions regarding person, place, and time. However, it is necessary to elicit an "embroidered" or specific history from the patient to facilitate the detection of subtle changes over time. Patients may learn to answer the same questions correctly because of repetition, but may still exhibit confusion when questioned further. For example, instead of asking the patient to state where he or she is, the nurse can ask the patient to recall what type of place he or she is in, or ask the name of the hospital, the city, and the state. Asking the patient to name his or her children, spouse, or close family members is also helpful.

ASSESSMENT OF LEVEL OF AROUSAL

In assessing arousal in the head-injured patient, a maximum stimulus must be applied in a systematic and escalating fashion to effectively elicit the patient's best, or maximum, response. Clinicians first attempt to arouse the patient simply by speaking (in the same manner as you would try to wake a person who is sleeping), then by shouting (as you would to wake a "sound sleeper"), next by shaking, and then by applying pain. This staged approach affords the patient the opportunity to demonstrate increasing wakefulness or his or her best response. If a patient wakes readily, his ability to follow simple commands should be assessed by asking him to move the extremities or show two fingers. When asking a patient to grip or squeeze the evaluator's hand, it is important to make sure that the person can both squeeze and release the grip. Patients with injury to the frontal lobe may have damaged the area of grasp inhibition, which develops after infancy. In this instance, the patient would grasp because of a reflex instead of a voluntary action.

If a painful stimulus must be applied, the following techniques are useful: Squeeze the belly of the trapezius muscle with the thumb and first finger where the neck and shoulder meet, apply pressure over the supraorbital notch, or perform a sternal rub (Fig. 36-5). The sternal rub should be performed less often because of severe bruising when patients are repeatedly examined. If a response is not elicited with these maneuvers, then pressure may be applied to the nailbeds of the patient's fingers or toes by placing a pencil on the nail and rolling it back and forth while applying pressure. Movement elicited by nailbed pressure may be reflexive. A painful stimulus should be applied for 15 to 30 seconds before the patient is considered not to have a motor response because patients with brain injury may exhibit delayed responses to stimuli.

ASSESSMENT OF THE EYES

Assessment of the eyes includes evaluation of the pupils and extraocular movements, which assists in localizing regions of the brain dysfunction.

Testing of cranial nerve II (the optic nerve) in the acute care setting involves detection of gross visual field defects and visual acuity. Visual fields can be adequately assessed by the patient's ability to detect movement of the evaluator's finger in each field of vision (see Chapter 33 for technique). Visual acuity can be grossly assessed by asking the patient to read printed words on a page or by using a Snellen eye chart. If there is concern about optic nerve impairment, a full evaluation by an ophthalmologist is recommended.

Evaluation of the third cranial nerve (the oculomotor nerve) involves inspection of the pupil, including size, shape, equality, and reaction to light. Increased ICP can cause irregularities in shape, pupillary inequality (anisocoria), and sluggish or absent reaction to light. Patients with increased ICP may also exhibit a pupillary response called *hippus*, in which the pupils dilate and contract continuously when light is shown on them.

Cranial nerves III, IV, and VI (the oculomotor, trochlear, and abducens nerves) are often grouped together for assessment purposes because these nerves enable movement of the eyes. Cranial nerves III and IV exit at the level of the midbrain, and cranial nerve VI exits at the level of the pons. Assessment of these nerves is accomplished by asking the patient to follow the evaluator's finger while it is moved in an "H" pattern. Double vision (diplopia) is a sign of eye muscle weakness and cranial nerve impairment.

In the comatose patient, the following tests are performed to evaluate cranial nerves III, VI, and VIII (the oculomotor and abducens nerves, and the vestibular portion of the acoustic nerve). The oculocephalic reflex (i.e., the "doll's eyes" phenomenon; see Chapter 33, Fig. 33-6) is tested by moving the head from side to side in a horizontal plane (after confirming the absence of cervical spinal fracture). If the oculocephalic response is present, the eyes will move together in the opposite direction of the head as it is turned from side to side. Absence of eye movement on head turning reflects brainstem dysfunction. The oculovestibular reflex (see Chapter 33, Fig. 33-7) is tested by instilling cold water into each ear and observing the eyes for movement. A normal oculovestibular response is characterized by movement of the eyes toward the stimulus with nystagmus. The absence of movement signals loss of function of the vestibular portion of the eighth cranial nerve as well as the brainstem.

ASSESSMENT OF BRAINSTEM RESPONSES

The brainstem can be further assessed in the unconscious patient by testing corneal, cough, and gag reflexes. The corneal reflex reflects function of both the fifth and seventh cranial nerves (the trigeminal and facial nerves), which exit the brain at the level of the midbrain and pons,

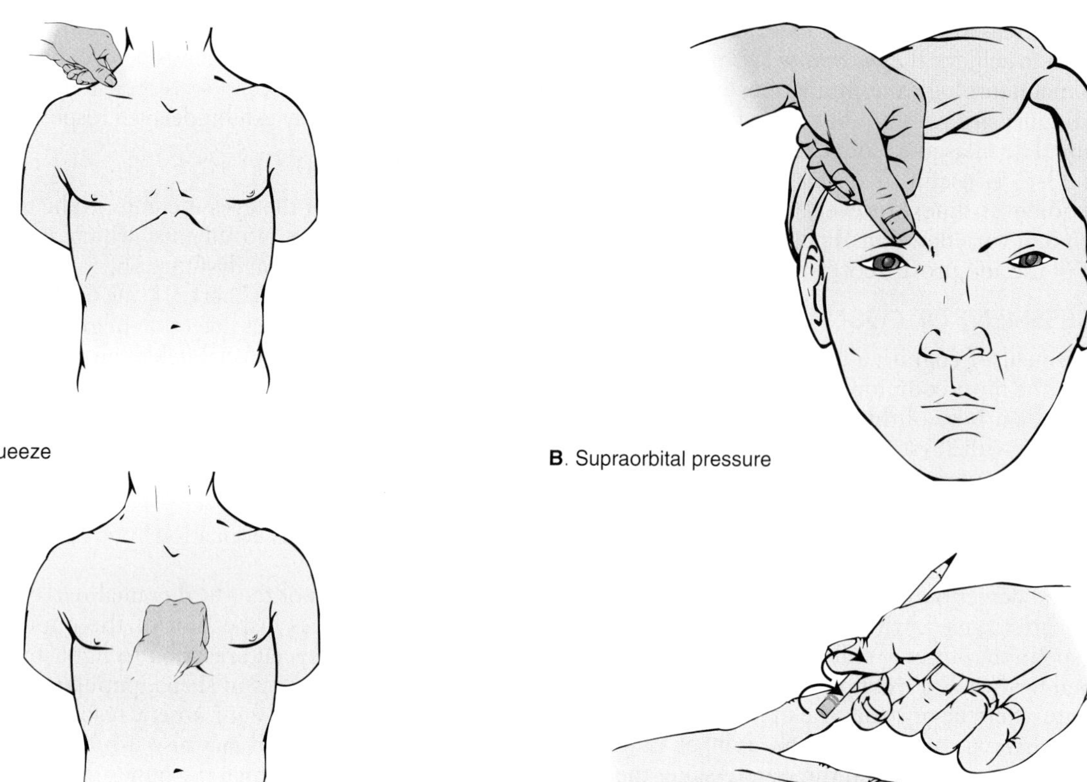

figure 36-5 Methods of applying a painful stimulus. (**A**) Trapezius squeeze. (**B**) Application of supraorbital pressure. (**C**) Sternal rub. (**D**) Application of pressure to the nailbed.

respectively. This reflex is tested by passing a wisp of cotton over the lower conjunctiva of each eye. Flickering or blinking of the lower lid indicates the presence of the reflex. Sensation of the irritating stimulus represents gross function of one branch of the trigeminal nerve, and movement of the lower lid represents motor function of the facial nerve. Care must be taken in testing the corneal reflex to avoid causing abrasions to the cornea.

Cranial nerves IX and X (the glossopharyngeal and vagus nerves) exit at the level of the medulla and are responsible for the cough and gag reflexes and protection of the airway from aspiration. The cough and gag reflexes should be evaluated in both the awake and unconscious patient.

ASSESSMENT OF MOTOR FUNCTION

Motor function is evaluated by using the staged approach described earlier. Further detailed assessment of motor function is tested in the awake and cooperative patient by having the patient move his or her extremities against gravity and with passive resistance, grading the movement on a scale of 1 to 5 (see Chapter 33).

The unresponsive patient may exhibit localization, withdrawal, or flexor or extensor posturing in response to noxious stimuli. Localization of a painful stimulus is observed as a purposeful response in which the patient is able to locate the source of pain and move toward it with one or both extremities crossing the midline of the body. A patient may try to remove the evaluator's hand when he or she performs a trapezius squeeze, or the patient may attempt to grab his or her endotracheal tube. A withdrawal response is characterized by movement away from a painful stimulus. Flexor posturing, also known as decorticate posturing, occurs as a result of diffuse cortical injury and is characterized by the bending or flexing of the upper extremities and extension of the lower extremities and feet. Extensor posturing or decerebrate posturing indicates injury to the brainstem and is observed as extension and internal rotation of the upper extremities and extension of the lower extremities and feet (see Chapter 33, Fig. 33-1). It is important to note that a patient may exhibit one type of movement in one extremity and another type of movement in another extremity. Presence of Babinski's reflex (upward fanning of the toes) is also observed in the patient with severe brain injury.

ASSESSMENT OF RESPIRATORY FUNCTION

Assessment of respiratory function and patterns of respiration are important in detecting worsening neurological injury and the need for mechanical support. Numerous locations in both cerebral hemispheres regulate voluntary control over the muscles used in breathing, with the cerebellum synchronizing and coordinating the muscular effort. The cerebrum also has some control over the rate and rhythm of respiration. Nuclei in the pons and midbrain areas of the brainstem regulate the automaticity of respiration.

Cheyne-Stokes breathing is periodic breathing in which the depth of each breath increases to a peak and then decreases to apnea (Fig. 36-6). The hyperpneic phase usually lasts longer than the apneic phase. Cheyne-Stokes breathing patterns may be a normal result of aging when they occur in an older person during sleep. The pattern also may be seen in patients with bilateral lesions located deep in the cerebral hemispheres. This herniation also can cause compression of the midbrain, and *central neurogenic hyperventilation* will be observed. Hyperventilation is sustained, regular, rapid, and deep. It usually is caused by a lesion above the midbrain. *Apneustic breathing* is characterized by respiration with a long pause at full inspiration or full expiration. The etiology of this pattern is loss of all cerebral and cerebellar control of breathing, with respiratory function at the brainstem level only. *Cluster breathing* may be seen in a patient when the lesion is high in the medulla or low in the pons. This pattern of respiration is seen as gasping breaths with irregular pauses.

The critical centers of inspiration and expiration are located in the medulla oblongata. Any rapidly expanding intracranial lesion, such as cerebellar hemorrhage, can compress the medulla, and *ataxic breathing* results. This irregular breathing consists of both deep and shallow breaths with irregular pauses. This pattern of respiration signals the need for definitive airway control through endotracheal intubation.

ASSESSMENT OF OTHER BODY SYSTEMS

In addition to the thorough assessment of the central nervous system, comprehensive assessment of all other body systems is crucial in the early identification of complications and sequelae in patients with brain injury.

Diagnostic Testing

Computed tomography (CT) scan is the most common initial test in the setting of head injury because it can be quickly performed and is sensitive to bleeding. One disadvantage of the CT scan is that it is unable to adequately capture the structures in the posterior fossa. Magnetic resonance imaging (MRI) is useful because artifact from bone is minimized so that structures in the base of the skull and the spinal cord are better visualized and neuronal changes caused by DAI can be visualized. Also, MRA can be used to evaluate cerebral vascular injuries in a noninvasive manner.

Cerebral angiography is a useful tool in assessing for blood vessel dissection and the absence of cerebral blood flow in patients with suspected brain death. The risks of this procedure include rupture of blood vessels, stroke from embolized debris, allergic reaction from radiopaque dye, acute renal failure from the intravenous (IV) dye, and retroperitoneal bleeding from the sheath insertion site after removal.

Transcranial Doppler (TCD) ultrasonography indirectly evaluates cerebral blood flow and autoregulatory mechanisms by measuring the velocity at which blood travels through blood vessels. The ability of this test to provide information about cerebral autoregulation may have implications in the management of intracranial dynamics in the head-injured patient in the future.

Neurophysiological tests include the electroencephalogram (EEG), brainstem auditory evoked responses (BAERs), and somatosensory evoked potentials (SSEPs). The EEG measures brain wave activity in all regions of the cortex and is useful in diagnosing seizures and correlating the abnormal neurological examination to abnormal cortical function. The EEG is necessary in ruling out subclinical or nonconvulsive seizures. The EEG has also been used as a confirmatory test in brain death. The most common finding in the head-injured patient is a slowing of electrical

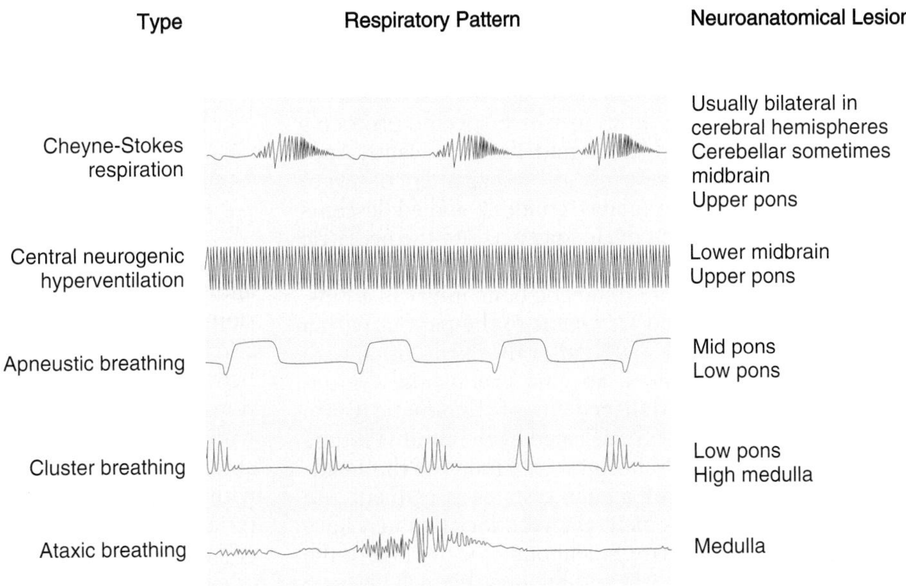

figure 36-6 Injury to the brainstem can result in various abnormal respiratory patterns.

wave activity in the area of injury. The BAER and SSEP are useful prognostic tests in head-injured patients. Abnormal results of either of these tests can help confirm a diagnosis of severe brainstem or cortical dysfunction that will not result in meaningful functional recovery.

Another type of physiological monitoring used in the critically ill patient with a head injury is the jugular bulb catheter, which measures venous oxygen saturation. The level of jugular bulb venous oxygen saturation is reflective of global oxygen delivery and consumption in the brain. The catheter is inserted in a similar manner as an internal jugular central line; however, the tip of the catheter is directed up toward the brain in an anatomical location called the jugular bulb. The average jugular venous oxygen saturation in patients without head injury is 62% (range, 55% to 71%). In head-injured patients, a sustained saturation of 50% to 55% requires investigation of the cause of desaturation.[15]

Contraindications to this catheter include cervical spine injuries, bleeding diathesis, local infection, and impairments of cerebral venous drainage. Because of the increased potential for infection, the presence of a tracheostomy is considered a relative contraindication. Measurement of oxygen delivery and extraction in brain tissue using an oxygen sensor placed in the deep white matter is currently used in institutions as an adjunct to ICP and cerebral perfusion pressure monitoring. Early goal-directed therapies aimed at keeping the partial pressure of brain tissue oxygen ($PbtO_2$) greater than 20 mm Hg in conjunction with ICP and cerebral perfusion pressure management may optimize patients' chances for maximum functional recovery.[16]

MANAGEMENT

Guidelines for the management of severe head injury were developed by the Brain Trauma Foundation and the American Association of Neurological Surgeons in 1995 and updated in 2000 to disseminate the most current scientifically supported recommendations.[17] The widespread dissemination of these guidelines sought to create a consistent standard of care for the treatment of head-injured patients.[18] Several studies have evaluated the effect these guidelines have had on increased positive outcomes in patients cared for in facilities in which specific protocols were implemented based on the guidelines.[19] Recently, specific guidelines for the acute medical management of severe traumatic brain injury in infants, children, and adolescents were published, outlining the unique needs of the pediatric population.[20] The focus of the discussion in this chapter is the management of severe traumatic brain injury in adults.

Initial assessment and treatment of the patient with a head injury begins immediately after the insult, often with prehospital care providers. Specific Prehospital Guidelines for Prehospital Management of Traumatic Brain Injury were developed and published by the Brain Trauma Foundation in 2002. Prehospital treatment of the head-injured patient focuses on a rapid systems assessment and definitive airway management, interventions that may have a positive effect on ultimate patient outcome because of the early correction of hypoxia and hypercarbia, which have been shown to cause and exacerbate secondary brain injury[10,11,21] (Fig. 36-7).

Airway management is a crucial initial step in providing care to the head-injured patient because hypoventilation is common with a decreased level of consciousness, and hypoxia and hypercarbia are extremely detrimental to the patient in the early stages of injury. Initial mechanical ventilation strategies aim to maintain normal ventilation or a partial pressure of carbon dioxide ($PaCO_2$) within normal limits (35 to 45 mm Hg). Further evaluation of neurological status may reveal the need for hyperventilation therapy if signs of cerebral herniation are present and not controlled by other initial pharmacological treatments; however, further monitoring of cerebral blood flow or tissue oxygenation may be warranted to prevent further cerebral ischemia. Hyperventilation should be avoided if at all possible in the first 24 hours after brain injury.[17]

Management of circulation in patients with head injuries aims to promote adequate cerebral perfusion through fluid resuscitation and the use of vasopressors if necessary. Management of cerebral perfusion is a twofold process—that is, concomitant management of ICP is necessary to decrease intracranial resistance to blood flow. Cerebral perfusion pressure is measured with an ICP monitoring device in place as well as an arterial line for accurate minute-to-minute blood pressure measurement; however, cerebral perfusion pressure should be kept in mind even in the initial resuscitation phases when these devices may not be in place. Understanding the concept of cerebral perfusion pressure leads the clinician to perform careful neurological assessment to detect signs of increasing ICP and to intervene rapidly to support a falling blood pressure.

Diagnostic testing is performed to evaluate the need for additional medical therapies or immediate surgical intervention. Essential radiographic imaging includes x-rays of the cervical spine and a CT scan, which is useful in diagnosing mass lesions that may require surgical intervention.

Continuing management seeks to control ICP, promote cerebral perfusion, and correct the primary pathological process. Examples of nursing diagnoses and collaborative problems for the patient with a head injury are given in Box 36-3. General management of the patient with a head injury requires a holistic, multisystem, multidisciplinary approach that is based on the primary pathology, taking into consideration the unique physiological and psychosocial characteristics of the individual (Box 36-4).

Monitoring and Controlling Intracranial Pressure

ICP monitoring, which is discussed in depth in Chapter 34, allows the health care team to make rapid treatment decisions based on pressure displays and ICP waveform analysis. ICP monitors are inserted by neurosurgeons at the bedside or in the operating room, depending on institutional policy. ICP monitoring is recommended for patients with severe head injury (a GCS score of 3 to 8) and CT scan abnormalities on admission. Severely head-injured patients with a negative CT scan who meet one of the following criteria—the patient must be older than 40 years, have unilateral or bilateral posturing, or have a systolic blood pressure of less than 90 mm Hg—should also have an ICP monitoring device. ICP monitoring may also be considered in other situations at the physician's discretion.[17]

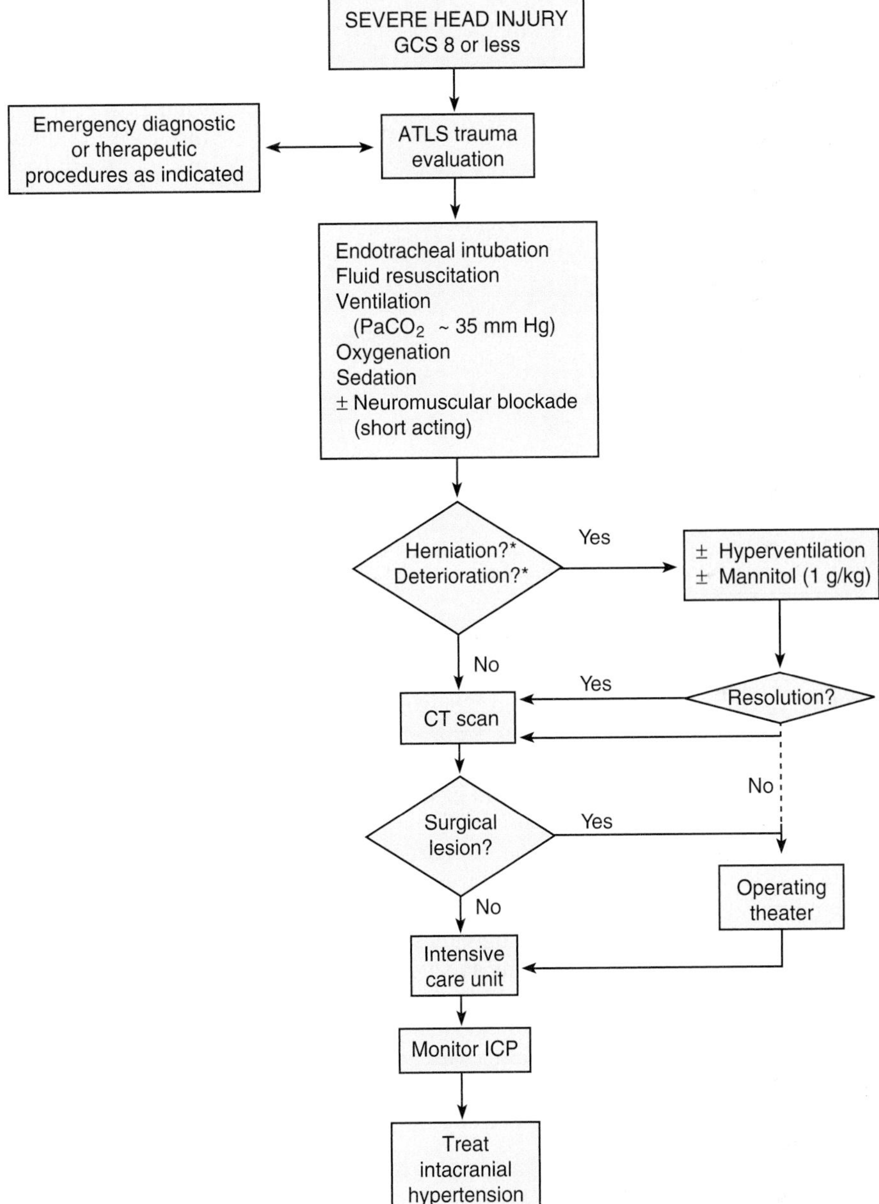

figure 36-7 Flowchart for resuscitation of the patient with a severe head injury before intracranial pressure (ICP) monitoring. *Presence or signs of herniation (pupillary dilation or motor posturing) or progressive neurological deterioration are not attributable to external factors. *GCS,* Glasgow Coma Scale; *ATLS,* Advanced Trauma Life Support; *CT,* computed tomography; *ICP,* intracranial pressure. (Used with permission from Chestnut RM: Medical management of severe head injury: Present and future. New Horiz 3[3]:583, 1995.)

Nursing interventions to manage increased ICP include maintenance of body alignment, avoiding sharp turning of the head to one side and sharp hip flexion. It is also thought that turning of the head to one side may cause compression of the jugular vein, preventing drainage of venous blood from the head and increasing ICP. Sharp hip flexion may also cause an increase in intra-abdominal pressure, preventing normal venous overflow and causing an increase in ICP.

Maintaining Cerebral Perfusion

Cerebral perfusion pressure can be managed either by decreasing ICP or increasing the mean arterial blood pressure. Evidence suggests that maintaining a cerebral perfusion pressure of greater than 60 mm Hg may reduce morbidity and mortality.[9,11,17,22] Aggressive management of increased ICP is attempted with the overall goal of maintaining the cerebral perfusion pressure. It is important that clinicians not get distracted by one single variable, either ICP or mean arterial blood pressure, but rather consider overall perfusion of the brain. For example, blood pressure augmentation may have to be undertaken while measures to decrease ICP are attempted; after ICP is adequately controlled, blood pressure support can be incrementally decreased.

Preventing and Treating Seizures

Post-traumatic seizures occurring in the 7-day period after injury are called *early post-traumatic seizures.* Seizures during this period can have severe negative effects on ICP and

box 36-3 *Examples of Nursing Diagnoses and Collaborative Problems for the Patient With a Head Injury*

- Impaired Cerebral Tissue Perfusion related to cerebral edema
- Ineffective Airway Clearance related to diminished airway protective reflexes
- Risk for Infection related to multiple indwelling monitoring devices
- Impaired Skin Integrity related to physical immobilization
- Imbalanced Nutrition: Less Than Body Requirements related to increased energy expenditure
- Acute Pain related to injury agents
- Disturbed Sleep Pattern related to ICU routine care and environment
- Interrupted Family Processes related to acute crisis
- Anticipatory Grieving related to uncertain prognosis and critical illness

cerebral metabolic demands. Therefore, the guidelines on the management of severe head injury support use of seizure prophylaxis in the early acute period.[17] Seizures that occur after this initial period are called *late post-traumatic seizures.* Multiple studies suggest that continuing anticonvulsant therapy beyond the initial injury period (i.e., the first 7 days) does not prevent late post-traumatic seizures.[17,23]

Phenytoin is one of the most common drugs used in the acute period.[23] Phenytoin is usually given as a bolus dose parenterally, followed by a maintenance dosing schedule. Patients are monitored closely for hypotension, bradycardia, rashes, and IV infiltration during and after administration. Hypotension can be mitigated by administering the drug slowly (no greater than 50 mg/minute). Truncal rashes with varying severity can occur with administration of phenytoin; therefore, careful assessment of the patient's skin is important. The drug should be discontinued with the appearance of rash.

General treatment of seizures in the setting of head injury focuses on stopping the seizure as soon as possible and maintaining patient safety. The patient is turned to the side after the seizure has stopped to facilitate drainage of oral secretions, side rails are padded, and objects are *not* inserted into the patient's mouth. Suction devices and supplemental oxygen should be readily available if the patient is not already intubated. The agents of choice for the rapid control of seizure activity are lorazepam, or diazepam. These drugs are likely to produce respiratory depression, so careful monitoring of respiratory rate and depth are important. (See Chapter 35 for a full discussion of seizure disorders and status epilepticus.)

Fever in the patient with severe traumatic brain injury may increase cerebrometabolic demands and compound secondary brain injury. Careful monitoring of body temperature is necessary to prevent further injury. Infection should be ruled out as the etiology of fever and cooling methods should be employed to maintain a normal body temperature. Therapeutic hypothermia has not been proven to improve outcome in head injury and may have deleterious effects.

Monitoring Fluid and Electrolyte Status

Patients with head injuries may experience derangements of fluid and electrolyte balance for a variety of reasons, such as the administration of osmotic diuretics, increased insensible fluid loss, and pituitary gland dysfunction causing sodium imbalance. The critical care nurse must take all variables into consideration when evaluating a patient's fluid and electrolyte imbalance.

Fluid imbalance in a patient with a head injury can be caused by mannitol therapy with inadequate fluid replacement, insensible losses in excess of daily IV fluid replacement, blood loss from coexisting injuries, gastrointestinal bleeding, and diabetes insipidus. After administering mannitol therapy for increased ICP, total fluid balance and central venous pressure readings may guide the health care team in prescribing adequate fluid replacement with isotonic fluids. Head-injured patients often exhibit periods of hyperpyrexia, which increases insensible losses in addition to other usual sources of insensible loss in the critically ill patient. Bleeding should always be ruled out in the setting of hypovolemia, especially in the trauma population. It is important to realize that trauma patients may present with bleeding or hematomas from occult injuries that were not visible on initial diagnostic examinations. Gastrointestinal bleeding is also a common culprit of volume loss in the critically ill population that must be considered.

Disorders of sodium imbalance are common in the head-injured patient (Table 36-4). Hyponatremia most commonly occurs as a result of syndrome of inappropriate antidiuretic hormone secretion (SIADH), in which antidiuretic hormone (ADH) is released continuously, causing constant reabsorption of water and expansion of intravascular volume. Expansion of intravascular volume creates hemodilution, which leads to a lower concentration of sodium in the blood or relative hyponatremia. SIADH often is a transient phenomenon that can be treated with fluid restriction and judicious sodium replacement.

Cerebral salt-wasting syndrome may also cause hyponatremia. Cerebral salt-wasting syndrome is not fully understood, but involves a primary loss of sodium through the kidneys and intravascular volume contraction. Treatment for this disorder requires fluid and sodium replacement in amounts that equal losses.[24]

Diabetes insipidus is a cause of hypernatremia and hypovolemia that occurs commonly in the patient whose condition has progressed to brain death or in patients with injury or ischemia in the region of the pituitary gland. Diabetes insipidus is diagnosed by an increasing serum sodium level with a low urine specific gravity, because the pituitary gland is either not releasing ADH or is not releasing the hormone in adequate amounts. Treatment for this disorder includes aggressive fluid replacement that matches hourly fluid losses as well as subcutaneous or IV administration of vasopressin. In long-term management of diabetes insipidus, vasopressin can also be administered intranasally.

Finally, hyperglycemia is common in this critically ill population; however, recent animal and clinical studies suggest that hyperglycemia surrounding brain injury, especially in the acute period, exacerbates cerebral ischemia and promotes anaerobic metabolism.[25,26] A study in surgical critical care patients demonstrated an overall improvement in outcome for patients whose glucose was tightly con-

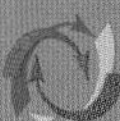 **box 36-4** collaborative care guide
for the Patient With a Head Injury

OUTCOMES	INTERVENTIONS
Oxygenation/Ventilation	
Patient will maintain a patent airway. Lungs will be clear to auscultation. Arterial pH, Pao_2, and Sao_2 will be maintained within normal limits. $ETCO_2$ or Pco_2 will be maintained within prescribed range. There will be no evidence of atelectasis or pneumonia on chest x-ray.	■ Auscultate breath sounds every 2–4 hours and PRN. ■ Hyperoxygenate before and after each suction pass. ■ Avoid suction passes greater than 10 seconds. ■ Monitor ICP and cerebral perfusion pressure (CPP) during suctioning and chest physiotherapy. ■ Provide meticulous oral hygiene. ■ Monitor for signs of aspiration. ■ Encourage nonintubated patients to use incentive spirometer, cough, and deep breathe every 4 hours and PRN. ■ Turn side-to-side every 2 hours. ■ Move patient out of bed to chair one to two times per day when ICP has been controlled.
Circulation/Perfusion	
Patient will exhibit normal sinus rhythm without ectopy or ischemic changes. Patient will not experience thromboembolic complications.	■ Monitor for myocardial ischemia and dysrhythmias due to sympathetic activation and catecholamine surges. ■ Prevent DVT with the use of pneumatic compression devices, antiembolic stockings, and subcutaneous heparin. ■ Implement early mobilization. Facilitate moving to a chair one to two times per day. ■ Monitor blood pressure continuously by arterial line or frequently by noninvasive cuff. ■ Monitor oxygen delivery (hemoglobin, Sao_2, cardiac output). ■ Administer red blood cells, inotropes, intravenous fluids as indicated.
Cerebral Perfusion/Intracranial Pressure	
CPP will be greater than 60 mm Hg. ICP will be less than 20 mm Hg. Patient will not experience seizure activity.	■ Monitor ICP and CPP every hour. ■ Make neurological checks every 1–2 hours. ■ Elevate the head of bed to 30° unless contraindicated. ■ Maintain proper body alignment, keeping the head in a neutral position, and avoiding sharp hip flexion. ■ Maintain normothermia. ■ Maintain a quiet environment, cluster care, and provide rest periods. ■ Provide sedation as necessary and as prescribed. ■ Administer prophylactic antiepileptic agents as prescribed to prevent seizure activity.
Fluids/Electrolytes	
Serum electrolytes will be within normal limits. Serum osmolality will remain within prescribed range.	■ Strict documentation of input/output, consider insensible losses due to intubation, fever, and the like. ■ Monitor serum electrolytes, glucose, and osmolality as ordered. ■ Consider need for electrolyte replacement therapy and administer per physician order or protocol.

(continued)

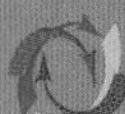

box 36-4 collaborative care guide *for the Patient With a Head Injury (Continued)*

OUTCOMES	INTERVENTIONS
Mobility/Safety	
There will be minimal and transient changes in ICP/CPP during treatments or patient care activities. ICP/CPP will return to baseline within 5 min. Patient will not experience complications related to prolonged immobilization (e.g., DVT, pneumonia, ankylosis). Patient will not harm self by dislodging medical equipment or falling.	▪ Provide range of motion and functional splinting for paralyzed limbs or patients in a coma. ▪ Position patient off of pressure points at least every 2 hours. ▪ Consider use of specialty mattresses based on skin and risk factor assessments. ▪ Keep bed rails in the upright position. ▪ Provide restraints if necessary to prevent dislodgement of medical devices as hospital policies permit.

trolled at levels of 70 to 110 mg/dL.[27] An observational study by Walia and Sutcliffe suggests that hyperglycemia in patients with brain injury independently increases mortality; however, additional studies are required.[28]

Managing Cardiovascular Complications

Initial injury to the brain is thought to cause a massive catecholamine response, which may produce myocardial damage and subsequent electrocardiographic changes. Inversion of T waves and ST segment elevation or depression may be noted on admission or in subsequent hours. It is essential to exclude myocardial damage as a cause for electrocardiographic changes by evaluating cardiac enzymes.

Invasive hemodynamic monitoring, such as arterial blood pressure and central venous pressure monitoring, is integral to the optimization of medical therapies in the critical phases of head injury. Monitoring pulmonary artery pressures and cardiac output may be useful if the patient demonstrates shock syndrome or multisystem failure.

Disorders of coagulation are a significant concern in patients with head injury because large amounts of thromboplastin can be produced and released in response to brain injury, causing disseminated intravascular coagulation (DIC).

Prophylaxis of deep venous thrombosis (DVT) is an essential component to the care of these patients, who are often immobile for extended periods. Sequential compression sleeves provide intermittent pulsatile pressure to the lower extremities, increasing venous return and promoting systemic fibrinolysis. Antiembolic stockings, subcutaneous heparin, and early mobilization help prevent DVT and pulmonary emboli.

Managing Pulmonary Complications

Pulmonary complications in the patient with head trauma include pneumonia, acute respiratory distress syndrome (ARDS), neurogenic pulmonary edema, and pulmonary embolus. Aspiration pneumonia is a common pulmonary complication in this population because of the loss or impairment of airway protective reflexes. Aspiration may occur at the time of the traumatic episode secondary to vomiting of gastric contents or blood, or may occur sometime during the course of hospitalization. It is easy to derive a false sense of security that the airway is completely protected because a patient is intubated; however,

table 36-4 Disorders of Sodium Imbalance: Comparison of Diabetes Insipidus, the Syndrome of Inappropriate Antidiuretic Hormone Secretion, and Cerebral Salt-Wasting Syndrome

	Diabetes Insipidus	Syndrome of Inappropriate Antidiuretic Hormone Secretion	Cerebral Salt-Wasting Syndrome
Urinary output	Increased	Decreased	Increased
Specific gravity	Decreased	Increased	Decreased
Volume status	Decreased	Mildly increased	Decreased
Serum sodium	Increased	Decreased	Decreased
Treatment	Administration of exogenous vasopressin, fluid replacement	Fluid restriction, judicious sodium replacement	Fluid and sodium replacement

these patients may continue to aspirate because of inadequate cuff inflation or pooling of secretions around the cuff that can continue to enter the trachea.[29] Pulmonary toilet, vigilant oral hygiene, and monitoring of endotracheal tube cuff pressure is necessary to prevent nosocomial pneumonia and mitigate most pulmonary complications in patients with head injury who require prolonged mechanical ventilation. The influence of suctioning on ICP and potential hypoxia should also be considered. Preoxygenation, administration of lidocaine, and administration of sedation before suctioning may blunt rises in ICP and decrease associated complications. Proper management of enteral feedings is critical in preventing aspiration. The following measures should be taken:

- Elevate the patient's head of bed to 30 degrees at all times.
- Monitor gastric residuals and consider administration of a prokinetic agent.
- Turn the patient onto the right side to facilitate gastric emptying.

Early mobility is critical in facilitating pulmonary toilet, preventing atelectasis, and preventing pulmonary emboli due to DVT.

ARDS is a hypoxic lung disease resulting from the activation of the inflammatory cascade, causing leakage of protein-rich fluid from the pulmonary capillaries into the interstitium of the lungs as well as destruction of alveolar cells. There are many causes of ARDS in patients with head injury, including concomitant pulmonary contusion, aspiration pneumonia, sepsis, and massive blood transfusion. Medical management of ARDS may involve the use of pressure modes of mechanical ventilation to decrease the volume needed to deliver each breath (high volumes have been implicated in furthering alveolar injury); see Chapter 27 for a complete discussion of the management of ARDS.

Neurogenic pulmonary edema may result from injury to the brainstem, increased ICP, or an increase in sympathetic tone that causes a catecholamine surge at the time of trauma. Neurogenic pulmonary edema often presents as "flash pulmonary edema" because it has a sudden onset. This type of pulmonary edema is thought to be caused by massive vasoconstriction secondary to increased circulating catecholamines, which cause a marked increase in left ventricular afterload and subsequent left ventricular failure. Pulmonary edema due to left ventricular failure is exacerbated by an increase in pulmonary capillary permeability, causing further edema.[29] Treatment includes judicious use of low-dose diuretics, considering the importance of maintaining adequate cerebral perfusion pressure. The condition is typically self-limiting in patients without comorbid cardiac disease.

Multidisciplinary care of the head-injured patient with respect to pulmonary complications must include the nursing team; the physician team; a respiratory therapist; an occupational therapist, a physical therapist (for early mobilization); and a speech–language pathologist (to address continued issues with aspiration).

Ensuring Optimal Nutrition

Nutrition is all too often placed as a lower priority in patients whose hemodynamic and neurological instability takes center stage; however, failure to meet nutritional requirements in a critically ill patient with a head injury may significantly increase morbidity and mortality.[17,30] Multidisciplinary collaboration with nutrition support teams is essential for optimal nutritional management of the patient with head injury.

Head injury is thought to cause hypermetabolic and hypercatabolic states as well as a decrease in immune competency.[30] This state of increased energy expenditure may be caused in part by muscle rigidity during posturing as well as hyperpyrexia, which is often experienced in the acute phase of injury. Patients with head injury treated with standard enteral or parenteral regimens were subsequently found to have a 169% greater energy requirement than expected.[23] Accurate measures of resting energy expenditure (REE) are obtained through indirect calorimetry using a machine (metabolic cart) interfaced with the ventilator, which measures oxygen consumption and carbon dioxide production. Indirect calorimetry is useful in hypermetabolic patients who fall outside of the typical calculations for REE.[30]

Head-injured patients should be fed as early as possible to achieve the goal rate within 7 days of the injury.[17] Enteral feeding may prevent the translocation of bacteria from the gut to the bloodstream, prevent the exacerbation of hyperglycemia, and prevent gastrointestinal ulceration and bleeding.[30] Current recommendations suggest replacement of 140% of a patient's REE who is not paralyzed and 100% of REE in patients who are paralyzed with formulas that contain 15% of calories as protein.[17] Recognition of the importance of nutrition, especially in the head-injured patient, is essential in optimizing patient outcome.

Managing Musculoskeletal and Integumentary Complications

Comprehensive care of the head-injured patient necessitates continued assessment of both the musculoskeletal system and integument for impairment. Collaboration with other disciplines, such as occupational and physical therapy, is helpful in protecting patients from contracture and skin breakdown. Splinting of the hands and feet, especially in an unresponsive patient, is necessary to preserve musculoskeletal function and promote the best conditions for future rehabilitation. Functional splinting and range-of-motion exercises also help reduce dependent edema in nonmoving extremities. Frequent turning of patients, even in the critical phase of the illness, is integral in maintaining skin integrity and facilitating pulmonary drainage.

Caring for the Family

Caring for families in crisis as well as coordinating available services (such as social work and pastoral care) is an integral function of the critical care nurse. Contemporary crisis theory emphasizes the importance of helping families identify coping mechanisms and support systems that enable them to return to a precrisis level of functioning within 24 hours.[31] Bond and colleagues surveyed the needs of family members of patients with severe traumatic brain injury and found the following four needs:

- The need for specific truthful information
- The need for information to be consistent

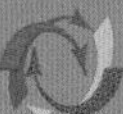

box 36-5 nursing interventions for *Sensory Stimulation*

Sound

- Explain to the patient what you are going to do.
- Play the patient's favorite television or radio program for 10–15 minutes. Alternatively, play a tape recording of a familiar voice of a friend or family member.
- During the program, do not converse with others in the room or perform other activities of patient care. The goal is to minimize distractions so the patient may learn to attend to the stimulus selectively.
- Another approach is to clap your hands or ring a bell. Do this for 5–10 seconds at a time, moving the sound to different locations around the bed.

Sight

- Place a brightly colored object in the patient's view. Present only one object at a time.
- Alternatively, use an object that is familiar, such as a family photo or favorite poster.

Touch

- Stroke the patient's arm or leg with fabrics of various textures. Alternatively, the back of a spoon can simulate smooth texture and a towel rough texture.
- Rubbing lotion over the patient's skin will also stimulate this sense. For some, firm pressure may be better tolerated than very light touch.

Smell

- Hold a container of a pleasing fragrance under the patient's nose. Use a familiar scent, such as perfume, aftershave, cinnamon, or coffee.
- Present this stimulation for very short periods (1–3 minutes maximum).
- If a cuffed tracheostomy or endotracheal tube is in place, the patient will not be able to appreciate this stimulation fully.

- The need to be actively involved in the care
- The need to make sense of the entire experience[32]

Critical care nurses have an opportunity to meet all of these specific needs, and to change unit culture to meet these needs. Encouraging family members to touch the patient despite the tangle of tubes and wires or allowing family members to assist in providing sensory stimulation (Box 36-5) may be helpful and comforting to some family members. For family members of a comatose patient, the Ranchos Los Amigos Scale can be used as an educational tool that describes stages of coma as they relate to rehabilitative methods (Table 36-5). Attention should be given to including both spiritual and cultural needs in the plan of care.

Patients with head injuries may be discharged to their homes or a rehabilitation program, depending on the degree of injury and the severity of deficits. Therefore, families must be educated about the expected course of events, including possible behavioral changes that may occur when the patient attempts to return to his or her former life. Reduced attention span as well as impulsivity and emotional lability may be exhibited, which may be difficult for both the family members and the patient. Careful observation by the family for behavioral changes and difficulties with tasks is valuable in the recognition of subtle difficulties and deficits.

BRAIN DEATH

The patient's condition may be so severe that brain death is the final outcome. The critical care nurse provides essential nursing care to such a patient as treatment is continued or life support measures are withdrawn. The nurse may be involved in determining whether the patient has suffered brain death, although a physician legally must make the final determination.

In the past, the declaration of brain death was controversial with regard to the standardization of tests needed to make the decision and ethical considerations. The Uniform Determination of Death Act was developed in 1981 by the President's Commission for the Study of Ethical Problems in Medicine and Biomedical Behavior Research and adopted by all 50 states. This act states: "An individual, who has sustained either (1) irreversible cessation of circulatory and respiratory functions, or (2) irreversible cessation of all functions of the entire brain, including the brainstem, is dead. A determination of death must be made in accordance with accepted medical standards."[33]

The brain death examination seeks to confirm the following three cardinal findings: coma or unresponsiveness, absence of brainstem reflexes, and apnea.[34] Tests specific for brain death include, but are not limited to, motor testing; evaluation of pupillary responses; evaluation of the oculocephalic reflex ("doll's eyes" phenomenon); evaluation of the oculovestibular reflex (caloric ice-water test); evaluation of the corneal, cough, and gag reflexes; and apnea testing. Apnea testing is performed by removing the patient from the ventilator and inspecting the chest for spontaneous respiratory effort while providing supplemental oxygen. An arterial blood gas (ABG) is sent after 8 minutes. A $PaCO_2$ greater than 60 mm Hg or an increase in the $PaCO_2$ of 20 mm Hg or more above the patient's baseline $PaCO_2$ is regarded as a positive test, supporting the diagnosis of brain death.[34] The patient is simultaneously observed for spontaneous respiration and hemodynamic instability, which would cause the test to be aborted. In the case of hemodynamic instability (e.g., a systolic blood pressure less than 90 mm Hg or cardiac arrhythmia), an ABG is drawn very quickly and the patient is placed back on the ventilator. An increased carbon dioxide level is the single strongest stimulus for the initiation of breathing; therefore, the absence of respiratory effort in the presence of severe hypercarbia constitutes strong evidence of brain death. Confirmatory

table 36-5 Ranchos Los Amigos Scale

Level	Guidelines for Interacting With Patient
1. **No response** to any stimuli occurs. 2. **Generalized response.** Stimulus response is incoherent, limited, and nonpurposeful with random movements or incomprehensible sounds. 3. **Localized response.** Stimulus response is specific but inconsistent; patient may withdraw or push away, may make sounds, may follow some simple commands, or may respond to certain family members.	• Assume that the patient can understand all that is said. Converse *with,* not *about,* the patient. • Do not overwhelm the patient with talking. Leave some moments of silence between verbal stimuli. • Manage the environment to provide only one source of stimulation at a time. If talking is taking place, the radio or television should be turned off. • Provide short, random periods of sensory input that are meaningful to the patient. A favorite television program or tape recording or 30 minutes of music from the patient's favorite radio station will provide more meaningful stimulation than constant radio accompaniment, which becomes as meaningless as the continual bleep of the cardiac monitor.
4. **Confused–agitated.** Stimulus response is primarily to internal confusion with increased state of activity; behavior may be bizarre or aggressive; patient may attempt to remove tubes or restraints or crawl out of bed; verbalization is incoherent or inappropriate; patient shows minimal awareness of environment and absent short-term memory.	• Be calm and soothing when handling the patient. Approach with gentle touch to decrease the occurrence of defensive emotional and motor reflexes. • Watch for early signs that the patient is becoming agitated (e.g., increased movement, vocal loudness, resistance to activity). • When the patient becomes upset, do not try to reason with him or her or "talk him or her out of it." Talking will be an additional external stimulus that the patient cannot handle. • If the patient remains upset, either remove him or her from the situation or remove the situation from him or her.
5. **Confused, inappropriate–nonagitated.** Patient is alert and responds consistently to simple commands; however, patient has a short attention span and is easily distracted; memory is impaired and patient exhibits confusion of past and present events; patient can perform previously learned tasks with maximal structure but is unable to learn new information; may wander off with vague intention of "going home." 6. **Confused–appropriate.** Patient shows goal-directed behavior but still needs external direction; can understand simple directions and reasoning; follows simple directions consistently and requires less supervision for previously learned tasks; has improved past memory depth and detail and basic awareness of self and surroundings.	• Present the patient with only one task at a time. Allow time to complete it before giving further instructions. • Make sure that you have the patient's attention by placing yourself in view and touching the patient before talking. • If the patient becomes confused or resistant, stop talking. Wait until he or she appears relaxed before continuing with instruction or activity. • Use gestures, demonstrations, and only the most necessary words when giving instructions. • Maintain the same sequence in routine activities and tasks. Describe these routines to the patient and relate them to time of day.
7. **Automatic–appropriate.** Patient is able to complete daily routines in structured environment; has increased awareness of self and surroundings but lacks insight, judgment, and problem-solving ability.	• Supervision is still necessary for continued learning and safety. • Reinforce the patient's memory of routines and schedules with clocks, calendars, and a written log of activities.
8. **Purposeful–appropriate.** Patient is alert, oriented, and able to recall and integrate past and recent events; responds appropriately to environment; still has decreased ability in abstract reasoning, stress tolerance, and judgment in emergencies or unusual situations.	• The patient should be able to function without supervision. • Consideration should be given to job retraining or a return to school.

tests for brain death, such as cerebral angiography (to test for the absence of cerebral blood flow), electroencephalography, TCD ultrasonography, BAERs, and SSEPs, can be used if any doubt exists after a full clinical examination has been completed.

The American Academy of Neurology recommends repeating the clinical evaluation for brain death after 6 hours.[35] Time of death is recorded at the time that brain death is declared, not when supportive measures are removed. Different institutions specify requirements based on state laws and statutes for physicians declaring brain death and the responsibilities of health care providers. Brain death determination in pediatric patients differs from the standards set forth for adults because of the increased viability of the immature brain.[36] Specific guidelines for the determination of brain death in children were developed by a federal task force in 1987. These guidelines delineate physical examination features unique to pediatric patients, as well as specific time frames for observation when brain death is suspected, depending on the age of the child.[37]

The concept of brain death is often confusing for families because death is so commonly associated with cardiopulmonary death, so the language that is used in discussions is very important. It is helpful to refer to the patient as "dead" (as opposed to "brain dead") after the declaration is made, because the term "brain dead" can be interpreted to mean that the rest of the body can continue to live.[38] The discussion of brain death should be separated in time from conversations regarding the opportunities for organ donation. In fact, it is helpful if a separate specialist in organ procurement is brought in to present and explain the option of organ donation. This method of communication is referred to *decoupling;* it helps to avoid the perception or appearance of a conflict of interest.

case study ■ HEAD TRAUMA

Mr. J., a 23-year-old man, is admitted to the intensive care unit (ICU) after an assault. During a robbery, he was struck in the back of the head with a baseball bat. Paramedics noted extensor posturing of both arms to sternal rub, without any verbalization or eye opening. On further assessment, the patient's respirations were sonorous at a rate of 6 breaths/minute, and his right pupil was dilated and fixed. Paramedics applied full spinal immobilization, intubated the patient, placed an IV line, and quickly transported him to the nearest trauma center. In the emergency department, the patient was noted to have abnormal flexion of the left arm and leg with localization on the right and no spontaneous eye opening. The patient was given 75 g of mannitol IV (based on the patient's weight of 75 kg), radiographs of the cervical spine were obtained, and a computed tomography (CT) scan was performed, which revealed a large right temporoparietal epidural hematoma. Neurosurgeons decided to emergently evacuate the epidural hematoma and place a subarachnoid bolt for intracranial pressure (ICP) monitoring. After surgery, Mr. J. is admitted to the ICU for further management.

Mr. J.'s neurological examination reveals a sluggishly reactive right pupil (5 mm) and a briskly reactive left pupil (4 mm), localization of the right upper and lower extremities and flexion of the left upper and lower extremities, and present brainstem reflexes. The following medical orders are written:

- 25% mannitol, 0.5 g/kg IV every 6 hours PRN for ICP >20 mm for >5 minutes and serum osmolality <320 mOsm
- Notify MD if sustained ICP >20 mm for >5 minutes
- Vital sign and neurological checks every hour
- Foley catheter to straight drainage
- Nasogastric tube to suction
- Head of bed (HOB) elevated 30 degrees
- Phenytoin 1,275 mg IV load (17 mg × 75 kg = 1,275 mg) and then 100 mg IV every 8 hours
- Acetaminophen 650 mg per nasogastric tube PRN for temperature greater than 100.4°F (38°C)
- Ventilator settings of fraction of inspired oxygen (FIO_2) = 0.5; tidal volume (VT) = 700 mL; intermittent mandatory ventilation (IMV) = 14; positive end-expiratory pressure (PEEP) = 5
- End-tidal CO_2 monitor; maintain CO_2 35 to 40 mm Hg
- IV of 0.9% saline with 20 mEq of potassium chloride at 100 mL/hour
- Monitor serum osmolality every 6 hours and notify MD for serum osmolality of >320 mOsm
- Maintain cervical immobilization with Philadelphia collar

The following assessment data are obtained on postoperative day 1, 24 hours after admission:

- ABG: pH 7.36, CO_2 40 mm Hg, PaO_2 154 mm Hg, HCO_3 22 mEq/L
- Blood pressure 200/68 mm Hg; mean arterial blood pressure 112 mm Hg; pulse 42 beats/minute; respiratory rate 18 breaths/minute; temperature 102.5°F (39.2°C)
- ICP: 40 mm Hg; CPP: 72 mm Hg
- Serum osmolality: 300 mOsm
- Right pupil dilated to 6 mm and fixed, left pupil sluggish and 4 mm
- Extensor posturing is noted on the left upper and lower extremity and flexion on the right upper and lower extremity

At this time, the patient is exhibiting signs of herniation syndrome, requiring rapid and aggressive action. Manual hyperventilation is ordered to decrease the carbon dioxide level and promote cerebral vasoconstriction, thereby reducing intracranial contents. At the same time, mannitol is ordered to promote osmotic diuresis and decrease brain water. The nurse ensures that the head of the patient's bed is elevated to 30 degrees and that the patient's head is positioned in midline.

Possible causes for this episode include the following: reaccumulation of the epidural hematoma, cerebral edema, or expansion of the intracerebral hematoma. A CT scan is obtained to guide further treatment. The second set of images reveals diffuse cerebral edema and uncal herniation.

On arrival back to the ICU, the patient's neurological examination shows sluggishly reactive pupils (right greater than the left) and flexion of the left upper and lower extremities to central pain. The right side of the body localizes central pain. Cough, gag, and corneal reflexes are preserved. Mr. J. does not exhibit eye opening and remains intubated. The medical and nursing teams are able to maximize therapy by increasing serum osmolality to 320 mOsm and maintaining the $PaCO_2$ in the range of 30 to 35 mm Hg. Despite optimization of these therapies, the patient's ICP continues to spike into the 40 to 50 mm Hg range for extended periods. Next, the team tries to control the ICP with bolus doses of thiopental, a barbiturate, to "quiet" the brain and decrease overall cerebral metabolic demands. This therapy works temporarily, but the patient again exhibits increased ICP and signs of impending herniation. Neurosurgeons are again consulted and decide to perform a hemicraniectomy, removing the right side of the skull. When the patient is returned to the ICU after the surgery, the nurse posts signs clearly stating the absence of bone on the right side of the patient's head. Alterations in general care include caution when turning the patient from side to side; eventually a helmet will be ordered when Mr. J. enters rehabilitation. The patient does not experience any further episodes of sustained increased ICP after surgery.

The patient receives a tracheostomy and percutaneous gastrostomy (PEG) tube on day 8 in the ICU for long-term airway and nutritional management. On transfer to an intermediate care unit on day 14, the patient is localizing to noxious stimuli on the left side of his body and holding up two fingers and wiggling his toes on the right side. The patient is also able to open his eyes and track family and friends as they move in front of him. After 4 weeks in the hospital, the patient is weaned from the ventilator to a tracheostomy collar with supplemental oxygen and transferred to a rehabilitation facility specializing in traumatic brain injury. ■

clinical applicability challenges

Self-Challenge: Critical Thinking

1. *Based on the initial assessments of the paramedics and the emergency department team, calculate Mr. J.'s score on the Glasgow Coma Scale (GCS).*
2. *Using the radiological findings and your knowledge regarding the pathophysiology of head injury, explain why Mr. J.'s right pupil was dilated and fixed. (Hint: State which cranial nerve was affected.)*

Study Questions

1. *Which of the following actions are appropriate for the acute care of the head-injured patient?*
   a. *Remove any cervical immobilization device after radiographs show the absence of fracture or dislocation.*
   b. *Maintain the cerebral perfusion pressure less than 60 mm Hg to avoid hyperemia.*
   c. *Elevate the head of bed to 30 degrees to promote venous drainage from the head.*
   d. *Do not turn the head-injured patient from side to side because any movement could cause a disproportionate spike in intracranial pressure (ICP).*
2. *Which cranial nerves are assessed when evaluating the oculovestibular response?*
   a. *Cranial nerves III, IV, and VI*
   b. *Cranial nerves I, XI, and XII*
   c. *Cranial nerves V and VII*
   d. *Cranial nerves III, VI, and VIII*
3. *The syndrome of inappropriate antidiuretic hormone secretion (SIADH) is characterized by which of the following sets of criteria?*
   a. *Increased sodium, increased urinary output, high urine specific gravity*
   b. *Decreased sodium, increased urinary output, low urine specific gravity*
   c. *Increased sodium, decreased urinary output, low urine specific gravity*
   d. *Decreased sodium, decreased urinary output, high urine specific gravity*
4. *The nurse suspects a basilar skull fracture in which of the following areas if there is ecchymosis behind the left ear?*
   a. *The base of the anterior fossa*
   b. *The left orbit*
   c. *The base of the middle fossa*
   d. *The base of the posterior fossa*

REFERENCES

1. Centers for Disease Control and Prevention: Traumatic Brain Injury in the United States: A Report to Congress, 1999. Available at www.cdc.gov/doc.do/id/0900f3ec8001011c.
2. Kaufman BA, Tunkel AR, Pryor JC, et al: Meningitis in the neurosurgical patient. Infect Dis Clin North Am 4(4):677–701, 1990
3. Dagi TF, Meyer FB, Poletti CA: The incidence and prevention of meningitis after basilar skull fracture. Am J Emerg Med 1(3):295–298, 1983
4. Mattioli C, Beretta L, Gerevini S, et al: Traumatic subarachnoid hemorrhage on the computerized tomography scan obtained at admission: A multicenter assessment of the accuracy of diagnosis and the potential impact on patient outcome. J Neurosurg 98(1):37–42, 2003
5. Servadei F, Murray GD, Teasdale GM, et al: Traumatic subarachnoid hemorrhage: Demographic and clinical study of 750 patients from the European Brain Injury Consortium survey of head injuries. Neurosurgery 50(2):261–267, 2002
6. Miller P, Fabian T, Bee T, et al: Blunt cerebrovascular injuries: Diagnosis and treatment. J Trauma 51(2):279–286, 2001
7. Zuccarelli L: Altered cellular anatomy and physiology of acute brain injury and spinal cord injury. Crit Care Clin North Am 12(4): 403–411, 2000
8. Yundt K, Diringer M: The use of hyperventilation and its impact on cerebral ischemia in the treatment of traumatic brain injury. Crit Care Clin 13(1):163–183, 1997
9. Geocadin R, Williams M, Hanley D: Intracranial hypertension. In O'Donnell JM, Nacul FE (eds): Surgical Intensive Care Medicine, pp 259–274. Boston, Kluwer, 2001
10. Jeremitsky E, Omert L, Dunham CM, et al: Harbingers of poor outcome the day after severe brain injury: Hypothermia, hypoxia, and hypoperfusion. J Trauma 54(2):312–319, 2003
11. Chestnut R: Secondary brain insults after head injury: Clinical perspectives. New Horiz 3(3):366–375, 1995
12. Davis AE: Cognitive impairments following traumatic brain injury. Crit Care Clin North Am 12(4):447–456, 2000
13. Hickey JV: The Clinical Practice of Neurological and Neurosurgical Nursing (5th Ed), pp 291–294. Philadelphia, Lippincott Williams & Wilkins, 2002
14. Quality Standards Subcommittee of the American Academy of Neurology: Practice parameters: Assessment and management of patients in the persistent vegetative state (summary statement). Report of the Quality Standards Subcommittee of the American Academy of Neurology. Neurology 45:1015–1018, 1995
15. Kidd KC, Criddle L: Using jugular venous catheters in patients with traumatic brain injury. Crit Care Nurse 21(6):17–22, 2001
16. Littlejohns LR, Bader MK, March K: Brain tissue oxygen monitoring in severe brain injury I. Crit Care Nurse 23(4):17–27, 2003
17. Bullock R, Chestnut R, Clifton G, et al: Guidelines for the Management of Severe Traumatic Brain Injury. New York, Brain Trauma Foundation/American Association of Neurological Surgeons, 2000
18. Bader M, Sylvain P: Keeping the brain in the zone: Applying the severe head injury guidelines to practice. Crit Care Clin North Am 12(4):413–426, 2000
19. McIlvoy L, Spain DA, Raque G, et al: Successful incorporation of the severe head injury guidelines into a phased-outcome clinical pathway. J Neurosci Nurs 33(2):72–78, 2001
20. Society of Critical Care Medicine: Guidelines for the acute medical management of severe traumatic brain injury in infants, children, and adolescents. Crit Care Med 31(6 Suppl):407–491, 2003
21. Robertson CS, Valadka AB, Hannay J, et al: Prevention of secondary ischemic insults after severe head injury. Crit Care Med 27(10): 2086–2095, 1999
22. Bullock R, Chestnut R, Clifton G, et al: Guidelines for the Management of Severe Traumatic Brain Injury Update: Cerebral Perfusion Pressure. New York, Brain Trauma Foundation, 2003
23. Chang BS, Lowenstein DH: Practice parameter: Antiepileptic drug prophylaxis in severe traumatic brain injury. Report of the Quality Standards Subcommittee of the American Academy of Neurology. Neurology 60(1):10–16, 2003
24. Hickey J: Fluid and electrolyte management in neuroscience patients. In Hickey J: The Clinical Practice of Neurological and Neurosurgical Nursing (4th Ed), pp 179–186. Philadelphia, Lippincott-Raven, 1997

25. Diaz-Parejo P, Stahl N, Xu W, et al: Cerebral energy metabolism during transient hyperglycemia in patients with severe brain trauma. Intensive Care Med 29(4):544–550, 2003
26. Song EC, Chu K, Jeong SW, et al: Hyperglycemia exacerbates brain edema and perihematomal cell death after intracerebral hemorrhage. Stroke 34(9):2215–2220, 2003
27. Van Den Berghe G, Wouters P, Weekers F, et al: Intensive insulin therapy in critically ill patients. N Engl J Med 19:1359–1367, 2001
28. Walia S, Sutcliffe AJ: The relationship between blood glucose, mean arterial pressure and outcome after severe head injury: An observational study. Injury 33(4):339–344, 2002
29. Munro N: Pulmonary challenges in neurotrauma. Crit Care Nurs Clin North Am 12(4):457–464, 2000
30. Donaldson J, Borzatta MA, Matossian D: Nutrition strategies in neurotrauma. Crit Care Nurs Clin North Am 12(4):465–475, 2000
31. Mitchell JW: Crisis intervention. In Mitchell JW: The Dynamics of Crisis Intervention, pp 3–5. Springfield, IL, Charles C Thomas, 1999
32. Bond AE, Draeger CRL, Mandleco B, et al: Needs of family members of patients with severe traumatic brain injury: Implications for evidenced-based practice. Crit Care Nurse 23(4):63–71, 2003
33. Uniform Determination of Death Act. Presented and approved at the 89th Annual Conference of Commissioners of Uniform State Laws, July 26–August 1, 1980, Kauai, Hawaii. Chicago, IL, National Conference of Commissioners on Uniform State Laws, 1980.
34. Wijdicks EFM: Determining brain death in adults. Neurology 45:1003–1011, 1995
35. Quality Standards Subcommittee of the American Academy of Neurology: Practice parameters for determining brain death in adults (summary statement). Report of the Quality Standards Subcommittee of the American Academy of Neurology. Neurology 45:1012–1014, 1995
36. Lovasik D: Brain death and organ donation. Crit Care Nurs Clin North Am 12(4):531–538, 2000
37. Task Force for the Determination of Brain Death in Children: Guidelines for the determination of brain death in children. Arch Neurol 44(6):587–588, 1987
38. Sullivan J, Seem DL, Chabalewski F: Determining brain death. Crit Care Nurse 19(2):37–45, 1999

OTHER SELECTED READING

Bader MK, Littlejohns LR, Mack K: Brain tissue oxygen monitoring in severe brain injury, II: Implications for critical care teams and case study. Crit Care Nurse 23(4): 29–44, 2003

Bond AE, Draeger CR, Mandleco B, Donnelly M: Needs of family members of patients with severe traumatic brain injury: Implications for evidence-based practice. Crit Care Nurse 23(4):63–72, 2003

Brain Trauma Foundation: Guidelines for the Prehospital Management of Traumatic Brain Injury. New York, Brain Trauma Foundation, 2000

Day L: How nurses shift from care of a brain-injured patient to maintenance of a brain-dead organ donor. Am J Crit Care 10(5):306–312, 2001

Kidd KC, Criddle L: Using jugular venous catheters in patients with traumatic brain injury. Crit Care Nurse 21(6):16–22, 2001

LeJune GM, Howard–Fain T: Nursing assessment and management of patients with head injuries. Dim Crit Care Nurs 21(6):226–229, 2002

Littlejohns LR, Bader MK: Guidelines for the management of severe head injury: Clinical application and changes in practice. Crit Care Nurse 21(6):48–65, 2001

Littlejohns LR, Bader MK, March K: Brain tissue oxygen monitoring in severe brain injury, I: Research and usefulness in critical care. Crit Care Nurse 23(4):17–25, 2003

Sommargren CE. Electrocardiographic abnormalities in patients with subarachnoid hemorrhage. Am J Crit Care 11(1):48–56, 2002

chapter

37

Spinal Cord Injury

KATHY A. HAUSMAN

objectives

Based on the content in this chapter, the reader should be able to:

- Describe the mechanism of spinal cord injury.
- Discuss the various classification systems for spinal cord injuries.
- Differentiate between the following syndromes: Brown-Séquard syndrome, central cord syndrome, anterior cord syndrome, and posterior cord syndrome.
- Perform an assessment of a patient with a spinal cord injury.
- Describe typical complications that occur after a spinal cord injury.
- Differentiate between spinal shock and neurogenic shock.
- Describe immediate nursing actions to take after autonomic dysreflexia is recognized.
- Develop a collaborative plan of care for a patient with an acute spinal cord injury.

Each year in the United States, there are approximately 11,000 new spinal cord injuries.[1] Fortunately, progress in neurological research and advances in technology have led to a dramatic increase in the number of people who survive a traumatic spinal cord injury. The number of people alive today who have a spinal cord injury is estimated at between 183,000 and 230,000.

Spinal cord injury is most common in young adults between the ages of 16 and 30 years. Among this age group, spinal cord injury is more common in men (82%) than in women (18%). The most common causes of spinal cord injuries include motor vehicle crashes (MVCs; 39%), falls (22%), acts of violence (25%), and sports 7%.[1] Approximately 20% of older adults experience a spinal cord injury. Among this age group, most injuries are due to falls.[2]

Slightly more than one-half of all new injuries to the cervical region of the spinal cord result in tetraplegia (the condition formerly referred to as *quadriplegia*). Paraplegia can result from lesions in the thoracic, lumbar, or sacral regions of the spinal cord. Recent trends indicate an increasing proportion of people with incomplete paraplegia and a declining number of people with complete tetraplegia. The overwhelming majority of people with spinal cord injury discharged from the health care system return home or to noninstitutional settings.

Many of those discharged home require partial or total care. The economic consequences of this type of injury, especially if there are repeated hospitalizations, can be staggering. The average lifetime costs depend on the level and severity of injury. A person who is tetraplegic may incur costs of $417,000 the first year after injury and approximately $74,000 each subsequent year of life.[2] A person who is paraplegic may incur costs of $152,000 the first year and $15,000 each subsequent year.[3]

CLASSIFICATION OF INJURY

Spinal cord injuries can be classified by mechanism, type of vertebral injury, level of injury, or cause. Spinal cord injuries occur as a result of penetrating injury or mechanical forces. Penetrating injuries, which are most often caused by gunshot or stab wounds, damage the spinal cord and cause loss of neurological functioning.

Mechanism of Injury

Mechanical forces that can result in spinal cord injury include hyperflexion, hyperextension, axial loading (compression), and rotational forces (Fig. 37-1):

- Hyperflexion, depicted in Figure 37-1A, is caused by a sudden deceleration of the head and neck. Hyperflexion injuries are often seen in patients who have sustained trauma from a head-on MVC or diving accident. The cervical region is most often involved, especially at the C5–C6 level.
- Hyperextension (see Fig. 37-1B) is the most common type of injury. Hyperextension injuries can be caused by a fall, a rear-end MVC, or getting hit in the head (e.g., during a boxing match). Hyperextension of the head and neck may cause contusion and ischemia of the spinal cord without vertebral column damage. Whiplash injuries are the result of hyperextension.
- Axial loading, also known as compression (see Fig. 37-1C), typically occurs when a person lands on the feet or buttocks after falling or jumping from a height. The vertebral column is compressed, causing a fracture that results in damage to the spinal cord.
- Rotational injuries result from forces that cause extreme twisting or lateral flexion of the head and neck (see Fig. 37-1D). Fracture or dislocation of vertebrae may also occur.

Type of Vertebral Injury

Mechanical forces can result in fracture or dislocation of vertebrae, or both. If vertebral injury occurs, the type of vertebral injury can be used to describe the person's spinal cord injury. Types of fractures and dislocations are defined in Box 37-1.[4] A fracture may be considered unstable if the posterior ligaments are torn.

Level of Injury

Spinal cord injuries can also be classified according to the segment of the spinal cord that is affected:

- Upper cervical (C1–C2) injuries (atlas fractures, atlantoaxial subluxation, odontoid fractures, and hangman's fractures)
- Lower cervical (C3–C8) injuries
- Thoracic (T1–T12) injuries
- Lumbar (L1–L5) injuries
- Sacral (S1–S5) injuries

The degree of functional recovery depends on the location and extent of the injury. The level of spinal cord injury is determined by the effect of the injury on sensory and motor function (Table 37-1). Retention of all or some of the motor or sensory function below the level of injury implies that the lesion is incomplete. Total loss of voluntary muscle control and sensation below the level of injury suggests that the lesion is complete. Complete lesions involving spinal cord regions C1 to T1 result in tetraplegia (Fig. 37-2). Complete lesions involving spinal cord regions T2 to L1 result in paraplegia (see Fig. 37-2). A person with a complete cord injury follows the dermatome pathways for the level of sensory loss shown in Figure 37-3.

Cause of Injury

Spinal cord injuries can also be classified according to the cause of injury. Causes of spinal cord injury include concussion or jarring injuries; compression of the neural elements by bony fragments or hemorrhage; contusion (bruising) of the spinal cord; and laceration, transection, or blockage of the blood vessels that supply the cord.

SPINAL CORD SYNDROMES

Incomplete cord injuries often cause recognizable neurological syndromes that are classified according to the area damaged (Fig. 37-4).

Central Cord Syndrome

Damage to the spinal cord in this syndrome is centrally located. Hyperextension of the cervical spine often is the mechanism of injury, and the damage is greatest to the cervical tracts supplying the arms. Clinically, the patient may present with paralyzed arms but with no deficit in the legs or bladder (see Fig. 37-4A).

Brown-Séquard Syndrome

The damage in this syndrome is located on one side of the spinal cord. The clinical presentation is one in which the patient has either increased or decreased cutaneous sensation of pain, temperature, and touch on the same side of the spinal cord at the level of the lesion. Below the level of the lesion on the same side, there is complete motor paralysis. On the patient's opposite side, below the level of the lesion, there is loss of pain, temperature, and touch because the spinothalamic tracts cross soon after entering the cord. The posterior columns are interrupted ipsilaterally, but this

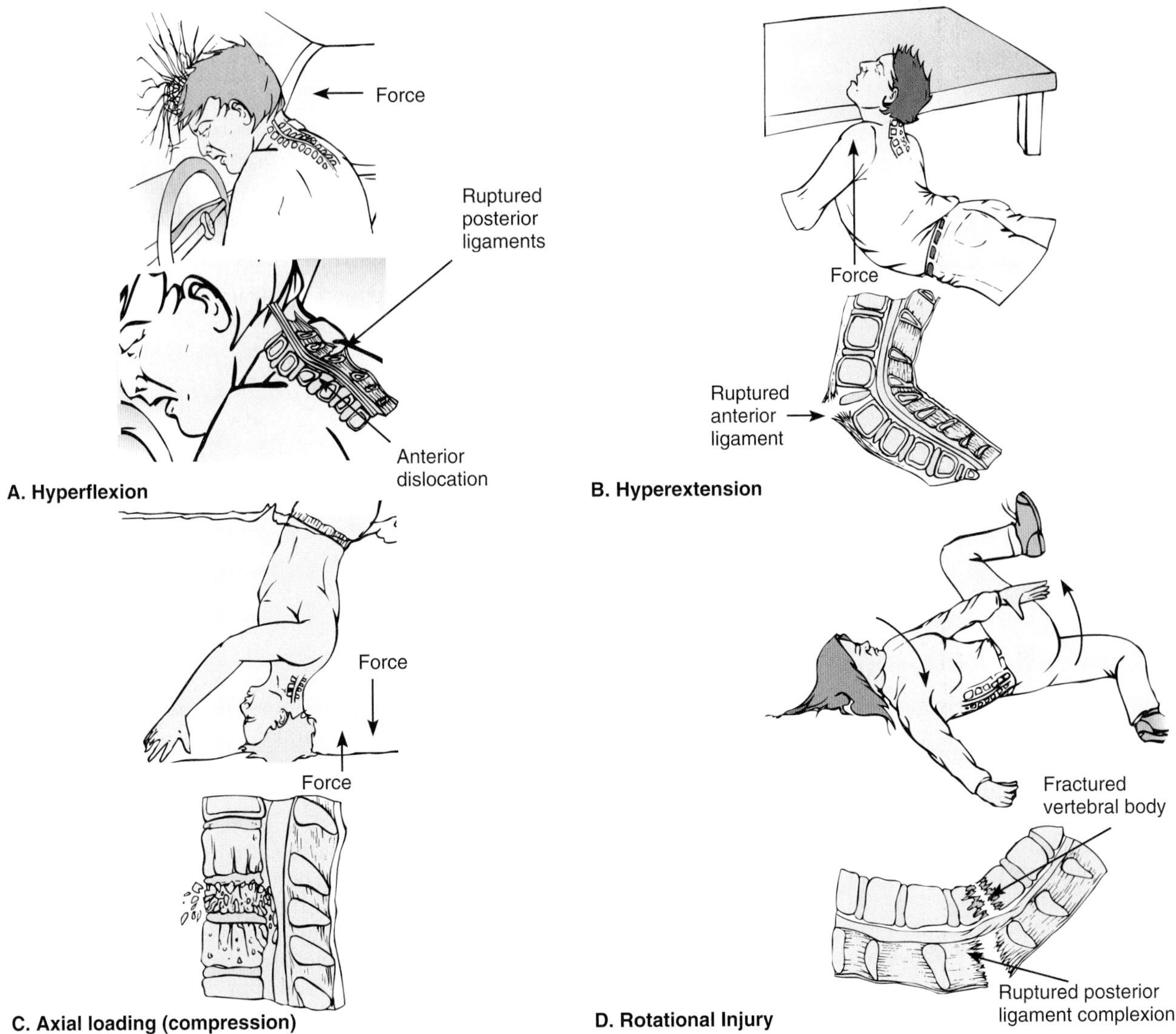

figure 37-1 Spinal cord injuries can be classified according to the mechanism of injury. (**A**) With hyperflexion to the cervical spine, there may be tearing of the posterior ligamentous complex, resulting in anterior dislocation. (**B**) Hyperextension injury can result in rupture of the anterior ligament. (**C**) Axial loading (compression) of the spine results in fracture and subsequent spinal cord damage. (**D**) When rotational force occurs, there is concurrent fracture and tearing of the posterior ligamentous complex. (From: Hickey JV: The Clinical Practice of Neurological and Neurosurgical Nursing [5th Ed.], pp 409–412. Philadelphia, Lippincott Williams & Wilkins, 2003.)

does not cause a major deficit because some fibers cross instead of running ipsilaterally. Clinically, the patient's limb with the best motor strength has the poorest sensation. Conversely, the limb with the best sensation has the poorest motor strength (see Fig. 37-4B).

Anterior Cord Syndrome

The area of damage in this syndrome is, as the name suggests, the anterior aspect of the spinal cord. Clinically, the patient usually has complete motor paralysis below the level of injury (corticospinal tracts) and loss of pain, temperature, and touch sensation (spinothalamic tracts), with preservation of light touch, proprioception, and position sense (see Fig. 37-4C).

Posterior Cord Syndrome

Posterior cord syndrome is usually the result of a hyperextension injury at the cervical level and is not commonly seen. Position sense, light touch, and vibratory sense are lost below the level of the injury.

AUTONOMIC NERVOUS SYSTEM SYNDROMES

Spinal Shock

Spinal shock is a condition that occurs immediately or within several hours of a spinal cord injury and is caused by the sudden cessation of impulses from the higher brain

box 37-1
Types of Vertebral Fractures and Dislocations

Fractures

Simple fracture: single fracture; alignment of the vertebrae is intact and neurological deficits do not occur

Compression fracture: fracture caused by axial loading and hyperflexion

Wedge compression fracture: a stable fracture that involves compression of the vertebral body in the cervical area

Teardrop fracture: an unstable fracture that involves a piece of bone breaking off the vertebra; seen in wedge fractures

Comminuted fracture: the vertebra is shattered into several pieces; bone fragments may be driven into spinal cord

Dislocations

Dislocation: one vertebra overrides another

Subluxation: partial or incomplete dislocation

Fracture–dislocation: fracture and dislocation

centers (Fig. 37-5). It is characterized by the loss of motor, sensory, reflex, and autonomic function below the level of the injury, with resultant flaccid paralysis (Box 37-2). Loss of bowel and bladder function also occurs. In addition, the body's ability to control temperature (poikilothermia) is lost and the patient's temperature tends to equilibrate with that of the external environment. There is no treatment for spinal shock.

If the spinal cord injury produces an incomplete transection, the suppression of function below the level of injury is temporary, lasting a few days, to weeks or months. The duration of spinal shock is variable, depending on the severity of the insult and the presence of other complications. The return of perianal reflex activity signals the end of the period of spinal shock. Reflexes associated with the area surrounding the injured cord return last. The skeletal muscles become spastic and there is increased muscle tone and exaggerated flexor muscle movement.

Neurogenic Shock

Neurogenic shock, a form of distributive shock, is a condition seen in patients with severe cervical and upper thoracic injuries. It is caused by the loss of sympathetic input to the systemic vasculature of the heart and subsequent decreased peripheral vascular resistance. Signs and symptoms include hypotension, severe bradycardia, and loss of the ability to sweat below the level of injury. The same clinical findings pertaining to disruption of the sympathetic transmissions in spinal shock occur in neurogenic shock.

Orthostatic Hypotension

Orthostatic hypotension may occur in a patient with a spinal cord injury because the patient is unable to compensate for changes in position. The vasoconstricting message from the medulla cannot reach the blood vessels because of the cord injury.

PATHOPHYSIOLOGY

The spinal cord extends from the base of the brain to approximately the level of the first or second lumbar vertebra. Blood is supplied to the cord by the anterior and posterior spinal arteries. Extending off of the spinal cord are the spinal nerve roots. The spinal cord is enclosed in the vertebral canal, which consists of 33 vertebrae: 7 cervical, 12 thoracic, 5 lumbar, 5 sacral (fused), and 4 coccygeal (fused). The vertebrae are held in place by ligaments, muscles, and other supporting structures.

Primary Injury

Injury to the spinal cord that occurs at impact is referred to as the primary injury. Damage to the spinal cord is most often associated with damage to the vertebral column. The vertebrae may be fractured, dislocated, or compressed. The more mobile areas of the vertebral column (such as the cervical area) are most frequently involved. As a result of the injury to the vertebral column, the spinal cord itself may be contused, compressed, or dislocated.

Secondary Injury

Equally destructive is the injury or damage to the spinal cord that continues for hours after the trauma. Secondary injuries result in additional axonal damage and further neurological deficit. Mechanisms of secondary injury include the following:

- Immune cells, which normally do not enter the spinal cord, engulf the area after a spinal cord injury. These immune cells respond as they normally would to inflammation in other parts of the body. However, some of the immune cells release regulatory chemicals, some of which are harmful to the spinal cord. Highly reactive oxidizing agents (free radicals) are produced, which damage the cell membrane and disrupt the sodium–potassium pump.
- Hypoperfusion of the spinal cord from microscopic hemorrhage and edema leads to ischemia. Ischemic areas develop at the injury site as well as one or two segments above and below the level of injury.
- The release of catecholamines and vasoactive substances (norepinephrine, serotonin, dopamine, and histamine) contributes to decreased circulation and cellular perfusion of the spinal cord.
- The release of excess neurotransmitters results in overexcitation of the nerve cells. Excitotoxicity allows high levels of calcium to enter the cells, causing further oxidative damage and damage to mitochondria. Excitotoxicity is thought to damage oligodendrocytes (the cells that produce myelin), leading to demyelinated axons that are unable to conduct impulses.

INITIAL ASSESSMENT AND MANAGEMENT

Prehospital Management

A spinal cord injury should be suspected at the scene of an accident any time the patient has decreased or absent movement or sensation. An unconscious patient is treated

table 37-1 Functional Loss From Spinal Cord Injury (Based on Complete Lesions)

Level of Spinal Injury	Motor Function	Deep Tendon Reflexes	Sensory Function	Respiratory Function	Voluntary Bowel and Bladder Function	Rehabilitative Potential
C1–C4	Quadriplegia: loss of all motor function from the neck down	All lost	Loss of all sensory function in the neck and below (C4 supplies the clavicles)	Loss of involuntary (phrenic) and voluntary (intercostals) respiratory function; ventilatory support and a tracheostomy needed	No bowel or bladder control	May be discharged home on a ventilator with home care
C5	Quadriplegia: loss of all function below the upper shoulders **Intact:** sternomastoids, cervical paraspinal muscles, and the trapezius; can control head	C5, C6 biceps	Loss of sensation below the clavicle and most portions of arms, hands, chest, abdomen, and lower extremities **Intact:** head, shoulders, deltoid, clavicle, portion of forearms (C5 supplies the lateral aspect of the arm)	Phrenic nerve intact, but not intercostal muscles	No bowel or bladder control	Use of extremity-powered devices to achieve some upper limb control Head control facilitates wheelchair (W/C) balance Adaptive tools, held in mouth, for typing and writing Some adaptive tools and use of special computer technology
C6	Quadriplegia: loss of all function below the shoulders and upper arms; lacks elbow, forearm, and hand control **Intact:** deltoid, biceps, and external rotator muscles of shoulders	C5, C6 brachioradials	Loss of everything listed for a C5 lesion, but greater arm and thumb sensation **Intact:** head, shoulders, arms, palms of hands, and thumbs (C6 supplies the forearm and thumb)	Phrenic nerve intact, but not intercostal muscles	No bowel or bladder control	Needs assistive devices to use arms (may be able to help feed, groom, and dress self) Needs a motorized W/C Dependent for all transfers
C7	Quadriplegia: loss of motor control to portions of the arms and hands **Intact:** voluntary strength in shoulder depressors, shoulder abductors, internal rotators, and radial wrist extensors	C7, C8 triceps	Loss of sensation below the clavicle and portions of arms and hands **Intact:** head, shoulders, most of arms and hands (C7 supplies the middle finger)	Phrenic nerve intact, but not intercostal muscles	No bowel or bladder function	Can perform some activities of daily living (ADLs) Can use wrist extensor with a special splint to induce finger flexion Can push a W/C with special handgrasps May be able to drive a specially equipped car

(continued)

table 37-1 Functional Loss From Spinal Cord Injury (Based on Complete Lesions) (Continued)

Level of Spinal Injury	Motor Function	Deep Tendon Reflexes	Sensory Function	Respiratory Function	Voluntary Bowel and Bladder Function	Rehabilitative Potential
C8	Quadriplegia: loss of motor control to portions of the arms and hands **Intact:** some voluntary control of elbow extensors, wrist, finger extension, and finger flexors		Loss of sensation below the chest and in portions of hands **Intact:** sensation to face, shoulders, arms, hands, and part of chest (C8 supplies the little finger)	Phrenic nerve intact, but not intercostal muscles	No bowel or bladder function	Able to push-up in the W/C Improved sitting tolerance Can grasp and release hands voluntarily Independent in most ADLs from W/C Independent in use of W/C Can use hands for catheterization and rectal stimulation for bowel movements
T1–T6	Paraplegia: loss of everything below the midchest region, including the trunk muscles **Intact:** control of function to the shoulders, upper chest, arms, and hands		Loss of sensation below the midchest area **Intact:** everything to the midchest region, including the arms and hands (T1 and T2 supply the inner aspect of the arm; T4 supplies the nipple area)	Phrenic nerve functions independently Some impairment of intercostal muscles	No bowel or bladder function	Full control of upper extremities and completely independent in W/C Full-time employment possible Independent in managing urinary drainage and inserting suppositories Able to live in a dwelling without major architectural changes
T6–T12	Paraplegia: loss of motor control below the waist **Intact:** shoulders, arms, hands, and long trunk muscles		Loss of everything below the waist **Intact:** shoulders, chest, arms, and hands (T10 supplies the umbilicus; T12 supplies the groin area)	No interference with respiratory function	No bowel or bladder control	In addition to the previously described capabilities, there is complete abdominal and upper back control. Good sitting balance (allows for greater ease of W/C operation and athletics)
L1–L3	Paraplegia: loss of most control of legs and pelvis **Intact:** shoulders, arms, hands, torso, hip rotation and flexion, and some leg flexion	L2–L4 (knee jerk)	Loss of sensation to the lower abdomen and legs **Intact:** all of the above plus some sensation to the inner and anterior thigh (L3 supplies the knee)	No interference with respiratory function	No bowel or bladder control	Independent for most activities from W/C

(continued)

table 37-1 Functional Loss From Spinal Cord Injury (Based on Complete Lesions) (Continued)

Level of Spinal Injury	Motor Function	Deep Tendon Reflexes	Sensory Function	Respiratory Function	Voluntary Bowel and Bladder Function	Rehabilitative Potential
L3–L4	Paraplegia: loss of control of portions of lower legs, ankles, and feet **Intact:** all of the above, plus increased knee extension		Loss of sensation to portions of the lower legs, feet, and ankles **Intact:** all of the above, plus sensation to the upper legs	No interference with respiratory function	No bowel or bladder control	Voluntary control of hip extensors; weak abductors Walking with braces possible
L4 to S5	Paraplegia: incomplete Segmental motor control L4 to S1: abduction and internal rotation of hip, ankle dorsiflexion, and foot inversion L5 to S1: foot eversion L4 to S2: knee flexion S1–S2: plantar flexion S1–S2: (ankle jerk) S2–S5: bowel/bladder control	S1–S2 (ankle jerk)	Lumbar sensory nerves innervate the upper legs and portions of the lower legs L5: medial aspect of foot S1: lateral aspect of foot S2: posterior aspect of calf/thigh Sacral sensory nerves innervate the lower legs, feet, and perineum	No interference with respiratory function	Bowel and bladder control possibly impaired S2–S4 segments control urinary continence S3–S5 segments control bowel continence (perianal muscles)	Can walk with braces or may use W/C Can be relatively independent

From Hickey JV: The Clinical Practice of Neurological and Neurosurgical Nursing (5th Ed), pp 424–425. Philadelphia, Lippincott Williams & Wilkins, 2003.

as though a spinal cord injury has occurred until proven otherwise. Because elapsed time from injury significantly affects prognosis, the patient with a spinal cord injury should be transported as safely and rapidly as possible to a specialized unit or a hospital with adequate diagnostic and treatment facilities to handle such trauma. A primary survey done at the scene of an accident includes a rapid assessment of airway, breathing, and circulation (ABCs). Airway patency is assessed, and the cervical spine is immobilized and stabilized. A neurological assessment is conducted and documented. This serves as a baseline for future comparison. The patient is assessed for other signs of life-threatening injuries (e.g., traumatic brain injury, chest contusion, or multiple fractures) and appropriate stabilization and treatment are initiated. Intravenous fluids are started as indicated. Special precautions are taken to extricate the person from the accident scene to prevent further injury to the spinal cord and other injured structures.

In-Hospital Management

The emergency department admission priority is the assessment of the patient's ventilation status. Based on assessment findings, appropriate ventilation support is promptly initiated. Ventilation support may include elective intubation and mechanical ventilation. The second priority is to establish the extent of the injury and begin definitive treatment. Finally, the emergency department staff stabilizes the patient before transfer to the intensive care unit (ICU) or a specialized trauma center.

High-dose methylprednisolone is often given in the emergency department if the injury occurred less than 8 hours before admission. Methylprednisolone reduces swelling and helps to minimize secondary injury by reversing the intracellular accumulation of calcium, reducing the risk of cord degeneration and ischemia. Box 37-3 summarizes the administration protocol for methylprednisolone, along with indications and relative contraindications for its use. Recent studies do not support the use of this medication as an evidence-based standard of care.[5]

PHYSICAL EXAMINATION

Respiratory Assessment

The patient's respiratory rate and arterial oxygen saturation (by pulse oximetry) are assessed and recorded. Clinical manifestations other than those associated with concomitant injuries may include hypoventilation or respiratory failure,

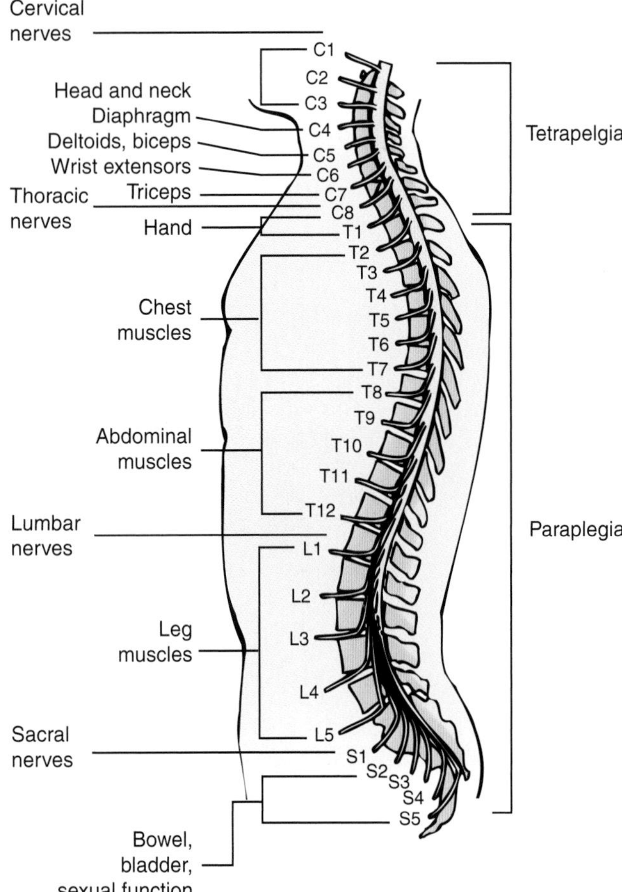

figure 37-2 The level of spinal cord injury relates to functional loss. The higher the spinal cord injury, the more motor, sensory, and autonomic functional losses are incurred. (From: Hickey JV: The Clinical Practice of Neurological and Neurosurgical Nursing [5th Ed.], p 408. Philadelphia, Lippincott Williams & Wilkins, 2003.)

particularly with high cervical injuries. Hypoventilation from inadequate innervation of respiratory muscles is a common problem after spinal cord injury. It is important to assess whether the intercostal muscles are functioning, or whether the patient has only diaphragmatic breathing. Spinal cord edema can act like an ascending lesion and may compromise function of the diaphragm. Assessment of tidal volume and vital capacity and auscultation of breath sounds are performed frequently.

The patient with a spinal cord injury may have additional respiratory compromise because of pre-existing pulmonary disease or coexistent chest, laryngeal, tracheal, or esophageal injuries. Major cranial nerves and surrounding arteries and veins may also be injured. Alveolar ventilation may be affected directly by the pulmonary collapse or by consolidation from retained secretions or aspiration of vomitus. Pulmonary edema may also result from incorrect management of intravenous fluids. Paralytic ileus and gastric dilation may increase the pressure on the diaphragm and cause further respiratory embarrassment. Consequently, a nasogastric tube may be inserted. A decreased cough reflex may combine with fluid imbalance to impair the airways.

Cardiovascular Assessment

The patient is immediately placed on a cardiac monitor. Vital signs are taken and a cardiovascular assessment is completed. Hypotension and bradycardia may be due to neurogenic shock or hemorrhage shock. Hemorrhagic shock (manifested by hypotension, tachycardia, and cold, clammy skin) may be caused by intrathoracic, intra-abdominal, or retroperitoneal injury, or pelvic or long bone fractures. The patient is examined to determine if other injuries are present. The rate of intravenous infusion is adjusted based on the patient's presenting signs and symptoms and past medical history. An indwelling Foley catheter is inserted and the patient's intake and output is strictly monitored. Chest injury often accompanies thoracic spinal cord trauma. The chest, head, and abdomen are examined for evidence of concomitant injuries.

Neurological Assessment

Neurological status is assessed frequently to determine the extent of the spinal cord injury, monitor for changes in level of consciousness that may occur secondary to traumatic brain injury, and detect damage to the cranial nerves. The patient's level of consciousness is determined using the Glasgow Coma Scale. The Glasgow Coma Scale is especially important to use if a confirmed or suspected traumatic brain injury occurred. Most spinal cord injury centers use a specialized flow sheet, such as the Standard Neurological Classification of Spinal Cord Injury flow sheet, to assess and document the patient's level of functioning (Fig. 37-6). Cranial nerve testing is done, particularly if the cause of the injury was penetrating trauma or involved a head injury.

During the early assessment of the patient with a spinal cord injury, a digital rectal examination is important to determine whether the injury is incomplete or complete. The lesion is incomplete if the patient can feel the palpating finger or can contract the perianal muscles around the finger voluntarily. Sensation may be present in the absence of voluntary motor activity. Sensation seldom is absent when voluntary perianal muscle contraction is present. In either case, the prognosis for further motor and sensory return is good. Preservation of sacral function might be the only finding that indicates an incomplete lesion, and significant neurological recovery may occur in the patient with an incomplete cord injury. Rectal tone by itself, without the presence of voluntary perianal muscle contraction or rectal sensation, is not evidence of an incomplete cord injury.

Bowel and Bladder Assessment

Incontinence of urine and possibly feces may have occurred at the scene of the accident. An indwelling urinary catheter is inserted to prevent the bladder from becoming distended secondary to an atonic bladder. There may be an imbalance between parasympathetic and sympathetic innervation to the bowel and therefore a loss of voluntary control.

DIAGNOSTIC STUDIES

Once the patient is stabilized, definitive diagnostic tests can be safely performed. The diagnostic workup consists of radiographs of the spine, chest, and other structures as clinically indicated. A computed tomography (CT) scan provides additional information concerning bony structures

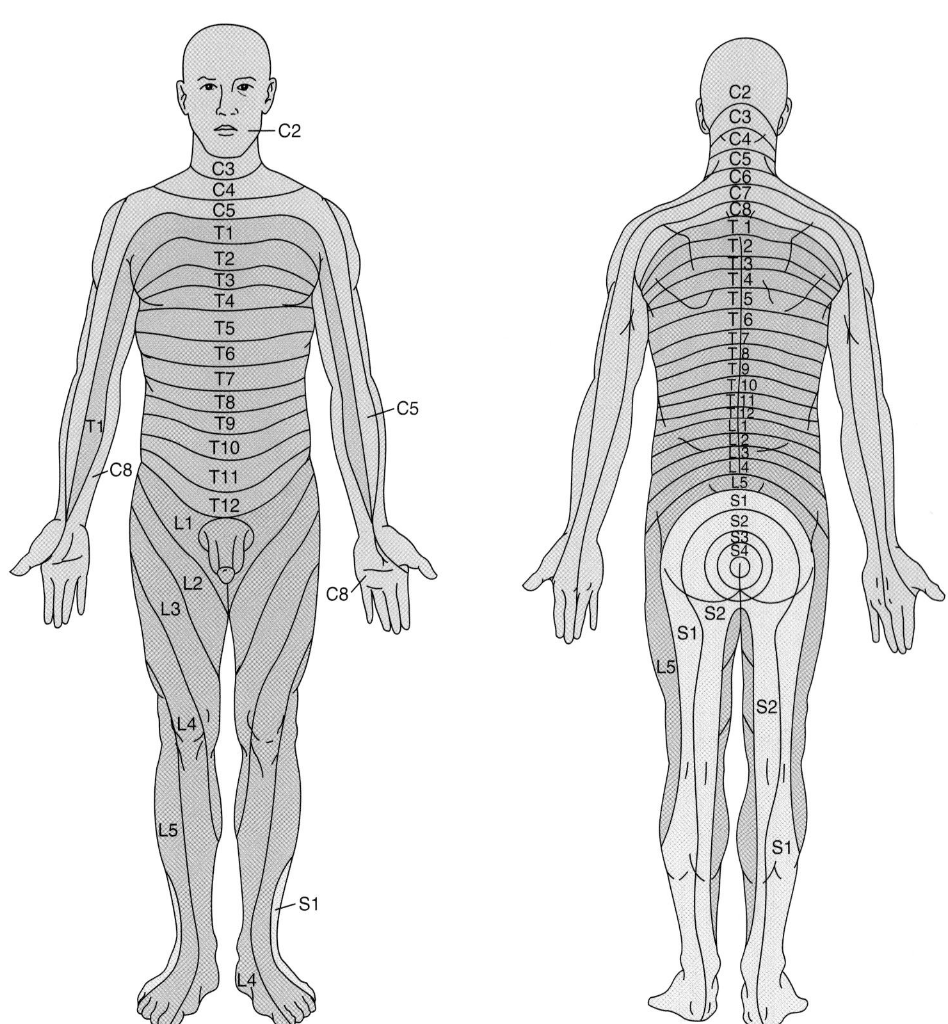

figure 37-3 A person with complete spinal cord injury follows the dermatome pathways for the level of sensory loss. (From: Smeltzer SC, Bare BG: Brunner & Suddarth's Textbook of Medical-Surgical Nursing [10th Ed.], p 1829. Philadelphia, Lippincott Williams & Wilkins, 2004.)

and fractures. Soft tissue injury is more easily diagnosed with magnetic resonance imaging (MRI). Somatosensory evoked potentials (see Chapter 33) are often obtained once the patient is in the critical care or acute care environment. This test measures the ability of the spinal cord to carry messages along the neural pathways to the higher centers in the brain, and is used as a tool to help determine treatment and patient outcome. In this test, a peripheral nerve in the arm or leg below the level of injury is stimulated and the neurological response (evoked potential) is recorded. If the injury is complete, there is no response. In incomplete injuries, a varying response occurs. Typical laboratory tests ordered include a complete blood count (CBC), electrolytes, glucose, blood urea nitrogen (BUN), creatinine, blood type and crossmatch, arterial blood gases (ABGs), and coagulation studies.

ONGOING ASSESSMENT AND MANAGEMENT

Examples of nursing diagnoses and collaborative problems for the patient with a spinal cord injury are given in Box 37-4. Based on the assessment data, an individual treatment plan is developed by the interdisciplinary team (Box 37-5). Management of the patient is based on the type and severity of injury. Collaboration of all health care disciplines is necessary to enable the patient to achieve his or her fullest potential after injury. The goals of ongoing management are to realign or stabilize the spine to prevent further neurological deterioration, to prevent complications, and to initiate prompt interventions to treat any complications that do occur.

Realignment and Stabilization of the Spine

Decompression of the cord by realignment of the spinal canal is of initial concern. This can be accomplished through medical or surgical management.

MEDICAL MANAGEMENT

Closed reduction of a cervical fracture is often accomplished with skeletal traction. Cervical traction is used when the fracture is unstable or if subluxation has occurred. Gardner-Wells, Vinke, or Crutchfield tongs are common forms of cervical traction; however, because of the complications that accompany prolonged immobility, long-term traction with tongs is seldom used, especially since the advent of the halo vest (Fig. 37-7). Collaborative care guides

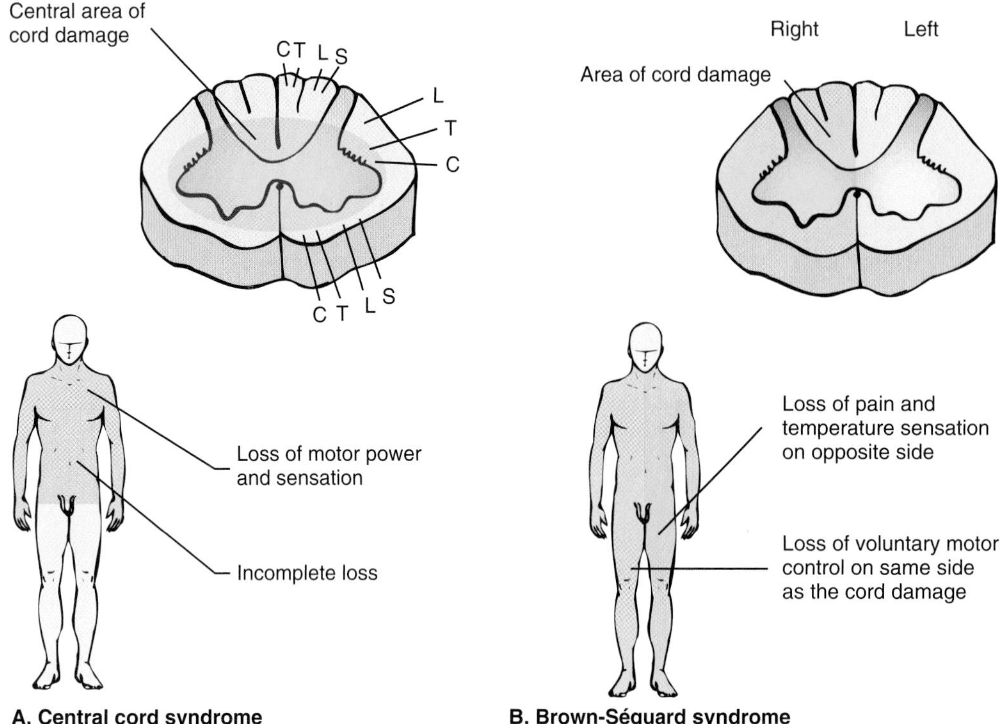

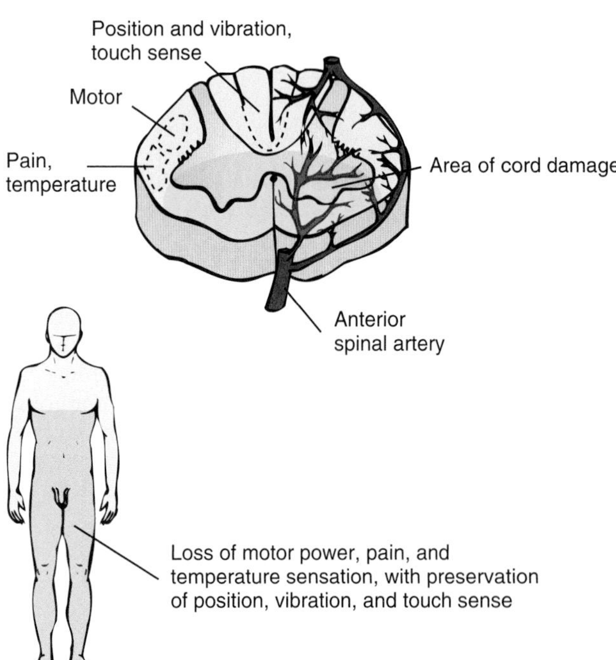

figure 37-4 Selected syndromes related to spinal cord injury. *C,* cervical; *L,* lumbar; *S,* sacrel: *T,* thoracic. (From: Hickey JV: The Clinical Practice of Neurological and Neurosurgical Nursing [5th Ed.], pp 420–421. Philadelphia, Lippincott Williams & Wilkins, 2003.)

for the patient in cervical traction and for the patient in a halo vest are given in Boxes 37-6 and 37-7, respectively.

Medical management of thoracic and lumbar injuries is accomplished by using a fiberglass or plastic vest, canvas corset, or Jewett brace.[5] Each of these devices is fitted to the patient to provide support and stabilization of the spine. Surgical stabilization may also be required. Bed rest is the recommended treatment for sacral and coccygeal injuries.

SURGICAL MANAGEMENT

The goal of surgical management is to stabilize and support the spine. Emergency surgery may be necessary to remove bone fragments, a hematoma, or a penetrating object such as a bullet. If the patient's neurological status continues to decline, a laminectomy may be performed to allow for swelling of the spinal cord secondary to edema. Surgical stabilization is accomplished by placement of rods, laminec-

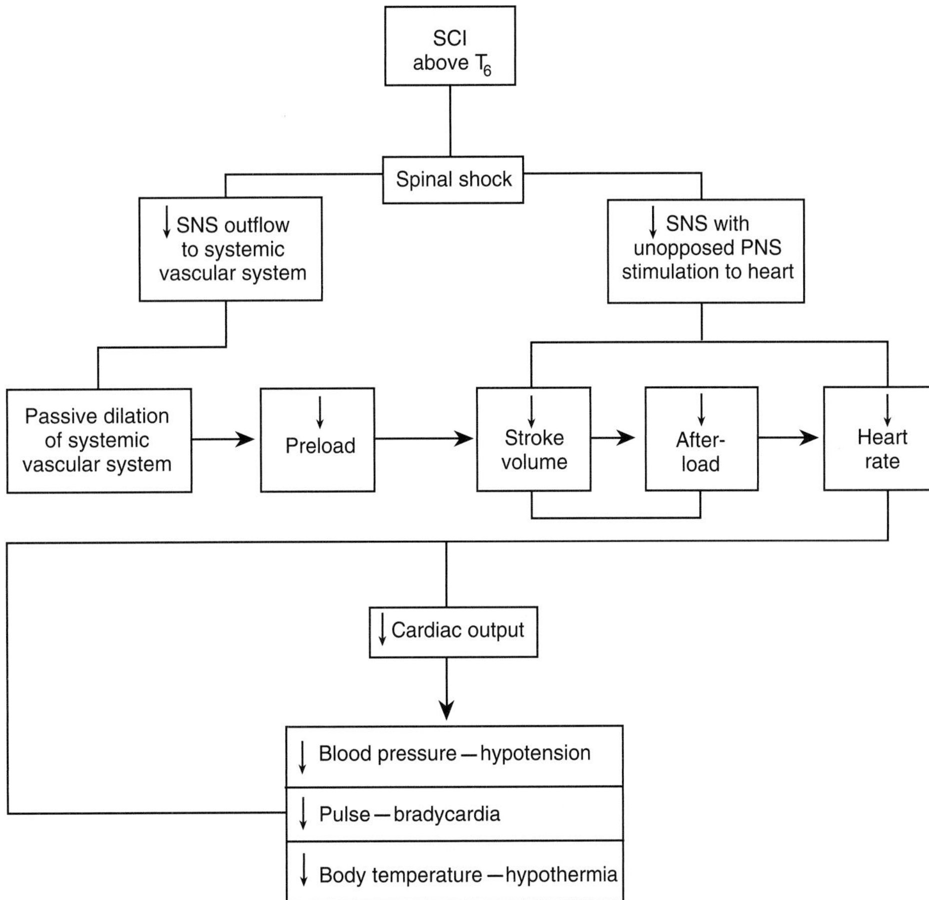

figure 37-5 Mechanisms involved in spinal shock. *SNS,* sympathetic nervous system; *PNS,* parasympathetic nervous system. (From: Zejdlik C: Management of Spinal Cord Injury. Boston, Jones and Bartlett Publishers, 1992.)

tomy and fusion, or by anterior fusion. Bone for fusion is usually taken from the iliac crest, tibia, or ribs.

After surgery, routine postoperative care is implemented. The patient's neurological status is monitored at least every hour for the first 24 hours and then every 4 hours. The surgeon is notified immediately if deterioration in neurological status occurs.

Prevention of Respiratory Problems

Patients with a spinal cord injury, especially injuries above T6, are at risk for respiratory problems such as ineffective airway clearance, ineffective breathing patterns, and impaired gas exchange. The degree of respiratory compromise is determined primarily by the level of the

box 37-2
Clinical Manifestations of Spinal Shock

- Flaccid paralysis below the level of injury
- Absence of cutaneous and proprioceptive sensation
- Hypotension and bradycardia
- Absence of reflex activity below the level of injury; may cause urinary retention, bowel paralysis, and ileus
- Loss of temperature control; vasodilation and inability to shiver make it difficult for the patient to conserve heat in a cool environment, and the inability to perspire prevents normal cooling in a hot environment

box 37-3
Methylprednisolone Administration Protocol for Patients With Spinal Cord Injury

Dosage

- Loading dose: 30 mg/kg IV over 15 min
- Pause for 45 min; infuse normal saline or other IV fluid
- Maintenance dose:
  - 5.4 mg/kg/h IV for 23 h if loading dose given within 3 h of injury
  - 5.4 mg/kg/h IV for 47 h if loading dose given within 3–8 h of injury

Administration

- Loading dose must be given within 8 h of injury.
- Maintenance dose must begin within 1 h of loading dose.

Indications

- Evidence of cord injury, including penetrating injuries
- Injury less than 8 h old

Relative Contraindications

- Pregnancy
- Uncontrolled diabetes mellitus
- Medication allergy
- Severe comorbidity
- Injury greater than 8 h old

*Based on National Association Spinal Cord Injury Study (NASCIS) 2. Source: Hickey J (ed): Vertebral and spinal cord injuries. In The Clinical Practice of Neurological and Neurosurgical Nursing (5th Ed), pp 407–450. Philadelphia, Lippincott Williams & Wilkins, 2002.

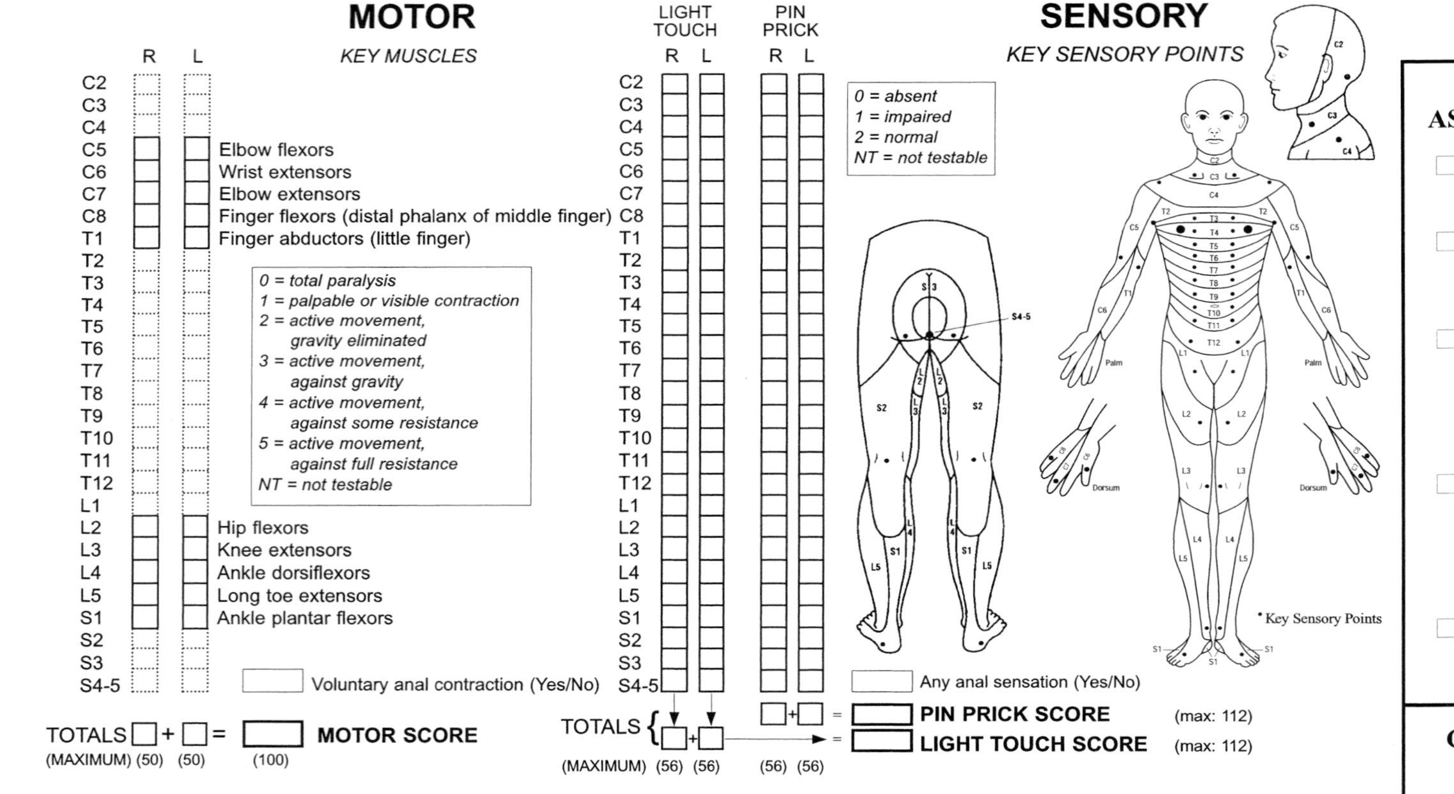

ASIA

STANDARD NEUROLOGICAL CLASSIFICATION OF SPINAL CORD INJURY

MOTOR

KEY MUSCLES

	R	L	
C2			
C3			
C4			
C5			Elbow flexors
C6			Wrist extensors
C7			Elbow extensors
C8			Finger flexors (distal phalanx of middle finger)
T1			Finger abductors (little finger)
T2			
T3			
T4			
T5			
T6			
T7			
T8			
T9			
T10			
T11			
T12			
L1			
L2			Hip flexors
L3			Knee extensors
L4			Ankle dorsiflexors
L5			Long toe extensors
S1			Ankle plantar flexors
S2			
S3			
S4-5			

0 = total paralysis
1 = palpable or visible contraction
2 = active movement, gravity eliminated
3 = active movement, against gravity
4 = active movement, against some resistance
5 = active movement, against full resistance
NT = not testable

Voluntary anal contraction (Yes/No)

TOTALS ☐ + ☐ = ☐ **MOTOR SCORE**
(MAXIMUM) (50) (50) (100)

SENSORY

KEY SENSORY POINTS

	LIGHT TOUCH R	LIGHT TOUCH L	PIN PRICK R	PIN PRICK L
C2				
C3				
C4				
C5				
C6				
C7				
C8				
T1				
T2				
T3				
T4				
T5				
T6				
T7				
T8				
T9				
T10				
T11				
T12				
L1				
L2				
L3				
L4				
L5				
S1				
S2				
S3				
S4-5				

0 = absent
1 = impaired
2 = normal
NT = not testable

Any anal sensation (Yes/No)

TOTALS { ☐ + ☐ = **PIN PRICK SCORE** (max: 112)
☐ + ☐ = **LIGHT TOUCH SCORE** (max: 112)
(MAXIMUM) (56) (56) (56) (56)

NEUROLOGICAL LEVEL *The most caudal segment with normal function* — SENSORY R ☐ L ☐; MOTOR R ☐ L ☐

COMPLETE OR INCOMPLETE? ☐ *Incomplete = Any sensory or motor function in S4-S5*

ASIA IMPAIRMENT SCALE ☐

ZONE OF PARTIAL PRESERVATION *Caudal extent of partially innervated segments* — SENSORY R ☐ L ☐; MOTOR R ☐ L ☐

This form may be copied freely but should not be altered without permission from the American Spinal Injury Association.

2000 Rev.

ASIA IMPAIRMENT SCALE

☐ A = **Complete:** No motor or sensory function is preserved in the sacral segments S4-S5.

☐ B = **Incomplete:** Sensory but not motor function is preserved below the neurological level and includes the sacral segments S4-S5.

☐ C = **Incomplete:** Motor function is preserved below the neurological level, and more than half of key muscles below the neurological level have a muscle grade less than 3.

☐ D = **Incomplete:** Motor function is preserved below the neurological level, and at least half of key muscles below the neurological level have a muscle grade of 3 or more.

☐ E = **Normal:** motor and sensory function are normal

CLINICAL SYNDROMES

☐ Central Cord
☐ Brown-Sequard
☐ Anterior Cord
☐ Conus Medullaris
☐ Cauda Equina

figure 37-6 This Standard Neurological Classification of Spinal Cord Injury flow sheet defines key motor and sensory impairments and clinical syndromes and also includes a functional assessment scale. Motor movement of the major muscle groups is scored on a scale of 0 to 5, with 0 indicating total paralysis and 5 indicating active movement against full resistance or normal movement. Sensation testing is done starting at the area of absent or decreased sensation and proceeding to the area of normal sensation, following the sensory distribution of the skin dermatones. Each spinal cord segment is tested for sensation and is scored as 0 for absent, 1 for impaired, or 2 for normal. (From: American Spinal Injury Association.)

box 37-4 *Examples of Nursing Diagnoses and Collaborative Problems for the Patient With Spinal Cord Injury*

Respiratory
- Impaired Gas Exchange
- Ineffective Airway Clearance
- Ineffective Breathing Pattern

Cardiovascular
- Cardiac Output, Decreased

Neurological
- Acute Pain
- Autonomic Dysreflexia, Risk for
- Body Temperature, Risk for Imbalanced
- Impaired Comfort
- Impaired Mobility, Wheelchair
- Tissue Perfusion, Ineffective

Gastrointestinal/Genitourinary
- Bladder Incontinence
- Bowel Incontinence
- Constipation

Psychosocial
- Anxiety
- Body Image Disturbance, Risk for
- Fear
- Impaired Adjustment, Risk for
- Ineffective Coping: Individual and Family

Activities of Daily Living
- Activity Intolerance, Risk for
- Nutrition, Imbalanced: Less than Body Requirements
- Impaired Skin Integrity, Risk for Complications
- Infection, Risk for
- Injury, Risk for
- Self Care Deficit, Bathing/Hygiene
- Self Care Deficit, Dressing/Grooming
- Self Care Deficit, Feeding
- Self Care Deficit, Toileting
- Sexual Dysfunction, Ineffective Sexuality Pattern

Collaborative Problems
- Potential for atelectasis, pneumonia
- Potential for deep vein thrombosis
- Potential for hypoxemia
- Potential for sepsis

injury, although not entirely. For example, a 28-year-old patient with C5 tetraplegia with no lung disease may have better ventilation than a 65-year-old patient with C8 tetraplegia with a long history of smoking and chronic obstructive pulmonary disease (COPD).

Normally, ventilation is accomplished through a complex interaction between muscles of the chest, the abdominal wall, and the diaphragm. A spinal cord injury results in paralysis of the inspiratory and expiratory muscles. Dysfunction of the intercostal and accessory muscles decreases ventilation and predisposes the patient to atelectasis. Dysfunction of the abdominal muscles and expiratory intercostal muscles diminishes the patient's ability to generate a cough to clear secretions. The intercostal muscles also normally provide support to the lateral chest wall. When the intercostals are impaired, this part of the chest wall collapses during inspiration as the abdomen expands. This breathing pattern is easily discernible and results in ineffective ventilation.

Respiratory complications are the leading cause of death in the acute and chronic phases of spinal cord injury, especially among tetraplegic patients. The nurse and respiratory therapist auscultate breath sounds and measure respiratory parameters (e.g., tidal volume and vital capacity) frequently. Respiratory failure should be anticipated if the patient's vital capacity is less than 15 to 20 mL/kg and the respiratory rate is above 30 breaths/minute. Other interventions include measuring the patient's pulse oximetry; if it is less than 80 mm Hg or if the arterial carbon dioxide tension ($PaCO_2$) is above 45 mm Hg, intubation may be required. Other interventions include oxygen per nasal canula and ensuring that the patient is well hydrated.

The patient is encouraged to take deep breaths and to use an incentive spirometer every 2 hours, or more frequently if tolerated. For example, every time there is a television or radio commercial, the patient can take four to five deep breaths or use the incentive spirometer independently or with the assistance of the nurse or a family member. Assisting the patient with the quad coughing technique may help clear airways more effectively despite weakness or loss of the respiratory muscles that produce the automatic cough reflex. With the quad coughing technique, the sides of the patient's chest (if patient is on his or her side or abdomen) or the diaphragm (if the patient is supine) are compressed during exhalation. This technique often is most helpful after postural drainage or vibration of the chest.

Suctioning may be necessary if the patient's airway cannot be cleared effectively with other techniques. Nurses should remember that suctioning (or nasogastric tube insertion) might trigger an abnormal vasovagal response, resulting in bradycardia.

When turning a patient to the prone position on a Stryker frame, the nurse needs to remain at the bedside for the first few turns to evaluate the patient's respiratory tolerance of the turn. Patients with high-level tetraplegia can experience respiratory arrest in the prone position because movement of the diaphragm is compromised. Bradycardia in the prone position also is common.

Restoration of Hemodynamic Stability

Continuous hemodynamic monitoring is essential to measure cardiac output and systemic perfusion. A pulmonary artery catheter and central venous line may be inserted if this was not done in the emergency department. The patient is at risk for cardiovascular compromise because of disruption in the autonomic nervous system. Bradycardia, hypotension, and dysrhythmias may occur. Hypotension and tachycardia may indicate hemorrhage from intra-abdominal bleeding or bleeding around fracture sites. Sequential compression devices, antiembolism stockings, or an abdominal binder may be used to promote venous return.

Left ventricular dysfunction may occur secondary to release of beta-endorphins. Cardiac enzymes should be obtained if there are electrocardiographic (ECG) changes. Dysrhythmias and heart block may occur. Adequate tissue perfusion to the spinal cord and other vital organs, such as

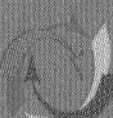

box 37-5 collaborative care guide *for the Patient With Spinal Cord Injury*

OUTCOMES	INTERVENTIONS
Oxygenation/Ventilation	
Arterial blood gas values will be within normal limits. No evidence of atelectasis is demonstrated.	■ Assess need for mechanical ventilation. ■ Provide routine pulmonary toilet, including: Airway suctioning Chest percussion, couth and deep breathing Incentive spirometer, nebulizer treatment ■ Turn frequently. ■ Mobilize out of bed to chair. ■ Apply abdominal binder when out of bed. ■ Consult pulmonologist as needed. ■ Obtain pulmonary function tests.
Circulation/Perfusion	
There will be no evidence of neurogenic (spinal) shock (T10 injuries and higher).	■ Monitor for bradycardia, vasodilation, and hypotension. ■ Assess for arrhythmias.
Blood pressure will be adequate to maintain vital organ function.	■ Prepare to administer intravascular volume, vasopressors, and positive chronotropic agents.
There will be no development of deep venous thrombosis (DVT) or pulmonary embolism.	■ Begin DVT prophylaxis on admission (e.g., external compression device, low-dose heparin). ■ Measure calf and thigh circumference daily and at same location; report increase. ■ Apply Ace wraps to lower extremities before mobilizing out of bed.
There will be no evidence of orthostatic hypotension.	■ Monitor for orthostatic hypotension when raising head of bed and getting out of bed. ■ Consult cardiology as needed.
Neurological	
There will be no evidence of deterioration in neurological status.	■ Perform neurological check and spinal cord function checks every 2–4 hours. ■ Monitor for deterioration in neurological status and report to the physician or nurse practitioner. ■ Monitor for and prevent complications. ■ Provide patient and family education concerning injury, effects of injury, and rehabilitation.
Fluids/Electrolytes	
Serum electrolytes will be within normal limits.	■ Monitor laboratory studies as indicated by patient condition. ■ Assess for dehydration. ■ Administer mineral/electrolyte replacement as ordered.
Fluid balance will be maintained as evidenced by stable weight, absence of edema, normal skin turgor.	■ Monitor gastrointestinal and insensible fluid loss. ■ Make accurate daily fluid intake and output measurements. ■ Weigh weekly. ■ Monitor results of laboratory studies, particularly albumin and electrolyte levels.
Mobility/Safety	
Joint range of motion will be maintained and contractures prevented. Skin integrity will be maintained under or around stabilization devices (e.g., cervical collar, Yale brace, halo vest).	■ Position in correct alignment. ■ Consult with wound care specialist to determine correct type of bed. ■ Begin range-of-motion exercises early after admission. ■ Use high-top tennis shoes, moon boots, extremity splints routinely. ■ Consult with physical and occupational therapists.

(continued)

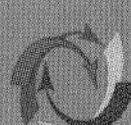

box 37-5 collaborative care guide *for the Patient With Spinal Cord Injury (Continued)*

OUTCOMES	INTERVENTIONS
	■ Maintain splint, brace, and adaptive device schedule; check for pressure ulcers every 4 hours or more often if indicated. ■ Monitor skin or pin sites of stabilization devices. ■ Use meticulous skin care/pin care under or around stabilization devices.
Skin Integrity Skin will remain intact.	■ Consult with wound care specialist to determine correct type of bed. ■ Reposition at least every 2 hours while in bed. ■ Position to prevent pressure on bony prominences. ■ Use upright, straight-backed chair when out of bed (not a reclining chair). Use felt pad on chair seat. ■ Reposition/shift weight every hour when sitting upright. ■ Use Braden Scale to monitor risk of skin breakdown.
Nutrition Protein, carbohydrate, fat, and calorie intake will meet minimum daily requirements.	■ Consult dietitian. ■ Encourage fluids, high-fiber diet. ■ Monitor fluid intake and output, calorie count. ■ Administer parenteral and enteral nutrition as appropriate. ■ Assist with feeding/feed as needed.
Comfort/Pain Pain will be less than "4" on visual analog scale.	■ Assess and differentiate pain from anxiety or stress response. ■ Administer appropriate analgesic or sedative to relieve pain and monitor patient response. ■ Use nonpharmacological pain relief techniques (e.g, distraction, music, relaxation therapies).
Psychosocial Patient will adapt to loss of motor and sensory function.	■ Provide emotional support by: Encouraging ventilation of sadness, fears, and the like. Arranging for social services, clergy, neuropsychologist, or support groups to see patient.
Therapeutic strategies will be used to cope with anxiety and chronic pain syndrome.	■ Provide information and counseling regarding: Personal resources Nonpharmacological pain management techniques Stress management strategies Appropriate use of prescribed pharmacological agents
Integration will be made into prior social role.	■ Provide patient/family counseling regarding: Stages of grief Sexual function and management techniques Social services and community resources
Teaching/Discharge Planning Patient will adapt to loss of bowel/bladder control. Patient will participate in bowel and bladder program.	■ Teach patient/family: Bowel program and training Dietary habits to maintain bowel function Bladder training/intermittent catheterization Prevention of, and signs/symptoms of autonomic dysreflexia
Complications of immobility will be prevented.	■ Teach patient/family: Positioning to prevent skin breakdown Physical therapy exercises Pulmonary toilet
Patient will be placed in appropriate postacute setting.	■ Consult rehabilitation/discharge planner/social services early after admission to initiate placement arrangements.

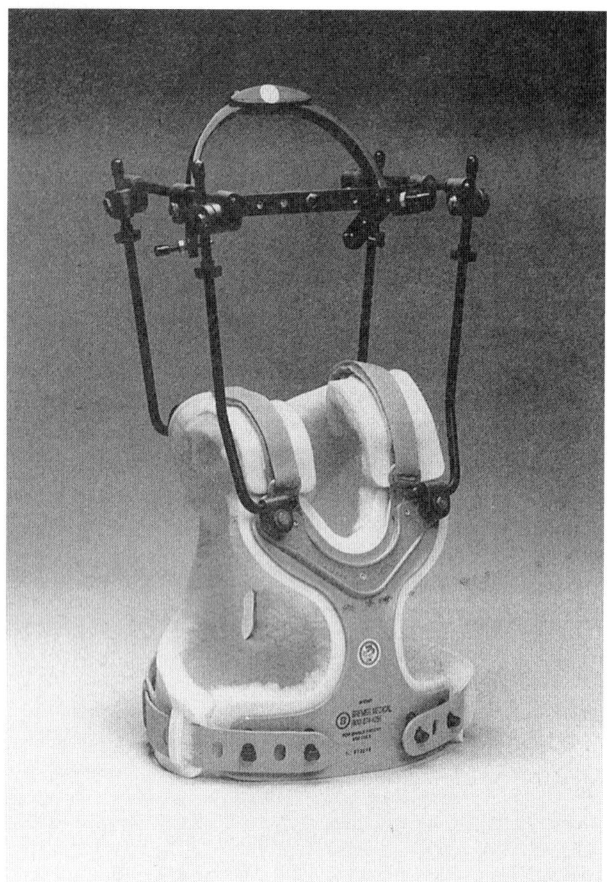

figure 37-7 A lightweight fleece-lined vest with a halo may be used to stabilize the cervical vertebrae. Note that the vest comes in various sizes and does not need to be removed for magnetic resonance imaging studies. (Courtesy of Bremer Medical, Inc., Dawin Road, Jacksonville, FL 32207).

the kidneys, needs to be addressed. Careful intravenous fluid replacement provides hydration without fluid overload. Vasopressors may not be needed to maintain blood pressure during spinal shock, but when the blood pressure is not high enough to sustain vital organ perfusion, usually low-dose dopamine is used. Bradycardia also may not need treatment but, if necessary, atropine may be used to speed up the heart rate. A transcutaneous or transvenous pacemaker may be need to be placed if the patient remains bradycardic despite atropine.[4]

Neurological Management

While in the ICU, the patient should have neurological assessments completed every hour until stable, then every 4 hours. Particular attention is paid to the patient's motor and sensory states. If there is any deterioration in the patient's condition, the frequency of assessment is increased and the physician or nurse practitioner is notified.

Pain Management

As a rule, sensation in the patient with a spinal cord injury is limited. Intractable pain may be present after spinal shock and is due to nerve root damage. Abnormal sensation may occur at the level of the lesion in injuries causing diverse nerve root damage, such as occurs with gunshot or knife wounds. Pain resulting from either the spinal cord injury, surgery, or both is treated aggressively following institutional protocol and within the pain management standards of the Joint Commission on Accreditation of Health Care Organizations.

Medication Administration

Medications used in the treatment of the patient with spinal cord injury are listed in Table 37-2. Nurses administering medications to patients with spinal cord injuries must take into account several special considerations. Subcutaneous and intramuscular injections are not absorbed well because of the lack of muscle tone. Sterile abscesses may result, causing autonomic dysreflexia or an increase in spasms. Injection sites are the deltoid area, the anterior thigh, and the abdominal area. These sites should be rotated, and the volume injected should not exceed 1 mL at any one site.

Nurses often start peripheral intravenous lines, but the intravenous site of choice is the subclavian vein. In this area of high blood flow, there is less chance of thrombosis secondary to vasomotor paralysis, especially during spinal shock. For this reason, the veins of the lower extremities should never be used for intravenous administration.

Thermoregulation

Ineffective thermoregulation is a common problem seen in patients with spinal cord injuries above the thoracolumbar area. Interruption of the sympathetic nervous system prevents the thalamic thermoregulatory mechanisms. As a result, the patient fails to sweat to get rid of body heat, and there is an absence of vasoconstriction, resulting in an inability to shiver to increase body heat. The degree of thermal control and dysfunction is directly proportional to the extent of body area with loss of thermal regulation. Hence, a tetraplegic patient has more difficulty with thermoregulation than a paraplegic patient.

Hypothermia is usually managed by using warmed blankets. The room temperature is adjusted to maintain patient comfort. Electric heating blankets or hot water bottles may present a danger for body parts with no sensation. An attempt is made to stabilize the patient's temperature above 96.5°F (35.8°C). Ideally, the patient is placed in a private room so the room temperature does not adversely affect the other patient in the room. Over the long term, thermal control can be facilitated by use of clothing appropriate for the weather conditions.

Nutrition

The possibility of inadequate nutrition is of significant concern even during the acute phase of injury, and must not be overlooked while hemodynamic stability is being addressed. Optimal nutrition is necessary for this stability to be achieved. A negative nitrogen balance contributes to skin breakdown, poor wound healing, and lack of energy for rehabilitative efforts. Caloric requirements must be calculated to ensure adequate, but not excessive, nutritional support. After collaboration with the dietitian, a caloric count may be instituted.

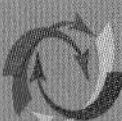

box 37-6 collaborative care guide *for the Patient in Cervical Traction*

OUTCOMES	INTERVENTIONS
Equipment Management	
The orthopedic frame will remain intact. Tongs will not slip. Traction weights will hang freely. There will not be any extension of cord injury secondary to slippage of the traction apparatus.	■ Check the orthopedic frame and traction daily to ensure that nuts and bolts are secure. ■ Check tongs daily to be sure that they are secure. ■ Be sure that traction weights are hanging freely and not resting on the floor or frame. (Releasing the traction is dangerous because cord injury could be extended.)
Oxygenation/Ventilation	
Airway patency will be maintained. The patient will not aspirate. The patient will not develop a respiratory infection.	■ Have suction available to maintain a patent airway. ■ Provide respiratory care. ■ Provide for deep-breathing, assistive coughing, and incentive spirometer exercises every 1 to 2 hours.
Circulation/Perfusion	
Air boots and thigh-high elastic hose (TEDs) will be worn at all times. Vital signs will be maintained within normal limits. The patient will be observed for deep venous thrombosis (DVT) and pulmonary emboli.	■ Maintain TEDs and sequential compression boots. ■ If the patient is receiving heparin, observe for signs and symptoms of bleeding. ■ Monitor for DVT and pulmonary emboli. (May be receiving minidoses of subcutaneous heparin every 12 hours, if not contraindicated.)
Mobility/Safety	
The patient will be free from pain. Contractures will not develop. Strategies will be used to manage spasticity if it occurs.	■ Provide comfort measures. ■ Provide range-of-motion exercises four times per day. ■ Position the patient in proper body alignment. ■ Reposition the patient frequently. ■ Stretch the patient's heel cord with exercises.
Skin Integrity	
The pin site will remain free of infection. Skin integrity will be maintained. The vertebral column will be maintained in a neutral position and in proper alignment.	■ Inspect tong sites, and clean and dress daily as ordered (may be referred to as "pin care"). ■ Turn the patient every 2 hours from side to back to other side using a triple log-roll technique as described below if a patient is on a regular hospital bed: Nurse #1 stands behind the head of the bed and places hands firmly on the patient's head and neck, maintaining it in a neutral position; the head and neck are turned as a unit. Nurse #2 stands at the patient's side and moves the patient's shoulders. Nurse #3 stands at the patient's side and moves the patient's hips and legs. Plan ahead, identifying desired position and pillow placement *before* moving the patient. When all three nurses are ready, turn the patient as a log on the count of three. Leave the patient positioned in the middle of the bed (if not, he or she will be uncomfortable); use pillows to support the patient's body in alignment. Nurse #1 should hold the head and neck until the patient is supported adequately (if traction slips, manual traction can be supplied by Nurse #1).

(continued)

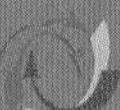

box 37-6 collaborative care guide *for the Patient in Cervical Traction (Continued)*

OUTCOMES	INTERVENTIONS
Nutrition	
A diet high in protein and carbohydrates, which includes a fluid intake of up to 3000 mL, will be provided. Aspiration will be prevented.	■ Encourage an adequate diet. ■ Ask the dietitian to see the patient. ■ Provide for adequate fluid intake up to 3000 mL daily. ■ Encourage the patient to take small portions of food into the mouth and chew well to prevent aspiration. ■ Keep suction equipment handy.
Elimination	
Pattern of bowel evacuation every 1 to 2 days will be established. Intake will be 3000 mL unless contraindicated. Postvoid residuals will be less than 100 mL. Strict aseptic technique will be used for catheter protocols.	■ Institute a bowel retraining program. ■ Auscultate the abdomen for bowel sounds. ■ Record the frequency and consistency of stool. ■ Monitor intake and output. ■ Force fluids. ■ If an intermittent catheterization protocol is initiated, use aseptic technique. ■ If the patient is voiding on his or her own, monitor postvoid residuals.
Psychosocial	
The patient's mental health will be supported. Social interaction and diversion will be provided based on the patient's ability to participate. A positive body image will be supported. Necessary information will be provided. Sexual function and spinal cord injury are discussed with the patient when he or she is ready.	■ Provide for social interaction and diversion based on the patient's functional level. ■ Reinforce a positive self-image. ■ Allow the patient to participate in decision making as much as possible. ■ Provide for patient teaching. ■ Provide information about sexual function.

Patients with spinal cord injuries often have increased energy needs owing to metabolic stress response. This can lead to a severe catabolic state and malnutrition. It is not unusual to see a 7-kg weight loss within the first few days of injury.[4] Total parental nutrition or enteral feedings are instituted until the patient is able to start on an oral diet. The patient's intake is strictly monitored.

Ensuring adequate nutrition is a collaborative problem involving the patient, family, dietitian, occupational therapist, and nurse. The dietitian meets with the patient and family to identify the foods the patient enjoys and develop a menu that incorporates patient preference into the required dietary plan. The family is taught what foods can be brought from home that are included in the patient's prescribed diet. The occupational therapist assesses the patient's need for assistive devices to use during mealtimes and teaches the patient and family how to use the adapted silverware. The nurse reinforces the information provided by the dietitian and occupational therapist. The nurse may teach family and friends how to assist the patient with meals and about the importance of allowing the patient as much independence as possible at mealtime. Unless contraindicated, fluids are encouraged along with a high-roughage diet. Before meals, the nurse assists the patient with mouth care and ensures that the patient has not been incontinent.

Mobilization and Skin Care

Rehabilitation begins in the ICU and is a collaborative effort involving the patient, physician, physical therapist, occupational therapist, nurse, and the patient's family. Initially, the nurse assists the patient with range-of-motion exercises. When the patient is stable, family members may be taught to assist the patient with these exercises. Based on their assessment findings, the physical therapist and occupational therapist develop an individualized treatment plan to begin mobilization of the patient.

Pressure is a common cause of structural damage to a muscle and its peripheral nerve supply. There is a definite time–pressure relationship in the development of pressure ulcers. Microscopic tissue changes secondary to local ischemia occur in less than 30 minutes. Pressure interferes with arteriolar and capillary blood flow. When the pressure is prolonged, there is definite damage to superficial circulation and tissue. The damage may be associated with congestion and induration of the area or blistering and loss of the superficial epidermal layers of the skin. As the pressure continues, the deeper skin layers are lost, leading to necrosis and ulceration. Serous drainage from such ulceration can constitute a continuous protein loss of as much as 50 g/day. Prolongation of the pressure results in deep penetrating necrosis of the skin, subcutaneous tissue,

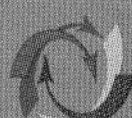

box 37-7 collaborative care guide *for the Patient in a Halo Vest*

OUTCOMES	INTERVENTIONS
Equipment Management	
The patient will be comfortable and without signs of skin irritation. Proper body alignment will be maintained.	■ Check the pins on the halo ring to be sure they are secure and tight. ■ Check the edges of the fiberglass vest for comfort and fit by inserting the small finger or index finger between the vest and the patient's skin. If the vest is too tight, skin breakdown, edema, and possible nerve injury can occur. ■ The vest should be supported while the patient is in bed. ■ Place a rubber cork over the tips of the halo device to diminish magnification of sound if the pin is bumped.
Oxygenation/Ventilation	
The patient will not develop a respiratory infection.	■ Provide for deep-breathing exercises at least four times daily.
Circulation/Perfusion	
Risk for thrombus or embolus formation will be decreased.	■ Apply thigh-high elastic hose (TED) to the legs to improve blood return to the heart. ■ Observe the legs for development of thrombophlebitis or deep venous thrombosis (DVT).
Mobility/Safety	
The patient will maintain muscle tone. The patient will ambulate in a safe manner to the best of his or her ability.	■ If the patient's neurological function is intact, he or she will be able to ambulate in the halo vest. ■ Start to assess the patient's tolerance of the upright position by having him or her sit on the edge of the bed ("dangle"). Check vital signs. (Orthostatic hypotension may be a problem to overcome in the early stages.) ■ Teach the patient to compensate for lost head and neck movement by making increased use of eye movement to scan the area. ■ Accompany patients when ambulating because they are more accident prone owing to a displaced center of gravity, a tendency for loss of balance, and decreased peripheral vision. ■ Consider the patient's use of a walker for ambulation as a means of support and greater safety.
Skin Integrity	
The patient will maintain skin integrity. The patient will maintain proper body alignment without injuries. Early signs of skin irritation or breakdown will be detected.	■ Inspect and cleanse the pin site once or twice daily, as prescribed, to prevent infection. ■ Turn the patient in bed every 2 hours by means of the triple log-roll technique to prevent the development of hypostatic pneumonia, atelectasis, and skin breakdown. ■ Provide sponge pads to prevent pressure on prominent body areas, such as the forehead and shoulder, while the patient is in bed. ■ Inspect under the vest, and keep all areas of skin dry.
Elimination	
Pattern of bowel elimination every 1 to 2 days will be established. Intake will be 3000 mL unless contraindicated; postvoid residuals will be less than 100 mL.	■ Institute a bowel retraining program. ■ Monitor intake and output.

(continued)

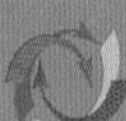

box 37-7 collaborative care guide *for the Patient in a Halo Vest (Continued)*

OUTCOMES	INTERVENTIONS
Comfort/Pain Control	
The patient will be comfortable, with pain controlled.	■ Administer mild analgesics to control headache and discomfort, which are common, around the pin site. ■ Provide a soft diet, because many patients have jaw pain if they attempt to chew.
Psychosocial	
The patient's emotional well-being will be supported.	■ Help the patient adjust to the distorted body image that the halo device can create. ■ Encourage self-care as much as possible.
Teaching/Discharge Planning	
The patient will be provided the necessary information to ensure competent home care. The patient will use equipment in a safe manner.	■ If the patient is to go home with the halo vest, begin a patient and family teaching plan using a booklet or other printed material. Review any written material prepared by the manufacturer for accuracy before giving it to the patient or family.

fascia, and muscle. The destruction may progress to gangrene of the underlying bony structure. Pressure necrosis can begin from within the tissue over a bony prominence, where the body weight is greatest per square inch.

A turn schedule for the patient is important. Turning is carried out a minimum of every 2 hours. Use of an air or egg-crate mattress does not preclude the need to turn. The condition of the skin is checked before and after the position change. Particular attention is paid to the patient's earlobes, back of head, elbows, inner aspects of the knees, and sacral area. Any change in skin integrity is documented. The wound care specialist is notified and a plan of care implemented to treat the pressure ulcer and prevent further deterioration in skin integrity. Numerous kinetic beds and airbeds are available for patient comfort. They are helpful for mobilizing pulmonary secretions, improving gas exchange, and preventing skin breakdown. These beds are useful for preventing and treating complications of immobility.

Together with the physical and occupational therapist, the nurse develops a plan to prevent foot drop. Frequently, high-top tennis shoes are worn. It is important to ensure that the shoes are the correct size, to check for signs of skin breakdown, and to ensure that the patient's feet are dry. An "on and off" schedule should be developed with the physical therapist. When the shoes are off, careful attention should be paid to foot positioning and assessing for pressure ulcers.

The occupational therapist determines the need for splints or braces for the patient's wrists and hands. The patient's skin must be assessed frequently to identify pressure areas early. If necessary, the splints are modified to prevent skin breakdown.

Urinary Management

Acute tubular necrosis (ATN) may occur within 48 hours of injury as a result of hypotension. An indwelling urinary catheter is necessary to allow for hourly measurement of urinary output during this phase, with the goal of keeping it at least 30 mL/hour. Fluid and electrolyte balance must be monitored closely. Removal of the indwelling catheter as soon as spinal shock has resolved reduces the risk of infection.

The long-range objective of bladder management, regardless of the level of the injury, is to achieve a means whereby the bladder consistently empties, the urine is sterile, and the patient remains continent. The ultimate goal is to have the patient catheter free, with consistent low residual urine checks, no urinary tract infection, and no evidence of damage to the upper urinary tract structures.

One method of bladder management is accomplished by intermittent catheterization, and it may begin in the early recovery phase after spinal shock is resolved. The purpose of this program is to exercise the detrusor muscle, again with the goal of keeping the patient catheter free. The advantage of this method is that no irritant remains in the bladder; consequently, the risk of urinary tract infection, periurethral abscess, and epididymitis is reduced.

Bowel Management

Before the initiation of a bowel program, a systematic, comprehensive evaluation of bowel function, impairment, and possible problems is performed. This includes an abdominal assessment, a rectal examination, and evaluation of anal sphincter tone. In addition, the anocutaneous and bulbocavernosus reflexes are assessed to determine if the patient has upper motor neuron or lower motor neuron dysfunction.

Simple steps can be taken to prevent constipation and begin progress toward bowel continence. Appropriate intake is maintained, either through intravenous or oral fluids and diet. Bowel movements are recorded in an area that is easily accessible for review. Stool softeners are administered daily. A consistent schedule for the bowel program is established. The program is usually timed for after meals to coincide with peristalsis that

table 37-2 ■ Drugs Used in the Treatment of the Patient With a Spinal Cord Injury

Drug	Description	Administration*
Drugs to Minimize Injury		
Methylprednisolone	Synthetic adrenal corticosteroid used as an anti-inflammatory agent	Loading dose: 30 mg/kg IV over 15 min Pause for 45 min; infuse normal saline or other IV fluid Maintenance dose: 5.4 mg/kg/h IV for 23 h if loading dose given within 3 h of injury 5.4 mg/kg/h IV for 47 h if loading dose given within 3–8 h of injury Loading dose must be given within 8 h of injury. Maintenance dose must begin within 1 h of loading dose.
Tirilazad	Used as an anti-inflammatory agent; inhibits lipid peroxidation without glucocorticoid activity; associated with a lower incidence of sepsis and pneumonia (compared with methylprednisolone)	Dosage: 25 mg/kg bolus infusion every 6 h for 48 h Limit use to those patients who received an initial bolus of methylprednisolone 3–8 h after injury
Drugs for Cardiovascular Stabilization		
Atropine	Anticholinergic used to treat symptomatic bradycardia	Dosage: 0.4–1.0 mg IV slowly; maximum dose 2 mg
Dobutamine (Dobutrex)	Beta-adrenergic agent that enhances myocardial contractility, stroke volume, and cardiac output; improves perfusion to the spinal cord	Dosage: 2.5–10 μg/kg/min up to maximum dosage of 40 μg/kg/min; usually given for a total of 72 h if needed
Dopamine (Intropin)	Alpha- and beta-adrenergic agent used to treat hypotension related to neurogenic shock	Dosage: 3–5 μg/kg/min; increase gradually at 10- to 30-minute intervals up to 20–50 μg/kg/min until optimum blood pressure achieved Start the older adult on lower doses; use with caution if the patient is on a monoamine oxidase (MAO) inhibitor
Drugs for Paralytic Ileus and Stress Ulcers		
Proton pump inhibitors (lansoprazole, omeprazole, pantoprazole)	Suppress gastric acid secretion; used to prevent or treat gastric ulcers	Dosage: dependent on medication prescribed
Histamine blockers (cimetidine, famotidine, nizantine, ranitidine hydrochloride)	Inhibit histamine action at H_2 receptor sites; used to treat and prevent ulcers and gastric reflux	Dosage: dependent on medication prescribed
Drugs for Autonomic Hyperreflexia		
Nitroglycerin	Organic nitrate used if systolic blood pressure above 140 mm Hg	Dosage: 1 inch of nitroglycerin paste placed above the level of injury
Nifedipine (Procardia)	Calcium channel blocker used to decrease systemic vascular resistance and blood pressure	Dosage: 10–20 mg PO every 20–30 min if necessary
Hydralazine, trimethaphan, diazoxide	Antihypertensive agents	Dosage: dependent on medication prescribed Trimethaphan: dilute per hospital protocol (usually 500 mg in 500 mL D_5W); usual dose 0.5–1 mg/min Hydralazine: 25 mg PO four times per day or 10–20 mg IV every 4–6 h Diazoxide: 1–3 mg/kg, up to 150 mg, IV; repeat at 5- to 15-min intervals if needed

(continued)

table 37-2 ■ Drugs Used in the Treatment of the Patient With a Spinal Cord Injury (Continued)

Drug	Description	Administration*
Drugs for Skeletal Muscle Spasm		
Dantrolene (Dantrium)	Skeletal muscle relaxant used to treat spasticity	Dosage: Initial dose 25 mg/day; increase to 25 mg two to four times per day; may increase up to 100 mg two to four times per day over 4–7 days
Baclofen (Lioresal)	Skeletal muscle relaxant used to treat spasticity	Dosage: Initially 5 mg two to three times per day; may increase slowly to range of 40–80 mg per day; total dose not to exceed 80 mg/day
Tizanidine hydrochloride (Zanaflex)	Central acting skeletal muscle relaxant used to treat acute and intermittent increased muscle tone associated with spasticity	Dosage: Initially 4 mg; gradually increase to 8 mg every 6–8 h for a maximum dose of 36 mg/24 h
Investigational Drugs		
Fampridine-SR ("4-AP," "4-aminopyridine")	In previous phase II studies, evidence of benefit has been seen in several areas—reduced muscle spasticity, improved sexual function, increased bladder control and bowel function	

*Follow hospital protocol. Refer to an up-to-date drug guide for updated information. Doses listed here are guidelines only.

occurs after meals to move food through the gastrointestinal tract. Rectal stimulation may be needed to trigger defecation.

Psychological Support

Psychological adjustment to the loss of previous physical abilities is unique to each person. The rate at which a person works through this process varies, and none of the stages is static. A person can move back and forth between stages. The emotions felt and displayed by someone with a cord injury are no different from the emotions felt by everyone at one time or another, and recognition of that fact may help promote empathy with the patient. Whatever names are given to the stages of grief, certain emotions are felt after a cord injury (Box 37-8).

All staff should have an understanding of the types of feelings and reactions the patient with a spinal cord injury may exhibit. This process of recovery can be shared with family members in helping them to support the injured person and participate in recovery. Psychological support is provided for family members as well. They no doubt have many concerns, such as finances, role changes, long-term outcomes, and more. It is important to be supportive of them and help them and the patient with coping strategies.

Addressing Concerns About Sexuality

After a spinal cord injury, patients are concerned about their ability to function sexually, although they may not verbalize this concern immediately. It is essential that nurses address this area of concern. Although nurses in the ICU probably will not deal with this problem specifically, it is important for them to have some knowledge of the functional potential of the patient to begin to deal with the patient's fears and concerns in this area early on. By avoiding discussion of this important issue, professionals validate the patient's fear that there can be no sex after a spinal cord injury, which is certainly not true.

MALE SEXUALITY

Many cord-injured men believe that their total sexuality is tied to erection and ejaculation. There are three general types of erection in men: psychogenic, reflexogenic, and spontaneous. A psychogenic erection can result from sexual thoughts. The area of the cord responsible for this type of erection is between T11 and L2. Therefore, if the lesion is above this level, the message from the brain cannot get through the damaged area.

Reflexogenic erections are a direct result of stimulation to the penis. Some patients may get this type of erection when changing their catheter or pulling the pubic hairs. The length of time the erection can be maintained is variable; therefore, its usefulness for sexual activity is variable. Reflexogenic erections are better with higher cervical and thoracic lesions. Damage to lumbar and sacral regions may destroy the reflex arc.

The third type of erection is spontaneous. This may occur when the bladder is full, and it comes from some internal stimulation. How long the spontaneous erection lasts will determine its usefulness for sexual activity. The ability to achieve a reflexogenic or spontaneous erection comes from nerves in the S2, S3, and S4 segments of the cord.

FEMALE SEXUALITY

In 50% of women with a spinal cord injury, the menstrual pattern is interrupted for approximately 6 months after injury, but then is reestablished. Women with spinal cord injuries are able to become pregnant and seem to have no increase in rate of miscarriage. There are potential complications for the pregnant woman with a spinal cord injury,

box 37-8
Stages of Grief in a Patient With a Spinal Cord Injury

STAGE	DESCRIPTION	IMPLICATIONS FOR THE NURSE
1. **Shock and disbelief**	During this phase, the patient does not request an explanation of what has happened. The patient is overwhelmed by the injury. There may be more concern with whether he or she will live than with whether he or she will walk again. This period may result in extreme dependence on the staff members.	The nurse may feel that the patient does not understand the ramifications of the injury. The nurse may identify with the feelings of being overwhelmed because he or she is often overwhelmed with the acute medical management of this catastrophic illness.
2. **Denial**	The process of denial is an escape mechanism. Usually, the whole disability is not denied, but particular aspects of it are. For instance, the patient may say he or she cannot walk now but will be able to in 6 months. Bargaining, instead of being a separate stage, can be considered a form of denial. Bargains with God may be in the form of offering Him the legs if He will just return function of the arms.	The nurse often finds it difficult to deal with patients in this stage. A helpful approach is to focus on the present problems. This is not the stage to discuss long-term changes, such as ordering a wheelchair or making modifications to the home. More appropriate matters to deal with would be skin care and range-of-motion exercises.
3. **Reaction**	During this stage, instead of denying the impact of the injury, the patient expresses this impact. There may be severe depression and loss of motivation and involvement. Previous hobbies or interests lose their meaning. There is great helplessness during this period, and there may be suicidal statements.	The nurse can help at this stage by listening to the patient as feelings are verbalized. The nurse should avoid setting up failure situations, which could happen if he or she pushes the patient too fast. It is important to note that both the sudden absence of muscular activity and sensations in the patient with a spinal cord injury and the mental state of helplessness appear to alter central nervous system metabolism. Depression coincides with a fall in a brain metabolite excreted in the urine as tryptamine. Thus, it is important for the nurse to understand that depression in some patients with spinal cord injury might have a metabolic basis and that a trial of pharmacological therapy might be beneficial.
4. **Mobilization**	Problem-solving behavior is seen during this stage. The patient is looking toward the future and wants to learn about self-care. In fact, the patient may become very possessive of the therapist or nurse and resent the time spent with other patients. This is a time of sharing and planning between patient and staff.	
5. **Coping**	Some authorities think that patients do not accept the disability *per se* but instead learn to cope with it. Disability still is an inconvenience, but it is no longer the center of the patient's life. Life is again meaningful to the patient, and the patient is again involved with others.	

such as urinary tract infection, pressure sores, and anemia, but with careful medical attention, complications usually can be avoided or minimized.

Labor may be painless, or the woman may experience other signs that indicate labor is occurring (e.g., abdominal or leg spasms, back pain, difficulty breathing). Autonomic dysreflexia is a complication of labor in women with injuries above T4 to T6 and should be anticipated so it can be controlled. Women with spinal cord injuries can breast-feed if desired.

COMPLICATIONS

Autonomic Dysreflexia

Autonomic dysreflexia, or hyperreflexia, is a syndrome that sometimes occurs after the acute phase in patients with a spinal cord lesion at T7 or above. Autonomic dysreflexia constitutes a medical emergency. The syndrome presents quickly and can precipitate a seizure or stroke. Death can occur if the cause is not relieved.

box 37-9
Precipitating Factors in Autonomic Dysreflexia

- Bladder distension or urinary tract infection
- Bladder or kidney stones
- Distended bowel
- Pressure areas or decubitus ulcers
- Thrombophlebitis
- Acute abdominal problems (e.g., ulcers, gastritis)
- Pulmonary emboli
- Menstruation
- Second stage of labor
- Constrictive clothing
- Heterotopic bone
- Pain
- Sexual activity; ejaculation by a man
- Manipulation or instrumentation of bladder or bowel
- Spasticity
- Exposure to hot or cold stimuli

Autonomic dysreflexia can be triggered by bladder or intestinal distention, spasticity, pressure ulcers, or stimulation of the skin below the level of the injury. In men, ejaculation can initiate the reflex, as can strong uterine contractions in a pregnant woman. Potential precipitating factors are listed in Box 37-9.

These stimuli produce a sympathetic discharge that causes a reflex vasoconstriction of the blood vessels in the skin and splanchnic bed below the level of the injury. The vasoconstriction produces extreme hypertension and a throbbing headache. Vasoconstriction of the splanchnic bed distends the baroreceptors in the carotid sinus and aortic arch. They in turn stimulate the vagus nerve, producing a bradycardia, in an attempt to lower the blood pressure. The body also attempts to reduce the hypertension by superficial vasodilation of vessels above the spinal cord injury. As a result, there is flushing, blurred vision, and nasal congestion. Because the spinal cord injury interrupts transmission of the vasodilation message below the level of the injury, the vasoconstriction continues below the level of the injury until the stimulus is identified and interrupted. The vasoconstriction results in pallor below the injury, whereas flushing occurs above the injury. Signs and symptoms of autonomic dysreflexia are summarized in Box 37-10.

When autonomic dysreflexia is recognized, there are several things the nurse can do quickly and can teach the patient to do. The head of the bed is elevated and frequent checks of blood pressure made. The bladder drainage system is checked quickly for kinks in the tubing. The urine collection bag should not be overly full. Some protocols for checking the patency of the urinary drainage system include irrigating the catheter with 10 to 30 mL of irrigating solution. Absolutely no more than that amount is used because the addition of the fluid may aggravate the massive sympathetic outflow already present. If the symptoms persist after these checks are made, the catheter is changed so that the bladder can empty. If the patient did not have a catheter in place when the hyperreflexia began, one is inserted.

box 37-10 ***Signs and Symptoms of Autonomic Dysreflexia***

- Paroxysmal hypertension
- Pounding headache
- Blurred vision
- Bradycardia
- Profuse sweating above the level of the injury
- Flushing or splotching of the face and neck
- Piloerection
- Nasal congestion
- Nausea
- Pupil dilation

If the urinary system does not seem to be the cause of the stimulus, the patient is checked for bowel impaction. The impaction is not removed until the symptoms subside. Dibucaine or lidocaine ointment can be applied to the rectum to anesthetize the area until symptoms subside. If the patient's blood pressure does not return to normal, sublingual nifedipine (Procardia) may be very effective. A sympathetic ganglionic blocking agent such as atropine sulfate, guanethidine sulfate (Ismelin), reserpine (Reserfia), or methyldopa (Aldomet) may be used. Hydralazine (Apresoline) and diazoxide (Hyperstat) also may be used. Nursing intervention guidelines for managing autonomic dysreflexia are given in Box 37-11.

Pulmonary Complications

Pulmonary complications are the most common cause of death in people with spinal cord injury, both in the acute and chronic phases. These pulmonary complications are especially prevalent in people injured above T10. If there is concomitant chest trauma or pre-existing pulmonary disease, a history of smoking, or older age, there is higher risk for these complications.

ATELECTASIS AND PNEUMONIA

Atelectasis is possible in any immobilized patient. Early mobilization, ensuring the airways are clear of secretions, and bronchial hygiene may be useful in minimizing or preventing atelectasis. Pneumonia may also result from hypoventilation and an inability to keep the airways clear. Adequate hydration helps keep secretions liquefied for ease of removal, and bronchoscopy may be necessary to remove mucus plugs. Supplemental oxygen administration is used to treat hypoxia. Ventilator-dependent patients need exquisite pulmonary care (see Chapter 25).

PULMONARY EMBOLUS

Especially during the acute phase of spinal cord injury, pulmonary embolus is a potential problem. Patients particularly at risk for a fat embolus are those with long bone fractures. Signs of chest or neck petechiae and low-grade fever may be early indications.

Many emboli originate from a deep venous thrombosis (DVT). Measures to prevent DVT may include the administration of low-dose heparin or low–molecular-weight

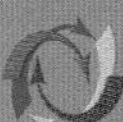

box 37-11 nursing interventions for *Managing Autonomic Dysreflexia*

1. Elevate the head of bed.
2. Apply blood pressure cuff, and check blood pressure every 1 to 2 minutes.
   - If BP is above 180/90, proceed to step 5.
   - If BP is below 180/90, proceed as follows.
3. Quickly insert bladder catheter or check bladder drainage system in place to detect possible obstruction.
   - Check to make sure plug or clamp is not in catheter or on tubing.
   - Check for kinks in catheter or drainage tubing.
   - Check inlet to leg bag to make sure it is not corroded.
   - Check to make sure leg bag is not overfull.
   - If none of these are evident, proceed to step 4.
4. Determine if catheter is plugged by irrigating the bladder slowly with no more than 30 mL of irrigation solution. Use of more solution may increase the massive sympathetic outflow already present. If symptoms have not subsided, proceed to step 5.
5. Change the catheter and empty the bladder.
6. When you are sure the bladder is empty and if BP is:
   - Above 180/90, call physician immediately.
   - Below 180/90, proceed as follows: Give sublingual nifedipine (Procardia) if protocol calls for it. Give atropine according to physician's order. If BP rises or fails to subside, call physician immediately. Guanethidine monosulfate (Ismelin), hydralazine (Apresoline), or inhaled amyl nitrate may then be ordered by the physician. Dibenzylene may be used for chronic dysreflexia.
7. Ideally, this procedure requires three people: one to check the BP, one to check the drainage system, and one to notify the physician.

If bladder overdistension does not seem to be the cause of the dysreflexia,

- Check for bowel impaction. Do not attempt to remove it, if present. Apply Nupercainal ointment or Xylocaine jelly to the rectum and anal area. As the area is anesthetized, the BP should fall. After the BP is again stable, using a generous amount of anesthetizing ointment or jelly, manually remove impaction.
- Change the patient's position. Pressure areas may be the source of dysreflexia.

heparin and the use of antiembolic stockings. During the acute phase, devices that sequentially compress the lower extremities may be used. Many centers that specialize in the treatment of spinal cord injury use prophylactic anticoagulation or low–molecular-weight heparin; others rely on passive range-of-motion exercises and early mobilization. A kinetic bed can also be used to prevent DVT; this device works by keeping the patient in continuous motion.

Leg veins should not be used as sites from which to draw blood, lest the trauma to the vessel wall enhance platelet aggregation and clot formation. Smokers should be encouraged to quit because nicotine causes vasoconstriction, thereby slowing blood flow through the periphery.

There is some controversy about the effectiveness of serial leg measurements in monitoring for DVT. If leg measurements are used, a standard measurement protocol should be established and followed by all staff. For example, use a special measuring tape rather than a sewing tape, mark the area where the tape is placed, and use running averages.[4]

Paralytic Ileus and Stress Ulcers

Early medical management for paralytic ileus and stress ulcers includes NPO status, particularly for cervical spinal cord–injured patients. Nasogastric tube placement with intermittent suction is used to treat the paralytic ileus that frequently accompanies spinal cord injury. Nasogastric tube placement is also used to decrease the risk of aspiration and decrease abdominal distension. Peristalsis should be stimulated as soon as bowel sounds are present. This may be done safely with stool softeners, mild laxatives, or suppositories. Enemas, other than the oil-retention type, should be avoided because the risk of intestinal perforation is high.

Patients with cervical injuries are more likely to experience gastrointestinal bleeding as a result of stress ulcers. Medical treatment includes histamine type 2 receptor (H_2) blockers, proton pump inhibitors, antacids, or a combination of the three.

Heterotropic Ossification

Calcification around a joint, especially the hip joint, may occur within 12 weeks of injury. Clinical manifestations include limited range of motion, swelling of the affected joint, and an elevated alkaline phosphatase (AP) level. Pain may or may not be present. The goal of treatment is to prevent further damage and progression. Additional treatment includes irradiation, nonsteroidal anti-inflammatory drugs (NSAIDs), and disodium etidronate.

Spasticity

Spasticity develops after recovery from the period of spinal shock and affects the flexor muscles of the arms and the extensor muscles of the legs. An interdisciplinary approach is the hallmark of treatment. Physical therapy is consulted to develop an exercise, stretching, and positioning program for the patient. A variety of medications may be used such as baclofen, dantrolene sodium, diazepam, and clonidine.

PATIENT TEACHING AND DISCHARGE PLANNING

Usually, the patient is discharged to a rehabilitation setting to learn the skills needed for activities of daily living and, when possible, independent living. The nurse assists the family to find a rehabilitation program specific for patients with spinal cord injury. When searching for an appropriate rehabilitation program, the family should obtain answers to the following questions[6]:

- How many patients with spinal cord injury are treated in the program each year?
- What is the average age of the patients in the program?
- Will the treatment plan identify both long-term and short-term goals?
- Will the patient be assigned an experienced case manager to coordinate the transition between the rehabilitation center and home?
- How much time is spent teaching the patient and family about sexuality, bowel and bladder care, and other activities of daily living?

The family should also ask if the staff has specialized training in spinal cord injury. Rehabilitation therapies should be available a minimum of 3 hours per day. There should be activities or programs for the patients on weekends and in the evenings. Most important, the facility should have 24-hour staffing with registered nurses and respiratory therapists. Box 37-12 contains a discharge planning guide for a person with a spinal cord injury. Box 37-13 provides a patient teaching guide for patients living with a spinal cord injury.

case study ■ SPINAL CORD INJURY

John Smith, a 20-year-old college student, was injured in a motor vehicle accident. Paramedics arrived at the scene of the accident within 10 minutes. The patient was unable to move any extremities and complained of neck pain rated at a 6 of 10 on the pain scale. The patient was awake, alert, and oriented to his current location, the date and day of the week, and details of the accident. His pupils were equal and reactive to light. He showed no other signs of injury except for a cut on his forehead. Vital signs were blood pressure 110/72 mm Hg; pulse rate 86 beats/minute; respirations 18 breaths/minute, unlabored and regular. The paramedics applied a cervical collar, placed the patient on a backboard, and transported him to the medical center by helicopter. He arrived in the emergency department within 45 minutes of his accident.

On initial examination, the patient's vital signs were blood pressure 100/60 mm Hg; pulse rate 68 beats/minute; respirations 24 breaths/minute and somewhat shallow; temperature 99.8°F (37.7°C). The patient's color was dusky, and his skin was warm and dry. His arm veins were quite distended. He had no motor function or sensation below the mid-axillary level. He could tighten his biceps but could not overcome gravity to raise his arms. Deep tendon reflexes were absent. He was given intravenous methylprednisolone to improve motor and sensory function. He was noted to be in spinal shock.

Full spine, skull, and chest radiographs were done. Intravenous lactated Ringer's solution was started, and a Foley catheter was inserted into the patient's bladder. A nasogastric tube was inserted and connected to low intermittent suction. The radiographs revealed that the patient had a dislocated fracture of C5 and C6. The chest film showed a lack of full lung field expansion. Blood work results were normal with the exception of arterial blood gases, which showed respiratory acidosis (pH 7.30).

The patient was admitted to the critical care unit and placed in a halo fixation device to realign the cervical vertebrae and stabilize the fracture. Spinal shock treatment included careful intravenous fluid replacement to avoid overhydration, the use of dopamine or a similar drug when hypotension compromised adequate perfusion of vital organs, and atropine to correct bradycardia if the patient became symptomatic.

Nursing interventions included monitoring neurological signs and vital signs every hour for the first 24 hours, then every 2 hours until stabilized. Particular attention was paid to the patient's respiratory status. He was at risk for respiratory failure due to spinal cord edema. He was turned every 2 hours. The output of his Foley catheter and nasogastric tube were measured and recorded every 4 hours. Every effort was made to prevent complications of immobility, both in the critical care and acute care units. Physical and occupation therapy were consulted and an initial treatment plan initiated. Once past the acute phase of his injury, the patient was transferred to a rehabilitation facility for further recovery and adaptation to his injury. ■

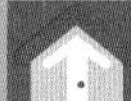

box 37-12 *Spinal Cord Injury*

- Arrange for representatives from physical and occupational therapy to evaluate the patient's home for the following:
  - Wheelchair accessibility
  - Clearance for maneuvering a wheelchair within the home
  - Necessary adaptations to the bedroom, bathroom, and kitchen
  - Smoke and fire alarms
- Obtain needed equipment for home care, depending on patient's level of injury. Be sure the equipment is delivered before the patient leaves the rehabilitation facility. Also be sure that the patient and his or her family members know how to operate the equipment.
- Make arrangements for home health care, physical therapy, occupational therapy, and job training or vocational rehabilitation, as necessary.
- Notify the electric company if there will be life-saving equipment in the home, such as a respirator.
- Carry out patient and family education (see Box 37-13).
- Locate community support groups.

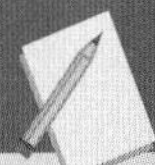

box 37-13
Living With a Spinal Cord Injury

Nutritional Management

- Eat a well-balanced diet that includes protein (lean meat, dairy foods, legumes), fresh fruits, vegetables, and liquids.
- Maintain ideal body weight.

Skin Management

- You and your helper should check your skin twice a day. Look for redness, bruises or scrapes, blisters, and rashes. Pay particular attention to bony areas. Check your groin for rashes and reddened areas.
- Keep your skin clean and dry, especially in areas where skin touches skin (e.g., between the toes, underneath the breasts). Do not use antimicrobial or harsh soaps. Apply moisturizing lotion. Avoid lotions or creams that dry the skin.
- Check your feet whenever you wear new shoes. Check for ingrown toenails. Keep your nails trimmed and filed smooth, and have calluses treated by a podiatrist.
- Use the wheelchair and cushion prescribed by your physical therapist.
- Change positions frequently to relieve pressure on bony areas.
- Be sure you are not sitting or lying on anything. Avoid putting objects in your pockets.
- Check to be sure braces, leg bags, and other adaptive equipment is not too tight.
- When in bed, use padding over bony areas. Use a firm mattress. If possible, sleep on your stomach.
- Notify your health care provider of any skin breakdown.

Urinary Tract Management

- Follow the bladder program developed by the rehabilitation team.
- Drink plenty of fluids unless contraindicated.
- If you have a Foley catheter, keep it free of kinks and change it as directed by your health care provider.
- Watch for signs and symptoms of urinary tract infection (e.g., cloudy urine with a foul odor, sediment in the urine).

Bowel Management

- Follow the bowel program developed by your rehabilitation team. Avoid the regular use of laxatives. Schedule sufficient time to complete the required activities. Notify your health care provider if you have not had a bowel movement in 3 or 4 days.
- Drink plenty of fluids, unless contraindicated.
- Monitor your diet to see what foods cause constipation and diarrhea.
- Prevent constipation through diet and fluid intake and medications as needed.
- Avoid foods that cause gas, such as beans, corn, and apples.
- Be aware of the potential for the development of autonomic dysreflexia during your bowel program.

Respiratory Management

- Cough and deep breathe routinely.
- Drink plenty of fluids, unless contraindicated.
- Use postural drainage or chest physiotherapy.
- Because you are at risk for pneumonia, be careful around anyone with a cold and get an annual influenza vaccination.

Complications

Autonomic Dysreflexia

- This complication occurs in patients with injury at T5 or above.
- The most common cause is overfilling of the bladder. Other causes include constipation or gas, skin irritations, pressure sores, wounds, and ingrown toenails.
- Autonomic dysreflexia it can be a life-threatening emergency. You or a helper must take immediate action to correct this problem.
- Signs and symptoms include a severe headache, nasal congestion, goose pimples, and restlessness.
- Be sure your head is up. If you are sitting in a chair, stay there; if you are in bed, get your head elevated.
- If you have an indwelling catheter:
  Check for kinks along the tubing.
  Empty the Foley bag; if there is no drainage, the Foley may be obstructed—change the Foley.
  Check the catheter and drainage bag for deposits.
  Check urine for color.
- If you are on intermittent catheterization, catheterize yourself.
- If the problem is related to the bowel, perform a digital stimulation and empty the bowel.
- If it is not related to a bladder or bowel problem, check for a pressure sore, ingrown toenail, or possible bone fracture.
- If none of the above actions relieve the signs and symptoms, get emergency medical treatment.

Deep Venous Thrombosis (DVT)

- Prevention is important.
- Signs and symptoms include leg swelling, chest pain, and cough.
- Call your health care provider immediately if signs or symptoms develop.

Hypothermia and Hyperthermia

- To prevent hyperthermia:
  Drink lots of fluids.
  Dress according to the temperature you will be in.
  Watch for signs and symptoms of hyperthermia.
  Use sun block.
- To prevent hypothermia:
  Dress appropriately for the weather.
  Watch for signs and symptoms of hypothermia and frostbite.

Heterotopic Ossification

- Check for development of abnormal bone in soft tissue, usually around the hip or knee.
- Signs and symptoms include a change in range of motion, decreased ability to perform activities of daily living, swelling, warmth, redness over the hip or knee, spasticity, and fever.

(continued)

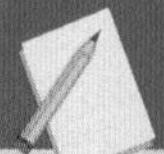

box 37-13
Living With a Spinal Cord Injury (Continued)

- Notify your health care provider immediately if any of these signs or symptoms develop.

Medication-Related Complications
- Select a pharmacy that will keep your medication profile on record, including any allergies you may have.
- Be sure the pharmacy has a system to check for and identify drug and food interactions.
- Have all of your prescriptions filled at the same pharmacy.
- Follow the directions on the label.
- Take all the medication that is ordered.
- Keep a current list of all medication.
- Know the important side effects of the medication; if any occur, notify your health care provider.

Pain
- Prevention of other problems such as pressure ulcers, stress ulcers, and infections is important.
- Maintain your activity program, range-of-motion exercises, and a healthy diet.
- Notify your health care provider of the type of pain you are experiencing.
- Medications and stress reduction techniques may be used.

Orthostatic Hypotension
- Know that this is a drop in blood pressure when you first sit up.
- Wear elastic hose or an abdominal support.
- Sit up slowly.
- If you experience orthostatic hypotension while you are sitting up, ask someone to tilt your wheelchair back until your head is parallel to the floor.
- Be sure to drink plenty of fluids.

Spasticity
- Prevention is crucial. Watch for and immediately treat skin problems such as an ingrown toenail. Prevent pressure ulcers. Maintain your bowel and bladder program.
- Notify your health care provider if spasticity develops.

clinical applicability challenges

Self-Challenge: Critical Thinking

1. *John Smith, the patient discussed in the case study, is engaged to be married. What information does he need about sexuality? What factors must be included in a teaching plan for Mr. Smith and his fiancée?*
2. *Mr. Jones is a 42-year-old married father of two children. He fell off of a ladder 1 week ago and sustained a C8 fracture and spinal cord injury. He is tetraplegic. What are three priorities of care and what are the required nursing interventions?*
3. *Formulate a teaching plan that will discuss autonomic dysreflexia with a patient with a new C5 to C6 spinal cord injury. Include causes, prevention, and treatment.*

Study Questions

1. *The patient arrives in the emergency department with a suspected cervical spinal cord injury. Which of the following is an assessment priority?*
   a. *Abdominal assessment*
   b. *Cardiac assessment*
   c. *Neurological assessment*
   d. *Respiratory assessment*
2. *Which of the following assessment findings are indicative of spinal shock?*
   a. *Hypertension, headache, blurred vision*
   b. *Hypotension and bradycardia*
   c. *Pink, warm, dry skin and vasodilation*
   d. *Pale, cool, clammy skin and vasoconstriction*
3. *The patient arrives in the intensive care unit (ICU) with a continuous intravenous infusion of methylprednisolone at a rate of 5.4 mg/kg/hour. All of the following are potential adverse effects except*
   a. *euphoria.*
   b. *hyperglycemia.*
   c. *heart failure.*
   d. *osteoporosis.*
4. *A patient with a cervical cord injury has been placed in cervical traction. The nurse discovers that the weights are resting on the floor. What is the nurse's best action?*
   a. *Do nothing—this is an expected finding*
   b. *Notify the physician*
   c. *Reposition the patient in the bed until the weights are off the floor*
   d. *Release the traction*
5. *The patient has a stage I pressure ulcer on the left ankle. What is the nurse's best response?*
   a. *Assess the area for blanching*
   b. *Do nothing—it is an expected finding*
   c. *Begin wet to dry dressing every 4 hours*
   d. *Rub the area with skin lotion*
6. *All of the following are interventions for the patient with ineffective thermoregulation except*
   a. *Adjust room temperature.*
   b. *Cover the patient with a warm blanket.*
   c. *Cover the patient's head with a hat or scarf.*
   d. *Use a heating pad.*
7. *A patient who experienced a cervical spinal cord injury 1 month ago has developed spasticity that is becoming increasingly severe. The patient thinks this means that he will walk again. Which of the following is the best interpretation of the data?*
   a. *Spasticity is the return of spinal reflex activity; there is no voluntary control of motor activity.*
   b. *Spasticity is a sign of autonomic hyperreflexia and must be treated immediately.*
   c. *Spasticity is an indicator that voluntary reflex activity has returned.*
   d. *Spasticity is an indicator that the patient has an excellent chance of a full recovery.*

8. *The nurse is called to the room of a patient who is paraplegic as a result of a thoracic spinal cord injury. The nursing assistant reports the patient's blood pressure is 240/104 mm Hg. The patient is complaining of headache and nasal congestion. What is the nursing priority?*
   a. *Administer nifedipine, which is ordered prn.*
   b. *Notify the health care provider immediately.*
   c. *Palpate the abdomen for distension.*
   d. *Raise the head of the bed.*

REFERENCES

1. The National Spinal Cord Injury Statistical Center: SCI: Facts and figures at a glance. Available at: http://www.spinalcord.uab.edu/docs/factsfig.htm. Accessed 2001
2. Sands J: Spinal cord and peripheral nerve problems. In Phipps WJ, Monahan FD, Sands JK, et al (eds): Medical–Surgical Nursing: Health and Illness Perspectives. St. Louis, CV Mosby, 2002
3. Neurotrauma Law Nexus: Understanding spinal cord injury. Available at: http://www.neurolaw.com/spine.htlm. Accessed 2000
4. Hickey J (ed): The Clinical Practice of Neurological and Neurosurgical Nursing (5th Ed), pp 407–450. Philadelphia, Lippincott Williams & Wilkins, 2003
5. Hugenholtz H: Methylprednisolone for acute spinal cord injury: Not a standard of care. CMAJ 168:1145–1146, 2003
6. Jastremski C: Spinal cord injury. In Bucher L, Melander S (eds): Critical Care Nursing. Philadelphia, WB Saunders, 1999

OTHER SELECTED READING

Belaval E: Cervical spine fractures. Available at: www.emedicine.com. April 29, 2002. 3(4), 2002

Davis K Jr, Johannigman JA, Campbell RS, et al: Crit Care 5(2):81–87, 2001

Guin PR: Advances in spinal cord injury care. Crit Care Nurs Clin North Am 13(3):399–409, 2001

Karlet MC: Acute management of the patient with a spinal cord injury. Int J Trauma Nurs (2):43–4, 2001

Levy D: Neck trauma. Available at: www.emedicine.com. June 21, 2002 2(6)

Lohne V: Hope in patients with spinal cord injury: A literature review related to nursing. J Neurosci Nurs (6):317–325, 2001

McEllvoy L, Meyer K, Vitaz T: Use of an acute spinal cord injury clinical pathway. Crit Care Nurs Clin North Am 12(4):521–530, 2000

Munro N: Pulmonary challenges in neurotrauma. Crit Care Nurs Clin North Am 12(4):457–464, 2000

McBride KE, Rines B: Sexuality and spinal cord injury: a road map for nurses. Spinal Cord Inj Nurs 17(1):8–13, 2000

McDonald JW, Sadowsky C: Spinal cord injury. Lancet 359:417, 2002

National Institute of Neurologic Disorders and Stroke: New strategies in spinal cord injury. Spinal Cord Injury: Emerging Concepts. NINDS Workshop on New Strategies in Spinal Cord Injury. Available at: www.ninds.nih.gov/health_and_medical/pubs/sci_report

National Institute of Neurologic Disorders and Stroke: Roles of the immune system in spinal cord injury. Notes from Spinal Cord Injury: Emerging Concepts. NINDS Workshop on New Strategies in Spinal Cord Injury. Available at: www.ninds.nih.gov/news

Prendergast V, Sullivan C: Acute spinal cord injury: Nursing considerations for the first 72 hours. Crit Care Nurs Clin North Am 14(4):499–508, 2002

Sphritz DW: Interventions for clients with problems of the central nervous system. In Ignatavicius D, Workman L (eds): Medical Surgical Nursing: Critical Thinking for Collaborative Care (4th Ed). Philadelphia, WB Saunders, 2002

Stinson-Kidd P: Spinal cord injury. In Kidd PS, Wagner KD (eds): High Acuity Nursing (3rd Ed). Englewood Cliffs, NJ, Prentice Hall, 2002

Villanueva NE: Spinal cord injury in the elderly. Crit Care Nurs Clin North Am 12(4):509–519, 2000

PART
one
two
three
four
five
six
seven
eight
nine
ten
eleven
twelve

Gastrointestinal System

INTERNET RESOURCES

Topic	Web Page Address
American College of Gastroenterology	www.acg.gi.org
American Gastroenterological Association	www.gastro.org
American Diabetes Association	www.diabetes.org
American Liver Foundation	www.liverfoundation.org
American Society of Gastrointestinal Endoscopy	www.asge.org
American Society for Clinical Nutrition	www.ascn.org
American Society for Parenteral and Enteral Nutrition	www.clinnutr.org
Canadian Enteral-Parenteral Nutrition Association	www.cpena.ca
The Centers for Disease Control and Prevention	www.cdc.gov
Center for Science in the Public Interest	www.cspinet.org
Children's Liver Disease Foundation	www.childliverdisease.org
The Combined Health Information Database	www.chid.nih.gov
The Digestive Disorders Foundation	www.digestivedisorders.org.uk
Electronic Enteral and Parenteral Nutrition	http://epen.kumc.edu
Hepatitis Foundation International	www.hepfi.org
The Hepatitis Information Network	www.hepnet.com
The Hepatitis Network	www.hepatitisnetwork.com
Medline Plus Website	www.nlm.nih.gov/medlineplus
The National Pancreas Foundation	www.pancreasfoundation.org
National Institute of Diabetes, Digestive and Kidney Diseases	www.niddk.nih.gov
The Nutrition Source	www.hsph.harvard.edu/nutritionsource
Pancreatitis Information	www.pancreatitis.org.uk
Society of Gastroenterology Nurses and Associates	www.sgna.org
Texas Virtual Clinic	http://utsurg.uth.tmc.edu/digestive
Virtual Hospital	www.vh.org

chapter

38

Anatomy and Physiology of the Gastrointestinal System

ALLISON G. STEELE ■ VALERIE K. SABOL

objectives

Based on the content in this chapter, the reader should be able to:

- Describe the functions of the major structures of the gastrointestinal system.
- Examine the processes of ingestion, digestion, absorption, and elimination.
- Explain digestion and absorption of carbohydrates, proteins, fats, vitamins, and minerals.
- Compare and contrast the processes involved in emesis and defecation.
- Describe bile production, secretion, and excretion.

The gastrointestinal system consists of the gastrointestinal tract and the accessory glandular organs that produce secretions. The major structures of the gastrointestinal tract are the mouth, pharynx, esophagus, stomach, small intestine (duodenum, jejunum, ileum), and large intestine (colon, rectum, anus). The accessory glandular organs include the salivary glands, liver, gallbladder, and pancreas.

The primary physiological functions of the gastrointestinal system are to provide nutrients for cell maintenance and growth and to eliminate waste. These functions are accomplished through the processes of ingestion (taking in food), motility (mixing and propelling food through the gastrointestinal tract), digestion (breaking down food), and absorption (movement of food particles into the bloodstream). Elimination is the process by which waste is eliminated from the body.

Gastrointestinal function is regulated and coordinated by the autonomic nervous system and a variety of peptides, which are further classified as endocrines (hormones), paracrines, and neurocrines. Endocrines are released in the general circulation and reach all tissues. Endocrine cells release paracrines, which target specific tissues. Neurocrines, or neurotransmitters, diffuse across a synaptic gap and can therefore stimulate or inhibit the release of endocrines and paracrines.

STRUCTURE OF THE GASTROINTESTINAL SYSTEM

Macroscopic Anatomy of the Gastrointestinal System

The gastrointestinal system is composed of the gastrointestinal tract, a hollow tube about 8 m (25 ft) long that begins at the mouth and ends at the anus (Fig. 38-1). The accessory glands (e.g., salivary glands) and organs (e.g., liver and pancreas) release products into the gastrointestinal tract.

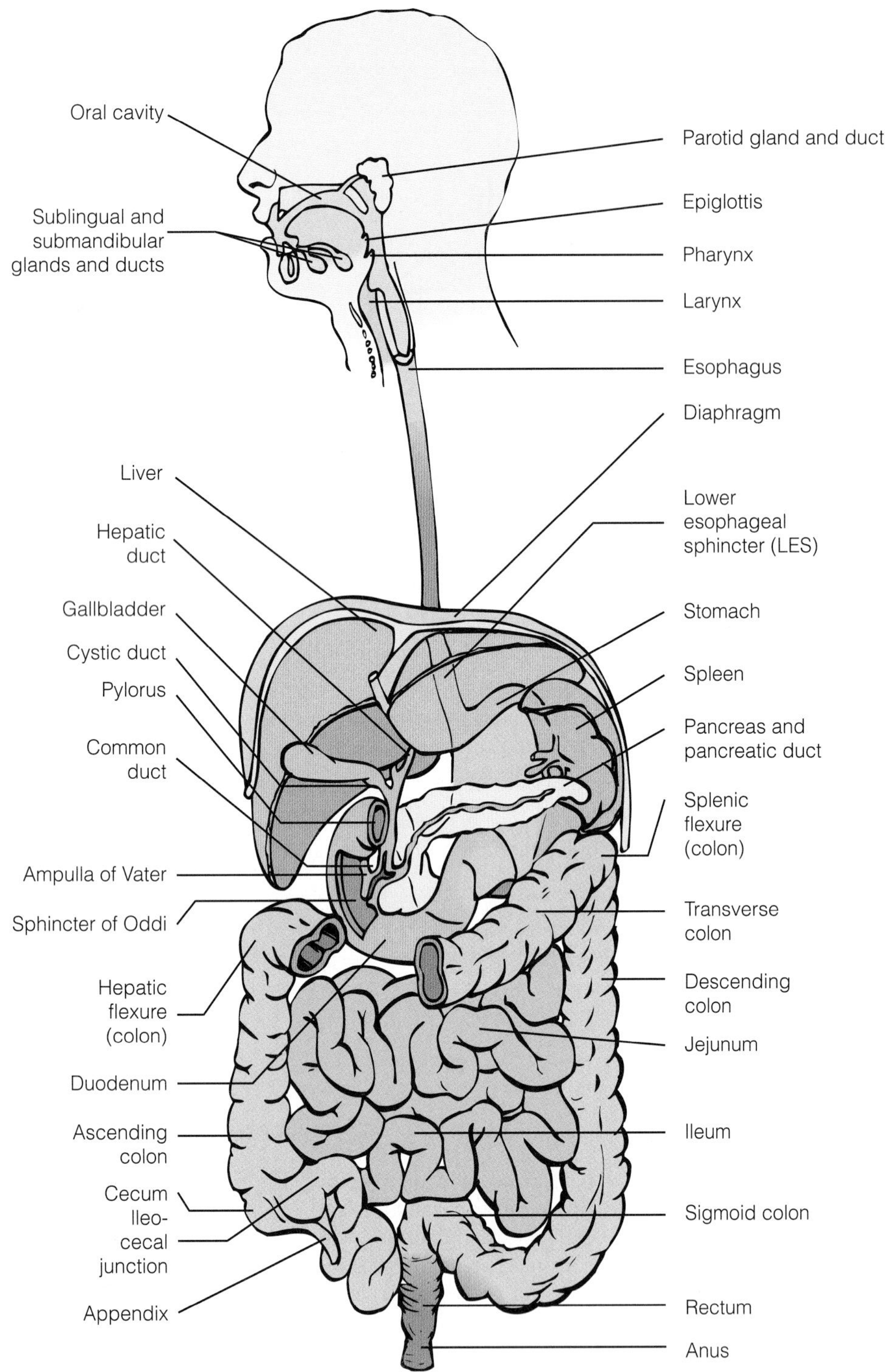

figure 38-1 The gastrointestinal tract.

The oral cavity opens into the pharynx, a structure that allows the passage of nutrients and air. The anterior pharynx, divided into the oropharynx and nasopharynx, connects the oral and nasal cavities. The posteroinferior end of the pharynx (at about the level of the sixth cervical vertebra) connects to the esophagus and larynx. The epiglottis, a thin cartilaginous flap covered by soft tissue, reflexively covers the larynx during swallowing and prevents the passage of food and water into the trachea.

The esophagus, a 25-cm (10-in) collapsible tube, connects the pharynx to the stomach at the cardiac orifice (Fig. 38-2). The esophagus is posterior to the trachea, in the posterior mediastinum, and crosses the diaphragm. Its main function is to deliver food to the stomach. Two muscular rings, the upper and lower esophageal sphincters, border the esophagus. The upper esophageal sphincter prevents aspiration and swallowing of excessive air. The lower esophageal sphincter (LES), a muscular ring at the

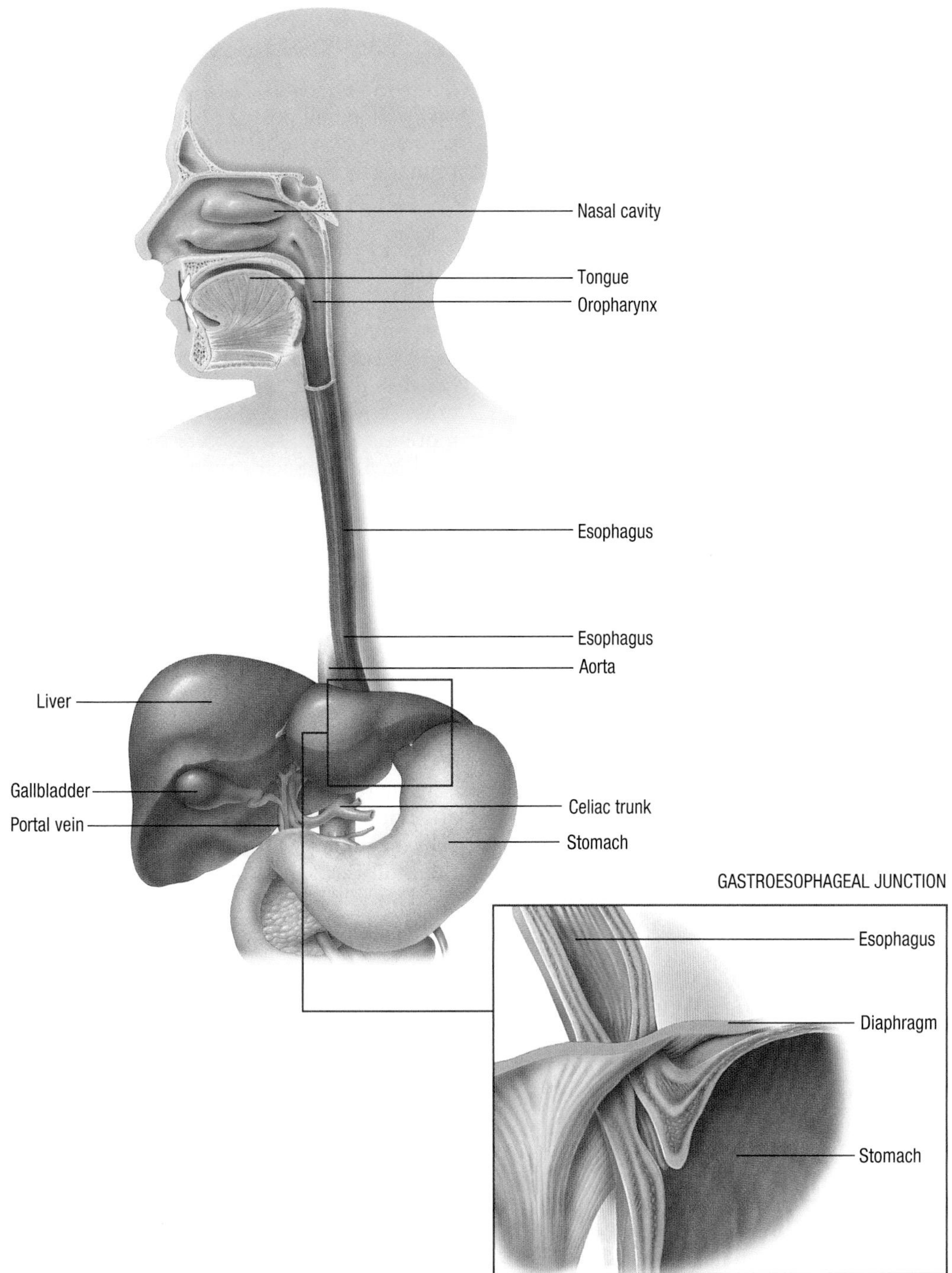

figure 38-2 Gastroesophageal junction. (Source: Anatomical Chart Company: Atlas of Human Anatomy, p 203. Springhouse, PA, Springhouse, 2001.)

gastroesophageal junction, prevents reflux of gastric contents into the esophagus.

The stomach is a flask-shaped organ that lies in the upper abdomen below the diaphragm (Fig. 38-3). The stomach serves several functions: it acts as a reservoir for chewed food, mixes ingested food with gastric secretions to form a semisolid liquid called *chyme*, and regulates the release of chyme into the duodenum at a controlled rate. The esophagus joins the stomach at the cardia of the stomach. The cells of the cardia secrete mucus that helps to protect the esophagus from the acidic secretions of the stomach. The dome-shaped fundus, located to the left of the cardia, acts as a reservoir. The body and the fundus have coarse folds called *rugae*. Gastric pits, which contain the acid-secreting cells of the stomach, are located mainly in the body of the stomach. The antrum, the most distal area of the stomach, is the site of G cells, which secrete gastrin. The antrum narrows into the pyloric channel, or pylorus,

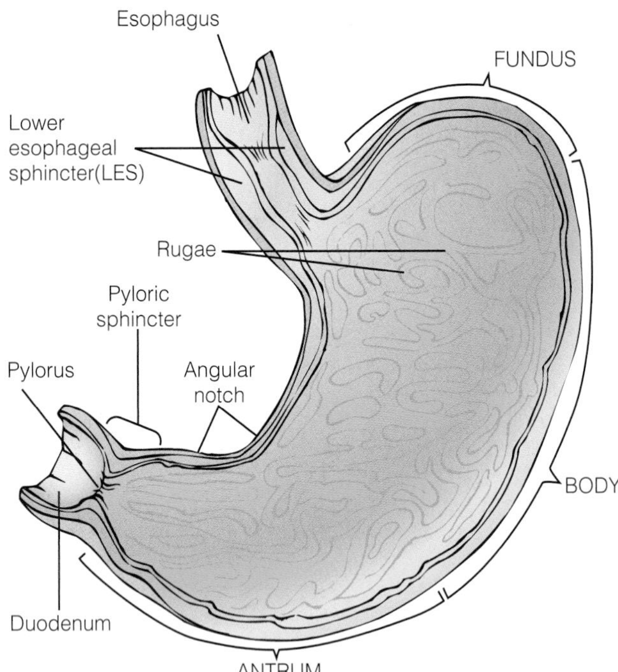

figure 38-3 Anatomy of the stomach.

ending in the gastroduodenal junction at the pyloric sphincter. The pyloric sphincter, a muscular structure between the stomach and the duodenum, minimizes intestinal reflux.

Most digestion and absorption take place in the small intestine. The duodenum, the first 25 to 30 cm (10 to 12 in) of the small intestine, begins at the pylorus. The common bile duct opens into the duodenum at the duodenal papilla through the ampulla of Vater. The next 2.6 m (8.5 ft) of the small intestine is the jejunum. The ileum, the last 1.1 m (3.6 ft) of the small intestine, connects to the colon (cecum) at the ileocecal valve, which prevents reflux of colonic contents into the ileum.

The colon is traditionally divided into six sections. The cecum is the most proximal section and is the location of the ileocecal valve. The vermiform appendix, a blind-ended 2.5- to 20-cm (1- to 8-in) tube, protrudes posteriorly from the cecum. The ascending colon extends superiorly from the cecum to the hepatic flexure. The transverse colon lies between the hepatic and splenic flexures. The descending colon extends from the splenic flexure to the level of the iliac crest. At the iliac crest, the colon becomes the sigmoid colon. The sigmoid colon continues downward to the pelvic floor as the rectum. The last 2.5 cm (1 in) or so of the rectum, the anal canal, passes between the levator ani muscles of the pelvic floor and opens to the exterior body surface as the anal orifice. Two sphincters, which work to provide fecal continence, guard this orifice: an internal sphincter composed of smooth muscle and an external sphincter composed of skeletal muscle. The colon, although not necessary for life, is responsible for the reabsorption of electrolytes and fluid, thus allowing the body to maintain fluid and electrolyte balance with less fluid intake.

Microscopic Anatomy of the Gastrointestinal System

The structure of the gastrointestinal tract varies depending on location, but possesses common features. The lumen, a central hollow tube through which food passes, is surrounded by four layers of tissue. From the lumen outward, these layers are the mucosa, submucosa, muscularis propria, and serosa (Fig. 38-4).

MUCOSA

The mucosa is composed of three layers: the epithelium, the lamina propria, and the muscularis mucosae. A single layer of epithelial cells lines the mucosa. The tight junctions between the epithelial cells act as a barrier to bacteria and other large molecules. In the small intestine this layer is more convoluted and possesses finger-like projections (villi; see Fig. 38-4). Such structural modifications dramatically increase the surface area of the small intestine, thereby facilitating absorption. The lamina propria, a layer of connective tissue, contains capillaries and lymph vessels. The muscularis mucosae, the innermost layer, is composed of two layers of smooth muscle. The mucosa contains cells that produce gastrointestinal secretions and cells that are sensitive to chemical and mechanical stimuli.

SUBMUCOSA

The submucosa contains blood vessels, nerve networks, and connective tissue. The submucosa of the small intestine contains aggregates of lymphatic tissue (Peyer's patches), which are especially numerous in the ileum. Specialized mucosal cells that lie superiorly to the patches of lymphatic tissue in the small intestine absorb viral and bacterial antigens. These specialized cells sensitize the lymphatic cells to antigens and manufacture and secrete antibodies of immunoglobulin class A (IgA). The antibodies protect the body from the antigen the next time (or times) it enters the small intestine.

MUSCULARIS PROPRIA

The muscularis propria consists of two layers of smooth muscle, an inner circular muscle layer and an outer longitudinal layer. The two smooth muscle layers function in the two major types of gastrointestinal motility: propulsive motion and mixing movements. The stomach has an additional layer of smooth muscle to facilitate its food-mixing movements.

SEROSA

The serosa, or adventitia, is the outermost layer of the gastrointestinal tract. The serosa is continuous with the mesentery and forms part of the visceral peritoneum.

Innervation

The gastrointestinal tract is innervated by the autonomic nervous system (ANS). The ANS can be divided into the extrinsic nervous system and the intrinsic (enteric) nervous system.

EXTRINSIC NERVOUS SYSTEM

The extrinsic nervous system is further divided into parasympathetic and sympathetic branches (Fig. 38-5). Supplied primarily by the vagus and pelvic nerves, para-

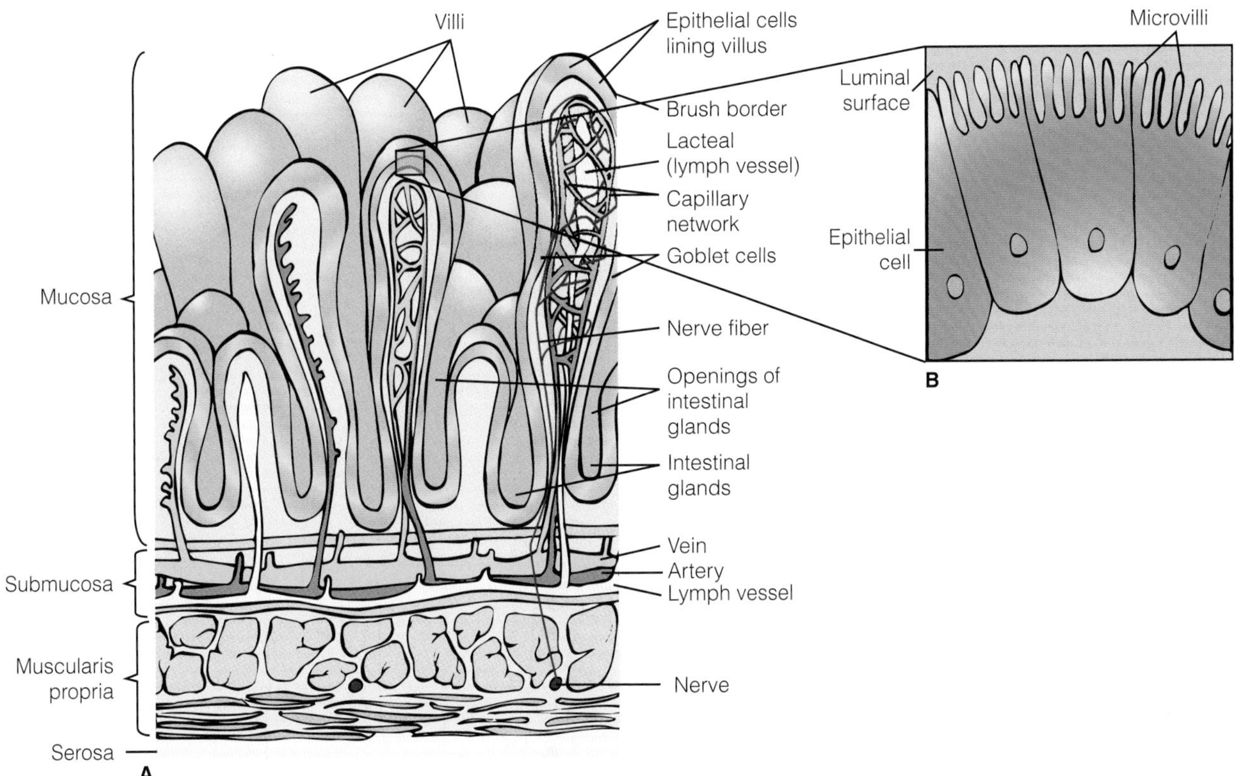

figure 38-4 (**A**) Layers of tissue in the gastrointestinal tract. (**B**) Microvilli on the luminal surface of intestinal epithelial cells.

sympathetic stimulation increases gastrointestinal activity through sensory and motor fibers to promote motility, relax sphincters, and promote secretion. Activation of the sympathetic nerves usually inhibits the motor and secretory activities of the gastrointestinal system.

Parasympathetic Branch

Parasympathetic efferents (motor) fibers of the gastrointestinal tract are preganglionic fibers carried primarily by the vagus and pelvic nerves. Vagal parasympathetic efferent preganglionic fibers richly innervate the gastrointestinal tract, including the esophagus, stomach, and small intestine. It is generally accepted that vagal efferents innervate the colon, but their distribution and function are controversial. Cell bodies for the vagal efferents are located primarily in the dorsal motor nucleus of the vagus. Vagal efferents synapse onto neurons in the myenteric plexus, or Auerbach plexus, which lies between the circular and longitudinal layers of smooth muscle cells in the muscularis propria. Postganglionic fibers then synapse with secretory and smooth muscle cells.

Vagal afferent (sensory) fibers originate in the esophagus, stomach, small intestine, and possibly the large intestine. The cell bodies are located in the nodose ganglion (in the neck) and join the vagus high in the neck. Afferent fibers relay information about pain and distension to the brain and spinal cord.

The pelvic nerve, issuing from spinal routes S2 to S4, carries parasympathetic afferent and efferent fibers to innervate the rectum and descending colon. For sacral efferents, the cell bodies are located in the spinal cord. Afferent cell bodies are in the corresponding dorsal root ganglia.

Sympathetic Branch

Sympathetic efferent fibers exit the spinal cord and synapse on ganglia near the spinal cord. Then, long postganglionic fibers travel to the gut and synapse on blood vessels, myenteric plexus ganglia, and secretory cells. The esophagus receives rich sympathetic innervation, but the origin and course of the fibers are not clear. Interestingly, although the muscle of the upper esophagus is primarily striated (e.g., skeletal voluntary muscle), the area receives dense sympathetic innervation. Stress-related impaired swallowing may be elicited by these fibers. Sympathetic fibers to the stomach and duodenum exit T6 to T9, synapse in the celiac ganglion, then travel along the celiac artery. Sympathetic fibers exiting at T9 and T10 synapse in the superior mesenteric ganglion and then travel with the celiac artery to the large and small intestine. Fibers terminate on enteric neurons and blood vessels; a few fibers innervate the muscle layers.

INTRINSIC (ENTERIC) NERVOUS SYSTEM

The intrinsic (enteric) nervous system coordinates gastrointestinal motility and secretion. The intrinsic (enteric) nervous system is grouped into several nerve plexuses, with the myenteric and submucosal plexuses being the most prominent. The nerves in these plexuses receive input from receptors in the gastrointestinal tract and from the extrinsic nervous system. When integrated into the

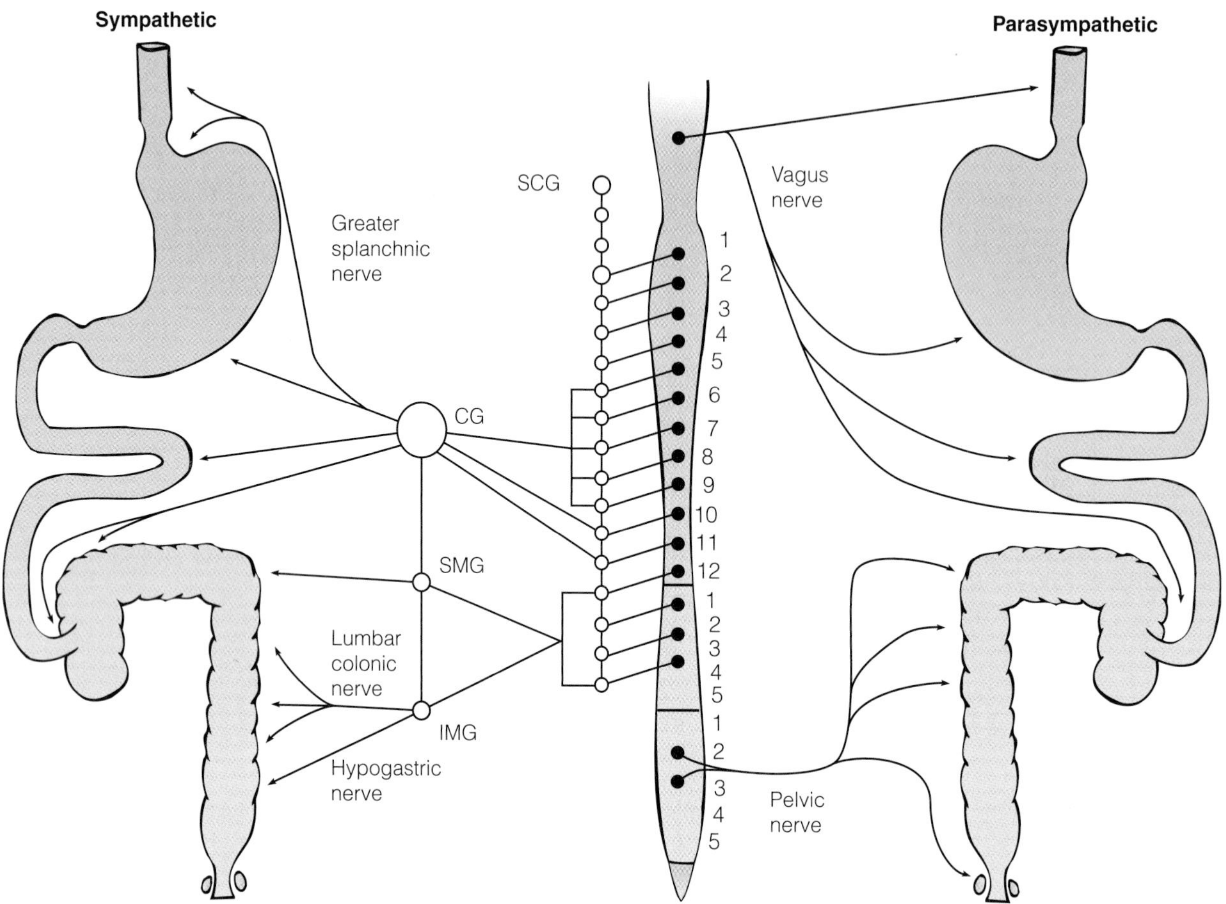

figure 38-5 Extrinsic efferent innervation of the gastrointestinal tract. SCG, superior cervical ganglion; CG, celiac ganglion; SMG, superior mesenteric ganglion; IMG, inferior mesenteric ganglion. (Redrawn with permission from Johnson LR [ed]: Physiology of the Gastrointestinal Tract, p 508. New York, Raven Press, 1987)

intrinsic system, this input helps coordinate function. Peripheral fibers innervate the voluntary muscles responsible for chewing, swallowing, and defecating.

The intrinsic (enteric) nervous system is a complex network embedded in the wall of the gastrointestinal tract from the pharynx to the anus. It includes intrinsic neurons (enteric neurons) and the processes of afferent and efferent extrinsic neurons. There are two main ganglionic plexuses containing the cell bodies of enteric neurons: the myenteric plexus (between the longitudinal and circular muscle layers) and the submucosal plexus, or Meissner plexus (between the circular muscle and the mucosa). From these two ganglionic plexuses emerge smaller bundles of fibers forming nonganglionic plexuses in longitudinal and circular muscle, around blood vessels, in the muscularis mucosae, at the base of mucosal glands, and within the villi.

Enteric neuronal neurotransmitters include acetylcholine, norepinephrine, serotonin, and dopamine. Neuropeptides form the largest group of potential enteric neurotransmitters. These include substance P, vasoactive intestinal polypeptide (VIP), gastric inhibitory peptide (GIP), and opioid peptides. There is evidence that this group of substances participates in the control of all gastrointestinal functions (secretion, motility, and absorption). How actions of these substances integrate with those of more classic neurotransmitters is an important aspect of current investigative work.

Circulation

Blood supply to the gastrointestinal tract and spleen is called the *splanchnic circulation.* The esophageal artery branches from the thoracic aorta and perfuses the esophagus. Three branches of the abdominal aortic artery perfuse the gastrointestinal organs:

- The celiac axis (consisting of the left gastric artery, the common hepatic artery, and the splenic artery) perfuses the lower esophagus, stomach, duodenum, gallbladder, and liver.
- The superior mesenteric artery perfuses the small intestine to transverse colon.
- The inferior mesenteric artery perfuses the descending colon, sigmoid colon, and rectum.

The areas of perfusion overlap, providing some protection against ischemia.

Venous drainage of the stomach and small and large intestines is primarily through the portal vein to the liver. The blood supply from the lower rectum and the lower esophagus bypasses the portal system. Blood from the rectum drains into the inferior vena cava through the rectal veins, which empty into the external iliac vein. Blood from the esophagus drains through the hemiazygos and azygos veins into the inferior vena cava.

The blood supply of the liver is unique. The liver receives its blood supply from both venous and arterial sources. The venous blood is supplied by way of the portal vein, which drains most of the blood from the gastrointestinal tract (Fig. 38-6). The portal vein forms behind the spleen at the confluence of the superior mesenteric and splenic veins and leads to the liver. The arterial supply is by the common hepatic artery, which branches from the celiac trunk near the aorta and then perfuses the liver. Both sets of vessels form capillaries and then drain into the hepatic vein, which in turn feeds into the inferior vena cava.

The gastrointestinal system receives about one fourth of the resting cardiac output, more than any other organ system. When circulation is impaired (as in shock), perfusion to the splanchnic bed is shunted to the systemic circulation. Because splanchnic organs normally extract only about 20% of the oxygen from the perfusing blood, splanchnic perfusion can be reduced without compromising the organs. However, a severe reduction in splanchnic perfusion can damage the mucosal lining of the gut.

FUNCTION OF THE GASTROINTESTINAL SYSTEM

The main function of the gastrointestinal tract is to break down nutrients into a form of energy. Therefore, each section of the gastrointestinal tract is discussed in terms of the secretions and motility that make digestion possible.

Oropharynx

SECRETIONS

The salivary glands of the oropharynx produce saliva. There are three pairs of salivary glands: the submaxillary glands, the sublingual glands, and the parotid glands. Saliva is composed of mucus (a lubricant that facilitates swallowing), lingual lipase (a fat-digesting enzyme secreted by tongue glands), salivary amylase (an enzyme that breaks down starch), and class A (IgA) antibodies (which provide a first line of defense against bacteria, viruses and bacteriostatic and carcinogenic chemicals; Table 38-1). Lingual lipase is estimated to digest about 30% of the dietary fat in the stomach. The salivary glands secrete about one half of the digestive amylase used in digestion; the rest is secreted by the pancreas.

Saliva production is elicited by multiple stimuli, including the sight, smell, or thought of food, and by the pleasant taste or smooth texture of food in the mouth. Rough, bad-tasting, unpleasant-smelling foods reduce salivary gland secretions. Stimuli are received by the two salivary centers in the medulla of the brainstem, which then send impulses to the salivary glands through the seventh and ninth cranial nerves (parasympathetic fibers) and the first and second thoracic nerves (sympathetic

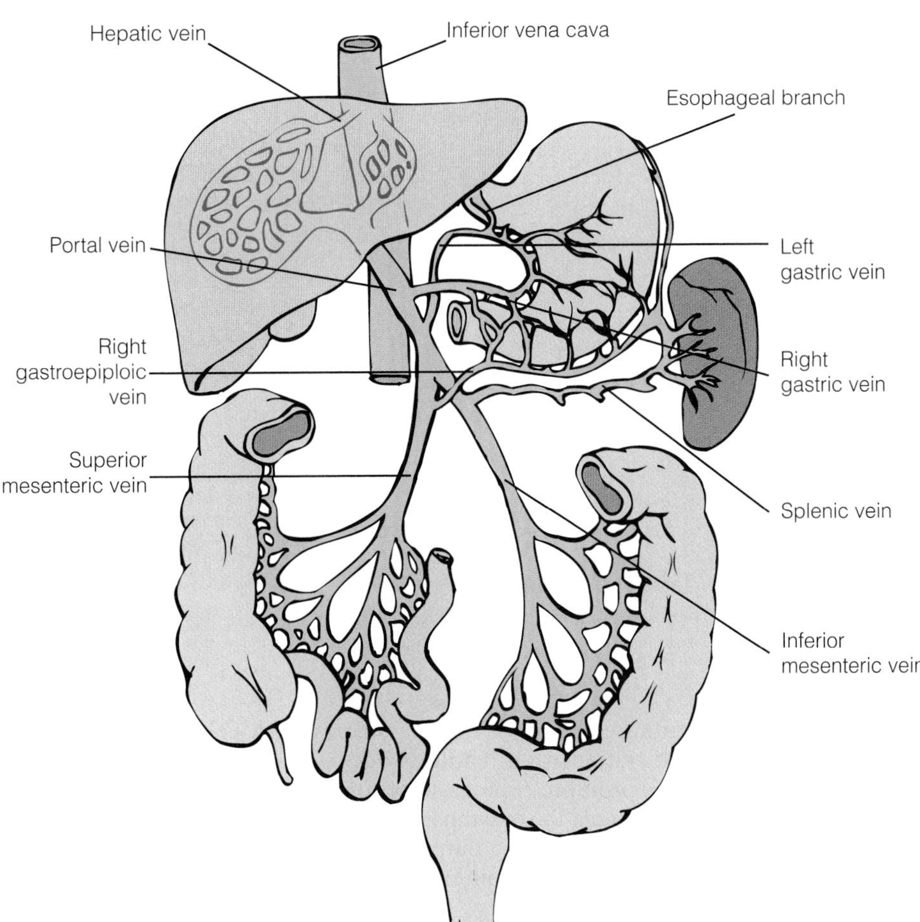

figure 38-6 Portal circulation. Blood from the gastrointestinal tract, spleen, and pancreas travels to the liver by way of the portal vein before moving into the inferior vena cava for return to the heart.

table 38-1 Major Gastrointestinal Secretions

Location	Daily Volume	Composition and (Action)
Mouth	1,000–2,000 mL	Amylase (carbohydrate digestion) Lipase (fat digestion) Immunoglobulins Mucus Water, electrolytes
Esophagus	300–800 mL	Mucus
Stomach	2,000 mL	Intrinsic factor (vitamin B_{12} absorption) Hydrochloric acid (activates pepsinogen) Pepsinogen (protein digestion) Mucus Water, electrolytes Gastrin (stimulates hydrochloric acid release; trophic effects on mucosa, especially in stomach)
Pancreas	1,200–1,800 mL	Enzymes • Amylase (carbohydrate digestion) • Trypsinogen (protein digestion) • Chymotrypsin (protein digestion) • Elastase (protein digestion) • Carboxypeptidase (protein digestion) • Lipase (fat digestion) • Colipase (fat digestion) • Esterase (cholesterol digestion) • Phospholipase (phospholipid digestion) • Nucleases (RNA and DNA digestion) Bicarbonate (protects lumenal wall by neutralizing acid) Water, electrolytes
Liver	500–1,000 mL	Bile salts (emulsifies fats) Bilirubin (excretory end-product of hemoglobin breakdown) Water, electrolytes
Small intestine	3,000–4,000 mL	Enzymes • Enterokinase (activates trypsinogen) • Lipase (fat digestion) • Enteropeptidase (protein digestion) • Peptidase (protein digestion) • Nucleases (RNA and DNA digestion) • Maltase (carbohydrate digestion) • Lactase (carbohydrate digestion) • Sucrase (carbohydrate digestion) Mucus Bicarbonate Water, electrolytes Cholecystokinin (CCK) into blood (stimulates pancreatic secretion and gallbladder contraction) Glucose-dependent insulinotropic peptide into blood (stimulates insulin release and gastric motility, secretion) Gastrin (stimulates gastric acid secretion)
Large intestine	Variable	Mucus

fibers). Parasympathetic stimulation, or the administration of drugs that mimic stimulation (cholinergics) or enhance it (neostigmine), promote copious secretion of watery saliva. Sympathetic stimulation or sympathomimetic drug administration produces a scanty output of thick saliva. Cholinergic blockers (e.g., atropine) also inhibit salivation.

MOTILITY

In the mouth, chewing mechanically breaks down food into smaller particles. This produces a bolus of food held together and lubricated by saliva that can then be propelled into the stomach by the process of swallowing. Swallowing is a complex process that has several phases (Fig. 38-7). During the oral phase, the tongue propels the food or fluid

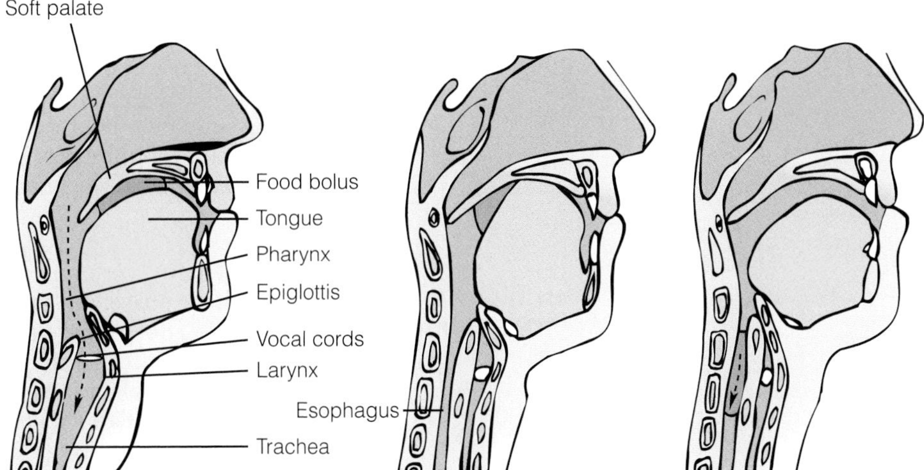

figure 38-7 Swallowing. Passage of bolus of food from the mouth through the pharynx. (From Rhoades RA, Pflanzer RG: Human Physiology [3rd Ed], p 675. Pacific Grove, CA, Brooks/Cole, 1996. Reprinted with permission of Brooks/Cole, a division of Thomson Learning)

bolus to the posterior pharynx. This is a voluntary process. During the involuntary pharyngeal phase, the presence of food or fluid in the pharynx stimulates pharyngeal sensory receptors that initiate impulses through cranial nerve V (the trigeminal nerve) to the swallowing center in the medulla. Sensory impulses reflexively trigger the outflow of impulses down motor fibers in cranial nerve IX (the glossopharyngeal nerve) and cranial nerve X (the vagus nerve) to pharyngeal and laryngeal structures. This causes the following coordinated events, which propel the solid or fluid substance into the esophagus:

1. The soft palate elevates and retracts, sealing off the nasopharynx to prevent regurgitation.
2. The vocal cords close and the epiglottis closes over the larynx to prevent aspiration.
3. The upper esophageal sphincter relaxes.
4. The larynx pulls up and increases the opening of the esophagus and upper esophageal sphincter.
5. The pharyngeal muscles contract, propelling food or fluid into the opened esophagus.

During this phase, respiration is reflexively inhibited. Damage to sensory or motor fibers (in cranial nerves V, IX, or X) or to the swallowing center in the brainstem weakens or eliminates the ability to swallow or causes poorly coordinated swallowing, wherein food or fluid enters the nasopharynx or larynx, or both.

Esophagus

SECRETIONS

Esophageal mucosal cells secrete mucus (see Table 38-1). The mucus protects the esophageal lining from damage by gastric secretions or food and acts as a lubricant to facilitate the passage of food.

MOTILITY

The esophageal phase of swallowing begins once food or fluid enters the esophagus (Fig. 38-8). Swallowing-induced contractions of the esophagus are called *primary peristalsis.* The wave of peristalsis causes the LES to relax, thereby allowing food to enter the stomach. If primary peristalsis is unable to clear the esophagus, food or fluid distends the esophagus. This distension stimulates stretch receptors that reflexively promote both relaxation of the esophageal muscles ahead of the area of distension, and contraction of the esophageal muscles in and behind it. This propels the food or fluid ahead into the newly relaxed area, which then becomes distended. This is called *secondary peristalsis.* The peristalsis reflex repeatedly recurs until the food or fluid arrives at the LES.

Tonus of the LES can be altered by a variety of agents (Table 38-2). Some people suffer from a hypertrophic

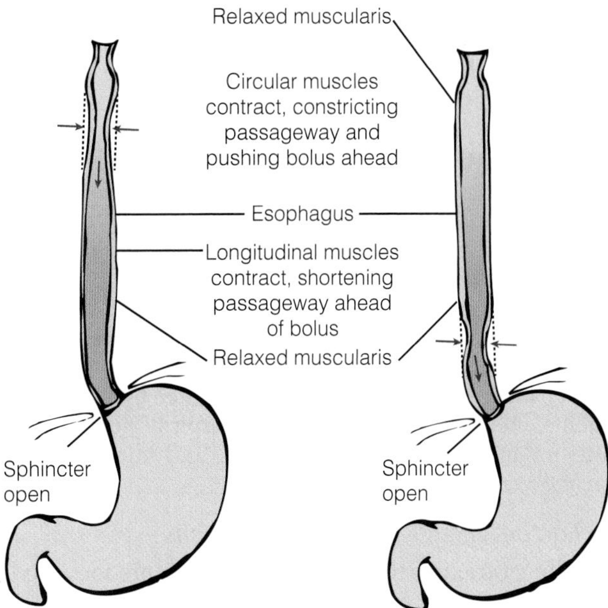

figure 38-8 Movement of a bolus of food through the esophagus by a peristaltic contraction. (From Rhoades RA, Pflanzer RG: Human Physiology [3rd Ed], p 675. Pacific Grove, CA, Brooks/Cole, 1996. Reprinted with permission of Brooks/Cole, a division of Thomson Learning)

table 38-2 Factors Influencing Lower Esophageal Sphincter (LES) Tone

Increased Tone	Decreased Tone
Food substances:	Food substances:
Protein	Fats
Drugs:	Coffee
Metoclopramide	Chocolate
Some prostaglandins (F_2)	Alcohol
	Cholecystokinin (CCK)
	Progesterone (as in pregnancy)
	Somatostatin
	Dopamine
	Some prostaglandins (E_2, A_2)
	Cigarette smoking

LES, which impedes esophageal emptying (and can lead to overdistension of the lower esophagus), whereas others have an incompetent LES, which results in repeated episodes of gastric reflux (which can lead to lower esophageal strictures).

Stomach

SECRETIONS

The major secretions of the stomach are hydrochloric acid, intrinsic factor, pepsinogen, gastrin, and mucus (see Table 38-1).

Parietal cells secrete hydrochloric acid and intrinsic factor. Intrinsic factor is necessary for the absorption of vitamin B_{12} in the small intestine. Hydrochloric acid converts pepsinogen, which is secreted by the chief cells of the stomach, to pepsin, a proteolytic enzyme. The hydrochloric acid provides an ideal pH for the activity of pepsin; together, hydrochloric acid and pepsin begin the digestion of protein. The chemical action of hydrochloric acid also breaks down food molecules, and helps to protect the gastrointestinal tract from bacterial invasion.

G cells, located in the gastric antrum, secrete the hormone gastrin, which promotes the secretion of the chief and parietal cells and promotes the growth of the gastric mucosa (Table 38-3).

Gastric mucosal cells continuously secrete a thin coat of mucus. Mucus, a lubricant, works together with bicarbonate to neutralize acid, protecting the stomach wall from damage. This barrier can be disrupted by a variety of agents, including bile salts, alcohol, aspirin, nonsteroidal anti-inflammatory drugs (NSAIDs), and infection with *Helicobacter pylori.*

Factors Affecting Gastric Secretions

The gastric parietal cells contain receptors for acetylcholine, histamine, and gastrin. Stimulation of these receptors prompts the parietal cells to secrete hydrochloric acid. Hydrochloric acid secretion is inhibited by chemicals that block the histamine receptors (e.g., H_2 receptor antagonists) or the acetylcholine receptors (e.g., atropine). Proton pump inhibitors inhibit the H^+/K^+-adenosine triphosphatase (ATPase) enzyme pathway, the final common step in the acid secretory pathway. Some prostaglandins also inhibit hydrochloric acid secretion.

Factors that stimulate gastric secretions include alcohol, caffeine, and hypoglycemia. The first two factors act directly by way of gastric chemoreceptors and the intramural nerve plexuses in the stomach wall. Hypoglycemia acts by way of the brainstem and vagal fibers.

Control of Gastric Secretions

Gastric secretions are regulated in three phases: the cephalic phase, the gastric phase, and the intestinal phase (Table 38-4). These phases are controlled by neural and hormonal mechanisms.

In the cephalic phase, the sight, smell, taste, or thought of food stimulates brainstem centers, reflexively prompting parasympathetic (vagal) stimulation of salivation, pancreatic secretion, bile release, and gastric secretions of pepsinogen and hydrochloric acid by the chief and parietal cells, respectively. Sympathetic stimulation can alter the cephalic phase response. This is the mechanism by which emotions can influence gastrointestinal secretions. Fear, anger, and depression decrease secretions.

During the gastric phase, distension of the stomach by food stimulates stretch receptors in the stomach wall. Chemicals, mainly proteins, stimulate chemoreceptors in the mucosa. The stretch receptors and chemoreceptors in turn activate neurons in the submucosal plexus, which then stimulate neurons in the myenteric plexus, which in turn stimulate secretion by the parietal and chief cells. Proteins in the chyme also directly promote gastrin secretion by G cells; the gastrin provides an additional stimulus for parietal and chief cell secretion. The gastric phase is eventually halted by a combination of events: the stretch receptors and chemoreceptors in the wall of the stomach become refractory to stimulation, the acidity of the chyme inhibits further gastrin secretion, and GIP decreases hydrochloric acid secretion and gastric motility.

The intestinal phase begins after chyme reaches the duodenum. The acidity of the chyme stimulates duodenal mucosal cells to release secretin into the bloodstream; proteins and fat trigger the release of cholecystokinin (CCK) into the blood from similar cells, and glucose and fat stimulate the secretion of GIP. Secretin and CCK cause pancreatic secretion and release of gallbladder contents into the duodenum. GIP stimulates the release of insulin from the islets of Langerhans and decreases gastric motility and secretions (see Table 38-3). Stretch receptors in the duodenum trigger peristalsis so that chyme is degraded, mixed with enzymes and diluents, and moved past the highly absorbent small intestinal lumen. If the chyme is less acidic, gastrin is released. Under neural control, motilin is another hormone that is cyclically released during fasting. Motilin stimulates stomach and small intestine motility.

MOTILITY

The passage of food from the esophagus into the stomach reflexively initiates receptive relaxation. After the stomach has filled with food, peristaltic contractions mix the food and propel gastric contents toward the pylorus, where small amounts enter the duodenum. The pyloric sphincter plays a minor role in gastric emptying; its main function is to prevent duodenal reflux. The bile acids in the chyme that re-

table 38-3 Hormones Controlling Secretion and Motility

Hormone	Source	Stimulation of Release	Major Function
Gastrin	Stomach, small intestine	Gastric distension, presence of partially digested protein near pylorus	Stimulates • Gastric acid secretion • Gastric intrinsic factor secretion • Gastric motility • Intestinal motility • Mucosal growth • Pancreatic growth • Pancreatic insulin release • Lower esophageal tone
Secretin	Small intestine	Acid entering small intestine	Stimulates • Pancreatic bicarbonate secretion • Pancreatic enzyme secretion • Pancreatic growth • Gastric pepsin secretion • Bile bicarbonate secretion • Gallbladder contraction Inhibits • Gastric emptying • Gastric motility • Intestinal motility
Cholecystokinin (CCK)	Small intestine	Fatty acid and amino acids in small intestine	Stimulates • Gastric acid secretion • Gastric motility • Intestinal motility • Colonic motility • Gallbladder contraction and sphincter of Oddi relaxation (thus increasing bile flow into small intestine) • Pancreatic bicarbonate secretion • Pancreatic enzyme release • Pancreatic growth Inhibits • Lower esophageal tone • Gastric emptying
Gastric inhibitory peptide (GIP)	Small intestine	Fatty acids and lipids in small intestine	Inhibits • Gastric acid secretion • Gastric emptying • Gastric motility Stimulates • Insulin release • Intestinal motility
Motilin	Small intestine	Acid and fat in small intestine	Stimulates • Gastric motility • Intestinal motility

enters the stomach through duodenal reflux damage the chemical barrier that coats the surfaces of gastric mucosal cells. Mild peristaltic contractions that persist after the stomach has completely emptied are called *hunger contractions;* however, they play no role in appetite regulation. Gastric emptying can be retarded by vagotomy; by the presence of fats, proteins, or hydrochloric acid in the duodenal chyme; by duodenal distension; and by intestinal hormones.

Emesis, or vomiting, is the regurgitation of food from the stomach through the mouth. During vomiting, the abdominal muscles and diaphragm contract, and the LES relaxes, allowing reflux of gastric content into esophagus and propulsion of gastric contents out of the mouth. The reflex elevation of the palate prevents expulsion through the nasopharynx. Respiratory inhibition and closure of the glottis prevent pulmonary aspiration. In addition, irritation of the small intestine (by materials in the chyme, by inflammation, or by a disease process) can cause reverse peristalsis. These movements move chyme toward the pyloric valve. If strong enough to force open the pylorus, intestinal contents may be vomited. When yellow bile from the duodenum is exposed to acid in the stomach, the interaction

table 38-4 Phases of Gastric Secretion

Phase	Stimulus to Secretion	Effect
Cephalic (neuronal)	Sight, smell, taste of food initiates central nervous system impulse mediated by vagus	Gastric effects: Hydrochloric acid (from parietal cells) Pepsinogen (from chief cells) Mucus secretion Other effects: Salivation Pancreatic secretion Bile release
Gastric (neuronal and hormonal)	Food in antrum initiates central nervous system impulse mediated by vagus	Gastrin release Hydrochloric acid release Pepsinogen release
Intestinal (hormonal)	Chyme in small intestine	pH of chyme <2: release of secretin, gastric inhibitory polypeptide (GIP), cholecystokinin (decreases gastric acid secretion) pH of chyme >3: release of gastrin (increases gastric acid secretion)

turns the vomitus green. Occasionally, vomiting of intestinal contents can be so rapid that the vomitus contains yellow bile. When blood is exposed to acid in the stomach, the exposure results in a brownish-black "coffee-ground" emesis. If the rapidity of vomiting does not allow sufficient time for this interaction between acid and blood to occur, blood in the vomitus has its normal red color (hematemesis).

Pancreas

The pancreas is composed of both exocrine tissue and endocrine tissue. The islets of Langerhans, endocrine tissue scattered throughout the pancreas, secrete insulin, glucagons, and pancreatic polypeptide hormones, which aid in the digestive process. The exocrine pancreas is composed of acinar cells, which are arranged in lobules. The acinar cells empty secretions into an internal pancreatic ductal system (Fig. 38-9). These internal ducts drain into progressively larger ducts that terminate in the duct of Wirsung, the main pancreatic duct. This pancreatic duct then joins the common bile duct to form a shared short duct called the *ampulla of Vater.* This ampulla, carrying bile and pancreatic secretions, opens into the duodenum. A smooth muscle ring, the sphincter of Oddi, encircles the ampulla. Because of the anatomical arrangements between the common bile duct and the duct of Wirsung, a gallstone that obstructs the ampulla of Vater can obstruct the normal flow of bile and pancreatic secretions. (Such obstruction, although rare, can lead to a stasis of pancreatic secretion, resulting in acute pancreatitis.) Some people have a second external pancreatic duct (duct of Santorini) that opens into the duodenum near the pylorus.

The exocrine acinar cells secrete both a watery alkaline bicarbonate solution and enzymes (see Table 38-1). The large amount of water secreted by the pancreas is instrumental in diluting chyme before absorption. In addition, the bicarbonate neutralizes the highly acidic chyme from the stomach. The pancreatic enzymes digest proteins (trypsin, chymotrypsin, elastase, and carboxypeptidase), fats (lipase, calipase, and esterase), phospholipase and nucleic acids (nucleases), and starch (amylase). Although pancreatic enzymes require a pH close to neutrality for optimal activity, they are capable of nearly completing the digestion of food in the absence of all other digestive secretions.

The pancreatic enzymes are secreted from the pancreas in inactive forms. Trypsin inhibitor prevents the premature activation of trypsin. Once the pancreatic secretions arrive in the duodenum, inactive trypsin (trypsinogen) is activated by an intestinal mucosal enzyme, enterokinase. Active trypsin then activates the other pancreatic enzymes.

Regulation of pancreatic secretion occurs by neural and hormonal means. Vagal stimulation results in the secretion of pancreatic enzymes. Hormonal regulation occurs as a result of duodenal mucosal responses to chyme, and is discussed later.

Gallbladder

In the duodenum, chyme mixed with pancreatic secretions is watery. The fat in chyme is not water soluble and requires a solvent enzyme mixture from the liver to render it absorbable by intestinal cells. Hepatocytes, among many other metabolic functions, make bile. Bile is a mixture of bile salts, cholesterol, bilirubin, and acids suspended in water. This solution emulsifies the fat in chyme, breaking the fat into small globules that can be absorbed across the intestinal lumen. The action of bile ionizes fat-soluble vitamins into absorbable forms. Bile also suspends cholesterol, triglycerides, and multiple-density lipoproteins in the bloodstream, thus preventing precipitation and deposition of these molecules in the vasculature until they can be catabolized.

Bile is stored and concentrated in the gallbladder. Gallbladder secretion is greatest during the intestinal phase of digestion. This activity is stimulated by CCK. CCK causes gallbladder contraction and relaxation of the sphincter of

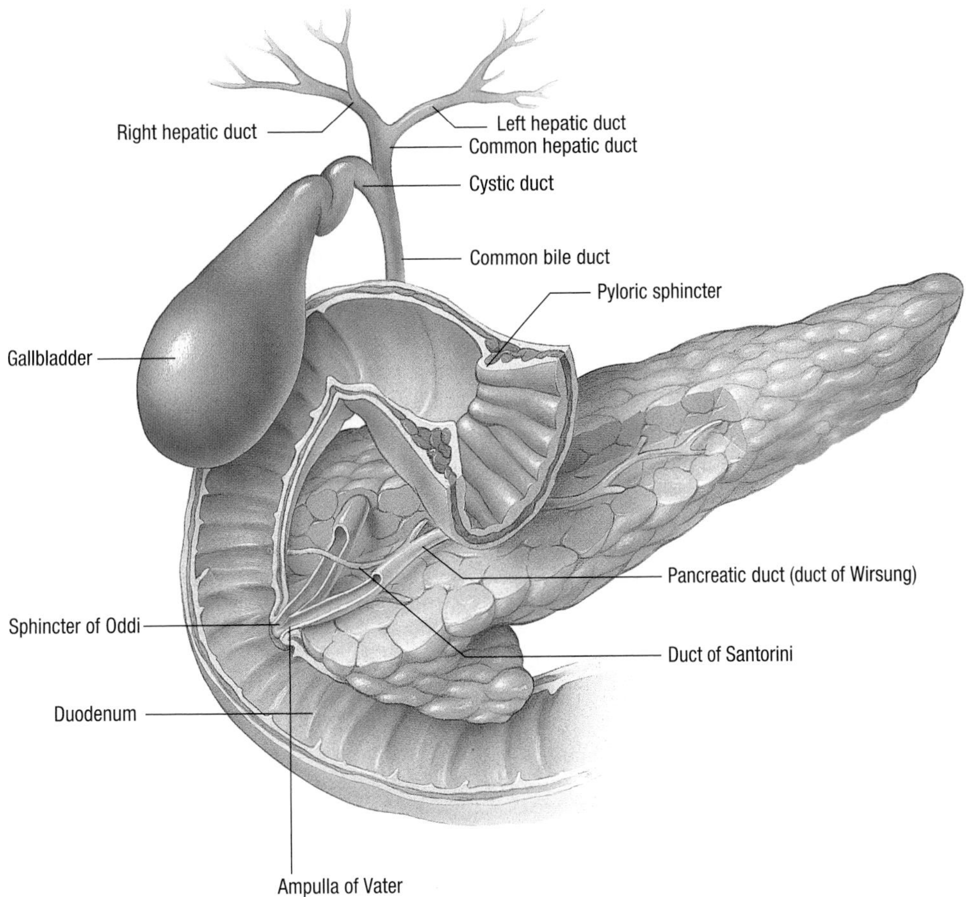

figure 38-9 Biliary system. (Source: Anatomical Chart Company: Atlas of Human Anatomy, p 217. Springhouse, PA, Springhouse, 2001.)

Oddi, allowing the release of bile into the duodenum to mix with chyme.

Small Intestine

SECRETIONS

In the duodenum, chyme mixes with pancreatic digestive enzymes, alkaline substances, water, mucus, and bile. The intestinal enzymes secretin, CCK, and enterokinase are added to this mixture, along with more mucus, more bicarbonate, and more water.

MOTILITY

The small intestine has two types of characteristic movements, propulsive and mixing. The intramural plexuses initiate and coordinate these movements, but the movements can be enhanced or retarded by extrinsic autonomic stimulation, as discussed previously. Propulsive movements propel food forward, allowing for digestion and absorption. This peristalsis is stimulated by distension. During mixing movement, localized concentric contractions of the intestinal wall called *segmentation* promote mixing of food particles. These segments have the appearance of linked sausages. Repetition of this process continually kneads the chyme, thereby eventually exposing all molecules of this material to the absorptive surfaces of the intestinal mucosa.

Emptying of the small intestine into the colon occurs in the same way as gastric emptying. Peristaltic waves build up pressure in the ileum behind the ileocecal valve and push the chyme through the valve into the colon. The ileocecal valve then prevents backflow. Ileal emptying can be retarded by intramural reflexes, which are initiated by a full (distended) colon.

ABSORPTION

The major functions of the small intestine are absorption and digestion, which are facilitated by secretions from the pancreas, liver, and gallbladder. The mucosal layer of the small intestine has many folds (valvulae conniventes) covered with numerous finger-like projections (villi) and microvilli, which dramatically increase the absorptive surface area of the small intestine.

Carbohydrates

The three major sources of carbohydrates in the human diet are sucrose, lactose, and starch. The breakdown of carbohydrates begins in the mouth when food mixes with salivary amylase during chewing. The digestion continues in the duodenum. Conversion to simple sugars continues in the small intestine by intestinal enzymes. Both active and passive transport are used to absorb sugars across the intestinal lumen into the bloodstream.

Proteins

Protein degradation is initiated in the stomach through the actions of hydrochloric acid and pepsin. However, in the absence of pepsin and hydrochloric acid, the small intestine is capable of fully digesting all available protein. Most digestion occurs in the duodenum and jejunum by proteolytic pancreatic enzymes. Polypeptides in the small intestine are degraded into peptide fragments and amino acids by trypsin, chymotrypsin, and carboxypeptidase. Amino acids are absorbed into the blood by active and passive diffusion.

Fats

Triglycerides, lipids, and phospholipids are first degraded in the small intestine. Bile salts, in a process called *emulsification*, facilitate the creation of small droplets of fats from larger globules. Pancreatic enzymes then degrade the fats into fatty acid chains and monoglycerides. These smaller molecules form into even smaller globules, called *micelles*. Fatty acids and monosaccharides are transported across the intestinal mucosa from a micelle passively, leaving bile behind.

In the submucosa, free fatty acids are passed into the blood directly, if small enough. If too large for direct passive diffusion, the free fatty acid is reorganized into a triglyceride, coupled with lipoproteins and cholesterol, and passed into the lymph fluid as chylomicron.

The bile left behind in the intestine after absorption of fats from a micelle is reabsorbed in the ileum. If bile salts enter the colon, they decrease the reabsorption of sodium and water, thereby increasing the liquidity of the undigested food residues in the colon. Most fat is absorbed by the time chyme reaches the middle of the jejunum.

Vitamins, Minerals, and Water

Most vitamins, whether they are fat or water soluble, diffuse across the intestinal mucosa and submucosa into the blood. Fat-soluble vitamin B_{12} couples with intrinsic factor, forming a larger molecule. In this form, vitamin B_{12} is absorbed.

Minerals and electrolytes vary in their absorption. Sodium and iron require active transport, whereas other minerals and electrolytes diffuse passively.

Water is absorbed passively throughout the stomach and small and large intestines. The gastrointestinal tract is highly permeable, in both directions, to water. Should a hypertonic solution enter the duodenum, osmosis occurs in the lumen. The converse is also true: a hypotonic chyme in the stomach and duodenum causes an extremely rapid movement of water into the bloodstream.

Large Intestine

SECRETION

The goblet cells of the colonic mucosa secrete mucus, which lubricates the passage of chyme (see Table 38-1). The production of mucus is stimulated by irritation and by cholinergic activation.

MOTILITY

Colonic movements include mixing and peristaltic movements. These operate as described for the small intestine. A third movement, unique to the colon, is mass movement. This consists of simultaneous contractions of colonic smooth muscle over large portions of the descending and sigmoid portions of the colon. Mass movement rapidly moves the undigested food residue (feces) from these areas into the rectum.

Humans cannot digest the cellulose, hemicellulose, or lignin in plant tissues. These plant materials form a large portion of the undigested food residue. They are usually termed *vegetable fiber* or *dietary bulk*. These fibers attract and hold water, creating a larger, softer stool. Low quantities of bulk result in a relatively inactive colon, leading to bowel movements that are relatively infrequent and feces that are relatively small, dry, and difficult to pass. Epidemiological reports suggest that high-fiber diets are associated with a decreased incidence of diverticulitis and colon cancer.

Filling of the rectum triggers the defecation reflex by stimulating stretch receptors in the rectal wall. Stimulation of the stretch receptors causes sensory (afferent) nerve fibers to transmit impulses to the lower spinal cord. Because of anatomical arrangements of neurons in this part of the cord, these afferent impulses reflexively cause nerve impulses to travel out of the cord along parasympathetic motor fibers that innervate the smooth muscles of the descending and sigmoid colon, the rectum, and the internal anal sphincter. The afferent impulses also reflexively cause nerve impulses to be sent out of the cord along somatic motor neurons that innervate the skeletal muscle of the external anal sphincter. The total effect of these events is to produce coordinated expulsive contractions of the colon and rectum, relaxation (opening) of the sphincters, and expulsion of feces from the anus.

The urge to defecate begins after the pressure within the rectum reaches 18 torr. After intrarectal pressure reaches 55 torr, reflex bowel evacuation occurs. This defecation reflex is inhibited in a continent person by descending neuronal impulses from higher brain centers that inhibit the actions of the somatic motor neurons that innervate the external sphincter. Such inhibition keeps the external anal sphincter closed, thereby averting inappropriate defecation. After a few minutes, the defecation reflex subsides, but it usually becomes active again a few hours later. Defecation is a spinal cord reflex that does not require intact pathways between the sacral cord and the brain. In the early posttraumatic phase of spinal shock, the reflex does not work. After cord shock is ended, reflex defecation occurs once again, but voluntary inhibition is not possible (neurogenic bowel).

ABSORPTION

In the large intestine, most of the water and potassium are absorbed from the chyme. This produces a semisolid residue of undigested food (feces) that can be eliminated from the body. Diarrhea can reduce the transit time for chyme, thereby limiting such potassium and water reabsorption. This can result in hypokalemia and dehydration. Diarrhea also can be caused by materials that hold water in the chyme (e.g., magnesium sulfate), resulting in semiliquid stool.

At birth, the colon is sterile, but large colonic bacterial populations become established soon afterward. Some of these organisms produce vitamin K and a number of

B vitamins. Other bacteria produce ammonia, which is absorbed. Normally, this is removed from the blood once it reaches the liver. However, in people with seriously impaired liver function or with collateral circulatory routes that bypass the liver (usually the result of portal hypertension), such ammonia can remain in the circulation and lead to encephalopathy.

Liver

The liver lies in the right upper quadrant of the abdomen. It has two lobes (right and left) and lies just below the diaphragm, with its greatest portion located to the right side of the body. Its superior (rounded) surface fits into the curve of the diaphragm and is in contact with the anterior wall of the abdominal cavity. The inferior surface is molded over the stomach, the duodenum, the pancreas, the hepatic flexure of the colon, the right kidney, and the right adrenal gland.

The liver is covered with a thin layer of peritoneum over a thin fibrous coat called Glisson's capsule. This fibrous capsule encases and partitions the liver, sending inward fibrous sheets that divide the liver into functional units called *lobules*. Each lobule consists of sheets of hepatocytes organized around a core cluster of vessels called the *portal triad* (Fig. 38-10). The portal triad includes the two sets of afferent vessels (portal vein and hepatic artery) and a small bile duct. The afferent vessels lead to the liver sinusoids, which drain into the efferent hepatic vein, lying at the periphery of each lobule.

The lobule measures approximately 1.5 mm in diameter and 8 mm in length. Each lobe of the liver contains between 50,000 and 100,000 lobules. Rows of hepatocytes radiate from a central venule like spokes of a wheel. Branches of the hepatic artery and the hepatic portal vein lie at the periphery of the wheel. Blood from these branches is poured into open channels (hepatic sinuses) that run between alternate rows of hepatocytes. Kupffer's cells, specialized white cells of the reticuloendothelial system, phagocytize bacteria, debris, and other foreign matter in the sinus blood. The sinuses drain into the central venule, which in turn carries blood to the hepatic vein.

Blind-ended bile canaliculi arise between the other rows of hepatocytes. They carry newly secreted bile to larger ducts located at the periphery. These smaller ducts eventually drain into the common bile duct. Bile that is leaving the liver is concentrated and stored in the gallbladder. Fluid and electrolyte reabsorption in the gallbladder can

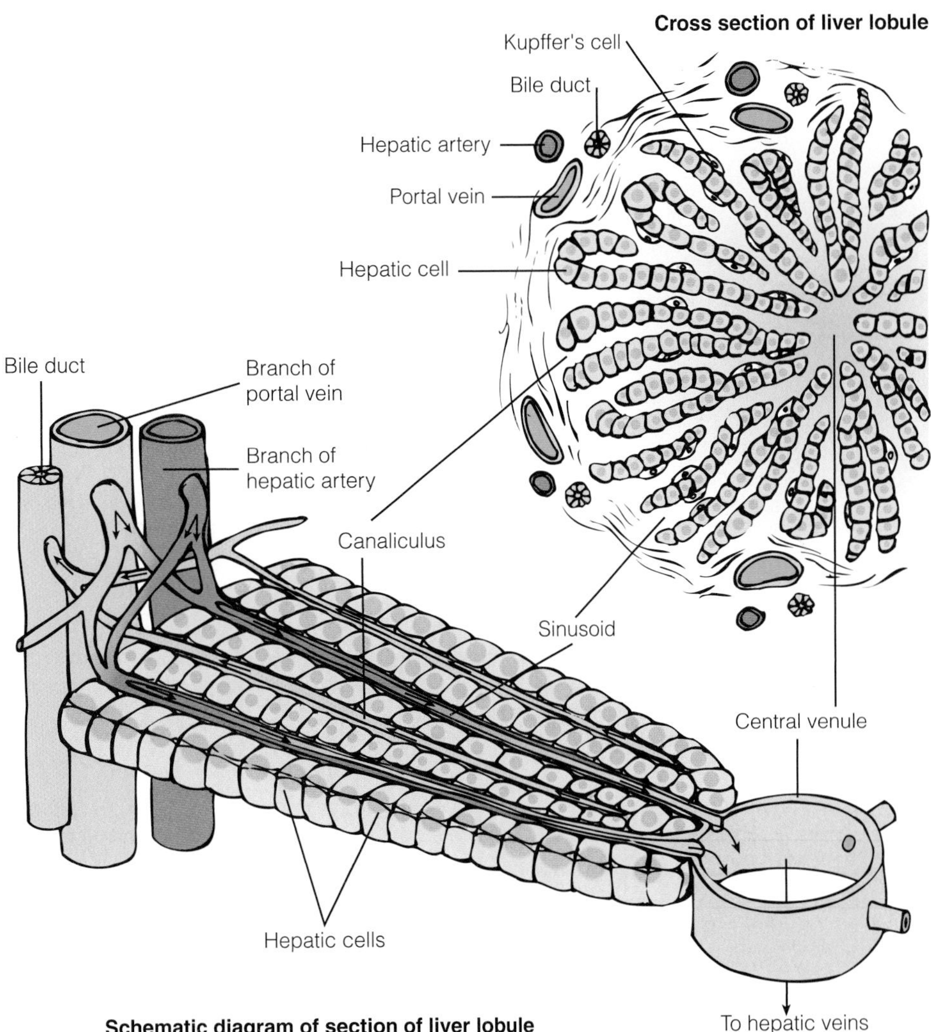

figure 38-10 A section of the liver lobule showing the location of the haptic veins, hepatic cells, liver sinusoids, and branches of the portal vein and hepatic artery.

increase the concentration of bile salts, cholesterol, and bilirubin 12-fold.

The gallbladder has a maximum capacity of 50 mL and can hold a 24-hour output of bile (600 mL) from the liver. The intestinal hormone CCK (secreted by the duodenal mucosa) and vagus nerve activity stimulate gallbladder contraction as a part of food digestion, particularly lipids. CCK and local reflexes initiated by duodenal peristalsis open the sphincter of Oddi. These events permit an outflow of bile down the common bile duct into the duodenum.

The common bile duct and the main duct from the pancreas usually unite just before the duct enters the lumen of the duodenum. There is often a dilatation of the tube after this junction (the ampulla of Vater). The opening of the common bile duct in the duodenum is about 8 to 10 cm from the pylorus.

The liver cells perform many vital functions, as described in the sections that follow and summarized in Table 38-5.

CARBOHYDRATE METABOLISM

The liver participates in carbohydrate metabolism. The liver and skeletal muscle are the two primary sites of glycogen storage. Serum glucose levels are maintained by hepatic glycostatic function, involving two mechanisms. When plasma glucose levels are high, hepatocytes remove glucose from the plasma. Some of this glucose is then stored in the liver as glycogen. If plasma glucose levels decline, hepatocytes convert the glycogen back into glucose through a process called *glycogenolysis,* and the glucose is released into the bloodstream. Although many body tissues have the requisite cellular enzymes for glycogenolysis, hepatocytes are one of the few cell types that can release this intracellular glucose into the bloodstream. Hepatocytes do not simply respond directly to plasma glucose. These glycostatic functions are mediated by several hormones; some (e.g., insulin) promote hepatic glucose uptake, and others (e.g., glucagon, growth hormone, and epinephrine) stimulate glycogenolysis and the release of glucose from liver cells.

The liver does not contain enough glycogen reserves to be able to buffer plasma glucose during prolonged fasting or severe exercise. During these times, low plasma glucose levels stimulate the secretion of one or more hormones (glucagon, glucocorticoids, or thyroxine) that trigger the biochemical conversion of intracellular fatty and amino acids into glucose (gluconeogenesis), which the liver cell can then release into the bloodstream or store as glycogen. Only hepatocytes possess the enzyme that is critical for gluconeogenesis. Glycogen storage is important for other functions of liver cells. A glycogen-rich hepatocyte conjugates bilirubin at a faster rate and is more resistant to toxins and infectious agents.

table 38-5 Hepatic Function

General Category	Specific Description
Carbohydrate metabolism	Glycogenesis (conversion of glucose to glycogen) Glycogenolysis (breakdown of glycogen to glucose) Gluconeogenesis (formation of glucose from amino acids or fatty acids)
Protein metabolism	Synthesis of nonessential amino acids Synthesis of plasma proteins (albumin, prealbumin, transferrin, clotting factors, complement factors; not gamma globulin or immunoglobulins) Urea formation from NH_3 (NH_3 formed by deamination of amino acids in liver and by action of colonic bacteria on proteins)
Lipid and lipoprotein metabolism	Synthesis of lipoproteins Breakdown of triglycerides into fatty acids and glycerol Formation of ketone bodies Synthesis of fatty acids from amino acids and glucose Synthesis and breakdown of cholesterol
Bile acid synthesis and excretion	Bile formation (containing bile salts, bile pigments [bilirubin, biliverdin]), cholesterol Bile excretion (about 1 L/d)
Storage	Glucose (as glycogen) Vitamins (A, D, E, K, B_1, B_2, B_{12}, folic acid) Fatty acids Minerals (Fe, Cu) Amino acids (as albumin, beta globulins)
Biotransformation, detoxification, excretion of endogenous and exogenous compounds	Inactivation of drugs and excretion of the breakdown products Clearance of procoagulants, activated clotting factors, byproducts of coagulation
Removal of pathogens	Clearance of microorganisms by macrophages
Steroid catabolism	Conjugation and excretion of gonadal steroids Conjugation and excretion of adrenal steroids (cortisol, aldosterone)

PROTEIN METABOLISM

The liver plays an essential role in the metabolism of proteins. The amino acids that result from the breakdown of proteins are deaminated to form ammonia by the liver, and then converted to urea. The liver also synthesizes plasma proteins, including albumins, globulins, fibrinogens, plasma lipoproteins, and other proteins involved in clotting. The albumins maintain normal plasma oncotic pressure. A fall in this pressure leads to edema (both systemic and pulmonary) and contributes to ascites. The globulins bind thyroid and adrenal hormones. Bound, the hormones are inactive. Decreased hepatic protein levels can lead to a clinical excess of these hormones.

LIPID AND LIPOPROTEIN METABOLISM

The liver contributes to adipose stores through the metabolism of triglycerides, fatty acids, and cholesterol. During fasting, triglycerides from adipose tissue are catabolized by the liver into fatty acids and glycerols. The free fatty acids in prolonged fasting are further catabolized into acetyl coenzyme-A and then into ketone bodies. Ketone bodies provide an energy source for some (non-neuronal) tissues.

BILE ACID SYNTHESIS AND EXCRETION

Hepatocytes make bile, which contains water, bile salts, cholesterol, bilirubin, gluconate, and inorganic acids. Bile salts aid digestion by emulsifying dietary fats and fostering their absorption and the absorption of fat-soluble vitamins through the intestinal mucosa. They also prevent the cholesterol in the bile from precipitating out of solution and forming calculi. More than 90% of the daily output of bile is reabsorbed for recycling by an active transport process of the ileal mucosa.

Another hepatic function is elimination of bilirubin from the body. Old or defective erythrocytes are phagocytosed by large reticuloendothelial cells that line the large veins and the sinuses of the liver and spleen. These phagocytes degrade the hemoglobin of these cells into biliverdin, iron, and globulin molecules. The last two components are recycled by the body and used for future erythropoiesis. The biliverdin is almost immediately converted to free bilirubin. Because free bilirubin is an insoluble compound, it is transported bound to plasma albumin molecules. The hepatocytes convert this insoluble bilirubin into a soluble (and thus excretable) form by conjugating it with glucuronic acid to form bilirubin gluconate. This soluble form of bilirubin is then added to the bile and is eliminated from the body by the feces. Bilirubin gluconate gives the bile its normal golden yellow color. Organisms in the intestine convert most of the bilirubin gluconate into a darker brown compound, urobilinogen, which gives the feces its natural brown color. Because it is soluble in water, urobilinogen can also be absorbed from the colon back into the bloodstream and be excreted by the kidneys. Excess plasma levels of either conjugated (direct) or unconjugated (indirect) bilirubin produce jaundice. Excess unconjugated bilirubin can cross the immature or damaged blood–brain barrier and bind with the basal ganglia, resulting in kernicterus.

STORAGE

Fat-soluble vitamins and many minerals are stored in the liver. These vitamins and minerals are released under the influence of hormones and serum concentrations of inorganic elements.

BIOTRANSFORMATION

Hepatocytes possess a mixed-function oxidase (MFO) system of enzymes that degrade certain drugs, including alcohol, benzodiazepines, tranquilizers, phenobarbital, phenytoin, and sodium warfarin, among others. This system operates in addition to other intracellular systems that also degrade some of these drugs. Its clinical significance lies in the nature of the drugs that this system catabolizes and in the fact that MFO system activity can be either inhibited or augmented (induced) by these same drugs, depending on when they are taken.

Administration of two MFO system–catabolized drugs within a few hours of one another or together causes each agent to act competitively, slowing down the degradation of the other. For example, simultaneous ingestion of diazepam (Valium) and alcohol can result in slower degradation of each drug. The outcome is higher blood levels of both chemicals for a longer time after administration.

The repeated administration of one MFO system–catabolized drug for several days causes the MFO system to enlarge physically and to possess more enzymes. This is called *induction.* Once induced, the MFO system degrades drugs more rapidly (including the drug that initiated the induction). If administration of a second MFO system–catabolized drug is begun after MFO system induction, a larger dose of this drug will be required to produce a given effect. For example, induction of the MFO system by diazepam increases the dosage of warfarin needed to produce a given therapeutic effect. Other drugs are degraded by various hepatic systems.

STEROID CATABOLISM

The liver cells degrade steroid hormones, thereby preventing excess serum levels of estrogen, testosterone, progesterone, aldosterone, and glucocorticosteroids.

clinical applicability challenges

Self-Challenge: Critical Thinking

1. *A 35-year-old nurse has complaints of epigastric burning during the end of her very busy shift. She reports that this has happened on a regular basis during the past 2 weeks, often occurs 1 to 2 hours after meals, and is relieved by antacids. A visit with her primary physician resulted in the following treatment plan: prescription for a proton pump inhibitor, antacids as needed, dietary changes, avoidance of nonsteroidal anti-inflammatory medications, and stress reduction therapy.*
   a. *What is the most likely reason for her symptoms?*
   b. *Give rationale for each of the therapies prescribed.*
2. *Compare and contrast the effects of extrinsic and intrinsic components of the autonomic nervous system (ANS) on*

motor and sensory function for one gastrointestinal function (e.g., swallowing, defecation).

3. *Explore the mechanisms by which digestive enzymes are regulated in the stomach and small intestine.*

Study Questions

1. *Which organ secretes enzymes capable of digesting food in the absence of all other digestive enzymes?*
   a. *Parotid salivary gland*
   b. *Stomach*
   c. *Liver*
   d. *Pancreas*
2. *Regulation of gastric hydrochloric acid secretion is regulated by all the following phases except*
   a. *the cephalic phase.*
   b. *the gastric phase.*
   c. *the intestinal phase.*
   d. *the colonic phase.*
3. *Which hormone released from the mucosa of the duodenum stimulates the gallbladder to contract and release bile to aid in the digestion of lipids?*
   a. *Cholecystokinin (CCK)*
   b. *Secretin*
   c. *Gastrin*
   d. *Gastric inhibitory peptide (GIP)*
4. *Reflux of gastric contents back into the esophagus is prevented by the*
   a. *effects of gravity.*
   b. *lower esophageal sphincter (LES).*
   c. *epiglottis.*
   d. *pyloric sphincter.*
5. *Which one of the following is unique to the colon?*
   a. *Peristaltic contractions*
   b. *Segmental contractions*
   c. *Mass movement*
   d. *Retropulsion*

OTHER SELECTED READING

Brandt LJ, Daum F, Friedman LS, et al. (eds): Clinical Practice of Gastroenterology (Vols. 1 and 2). Philadelphia, Current Medicine, 1999

Braunwald E, Fauci AS, Kasper DL, et al. (eds): Harrison's Principles of Internal Medicine (15th Ed), pp 1631–1788. New York, McGraw-Hill, 2001

Guyton AC, Hall JE: Textbook of Medical Physiology (10th Ed), pp 718–770. Philadelphia, WB Saunders, 2000

Yamada T, Alpers DH, Laine L, et al. (eds): Textbook of Gastroenterology (3rd Ed). Philadelphia, Lippincott Williams & Wilkins, 1999

chapter
39

Patient Assessment: Gastrointestinal System

JoAnn Coleman

objectives

Based on the content in this chapter, the reader should be able to:

- Discuss important health history components that provide information about gastrointestinal system status.
- Describe a systematic approach for conducting a complete gastrointestinal physical examination.
- Differentiate between normal and abnormal findings detected on physical assessment of the gastrointestinal system.
- Discuss the importance of referred pain patterns in an abdominal assessment.
- Identify the data used to make judgments about nutrition and metabolism in a critical care patient.
- Discuss appropriate studies and procedures used to diagnose gastrointestinal disorders.
- Explain the nursing role in assessing the critical care patient with gastrointestinal compromise.

The gastrointestinal system is a long tube with glands and accessory organs (salivary glands, liver, gallbladder, and pancreas). The gastrointestinal tract begins at the mouth, extends through the pharynx, esophagus, stomach, small intestine, colon, and rectum, and ends at the anus. It is an unsterile system filled with bacteria and other flora. These organisms can cause superinfection from antibiotic therapy, and they can infect other systems when an organ of the gastrointestinal tract ruptures. A malfunction along the gastrointestinal tract can produce a variety of metabolic effects, which eventually may be life threatening.

Assessment of the gastrointestinal system in a critically ill patient provides essential information. Early identification and treatment of gastrointestinal disorders is necessary and serves as a foundation for developing a holistic plan of care for the patient. Ongoing assessment of the gastrointestinal system of the critical care patient can help identify new complications. The ability to complete a comprehensive assessment of the gastrointestinal system depends on the status of the patient. In an intensive care environment, the dynamic nature of the patient may dictate a more focused assessment of the patient. The nurse must be perceptive in obtaining information and timely in soliciting critical information. For example, a ventilated patient cannot converse in an intensive care area, and a comprehensive assessment of the gastrointestinal system cannot be obtained, nor would it be necessary at that time.

When a patient is critically ill, assessment of the gastrointestinal system helps determine whether assessment findings relate to the current clinical problem or herald a new complication. The nurse correlates and integrates presenting gastrointestinal signs and symptoms, whether they are isolated entities or related to another underlying problem: Is the bright red blood in the stool a result of gastrointestinal bleeding or from external bleeding hemorrhoids? Is the abdominal pain due to recent bowel surgery or to a distended stomach? The nurse must be aware of the patient's changing metabolic state and nutritional status because this information may directly affect other health outcomes such as length of stay, morbidity, and even mortality.[1]

HISTORY

Unless emergency conditions require immediate action to preserve life, an assessment of the gastrointestinal system begins with the history. A thorough and accurate history greatly enhances the assessment process. The patient's history provides information that can lay the foundation and set the direction for the rest of the assessment.

The history is the major subjective data source about a patient's health status and provides insight into actual or potential health problems. It guides the physical assessment. The history organizes pertinent physiological, psychological, cultural, and psychosocial information as it relates to the patient's current health status, and accounts for factors such as lifestyle, family relationships, and cultural influences.[2] Box 39-1 lists elements for a comprehensive gastrointestinal history.

The initial presentation of the patient in the intensive care area determines how quickly the history will be obtained, as well as the focus of the interview. If the patient is in acute distress, the history must focus on obtaining answers to pertinent questions about the patient's chief complaint and precipitating events. Information may be more readily obtained from family members or friends. The nurse can obtain a more thorough history from a patient in no obvious distress by focusing on the patient's current symptoms, medical history, and family history. Information that is fixed and needs to be obtained only once includes data about personal health, pre-existing gastrointestinal conditions, previous gastrointestinal or abdominal surgeries or injuries, and hospitalizations. The critical care nurse must also consider the present nutritional status of the patient, the projected length of illness, and its impact on future nutritional needs or adjustments.[3]

The gastrointestinal assessment may change over the course of the illness. The data gathered during the initial history may have focused on the pressing issues facing the patient at that time, but these issues can change in a short or protracted amount of time. The critical care nurse must be vigilant and is challenged to maintain data and incorporate additional information to provide individualized and holistic nursing care, as the status of the patient continually evolves.

Because pain is often the chief complaint of patients presenting with abdominal disorders, it must be dealt with in detail.[4] A thorough assessment of pain must include details about the onset, progression, migration, character, localization and radiation, and duration of the pain, as well as information about factors that exacerbate or alleviate the pain. Box 39-2 summarizes common causes of pain by location.

box 39-1
Comprehensive Gastrointestinal History

Present Gastrointestinal Problem

Type, onset, location, duration, frequency, severity/intensity, character, associated factors (events or activities), associated symptoms, exacerbating or relieving factors

Abdominal Pain

- *Onset and duration:* when it began; sudden or gradual; persistent, recurrent, intermittent
- *Character:* dull, sharp, burning, gnawing, stabbing, cramping, aching, colicky
- *Location:* of onset, change in location over time, radiating to another area, superficial or deep
- *Associated symptoms:* vomiting, diarrhea, constipation, passage of flatus, belching, jaundice, change in abdominal girth
- *Relationship to:* menstrual cycle, abnormal menses, urination, defecation, inspiration, change in body position, food or alcohol intake, stress, time of day, trauma
- *Recent stool characteristic:* color, consistency, odor, frequency
- *Urinary characteristics:* frequency, color, volume congruent with fluid intake, force of stream, ease of starting stream, ability to empty bladder
- *Medications:* prescription or nonprescription; high doses of aspirin, acetaminophen; steroids; nonsteroidal anti-inflammatory drugs

Past Medical History

- Major chronic illnesses (diabetes, cancer, hypertension, coronary artery disease)
- Inflammatory bowel disease (Crohn's disease, ulcerative colitis, irritable bowel syndrome, diverticulitis)
- Peptic ulcer
- Gallstones
- Polyps
- Pancreatitis
- Hepatitis or cirrhosis of the liver
- Previous gastrointestinal bleeding
- Previous gastrointestinal surgeries (mouth, pharyngeal, esophageal, stomach, small intestine, colon, liver, gallbladder, pancreas)
- Cancers or tumors of the gastrointestinal tract
- Abdominal surgeries or trauma
- Drugs (including prescription, over-the-counter, recreational drug use, aspirin, steroids, anticoagulants)
- Herbal therapies, preparations, or medications
- Smoking or chewing tobacco
- Vaccinations (hepatitis, flu, pneumococcal)
- Prior gastrointestinal examinations (upper endoscopy, colonoscopy)
- Spinal cord injury
- For women: episiotomy or fourth-degree laceration during delivery

box 39-1
Comprehensive Gastrointestinal History (Continued)

- Previous blood transfusions
- Depression, anxiety, or recent emotional upset

Family Medical History
- Inflammatory bowel disease
- Hirschsprung's disease, aganglionic megacolon
- Malabsorption syndrome: cystic fibrosis, celiac disease
- Gallbladder disease
- Polyposis syndromes: Peutz-Jeghers syndrome, familial multiple polyposis
- Familial Mediterranean fever (periodic peritonitis)
- Any cancers of the gastrointestinal tract

Personal and Social History
- Dietary habits
- Bowel habits (use of laxatives, stool softeners)
- Exercise patterns
- Oral hygiene (dental status, pattern of dental care, braces, dentures, bridges, crowns, caries)
- Alcohol use (type, usual amount, frequency)
- Use of street drugs
- Exposure to infectious diseases: hepatitis, flu, travel history, overseas military duty
- Occupation
- Lifestyle
- Recent stressful life events: physical or psychological changes

Gastrointestinal System Review
- Anorexia
- Indigestion (heartburn)
- Dysphagia
- Eructations
- Nausea
- Vomiting
- Hematemesis
- Pain
- Fever and chills
- Jaundice
- Hepatitis
- Constipation
- Diarrhea
- Flatulence
- Change in color of stool or contents (clay colored, tarry, bright red blood, mucus, undigested food)
- Bleeding
- Hemorrhoids
- Change in appetite
- Recent weight gain or loss (usual height and weight)
- Mouth lesions
- Ulcers
- Gallstones
- Polyps
- Tumors of the gastrointestinal tract
- Anal discomfort
- Fecal incontinence
- Exposure to infectious agents (foreign travel, military duty, water source)

Nutrition History
- Dietary habits/intake
- Changes in appetite
- Food allergies
- Food intolerances
- Special diet
- Taste sensations
- Heartburn
- Coffee intake
- Alcohol intake
- Vitamins or nutritional supplements

With many gastrointestinal problems, the pain is referred, which makes diagnosis especially difficult. Referred pain is pain felt at a site different from that of the involved organ. Pain results because nerves that supply an organ also supply the body surface.[4] Figure 39-1 identifies common sites of referred abdominal pain.

PHYSICAL EXAMINATION

The physical examination helps establish baseline information about the physical dimensions of the patient's present situation. The physical assessment begins by observing the patient's overall appearance. Motor activity, body position, gait, hair (pattern, loss), skin color (jaundice, cyanosis, pallor) and quality (edema), facial expression, level of consciousness, and signs of depression, anxiety, confusion, or irritability are noted. It is important to note that changes in fluid and electrolyte balance, severe infection, drug toxicity, and hepatic disease may cause abnormal behavior. Next, a focused examination of the gastrointestinal system is performed. A focused examination of the gastrointestinal system includes evaluation of the oral cavity and throat, abdomen, and rectum. Assessment of the abdomen includes assessment of the liver, gallbladder, and pancreas.[5]

Oral Cavity and Throat

Adequate nutrition is related to good dental health and the general condition of the mouth. Any disorders of the upper gastrointestinal tract (lips, mouth, teeth, pharynx, and esophagus) can prevent adequate nutritional intake. Changes in the oral cavity may influence the type and amount of food ingested and the extent to which food is properly mixed with salivary enzymes. Esophageal problems can also adversely affect food and fluid intake, jeopardizing a patient's health.

The oral cavity is examined by inspection and palpation using a good light source, a tongue depressor, an examining glove, and a mask. The nurse should explain the procedure

box 39-2
Common Causes of Pain by Location

Right Hypochondriac
Cholecystitis/cholangitis
Hepatitis
Metastatic disease to the liver
Pleurisy, lower lobe pneumonia, or pneumothorax
Congestive hepatomegaly
Pyelonephritis
Renal colic
Duodenal ulcer

Epigastric
Duodenal or gastric ulcer
Duodenitis or gastritis
Pancreatitis
Myocardial infarction or angina
Pericarditis
Gastroenteritis
Mesenteric embolus or thrombus
Small bowel obstruction

Left Hypochondriac
Pleurisy, lower lobe pneumonia, or pneumothorax
Myocardial infarction or angina
Pericarditis
Pyelonephritis
Renal colic
Splenic injury

Right Lumbar
Pancreatitis
Pyelonephritis
Renal colic
Colon obstruction/gangrene

Umbilical
Appendicitis
Small bowel obstruction
Rectus sheath hematoma
Gastroenteritis
Umbilical hernia
Abdominal aortic aneurysm
Aortic dissection
Mesenteric embolus or thrombus

Left Lumbar
Pancreatitis
Pyelonephritis
Renal colic
Sigmoid diverticulitis
Colon obstruction/gangrene

Right Inguinal
Meckel's diverticulum
Appendicitis
Cecal perforation
Groin hernia
Colon obstruction/gangrene
Ectopic pregnancy
Spigelian hernia
Regional enteritis

Suprapubic or Hypogastric
Rectus sheath hematoma
Salpingitis
Ectopic pregnancy
Tubo-ovarian torsion
Mittelschmertz
Regional enteritis
Endometriosis
Abdominal aortic aneurysm

Left Inguinal
Sigmoid diverticulitis
Groin hernia
Colon obstruction/gangrene
Ectopic pregnancy
Spigelian hernia
Regional enteritis

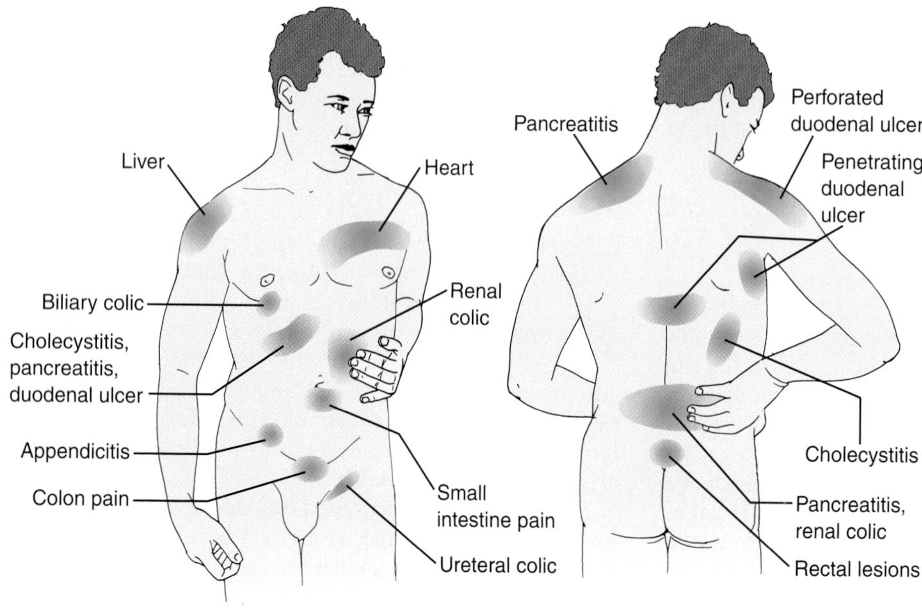

figure 39-1 Common sites of referred abdominal pain. (Source: Smeltzer SC, Bare BG: Brunner and Suddarth's Textbook of Medical–Surgical Nursing [10th Ed], p 945. Philadelphia, Lippincott Williams & Wilkins, 2004.)

to the patient. The patient assumes a comfortable position that facilitates examination. Sitting upright is the best position for this part of the examination.

The lips and jaws are inspected for abnormal color, texture, lesions, symmetry, and swellings. The temporomandibular joints are palpated for mobility, tenderness, and crepitus. The nurse retracts the lips to allow adequate visualization. Dentures are inspected for fit, and they are removed for the oral examination. The nurse should use a good light source to inspect all structures inside the mouth and the buccal mucosa. Missing, broken, loose, and decayed teeth are identified, while the nurse notes redness, pallor, white patches, plaques, ulcers, petechiae, bleeding, and masses. A pool of saliva under the tongue helps assess hydration. The parotid and submaxillary ducts are palpated. The nurse palpates suspect areas with a gloved finger to determine tenderness or induration. The patient should stick out his or her tongue, while the nurse checks for symmetry of movement, swelling, lesions, and any abnormal coating. While depressing the tongue with a tongue blade, the nurse observes the movement of the soft palate and uvula as the patient says "ah." These structures should rise symmetrically. This is a good time to inspect the hard and soft palates, the uvula, the tonsils, the pillars, and the posterior pharynx. Note decreased or absent gag reflex, which suggests possible neurological dysfunction and increases the patient's risk of aspiration. Deviation of the uvula to one side when the patient says "ah" may indicate pathology of cranial nerve IX (the glossopharyngeal nerve) or cranial nerve X (the vagus nerve).[5] Unusual breath odors may indicate serious gastrointestinal disease, such as an esophageal cancer. Fecal breath odor may be caused by a bowel obstruction or hepatic failure; a fruity breath odor may be the result of diabetic or starvation ketoacidosis. Table 39-1 reviews oral assessment, normal and abnormal findings, and possible causes of abnormal findings.

Examination of the oral cavity in an intubated patient is very important, even though the tube may hinder vision during the assessment. The condition of the mouth of a critically ill patient can change rapidly and the nurse must conduct a periodic assessment to initiate treatment and intervene to prevent complications. The presence of any secretions, oral odor, or changes in odors coming from the oral cavity should be promptly assessed. Studies suggest there may be a relationship between pneumonia and mouth colonizations in patients who are intubated. An intubation tube can be a source of odorous fluid if it leaks; this fluid can cause corrosion of oral structures.[6]

The patient with a nasogastric, orogastric, or long tube for intestinal decompression warrants close observation because these tubes prevent the lower esophageal sphincter (LES) from completely closing. Gastric reflux or even reflux into the oropharynx may occur, which can cause erosive damage to the esophagus as well as a noxious odor in the mouth. Delayed gastric emptying may also exacerbate the reflux.

Abdomen

The patient's comfort should be preserved as the nurse performs the abdominal examination. The patient should empty his or her bladder before the examination. A supine position with arms down and knees slightly bent is preferred because this position relieves tension on the abdominal wall. Draping exposes the abdomen and protects the patient's modesty.[5] This is the ideal situation for performing an abdominal examination, but it may not always be possible in a critically ill patient. The nurse must assess the circumstances and prioritize for the individual patient at that time. If the patient is experiencing any or severe pain, the need for an examination may be reevaluated. Likewise, if the procedure increases discomfort or intensity of pain, the examination is stopped. An abdominal examination is not conducted if the patient has appendicitis, a dissecting abdominal aortic aneurysm, polycystic kidneys, or an organ transplant.

The order of the abdominal examination is inspection, auscultation, percussion, and palpation. Auscultation precedes percussion and palpation because the latter can alter the frequency and quality of bowel sounds. Likewise, if the painful area is palpated first, the patient may tense the abdominal muscles, making assessment difficult or impossible.

The abdomen is usually divided into four quadrants by imaginary lines crossing at the umbilicus: right upper, right lower, left upper, and left lower quadrants. Another way to view the abdomen is to divide it into nine sections. Figure 39-2 shows the abdominal organs and their relationship to these two methods of identifying abdominal landmarks.

INSPECTION

The examination begins with the nurse standing at the foot of the patient's bed and inspecting for symmetry of the abdomen, visible masses, and pulsations. The nurse inspects the skin of the abdomen for tense, shiny skin, any areas of discoloration, rashes, striae (lines resulting from rapid or prolonged skin stretching), ecchymoses, lesions, scars, and prominent or dilated veins. Then the nurse moves to the patient's side and assumes a position to obtain an eye-level view across the abdomen. Size, shape, asymmetry, and movements from respirations, peristalsis, vascular pulsations, and exaggerated movement are noted. The umbilicus is inspected for position, contour, and color. Pulsation of the aorta is normally seen in the epigastric area. In a thin person, the femoral pulses may be visible. When ascites or abdominal bleeding is suspected, the nurse should measure the abdominal girth.[5] Table 39-2 lists common abnormal abdominal findings.

AUSCULTATION

Auscultation provides information on bowel motility and the vessels and organs that lie beneath the abdominal wall. The nurse applies light pressure on the diaphragm of the stethoscope when auscultating the four quadrants of the abdomen. The nurse starts below and to the right of the umbilicus and proceeds in a methodical direction through all four quadrants. To prevent contraction of the abdominal muscles that can obscure sounds, the nurse lifts the stethoscope completely off the abdominal wall when changing its location. Normally, air and fluid moving through the bowel by peristalsis create a soft, bubbling sound with no regular pattern, often with soft clicks and gurgles interspersed, approximately every 5 to 15 seconds. Colonic sounds are low pitched with a rumbling feature. A

table 39-1 Oral Assessment

Structure	Normal	Abnormal Findings	Possible Cause
Lips	Smooth, pink, and moist	Dry or cracked	Febrile illness
		Asymmetrical, cracked, fissured, or bleeding	Cheilitis
		Cyanotic	Cold or hypoxia
		Cracks at corner of lips	Possible vitamin B deficiency or poor hygiene
Tongue	Pink, moist with papillae present	Coated or loss of papilla and a shiny appearance (with or without redness); blistered or cracked; altered taste	Infection
		Deviation to one side	Cranial nerve XII (hypoglossal nerve) problem
		Nodules or ulcers on base of tongue	Cancerous lesion
Saliva	Watery	Thick, ropy, or absent	
Mucous membranes	Pink and moist	Reddened without ulcerations	Infection
		Ulcerations with or without bleeding	Poor nutrition
		Inflammation	Ill-fitting dentures
		Leukoplakia on buccal membrane	Precancerous lesion
		Cyanosis	Hypoxia
		Pale mucosa	Anemia
		Small areas of white scar tissue	Chronic irritation from friction of irregular tooth surfaces or biting when chewing
		Inflamed or painful Stensen's duct opening	Parotid gland infection
Gingiva	Pink, stippled, and firm	Edematous with or without redness; spontaneous bleeding or bleeding with pressure; soreness	Gingivitis
Teeth or dentures	Clean without debris	Plaque or debris in between teeth; plaque or debris along gum line or denture-bearing area	
		Toothache, tooth abscess	
		Misfit of dental appliances	
		Absent or broken teeth, cavities	
		Malocclusion, worn or flattened tooth edges	Bruxism
Voice	Normal	Deeper or raspy; difficulty talking or painful to talk	Vocal cord paralysis
Throat/swallowing	Normal	Some pain on swallowing or unable to swallow; sore throat	Cancerous lesion
Glands	Nonpalpable	Inflammation and lumps	Stones or cysts

hungry patient may exhibit a "growling stomach" resulting from hyperperistalsis, called *borborygmi*. High-pitched, rapid, loud, and gurgling bowel sounds are hyperactive and may occur in a hungry patient. Bowel sounds that occur once every minute or less frequently are hypoactive and usually occur after bowel surgery or when feces fills the colon.[6]

Edema of the abdominal wall can be detected when an imprint of the diaphragm remains after light auscultation. The nurse uses the bell of the stethoscope to listen for vascular sounds over the abdominal aorta and the renal and femoral arteries. Figure 39-3 illustrates auscultation of the abdomen for vascular sounds. If a bruit (a continuous purring, blowing, or humming sound) is heard, percussion and palpation are not performed. If a bruit is a new finding, the physician is notified. Table 39-3 describes abnormal abdominal sounds.

PERCUSSION

Abdominal percussion helps identify air, gas, and fluid in the abdomen and helps determine the size and location of abdominal organs. The percussion sound depends on the density of the underlying structure. A dull sound is heard over solid organs (such as the liver), a stool-filled colon, abdominal masses, or pleural effusions. A tympanic sound is heard over air, as in the gastric bubble or air-filled intes-

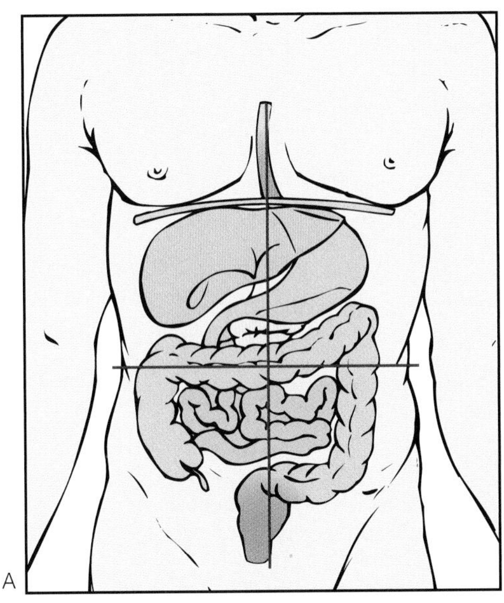

Right upper quadrant (RUQ)	Left upper quadrant (LUQ)
Liver and gallbladder Pylorus Duodenum Head of pancreas Hepatic flexure of colon Portions of ascending and transverse colon	Left liver lobe Stomach Body of pancreas Splenic flexure of colon Portions of transverse and descending colon
Right lower quadrant (RLQ)	**Left lower quadrant (LLQ)**
Cecum and appendix Portion of ascending colon	Sigmoid colon Portion of descending colon

A

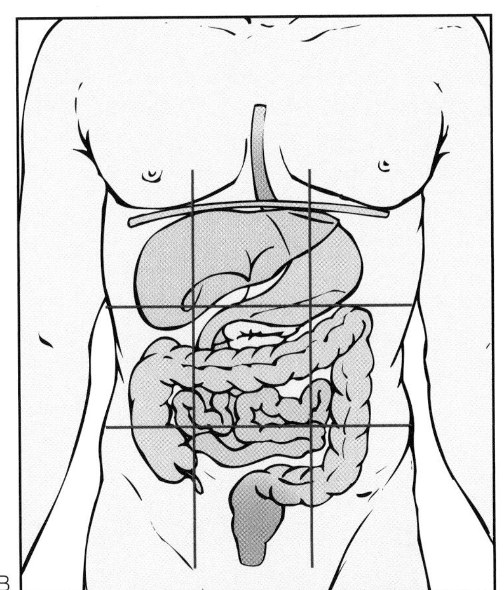

Right hypochondriac	Epigastric	Left hypochondriac
Right liver lobe Gallbladder	Pyloric end of stomach Duodenum Pancreas Portion of liver	Stomach Tail of pancreas Splenic flexure of colon
Right lumbar	**Umbilical**	**Left lumbar**
Ascending colon Portions of duodenum and jejunum	Omentum Mesentery Lower part of duodenum Jejunum and ileum	Descending colon Portions of jejunum and ileum
Right inguinal	**Suprapubic or hypogastric**	**Left inguinal**
Cecum Appendix Lower end of ileum	Ileum	Sigmoid colon

B

figure 39-2 To aid accurate abdominal assessment and documentation of findings, the nurse can mentally divide the patient's abdomen into regions. (**A**) The quadrant method. (**B**) The nine regions method.

tine. The size of the liver is determined by percussing along the right mid-clavicular line. One method is to begin at the iliac crest and work upward. The point at which the sound becomes dull is marked. Percussion is performed down from the clavicle. The dull sound of the rib should not be mistaken for the superior edge of the liver. After marking the superior edge, the nurse measures the distance between the marks in centimeters. The normal liver measures 6 to 12 cm in height at the mid-clavicular line.[5] Systematic percussion of the abdomen is illustrated in Figure 39-4.

Performing abdominal percussion on a critically ill patient may be postponed, especially if there is abdominal guarding. Areas where the patient is not experiencing pain should be percussed before painful areas are examined. Abdominal percussion or palpation is contraindicated in a patient with suspected abdominal aortic aneurysm or in a patient who has received an abdominal organ transplant. Likewise, percussion and palpation should be performed cautiously in a patient with suspected appendicitis.[4]

PALPATION

Abdominal palpation is performed to establish the character of the abdominal wall, including the size, condition, and consistency of abdominal organs; the presence of abdominal masses; and the presence, location, and degree

table 39-2 Abnormal Abdominal Findings

Finding	Characteristic	Possible Cause
Abdominal contour	Concave (scaphoid)	Malnutrition
	Distension	Tumor; excessive fluid (ascites, perforation); gas accumulation; severe malnutrition
Skin abnormalities	Bulging around old scar	Incisional hernia
	Striae	Obesity; pregnancy; abdominal tumor; Cushing's syndrome (purple striae)
	Pink or blue	Recently developed striae
	White or silver	Older striae
	Tense, glistening	Ascites
	Dilated, tortuous veins	Inferior vena cava obstruction
Umbilicus	Everted	Increased intra-abdominal pressure
	Bluish ecchymosis surrounding umbilicus (Cullen's sign)	Intra-abdominal bleeding; pancreatitis; ectopic pregnancy
Peristaltic wave	Strong	Intestinal obstruction
Abdominal aortic pulsations	Obvious and pronounced	Increased intra-abdominal pressure (from tumor or ascites)
Murphy's sign	Sharp pain that stops respiration when palpating under liver border	Cholecystitis
Grey Turner's sign	Flank ecchymosis	Intra-abdominal bleeding; hemorrhagic pancreatitis
Blumberg's sign	Rebound tenderness	Peritoneal irritation; inflamed or perforated appendix
Iliopsoas muscle	Right lower quadrant pain when right leg elevated against tension	Inflamed or perforated appendix from inflamed psoas muscle
Obturator muscle	Abdominal pain when right leg rotated at hip (internal or external rotation)	Inflamed or perforated appendix

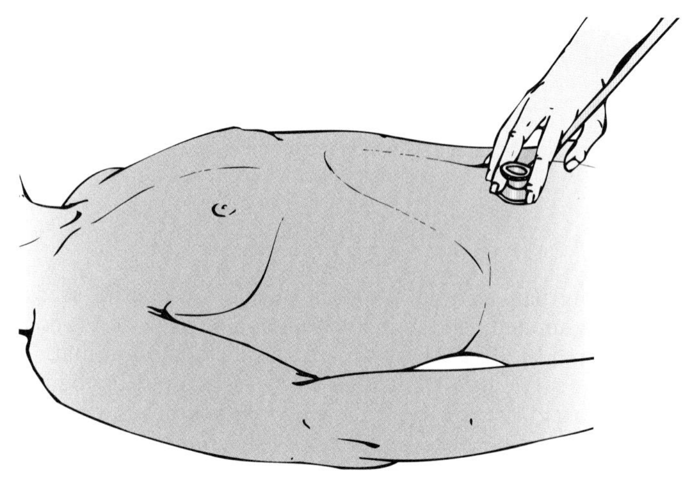

A. Stethoscope placement for auscultation of bowel sounds

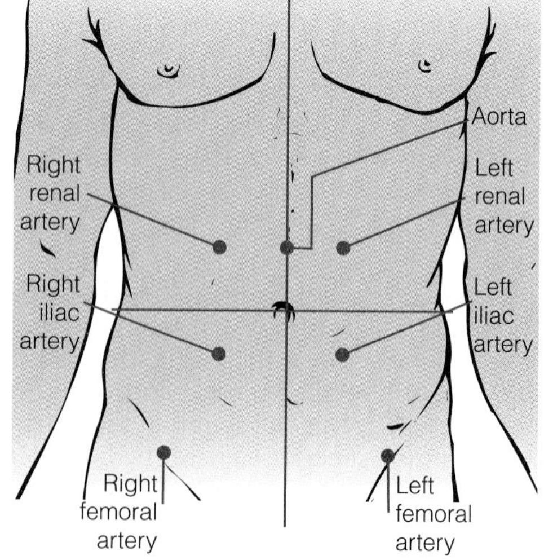

B. Auscultation sites for vascular sounds

figure 39-3 Auscultating the abdomen. Before using a stethoscope to auscultate the abdomen, warm your hands and the stethoscope to prevent muscular contraction, which can alter auscultatory findings. (**A**) First, use the diaphragm of the stethoscope to auscultate for bowel sounds throughout all four quadrants. (**B**) Then use the bell of the stethoscope to listen for vascular sounds in the sites shown.

table 39-3 Abnormal Abdominal Sounds

Sound and Description	Location	Sound	Possible Cause
Bowel sounds	All four quadrants	Hypoactive sounds unrelated to hunger	Diarrhea or early intestinal obstruction
		Hypoactive, then absent, sounds	Paralytic ileus or peritonitis
		High-pitched "tinkling" sounds	Intestinal air and fluid under tension in a dilated bowel; early intestinal obstruction
		High-pitched "rushing" sounds coinciding with an abdominal cramp	Intestinal obstruction
		Hyperactive sounds, long and prolonged (borborygmi)	Hunger, gastroenteritis
		Absence of sounds over 5 min in all four quadrants	Temporary loss of intestinal motility; occurs with ileus
Systolic bruits (vascular "blowing"sounds resembling cardiac murmurs)	Abdominal aorta	Partial arterial obstruction or turbulent blood flow	Dissecting abdominal aneurysm
	Renal artery		Renal artery stenosis
	Iliac artery		Hepatomegaly
Venous hum (continuous, medium-pitched tone created by blood flow in a large, engorged vascular organ such as the liver)	Epigastric area and umbilicus	Increased collateral circulation between portal and systemic venous systems	Hepatic cirrhosis
Friction rub (harsh, grating sound resembling two pieces of sandpaper rubbing together)	Hepatic	Inflammation of the peritoneal surface of an organ	Liver mass

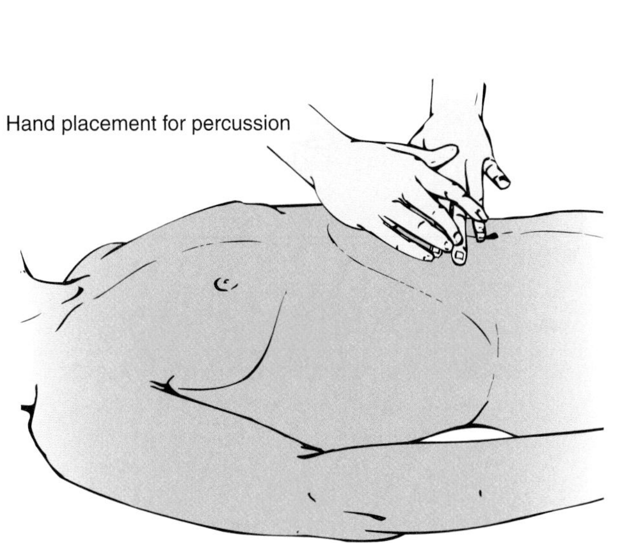

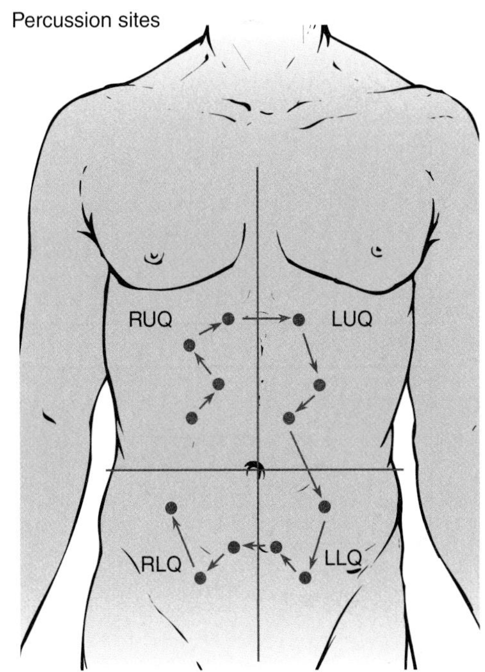

figure 39-4 Percussing the abdomen. Percuss the abdomen systematically, starting with the right upper quadrant and moving clockwise to the percussion sites in each quadrant. If the patient complains of pain in a particular quadrant, adjust the percussion sequence to percuss that quadrant last. Remember when tapping to move your right finger away quickly so you do not inhibit vibrations.

of abdominal pain. Abdominal palpation includes light palpation, deep palpation, and ballottement.

Light palpation should be performed first; it identifies muscular resistance and areas of tenderness. Fingertips are used to depress the abdominal wall 1 cm (0.5 in). The nurse notes skin temperature, muscle resistance, tender areas, and masses. The femoral artery is palpated bilaterally. A symptomatic area is always palpated last to ensure patient cooperation and relaxed muscles.

When disease is present, palpation may result in somatic or organ pain. Somatic pain is localized and reflects inflammation of the skin, fascia, or abdominal surfaces. Guarding of the abdominal muscles accompanies somatic pain. Organ pain is visceral in nature and is usually dull, diffuse, and generalized.

Deep palpation is used to locate organs (enlarged spleen, edge of the liver, poles of the right and left kidney) and large masses. The fingertips are used to depress the abdominal wall firmly to a depth of 7.5 cm (3 in). Palpation is performed in the epigastric area for the pulse of the aorta. If an area of tenderness is found with light palpation, rebound tenderness should be checked by quickly withdrawing the fingertips after depression. Rebound tenderness usually indicates an inflammation of the peritoneum from an abdominal process such as an organ inflammation, infection, abscess formation, or perforated bowel (release of bowel contents into the abdomen). If a mass is palpated, the nurse notes its location, size, shape, consistency, type of border, degree of tenderness, presence of pulsations, and degree of mobility (fixed or mobile).[5]

The liver is most easily palpated by placing one hand under the patient at the level of the 11th rib, while the other hand is placed on the abdomen at the level of the percussed liver edge dullness. With the abdominal fingers pointing upward to lift the organ, the upper hand pushes down and upward to palpate the lower border of the liver. The liver edge should be firm and smooth. An enlarged, nodular, or irregularly shaped liver should be reported. Figure 39-5 illustrates assessment of the liver.

Ballottement is the light, rapid tapping of the fingertips against the abdominal wall. This is used to elicit abdominal muscle resistance or guarding that may be missed with deep palpation, or to detect the movement or bounce of a movable mass. In a patient with ascites, deep ballottement may be performed. The fingertips are rapidly pushed deeply inward in a rapid movement, then quickly released, maintaining fingertip contact with the abdominal wall. Any movement of an organ lying beneath will be felt or a movable mass will move toward the fingertips.[6]

Anus and Rectum

The anus is assessed by inspection and palpation. The skin around the anus is normally darker than the surrounding area. The nurse should inspect for inflammation, lesions, skin tags or warts, obvious fissures, and hemorrhoids. The

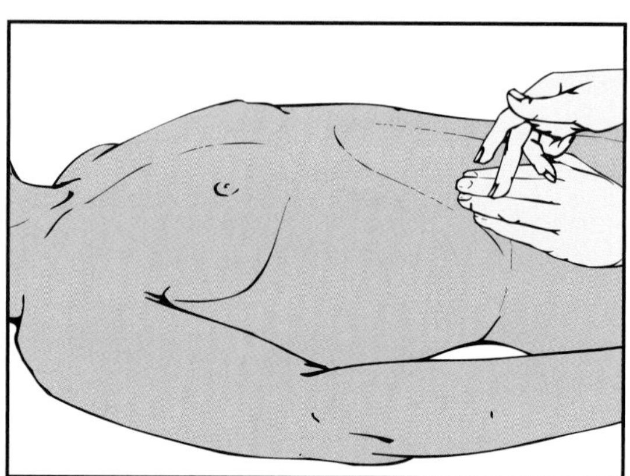

A. Percussion

B. Palpation

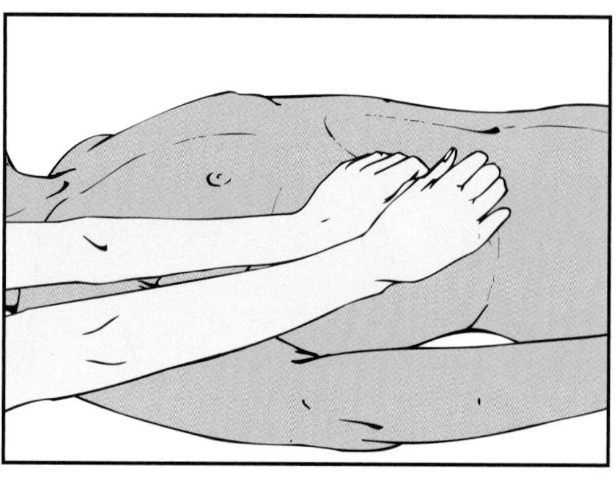

C. Hooking

figure 39-5 Assessing the liver. To assess the liver, the nurse should percuss and attempt to palpate or hook the liver.

area should be palpated with a well-lubricated gloved finger for outpouchings, nodules, tenderness, irregularities, and fecal impaction. Alteration in elimination due to immobility, limited or no gastrointestinal intake, opioids, or decreased intestinal peristalsis may result from a patient's disease or its treatment. Constipation may compound matters and, if left untreated, can lead to fecal impaction.[2] Astute nursing assessment is critical in preventing and treating constipation or fecal impaction in any patient.

Anal sphincter tone can be assessed by palpation. A gloved hand and well-lubricated tip of the index finger can be slipped into the anal canal. A patient who can cooperate is asked to bear down to tighten the external sphincter around the inserted finger. The tone is assessed; it should tighten, exert even pressure all around, feel smooth, and cause no discomfort to the patient. A lax sphincter may indicate a neurological deficit. A very tight sphincter may result from scarring, spasticity caused by a fissure or other lesion, inflammation, or from anxiety about the examination. Inserting the finger farther allows palpation of the walls of the rectum. The walls are assessed for any nodules, masses, irregularities, polyps or tenderness. The wall should feel smooth, even, and uninterrupted.[5]

NUTRITIONAL ASSESSMENT

A critically ill patient's nutritional status may fall anywhere on a continuum ranging from optimum nutrition to malnutrition. The critical care patient may have an inadequate dietary intake because of illness or the disorder that caused the hospitalization, particularly if the disorder is gastrointestinal. In addition, critically ill patients are at risk for gastrointestinal problems due to treatments that cause damage to the gastrointestinal system and reduce the body's ability to absorb nutrients. Optimum nutrient intake provides adequate energy and can protect from complications of disease.[7]

The nurse plays an important role in evaluating the nutritional status of the patients under his or her care. Certain signs and symptoms that suggest possible nutritional deficiency are easy to note because they are specific. Conversely, fluid changes, such as edema or effusions, can mask protein and fat loss. The fact that nutritional disturbances can be subtle and are frequently nonspecific makes the need for assessment important.

An initial nutritional screening may begin with cursory data, as dictated by the patient's condition.[7] A registered dietitian or nutritionist or a nutritional support team may perform a more comprehensive assessment. The parameters of the nutritional assessment include anthropometric measurement, laboratory studies, physical examination, and dietary evaluation (Box 39-3).

Serial weight measurement is perhaps the single most important indicator of nutritional status and is the evaluation that the nurse performs most often. In addition, a number of quick and efficient screening instruments have been developed. The Subjective Global Assessment (SGA) is an example of a screening instrument (Fig. 39-6).

An important factor that influences nutritional status is nitrogen balance, a sensitive indicator of the body's gain or loss of protein. An adult is in nitrogen balance when the nitrogen intake equals the nitrogen output (in urine, feces, and perspiration). Nitrogen balance is a sign of health. A positive nitrogen balance exists when nitrogen intake exceeds nitrogen output and indicates tissue growth, such as occurs during recovery from surgery, and rebuilding of wasted tissue. A negative nitrogen balance indicates that the tissue is breaking down faster than it is being replaced. In the absence of an adequate intake of protein, the body converts protein to glucose for energy. This can occur with fever, starvation, surgery, burns, and debilitating diseases. Malnutrition occurs when a patient is in negative nitrogen balance. Malnutrition, in turn, interferes with wound healing, increases susceptibility to infection, and contributes to an increased incidence of complications, a protracted hospitalization, and an extended bed confinement.[7]

The nutritional assessment directs the nutritional prescription and assists in the development of the interventions. Enteral or parenteral nutrition may be initiated if oral intake is prohibited or threatened for longer than a week. If the gastrointestinal tract of the patient is functioning, enteral feeding is the intervention of choice. For individuals without a functioning gastrointestinal tract, total parenteral nutrition may be the nutritional treatment of choice. The level of interventions is dictated by the patient's baseline nutritional state, disease status, risks for malnutrition from treatment, and anticipated response to therapy.

box 39-3
Nutritional Assessment

Anthropometrics Measurement
- Height
- Weight
- Body mass index
- Triceps skinfold thickness, midarm and arm muscle circumference

Laboratory Studies
- Albumin
- Transferrin
- Prealbumin
- Retinol-binding protein
- Total lymphocyte count
- Electrolyte levels
- Creatinine/height levels

Physical Examination
- Patient's appearance
- Normal body weight with respect to height, body frame, and age
- Hair, skin, teeth, gums, mucous membranes, mouth and tongue, skeletal muscles, abdomen, lower extremities, thyroid gland
- Skin assessment for turgor, edema, elasticity, dryness, tone, condition of wounds and ulcers, purpura, and bruises

Dietary Evaluation
- Quantity and quality of the diet
- Food record
- 24-hour recall (must consider culture and religious beliefs)

(Select appropriate category with a checkmark, or enter numerical value where indicated by "#.")

A. History
1. Weight change
   Overall loss in past 6 months: amount = #______kg; % loss = #______
   Change in past 2 weeks ______increase,
   ______no change,
   ______decrease.
2. Dietary intake change (relative to normal)
   ______No change
   ______Change ______duration = #______weeks.
   ______type: ______suboptimal solid diet, ______full liquid diet,
   ______hypocaloric liquids, ______starvation.
3. Gastrointestinal symptoms (that persisted for > 2 weeks)
   ______none, ______nausea, ______vomiting, ______diarrhea, ______anorexia.
4. Functional capacity
   ______No dysfunction (e.g., full capacity)
   ______Dysfunction ______duration = #______weeks.
   ______type: ______working suboptimally,
   ______ambulatory,
   ______bedridden.
5. Disease and its relation to nutritional requirements
   Primary diagnosis (specify)____
   Metabolic demand (stress): ______no stress, ______low stress,
   ______moderate stress, ______high stress.

B. Physical (for each trait specify: 0 = normal, 1+ = mild, 2+ = moderate, 3+ = severe)
#______loss of subcutaneous fat (triceps, chest)
#______muscle wasting (quadriceps, deltoids)
#______ankle edema
#______sacral edema
#______ascites

C. SGA rating (select one)
______A = Well-nourished
______B = Moderately (or suspected of being) malnourished
______C = Severely malnourished

figure 39-6 The Subjective Global Assessment (SGA), used to assess nutritional status. The final SGA rating is based on clinical judgment of the items and not a specific number. (Reprinted with permission from the American Society for Parenteral and Enteral Nutrition [ASPEN] from the following: Journal of Parenteral Enteral Nutrition 11 [1]:8–13, 1987. ASPEN does not endorse the use of this material in any form other than its entirety.)

LABORATORY STUDIES

Because the oral cavity is the only part of the gastrointestinal tract that is visible, it is essential to combine the information gleaned from the history and physical examination with the results of laboratory and diagnostic studies to assess the rest of the gastrointestinal tract. Many laboratory studies help in the diagnosis of gastrointestinal and abdominal disorders in the critically ill patient. Parameters evaluated include serum electrolytes; levels of end products of metabolism, enzymes, and proteins; and hematological parameters.

Laboratory Studies Relating to Liver Function

The liver is responsible for many functions, the most significant being bile formation and secretion, protein and fat metabolism, detoxification of many substances, and the production of clotting factors and enzymes. Table 39-4 summarizes common laboratory studies relating to liver function.

A single laboratory test or single value from any laboratory test does not give an accurate assessment of an organ's function. A series of values from a laboratory study and combinations of studies provide a more precise picture. For example, when a patient's liver enzymes and bilirubin are elevated but the alkaline phosphatase (AP) level is normal, this usually indicates injury to the hepatocytes, such as in hepatitis and cirrhosis. If the liver enzymes are within normal range and the bilirubin and AP levels are elevated, this usually indicates an extrahepatic biliary obstruction, as in distal bile duct obstruction from pancreatic cancer or a clip occluding the common bile duct from a laparoscopic cholecystectomy misadventure.

Laboratory Studies Relating to Pancreatic Function

Serum laboratory tests that relate to pancreatic function are listed in Table 39-5. Amylase and lipase are digestive enzymes secreted by the pancreas. Serum amylase is found in the pancreas, parotid glands, intestine, liver, and fallopian tubes. Lipase is found primarily in the pancreas. In acute pancreatitis, serum amylase and lipase can be elevated four to six times the normal level, whereas in chronic pancreatitis, serum amylase and lipase levels may be normal or very low because the pancreas may no longer be producing the enzymes.

The pancreas produces insulin and glucagons, hormones that aid in the regulation of serum glucose levels. When there is a disruption in normal pancreatic function or in the presence of a tumor, the production of these hormones may be altered. Frequent blood glucose monitoring is warranted. Any elevation in the serum and urine glucose levels has a cascading effect on multiple body systems, which in turn affects the patient's overall condition.[8]

table 39-4 Laboratory Studies Used to Evaluate Liver Function

Study	Normal Findings	Clinical and Nursing Significance
Bile Formation and Secretion		
Serum bilirubin		
Direct (conjugated)—soluble in water	0–5.1 μmol/L	Abnormal in biliary and liver disease; causes clinical jaundice
Indirect (unconjugated)—insoluble in water	0–14 μmol/L	Abnormal in hemolysis and in functional disorders of uptake or conjugation
Urine bilirubin	0	Urine is mahogany in color; shaking the specimen results in a light yellow foam; confirmed with Ictotest tablet or dipstick; false-positive results possible if patient is taking phenazopyridine (Pyridium)
Urobilinogen		Increased in cirrhosis; biliary obstruction with biliary tract infection; hemorrhage; and hepatoxicity; decreased in biliary obstruction without biliary tract infection; hepatocellular damage; and renal insufficiency
Urine urobilinogen	Up to 0.09–4.23 μmol/24 h	Urine specimen is collected over a 2-h period after lunch; must be placed in a dark brown container and sent to the laboratory immediately to prevent decomposition
Fecal urobilinogen	Up to 0.068–0.34 mmol/24 h	
Protein Studies		
Albumin	35–55 g/L	Decreased in cirrhosis, chronic hepatitis
Globulin	15–30 g/L	Increased in cirrhosis, chronic obstructive jaundice, viral hepatitis
Albumin:globulin ratio	1.5:1 to 2.5:1	Ratio reverses with chronic hepatitis or other chronic liver disease
Total serum protein	60–80 g/L	Individual protein measurements are of greater significance than total protein measurements
Transferrin	220–400 μg/dL	Decreased in cirrhosis, hepatitis, and malignancy; increased in severe iron deficiency anemia
Prothrombin time (PT)	11.0–14.0 sec or 100% of control	Prolonged PT in liver disease will not return to normal with vitamin K administration, whereas prolonged PT resulting from malabsorption of fat and fat-soluble vitamins will return to normal with vitamin K administration
Partial thromboplastin time (PTT)	25.0–36.0 sec	Increased with severe liver disease or therapy with heparin or other anticoagulants
α-Fetoprotein (AFP)	6–20 ng/mL	Elevated in primary hepatocellular carcinoma
Fat Metabolism		
Cholesterol	< 200 mg/dL (adults)	Decreased in parenchymal liver disease; increased in biliary obstruction
High-density lipoprotein (HDL)		
Men	35–70 mg/dL	
Women	35–85 mg/dL	
Low-density lipoprotein (LDL)	<130 mg/dL	
Very–low-density lipoprotein (VLDL)	25%–50%	
Liver Detoxification		
Serum alkaline phosphatase (AP)	20–90 U/L at 30°C	Level is elevated to more than three times normal in obstructive jaundice, intrahepatic cholestasis, liver metastasis, or granulomas; also elevated in osteoblastic diseases, Paget's disease, and hyperparathyroidism
Ammonia	15–49 μg/dL	An elevation indicates hepatocyte damage (liver converts ammonia to urea)

(continued)

table 39-4 Laboratory Studies Used to Evaluate Liver Function (Continued)

Study	Normal Findings	Clinical and Nursing Significance
Enzyme Production		
Aspartate aminotransferase (AST)	8–20 U/L	Any elevation indicates hepatocyte damage
Alanine aminotransferase (ALT)	10–32 U/L	Any elevation indicates hepatocyte damage
Lactate dehydrogenase (LDH)	200–500 U/L	Any elevation indicates hepatocyte damage
Gamma-glutamyl transferase (GGT)	0–30 U/L at 30°C	An elevation in GGT along with an elevated AP usually indicates biliary disease; helpful in the diagnosis of chronic liver disease

Other Laboratory Studies

Table 39-6 provides information about other selected laboratory studies that are used in the evaluation of gastrointestinal disorders.

DIAGNOSTIC STUDIES

The nurse caring for the critically ill patient coordinates the preparation, and possibly the timing, for many diagnostic tests. The nurse prepares the patient, the family members, or both for the test by providing a thorough explanation of how the test is performed and what information the test is expected to yield. In addition, the nurse explains the need for informed consent to perform the test, and answers any questions the patient or family members may have about the test. Diagnostic studies for evaluating the gastrointestinal tract can be divided into two categories, noninvasive and invasive, and are summarized in Table 39-7.

Radiological and Imaging Studies

Body tissue has different densities that produce different shades of black and white on an x-ray: bone tissue is high in density and appears white on an x-ray; air appears black;

(text continues on page 929)

table 39-5 Laboratory Studies Used to Evaluate Pancreatic Function

Study	Normal Findings	Clinical and Nursing Significance
Serum amylase	25–125 U/L	In acute pancreatitis, the serum levels peak between 4–8 h after onset of condition, then fall to normal within 48–72 h; low levels usually indicate pancreatic insufficiency.
Urine amylase	2 h: 2–34 units 24 h: 24–408 units	Urine values 6–10 h behind serum values; low levels indicate pancreatic insufficiency.
Serum lipase	10–40 U/L (adults)	Elevated only in pancreatitis, markedly in acute pancreatitis and pancreatic duct obstruction; remains elevated after amylase returns to baseline.
Serum glucose	65–110 mg/dL (fasting)	Patient must fast for 12 h before drawing of specimen.
Serum triglycerides	50–250 mg/dL	Patient must fast for 12 h before drawing of specimen; levels increased in alcoholic cirrhosis, diabetes mellitus (untreated), high-carbohydrate diet, hyperlipoproteinemia, and hypertension; levels decreased in malnutrition, vigorous exercise.
Serum calcium		
Total	8.2–10.2 mg/dL	High total calcium levels seen in cancer of the liver, pancreas, and other organs.
Ionized	4.65–5.28 mg/dL	Useful in tracking the course of disorders such as cancer and acute pancreatitis.
Fecal fat	2–5 g/24 h	Content of greater than 6 g/24 h is suggestive of a decrease in the body's ability to absorb foods; indicative of pancreatic exocrine insufficiency as in chronic pancreatitis.

table 39-6 Other Selected Laboratory Studies Used in the Diagnosis of Gastrointestinal Disorders

Study	Normal Findings	Clinical and Nursing Significance
Stool specimen		
Occult blood	None	Positive test suggests possible malignancy.
Fat	2–5 g/24 h	Screening test for steatorrhea when malabsorption syndrome or pancreatic insufficiency is suspected.
Ova and parasites	None	Positive test suggests infection.
Pus	None	Increased amount of pus may indicate ulcerative colitis, abscess, or anal or rectal fissure.
Pathogens	None	Common pathogens are *Salmonella typhi* (typhoid fever), *Shigella* (dysentery), *Vibrio cholerae* (cholera), *Yersinia* (enterocolitis), *Escherichia coli* and *Aeromonas* (gastroenteritis), *Staphylococcus aureus, Clostridium botulinum,* and *Clostridium perfringens* (food poisoning).
Urea breath test	Negative	Detects the presence of *Helicobacter pylori*
Hydrogen breath test	Negative	Determines the amount of hydrogen expelled in the breath after it is produced in the colon and absorbed into the blood; aids in the diagnosis of bacterial overgrowth in the intestine and short bowel syndrome.

table 39-7 Diagnostic Studies Used to Evaluate the Gastrointestinal Tract

Study	Description	Indications	Invasiveness	Preparation	Contrast
Abdominal film "flat plate of the abdomen"	Radiology test used to visualize a single flat plane; shows organ size, position, intactness, and normal gas patterns in the stomach, small intestine, and colon	Aids in diagnosis of intestinal obstruction, organ rupture, masses, foreign bodies, abnormal fluid or air ("stones, bones, gas, masses")	Noninvasive	None	No
Upper gastrointestinal (GI) series (barium swallow)	Radiology test used to visualize the esophagus, stomach, and duodenum; barium enhances image; double-contrast study administers barium first followed by a radiolucent substance, such as air, to help coat bowel mucosa for better visualization of any type of lesion	Aids in diagnosis of hiatal hernia, ulcers, tumors, foreign bodies, bowel obstruction	Noninvasive	NPO	Yes
Upper GI series with small bowel follow-through	Radiology test used to visualize the jejunum, ileum, and cecum	Aids in the diagnosis of tumors, Crohn's disease, Meckel's diverticulum	Noninvasive	NPO	Yes

(continued)

table 39-7 Diagnostic Studies Used to Evaluate the Gastrointestinal Tract (Continued)

Study	Description	Indications	Invasiveness	Preparation	Contrast
Enteroclysis	Radiology test used to visualize entire small intestine; continuous infusion (through a duodenal tube) of air in a barium sulfate suspension along with methylcellulose fills the intestinal loops; transit of contrast filmed at intervals for progress through jejunum and ileum	Aids in diagnosis of partial bowel obstruction or diverticula	Invasive	NPO	Yes
Barium enema	Radiology test used to visualize the colon; barium enhances image; air may be introduced after the barium to provide a double-contrast study	Aids in diagnosis of polyps, tumors, fistulas, obstruction, diverticula, and stenosis	Noninvasive	Bowel cleansing	Yes
Gastric lavage	Aspiration of stomach contents and washing out of the stomach by a large gastric tube	Aids in diagnosis of upper GI bleeding, also used to arrest hemorrhage and prepare for further tests	Invasive	None	No
Paracentesis	Aspiration of peritoneal fluid	Laboratory studies (such as amylase and lipase to assess for pancreatitis); cytologic studies (to detect tumors); comfort measure (to alleviate accumulation of ascitic fluid)	Invasive	None	No
Peritoneal lavage	Irrigation of peritoneal cavity to examine irrigating fluid for blood	Blunt or penetrating trauma to the abdomen	Invasive	None	No
Biopsy					
Percutaneous	A needle is placed through the skin to obtain tissue specimen for pathology evaluation	Aids in diagnosis of malignancy	Invasive	NPO	No
Fine-needle aspiration (FNA)	A thin needle is used to obtain cells or minute tissue fragments from a suspect area for examination by light microscopy; usually guided by radiologists with fluoroscopy, ultrasound, computed tomography, or magnetic resonance imaging	Aids in diagnosis of malignancy	Invasive	NPO	No

(continued)

table 39-7 Diagnostic Studies Used to Evaluate the Gastrointestinal Tract (Continued)

Study	Description	Indications	Invasiveness	Preparation	Contrast
Ultrasonography (sonogram)	Use of high-frequency sound waves over an abdominal organ to obtain an image of the structure	Aids in diagnosis of masses, dilated bile ducts, gallstones, and ascites	Noninvasive	NPO	No
Hepatobiliary scan	Intravenously injected radioisotope is primarily taken up by the liver and then secreted into the bile, allowing visualization of the biliary system, gallbladder, and duodenum (size, function, vascularity, and blood flow)	Aids in the diagnoses of common bile duct obstruction, acute and chronic cholecystitis, bile leaks, biliary dyskinesia, and biliary atresia; also used to evaluate liver transplant function	Noninvasive	NPO	Yes
Tagged red blood cell scan (technetium-labeled red blood cell scintigraphy)	Red blood cells are labeled with technetium and injected intravenously; images are obtained with a gamma camera that can identify areas of increased radioactivity as a site of slow or intermittent GI hemorrhage	Aids in the diagnosis of GI bleeding	Noninvasive	None	Yes
Computed tomography (CT) scan	A radiological procedure that uses narrow x-ray beams to produce cross-sectional images of organs and tissues; can be performed with or without contrast medium; fast-spin, spiral, three-dimensional CT scans now provide more exact information	Excellent for visualizing the abdomen, retroperitoneal structures, tumors, cysts, collection of fluid, air in a cavity, bleeding or pulmonary embolism	Noninvasive	NPO	Yes/No
Magnetic resonance imaging (MRI)	Diagnostic study that does not use radiation; obtains images by passing the patient through a tubular device that generates a powerful electromagnetic field; radiofrequency waves are transmitted into the patient in a controlled manner so that the patient's hydrogen ions (protons) emit radiofrequency signals that are processed by a computer to produce an image	Useful in evaluating abdominal soft tissue and blood vessels, abscesses, fistulas, tumors, and sources of bleeding	Noninvasive	No metal devices attached to or implanted in the patient; patient must be able to lie quietly for a period of time	No

(continued)

table 39-7 Diagnostic Studies Used to Evaluate the Gastrointestinal Tract (Continued)

Study	Description	Indications	Invasiveness	Preparation	Contrast
Magnetic resonance cholangiopancreatography (MRCP)	Similar to MRI; because no contrast agent is required, MRCP is ideal for patients with allergies to iodine-based contrast medium	Aids in the diagnosis of disorders affecting the pancreatic ducts and biliary tree	Noninvasive	No metal devices attached to or implanted in the patient	No
Percutaneous transhepatic cholangiography (PTC)	Radiological procedure done under fluoroscopy to examine the intrahepatic and extrahepatic biliary ducts after injection of contrast medium into the biliary tree through percutaneous needle injection	Helps to distinguish obstructive jaundice caused by liver disease from jaundice caused by biliary obstruction (e.g., from a tumor, common bile duct injury, stones within the bile ducts, or sclerosing cholangitis)	Invasive	NPO	Yes
Percutaneous transhepatic biliary drainage (PTBD)	A biliary catheter is placed during a PTC; the biliary catheter may be placed to the obstruction or it may bypass the obstruction to allow the free flow of bile; catheter relieves jaundice and pruritus; improves nutritional status; allows easy access into the biliary tree for further procedures; can be used as an anatomical landmark and stent at the time of surgery	Biliary obstruction resulting in jaundice, cholangitis, sepsis, or pain	Invasive	NPO	Yes
Positron emission tomography (PET)	A computerized radiographic technique that uses radioactive substances to examine the metabolic activity of body structures	Useful for precisely locating a tumor	Noninvasive	None	Yes
Angiography	A radiographic study of selected arteries and veins to see defects in the walls of the vessels; also used to evaluate blood flow through the vessels	Usually done when initial, noninvasive procedures are insufficient in revealing the cause of a suspected vascular defect	Invasive	NPO	Yes

and soft tissue results in shades of gray. The stomach and intestines usually contain some air and appear darker on an x-ray. Solid organs, such as the pancreas, spleen, kidneys, or liver, appear grayer on an x-ray.[9]

Endoscopic Studies

The use of an endoscope is an important adjunct to radiographic studies because it allows direct observation of portions of the intestinal tract. A flexible fiberoptic endoscope, designed with a moveable tip, can be manipulated through the intestinal tract by the operator. It also includes an instrument channel that allows for biopsy of lesions, such as tumors, ulcers, or areas of inflammation. Fluids can be aspirated from the lumen of the intestinal tract, and air can be insufflated to distend the intestinal tract for better observation. Cytology brushes and electrocautery snares can be passed through the scope. Special studies of the common bile duct and the pancreatic duct, or endoscopic retrograde cholangiopancreatography (ERCP), use a side-viewing upper intestinal endoscope.[10] Table 39-8 describes endoscopic procedures used to evaluate the gastrointestinal tract.

Other Diagnostic Studies

In addition to radiological and imaging studies and endoscopic procedures, there are other studies specifically designed to aid in the diagnosis of gastrointestinal disorders.[11] Table 39-9 provides information about selected diagnostic studies used to diagnose specific gastrointestinal disorders.

table 39-8 Endoscopic Studies Used to Evaluate the Gastrointestinal Tract

Study	Description	Indications	Invasiveness	Preparation	Contrast
Esophagogastroduodenoscopy (EGD)	Endoscope passed through the mouth and advanced to visualize the esophagus, stomach, and duodenum; any abnormalities can be photographed and biopsied; bleeding areas may be cauterized and varices may be injected with sclerosing agents	Helps to diagnose acute or chronic upper GI bleeding, esophageal or gastric varices, polyps, tumors, ulcers, esophagitis, gastritis, esophageal stenosis, and gastroesophageal reflux	Invasive	NPO	No
Colonoscopy	Flexible fiberoptic endoscope passed through the rectum and advanced to visualize the large intestine; any abnormalities can be photographed and biopsied; polyps can be removed and bleeding areas may be cauterized	Helps to diagnose bleeding, diverticulosis, polyps, stricture, tumor, or inflammatory bowel disease (Crohn's disease or ulcerative colitis)	Invasive	Bowel cleansing	No
Proctoscopy (anoscopy)	Rigid scope passed through the rectum to visualize the mucosal surface of the anus and rectum	Helps to diagnose polyps, bleeding, tumors, and other defects	Invasive	None	No
Sigmoidoscopy	Flexible fiberoptic endoscope passed through the rectum and advanced to visualize the rectum, sigmoid colon, and proximal colon; any lesions can be biopsied	Helps to diagnose tumors, polyps, diverticula, or bleeding	Invasive	Enema	No

(continued)

table 39-8 Endoscopic Studies Used to Evaluate the Gastrointestinal Tract (Continued)

Study	Description	Indications	Invasiveness	Preparation	Contrast
Endoscopic retrograde cholangiopancreatography (ERCP)	Flexible fiberoptic endoscope inserted into the esophagus, passed through the stomach, and into the duodenum to visualize the common bile duct, hepatic bile ducts, and pancreatic ducts; the common bile duct and pancreatic duct are cannulated and contrast medium is injected into the ducts, permitting visualization and radiographic evaluation	Can detect extrahepatic biliary obstruction (e.g., from stones, tumors of the bile duct, strictures or injuries to the bile duct); intrahepatic biliary obstruction caused by stones or tumor; and pancreatic disease, such as chronic pancreatitis, pseudocysts, or tumors	Invasive	NPO	Yes
Endoscopic ultrasonography	Endoscopy and ultrasonography are used to visualize the GI tract; an ultrasonic transducer built into the distal end of the endoscope allows for high-quality resolution of the walls of the GI tract	Useful in evaluating and staging tumors of the GI tract	Invasive	NPO	No

table 39-9 Other Selected Diagnostic Studies Used in the Diagnosis of Gastrointestinal Disorders

Study	Description	Normal Findings
Gastric emptying studies	Liquid and solid components of a meal are tagged with a radionuclide marker. After ingesting the meal, the rate of passage of the radioactive substance out of the stomach is measured by a scintiscanner. Useful in diagnosing gastric motility disorders	Normal transit
Gastric analysis	Analysis of gastric juice yields information about the secretory activity of the gastric mucosa and the presence or degree of gastric retention, which is useful to help diagnose patients with pyloric or duodenal obstruction.	Normal contents
Gastric acid stimulation (usually performed in conjunction with gastric analysis)	Histamine or pentagastrin is given subcutaneously to stimulate gastric secretions. Gastric specimens are collected at intervals for analysis. Helps to determine the presence or absence of malignant cells.	11–20 mEq/h after stimulation
Manometry	Measurement of pressures using a water-filled catheter connected to a transducer passed into the esophagus, stomach, colon, or rectum to evaluate contractility; useful in detecting motility disorders of the esophagus and lower esophageal sphincter (LES); gastroduodenal, small intestine, and colonic manometry are used to evaluate delayed gastric emptying and gastric and intestinal motility disorders such as irritable bowel syndrome or atonic colon; anorectal manometry measures the resting tone of the internal anal sphincter and the contractility of the external anal sphincter, which is helpful in evaluation of chronic constipation or fecal incontinence	Values differ at various levels of the intestine

clinical applicability challenges

Self-Challenge: Critical Thinking

1. *A female patient complains of acute abdominal pain. What critical history should be elicited and how should the physical examination proceed?*
2. *An elderly, cachectic male patient has sustained multiple injuries as a result of a motor vehicle accident. What factors should be included in the initial nutritional assessment?*

Study Questions

1. *The anthropometric measurement that reflects the status of the body's fat stores is*
   a. *weight.*
   b. *midarm circumference.*
   c. *midarm muscle circumference.*
   d. *triceps skinfold.*
2. *Which of the following would be considered a normal finding when elicited during abdominal percussion?*
   a. *Dullness of the left upper outer quadrant during deep inspiration*
   b. *Hyperresonance over the liver*
   c. *Tympany over the stomach*
   d. *Dullness predominating over the lower quadrants*
3. *Which of the following sounds is most likely to be heard over the abdomen in a patient with early intestinal obstruction?*
   a. *Intermittent soft gurgling sounds at the rate of 20 per minute*
   b. *Loud, high-pitched, tinkling bowel sounds*
   c. *Hypoactive sounds due to intestinal muscle weakness*
   d. *Peritoneal friction rubs*
4. *Which of the following is an enzyme produced in the liver that is the end product of protein metabolism and an important indicator of liver function?*
   a. *Ammonia*
   b. *Gamma-glutamyl transpeptidase (GGT)*
   c. *Bilirubin*
   d. *Albumin*
5. *The invasive study that best visualizes the common bile duct and pancreatic duct as well as permitting diagnostic and therapeutic procedures is*
   a. *an abdominal plain film.*
   b. *computed tomography (CT) scan.*
   c. *endoscopic retrograde cholangiopancreatography (ERCP).*
   d. *magnetic resonance cholangiopancreatography (MRCP).*

REFERENCES

1. Ignatavicius DD, Workman ML: Medical-Surgical Nursing: Critical Thinking for Collaborative Care (4th Ed). Philadelphia, WB Saunders, 2002
2. Fuller J, Schaller-Ayers J: Health Assessment: A Nursing Approach (3rd Ed). Philadelphia, Lippincott Williams & Wilkins, 1999
3. Case KO, Cuddy PG, Dooling McGurk EP: Nutrition support in the critically ill patient. Crit Care Nurs Q 22(4):75–89, 2000
4. Silen W: Cope's Early Diagnosis of the Acute Abdomen (20th Ed). Oxford, Oxford University Press, 2000
5. Bickley LS, Szalagyi PS, Stackhouse JG: Bates' Guide to Physical Examination and History Taking (8th Ed). Philadelphia, Lippincott Williams & Wilkins, 2002
6. Orient JM: Sapira's Art and Science of Bedside Diagnosis (2nd Ed). Philadelphia, Lippincott Williams & Wilkins, 2000
7. Quirk J: Malnutrition in critically ill patients in intensive care units. Br J Nurs 9(9):537–541, 2000
8. Segen JC: The Patient's Guide to Medical Tests (2nd Ed). New York, Facts On File, 2002
9. Fleckenstein P, Tranum-Jensen J: Anatomy in Diagnostic Imaging. Philadelphia, WB Saunders, 2001
10. Ogilvie J, Norwitz L, Kalloo AN: Johns Hopkins Manual for Gastrointestinal Endoscopy Nursing. Thorofare, NJ, Slack, 2002
11. Gore RM, Levine MS: Textbook of Gastrointestinal Radiology (2nd Ed). Philadelphia, WB Saunders, 2000

OTHER SELECTED READING

Brant WE, Helms CA: Fundamentals of Diagnostic Radiology. Philadelphia, Lippincott Williams & Wilkins, 1999

Braunwald E: Harrison's Principles of Internal Medicine (15th Ed). New York, McGraw-Hill, 2001

Dambro M, Griffith J: Griffith's 5 Minute Clinical Consult (7th Ed). Baltimore, Williams & Wilkins, 2001

Heyland DK, Novak F, Drover JW, et al: Should immunonutrition become routine in critically ill patients? A systematic review of the evidence. JAMA 286(8):944–953, 2001

Swanson RW, Winkelman C: Exploring the benefits and myths of enteral feeding in the critically ill. Crit Care Nurs Q 24(4):67–74, 2002

Swartz MH: Textbook of Physical Diagnosis: History and Examination (4th Ed). Philadelphia, WB Saunders, 2001

Tierney L, McPhee S, Papadaris M: Current Medical Diagnosis and Treatment (42nd Ed). Old Tappan, NJ, Appleton & Lange, 2002

chapter

40

Patient Management: Gastrointestinal System

VALERIE K. SABOL ■ ALLISON G. STEELE

objectives

Based on the content in this chapter, the reader should be able to:

- Explain how physiological stresses of illness and injury alter the body's needs for energy.
- Identify and describe the different forms of malnutrition.
- Identify and describe enteral and parenteral nutrition with regard to indications, assessment, management, and complications.

Health and nutrition have a symbiotic relationship. Physiological stressors, such as illness and injury, alter the body's metabolic and energy demands. Although early identification and nutritional intervention can lessen morbidity and mortality risks in critically ill patients, it is often the underlying disease process that must be identified and corrected before the body can reverse abnormal nutrient metabolism.[1,2] This chapter presents an overview of physiological stress and its effect on metabolism, types of malnutrition, and the indications, assessment, and management of enteral and parenteral nutrition support therapies and the complications associated with these therapies.

In addition to the variety of macronutrients and micronutrients that are discussed later in this chapter, it is important to understand the variety of medications administered to the critically ill to combat disease processes and their associated side effects. Table 40-1 summarizes many of the common gastrointestinal medications administered to critically ill patients who are concurrently receiving nutrition support therapy.

According to the laws of thermodynamics, energy can be neither created nor destroyed. Through the processes of metabolism, people obtain energy from the foods (or organic fuels) they consume. Metabolism has two parts: anabolism and catabolism. Anabolism is a building-up and repair process that requires energy. Catabolism consists of breaking down food and body tissues for the purpose of liberating energy.

Glucose is the obligatory fuel of the body, and of the brain and nervous system in particular. The nervous system cannot store or synthesize glucose as a fuel source, so it relies on glucose extraction from the bloodstream. The brain and nervous system depend on glucose to meet their metabolic requirements. The liver regulates glucose entry into the circulatory system because it has the ability to both store and synthesize glucose. Excess glucose is converted and stored as either glycogen or fatty acids (triglycerides). Although glucose can be converted to fatty acids for storage, there is no pathway for converting fatty acids back to glucose. Instead, fatty acids are used directly as a fuel source or are converted to ketones by the liver. After prolonged starvation, the body adapts to preserve vital proteins by using ketones, rather than glucose, as energy. Ketoacidosis occurs when ketone production exceeds utilization.

The pancreatic hormones glucagon and insulin have opposing functions in metabolic processes. Glucagon stimulates glycogenolysis (glycogen breakdown) and gluconeogenesis (the process of glucose synthesis from other

(text continues on page 937)

table 40-1 ■ **Mechanisms of Action, Indications, Common Adverse Effects, and Comments for Common Gastrointestinal Medications**

Agent	Mechanism of Action	Indication	Common Adverse Effects	Comments
Antacids				
Aluminum carbonate	Neutralization of gastric acid; binding phosphates in the gastrointestinal tract	Symptomatic relief of gastric irritation, prevention of urinary phosphate stone development, binding of phosphate in chronic renal failure	Fecal impaction, cramps, constipation, hypophosphatemia (when given in excessive doses)	Monitor phosphorus levels.
Aluminum hydroxide (Amphojel, AlternaGEL)	Neutralization of gastric acid; binding phosphates in the gastrointestinal tract	Symptomatic relief of gastric irritation, hyperphosphatemia in chronic renal failure	Constipation, hypophosphatemia (when given in excessive doses)	Less phosphate binding than aluminum carbonate. Monitor phosphorus levels.
Calcium carbonate (Tums, Caltrate)	Neutralization of gastric acid	Symptomatic relief of gastric irritation, calcium supplementation	Headaches	Usually well tolerated. Monitor calcium and phosphorus levels.
Magnesium hydroxide (Milk of Magnesia)	Neutralization of gastric acid	Symptomatic relief of gastric irritation, hypomagnesemia, constipation	Hypermagnesemia, abdominal cramping and diarrhea (with high doses)	Monitor magnesium levels.
Dihydroxyaluminum, sodium carbonate (Rolaids)	Neutralization of gastric acid; reduction of pepsin	Symptomatic relief of gastric irritation	Constipation	Use with caution in sodium-restricted patients.
Histamine Type 2 (H_2) Receptor Antagonists				
Cimetidine (Tagamet)	Inhibition of histamine at H_2 receptor sites on gastric parietal cells, which inhibits gastric acid secretion	GERD, PUD, acid hypersecretory states	Confusion, headaches, diarrhea	May cause rare blood dyscrasias. Monitor CBC.
Ranitidine (Zantac)	Inhibition of histamine at H_2 receptor sites on gastric parietal cells, which inhibits gastric acid secretion	GERD, PUD, acid hypersecretory states	Headaches, dizziness, constipation	May cause hepatotoxicity and rare blood dyscrasias.
Famotidine (Pepcid)	Inhibition of histamine at H_2 receptor sites on gastric parietal cells, which inhibits gastric acid secretion	GERD, PUD, acid hypersecretory states	Headaches, dizziness	May cause seizures, bronchospasm, constipation, or thrombocytopenia. Monitor CBC.
Nizatidine (Axid)	Inhibition of histamine at H_2 receptor sites on gastric parietal cells, which inhibits gastric acid secretion	GERD, PUD, acid hypersecretory states	Dizziness, headaches, diarrhea	
Proton Pump Inhibitors				
Omeprazole (Prilosec), lansoprazole (Prevacid), rapeprazole (Aciphex), pantoprazole (Protonix), esomeprazole (Nexium)	Suppression of gastric acid secretion by inhibition of H^+, K^+-ATPase pump (proton pump) of parietal cells, blocking final step in acid production	Reflux esophagitis, treatment of gastric and duodenal ulcers, pathological hypersecretory states (Zollinger-Ellison syndrome)	Headaches, diarrhea, abdominal pain	Less common side effects include nausea, vomiting, and dizziness.

(continued)

table 40-1 ■ Mechanisms of Action, Indications, Common Adverse Effects, and Comments for Common Gastrointestinal Medications (Continued)

Agent	Mechanism of Action	Indication	Common Adverse Effects	Comments
Pancreatic Enzymes				
Pancreatin (Creon, Donnazyme, Ultrase)	Assistance in the digestion of carbohydrates, fats, and proteins	Replacement in pancreatic enzyme deficiencies, cystic fibrosis	Nausea, diarrhea, cramping, anorexia, hypersensitivity reactions, perianal irritation	
Pancrealipase (Pancrease, Viokase)	Assistance in the digestion of carbohydrates, fats, and proteins	Replacement in pancreatic enzyme deficiencies, steatorrhea of malabsorption, cystic fibrosis, postgastrectomy, or postpancreatectomy	Nausea, diarrhea, cramping, anorexia, hypersensitivity reactions, perianal irritation	
Antidiarrheals				
Attapulgite (Kaopectate)	Absorption of toxins produced by bacterial and gastrointestinal irritants; decrease in gastric motility and stool water content	Diarrhea	Increased potassium loss, interference with absorption of medications	
Bismuth subsalicylate (Pepto Bismol)	Slowing of motility; antimicrobial activity against gastrointestinal microbes; antisecretory sensitivity	Diarrhea, prophylaxis of traveler's diarrhea	Tongue discoloration, dark stools	Assess electrolytes if diarrhea persists. Use cautiously in patients using other salicylates.
Cholestyramine (Questran)	Absorption of bile salts, which can cause diarrhea; absorption of *Clostridium difficile* toxin	Diarrhea caused by bile salts or *C. difficile*	Constipation	Because it may alter absorption of other medications, administer other medications at least 1 h before cholestyramine.
Loperamide (Imodium)	Slowing intestinal motility, including peristalsis	Acute and chronic diarrhea	Abdominal distension, constipation, drowsiness, dizziness, nausea, vomiting	
Tincture of opium (Paragoric, DTO)	Decrease in gastrointestinal motility and peristalsis, decrease in digestive secretions	Acute diarrhea, relief of abdominal cramping	Drowsiness, lightheadedness, bradycardia	Side effects are related to opioid content. Other possible reactions include allergic reactions, vomiting, dizziness, sweating, constipation, and habituation.
Laxatives				
Bowel Evacuants				
Polyethylene glycol with electrolytes (Colyte, NuLytely, GoLYTELY)	Nonabsorbable solution that acts like an osmotic agent	Bowel cleansing before colonoscopy or bowel surgery	Transient bloating, nausea, cramping	
Bulk-Forming Agents				
Calcium polycarbophil (Fibercon), methylcellulose (Citracel), psyllium (Metamucil)	Nondigestable plant cell wall draws water into the feces and softens stool; absorption of excess water in the stool	Diarrhea, constipation	Flatulence, impaction (if feces is obstructed)	Generally well tolerated.

(continued)

table 40-1 ■ Mechanisms of Action, Indications, Common Adverse Effects, and Comments for Common Gastrointestinal Medications (Continued)

Agent	Mechanism of Action	Indication	Common Adverse Effects	Comments
Lactulose (Cephulac, Enulose)	Hyperosmolality draws water into the intestinal lumen, increasing stool water content and softening stool; prevention of absorption of ammonia in the colon	Constipation, prevention and treatment of hepatic encephalopathy	Flatulence, cramping, impaction (if feces is obstructed)	For use in prevention and treatment of hepatic encephalopathy, titrate dose to two to three loose stools a day. Monitor serum ammonia levels.
Polyethylene glycol (MiraLax)	Nonabsorbable solution that acts like an osmotic agent	Constipation	Nausea, abdominal bloating, cramping, diarrhea	
Saline Laxatives				
Magnesium citrate (Citrate of Magnesium)	Magnesium and sodium salts are poorly absorbed, drawing water into the intestinal lumen	Constipation, cleansing of the colon before examination	Cramps, flatulence, nausea, vomiting	Do not use in renal disease. Observe for hypermagnesemia (watching for thirst, drowsiness, dizziness).
Sodium biphosphate (Fleet Phospha-soda, Fleet Enema)	Increase in water absorption in the small intestine through osmosis	Constipation, acute bowel evacuation before a bowel or colon examination	Nausea, cramps	May precipitate or exacerbate cardiac, renal, or seizure shock disorder.
Stimulants				
Bisacodyl (Dulcolax)	Increase in peristalsis by direct effect on nerve endings in colonic mucosa	Constipation, evacuation of bowel before examination		Can cause habituation with gradual lessening effect in long-term use. PO onset is 6 to 10 h; PR onset is 15 to 60 min.
Cascara	Increase in propulsive movements through chemical irritation of the colon	Constipation	Discoloration of urine (red or yellow-brown)	May cause habituation. Onset is 6 to 10 h.
Senna (Senokot, SenokotXTRA)	Stimulation of propulsion	Constipation	Discoloration of urine	Natural product from cassia
Phenolphthalein (Ex-Lax)	Stimulation of peristalsis (similar to bisacodyl)	Constipation		May cause an allergic reaction; discontinue use if rash develops.
Stool Softeners				
Docusate sodium (Surfak, Colace)	Increase in the penetration of the feces by water and fat; softening of the stool	Constipation	Cramping, diarrhea	Prolonged or excessive use may cause habituation or electrolyte abnormalities.
Stimulant/Stool Softeners				
Glycerin	Drawing water into the colon (by high osmotic pressure)	Constipation	Headaches, nausea, vomiting	
Antiemetics				
Trimethobenzamide (Tigan)	Inhibition of the chemoreceptor trigger zone, which then inhibits the vomiting center	Symptomatic relief of nausea and vomiting	Hypersensitivity, drowsiness, hypotension, diarrhea, depression, vertigo	

(continued)

table 40-1 Mechanisms of Action, Indications, Common Adverse Effects, and Comments for Common Gastrointestinal Medications (Continued)

Agent	Mechanism of Action	Indication	Common Adverse Effects	Comments
Prochlorperazine (Compazine)	Blocking of dopamine receptors in the chemoreceptor trigger zone in the brainstem	Nausea, vomiting	Extrapyramidal side effects such as drowsiness, blurred vision, tachycardia, and respiratory depression	
Promethazine (Phenergan)	Competition with histamine in blood vessels and gastrointestinal and respiratory systems to decrease allergic responses	Nausea, vomiting, motion sickness, sedation	Dizziness, drowsiness, constipation, urinary retention	Other reactions may include thrombocytopenia, agranulocytosis, and hemolytic anemia.
Dolasetron (Anzemet)	Blocking serotonin ($5\text{-}HT_3$) receptors in the chemoreceptor trigger zone and gastrointestinal tract	Nausea and vomiting associated with chemotherapy, prevention and treatment of postoperative nausea and vomiting	ECG changes, hypertension, abdominal pain, diarrhea, urinary retention	
Granisetron (Kytril)	Blocking serotonin ($5\text{-}HT_3$) receptors in the chemoreceptor trigger zone and gastrointestinal tract	Nausea and vomiting associated with chemotherapy and radiation	Headache, constipation, asthenia	Use with caution in patients with liver disease.
Ondansetron (Zofran)	Blocking serotonin ($5\text{-}HT_3$) receptors in the chemoreceptor trigger zone and gastrointestinal tract	Nausea and vomiting associated with chemotherapy, prevention of postoperative nausea and vomiting	Diarrhea, bronchospasm, fatigue, constipation	
Other				
Sucralfate (Carafate)	Formation of a protective covering at ulcer site	Short-term treatment of peptic ulcers	Constipation	Because it may alter absorption of other medications, patient should take other medications at least 2 h before sucralfate.
Metoclopramide (Reglan)	Stimulation of upper gastrointestinal motility; decrease in inhibitory tone	Diabetic gastroparesis, delayed gastric emptying, short-term treatment of GERD, prevention of postoperative nausea and vomiting, facilitation of small bowel feeding tube placement	Diarrhea, constipation, drowsiness, restlessness	May occasionally have extrapyramidal side effects.
Misoprostol (Cytotec)	Prostaglandin analog increases bicarbonate and mucus release and decreases acid secretions	Prevention of aspirin- and NSAID-induced ulcers	Diarrhea, nausea, vomiting, flatulence	Use with caution in pregnant women and in women of childbearing age; it increases uterine contractions, which may cause abortion.

(continued)

table 40-1 ■ Mechanisms of Action, Indications, Common Adverse Effects, and Comments for Common Gastrointestinal Medications (Continued)

Agent	Mechanism of Action	Indication	Common Adverse Effects	Comments
Octreotide (Sandostatin)	Synthetic analog of somostatin, inhibition of the secretion of gastrin, vasoactive intestinal peptide (VIP), insulin, glucagon, motilin, secretin, and pancreatic polypeptides	Secretory diarrhea, acute variceal hemorrhage	Edema, flushing, dizziness, headache, abdominal pain, constipation, diarrhea, hyperglycemia, hypoglycemia	Monitor blood sugars and adjust insulin requirements.

CBC, complete blood count; *GERD*, gastroesophageal reflux disease; *NSAIDs*, nonsteroidal anti-inflammatory drugs; *PUD*, peptic ulcer disease.

sources such as proteins), and increases lipolysis (fat breakdown and mobilization). Insulin, in contrast, helps transport glucose for storage into the cells and tissues, prevents fat breakdown, and increases protein synthesis.

Glycogenolysis is controlled by the hormone glucagon and the catecholamines epinephrine and norepinephrine (which are released from the adrenal medulla in times of stress). Once glucose and glycogen stores have been exhausted (usually within 8 to 12 hours), hepatic gluconeogenesis increases dramatically to meet metabolic demands.[3] Hormones that stimulate gluconeogenesis include glucagon and the glucocorticoid hormone, cortisol. If catabolic processes continue without the support of energy, amino acids, and essential nutrients, depletion of existing body stores compromises overall bodily health and function, and the patient progresses toward a malnourished state.

Approximately 15% to 20% of hospitalized patients have evidence of malnutrition.[3] The most important reason to properly nourish patients is to prevent the immunosuppression and impairment of physiological organ function that result from malnutrition. Malnutrition from starvation alone can usually be corrected by replacing body stores of essential nutrients. However, malnutrition resulting from critical illness and disease processes that alter metabolism is not as easily rectified.

The degree of starvation and physiological stress determines the extent and type of malnutrition. The three major types of protein-energy malnutrition are marasmus, kwashiorkor, and protein–calorie malnutrition. Marasmus is a more severe, cachectic process, whereby virtually all of the available fat stores have been exhausted from prolonged calorie deficiency and severe muscle wasting is evident. Despite this, albumin, a visceral protein measurement, may be within normal limits or only slightly reduced.[3] Treatment requires slow initiation of nutrition and fluid volume to prevent the complications associated with sudden fluid shifts, electrolyte abnormalities, and cardiorespiratory failure.

In contrast to the adaptive response of relative protein sparing of marasmus, kwashiorkor and protein-calorie malnutrition are typically caused by an acute, life-threatening illness, such as surgery, trauma, or sepsis. Kwashiorkor tends to be seen in children in developing countries who have had prolonged periods of protein malnutrition, whereas protein-calorie malnutrition is more commonly seen in developed countries and is due to depletion of fat, muscle wasting, and micronutrient deficiencies from acute and chronic illness. Typically, during periods of high acuity when the patient is relegated to NPO status (*nil per os*, nothing by mouth) for surgery, diagnostic testing, or a number of other medical complications, hypermetabolism increases protein and energy demands. Although the critically ill patient may appear nourished, this is often due to the masking effects of generalized edema—the result of extracellular fluid shifts caused by low-protein oncotic pressures in the intravascular space. Other than edema, clinical signs of protein malnutrition include skin breakdown, poor wound healing, surgical dehiscence, or a combination of the three. Additionally, hair can easily be plucked, and hair remnants are often noted on the patient's pillowcase and sheets. Laboratory data reveal low serum albumin levels, and treatment requires aggressive repletion of protein stores.[3] The fact that protein malnutrition is much easier to prevent than to treat reinforces intense nursing vigilance over the patient's nutrition status.

Both marasmus and kwashiorkor can coexist. Typically, this is seen when a marasmic patient is exposed to an acute stressor such as surgery, trauma, or sepsis. Although each situation must be evaluated individually, aggressive protein and calorie replacement is often indicated. Regardless of the type, or types, of malnutrition, vigilant monitoring is crucial to the success of nutrition therapy.

A nutritional assessment should be completed on all critically ill or injured patients early in their hospitalization to determine the need for nutritional support. Goals of care in nutritional support include the following: prevention and treatment of macronutrient and micronutrient deficiencies, maintenance of fluid and electrolyte balance, prevention of infection and other complications associated with nutritional support, and improvement of patient morbidity and mortality. Meeting these goals involves a multidisciplinary approach that includes the nurse, physician, dietitian, and pharmacist. Sample nursing diagnoses and collaborative problems are given in Box 40-1. After a dietitian determines nutritional needs, a method of delivering nutritional

box 40-1 *Examples of Nursing Diagnoses and Collaborative Problems for the Patient With Gastrointestinal Problems*

- Imbalanced Nutrition: Less than Body Requirements
- Imbalanced Nutrition: More than Body Requirements
- Risk for Aspiration related to reduced level of consciousness, depressed cough and gag reflexes, incompetent lower esophageal sphincter, delayed gastric emptying, displaced feeding tube
- Diarrhea related to altered dietary intake, malabsorption, concomitant drug therapy, type of formula, bacterial contamination, stress/anxiety
- Risk for Infection related to invasive procedure and delivery of high concentrations of glucose parenterally

supplementation must be selected. In patients unable to meet their nutritional needs with oral intake, nutritional supplementation may be delivered by either enteral or parenteral routes. Figure 40-1 outlines the decision-making process. Considerations for special populations are given in Boxes 40-2 and 40-3.

ENTERAL NUTRITION

Enteral nutrition refers to any form of nutrition delivered to the gastrointestinal tract. For those patients with an intact gastrointestinal tract, the enteral route is the preferred method of nutritional support. A clinical rule of thumb is, "if the gut works, use it."

The gastrointestinal mucosa depends on nutrient delivery and adequate blood flow to prevent atrophy, thereby maintaining the absorptive, barrier, and immunological functions of the intestine.[4–6] Enterocytes are tightly packed epithelial cells that line the intestinal lumen and function as a barrier to bacterial invasion. Gut-associated lymphoid tissue (GALT) lines the gastrointestinal tract and is associated with maintenance of the immunological function of the mucosa.[4] GALT produces immunoglobulin A (IgA), which is secreted across the gastrointestinal mucosa, preventing bacterial adherence to the enterocytes.[4,7] Without food, the gastrointestinal mucosa atrophies. As a result of atrophy, the tissue available to absorb nutrients decreases, and GALT is impaired. Preservation of the intestinal mucosal integrity is also essential to preserve its function as a barrier. With atrophy, there is a loss of the tight junctions between enterocytes, resulting in increased mucosal permeability and decreased barrier function.[4,7,8] This decreased barrier function can allow resident gastrointestinal bacteria and endotoxins to enter the systemic circulation. This process, called *bacterial translocation*, can trigger immune and inflammatory responses that can lead to infection, sepsis, and multisystem organ failure.[4,9] In addition to its trophic effects on the gastrointestinal tract, enteral nutrition is associated with enhanced utilization of nutrients, decreased infectious complications, ease and safety of delivery, and lower cost.

Enteral nutrition is considered when the patient cannot or should not eat, intake is insufficient or unreliable, the patient has a functional gastrointestinal tract, and access can be safely achieved. Mechanical obstruction is the only absolute contraindication to enteral feedings. Relative contraindications include severe hemorrhagic pancreatitis, necrotizing enterocolitis, prolonged ileus, severe diarrhea, protracted vomiting, enteric fistulas, and intestinal dysmotility.[8] Each situation should be evaluated individually.

Enteral nutrition can be delivered through feeding tubes placed into the stomach or the small intestine. The expected duration of nutritional support, the patient's overall condition, risk of aspiration, function of the gastrointestinal tract, and placement technique should all be considered when deciding on which type of feeding tube to place. Oral enteric tubes are a good choice for neonates who are obligate nose breathers to avoid airway compromise, but for most other patient populations, nasoenteric tubes are more widely used.[10]

Methods of Enteral Nutrition Delivery

NASOENTERAL FEEDING TUBES

A nasoenteric tube is indicated for short-term use, usually less than 30 days. Nasoenteral tubes are inserted through the nose and advanced through the esophagus into the stomach (nasogastric tube), the duodenum (nasoduodenal tube), or jejunum (nasojejunal tube). The tube is identified by the distal location of its tip. Most nasoenteric tubes are soft, flexible, small-bore polyurethane or silicone tubes that are 8 to 14 French in diameter, 20 to 60 inches in length, and radiopaque to allow for radiographic confirmation of placement. The shorter lengths are used for nasogastric feedings, and the longer for nasoduodenal or nasojejunal feedings. As a general rule, the smallest-diameter tube of appropriate length is preferred because the smaller diameter has been associated with less complications and increased patient comfort. Small-diameter tubes may help to prevent reflux and lessen the risk of aspiration because the small diameter lessens compromise of the lower esophageal sphincter (LES). In addition, small-diameter tubes cause less inhibition of swallowing, which is more comfortable for patients. Tubes made of polyvinyl chloride are less desirable because, over time, they can stiffen in the presence of acid, which can lead to patient discomfort and increased complications (such as tube perforation).[10] Any nasally placed tube can cause sinusitis, erosion of the nasal septum or esophagus, epistaxis, or distal esophageal strictures, which may limit long-term use. Small, soft-bore tubes are less likely to cause these complications.

Most nasoenteric tubes have multiple ports staggered along their sides and tip, which minimize clogging and maximize flow. Many devices also have weighted tips and a stylet, which stiffens the tube to assist in placement. Another common feature of many nasoenteric tubes is a "Y port" at the proximal tip, which allows for the administration of medications and irrigation without interrupting tube feeding.

Types of Nasoenteric Tubes

Nasogastric Tubes. Gastric feedings through a nasogastric tube are appropriate for patients who have intact gag and cough reflexes and adequate gastric emptying.

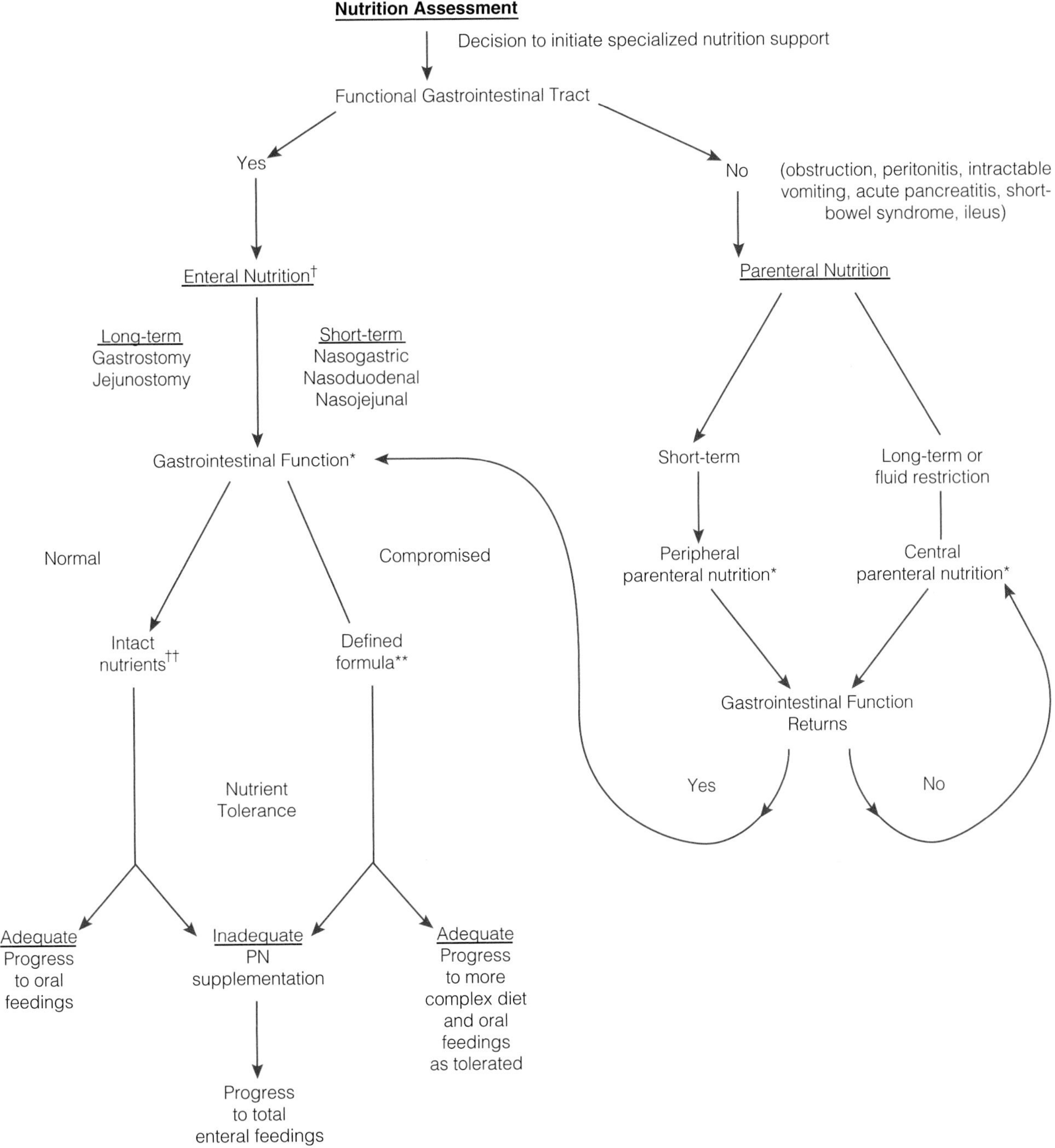

figure 40-1 Route of administration of specialized nutrition support. Adapted from ASPEN Clinical Pathways and Algorithms for Delivery of Parenteral and Enteral Nutrition Support in Adults. (Source: Jacobs D (ed): Section II: Nutrition Care Process. Journal of Parenteral and Enteral Nutrition 26 (1 Suppl): 85A, 2002.)
*Formulation of enteral and parenteral solutions should be made considering organ function (e.g., cardiac, renal, respiratory, hepatic).
†Feeding may be more appropriate distal to the pylorus if the patient is at increased aspiration risk.
**Elemental low-/high-fat content, lactose-free, fiber-rich, and modular formulas should be provided according to the patient's gastrointestinal tolerance.
‡Polymeric, complete formulas, or pureed diets are appropriate.

Nasogastric tubes usually range from 8 to 12 French in diameter and 30 to 36 inches in length. Small-caliber nasogastric tubes are used solely for feeding, whereas large-caliber tubes can be used to decompress the stomach, monitor gastric pH, and deliver medications and feedings. Large-caliber nasogastric tubes are usually made of stiffer material and are often less comfortable for patients, possibly triggering self-extubation. These tubes are usually used to decompress and drain the stomach temporarily and are therefore typically for short-term use.

Advantages to gastric feeding include the ease of placement, the ease of checking residuals, and patient tolerability

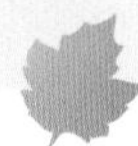

box 40-2

Nutritional Care of the Pediatric Patient

- Address all the child's questions and explain all the procedures according to the child's developmental level.
- Involve the child (if old enough) in his or her nutritional care.
- Allow the parents to assist as much as possible.
- Pediatric patients have a greater need for many nutrients, so consider age, weight, size, activity level, and development when administering solution components.
- Pediatric patients are particularly susceptible to fluid overload; therefore, be careful to administer the correct volume and infusion rate.
- Monitor intake and output and weight daily.
- Provide written educational material for the parents for review and reinforcement.

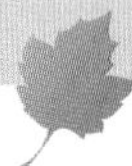

box 40-3

Nutritional Requirements in the Older Patient

- The risk for malnutrition increases as functional abilities decrease.
- The caloric needs of the elderly are generally less, secondary to decreased metabolism.
- Although protein requirements remain the same, it is important to monitor renal function.
- There is decreased ability to tolerate glucose loads.
- Atrophic gastritis occurs frequently in the elderly, which can result in decreased gastric acid secretion. The resultant achlorhydria or hypochlorhydria can lead to bacterial overgrowth and altered absorption of iron, vitamin B_{12}, folate, calcium, vitamin K, and zinc.
- Lactose intolerance increases with age; this intolerance to dairy products can contribute to osteopenia.
- Vitamin D deficiency in the elderly can be due to decreased dietary intake, decreased synthesis, or decreased exposure to sunlight.
- The elderly have less ability to regulate fluid balance, which places them at an increased risk for dehydration or overhydration.
- Encourage increased dietary fiber, fluids, and exercise to reduce the incidence of constipation.
- Decreased gastrointestinal motility, exocrine function, and digestion or absorption may occur in the elderly.
- Physical changes in the jaw, including poor dentition or poorly fitting dentures, may interfere with mastication and adequate food intake.
- Swallowing may be more difficult because of decreased esophageal motility and decreased saliva production.
- Multiple medications or concomitant disease may contribute to anorexia or diminished sense of taste.

during enteral infusions. However, patients with nasogastric tubes are at the greatest risk for aspiration, especially when they are unconscious, mechanically ventilated, or otherwise unable to protect their airway. In a conscious patient, the mere physical appearance of the tube and associated discomfort may limit the clinical use of nasogastric tubes.

Nasoduodenal Tubes and Nasojejunal Tubes. Nasoduodenal tubes and nasojejunal tubes are thought to be better suited for long-term use than nasogastric tubes. Nasoduodenal tubes and nasojejunal tubes are advanced through the stomach, past the pylorus, and into the small intestine, usually in the third portion of the duodenum beyond the ligament of Treitz. In theory, the pyloric sphincter provides a barrier that lessens the risk of aspiration or regurgitation.

Many critically ill patients and those with medical issues, such as diabetes, renal dysfunction, or spinal cord injuries, may have delayed gastric emptying. Transpyloric feeding can be given without regard to gastric emptying, providing an additional advantage over intragastric feeding. Candidates for transpyloric feedings include critically ill patients with a prior history of gastric aspiration, patients at risk for aspiration (such as ventilated patients), and patients with neurological conditions who are unable to protect their airway.

A common misconception is that enteral feedings should not be started if bowel sounds are absent. Bowel sounds are an indication of gastrointestinal motility, not of absorption. Postinjury and postoperatively, bowel sounds may not be detected for 3 to 5 days owing to gastric atony. The small bowel is less prone to ileus than the stomach or the colon and retains its absorptive and digestive capabilities, making it possible to accept enteral feedings immediately after surgery or trauma.[11]

Nasoduodenal tubes and nasojejunal tubes range from 8 to 14 French in diameter and 46 to 60 inches in length. The length and diameter make it more difficult to check feeding residual because the lumen is smaller and tends to collapse on itself when aspirated. In addition, clogging of medications is more common than with nasogastric tubes. The primary disadvantage associated with nasoduodenal and nasojejunal tubes relates to the difficulty in initially placing the tubing tip past the pyloric sphincter.

Placement of Nasoenteric Tubes

In most intensive care units (ICUs), trained nurses or physicians routinely place nasoenteric tubes. Before placing a feeding tube, the nurse refers to institution policy and protocol because nasoenteric tube placement has many potential complications. Patients with a decreased level of consciousness, poor cough or gag reflex, or an inability or unwillingness to cooperate are at increased risk for pulmonary intubation. When a patient cannot cooperate or cough when the tube enters the bronchial tree, the nurse must take extra precautions to ensure proper placement. Feeding tubes placed in the bronchial tree can cause pulmonary hemorrhage or pneumothorax. Never assume a cuffed endotracheal tube precludes accidental pulmonary intubation. Nasoenteric tubes can also be accidentally placed in the esophagus or, in patients with basilar skull fractures, in the intracranial space.

Nasogastric tube placement is usually easier than nasoduodenal or nasojejunal tube placement. When placing a nasoenteric feeding tube in the stomach, determine the length of tube insertion by measuring the distance from the tip of the nose, to the earlobe, to the tip of the xiphoid process. Before insertion, consider using a topical anesthetic or water-soluble lubricant to assist in placement. After placing the patient's bed in a high Fowler's position, slightly flex the patient's head (if not clinically contraindicated), and pass the lubricated tip through the nares into the nasopharynx. Ask the patient to swallow repeatedly while advancing the tube. Having the patient sip water through a straw may also assist in tube placement (if not clinically contraindicated). Rotating the tube as it is advanced may also ease advancement.

When attempting to pass the nasoenteric tube tip past the pylorus, follow the same procedure described previously, then turn the patient to the right lateral decubitus position to take advantage of gravity and peristalsis. To get the tip of the feeding tube past the pylorus into the small bowel, the length of the tube should be at least 40 inches.[12] Nasoduodenal and nasojejunal tubes depend on gastric motility to carry the tip through the pylorus, but have a tendency to coil in the stomach. Some nasoduodenal tubes and nasojejunal tubes have weights to aid in passage through the pylorus; however, the utility of the weighted tip is dubious. A promotility agent such as metoclopramide or erythromycin may be ordered before insertion. These medications increase upper gastrointestinal motility while relaxing the pylorus. Air insufflation, the process of inserting large amounts of air into the stomach, may also be helpful by distending the stomach and facilitating tube passage though the pylorus.[9] If passage of a nasoduodenal or nasojejunal tube does not occur within 24 hours, endoscopic or radiological assistance should be sought to advance the tip of the tube.

Before initiating tube feeding, proper tube placement must be confirmed by an abdominal radiograph. Feeding tubes placed surgically, by endoscopy, or under fluoroscopy do not require radiographic confirmation of placement. The external length of the tube is documented after placement is confirmed. Mark the tube with tape or indelible ink at the point it enters the nares. Recheck tube placement before initiating intermittent feedings or medication administration, and at least once each shift. Monitor tube placement during continuous tube feeding according to the institution's policy.

Auscultation, aspiration and inspection of aspirate, and pH testing may all be used to monitor tube placement after initial placement is confirmed by an abdominal radiograph. No one method is infallible, so using a combination of these methods is advised.[4] Injecting air into the tube and auscultating the gastric bubble, although commonly used, is not an accurate method to verify initial tube placement. An air bubble sound can be transmitted to the epigastrium when the tube is in the esophagus. Although auscultation of insufflated air is not a reliable method to confirm initial feeding tube placement, it may still provide useful information. If no resistance is met, the tube is unlikely to be kinked, and, if the patient immediately burps back air, the tip of the tube is probably in the esophagus.[12]

Aspiration and inspection of the aspirate may help to differentiate between gastric and intestinal placement, but not between intestinal and pulmonary placement. Fluid aspirated from the stomach is usually cloudy green, tan, brown, or bloody.[4,10,11] Small intestinal aspirate is usually yellow, clear, or bile colored. Pulmonary fluid is usually tan, white, clear, or pale yellow and can closely mimic gastric or intestinal aspirates.[4,10,11]

Measuring the pH of fluid aspirated from the feeding tube is another method of monitoring tube placement. Keep in mind that the diameter of small intestinal tubes may not allow withdrawal to check aspirate. Aspirate with a pH of less than 4.0 is highly predictive of gastric placement.[12,13] However, the pH of gastric aspirate can be elevated with the infusion of enteral formulas, the use of acid-modifying medications, and the presence of bile reflux. The pH of both small intestinal aspirate and pulmonary fluid is usually greater than 6.0; therefore, if the pH of the aspirate is greater than 4.0, tube position cannot be determined based on pH alone.[12,13]

Suctioning and patient movement or coughing may potentially dislodge a feeding tube. If at any time tube location is in question, hold the tube feeding and obtain an abdominal radiograph to confirm placement.

Securing Nasoenteric Tubes

Before securing any feeding tube, clean the skin with alcohol to remove oils and dirt and consider applying a skin protectant to maintain skin integrity. Nasoenteric tubes should be secured in a way that avoids irritation or pressure of the nares, thus preventing necrosis. Allow the tube to hang straight from the nares and secure it to the bridge of the nose or the cheek with tape (or one of the many commercially available devices). For agitated or uncooperative patients, consider soft wrist restraints or mitts to avoid accidental self-extubation. The institution's policy and procedure should be referred to regarding the use of restraints. The skin and nostrils should be inspected every 4 to 8 hours for signs and symptoms of irritation, erythema, or skin breakdown. Patient comfort can be maximized by providing frequent mouth care and moistening of the nares.

ENTEROSTOMAL FEEDING TUBES

If therapy is expected to last a month or more, a more permanent enterostomal device can be inserted through the abdomen into the stomach (gastrostomy) or jejunum (jejunostomy; Fig. 40-2). Enterostomal feeding tubes are also indicated when the nasal route is contraindicated and in patients with impaired swallowing or obstruction of the oropharynx, the larynx, or esophagus. Enterostomal tubes are made of silicone and polyurethane and are very durable.

Types of Enterostomal Feeding Tubes

Gastrostomy Tubes. Gastrostomy tubes may be used temporarily or for permanent feeding. If a gastrostomy tube is intended for permanent feedings, it may need to be replaced as the tube material deteriorates over time. Gastrostomy tubes may also be used for chronic gastric decompression. A low-profile gastrostomy device (LPGD), often referred to as a button, may be used to replace gastrostomy tubes in a mature gastrostomy tract, usually 3 to 6 months after initial placement or as an initial placement.[10] LPGDs are anchored in the stomach and protrude through the

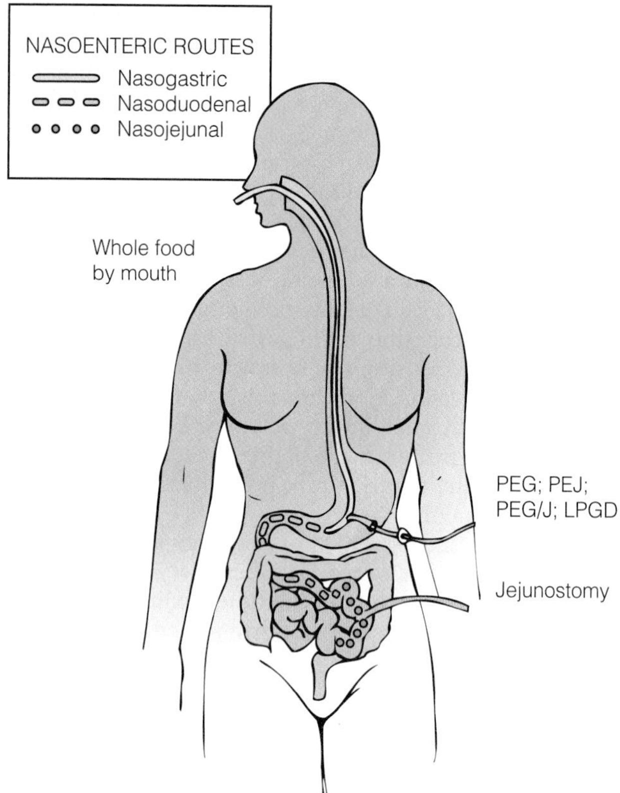

figure 40-2 Possible routes for feeding. *PEG*, percutaneous endoscopic gastronomy; *PEG/J*, PEG modified with a jejunal extension tube; *PEJ*, percutaneous endoscopic jejunostomy; *LPGD*, low-profile gastrostomy device.

abdomen, flush with the skin. These devices require a special extension adapter to connect with the tube-feeding bag, to check for residuals, and to use for decompression. This adapter may then be removed after use. Some LPGDs are equipped with a one-way antireflux valve to prevent leakage of gastric contents onto the skin. These devices are usually well accepted because they are durable, unlikely to irritate the skin, and difficult to dislodge. With agitated or confused adults who have a tendency to pull on their tubes, these advantages may be of benefit.

Jejunostomy Tubes. When gastric feedings are not possible or desired, jejunostomy tubes (J-tubes) are preferred for long-term feeding. J-tubes deliver enteral formula past the duodenum into the jejunum, decreasing pancreatic stimulation. J-tubes are indicated in patients who will benefit from jejunal feeding, such as those with gastric disease, abnormal gastric emptying, upper gastrointestinal obstruction or fistula, pancreatitis, or decreased gag reflex with significant risk of aspiration. J-tubes are contraindicated in patients with primary diseases of the small bowel (such as Crohn's disease) or radiation enteritis because they may increase the risk of enterocutaneous fistula formation.[11] A limitation of J-tubes is the potential for obstruction due to the small diameter of the lumen.

Placement of Enterostomal Tubes

Percutaneous endoscopic, open surgical, laparoscopic, and fluoroscopic techniques may be used to place a gastrostomy tube. J-tubes may be placed by percutaneous endoscopy or surgical methods. The patient's underlying disease and physician expertise need to be considered when selecting the appropriate placement technique.

Percutaneous Endoscopic Gastrostomy. Percutaneous endoscopic gastrostomy (PEG) has rapidly become the preferred method for placement of gastrostomy devices. A PEG may be done at the bedside or in the endoscopy suite, using minimal sedation. Other advantages of PEG placement include increased comfort, decreased cost, and decreased recovery time. A candidate for a PEG must have an intact oropharynx and an esophagus free from obstruction. The only absolute contraindication to PEG placement is the inability to bring the gastric wall into apposition with the abdomen. Prior abdominal surgeries, ascites, hepatomegaly, and obesity may impede gastric transillumination and preclude the placement of a PEG.

Complications of PEG are infrequent but include wound infection, necrotizing fasciitis, peritonitis, and aspiration. Pneumoperitoneum, a common finding after PEG placement, is not clinically significant unless accompanied by signs and symptoms of peritonitis.[6] Prophylactic antibiotics are usually given 30 to 60 minutes before procedure. Correct placement is then verified by endoscopy.

In patients with severe gastroesophageal reflux disease, gastroparesis, or aspiration related to tube feeding, a PEG can be modified with a jejunal extension tube known as a PEG/J tube. The gastric lumen of a PEG/J tube is usually used for gastric decompression, and the jejunal lumen is used for the simultaneous delivery of enteral feeding. PEG/J tubes may decrease the risk of gastric aspiration; however, they do not necessarily provide the same protection against aspiration as jejunal tubes because the pylorus is compromised by the large catheter.[11] The jejunal portion of a PEG/J tube may migrate back into the stomach and increase the risk of occlusion, gastric reflux, or aspiration. Both PEG and PEG/J tubes are held in place by internal and external retention devices. The internal device rests in the stomach, which prevents migration and leakage of gastric contents. The external retention device anchors the tube to the abdomen.

Surgical Gastrostomy. Surgical gastrostomy tubes are inserted through an incision in the abdominal wall under general anesthesia. The stomach is usually sutured to the abdominal wall to create a permanent connection between the gastric and abdominal wall. Surgical placement of a gastrostomy is usually chosen if the surgeon wants to view the gastric anatomy clearly or as a secondary procedure during abdominal surgery. Disadvantages of surgical placement include increased recovery time, decreased comfort, and increased cost.

Laparoscopic Gastrostomy. A laparoscopically placed gastrostomy tube also requires general anesthesia or intravenous (IV) conscious sedation. Laparoscopic placement is usually reserved for patients with head, neck, or esophageal cancer. It is less invasive, less painful, and usually involves less complications than a surgical gastrostomy.

Fluoroscopic Gastrostomy. Direct percutaneous catheter insertion of a gastrostomy tube under fluoroscopy is indicated with high-grade pharyngeal or esophageal obstruction. Disadvantages to the use of fluoroscopy to place enterostomal devices include the inability to detect mucosal disease, the potential for prolonged exposure to radiation, the necessity of transport to the fluoroscopy suite, and increased cost.

Securing Enterostomal Tubes and Caring for the Enterostomy Site

Enterostomal tubes are secured to the abdominal wall to prevent dislodgment or migration of the tube, to avoid tension on the tubing, and to prevent the external retention device from digging into the skin. The length of the external tubing is documented to monitor for migration of the tubing.

To avoid maceration, the insertion site is kept clean and dry by leaving it open to air (unless draining), and lifting or adjusting the tube is avoided for several days after the initial insertion. To avoid pulling the internal retention device taut against the gastric or intestinal mucosa, the amount of dressing between the device and the skin is limited. A cotton-tipped applicator is used to clean any accumulated drainage with half-strength peroxide.[11,12] If no drainage is present, cleansing with soap and water is adequate. The skin around the insertion site and the retention device is assessed at least daily for skin breakdown, erythema, or drainage. The tissue usually heals within a month.[11]

In-and-out play on the tubing is checked; it should be able to move one quarter of an inch to prevent erosion of gastric or abdominal tissue.[11,12] If the anchor is too tight, the nurse should notify the physician immediately because this may indicate "buried bumper syndrome," a situation where the retention device is imbedded in the tissue, thereby leading to mucosal or skin erosion. If a gastrostomy tube becomes accidentally dislodged, the nurse should notify the physician immediately so the tube can be reinserted quickly before the tract closes.

Types and Delivery of Enteral Formulas

When selecting a tube feeding formula, nutrient requirements, the patient's clinical status, location of enteral access, gastrointestinal function, cost, and duration must all be considered. There are numerous tube feeding solutions available for enteral nutrition, with many designed to assist in the management of specific disease processes; however, no single formula is ideal for all patients. All contain proteins, carbohydrates, fats, vitamins, and trace minerals. The difference lies in how these nutrients are structured and delivered. The dietary formula selected is based on the patient's ability to digest and absorb major nutrients, the total nutrient requirements, and fluid and electrolyte restrictions. Classifications of enteral formulas include polymeric, peptide (elemental), and modular:

- Polymeric solutions are isotonic, and can provide enough protein, carbohydrate, fat, vitamins, trace elements, and minerals to prevent nutritional deficiencies. They are considered nutritionally complete if given in enough volume to meet caloric needs.[14] Standard formulas deliver 1 kcal/mL, but some concentrated formulas may provide 2 kcal/mL.[8,14,15] The carbohydrates in polymeric solutions are oligosaccharides and polysaccharides that require pancreatic enzymes for digestion.[15] All polymeric solutions contain intact proteins (most often meat, whey, milk, or soy proteins) that require normal pancreatic enzymes for digestion.[8,14,15]
- Peptide (elemental) formulas provide proteins as dipeptides, tripeptides, or oligopeptides and free amino acids from hydrolysis of whey, milk, or soy proteins.[14] These proteins do not require pancreatic enzymes for digestion.[14] Elemental solutions are used when digestion is impaired, as in pancreatic insufficiency, radiation enteritis, Crohn's disease, or short bowel syndrome secondary to surgical resection.[8,14] Elemental solutions have no proven advantage in patients with normal gut function, are usually more expensive than polymeric formulas, and have an unpleasant taste.[14,15]
- Modular formulas contain individual nutrient components that can be mixed or added to other formulas to individualize feedings to a patient's specific nutritional needs. The involvement of a dietitian is essential in the preparation of these formulas because improper mixing can result in metabolic abnormalities.

When initiating enteral tube feedings, most clinicians recommend beginning with an isotonic formula at a slow rate and increasing the rate incrementally every 8 to 12 hours until the goal rate is achieved. Dilution of formula may help assist in tolerance but is not recommended because this may increase the time needed to meet the nutritional requirements.

Enteral feedings can be administered by bolus, gravity infusion, intermittent infusion, continuous infusion, or cyclic infusion. The tube tip location and tolerance generally dictate formula delivery. Gastric feedings are appropriate for patients who have intact gag and cough reflexes and adequate gastric emptying.

BOLUS FEEDINGS

Bolus feedings, considered the most natural method physiologically, are given by a large syringe in volumes as high as 400 mL over 5 to 10 minutes, five to six times a day.[4,8] The stomach is the preferred site for bolus feedings. The stomach and pyloric sphincter regulate the outflow of feeding from the stomach. Bolus feedings allow for increased patient mobility because the patient is free from a mechanical device between feedings. Unfortunately, as a result of high residuals, bolus feedings are usually not well tolerated and are often accompanied by nausea, bloating, cramping, diarrhea, or aspiration.

INTERMITTENT FEEDINGS

Intermittent feedings of 300 to 400 mL are administered by slow gravity drip or infusion four to six times a day over a period of 30 to 60 minutes. The stomach is the preferred site for intermittent infusion because of its capacity. Intermittent feedings are associated with a decreased risk of osmotic diarrhea. Disadvantages of intermittent feedings include the dependence on a mechanical device and a power source, which can increase cost and decrease patient mobility.

CONTINUOUS FEEDINGS

If the tip of the nasoenteric tube is in the duodenum or jejunum, tube feedings must be delivered by infusion. Continuous infusions are administered over 24 hours with the aid of a feeding pump to ensure a constant flow rate. Continuous pump feedings are the preferred method for intestinal feeding because delivery that is too rapid may lead to "dumping syndrome," characterized by osmotic diarrhea, abdominal distension, cramps, hyperperistalsis, lightheadedness, diaphoresis, and palpitations.[11,12] When the tube is placed in the third portion of the duodenum, past the ligament of Treitz, continuous pump feedings are associated with decreased risk of aspiration. If the feeding is advanced slowly, the small bowel can usually tolerate feedings at a rate of 150 mL/hour.[10] The continuous method is best suited to the critically ill patient because it allows more time for nutrients to be absorbed in the intestine. Continuous infusion is also often used in the ICU because there is decreased incidence of gastric distension and potential for aspiration.[6] Continuous-infusion tube feeding may also act prophylactically to prevent stress ulcers and metabolic complications. As with intermittent feedings, disadvantages include the dependence on a mechanical device and a power source.

CYCLIC FEEDINGS

Cyclic feedings are continuous feedings that deliver the total daily nutritional requirements in a shorter time frame, typically over 8 to 12 hours, to allow the patient freedom from 24-hour continuous feedings.[4] Cyclic feedings of high density and high volume are typically given at night. This schedule may assist the patient in progressing from enteral to oral consumption.

The ultimate goal is for patients to resume adequate oral intake. Enteral feeding may be discontinued when patients can drink enough liquid to maintain hydration and can eat two thirds of their nutritional requirements.

Complications of Enteral Nutrition

Although enteral nutrition is in general associated with fewer complications than parenteral nutrition, complications still may occur. These complications generally fall into gastrointestinal, mechanical, metabolic, and infectious categories. Many of these complications can be prevented or treated by closely observing residuals and watching for signs and symptoms of gastric intolerance.

GASTROINTESTINAL COMPLICATIONS

The patient's tolerance to enteral feeding depends on the rate of flow and the osmolality of the formula. Signs and symptoms of gastrointestinal intolerance to enteral feeding include diarrhea, nausea, vomiting, abdominal discomfort, distension, and high residual returns. Food normally passes through the stomach at a rate of 2 to 10 mL/minute; however, gastric emptying is delayed or absent in many critically ill patients.[13] Unlike the stomach, the small intestine cannot act as a reservoir. If large residuals are withdrawn through a nasoduodenal tube or nasojejunal tube, the tube may have moved back into the stomach, and placement should be confirmed with an abdominal radiograph.

High Residuals

High gastric residuals can also be problematic; however, consensus about what constitutes a high gastric residual varies. Recommendations for the cessation of tube feeding for high gastric residuals also vary widely. Many clinicians stop tube feeding inappropriately, based on a single high residual of greater than 200 mL from a nasogastric tube or greater than 100 mL from a gastrostomy tube.[4,8,13] Although this should raise suspicion of intolerance, one high residual does not mean feeding failure, and automatic cessation of feeding can delay the patient's ability to meet his or her nutritional goals. Be sure to evaluate the clinical status of your patient before stopping tube feeding solely on the basis of one high residual; the key is to monitor subsequent volume residuals.

If cessation of tube feedings for high residuals is necessary, a common intervention involves holding the feeding for 1 to 2 hours and rechecking the residual every 1 to 2 hours until the residual is less than 200 mL from a nasogastric tube or less than 100 mL from a gastrostomy tube, at which point feedings can be resumed. This allows time for normal gastric emptying and reduces the risk for aspiration. Remember that high infusion rates result in higher residual volumes. The institution's policy and protocol regarding high gastric residuals should be checked.

Nausea, Vomiting, and Bloating

Nausea, vomiting, and bloating are commonly associated with enteral feedings. Medications, rapid infusion rate, or improper tube placement may cause both nausea and vomiting. Nausea, vomiting, and bloating are most likely to occur when gastric emptying is delayed. A careful assessment of medications that may contribute to these symptoms should be undertaken, and the medication should be eliminated, if possible. A change of formula, reduction in rate, or addition of a prokinetic agent may also help in the management.

Diarrhea

Diarrhea is the most common complication of enteral feedings; however, it is important to consider other etiologies before assuming that enteral feedings are the cause of diarrhea. Diarrhea in a patient receiving enteral feeding may result from the use of antibiotics or other diarrhea-inducing medications; altered bacterial flora; formula composition; intolerance to lactose, fat, or osmolality; a rate of infusion that is too high; hypoalbuminemia; or enteral formula contamination.

The liquid form of many medications may contain hypertonic sorbitol, which can have laxative effects. Antibiotics, antacids, magnesium, and prokinetic medications can also contribute to diarrhea.[7] Antibiotics can contribute to diarrhea by causing bacterial overgrowth of *Clostridium difficile*. To assess for *C. difficile* infection, a stool sample should be assessed for *C. difficile* toxin. Treatment options include antibiotic therapy with oral metronidazole, vancomycin, or cholestyramine (a bile acid sequestrant that binds the toxin). A patient who has received antibiotics should not receive antidiarrheals until *C. difficile* infection has been ruled out because diarrhea helps eliminate the toxin from the intestinal mucosa.

Bacterial overgrowth may cause diarrhea. Reduced gastric and small bowel motility may lead to small intestinal overgrowth, which can alter intestinal microflora. Acid suppression may also permit bacterial overgrowth because bacteria can colonize the gastrointestinal tract when the gastric pH is greater than 4.0.[8]

Infusing of enteral feedings too rapidly may cause diarrhea. Intolerance of lactose, fat, or osmolality may also lead to diarrhea. Reducing the infusion rate, changing to a peptide-based formula that is easier to digest, and giving an absorbing product, such as Metamucil, may help. The use of a fiber-containing formula may be useful in bulking stools and correction of the diarrhea. Diarrhea can also be caused by bacterial contamination of the solution or administration set. The nurse checks the expiration date of the formula and discards the formula if it is expired. Breaks in the system are minimized, and the use of a closed, prefilled, ready-to-hang solution should be considered. To prevent bacterial contamination, no more than 4 hours of feeding solution should be hung in the container at one time; any open solution should be used within 24 hours; administration sets should be changed daily; rinsing should occur between bolus feedings; and good handwashing technique should be used when handling equipment.

In patients receiving enteral feedings, a hyperosmotic formula may also contribute to diarrhea. If diarrhea decreases when the feedings are held, the formula may be the cause. After consultation with the dietitian, the nurse should consider changing the formula. Also, a stool sample should be collected to evaluate for an osmotic gap; this may help identify osmotic diarrhea.

Hypoalbuminemia may predispose patients to diarrhea by decreasing the osmotic pressure gradient.[13] This decrease may lead to bowel edema and malabsorption. Any formula that is not absorbed may contribute to the diarrhea.[13] The prealbumin should be monitored because it is a more reliable indicator of current nutritional status than serum albumin.

Constipation

Constipation associated with enteral feedings may be related to poor hydration, lack of fiber, bed rest, impaction, obstruction, and narcotics. Adequate hydration should be ensured, and adding a stool softener should be considered, along with minimizing narcotics, encouraging ambulation, and considering the addition of fiber to relieve constipation.

MECHANICAL COMPLICATIONS

Mechanical complications occur when the tube becomes dislodged, occluded, or malpositioned.

Tube Dislodgement

Tube dislodgment by either patients or staff accounts for most tube removals. Soft restraints or hand mitts should be considered for agitated patients to prevent accidental self-extubation.

Tube Clogging

Precipitation of medications, clogging of pill fragments, or coagulation of formula may cause obstruction of any feeding tube, delaying the administration of nutrients and medications. To avoid clogging, enteral feeding tubes are flushed every 4 to 6 hours during continuous feeds, before and after medication administration, after checking residuals, and when turning off feedings. Nasoenteric tubes should always be flushed with a large, 30- to 60-mL syringe to avoid rupturing the tube with excessive pressure. They should be irrigated with 20 to 30 mL of tepid water.

The enteral solution container should be checked frequently for precipitation. Crushed tablets may leave a residual that blocks the tube. To prevent clogging, liquid medications should be administered when available. Flushing the tube before and after each medication administration also helps to avoid incompatibilities between medications and feedings and reduces the incidence of clogging.

An obstruction is suspected if the formula does not flow by gravity, flushing an aspirate from the tube is not possible, or the occlusion alarm of the feeding pump sounds repeatedly. If an occlusion is suspected, the nurse uses a large piston syringe to flush the tube with warm water, using a gentle push–pull motion. Although many solutions have been proposed to assist in clearing an obstructed feeding tube, they offer no demonstrable benefit over tap water.[4,10,12] A stylet should never be used to unclog a tube because of the risk of rupturing the feeding tube and perforating the esophagus, stomach, or small intestine. Recent studies have shown that the pancreatic enzyme, pancrelipase, has been effective in unclogging a tube when water is unsuccessful.[4,10]

METABOLIC COMPLICATIONS

Multiple metabolic complications can accompany enteral nutrition. Fluid and electrolyte imbalance may occur because of fluid excess, fluid depletion by gastrointestinal or renal losses, wound drainage, diuresis, fever, or inadequate free water intake. If dehydration is due to inadequate fluid intake, extra fluid may need to be given by bolus or by automatic flush using specialized feeding pumps. The average patient with good renal function needs 30 to 35 mL/kg of free water per day, if not otherwise medically contraindicated.[4,8,16] Conversely, if cardiac or hepatic function is impaired, overhydration from enteral feedings may occur. The determination of the patient's baseline fluid requirements and accurate measurement of intake and output can help to maintain fluid balance. Keep in mind that many of the patients seen in the ICU are often unable to convey feelings of thirst, secondary to diminished levels of consciousness or intubation.

Hyperglycemia may occur if patients are being overfed, during hypermetabolic states, and as a result of steroid medications. Blood glucose should be monitored during enteral therapy; a decrease in formula rate or concentration may help if hyperglycemia occurs. Bolus feeding may exacerbate hyperglycemia in patients with diabetes. If feedings are abruptly stopped, hypoglycemia should be assessed, especially in patients receiving insulin.

INFECTIOUS COMPLICATIONS

Aspiration of enteral formulas into the lung is a potentially fatal complication. Loss of consciousness, mechanical ventilation, and many medications used in critically ill patients increase the risk of aspiration. To limit this risk, the head of the bed should be maintained at a 30- to 45-degree angle during feeding and 1 hour after use; intermittent or continuous feedings should be used rather than rapid boluses; gastric residuals should be checked frequently; and signs of feeding intolerance should be assessed. Feedings should be discontinued at least 30 minutes before any procedure for which the patient must lay flat.

Pulmonary aspiration, although often subclinical, may be indicated by a low-grade fever, coughing, shortness of breath, rhonchi during or after enteral feeding infusions, and presence of a "sweet" formula odor emanating from the tracheal or oral secretions during suctioning. If the patient is at high risk for aspiration or if there is a clinical suspicion of aspiration, addition of blue dye to the enteral feeding formula is suggested to help visually identify aspirated feeding formula. The institution's policy and protocol should be checked regarding blue dye administration. Checking tracheal suction fluid with a glucose strip and glucometer tests formula aspiration. If the reading is greater than 20 mg/dL or is blue-tinged, aspiration is suggested.[13]

PARENTERAL (INTRAVENOUS) NUTRITION

There are two types of parenteral (IV) nutrition: central and peripheral. Central parenteral nutrition, also known as *total parenteral nutrition* (TPN), is infused through a large central vein (Fig. 40-3). Peripheral parenteral nutrition (PPN) can be infused into a smaller, peripheral vein owing to the lower osmolarity concentrations. TPN has sometimes been referred to as *hyperalimentation* or "hyperal." This is not a preferred term because it implies that parenteral nutrition gives more nutrients than the patient may actually require.

Parenteral nutrition is indicated when oral or enteral nutrition is not possible or when absorption or function of the gastrointestinal tract is not sufficient (or is unreliable) to meet the nutritional needs of the patient. Since the inception of parenteral nutrition in the early 1960s, bowel rest was thought to be the cornerstone of treatment for many gastrointestinal disorders. Today, except in cases of severe hemorrhagic pancreatitis, necrotizing enterocolitis, prolonged ileus, and distal bowel obstruction, some enteral nutrition is recommended to maintain gut integrity and function.[3] If the patient has a functioning gastrointestinal tract, if the treatment is anticipated to last for less than 5 days, or if prognosis does not warrant aggressive nutrition support, an alternative form of nutritional therapy is suggested.

Methods of Parenteral Nutrition Delivery

TOTAL PARENTERAL NUTRITION

TPN differs from standard IV fluids in that *all* of the *daily* required nutrients (carbohydrates, proteins, fats, vitamins, minerals, and trace elements) are delivered to the patient. The solution is infused at a constant rate over a 24-hour period to achieve maximum assimilation of the nutrients and to prevent hyperglycemia (or hypoglycemia). The aim of treatment is a continuous infusion that meets the caloric and nutritional requirements of the patient.

The high osmolarity of TPN formulas requires delivery through a central venous catheter so that the higher blood volumes in larger central veins are able to dilute and disperse the solution. The superior vena cava is an excellent site for such delivery. Passage of the catheter, by way of the subclavian vein into the superior vena cava, is the route of choice because it allows the patient the greatest freedom of movement without disturbing the insertion site. Jugular veins can also be used, but they are not as comfortable because of the limitations in neck movement.

Critically ill patients often have issues with reliable IV access. Because the TPN formula must be infused separately owing to the high risk of precipitation and the risk of contamination from increased handling, the introduction of multiple-lumen catheters has greatly facilitated the care

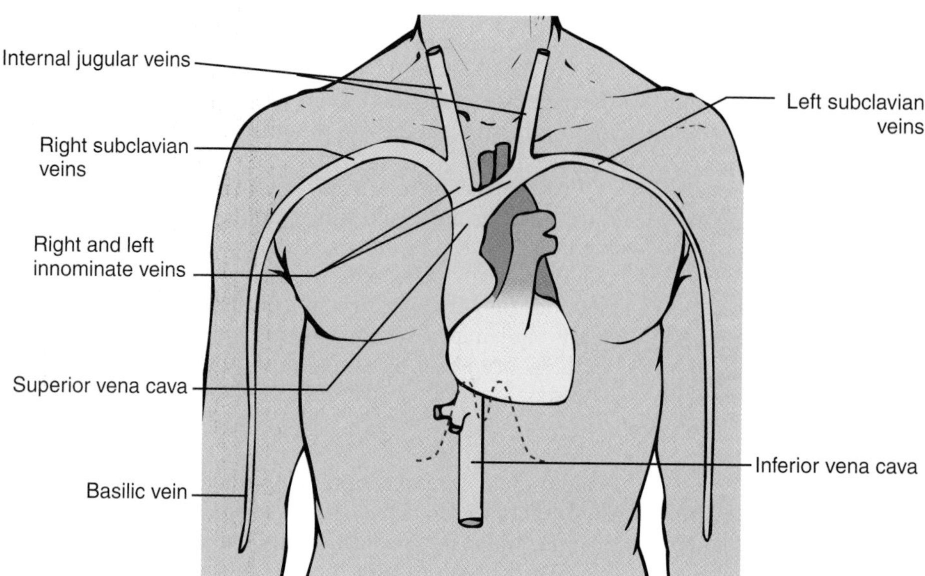

figure 40-3 Venous anatomy for hyperalimentation routes.

of patients who require multiple IV therapies. These catheters provide separate infusion ports and corresponding distal exit sites along the catheter tubing. This prevents direct mixing of solutions before they are diluted by the high blood volumes of the central veins. Therefore, one port can be dedicated to exclusive use of TPN, while the remaining ports can be used for the administration of IV antibiotics, medications, and blood products, and for blood sampling. When the central line is a single lumen, this lumen should be used exclusively for the infusion of TPN.

TPN formulas typically contain three primary macronutrients: carbohydrates, lipids (fats), and amino acids (protein). This combination is called a *mixed fuel source.* When all three fuel sources are combined together in one TPN bag, this is often referred to as a "3 in 1" admixture. The desired proportions of these nutrients are prepared by a pharmacist under a laminar flow hood to maintain strict sterility. Because of differences in pharmacy equipment to compound TPN, some agencies infuse lipids separately, usually in a glass bottle. Medications are *not* to be added to a TPN bag after it has been prepared by the pharmacist because of the risk of contamination or precipitation of its contents. The current trend for TPN formulation is based on the specific needs of each patient; standard formulas are no longer widely prescribed.

Macronutrients

Carbohydrates. The primary source of energy in the body is carbohydrates. This macronutrient usually provides 40% to 60% of daily caloric requirements and is essential to central nervous system function. The most common and preferred source of carbohydrates is dextrose (D-glucose) because it is readily metabolized, stimulates the secretion of insulin, and is usually well tolerated in large quantities. Dextrose provides 3.4 kcal/g in IV form and contributes to most of the osmolality (or concentration) of the TPN solution. Initial concentrations of dextrose may range from 50% to 70%, but final concentration is diluted to approximately 25% after the addition of amino acids, lipid emulsions, and water.[3] This final dilution, however, remains very hypertonic, which can be caustic to smaller blood vessels. To reduce the risk of phlebitis, TPN needs to be infused through a large central vein in which the TPN solution can be diluted by higher blood volumes.

The amount of dextrose prescribed in TPN is based on metabolic needs, which, once met, allow utilization of amino acids for protein synthesis rather than solely as an energy source. One of the most common metabolic side effects of high dextrose concentrations is hyperglycemia, which often requires the use of insulin. In addition, high dextrose concentrations may put certain patients, such as those with pulmonary compromise, at risk for carbon dioxide retention and subsequent respiratory acidosis. Because one of the end products of dextrose metabolism is carbon dioxide, elevated levels may increase minute ventilation and hence the work of breathing. Overfeeding carbohydrates may make ventilator weaning difficult, if not impossible.

Lipids. Intravenous lipids, or fat emulsions, are long-chain triglycerides from vegetable oils (safflower or soybean oils) that are rich in essential and nonessential amino acids. Lipids provide a concentrated source of calories and are important in the maintenance of connective tissue integrity and prevention of fatty acid deficiency. Symptoms of fatty acid deficiency include dry skin, hair loss, poor wound healing, and diarrhea.[17] Lipid concentrations are available in 10%, 20%, and 30% solutions, providing 1.0, 2.0, and 3.0 kcal/mL, respectively. The benefit of higher concentrations is that they provide a greater concentration of calories in less total volume, an important consideration in many patients. The usual dose is 0.5 to 1 g/kg/day to supply up to 30% of the patient's calorie intake; fats are a concentrated energy source providing 9 kcal/g. When additional lipid sources such as propofol (Diprivan), a sedative that is delivered as a lipid emulsion, are added, TPN lipid concentrations or quantities may need to be adjusted. Because lipid emulsions contain egg phospholipids as an emulsifying agent, the nurse checks for any egg allergies before infusion. Other adverse reactions include fever, chills, chest tightness, dyspnea, tachycardia, headache, nausea, and vomiting.[18] If such reactions occur, the infusion is stopped immediately and the reaction is reported to the physician and pharmacist. Before infusion, TPN solutions containing lipids are inspected for separation of the lipid solution, also know as *cracking* and *coalescence.* This loss of emulsion can be identified by yellow-brown marbling of the entire solution or a layering of oil at the surface. Such solutions are not safe for infusion and should be returned to the pharmacy for replacement.

Lipid solutions are isotonic and therefore help to reduce the osmolality of high dextrose concentrations when mixed together in a "3 in 1" admixture. Because of the expense of the equipment needed to compound lipids into the TPN solution, some facilities opt to infuse lipids separately by IV piggyback. Regardless of the method of delivery, weekly triglyceride trends monitor tolerance. If serum triglyceride levels exceed 500 mg/dL, lipids are often held until levels return to normal.[18] Use of a filter, no smaller than 1.2 μm, can reduce the incidence of particulates and air being transfused, thus reducing the risk of pulmonary embolism. There is no evidence, however, to suggest that these filters reduce the risk of infection.[19,20]

Amino Acids. All tissues require protein to maintain structure and facilitate wound healing. If protein intake is inadequate, the body becomes catabolic, seeking protein from skeletal muscle and vital organs. In TPN, protein is provided as a mixture of essential and nonessential crystalline acids, which are available in concentrations ranging from 5% to 15%. Standard amino acid solutions contain approximately 50% amino acids and 50% nonessential plus semiessential amino acids. For patients with renal disease, there are solutions available with a higher concentration of essential amino acids. For patients with hepatic failure or hypercatabolic conditions, there are formulas with branched amino acids, which spare the breakdown of other muscle proteins to use as energy, possibly reducing the incidence of hepatic encephalopathy.

Micronutrients

Vitamins, minerals, and trace elements are considered micronutrients. Unfortunately, the U.S. Recommended Dietary Allowance requirements do not apply to parenteral nutrition for multiple reasons. First, the liver and gastrointestinal tract absorptive processes are bypassed, resulting in elimination of these micronutrients through the urine without their being utilized. Second, many diseases alter the gut's ability to absorb fat-soluble vitamins and vitamin B_{12}. Finally, many nutrients adhere to the plastic tubing and IV solution bags or are destroyed by light and oxygen exposure (especially vitamin A) before reaching the bloodstream.[3] With these factors in mind, standard aqueous multivitamin preparations have been created. However, in hypermetabolic conditions, deficiencies that require close monitoring and potential supplementation can occur. Vitamin K is the only vitamin not included in the multivitamin preparation; it is provided by adding up to 10 mg/week of the vitamin to the TPN solution, unless contraindicated by anticoagulation treatment.

Trace elements also come in a variety of commercial mixtures but typically include chromium, copper, manganese, zinc, and selenium. Iron and iodine are not routinely added to TPN solutions and may need to be supplemented in long-term therapy.

Most electrolyte mixtures contain sodium, chloride, potassium, magnesium calcium, and phosphorus. Depending on the patient's underlying disease process and physical assessment findings, specific electrolyte concentrations can be adjusted daily in the TPN solution. If an electrolyte deficiency is detected after the TPN solution has already been prepared or while infusing, additional IV supplements can be given as a separate IV piggyback. Supplements and medications should never be added to the TPN bag after the pharmacist has formulated it because this would break the sterility of the solution and may cause the solution to precipitate.

Medications

During the process of compounding the TPN solution, the pharmacist can add medications, many of which are often necessitated by the TPN therapy itself. For instance, insulin is commonly added to the solutions because of the increased incidence of hyperglycemia during TPN infusion. Also, heparin is often added to reduce fibrin buildup along the catheter tip. Various medications are often added to treat underlying disease processes and their associated complications that necessitate the need for TPN therapy.

PERIPHERAL PARENTERAL NUTRITION

Patients who need temporary nutritional support or who need to supplement the nutrient intake they are consuming orally or by tube feedings are optimal candidates for PPN. To decrease the incidence of phlebitis, an osmolarity of less than 800 mOsm/L is the goal to infuse PPN safely by a peripheral vein.[21] This osmolarity can be attained only by limiting the dextrose concentration and by increasing the overall fluid volume and lipid concentration. Higher fluid volumes and reduced caloric/nutritional content limit PPN to short-term use, usually no more than 5 to 7 days. Therefore, goals of PPN are thought of in terms of preventing malnutrition, as opposed to correcting existing deficits. PPN may be infused through a standard peripheral cannula or through long-term peripheral access devices. PPN can be reduced or discontinued once the patient begins to tolerate oral or enteral feedings.

PPN requires good venous access, such as the basilic vein (see Fig. 40-3). The use of peripherally inserted central catheter lines increases patient comfort and improves the ability to provide nutrition through this access.

Complications of Parenteral Nutrition

Complications can be divided into four main categories: gastrointestinal, mechanical, metabolic, and infectious.

GASTROINTESTINAL COMPLICATIONS

Hepatic dysfunction may be seen in patients receiving lipid infusions; this is often related to the infusion amount and flow rate. Complications include hepatic steatosis (fatty liver), intrahepatic and extrahepatic cholestasis (suppression of bile flow), and cholelithiasis (formation of gallstones). Although the exact mechanism for these hepatic disorders is still not completely understood, it has been observed that cholestasis is less likely to occur if some form of enteral feeding is maintained.[3]

Gastrointestinal atrophy, and all of its associated complications, may occur from disuse. If not contraindicated, oral or enteral feedings should be initiated as soon as possible.

MECHANICAL COMPLICATIONS

Mechanical complications include those associated with central venous catheterization insertion, such as trauma to the vessel, pneumothorax, catheter occlusion, thrombosis, and venous air embolism. After insertion of a central catheter, a chest radiograph is the standard of care to confirm correct placement. If there is a clinical suspicion of catheter tip migration or other potential complications, further diagnostic testing is indicated.

Trauma to vessels and pneumothorax are complications that may warrant surgical intervention, insertion of a chest tube or tubes, or both. Catheter occlusion can simply be a result of the catheter tip lodging against the vessel wall or being physiologically "pinched" between the clavicle and first rib. Occlusion can also occur from fibrin buildup (which accounts for 70% of occurrences of occlusion), blood or lipid deposition, drug precipitates, and catheter breakage.[22] Another type of occlusion, "withdrawal occlusion," is an occlusion that allows infusion of a solution but prevents blood withdrawal. Although more research is needed to determine optimal methods for catheter maintenance and patency during parenteral nutrition infusions, routine flushing of catheters with diluted heparin (10 to 100 units/mL in those without heparin sensitivities) is recommended.[17]

Thrombosis formation in the lumen of the vessel often results from mechanical irritation (such as from traumatic catheter insertion), a small lumen, an extended duration of catheter use, the catheter material, or malpositioning. The reported rate of occurrence of subclavian thrombosis is 2%, whereas the incidence of subclinical venous thrombosis is near 50%.[23] Therefore, nurses need to be aware that patients may have a thrombosis and may be asymptomatic, yet complain of vague head and eye swelling on the affected side.[17] Vigilant assessments during parenteral nutrition administration are recommended. Treatment includes catheter removal, systemic anticoagulation, and thrombolytic therapy.

A venous air embolism is another serious complication, with a mortality rate of up to 50%.[17] Any disruption of the closed catheter system (usually during line connection changes, when hanging a new bag of TPN, or in an accidental tubing disconnection) can increase the risk for an air embolism. If such an incident occurs, the patient will most likely experience acute, centrally located chest pain, dyspnea, and hypotension. Immediate nursing interventions include clamping the tubing of the catheter or occluding the catheter hub, attempting to aspirate air directly from the venous line, administering 100% oxygen, and placing the patient in steep Trendelenburg's position with the left lateral side down (because this position allows air to rise to the level of the right ventricle, away from the pulmonary vasculature).[17,23] Prevention of an air embolism can be facilitated by having the patient perform the Valsalva maneuver or simply hum audibly during line changes. In ventilator-dependent patients, positive intrathoracic pressure can be created by initiating mechanical lung inflations or "breaths." Finally, use of sterile occlusive dressings (e.g., petroleum gauze) over the catheter entrance site is an effective measure in preventing air from entering the track after the catheter has been discontinued.[17]

METABOLIC COMPLICATIONS

Checking each bag of parenteral nutrition solution for transcription accuracy, monitoring the IV pump for infusion accuracy, and monitoring the patient's response to therapy are all paramount in preventing serious metabolic complications. It is important to understand that many metabolic complications stem from the patient's underlying disease processes or from imprudent formula administration. Metabolic laboratory abnormalities, such as hyperglycemia and hypokalemia, can be treated by adjusting the formula's concentration of macronutrients, micronutrients, electrolytes, and insulin.

Virtually any metabolic disturbance can occur during parenteral nutrition infusion. Glucose intolerance or hyperglycemia, hypophosphatemia, hypokalemia, hypomagnesemia, and hypocalcemia are among the most common metabolic complications. Many of these metabolic disturbances, coupled with fluid imbalances, may lead to refeeding syndrome.

Hyperglycemia

Hyperglycemia, or a blood sugar elevated over 220 mg/dL, can occur if the pancreas does not respond to the increased glucose load. Although it can be caused by either enteral or parenteral feedings, it is more commonly seen in patients receiving parenteral nutrition. Even slightly elevated blood glucose levels can impair the function of lymphocytes, leading to immunosuppression and increased infection risk. Elevated glucose concentrations have been shown to reduce neutrophil chemotaxis and phagocytosis and may be an independent risk factor for short-term infections.[3] If the renal threshold for glucose reabsorption is exceeded, osmotic diuresis results in subsequent dehydration and electrolyte imbalances. While compounding the TPN solution under sterile conditions, a pharmacist can add insulin to the solution. Glycemic control can be achieved by increasing the amount of insulin in the TPN solution, by maintaining a continuous insulin drip during TPN administration, or by administering sliding-scale insulin subcutaneously at regular intervals. Once TPN is discontinued, insulin requirements will be notably less or nonexistent. When new TPN solution is temporarily unavailable, administration of 10% dextrose in water ($D_{10}W$) is recommended to prevent rebound hypoglycemia. In addition, if a solution is "behind schedule," it is not recommended that the infusion rate be increased to make up time; this may cause sudden metabolic fluctuations and fluid overload.

Refeeding Syndrome

In situations where a patient may be severely malnourished, initiation of TPN may induce a phenomenon called *refeeding syndrome.* This is characterized by rapid changes in electrolytes (phosphorus, potassium, magnesium, calcium), glucose, and volume status within hours to days of nutrition implementation. Despite relatively normal serum phosphorus levels, intracellular stores are markedly depleted in malnourished catabolic patients. Glucose loads stimulate insulin release, which in turn stimulates intracellular uptake of phosphorus, glucose, and other electrolytes for anabolic processes. Severe hypophosphatemia (<1 mg/dL) can lead to neuromuscular, respiratory, and cardiac dysfunction.[3] Low serum levels of potassium, magnesium, and calcium can precipitate cardiac arrhythmias. The increased intravascular fluid volumes, associated with parenteral nutrition in particular, can strain the viscerally depleted heart and possibly induce heart failure and myocardial damage.

Prevention and management of refeeding syndrome include correction of pre-existing glucose and electrolyte abnormalities before institution of nutritional therapy. Total volume and rate are titrated slowly to evaluate for fluid overload and potential cardiac decompensation. Accurate intake and output measurements and daily weights are of paramount importance because adequate parenteral nutrition often means giving 1.5 to 3 L of fluid per day in addition to other therapies. If the patient has impaired cardiac or renal function, this could lead to fluid overload and congestive heart failure; a progressive weight gain could be an early indicator of poor fluid tolerance.

INFECTIOUS COMPLICATIONS

Both the solution and the indwelling catheter are prime sites for infection owing to the high glucose content. Any break in the system is a nidus for infection that can progress to a systemic infection if left unchecked. Therefore, the solutions are prepared by a pharmacist under a laminar flow hood to ensure a particle-free, sterile environment. After initial preparation, the access hubs are often covered with tape as a reminder that no additional solutions or medications are to be added.

At the bedside, the solution bag and tubing are changed according to institution policy, usually every 24 hours. The catheter insertion site is redressed per institution policy, usually every 24 to 72 hours, using either a sterile transparent or gauze dressing. Although transparent dressings allow for easier observation of the catheter entrance site, these dressings have a tendency to trap more moisture and hence have a higher incidence of infection and sepsis than traditional, sterile dry gauze dressings; however, this is still under investigation.[3] At the time of the dressing change, the site should be examined for signs of leakage, erythema, edema, and inflammation. The skin must be cleansed well with an antibacterial solution to remove pathogenic organisms. Chlorhexidine solution has been shown to be a more effective local antiseptic than iodophor or alcohol.[24] The presence of a tracheostomy or other open draining wounds near the IV insertion site requires special precautions to prevent site contamination.

Potential for infection can be minimized by meticulous catheter care. In critically ill patients, catheter-related infections range from local inflammation to systemic bloodstream infection and sepsis. Systemic catheter-related infections are associated with a 35% mortality rate, and hospital stays are reportedly longer and more expensive as a result of complications and associated treatment.[3,25,26] If fever, rigors, or chills coincide with parenteral infusion, catheter-related sepsis should be suspected; slowing or stopping the infusion may cause defervescence.[3] Treatment of an infection may involve local topical antibiotics, systemic antibiotics, and, in many cases, catheter removal. If catheter sepsis is suspected, the catheter tip is usually cultured to identify the offending organism for appropriate antibiotic coverage.

Terminating Parenteral Nutrition

Tapering or cycling (bedtime) TPN is often given in those patients who are able safely to resume (and tolerate) oral or enteral nutrition. In such instances, a calorie count is essential to ascertain that the patient's nutritional needs are being met. Before discontinuation of parenteral nutrition, the infusion rate is decreased by half for 30 to 60 minutes to allow for a plasma glucose response and prevention of rebound hypoglycemia.[27] Checking blood sugars within a 30- to 60-minute window after discontinuation helps the nurse identify and manage immediate glucose abnormalities.

In situations where poor prognosis does not warrant aggressive nutritional support, emotional and ethical dilemmas may surface for many nurses because feeding and hydration have long been basic tenets of nursing care. Although many institutions may have protocols in place regarding parenteral nutrition, treatment decisions and plan of care should be discussed on an individual basis; frequent, ongoing discussions between the patient, family, and the health care team are imperative to providing the best possible care to each patient.

ROLE OF THE NURSE IN NUTRITIONAL SUPPORT

Nurses are responsible for obtaining initial "dry weight" and weekly weight measurements, vital signs, intake and output measurements, and laboratory data, and for providing enteral tube and IV catheter care throughout the duration of nutrition support therapies. Many complications, whether from enteral or parenteral nutrition, can be prevented by vigilant observation and care. If the patient is awake and alert, the patient's subjective assessment of tolerance can be very informative. More objective signs of feeding tolerance are obtained through abdominal examinations, which assess bowel sounds and changes in abdominal girth. Volume and frequency of both urine and stool are monitored and recorded.

The nurse must also monitor for clinical signs of dehydration (thirst, dry mucous membranes, tachycardia, and poor skin turgor), and fluid excess (peripheral edema and adventitious lung sounds). Early detection and subsequent interventions may prevent the occurrence of excessive fluid shifts and cardiac compromise. This is of special concern if the patient is severely malnourished, which may precipitate refeeding syndrome and other untoward complications. Meticulous feeding tube and IV catheter care is critical to preventing local and systemic forms of infection.

Care also includes providing information and emotional support to the patient and family. Examples include explaining the procedure, what to expect, risks, and expected outcomes (Box 40-4). Guidelines for discharge planning are given in Box 40-5.

clinical applicability challenges

Self-Challenge: Critical Thinking

1. *An elderly man is status post-right cerebral vascular accident, resulting in left hemiparesis and severe dysphagia. Despite daily work with a speech and swallowing specialist, oral feeding is contraindicated because of high risk for aspiration. His wife gives consent for surgical placement of a percutaneous endoscopic gastrostomy (PEG) tube for long-term management of nutrition and hydration. Explore why this tube placement was chosen.*
   a. *Is this an appropriate intervention for this patient? Why or why not?*
   b. *What are the alternatives?*

Study Questions

1. *The most accurate method of determining initial nasogastric feeding tube placement is*
   a. *auscultating for air over the gastric region.*
   b. *aspirating secretions and checking the pH.*
   c. *abdominal radiography.*
   d. *both a and b.*
2. *Immediately after an open cholecystectomy, a patient is started on enteral tube feedings at goal rate. Twelve hours after surgery, the patient has had four episodes of diarrhea, approximately 475 mL. Bowel sounds are present. The most appropriate and initial nursing action would be to*
   a. *request that the patient be changed to parenteral nutrition.*
   b. *request that the patient be changed to maintenance intravenous IV fluids only.*
   c. *reduce the rate of the enteral feeding infusion.*
   d. *send stool for* Clostridium difficile *cultures.*
3. *A patient has a duodenal feeding tube placed endoscopically past the pylorus. The nurse giving you the report tells you that the patient is receiving enteral nutrition at goal rate of infusion of 60 mL/hour; however, he is concerned that the residual 1 hour ago was 125 mL. An abdominal film*

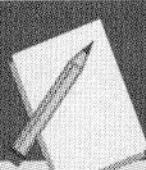

box 40-4 Living With Nutritional Support

General Care: Enteral Nutrition

- Administer enteral formulas as prescribed.
- Know potential complications and appropriate treatments.
- Avoid activities that may result in high impact or stress at the insertion site and report any activity that may have damaged the enteral access site.
- Return to previous activities (e.g., work, leisure, sexual activity) after obtaining physician consent.

General Care: Parenteral Nutrition

- Administer parenteral formulas as prescribed.
- Monitor blood sugars closely to help determine tolerance of parenteral solutions.
- Know the potential complications and appropriate treatments.
- Avoid activities that may result in high impact or stress at the insertion site and report any activity that may have damaged the parenteral access site.
- Return to previous activities (e.g., work, leisure, sexual activity) after obtaining physician consent.

Signs of Infections

- Understand the rationale for aseptic technique.
- Notify the nurse of symptoms of fever, localized warmth, redness, pain, or drainage at the feeding tube or intravenous insertion site.

Medications

- Follow instructions regarding medications.
- Know the names of medications and the dose, frequency of administration, side effects, and use of each medication.
- Know the proper technique of administering medications through the feeding tube and proper flushing technique.
- Never add medications to TPN solutions—they should be added by the supplier because of risk of contamination or precipitation of the formula.

Safety Measures

- Inform other health care providers of either enteral or parenteral access devices and notify them of any medications that the patient may be taking.

Follow-up Care

- Report any problems to the home care nurse.
- Adhere to schedule for follow-up visits with patient's physician or clinic.

confirms correct placement. The most appropriate nursing action is to

a. *hold tube feedings for 2 hours and restart at a lower rate.*
b. *resume tube feedings as ordered and monitor for nausea/vomiting; residuals postpyloric may be misleading.*
c. *discontinue enteral feedings and request parenteral nutrition be initiated.*
d. *hold tube feedings for 4 hours and restart after diluting with water.*

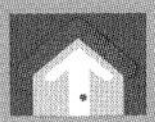

box 40-5 Nutritional Therapy

- Assess patient/caregiver ability to deliver home nutritional therapy, including physical and cognitive abilities.
- Identify health care team members who will be responsible for the management of home therapy.
- Assess patient's home environment for safety.
- Evaluate support system available in home.
- Identify an in-home caretaker who is willing and able to learn and carry out the home care regimen. If the patient does not have a caretaker at home and there are concerns about patient's ability to become independent, reevaluate discharge plan.
- Ensure that patient/caregiver learning includes determining procedures and risks, picking up patient and equipment problems early, troubleshooting, and following up with the health care provider.
- Refer to and communicate with home care services.
- Provide written instructions for patient.
- If possible, do not change the amount or rate of nutrition support on the day of discharge to home.

4. *Which of the following macronutrients in parenteral nutrition may need to be increased in a patient who has large, nonhealing wounds?*
   a. *Carbohydrates*
   b. *Lipids*
   c. *Trace elements*
   d. *Protein*

REFERENCES

1. Souba WW: Nutritional support. N Engl J Med 336(1):41–48, 1997
2. Braunschweig C, Gomez S, Sheean PM: Impact of declines in nutritional status outcomes in adult patients hospitalized for more than 7 days. J Am Diet Assoc 100(11):1316–1324, 2000
3. Braunwald E, Fauci AS, Kasper DL, et al: Enteral and parenteral nutrition therapy. In Harrison TR (ed): Principles of Internal Medicine (15th Ed), pp. 470–478. New York, McGraw-Hill, 2001
4. Marian MJ, Allen P: Nutrition support for patients in long-term acute care and subacute care facilities. AACN Clin Issues 9(3):427–440, 1998
5. Cerra FB, Blackburn GL, Jeejeebhoy K, et al: Applied nutrition in ICU patients: A consensus statement of the American College of Chest Physicians. Chest 111(3):769–778, 1997
6. Guenter P, Jones S, Ericson M: Enteral nutrition therapy. Nurs Clin North Am 32(4):651–668, 1997
7. Bliss DZ, Lehmann S: Tube feeding administration tips. RN 62(8): 29–32, 1999
8. Kirby DF, Delegge MH: American Gastroenterological Association medical position statement: Guidelines for the use of enteral nutrition. Gastroenterology 108(4):1280–1301, 1995
9. Stone SJ, Pickett JD, Jesurum JT: Bedside placement of postpyloric feeding tubes. AACN Clin Issues 11(4):517–530, 2000
10. Grant MC, Martin S: Delivery of enteral nutrition. AACN Clin Issues 11(4):507–516, 2000
11. Bowers S: All about tubes: Your guide to enteral feeding devices. Nursing 2000 30(12):41–48, 2000
12. Lord LM: Enteral access devices. Nurs Clin North Am 32(4): 685–704, 1997
13. Loan T, Magnuson B, Williams S: Debunking six myths about enteral feeding. Nursing 98 28(8):43–49, 1998

14. Weinstein DS, Furman J: Enteral formulas. Nurs Clin North Am 32(4):669–683, 1997
15. DeWitt RC, Kudsk KA: Enteral nutrition. Gastroenterol Clin North Am 7(2):371–386, 1998
16. Morrisson SG: Feeding the elderly population. Nurs Clin North Am 32(4):791–812, 1997
17. Worthington P, Gilbert KA, Wagner BA: Parenteral nutrition for the acutely ill. AACN Clin Issues 11(4):559–579, 2000
18. Heimburger DC, Weinster RL: Handbook of Clinical Nutrition (3rd Ed). St. Louis, Mosby, 1997
19. A.S.P.E.N. Board of Directors: Safe practices for nutrition formulations. JPEN J Parenter Enteral Nutr 22:49–66, 1998
20. U.S. Food and Drug Administration: Safety Alert: Hazards of precipitation associated with parenteral nutrition. Am J Hosp Pharm 51:1427–1442, 1994
21. Semrad CE: Parenteral nutrition. Clin Perspect Gastroenterol 3(6): 307–313, 2000
22. Wickham RS: Advances in venous access devices and nursing management strategies. Nurs Clin North Am 25:345–364, 1990
23. Hinke DH, Zandt-Stastny DA, Goodman LR, et al: Pinch-off sign: A complication of implantable subclavian access devices. Radiology 177:353–356, 1990
24. Maki DG, Ringer M, Alvarado CJ: Prospective randomized trial of povidone-iodine, alcohol, and chlorhexidine for prevention of infection associated with central venous and arterial catheters. Lancet 338:339, 1991
25. Krzywda EA, Andris DA, Edminston CE: Catheter infections: Diagnosis, treatment, and prevention. Nutr Clin Pract 14:178–190, 1999
26. U.S. Department of Health and Human Services, Public Health Service, Centers for Disease Control and Prevention: Guideline for prevention of intravascular device-related infections. Am J Infect Control 24:262–293, 1996
27. Krzydwa EA, Andris DA, Whipple JA, et al: Glucose response to abrupt initiation and discontinuation of total parenteral nutrition. JPEN J Parenter Enteral Nutr 17:64–67, 1991

OTHER SELECTED READING

Adams GF, Guest DP, Ciraulo DL, et al: Maximizing tolerance of enteral nutrition in severely injured trauma patients: A comparison of enteral feedings by means of percutaneous endoscopic gastrostomy versus percutaneous endoscopic gastrojejunostomy. J Trauma 48(3):459–465, 2000

American Society for Gastrointestinal Endoscopy: The role of PEG/PEJ in enteral feeding. Gastrointest Endosc 48(6):699–701, 1998

Braunschweig CL, Levy P, Sheean PM, et al: Enteral compared with parenteral nutrition: A meta analysis. Am J Clin Nutr 74:534–542, 2001

Dimick J, Swoboda S, Talamini M, et al: Risk of colonization for central venous catheters: Catheters for total parenteral nutrition versus other catheters. Am J of Crit Care 12(4):328–335, 2003

Dranoff JA, Angood PJ, Topazian M: Transnasal endoscopy for enteral feeding tube placement in critically ill patients. Am J Gastroenterol 94(10):2902–2904, 1999

Evans-Stoner N: Guidelines for care of the patient on home nutrition support: An appendix. Nurs Clin North Am 32(4):769–775, 1997

Garrett K, Tsuruta K, Walker S, et al: Managing nausea and vomiting: Current strategies. Criti Care Nurse 23(1):31–52, 2003

Hammond K: Physical assessment: A nutritional assessment. Nurs Clin North Am 32(4):779–790, 1997

Horn D, Chaboyer W: Gastric feeding in critically ill children: A randomized controlled trial. Am J of Crit Care 12(5):461–468, 2003

Karch AM: 2002 Lippincott's Nursing Drug Guide. Philadelphia, Lippincott Williams & Wilkins, 2002

Kohn-Keeth C: How to keep feeding tubes flowing freely: How to clear the way if clogging occurs. Nursing 2000 30(3):58–59, 2000

Kudsk KA, Croce MA, Fabian TC, et al: Enteral versus parenteral feeding: Effects on septic morbidity after blunt and penetrating abdominal trauma. Ann Surg 215:503–511, 1992

Lacy CF, Armstrong LL, Golman MP, et al: Drug Information Handbook (9th Ed). Hudson, OH, Lexi-Comp, 2001

Lenart S, Polissar NL: Comparison of 2 methods for postpyloric placement of enteral feeding tubes. Am J of Crit Care 12(4):357–360, 2003

Loan T, Kearney P, Magnuson B, et al: Enteral feeding in the home environment. Home Healthcare Nurse 15(8):531–538, 1997

Marino PL: The ICU Book (2nd Ed). Baltimore, Williams and Wilkins, 1998

Marshall AP, West SH: Gastric tonometry and enteral nutition: A possible conflict in critical care nursing practice. Am J of Crit Care 12(4):349–356, 2003

Medical Economics Staff: PDR: Physicians Desk Reference (56th Ed). Montvale, NJ, Medical Economics, 2002

Medical Economics Staff: Physician's Desk Reference for Nonprescription Drugs and Dietary Supplements (22nd Ed). Montvale, NJ, Medical Economics, 2001

Metheny NM: Fluid and Electrolyte Balance: Nursing Considerations (4th Ed). Philadelphia, Lippincott Williams & Wilkins, 2000

Olsen J: Clinical Pharmacology Made Ridiculously Simple (2nd Ed). Miami, Medmaster, 2001

Parrish CR: Protocols for practice: Applying research at the bedside. Crit Care Nurse 19(1):91–94, 1999

Powers J, Chance R, Bortenschlager L, et al: Bedside placement of small-bowel feeding tubes in the intensive care unit. Crit Care Nurse 23(1):16–24, 2003

Reddy P, Malone M: Cost and outcome analysis of home parenteral and enteral nutrition. JPEN J Parenter Enteral Nutr 22(5):302–310, 1998

Roberts SR, Kennerly DA, Keane D, George C: Nutrition support in the intensive care unit: Adequacy, timeliness, and outcomes. Crit Care Nurse 23(6):49–57, 2003

Schiff L (ed): Enhanced enteral feeding formulas. RN 63(9):77–79, 2000

chapter

41

Common Gastrointestinal Disorders

ALLISON G. STEELE ■ VALERIE SABOL

objectives

Based on the content in this chapter, the reader should be able to:

- Examine the pathophysiological concepts that help define acute gastrointestinal bleeding, obstruction and ileus, acute pancreatitis, hepatitis, and cirrhosis.
- Compare and contrast the pertinent history, physical examination, and diagnostic study findings for acute gastrointestinal bleeding, obstruction and ileus, acute pancreatitis, hepatitis, and cirrhosis.
- Discuss laboratory studies that are useful in the diagnosis and management of acute gastrointestinal bleeding, obstruction and ileus, acute pancreatitis, hepatitis, and cirrhosis.
- Analyze the similarities and differences in caring for patients with acute gastrointestinal bleeding, obstruction and ileus, hepatitis, and cirrhosis.
- Explore the nursing role in assessing, managing, and evaluating a plan of care for patients with acute gastrointestinal bleeding, obstruction and ileus, acute pancreatitis, hepatitis, and cirrhosis.

ACUTE GASTROINTESTINAL BLEEDING

Acute gastrointestinal bleeding is a common, and potentially lethal, medical emergency seen in people admitted to the intensive care unit (ICU). There are 300,000 hospital admissions each year in the United States as a result of acute gastrointestinal bleeding.[1] The 10% mortality rate associated with acute gastrointestinal bleeding has remained constant over the past half century despite advances in diagnosis and treatment.[1,2] The cause of death is rarely from exsanguination but rather from the exacerbation of other medical illnesses. Prompt recognition and treatment of the patient experiencing an acute gastrointestinal bleed requires a team approach.

Acute gastrointestinal bleeding is differentiated into upper and lower gastrointestinal bleeding. The ligament of Treitz at the junction of the duodenum and jejunum is the anatomic division between the upper and lower gastrointestinal tracts. An upper gastrointestinal bleed occurs from a source in the esophagus, stomach, or duodenum. A lower gastrointestinal bleed occurs from a source in the jejunum, ileum, colon, or rectum.

Upper Gastrointestinal Bleeding

ETIOLOGY

The possible causes of acute upper gastrointestinal bleeding are listed in Box 41-1. A complete discussion of this list is beyond the scope of this chapter. The most commonly

box 41-1
Common Causes of Acute Gastrointestinal Bleeding

Upper Gastrointestinal Bleeding

Esophageal Source
- Varices
- Esophagitis
- Ulcers
- Tumors
- Mallory-Weiss tears

Gastric Source
- Peptic ulcers
- Gastritis
- Tumors
- Angiodysplasia
- Dieulafoy's lesions

Duodenal Source
- Peptic ulcers
- Angiodysplasia
- Crohn's disease
- Meckel's diverticulum

Lower Gastrointestinal Bleeding
- Malignant tumors
- Polyps
- Ulcerative colitis
- Crohn's disease
- Ischemic colitis
- Infectious colitis
- Angiodysplasia
- Diverticulosis
- Hemorrhoids
- Massive upper gastrointestinal hemorrhage

seen causes of acute gastrointestinal bleeding in the ICU are discussed.

Peptic Ulcer Disease

Peptic ulcer disease, which includes both gastric and duodenal ulcers, accounts for approximately 50% of acute upper gastrointestinal bleeding.[1] The epithelial cells of the gastroduodenal mucosa are protected from the potentially damaging effects of gastric secretions, medications, alcohol, and bacteria by several protective mechanisms. These cells secrete mucins, phospholipids, and bicarbonate that create a pH gradient between the acidic gastric lumen and the cell surface. Prostaglandins enhance this mucosal protection by increasing mucosal secretion, increasing bicarbonate production, maintaining mucosal blood flow, and enhancing the resistance of gastroduodenal cells to injury. In addition, the tight junctions of the epithelial cells resist diffusion. When these protective factors are overwhelmed by aggressive factors, the integrity of the gastric or duodenal mucosal is interrupted, which can result in peptic ulcer disease. Bleeding from peptic ulcer disease occurs when the ulcer erodes into the wall of a blood vessel.

The primary risk factor for peptic ulcer disease is infection with the bacterium *Helicobacter pylori*. *H. pylori* infection has been associated with 90% of duodenal ulcers and 75% of gastric ulcers. *H. pylori* is a gram-negative, spiral, flagellated rod that colonizes the mucus layer overlying the gastric epithelium. The flagellum of *H. pylori* facilitates the bacterium's ability to move and adhere to the mucus layer. *H. pylori* produces urease, which converts urea to ammonia and carbon dioxide. The ammonia buffers the acid surrounding the bacterium, creating a more hospitable environment that allows the bacterium to thrive in the acidic stomach. *H. pylori* infection predisposes the mucosa to damage by disrupting the mucus layer, liberating enzymes and toxins, and adhering to the epithelium. Inflammation is furthered by a host immune response. This chronic inflammation usually results in an asymptomatic chronic gastritis. However, in some instances ulceration develops.

In the absence of *H. pylori* infection, the ingestion of aspirin or nonsteroidal anti-inflammatory drugs (NSAIDs) account for most cases of peptic ulcer disease. The ingestion of aspirin and NSAIDs may directly injure the mucosal layer. Ingestion enhances mucosal permeability and allows back-diffusion of acid. Systemic effects of chronic aspirin or NSAID use include inhibition of prostaglandin synthesis by the gastroduodenal mucosa, which decreases mucus and bicarbonate production, as well as mucosal blood flow. This alteration in mucosal cytoprotection may lead to the development of an ulcer. Cigarette smoking may also predispose to peptic ulcer disease, and is linked to prolonged healing rates and high ulcer reoccurrence.

Stress-Related Erosive Syndrome

Stress-related erosive syndrome, also called *erosive gastritis*, *stress ulceration*, and *hemorrhagic gastritis*, is a common cause of acute gastrointestinal bleeding in critically ill patients. Stress ulcers are different from the ulcers of peptic ulcer disease; they tend to be more numerous, more shallow, and more diffuse. These ulcers may develop in the stomach, duodenum, and esophagus within hours of injury. They are usually shallow and cause oozing from superficial capillaries, but may erode into the submucosa and cause massive hemorrhage.

The risk for development of a stress ulcer depends on the severity and type of illness (Box 41-2). The common

box 41-2 ***Risk Factors for Stress-Related Erosive Syndrome***

- Hypotension or shock
- Coagulopathy
- Respiratory failure requiring mechanical ventilation
- Sepsis
- Hepatic failure
- Renal failure
- Multiple or severe trauma
- Burns over 35% of the total body surface area (TBSA)
- Post–organ transplant status
- Head or spinal cord injury
- History of peptic ulcer disease or upper gastrointestinal bleeding
- Prolonged stay in intensive care unit (ICU)

feature of these risk factors is the relationship to physiological stress. Decreased perfusion of the stomach mucosa is probably the main mechanism of ulcer development. This contributes to impaired mucus secretion, low mucosal pH, poor mucosal cell regeneration, and decreased tolerance to acid gastric secretions. Acute gastrointestinal bleeding from stress-related erosive syndrome is associated with a high mortality rate.[1]

Esophageal Varices

Portal hypertension usually develops as a result of cirrhosis, from increased resistance in the portal venous system caused by disruption of the normal liver lobular structure. This resistance impedes blood flow into, through, and out of the liver. In response to portal hypertension, collateral veins develop to bypass the increased portal resistance in an attempt to return blood to systemic circulation. As pressure rises in these veins, they become tortuous and distended, forming varicose veins or varices.

Varices may develop in the esophagus, stomach, duodenum, colon, rectum, or anus. The most clinically significant site of varices is the gastroesophageal junction because of the propensity of varices in this area to rupture, resulting in massive gastrointestinal hemorrhage. Esophageal varices account for 10% to 15% of all cases of acute upper gastrointestinal bleeding.[1] In patients with cirrhosis, 60% of upper gastrointestinal bleeds are the result of varices.[1] The mortality rate associated with variceal bleeding is 40%.[1]

Mallory-Weiss Tears

Mallory-Weiss tears account for approximately 10% to 15% of acute upper gastrointestinal bleeds.[1] Mallory-Weiss tears are lacerations that occur in the distal esophagus, at the gastroesophageal junction, and the cardia of the stomach. Bleeding from Mallory-Weiss tears occurs when the tear involves the underlying venous or arterial bed. Mallory-Weiss tears are strongly associated with heavy alcohol use or recent binge drinking and a prior history of forceful vomiting or retching, or violent coughing. Patients with portal hypertension have an increased risk of bleeding from Mallory-Weiss tears.

Dieulafoy's Lesions

Dieulafoy's lesions are vascular malformations of unusually large submucosal arteries, which lie in close contact with the mucosal surface. They can be found anywhere in the gastrointestinal tract but are most likely to be found in the proximal stomach. Because of the large size of the artery, bleeding from a Dieulafoy's lesion may be massive and recurrent. When bleeding ceases, a Dieulafoy's lesion can be difficult to identify because there is no associated ulcer.

CLINICAL PRESENTATION

Regardless of the cause, patients with acute upper gastrointestinal bleeding have a clinical presentation consistent with the amount of blood loss. Patients with minimal loss may present with anemia and no further symptoms, whereas those patients with rapid and severe loss may present with signs and symptoms of shock. If blood loss is moderate, the sympathetic nervous system responds with a release of the catecholamines epinephrine and norepinephrine, which initially cause an increase in heart rate and peripheral vascular vasoconstriction in an attempt to maintain an adequate blood pressure. In this setting, orthostatic changes may be present (a decrease in blood pressure greater than 10 mm Hg with a corresponding heart rate increase of 20 beats/minute in the sitting or standing position). Orthostatic hypotension indicates blood loss of greater than 1,000 mL.

The patient's response to blood loss depends on the amount and rate of blood loss, his or her age, the degree of compensation, and the rapidity of treatment. With severe blood loss, signs and symptoms of shock appear. The release of catecholamines triggers the blood vessels in the skin, lungs, intestines, liver, and kidneys to constrict, thereby increasing the volume of blood flow to the brain and heart. Because of the decreased flow of blood in the skin, the person's skin is cool to the touch. With decreased blood flow to the lungs, hyperventilation occurs to maintain adequate gas exchange.

The classic hallmarks of gastrointestinal bleeding are hematemesis, hematochezia, and melena. Patients with upper gastrointestinal bleeding usually present with hematemesis, the vomiting of fresh, unaltered blood or "coffee-ground" material; melena, the passage of black, tarry, sticky stool; or both. A patient who presents with hematemesis is usually bleeding from a source above the ligament of Treitz. Reverse peristalsis is seldom sufficient to cause hematemesis if the bleeding point is below this area. The classic "coffee-ground" emesis associated with upper gastrointestinal bleeds results from the partial decomposition of the blood from contact with gastric secretions. Gastric acid converts bright red hemoglobin to brown hematin, accounting for the coffee-ground appearance of the drainage. Maroon or bright red blood results from profuse bleeding and little contact with gastric juices.

Melena is black from the breakdown of the blood in transit and suggests a long transit time through the gastrointestinal tract. Melena is indicative of an upper gastrointestinal bleed in 90% of cases. It may take several days after bleeding cessation for melenic stools to clear. After an upper gastrointestinal bleed, stool may remain hemoccult-positive for 1 to 2 weeks. Hematochezia, the passage of maroon or bright red blood, usually indicates bleeding from a lower gastrointestinal source. Uncommonly, hematochezia can occur in the setting of massive, rapid hemorrhage from the upper gastrointestinal tract, where the large amount of blood acts as a cathartic and result in rapid transit through the gastrointestinal tract.

ASSESSMENT

History

Patients may present with hematemesis, hematochezia, or melena suggestive of an upper gastrointestinal bleed, or hematochezia suggestive of a lower gastrointestinal bleed. A prompt, careful, focused history may suggest the underlying cause. A history of epigastric pain, dyspepsia, or a past medical history of peptic ulcer disease is suggestive of peptic ulcer disease. A past medical history of gastrointestinal bleeding should be elicited because 60% of upper gastrointestinal bleeds rebleed from the same site.[1] Heavy alcohol use increases the likelihood of cirrhosis and bleeding from esophageal varices. Patients with a history of tobacco use have a greater risk for duodenal ulcers. Underlying medical conditions may suggest an underlying cause; patients with renal failure frequently bleed from arteriovenous malformations. Vomiting, coughing, or retching before bleeding suggests a Mallory-Weiss tear. Prior use of NSAIDs or aspirin increases the risk of gastroduodenal ulcers, and the likelihood of bleeding from these ulcers.

Physical Examination

The physical examination should be directed initially to the assessment of hemodynamic stability. Tachycardia and orthostatic hypotension indicate dehydration secondary to blood loss or vomiting. Orthostatic hypotension is suggestive of a greater than 15% blood volume loss, and tachycardia usually occurs when greater than 15% of blood volume is lost.[1] If 40% of blood volume is lost, hypovolemia may occur.[1] Therefore, assessing for signs and symptoms of poor tissue perfusion such as angina, cyanosis, and altered mental status is important. A baseline electrocardiogram is critical in patients with known cardiac disease because blood loss may precipitate cardiac ischemia. A loss of circulating blood volume may result in decreased cerebral perfusion. The nurse should be alert to signs of agitation or confusion, which may signal cerebral hypoperfusion. The abdomen should be assessed for bowel sounds; abdominal tenderness; the presence of guarding, rigidity, abdominal masses; and the stigmata of liver disease. A tender, boardlike abdomen is suggestive of peritonitis, possibly as a result of perforation. A rectal examination is essential to assess for hematochezia and melena.

Laboratory Studies

Laboratory studies can help determine the extent of bleeding, and can often provide a clue to the etiology. Common laboratory abnormalities for the patient with acute gastrointestinal bleeding are listed in Box 41-3. The initial hematocrit and hemoglobin may not accurately reflect initial blood loss because plasma volume is lost in the same proportion as red blood cells. Within 24 to 48 hours of the initial bleed, redistribution of plasma from the extravascular to the intravascular space results in a decreased hematocrit. Fluids administered during resuscitation contribute to the hemodilution. Leukocytosis and hyperglycemia may reflect the body's response to stress. Hypokalemia and hypernatremia may result from loss through emesis. An elevated blood urea nitrogen (BUN) level reflects a large protein load from the breakdown of blood. A high BUN-to-creatinine ratio suggests an upper gastrointestinal source of bleeding.[1] Coagulopathy with a prolonged prothrombin time (PT) can indicate liver disease or concurrent long-term anticoagulant therapy. Thrombocytopenia may be present in patients with cirrhosis and portal hypertension with splenomegaly. If large amounts of blood are lost, metabolic acidosis occurs as a result of anaerobic metabolism. Severe blood loss can result in hypoxemia because of decreased circulating hemoglobin with impairment of oxygen transport to cells.

box 41-3
Typical Laboratory Abnormalities in a Patient With Acute Gastrointestinal Bleeding

- Decreased hemoglobin and hematocrit
- Mild leukocytosis and hyperglycemia
- Elevated blood urea nitrogen (BUN) level
- Hypernatremia
- Hypokalemia
- Prolonged prothrombin time (PT)/partial thromboplastin time (PTT)
- Thrombocytopenia
- Hypoxemia

MANAGEMENT

Resuscitation

The initial management of any patient with an acute gastrointestinal bleed is directed at fluid resuscitation to reverse the effects of blood loss. Supplemental oxygen is provided to any patient with an acute gastrointestinal bleed to promote oxygen saturation and transport. Intubation may be required for actively bleeding patients at high risk of aspiration, those with a diminished mental status, and those in respiratory distress. Patients with acute upper gastrointestinal bleeding should be made NPO because urgent endoscopy or surgery may be required. A Foley catheter is inserted to monitor urine output as an indication of the adequacy of fluid resuscitation. All patients with hemodynamic instability, a drop in hematocrit, transfusion requirements greater than 2 units of packed red blood cells (PRBCs), or active bleeding warrant an ICU admission.

Volume Resuscitation. Patients with acute gastrointestinal bleeding require immediate intravenous (IV) access with at least two large-bore (14- to 16-gauge) IV catheters or central access. A type and cross-match should be sent early in the course of the bleed because blood losses of greater than 1,500 mL require blood replacement in addition to fluids. While awaiting cross-matched blood, Ringer's lactate or normal saline is infused to restore circulating volume and to prevent the progression to hypovolemic shock. Packed red blood cells are often transfused to reestablish the oxygen-carrying capacity of the blood. Other blood products, such as platelets and clotting factors, are ordered according to results of laboratory tests and the patient's underlying condition. Calcium replacement may be necessary if large numbers of banked red blood cells are transfused because the citrate in banked blood products can bind calcium and lead to hypocalcemia. A pulmonary artery catheter or central venous catheter may be useful to help avoid over-resuscitation in patients with underlying renal or cardiac disease. In patients with a coagulopathy, vitamin K can be given in the form of phytonadione (AquaMEPHYTON), 10 mg intramuscularly or very slowly intravenously, in an attempt to restore the PT to normal. Fresh frozen plasma is ordered to correct the abnormality if rapid correction of the abnormality is warranted.

Rarely, vasoactive drugs are used until fluid balance is restored to maintain blood pressure and perfusion to vital body organs. Dopamine, epinephrine, and norepinephrine are drugs that may be ordered to stabilize the patient until definitive treatment can be undertaken.

Nasogastric Intubation. A large-bore nasogastric tube is placed in all patients with gastrointestinal bleeding to aspirate and lavage gastric contents. A nasogastric tube documents the presence and activity of bleeding. The color of gastric aspirate is prognostically significant. "Coffee-ground" or black nasogastric drainage with melenic stools indicates a slow bleed, and has a corresponding 9% mortality rate, whereas bright red nasogastric drainage and bright red blood in the stools signify a rapidly bleeding upper gastrointestinal source, with a corresponding mortality rate of 30%.[1]

A nasogastric tube is also useful for decompression and lavage. Lavage helps to clear blood from the stomach, which assists in identifying the source of bleeding during endoscopy. Iced lavage should be avoided because it is uncomfortable, fails to control bleeding, can significantly decrease core body temperature, and can trigger cardiac dysrhythmias. Lavage should be performed with tap water or saline—250 to 500 mL is instilled through the nasogastric tube and then removed with a syringe or by intermittent wall suction until gastric secretions are clear. Nasogastric tubes are usually removed after lavage of stomach contents unless the patient is actively bleeding or is experiencing severe nausea and vomiting, because a nasogastric tube may injure the gastric mucosa and contribute to bleeding.

Acid-Suppressive Therapy. Patients with acute upper gastrointestinal bleeding are often treated with acid-suppressive therapy to decrease the risk of recurrent bleeding, particularly from peptic ulcers. The use of high-dose proton pump inhibitors (omeprazole, lansoprazole, esomeprazole, pantoprazole, rabeprazole) to maintain a gastric pH greater than 4 has been shown to be beneficial in this setting.[2] Acid-suppressive therapy with histamine (H_2)-antagonistic drugs (cimetidine, ranitidine, famotidine, nizatidine) may be used as prophylactic therapy in patients at high risk for stress-related erosive syndrome.

Antacids are also ordered. Antacids act as a direct alkaline buffer and are administered to control gastric pH. Sucralfate, a basic aluminum salt of sucrose octasulfate, acts locally as a cytoprotective drug and can be ordered for stress-related erosive syndrome prophylaxis.

Pharmacotherapy for Decreasing Portal Hypertension. Even before a bleeding source is identified, decreasing portal pressure with vasopressin or octreotide should be considered in patients for whom variceal hemorrhage is suspected. Vasopressin (Pitressin) decreases portal hypertension by constriction of the splanchnic arteries, which reduces blood flow. Vasopressin is administered through a central line at a rate of 0.4 to 1 U/minute. Complications of vasopressin therapy can limit its use. Vasopressin reduces coronary blood flow and increases blood pressure, which increases oxygen demand, and causes coronary artery constriction, which can potentially result in multiple cardiac dysrhythmias. Because vasopressin also reduces blood flow to the mesenteric circulation, bowel ischemia can develop. To minimize these potential side effects, vasopressin should be given with concomitant use of IV, sublingual, or topical nitroglycerin to minimize the systemic effects.

Somatostatin is a natural polypeptide that lowers portal venous pressure by vasoconstriction of splanchnic circulation. Somatostatin causes selective vasoconstriction of the splanchnic circulation and is associated with fewer systemic side effects than vasopressin. IV infusion is necessary because of its short half-life.

Octreotide (Sandostatin) is a synthetic analog of somatostatin with similar hemodynamic properties but a longer half-life. Octreotide causes a 25% decrease in splanchnic blood flow and a 30% to 35% decrease in intravariceal pressure.[3] Octreotide is usually given as a 50-μg IV bolus followed by 50 μg/hour for 3 to 5 days. The effects of octreotide are similar to vasopressin with nitroglycerin infusion without the impact on hemodynamics or cardiac output.[3]

Definitive Diagnosis

After patents with acute upper gastrointestinal bleeding are resuscitated, endoscopy is considered. Endoscopy can be performed urgently at the bedside and is the procedure of choice for the diagnosis and potential treatment of acute upper gastrointestinal bleeding. Endoscopy within 12 to 24 hours of the initial bleed has the best results. When endoscopy is performed soon after bleeding, it has 90% to 95% accuracy in diagnosis.[1] Early endoscopy is essential in gastrointestinal bleeding from esophageal varices because the treatment is different. Endoscopy allows the identification of the site of the bleed because direct mucosal inspection is possible. The endoscopic appearance provides prognostic value for the risk of rebleeding based on the presence of stigmata of recent bleeding and the patient's hemodynamic status.[1] Vital signs must be monitored closely during endoscopy. The left lateral decubitus position decreases the risk of aspiration from active bleeding.

When diagnostic endoscopy is unsuccessful due to massive hemorrhage, angiography can be used to define the site of bleeding or abnormal vasculature. Angiography can detect bleeding rates as low as 0.5 to 1 mL/minute.[4]

Barium studies, such as an upper gastrointestinal series, are not of any value in acute upper gastrointestinal bleeding. These studies lack therapeutic capability and preclude endoscopy and angiography because of retained barium.[4] Barium studies are also often inconclusive if there are clots in the stomach or if there is superficial bleeding.

Therapeutic Intervention

Endoscopy. In addition to its use in diagnosis, endoscopy is the procedure of choice for the treatment of a gastrointestinal bleed. Multiple therapeutic options are available, including injection sclerotherapy, thermal coagulation, the placement of hemostatic clips, and endoscopic variceal ligation (EVL). The optimal technique depends on multiple variables, including the type and appearance of the lesion and the experience of the endoscopist.

The primary methods of endoscopic control of upper gastrointestinal hemorrhage from peptic ulcers include injection therapy and thermal methods. Injection therapy consists of the injection of an agent such as epinephrine around and into the bleeding vessel. Thermal methods include heater probe and bipolar electrocoagulation (where a probe is applied with pressure to heat and seal the bleeding vessel).[5] Hemostatic clips, called *endoclips*, have also been used successfully to ligate bleeding blood vessels within a lesion.

EVL is the treatment of choice for the treatment of variceal bleeding. In EVL, a rubber band is placed endoscopically around the base of each varix. This causes coagulative necrosis and sloughing of thrombosed varices. EVL can control acute variceal bleeding in 90% of cases with a reduction in the rate of rebleeding to 30%.[1] An alternative to EVL is sclerotherapy. Injection sclerotherapy involves injecting the varices with a sclerosing agent to stop the bleeding. These agents cause local tamponade and vasoconstriction, causing necrosis and eventual sclerosis of the bleeding vessel. Acute hemostasis rates are similar to those with EVL, but sclerotherapy is associated with a higher complication rate.

Angiography. Most cases of gastrointestinal bleeding resolve spontaneously or can be controlled during endoscopy. However, those patients with persistent bleeding may require angiography to control the source of bleeding. During angiography, arterial gastrointestinal bleeding can be controlled by the infusion of intra-arterial vasopressin or by the embolization of the artery by an interventional radiologist. If therapeutic endoscopy fails this is a useful therapeutic option, particularly in those who are critically ill and poor surgical candidates.

Intra-arterial vasopressin causes a generalized vasoconstriction that produces a rapid reduction in local blood flow. Patients should be monitored closely for dysrhythmias and fluid retention with resultant hyponatremia. Repeat angiography is performed after the initial infusion and the dose can then be titrated as needed. Once bleeding is controlled, this infusion may be continued in the ICU for 24 to 36 hours and then tapered over 24 hours.[4] Patients should have cardiac monitoring during vasopressin therapy to watch for cardiac dysrhythmias. Nitroglycerin patches or drips may be used to counteract any ischemic changes.

Embolization of a bleeding vessel consists of occluding the vessel with material that can be either temporary or permanent. Biodegradable long-acting gelatin sponges are commonly used. These sponges cause hemostasis on contact when injected into the vessel. Steel coils, balloons, and silk thread can be used to block an artery mechanically, resulting in permanent occlusion.

Balloon Tamponade. Variceal bleeding unresponsive to endoscopic therapy can be temporarily controlled with balloon tamponade in 60% to 90% of cases.[1] Most esophagogastric tubes have two balloons, one for the stomach and one for the esophagus, and a distal port for gastric drainage. The Sengstaken-Blakemore tube is the most widely used (Fig. 41-1).

With the use of balloon tamponade, pressure is exerted on the cardia of the stomach and against the bleeding varices. The tube is inserted to at least 50 cm to ensure gastric intubation. The gastric balloon is then slowly inflated with 250 to 300 mL of air, and gentle traction is applied, until the gastric balloon fits snugly against the cardia of the stomach. Position is then confirmed by x-ray. Traction is then placed on the tube where it enters the patient by means of a piece of sponge rubber, as shown in Figure 41-1, or by traction fixed to a head helmet device or the foot of bed. If chest pain occurs, the gastric balloon must be deflated immediately because it may have shifted into the esophagus.

If bleeding continues, the esophageal balloon is inflated to a pressure of 25 to 40 mm Hg and maintained at this pressure for 24 to 48 hours. Although pressure for longer than 24 hours may be needed to control bleeding, it can cause edema, esophagitis, ulcerations, or perforation of the esophagus. After bleeding is controlled, the balloon is maintained and inflated for no longer than 12 to 24 hours to decrease the risk of gastric ischemia and necrosis. Unfortunately, rebleeding often occurs after balloon deflation unless additional therapeutic measures are taken.

A nasogastric tube should be placed in patients with a Sengstaken-Blakemore tube to aspirate oral and nasopharyngeal secretions that collect above the esophageal balloon, preventing aspiration of these secretions into the lungs. The Minnesota esophagogastric tamponade tube (see Fig. 41-1) has a suction port above the esophageal balloon in addition to the usual ports (two balloon, one gastric suction) of the Sengstaken-Blakemore tube. Nursing interventions for the patient with an esophageal tamponade tube are given in Box 41-4.

Transjugular Intrahepatic Portosystemic Shunt. A transjugular intrahepatic portosystemic shunt (TIPS) is a radiologic procedure that creates an intrahepatic shunt in an attempt to decrease portal pressure. The placement of a TIPS may be considered if other methods of managing esophageal varices fail.

Surgery. In the era of endoscopic therapy and proton pump inhibitors, surgery is rarely used for the control of gastrointestinal bleeding. The indications for surgical intervention are severe hemorrhage unresponsive to initial resuscitation, massive bleeding that is immediately life-threatening, unavailable or failed endoscopic therapy, perforation, obstruction, suspicion of malignancy, or continued bleeding despite aggressive medical therapies.[6]

Surgical options for a bleeding peptic ulcer depend on the age and the condition of the patient, as well as on the location, size, and anatomy of the bleeding source. Emergency surgery of a bleeding duodenal ulcer may be a simple suturing (e.g., oversew) of the ulcer. Bleeding duodenal ulcers can also be treated using one of the following procedures:

- Truncal vagotomy and pyloroplasty with suture ligation of the ulcer
- Truncal vagotomy and antrectomy with resection or suture ligation of the ulcer
- Proximal gastric vagotomy with duodenotomy and suture ligation of the ulcer[6]

Bleeding gastric ulcers are commonly treated with one of the following procedures:

- Truncal vagotomy and pyloroplasty with wedge resection of the ulcer
- Antrectomy with wedge excision of the proximal ulcer
- Distal gastrectomy with or without truncal vagotomy
- Wedge resection of the ulcer[6]

A vagotomy involves severing the vagus nerve, which innervates the gastric cells. This results in decreased gastric acid secretion. A truncal (gastric) vagotomy selectively cuts the vagus distribution to the stomach. A pyloroplasty is necessary in conjunction with the vagotomy because

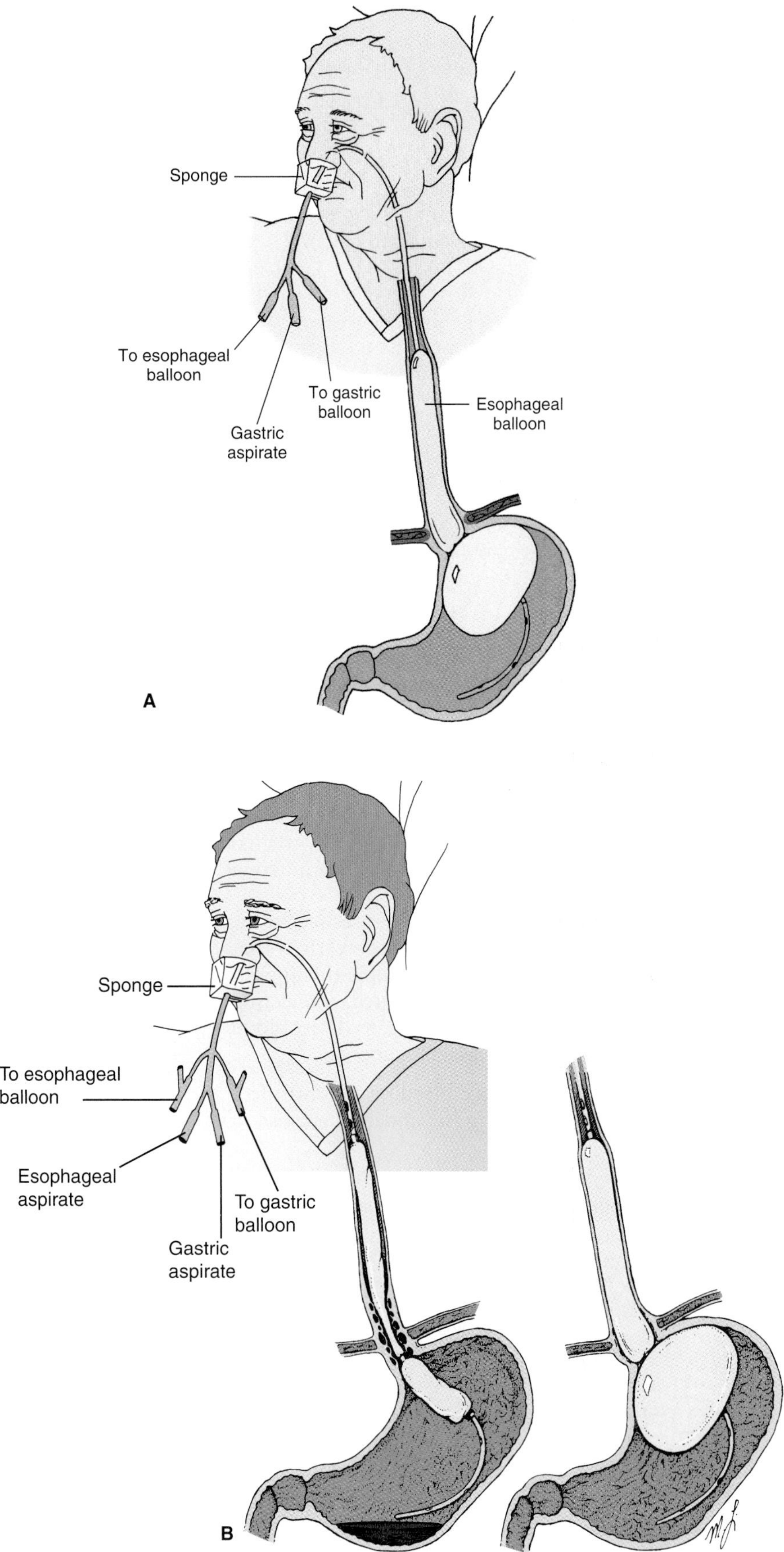

figure 41-1 Comparison of two types of esophageal tamponade tubes. (**A**) The Sengstaken-Blakemore tube is the best known. An additional tube must be placed in the proximal esophagus. (**B**) The Minnesota esophagogastric tamponade tube includes an esophageal aspirate lumen.

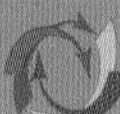

box 41-4 nursing interventions for the Patient With an Esophagogastric Balloon Tamponade Tube

- Explain the purpose of the tube and the procedure to the patient.
- Lubricate and chill the tube as directed by the manufacturer.
- Identify and label the lumens of the tube.
- Check the patency of each lumen before insertion of the tube.
- Lavage the patient's stomach before insertion of the tube.
- Monitor the patient while the physician inserts the tube.
- Elevate the head of the bed to 30 degrees to prevent reflux.
- When a Sengstaken-Blakemore tube is in place, perform oropharyngeal suction frequently to prevent aspiration, *or* place a second nasogastric tube if ordered above the esophageal balloon to control secretions and prevent aspiration.
- Suction the esophageal port when a Minnesota tube is used.
- Maintain balloon pressure and traction.
- Maintain balloon position.
- Clean and lubricate the patient's nostrils frequently to prevent tube-caused pressure areas.
- Irrigate the nasogastric port every 2 hours to ensure patency and to keep the stomach empty.
- Teach the patient to avoid coughing or straining, which increases intra-abdominal pressure and predisposes to further bleeding.
- Have a second nasogastric tube, suction, and scissors available at the bedside.
- If the gastric balloon ruptures, the tube can rise into the nasopharynx, obstructing the airway. If this occurs, cut the tube immediately to deflate the balloon rapidly.
- Cut and remove the tube whenever there is a question of respiratory insufficiency or aspiration.
- Restrain the patient's arms if the patient is at risk for pulling out the tube. Agitation, confusion, and restlessness are risk factors.
- Assess for complications, including rupture or deflation of the balloon, pulmonary aspiration, and esophageal rupture.

denervation of the vagus nerve affects gastric motility. A pyloroplasty allows for continued gastric emptying. An antrectomy removes acid-producing cells in the stomach. A Billroth I procedure includes a vagotomy and antrectomy with anastomosis of the stomach to the duodenum. A Billroth II procedure involves a vagotomy, resection of the antrum, and anastomosis of the stomach to the jejunum (Fig. 41-2). A gastric perforation can be surgically treated by simple closure or use of a patch to cover the mucosal hole.

Surgical decompression of portal hypertension can be used in patients with esophageal or gastric varices that are unresponsive to medical and endoscopic therapy. In this surgery, a portosystemic shunt is created, connecting the portal vein and the inferior vena cava to divert blood flow into the vena cava to decrease pressure.

Medical Management. Once bleeding is controlled, management focuses on treating the underlying cause of the acute upper gastrointestinal bleeding. For patients with peptic ulcer disease, eradication of *H. pylori* and elimination of NSAID use increases the healing rate and markedly reduces the recurrence of a rebleed. Esophageal varices can be obliterated in subsequent endoscopy sessions, and beta-blockade with propanolol (Inderal) or nadolol (Corgard) can be instituted to decrease the rebleeding rate. The dose should be titrated to achieve a 25% decrease in resting heart rate or a heart rate around 60 beats/minute as the desired end point.[7,8] Cessation of alcohol ingestion is imperative. See Box 41-5 for nursing interventions in the care of the patient with acute gastrointestinal bleeding.

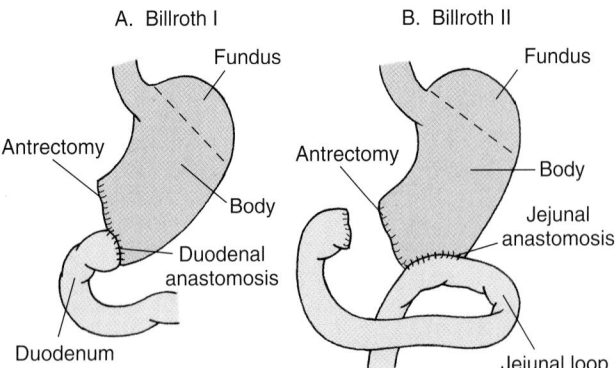

figure 41-2 (**A**) The Billroth I procedure includes a vagotomy and antrectomy with anastomosis of the stomach to the duodenum. (**B**) The Billroth II procedure includes a vagotomy, antrectomy, and anastomosis of the stomach to the jejunum.

Lower Gastrointestinal Bleeding

ETIOLOGY

Common causes of lower gastrointestinal bleeding are listed in Box 41-1. Most cases of acute lower gastrointestinal bleeding that require ICU admission result from diverticulosis or angiodysplasia, although bleeding from neoplasm, colitis, inflammatory bowel disease, and hemorrhoids is also seen.

Diverticulosis

Diverticula are saclike protrusions in the colon wall that usually develop at the point where arteries penetrate the colon wall. These vessels are separated from the bowel lumen only by the mucosa and are subsequently prone to injury. Diverticular bleeding accounts for 30% to 50% of all cases of acute lower gastrointestinal bleeds.[9] In the elderly, colonic diverticula account for 42% to 55% of all cases of acute lower gastrointestinal bleeding.[10] Diverticular bleeding may be massive, resulting in hemorrhage. Risk factors for diverticular bleeding include a diet low in fiber, aspirin and NSAID use, advanced age, and constipation.

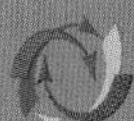

box 41-5 nursing interventions for *the Patient With Acute Gastrointestinal Bleeding*

- Maintain a patent airway, elevate the head of the bed, and have suction available at the bedside to prevent aspiration of emesis or blood.
- Administer oxygen therapy to treat hypoxia that may result from decreased hemoglobin levels.
- Monitor pulse oximetry.
- Assess and document signs and symptoms of shock, such as restlessness; diminished peripheral pulses; or cool, pale, or moist skin. Assess and document vital signs, urinary output, hemodynamic values, and oxygen saturation (Sao_2).
- Assess and document electrocardiographic monitoring and heart, lung, and bowel sounds.
- Assist with the placement of a central venous pressure catheter or a pulmonary artery catheter.
- Monitor and document central venous pressure (CVP), pulmonary artery pressure (PAP), pulmonary artery wedge pressure (PAWP), cardiac output, and systemic vascular resistance (SVR).
- Maintain IV access and administer IV fluids and blood products as ordered.
- Insert a nasogastric tube and lavage as ordered.
- Monitor gastric pH; consult with physician about specific pH range and antacid administration.
- Administer antisecretory medications as ordered to reduce gastric acid secretion.
- Administer vasopressin or octreotide as ordered.
- Maintain accurate intake and output every 1 to 2 hours and PRN.
- Record urine, nasogastric drainage, and emesis.
- Monitor electrolytes, which may be lost with fluids or altered due to fluid shifts, and report abnormal values.
- Monitor hemoglobin, hematocrit, red blood cell count, prothrombin time (PT), partial thromboplastin time (PTT), and blood urea nitrogen (BUN) level and report abnormal values.
- Provide mouth care as needed.
- Explain all procedures to the patient.
- Prepare the patient for diagnostic procedures and therapeutic interventions.
- Monitor the patient for potential complications of endoscopy or colonoscopy, which include perforation, sepsis, pulmonary aspiration, and induced bleeding.
- Teach the patient the importance of seeking medical intervention if signs or symptoms of bleeding recur.
- Encourage smoking cessation and avoidance of alcohol.

Angiodysplasia

Angiodysplasia, also called *arteriovenous malformation* or *angioma*, is the term used to describe dilated, tortuous submucosal veins, small arteriovenous communications, or enlarged arteries. The walls of the vessels lack smooth muscle and are composed of endothelial cells. The incidence of angiodysplasia increases with age due to the degeneration of the vessel walls; most occur in people older than 50 years and two thirds occur in those older than 70 years.[10] Acute lower gastrointestinal bleeding from angiodysplasia accounts for 20% to 30% of cases.[9] Angiodysplasia can occur anywhere in the colon, although it most often occurs in the cecum or ascending colon. As opposed to bleeding from diverticula, bleeding from angiodysplasia may be venous or arteriovenous in nature and is therefore usually less severe than bleeding from diverticular disease, which is arterial. Angiodysplasia is a common cause of lower gastrointestinal bleeding in patients with renal disease.

CLINICAL PRESENTATION

Acute lower gastrointestinal bleeding is defined by the presence of hemodynamic instability and the passage of hematochezia. Patients with diverticular bleeding usually describe the sudden onset of painless maroon or bright red hematochezia, although melena can rarely occur. Diverticular bleeding is often painless, although patients may complain of cramping (which results from colonic spasm secondary to intraluminal exposure to blood). Blood loss from angiodysplasia usually presents as painless hematochezia.

If lower gastrointestinal bleeding is chronic, patients may present with iron-deficiency anemia and symptoms related to the anemia, such as weakness, fatigue, or dyspnea on exertion. Massive bleeding from hemorrhoids is rare but can occur in patients with rectal varices from portal hypertension.

ASSESSMENT

History

Relevant findings in the past medical history include abdominal surgery; a previous bleeding episode; peptic ulcer disease; inflammatory bowel disease; radiation to the abdomen or pelvis; or cardiopulmonary, renal, or liver disease. Knowledge of the patient's current medications and the existence of any allergies can also assist in diagnosis. A history of associated symptoms, including abdominal pain, fever, rectal urgency, tenesmus, weight loss, a change in bowel habits, and the color and consistency of the stool should be elicited. The age of the patient may give a clue to diagnosis because the risk of bleeding from diverticula and angiodysplasia increases with age.

Physical Examination

The physical examination is often unremarkable. Vital signs are closely monitored to assess for hemodynamic instability. A palpable mass may reveal a neoplasm. A rectal examination is essential to assess for hematochezia and melena and exclude the possibility of bleeding hemorrhoids, which can occasionally present as a hemorrhage.

Laboratory Studies

The initial laboratory studies include a complete blood count, serum electrolytes, BUN and creatinine levels, and PT and partial thromboplastin time (PTT). Type and cross-match is mandatory before red blood cell transfusion, as in acute upper gastrointestinal bleeding.

MANAGEMENT

Resuscitation

The management of acute lower gastrointestinal bleeding requires aggressive fluid resuscitation as described for acute upper gastrointestinal bleeding. Patients with hematochezia should have a nasogastric tube inserted to exclude an upper gastrointestinal source of bleeding because 10% of suspected lower gastrointestinal bleeding occurs from upper gastrointestinal sources.[11] The presence of bloody aspirate confirms an upper gastrointestinal source of bleeding. However, the absence of blood does not exclude an upper gastrointestinal source because bleeding from a site in the duodenum may not reflux into the stomach. Nasogastric aspirate that reveals bile without blood is unlikely in bleeding from an upper gastrointestinal source. Once it is determined that bleeding is coming from a lower gastrointestinal source, colonoscopy is the procedure of choice for both diagnosis and treatment.

Definitive Diagnosis

Endoscopy. Colonoscopy is the test of choice for the evaluation of lower gastrointestinal bleeding. Colonoscopy has a diagnostic accuracy of 70% to 80% in patients with lower gastrointestinal bleeding.[11] Other advantages of colonoscopy are the ability to precisely locate the source of the bleeding, the ability to take biopsies, and the potential for therapeutic intervention. Before colonoscopy, the colon needs to be cleansed with 4 L of polyethylene glycol solution given orally or by nasogastric tube until the waste is clear. For those patients in whom bleeding has stopped, it is reasonable to perform colonoscopy on an elective rather than emergent basis. If a source of bleeding is identified during colonoscopy, therapeutic options include thermal coagulation or injection with epinephrine or other sclerosants, as discussed previously. Upper endoscopy should be performed if colonoscopy is unable to distinguish a lower gastrointestinal source.

Radionucleotide Imaging. When colonoscopy fails to identify a bleeding source, radionucleotide scanning can detect bleeding that occurs at rates of 0.1 to 0.5 mL/minute. This is more sensitive than angiography but less specific than either colonoscopy or a positive angiogram. The two types of scanning available are the technetium (^{99m}Tc)–sulfur colloid and ^{99m}Tc pertechnetate–labeled autologous red blood cells. Unfortunately, both of these techniques provide poor localization because of the peristaltic action of the bowel. However, these scans may be useful before angiography because those patients with a negative scan are likely to have negative angiograms.

Angiography. Angiography is reserved for patients with massive, ongoing bleeding where endoscopy is not an acceptable option, or in the case of recurrent or persistent bleeding from a source not identified on colonoscopy. Angiography requires the active blood loss of 0.5 to 1.5 mL/minute to visualize a bleeding site.[6] A positive angiogram is associated with a high likelihood for surgical intervention. When an active source is identified, arteriographic intervention with intra-arterial vasopressin or embolization may be used. The critical care nurse must be aware of the potential complications associated with arteriography, which include allergy to contrast, contrast-induced renal failure, bleeding from the arterial puncture site, and even embolism from thrombus.

Surgical Intervention

Surgical management of lower gastrointestinal bleeding is less likely to be an emergent procedure. An exploratory laparotomy to identify the source of the bleeding is often performed. A segmental bowel resection with a primary anastomosis is often done for definitive treatment of lower gastrointestinal bleeding. In patients who are unstable, a stoma and mucus fistula may be created. In those patients with severe lower gastrointestinal bleeding without a localized source, a blind total colectomy may be the operative choice.[6] Surgical management of diverticular bleeding is indicated if bleeding is not controlled with endoscopic or angiographic means or in patients with recurrent bleeding from the same segment.[6]

INTESTINAL OBSTRUCTION AND ILEUS

Intestinal obstruction occurs when the passage of intestinal contents through the lumen is impaired. This can result from either mechanical (anatomical) or nonmechanical causes. Ileus is the failure of passage of intestinal contents in the absence of mechanical obstruction. Intestinal obstruction is classified as either partial or complete, depending on the degree of obstruction. In a simple obstruction there is no ischemia, whereas in cases of strangulated obstruction, ischemia is present. A closed-loop obstruction describes a mechanical obstruction with a proximal and distal occlusion of the affected intestinal segment.

Bowel obstruction can occur in both the small and large bowel. The small bowel is most commonly affected, with the ileum as the most common site of obstruction. Large bowel obstruction accounts for only 15% of cases of bowel obstruction and the sigmoid colon is the most common site of obstruction. The location of the obstruction, the degree of obstruction, and the presence of ischemia are important distinctions because treatment varies. Prompt recognition of bowel obstruction is important for the critical care nurse because intestinal obstruction can progress to bowel strangulation, infarction, and perforation and result in potentially life-threatening peritoneal and systemic infection. The mortality rate associated with a strangulated obstruction is 30%.[12,13]

The causes of mechanical obstruction are varied and classified as extrinsic, intrinsic, and intraluminal (Box 41-6). Extrinsic lesions occur outside of the bowel. Examples of extrinsic lesions are adhesions, hernias, volvulus, and masses. Intrinsic lesions extend into the bowel wall. Diverticulitis, neoplasms, and radiation enteritis are examples of intrinsic lesions. Intraluminal causes of obstruction can

box 41-6
Causes of Mechanical Obstruction

Extrinsic Lesions
- Adhesions and congenital bands
- Hernias
  - External hernias
  - Internal hernias
  - Diaphragmatic hernias
  - Pelvic hernias
- Volvulus
  - Gastric
  - Midgut
  - Cecal
  - Sigmoid
- Extrinsic masses
  - Benign or malignant tumors
  - Abscesses
  - Aneurysms
  - Hematomas
  - Endometriosis

Intrinsic Lesions
- Benign and malignant neoplasms
  - Adenocarcinomas
  - Lymphomas, lymphosarcomas
  - Carcinoid tumors
- Inflammatory conditions
  - Tuberculous enteritis, Crohn's disease
  - Strictures secondary to Potassium chloride, nonsteroidal anti-inflammatory drugs, and ischemia
  - Radiation injury, caustic ingestants
  - Eosinophilic gastroenteritis, ameboma
  - Diverticulitis, pelvic inflammatory disease
- Intussusception
- Congenital defects
  - Hypertrophic pyloric stenosis, annular pancreas
  - Intestinal atresia/agenesis
  - Malrotation/volvulus
  - Intestinal duplication, mesenteric cysts
  - Meckel's diverticulum
  - Hirschsprung's disease
- Hematoma
  - Abdominal trauma
  - Thrombocytopenia
  - Henoch-Schönlein purpura

Intraluminal Causes
- Meconium ileus
- Barium impaction
- Fecal impaction
- Gallstone ileus
- Gastric bezoars
- Foreign bodies

From Yamada T, Alpers DH, Laine L, et al (eds): Textbook of Gastroenterology (4th Ed), p 834. Philadelphia, Lippincott Williams & Wilkins, 2003.

result from the ingestion of foreign bodies, intussusception, and neoplasms.

Small Bowel Obstruction

ETIOLOGY

Adhesions are the most common cause of small bowel obstruction in adults and account for 66% to 75% of obstructions.[14] Adhesions most commonly occur after laparotomy for colectomy, appendectomy, or gynecological procedures. Adhesions can also develop after abdominal radiation, ischemia, or infection, or as the result of foreign bodies. Adhesions may develop only days after surgery and as late as 10 to 20 years later. Adhesive bands can form and contract and, in time, may entrap a loop of bowel.

Hernias are the second most common cause of small bowel obstruction and account for 25% of cases.[14] Small bowel obstruction secondary to hernia carries a high risk of complete obstruction and strangulation. The herniation of a portion of the bowel after laparotomy is called a Richter's hernia. The occurrence of a small bowel obstruction in the absence of previous laparotomy should suggest hernia as the cause. Tumors are uncommon in the small bowel, although luminal compression by gastric, pancreatic, colonic, and gynecological cancers can cause extrinsic compression in approximately 10% of small bowel obstruction.[14] Primary neoplasms of the small bowel account for less than 3% of small bowel obstruction.[14]

PATHOPHYSIOLOGY

In small bowel obstruction, large amounts of fluid and swallowed air accumulate in the intestinal lumen proximal to the obstruction, causing distension (Fig. 41-3). Fluid accumulates from oral intake; swallowed saliva; and gastric, biliary, and pancreatic juices. Swallowed air has a high nitrogen content and is poorly absorbed from the lumen.[15]

As the obstruction continues, the bowel wall and lumen become edematous and distended. Increased intraluminal pressure leads to increased capillary permeability and movement of fluid and electrolytes into the abdominal cavity. This extravasation of fluid and electrolytes into the peritoneal cavity combined with fluid lost through vomiting can lead to hypovolemia, hypokalemia, and hyponatremia. Peristalsis decreases and the normal functions of the intestine decrease or halt. In the absence of normal intestinal motility, bacterial overgrowth occurs. If oral intake continues, bacterial fermentation can contribute to gas accumulation. Within hours of acute obstruction, the contents of the lumen proximal to obstruction become malodorous and feculent because of this bacterial overgrowth.

CLINICAL PRESENTATION

The severity of symptoms is related to the site and degree of obstruction (Table 41-1). Patients with small bowel obstruction usually complain of the acute onset of intermittent, crampy abdominal pain. Bursts of peristalsis above the obstruction cause pain. The pain is often more severe the more proximal the obstruction. Patients with an incomplete obstruction often describe crampy abdominal pain after meals. The pain in incomplete obstruction may be exacerbated by the ingestion of high-fiber meals. In proximal small bowel obstruction, vomiting occurs frequently and early in the course of obstruction. The emesis is usually bilious and vomiting often relieves the pain. Minimal abdominal distension usually accompanies proximal small bowel obstruction.

Distal small bowel obstruction often presents with moderate abdominal distension and intermittent or constant pain. Vomiting is intermittent. In ileal small bowel obstruction, the emesis may be feculent secondary to bacterial overgrowth.

In strangulated obstruction, the pain is more localized and may be steady and severe. When vomiting is protracted, dehydration and hypovolemia may occur.

Fever may be present secondary to an inflammatory process or in response to bowel ischemia or perforation. Constipation is also a common complaint, although patients may continue to pass gas and stool as the bowel distal to the obstruction empties. Depending on the duration

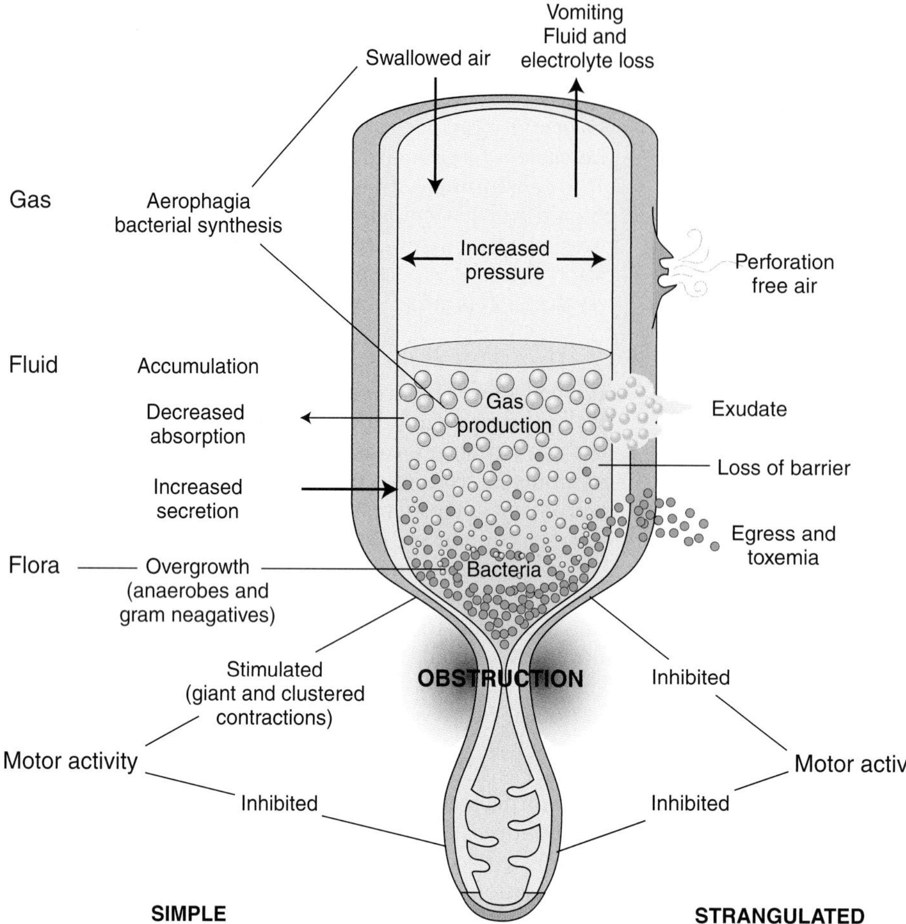

figure 41-3 The pathophysiology of simple obstruction (*left*) and strangulated obstruction (*right*) in the small intestine. (Used with permission from Yamada T, Alpers DH, Laine L et al [eds]: Textbook of Gastroenterology [4th Ed], p 830. Philadelphia, Lippincott Williams & Wilkins, 2003).

and severity of the obstruction, hemodynamic instability may develop as a result of massive fluid trapping in the lumen with leakage into the peritoneum.

ASSESSMENT

History

A careful history provides clues to etiology. A past medical history of previous abdominal surgery or trauma increases the risk of adhesions. Other pertinent past medical history findings include inflammatory bowel disease, diverticulitis, abdominal or pelvic radiation, peptic ulcer disease, pancreatitis, and previous obstruction or cancer. Correlation to menses suggests endometriosis. A complete medication history is also essential. Patients with a psychiatric history should be questioned about ingestion of foreign objects.

table 41-1 Clinical Features of Ileus and Obstruction Dependent on Anatomic Site

	Site of Obstruction				
	Ileus	***Gastric Outlet***	***Distal Duodenum***	***Jejunoileal***	***Colon***
Pain	Mild	Mild	Mild	Moderate	Severe
Distension	Moderate to severe	Mild	Mild	Moderate	Severe
Emesis					
Amount/frequency	Small, infrequent	Copious, frequent	Copious, frequent	Smaller/less frequent	Uncommon
Nature	Sour, bilious	Clear, sour, HCl, KCl	Bile-stained, bitter, NaCl, $NaHCO_3$	Malodorous, feculent	Variable
Acid–base imbalance	Variable	Metabolic alkalosis	Metabolic acidosis	Dehydration, hypotension	Usually not severe

HCl, hydrogen chloride; KCl, potassium chloride; $NaHCO_3$, sodium bicarbonate; NaCl, sodium chloride.
From Yamada T, Alpers DH, Laine L, et al (eds): Textbook of Gastroenterology (4th Ed), p 833. Philadelphia, Lippincott Williams & Wilkins, 2003.

Physical Examination

Inspection of the abdomen often reveals visible peristalsis and distension. Patients with a proximal small bowel obstruction may have epigastric or periumbilical tenderness, whereas those with distal small bowel obstruction often have more diffuse tenderness. Bowel sounds are usually hyperactive in the early course of the obstruction, then high-pitched and tinkling with loud rushes as peristaltic waves attempt to push intestinal contents past the obstruction. Skin turgor and mucous membranes may show signs of dehydration. A palpable mass may represent a neoplasm or volvulus. A rectal examination is performed to assess for blood. Inspection may reveal scars and external hernias. Hepatomegaly, liver masses, or other abdominal masses suggest malignancy. Abdominal tenderness and palpable masses may suggest abscess. Fever, rigors, and declining clinical status suggest bowel strangulation. Patients with a closed-loop obstruction may describe pain out of proportion to physical findings. Borborygmi are often audible and may correlate with abdominal cramping. If rebound tenderness is present, observe for signs and symptoms of shock because perforation is a possibility. Percussion of the abdomen may reveal resonance or tympany from fluid trapped in the intestine. Shifting dullness indicates ascites. Palpate for inguinal, femoral, and umbilical hernias. A tender mass at the site of a hernia suggests the etiology. Erythema overlying the skin may result from strangulation.[14] Tachycardia, tachypnea, altered mental status, oliguria, and hypotension may all be present in hypovolemia.

Laboratory Studies

Although there is no single laboratory value that is diagnostic for small bowel obstruction, laboratory values are important in the management of small bowel obstruction. Mild leukocytosis is present with simple obstructions, whereas white blood cell elevations from 15,000 to 25,000/µL accompany strangulation.[12] Mesenteric occlusion and perforation result in white blood cell elevations of 25,000/µL or more.[12] In proximal obstruction, potassium, sodium, hydrogen, and chloride may be lost in emesis, resulting in metabolic alkalosis. BUN, creatinine, sodium, and osmolality levels reflect the fluid and electrolyte shifts that occur as fluid leaks out of the intestine and electrolytes are either reabsorbed or lost. As dehydration increases, the hemoglobin and hematocrit level is elevated, reflecting hemoconcentration. In ischemia or strangulation, amylase, lipase, alkaline phosphatase, creatine phosphokinase (CPK), aspartate aminotransferase (AST), alanine aminotransferase (ALT), and lactate dehydrogenase (LDH) levels may rise.[14] Heme-positive stools are often present in ischemia or carcinoma. Metabolic acidosis suggests severe hypoxemia due to hypoperfusion, and metabolic acidosis refractory to fluid resuscitation suggests strangulation.[14]

Imaging Studies

Radiography. When a small bowel obstruction is suspected, abdominal x-rays with the patient in upright, flat, and side-lying positions can confirm the diagnosis of obstruction, localize the site of obstruction, and assist in determining if the obstruction is complete or partial. Normally there is little air in the small bowel. In complete small bowel obstruction, gas and fluid accumulate proximal to the obstruction. Multiple air–fluid levels may be visible, with a stepladder pattern that demonstrates multiple loops of bowel with different air levels. Distal to the obstruction, the bowel lumen empties and collapses within 12 to 24 hours. Successive films may also confirm the diagnosis.

Barium studies may be helpful in the diagnosis of obstruction if plain films are nondiagnostic. Contrast studies can differentiate between a complete or partial obstruction. Barium is the agent of choice if small bowel obstruction is suspected because it provides a better contrast than water-soluble material. In small bowel obstruction, the large amount of water present proximal to the obstruction dilutes water-soluble contrast. However, if there is any question about bowel perforation, barium should be avoided because free barium in the peritoneum can cause significant inflammation. If colonic obstruction is suspected, a limited barium enema is used for diagnosis before barium is given by mouth.

Computed Tomography. Abdominal computed tomography (CT) scans can help to identify obstructive lesions and signs of ischemia. Abdominal CT with oral or IV contrast can help to differentiate mechanical obstruction from pseudo-obstruction. A transition zone may be visible between dilated and collapsed loops of bowel, suggesting the point of obstruction.

Endoscopy. Direct visualization with endoscopy may confirm the obstruction in the colon or proximal small bowel and aid in determining the type (mechanical, strangulated, paralytic).

MANAGEMENT

Medical Management

When possible, obstructions, especially incomplete obstructions, are treated medically rather than surgically. Oral food and fluid are withheld (i.e., the patient is put on NPO status) and a nasogastric tube is placed to decompress the stomach or duodenum. Fluid and electrolytes are repleted intravenously with Ringer's lactate or saline solution based on central venous pressure (CVP) readings and electrolyte results. Where possible, the underlying causes are treated. Total parenteral nutrition may be required to provide nutritional support. A Foley catheter is inserted to allow continual assessment of the fluid replacement. In patients with renal or cardiac disease, a CVP or pulmonary artery catheter may guide fluid replacement.

If patients continue to pass gas and stool, supportive management is continued. If patients show no improvement within 24 to 48 hours, or if fever or rebound tenderness occurs, a surgical evaluation is indicated. All patients with intestinal obstruction should be watched closely for signs and symptoms that reflect sepsis, perforation, ischemia, necrosis, or gangrene. Broad-spectrum antibiotics are started immediately when strangulation or sepsis is suspected. The mortality rate associated with bowel ischemia resulting from obstruction is high.

Surgical Management

Acute complete obstruction is a surgical emergency. Acute complete obstruction is suspected when the patient fails to pass gas and stool, and gas is not evident in the distal intestine on x-ray. An acute complete obstruction is accompanied by the risk of bowel strangulation. Patients with strangulated bowel, volvulus, and incarceration of bowel loop in a hernia or a closed-loop obstruction require immediate surgery. In addition, those patients who fail conservative therapy or experience a decline in clinical status warrant surgical intervention.

Surgical procedures include laparoscopic lysis of adhesion, reduction of volvulus, bowel resection of the involved and surrounding area of bowel with impaired blood supply, bowel decompression, and possible ostomy. These patients may require a second surgery to assess bowel viability.

case study ■ SMALL BOWEL OBSTRUCTION

Mrs. Kane is 82 years old, with a history of hypertension, cholecystitis, status post (S/P) open cholecystotomy in 1960; endometrial cancer, S/P radiation therapy, and abdominal hysterectomy with bilateral salpingo-oophorectomy in 1981, admitted to critical care with a 3-day history of abdominal pain, nausea, and vomiting. The patient was in her usual state of health until 3 days before admission when she awoke from sleep at 4 A.M. with severe, crampy abdominal pain. The pain, located in the right upper quadrant (RUQ), resolved after several minutes, and the patient returned to bed. The following day she experienced intermittent, crampy abdominal pain, accompanied by nausea and several episodes of the "dry heaves." She stayed in bed convinced she had a stomach virus, drank fluids, and ate no solids. She had several small solid bowel movements without relief of the abdominal pain, and passed small amounts of flatus throughout the day. She awoke from sleep that night with increased pain, and vomited a small amount of brownish emesis with partial relief of the abdominal pain. The following day the abdominal pain increased in intensity and frequency, the nausea persisted, and she vomited feculent emesis multiple times. That evening she was persuaded by her husband to go to the emergency department.

Physical examination on presentation to the emergency department revealed an alert, oriented, well-groomed, well-nourished, pleasant elderly woman in mild distress. Vital signs while supine were as follows: blood pressure 102/60 mm Hg; heart rate 115 beats/minute; respiratory rate 16 breaths/minute; temperature 37.9°C. While standing, the patient's blood pressure was 90/55 mm Hg and her pulse was 125 beats/minute. Examination of the oral cavity revealed no exudates or lesions and pink, dry mucous membranes. Cardiovascular examination revealed S_1S_2, without audible murmur, rub, or gallop, with a regular rate and rhythm. No ectopy was noted on cardiac monitor. The lungs were clear to auscultation and chest expansion was equal. The patient's abdomen was round and mildly distended, without visible peristalsis. Well-healed surgical incisional scars in the RUQ and midline were noted, consistent with the patient's previous cholecystectomy and hysterectomy. Bowel sounds were hyperactive, high-pitched, and tinkling in all four quadrants, with audible borborygmi. The patient's abdomen was diffusely tympanitic to percussion with diffuse mild tenderness to deep palpation, without rebound or guarding. A large ventral hernia, easily reducible, was noted. There were no palpable masses or bruits. Rectal examination revealed normal sphincter tone, without palpable masses or lesions. Heme-negative brown stool was detected in the rectal vault.

Laboratory studies revealed the following: Na^+ 132 mEq/L; K^+ 3.2 mEq/L; Cl^- 93 mmol/L; BUN 24 mg/dL; glucose 172 mg/dL; alkaline phosphatase 81 µg/L, AST 40 µg/L; ALT 37 µg/L; amylase 72, lipase 39, white blood cell (WBC) count 10.6 K/µl, hemoglobin and hematocrit 16.5 g/dL and 49.0%. Flat and upright abdominal films revealed stool in the colon, and several air-filled and distended loops of small bowel. There was no evidence of intraperitoneal air. A diagnosis of small bowel obstruction was made, and the patient was admitted to critical care for further evaluation and management.

On arrival to the intensive care unit, the patient was made NPO and a nasogastric tube was placed. Maintenance IV fluids were initiated after successful IV line insertion. Medications prescribed included antiemetics. Frequent abdominal assessments were performed and included inspection, auscultation, percussion, and palpation. Serial radiographs (flat and upright) were taken daily without resolution of the small bowel obstruction. On hospital day 4, the patient was taken to surgery for laparoscopic lysis of adhesions and small bowel resection. On postoperative day 1, the patient was nausea-free and was tolerating a clear liquid diet, which was advanced as tolerated. She was hemodynamically stable and discharged to the floor with no further complications. The patient was subsequently discharged to home and was given discharge instructions to follow up with her primary care physician and surgeon in 1 month. ■

Colonic Obstruction

ETIOLOGY

Carcinoma, sigmoid diverticulitis, and volvulus are the three most common causes of colonic obstruction and together account for 90% of cases. Malignancy is the most common cause of colonic obstruction in the United States and accounts for approximately 50% of cases.[14] Diverticulitis can cause strictures in the colon that can lead to mechanical obstruction. Obstruction from diverticulitis accounts for approximately 10% of cases of colonic obstruction. Volvulus (twisting of a segment of the bowel upon itself) causes 10% to 15% of colonic obstructions.[14] A closed-loop obstruction is usually produced with volvulus and carries a high incidence of strangulation.[14] A history of laxative use and constipation is common in patients with volvulus.

PATHOPHYSIOLOGY

When the ileocecal valve is competent, a closed-loop obstruction can occur because the cecum does not allow decompression of fluid and gas into the small bowel. As fluid and gas accumulate, the intraluminal pressure increases and the colonic wall can become ischemic if this pressure exceeds the capillary pressure.[14] Dehydration results when secretions are sequestered in the colon.

Patients with colonic obstruction have changes in intestinal flora and translocation of bacteria in mesenteric lymph nodes. This is the most likely cause of septic complications of colonic obstruction. In some cases, the cecum may become so severely distended that it inhibits intramural blood flow, which can result in necrosis and gangrene.[14] In colonic obstruction, the normal colonic flora produces methane and ammonia, which contribute to the distension.

CLINICAL PRESENTATION

The clinical presentation of patients with colonic obstruction depends on the degree of obstruction, the cause, the presence of comorbidity, the presence of closed-loop obstruction, and the competency of the ileocecal valve. Patients with colonic obstruction typically present with abdominal pain and distension. The pain may be colicky or severe and unremitting if peritonitis is present. Severe, constant pain suggests gangrenous bowel. If vomiting occurs, it tends to be late in the course of obstruction, especially in patients with a competent ileocecal valve. Patients with volvulus may present with a sudden onset of marked abdominal distension.[16] Patients with obstruction from colon cancer may describe altered bowel habits or a change in stool caliber. Dehydration results when secretions become sequestered in the colon. Patients with a competent ileocecal valve may have greater distension, which increases the risk for ischemia and perforation because an incompetent ileocecal valve allows decompression into the small intestine. Most patients with colonic obstruction complain of constipation; however, diarrhea may be present if stool is leaking past an obstruction. Patients may complain of dyspnea if diaphragmatic excursion is compromised by abdominal distension.

ASSESSMENT

History

A history of altered bowel movements or blood in the stool is suggestive of carcinoma. Diverticulitis typically presents with left lower quadrant pain and associated fever. There may be a change in bowel habits as well. Bleeding is not usually associated with diverticulitis.

Physical Examination

Abdominal distension is common. Signs of dehydration may be seen. Abdominal masses and signs of peritoneal irritation may be elicited. Bowel sounds may be altered. Ascites and hepatomegaly may be present in patients with colon cancer with liver metastasis. A rectal examination may be helpful in identification of rectal cancer. High fever and tachycardia regardless of rehydration or the presence of peritoneal signs suggests strangulation and warrants urgent surgical evaluation.

Laboratory Studies

Iron deficiency anemia may be present if obstruction results from neoplasm. Marked leukocytosis suggests diverticulitis, ischemia, or perforation.

Imaging Studies

Plain abdominal films can reveal findings suspect for the diagnosis of colonic obstruction but may not be able to identify the site or its cause. Obstruction in patients with a competent ileocecal valve causes dilation confined to the colon.

Barium should never be given orally unless a barium enema, CT scan, or colonoscopy has ruled out colonic obstruction. Oral barium accumulates proximal to the colonic obstruction and water will continually be extracted, causing a barium impaction.

MANAGEMENT

Medical Management

The medical management of the patient with acute colonic obstruction is similar to that for the patient with a small bowel obstruction. Medical management focuses on fluid and electrolyte replacement. Oral intake is limited or the patient is placed on NPO status. Nasogastric suction may assist in decompression of abdominal distension.

Surgical Management

Colonic obstruction usually requires surgery. Colonic decompression in the setting of a volvulus can be attempted by colonoscopy. Surgical management of the colonic obstruction is warranted if the patient fails to improve with medical management, the patient's clinical status deteriorates, or the patient has a complete colonic obstruction with a competent ileocecal valve. For obstruction of the left colon, operative decompression followed by primary anastomosis after intraoperative lavage is the treatment of choice. For obstruction in the transverse and right colon, primary resection and anastomosis can also be performed safely. Colonic stents that are placed endoscopically can be used as a temporary measure before surgical resection of obstruction from malignancy or as a palliative measure in nonoperative colorectal cancer.[13,16]

Ileus

Ileus, often called *paralytic* or *adynamic* ileus, is the failure of intestinal contents to pass in the absence of mechanical obstruction. Ileus can have an intra-abdominal or extra-abdominal cause (Box 41-7), many of which are likely to be seen in the ICU setting. Acute colonic pseudo-obstruction, also called *Ogilvie's syndrome*, implies nonmechanical obstruction of the colon that is temporary and reversible.

ETIOLOGY

Postoperative ileus (a transient inhibition of normal gastrointestinal motility that usually lasts for 3 to 5 days after surgery) is very common. Other causes of acute ileus include metabolic abnormalities (electrolyte disturbances, uremia, heavy metal poisoning), drugs (narcotics, catecholamines, adrenocorticotropic hormones, anticholinergics), and local or systemic inflammation (peritonitis, ischemia, pancreatitis). Ileus may also be present after spinal cord injury. Bloodborne toxins, abnormalities in acid–base balance, electrolyte disturbances, and decreased oxygen supply are all possible causes of ileus.[13]

box 41-7
Causes of Adynamic Ileus and Acute Colonic Pseudo-Obstruction

Intra-abdominal Causes	Extra-abdominal Causes
Reflex inhibition	Reflex inhibition
Laparotomy	Craniotomy
Abdominal trauma	Rib, spine, or pelvic fractures
Renal transplantation	Myocardial infarction
Inflammatory conditions	Coronary bypass
Perforated viscus or penetrating wounds	Open heart surgery
Bile peritonitis	Pneumonia, pulmonary embolus
Chemical peritonitis	Burns
Intraperitoneal hemorrhage	Black widow spider bites
Toxic megacolon	Drug-induced
Familial Mediterranean fever	Anticholinergic/ ganglionic antagonists
Acute pancreatitis	Opiates
Acute cholecystitis	Chemotherapeutic agents
Celiac disease	Tricyclic anti-depressants
Inflammatory bowel disease	Phenothiazines
Acute irradiation injury	Metabolic abnormalities
Abdominal irradiation	Septicemia
Infectious processes	Electrolyte imbalance
Bacterial peritonitis	Heavy metal poisoning (lead, mercury)
Appendicitis	Porphyria
Diverticulitis	Uremia
Herpes zoster virus	Diabetic ketoacidosis
Anorectal herpes simplex virus	Sickle cell disease
Ischemic processes	Pulmonary failure
Arterial insufficiency	
Venous thrombosis	
Mesenteric arteritis	
Strangulation obstruction	
Retroperitoneal processes	
Ureteropelvic stones	
Pyelonephritis	
Retroperitoneal hemorrhage	
Pheochromocytoma	
Malignancy (Ogilvie's syndrome)	

From Yamada T, Alpers DH, Laine L, et al (eds): Textbook of Gastroenterology (4th Ed), p 836. Philadelphia, Lippincott Williams & Wilkins, 2003.

PATHOPHYSIOLOGY

Although the etiology of ileus can be defined, the pathophysiology of ileus is poorly understood. Postoperative ileus has been widely studied, and multiple mechanisms are thought to play a role, including sympathetic neural reflexes, local and systemic inflammatory mediators, and changes in neural and hormonal transmitters.[17] The effects of anesthesia combined with inflammation or ischemia in the operative area may also interfere with nerve conduction. Opioid narcotics may also contribute to postoperative ileus because they decrease propulsive motility of the intestine.

In ileus, peristalsis ceases and distension of the intestine occurs as fluid and electrolytes accumulate in a process similar to that seen in mechanical obstruction.

CLINICAL PRESENTATION

Patients may complain of diffuse abdominal discomfort and distension (see Table 41-1). Nausea and vomiting are often predominant in patients with postoperative ileus. Vomiting is frequent, and the emesis usually contains gastric contents and bile. The vomiting of feculent material is rare. The pain is usually less intense than in small bowel or colonic obstruction. The patient with ileus also complains of constipation and usually denies the passage of flatus. Other common symptoms are nausea, anorexia, hiccups, and bloating.

ASSESSMENT

History

A history of thyroid or parathyroid disease, heavy metal exposure, diabetes mellitus, and scleroderma should be elicited to identify underlying causes.[13]

Physical Examination

Abdominal distension is often prominent in ileus. Auscultation of the abdomen usually reveals infrequent or absent bowel sounds. The abdomen is usually resonant to percussion secondary to air in the dilated loops of intestine. Abdominal girth is assessed at frequent intervals. Signs of peritoneal irritation or sepsis are also sought during the abdominal examination.

Laboratory Studies

Electrolyte abnormalities commonly associated with ileus are similar to those seen in patients with mechanical obstruction.

Imaging Studies

In ileus, gas and fluid accumulate in loops of mildly dilated bowel proximal or adjacent to the site of an acute inflammatory process like appendicitis or pancreatitis. These loops are involved in localized ileus and are called *sentinel loops.*[13] In acute colonic pseudo-obstruction, the entire colon becomes dilated, with the cecal diameter the greatest. Chest x-rays may help to identify pneumonia or other causes of ileus. Contrast studies can be used to differentiate complete obstruction from partial obstruction and ileus. CT scan of the abdomen may identify causes that can contribute to ileus. Ultrasonography has no role in the diagnosis of ileus because the dilated loops of bowel prevent imaging.

MANAGEMENT

Treatment of ileus focuses on management of underlying causes. Because ileus may present in much the same way as mechanical obstruction, exclusion of mechanical causes is necessary. Treatment usually consists of supportive care. Patients with ileus are usually placed on NPO status. Fluid and electrolyte replacement is directed by clinical status and laboratory values as needed. Nasogastric suction limits the collection of swallowed air that can contribute to abdominal distension. Medications that can adversely affect colonic motility are halted where possible. Laxative use is avoided because these agents can provide a substrate for bacterial fermentation, which results in further gas accumulation. If the patient shows no improvement in 3 to 5 days, a further search for underlying causes is initiated. Neostigmine has been effective in the treatment of colonic ileus not responsive to conservative therapy.[13] Prokinetic medications, such as metoclopramide (Reglan) and erythromycin, have not been found to be effective in the treatment of ileus.[17] Therapeutic interventions for the decompression of the colon include colonoscopy, open or percutaneous cecostomy, and a decompression colostomy.[16]

ACUTE PANCREATITIS

Acute pancreatitis is defined as acute inflammation of the pancreas that can also involve surrounding tissues, remote organs, or both. Acute pancreatitis can be mild or severe. In mild acute pancreatitis, there are areas of fat necrosis in and around pancreatic cells, along with interstitial edema. Mild pancreatitis is not associated with organ dysfunction or complications, and recovery is usually uneventful. In severe acute pancreatitis, also called *necrotic* or *hemorrhagic* pancreatitis, there is extensive fat necrosis in and around the pancreas, pancreatic cellular necrosis, and hemorrhage in the pancreas. Severe acute pancreatitis is associated with local and systemic complications. The incidence of acute pancreatitis varies among populations based on the prevalence of precipitating factors such as alcohol use and gallstone disease. The incidence of acute pancreatitis is 1 to 5/10,000 in the United States.[18] The mortality rate associated with acute pancreatitis is approximately 10%.[19]

Etiology

There are multiple causes of acute pancreatitis (Box 41-8). Gallstones and excessive alcohol use together account for 70% to 80% of cases.[20] Gallstone pancreatitis is more common in women and alcoholic pancreatitis is more common in men. Acute pancreatitis often follows the ingestion of a large meal or drinking episode. Biliary stones and biliary sludge may also precipitate acute pancreatitis as they are passed through the ampulla of Vater. Many drugs, including diuretics, sulfonamides, metronidazole, aminosalicylates, and estrogen, can precipitate acute pancreatitis as a result of toxic metabolites or a drug reaction. Hypercalcemia and hypertriglyceridemia are metabolic causes of acute pancreatitis. Idiopathic pancreatitis is associated with pregnancy, the administration of total parenteral nutrition, or major surgery. Pancreatitis has also occurred after blunt or penetrating abdominal trauma or after endoscopic manipulation of the ampulla of Vater. Other possible precipitating factors include infectious processes, such as mumps, staphylococcal infection, scarlet fever, and viral infections, as well as the congenital variant of pancreas divisum. Pancreatitis may occur as an isolated event, or the patient may suffer repeated attacks.

box 41-8
Major Causes of Acute Pancreatitis

- Biliary disease: gallstones or microlithiasis, common bile duct obstruction, biliary sludge
- Pancreas divisum
- Alcohol abuse
- Drugs: thiazide diuretics, furosemide, procainamide, tetracycline, sulfonamides, azathioprine, 6-mercaptopurine, angiotensin-converting enzyme (ACE) inhibitors, valproic acid
- Hypertriglyceridemia
- Hypercalcemia
- Idiopathic
- Miscellaneous (postoperative, ectopic pregnancy, ovarian cyst, total parenteral nutrition)
- Abdominal trauma
- Endoscopic retrograde cholangiopancreatography (ERCP)
- Infectious processes

Pathophysiology

The acinar cells of the pancreas synthesize and secrete digestive enzymes to assist in the breakdown of starch, fat, and proteins. Under normal circumstances these enzymes remain inactive until they enter the duodenum. Acute pancreatitis develops when pancreatic enzymes become prematurely activated in the pancreas. This premature activation results in autodigestion of the pancreas and peripancreatic tissue. The exact mechanism by which pancreatic enzymes become activated and initiate autodigestion is not fully understood, but the activation of trypsinogen into its active form trypsin appears to promote activation of other enzymes, including elastase, kinases, and phospholipase A. Elastase can cause dissolution of elastic fibers in blood vessels. Activated kinins cause systemic vasodilatation and increased vascular permeability, which promotes edema.[18,21] Phospholipase A causes necrosis of the pancreas and the surrounding fatty tissue. Pancreatic enzymes, vasoactive substances, and hormones released from the injured pancreas cause a cascade of events that can lead to systemic effects and multiple complications.

Clinical Presentation

Abdominal pain is the hallmark of acute pancreatitis. The severity of the pain correlates to the degree of pancreatic involvement. The pain is usually mid-epigastric or periumbilical, with radiation to the back, but may radiate to the spine, flank, or left shoulder. The pain usually begins abruptly, often after a large meal or large intake of alcohol. It may be steady and severe, or increase in intensity over several hours. The pain is usually exacerbated when the patient lies supine and is usually relieved when the patient sits and leans forward or lies in a fetal position. Nausea, vomiting without pain relief, tachycardia, abdominal distension, and hypotension are other common symptoms. A low-grade fever may or may not be present. A persistent fever may indicate complications, such as peritonitis, cholecystitis, or intra-abdominal abscess.

The diagnosis of acute pancreatitis is often challenging because acute pancreatitis can mimic many other conditions. The differential diagnosis includes gastritis, perforated duodenal or gastric ulcers, acute small bowel obstruction, ruptured ectopic pregnancy, sickle cell crisis, acute cholecystitis, mesenteric artery occlusion, and ruptured aortic aneurysm. Diagnosis is made on the basis of the patient's clinical presentation, history, and physical examination findings, and the results of laboratory and radiographic studies (Box 41-9).

Assessment

HISTORY

A careful history can provide important clues to diagnosis. A history of biliary tract disease, alcohol intake, and medication use should be elicited to identify precipitating causes. A family history of acute pancreatitis may suggest hereditary causes. The patient may report anorexia, weight loss, nausea, vomiting, or abdominal distension. Assessment of the location, duration, quality, quantity, and precipitating factors of pain is important to help identify potential causes.

PHYSICAL EXAMINATION

Diffuse abdominal tenderness and guarding may be present during abdominal palpation. The upper abdomen may be distended and tympanic to percussion. Bowel sounds may be hypoactive or absent due to decreased intestinal mobility or paralytic ileus. Jaundice may be present in gallstone disease or from obstruction of the biliary tree from pancreatic edema. Ascites or palpable abdominal masses may be present. Patients with severe acute hemorrhagic pancreatitis may have signs of dehydration and hypovolemic shock. These signs may worsen when fluid is lost into the bowel lumen due to a paralytic ileus. The presence of a bluish discoloration of the lower abdominal flanks (Grey Turner's sign) or around the umbilical area (Cullen's sign) indicates hemorrhagic pancreatitis and an accumulation of blood in these areas. These uncommon signs usually do not appear until 48 hours or more after onset of symptoms.[22]

box 41-9
Clinical Manifestations of Acute Pancreatitis

Physical Examination Findings
- Abdominal pain
- Low-grade fever
- +/– Jaundice
- Abdominal guarding or distension
- Paralytic ileus
- Grey Turner's sign
- Cullen's sign
- Nausea or vomiting without relief

Laboratory Findings
- Elevated serum and urine amylase
- Elevated serum lipase
- Elevated white blood cell count
- Hypokalemia
- Hypocalcemia
- Elevated bilirubin, aspartate aminotransferase (AST), and prothrombin time (PT) (with liver disease)
- Elevated alkaline phosphatase level (with biliary disease)
- Hypertriglyceridemia
- Hyperglycemia
- Hypoxemia

LABORATORY STUDIES

No single laboratory study is diagnostic of acute pancreatitis; however, elevations of serum amylase and lipase enzymes are often seen in acute pancreatitis. These enzymes are released as the pancreatic cells and ducts are destroyed. Serum amylase levels rise within 2 to 12 hours of the onset of symptoms and gradually return to baseline within 3 to 5 days in acute pancreatitis.[23] In mild pancreatitis, amylase levels can be close to normal. If a few days have elapsed since symptoms began, amylase values can also be normal even with an active inflammatory process in the pancreas. The sensitivity of serum amylase is limited in patients with elevated serum triglycerides and in acute pancreatitis related to alcohol.[23] The specificity of serum amylase is decreased in biliary tract disease, tumors, salivary gland lesions, cerebral trauma, gynecological disorders, and renal failure. However, the specificity for serum amylase in the diagnosis of acute pancreatitis is increased if levels are more than two to three times the upper limits of normal.[19,23]

Compared with serum amylase levels, serum lipase levels rise later and remain elevated. Serum lipase levels usually rise within 4 to 8 hours of the onset of symptoms, peak at 24 hours, and return to normal at 8 to 14 days.[23] Because serum lipase stays elevated longer, it is a useful test in diagnosis if there is a delay in examination. Like amylase, serum lipase levels may be elevated in patients who have intra-abdominal inflammation or renal insufficiency.

Elevations of isoenzymes, urinary amylase, and the amylase values of pleural fluid and paracentesis drainage support the presence of acute pancreatitis. Leukocytosis, hypokalemia, hypocalcemia, and hypertriglyceridemia may be present but are not specific to acute pancreatitis. Leukocytosis may result from infection, stress, or dehydration. Persistent vomiting may result in hypokalemia. Hypocalcemia may indicate the presence of pancreatic fat necrosis because calcium binds with fatty acids during tissue necrosis. In addition, trypsin inactivates parathyroid hormone, which is needed for calcium absorption. Hyperglycemia may result from decreased insulin release, increased glucagon release, and the stress response. Hemoconcentration may occur, as fluid is lost into the peritoneal space. Elevations in serum bilirubin, AST, and PT are common in the presence of concurrent liver disease. A greater than threefold elevation in ALT suggests biliary pancreatitis.[24] Alkaline phosphatase is elevated with biliary tract disease. Triglyceride levels associated with acute pancreatitis are usually greater than 800 to 1,000 mg/dL.[23]

IMAGING STUDIES

Radiographs of the chest and abdomen are useful to exclude other causes of abdominal pain, including intestinal ileus, perforation, pericardial effusion, and pulmonary disease.

Abdominal ultrasound is of limited use in visualization of the pancreas due to intestinal gas and adipose tissue. Abdominal ultrasound is useful to evaluate the biliary tree for gallstones, sludge, or ductal dilation.[25]

CT is helpful in confirming the clinical diagnosis and determining the severity of acute pancreatitis. CT can visualize the size of the pancreas and identify the presence of peripancreatic fluid, pancreatic pseudocysts, and abscesses. Dynamic CT done with contrast can help to identify areas of necrosis in the pancreas. CT findings of extensive necrosis have correlated with a high risk for pancreatitis-related infection and death.[25] Sequential CT allows for assessment of progressive disease or resolution. CT can also demonstrate fluid collection and areas of necrosis and can be used to guide percutaneous needle aspiration for culture.

Magnetic resonance cholangiopancreatography (MRCP) may have a sensitivity of more than 90% for bile duct stones. Endoscopic retrograde cholangiopancreatography (ERCP) plays a role in locating and removing stones in the common bile duct if gallstone pancreatitis is present.

TOOLS FOR PREDICTING SEVERITY

Acute pancreatitis is self-limiting and mild in 80% to 90% of patients, resolving spontaneously within 5 to 7 days.[22] These patients usually require conservative care. The mortality rate for severe acute pancreatitis is 10%; however, this rises to 50% or more when there are complications. Multiple assessment tools have been developed in attempts to identify patients who are likely to develop severe acute pancreatitis so that aggressive treatment and surveillance can decrease complications and mortality.

Ranson's criteria have been widely used to assess the severity of acute pancreatitis (Box 41-10). Ranson's criteria consist of multiple clinical criteria used to identify those patients at risk for increased morbidity and mortality. Three or more signs identified at the time of admission or during the initial 48 hours are predictive of severe acute pancreatitis, with an associated mortality rate of 10% to 20%.[19] Ranson's criteria have a greater than 90% accuracy rate and are useful clinically in identifying high-risk patients. The primary disadvantage to Ranson's criteria is the 48-hour delay before the assessment is completed.

The Acute Physiology and Chronic Health Evaluation II (APACHE II) score has also been studied and found to be useful in predicting severity of acute pancreatitis (Table 41-2). The APACHE II uses the worst values of physiological measures, age, and previous health status at admission, at 24 hours, and at 48 hours to predict severity of acute pancreatitis. An APACHE II score on admission of 8 or more predicted 68% of severe attacks.[22] An advantage to the use of the APACHE II score is that it can be used daily. Both Ranson's criteria results and APACHE II scores are comparable at 48 hours.

The use of serum markers to prognosticate severity has been tested. The most promising have been quantification of C-reactive protein (CRP), leukocyte elastase, and trypsinogen active peptide (TAP). CRP rises in relation to severity, is inexpensive, and readily available. Unfortunately, CRP does not become significantly elevated until 48 hours after inflammation, which limits its use in diagnosis of acute pancreatitis.[22] TAP is released when trypsinogen is activated into trypsin, which makes this an attractive marker for acute pancreatitis; however, false-negative and false-positive responses remain a concern.[22]

box 41-10
Ranson's Criteria for Acute Pancreatitis

Evaluate on admission or on diagnosis:

- Age >55 years
- Leukocyte count >16,000/μL
- Serum glucose >200 mg/dL
- Serum lactate dehydrogenase (LDH) >350 IU/mL
- Serum aspartate aminotransferase (AST) >250 IU/dL

Evaluate during initial 48 hours:

- Fall in hematocrit >10%
- Blood urea nitrogen (BUN) level rise >5 mg/dL
- Serum calcium <8 mg/dL
- Base deficit >4 mEq/L
- Estimated fluid sequestration >6 L
- Arterial Pao_2 <60 mm Hg

Complications

The local and systemic complications of acute pancreatitis are summarized in Box 41-11.

LOCAL COMPLICATIONS

The local effects of pancreatitis include inflammation of the peritoneum around the pancreas and fluid accumulation in the peritoneal cavity. These changes can lead to pancreatic pseudocyst, pancreatic abscess, and acute gastrointestinal hemorrhage. Pancreatic pseudocysts occur in up to 20% of all cases of acute pancreatitis and are a part of the necrotizing process. A pseudocyst is a collection of inflammatory debris and pancreatic secretions. The pseudocyst can rupture and hemorrhage or become infected, causing bacterial translocation and sepsis. A pseudocyst is suspected in any patient who has persistent abdominal pain with nausea and vomiting, a prolonged fever, and elevated serum amylase. Surgery may also be indicated for pseudocysts; however, it is usually delayed because some pseudocysts have been known to resolve spontaneously. Surgical treatment of the pseudocyst can be done through internal or external drainage or needle aspiration. Acute surgical intervention may be required if the pseudocyst becomes infected or perforates.

Pancreatic abscess is a walled-off collection of purulent material in or around the pancreas. Signs and symptoms of an abdominal abscess or infected pancreatic necrosis include increased WBC count, fever, abdominal pain, and vomiting.[24] Pancreatic infection from an abscess, pseudocyst, or necrotic tissue may be present whenever a patient has a temperature greater than 39°C (102.2°F), tachycardia, or leukocytosis greater than 20,000 cells/mL, or shows other signs of clinical deterioration. Infections after the onset of pancreatitis, if untreated, are often fatal. Broad-spectrum antibiotics are given to those patients with suspected infection.

Gastrointestinal complications of acute pancreatitis include gastrointestinal bleeding and bacterial translocation. Gastrointestinal bleeding, the most common gastrointestinal complication of acute pancreatitis, includes bleeding from peptic ulcers, hemorrhagic gastroduodenitis, stress ulcers, and Mallory-Weiss syndrome. Decreased peristalsis can lead to bacterial translocation.

table 41-2 The Acute Physiology and Chronic Health Evaluation II (APACHE II) Classification System

Physiologic Variable	High Abnormal Range								Low Abnormal Range
	+4	*+3*	*+2*	*+1*	*0*	*+1*	*+2*	*+3*	*+4*
Temperature rectal (°C)	≥41	39–40.9		38.5–38.9	36.0–38.4	34–35.9	32–33.9	30–31.9	≤29.9
Mean arterial pressure = (2 × diastolic + systolic)/3	≥160	130–159	110–129		70–109		50–69		≤49
Heart rate (ventricular response)	≥180	140–179	110–139		70–109		55–69	40–54	≤39
Respiratory rate (nonventilated or ventilated)	≥50	35–49		25–34	12–24	10–11	6–9		<5
Oxygenation A-aDO_2 or PaO_2 (mm Hg); FIO_2 >0.5; record A-aDO_2;	≥500	350–499	200–349		<200				
FIO_2 <0.5, record only PaO_2					>70	61–70		55–60	<55
Arterial pH (if no arterial blood gases [ABGs] record serum HCO_3 below)*	≥7.7	7.6–7.69		7.5–7.59	7.33–7.49		7.25–7.32	7.15–7.24	<7.15
Serum sodium	≥180	160–179	155–159	150–154	130–139		120–129	111–119	≤110
Serum potassium	≥7	6–6.9		5.6–5.9	3.5–5.4	3–3.4	2.5–2.9		<2.5
Serum creatinine (mg/dL) (double point for acute renal failure)	≥3.5	2–3.4	1.5–1.9		0.6–1.4		<0.6		
Hematocrit (%)	≥60		50–59.9	46–49.9	30–45.9		20–29.9		<20
White blood count	≥40		20–39.9	15–19.9	3–14.9		1–2.9		<1
Glasgow coma scale (GCS) (score = 15 minus actual GCS)†	15 – GCS =								
A Total acute physiology score (APS)	Sum of the 12 individual variable points =								
*Serum HCO_3 (venous mmol/L) (not preferred, use if no ABGs)	<52	41–51.9		32–40.9	22–31.9		18–21.9	15–17.9	<15

†Glasgow Coma Scale (Circle Appropriate Response)

Eyes open
- 4 - spontaneously
- 3 - to verbal command
- 2 - to painful stimuli
- 1 - no response

Motor response
- 6 - to verbal command
- 5 - localizes to pain
- 4 - withdraws to pain
- 3 - decorticate
- 2 - decerebrate
- 1 - no response

Verbal—*nonintubated*
- 5 - oriented and controversed
- 4 - disoriented and talks
- 3 - inappropriate words
- 2 - incomprehensible sounds
- 1 - no response

Verbal—*intubated*
- 5 - seems able to talk
- 3 - questionable ability to talk
- 1 - generally unresponsive

B (Age and Points)

Age	Points
<44 y	0
45–54 y	2
55–64 y	3
65–74 y	5
>75 y	6

Age points =

C (Chronic Health Points)

If any of the 5 CHE categories is answered with yes give +5 points for nonoperative or emergency postoperative patients

Liver	Cirrhosis with portal hypertension or encephalopathy
Cardiovascular	Class IV angina or at rest or with minimal self-care activities
Pulmonary	Chronic hypoxemia or hypercapnia or polycythemia or pulmonary hypertension >40 mm Hg
Kidney	Chronic peritoneal or hemodialysis
Immune	Immune-compromised host

Chronic health points =

Credit given to Nick Mendel, Kiev, Ukraine, for producing this document.
APACHE II score **(sum of A + B + C)**: **A** APS points + **B** age points + **C** chronic health points = total APACHE II.
From Triester SL, Kowdley KV: Prognostic factors in acute pancreatitis. J Clin Gastroenterol 34(2):167–176, 2002.

box 41-11
Major Complications of Acute Pancreatitis

Local
- Pancreatic necrosis
- Pancreatic pseudocyst
- Pancreatic abscess

Pulmonary
- Atelectasis
- Acute respiratory distress syndrome
- Pleural effusions

Cardiovascular
- Hypotensive shock
- Septic shock
- Hemorrhagic shock

Renal
- Acute renal failure

Hematological
- Disseminated intravascular coagulation (DIC)

Metabolic
- Hyperglycemia
- Hypertriglyceridemia
- Hypocalcemia
- Metabolic acidosis

Gastrointestinal
- Gastrointestinal bleed

PULMONARY COMPLICATIONS

The release of enzymes (e.g., phospholipase) is thought to cause the many pulmonary complications associated with acute pancreatitis. These include arterial hypoxemia, atelectasis, pleural effusions, pneumonia, acute respiratory failure, and acute respiratory distress syndrome (ARDS). Arterial hypoxemia can occur in patients with mild disease without clinical or radiographic findings to support the pulmonary dysfunction. In severe acute pancreatitis, arterial blood gases should be drawn every 8 hours for the first few days to detect this complication. Treatment for hypoxemia includes vigorous pulmonary care (e.g., deep breathing and coughing) and frequent position changes. Oxygen therapy can also be used to improve overall oxygenation status. Careful fluid administration is also necessary to prevent fluid overload and pulmonary congestion. Patients with acute respiratory compromise may require mechanical ventilatory support. Abdominal distension and diminished diaphragmatic excursion may also contribute to atelectasis seen in acute pancreatitis.

CARDIOVASCULAR COMPLICATIONS

Hemodynamically significant fluid sequestration is characteristic of fulminant pancreatitis. Another major systemic effect of enzyme release into the circulatory system is peripheral vasodilation, which in turn can cause hypotension and shock.

Decreased perfusion to the pancreas itself can result in the release of myocardial depressant factor (MDF). MDF decreases heart contractility and affects cardiac output. Perfusion of all body organs can then become compromised. Early and aggressive fluid resuscitation is thought to prevent the release of MDF. Trypsin activation causes abnormalities in blood coagulation and clot lysis. This promotes the development of disseminated intravascular coagulation (DIC) with its associated bleeding (see Chapter 49).

RENAL COMPLICATIONS

Acute renal failure is thought to be a consequence of hypovolemia and decreased renal perfusion. Death during the first 2 weeks of acute pancreatitis usually results from pulmonary or renal complications.

METABOLIC COMPLICATIONS

Metabolic complications of acute pancreatitis include hypocalcemia and hyperlipidemia, which are thought to be related to areas of fat necrosis around the inflamed pancreas. Hyperglycemia may occur as a result of damage to the cells of the islets of Langerhans; metabolic acidosis can result from hypoperfusion and activation of anaerobic metabolism.

Management

MEDICAL MANAGEMENT

Conventional care of the patient with acute pancreatitis focuses on fluid and electrolyte replacement to maintain or replenish vascular volume and electrolyte balance, pain management, resting the pancreas in an effort to prevent the release of pancreatic secretions, and maintaining the patient's nutritional status Box 41-12. Close observation and clinical judgment are the basis for therapy and management.

Fluid and Electrolyte Replacement

Most patients with acute pancreatitis require the infusion of IV fluids to replace fluid lost through third-spacing and intravascular volume depletion. Patients with severe acute pancreatitis may have up to 12 L of fluid sequestration in the retroperitoneal space or peritoneal cavity. The goal is to administer enough fluid to obtain a circulating volume sufficient to maintain organ and tissue perfusion and prevent end-stage shock. Hypovolemia and shock are major causes of death early in the disease process when aggressive fluid resuscitation fails to reverse the shock process.

Colloid and crystalloid solutions, such as albumin and Ringer's lactate solution, are used for volume replacement. Patients with acute hemorrhagic pancreatitis may also need packed red blood cells to restore volume. Fluid replacement is evaluated by monitoring intake and output and daily weights. Patients with more severe disease may require hemodynamic monitoring with measurement of pulmonary capillary wedge pressure (PCWP) or central venous pressure (CVP).

Patients with severe disease whose hypotension fails to respond to fluid therapy may need medications to support blood pressure. The drug of choice is dopamine, which can be started at a low dose (2 to 5 µg/kg/minute). An advantage of this drug is that at low doses it maintains renal perfusion while supporting blood pressure.

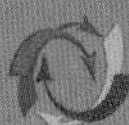

box 41-12 collaborative care guide *for the Patient With Pancreatitis*

OUTCOMES	INTERVENTIONS
Oxygenation/Ventilation	
Arterial blood gases are maintained within normal limits.	■ Assist patient to turn, deep breathe, cough, and use incentive spirometer q4h and PRN. Provide chest physiotherapy. ■ Assess for hypoventilation, rapid and shallow breathing, and respiratory distress. ■ Monitor pulse oximetry, end-tidal CO_2, and arterial blood gases. ■ Administer analgesics if splinting is reducing effective ventilation. ■ Provide supplemental oxygen as needed.
The patient's lungs are clear. The patient has no evidence of atelectasis, pneumonia, or acute respiratory distress syndrome (ARDS).	■ Auscultate breath sounds q2–4h and PRN. ■ Suction only when rhonchi are present or secretions are visible in endotracheal tube. ■ Hyperoxygenate and hyperventilate before and after each suction pass.
Circulation/Perfusion	
Blood pressure, heart rate, and hemodynamic parameters are within normal limits.	■ Monitor vital signs q1–2h. ■ Monitor pulmonary artery pressures and right atrial pressure q1h and cardiac output, systemic vascular resistance (SVR), and peripheral vascular resistance (PVR) q6–12h if pulmonary artery catheter is in place. ■ Maintain patent IV access. ■ Administer intravascular volume as indicated by real or relative hypovolemia, and evaluate response.
Serum lactate will be within normal limits.	■ Monitor lactate qd until it is within normal limits. ■ Administer red blood cells, positive inotropic agents, colloid infusion as ordered to increase oxygen delivery.
Patient will not experience bleeding related to acute gastrointestinal hemorrhage, coagulopathies, or disseminated intravascular coagulation (DIC).	■ Monitor PT, PTT, CBC daily or PRN. ■ Assess for signs of bleeding. Observe for Cullen's or Grey Turner's signs. ■ Administer blood products as indicated.
Fluids/Electrolytes	
Patient is euvolemic.	■ Maintain patent IV access. ■ Monitor daily weights. ■ Monitor intake and output. ■ Measure abdominal girth q8h at the same location on the abdomen.
No evidence of electrolyte imbalance or renal dysfunction.	■ Monitor electrolytes daily and PRN. ■ Assess for signs of lethargy, tremors, tetany, and dysrhythmias. ■ Replace electrolytes as ordered. ■ Monitor BUN, creatinine, serum osmolality, and urine electrolytes daily.
Mobility/Safety	
No evidence of complications related to bed rest and immobility.	■ Initiate deep venous thrombosis prophylaxis. ■ Reposition frequently. ■ Ambulate to chair when acute phase is past, hemodynamic stability and hemostasis achieved.
Patient achieves or maintains ability to conduct activities of daily living (ADLs) and mobilize self.	■ Consult physical therapist. ■ Conduct range-of-motion and strengthening exercises.

(continued)

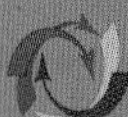

box 41-12 collaborative care guide *for the Patient With Pancreatitis (Continued)*

OUTCOMES	INTERVENTIONS
No evidence of infection, WBC within normal limits.	■ Monitor SIRS (systemic inflammatory response syndrome) Criteria: increased WBC count, increased temperature, tachypnea, tachycardia. ■ Use strict aseptic technique during procedures. ■ Maintain invasive catheter tube sterility. ■ Change invasive catheters, culture blood, line tips, or fluids, etc., according to hospital protocol.
Skin Integrity Skin will remain intact.	■ Assess skin q8h and each time patient is repositioned. ■ Turn q2h. ■ Consider pressure relief/reduction mattress.
Nutrition Caloric and nutrient intake meet metabolic requirements per calculation (e.g., basal energy expenditure).	■ Provide parenteral feeding. ■ Maintain NPO. ■ Consult dietitian or nutritional support service. ■ Fat or lipid restriction. ■ Provide small, frequent feedings.
Evidence of metabolic dysfunction is minimal.	■ Monitor albumin, prealbumin, transferrin, cholesterol, triglycerides, glucose.
Comfort/Pain Control Patient will have minimal pain, < 5 on pain scale.	■ Assess pain and discomfort using objective pain scale q4h PRN and after administration of pain medication. ■ Administer analgesics and monitor patient response. ■ Use nonpharmacological pain management techniques (e.g., music, distraction, touch) as adjunct to analgesics.
Patient will have minimal nausea.	■ Maintain nasogastric tube patency. ■ Monitor nausea and vomiting. ■ Administer antiemetic as ordered.
Psychosocial Patient demonstrates decreased anxiety.	■ Listen to patient's worries and fears. ■ Assess patient's response to anxiety. ■ Support effective coping behaviors. ■ Teach alternative behaviors for those that are not helpful. ■ Help patient increase sense of control by providing information and explanation. ■ Allow choices when possible. ■ Provide as much predictability in routine as possible.
Teaching/Discharge Planning Patient/significant others understand procedures and tests needed for treatment.	■ Prepare patient/significant others for procedures such as paracentesis, pulmonary artery catheter insertion, or laboratory studies.
Significant others understand the severity of the illness, ask appropriate questions, anticipate potential complications.	■ Explain the widespread effects of pancreatitis and the potential for complications such as sepsis or ARDS. ■ Encourage significant others to ask questions related to pathophysiology, monitoring, treatments, etc. ■ Instruct patient and family in discharge regimen that may include wound care, medications, and dietary limitations.

Urinary output is a sensitive measure of the adequacy of fluid replacement, and it should be maintained at greater then 30 mL/hour or 0.6 mL/kg/hour. Blood pressure and heart rate are also sensitive measures of volume status.

Patients with severe hypocalcemia are placed on seizure precautions with respiratory support equipment on hand. The nurse is responsible for monitoring calcium levels, administering replacement solutions, and evaluating the patient's response to any calcium supplementation. Calcium replacements are infused through a central line because peripheral infiltration can cause tissue necrosis. The patient also needs to be monitored for calcium toxicity; symptoms include lethargy, nausea, shortening of the QT interval, and decreased excitability of nerves and muscles. Hypomagnesemia may also be present, so magnesium may need to be replaced as well. Serum magnesium levels usually need to be corrected before calcium levels can return to normal. Potassium may need to be replaced early in the treatment regimen because it is lost through vomiting and sequestration of potassium-rich pancreatic juices.

Hyperglycemia is related to impaired secretion of insulin, an increased release of glucagon, or increased stress response. In some cases, hyperglycemia can be associated with dehydration or other electrolyte imbalances. Sliding-scale regular insulin may be ordered; it needs to be administered very cautiously because glucagon levels are only transiently elevated in acute pancreatitis. Successful fluid replacement is marked by return of alert mental status, urine output, cardiac output, stable hemodynamic values, and a normal serum lactate level.

Pain Management

Pain control is a nursing priority for patients with acute pancreatitis, not only because of the extreme discomfort, but because pain increases pancreatic enzyme secretion. Pain is related to the degree of pancreatic inflammation, can be severe and constant, and can last for many days.

Adequate pain control with the use of IV narcotics, preferably delivered by patient-controlled analgesia (PCA), is essential in the treatment of acute pancreatitis. Meperidine has traditionally been the analgesic of choice because of the potential for sphincter of Oddi spasm that can accompany opioid use. However, meperidine is not always effective and other analgesics (including opioids) should not be withheld. Fentanyl citrate (Sublimaze), although an opiate, has been used successfully to control the pain of acute pancreatitis.

Analgesia should be routinely administered at least every 3 to 4 hours to prevent uncontrollable abdominal pain. Use of a pain rating scale is recommended for evaluating the patient's response to medication. Be alert to the patient's respiratory status because narcotics can induce respiratory depression. A nasogastric tube attached to low intermittent suction can help ease pain considerably, although the use of a nasogastric tube is controversial in patients without vomiting. Patient positioning can also relieve some of the discomfort.

Resting the Pancreas

In some patients with acute pancreatitis, nasogastric suction is used to decompress the stomach and decrease stimulation of secretin. Secretin, which stimulates production of pancreatic secretions, is released in response to acid in the duodenum. Nausea, vomiting, and abdominal pain may decrease when a nasogastric tube is placed and connected to suction early in treatment. A nasogastric tube is also necessary in patients with severe gastric distension or a paralytic ileus. Patients with acute pancreatitis should be placed on NPO status until the abdominal pain subsides and serum amylase levels have returned to normal. Starting oral intake sooner can cause the abdominal pain to return and can induce further inflammation of the pancreas by stimulating the autodigestive disease process.

Nutritional Support

Total parenteral nutrition is recommended for patients with fulminant acute pancreatitis who are being kept on prolonged NPO status with nasogastric suction because of paralytic ileus, persistent abdominal pain, or pancreatic complications. Lipid administration is avoided to prevent increasing triglyceride levels, which can exacerbate the inflammatory process. In the patient with mild acute pancreatitis, oral fluids can usually be restarted within 3 to7 days, with solid food introduced slowly and as tolerated.

Prolonged NPO status is often difficult for patients. Frequent mouth care and proper positioning of the nasogastric tube are important to maintain skin integrity and maximize patient comfort. Bed rest is prescribed to decrease the patient's basal metabolic rate; this, in turn, decreases the stimulation of pancreatic secretions.

PERITONEAL LAVAGE

Peritoneal lavage has been used since the 1960s for the treatment of systemic complications of pancreatitis. The rationale for this therapy is that peritoneal lavage removes the toxic substances released by the damaged pancreas into the peritoneal fluid before systemic effects can be initiated. Lavage may be used if standard therapies have not been effective during the first days of hospitalization.

The procedure for peritoneal lavage involves placement of a peritoneal dialysis catheter. Isotonic solutions with dextrose, heparin, and potassium are added. An antibiotic may also be used in the solution. Two liters of solution is infused over 15 to 20 minutes and then is drained by gravity. This cycle is repeated every 1 to 2 hours for 48 to 72 hours. If peritoneal lavage is effective, the hemodynamic response by the patient is usually immediate.

Respiratory status must be closely monitored during peritoneal lavage because accumulation of fluid in the peritoneum causes restricted movement of the diaphragm. Hyperglycemia can be another effect of this therapy because dextrose can be absorbed from the fluid into the bloodstream.

SURGICAL MANAGEMENT

A pancreatic resection for acute necrotizing pancreatitis can be performed to prevent systemic complications of the disease process. In this procedure, dead or infected pancreatic tissue is surgically removed. In some cases, the entire pancreas is removed. Broad-spectrum antibiotics are given to patients who require surgical debridement of necrotic tissue.

Surgery may also be performed if gallstones are thought to be the cause of the acute pancreatitis. A cholecystectomy or ERCP and endoscopic sphincterotomy are performed.

HEPATITIS

Etiology

Diffuse inflammation of the liver, otherwise known as *hepatitis*, can be noninfectious or infectious in origin (Box 41-13). Acute hepatitis lasts less than 6 months, and either resolves completely with return of normal liver function, or can progress to chronic hepatitis, then cirrhosis, and possibly liver failure. Chronic hepatitis is an inflammatory process that lasts longer than 6 months, and may also progress to cirrhosis and possibly liver failure.

box 41-13
Selected Causes of Hepatic Inflammation

Infectious Diseases
- Viral hepatitis (A, B, C, D, E)
- Epstein-Barr virus (EBV)
- Cytomegalovirus (CMV)
- Herpes simplex virus (HSV)
- Coxsackievirus B
- Toxoplasmosis
- Adenovirus
- Varicella-zoster virus (VZV)

Drugs and Toxins
- Alcohol
- Acetaminophen
- Isoniazid
- Salicylates
- Anticonvulsants
- Antimicrobials
- HMG-CoA reductase inhibitors
- Alpha-methyldopa
- Amiodarone
- Estrogens
- *Amanita phalloides* mushrooms
- Ecstasy (methylenedioxymethamphetamine)
- Herbal medicines (ginseng, comfrey tea, pennyroyal oil, *Teucrium polium*)

Autoimmune Diseases
- Autoimmune hepatitis
- Primary biliary cirrhosis
- Primary sclerosing cholangitis

Congenital Diseases
- Hemochromatosis (iron overload)
- Wilson's disease (copper deposition)
- α_1-Antitrypsin deficiency

Miscellaneous Causes
- Nonalcoholic fatty liver
- Fatty liver of pregnancy
- Severe right-sided congestive heart failure
- Budd-Chiari syndrome (vascular obstruction)

NONINFECTIOUS HEPATITIS

Noninfectious hepatitis can be caused by excessive alcohol consumption, autoimmune disorders, metabolic or vascular disorders (including right-sided heart failure), acute biliary obstruction, and many individual drugs and drug classes (depending on the amount ingested and length of exposure). Examples include but are not limited to acetaminophen, isoniazid, HMG-CoA reductase inhibitors, anticonvulsants, antimicrobials, alpha-methyldopa, amiodarone, and estrogens. Ten to 15% of patients using alcohol for prolonged periods acquire hepatitis.[26]

Other toxins include *Amanita phalloides* (poisonous mushrooms), ecstasy (methylenedioxymethamphetamine), and some herbal medicines (ginseng, comfrey tea, pennyroyal oil, and *Teucrium polium*).[27] Autoimmune hepatitis, a condition in which the patient's own immune system attacks the liver, causes inflammation and hepatocyte injury or death. Autoimmune hepatitis can be mistaken for an acute viral hepatitis if the patient presents with severe symptoms.

INFECTIOUS HEPATITIS

Viral hepatitis is a highly contagious inflammatory condition and is the leading cause of liver transplantation in the United States.[28] Just like noninfectious hepatitis, infectious hepatitis can be acute and chronic, with 6 months as the delineating time frame. Viral infections of the liver parenchyma have been classified according to their specific infecting agent and corresponding serology markers. Hepatitis A, B, C, D, and E are summarized in Table 41-3. Other viral causes of hepatitis include herpes simplex virus (HSV), Epstein-Barr virus (EBV), cytomegalovirus (CMV), adenovirus, coxsackievirus B, and varicella-zoster virus (VZV). Typically patients with viral hepatitis present with similar nonspecific, flulike symptoms such as malaise, nausea, vomiting, diarrhea, loss of appetite, mid-epigastric abdominal discomfort, and low-grade fever. In patients with hepatitis B, symptoms may be more severe.

Hepatitis A

Hepatitis A is caused by an RNA enterovirus transmitted through the oral–fecal route, predominantly by contaminated water or raw or partially cooked shellfish. In most patients, symptoms of hepatitis A virus (HAV) infection are either relatively mild or nonexistent, although an older person is at greater risk of having more severe symptoms. The incubation period ranges from 15 to 45 days after exposure. HAV infection causes only acute liver disease; recovery is usually complete and does not lead to chronic hepatitis or cirrhosis. In rare instances, HAV infection can lead to fulminant liver failure; approximately 100 people in the United States die annually from HAV infection, with more than 70% of the reported deaths in those older than 49 years.[29] Blood tests usually reveal elevations in the aminotransferases (ALT and AST), bilirubin concentrations, and alkaline phosphatase level. In severe cases, the PT may be prolonged. Diagnosis can be made with serology antibody testing. Anti-HAV immunoglobulin G (IgG) antibodies can be found in individuals who have had hepatitis A in the past, but are not helpful in diagnosing an acute infection. Instead, a positive anti-HAV IgM serology marker indicates HAV infection within

table 41-3 Summary of Types of Hepatitis

	Hepatitis A	Hepatitis B	Hepatitis C	Hepatitis D	Hepatitis E
Incubation (days)	15–45	30–180	15–160	30–180	14–60
Onset	Acute	Insidious	Insidious	Acute or insidious	Acute
Transmission	Fecal/oral Contaminated food, water	Blood Sexual Perinatal Percutaneous	Blood Maybe sexual	Blood Sexual (comorbid infection with HBV)	Fecal/oral Contaminated food, water
Severity	Mild	Often severe	Moderate	May be very severe	Virulent, especially in pregnant women
Prognosis	Generally good	Worse with age, debility	Moderate	Fair, worse with chronic disease	Good, unless pregnant
Diagnosis					
Acute	Anti-HAV IgM	HBsAG Anti-HBc (IgM) HBeAg	HCV ELISA Anti-HCV recombinant strip immunoblot assay (RIBA) HCV RNA	HDV Ag	Clinical
Chronic	—	Anti-HBc (IgG)	Anti-HCV	Anti-HDV	—
Prophylaxis (adults)	Immune globulin	Hepatitis B vaccine Immune globulin	?Immune globulin	None available	None available
Carrier	No	Yes	?	Yes	No

the preceding 6 months. HAV infection does not induce a carrier state.

Early in the course of the disease, there is an incubation period during which the patient is asymptomatic but highly contagious, particularly with high HAV levels in the stool. After symptoms are apparent, the hepatitis infection can be misdiagnosed because many of the symptoms are similar to those of the flu. Some patients seek medical attention because they become jaundiced; the two most common physical examination findings are jaundice and hepatomegaly, which occur in 70% and 80% of symptomatic patients, respectively.[30] Acute symptoms can progress or disappear once jaundice is present. By the time symptoms occur, the virus is no longer shed in the stool, and the patient is usually not infectious. Recovery is signaled by liver function test results returning to normal.

After exposure to HAV, passive immunization can be achieved through the use of immune serum globulin. Most preparations of immune serum globulin contain adequate quantities of anti-HAV. The immune serum globulin may not entirely abort an infection, but it significantly ameliorates the symptoms. It is usually given to intimate contacts of patients with hepatitis A.

Hepatitis B

Hepatitis B virus (HBV) is a DNA virus of the Hepadnaviridae family that replicates by reverse transcription. Infection causes both acute and chronic hepatitis and the incubation period is 30 to 180 days, with the average at 12 weeks. HBV is spread by contact with blood or blood products. Hepatitis B can be transmitted parenterally through blood transfusions, occupational needlestick injuries, and the use of contaminated needles (e.g., in illicit drug use). However, a significant number of patients contract HBV through nonparenteral routes. The antigen has been identified in body secretions, such as semen, mucus, and saliva; sexual exposure to a person with HBV is a common mode of transmission. Maternal perinatal transmission also occurs. It appears that a break in the skin or the mucous membrane is necessary for the transmission to occur.

Incorrect interpretation of HBV serologic markers is common. Familiarity with the serology testing is important for the critical care nurse who is assisting in the diagnostic evaluation of a suspected case of viral hepatitis to prevent inappropriate laboratory testing and patient discomfort. Hepatitis B surface antigen (HBsAg) is a protein that coats the outer surface of the HBV and is produced in great excess during viral replication. HBsAg is the single most important test to detect infection with HBV. A positive result indicates that a patient is infected with HBV. If the presence of HBsAg is associated with an acute illness and a marked rise in the aminotransferases as well as the presence of hepatitis B core IgM antibody, the patient has acute hepatitis B. If HBsAg disappears from the blood within 6 months, there is resolution of infection and the patient does not advance to chronic disease. Patients with acute HBV infection who overcome their infection and eradicate the virus develop antibodies against hepatitis B surface antigen (anti-HBs). In some laboratories, these results may be reported as hepatitis B surface antibody (HBsAb) instead of anti-HBs. Regardless of the form of documentation, these individuals are protected against future HBV infection. A person who receives the hepatitis B vaccine also develops HBsAb.

Acute hepatitis B can lead to fulminant liver failure. The mortality rate from HBV infection is approximately 1%; chronic active hepatitis B is seen in 5% to 10% of the patients.[30] These patients continue to have high levels of HBsAg and can be infectious to others. Anti-hepatitis B core (anti-HBc) also appears early in the course of infection and may persist for many years, but it is helpful in evaluating an acute versus chronic infection because anti-HBc can be further divided into two subtypes. Anti-HBc (IgM) is the initial response to infection and lasts for 6 to 18 months after recovery from infection. Therefore, high titers of anti-HBc (IgM) indicate the presence of acute infection and low titers indicate chronic liver infection. Anti-HBc (IgG) is the second subtype and is positive in patients who are either chronically infected or previously infected, persisting in the bloodstream for a lifetime. Once an infection of HBV is established with HBsAg and anti-HBc, further serological testing can be ordered. For instance, the presence of the hepatitis Be antigen (HBeAg) indicates active viral replication, and helps in diagnosing disease severity, prognosis, and treatment options. Those patients who have a positive HBeAg are considered highly infectious. The degree of liver impairment in chronic active hepatitis is variable from mild to serious and can progress to cirrhosis.

Clinical signs and symptoms for HBV infection during the acute phase are the same as with HAV infection, although arthralgia, high fever, and rash are hallmark signs of HBV infection. There is, however, a greater risk for the development of fulminant hepatic failure in patients with HBV infection, which is characterized by jaundice, hepatic encephalopathy, and rapidly deteriorating hepatic synthetic function.

HBV exposure is associated with high risk. After accidental exposure, such as an inadvertent needlestick, passive immunoprophylaxis can be achieved by using high anti-HBs titer hepatitis B immune globulin. This is a pooled serum containing high titers of the anti-hepatitis B immune globulin. It is recommended only for postexposure inoculations of high-risk patients.

Fortunately, a vaccine exists for active immunization against hepatitis B (Recombivax-HB, Engerix-B). This vaccine, administered prophylactically over a 6-month period, provides active immunization against hepatitis B. It is highly recommended for health care personnel at risk of infection with hepatitis B. It is also recommended for people who have had intimate contacts with people already infected with hepatitis B. Precautions to protect against exposure to bloodborne pathogens must be followed. In the United States, children are being universally vaccinated against HBV.

Hepatitis C

As diagnostic tests improved, hepatitis C virus (HCV), formally called non-A, non-B hepatitis, was identified in 1989. HCV is a single-stranded RNA virus related to the flavivirus family. It is a bloodborne virus that can cause both acute and chronic hepatitis. HCV chronicity can occur in as many as 85% of patients[28] and is the leading cause of liver transplantation in the United States.[28] Many people acquired HCV through blood transfusions before 1992 (when testing for HCV was mandated). Other risk factors include illicit drug use with shared contaminated needles, and occupational needlestick exposure. There are indications that the virus might also be transmitted through perinatal, sexual, and household contacts, although not commonly. Incubation of HCV is 15 to 160 days, with an average of 7 weeks. The hepatitis C antibody does not confer immunity, and approximately 50% to 70% of those infected progress to chronic disease, with cirrhosis or liver cancer developing in 20% to 30%.[31]

Fatigue, anorexia, weight loss, and abdominal pain are the most common symptoms of HCV infection. Diagnostic evaluation for HCV infection includes an HCV enzyme-linked immunosorbent assay (ELISA; ordered when the aminotransferase levels are elevated and for screening patients on hemodialysis), an anti-HCV recombinant strip immunoblot assay (RIBA; ordered to confirm a positive HCV test or if a patient presents with symptoms of hepatitis), or an HCV RNA test (ordered when HCV RIBA findings are indeterminate, but there remains a high index of suspicion for HCV). HCV RNA, which tests for the presence of the virus in the blood (rather than antibodies against the virus), is the gold standard for detecting HCV in the serum or liver tissue. HCV RNA levels are also helpful in following disease progression and monitoring therapy results.[32]

The only approved treatment for HCV infection is the used of interferon-alpha but, unfortunately, as much as 70% to 80% of patients who go into remission from the disease relapse into active disease within 6 to 12 months after discontinuing treatment.[31] HCV infection is rarely diagnosed as the acute infection. However, if a patient with acute hepatitis C is treated with interferon, the response rate approaches 98%.[33]

Hepatitis D

Hepatitis D (delta hepatitis) always occurs in the presence of hepatitis B. Hepatitis D virus (HDV) relies on HBV to replicate. HDV infection may occur as a superinfection in the patient who has chronic hepatitis B, or it may occur simultaneously with HBV infection. Hepatitis D can progress to fulminant hepatitis and chronic disease. In the United States, HDV infection occurs primarily among individuals receiving multiple transfusions and those abusing IV drugs. Early in the disease, the hepatitis D antigen (HDV Ag) is present in the blood. Later in the disease, antibodies to the hepatitis D virus are present (anti-HDV).

Because this disease coexists with hepatitis B, patients with hepatitis D have symptoms similar to those of acute or chronic hepatitis B, but symptoms may be more pronounced.

Hepatitis E

Hepatitis E virus (HEV) is a single-stranded RNA virus similar to HAV. It is transmitted by the oral–fecal route from contaminated water and food. The incubation period is 14 to 60 days. HEV has been implicated in epidemics in India, Southeast Asian countries, and parts of Africa and Mexico, and is associated with an overall low mortality rate of approximately 0.5%. For reasons still unclear, hepatitis E often progresses to fulminant liver failure in pregnant women, with mortality rates up to 20%.[34] Because the incidence of HEV infection is less than 1% in the United States, the critical care nurse should pay careful attention if a patient presents with symptoms of hepatitis and has recently traveled or lived in endemic areas.

Pathophysiology

To improve patient outcomes, it is important that critical care nurses have a solid knowledge base regarding the underlying pathophysiology, assessment, and management of acute and chronic liver disease. Hepatocytes, the metabolic functional cells of the liver, perform many essential functions. The most essential of these functions include the metabolism of nutrients (e.g., glucose, proteins, lipids, vitamins) and the detoxification of medications, alcohol, ammonia, toxins, and hormones. In addition, hepatocytes are responsible for synthesis of clotting factors, conjugation and secretion of bilirubin, and synthesis of bile salts. Abnormal liver function is usually not apparent unless a significant acute insult occurs or chronic liver disease is fairly advanced. Liver failure occurs when there is a loss of 60% of the hepatocytes, and symptoms are usually detectable after 75% or more of the hepatocytes are injured or killed. Liver function testing and evaluation begins with a complete history and physical examination. Interpretation of liver serum enzymes, synthetic function, and cholestasis (or excretory function) tests are important for the critical care nurse to understand and are discussed later in this chapter.

Acute liver disease, typically caused by viral or chemical insults, occurs suddenly and resolves, becomes chronic, or results in a patient's death. Chronic liver disease leading to cirrhosis, typically more insidious in nature, is the 12th leading cause of death in the United States.[35] Disease processes in the liver can affect the hepatocytes, the blood vessels, and Kupffer cells, which are responsible for uptake and subsequent degradation of foreign and potentially harmful substances in the body. If the injury is mild and reversible, hepatocytes may regenerate and liver function may return to normal. However, if the injury is more severe or sustained, regeneration may be incomplete or the healing process may cause fibrosis. Fibrotic changes alter the liver architecture and can lead to cirrhosis and impediment of blood flow through the liver. An acute insult to the liver can progress to fulminant liver failure, which is defined as hepatic encephalopathy occurring within 8 weeks of jaundice. Hepatic encephalopathy is a state of abnormal mental functioning as a result of the inability of the liver to remove ammonia and other toxins from the blood. If liver function does not return and liver transplantation is unavailable, fulminant liver failure can progress to cerebral edema, coma, and death from brain herniation.

Assessment

HISTORY

Questions regarding the patient's alcohol consumption and illicit drug use, use of prescription and over-the-counter medications, use of herbal supplements, surgical and transfusion history, occupational or travel exposure history, and sexual history may be helpful in determining the diagnosis, nursing plan of care, and teaching needs of the patient. In acute hepatitis, most patients are asymptomatic except for mildly elevated liver enzymes. Constitutional symptoms vary widely but typically include malaise, fatigue, low-grade fever, nausea, vomiting, and sometimes diarrhea.

PHYSICAL EXAMINATION

When cirrhosis and portal hypertension resulting from chronic hepatitis are present, jaundice (yellow staining of the skin and mucous membranes as a result of bilirubin pigments) may be noted. Hepatomegaly (enlargement of the liver) may result in right upper quadrant tenderness and is a result of portal hypertension or congestion in the liver from altered blood flow due to cirrhosis. The liver edge is often noted to be firm and nodular. In advanced cirrhosis, the liver size is often decreased and difficult to palpate. Dullness of percussion over the liver span can provide serial observations of resolution of hepatitis or progression of cirrhosis. Splenomegaly as a result of portal hypertension and sequestration of fluid in the spleen may result in left upper quadrant tenderness. Muscle wasting and abdominal ascites may develop as a result of malnutrition, portal hypertension, and hypoalbuminemia due to the liver's impaired ability to synthesize proteins. Peripheral edema may result from hypoalbuminemia and from ascites obstructing blood return from the lower extremities. Vitamin deficiencies may result in glossitis of the tongue and cheilosis of the lips. Bruising and bleeding tendencies may develop as a result of impaired production of clotting factors and sequestration of platelets in the spleen. Other manifestations include telangiectasis or spider nevi (usually of the upper half of the body). These lesions consist of a pulsating arteriole from which smaller vessels radiate. Palmar erythema, or redness of the palms, is a result of increased blood flow from hyperdynamic cardiac dysfunction associated with hepatitis (with ascites). In men, there may be a loss of body hair, testicular atrophy, and gynecomastia. These changes are thought to be related to altered hormone metabolism and estrogen excess in the liver.

Physical examination may also reveal abdominal wall vein dilatation around the umbilicus, known as caput medusae. This is the result of portal hypertension and congestion and collateral vessel development (Fig. 41-4). This congestion may be auscultated as an arterial bruit (systolic phase) or a venous hum (both systolic and diastolic phases) over the liver and epigastrium. Encephalopathy, ascites, and peripheral edema, reflective of advanced disease, may be present. Other observable assessment findings include frothy, dark amber urine and clay-colored stools as a result of alterations in bilirubin excretion. Common signs and symptoms for noninfectious and infectious hepatitis are summarized in Table 41-4. Patients with signs and symptoms of hepatic decompensation (e.g., portal hypertension, ascites, encephalopathy, and coagulopathy) should be hospitalized, evaluated, and treated more expeditiously than those patients who demonstrate adequate hepatic compensation and stability.

LABORATORY STUDIES

Tests for Evaluating Hepatocellular Injury

The clinical significance of any liver chemistry must be evaluated in the context of the patient's history and clinical

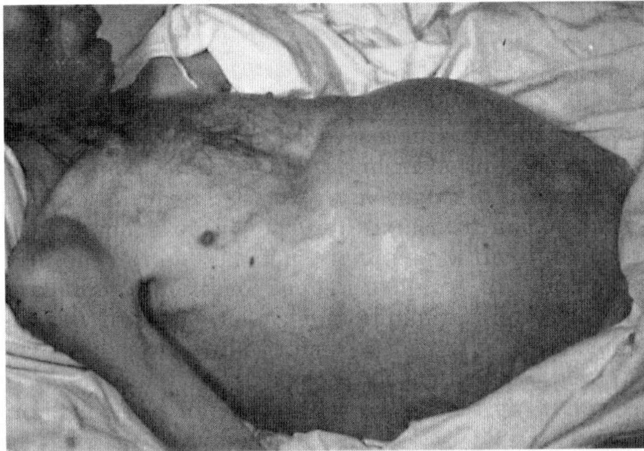

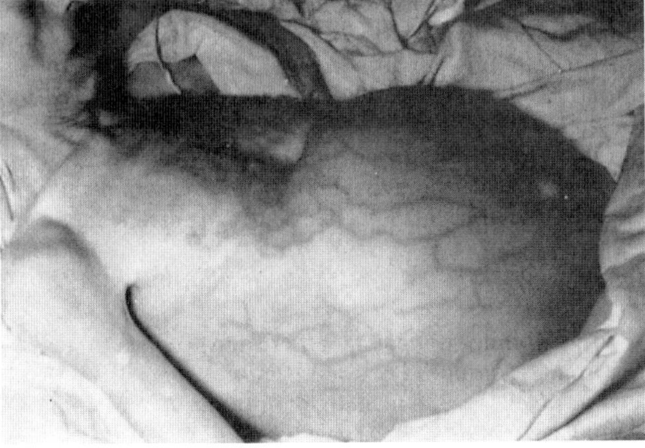

figure 41-4 Collateral abdominal veins on the anterior abdominal wall in a patient with alcoholic liver disease as recorded by black and white photography (*top*) and infrared photography (*bottom*). (From Schiff L: Diseases of the Liver. Philadelphia, J. B. Lippincott, 1982).

situation. The term *liver function tests* is commonly used, but is not an entirely accurate term. Some laboratory tests do measure liver synthetic function and these include albumin, PT, and total bilirubin. Other laboratory tests, however, are markers of hepatocellular injury and include AST, previously known as serum glutamic oxaloacetic transaminase (SGOT), and ALT, previously known as serum glutamic pyruvic transaminase (SGPT).

The aminotransferases are enzymes present inside the hepatocytes. When hepatocytes are injured or die, they release AST and ALT into the serum. Therefore, the presence of these enzymes in the blood signals the presence of hepatocyte injury. However, AST and ALT lack sensitivity (for a particular diagnosis) in evaluating chronic liver injury for two reasons. First, AST and ALT are also found in the skeletal muscle and, as such, elevations may be related to a skeletal muscle injury or overexertion; this is particularly true for AST because ALT is almost exclusively present in hepatocytes and is the most specific test for hepatocellular damage. Second, it is thought that dying hepatocytes synthesize less AST and ALT enzymes than healthy ones. Therefore, despite inflammation detected on a liver biopsy, patients with chronic hepatitis may have relatively normal levels of AST and ALT.

Despite these difficulties in laboratory interpretation, elevations of AST and ALT are often helpful in evaluating acute liver injury, response to treatment, and monitoring those at risk for liver disease due to medical interventions. Elevations of these enzymes suggest hepatocyte death and the degree of elevation roughly approximates the amount of liver cell death. AST and ALT elevate at relatively equal levels, but an exception occurs in alcoholic hepatitis, in which AST levels tend to be higher than ALT levels. This is thought to be due to the depletion of vitamin B_6 (pyridoxine) in patients with chronic alcoholism; ALT synthesis is more strongly inhibited by pyridoxine deficiency than AST synthesis. In chronic hepatitis, AST and ALT levels are usually less than 10 times normal. However, in acute viral, toxin-induced, or ischemic hepatitis, these elevations may be greater than 1,000 U/L. In addition, alcoholic hepatitis causes smaller elevations (less than 300 U/L). An AST:ALT ratio of greater than 2 is suggestive of alcohol-induced hepatic injury.[36] Unfortunately, AST and ALT levels have low prognostic value.

Tests for Evaluating Liver Synthetic Function

As mentioned earlier, albumin, total protein, and PT are measures of actual liver synthetic function. Because proteins are synthesized by the liver, albumin and other proteins are an index of liver function. Albumin is the predominant protein in the serum; those patients with advanced liver disease and cirrhosis tend to have low serum concentrations (hypoalbuminemia). Because albumin is responsible for colloid osmotic pressure, low concentrations lead to leakage of intravascular fluids into interstitial spaces and peripheral edema. Because albumin levels are also influenced by poor nutrition and renal disease, care must be taken when interpreting laboratory test results.

The PT is a measure of the liver's capacity to synthesize clotting factors. The liver synthesizes blood clotting factors II, V, VII, IX, and X. An elevation in PT values is not seen until more than 80% of hepatocyte function is lost. However, because of the short half-life of factor VII, a PT is helpful in evaluating acute liver failure. Evaluation for vitamin K deficiency is performed because malabsorption or poor nutritional intake must be excluded in a patient who is hypoprothrombinemic. Failure of improvement in a PT level after vitamin K supplementation (5 to 10 mg orally for 3 days) may indicate intrinsic liver disease.

Tests for Evaluating Cholestasis (Excretory Function)

Tests for cholestasis (lack of bile flow) help determine what is happening in the bile ducts. Obstruction of bile flow may be extrahepatic (e.g., gallstones, postsurgical stricture, or malignancy) or intrahepatic (e.g., poor hepatocyte function or damage to the small septal or intralobular bile ducts). Present in the biliary epithelium, elevated alkaline phosphatase and gamma-glutamyltransferase (GGT) levels reflect damage to the bile ducts or obstruction of bile flow.

An elevated serum bilirubin level is roughly proportional to the amount of liver dysfunction or disease severity. Bilirubin is the major source of hemoglobin metabolism from the destruction of adult red blood cells. The unconjugated (indirect) form of bilirubin is not water soluble and is bound to albumin as a means of transport to the liver for conjugation and subsequent excretion in the bile.

table 41-4 Common Signs and Symptoms of Hepatitis

Signs and Symptoms	Cause
Constitutional	
Fever, chills	Immune response to viral infection
Generalized weakness, malnutrition	Inability to metabolize nutrients
Gastrointestinal	
Right upper quadrant pain	Hepatomegaly
Left upper quadrant pain	Splenomegaly
Loss of appetite	Ascites, fatigue
Abdominal distension	Ascites
Nausea, vomiting/hematemesis	Portal hypertension
Clay-colored feces	Inability to excrete conjugated bilirubin
Diarrhea	Impaired fat metabolism
Melena, hematochezia	Portal hypertension
Pulmonary	
Shortness of breath Increased work of breathing Decreased oxygen saturation Decreased partial pressure of oxygen	Ascites, decreased lung and diaphragmatic expansion
Cardiac	
Increased heart rate Decreased blood pressure	Hypotension, sequestration of fluid in the liver and spleen, third-spacing in the peripheral extremities from decreased protein metabolism/low albumin levels
Dysrhythmias	Electrolyte disturbances
Peripheral edema	Impaired protein metabolism
Neurological	
Headache Depression/irritability Asterixis	Impaired metabolism of ammonia and other circulating toxins
Genitourinary	
Decreased urinary output	Decreased circulating volume and impaired glomerular filtration rate
Frothy, dark amber urine	Excretion of conjugated bilirubin (water-soluble bile)
Integumentary	
Jaundice	Impaired excretion of bile
Pruritus, dry skin	Impaired excretion of bile
Bruising, ecchymosis	Impaired ability to synthesize clotting factors
Spider nevi, caput medusae	Portal hypertension
Palmar erythema	Portal hypertension
Hair loss	Impaired metabolism of circulating hormones
Endocrine	
Hypoglycemia	Impaired glucose metabolism and storage
Increased weight	Ascites, third-spacing of fluid
Gynecomastia, testicular atrophy (in men)	Inability to metabolize hormones (e.g., estrogens)
Immune	
Infection, spontaneous bacterial peritonitis	Impaired Kupffer cell function, splenomegaly

In the hepatocytes, unconjugated bilirubin is combined with glucuronic acid to make it water soluble (or conjugated) for excretion into the bile and feces. Cholestasis causes reflux of conjugated bilirubin into the blood (a condition called *conjugated hyperbilirubinemia*), so that the conjugated bilirubin is instead excreted through the kidneys. The urine becomes frothy and very dark amber in color from bilirubin pigments. The critical care nurse may be asked to perform a dipstick test on the urine for bilirubin to confirm this clinical suspicion. Unconjugated hyperbilirubinemia results from a poor nutritional state (e.g., decreased albumin available for transport of bilirubin to the liver) or hepatocyte dysfunction in the conjugation process. Jaundice is usually present when the serum bilirubin level is greater than 2 to 3 mg/dL.

Management

The primary treatment of acute hepatitis of any type is primarily supportive. Measures include providing rest and adequate nutrition and preventing further liver injury by the avoidance of hepatotoxic medications and substances. Hospitalization is rarely required but is needed in cases of disease complicated by hemodynamic instability, failure to maintain adequate nutrition and fluid intake, encephalopathy, blood coagulopathies, and renal failure.

In situations of hemodynamic instability, monitoring of blood pressure, heart rate, cardiac dysrhythmias, and urine output is essential. IV fluids will most likely need to be provided. It is important to avoid lactated Ringer's solutions because of the inability of the impaired liver to metabolize lactate, which could induce or exacerbate a metabolic acidosis. Frequent monitoring of hepatic enzymes and synthetic function will be requested to evaluate disease progression and response to treatment interventions. Altered electrolyte, nutrient, and vitamin abnormalities from disease progression, malnutrition, and nausea and vomiting require repletion. The critical care nurse may have to assist in invasive treatments or procedures, such as placement of a Sengstaken-Blakemore tube for control of bleeding esophageal varices, paracentesis for ascites, and liver biopsy. In the event of fluid volume overload, diuretics, albumin, and protein supplements may be prescribed. Accurate intake and output, daily weight, and abdominal girth measurements may alert the critical care nurse to significant volume shifts and potential hemodynamic or respiratory issues.

Maintaining adequate nutrition is a priority. Small, frequent meals and antiemetics are administered as needed. A high-calorie, low-protein diet is recommended to prevent complications associated with impaired protein and ammonia metabolism associated with acute hepatic encephalopathy. However, a low-protein diet is used only in the short term because seriously ill patients actually have increased protein requirements to build and maintain muscle mass and to assist in healing and repair. IV feedings are needed only if oral intake is impaired by intractable nausea and vomiting. Patients with severe fatigue require frequent rest and spacing of activities.

Because of the patient's risk for coagulopathies, the critical care nurse must monitor for bleeding gums, epistaxis, ecchymosis, petechiae, hematemesis, hematuria, and melena. Vitamin K may be prescribed to help reduce the effects of bleeding tendencies, and a PT may be ordered to monitor the efficacy of treatment.

Avoidance of alcohol, narcotics, barbiturates, and medications that are metabolized by the liver is recommended. Careful observation and documentation of patient responses (e.g., mental status, level of consciousness) to medications and treatment regimens is recommended. Due to the liver's inability to metabolize or detoxify many foods, drugs, and toxins, the critical care nurse may be asked to administer frequent medications such as lactulose, neomycin sulfate, and metronidazole to treat hepatic encephalopathy. Lactulose is a laxative that acidifies the colon to prevent the absorption of ammonia. The dose of lactulose is titrated so that the patient has two to three soft stools per day without diarrhea. Neomycin and metronidazole act as antibiotics to clear the colon of bacteria that make ammonia.

If there is severe pruritus from jaundice, a bile salt sequestering agent (such as cholestyramine), a topical emollient, or both can be used to help alleviate this symptom. Mittens may need to be used to prevent excessive scratching and subsequent skin breakdown in a confused patient.

Patient teaching for the patient with hepatitis includes measures to prevent infection and transmission, dietary limitations and alcohol avoidance, and the necessity for follow-up care. The patient is advised to monitor activity tolerance and fatigue. If signs and symptoms persist and liver enzymes remain elevated for greater than 6 months, the patient will progress to chronic disease. This is more common in HBV and HCV infection and is confirmed by liver biopsy.

COMPLICATIONS OF LIVER DISEASE

Complications of advanced liver disease include cirrhosis, hepatic encephalopathy, hepatorenal syndrome, and spontaneous bacterial peritonitis.

Cirrhosis

ETIOLOGY

Cirrhosis of the liver can result from a number of diseases. In the United States, alcohol abuse is the most common cause of cirrhosis.[26] Other causes of cirrhosis include chronic active hepatitis and diseases causing biliary obstruction.

PATHOPHYSIOLOGY

Cirrhosis, which develops over time, can cause severe alterations in the structural architecture of the liver and function of the hepatocytes. These changes are characterized by inflammation and liver cell necrosis, which can be focal or diffuse. Necrosis is followed by regeneration of liver tissue, but not in a normal fashion. Fibrous tissue and regenerative nodules are laid down over time, which distorts the normal architecture of the liver lobule and alters blood flow. These fibrotic changes are irreversible, resulting in chronic liver dysfunction and eventual liver failure. Fatty deposits in the parenchymal cells may be seen initially. The cause of the fatty changes is unclear, but it may be a response to alterations in enzymatic function responsible for normal fat metabolism. Eventually, all of the liver's metabolic processes are altered.

Inflammation, fibrotic changes, and increased intrahepatic vascular resistance cause compression of the liver lobule, leading to increased resistance or obstruction of normal blood flow through the liver, which is normally a low-pressure system. This portal hypertension results in significant venous congestion and dilatation (Fig. 41-5). Subsequently, nutrient-rich blood from the gastrointestinal tract is shunted away from the liver, the first site of metabolism for many nutrients, drugs, and toxins. Pressure builds up in the systemic venous circulation, causing congestion where the portal and systemic venous systems connect: the esophagus, stomach, and rectum. These vascular changes result in varicose veins, or varices. Esophageal varices and gastric varices are of particular concern in the care of these patients because they are extremely friable; rupture from these varices can result in massive internal bleeding that may be life-threatening. Portal hypertension also promotes increased collateral circulation and allows blood to flow from the intestines directly

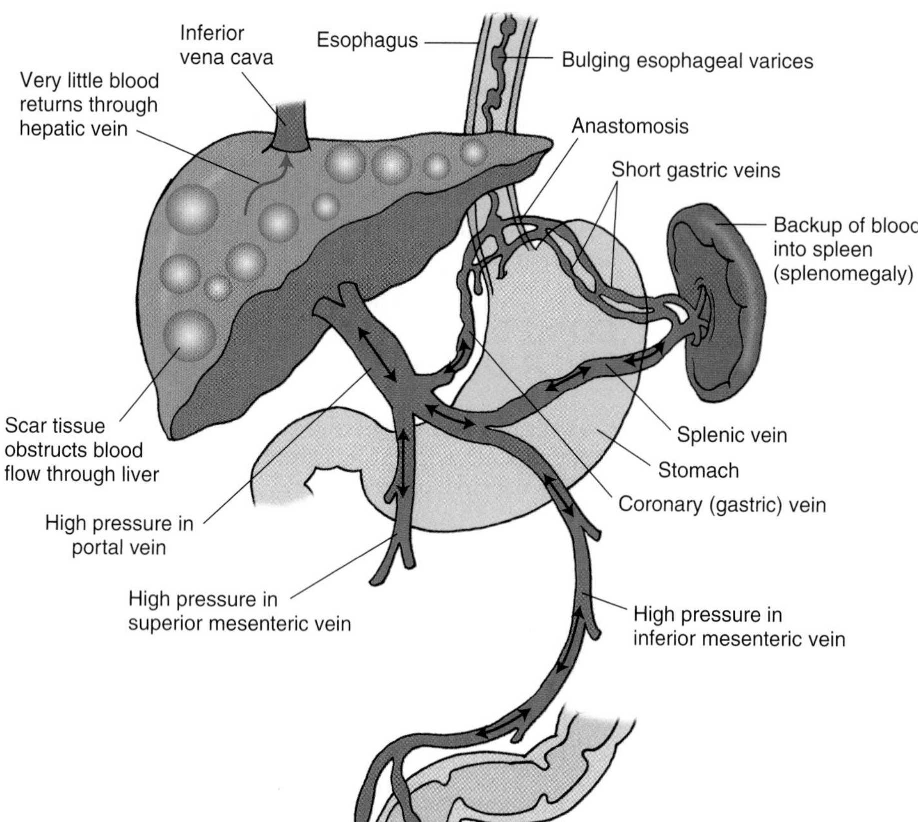

figure 41-5 Esophageal varices develop from increased portal pressure. In an attempt to return blood to the systemic circulation, collateral veins develop to bypass increased portal resistance. These collateral vessels become tortuous and distended and are called *varices*.

to the vena cava; this congestion is often seen as a collection of prominent vessels on the surface of the abdomen and is known as caput medusae. Splenomegaly results from the sequestration of trapped blood from portal hypertension. Of particular concern is the trapping of platelets, which can be seen clinically by bleeding tendencies and a thrombocytopenia on laboratory evaluation. Bleeding from esophageal and gastric varices can cause stools to be black and tarry, known as melena. Hemorrhoidal varices, or hemorrhoids, can also result from portal hypertension. Finally, portal hypertension may result in abdominal fluid accumulation, known as ascites. As liver disease progresses and cirrhosis develops, mild to moderate high-output cardiac dysfunction may occur. This hyperdynamic dysfunction is characterized by splanchnic and systemic vasodilation, an afterload effect that decreases cardiac work and elevates cardiac output.[37] Clinically, it is seen as hypotension, tachycardia, and cardiac flow murmurs. As hepatic cirrhosis progresses, these clinical findings become more pronounced.[38] Figure 41-6 illustrates clinical effects of cirrhosis.

ASSESSMENT

In some patients, cirrhosis may be subclinical. However, history and physical examination findings may reveal clues to altered liver function. For example, altered carbohydrate metabolism can result in unstable blood sugars. Altered fat metabolism can cause fatigue and decreased activity tolerance. Altered protein metabolism results in a decreased synthesis of albumin. Albumin is necessary for colloid osmotic pressure, which holds fluid in the intravascular space. A decrease leads to interstitial tissue edema and decreased plasma volume. Globulin, another protein, is essential for normal blood clotting. This, coupled with a decreased synthesis of many blood clotting factors and decreased metabolism of vitamins and iron, predisposes the patient to hematological complications that range from bruising to hemorrhage. A low-grade disseminated intravascular coagulopathy (DIC) also may develop. Portal hypertension, ascites, and lower extremity edema cause hypotension. Initially, the patient may have flushed skin and bounding pulses from the vasodilation in the portal venous system, which leads to a hyperdynamic state with peripheral circulation vasodilation and hypotension. Table 41-5 summarizes laboratory findings in patients with cirrhosis and impending liver failure.

MANAGEMENT

Management goals include the prevention of additional stress on liver function and early recognition and treatment of complications. Liver functions under stress include nutritional metabolism, clearing medication and metabolic waste products, and formation of clotting factors. Interventions include monitoring nutritional markers and providing nutrition; monitoring fluid balance, urinary output, electrolyte and chemistry studies, drug type, and dose requirements; monitoring bleeding times, platelet function, and hematocrit; and detecting signs of bleeding (Box 41-14). Bowel cleansing regimens may be ordered. The early recognition of complications includes detecting signs of impending liver failure: changes in neurological and mental status, increasing ascites, and hepatorenal syndrome.

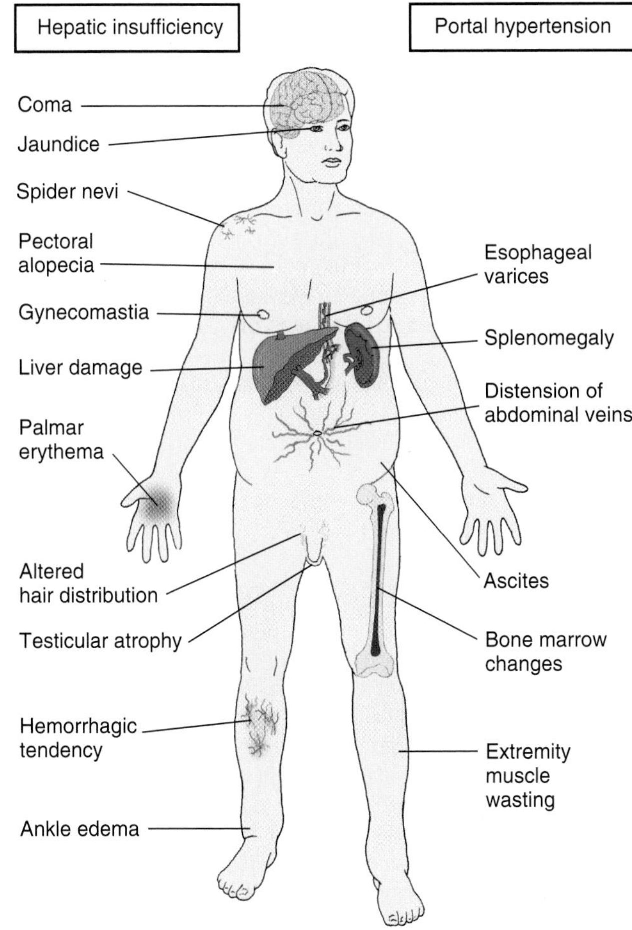

figure 41-6 Clinical effects of cirrhosis of the liver. (From Bullock BL: Pathophysiology: Adaptations and Alterations in Function [4th Ed]. Philadelphia, Lippincott-Raven, 1996.)

The critically ill patient in liver failure is often in some state of unconsciousness, with jaundiced skin and sclera. Coagulation times are prolonged, so bleeding is apt to occur from many sources. There is a risk for sores and skin breakdown because of the patient's debilitated state.

Maintaining fluid and electrolyte balance requires ongoing nursing assessment. Imbalance can result from replacement therapy, malnutrition, gastric suction, diuretics, vomiting, diaphoresis, ascites, diarrhea, inadequate fluid intake, and elevated aldosterone levels. The patient may complain of headache, weakness, numbness and tingling of extremities, muscle twitching, thirst, nausea, or muscle cramps and may become confused. Monitor weight and CVP to help determine fluid retention and vascular loading. Monitor for an increase or decrease in urinary output, cardiac dysrhythmias, changes in mental status and level of consciousness, prolonged vomiting or frequent liquid stools, muscle tremors, spasms, edema, or poor skin turgor.

Impaired handling of salt and water by the kidney and other abnormalities in fluid homeostasis predispose the patient to an accumulation of fluid in the peritoneum (i.e., ascites). This complication can be problematic because it can restrict movement of the diaphragm, causing impairment of the patient's breathing pattern. Therefore, monitoring respiratory status is critical. Ascites is managed through bed rest, a low-sodium diet, fluid restriction, and diuretic therapy. A sodium restriction of 2 g/day (88 mEq/day) seems to be commonly cited because it allows a patient to follow the diet without purchasing specialty foods.[39] It has been demonstrated that ascites absorption has an upper limit of 700 to 900 mL/day during diuresis therapy; if diuresis exceeds this limit, it may be at the expense of the intravascular volume and may potentiate hemodynamic instability.[39] Diuresis with spironolactone, an aldosterone antagonist, is first-line diuretic therapy

table 41-5 Laboratory Studies for Hepatic Injury and Function

Parameter	Normal	Increased	Decreased
Hepatocellular Injury			
ALT	5–35 IU/L	Acute viral hepatitis (ALT > AST)	Vitamin B deficiency
AST	5–40 IU/L	Biliary tract obstruction	
		Alcoholic hepatitis (AST > ALT)	
		Ischemia or hypoxia ("shock liver")	
		Drug toxicity	
		Right-sided heart failure	
		Liver cancer	
Liver Synthetic Function			
Albumin	3.4–4.7 g/dL	Dehydration, shock	Chronic liver disease, malnutrition, malabsorption
Total protein	6.0–8.0 g/dL		
PT	11–15 sec	Liver disease	N/A
International normalized ratio (INR)	0.8–1.2 sec	Vitamin K deficiency	
		Anticoagulants	
Cholestasis or Excretory Function			
Total bilirubin	0.2–1.3 mg/dL	Viral hepatitis	N/A
Conjugated (direct)	0.1–0.3 mg/dL	Alcoholic hepatitis	
Unconjugated (indirect)	0.2–0.7 mg/dL	Obstructive jaundice	
Alkaline phosphatase	30–115 IU/L	Primary biliary cirrhosis	
GGT	9–85 U/L		

N/A, not applicable.

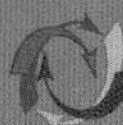

box 41-14 collaborative care guide
for the Patient With Cirrhosis and Impending Liver Failure

OUTCOMES	INTERVENTIONS
Oxygenation/Ventilation	
The patient's arterial blood gases will be within normal limits.	• Monitor pulse oximetry and arterial blood gases, respiratory rate and pattern, and ability to clear secretions. • Validate significant changes in pulse oximetry with cooximetry arterial saturation measurement.
The patient has no evidence of pulmonary edema or atelectasis. Breath sounds are clear bilaterally.	• Assist patient to turn, cough, deep breath, and use incentive spirometer q2h. • Provide chest percussion with postural drainage if indicated q4h. • Monitor effect of ascites on respiratory effort and lung compliance. • Position on side and with head of bed elevated to improve diaphragmatic movement.
Circulation/Perfusion	
Patient will achieve or maintain stable blood pressure and oxygen delivery.	• Monitor vital signs, including cardiac output, systemic vascular resistance, oxygen delivery, and oxygen consumption.
Serum lactate will be within normal limits.	• Monitor lactate qd until it is within normal limits. • Administer red blood cells, positive inotropic agents, colloid infusion as ordered to increase oxygen delivery.
Patient will not experience bleeding related to coagulopathies, varices, hepatorenal syndrome.	• Monitor PT, PTT, CBC daily. • Assess for signs of bleeding (e.g., blood in gastric contents, stools or urine); observe for petechiae, bruising. • Administer blood products as indicated. • Assist with insertion and manage the esophageal tamponade balloon tube. • Perform gastric lavage as needed.
Fluids/Electrolytes	
Patient is euvolemic.	• Daily weights.
Patient will not gain weight due to fluid retention.	• Monitor intake and output. • Monitor electrolyte values. • Measure abdominal girth daily at the same location on the abdomen. • Monitor signs of volume overload: Cardiac gallop Pulmonary crackles Shortness of breath Jugular vein distension Peripheral edema • Administer diuretics as ordered.
Mobility/Safety	
Patient is alert and oriented.	• Assess serum ammonia level. • Administer lactulose as ordered.
Ammonia level is within normal limits.	• Monitor level of consciousness, orientation, thought processing. • Assess asterixis. • Take precautions to prevent falls.
Patient achieves or maintains ability to conduct activities of daily living (ADLs) and mobilize self.	• Consult physical therapist. • Conduct range-of-motion and strengthening exercises.
No evidence of infection, WBC within normal limits.	• Monitor SIRS (systemic inflammatory response syndrome) criteria: increased WBC, increased temperature, tachypnea, tachycardia. • Use aseptic technique during procedures and monitor others.

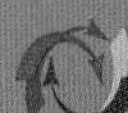

box 41-14 collaborative care guide
for the Patient With Cirrhosis and Impending Liver Failure (Continued)

OUTCOMES	INTERVENTIONS
	• Maintain invasive catheter tube sterility. • Change invasive catheters, culture blood, line tips, or fluids, provide site care, etc., according to hospital protocol.
Skin Integrity	
Skin will remain intact.	• Assess skin q8h and each time patient is repositioned. • Turn q2h. Assist or teach patient to shift weight or reposition. • Consider pressure relief/reduction mattress.
Nutrition	
Caloric and nutrient intake meet metabolic requirements per calculation (e.g., basal energy expenditure).	• Provide nutrition by oral, enteral, or parenteral feeding. • Sodium, protein, fat, or fluid restriction may be necessary. • Consult dietitian or nutritional support service to evaluate nutritional needs and restrictions. • Provide small, frequent feedings.
Evidence of metabolic dysfunction is minimal.	• Monitor albumin, prealbumin, transferrin, BUN, cholesterol, triglycerides, bilirubin, AST, ALT. • Administer cleansing enemas and cathartics if ordered.
Comfort/Pain Control	
Patient will have minimal pain.	• Assess pain and discomfort from ascites, bleeding, pruritus.
Patient will have minimal pruritus.	• Administer analgesics cautiously and monitor patient response. • Bathe with cool water, blot dry. • Lubricate skin. • Administer antipruritic medication; apply to skin PRN as ordered.
Psychosocial	
Patient demonstrates decreased anxiety.	• Assess patient's response to illness. Provide time to listen. • Assess effect of critical care environment on the patient. • Minimize sensory overload. • Provide adequate time for uninterrupted sleep. • Encourage flexible visiting hours for family. • Plan for consistent caregiver.
Teaching/Discharge Planning	
Patient/significant others understand procedures and tests needed for treatment of hepatic dysfunction.	• Prepare patient/significant others for procedures such as paracentesis or laboratory studies. • Teach patient and family information regarding sodium, protein, and fluid restrictions. Give written materials.
Patient/significant others are prepared for home care.	• Teach signs and symptoms of progressing hepatic failure (e.g., change in mentation, skin coloration, ascites). • Teach signs and symptoms of occult bleeding and respiratory infection. • Teach home medication regimen. • Teach comfort measures.

for ascites, although combination therapy with furosemide is more effective. Monitoring for electrolyte imbalance, particularly hypokalemia, is essential. In addition to strict intake and output balance and daily weights, abdominal girth should be measured daily.

Paracentesis is also used to treat ascites in patients unresponsive to salt restriction and diuretic therapy, which occurs in 10% of cirrhotic patients.[39] In this procedure, ascitic fluid is withdrawn from the abdomen through a percutaneous needle aspiration. As much as 4 to 6 L/day of ascitic fluid could be withdrawn, and therefore close monitoring of vital signs is important during this procedure. A sudden loss of intravascular pressure may precipitate hypotension, decreased renal perfusion, and tachycardia. If a patient requires multiple invasive paracentesis procedures, there is an increased risk of infection.

Venous-peritoneal shunt (VP shunt) is a surgical procedure used to relieve ascites that is resistant to other therapies. The LeVeen shunt (Fig. 41-7) is inserted by placing the distal end of a tube in the abdominal cavity and tunneling the other end into a central vein (e.g., the superior vena cava). This perforated intra-abdominal tube allows for ascitic fluid to flow into the central vein. Complications related to placement and use include sepsis, peritonitis, DIC, thrombi formation, and variceal hemorrhage. It is not recommended for patients with infected ascites, encephalopathy, or renal failure. Although the VP shunt controls ascites better than paracentesis, there is a 40% to 60% occlusion rate within the first year of placement.[39] Because of the aforementioned complications, these shunts are rarely placed in current hepatology practice.

A nonsurgical approach to managing ascites and acute variceal hemorrhage is the transjugular intrahepatic portosystemic shunt (TIPS), illustrated in Figure 41-8. At least 90% of patients stop bleeding after a TIPS procedure,[40] and it may prevent rebleeding when other methods of managing esophageal varices fail. Using an angiographic catheter, a guidewire with a dilating balloon is inserted into the internal jugular vein and is advanced through the liver parenchyma to connect the portal vein, where most of the blood flowing to the liver enters, to the hepatic vein, which empties blood into the inferior vena cava. A stent is then placed to create a conduit between the hepatic and portal vein, which decreases portal pressure. Complications include hepatic encephalopathy in 25% of cases, shunt stenosis in 60% of cases, and shunt occlusion in 30% of cases.[39,41] Hepatic encephalopathy increases after a TIPS procedure because this portacaval shunt diverts portal blood flow away from the liver parenchyma. Risk factors that worsen hepatic encephalopathy post-TIPS procedure include age greater than 60 years, severity of liver disease, nonalcoholic liver disease, and history of previous hepatic encephalopathy.[41]

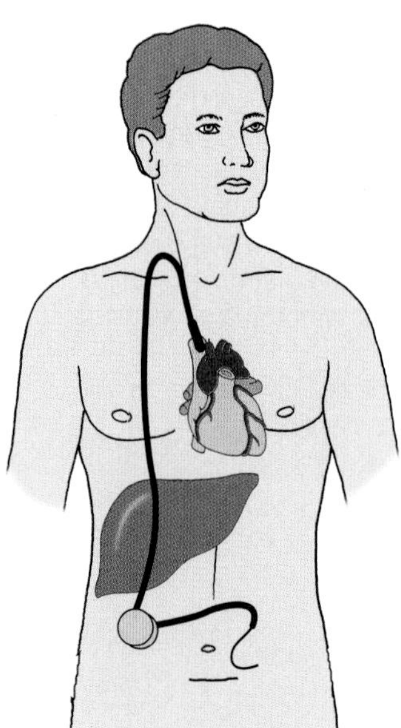

figure 41-7 The distal end of the Leveen shunt is tunneled into a central vein. The shunt allows ascites fluid to drain from the abdominal cavity.

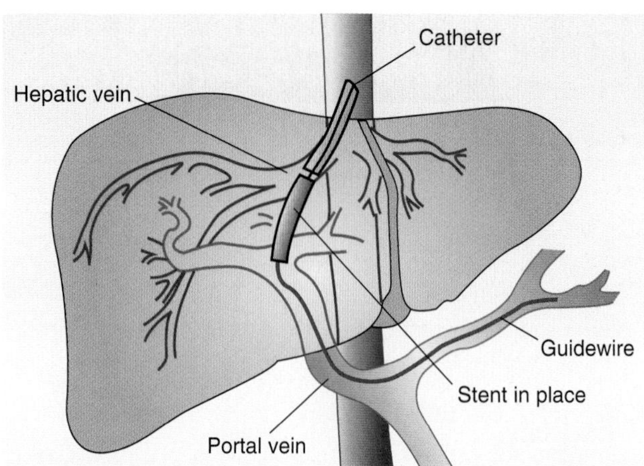

figure 41-8 Transjugular intrahepatic portosystemic shunt (TIPS). A stent is inserted through a catheter to the portal vein to divert blood flow and reduce portal hypertension. (From Smeltzer SC, Bare BG: Brunner and Suddarth's Textbook of Medical–Surgical Nursing [10th Ed], p 1089. Philadelphia, Lippincott Williams & Wilkins, 2004.)

Hepatic Encephalopathy

Patients with severe liver disease can progress to hepatic encephalopathy. Clinical manifestations start with cognitive changes, irritability, reversal of day and night schedules, and somnolence, which can progress to a terminal coma. Sometimes patients become very agitated and difficult to manage. Asterixis (a flapping tremor, usually of the hands) is a very early sign of hepatic encephalopathy. To test for this, ask the patient to hold an arm and hand out, with fingers spread, as if stopping traffic and look for involuntary hand "flapping." Other signs are hyperreflexia and muscle rigidity.

The cause of the hepatic encephalopathy is thought to be related to the accumulation of toxic agents absorbed from the intestinal tract. These substances accumulate because the liver has lost the ability to metabolize and detoxify these substances. Elevated serum ammonia, a byproduct of protein and amino acid metabolism, is one of the suspected neurotoxins. Normally, ammonia is metabolized into urea before entering the systemic circulation, and the urea is then excreted. If the liver is unable to perform this detoxification or if a good portion of the portal blood is shunted around the liver, the circulating level of ammonia rises. If ammonia and the other toxic agents can be reduced through effective therapy, the encephalopathy gradually clears. Although arterial ammonia levels are more reliable than venous samples, it is often more difficult to obtain and more painful for the patient. In addition, symptoms of hepatic encephalopathy may lag behind ammonia level elevations, and improvements in hepatic encephalopathy symptoms may occur before any improvement in ammonia levels.

Unfortunately, bypassing the clearance function of the liver with any kind of stent or shunt may result in decreased clearance and increased accumulation of toxins. Hepatic encephalopathy can develop quite rapidly in those with portosystemic shunts. People with portal hypertension can hemorrhage from esophageal varices or other sites in the gastrointestinal tract. The hemorrhage produces a significant nitrogenous load to the intestinal tract in the form of blood, from which bacterial deamination produces the ammonia. Protein intake is limited to 20 to 40 g/day for the treatment of acute hepatic encephalopathy. Lactulose is used to facilitate bowel movements and clearance of nitrogenous products. Neomycin or metronidazole may be given to clear the gut of bacteria that promote nitrogenous production. Lactulose decreases the colonic pH to prevent the absorption of ammonia. Nursing measures to protect the patient with mental status changes from harm are a priority.

Hepatorenal Syndrome

Acute renal failure that occurs with liver failure is called *hepatorenal syndrome.* It is characterized by impaired renal function during the terminal stages of liver failure (with ascites) in a patient without previous or coexistent intrinsic renal disease.[42] After the onset of ascites, the probability for development of hepatorenal syndrome was noted in one study to be 18% after 1 year, and 39% after 5 years.[43] This failure of the kidneys is the result of extreme vasodilatation, which decreases the effective blood volume and leads to maximal vasoconstriction, renal vasoconstriction, and renal failure. Ascites, jaundice, hypotension, and oliguria are clinical findings; laboratory findings typically include azotemia, elevated serum creatinine, urine sodium less than 10 mEq/L, and hyponatremia.[42] The prognosis for the patient is generally poor once renal failure is evident. Management goals include therapies to support liver and kidney functions, but liver transplantation is the treatment of choice.

Spontaneous Bacterial Peritonitis

Patients with liver disease may be more susceptible to infection because the hepatic Kupffer cells, which are responsible for uptake and subsequent degradation of foreign and potentially harmful substances in the body, do not function as efficiently. Spontaneous bacterial peritonitis occurs when there is a large accumulation of ascites without an identifiable intra-abdominal source of infection. It may be triggered during endoscopy or when a nasogastric tube, IV line, or indwelling bladder catheter is placed. *Escherichia coli, Klebsiella* species, and *Streptococcus pneumoniae* are the most common causes. The patient may complain of fever, abdominal pain, and tenderness with palpation. Approximately 20% of hospitalized patients with cirrhosis and ascites have spontaneous bacterial peritonitis,[44] and 30% of these are without symptoms.[45] If spontaneous bacterial peritonitis is suspected, the ascitic fluid is evaluated for cell count, differential, and culture. The patient is treated with broad-spectrum antibiotic coverage until the results of these tests are returned. Spontaneous bacterial peritonitis must be differentiated from peritonitis secondary to an abscess or perforation because the latter needs immediate surgical treatment.

Common nursing diagnoses for the patient with a gastrointestinal disorder are listed in Box 41-15. A discharge planning guide for the patient with a gastrointestinal disorder is given in Box 41-16.

box 41-15 Examples of Nursing Diagnoses for the Patient With a Gastrointestinal Disorder

- Impaired Nutrition: Less than Body Requirements related to altered pancreatic or liver function, impaired digestion from inadequate bile or pancreatic enzyme production, poor eating habits, excessive alcohol intake, nausea, vomiting, or anorexia
- Excess Fluid Volume related to extravascular ascites, portal hypertension, and hypoalbuminemia
- Risk for Deficient Fluid Volume related to overly aggressive diuresis, gastrointestinal bleeding and coagulopathies, and peritoneal sequestration of intra-abdominal fluids
- Risk for Electrolyte Imbalance related to anorexia, nausea, and vomiting
- Risk for Aspiration related to delayed gastric emptying, intestinal obstruction, ileus, or gastrointestinal bleeding
- Risk for Impaired Gas Exchange related to decreased diaphragmatic excursion secondary to abdominal distension and potential for aspiration
- Risk for Decreased Cardiac Output related to hepatic portal hypertension or blood loss from gastrointestinal bleeding
- Acute Pain or Discomfort related to nasogastric tube irritation, pruritus related to accumulation of bilirubin pigment and salts, inflammation of the pancreas and surrounding tissues, and local peritonitis
- Risk for Disturbed Sensory Perception related to hepatic encephalopathy and delirium tremens (in cases of alcohol abuse)
- Risk for Ineffective Therapeutic Regimen Management related to insufficient knowledge of disease process, treatments, contraindications, dietary management, and follow-up care

box 41-16 *Common Gastrointestinal Disorders*

- Explain signs and symptoms of gastrointestinal bleeding: hematemesis, tarry stools, melena.
- Explain signs and symptoms of recurrent ileus: nausea or vomiting, abdominal distension.
- Explain signs and symptoms of acute or recurrent pancreatitis: severe left upper quadrant pain, especially after a large meal or alcohol intake. The pain may be intermittent or constant in the epigastric area and accompanied by nausea and anorexia.
- Explain signs and symptoms of acute or worsening chronic hepatitis: generalized fatigue or malaise, right upper quadrant abdominal pain and distension, clay-colored stools or diarrhea, change in mental status, and jaundice.
- Explain the importance of monitoring for fever, chills.
- Explain how to check weight daily (same time of day) to monitor for increased ascites.
- Review and provide written instructions for medications and treatments.
- Discuss potential side effects of medications and treatments.
- Encourage follow-up care.
- Provide the patient and family with information regarding smoking cessation and alcohol and drug treatment programs as necessary.

clinical applicability challenges

Self-Challenge: Critical Thinking

1. *What is the most likely etiology of a small bowel obstruction?*
2. *Describe the potential complications of a small bowel obstruction.*
3. *What is the most common cause of acute pancreatitis?*
4. *Name three risk factors for the development of gallstone-induced pancreatitis.*
5. *What are the two most common causes of peptic ulcer disease?*
6. *Describe the potential for long-term sequelae of hepatitis.*
7. *What discharge instructions would you recommend for a patient who is being discharged to home after an episode of upper gastrointestinal bleeding?*

Study Questions

1. *Mr. Johnson, a 43-year-old man with a history of esophageal varices from prolonged alcohol abuse, is admitted with severe upper gastrointestinal bleeding. To maintain hemodynamic stability, intravenous volume replacement is initiated and he is placed on a vasopressin (Pitressin) drip. Endoscopy is ordered for evaluation of the varices and sclerotherapy is successfully performed. One hour later, Mr. Johnson complains of chest pressure. The most likely etiology of his chest pressure is*
   a. *esophageal variceal spasms.*
   b. *gastroesophageal reflux disease (GERD).*
   c. *myocardial ischemia.*
   d. *pancreatitis.*
2. *Mr. Johnson, the patient in question 1, continues to have chest pain and his vasopressin drip is discontinued. He subsequently experiences recurrent bleeding of his esophageal varices and a Sengstaken-Blakemore tube is successfully placed. The bleeding is controlled and hemodynamic stability is restored. Later that day, sudden respiratory distress develops in Mr. Johnson. What is the critical care nurse's first responsibility?*
   a. *To call the physician and ask for a stat chest x-ray*
   b. *To check a stat pulse oximetry reading*
   c. *To cut and remove the Sengstaken-Blakemore tube*
   d. *To raise the head of the bed and apply oxygen*
3. *Acute pancreatitis is associated with*
   a. *elevated serum amylase, elevated serum lipase, decreased serum calcium, and decreased serum albumin.*
   b. *elevated serum amylase, decreased serum lipase, decreased serum calcium, and decreased serum albumin.*
   c. *decreased serum amylase, elevated serum lipase, decreased serum calcium, and decreased serum albumin.*
   d. *decreased serum amylase, elevated serum lipase, increased serum calcium, and increased serum albumin.*
4. *A patient with acute pancreatitis is noted to have facial twitching when the facial nerve is tapped. In addition, the patient's arm spasms during blood pressure measurements. This is because*
   a. *elevated serum amylase and lipase enzymes are very irritating to the nerves.*
   b. *decreased serum lipase levels cause hypoglycemia and seizure activity.*
   c. *decreased serum calcium levels result in muscle tetany.*
   d. *hypoalbuminemia causes muscle weakness and spasms.*
5. *The critical care nurse's first priority in a patient with acute pancreatitis is*
   a. *insertion of a nasogastric tube.*
   b. *insertion of a Foley catheter.*
   c. *administration of intravenous fluids and electrolyte repletion.*
   d. *encouragement of oral fluid intake.*
6. *Hypoactive bowel sounds may be associated with*
   a. *diarrhea.*
   b. *an early intestinal obstruction.*
   c. *portal hypertension.*
   d. *an ileus.*
7. *A 65-year-old woman had a total abdominal hysterectomy 2 months ago. She presents to the emergency department with severe, colicky abdominal pain and feculent vomiting for the past 12 hours. What is the most likely diagnosis for this patient?*
   a. *Gastroesophageal reflux disease*
   b. *Acute pancreatitis*
   c. *Small bowel obstruction*
   d. *Hepatitis*
8. *Cholestasis may precipitate which of the following problems?*
   a. *Acute small bowel obstruction*
   b. *Acute hepatitis*
   c. *Acute pancreatitis*
   d. *Both b and c*

9. *Mr. Moore is a 34-year-old man admitted to the critical care unit with a history of intravenous drug abuse. He reports a 4-week history of "flulike symptoms," malaise, and right upper quadrant tenderness. The nurse notes that the patient has scleral and generalized jaundice. A battery of serological diagnostic tests has been ordered. As expected, the patient's total bilirubin level is elevated at 2.4 mg/dL. Other results reveal an elevated ALT of 980 mg/dL, an elevated AST of 760 mg/dL, and an elevated alkaline phosphatase of 143 mg/dL. The hepatitis serology markers are as follows: human immunodeficiency virus (HIV) is negative; anti-HAV IgM (anti-hepatitis A virus antibody) is negative; HBsAg (hepatitis B surface antigen) is positive; anti-HBc IgM (hepatitis B core antibody) is positive; HBeAg (hepatitis B core antigen) is positive; and anti-HCV (anti-hepatitis C virus antibody) is negative. As the critical care nurse, what is the correct interpretation of these serology markers?*
   a. *The patient has acute hepatitis A virus (HAV) infection.*
   b. *The patient has acute hepatitis B virus (HBV) infection.*
   c. *The patient has been exposed to hepatitis B virus (HBV) but does not have active disease.*
   d. *The patient has hepatitis C virus (HCV) infection.*

REFERENCES

1. Kupfer Y, Cappell MS, Tessler S: Acute gastrointestinal bleeding in the intensive care unit: The intensivist's perspective. Gastroenterol Clin North Am 29(2):275–307, 2000
2. Beejay U, Wolfe MM: Acute gastrointestinal bleeding in the intensive care unit. Gastroenterol Clin North Am 29(2):309–336, 2000
3. Cello JP: Octreotide. Clin Perspect Gastroenterol 3(6):349–352, 2000
4. Lefkovitz Z, Cappell MS, Kaplan M, et al: Radiology in the diagnosis and therapy of gastrointestinal bleeding. Gastroenterol Clin North Am 29(2):489–512, 2000
5. Savides TJ, Jensen DM: Therapeutic endoscopy for nonvariceal bleeding. Gastroenterol Clin North Am 29(2):465–488, 2000
6. Stabile BE, Stamos MJ: Surgical management of gastrointestinal bleeding. Gastroenterol Clin North Am 29(1):189–222, 2000
7. Luketic VA, Sanyal AJ: Esophageal varices: II. TIPS (transjugular intrahepatic portosystemic shunt) and surgical therapy. Gastroenterol Clin North Am 29(2):337–386, 2000
8. Shah VH, Kamath PS: New developments in portal hypertensive bleeding. Clin Perspect Gastroenterol 5(1):17–22, 2002
9. Gostout CJ, Wang KK, Ahlquist DA, et al: Acute gastrointestinal bleeding: Experience of a special management team. J Clin Gastroenterol 14(3):267–271, 1992
10. Farrell JJ, Friedman LS: Gastrointestinal bleeding in older people. Gastroenterol Clin North Am 29(1):1–36, 2000
11. Zuccaro G: Management of the adult patient with acute lower gastrointestinal bleeding. Am J Gastroenterol 93(8):1202–1208, 1998
12. Shelton BK: Intestinal obstruction. AACN Clin Issues 10(4): 478–491, 1999
13. Summers RW: Approach to the patient with ileus and obstruction. In Yamada T, Alpers DH, Kaplowitz N, et al (eds): Textbook of Gastroenterology (4th Ed), vol I, pp 829–843. Philadelphia, Lippincott Williams & Wilkins, 2003
14. Turnage RH, Bergen PC: Intestinal obstruction and ileus. In Feldman M, Friedman LS, Sleisenger MH (eds): Sleisenger & Fortran's Gastrointestinal and Liver Disease: Pathophysiology, Diagnosis and Management (7th Ed), pp 2113–2128. Philadelphia, WB Saunders, 2002
15. Silen W: Acute intestinal obstruction. In Braunwald E, Fauci AS, Kasper DL, et al (eds): Harrison's Principles of Internal Medicine (15th Ed), pp 1703–1705. New York, McGraw-Hill, 2001
16. Lopez-Kostner F, Hool GR, Lavery IC: Management and causes of acute large-bowel obstruction. Surg Clin North Am 77(6): 1265–1290, 1997
17. Behm B, Stollman N: Postoperative ileus. Practical Gastroenterol 26(12):13–24, 2002
18. Topazian M, Gorelick FS: Acute pancreatitis. In Yamada T, Alpers DH, Kaplowitz N, et al (eds): Textbook of Gastroenterology (4th Ed), vol II, pp 2026–2060. Philadelphia, Lippincott Williams & Wilkins, 2003
19. Banks PA: Practice guidelines in acute pancreatitis. Am J Gastroenterol 92(3):377–386, 1997
20. Conwell DL: Acute and chronic pancreatitis. Practical Gastroenterol 25(12):47–55, 2001
21. Schaplman N: Spotting acute pancreatitis. RN 64(11):54–59, 2001
22. Triester SL, Kowdley KV: Prognostic factors in acute pancreatitis. J Clin Gastroenterol 34(2):167–176, 2002
23. Smotkin J, Tenner S: Laboratory diagnostic tests in acute pancreatitis. J Clin Gastroenterol 34(4):459–462, 2002
24. Grendell JH: Acute pancreatitis. Clin Perspect Gastroenterol 3(6): 327–333, 2000
25. Greenberger NJ, Toskes PP: Acute and chronic pancreatitis. In Braunwald E, Fauci AS, Kasper DL, et al (eds): Harrison's Principles of Internal Medicine (15th Ed), pp 1792–1804. New York, McGraw-Hill, 2001
26. Rodes I, Kamath P: Pathogenesis and treatment of ascites. J Intern Med 240:111–114, 1996
27. Vargas HI: Hepatobiliary disease. In Bongard FS, Sue DY (eds): Current Critical Diagnosis and Treatment (2nd Ed), pp 768–776. New York, McGraw-Hill, 2002
28. Sahara AI: Chronic hepatitis C. South Med Rev 90(9):872–877, 1997
29. Marcus EL, Tur-Kaspa R: Viral hepatitis in older adults. J Am Geriatr Soc 45:755–763, 1997
30. Dienstag JL, Isselbacher KJ: Acute viral hepatitis. In Braunwald E, Fauci AS, Kasper DL, et al (eds): Harrison's Principles of Internal Medicine (15th Ed), pp 1721–1736. New York, McGraw-Hill, 2001
31. King RR: Hepatitis C: Past, present, and future issues. Adv Nurse Practitioners 5(3):51–56, 1997
32. Urdea MS, Wuestehube LJ, Laurenson PM, et al: Hepatitis C: Diagnosis and monitoring. Clin Chem 43(8[B]):1507–1511, 1997
33. Jaeckel E, Cornberg M, Wedemeyer H, et al: Treatment of acute hepatitis C with interferon alfa-2b. N Engl J Med 345(20):1452–1457, 2001
34. Janisch T, Preiser W, Berger A, et al: Emerging viral pathogens in long-term expatriates: Hepatitis E virus. Trop Med Int Health 2(9):885–891, 1997
35. Miniño AM, Arias E, Kochanek KD, et al: National Vital Statistics Report, Deaths: Final Data for 2000, 50(15) Electronic Version. Available at: http://www.cdc.gov/nchs/data/nvsr/nvsr50/nvsr50_15.pdf. Accessed June 27, 2003
36. Reichling JJ, Kaplan MM: Clinical use of serum enzymes in liver disease. Dig Dis Sci 33:1601, 1988
37. Ma Z, Lee S: Cirrhotic cardiomyopathy: Getting to the heart of the matter. Hepatology 24:451, 1996
38. Le Moine O, Soupison T, Sogni T, et al: Plasma endotoxin and tumor necrosis factor-alpha in the hyperkinetic state of cirrhosis. J Hepatol 23:391, 1995
39. Bass M: Fluid and electrolyte management of ascites in patients with cirrhosis. Crit Care Nurs Clin North Am 10(4):459–467, 1998
40. Shiffman ML, Jeffers L, Hoofnagle JH, et al: The role of transjugular intrahepatic portosystemic shunt (TIPS) for treatment of portal hypertension and its complications. Hepatology 22:1591, 1995
41. Grace N: The side-to side portacaval shunt revisited. N Engl J Med 330:208, 1994
42. Roberts LR, Kamath PS: Ascites and hepatorenal syndrome: Pathophysiology and management. Mayo Clin Proc 71:874–881, 1996
43. Gines A, Escorsell A, Gines P, et al: Incidence, predictive factors, and prognosis of the hepatorenal syndrome in cirrhosis with ascites. Gastroenterology 105:229–236, 1993
44. Runyon BA: Ascites. In Schiff ER (ed): Diseases of the Liver (7th Ed), pp 990–1015. Philadelphia, JB Lippincott, 1993

45. Gilbert JA, Kamath PS: Spontaneous bacterial peritonitis: An update. Mayo Clin Proc 70:365–370, 1995

OTHER SELECTED READING

American Gastroenterology Association: American Gastroenterology Association Medical Position Statement: Evaluation of liver chemistry tests. Gastroenterology 123:1364–1366, 2002

Cole L: Unraveling the mystery of acute pancreatitis. Nursing 31(12): 58–64, 2001

Fishchbach F: Nurses' Quick Reference to Common Laboratory and Diagnostic Tests (3rd Ed). Philadelphia, Lippincott Williams & Wilkins, 2002

Garcia-Tsao G: Portal hypertension. Curr Opin Gastroenterol 19(3): 250–258, 2003; also available at: http://www.medscape.com/viewarticle/452729. Accessed May 5, 2003

Go MF, Vakil N: *Helicobacter pylori* infection. Clin Perspect Gastroenterol 2(3):143–153, 1999

Hoerner M, Schumann L: Diagnosis and management of acute pancreatitis. J Am Acad Nurse Practitioners 10(10):471–480, 1998

Johnston DE: Special considerations in interpreting liver function tests. Am Fam Physician 59(8):2223–2230, 1999

McNally PR: Gastrointestinal/Liver Secrets (2nd Ed). Philadelphia, Hanley & Belfus, 2001

Morton PG (ed): Gastrointestinal Disorders. AACN Clin Issues 10(4): 433–441, 455–463, 465–477, 478–491, 1999

Saunders MD, Kimmey MB: Acute colonic pseudo-obstruction. Clin Perspect Gastroenterol 3(3):156–162, 2000

PART
one
two
three
four
five
six
seven
eight
nine
ten
eleven
twelve

Endocrine System

INTERNET RESOURCES

Topic	Web Page Address
American Association of Clinical Endocrinologists	www.aace.com
American Association of Diabetes Educators	www.aadenet.org
American Diabetes Association	www.diabetes.org
American Dietetic Association	www.eatright.org
American Thyroid Association	www.thyroid.org
Canadian Diabetes Association	www.diabetes.ca
Centers for Disease Control and Prevention	www.cdc.gov/diabetes
Diabetes Action Research and Education Foundation	www.diabetesaction.org
Diabetes Exercise and Sports Association	www.diabetes-exercise.org
Endocrine Disorders and Endocrine Surgery	www.endocrineweb.com
Endocrine Nurses' Society	www.endo-nurses.org
Endocrine Online	www.endocrineonline.org
The Endocrine Society	www.endo-society.org
Endocrine Surgery Website by Johns Hopkins Hospital	http://www.path.jhu.edu/endocrine/
European Federation of Endocrine Societies	www.euro-endo.org
Federation of European Nurses in Diabetes	www.fend.org
International Association of Endocrine Surgeons	www.iaes-endocrine-surgeons.com
International Diabetes Federation	www.idf.org
Joslin Diabetes Center	www.joslin.org
Juvenile Diabetes Research Foundation International	www.jdrf.org
National Adrenal Diseases Foundation	www.medhelp.org/nadf/
National Kidney Foundation	www.kidney.org
National Institute of Diabetes and Digestive and Kidney Disorders	www.niddk.nih.gov
Thyroid Federation International	www.thyroid-fed.org
Thyroid Foundation of America	www.allthyroid.org

chapter 42

Anatomy and Physiology of the Endocrine System

JANE KAPUSTIN

objectives

Based on the content in this chapter, the reader should be able to:

- Describe the production, action, and regulation of antidiuretic hormone, growth and thyroid hormones, insulin, and glucagon.
- Identify how activated vitamin D, parathyroid hormone, and calcitonin each influence calcium concentrations in the blood.
- Explain how glucocorticoids are secreted.
- Summarize the renin–angiotensin mechanism for regulating mineralocorticoid secretion.
- List the significant effects of glucocorticoid medications.

Communication between systems in the body is accomplished in three ways. One method of communication is the nervous system. A second method is the cellular secretion of chemicals that are released into the interstitial fluid. Examples of this method of communication include the chemicals that trigger a local inflammatory response, such as histamine, complement, and prostaglandins. The third method of communication is the cellular secretion of chemicals that are circulated through the bloodstream. This communication is known more commonly as the *endocrine system* (Fig. 42-1, Table 42-1). The secretions of endocrine cells are termed *hormones*. Hormones are molecules synthesized and secreted by specialized cells and released into blood vessels to exert biochemical effects on target cells distant from the site of origin. They control metabolism, transport of substances across the cell membrane, fluid and electrolyte balance, growth and development, adaptation, and reproduction.

Hormone action is specific and depends on linkage with a specialized hormone receptor on the target cell. This hormone–receptor complex is responsible for a series of biological responses. Hormones are either stimulatory or inhibitory. Their actions are either very organ specific, such as prolactin (which only affects the mammary glands), or their effects are generalized, such as the action of insulin (which affects most cellular functions of the body).

Hormone production is maintained by a feedback loop mechanism involving the hypothalamic–pituitary axis system (Fig. 42-2). Release of a specific hormone is made possible when the circulating level of that hormone is low (positive feedback). Conversely, when the circulating level of a hormone is high, the release of more hormone is inhibited (negative feedback) until a lower level is reached. This system is regulated by specialized sensors in the hypothalamus that continuously monitor hormone assays to maintain self-regulated homeostasis. Theoretically, this system prevents the overproduction of hormones.

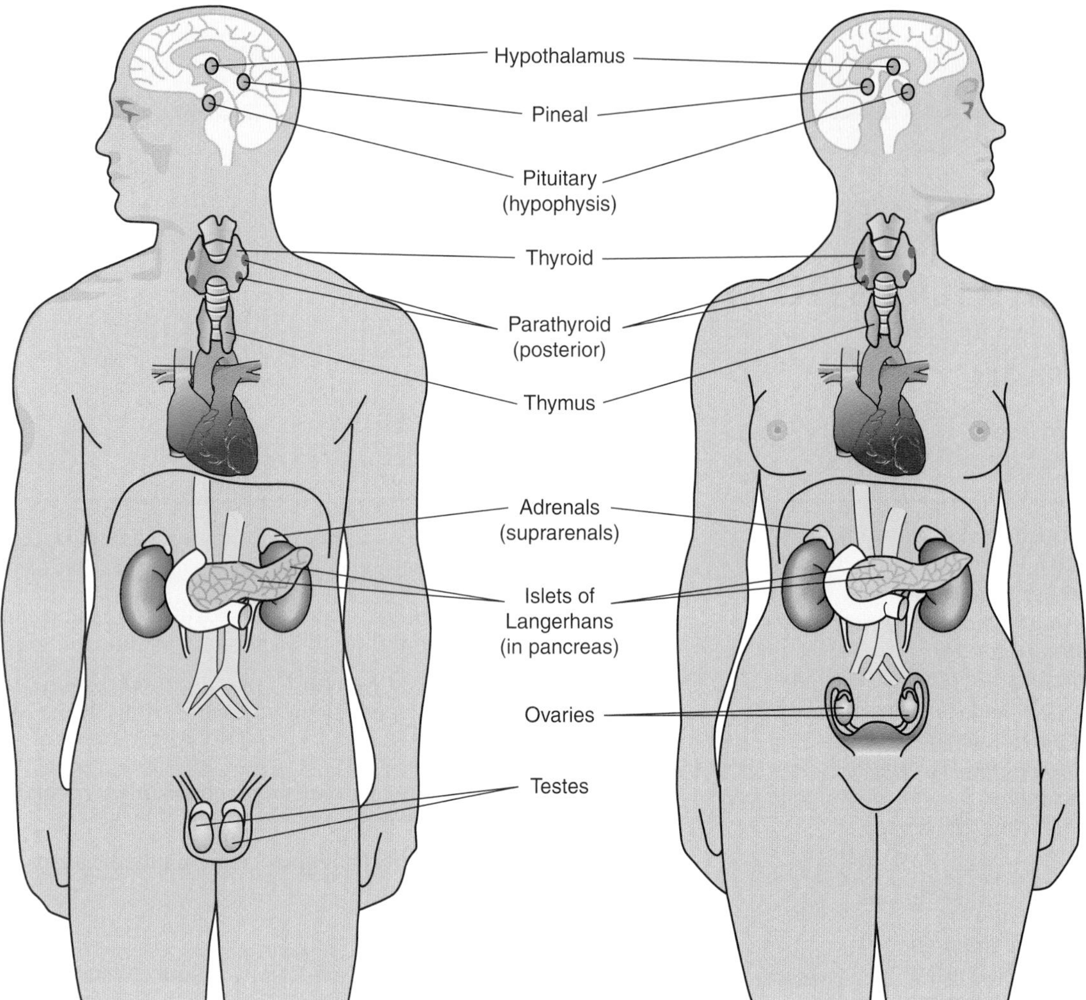

figure 42-1 The endocrine system. (Source: Smeltzer SC, Bare BG: Brunner & Suddarth's Textbook of Medical–Surgical Nursing [9th Ed], p 1029. Philadelphia, Lippincott Williams & Wilkins, 2000.)

The effects of aging can influence the endocrine system as well (Box 42-1). As humans age, target organ sensitivity decreases. The target organs demonstrate the effects of aging by either increasing in pigmentation or shrinking in size. This, in effect, decreases hormone receptor binding. This phenomenon explains why older patients are at higher risk for development of hypothyroidism—aging can decrease production of triiodothyronine (T_3) and thyroxine (T_4) and can lead to thyroid gland atrophy.

Endocrine dysfunction can be identified as belonging to one of five major categories:

- Subnormal hormone production as a result of gland destruction or malformation
- Hormone excess
- Production of abnormal hormone resulting from gene mutation
- Hormone receptor disorders resulting from autoimmune processes
- Disorders of hormone transport or metabolism, resulting in increased levels of "free" hormones in the blood

THE HYPOTHALAMUS AND PITUITARY GLAND

The key to understanding the physiology of the hormones of the pituitary gland lies in visualizing the anatomy of the gland and its blood supply. Together, the hypothalamus and pituitary gland form a unit that controls the thyroid gland, the adrenal glands, and the gonads, and exerts control over the growth and metabolism of the organism. Because of the control it exerts over all body functions, the pituitary gland is often referred to as the *master gland.* It is located at the base of the skull in the sphenoid bone at a site referred to as the *sella turcica.* This well-protected gland is difficult to reach surgically because it is so deeply embedded in the skull. Despite being well protected, the pituitary is still susceptible to injury as a result of head or facial trauma, edema, or surgical complications. Because it is so vascular, the pituitary is extremely vulnerable to injury from ischemia and infarction.

The hypothalamus is a small area at the base of the brain connected to the posterior pituitary (also known as the *neurohypophysis*) by the pituitary stalk. This stalk is a direct

table 42-1 Endocrine System in Summary

Endocrine Gland and Hormone	Principal Site of Action	Principal Processes Affected
Pituitary Gland		
Anterior Lobe		
Growth hormone (GH, somatotropin)	General	Growth of bones, muscles, and other organs
Thyroid-stimulating hormone (TSH)	Thyroid	Growth and secretory activity of thyroid gland
Adrenocorticotropic hormone (ACTH)	Adrenal cortex	Growth and secretory activity of adrenal cortex
Follicle-stimulating hormone (FSH)	Ovaries	Development of follicles and secretion of estrogen
	Testes	Development of seminiferous tubules, spermatogenesis
Luteinizing hormone (LH) or interstitial cell-stimulating hormone (ICSH)	Ovaries	Ovulation, formation of corpus luteum, secretion of progesterone
Prolactin (luteotropic hormone, LTH)	Testes	Secretion of testosterone
Melanocyte-stimulating hormone (MSH)	Mammary glands and ovaries	Secretion of milk; maintenance of corpus luteum
β-lipotropin	Skin	Pigmentation
Posterior Lobe		
Antidiuretic hormone (ADH, vasopressin)	Kidney	Reabsorption of water; water balance
	Arterioles	Blood pressure
Oxytocin	Uterus	Contraction
	Breast	Expression of milk
Pineal Gland		
Melatonin	Gonads	Sexual maturation
Thyroid Gland		
Thyroxine (T_4) and triiodothyronine (T_3)	General	Metabolic rate; growth and development; intermediate metabolism
Calcitonin	Bone	Inhibits bone resorption; lowers blood level of calcium
Parathyroid Glands		
Parathyroid hormone (PTH)	Bone, kidney, intestine	Promotes bone resorption; increases absorption of calcium; raises blood calcium level
Adrenal Glands		
Cortex		
Mineralocorticoids (eg, aldosterone)	Kidney	Reabsorption of sodium; elimination of potassium
Glucocorticoids (eg, cortisol)	General	Metabolism of carbohydrate, protein, and fat; response to stress; anti-inflammatory
Sex hormones	General	Preadolescent growth spurt
Medulla		
Epinephrine	Cardiac muscle, smooth muscle, glands	Emergency functions: same as stimulation of sympathetic nervous system
Norepinephrine	Organs innervated by sympathetic nervous system	Chemical transmitter substance; increases peripheral resistance
Islet Cells of Pancreas		
Insulin	General	Lowers blood sugar; utilization and storage of carbohydrate; decreases gluconeogenesis
Glucagon	Liver	Raises blood glucose; glycogenolysis
Somatostatin	General	Lowers blood glucose by interfering with release of growth hormone and glucagon
Testes		
Testosterone	General	Development of secondary sex characteristics
	Reproductive organs	Development and maintenance; normal function
Ovaries		
Estrogens	General	Development of secondary sex characteristics
	Mammary glands	Development of duct system
	Reproductive organs	Maturation and normal cyclic function
Progesterone	Mammary glands	Development of secretory tissue
	Uterus	Preparation for implantation; maintenance of pregnancy

(continued)

table 42-1 Endocrine System in Summary (Continued)

Endocrine Gland and Hormone	Principal Site of Action	Principal Processes Affected
Gastrointestinal Tract		
Gastrin	Stomach	Production of gastric juice
Enterogastrone	Stomach	Inhibits secretion and motility
Secretin	Liver and pancreas	Production of bile; production of watery pancreatic juice (rich in $NaHCO_3$)
Pancreozymin	Pancreas	Production of pancreatic juice rich in enzymes
Cholecystokinin	Gallbladder	Contraction and emptying

Source: Smeltzer SC, Bare BG: Brunner & Suddarth's Textbook of Medical-Surgical Nursing (9th Ed), p 1030. Philadelphia, Lippincott Williams & Wilkins, 2000.

outgrowth of the neuroectoderm of the base of the brain that drops during development of the gland into the bony sella turcica. This is in direct contrast to the anterior pituitary (adenohypophysis), which arises from the buccal endothelium and develops separately in the same bony structure. Besides being embryogenically separate, the blood supplies of the anterior and posterior pituitary differ.

The anterior pituitary hormones are controlled by factors that are released from the hypothalamus, called *hypophysiotropic hormones* (releasing factors). The hypophysiotropic hormones are secreted into the primary capillary plexus near the median eminence that supplies blood to the anterior pituitary (Fig. 42-3). This blood may also travel in a retrograde fashion and may be responsible for one level of feedback control of the anterior pituitary and hypophysiotropic hormones. A given hypophysiotropic hormone regulates the secretion of one or two anterior pituitary hormones. Both growth hormone (GH, somatotropin) and prolactin are dually controlled by a stimulatory and an inhibitory hypophysiotropic hormone. The posterior pituitary is a direct neural extension of the hypothalamus, and the controlling factors reside in the neural chiasma of the hypothalamus; they are secreted by those cells into the posterior pituitary (see Fig. 42-3). In addition to controlling the pituitary gland through releasing factors, the hypothalamus controls other endocrine roles through releasing factors that control appetite, thirst, emotions, sleep–wake cycles, and cognition.

Such hypothalamic regulation of pituitary functioning can be disrupted by hypothalamic lesions. This can lead to oversecretion or undersecretion of one or more hormones released from the anterior or posterior pituitary. The hypothalamus also receives input from various higher and lower brain centers. These neural connections, together with the influence of the hypothalamus on the pituitary, provide the biological basis for the construction of conceptual models that describe how stress, emotions, environmental stimuli, and perceptions affect endocrine functions.

Posterior Pituitary (Neurohypophysis) Hormones

The posterior pituitary (neurohypophysis) comprises 25% of the gland. The two major hormones of the posterior pituitary gland are antidiuretic hormone (ADH, vasopressin) and oxytocin (see Table 42-1).

ANTIDIURETIC HORMONE (VASOPRESSIN)

The two major actions of ADH are to concentrate the urine (by permitting only water reabsorption from the hypotonic tubular fluid in the distal nephron) and to constrict smooth muscles in the arterial wall. ADH binds to specific receptors in the distal renal tubules to increase their permeability to water. This results in increased water reabsorption but without electrolyte reabsorption. This reabsorbed water increases the volume and decreases the osmolality of the extracellular fluid (ECF). At the same time, it decreases the volume and increases the concentration of the urine excreted. Without ADH, the distal convoluted tubule would be impermeable to water. In the presence of ADH, the tubule and collecting duct are permeable to water, which diffuses from the hypotonic tubular fluid to the hypertonic tissue surrounding the tubules. This concentrates the tubular fluid and ultimately the urine.

The term *vasopressin* originated from the observation that large, supraphysiological dosages of ADH act on arteriole smooth muscle to elevate blood pressure. Although this pressor action of ADH does not appear to play a role in the normal homeostasis of blood pressure, it does counteract a fall in blood pressure that results from hemorrhagic or other drastic hypovolemic states.

The half-life of ADH is 18 minutes. It is degraded principally by the liver and kidneys. Metabolic clearance of ADH is augmented from the 10th week of gestation to midterm pregnancy. This phenomenon is the result of an increase in plasma vasopressinase, an enzyme aminopeptidase specific for ADH.

There are three major stimuli for the regulation of ADH secretion. The first is plasma osmolality, which is monitored by osmoreceptors in the anterior hypothalamus. An increase above the normal osmolality of plasma (290 mOsm/kg) results in neural stimuli from these receptors to the ADH-secreting cells, increasing ADH secretion. This increases water retention, thereby diluting the ECF and lowering the plasma osmolality back to normal. Similarly, a fall in plasma osmolality triggers a decrease or cessation in ADH secretion. This allows more water excretion, thereby raising the ECF osmolality. ADH secretion can be altered by changes in osmolality of less than 1%. This osmoreceptor-mediated reflex arc functions in maintaining osmotic homeostasis of the ECF.

The second stimulus consists of changes in ECF volume. Stretch receptors in the low-pressure portion of the

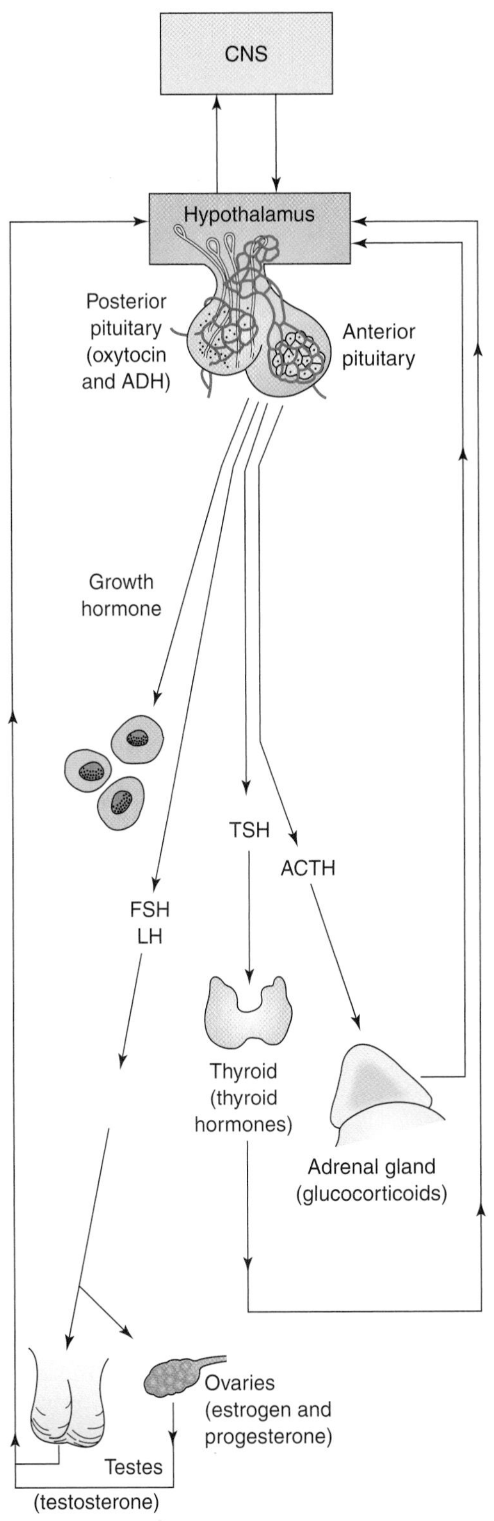

figure 42-2 The feedback loop mechanism that controls hormone production. Sensors in the hypothalamus monitor hormone levels and initiate or suppress production accordingly. *ACTH,* adrenocorticotropic hormone; *ADH,* antidiuretic hormone; *CNS,* central nervous system; *FSH,* follicle-stimulating hormone; *LH,* luteinizing hormone; *TSH,* thyroid-stimulating hormone. (Source: Porth CM: Pathophysiology: Concepts of Altered Health States [6th Ed], p 899. Philadelphia, Lippincott Williams & Wilkins, 2002.)

cardiovascular system (e.g., the vena cava, the right side of the heart, and the pulmonary vessels) monitor blood volume. Stimuli from these receptors are conducted by afferent fibers to the hypothalamus (by way of the brainstem). A decrease in blood volume stimulates ADH secretion. The resultant increase in water retention elevates the blood volume without affecting arterial blood pressure. An increase in blood volume stops ADH secretion. This halts water retention, thereby restoring the normal volume of the ECF compartment. This mechanism alters ADH secretion in response to changes in body position. Movement from the recumbent to the upright position causes a temporary decrease in the stimulation of volume receptors because blood pools in the legs. This results in an increase in ADH secretion. Recumbency increases venous return from the legs. The increased volume triggers a decrease in ADH secretion, thereby increasing the volume of urine excreted.

The third stimulus, changes in arterial blood pressure, also can regulate ADH secretion. The hypothalamus receives information from pressure receptors located in the carotid sinuses and aorta. A fall in arterial pressure increases ADH secretion. The water retention thereby produced increases the plasma volume and pressure. A rise in arterial pressure produces the opposite effect. This mechanism is most important in compensating for large changes in arterial blood pressure (e.g., impending or actual shock).

Various other stimuli have been shown to influence ADH secretion. Increased ADH secretion can be prompted by angiotensin II, pain, increased serum osmolality, hypovolemia, nausea, hypoglycemia, stress, acute infections, malignancies, and trauma to the hypothalamic–hypophyseal system. Secretion of ADH is inhibited by decreased serum osmolality, hypervolemia, cold, trauma to the hypothalamic–hypophyseal system, carbon dioxide inhalation, and alcohol ingestion. Many drugs affect ADH secretion (Box 42-2).

OXYTOCIN

Oxytocin is stored as insoluble complexes with specific proteins called *neurophysins.* These neurophysins are specific for the proteins to which they are bound. Oxytocin stimulates contraction of the myoepithelial cells that line the milk ducts of the breast. This causes milk to be squeezed into the sinuses, leading to the nipple surface. Oxytocin secretion is triggered by the hypothalamic receipt of afferent impulses from touch receptors around the nipples and

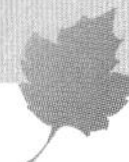

box 42-1

Physiological Changes in the Endocrine System That Occur With Aging

- Production of thyroid hormone, cortisol, and aldosterone decreases with age.
- Levels of somatostatin, triiodothyronine (T_3), thyroxine (T_4), aldosterone, renin, calcitonin, and vasopressin decrease with age, as does glucose tolerance.
- Levels of norepinephrine, parathyroid hormone (PTH), atrial natriuretic peptide (ANP), insulin, and glucagon increase with age.

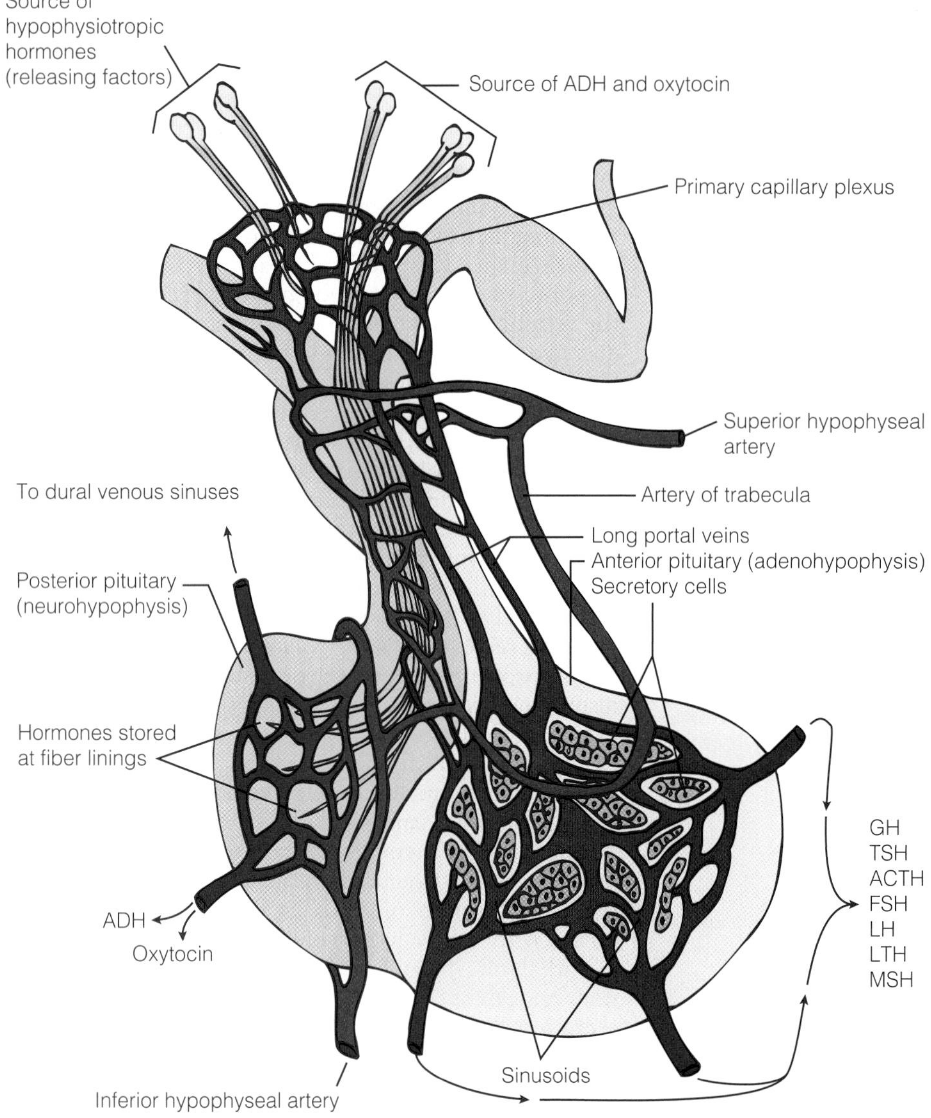

figure 42-3 Highly diagrammatic and schematic representation of hypophyseal nerve fiber tracts and the portal system in the hypothalamus and pituitary gland. Releasing factors (hypophysiotropic hormones) produced by cell bodies in the hypothalamus trickle down axons to the proximal part of the stalk, where they enter the primary capillary plexus and are transported via portal vessels to sinusoids in the anterior lobe of the pituitary gland (i.e., the adenohypophysis) for control of secretions. Antidiuretic hormone (*ADH*) and oxytocin, produced by other cell bodies in the hypothalamus, trickle down axons for storage in the posterior lobe of the pituitary gland (i.e., the neurohypophysis) until they are needed. *ACTH*, adrenocorticotropic hormone; *FSH*, follicle-stimulating hormone; *GH*, growth hormone; *LH*, luteinizing hormone; *LTH*, lactogenic hormone; *MSH*, melanocyte-stimulating hormone; *TSH*, thyroid-stimulating hormone.

box 42-2
Drugs That Influence Antidiuretic Hormone (ADH) Secretion

Drugs That Stimulate ADH Secretion
- Diuretics
- Barbiturates
- Glucocorticoids
- Tricyclic antidepressants
- Carbamazepine
- Chlorpropamide
- Anesthetics
- Acetaminophen

Drugs That Inhibit ADH Secretion
- Alcohol
- Phenytoin
- Narcotics
- Lithium
- Demeclocycline
- Norepinephrine
- Chlorpromazine

also by receipt of afferent optical and aural stimuli. Therefore, suckling by the newborn, manual stimulation of the nipples, or the sight or sound of a crying infant can trigger milk secretion. Oxytocin also causes contraction of the smooth muscles of the uterus. Such contractions play a role in labor and facilitate the transport of sperm from the cervix to the fallopian tubes. During pregnancy, oxytocin secretion is stimulated by cervical dilation and estrogen and inhibited by progesterone and alcohol.

Anterior Pituitary (Adenohypophysis) Hormones

This anterior lobe of the pituitary gland contains five morphologically different types of cells that secrete polypeptide hormones:

- Somatotrophs, which secrete growth hormone (GH, somatotropin)
- Mammotrophs, which secrete prolactin (luteotropic hormone, or LTH)
- Thyrotrophs, which secrete thyroid-stimulating hormone (TSH)

- Corticotrophs, which secrete adrenocorticotropic hormone (ACTH), β-lipotropin (β-LPH), β-endorphin, and melanophore-stimulating hormone (MSH)
- Gonadotrophs, which secrete luteinizing hormone (LH) and follicle-stimulating hormone (FSH)

Each type of cell is separately regulated by hypophysiotropic hormones (Fig. 42-4).

LTH, LH, and FSH act on cells of the gonads (ovaries and testes) to regulate gamete (sperm and egg) and hormone production. Their function is primarily determined by the timing, relative ratios, and pattern of secretion from the anterior pituitary gland. Melanin is a dark pigment contained in special structures called melanophores in the cells of the skin of lower vertebrates (e.g., fish, amphibians, and reptiles). MSH stimulates the dispersion of the melanin granules in these melanophores. This darkens the animal temporarily. The normal function of MSH in humans is not known, although there is some evidence that it can cause a darkening of certain areas of skin in humans with Addison's disease. In this condition, excess corticotropin (ACTH)-releasing hormone stimulates corticotrophs to secrete ACTH. The roles of MSH, LTH, LH, and FSH are not significant in the critical care arena and are not discussed further in this chapter. TSH, which stimulates cells of the thyroid gland to produce and secrete the two thyroid hormones, is discussed later in this chapter, and GH is described in the following section.

GROWTH HORMONE (SOMATOTROPIN)

The production and secretion of GH occurs in the anterior pituitary in response to growth hormone–releasing hormone (GHRH) produced in the hypothalamus. Growth-inhibiting hormone (GIH) inhibits the secretion of GH. GH acts both directly on target cells and indirectly by stimulating the liver and other as-yet-unidentified tissues to secrete various growth factors termed *somatomedins*. These growth factors are structurally similar to insulin. Direct actions of GH include increasing the breakdown of fats (lipolysis) in adipose cells and releasing the fatty acids produced by lipolysis into the bloodstream (this is termed its *ketogenic effect*); increasing hepatic glycolysis and thereby increasing plasma glucose levels; increasing the sensitivity of insulin-producing cells to certain stimuli; increasing the cellular uptake of amino acids; and stimulating erythropoiesis.

The various somatomedins exert growth-promoting activity in different types of tissues. Normally, the result of somatomedin-mediated GH activity consists of an increase in the formation of cartilage in the epiphyseal plates, which fosters the growth in length of long bones; an increase in other skeletal growth; and the growth of all other parts of the body (e.g., soft tissue and viscera). All GH actions operate together to produce growth (e.g., by cell division) and to provide the materials needed for this growth (i.e., amino acids for synthesis of protein cell structure, fatty acids and glucose to provide energy, and erythrocytes to increase the availability of oxygen).

Plasma concentrations of GH are controlled by the release of GRH and GIH from the hypothalamus. Several stimuli influence the secretion of GH. Age is the most important overriding variable, and the actions of many of these other stimuli are influenced by it. Factors that, at the appropriate age, can stimulate the secretion of GH include hypoglycemia, fasting, exercise, a protein meal, glucagon, stress (both physiological and psychological), deeper stages of sleep, and drugs that bind to dopamine receptors. Major stimuli that decrease the output of GH include rapid eye movement (REM) sleep (dreaming), elevated plasma levels of glucose or fatty acids, and cortisol. Fluctuations in the levels of GH are dramatic; the average serum level, however, is remarkably similar at all ages. Growth is facilitated by GH, but other factors, such as somatotropins, direct the rate of growth and the organs targeted for growth.

THE THYROID AND PARATHYROID GLANDS

The thyroid gland is a bilobed, richly vascularized structure. The lobes lie lateral to the trachea just beneath the larynx and are connected by a bridge of thyroid tissue, the isthmus, that runs across the anterior surface of the trachea

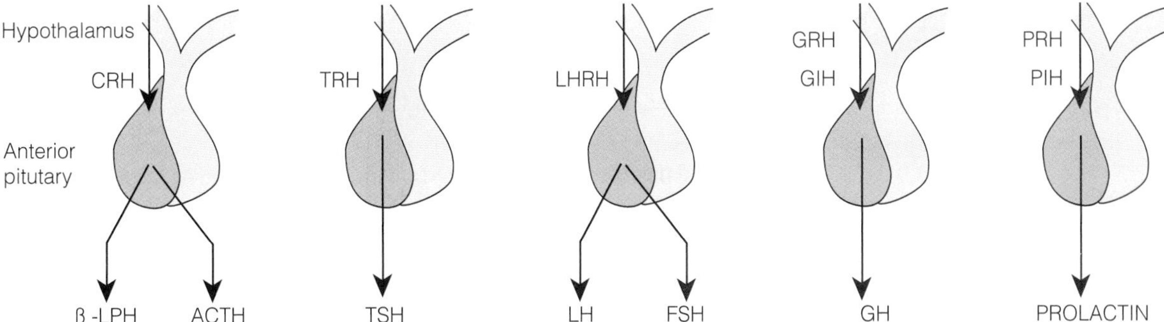

figure 42-4 Effects of the hypophysiotropic hormones on the secretion of anterior pituitary hormones. The hypophysiotropic hormones are corticotropin-releasing hormone (*CRH*), thyrotropin-releasing hormone (*TRH*), luteinizing hormone–releasing hormone (*LHRH*), growth hormone–releasing hormone (*GRH*), growth-inhibiting hormone (*GIH*), prolactin-releasing hormone (*PRH*), and prolactin-inhibiting hormone (*PIH*). CRH prompts the release of β-lipotropin (*β-LPH*) and adrenocorticotropic hormone (*ACTH*). TRH prompts the release of thyroid-stimulating hormone (*TSH*). LHRH prompts the release of luteinizing hormone (*LH*) and follicle-stimulating hormone (*FSH*). GRH and GIH promote and inhibit the secretion of growth hormone (*GH*), respectively. PRH and PIH promote and inhibit the secretion of prolactin, respectively.

(Fig. 42-5). Microscopically, the thyroid is composed primarily of spheroid follicles, each of which stores a colloid material in its center. The follicles produce, store, and secrete the two major thyroid hormones: T_3 and T_4. If the gland is actively secreting, the follicles are small and contain little colloid. Inactive thyroid tissue contains large follicles, each of which possesses a large quantity of stored colloid. Parafollicular cells (C cells), which produce the hormone calcitonin, are scattered between the follicles of the thyroid gland.

Each lobe of the thyroid gland typically contains two parathyroid glands: one in its superior pole and one in its inferior pole. Individual variation exists with respect to the number and distribution of parathyroid glands. Some people have more or fewer than four. Others have parathyroid tissue in the mediastinum. The parathyroid glands produce parathyroid hormone (PTH).

Thyroid Hormones

The follicular cells absorb tyrosine (an amino acid) and iodide from the plasma and secrete them into the central colloid portion of the follicle, where they are used in the synthesis of T_3 and T_4. (The subscript refers to the number of iodide molecules that each substance contains.) Two iodide molecules are attached, first one and then the other, to each tyrosine molecule. Two such doubly iodinated tyrosines are combined to form T_4. T_3, which is much more biologically active than T_4 and is the predominant form of thyroid hormone produced, is formed by the combination of a doubly iodinated tyrosine with a singly iodinated one. Because of the role of iodine in the manufacture of thyroid hormones, storage and release of small amounts of radioactive iodine by the thyroid can be used to measure the activity of this gland. Because the thyroid gland is virtually the only tissue of the body that absorbs and stores iodine, larger amounts of radioactive iodine can be used to destroy portions of the thyroid gland as a treatment for hyperthyroidism.

T_3 and T_4 are stored in the colloid until they are needed. When they are to be secreted, the follicular cells transport them from the colloid to the plasma. Less than 1% of the secreted T_3 and T_4 remains free and physiologically active in the plasma. The remainder is bound to plasma proteins. Most is bound to thyroxine-binding globulin (TBG), a molecule manufactured by the liver, and the remainder is bound to two types of plasma albumin. Such protein-bound hormone serves as a reservoir to replace free T_3 and T_4 that has been degraded, thereby maintaining stable blood levels of thyroid hormones. The plasma proteins involved in transporting T_3 and T_4 are manufactured in the liver. Consequently, liver damage that decreases the plasma levels of these proteins can produce a condition resembling thyroid hormone excess (i.e., hyperthyroidism). Plasma levels of these proteins can also be depressed by glucocorticoids, androgens, and L-asparaginase (an antineoplastic drug). They are elevated during pregnancy, and by estrogens, opiates, clofibrate, and major tranquilizers. Thyroid hormones are deiodinated and catabolized by the liver, kidneys, and various other tissues. A small amount of degraded hormone is added to the bile secreted by the liver and is excreted in the stool.

T_3 directly crosses target cell membranes, whereas T_4 is changed into T_3 by target cell membranes before crossing. T_3 binds with receptors on the cell nucleus. Through this interaction with the nucleus, these hormones can alter the cellular synthesis of various enzymes and thereby modify cellular operations. The actions of thyroid hormones are widespread and apparently arise from their stimulation of the basal metabolic rate (BMR) of most tissues (excluding tissues of the brain, anterior pituitary, spleen, lymph nodes, testes, and lung). The exact manner by which these hor-

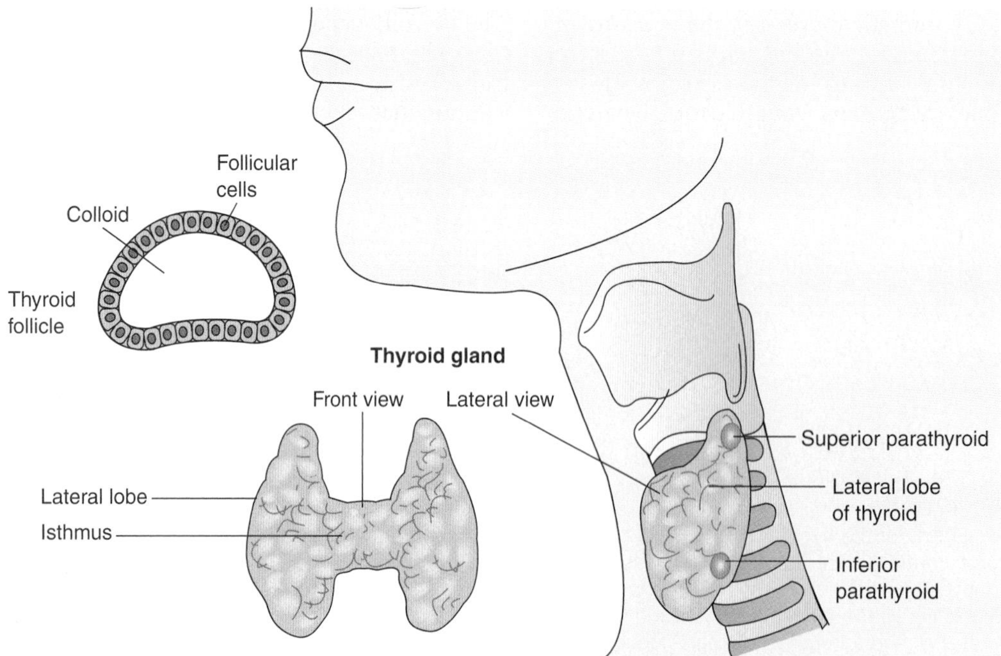

figure 42-5 The thyroid gland. (Source: Porth CM: Pathophysiology: Concepts of Altered Health States [6th Ed], p 909. Philadelphia, Lippincott Williams & Wilkins, 2002.)

mones act on cell metabolism is not clear. T_3 and, to a lesser extent, T_4 increase the activity of the mitochondrial enzyme systems involved in the oxidation of foodstuffs. The energy released by such oxidation is not efficiently stored in the high-energy bonds of adenosine triphosphate (ATP). Much is lost in the form of heat. This increases oxygen consumption of, and heat production by, these tissues (i.e., the BMR). This is termed *calorigenic action.*

Thyroid hormone increases the number of β_1- and β_2-adrenergic receptors in various tissues and the affinity of these receptors for catecholamines. This is why an increased heart rate and sweating often occur in hyperthyroidism. The catabolism of skeletal muscle proteins is increased by thyroid hormones to such a degree that pronounced muscle weakness results from prolonged hyperthyroidism (thyrotoxic myopathy). Thyroid hormones increase the rate of carbohydrate absorption from the small intestine and decrease circulating levels of cholesterol.

Thyroid hormones are essential for the normal growth and development of many body systems, notably the skeletal and nervous systems. These hormones stimulate the secretion of GH and potentiate its effect on various tissues. Thyroid hormones are also necessary for normal levels of neuronal functioning. Thyroid insufficiency leads to slowed reflexes, slowed mentation, and decreased level of consciousness (through decreased levels of reticular activating system activity). Hyperthyroidism lowers synaptic thresholds in the central nervous system (CNS), causing hyperreflexia and a silky skeletal muscle tremor. The effect of thyroid hormones on the nervous system is best illustrated by the cretinism resulting from congenital thyroid insufficiency.

The secretion of T_3 and T_4 by the thyroid gland is primarily regulated by the secretion of TSH from the anterior pituitary. TSH stimulates the manufacture and secretion of T_3 and T_4. A negative feedback regulatory loop exists whereby increased levels of free (unbound) T_3 and T_4 suppress TSH secretion. Decreased plasma TSH results in decreased thyroid function, which causes a fall in free plasma T_3 and T_4. Low T_3 and T_4 levels stimulate TSH secretion. If a TSH-induced increase in thyroid activity does not raise the plasma levels of free T_3 and T_4, the continued high levels of TSH eventually cause an increase in the size of the thyroid gland (nontoxic goiter). In this case, an enlarged thyroid is not associated with overproduction of hormone. This feedback loop maintains homeostasis of the daily secretion of TSH and thyroid hormones. In addition to being influenced by circulatory T_3 and T_4 levels, TSH secretion is regulated by a hypothalamic neurosecretory material termed *thyrotropin-releasing hormone* (TRH).

Calcitonin and Parathyroid Hormone

Calcitonin, which is secreted by the parafollicular cells of the thyroid gland, and PTH, which is produced and secreted by the parathyroid glands, exert a major influence on calcium metabolism in conjunction with 1,25-dihydroxycholecalciferol, which is produced by the action of the liver and the kidneys on vitamin D. Ultraviolet light changes 7-dehydrocholesterol provitamins in the skin to a group of compounds, collectively called vitamin D. One of these, D_3, can also be obtained from vitamin D–enriched and other foods. The liver converts D_3 to 25-hydroxycholecalciferol, which is then altered by kidney cells to a more active form, 1,25-dihydroxycholecalciferol. (The hypocalcemia seen in chronic renal disease results from an activated vitamin D deficiency.) Activated vitamin D acts on intracellular enzymes of the intestinal mucosal cells to increase calcium absorption. To a lesser extent, it also increases the active transport of calcium out of osteoblasts into the bloodstream. Both of these actions elevate plasma calcium levels. In vitamin deficiency states, the effect of decreased intestinal absorption outweighs any decrease in the mobilization of calcium from bone to produce an overall hypocalcia and poor mineralization of bone.

Vitamin D is synthesized in the skin, absorbed in the small intestine, and transported into the plasma bound to vitamin D–binding proteins. The metabolism of vitamin D is strictly regulated by phosphate concentration in the kidney and by PTH. Thus, the effect of a decrease in dietary phosphate or serum phosphate is to increase levels of 1,25-dihydroxycholecalciferol.

PARATHYROID HORMONE

PTH is a polypeptide produced and secreted by the chief cells of the parathyroid glands. This hormone is stored in secretory granules and released in response to a decrease in ionized calcium concentrations. It is cleaved into active form in the kidneys and liver. Plasma calcium and phosphate levels operate in a negative feedback loop to influence the activity of the renal enzyme system, which catalyzes the conversion of metabolically inactive vitamin D to the metabolically active form. High plasma calcium levels decrease this activation process, whereas low levels increase it. The formation of activated vitamin D is also facilitated by PTH and decreased by metabolic acidosis and hypoinsulinemia (diabetes mellitus).

PTH is transported free (unbound) in the plasma, has a half-life of less than 20 minutes, and is metabolically degraded by cells in the liver. A decrease in calcium concentration increases PTH secretion. PTH acts on two target tissues: bone cells and kidney tubules. In bone, it stimulates osteoclast activity and inhibits osteoblast activity. This results in bone reabsorption with consequent mobilization of calcium and phosphate from the bony matrix into the bloodstream. In the kidney, PTH increases the reabsorption of calcium by distal tubule cells and decreases the reabsorption of phosphate by proximal tubule cells. The effect of these multiple actions is elevation of plasma calcium levels and lowering of plasma phosphate levels.

Plasma calcium levels alter PTH secretion through a negative feedback loop. Secretion is inhibited by high plasma calcium levels and stimulated by low blood levels of calcium. The activated vitamin D deficiency–induced hypocalcemia, which occurs in chronic renal failure, typically produces a secondary hyperparathyroidism. Secretion of PTH by the parathyroid gland is also stimulated by hypomagnesemia, adrenergic agonists, and prostaglandins.

CALCITONIN

This polypeptide hormone is produced by the parafollicular cells (C cells) of the thyroid gland. It can also be secreted by nonthyroidal tissue (e.g., tissue of the lung, intestine, pituitary, and bladder). Calcitonin is transported unbound in the plasma. It has a half-life of 5 minutes and is predominantly metabolized in the kidney. Calcitonin lowers plasma calcium and phosphate levels by inhibiting osteoclastic bone reabsorption and increasing urinary phosphate and calcium excretion. Calcitonin levels are elevated during pregnancy and lactation, suggesting that calcitonin may help to protect the mother's skeleton from excess calcium loss during these periods of calcium drain.

Calcitonin does not function in the normal daily homeostasis of plasma calcium levels. It appears to serve more of an emergency function in that it is secreted only if the plasma calcium level exceeds 9.3 mg/dL. At high blood calcium levels, calcitonin secretion is stimulated by increased levels of plasma calcium. Calcitonin is also released by the action of gastrin, glucagon, and secretion of gastrointestinal hormones.

Table 42-2 summarizes the hormones secreted by the thyroid and parathyroid glands.

THE ENDOCRINE PANCREAS

The pancreas has both endocrine and exocrine functions under the control of different groups of cells. The endocrine portion is limited to clusters of glandular tissues, the islets of Langerhans, which secrete the peptide hormones involved in blood glucose regulation. The name *islets of Langerhans* refers to the more than 1 million ovoid islands (clusters) of cells that are scattered throughout the pancreas, predominantly in the tail. Because of this distribution of islet cells, acute attacks of pancreatitis, which usually spare the tail, tend to spare the islets. Episodes of chronic recurrent pancreatitis typically involve all of the pancreas. Consequently, these episodes cause islet cell destruction and diabetes mellitus.

Each cell cluster is richly supplied with capillaries, into which its hormones are secreted. The islets are composed of four types of cells: alpha cells, which secrete glucagon; beta cells, which secrete insulin; delta cells, which secrete somatostatin; and F cells, which secrete pancreatic polypeptide. The hormones secreted by the pancreas are summarized in Table 42-3.

table 42-2 Hormones of the Thyroid and Parathyroid Glands and Their Actions

Gland	Hormone	Action
Thyroid gland	Thyroxine (T_4)	Controls basic metabolic rate
	Triiodothyronine (T_3)	Induces growth and development Inhibits bone resorption
	Calcitonin	Inhibits calcium reabsorption in gastrointestinal tract Increases calcium excretion from kidney
Parathyroid gland	Parathyroid hormone	Promotes bone resorption Increases calcium reabsorption Increases calcium blood levels

Insulin

Insulin, an anabolic hormone, is regulated by a number of stimulatory and inhibitory factors. It is responsible for the control of blood glucose concentrations and storage of carbohydrate, proteins, and fats. Insulin facilitates the use of glucose as the main source of energy for most body tissues. Insulin is the only hormone with the ability to directly lower the blood glucose level. Also, insulin facilitates an increase in the cellular transport of glucose, amino acids, and fatty acids across cell membranes and modulates intracellular metabolic synthesis of nucleic acids.

The precursor of insulin, proinsulin, is manufactured in the beta cells of the islets of Langerhans. Proinsulin can be thought of as a "necklace" of amino acid beads and is stored as secretory granules in another cell structure. Proinsulin can be found in the plasma as a result of certain islet tumors or overstimulation of the beta cells. C-peptide is secreted into the bloodstream along with insulin. Because there is a 1:1 ratio between C-peptide and insulin, plasma C-peptide levels can be used to measure endogenous insulin secretion or degree of beta cell activity.

The actions of insulin are summarized in Box 42-3. In addition to facilitating glucose uptake by muscle and adipose cells, insulin facilitates glucose uptake by connective tissue, leukocytes, mammary glands, the lens of the eye, the aorta, the pituitary gland, and alpha islet cells. In general, insulin enables glucose to be readily available for aerobic oxidation in muscle, adipose, and connective tissue cells. Facilitation of the preferential use of glucose as cellular fuel means that the cells do not need to oxidize fatty or amino acids. Instead, these can be conserved. Protein synthesis and fat storage are increased in liver, muscle, and adipose tissue. Breakdown of fats and proteins is decreased. Hepatic gluconeogenesis also is decreased or halted, and glycogen synthesis is increased.

Insulin acts only on a few types of tissues. However, the membranes of nearly all types of body cells possess insulin receptors. Binding of insulin to the insulin receptors initiates the physiological action of insulin on the cell. After a molecule of insulin binds to a receptor, the insulin–receptor complex is taken into the cytoplasm of the cell by endocytosis and is destroyed within 14 to 15 hours by lysosomal enzymes. New receptors replace the destroyed ones in the cell membranes. Plasma insulin has a half-life of approximately 5 minutes. About 80% of all circulating insulin is catabolized by liver and kidney cells.

Insulin secretion is influenced by a variety of factors as listed in Box 42-4. Monosaccharides are the primary regulatory mechanism for insulin secretion. Elevated plasma levels of glucose act in a negative feedback loop to increase the secretion of insulin. Lower levels of glucose decrease insulin output. Glucagon, β-adrenergic agonists, and theophylline increase insulin secretion. Beta cells are also stimulated to secrete insulin by tolbutamide and other sulfonylurea derivatives; acetylcholine; impulses from vagal nerve branches

table 42-3 The Hormones of the Pancreas and Their Actions

Hormone	Cell	Stimulant	Response
Insulin	Beta	Glucose	Decreased glucose level Increased fat storage Increased protein synthesis Increased glucogenesis
Glucagon	Alpha	Decreased glucose level, exercise	Increased glucose level Increased gluconeogenesis Increased glycogenolysis
Somatostatin	Delta	Hyperglycemia	Increased glucose Increased glycogen
Pancreatic polypeptide	F	Acute hypoglycemia	Increased gallbladder contraction Increased pancreatic enzymes

to the islets; selected amino acids, such as arginine; and β-ketoacids. The mechanisms of action of these stimuli are as yet unclear. Insulin production is inhibited by α-adrenergic agonists, β-adrenergic blocking agents, diazoxide (Proglycem), thiazide diuretics, phenytoin (Dilantin), alloxan, agents that prevent glucose metabolism (2-deoxyglucose or mannoheptulose), somatostatin, and insulin itself.

Chronic stimulation of beta cells, such as by a high-carbohydrate diet for several weeks, can cause a limited amount of hypertrophy and subsequent increase in the insulin-producing capacity. Overstimulation, however, produces beta cell exhaustion. Stimulation of these exhausted cells produces beta cell death and depletes the beta cell reserve. Beta cell activity is also decreased by the administration of exogenous insulin. Such decreased activity enables the cells to rest and results in temporary hyperproduction after the withdrawal of exogenous insulin.

Insulin resistance, characteristic with type 2 diabetes, is the main defect seen with the development of hyperglycemia, hyperinsulinemia, and consequent beta cell exhaustion. The degree of obesity directly affects the resistance to insulin in most patients with type 2 diabetes. One principal mechanism involved may be a defect in insulin receptor function due to a genetic mutation of the insulin receptor gene. The quantity and activity of insulin receptors also can be regulated by various factors. Increased amounts of insulin, obesity, acromegaly, and excess glucocorticoids decrease the receptors' number or activity, or both. Exercise and decreased circulating levels of insulin increase the activity of insulin receptors.

Glucagon

This polypeptide hormone is manufactured and secreted by the alpha cells of the islets of Langerhans and is stimulated by pure protein meal ingestion that produces an aminoacidemia. The half-life of plasma glucagon is 5 to 10 minutes. Glucagon influences enzyme systems in liver, fat, and muscle cells and is degraded mainly by the liver.

The major function of glucagon, which stimulates the synthesis of the gluconeogenic enzyme fructose-

box 42-3
Major Actions of Insulin on Adipose and Muscle Cells

Muscle Cells	*Adipose Cells*
Increased glucose entry	Increased glucose entry
Increased K^+ uptake	Increased K^+ uptake
Increased glycogen synthesis	Increased fatty acid entry and synthesis
Increased amino acid entry	Increased fat deposition
Increased protein synthesis	Increased conversion of glucose to fatty acids
Decreased protein catabolism	Inhibition of lipolysis
Increased ketone entry into cells	

box 42-4
Factors Affecting Insulin Secretion

Stimulators
- Glucose
- Mannose
- Amino acids (leucine, arginine, others)
- Intestinal hormones (gastric inhibitory peptide [GIP], gastrin, secretin, cholecystokinin [CCK], glucagon, others?)
- β-Keto acids
- Acetylcholine
- Glucagon
- Cyclic adenosine monophosphate (AMP) and various cyclic AMP–generating substances
- β-Adrenergic-stimulating agents
- Theophylline
- Sulfonylureas

Inhibitors
- Somatostatin
- 2-Deoxyglucose
- Mannoheptulose
- α-Adrenergic-stimulating agents (norepinephrine, epinephrine)
- β-Adrenergic-blocking agents (propranolol)
- Diazoxide
- Thiazide diuretics
- Phenytoin
- Alloxan
- Microtubule inhibitors
- Insulin

1,6-biphosphate, is to elevate blood glucose levels and then to enable this plasma glucose to enter and be used by the cells of the body (e.g., the muscle cells) by stimulating the secretion of insulin. In this manner, glucagon prevents hypoglycemia between meals, during exercise, during the first few days of fasting, and after a high-protein meal. Dietary protein stimulates an increase in plasma insulin, which causes a rapid cellular uptake of absorbed dietary carbohydrates.

To elevate blood glucose levels, glucagon stimulates liver cells to perform glycogenolysis and gluconeogenesis. This increases the glucose concentration in liver cells, and because these cells can dephosphorylate intracellular glucose, this glucose can be released from the liver into the bloodstream. The fatty acids and amino acids needed for gluconeogenesis are supplied by the glucagon-stimulated breakdown of fats in adipose cells and the release of fatty acids into the bloodstream. If the supply of fatty acids is not sufficient, glucagon also stimulates the breakdown of proteins into amino acids in muscle cells and the release of amino acids into the plasma. These fatty acids and amino acids are then taken up by hepatocytes and used as raw materials in gluconeogenesis. Glucagon also elevates plasma ketone levels by increasing hepatic ketone production, and promotes the secretion of somatostatin and GH.

Although glucagon opposes the effects of insulin on blood sugar levels, it also stimulates the secretion of insulin. This apparent contradiction is actually a logical second step in the biological function of this hormone. It enables the increased plasma glucose to enter and be used by various tissues. An elevated plasma glucose level stimulates insulin secretion, but this takes a while. The direct action of glucagon on beta cells simply is faster.

As is the case with beta cells, alpha cells are stimulated by β-adrenergic agonists, theophylline, elevated plasma levels of dietary amino acids (primarily those used in gluconeogenesis), and vagal (cholinergic) stimulation. Glucagon secretion is also prompted by glucocorticoids (e.g., cortisol), cholecystokinin (CCK), and gastrin. Exercise, physical stress, and infections also increase alpha cell activity. Whereas the effects of exercise on glucagon secretion seem to be mediated by increased β-adrenergic activity, stress and infection probably operate by increasing plasma glucocorticoid levels. Dietary amino acids are believed to enhance glucagon secretion by their effects on CCK or gastrin, or both, because intravenous amino acids exert little or no effect on alpha cells.

Elevated plasma glucose levels enact a negative feedback loop to retard or halt the output of glucagon; however, plasma insulin must be present for this mechanism to operate. Like beta cell secretion, alpha cell secretion is inhibited by adrenergic agonists, phenytoin, and somatostatin. Fatty acids and ketone bodies in the plasma can inhibit glucagon secretion, but this inhibition must be weak because plasma glucagon levels can be quite elevated during diabetic ketoacidosis (DKA).

In addition to glucagon, other hormones—cortisol, epinephrine, and GH—have great influence on the regulation of glucose and insulin. These counter-regulatory hormones have a synergistic effect on glucose production as a mechanism to protect the body during stress. They act to inhibit insulin while increasing glucagon, producing an insulin-resistant state, and increasing overall serum glucose levels to produce sufficient energy levels during "fight-or-flight" responses.

Somatostatin

This tetradecapeptide is produced not only by the delta cells of the pancreas but by the hypothalamus, where it functions as an inhibitor of anterior pituitary GH secretion; neurons of the CNS, where it probably functions as a synaptic neurotransmitter agent; and delta cells in the gastric mucosa, where it inhibits the secretion of gastrin and other, lesser known gastrointestinal hormones. Islet cell somatostatin is secreted into the bloodstream and therefore functions as a hormone. Little is known of the metabolism of somatostatin because it is so tightly bound with the actions of GH.

Somatostatin inhibits the release of insulin and glucagons from the pancreas. Pancreatic somatostatin inhibits the activity of all other islet cells. The biological significance of this action is not yet known. The only clinical data of relevance concern delta cell tumors. These produce a clinical picture that resembles diabetes mellitus but that is reversible with tumor ablation. The secretion of somatostatin from islet cells is increased by glucose, certain amino acids, and CCK. Factors that inhibit islet somatostatin secretion are unknown.

Pancreatic Polypeptide

Not much is known about this islet hormone in humans. It is produced by the endocrine cells found in small clusters of cells located between the cells of the islets of Langerhans and the acinar cells of the pancreas. Its secretion in humans is enhanced by dietary protein, exercise, acute hypoglycemia, and fasting. Somatostatin and elevated plasma glucose levels decrease the secretion of this polypeptide. No definite actions of this hormone have been established for humans, but it appears to have a role in smooth muscle relaxation of the gallbladder.

THE ADRENAL GLANDS

An adrenal gland lies at the superior pole of each kidney. Each gland is composed of an inner core, the medulla, surrounded by an outer layer, the cortex (Fig. 42-6). Although they are structurally related, the medulla and cortex are

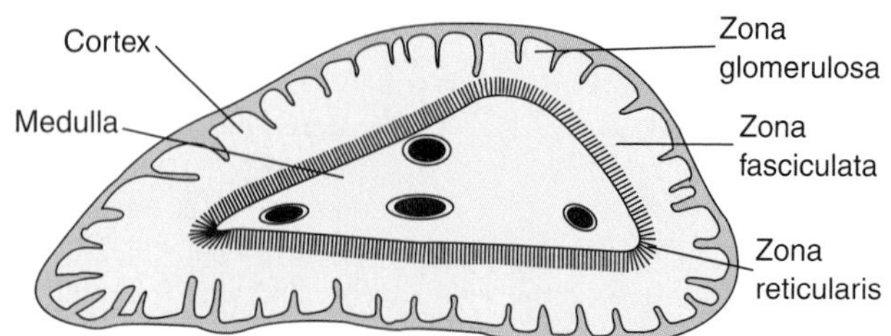

figure 42-6 The adrenal gland has a cortex and a medulla. (Source: Porth CM: Pathophysiology: Concepts of Altered Health States [6th Ed], p 916. Philadelphia, Lippincott Williams & Wilkins, 2002.)

derived from different embryological tissues and function as separate entities. The hormones produced by the adrenal glands are summarized in Table 42-4.

Medullary Hormones

The adrenal medulla is basically a modified sympathetic ganglion. The axons of preganglionic sympathetic neurons arrive from the thoracic cord by way of splanchnic nerves. They synapse in the adrenal medulla with modified postganglionic cells that have lost their axons and secrete chemicals directly into the bloodstream. Therefore, the adrenal medulla may appropriately be viewed as an endocrine extension of the autonomic nervous system.

Four chemicals are produced and secreted in the adrenal medulla by two morphologically different cell types:

- Dopamine, a precursor of norepinephrine
- Norepinephrine, the typical product of postganglionic sympathetic neurons
- Epinephrine, a methylated version of norepinephrine
- Opioid peptides (enkephalins)

Not much is known about the opioid peptides. The specific stimulus for their secretion has yet to be identified, and their physiological actions are unknown, as is their metabolism and fate. Dopamine, norepinephrine, and epinephrine are collectively termed *catecholamines.* They are stored in granules in the medullary cells. The secretion of these chemicals is triggered by stimulation of the preganglionic neurons that innervate the medulla. This causes the neurons to release acetylcholine, which in turn prompts the medullary cells to secrete. The half-life of plasma catecholamines is approximately 2 minutes. These compounds are rapidly degraded by plasma renal and hepatic catechol-*O*-methyltransferase enzymes into vanillylmandelic acid, metanephrine, and normetanephrine, which are excreted in the urine. Only small quantities of nondegraded catecholamines are found in normal urine.

Predictably, the epinephrine and norepinephrine secreted by the adrenal medulla mimic the effects of a mass discharge from sympathetic neurons. Apart from this, however, they produce several metabolic actions. First, they elevate blood sugar levels by activating an enzyme, phosphorylase, which promotes hepatic glycogenolysis. Because liver cells possess the enzyme glucose-6-phosphatase, the glucose produced by this glycogen breakdown is able to diffuse out of hepatocytes and into the bloodstream. These hormones also induce muscle cells to participate in elevating blood sugar levels, although this process is less direct. Phosphorylase in muscle cells also is activated by these catecholamines. However, the intracellular glucose thereby produced is unable to exit the muscle cells because they do not possess glucose-6-phosphatase. Instead, this glucose is catabolized to lactate, which can leave the muscle cells. Lactate then circulates to the liver, where it is converted to glucose that can enter the bloodstream. These hormones can also elevate plasma glucose levels by stimulating the secretion of glucagon and increase the uptake of glucose into body tissues by stimulating the secretion of insulin. Epinephrine and norepinephrine can also produce the opposite effects by stimulating α-adrenergic receptors on islet cells. Because of differential effects of both hormones on α- and β-adrenergic receptors, the result is that epinephrine elevates plasma glucose levels much more than does norepinephrine.

A second metabolic effect of catecholamines is promotion of lipolysis in adipose tissue. This elevates plasma free fatty acid levels and provides an alternative energy source for many body cells. Circulating catecholamines also increase alertness by stimulating the reticular activating system. Last, these hormones produce an increase in the metabolic rate of the body and a cutaneous vasoconstriction, both of which result in an elevation in body temperature. However, the accelerated metabolism requires the presence of the thyroid and adrenal cortex hormones.

Although the physiological action of adrenal medullary dopamine is unknown, exogenous dopamine is useful in combating certain shocks because it has a positive inotropic effect on the heart (by way of β receptors) and produces renal vasodilation and peripheral vasoconstriction. The overall effect of moderate dosages is elevation of systolic blood pressure (without an appreciable increase in diastolic blood pressure) together with retention or restoration of renal output.

Stimulation of the adrenal medulla glands is part of a general sympathetic–adrenal medulla (SAM) response to exercise and to perceived threats to biopsychological integrity and survival. (Cannon termed the latter the "fight-or-flight" response.) Hypoglycemia also stimulates increased adrenal medullary secretion. The results of the SAM response enable the body to perform vigorous physical exertion optimally. The heart rate and blood pressure are increased (increasing perfusion), and blood flow is shunted away from the skin and gastrointestinal tract to more vital organs for exertion, such as skeletal muscles, brain, and heart. The reticular activating system is stimulated, fostering alertness. Blood glucose and fatty acid levels are raised, thereby increasing the available energy sources for cells. Pupils are dilated, increasing the field of peripheral vision and the amount of light entering the eyes. Sweat glands are stimulated, cooling the body in advance of and during the time that the body temperature is elevated as the result of the physical exertion. Most of this SAM response is mediated by sympathetic nerve fibers to various body structures; circulating catecholamines play only a

table 42-4 Hormones of the Adrenal Gland and Their Actions

Gland	Hormone	Action
Adrenal gland cortex	Mineralocorticoids	Reabsorption of sodium Elimination of potassium
	Glucocorticoids	Responds to stress Decreases inflammation Alters metabolism of protein and fat
Medulla	Epinephrine	Stimulates sympathetic system
	Norepinephrine	Increases peripheral resistance

minor role. Furthermore, many tissue responses (e.g., those of muscle cells) to such sympathetic demands require the presence of glucocorticoids to enable the tissues to meet the demands of the SAM response, and the SAM response often accompanies the stress-induced secretion of adrenal steroids discovered by Seyle. (This and the endocrine response to physical and psychological stress are discussed in the section on cortical hormones.)

The SAM response is initiated by the perception of a stimulus or situation that a person evaluates on the basis of experience and current resources to be a threat to his or her well-being. This response involves the cerebral cortex. Impulses from the cortex travel by way of nerve fibers to the limbic system, where they are involved in generating an emotional response. Additional impulses from the cortex and the limbic system stimulate sympathetic centers in the diencephalon. These centers in turn discharge a specific pattern of impulses down descending fibers to various sympathetic neurons in the cord, bringing about the SAM response.

Cortical Hormones

The adrenal cortex is composed of three histologically different layers (see Fig. 42-6). Its exterior is covered by a capsule. The outermost layer, the zona glomerulosa, lies just beneath the capsule. It produces and secretes primarily mineralocorticoids, such as aldosterone. The inner two layers, the zona fasciculata and zona reticularis, manufacture and secrete glucocorticoids (cortisol and corticosterone) and adrenal androgens and estrogens. If these inner cortical layers are destroyed, they can be regenerated from zona glomerulosa cells.

Figure 42-7 depicts the metabolic pathways for synthesis of all adrenocortical hormones. Each of these metabolic steps is governed by a specific enzyme. Genetic deficiencies in one or more of these enzymes produce syndromes involving the underproduction or overproduction of various cortical hormones. Drugs that inhibit specific enzymes are used clinically to assess cortical function. One such drug is metyrapone, which inhibits cortisol synthesis.

After secretion, plasma cortisol and, to a lesser extent, corticosterone are bound to a plasma globulin called corticosteroid-binding globulin (CBG), or transcortin. Only the unbound hormones are physiologically active. The bound glucocorticoids serve as a hormone reservoir that is used to replace degraded unbound hormone. The half-lives of plasma corticosterone and cortisol are roughly 50 and 80 minutes, respectively. CBG is manufactured by liver cells. Therefore, decreased hepatic function (e.g., cirrhosis) can lead to subnormal quantities of plasma CBG, resulting in excess quantities of circulating unbound, active glucocorticoids. Only a small amount of aldosterone is bound to plasma proteins. Its half-life is approximately 20 minutes.

Adrenal steroids are degraded by the liver. Depressed hepatic function can retard the degradation of adrenal steroids, thereby producing a clinical picture of hormone excess. The soluble degraded steroid metabolites are excreted by the kidneys.

GLUCOCORTICOIDS

As the name *glucocorticoid* suggests, cortisol and corticosterone influence glucose metabolism. They elevate plasma glucose levels by promoting hepatic gluconeogenesis and glycogenolysis. To facilitate gluconeogenesis, these hormones cause the breakdown of fat and proteins and the release of fatty and amino acids into the bloodstream, which carries them to the liver. Glucocorticoids enable tissues to respond to glucagon and catecholamines; they also prevent rapid fatigue of skeletal muscle. Cortisol and corticosterone also act on the kidneys to permit the excretion of a normal water load in one of three ways: Glucocorticoids make distal or collecting tubules more permeable to the reabsorption of water independently of sodium reabsorption; they increase the glomerular filtration rate (GFR); or they reduce the output of ADH.

The effects of glucocorticoids on plasma components are mixed. They decrease the number of plasma eosinophils and basophils but increase the number of circulating neutrophils, platelets, and erythrocytes. By suppressing production and increasing destruction, glucocorticoids decrease the number of lymphocytes. They also decrease the size of

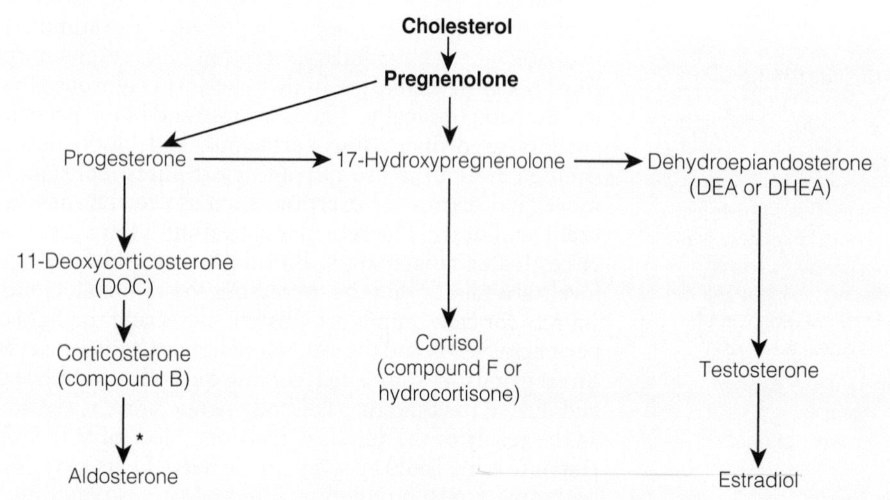

figure 42-7 Biosynthetic pathways for adrenal cortical hormones. Only cells of the zona glomerulosa can convert corticosterone to aldosterone (*). All of the other pathways can be carried out by cells in all three layers of the adrenal cortex.

lymph nodes. A major function of lymphocytes is to provide either humoral immunity (with antibodies) or cell-mediated immunity. Stress-induced elevations in glucocorticoid secretion and the resulting decrease in lymphocytes may explain the decrease in immunocompetence that often occurs in people who are under psychological or physical stress.

Other effects of physiological levels of glucocorticoids include decreasing olfactory and gustatory sensitivity. People with adrenal insufficiency can detect various chemicals (e.g., sugar, salt, urea, and potassium chloride) by either taste or smell with a sensitivity that is 40 to 120 times greater than normal.

The effects of pharmacological dosages of glucocorticoids are considered separately from those of normal physiological levels. In pharmacological dosages, glucocorticoids possess immunosuppressive anti-inflammatory and antihistaminic activity. Glucocorticoids suppress the immune system by inhibiting the production of interleukin-2 by T4 (helper) lymphocytes. Decreases in interleukin-2 reduce the proliferation of T8 (suppressor, cytotoxic) T cells and B lymphocytes. Glucocorticoids act in several ways to suppress the inflammatory response, including the influx of phagocytes and the activation of complement and kinins.

Conversely, glucocorticoids can be of great benefit in the treatment of certain noninfective inflammatory conditions (e.g., rheumatoid arthritis and systemic lupus erythematosus [SLE]). Glucocorticoids can also be beneficial in the treatment of certain allergies (e.g., asthma, hives, and minimal-change glomerular disease) because they prevent the release of histamines from mast cells. Their use as immunosuppressives enables patients to receive organ transplants. In any case, the potentially deleterious side effects of glucocorticoids usually require that they be used only after other treatments (e.g., nonsteroidal anti-inflammatory drugs [NSAIDs] or antihistamines) have failed or if the benefits clearly outweigh the risks (e.g., in renal disease or with organ transplants). In addition to immunosuppression, glucocorticoids trigger the development of all or part of Cushing's syndrome (e.g., diabetes, hypertension, protein wasting, and osteoporosis) and inhibit growth in infants and children. The pharmacological and physiological actions of glucocorticoids are summarized in Table 42-5.

Regulation of glucocorticoid secretion is outlined in Figure 42-8. The secretion of glucocorticoids is triggered by the release of corticotropin-releasing hormone (CRH), a neurosecretory material released by the hypothalamus. CRH stimulates the cells of the anterior pituitary to secrete ACTH. Without the stimulus of ACTH, the cells of the zona fasciculata and zona reticularis do not secrete glucocorticoids. Elevated plasma glucocorticoid levels function in a negative feedback loop to decrease or halt the secretion of CRH and thereby indirectly inhibit the secretion of ACTH as well.

There is a diurnal rhythm to the secretion of CRH that causes a similar rhythm in the output of ACTH and glucocorticoids. The result is that maximal glucocorticoid secretion occurs between 6:00 AM and 8:00 AM in people

table 42-5 Actions of Glucocorticoids

Major Influence	Effect on Body
Glucose metabolism	Stimulates gluconeogenesis Decreases glucose use by the tissues
Protein metabolism	Increases breakdown of proteins Increases plasma protein levels
Fat metabolism	Increases mobilization of fatty acids Increases use of fatty acids
Anti-inflammatory action (pharmacological levels)	Stabilizes lysosomal membranes of the inflammatory cells, preventing the release of inflammatory mediators Decreases capillary permeability to prevent inflammatory edema Depresses phagocytosis by white blood cells to reduce the release of inflammatory mediators Suppresses the immune response Causes atrophy of lymphoid tissue Decreases eosinophils Decreases antibody formation Decreases the development of cell-mediated immunity Reduces fever Inhibits fibroblast activity
Psychic effect	May contribute to emotional instability
Permissive effect	Facilitates the response of the tissues to humoral and neural influences, such as that of the catecholamines, during trauma and extreme stress

Source: Porth CM: Pathophysiology: Concepts of Altered Health States (6th Ed), p 919. Philadelphia, Lippincott Williams & Wilkins, 2002.

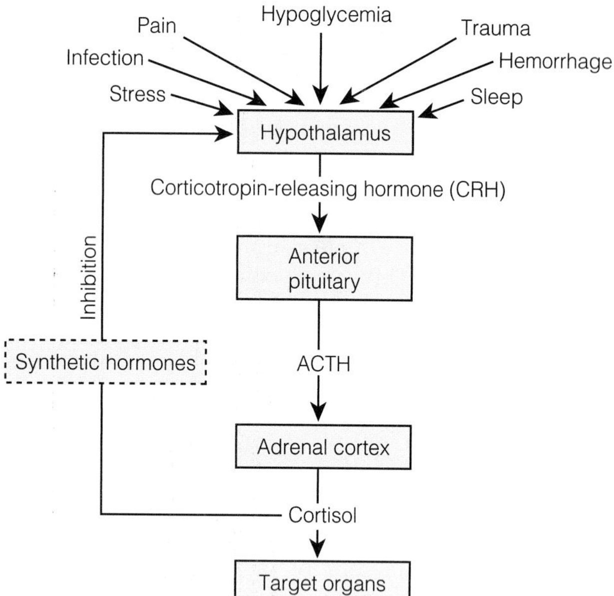

figure 42-8 The hypothalamic–pituitary–adrenal (HPA) feedback system that regulates glucocorticoid (cortisol) levels. Cortisol release is regulated by adrenocorticotropic hormone (*ACTH*). Stress exerts its effects on cortisol release through the HPA system and corticotropin-releasing hormone (*CRH*), which controls the release of ACTH from the anterior pituitary gland. Increased cortisol levels incite negative feedback inhibition of ACTH release. Pharmacological doses of synthetic steroids inhibit ACTH release by way of the hypothalamic CRH.

sleeping from midnight to 8:00 AM in a 24-hour day. Tumors that secrete CRH, ACTH, or glucocorticoids do not demonstrate such a rhythm, a fact that is useful in their diagnosis. The biological clock that regulates this and other diurnal, or circadian, rhythms is located in the hypothalamus, just above the area where the optic nerves cross (optic chiasma).

The beneficial functions of normal levels of glucocorticoids in enabling tissues to respond to glucagon and catecholamines are more than adequate to meet the needs of the SAM mechanism for a short time. If these needs continue, additional stress-induced glucocorticoid secretion is required. Eventually, if the stress continues unameliorated, exhaustion of the adrenal cortex occurs, glucocorticoid levels drop, tissues are no longer able to meet the demands of the SAM mechanism, muscle fatigue occurs, readily available cell energy sources (e.g., plasma glucose and fatty acid) are depleted, and vascular collapse and death result.

MINERALOCORTICOIDS

Aldosterone and glucocorticoids that have some mineralocorticoid function (e.g., 11-deoxycorticosterone) increase sodium reabsorption by the cells of the collecting ducts and distal tubules of the nephrons. Because of the cation exchange system in the distal tubule cells, such sodium reabsorption can increase potassium secretion and thereby foster potential hypokalemia. The reabsorption of sodium osmotically causes water reabsorption. This expands the volume of ECF. The increase in blood volume causes an elevation in blood pressure. Edema does not usually result, however. Above a certain level of aldosterone-induced sodium reabsorption, the expansion of the ECF compartment can trigger secretion of natriuretic hormone or decreased sodium reabsorption in the proximal tubule. Either of these effects opposes the action of aldosterone and sodium excretion.

The primary mechanism for regulating aldosterone secretion is the renin–angiotensin system (Fig. 42-9). Pituitary ACTH does not stimulate zona glomerulosa cells under normal conditions. Cells of the juxtaglomerular apparatus are wedged between the renal afferent arteriole as it enters the glomerulus and the distal tubule as it passes by this area. The juxtaglomerular apparatus contains baroreceptor cells that monitor the afferent arteriole blood pressure and other cells that monitor the sodium and chloride concentration in the urine in the distal tubule (the lower the concentration, the slower the formation of filtrate, if all other factors are equal). A decrease either in blood pressure or in the concentration of electrolytes stimulates the juxtaglomerular apparatus to secrete the glycoprotein hormone renin. The major classes of stimuli that trigger renin secretion are decreased renal perfusion (e.g., cardiac failure, dehydration, and hemorrhage) and low ECF salt concentrations (e.g., from excessive use of diuretics).

Renin converts a circulating plasma globulin into angiotensin I. As the blood passes through the lungs (and to a lesser extent in other parts of the circulatory system), angiotensin I is converted to angiotensin II. This physiologically active chemical acts on the zona glomerulosa to promote aldosterone secretion, which leads to retention of salt and water, and contraction of vascular smooth muscle, thereby stimulating profound vasoconstriction. The result of both actions of angiotensin II is elevation of systemic blood pressure, which, among other things, improves renal perfusion.

The juxtaglomerular apparatus contains β_2 receptors and can be stimulated by sympathetic fibers. Prostaglandins also stimulate the juxtaglomerular apparatus. All three stimulate the secretion of renin. Therefore, the secretion of renin can be pharmacologically decreased by β_2-blockers (e.g., propranolol or atenolol). Prostaglandin inhibitors (aspirin and NSAIDs) can exert a similar action. Angiotensin-converting enzyme (ACE) inhibitors (e.g., lisinopril) prevent the conversion of angiotensin I to angiotensin II. These effects have made ACE inhibitors and β_2-blockers useful as antihypertensive agents.

Aldosterone secretion is also stimulated by an increase in plasma potassium levels, but not by increased sodium levels. Another regulating factor for aldosterone secretion is posture. An upright body position increases aldosterone levels by increasing production and decreasing degradation. How this works is unclear, but because of this, aldosterone levels of bedridden patients are slightly subnormal. There also is a poorly understood diurnal rhythm of aldosterone secretion, with highest levels occurring in the early morning hours just before the person's awakening.

ATRIAL NATRIURETIC PEPTIDE (NATRIURETIC HORMONE)

Atrial natriuretic peptide (ANP) is manufactured by cells in the walls of the atria of the heart. The main stimulus for ANP secretion is atrial stretch. ANP increases renal excre-

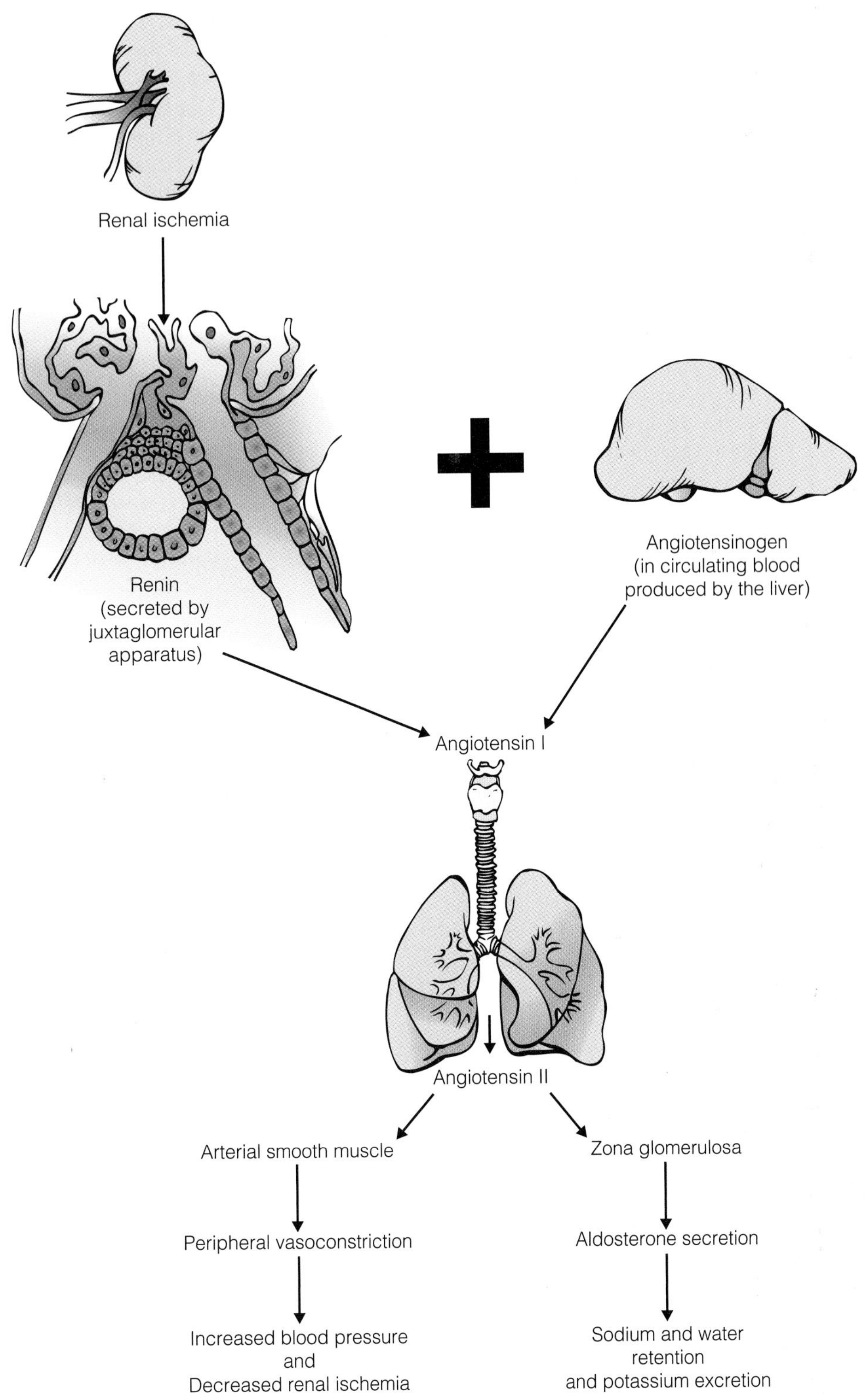

figure 42-9 The renin–angiotensin system induces aldosterone secretion and vasoconstriction, which in turn elevates the systemic blood pressure.

tion of salt and water. Some evidence suggests that ANP acts by increasing glomerular filtration. Other evidence indicates that ANP inhibits the membrane active transport mechanism responsible for the reabsorption of sodium by renal tubule cells. Decreased sodium reabsorption decreases the movement of water from the urine in the nephron back into the blood of the peritubular capillaries, thereby increasing the elimination of water and salt from the body. ANP also inhibits the secretion of renin by the juxtaglomerular apparatus, thereby lowering plasma angiotensin levels. In addition, ANP inhibits the membrane active transport mechanism responsible for pumping sodium out of vascular smooth muscle cells. The consequent rise in intracellular sodium inhibits the entry of calcium ions, thereby lowering the intracellular concentration of calcium ions. The decrease in the intracellular free calcium promotes vasodilation and a lowering of the systemic blood pressure.

ANP is secreted in response to an increase in ECF volume caused by the ingestion of salt and water. The exact stimulus appears to be a stretch of the muscle fibers in the atrial walls, which results from the increased venous return that is caused by the rise in ECF volume. As the natriuresis causes the ECF volume to fall back to normal, the secretion of ANP stops. The capability of ANP to increase the GFR, together with its direct effects on the collecting tubules, results in a profound natriuresis and diuresis.

The metabolic fate of ANP is unknown, but circulating levels of this hormone are elevated in patients with congestive heart failure, cirrhosis, or renal insufficiency and are low in those with nephrotic syndrome or volume depletion. These results suggest liver and kidney regulation.

clinical applicability challenges

Self-Challenge: Critical Thinking

1. *Explore physiological implications when there is faulty regulation of antidiuretic hormone (ADH) by the posterior pituitary.*
2. *Compare and contrast the feedback mechanisms that affect the synthesis and production of thyroxine (T_4) by the thyroid and cortisol by the adrenal cortex.*
3. *Compare and contrast the mechanisms by which glucagon and insulin regulate the body's glucose level.*

Study Questions

1. *Actions of glucocorticoids include*
   a. *glucose elevation by gluconeogenesis.*
   b. *suppression of the anti-inflammatory response.*
   c. *stimulation of histamine triggers.*
   d. *stimulation of water excretion in the kidney.*
2. *Blood glucose regulation is affected by which of the following hormones?*
   a. *Aldosterone*
   b. *Calcitonin*
   c. *Glucagon*
   d. *Antidiuretic hormone (ADH)*
3. *The renin–angiotensin–aldosterone system is stimulated under which condition?*
   a. *Hemorrhage*
   b. *Hypervolemia*
   c. *Hypertension*
   d. *Hyperventilation*
4. *Antidiuretic hormone (ADH) is secreted under which of the following stimuli?*
   a. *Low serum osmolality*
   b. *High urinary output*
   c. *Hypoxia*
   d. *Ethanol alcohol*
5. *Lower levels of T_3 and T_4 would be associated with which of the following?*
   a. *Hyperthyroidism*
   b. *Hyperadrenalism*
   c. *Hypothyroidism*
   d. *Hypoadrenalism*

OTHER SELECTED READING

Becker KL (ed): Principles and Practice of Endocrinology and Metabolism (3rd Ed). Philadelphia, Lippincott Williams & Wilkins, 2001

Brook CG, Marshall NJ: Essential Endocrinology (4th Ed). London, Blackwell Science, 2001

Constanti A, Bartke A, Khardori R: Basic Endocrinology for Students of Pharmacy and Allied Health Sciences. Australia, Harwood Academic Publishers, 1998

Greenspan FS, Gardner DG: Basic and Clinical Endocrinology (6th Ed). New York, Lange Medical Books/McGraw-Hill, 2001

Guyton AC, Hall JE: Textbook of Medical Physiology (10th Ed). Philadelphia, WB Saunders, 2000

Korenman SG: Atlas of Clinical Endocrinology. Volume IV: Neuroendocrinology and Pituitary Disease. Philadelphia, Blackwell Science, 2000

McCance KL, Huether SE: Pathophysiology: The Biologic Basis for Disease in Adults and Children (4th Ed). St. Louis, Mosby-Year Book, 2002

Porterfield SP: Endocrine Physiology. St. Louis, Mosby, 1997

Porth CM: Pathophysiology: Concepts of Altered Health States (6th Ed). Philadelphia, Lippincott Williams & Wilkins, 2002

Smeltzer SC, Bare BG. Brunner & Suddarth's Textbook of Medical-Surgical Nursing (10th Ed). Philadelphia, Lippincott Williams & Wilkins, 2004

chapter

43

Patient Assessment: Endocrine System

JANE KAPUSTIN

objectives

Based on the content in this chapter, the reader should be able to:

- Analyze the relationship between the physiological functions of the endocrine gland and the signs and symptoms that indicate endocrine dysfunction.
- Formulate a plan for collecting history and physical examination data when the patient may have an acute endocrine disorder.
- Differentiate between normal and abnormal findings for specific endocrine disorders.
- Explore laboratory tests used to diagnose acute endocrine disorders.

Endocrine disorders can affect all body systems and are usually caused by the overproduction or underproduction of *hormones*. This chapter presents an overview of the history, physical examination, and diagnostic studies that help diagnose the following specific endocrine disorders: thyroid crisis; myxedema coma; adrenal crisis; syndrome of inappropriate antidiuretic hormone excretion (SIADH); diabetes insipidus; diabetic ketoacidosis (DKA); hyperglycemic, hyperosmolar, and nonketotic coma (HHNC); and hypoglycemia. It builds on the content presented in Chapter 42, which explored the far-reaching effects of the endocrine system on body functions. This chapter also paves the way for specific applications described in Chapter 44, Common Endocrine Disorders.

Because the endocrine system affects so many general areas of the body, assessment must include a variety of signs and symptoms. General manifestations of disorders are evident through vital signs, energy level, fluid and electrolyte imbalances, and ability to carry out activities of daily living. Other parameters to be observed include heat or cold intolerance, changes in weight, fat redistribution, changes in sexual functioning, and altered sleep patterns. More specific manifestations are covered in more detail under each disorder. Box 43-1 summarizes the approach used to assess a patient suspected of having an acute endocrine disorder.

Because the endocrine system exerts control over the entire body, many laboratory tests that have been discussed in other chapters are applicable to the assessment of an acute endocrine disorder. For example, fluid and electrolyte problems accompany many acute endocrine disorders. Therefore, serum sodium, potassium, magnesium, and osmolality are assessed. Blood urea nitrogen (BUN) and creatinine levels may also help assess renal involvement (see

box 43-1
Assessment of Acute Endocrine Disorders

Factors Evaluated During the History and Physical Examination

- Presenting signs and symptoms
- Precipitating events
- Medical conditions
- Medications
- Nutrition
- Hydration
- Activity level
- Mental status

Sample Assessment Questions Related to Endocrine Disorders

- Has anyone in your family had high blood pressure, elevated fats, thyroid problems, or diabetes?
- What medications do you take? Do you take any others, such as over-the-counter pills like aspirin? Have you been able to take your medications every day?
- Have you had an infection, injury, or radiation treatment lately?
- Has your appetite increased or decreased lately?
- Have you lost or gained weight recently?
- Do you have constipation or frequent bowel movements?
- Have you been more thirsty than usual?
- How much urine have you been passing compared with your usual amount?
- Have you been as active as usual?
- Have you been more tired or weak?
- How have you been sleeping?
- Do you feel hot (or cold) before anyone else feels it?
- Have you felt nervous, irritable, or jumpy?
- Have you felt slowed down, lethargic, or sad?

Chapter 29). Arterial blood gases (ABGs), bicarbonate levels, and anion gap calculation may be necessary to diagnose acidosis. Laboratory studies specific to endocrine gland dysfunction are described in the following sections and summarized in Table 43-1.

Similarly, in the evaluation of endocrine disorders, it is often necessary to evaluate body systems other than the endocrine system using diagnostic studies. For example, electrocardiography and cardiac monitoring may be needed to diagnose cardiac problems, whereas a chest x-ray may be necessary to detect pulmonary problems, such as the pleural effusion that can occur in myxedema coma. Computed tomography (CT), magnetic resonance imaging (MRI), and ultrasound may be used to localize tumors.

THE HYPOTHALAMUS AND PITUITARY GLAND

Some of the hormones of the hypothalamus and the pituitary have a profound impact on the critically ill patient and are described in detail in this section (antidiuretic hormone [ADH], adrenocorticotropic hormone [ACTH], thyroid-stimulating hormone [TSH]). Those hormones that are mainly responsible for normal physiological functioning of the reproductive system are not significant in the care of the critically ill adult and therefore are not covered in this section (oxytocin, follicle-stimulating hormone [FSH], luteinizing hormone [LH], growth hormone [GH], melanophore-stimulating hormone [MSH]).

The pituitary gland hormones are under the control of the hypothalamus. The posterior lobe of the pituitary stores and secretes ADH (vasopressin) in response to serum osmolality. Because the primary function of ADH is to control water excretion by the kidney, attention must be focused on the patient's hydration status and serum and urine osmolality to acquire information about the general functioning of this part of the pituitary.

History and Physical Examination

The nurse obtains important information about the nature of endocrine disorders by conducting a thorough history. Because disorders of the pituitary that could result in critical care admission affect fluid and electrolyte balance, the nurse inquires about general hydration status. Parameters to be included are weight gain or loss, excessive urination, thirst, edema, and cognitive changes such as slowed mentation, fatigue, or memory impairment. A history of a head injury or neurological insult (e.g., stroke, aneurysm rupture, or concussion) is obtained because problems like these can lead to ADH secretion dysfunction.

Physical examination of the patient includes assessment of hydration status. Skin turgor, buccal membrane moisture, vital signs, and weight are assessed. A patient with hypovolemia (as seen in diabetes insipidus) would experience weight loss from excretion of large volumes of dilute urine. Eventually, the patient would experience tachycardia, hypotension, poor skin turgor, dry buccal membranes, and cognitive changes associated with dehydration and hypernatremia. Conversely, a patient with hypervolemia (as seen in SIADH) would display signs of water intoxication, such as edema, scant urinary output, weight gain, hypertension, moist buccal membranes, good skin turgor, and cognitive changes associated with hyponatremia.

For patients experiencing fluid balance alterations, the nurse needs to maintain strict measuring of intake and output. Urine specific gravity is measured routinely, noting the nature of the urine (color, concentration, and volume). In addition, critically ill patients with fluid imbalance often have advanced monitoring techniques in place such as central venous pressure (CVP) or hemodynamic monitoring with a Swan-Ganz line. Vigilant monitoring of the patient's fluid status needs to be maintained.

Laboratory Studies

SERUM ANTIDIURETIC HORMONE

The normal serum ADH level is 1 to 13.3 pg/mL. This radioimmunoassay level distinguishes between central diabetes insipidus and SIADH. Elevated serum ADH compared with low serum osmolality and elevated urine osmolality confirms the diagnosis of SIADH. Conversely, reduced levels of ADH with a correspondingly high serum

table 43-1 Sampling of Laboratory Studies Used to Assess Acute Endocrine Disorders

Test	Normal Adult Values	Abnormal Values
Total T_4	4–12 μg/dL	High in hyperthyroidism Low in hypothyroidism
Free T_4	0.8–2.7 ng/mL	High in hyperthyroidism Low in hypothyroidism
Free T_4 index	4.6–12 ng/mL	High in hyperthyroidism Low in hypothyroidism
Free T_3	260–480 pg/dL	Low in hypothyroidism
Thyroid-stimulating hormone (TSH)	260–480 pg/dL	High in hypothyroidism (primary) Low in hypofunction of anterior pituitary (secondary hypothyroidism)
Cortisol	8 AM 5–23 μg/dL 4 PM 3–16 μg/dL	High in Cushing's disease (increased ACTH secretion by pituitary) High in stress, trauma, and surgery Low in hyposecretion of ACTH by pituitary and adrenal insufficiency
Cortisol stimulation	Should increase to 18 μg/dL	Low or absent in adrenal insufficiency and hypopituitarism
Urine vanillylmandelic acid and catecholamines	VMA up to 2–7 mg/24 h Catecholamines: 270 μg/24 h	High in pheochromocytoma High in hypothyroidism and diabetic acidosis
Urine specific gravity	1.010–1.025 with normal hydration and volume	Low in diabetes insipidus High in diabetes mellitus with dehydration
Urine ketones	Negative	Positive in diabetic ketoacidosis

T_3, triiodothyronine; T_4, thyroxine.

osmolality, hypernatremia, and reduced urine concentration indicate central diabetes insipidus. Table 43-2 compares and contrasts laboratory values for diabetes insipidus and SIADH.

URINE SPECIFIC GRAVITY

Specific gravity reflects the kidneys' ability to dilute and concentrate urine. The range depends on hydration, urine volume, and the amount of solids in the urine. The specific gravity can be measured by using a multiple-test dipstick that has a reagent for specific gravity, or by using a refractometer or urinometer. Low specific gravity (1.001 to 1.010) is seen in diabetes insipidus and is accompanied by copious, dilute urine. Increased specific gravity (1.025 to 1.030) is seen in diabetes mellitus with dehydration; the urine in general is more concentrated with smaller volumes.

table 43-2 Comparison of Laboratory Values in Diabetes Insipidus and Syndrome of Inappropriate Antidiuretic Hormone (SIADH)

Laboratory Test	Diabetes Insipidus	SIADH
Antidiuretic hormone (ADH)	Decreased	Increased
Serum osmolality	Increased	Decreased
Sodium	Increased	Decreased
Urinary output	Increased	Decreased
Urine specific gravity	Decreased	Increased
Urine osmolality	Decreased	Increased

SERUM OSMOLALITY

Serum osmolality ranges from 270 to 300 mOsm/kg and measures the concentration of diluted particles in the bloodstream. Elevated serum osmolality (hemoconcentration) stimulates the release of ADH, which enhances the reabsorption of fluid and sodium at the nephron level. Through this process, extracellular fluid (ECF) volume is restored and the plasma becomes less concentrated (serum hemoconcentration).

Conversely, hemodilution or decreased serum osmolality inhibits ADH, causing excess fluid to be eliminated by the kidneys to maintain homeostasis. Concentration of the plasma is restored.

URINE OSMOLALITY

This test is a more exact measure of urine concentration. It is also a more useful test when done in conjunction with serum osmolality. It can be used to diagnose kidney function, diabetes insipidus, and psychogenic water drinking. The urine osmolality is increased in Addison's disease, SIADH, dehydration, and renal disease. It is decreased in diabetes insipidus and psychogenic water drinking. The normal range is 300 to 900 mOsm/kg per 24 hours and 50 to 1,200 mOsm/kg in a random sample.

WATER DEPRIVATION TEST

Water restriction is a useful test because healthy people respond with a rapid decrease in urine volume when water intake is withheld. However, people with diabetes insipidus have no decrease in urine volume in response to severe water restriction. This signifies that the normal mechanism of ADH release in the face of water restriction and dehydration is dysfunctional. This test is rarely performed in a critical care unit because the patient is too ill and fragile to withstand the rigors of severe dehydration. The preferred test is measurement of serum ADH to diagnose diabetes insipidus.

ANTIDIURETIC HORMONE ADMINISTRATION

One final laboratory test used to diagnose diabetes insipidus is ADH administration. Exogenous ADH (vasopressin or Pitressin) given subcutaneously to the person suspected of having diabetes insipidus causes a temporary increase in urine osmolality. For a brief time, the person displays the appropriate response to ADH by conserving water at the kidney level, and urine output slows down in an attempt to restore ECF. This test also helps distinguish between the two types of diabetes insipidus, nephrogenic and central. In nephrogenic diabetes insipidus, the person does not demonstrate a reaction to exogenous ADH because the kidney receptors in the collecting duct are unresponsive to ADH. People with central diabetes insipidus respond readily to the exogenous ADH.

Diagnostic Studies

Diagnostic imaging studies are frequently used for patients suspected of having pituitary or hypothalamic disorders. CT and MRI are essential in diagnosing primary diseases affecting this area of the brain. Examples of disorders that affect the pituitary–hypothalamic axis are brain tumors, aneurysms, edema from surgical exploration or traumatic injuries, and necrotic lesions. Imaging techniques are used to view the sella turcica and the surrounding structures, the pituitary within the bony encasement of the middle cranial fossa. Angiography assists with precise viewing of the vascular supply in the area. Figure 43-1 provides examples of MRI and CT scans of a pituitary tumor.

The critically ill patient requires monitoring at all times during these procedures. Quite often, the patient requires sedation to eliminate all patient motion in an effort to ensure clear images. Institutional policies and procedures need to be followed during diagnostic testing.

THE THYROID GLAND

The thyroid hormones are regulated by the hypothalamus and the pituitary gland in a negative feedback system as previously described. Low levels of triiodothyronine (T_3) and thyroxine (T_4) cause the hypothalamus to secrete thyrotropin-releasing hormone (TRH), which then stimulates the anterior pituitary gland to release thyroid-stimulating hormone (TSH). TSH stimulates the production and release of the thyroid hormones (Fig. 43-2).

Increased thyroid hormone production results in hyperthyroidism, which can lead to an extreme form of thyrotoxicosis. This is a rare, life-threatening illness necessitating critical care admission for management of the patient. Conversely, hypothyroidism can occur, resulting in a severe hypometabolic state. If hypothyroidism is untreated, myxedema coma can develop in the patient, which is most likely to be managed and treated in a critical care unit.

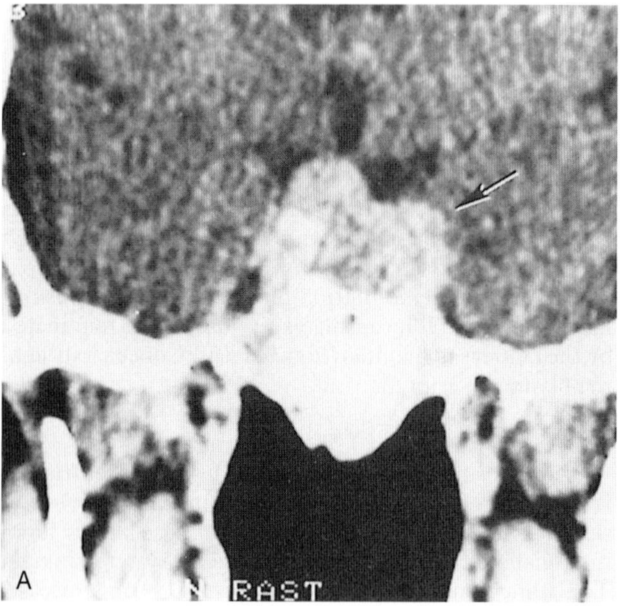

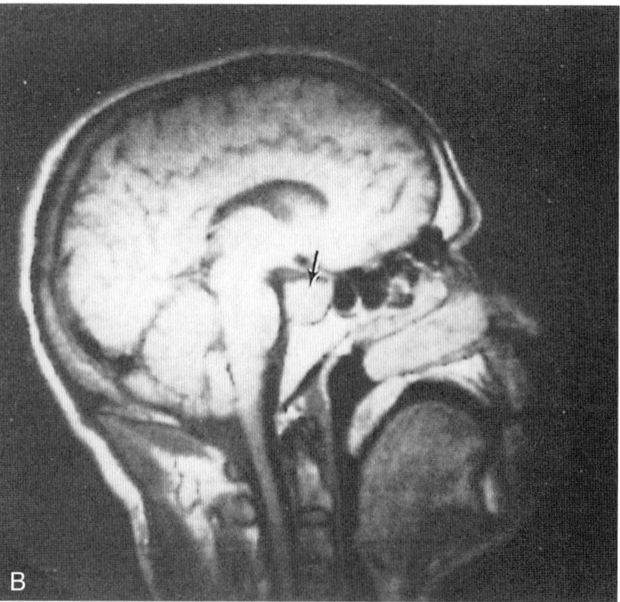

figure 43-1 (**A**) Computed tomography (CT) scan showing a suprasellar pituitary tumor (*arrow*) in a thyroid-toxic patient with a thyroid-stimulating hormone (TSH)–secreting pituitary tumor. (**B**) T_1-weighted magnetic resonance imaging (MRI) scan in the same patient showing a 2 × 2-cm pituitary tumor (*arrow*). T_1-weighted images are favorable for demonstrating anatomical detail. (Adapted from Smallridge RC: Thyrotropin-secreting pituitary tumors. Endocrinol Metab Clin North Am 16:3, 1987.)

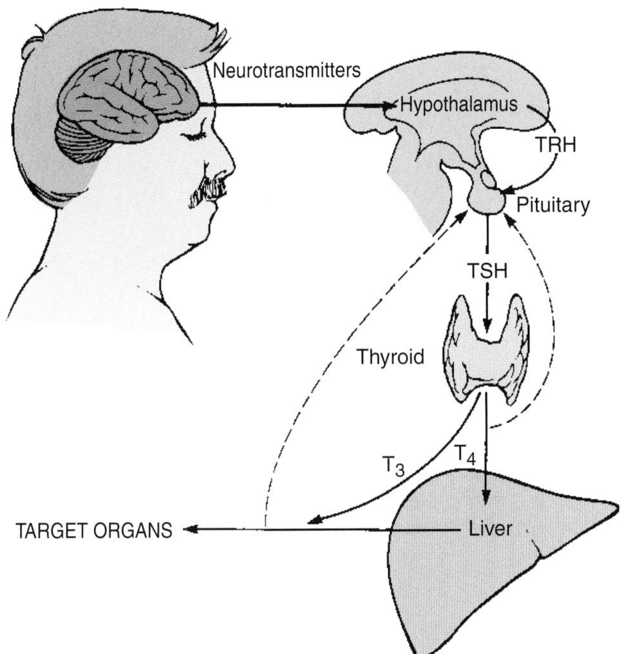

figure 43-2 The hypothalamic–pituitary–thyroid axis. Thyrotropin-releasing hormone (TRH) from the hypothalamus stimulates the pituitary gland to secrete thyroid-stimulating hormone (TSH). TSH stimulates the thyroid to produce thyroid hormone (T_3 and T_4). High circulating levels of T_3 and T_4 inhibit further TSH secretion and thyroid hormone production through a negative feedback mechanism (*dashed lines*). (Source: Smeltzer SC, Bare BG: Brunner & Suddarth's Textbook of Medical–Surgical Nursing [10th Ed], p 1213. Lippincott Williams & Wilkins, 2004.)

History and Physical Examination

Thyroid hormones affect nearly every cell and tissue in the body. Therefore, manifestations of these disorders are widespread. The typical course of disease progression is insidious, and the nurse needs to take a detailed history to uncover signs and symptoms of either hypothyroidism or hyperthyroidism.

History taking focuses on the variety of expected signs and symptoms associated with hypothyroidism and hyperthyroidism. Table 43-3 compares and contrasts the two disorders. Boxes 43-2 and 43-3 explore the incidence of thyroid disorders in the older patient and the pediatric patient, respectively.

Because of their deep, protected locations in the body, the endocrine glands are in general inaccessible to palpation, percussion, and auscultation. The exception is the thyroid gland, which can be examined physically when it is enlarged. Assessment begins with inspection of the area for enlargement, nodules, and symmetry of the gland. The patient is then asked to swallow while the nurse observes the thyroid rising. Next, the thyroid is palpated for size, shape, symmetry, and presence of tenderness. Thyromegaly (goiter) or thyroid nodules can be detected by palpation. Both lobes of the gland and the isthmus are palpated. The technique used to palpate the thyroid is specific (Fig. 43-3).

Occasionally, a thyroid bruit can be detected by listening over the gland with the bell of the stethoscope. A bruit is caused by excessive or turbulent blood flow associated with hyperthyroidism and the resultant hypermetabolic state.

table 43-3 Manifestations of Hypothyroid and Hyperthyroid States

Level of Organization	Hypothyroidism	Hyperthyroidism
Basal metabolic rate (BMR)	Decreased	Increased
Sensitivity to catecholamines	Decreased	Increased
General features	Myxedematous features Deep voice Impaired growth (child)	Exophthalmos Lid lag Decreased blinking
Blood cholesterol levels	Increased	Decreased
General behavior	Mental retardation (infant) Mental and physical sluggishness Somnolence	Restlessness, irritability, anxiety Hyperkinesis Wakefulness
Cardiovascular function	Decreased cardiac output Bradycardia	Increased cardiac output Tachycardia and palpitations
Gastrointestinal function	Constipation Decreased appetite	Diarrhea Increased appetite
Respiratory function	Hypoventilation	Dyspnea
Muscle tone and reflexes	Decreased	Increased, with tremor and fibrillatory twitching
Temperature tolerance	Cold intolerance	Heat intolerance
Skin and hair	Decreased sweating Coarse and dry skin and hair	Increased sweating Thin and silky skin and hair
Weight	Gain	Loss

Source: Porth CM: Pathophysiology: Concepts of Altered Health States (6th Ed), p 912. Philadelphia, Lippincott Williams & Wilkins, 2002.

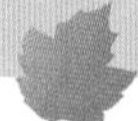

box 43-2

Endocrine Disorders in the Older Patient

- Expect a higher prevalence of hypothyroidism in the elderly population. Often, the older patient presents with atypical initial symptoms such as depression, apathy, and immobilization.
- Hyperthyroidism in the elderly is much less common; however, the older patient may present with a subclinical picture. Common complaints such as weight loss, fatigue, palpitations and tachycardia, mental confusion, and anxiety are typically attributed to "old age," thus making the disorder harder to detect. Worsening heart failure or unstable angina may result, and often the elderly patient presents with new-onset atrial fibrillation. For these reasons, the highly sensitive thyroid-stimulating hormone (TSH) test should be considered for the older patient with cardiovascular and neurological manifestations.
- The older adult experiences increased insulin resistance and hyperinsulinemia and is, therefore, at higher risk for developing type 2 diabetes.
- Hyperglycemic hyperosmolar state (HHS) affects the frail elderly population, with the acutely ill older patient at higher risk. Be suspicious of the older patient with diabetes and the new onset of acute illness, such as myocardial infarction, pancreatitis, pneumonia, or other serious infections or illnesses.
- Another expected result of aging is the decrease in secretion of aldosterone and cortisol. This can result in a diminished response to acute illness or trauma. The older patient may have a decreased ability to maintain appropriate fluid and electrolyte balance. In general, older adults display diminished responses to stressors such as critical illness or trauma.

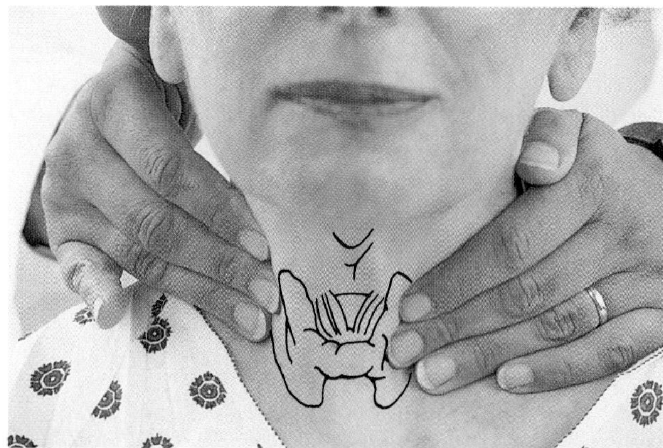

figure 43-3 The thyroid is examined from behind, with the patient in a sitting position, avoiding hyperextension of the neck. (From Timby BK, Smith NE: Introductory Medical–Surgical Nursing [8th Ed], p 162. Philadelphia, Lippincott Williams & Wilkins, 2003. © B. Proud.)

Other assessment parameters include noting vital sign changes, skin changes (including edema), neurological changes, and weight changes associated with either disorder. Hypothyroidism is frequently associated with hypotension, bradycardia, hypoventilation, and subnormal temperature. The patient often has dry, flaky skin; edema over the pretibial area; and a deep or husky voice. The patient displays slowed cognitive functioning with slower-than-normal verbal responses, slowed rapid alternating movements, and decreased deep tendon reflexes.

Patients with hyperthyroidism have more neurological manifestations such as tremor, nervousness, insomnia and restless movements, and hyperactive reflexes. Vital signs are characteristic: hypertension, tachycardia, tachypnea, and hyperthermia. The patient may have a goiter with detectible bruit. Also, the patient may have exophthalmos or proptosis of the eyes. The eyes may unilaterally or bilaterally protrude from the eye sockets, rendering the patient unable to close one or both eyes (Fig. 43-4).

box 43-3

Endocrine Disorders in the Pediatric Patient

- Thyroid hormone secretion is necessary for normal fetal growth and development, particularly for brain development. Maternal hypothyroidism is screened aggressively during the prenatal period. Congenital hypothyroidism is a rare but serious disorder that results in permanent abnormalities associated with cretinism. Therefore, all newborns are screened for hypothyroidism.
- Peak onset for type 1 diabetes is 11 to 13 years, suggesting a correlation with surges in growth hormone (GH). There is strong evidence for a genetic predisposition to developing this autoimmune form of diabetes.
- Patients with type 1 diabetes are at higher risk for diabetic ketoacidosis (DKA). Emotional factors and stress are suspected to contribute to the development of DKA in children.

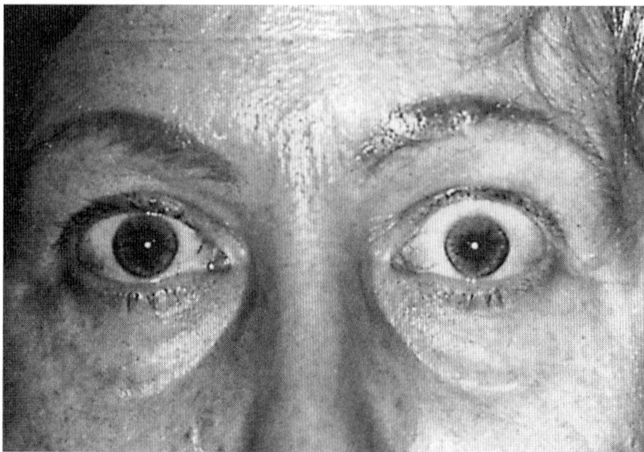

figure 43-4 A 38-year-old woman with Graves' disease (hyperthyroidism). Note the exophthalmos. (Source: Becker KL et al: Principles and Practice of Endocrinology and Metabolism [3rd Ed], p 429. Philadelphia, Lippincott Williams & Wilkins, 2001.)

Laboratory Studies

THYROID-STIMULATING HORMONE TEST (THYROTROPIN ASSAY)

The TSH test is a highly sensitive test used to diagnose hypothyroidism and hyperthyroidism. The third-generation immunometric assay (IMA) tests of TSH are 100 times more sensitive than the earlier methods for measuring TSH, and this test is the preferred method for diagnosing and monitoring progression of thyroid disease. Box 43-4 provides a review of common thyroid tests. Box 43-5 lists medications that may interfere with thyroid tests.

The TSH test measures circulating TSH from the anterior pituitary. TSH stimulates the release and distribution of the T_3 and T_4 stored in large amounts in the thyroid gland. Measuring TSH helps determine whether the hypothyroidism is primary (i.e., caused by dysfunction of the thyroid gland) or secondary (i.e., caused by hypofunction of the anterior pituitary gland). A high TSH level helps to diagnose primary hypothyroidism. Measuring the TSH level also helps to guide medication titrations for patients requiring exogenous thyroid hormone.

However, the levels of TSH and free T_4 are highly influenced by stress in critically ill patients owing to problems with protein levels that are often seen in critical care. Malnutrition, hepatic dysfunction, pregnancy, and drugs affect the TSH and free T_4 levels. Therefore, the results of the TSH test need to be analyzed carefully for the critically ill patient. The normal adult value for TSH is 0.4 to 5.4 mU/L.

box 43-4
Laboratory Evaluation of the Thyroid

Tests That Assess Thyroid Function
- Radioactive iodine uptake

Tests That Assess the Hypothalamic–Pituitary Axis
- Sensitive thyroid-stimulating hormone (TSH)
- TSH-releasing hormone stimulation test

Tests That Assess Thyroid Hormone Binding Peripherally
- Total thyroxine (T_4) and total triiodothyronine (T_3)
- Free T_4 and free T_3
- In vitro uptake tests (T_3 resin uptake)
- Thyroid hormone–binding ratios (free T_4 index)
- T_4-binding globulin

Diagnostic Studies
- Iodine-131, technetium-99m scans
- Ultrasound
- Computed tomography (CT)
- Magnetic resonance imaging (MRI)

Miscellaneous Tests
- Thyroid antibodies (thyroid peroxidase, thyroid-stimulating immunoglobulin)
- Thyroglobulin
- Calcitonin
- Basal metabolic rate (BMR)

box 43-5
Selected Medications That May Interfere With Thyroid Tests

- Phenytoin
- Propranolol
- Corticosteroids
- Aspirin
- Estrogen
- Furosemide
- Methadone
- Opioids
- Lithium
- Heparin
- Potassium iodide
- Amiodarone
- Sulfonamides
- Iodides

TOTAL THYROXINE

Total T_4 measures both the free T_4 and the portion carried by thyroxine-binding globulin (TBG). T_4 is increased in hyperthyroidism and decreased in hypothyroidism. Any factor that affects protein binding will affect the results of the total T_4. This includes pregnancy, estrogen or androgen therapy, and taking oral contraceptives, salicylates, or phenytoin. Normal values depend on the laboratory method used. The normal value declines with age and is 16.5 fg/dL in infants. Childhood norms are up to 15 fg/dL. Normal adult values range from 4 to 12 fg/dL and are higher during pregnancy. Older adults have lower values because plasma proteins decrease as people age.

FREE THYROXINE AND FREE THYROXINE INDEX

Free T_4 and free T_4 index measure the free part of T_4, the part that is not bound to protein. Free T_4 is the metabolically active form of the hormone that can be used by tissues. It makes up a small part of the total T_4. The free T_4 test is more useful than the total T_4 test in diagnosing hypofunction and hyperfunction of the thyroid gland because it helps diagnose thyroid function when people have abnormal binding globulin levels. This test can also evaluate thyroid replacement therapy. Radioisotopes can interfere with test results, and heparin can give false high readings. This test can be done by direct assay or by indirect measurement. The direct assay normal value is 0.8 to 2.7 ng/mL, whereas the free T_4 index is 4.6 to 12 ng/mL.

FREE TRIIODOTHYRONINE

Free T_3 measures the circulating T_3 that exists in the free state in the blood, unbound to protein. This is one measure to evaluate thyroid function. T_3 is about five times more potent than T_4 and is more metabolically active. Decreased values indicate hypothyroidism. Radioisotopes also affect results. Normal adult values are 260 to 480 pg/dL.

TRIIODOTHYRONINE RESIN UPTAKE TEST

The T_3 resin uptake test is an indirect measure of TBG available to bind T_3 and T_4. It is increased with thyrotoxicosis.

CALCITONIN

Calcitonin, or thyrocalcitonin, is a hormone secreted by the thyroid. It is secreted in response to high levels of calcium and reduces the calcium level by increasing its deposition in bone.

THYROID ANTIBODIES

Several autoimmune thyroid diseases produce detectable antibodies. Specifically, Graves' disease, Hashimoto's thyroiditis, and chronic autoimmune thyroid disease cause elevations in antithyroid antibodies, detectable by immunoassay techniques. These conditions can lead to severe hypothyroidism or hyperthyroidism if not treated.

THYROGLOBULIN

Thyroglobulin can be measured by radioimmunoassay and is elevated in most thyroid disorders. This test has limited diagnostic value because it is nonspecific. It is used clinically to follow the progression of disease in a patient being treated for thyroid cancer.

Diagnostic Studies

THYROID SCAN AND RADIOACTIVE IODINE UPTAKE

The radioactive iodine uptake test measures the rate of iodine uptake by the thyroid gland after the administration of iodine-123 tracer (by capsule, solution, or intravenous injection). A scintillation counter then measures gamma rays released from the breakdown of the tracer in the thyroid. This produces a visual representation of the radioactivity in the thyroid gland, neck, and mediastinum. Scan time is about 20 minutes. Normally, the radioactive iodine is evenly distributed in the thyroid gland, and the scan shows a normal size, position, and shape.

The thyroid scan may be done in conjunction with a radioactive iodine uptake study. After the patient takes the radioactive iodine, a count is made over the thyroid gland with a scintillation counter at specific times. These nuclear tests can indicate areas of increased and decreased function and provide data to diagnose hyperthyroidism, hypothyroidism, nodules, ectopic thyroid tissue, and cancer of the thyroid.

FINE-NEEDLE BIOPSY

Fine-needle biopsy is the diagnostic tool of choice for detecting malignancy for a thyroid nodule. It is often the initial test for evaluation of any thyroid mass. The test is safe, quick, and accurate, and results are usually available within hours to several days.

ULTRASOUND

Ultrasound of the thyroid gland uses high-frequency sound waves to produce an image of the gland. Ultrasound is an easy, noninvasive procedure that has no radiation risks and can be performed at the bedside. The test produces good images of structures and can detect masses, cysts, and enlargements of the gland.

THE PARATHYROID GLAND

The parathyroid gland produces parathyroid hormone (PTH), which maintains blood calcium and phosphorus levels, neuromuscular activity, blood clotting function, and cell membrane permeability. The four parathyroid glands are located just posterior to the thyroid gland and are sometimes damaged during thyroid surgery.

The output of PTH is regulated by the serum level of calcium under a negative feedback system. Overproduction of PTH results in hyperparathyroidism and is characterized by bone decalcification and the development of renal stones containing calcium.

Hypocalcemia as a result of hypoparathyroidism manifests neurologically. The patient manifests tetany (general muscular hypertonia, tremor, and spasmodic movements) as calcium levels dip below 5 to 6 mg/dL. The patient may complain of numbness, tingling, and cramps in the extremities. As the hypocalcemia worsens, the patient experiences bronchospasm, laryngeal spasm, carpopedal spasm (flexion of the elbows and wrists with extension of the carpophalangeal joints), dysphagia, photophobia, cardiac dysrhythmias, and seizures.

History and Physical Examination

The nurse ascertains a history of electrolyte imbalance, specifically calcium and phosphorus. Additional information includes a history of the following symptoms: apathy, fatigue, muscular weakness, nausea, vomiting, constipation, hypertension, and cardiac dysrhythmias. The patient may present with kidney stone symptoms such as severe flank pain, groin pain, frequent urination, hematuria, and nausea and vomiting. The patient may experience joint and bone pains and may sustain pathological fractures, especially of the spine. The nurse remains vigilant for signs of tetany (Fig. 43-5) and related complications.

Tetany can be assessed by evaluating the patient for Trousseau's sign or Chvostek's sign. Trousseau's sign is

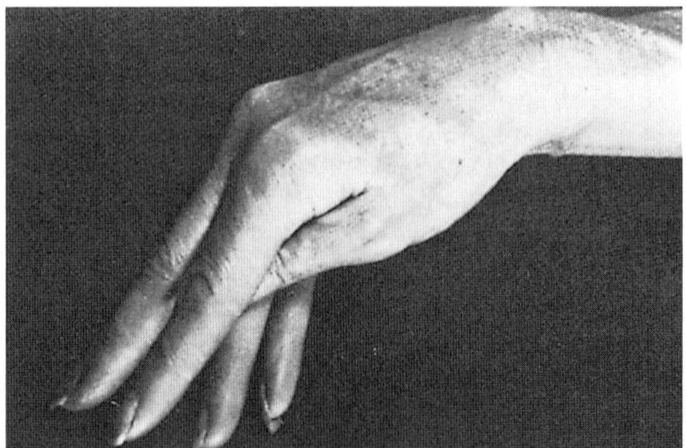

figure 43-5 Tetany is caused by tonic spasm of the intrinsic hand muscles. (Source: Spillane R: An Atlas of Clinical Neurology [3rd Ed], p 295. London, Oxford University Press, 1982.)

positive when carpopedal spasm is induced by occluding the blood flow to the arm for 3 minutes with the use of a blood pressure cuff. If tapping over the facial nerve just in front of the parotid gland causes twitching of the mouth or eye, the patient has a positive Chvostek's sign.

Laboratory Studies

SERUM CALCIUM LEVEL

Normal calcium levels range from 8.6 to 10.3 mg/dL. Most (99%) of body calcium is in the bone. The remaining 1% is in the ECF. Nearly 50% of serum calcium is ionized or free, whereas the remainder is bound to albumin. Changes in serum albumin alter total serum calcium concentration. Therefore, if albumin levels are also abnormal, clinical decisions regarding calcium should be based on the free calcium levels.

Marked serum calcium elevations are the most obvious manifestation of hyperparathyroidism. Calcium levels greater than 10.3 mg/dL are considered abnormally elevated. The common causes of hypercalcemia include primary hyperparathyroidism, malignancy, sarcoidosis, vitamin D toxicity, hyperthyroidism, and some medications such as thiazide diuretics and lithium.

Low serum calcium levels are the marker for hypoparathyroidism. Tetany develops at calcium levels of 5 to 6 mg/dL or lower. Common causes of hypocalcemia include hypoalbuminemia, renal failure, hypoparathyroidism, acute pancreatitis, tumor lysis syndrome, severe hypomagnesemia, and multiple citrated blood transfusions.

PARATHYROID HORMONE LEVEL

Radioimmunoassay reveals elevated PTH levels in hyperparathyroidism and decreased PTH levels in hypoparathyroidism. PTH regulates calcium and phosphorus metabolism. Increased secretion of PTH results in increased calcium absorption from the kidneys, intestines, and bones, thereby raising calcium levels. This hormone's actions are enhanced by the presence of vitamin D.

Diagnostic Studies

RADIOGRAPHIC STUDIES

Plain films, bone scans, MRI, ultrasound, or a combination of these modalities may be used to examine the parathyroid glands and evaluate the bone changes that have occurred as a result of the disease.

THE ENDOCRINE PANCREAS

Disorders of the endocrine pancreas are characterized by chronic hyperglycemia and result in major shifts of fluids and electrolytes as well as in blood glucose levels. The risk for developing diabetes increases with age. The two main types of diabetes are type 1 and type 2, and both forms of diabetes can lead to serious illnesses requiring critical care.

History and Physical Examination

A complete history is multisystem focused because glucose dysfunction affects every system of the body. The nurse inquires about a history of polydipsia, polyphagia, and polyuria. In addition, complaints of fatigue, a change in weight, blurred vision, chronic vaginitis, disorientation, nocturia, wounds that resist healing, and dental caries are noted. A good family history is obtained to document the role of familial patterns often seen in type 2 diabetes. The characteristics of patients at risk for developing type 2 diabetes are reviewed in Box 43-6.

For the patient with known diabetes who enters the critical care arena, the nurse focuses on gathering information about the extent of the disease and its duration, the onset of complications, the medications taken for the disease, and other past medical and surgical history. Chronic complications such as neuropathy, retinopathy, and nephropathy are explored, as well as the existence of other medical conditions such as hypertension, hyperlipidemia, obesity, and peripheral vascular disease.

Physical examination focuses on the severe fluid and electrolyte and neurological dysfunction seen with acute diabetes complications such as diabetic ketoacidosis (DKA), hyperglycemic hyperosmolar state (HHS), and hypoglycemia. Observation of fluid status and hydration is mandatory. Skin turgor, buccal membranes, weight, urine specific gravity, and vital signs are assessed. The nurse monitors the patient's neurological status frequently. The presence of a fruity odor on the breath (associated with ketonemia) should be noted. In addition, the patient may display Kussmaul's respirations as an attempt to rapidly exhale excess carbon dioxide. This respiratory pattern is characterized by deep, rapid breathing.

Laboratory Studies

FASTING BLOOD GLUCOSE LEVEL AND FINGERSTICK GLUCOSE ANALYSIS

The fasting blood glucose level provides a foundation for managing diabetes mellitus. Very high blood glucose levels can occur in DKA and HHS. In addition, elevated glucose

box 43-6 ***Risk Factors Associated With Developing Type 2 Diabetes***

- Family history of diabetes (parents, grandparents, siblings)
- Obesity (body mass index [BMI] greater than 27 kg/m^2)
- Race and ethnicity (African American, Native American, Hispanic American, Asian American, Pacific Islander)
- Age greater than 45 years
- History of impaired fasting glucose or impaired glucose tolerance
- Hypertension
- High-density lipoprotein (HDL) cholesterol less than 35 mg/dL
- Triglyceride level greater than 250 mg/dL
- History of gestational diabetes, the delivery of a baby greater than 9 pounds, or both

levels can occur in Cushing's syndrome, high-stress states, pancreatitis, and chronic renal and liver disease. Hypoglycemia can occur in Addison's disease, pancreatic tumors, starvation, and hypopituitary problems. The normal value for adults is 65 to 110 mg/dL. Two-hour postprandial blood glucose testing helps further evaluate carbohydrate metabolism, especially in people with diabetes mellitus. The normal value is 65 to 139 mg/dL. Criteria for diagnosing diabetes are given in Table 43-4.

Numerous drugs can interfere with glucose regulation, including corticosteroids, diuretics, lithium, phenytoin, beta-blockers, and estrogen. Hypoglycemic reactions can result from sulfonylureas, insulin, alcohol, beta-blockers, angiotensin-converting enzyme (ACE) inhibitors, and aspirin.

Fingerstick glucose testing can be used at the bedside for immediate feedback regarding the patient's glucose status. In addition, patients can be taught to use fingerstick devices at home to monitor their glucose levels and responses to medication. Standardization of the equipment must be ensured when these devices are used for patient monitoring.

In general, point-of-service testing such as this may not be appropriate for the critically ill patient because fingerstick testing requires adequate tissue perfusion for accuracy, and many critically ill patients do not have this required level of perfusion. Testing glucose from more direct sources of blood (i.e., veins, venous lines, central lines, arterial lines) may enhance accuracy.

GLYCOSYLATED HEMOGLOBIN

Glycosylated hemoglobin (HbA_{1c}) testing offers information about the average amount of glucose present in the patient's bloodstream for the 120-day life span of erythrocytes. This information is useful to assess data trends for a person who has been previously diagnosed with diabetes. The percentage result (normal: 4% to 7%) enhances accuracy because it controls for many variables such as stress, exercise, fasting state, interfering medications, and recent changes in patient compliance. In comparison with the highly variable, "snapshot view" that is provided by a fasting glucose level, HbA_{1c} testing provides insight into the patient's overall status over the previous 2 to 3 months.

INSULIN

This test helps measure abnormal carbohydrate metabolism by measuring the amount of circulating serum insulin in the fasting state. Insulin is released in response to serum glucose levels. When glucose is elevated, insulin levels should increase as well. Abnormally high levels of insulin may help diagnose insulinoma, a tumor of the islets of Langerhans. The normal adult value is 6 to 24 fU/mL.

A low insulin level helps to diagnose diabetes mellitus, especially in the presence of an abnormal glucose tolerance test (GTT). A fasting blood sample is tested. If the insulin test is done in conjunction with a GTT, blood samples are drawn at that time. Oral contraceptives and recent administration of radioisotopes interfere with results.

GLUCAGON

This hormone, produced in the alpha cells in the islets of Langerhans, controls the production, storage, and release of glucose. Normally, insulin opposes the action of glucagon. This test measures the production and metabolism of glucagon. A deficiency occurs when pancreatic tissue is lost because of chronic pancreatitis or pancreatic tumors. Increased levels occur in diabetes, acute pancreatitis, and catecholamine secretion (such as occurs with infection, high stress levels, or pheochromocytoma). Chronic renal failure and cirrhosis of the liver can also increase glucagon levels. Normal fasting values are 50 to 200 pg/mL.

SERUM KETONES

Measuring serum ketones reveals information about the use of fat metabolism in lieu of carbohydrates as seen in the critically ill person with diabetes. The normal serum ketone level is 2 to 4 mg/dL. Ketonemia (ketone bodies in the bloodstream) is manifested by Kussmaul's respirations and a fruity, sweet-smelling odor on the exhaled breath. These signs are the result of the patient's attempt to maintain a normal pH during extreme metabolic acidosis.

table 43-4 American Diabetes Association's Diagnostic Criteria for Diabetes Mellitus

	Normoglycemia	Impaired Fasting Glucose or Impaired Glucose Tolerance	Diabetes Mellitus*
Fasting plasma glucose	<110 mg/dL	>110 mg/dL and <126 mg/dL (impaired fasting glucose)	>126 mg/dL
2-Hour plasma glucose†	<140 mg/dL	>140 mg/dL and <200 mg/dL	>200 mg/dL
Random plasma glucose	—	—	>200 mg/dL

*A diagnosis of diabetes mellitus must be confirmed on a subsequent day by measurement of a fasting plasma glucose, a 2-hour plasma glucose, or a random plasma glucose (if symptoms are present). The fasting plasma glucose is usually preferred because of ease of administration, convenience, acceptability to patients, and lower costs. *Fasting* is defined as no caloric intake for at least 8 hours.

†The 2-hour plasma glucose test requires the use of a glucose load containing the equivalent of 75 g anhydrous glucose dissolved in water.

URINE KETONES

Ketones are not normally found in the urine. Ketones in the urine are associated with diabetes and other diseases of altered carbohydrate metabolism. People with diabetes should test for ketones whenever their urine or blood sugar is high. Because ketones appear in the urine before they can be detected in the blood, this test is often used in the emergency department when screening for acidosis. The test is performed by dipping a ketone reagent strip in a fresh urine sample. The presence of ketones in the urine results from lipolysis or fat breakdown in the absence of adequate insulin.

THE ADRENAL GLAND

The adrenal gland is anatomically and functionally divided into two distinct parts—the outer cortex and the inner medulla (see Chapter 42, Fig. 42-6). The two regions secrete different hormones. The cortex produces mineralocorticoids (e.g., aldosterone), glucocorticoids (e.g., cortisol), and androgens. The medulla secretes catecholamines such as epinephrine, norepinephrine, and dopamine. Disorders of the adrenal gland have widespread effects on the human body because these hormones regulate major body functions such as fluid and electrolyte balance, sympathetic nervous system responses, inflammation, and metabolism.

The secretion of hormones by the adrenal gland is regulated in a negative feedback system through the hypothalamic–pituitary axis. The hypothalamus releases corticotropin-releasing hormone (CRH), which in turn stimulates the release of ACTH from the anterior pituitary. ACTH then stimulates the adrenal cortex to secrete cortisol.

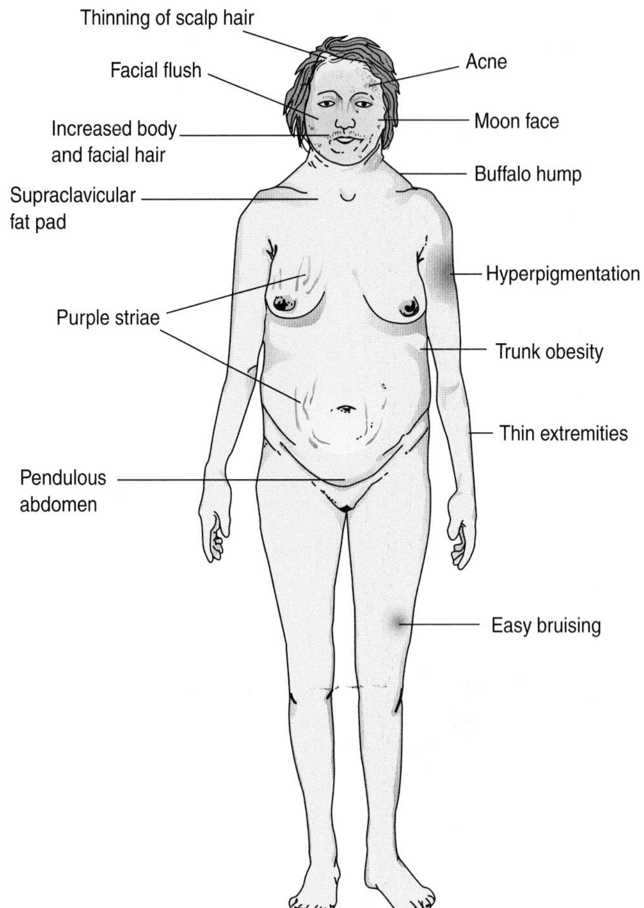

figure 43-6 Clinical manifestations of Cushing's syndrome. (Source: Smeltzer SC, Bare BG: Brunner & Suddarth's Textbook of Medical–Surgical Nursing [9th Ed], p 1061. Philadelphia, Lippincott Williams & Wilkins, 2000.)

History and Physical Examination

Clinical manifestations of adrenal gland dysfunction depend on the nature of the lesion and which hormone is adversely affected. Adrenal cortex lesions may affect the release of catecholamines and cause sudden, severe headache, diaphoresis, palpitations, and other symptoms associated with paroxysmal hypertension. One such lesion is pheochromocytoma, a benign adrenal cortex tumor that mediates this severe outpouring of catecholamines.

Another common pathology affecting the adrenal gland is a pituitary tumor that leads to hypersecretion of ACTH. The resulting disease, Cushing's syndrome, manifests as central obesity, unusual fat deposits, thin extremities, fragile skin, skin discoloration (striae), sleep disturbances, and catabolism (Fig. 43-6). The same clinical picture can result from chronic exogenous steroid use.

Adrenal insufficiency from autoimmune Addison's disease can lead to an adrenal crisis. The patient lacks adequate stimulation of the adrenal gland or the adrenal gland is rendered ineffective and stops secreting adequate levels of hormone. Consequently, the patient becomes lethargic, dehydrated, and unable to mount any stress response to handle acute illness or trauma. The critically ill patient often suffers from mild forms of adrenal insufficiency because the patient's normal stores of hormones are used quickly in response to the illness. Many require exogenous steroids to assist with recovery. A summary of the clinical manifestations of adrenal cortical insufficiency and glucocorticoid excess is given in Table 43-5.

Laboratory Studies

CORTISOL (HYDROCORTISONE)

This test evaluates the ability of the adrenal cortex to produce the glucocorticoid hormone cortisol. Cortisol is elevated in adrenal hyperfunction and decreased in adrenal hypofunction. Adrenal hyperfunction may be caused by excess secretion of ACTH by the pituitary gland (Cushing's syndrome), high stress, trauma, and surgery. Adrenal hypofunction may be the result of anterior pituitary hyposecretion, hepatitis, and cirrhosis.

Cortisol secretion is diurnal; it is normally higher in the early morning (6:00 AM to 8:00 AM) and lower in the evening (4:00 PM to 6:00 PM). This variation is lost in patients with adrenal hyperfunction and in people under stress. Serum samples are drawn between 6:00 AM and 8:00 AM and between 4:00 PM and 6:00 PM. Normal 8:00 AM values are 5 to 23 fg/dL or 138 to 635 mmol/L. Normal 4:00 PM values are 3 to 16 fg/dL or 83 to 441 mmol/L.

table 43-5 Manifestations of Adrenal Cortical Insufficiency and Excess

Parameter	Adrenal Cortical Insufficiency	Glucorticoid Excess
Electrolytes	Hyponatremia* Hyperkalemia*	Hypokalemia
Fluids	Dehydration* (e.g., elevated BUN)	Edema
Blood pressure	Hypotension Shock* Orthostatic hypotension	Hypertension
Musculoskeletal	Muscle weakness* Fatigue*	Muscle wasting Fatigue
Hair and skin	Skin pigmentation	Easy bruisability Hirsutism, acne, and striae (abdomen and thighs)
Inflammatory response	Low resistance to trauma, infection and stress	Decrease in eosinophils, lymphocytopenia
Gastrointestinal	Nausea, vomiting* Abdominal pain*	Possible gastrointestinal bleeding
Glucose metabolism	Hypoglycemia*	Impaired glucose tolerance Glycosuria Elevated blood sugar
Emotional	Depression and irritability	Emotional lability to psychosis
Other	Menstrual irregularity Decreased axillary and pubic hair in women	Oligomenorrhea Impotence in the male Centripetal obesity (moon face and buffalo hump)

*Occurs with acute adrenal insufficiency.
BUN, blood urea nitrogen.
Source: Porth CM: Pathophysiology: Concepts of Altered Health States (5th Ed), p 801. Philadelphia, Lippincott Williams & Wilkins, 1998.

CORTISOL (DEXAMETHASONE) SUPPRESSION

When healthy people receive a low dose of dexamethasone (chemically similar to cortisol), ACTH production is suppressed. However, people with adrenal hyperfunction and some with endogenous depression continue to produce ACTH and do not have a diurnal variation of cortisol.

For this test, dexamethasone is given at bedtime. Blood samples are taken the next day at 8 AM and 4 PM. Medications are discontinued for 24 to 48 hours before this test is started, especially estrogens, phenytoin, and cortisol-related preparations. Radioisotopes should not be given within 1 week of this test. This test is the test of choice to diagnose Cushing's syndrome.

CORTISOL STIMULATION

This test measures the response of the adrenal glands to an injection of cosyntropin (Cortrosyn, a synthetic ACTH preparation). A fasting 8 AM cortisol level is drawn before cosyntropin is administered, and then blood samples are taken 30 and 60 minutes after it is administered. The adrenal glands normally respond to the cosyntropin by synthesizing and secreting adrenocorticoids. The plasma cortisol level should increase to at least 18 fg/dL. The response to cosyntropin is decreased or absent in people with adrenal insufficiency or hypopituitarism. Long-term steroid therapy affects results. This test may be contraindicated in the presence of infections, inflammatory diseases, and cardiac disease. Cortisol stimulation is the preferred test to diagnose Addison's disease.

URINE VANILLYLMANDELIC ACID AND CATECHOLAMINE LEVELS

Urine vanillylmandelic acid is a metabolite of catecholamines. It has a high concentration in the urine and is easy to detect. Therefore, this 24-hour urine test is done when a person is suspected of having hypertension due to pheochromocytoma. Catecholamines can also be detected in the urine. Elevated levels of catecholamines can be found in patients with hypothyroidism, DKA, neuroblastomas, and ganglioneuromas.

Urine should not be collected when the patient is NPO. Test results are also affected by many drugs and foods, such as tea, coffee, vanilla, and fruit juice. Therefore, some laboratories restrict certain foods for 2 days before testing and on the day of testing. Certain drugs may also be discontinued for 4 to 7 days before testing. Normal adult values for urine vanillylmandelic acid are 2 to 7 mg/24 hours, and for catecholamines, 270 fg/24 hours.

URINE 17-KETOSTEROIDS AND 17-HYDROXYCORTICOSTEROIDS

These 24-hour urine collection tests reflect adrenal function by measuring the urinary excretion of steroids. They are used infrequently because they have been replaced by serum immunoassays.

Diagnostic Studies

ADRENAL SCAN

This scan is used to identify the site of certain tumors or sites that produce excessive amounts of catecholamines. The radionuclide iobenguane (^{131}I) is injected intravenously, and scans are done on days 2, 3, and 4. Sometimes only 1 day is needed, and other times imaging is needed on days 6 and 7. Normally tumors and sites of hypersecretion are absent.

clinical applicability challenges

Self-Challenge: Critical Thinking

1. *Compare and contrast the history, physical examination, and laboratory findings for diabetes insipidus and syndrome of inappropriate antidiuretic hormone secretion.*
2. *Analyze how the history, physical examination, and laboratory data help distinguish the mechanisms that cause decreased consciousness in myxedema coma.*
3. *Compare and contrast the physical findings in hyperthyroidism and hypothyroidism.*
4. *Evaluate the etiology of decreased level of consciousness in diabetic ketoacidosis and hyperosmolar hyperglycemic state.*
5. *Analyze the history, physical examination, and laboratory findings for adrenal crisis.*

Study Questions

1. *The expected serum osmolality for the patient with diabetes insipidus will be*
   a. *decreased.*
   b. *increased.*
   c. *completely normal.*
   d. *same as the urine osmolality.*
2. *The normal thyroid gland will have all the following characteristics except which one?*
   a. *It is slightly enlarged, enabling easy access for direct assessment.*
   b. *It is usually nonpalpable.*
   c. *It is easy to visualize when the patient is swallowing.*
   d. *It is preferable to palpate when located behind the patient.*
3. *Hypocalcemia leading to tetany is assessed by which one of the following parameters?*
   a. *Positive Hoffman's sign*
   b. *Positive Turner's sign*
   c. *Positive Trousseau's sign*
   d. *Positive Rovsing's sign*
4. *According to the American Diabetes Association, the diagnosis of type 2 diabetes is made by which one of the following?*
   a. *Positive results on glycosylated hemoglobin (HbA_{1c}) testing*
   b. *Two fasting glucose samples that are greater than 140 mg/dL*
   c. *Two fasting glucose samples that are greater than 126 mg/dL*
   d. *Any gestational diabetic event*
5. *The profound neurological signs in a patient with diabetic ketoacidosis (DKA) result from*
   a. *severe sepsis and fever.*
   b. *dehydration.*
   c. *systemic hypokalemia.*
   d. *neurologic hypoglycemia.*

OTHER SUGGESTED READING

Allen C, et al: Risk factors for frequent and severe hypoglycemia in type 1 diabetes. Diabetes Care 24(11):1878–1881, 2001

American Diabetes Association: Position statement: Hyperglycemic crises in patients with diabetes mellitus. Diabetes Care 25(Suppl): S100–S108, 2002

Becker KL (ed): Principles and Practice of Endocrinology and Metabolism (3rd Ed). Philadelphia, Lippincott Williams & Wilkins, 2001

Brook CGD, Marshall NJ: Essential Endocrinology (4th Ed). Oxford, Blackwell Science, 2001

Carson PP: Emergency: Adrenal crisis. Am J Nurs 100(7):49–50, 2000

Cypress M: Acute complications [Diabetes Update: CE Articles]. RN 64(4):26–28, 30–32, 2001

Czenis AL: Thyroid disease in the elderly. Adv Nurse Pract 7(9):38–46, 1999

Demester N: Diseases of the thyroid: A broad spectrum. Clin Rev 11(7):58–64, 2001

Fatourechi V: Demystifying autoimmune thyroid disease: Which disorders require treatment? Postgrad Med 107(1):127–134, 2000

Felner EI, White PC: Improving management of diabetic ketoacidosis in children. Pediatrics 108(3):735–740, 2001

Fischbach F: Common Laboratory and Diagnostic Tests (3rd Ed). Philadelphia, Lippincott Williams & Wilkins, 2002

Kacsoh B: Endocrine Physiology. New York, McGraw-Hill, 2000

Korenman SG (series ed): Atlas of Clinical Endocrinology (Vol IV). Philadelphia, Current Medicine, 2000

Miller CD, et al: Hypoglycemia in patients with type 2 diabetes mellitus. Arch Intern Med 161(13):1653–1659, 2001

Miller J: Management of diabetic ketoacidosis. J Emerg Nurs 25(6): 514–519, 578–582, 1999

Porth CM: Pathophysiology: Concepts of Altered Health States (6th Ed). Philadelphia, Lippincott Williams & Wilkins, 2002

Smeltzer SC, Bare BG: Brunner & Suddarth's Textbook of Medical-Surgical Nursing (10th Ed). Philadelphia, Lippincott Williams & Wilkins, 2004

Tkacs NC: Hypoglycemia unawareness: Your patient with diabetes won't always know when their blood sugar is low. Am J Nurs 102(2):34–41, 2002

Wilson JD, et al: Williams Textbook of Endocrinology (9th Ed). Philadelphia, WB Saunders, 1998

chapter 44

Common Endocrine Disorders

JANE KAPUSTIN

objectives

Based on the content in this chapter, the reader should be able to:

- Examine the pathophysiological principles that help explain thyroid crises, myxedema coma, adrenal crises, syndrome of inappropriate antidiuretic hormone secretion (SIADH), diabetes insipidus, diabetic ketoacidosis (DKA), hyperglycemic hyperosmolar state (HHS), and hypoglycemia.
- Distinguish key precipitating factors, history, and clinical manifestations for each disorder.
- Discuss five laboratory studies that are useful in diagnosing acute endocrine disorders.
- Analyze the similarities and differences in caring for patients with endocrine crises.
- Explore the nursing role in assessing, managing, and evaluating a plan of care for patients with endocrine crises.

Endocrine disorders have multisystem effects. At the same time, acute illness may lead to hypofunction and, less commonly, hyperfunction of the neuroendocrine system. Patients with acute illness who are at risk for endocrine dysfunction may have a pre-existing endocrine disorder. That disorder may be known, but many endocrine dysfunctions are not recognized before acute illness. For that reason, endocrine dysfunction should be considered in the assessment and management of all critically ill patients.

This chapter presents an overview of the pathophysiology, assessment, management, and complications of patients with acute endocrine disorders. These disorders are thyroid dysfunctions, adrenal gland dysfunctions, antidiuretic hormone (ADH) dysfunctions, and diabetic emergencies.

THYROID DYSFUNCTION

Thyroid dysfunction is a common clinical problem in the United States. Women are 5 to 10 times more likely than men to present with thyroid disease. The most common thyroid conditions are hyperthyroidism, hypothyroidism, and thyroid nodule. Clinical presentations may be quite subtle; therefore, patients with endocrine manifestations must be regarded with a high index of suspicion. Extremes of these two conditions are discussed in greater detail in this chapter. Figure 44-1 compares the signs and symptoms of hyperthyroidism and hypothyroidism.

Thyroid Crisis

Thyrotoxic crisis is a severe form of hyperthyroidism often associated with physiological or psychological stress. When the thyroid state worsens critically, it is called *thyroid crisis.* Rapid deterioration and death can occur if the condition is untreated. These patients must be admitted to the intensive care unit for supportive measures, antithyroid medications, steroids, and continuous nursing care. Consultation with an endocrinologist and cardiologist is essential. Even without pre-existing coronary artery disease (CAD), untreated thyroid crisis can cause angina pectoris and myocardial infarction, congestive heart failure, cardiovascular collapse, coma, and death. The condition may develop spontaneously, but it occurs most frequently in people who have undiagnosed or partially treated severe hyperthyroidism. By defini-

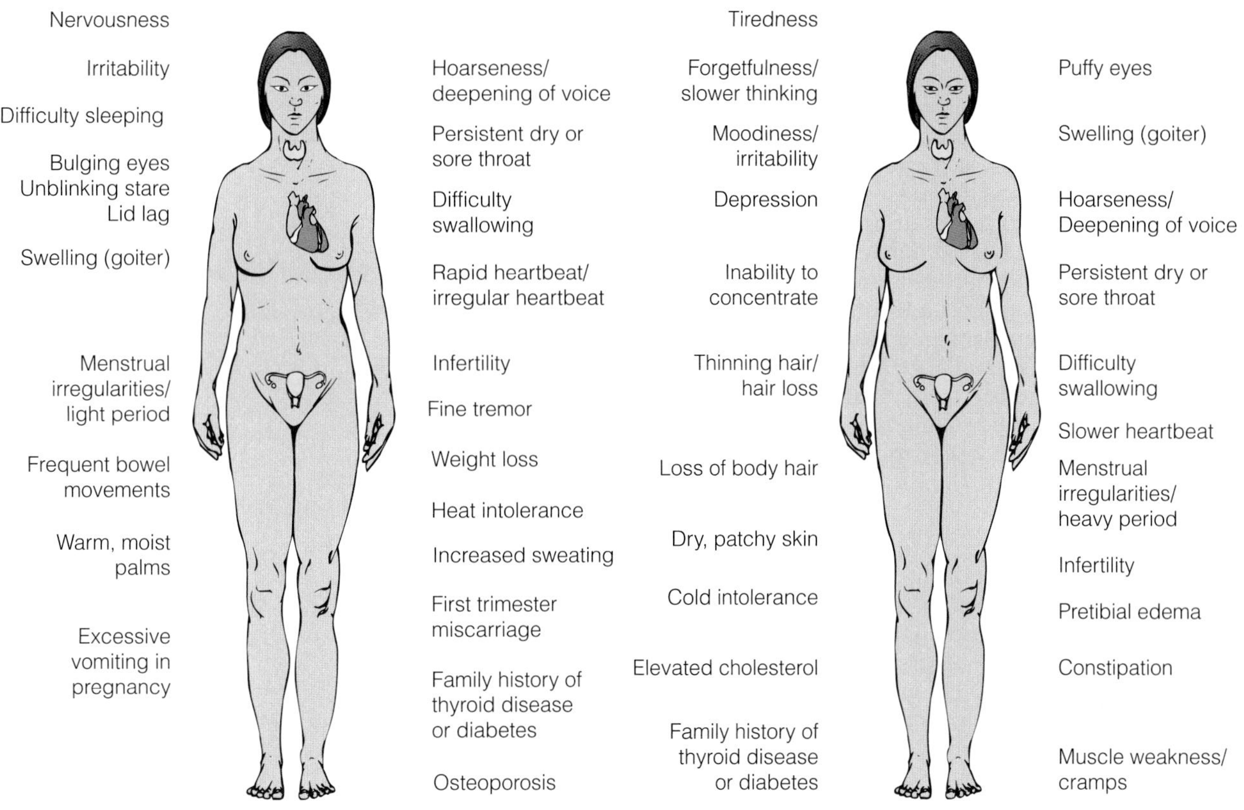

figure 44-1 Clinical manifestations of (**A**) hyperthyroidism and (**B**) hypothyroidism.

tion, hyperthyroidism is a condition in which the actions of the thyroid hormones result in greater-than-normal responses. Specific diseases that can cause hyperthyroidism include Graves' disease, exogenous hyperthyroidism, thyroiditis, toxic nodular goiter, toxic multinodular goiter, and thyroid cancer. Certain drugs, such as contrast material for radiographic procedures or amiodarone (an antidysrhythmic drug), may precipitate the thyrotoxic state because of their high iodine content. The conditions associated with hyperthyroidism are summarized in Box 44-1.

PATHOPHYSIOLOGY

The cause of thyroid crisis, often referred to as *thyroid storm* or *thyrotoxicosis*, is poorly understood. Physiological mechanisms that are thought to induce thyroid crises include the sudden release of large quantities of thyroid hormone, low tissue tolerance to triiodothyronine (T_3) and thyroxine (T_4), adrenergic hyperactivity, and excessive lipolysis and fatty acid production. The abrupt release of large quantities of thyroid hormone is thought to produce the hypermetabolic manifestations seen during thyroid crises. The many different endocrine, reproductive, gastrointestinal, integumentary, and ocular manifestations are caused by increased circulating levels of thyroid hormone and by stimulation of the sympathetic nervous system.

box 44-1
Conditions Associated With Hyperthyroidism or Thyrotoxicosis

Endocrine Disorders
- Graves' disease
- Nodular goiter
- Toxic multinodular adenoma
- Radiation-induced thyroiditis
- Subacute thyroiditis

Drugs
- Iatrogenic thyroid replacement
- Accidental or purposeful ingestion of thyroid medication
- Contrast media dye
- Amiodarone
- Beta blockers

Tumors
- Metastatic thyroid cancer
- Hypophyseal tumors
- Hypothalamus tumor
- Hydatidiform mole

Adrenergic hyperactivity is considered a possible link to thyroid crisis. Although thyroid hormone and catecholamines potentiate each other, catecholamine levels during thyroid crisis are usually within the normal range. It is uncertain whether the effects of hypersecretion of thyroid hormone or increased catecholamine levels cause heightened sensitivity and thyroid overfunction. Thyroid–catecholamine interactions result in an increased rate of chemical reactions, increased nutrient and oxygen consumption, increased heat production, alterations in fluid and electrolyte balance, and a catabolic state.

Another mechanism that may contribute to thyroid crisis is excessive lipolysis and fatty acid production. With excessive lipolysis, increased fatty acids are oxidized and produce an overabundance of thermal energy that is difficult to dissipate through vasodilation.

ASSESSMENT

History and Physical Examination

Accurate identification of the precipitating factor for thyroid storm allows for proper treatment to be initiated. Precipitating factors for people with recognized and unrecognized existing thyroid disease are listed in Box 44-2. Hyperthyroidism's most common form, Graves' disease, is an autoimmune condition caused by thyroid-stimulating immunoglobulins. It is not always apparent that the patient is suffering from this particular disease. Therefore, subtle clues need to be explored, such as the patient's exposure to iodine, prior or current use of thyroid hormone, anterior neck pain, thyroid enlargement, exophthalmos (i.e., protrusion of one or both eyes) or other eye symptoms, pregnancy, a history of goiter, and a family history of thyroid disease.

Signs and symptoms of hyperthyroidism affect all body systems and include sweating, heat intolerance, nervousness, tremors, palpitations, tachycardia, hyperkinesis, and increased bowel sounds. Extremes of these manifestations, specifically a temperature greater than 104°F (40°C) in the absence of an infection, tachycardia, and central nervous system (CNS) dysfunction, may be present in hyperthyroidism. CNS abnormalities include agitation, restlessness, delirium, seizures, or coma. Signs of thyroid emergencies are listed in Table 44-1.

As discussed in Box 44-3, older patients may not have the classic signs and symptoms of thyroid crisis, causing this condition to be overlooked. However, they frequently have suggestive signs and symptoms. In these circumstances, older patients are asked if they have heart disease and what medications they take. This can be important in determining whether there is underlying thyroid disease because beta blocker medication may mask cardiovascular clues.

Laboratory Studies

Laboratory studies may show elevated total T_4, free T_3, and free T_4 levels. The thyroid-stimulating hormone (TSH) level is extremely low in hyperthyroidism. TSH is suppressed because the levels of circulating hormones, T_3 and T_4, are so elevated. Recall that TSH is secreted when thyroid hormone levels are low.

Serum electrolytes, liver function tests, and complete blood counts, although not diagnostic, may help uncover abnormalities that require treatment. They may also help

box 44-2 ***Risk Factors for Development of Thyroid Crisis***

In the Presence of a Known Preexisting Condition

Precipitating factors

- Infection
- Trauma
- Stress
- Coexistent medical illness (e.g., myocardial infarction, pulmonary disease)
- Pregnancy
- Exposure to cold

Medications

- Chronic steroid therapy
- Beta blockers
- Narcotics, anesthetics
- Alcohol, tricyclic antidepressants
- Glucocorticoid therapy
- Insulin therapy
- Thiazide diuretics
- Phenytoin
- Chemotherapy agents
- Nonsteroidal anti-inflammatory agents (NSAIDs)

In the Presence of an Unknown Preexisting Condition

Precipitating factors

- Pituitary tumors
- Radiation therapy of the head and neck
- Autoimmune disease
- Neurosurgical procedures
- Metastatic malignancies (e.g., lung, breast)
- Surgery
- Long-term illness
- Shock
- Postpartum status
- Trauma

table 44-1 Possible Indications of Thyroid Emergencies

Thyroid Storm	Myxedema Coma
Tachycardia	Bradycardia
Hyperthermia	Hypothermia
Tachypnea	Hypoventilation
Hypercalcemia	Hyponatremia
Hyperglycemia	Hypoglycemia
Metabolic acidosis	Respiratory and metabolic acidosis
Cardiovascular collapse	Cardiovascular collapse
Cardiogenic shock	Decreased vascular tone
Hypovolemia	
Cardiac arrhythmias	
Depressed LOC	Depressed LOC
Emotional lability	Seizures, coma
Psychosis	—
Tremors, restlessness	Hyporeflexia

LOC, level of consciousness.

Data from Halloran T: Nursing responsibilities in endocrine emergencies. Critical Care Nursing Quarterly 13(3):74–81, 1990.

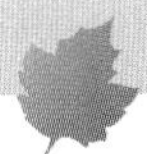

box 44-3

Hyperthyroidism in Older Adults

Elderly patients with hyperthyroidism often present with atypical signs and symptoms of the disorder. Apathetic hyperthyroidism, as seen in the older patient, manifests with a single symptom such as depression or muscle weakness. Thus, the elderly patient may present with palpitations, shortness of breath, tremor, and nervousness, but many other symptoms, as seen in younger patients, are masked. Much time can transpire until the patient deteriorates into full-blown thyroid storm.

identify the precipitating cause. Electrolyte imbalances due to dehydration, excessive bone resorption, and increased insulin degradation often occur. The serum calcium is often elevated, whereas potassium and magnesium are decreased, and liver function test values are increased. Hyperglycemia due to insulin resistance and breakdown of stored glucose often occurs.

Diagnostic Studies

Diagnostic tests include the radioactive iodine uptake test, which is usually increased. Electrocardiography and cardiac monitoring may show atrial fibrillation, supraventricular tachycardia, sinus bradycardia, heart block, conduction disturbances, and ventricular dysrhythmias, all reflective of the hypermetabolic state and the synergized catecholamines.

MANAGEMENT

Management goals for thyroid crises are fourfold: (1) treating the precipitating factor or factors, (2) controlling excessive thyroid hormone release, (3) inhibiting the thyroid hormone biosynthesis, and (4) treating the peripheral effects of thyroid hormone.

Antithyroid drugs (Table 44-2) are used to control thyroid release or biosynthesis. Propylthiouracil is the preferred agent, although it can be given only orally. Propylthiouracil is preferred because it blocks the conversion of T_4 to T_3 in peripheral tissues and binds iodine to prevent synthesis of the hormone. If the oral route is not possible, methimazole can be given rectally.

Iodine solutions, such as sodium iodide intravenously or potassium iodide (SSKI) or Lugol's solution orally, are given to block the release of thyroid hormone. These agents should not be given until 1 hour after the administration of antithyroid medications. Lithium is the choice for patients who are iodine sensitive. Glucocorticoids may be ordered because they also inhibit thyroid hormone release.

Emergency removal of excess circulating hormone replacement therapy can be accomplished by instituting plasmapheresis, dialysis, or hemoperfusion adsorption.

table 44-2 Pharmacologic Agents Used to Treat Hyperthyroidism

Drug	Dose	Action	Nursing Considerations
Propylthiouracil (PTU)	Loading: 800–1200 mg Maintenance: 100–400 mg every 4–6 h orally (PO)	Blocks synthesis of hormones (conversion of T_3 to T_4)	Monitor cardiac parameters. Observe for conversion to hypothyroidism. Must be given by mouth. Watch for rash, nausea, vomiting, agranulocytosis, lupus syndrome.
Methimazole	10–20 mg every 6–8 h PO	Blocks synthesis of thyroid hormone	More toxic than PTU. Watch for rash and other symptoms as for PTU.
Sodium iodide	1 g every 12 h intravenously (IV)	Suppresses release of thyroid hormone	Given 1 h after PTU or methimazole. Watch for edema, hemorrhage, gastrointestinal upset.
Potassium iodide	2–5 gtt every 8 h PO	Suppresses release of thyroid hormone	Discontinue for rash. Watch for signs of toxic iodinism.
SSKI	5–10 drops every 8 h PO	Suppresses release of thyroid hormone	Mix with juice or milk. Give by straw to prevent staining of teeth.
Dexamethasone	2 mg every 6 h IV	Suppresses thyroid hormone release	Monitor input and output. Monitor glucose. May cause hypertension, nausea, vomiting, anorexia, infection.
Beta blocker (e.g., propranolol)	13 mg every 1–4 h IV	Beta-adrenergic blocking agent	Monitor cardiac status. Hold for bradycardia or decreased cardiac output. Use with caution in patients with congestive heart failure.

Cholestyramine may be used to assist with oral absorption of excess hormone.

Cardiovascular decompensation, secondary to decreased stroke volume and reduced cardiac output, may be life-threatening. Beta blockers, specifically propranolol, are used to treat the symptoms of the hyperthyroidism rather than the primary thyroid disease. This therapy may be ordered to restore cardiac function by decreasing the catecholamine-mediated symptoms. The response to beta blockers is carefully monitored because intrinsic cardiac disease may worsen as a result of the negative inotropic effects. Digoxin, diltiazem (Cardizem), diuretics, or a combination of these agents may also be used to treat congestive heart failure or supraventricular tachydysrhythmias. Oxygen is delivered to address the additional metabolic requirements. The goal of therapy is to decrease myocardial oxygen consumption, decrease the heart rate (ideally to below 100 beats/minute), and increase cardiac output.

Management also focuses on monitoring multisystem effects from the hypermetabolism of thyroid crisis and the response to treatment. Cardiovascular function, fluid and electrolyte balance, and neurological status require close attention. Blood pressure, heart rate and rhythm, respiratory rate, and extra heart sounds are assessed every hour.

Fluid status and laboratory values are evaluated. Body temperature is monitored hourly because the patient is at risk for hyperthermia. Antipyretic agents, particularly acetaminophen, are recommended for fever control. Aspirin is not given because it increases free T_3 and T_4 levels. Tepid baths or a cooling blanket may be needed. Cooling to the point of shivering and piloerection is avoided because this may have a rebound effect of raising body temperature.

Neurological status is also assessed at least hourly. Seizure precautions and safety measures prevent injury. If the patient's level of consciousness decreases, airway patency and safety issues are assessed.

Energy and nutritional needs are heightened because of the hypermetabolism. Interventions include administering glucose-containing solutions, nutritional support, vitamin supplementation, and sedation if needed. Box 44-4 lists examples of nursing diagnoses for the patient in thyroid crisis.

Effective therapy can expect to result in clinical improvement within 24 to 48 hours. The patient's mental status is monitored carefully as well as stabilization of vital signs and normalization of body temperature. Patient follow-up to prevent another episode is necessary and may involve life-long medication or suppressive therapy with thyroid ablation.

box 44-4 ***Examples of Nursing Diagnoses and Collaborative Problems for the Patient in Thyroid Crisis***

- Deficient Fluid Volume related to hypermetabolic state
- Hyperthermia related to hypermetabolic state
- Decreased Cardiac Output related to hypermetabolic state and heart failure
- Impaired Cerebral Tissue Perfusion related to hypermetabolic state and heart failure
- Potential for Injury related to altered mental status

case study ■ GRAVES' DISEASE

Mrs. Clark was admitted to the medical intensive care unit (ICU) with an initial diagnosis of supraventricular tachycardia unresponsive to therapy. Her neurological status was depressed; she was arousable at times but disoriented. She did not recognize her family and could not remember that she was in the hospital. Mrs. Clark was recently diagnosed with hyperthyroid state due to Graves' disease. She had not been taking her medications. The initial complete blood count and chemistry laboratory values were normal. The physician ordered 5% dextrose in normal saline solution (D_5NSS) intravenously, to infuse at a rate of 100 mL/hour. The patient's initial vital signs were abnormal: temperature 102°F (38.8°C); heart rate 165 beats/minute; mean arterial blood pressure 70 mm Hg. The physician ordered serum thyroid tests. Propylthiouracil was started, as well as acetaminophen for the fever. Cardiac monitoring was also ordered to observe for signs and symptoms of congestive heart failure. Small doses of a beta blocker were titrated to control and reduce her heart rate, blood pressure, and her general level of circulating catecholamines. After 24 hours, the patient became more stable in response to the medications. ■

Myxedema Coma

Hypothyroidism is a common disorder with a broad clinical spectrum—patients may be asymptomatic, or they may be severely ill with myxedema coma. Hypothyroidism is more common among women and the incidence increases with age. Approximately 10% to 15% of elderly patients have elevated TSH associated with hypothyroidism, and routine screening of high-risk populations is often done in primary care settings.

Myxedema coma is a rare, life-threatening emergency brought on by extreme hypothyroidism. It usually is seen in older patients during winter months after certain precipitating factors such as stress, exposure to extreme cold temperatures, or trauma. In addition to coma, complications of myxedema coma include pericardial and pleural effusions, megacolon with paralytic ileus, and seizures. Death can result if severe hypoxia and hypercapnia are not reversed.

PATHOPHYSIOLOGY

Deficient production of thyroid hormone results in the clinical state termed *hypothyroidism.* Hypothyroidism, a chronic disease, is 10 times more common in women than in men. It occurs in all age groups but most commonly in those older than 50 years. It is more common than hyperthyroidism.

Hypothyroidism can be primary or secondary. Primary causes include congenital defects, loss of thyroid tissue after treatment for hyperthyroidism, defective hormone synthesis due to an autoimmune process, and antithyroid drug administration or iodine deficiency. Secondary causes include peripheral resistance to thyroid hormone, pituitary infarction, and hypothalamic disorders. Transient hypothyroidism can occur after withdrawal of prolonged T_4 or T_3 treatment. The common causes of hypothyroidism are summarized in Box 44-5.

Hypothyroidism usually affects all body systems. A low basal metabolic rate (BMR) and decreased energy metabolism and heat production are characteristic. The patient with chronic hypothyroidism may have myxedema, an alteration in the composition of the dermis and other tissues. The connective fibers are separated by an increased amount of protein and mucopolysaccharides. This binds water, producing nonpitting, boggy edema, especially around the eyes, hands, and feet; it is also responsible for thickening of the tongue and the laryngeal and pharyngeal mucous membranes, resulting in slurred speech and hoarseness.

ASSESSMENT

History and Physical Examination

Signs and symptoms of hypothyroidism include fatigue, weakness, decreased bowel sounds, decreased appetite, weight gain, and electrocardiographic (ECG) changes. Myxedema coma is a rare manifestation of hypothyroidism, characterized by severe depression of the sensorium, hypothermia, hypoventilation, hypoxemia, hyponatremia, hypoglycemia, hyperreflexia, hypotension, and bradycardia. Patients with myxedema coma do not shiver, although body temperatures below 80°F (26.6°C) have been reported. The diagnosis of myxedema coma depends on recognizing the clinical symptoms and identifying the underlying precipitating factor. The most common precipitating factor is pulmonary infection; others include trauma, stress, infections, drugs (e.g., narcotics or barbiturates), surgery, and metabolic disturbances (see Table 44-1).

Laboratory Studies

A decrease in T_4 and free T_4 is most common, whereas sodium is usually decreased and potassium is increased. TSH is markedly elevated in severe hypothyroidism. Arterial blood gases (ABGs) usually show a severe hypercapnia with a decreased arterial oxygen tension (PaO_2) and increased arterial carbon dioxide tension ($PaCO_2$).

box 44-5
Causes of Hypothyroidism

- Destruction of the thyroid gland (e.g., surgery, radioactive iodine, external radiation to the neck)
- Infiltrative disease (e.g., sarcoidosis, amyloidosis, lymphoma)
- Autoimmune disease (e.g., Hashimoto's disease, post-Graves' disease)
- Thyroiditis (e.g., viral, silent, postpartum)
- Drug induced (e.g., iodides, lithium, amiodarone)
- Hereditary hypothyroidism
- Thyrotropin-releasing hormone (TRH) deficiency
- Thyroid-stimulating hormone (TSH) deficiency

Diagnostic Studies

A chest radiograph detects pleural effusion. ECG changes include bradycardia, a prolonged PR interval, and decreased amplitude of the P wave and QRS complex. Heart block may develop.

MANAGEMENT

The most serious complication of hypothyroidism is progression to myxedema coma and death, if the condition is untreated. A multisystem approach must be used in treating this emergency. Mechanical ventilation is used to control hypoventilation, hypercapnia, and respiratory arrest. Intravenous hypertonic normal saline and glucose correct the dilutional hyponatremia and hypoglycemia. Fluid administration plus vasopressor therapy may be necessary to correct hypotension.

Pharmacological therapy includes the administration of thyroid hormone and corticosteroids. There are several approaches to this aspect of medical management. Initial drug therapy includes 300 to 500 µg T_4 intravenously to saturate all protein-binding sites and establish a relatively normal T_4 level. Subsequent doses may include 100 µg daily. Intravenous or oral T_3 is an alternative order. Guidelines to T_3 replacement are 25 µg intravenously every 8 hours for the first 24 to 48 hours. Oral T_3 doses every 8 hours are also ordered. Hormone replacement should be given slowly and the patient should be monitored continuously during treatment to avoid sudden increased metabolic demand and resultant myocardial infarction. Fluid replacement and rewarming of the patient should also be done methodically to avoid complications.

Additional interventions include treating abdominal distension and fecal impaction and managing hypothermia by gradually rewarming the patient using blankets and socks. Mechanical devices are not used. The patient is monitored for neurological status and changes in level of consciousness. Seizure precautions are implemented. When the patient is comatose, care includes preventing complications related to aspiration, immobility, skin breakdown, and infection. Cardiovascular and respiratory function is monitored. Fluid administration must also be monitored because there is a risk for fluid overload. An important aspect of care is to detect early signs of complications. As the patient recovers, interventions focus on patient self-care and education.

Patient follow-up includes a thorough investigation of how the severe hypothyroidism occurred and how it can best be avoided in the future. Patient teaching, family follow-up, medical alert activation, and involvement of community supports may be necessary for this complex patient.

ADRENAL GLAND DYSFUNCTION

Adrenal Crisis

PATHOPHYSIOLOGY

Adrenal insufficiency, also known as *hypoadrenalism* or *hypocorticism*, is a rare but life-threatening dysfunction of the adrenal cortex. Adrenal hormone insufficiency may be either primary (i.e., directly involving the adrenal gland) or secondary (i.e., due to hypothalamic–pituitary disease).

Primary adrenal insufficiency is termed *Addison's disease*. The most common cause of primary hypoadrenalism in the industrialized West is autoimmune adrenalitis. Autoimmune antibody formation leads to the gradual destruction of the adrenal gland, resulting in adrenal insufficiency. The second leading cause of primary adrenal insufficiency is destruction of the gland secondary to *Mycobacterium tuberculosis* infection. Worldwide, tuberculosis remains the most common cause of primary adrenal insufficiency. Other causes include bilateral hemorrhage of the glands secondary to bacterial infection with sepsis and shock, metastatic malignancies, acquired immunodeficiency syndrome (AIDS), fungal infections, surgical adrenalectomy, and sarcoidosis.

The most common cause of secondary adrenal insufficiency is iatrogenic, resulting from abrupt withdrawal of exogenous adrenocorticotropic hormone (ACTH) or as a complication of cortisol therapy. Suppressed ACTH secretion as a result of exogenous cortisol therapy disrupts the body's natural feedback loop that controls cortisol secretion, rendering the patient in an acute state of adrenal insufficiency. Other causes of secondary adrenal insufficiency include metastatic carcinomas of the lung or breast, pituitary infarction, surgery or irradiation, and CNS disturbances, such as basilar skull fractures or infections.

Acute adrenal insufficiency or adrenal crisis occurs when there is a change in the chronic condition or massive adrenal hemorrhage. In addition to the chronic disease, an infection, trauma, surgical procedure, or some extra stress occurs, precipitating acute adrenal crisis in the patient. The patient is therefore unable to meet the requirements for normal metabolic function or increased metabolic needs as necessary for stress or illness. Any stressed, critically ill patient can develop adrenal insufficiency as a result of suddenly imposed extraneous stressors. As the patient struggles to survive, he or she quickly depletes cortisol stores and may require exogenous replacement.

ASSESSMENT

History and Physical Examination

Symptoms of adrenal insufficiency are the same for primary and secondary disease. Because adrenal insufficiency affects both glucocorticoids and mineralocorticoids, many body functions are affected, including glucose metabolism, fluid and electrolyte balance, cognitive state, and cardiopulmonary status. Weakness, fatigue, anorexia, nausea, vomiting, diarrhea, and abdominal pain may be initial clues to adrenal crisis. These findings are nonspecific until linked with the history of a chronic condition requiring past or present corticosteroid use. Specifically, use of more than 20 mg of hydrocortisone or its equivalent, taken for longer than 7 to 10 days, has the potential for suppressing the hypothalamic–pituitary–adrenal axis.

Hyperpigmentation on areas of the elbows, knees, hands, or buccal mucosa is seen in primary adrenal insufficiency. The presence of hyperpigmentation, secondary to the deposition of melanin in the skin, strengthens the clinical picture of adrenal crisis. The most common physical changes include signs of severe dehydration, such as weight loss and orthostatic hypotension. Dehydration occurs secondary to the nephrons' insufficient ability to reabsorb sodium and water. Signs and symptoms of an impending adrenal crisis are summarized in Box 44-6.

box 44-6 *Indications of Impending Adrenal Crisis*

Aldosterone deficiency
- Hyperkalemia
- Hyponatremia
- Hypovolemia
- Elevated (BUN)

Cortisol deficiency
- Hypoglycemia
- Decreased gastric motility
- Decreased vascular tone
- Hypercalcemia

Generalized signs and symptoms
- Anorexia
- Nausea and vomiting
- Abdominal cramping
- Diarrhea
- Tachycardia
- Orthostatic hypotension
- Headache, lethargy
- Fatigue, weakness
- Hyperkalemic electrocardiographic changes
- Hyperpigmentation

Laboratory Studies

Laboratory values in acute conditions of glucocorticoid and mineralocorticoid deficiency show hyponatremia, hyperkalemia, decreased serum bicarbonate levels, and elevated blood urea nitrogen (BUN). Metabolic acidosis may occur because of dehydration. Hypoglycemia is usually present. Other abnormal laboratory findings include anemia and lymphocytosis with eosinophilia. In primary adrenal insufficiency, the patient presents with chronically elevated ACTH levels. ACTH levels are normal or decreased in the patient with secondary adrenal insufficiency.

Serum cortisol levels and cortisol stimulation (ACTH stimulation) tests are also used to confirm the diagnosis. In primary adrenal insufficiency, repeated injections of ACTH (or Cortrosyn) do not cause a rise in cortisol levels because the adrenal gland is dysfunctional. In secondary adrenal insufficiency, ACTH injections cause a normal but delayed response.

Diagnostic Studies

A computed tomography (CT) scan of the adrenal glands and the head may be done to detect tumors or other pathology of the adrenal and pituitary gland.

MANAGEMENT

The immediate goal of therapy is to administer the needed hormones and restore fluid and electrolyte balance. Hydrocortisone, 100 mg intravenously, is administered immediately, followed by 100 mg every 6 to 8 hours. Fluid resuscitation is also started immediately with normal saline and 5% dextrose solutions. The rate of fluid and electrolyte replacements is dictated by the degree of volume depletion, serum electrolyte levels, and clinical response to therapy. Associated medical or surgical problems may indicate the need for invasive blood pressure and hemodynamic monitoring.

Another management goal is to prevent complications. This includes monitoring signs and symptoms of electrolyte imbalance (hyponatremia and hypercalcemia) and respiratory and cardiovascular function. The nurse looks for changes in blood pressure, heart rate and rhythm, skin color and temperature, capillary refill time, and central venous pressure (CVP). There is a risk for orthostatic hypotension, bradycardia, and dysrhythmias. The nurse also monitors neuromuscular signs, such as weakness, twitching, hyperreflexia, and paresthesia.

Emotional support, a simple explanation, and a quiet environment are effective in assisting the patient emotionally through the physiological crisis. Once the acute crisis is over, patient education is a goal of care. Patient education is necessary because the ultimate prognosis depends on the patient's ability to understand and follow through with self-care. Self-care includes knowing the medication regimen, stress factors and their effect on the disease, and the signs of impending crisis; wearing a medical alert tag, bracelet, or carrying a wallet card; and taking medication as prescribed.

case study ■ ADDISON'S DISEASE

Mr. Cerelo, a 55-year-old man with Addison's disease, was seen in the emergency department with initial symptoms of generalized weakness, fever, orthostatic hypotension, tachycardia, and gastrointestinal complaints. A chest radiograph showed multiple infiltrates. Laboratory values indicated decreased serum sodium and increased serum potassium levels. The initial diagnosis was impending adrenal crisis precipitated by a lung infection.

Fluid resuscitation was started in the emergency department with D_5NSS at 200 mL/hour. An initial dose of hydrocortisone was also administered. The patient was awake and alert. Initial vital signs were stable; however, the patient remained tachycardic and tachypneic. Chemistry studies were to be completed in 2 hours to evaluate any changes in sodium and potassium values. A Foley catheter was inserted to monitor urine output. More hydrocortisone was given at regular intervals to replace the patient's steroid deficit. He became more stable as evidenced by fluid and electrolyte balance, normalization of vital signs, and improvement in cognition and energy levels. ■

ANTIDIURETIC HORMONE DYSFUNCTION

Two disorders involve antidiuretic hormone (ADH) dysfunction. One is an excess of ADH called syndrome of inappropriate antidiuretic hormone secretion (SIADH). The second, diabetes insipidus, involves a deficiency of ADH. Both of these disorders can produce severe fluid and electrolyte imbalances and adverse neurological changes. Recall that ADH is synthesized in the hypothalamus and stored in the posterior pituitary. It is released when stimulated by specific conditions and causes the renal tubules to reabsorb more water and sodium.

Syndrome of Inappropriate Antidiuretic Hormone Secretion

PATHOPHYSIOLOGY

In SIADH, there may be either increased secretion or increased production of ADH. This increase in ADH occurs despite the fact that the initial osmolality is normal. As a result, it causes an increase in total body water. SIADH is considered whenever the patient experiences hypotonic hyponatremia, the hallmark of the disorder.

The secretion of ADH is considered "inappropriate" in that it continues despite the decreased osmolality of the plasma. The normal feedback system regulating the release and inhibition of ADH fails, and ADH secretion continues. The circulating ADH acts on the renal tubules, causing reabsorption of water that is inconsistent with the body's needs. Other reasons for the continued secretion of ADH are also lacking. There is no hypokalemia and edema; cardiac, renal, and adrenal function are normal; and there is normal or expanded plasma and extracellular fluid (ECF) volumes.

Occasionally, SIADH is caused by a pituitary tumor, but more commonly it is caused by a bronchogenic (oat cell) or pancreatic carcinoma. These tumors actually secrete ADH but are independent of normal physiological controls. Other possible causes of SIADH include head injuries; other endocrine disorders; pulmonary diseases, such as pneumonia and lung abscesses; CNS infections or tumors; and drugs. Box 44-7 outlines the most common causes of SIADH.

ASSESSMENT

History and Physical Examination

SIADH is characterized by water retention and eventually water intoxication secondary to sustained ADH effect. The hyponatremia in SIADH has two components, an early dilutional component due to increased water and a later, clinically undetectable component, caused by the increased urinary sodium excretion.

The signs and symptoms produced by SIADH are predominantly neurological and gastrointestinal. The most common signs and symptoms are personality changes, headache, decreased mentation, lethargy, abdominal cramps, nausea, vomiting, diarrhea, anorexia, decreased tendon reflexes, disorientation, confusion, and, finally, seizures and coma. Many patients remain asymptomatic until the sodium level drops well below 125 mEq/L. Subtle neurological findings such as altered mental state, slight confusion, anorexia, inability to concentrate, and complaints of weakness may be the earliest indication of impending problems.

Hyponatremia is the clinical focus and probable cause of hospital admission. When the serum sodium falls to less than 120 to 125 mEq/L, more pronounced symptoms such as nausea and vomiting, muscular irritability, and seizures often result. If the condition develops acutely (i.e., within 24 hours), a mortality rate of 50% has been reported. Children and the elderly are more susceptible to hyponatremia because of their lower body water content.

box 44-7
Common Causes of Syndrome of Inappropriate Antidiuretic Hormone Secretion (SIADH)

Malignancies
- Bronchogenic carcinoma
- Pancreatic carcinoma
- Prostate or thymus cancer

Central Nervous System (CNS) Causes
- Neoplasm
- Hemorrhage
- Trauma
- Infection

Pulmonary Causes
- Mechanical ventilation
- Chronic obstructive pulmonary disease (COPD)
- Respiratory failure
- Lung abscess

Medications
- Nicotine
- Morphine
- Chlorpropamide
- Antineoplastics
- Tricyclic antidepressants
- Anesthetics
- Clofibrate

Other Causes
- Human immunodeficiency virus (HIV)/acquired immunodeficiency syndrome (AIDS)
- Senile atrophy
- Idiopathic

Physical evidence of hyponatremia includes dyspnea, jugular venous distension, restlessness, hypothermia, weight gain, edema, reduced and concentrated urine, and disorientation. The nurse often is the first to identify these early, subtle signs.

Laboratory Studies

The main laboratory abnormalities in SIADH are a plasma hyponatremia and hypo-osmolality. The urine simultaneously is hyperosmolar and there is a high excretion of urinary sodium. The urine specific gravity is high, usually greater than 1.025, and the overall urinary output is lower (less than 30 mL/hour). Other laboratory findings include low BUN, creatinine, and uric acid levels; hypocalcemia and hypokalemia; and decreased hemoglobin and hematocrit. The diagnosis can be confirmed by radioimmunoassay of plasma ADH. (See Chapter 43, Table 43-2 for a comparison of laboratory values in SIADH and diabetes insipidus.)

MANAGEMENT

There are three goals in the management of SIADH: (1) treating the underlying disease, (2) alleviating excessive water retention, and (3) providing the comprehensive care needed when the patient has a depressed level of consciousness.

Treatment of the underlying cause of SIADH may or may not be possible, depending on the pathological process. Surgical resection, radiation, or chemotherapy may alleviate some of the water retention caused by some cancers. No drug completely inhibits the release of ADH from the pituitary gland or a tumor. When the cause of the SIADH is unknown, the treatment consists of fluid restriction.

The first step in managing SIADH is to restrict fluid intake. In mild cases, fluid restriction is sufficient. It slows renal blood flow and glomerular filtration, enhancing proximal tubular reabsorption of salt and water; increases aldosterone secretion; and enhances distal tubule sodium reabsorption. As a general guideline, water intake should not exceed urinary output until the serum sodium concentration normalizes and symptoms abate. Fluid restriction is usually successful for the patient with sodium levels between 125 and 135 mEq/L.

In severely symptomatic patients, the administration of 3% hypertonic saline and furosemide is the treatment of choice to correct hyponatremia in an emergency situation. Hypertonic saline should be infused at 0.1 mg/kg/minute to prevent rapid volume overload and pulmonary edema. Usually, less than 1,000 mL is given at one time.

One major complication to avoid is central pontine myelinolysis. This may occur when correction of hyponatremia by hypertonic saline infusion is too rapid. Rapid correction of hyponatremia may lead to brain dehydration, cerebral bleeding, demyelination, neurological injury, or death. Initial signs and symptoms include seizures, movement disorders, akinetic mutism, quadriparesis, and unresponsiveness. The best plan is to replace sodium at a rate no faster than 1 to 2 mEq/L/hour to avoid the syndrome.

Other medications are effective by interfering with the ADH–renal tubule interaction. Demeclocycline, an antibiotic, has been effective because it interferes with the normal ADH effect in kidney tubules. Other medications that block the effects of ADH at the tubules include phenytoin (Dilantin), lithium, and fludrocortisone (Florinef).

Fluid and electrolyte balance, especially the serum sodium level, is monitored. The nurse evaluates intake and output, including hourly urine amounts, and observes for signs of fluid overload. Output should exceed intake.

Neurological status is evaluated. Rapid changes in sodium levels can result in neurological deterioration. When the serum sodium is less than 125 mEq/L, there is a significant risk of neurological symptoms, including disorientation and decreasing consciousness. Seizure precautions may be necessary. Complications of SIADH include neurological deterioration, leading to seizures, coma, and death.

Patients may find it difficult to limit their fluid intake. Mealtimes may also be difficult because menus are aimed at meeting nutritional needs without increasing fluid intake. Providing good oral care and offering substitutions for fluids (e.g., Toothettes, lemon-glycerin swabs) may be helpful for the persistently thirsty patient. Information, emotional support, and acknowledging the deprivation may help patients through this period.

case study ■ SYNDROME OF INAPPROPRIATE ANTIDIURETIC HORMONE SECRETION

A 65-year-old woman, Mrs. Perez, was admitted to the critical care unit (CCU) with an initial diagnosis of acute mental status changes and severe hyponatremia. Past medical history included recent pneumonia and a history of congestive heart failure related to CAD. The pneumonia was treated with antibiotics, and the patient takes a thiazide diuretic for the congestive heart failure.

Initially, the patient's level of consciousness was depressed, and she had decreased deep tendon reflexes. Laboratory tests showed hyponatremia and normal ABGs. Heart and lung sounds were normal, and her extremities were warm, adequately perfused, and without edema. The CT scan did not show any structural defect. Mrs. Perez had a generalized tonic–clonic seizure as she was admitted to the CCU. Laboratory values were as follows: sodium 115 mEq/L; potassium 4.5 mEq/L; chloride 90 mEq/L; plasma osmolality 260 mOsm/kg. Urine sodium levels were elevated.

To prevent further seizure activity, the patient was placed on immediate fluid restriction and hypertonic (3%) saline was initiated slowly to replace the sodium deficit. Seizure precautions were initiated and antiseizure medications were administered. The patient was monitored closely for cardiac compromise as a low-dose saline infusion was administered. As the patient's serum sodium level normalized, the saline infusion was stopped. The fluid restriction was continued until the patient was more stable. The underlying cause of the patient's SIADH was discovered and treated. ■

Diabetes Insipidus

PATHOPHYSIOLOGY

Diabetes insipidus is a disease characterized by water imbalance resulting from inadequate ADH or resistance to ADH, leading to water diuresis and dehydration. In diabetes insipidus, the kidneys excrete great quantities of dilute urine, at times up to 20 L/day. Normally, the posterior pituitary releases ADH, which then acts on the distal renal tubules to promote reabsorption of water. When there is an absence of or deficit in ADH, the kidneys lose their ability to reabsorb water and control fluid output (see Chapter 42).

Diabetes insipidus may manifest in two forms: central or nephrogenic. Central diabetes insipidus is the more common condition that results in ADH deficit and responds favorably to exogenous vasopressin administration. This type of diabetes insipidus is the disease most often encountered in the critical care environment. Nephrogenic diabetes insipidus is a very rare genetic disorder that results from the failure of the kidney to respond to ADH. Only central diabetes insipidus is discussed in this chapter.

Diabetes insipidus can be transient, temporary, partial, or permanent, depending on the initial cause and circumstances surrounding the patient illness or injury. The hypothalamus's osmolality sensors control ADH release from the posterior pituitary. As the osmolality increases, the osmoreceptors are stimulated, releasing more ADH. In the kidneys, ADH causes more water and sodium to be absorbed, restoring adequate fluid balance. In the absence of ADH, the renal tubules and collecting ducts are impermeable to water. Consequently, large volumes of dilute urine are excreted. Serum osmolality and sodium rise, and the patient continues to become progressively more dehydrated. The thirst sensation may or may not be affected, depending on the patient's level of consciousness. For patients with an impaired thirst mechanism, dehydration and hypovolemic shock will result more quickly if the condition is not corrected.

Diabetes insipidus can develop after any event that causes edema or direct damage to the neurohypophysis. After surgery, diabetes insipidus may occur when regions of the brain around the hypothalamus and pituitary are affected. It can occur after head injuries, gunshot wounds, and lesions that disrupt blood supply to the area. Damage to the sphenoid bone, maxillofacial injuries, hypothalamic tumors, and nasopharyngeal tumors that invade the base of the skull may also lead to the development of diabetes insipidus. Direct trauma or ischemic events involving the hypothalamus, such as hemorrhage, infection, or neoplasm, may result in diabetes insipidus. Also, diseases or drugs that affect the renal collecting tubules may lead to diabetes insipidus. There is also a psychogenic polydipsia, in which excessive water is consumed, resulting in excess output.

After trauma or surgery, diabetes insipidus can be transient until initial edema subsides. The neurohypophysis is very sensitive to extraneous pressure; consequently, these structures may be unable to produce, secrete, or release ADH as needed. The patient displays temporary signs of diabetes insipidus. As the edema abates, ADH secretion resumes its normal course and the diabetes insipidus eventually is corrected. In some cases of severe trauma or hemorrhage, the structures may be completely damaged and the patient may permanently develop diabetes insipidus.

The classic example of the transient type of disorder is illustrated by the patient undergoing a transsphenoidal approach for a hypophysectomy to remove a pituitary tumor. In most cases, the patient experiences temporary problems related to an inability to synthesize, store, or release ADH due to edema of the hypothalamus and pituitary. This patient requires close monitoring for the development of diabetes insipidus, and may need treatment. Figure 44-2 illustrates a transsphenoidal approach to a pituitary tumor.

ASSESSMENT

Polyuria, polydipsia, and dehydration are the hallmarks of diabetes insipidus. Patients can excrete from 3 to 20 L of urine per day. When patients are alert, they experience excessive thirst and excessive urinary output. They try to increase their fluid intake, but this can cause exhaustion and eventually result in dehydration. On the other hand, when people are not alert enough to detect thirst and increase their fluid intake, they can quickly become hypovolemic because of the fluid loss. If left untreated, this can lead to death.

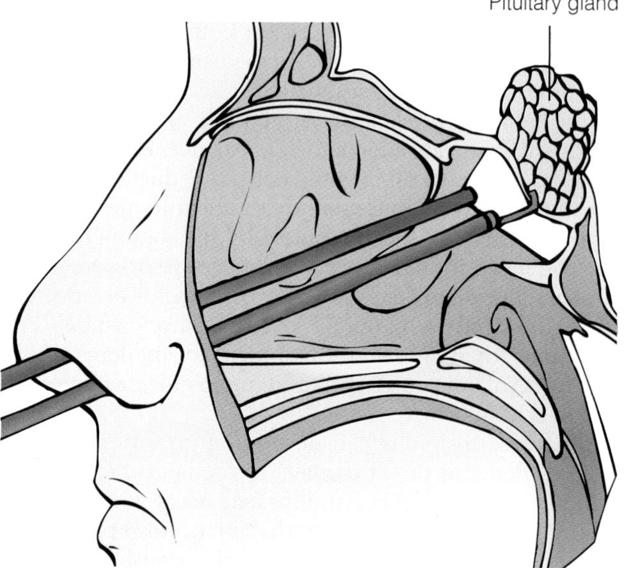

figure 44-2 The transsphenoidal approach to a pituitary tumor can lead to transient diabetes insipidus. The neurohypophysis is very sensitive to extraneous pressure; consequently, these structures may be unable to produce, secrete, or release antidiuretic hormone (ADH) as needed. The resultant diabetes insipidus resolves as the edema (from the surgery) resolves.

Signs of dehydration include dry skin, dry mucous membranes, confusion, sunken eyeballs, constipation, poor skin turgor, lethargy, muscle weakness, muscle pain, and pallor. Vital signs are adversely affected, with severe tachycardia, hypotension, low CVP, and a possible rise in body temperature. Weight loss may be apparent.

Recognizing diabetes insipidus may be more difficult when patients are recovering from surgery because steroids and cerebral dehydrating agents used before and during surgery promote diuresis for the first postoperative day or so. If awake, the patient complains of progressive thirst if diabetes insipidus is present. Urine output increases and persists regardless of the amount of fluid intake. Urine specific gravity falls or remains at about 1.001 to 1.005. Urine is copious, clear, and almost colorless. Plasma osmolality increases, often to levels greater than 300 mOsm/kg. Urine osmolality decreases to 50 to 100 mOsm/kg. The urine sodium is below normal, whereas the serum sodium is elevated (see Chapter 43, Table 43-2). The water deprivation test is also helpful to diagnose diabetes insipidus. These tests, combined with the constellation of signs and symptoms, lead to the diagnosis. Table 44-3 presents laboratory values for patients with diabetes insipidus.

MANAGEMENT

The objective of therapy is to prevent dehydration and electrolyte imbalance, while treating the underlying cause and preventing complications. Hypotonic intravenous solutions, such 0.45% sodium chloride, are administered to match the urine output. The volume of replacement fluids depends on the degree of dehydration and the amount needed to reverse hypovolemic shock.

A variety of replacement ADH (vasopressin) therapies are available. Desmopressin acetate (DDAVP) is synthetic ADH that can be administered intravenously or as a nasal spray. Aqueous vasopressin (Pitressin) may be given as an intravenous bolus, continuous infusion, or subcutaneously. The medications can be used for temporary or permanent ADH replacement. Permanent hormone replacement requires more patient and family education. In addition, the patient should obtain medical alert identification to wear at all times. Table 44-4 reviews the commonly administered drugs for diabetes insipidus.

Management also focuses on monitoring fluid and electrolyte balance. Fluid excesses or deficits can be detected by evaluating hourly intake and output, serum and urine electrolytes and osmolality results, and urine specific gravity. Changes in blood pressure, pulse, and respirations and the onset of pulmonary crackles, neck vein distension, peripheral edema, and increasing CVP and pulmonary artery wedge pressure are noted. The nurse observes skin turgor and mucous membranes and changes in alertness and cognition. Drowsiness, confusion, and headache may

table 44-3 Laboratory Values for Patients With Diabetes Insipidus

Value	Normal	Diabetes Insipidus
Serum antidiuretic hormone (ADH)	1–5 pg/mL	Decreased in central diabetes insipidus, may be normal with nephrogenic or psychogenic diabetes insipidus
Serum osmolality	285–300 mOsm/kg	>300 mOsm/kg
Serum sodium	135–145 mEq/L	>145 mEq/L
Urine osmolality	300–1,400 mOsm/kg	<300 mOsm/kg
Urine specific gravity	1.005–1.030	<1.005
Urine output	1–1.5 L/24 h	30–40 L/24 h
Fluid intake	1–1.5 L/24 h	>50 L/24 h

Source: Anatomical Chart Company: Atlas of Pathophysiology, p 269. Philadelphia, Lippincott Williams & Wilkins, 2002.

table 44-4 ■ Commonly Administered Medications for Diabetes Insipidus

Drug	Dosage	Route of Administration	Duration of Drug	Adverse Effects
Desmopressin (DDAVP)	5–20 μg each day	Nasal spray (cannot be given if nasal passages blocked)	8–24 h	Headache, chest pain, nausea, diarrhea, edema
Aqueous pitressin	2–4 units every 4–6 h	Intramuscularly, subcutaneously, intranasally	1–8 h	Headache, chest pain, nausea, diarrhea, edema
Pitressin tannate in oil	2.5–5 units	Intramuscularly	36–48 h	Headache, chest pain, nausea, diarrhea, edema
Lysine vasopressin nasal spray	5–20 units three to seven times daily; titrate to output	Intranasally	2–6 h	—
Chlorpropamide (Diabinese)	100–250 mg/day	By mouth	60–72 h	Hypoglycemia, headache, tinnitus, alcohol intolerance, gastrointestinal disturbances, diarrhea
Clofibrate	250–500 mg	By mouth	6–8 h	Gastrointestinal disturbances

indicate water intoxication. Weight is another indicator of fluid status.

COMPLICATIONS

Major complications of diabetes insipidus are cardiovascular collapse and tissue hypoxia. Seizures and encephalopathy can also result from fluid and electrolyte imbalance. Prognosis is excellent as long as the patient receives prompt and aggressive treatment.

DIABETIC EMERGENCIES

Diabetes is a complex and chronic metabolic disorder characterized by hyperglycemia and defects in insulin secretion. Figure 44-3 illustrates how chronic hyperglycemia is associated with long-term organ dysfunction, particularly of the eyes, kidneys, nerves, heart, and blood vessels. These long-term microvascular and macrovascular complications of retinopathy, neuropathy, nephropathy, and cardiovascular disease are the primary causes of morbidity and mortality in those affected with diabetes. Diabetes is the seventh leading cause of death in the United States.

The pathogenic processes associated with diabetes range from autoimmune destruction of the islet beta cells of the pancreas to insulin resistance. The derangements of carbohydrate, protein, and fat metabolism all result from deficient action of insulin on target tissues. The main effect is hyperglycemia. Hyperglycemia is manifested as polyuria, polydipsia, polyphagia, weight loss, and blurred vision. Acute, critical illnesses associated with diabetes are hyperglycemia with ketoacidosis and nonketotic hyperosmolar state.

The incidence of diabetes in the United States has risen dramatically, and diabetes morbidity and mortality are also increasing. Certain population subgroups (Native American, Hispanic American, African American) have prevalence rates approaching 50%. This rate is strongly related to the epidemic of obesity and the socioeconomic inequalities that plague our nation. Often almost half of patients with type 2 diabetes are not diagnosed until complications have already developed, and many suffer acute syndromes requiring emergency department evaluation, intensive care management, or both. The critical care nurse must be vigilant in identifying high-risk patients. Table 43-4 in Chapter 43 contains the American Diabetes Association's Position Statement on the diagnostic parameters for diabetes.

Most patients with diabetes can be classified into two main groups, those with type 1 diabetes and those with type 2 diabetes (Table 44-5). The cause of type 1 diabetes is an absolute deficiency of insulin secretion. This insulin secretion impairment results from autoimmune destruction of the beta cells of the pancreas. Markers of immune destruction include islet cell autoantibodies (ICAs). The rate of islet cell destruction is variable, and some children and adolescents present with ketoacidosis as the first manifestation of the disease. As the islet cell destruction occurs, the patient is rendered insulin dependent for survival. There may be genetic links to the predisposition for type 1 diabetes, and these patients are rarely obese. Type 1 diabetes accounts for approximately 10% to 20% of all cases of diabetes, and onset occurs mainly during childhood or at puberty.

Type 2 diabetes manifests as insulin resistance with relative, rather than absolute, insulin deficiency. Most of the patients with this form of diabetes do not require insulin,

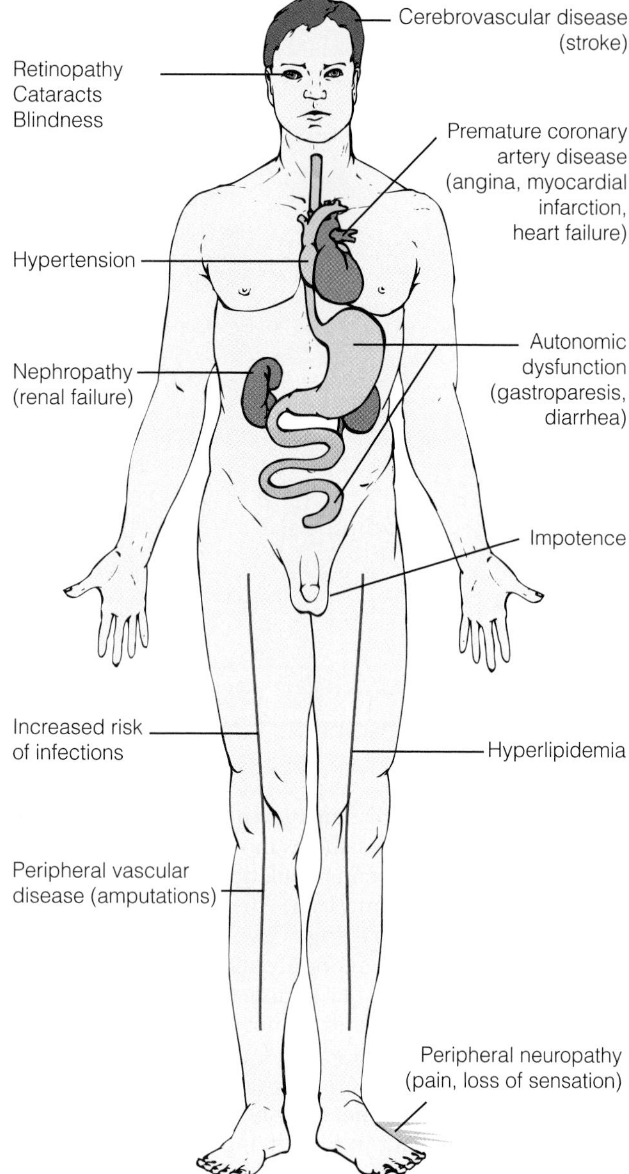

figure 44-3 The complications of diabetes can be widespread.

at least initially. The specific cause of insulin resistance is not known; however, these patients do not suffer from autoimmune destruction of the islet cells of the pancreas. Most patients are obese, and obesity itself can lead to insulin resistance. Ketoacidosis seldom occurs in this form of diabetes because the patient still secretes just enough insulin to avoid critical illness. When the patient does sustain severe complications associated with hyperglycemia, usually he or she has concomitant illness such as myocardial infarction, infection, or trauma. Because of the high incidence of insulin resistance and relative insulin deficiency, hyperglycemic hyperosmolar state (HHS) usually develops in patients with type 2 diabetes when they become critically ill.

Type 2 diabetes can go undiagnosed for many years because this disease progresses slowly. However, the patient is at high risk for developing macrovascular and microvascular complications. Quite often, these patients have normal to higher-than-normal insulin levels. Instead, insulin resistance develops because their circulating insulin is insufficient to prevent hyperglycemia. Insulin resistance is best treated with weight loss, exercise, and pharmacological management. The medications to treat type 2 diabetes range from insulin secretagogues to medications that affect insulin sensitivity. Refer to Table 44-6 and Figure 44-4 for a review of the commonly used oral medications for type 2 diabetes and their mechanisms of action. Eventually, many people with diabetes require insulin as their disease progresses. The risk for developing type 2 diabetes increases with age, obesity, sedentary lifestyle, and family history of type 2 diabetes. Its incidence varies with ethnicity.

Diabetic Ketoacidosis

PATHOPHYSIOLOGY

Diabetic ketoacidosis (DKA) is a critical illness that manifests with severe hyperglycemia, metabolic acidosis, and fluid and electrolyte imbalances. DKA results from severe insulin deficiency that leads to the disordered metabolism of proteins, carbohydrates, and fats. The concomitant elevation of counter-regulatory hormones such as growth hormone (GH), cortisol, epinephrine, and glucagon exacerbates the condition, leading to further hyperglycemia and hyperosmolality, ketoacidosis, and volume depletion. Figure 44-5 outlines these mechanisms and their interrelationships.

Three major physiological disturbances exist in DKA: (1) hyperosmolality due to hyperglycemia, (2) metabolic acidosis due to accumulation of ketoacids, and (3) volume depletion due to osmotic diuresis. Each of these three disturbances may be more or less severe in any patient. Furthermore, interactions among these disturbances may occur, aggravating (or possibly partially compensating for) one another.

Hyperglycemia and Hyperosmolality

The first major consequence of DKA is hyperosmolality due to hyperglycemia. The hyperglycemia seen in DKA is the result of excessive hepatic glucose production. With insulin deficiency, the plasma glucose level rises. As illustrated in Figure 44-6, the concomitant effects of the counter-regulatory hormones, particularly cortisol and catecholamines, further aggravate hyperglycemia by enhancing gluconeogenesis, insulin resistance, and lipolysis.

The central mechanism that protects against hyperosmolality is excretion of glucose by the kidneys. Glucose is filtered at the kidney glomerulus. With normal circulating blood volume and a normal glucose load, all this glucose is reabsorbed into the bloodstream. However, when the blood sugar exceeds the normal threshold of about 180 mg/dL, glucose begins to escape into the urine because the reabsorption capacity of the tubules is exceeded. As the glucose load to be filtered increases, glucose is lost rapidly in the urine. Eventually, nearly all of the additional glucose put into the circulation is lost into the urine. The renal "escape valve" serves as a protective device to prevent extreme accumulation of glucose in blood. Indeed, in people with diabetes whose circulating blood volume is well maintained, it is extremely unusual to find blood sugar

table 44-5 Comparison of Type 1 and Type 2 Diabetes Mellitus

	Type 1 Diabetes	Type 2 Diabetes
Etiology	Autoimmune destruction of islet cells	Insulin resistance
Incidence	10%	90%
Age of onset	Usually before 35 years	Usually after 35 years
Speed of onset	Usually rapid	Usually gradual
Nutritional state	Usually thin	Usually overweight, obese
Endogenous insulin	Absent	Low or high, rarely absent
Symptoms	Polyuria, polydipsia, polyphagia, weight loss	Same, plus blurred vision, fatigue
Ketosis	Frequently present with poor control	Infrequent
Treatment goal	Exogenous insulin management	Weight loss, exercise, improved insulin resistance
Treatment	Exogenous insulin, diet control, exercise, weight maintenance	Oral agents, diet control, exercise, weight loss

levels in excess of 500 mg/dL because of the intense glucose diuresis. Conversely, any patient whose blood sugar is higher than this level has either a severely reduced circulating blood volume, renal damage, or both.

Glycosuria is largely responsible for volume depletion. A vicious cycle occurs in a patient whose diabetes is badly out of control and who cannot take in enough sodium and water to compensate for urinary losses. Hyperglycemia leads to volume depletion, which in turn reduces urinary glucose losses and permits the blood sugar to rise even higher.

This hyperosmolality of body fluids and dehydration probably accounts for the lethargy, stupor, and, ultimately, the coma that occurs as DKA worsens. Diabetic patients who have ketoacidosis without hyperosmolality are less likely to have changes in consciousness.

Ketosis and Acidosis

The second major consequence of severe insulin deficiency is uncontrolled ketogenesis (see Fig. 44-6). As ketoacids enter the ECF, the hydrogen ion is stripped from the molecule and neutralized by combining with bicarbonate ion buffer, thereby protecting the pH of the ECF and leaving behind ketoacid anion residues. The resulting carbonic acid breaks down into water and carbon dioxide gas, which is exhaled.

As ketoacid anions accumulate, they progressively displace bicarbonate from the ECF. The usual laboratory determination of electrolytes does not measure ketoacid concentration directly. However, an excess of total measured cations (sodium plus potassium) over total measured anions (chloride plus bicarbonate) provides a clue to the presence of these so-called unmeasured anions. This excess, referred to as the *anion gap*, can serve as an indirect measure of the quantity of ketoacids present.

The following formula is used to calculate the anion gap:

$$(\text{Sodium}) - (\text{Chloride} + \text{Carbon Dioxide})$$

The normal value is less than 15 mEq/L. An abnormal result indicates metabolic acidosis. For example, if sodium = 144 mEq/L, chloride = 92 mEq/L, and carbon dioxide = 26 mEq/L, then the anion gap is 26 mEq/L, a value that indicates severe metabolic acidosis. As the ketoacids continue to accumulate, the serum bicarbonate falls and the anion gap increases. If this continues, the pH falls, and the acidosis becomes life-threatening.

Another cause of metabolic acidosis in DKA is the formation of lactic acidosis resulting from poor tissue perfusion and hypovolemia. This further exacerbates the anion gap, decreasing the serum bicarbonate level. Neutrality of body fluids is protected primarily by the bicarbonate buffering system, which determines the pH at all times by the ratio of bicarbonate anion to carbon dioxide in plasma. If bicarbonate anion is lost because of its displacement by ketoacid anions, excess carbon dioxide gas must be driven off at the level of the lung by hyperventilation. This process keeps the ratio at or close to its usual value of 20:1 and maintains the pH close to its physiological value of 7.4. Hyperventilation, which is gradual at first and then rapidly becomes more vigorous and more obvious as the arterial pH drops below 7.2, is a characteristic physical finding in DKA. This dramatic increase in ventilation, which occurs more by an increase in the depth than in the frequency of breathing, is known as Kussmaul's respirations. It is associated with the classic "fruity" odor of the breath in DKA. The presence of clear-cut Kussmaul's respirations is a signal that the ECF pH is at or below 7.2, a relatively severe degree of acidosis.

Volume Depletion

Ketoacids are excreted in the urine largely as sodium, potassium, and ammonium salts. This contributes to the third pathophysiological problem of DKA: volume depletion and fluid and electrolyte loss as a result of osmotic diuresis.

Although loss of glucose through the kidneys helps protect against the ravages of extreme hyperosmolality,

table 44-6 ■ Oral Pharmacologic Agents to Treat Diabetes Mellitus

Drug	Example	Action	Duration of Action	Nursing Considerations
First-generation sulfonylureas	Tolinase, Diabinese	Stimulates pancreatic insulin secretion	12–60 h	Side effects include hypoglycemia, gastrointestinal disturbances, and rash Contraindicated in pregnancy
Second-generation sulfonylureas	Glyburide, Glucotrol, Micronase	Stimulates pancreatic insulin secretion	10–24 h	Side effects include hypoglycemia, gastrointestinal disturbances, and rash Safer in elderly patients
Biguanides	Metformin (Glucophage)	Reduces hepatic glucose production, increases insulin sensitivity	8 h	Lactic acidosis is a serious side effect (stop when using contrast medium for x-rays); other side effects include gastrointestinal disturbances (e.g., flatulence, diarrhea) Use with caution in patients with renal disease Improves insulin resistance Promotes weight loss
Thiazolidinediones	Actos, Avandia	Enhances insulin's effects at receptor sites	12–24 h	Will not increase level of circulating insulin Side effects include edema, weight gain, and anemia Monitor liver function tests Improves lipid profile
Alpha-glucosidase inhibitors	Precose, Miglitol	Inhibits metabolism of carbohydrates in intestines	8 h	Take with meals Side effects include gastrointestinal symptoms (e.g., flatulence, abdominal pain, diarrhea, nausea) Use with caution in patients with renal disease
Meglitinides	Prandin	Stimulates beta cell insulin release		Side effects include hypoglycemia, upper respiratory infection, headache, and diarrhea Use with caution in patients with hepatic or renal disease
Amino acid derivatives (insulin secretagogue)	Starlix	Stimulates beta cell insulin release		Side effects include hypoglycemia, gastrointestinal disturbances (e.g., nausea), upper respiratory tract symptoms, and dizziness Use with caution in patients with hepatic disease
Combination therapy (Glucovance)	Glyburide and metformin	As above with each drug	As above with each drug	As above with each drug

the diabetic patient who develops ketoacidosis pays a price for this glycosuria. Glucose remaining in the glomerular filtrate after the renal tubules have reabsorbed all they can forces water to remain in the tubules. This glucose-rich filtrate then flows out of the body, carrying with it water, sodium, potassium, ammonium, phosphate, and other salts. This rapid urine flow and obligate loss of water and electrolytes is known as an *osmotic diuresis*. Salts of ketone bodies and the urea resulting from rapid protein breakdown and accelerated gluconeogenesis also contribute to the solute load in the renal tubule, further aggravating the diuresis. The average amounts of salts and water lost to the body through osmotic diuresis during the development of DKA have been measured. Overall water loss in a 70-kg adult patient with DKA can be 5 to 8 L, or 15% of total body water.

The fluid lost to the body is slightly hypotonic; it contains a slight excess of water compared with the volume of salts. This is expected from an osmotic diuresis due to glucose and urea. The fluid losses result from the combination of many different factors, including the intensity and duration of the hyperglycemia and osmotic diuresis; the amount of water and electrolyte replaced orally during this time; the presence of other fluid and electrolyte losses,

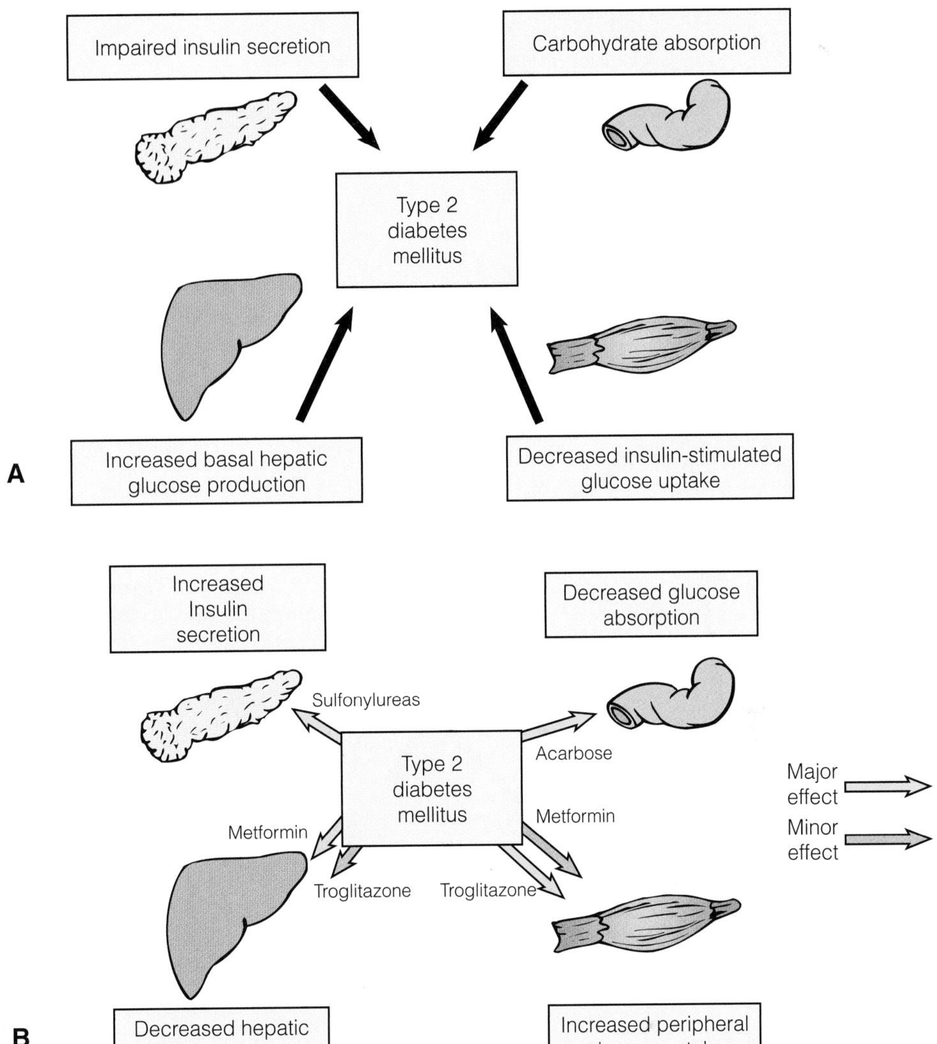

figure 44-4 (**A**) Factors leading to elevated blood glucose levels in type 2 diabetes mellitus. (**B**) Mechanisms of action of the oral hypoglycemic agents used in the treatment of type 2 diabetes mellitus. (Source: Porth CM: Pathophysiology: Concepts of Altered Health States [6th Ed], p 940. Philadelphia, Lippincott Williams & Wilkins, 2002).

such as vomiting, diarrhea, or sweating; and the integrity of renal function.

Sodium and water make up the central structure of the ECF, including the vascular volume. When large quantities of sodium and water are lost in the urine, the body perceives it as a serious threat to the maintenance of the circulation. A variety of compensatory mechanisms are called into play to prevent vascular collapse and shock. For example, an increase in pulse rate usually occurs, which helps maintain cardiac output in the face of shrinking intravascular volume.

At least as important, however, is a protective shift in body fluid brought about by the hyperglycemia. Because free glucose is limited almost entirely to the extracellular water, an osmotic pressure gradient is set up across the cell membrane, between the extracellular compartment and the interior of the cells. Therefore, the higher the blood sugar, the more water is drawn out of cells and into the extracellular space. Therefore, as sodium and water are lost into the urine, shrinking the ECF, they are "replaced" (at least as to their osmotic effect) by glucose entering from the liver and by water entering from all cells. This re-expands the ECF.

Although hyperosmolality produces damaging CNS effects and osmotic diuresis, it provides a temporary mechanism for preventing vascular collapse. Despite these compensatory mechanisms, circulatory volume falls as DKA progresses. This leads to decreased glomerular filtration, decreased tissue perfusion, metabolic acidosis, and shock.

As the vascular volume falls, glomerular filtration also falls. This decreasing renal function leads to increasing blood levels of glucose, potassium, urea nitrogen, and creatinine. The excretion of potassium by the kidney occurs through the exchange of potassium for sodium. Therefore, adequate sodium must be present at the exchange site in the kidney for the rate of potassium excretion to keep pace with the need for excretion. If renal perfusion falls, enough sodium may not be available for this exchange. As a result, despite a total body depletion of potassium, the serum potassium level may rise above normal, even to dangerously high levels.

A second major consequence of diminished vascular volume is a generalized decrease in tissue perfusion. Well before the drop in volume has reached the point at which blood pressure actually falls and full-blown shock occurs, blood is shunted away from many tissues, and the perfusion of nearly all tissues suffers. The resulting decrease in oxygen causes those tissues to shift to some degree of anaerobic glucose metabolism. This results in the increased production of lactic acid. The release of lactic acid into the

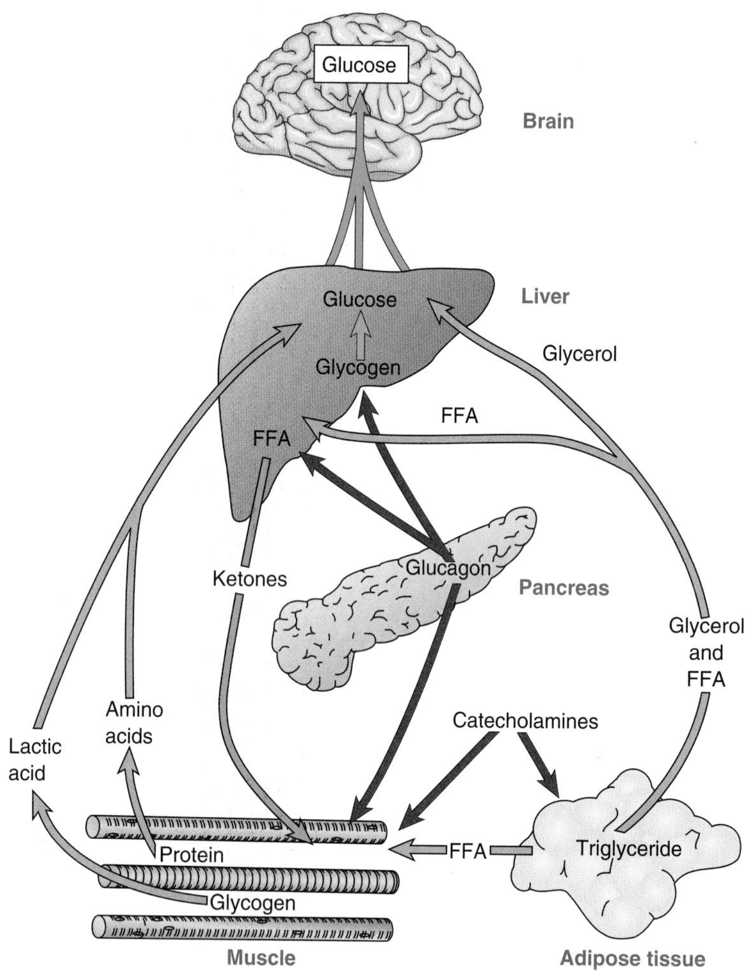

figure 44-5 Mechanisms of diabetic ketoacidosis (DKA). DKA is associated with very low insulin levels and extremely high levels of glucagon, catecholamines, and other counter-regulatory hormones. Increased levels of glucagon and catecholamines (*red arrows*) lead to mobilization of substrates (*blue arrows*) for gluconeogenesis and ketogenesis by the liver (*green arrows*). Gluconeogenesis in excess of that needed to supply glucose to the brain and other glucose-dependent tissues produces a rise in blood glucose levels. Mobilization of free fatty acids (FFA) from triglyceride stores in adipose tissue leads to accelerated ketone production and ketosis. (Source: Porth CM: Pathophysiology: Concepts of Altered Health States [6th Ed], p 943. Philadelphia, Lippincott Williams & Wilkins, 2002.)

circulation lowers the bicarbonate further, aggravating the already existing metabolic acidosis. Therefore, in patients with DKA, combined lactic acidosis and ketoacidosis is a common finding.

The loss of phosphate in the urine worsens tissue hypoxia. As body phosphate stores are depleted, circulating plasma phosphate levels fall quite low, depriving the red blood cells of organic phosphate compounds. Under these circumstances, the red blood cells become depleted of certain key phosphate derivatives, which in turn increases the tightness of oxygen binding to the hemoglobin in these cells. As these cells pass through poorly perfused tissues, less oxygen is given up, and tissue hypoxia worsens.

Finally, if vascular volume falls low enough, compensation mechanisms fail, blood pressure drops, and true shock supervenes. A rapidly worsening cycle of acidosis, tissue damage, and deepening shock may then occur, leading ultimately to irreversible vascular collapse and death. The full-blown syndrome of DKA is characterized by major contributions from all three major pathophysiological disruptions, each of which is primarily responsible for one of the major clinical features: coma, shock, and metabolic acidosis.

CAUSES

The most common cause of DKA is infection. Other precipitating factors include severe illness (cerebrovascular accident [CVA], myocardial infarction, pancreatitis), alcohol abuse, trauma, and drugs. In addition, many people with type 1 diabetes present with DKA on initial diagnosis. Also, many patients with type 1 diabetes suddenly discontinue their insulin and deteriorate; reasons for insulin omission in younger patients include fear of weight gain, fear of hypoglycemia, rebellion against authority, and the stress of chronic disease. Other reasons given for sudden discontinuation of insulin or oral medications include lack of knowledge and poor compliance related to lack of financial resources.

ASSESSMENT

Initial laboratory analysis should include an immediate glucose level using a venous sample and glucose meter measurement at the bedside to confirm the diagnosis. While these preliminary data are collected, an intravenous line is inserted and volume replacement is started. A more considered assessment follows, which begins with details of the history and physical examination, a search for precipitating causes, and more complete laboratory tests. Physical examination and laboratory findings in DKA are summarized in Box 44-8.

History and Physical Examination

If ketoacidosis is strongly suspected, an effort is made to establish the diagnosis quickly so that life-preserving

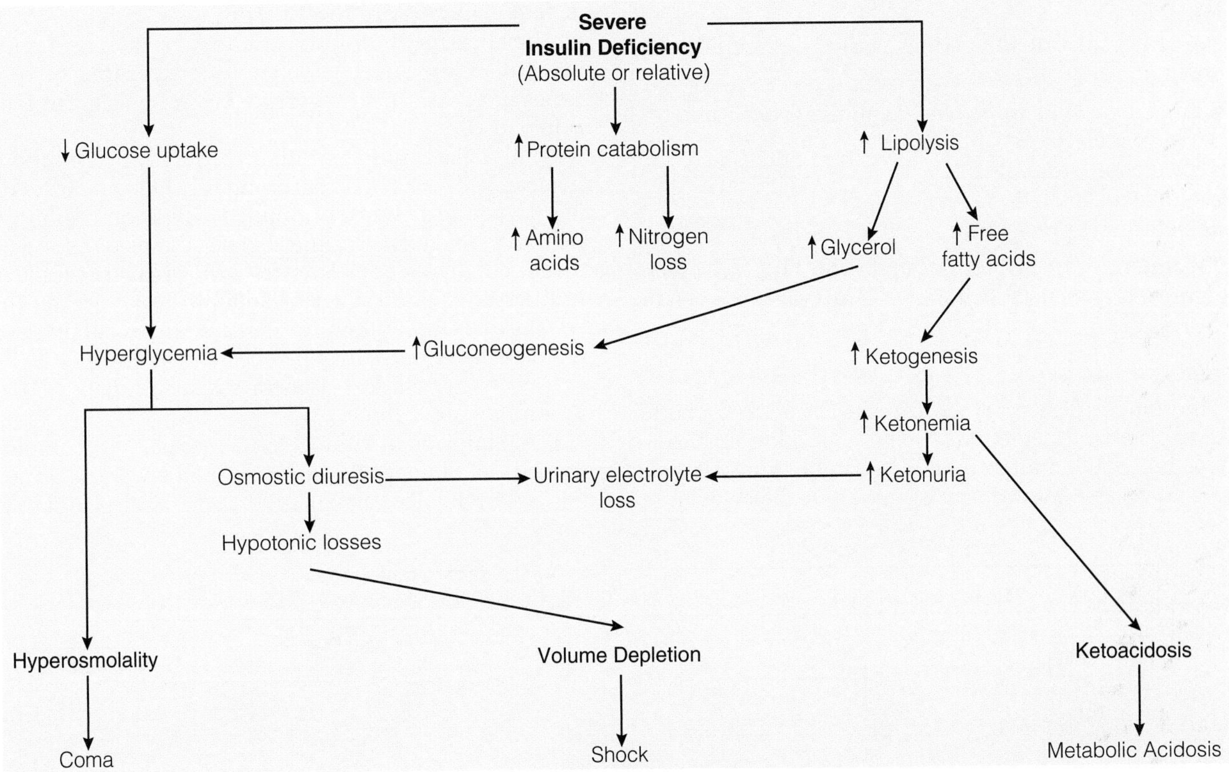

figure 44-6 The metabolic consequences of severe insulin deficiency and the interrelations of these consequences lead to diabetic ketoacidosis (DKA). (Adapted from Davidson MD: Diabetic ketoacidosis and hyperosmolar nonketotic syndrome. In Diabetes Mellitus: Diagnosis and Treatment [3rd Ed], pp 175–212. New York, Churchill Livingstone, 1991.)

therapy can be started. Initial data collection includes an abbreviated history from the family or friends of an unconscious patient, a search for a diabetic identification card, and rapid assessment for clinical clues of volume depletion. After asking about the diabetic regimen, medications, and recent changes in health, a review of systems is performed. Questions concern appetite, weight change, food and fluid intake, thirst, abdominal bloating and discomfort, bowel function, and urinary frequency and amount. Cognition and responsiveness can be observed while interviewing the patient. Possible findings include thirst, frequent urination, poor appetite, nausea and vomiting, abdominal cramps, fatigue, weakness, and drowsiness. The patient may also have symptoms related to urinary tract infection, upper respiratory infection, and chest symptoms because infection is often a precipitating factor.

The physical examination includes blood pressure, heart and respiratory rate, breathing pattern, heart sounds and rhythm, breath sounds, capillary refill, color and warmth of extremities, temperature, signs of hydration (e.g., skin turgor, mucus pool under tongue), deep tendon reflexes, level of consciousness, and an abdominal examination. Possible findings include hyperventilation, Kussmaul's respirations and fruity breath, dehydration, abdominal distension, dry mucous membranes, flushed skin, poor skin turgor and perfusion, hypotension, tachycardia, and varying degrees of responsiveness from lethargy to coma.

box 44-8
Signs of Diabetic Ketoacidosis (DKA)

- Hyperventilation
- Kussmaul's respirations and "fruity" breath
- Lethargy, stupor, coma
- Hyperglycemia
- Glycosuria
- Volume depletion
- Hyperosmolality
- Increased anion gap (>7 mEq/L)
- Decreased bicarbonate (<10 mEq/L)
- Decreased pH (<7.4)

Laboratory Studies

Laboratory studies include blood glucose, chemistries, osmolality, anion gap, pH, ABGs, urine acetone, and glucose. Possible findings include hyperosmolality, increased anion gap (>7 mEq/L), decreased bicarbonate (<10 mEq/L), and decreased pH (<7.4). The serum glucose may range from 300 mg/dL to 800 mg/dL or higher. Sodium, potassium, creatinine, and BUN are all elevated. Magnesium and phosphate may also be high.

Diagnostic Studies

Throat, urine, or blood cultures may also be done to determine the presence of infection. A chest x-ray should be obtained to rule out acute infection, and an ECG should be obtained.

MANAGEMENT

Treatment goals for the patient with DKA include the following:

- Improve circulatory volume and tissue perfusion
- Correct electrolyte imbalances
- Decrease serum glucose
- Correct ketoacidosis
- Determine precipitating events

Treatment protocols for the adult with DKA are given in Figure 44-7, and a Collaborative Care Guide is given in Box 44-9.

Fluid Replacement

The immediate threat to life in a critically ill ketoacidotic patient is volume depletion. After establishing an intravenous line, 0.9% (normal) saline is rapidly infused. The goal is to reverse the severity of the extracellular volume depletion and restore renal perfusion as soon as possible. The first liter may be infused in 1 hour in patients with normal cardiac function. This will replace only a fraction of the extracellular loss in the average patient, which can range from 6 to 10 L.

Fluid replacement continues at roughly 1 L/hour until the heart rate, blood pressure, and urine flow indicate that hemodynamic stability is attained. Hypotonic solutions, such as 0.45% normal saline, can be administered at a rate of 150 to 250 mL/hour after the intravascular volume has been restored, or if the serum sodium level is greater than 155 mg/dL. Other plasma expanders, such as albumin and plasma concentrates, may be necessary if low blood pressure and other clinical signs of vascular collapse do not respond to saline alone.

Rapid infusion of saline in DKA has possible complications. It can dilute plasma proteins and lower the osmotic pressure of the plasma. This allows fluid to leak out of the

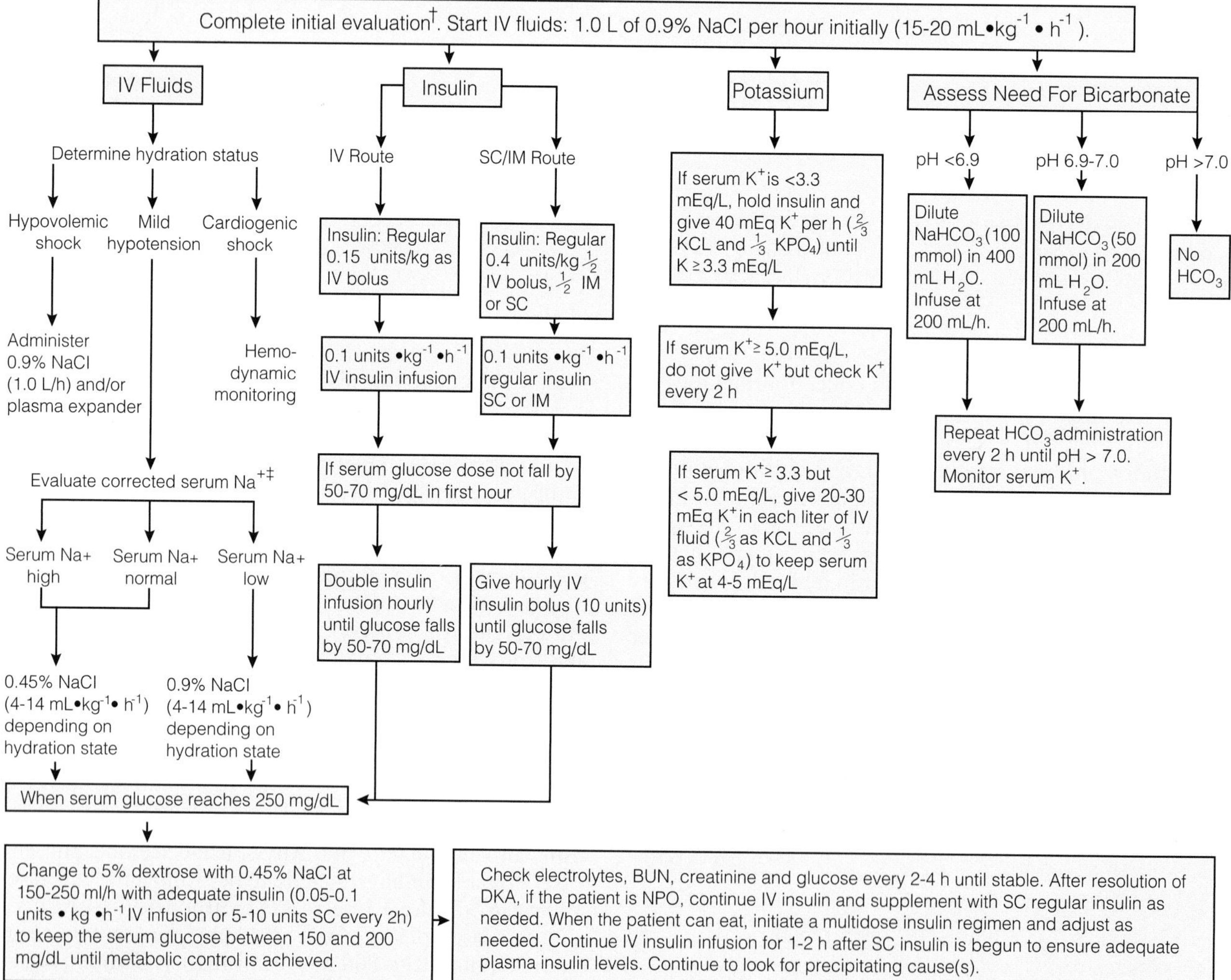

figure 44-7 Management of adults with diabetic ketoacidosis (DKA). *DKA diagnostic criteria: blood glucose >250 mg/dL, arterial pH <7.3, bicarbonate <15 mEq/L, and moderate ketonuria or ketonemia. †After history and physical examination, obtain arterial blood gases, complete blood count with differential, urinalysis, blood glucose, blood urea nitrogen (BUN), electrolytes, chemistry profile, and creatinine levels STAT as well as an electrocardiogram. Obtain chest X-ray and cultures as needed. ‡Serum Na should be corrected for hyperglycemia (for each 100 mg/dL glucose >100 mg/dL, add 1.6 mEq to sodium value for corrected serum sodium value). IM, intramuscular; IV, intravenous; SC, subcutaneous. Copyright © 2002 American Diabetes Association. (From Diabetes Care [Suppl 1]: S100–S108, 2002. Reprinted with permission from The American Diabetes Association.)

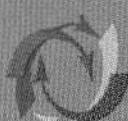

box 44-9 collaborative care guide *for the Patient With Diabetic Ketoacidosis (DKA)*

OUTCOMES	INTERVENTIONS
Oxygenation/Ventilation	
Arterial blood gases are maintained within normal limits. No evidence of acute respiratory failure.	■ Provide chest physiotherapy, turn, deep breath, cough, incentive spirometer q 4 h and PRN. ■ Continuously monitor patient's respiratory rate, depth, and pattern. Observe for Kussmaul's respiration, rapid and shallow breathing, and other signs of respiratory distress. ■ Monitor arterial blood gases, pulse oximetry and, if intubated, end tidal CO_2. ■ Provide supplemental oxygen. ■ Prepare for intubation and mechanical ventilation (see Collaborative Care Guide for Patient on Ventilator).
The patient's lungs are clear. There is no evidence of atelectasis or pneumonia.	■ Auscultate breath sounds q 2 h and PRN. ■ Take daily chest x-ray. ■ Provide chest physiotherapy q 4 h. ■ Mobilize out of bed as soon as patient is stabilized.
Circulation/Perfusion	
Blood pressure and heart rate are within normal limits. If PA catheter is in place, hemodynamic parameters are within normal limits.	■ Monitor vital signs q 1 h and PRN. ■ Assess for dehydration/hypovolemia: tachycardia, decreased CVP and PAWP. ■ Assess for hypervolemia: neck vein distension, pulmonary crackles and edema, increased CVP and PAWP. ■ Administer vasopressor agents if hypotension is related to vasodilation.
Patient is free of dysrhythmias.	■ Monitor ECG continuously. ■ Evaluate and treat the cause of dysrhythmias (eg, acidosis, hypoxia, hypokalemia/hyperkalemia).
Fluids/Electrolytes	
Evidence of rehydration without complications: —balanced intake and output —normal skin turgor —hemodynamic stability —intact sensorium	■ Infuse normal saline or lactated Ringer's, then 0.45% normal saline. ■ Monitor serum osmolality, urine output, neurological status, and vital signs closely during rehydration. Observe for complications of DKA (eg, shock, renal failure, decreased LOC and seizures). ■ Assess BUN, creatinine, urine for glucose and ketones.
Normal serum electrolytes and acid–base balance.	■ Assess and replace electrolytes, Mg, and PO_4, as indicated. ■ Closely monitor potassium fluctuations as serum glucose is decreased and acidosis reversed. ■ Assess arterial pH and bicarbonate level q 2–4 h during rehydration and insulin administration.
Serum glucose returns to normal range.	■ Monitor serum glucose q 30–60 min, then q 1–4 h after level <300 mg/dL. ■ Administer IV insulin bolus then continuous low dose infusion. ■ Infuse $D_5$1/2 normal saline or D_5W, after glucose is <300 mg/dL.
Mobility/Safety	
The patient will be free of injury related to altered sensorium or seizures.	■ Place on seizure and falls precautions. ■ Assess neurological status q 1 h, then q 2–4 h after initial rehydration phase.
Maintain muscle tone and joint range of motion.	■ Provide range-of-motion exercises q 4 h. ■ Reposition in bed q 2 h. ■ Mobilize to chair when condition stable. ■ Consult physical therapist.

(continued)

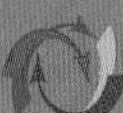

box 44-9 collaborative care guide
for the Patient With Diabetic Ketoacidosis (DKA) (Continued)

OUTCOMES	INTERVENTIONS
Skin Integrity	
Skin will remain intact.	■ Assess risk for skin breakdown using the Braden Scale. ■ Initially assess skin and circulation q 1–2 h for 12 h. ■ If risk for skin breakdown low, assess skin q 8 h and each time patient is repositioned. ■ Turn q 2 h. ■ Consider pressure relief/reduction mattress if at risk for skin breakdown.
Nutrition	
Calorie and nutrient intake meet metabolic requirements per calculation (eg, Basal Energy Expenditure).	■ Provide parenteral feeding if patient is NPO. ■ Provide clear, then full liquid diet, and assess patient response. ■ Progress to diabetic diet (ADA). ■ Consult dietitian or nutritional support service regarding special nutritional needs.
No evidence of metabolic dysfunction.	■ Monitor albumin, prealbumin, transferrin, cholesterol, triglycerides, glucose, and protein levels.
Comfort/Pain Control	
Patient will have minimal pain, <5 on pain scale.	■ Assess pain and discomfort. If pain present, use objective pain scale q 4 h PRN and following administration of pain medication. ■ If analgesics are needed, administer cautiously due to risk of respiratory and neurological complications. ■ Consider nonpharmacological pain management techniques (eg, distraction, touch).
The patient's nausea, vomiting, and abdominal pain or tenderness will resolve.	■ Maintain nasogastric tube patency. ■ Assess bowel sounds q 1–2 h. ■ Administer antiemetic as ordered. ■ Provide ice chips and frequent oral hygiene.
Psychosocial	
Patient demonstrates decreased anxiety.	■ Provide nonjudgmental atmosphere in which patient can discuss concerns and fears. ■ Provide patients who are intubated with a method to communicate. ■ Provide patients with decreased LOC with sensory input. ■ Provide for adequate rest and sleep.
Teaching/Discharge Planning	
Patient/significant others understand the tests needed for treatment.	■ Prepare patient/significant others for procedures such as EEG, ECG, and multiple laboratory studies.
Significant others understand the severity of the illness, ask appropriate questions, anticipate potential complications.	■ Explain the widespread effects of diabetes and the potential for complications of DKA such as seizures, renal failure or vascular collapse. ■ Encourage significant others to ask questions related to complications, pathophysiology, monitoring, treatments, etc.
Patient/significant others are prepared for home care.	■ Teach patient and family information needed to manage diabetes: diabetic diet, skin care, glucose monitoring, insulin administration, signs and symptoms of hypoglycemia and hyperglycemia and appropriate actions. ■ Discuss sick-day management and factors that can precipitate DKA. ■ Initiate contacts with diabetic support groups, social services and home health agency.

vascular space through the capillary walls and contributes to the development of pulmonary edema or cerebral edema, particularly in children and older adults. Therefore, patients must be observed carefully during the first 24 to 36 hours for signs of pulmonary or cerebral edema.

Volume losses continue throughout the first hours of treatment until the glycosuria and osmotic diuresis are controlled. The next step of fluid replacement can be based on an estimate of the patient's total body fluid loss. About 80% of the fall in blood sugar during treatment of DKA is due to glucose loss into the urine, rather than the result of insulin-induced changes in glucose production and consumption. Therefore, in the earliest phases of treatment, insulin therapy complements fluid and electrolyte replacement.

Insulin Therapy

Insulin is important in treating ketoacidosis for several reasons. It decreases the production of ketones by shutting off the supply of free fatty acids emerging from adipose tissue. It inhibits hepatic gluconeogenesis. This prevents further glucose from being added to the ECF. Simultaneously, hepatic ketogenesis is further reduced. Insulin also restores cellular protein synthesis. This effect occurs more slowly and permits the restoration of normal potassium, magnesium, and phosphate stores in tissues.

Blood sugar should not fall too fast or too far. Sudden and rapid lowering of the blood sugar with insulin allows water to move very rapidly back into the cells. This can potentially lead to vascular collapse. Instead, early volume replacement should include sodium and water either before or along with insulin therapy.

Low-dose insulin is given by continuous intravenous infusion rather than by intravenous bolus or subcutaneous doses. Intramuscular insulin injections are an alternative to intravenous insulin; however, they should be avoided in hypotensive patients because absorption is unpredictable. Guidelines for insulin administration are summarized in Box 44-10.

Insulin initially should be given as an intravenous bolus of regular insulin at 0.15 U/kg body weight followed by a continuous infusion of regular insulin at a dose of 0.1 U/kg/hour. When the plasma glucose reaches 250 mg/dL, the insulin infusion should be decreased and dextrose should be added to the intravenous fluids. Hypoglycemia should be avoided at this point to prevent cerebral edema that may occur when the blood–brain barrier is affected by extreme fluid shifts.

Potassium and Phosphate Replacement

The initial plasma potassium in patients with DKA can range from very low to very high. Therefore, potassium is not given until the laboratory report is available. Beginning intravenous potassium therapy in the presence of unrecognized hyperkalemia and inadequate renal mechanisms for handling potassium loads can be fatal. Although the ECG can provide clues to the presence of high or low potassium levels, potassium therapy should not be based on the ECG alone.

If the initial serum potassium level is low, intravenous potassium is usually started right away. This is particularly important because both insulin and saline drive the potassium even lower, possibly to dangerously low levels at which skeletal muscle paralysis and cardiac arrest may occur. If the initial potassium is normal or high, intravenous potassium is usually withheld until the level has begun to drop and urine flow is established. Potassium is usually replaced at concentrations of 20 to 40 mEq/L of intravenous fluid, depending on the serum potassium level. Failure of the potassium to fall can occur for the following reasons:

- Persistent, uncorrected acidosis (which drives potassium out of cells and into ECF)
- Hyperosmolality
- Intrinsically impaired renal function
- Insufficient circulating volume

Phosphate levels usually also drop during therapy, aggravating any pre-existing tendency of red blood cells to bind oxygen more tightly. Therefore, many patients receive phosphate in the middle and later phases of therapy. It is usually combined with potassium replacement in the form of potassium phosphate salts added to the intravenous infusion. Patients who are receiving intravenous phosphate therapy should be watched carefully for signs of tetany: tingling around the mouth or in the hands, neuromuscular irritability, carpopedal spasm, or even seizures. Tetany can occur because phosphate lowers the level of circulating calcium.

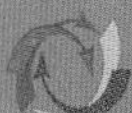

box 44-10 nursing interventions for *Insulin Administration*

- Administer insulin intravenously to the patient with diabetic ketoacidosis (DKA) to minimize the trauma of repeated injections.
- Use only human regular insulin in intravenous insulin infusions because it is less antigenic than animal (beef, pork) insulins.
- Administer the insulin infusion through an intravenous infusion pump. Flush tubing well with insulin mixture before infusing to patient to prevent tubing from absorbing too much insulin.
- When the serum glucose level reaches 250 mg/dL, the intravenous fluids should be changed to a glucose-based solution.
- Changes in blood sugar and clinical state should indicate a clear-cut beneficial response to insulin and fluid replacement. If blood sugar does not drop and blood pressure and urine output do not stabilize, insulin or fluid replacement may not be adequate.

Bicarbonate Replacement

Patients with mild or moderate ketoacidosis who are treated with salt, water, and insulin eventually excrete and metabolize the ketone bodies remaining in ECF. As this process continues, more bicarbonate anions are reabsorbed from the renal tubules, and the bicarbonate deficit is slowly repaired. Sometimes the large amounts of chloride administered along with the sodium in intravenous saline can produce a transient hyperchloremia; this delays the full return of the bicarbonate level to normal for several days.

Bicarbonate is administered to patients with severe acidosis as indicated by an arterial pH of 7.0 or less, whose bicarbonate levels are initially 5 mEq/L or lower. It should also be given when there is cardiac decompensation. The bicarbonate deficit can be calculated and replaced intravenously over several hours to raise the level at least to the 10 to 12 mEq/L range. Sodium bicarbonate should be administered by slow intravenous infusion over several hours. It is administered as a bolus injection only in the case of cardiac arrest. Sodium bicarbonate administration can cause a rapid reduction in plasma potassium concentration and sodium overload.

Reestablishing Metabolic Function

Gastric motility is greatly impaired in DKA. Gastric distension with dark, hemopositive fluid and vomiting is common. Abdominal pain, tenderness, and a paralytic ileus may also be due to DKA. The patient may need a nasogastric tube to decompress the stomach. This increases comfort and decreases the risk of aspiration. Patients should not eat or drink in this phase of illness. Ice chips may decrease thirst. Later, when distension lessens and motility returns, oral intake begins in order to provide the complex nutritional requirements for recovery.

Metabolic abnormalities should not be corrected too rapidly, especially in patients in whom DKA has been developing for a long time. The key risks during this phase are worsening stupor or coma, hypotension, and hyperkalemia. Osmotic or pH disequilibrium may occur when blood sugar or bicarbonate has been corrected too rapidly. The patient's mental state may worsen even though blood chemistries are improving. Rapid reduction of blood sugar without sufficient sodium and water replacement may be responsible for hypotension. However, sepsis, myocardial infarction, and other causes of shock may also cause hypotension. Hyperkalemia usually results from premature potassium infusion, persistent acidosis, and insufficient volume replacement. However, there may be an early occlusion of the arterial supply to a limb. This can cause large amounts of potassium to leak into the circulation. Therefore, limbs are monitored for asymmetrical pallor, coolness, and rubor.

Although patients begin to improve during the initial phase of treatment, recovery usually takes place over approximately 12 days. During this time, most metabolic abnormalities are reversed, and body stores of many nutrients (e.g., magnesium, protein, and phosphate) are replenished. Once recovery is well underway, it is time to help the patient and family understand how to prevent a recurrence.

PATIENT EDUCATION

Patients and families who are well informed about diabetes may be more likely to recognize early signs of complications, minimize their development, and seek help if they begin to occur. Although people usually understand the need for insulin injections when they are hungry and eating normally, they may not understand why they need their insulin when they are ill, have no appetite, are not eating, or are vomiting. Teaching points after an episode of DKA are given in Box 44-11. Box 44-12 presents a "sick day" plan for managing diabetes.

case study ■ COMPLICATIONS OF DIABETES MELLITUS

Ms. Smithson, age 23 years, was admitted to the hospital with the chief complaints of fatigue, cough, nausea, and vomiting for 4 days. She had been diagnosed as having diabetes mellitus 8 years before admission. Since that time, she had been maintained on 24 units of NPH and 9 units of regular insulin in the morning and 11 units of NPH and 6 units of regular insulin in the evening. Four days before admission, she began to cough, raising first clear, then brownish, sputum. She soon became fatigued, and then experienced some nausea and intermittent vomiting. For several days before admission, she omitted her evening insulin, and then took no further insulin the day before and the day of admission, "because she was not eating anything." On the day of admission, the patient's mother noted that she had become "less responsive and was breathing fast and deeply" and brought her to the emergency department.

On admission, the patient's rectal temperature was 38.1°C, her pulse was 132 beats/minute, her respirations were 32 breaths/minute and deep, and her blood pressure

box 44-11
Self-Management After Ketoacidosis

- A person with diabetes, as any other person, must have insulin, even if no food is being taken in.
- The amount of insulin required when the person with diabetes is not eating is about half the total needed when eating.
- The amount of insulin required when a person with diabetes is fasting must be spread out as an insulin "trickle" rather than as an insulin "burst."
- Illness generally increases the need for insulin so that even if the person with diabetes is not eating, he or she may actually require more than 50% of the usual daily dose.
- Always keep enough insulin on hand for daily injections.
- Know how to reach a health care provider for timely phone advice.
- When you are ill, adjustments for managing your diabetes may need to be made (see Box 44-12).

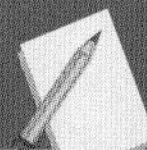

box 44-12
"Sick Day" Plan for Managing Diabetes

- Take your usual daily dose of insulin or oral hypoglycemic agent.
- Place an early call to your health care provider to inform him or her of your symptoms and actions.
- Monitor your blood glucose every 4 hours or a minimum of four times a day.
- Test your urine for ketones every 4 hours if your blood glucose level is 240 mg/dL or greater.
- Inject small, supplemental doses of short-acting insulin several times daily, if necessary, according to blood glucose test results until glucose levels come under control.
- Consume liberal amounts of fluids, such as water, tea, broth, apple and grape juice, and popsicles.
- Eat easily digested carbohydrates, such as custard, pudding, cream soup, saltine crackers, and toast, if you are unable to eat your normal diet.

was 98/52 mm Hg. She was oriented but lethargic, with coarse rales at both lung bases. She had been incontinent of urine.

Admission laboratory work revealed the following: hematocrit 48.6%; white blood cells 36,400/mm^3; glucose 910 mg/dL; sodium 128 mEq/L; potassium 6.7 mEq/L; chloride 90 mEq/L; bicarbonate 4 mEq/L; BUN 43 mg/100 mL; creatinine 2.3 mg/dL; serum ketones 4+; urine glucose and ketones 4+. ABGs revealed the following: arterial blood pH 7.06; PaO_2 112 mm Hg; $PaCO_2$ 13 mm Hg; bicarbonate 2.5 mEq/L. The admission chest film was positive for right lower lobe infiltrate, and sputum cultures on admission ultimately grew out *Haemophilus influenzae* and *Streptococcus pneumoniae.*

Initial therapy consisted of several liters of intravenous infusion of normal saline and 20 units regular insulin by intravenous push, followed by an infusion of insulin at 5 units per hour during the first 9 hours. The patient's mental status and sense of well-being improved rapidly. The flow sheet in Box 44-13 summarizes the biochemical changes over the first 15 hours.

Ms. Smithson remained febrile for several days and was treated with antibiotics. By the time of discharge 4 days later, she was eating well, her blood sugars were controlled on her usual doses of NPH insulin, and her cough had improved.

CASE ANALYSIS

- *Hyperglycemia and hyperosmolality.* Ms. Smithson presented with the classic findings of extreme hyperglycemia. As expected in this situation, the BUN and creatinine were elevated, indicating that renal perfusion was reduced, permitting less glucose to escape into the urine and allowing the blood sugar to reach these high levels. The patient's lethargic mental state was the result of the moderately severe hyperosmolality and dehydration.
- *Ketosis and acidosis.* For Ms. Smithson, the extremely low initial bicarbonate concentration of 2.5 to 4 signaled the consumption of nearly all the available buffering capacity of plasma, indicating the presence of severe metabolic acidosis. This conclusion was reinforced by the anion gap of 42 mEq/L ([128 + 7] – [90 + 3]), about 27 mEq/L above the usual anion gap upper limit of 15 mEq/L, indicating the presence of 27 mEq/L of "unmeasured anions." The serum ketones were strongly positive, confirming the presence of a large quantity of ketone bodies, which could account for most of the unmeasured anions. These findings confirmed the diagnosis of severe DKA. The patient's deep, rapid breaths represented Kussmaul's respirations, a critically important compensating mechanism that had reduced her arterial CO_2 level ($PaCO_2$) to about one-fourth its usual level and had helped keep her blood pH from falling below its already very low level of 7.06.
- *Volume depletion: fluid and electrolyte losses.* Ms. Smithson's history of increasing symptoms over at least 4 days suggests that this episode of ketoacidosis had been developing for a substantial period of time, sufficient for osmotic diuresis to produce extensive salt and water losses. Nausea prevented volume replacement by mouth, and vomiting further aggravated the losses. Ms. Smithson failed to realize the need to initiate sick day measures to control her serum glucose level or the need to consult her physician immediately. As this case illustrates, the diabetic patient with concomitant illness as severe as pneumonia must continue to take insulin because the body's needs for insulin actually increase during acute illness. This is due to the effects of the counter-regulatory hormones that prepare the body for a stressful event.

box 44-13
Biochemical Flow Sheet Indicating Diabetic Ketoacidosis in Ms. Smithson

TIME	SUGAR	pH	Na	K	Cl	HCO_3	BUN/CREATININE
1:00 PM	710	7.06	128	6.9	90	4	43/2.3
3:00 PM	492		132	6.8	101	6	41/1.7
5:15 PM	375	7.25	137	4.1	106	8	45/1.4
10:00 PM	303		139	4.7	114	15	27/1.2
4:00 AM	304		143	4.3	113	22	22/1.1

They exacerbate the hyperglycemia because excess catecholamines and epinephrine synergize gluconeogenesis and resultant hyperglycemia. The rapid pulse and low blood pressure on admission were further clues to the presence of significant hypovolemia. This was confirmed by the elevated BUN and creatinine, reflecting inadequate circulating blood volume to maintain renal perfusion. Finally, the elevated serum potassium (potassium = 6.7 mEq/L, normal = 3.5 to 4.8 mEq/L) indicated that not enough sodium was being filtered in the kidneys to permit adequate potassium exchange and potassium excretion.

- *Response to treatment.* Despite severe hyperglycemia, metabolic acidosis, and volume depletion, Ms. Smithson responded promptly to volume replacement with saline and low-dose intravenous insulin. Clinical and chemical signs indicated steady and progressive improvement over the first 15 hours of treatment. Rapid fluid infusion was possible because she was young and otherwise quite healthy. The blood sugar fell from 710 to 304 mg/dL over this time as glucose continued to be lost through the kidneys. The presence of insulin also decreased the hepatic production of glucose. The falling BUN and creatinine indicated that volume replacement had restored renal perfusion. The serum bicarbonate level rose from 4 to 22 mEq/L without the use of intravenous bicarbonate. The production of ketones was turned off by insulin; instead, the ketones were metabolized to bicarbonate, which was then reabsorbed by the kidney. Arterial blood pH was restored from its initial very low level of 7.06 to 7.25 as the bicarbonate buffer reappeared in plasma. Serum potassium fell from 6.9 mEq/L into the normal range as insulin drove potassium back into cells, pH improved, osmolality returned to normal, and improved renal perfusion permitted exchange of potassium for sodium. Finally, the serum chloride rose from the low initial value of 90 mEq/L (normal range, 96 to 103 mEq/L) to the abnormally high level of 114 mEq/L. The mechanism for this is not entirely understood but is partly due to the intravenous infusion of large amounts of chloride. Fortunately, despite Ms. Smithson's severe chemical abnormalities, she was lethargic rather than comatose. This may have been because she was young and otherwise healthy, and the ketoacidosis had developed over a short time. She did not need to be intubated or catheterized, and she tolerated the rapid shifts in volume, pH, and osmolality induced by therapy very well. Her rapid response resulted in a brief hospitalization. The slow replenishment of body constituents and readjustment of diabetic regimen—the fourth phase of therapy—could be safely carried out at home with nurse and physician supervision.
- *Preventing recurrence.* The precipitating causes of the ketoacidosis in Ms. Smithson were classic: the onset of respiratory infection and possibly some initial gastroenteritis and Ms. Smithson's failure to recognize the continuing need for insulin even in the absence of food intake. This episode of ketoacidosis could probably have been prevented if she had continued to take insulin, perhaps one-half to two-thirds her usual dose, with supplemental short-acting insulin as needed. If the nausea and vomiting had been controlled early, she might also have been able to continue oral fluid and sodium replacement. This situation points out the value of a "diabetes illness plan" and of early contact during an acute illness with a physician or a nurse familiar with diabetes management. ■

Hyperosmolar Hyperglycemic State

Sometimes a marked hyperglycemia and hyperosmolality without ketoacidosis develops in patients with diabetes. This is the syndrome of HHS. Patients are usually middle-aged or older with type 2 diabetes, sometimes not yet diagnosed. Ketosis is mild or absent.

HHS has a higher mortality rate than any other complication of diabetes, reflecting the higher morbidity associated with patients affected by this type of diabetic emergency. Often, these elderly, obese patients suffer from other severe medical conditions such as congestive heart failure or kidney disease. Extremely high levels of glucose coupled with severe dehydration in a vulnerable, elderly patient with other medical illnesses explain the higher mortality rate for this diabetic complication.

HHS is compared with DKA in Table 44-7.

PATHOPHYSIOLOGY

It is not known specifically why some people with diabetes develop HHS rather than DKA, although it is speculated that these patients may have just enough insulin to prevent ketosis. Pathophysiologically, the mechanisms of disease are the same as for DKA. A reduction in circulating insulin coupled with the effects of counter-regulatory hormones such as cortisol and epinephrine leads to the development of hyperglycemia and the extreme hyperosmolar state. Usually, the patient has coexisting impaired renal excretion of glucose and antecedent renal insufficiency or prerenal azotemia. Because basal insulin levels are unaffected, excessive ketone production does not occur. The acidosis that these patients develop is attributed to lactic acidosis from poor tissue perfusion instead of ketoacidosis.

Marked dehydration develops if the patient is unable to maintain an adequate fluid intake. As dehydration worsens, the patient develops increasing serum glucose and serum osmolality. The life-threatening cycle of hyperglycemia, hyperosmolality, osmotic diuresis, and profound dehydration triggers the sympathetic nervous system "fight-or-flight" response. The counter-regulatory hormones epinephrine and cortisol stimulate gluconeogenesis and increase hepatic glucose production. Dehydration worsens and leads to CNS dysfunction. Confusion and lethargy ensue quickly. Hemoconcentration of the blood increases the risk of clot formation, thromboemboli, and infarcts in major organs.

CAUSES

HHS may occur secondary to extreme stress associated with severe medical illness such as stroke, myocardial infarction, pancreatitis, trauma, sepsis, burns, or pneumo-

table 44-7 Comparison of Signs and Symptoms of Diabetic Ketoacidosis (DKA) and Hyperglycemic Hyperosmolar State (HHS)

	DKA	HHS
Onset	Gradual or sudden, usually less than 2 days	Gradual, usually more than 5 days
Previous history of diabetes mellitus	85% (15% have new onset)	60%
Type of diabetes mellitus	Type 1	Type 2
Age of patient	Usually younger than 40 years	Usually older than 60 years
Mortality risk	1%–15%	20%–40%
Drug history	Insulin	Steroids, thiazides, oral agents
Physical signs	Dehydration, Kussmaul's respirations, mental status changes, "fruity breath," febrile at times	Dehydration, obtundation, hypothermia, toxic appearance, Kussmaul's respirations absent
Glucose level	Mean, 600 mg/dL Range, 250–1200 mg/dL	Mean, 1100 mg/dL Range, 400–4000 mg/dL
Ketones	Present	Absent
Osmolarity	Mean, 320 mOsm/L	Mean, 400 mOsm/L
Arterial pH	Mean, 7.07	Mean, 7.26
Bicarbonate	Markedly low (<10 mEq/L)	Normal or >10 mEq/L
Anion gap	>12 mEq/L	<12 mEq/L

nia. Often, HHS results from excessive carbohydrate intake or exposure such as through dietary supplements, total enteral support with tube feedings, or peritoneal dialysis. Elderly people are at particularly high risk, especially those who have impaired cognition and who are in long-term chronic care facilities. Drugs such as corticosteroids, thiazide diuretics, sedatives, and sympathomimetics affect carbohydrate metabolism adversely and may lead to glucose impairment.

ASSESSMENT

History and Physical Examination

The nurse assesses the patient for precipitating or associated events. This syndrome can be iatrogenic (e.g., induced by certain medications, hemodialysis against hyperosmolar glucose solutions, or prolonged intravenous hypertonic glucose infusions such as those given for total parenteral nutrition). It can also be precipitated by serious medical illnesses such as pneumonia or pancreatitis.

Often family members or long-term care personnel report that the patient became a bit drowsy, took in less food and fluid over several days, and slept more until he or she became hard to awaken. The patient often arrives at the hospital with serious volume depletion and in a stupor or coma. The signs and symptoms of HHS are given in Table 44-7.

The clinical manifestations may take days to weeks to develop, and the patient often displays weakness, polyuria, polydipsia, and impaired mental state ranging from confusion to coma. Dehydration is manifested by tachycardia, hypotension, low cardiac output, poor skin turgor, rapid respirations without Kussmaul's breathing, and warm, flushed skin.

Laboratory Studies

Hyperglycemia in HHS is, by definition, a blood glucose level greater than 600 mg/dL. In addition to extracellular sodium and water losses, a large additional "free water" deficit exists, probably because patients do not become thirsty, causing them to take in decreasing amounts of fluid. As a result, patients have very high serum levels of sodium and glucose. Glucose can be in excess of 2,000 mg/dL. Serum osmolality is extremely high (>310 to 320 mOsm/kg). Patients may have some degree of ketosis as well, but usually are nonketotic. In HHS, the anion gap attributable to ketoacids usually is less than 7 mEq/L. The patient may present with azotemia, hyperkalemia, and lactic acidosis as well.

MANAGEMENT

Therapy for HHS is directed at correcting the volume depletion, controlling hyperglycemia, and identifying the underlying cause of HHS and treating it. The volume depletion is usually greater in HHS than in DKA. Rapid rehydration is more cautiously carried out owing to the fragile state of the patient, who often has comorbidities. Isotonic saline or hypotonic saline is administered initially to correct the fluid imbalance, and some patients may require as many as 9 to 12 L of fluid overall. The nurse should be vigilant for the signs of fluid overload during rehydration. Figures 44-8 and 44-9 provide algorithms for caring for people with HHS who are older than and younger than 20 years, respectively.

Critically ill patients require hemodynamic monitoring during fluid resuscitation, especially elderly patients with cardiac or renal disease. Careful monitoring of fluid intake, urine output, blood pressure, central pressures, pulse, and neurological status are some of the nurse's primary responsibilities. In addition, the patient requires frequent laboratory monitoring.

Patients receive low doses of insulin along with the fluid replacement. Low-dose insulin is given by continuous infusion (0.1 mg/kg/hour) because this population is vulnerable to the sudden loss of circulating blood volume that occurs with higher doses of insulin and a rapid blood sugar reduction. As the glucose level returns close to normal (250 to 300 mg/dL), the insulin infusion is stopped and dextrose is added to the intravenous fluids to prevent a sudden drop in the blood glucose level. At this point, insulin can be administered subcutaneously.

The underlying cause of HHS should be investigated and treated if possible. For example, underlying infection from pneumonia should be managed aggressively with antibiotics, chest physiotherapy, turning, and coughing/deep breathing or suctioning as needed to clear the infiltrate. Exogenous sources of glucose (tube feedings, peri-

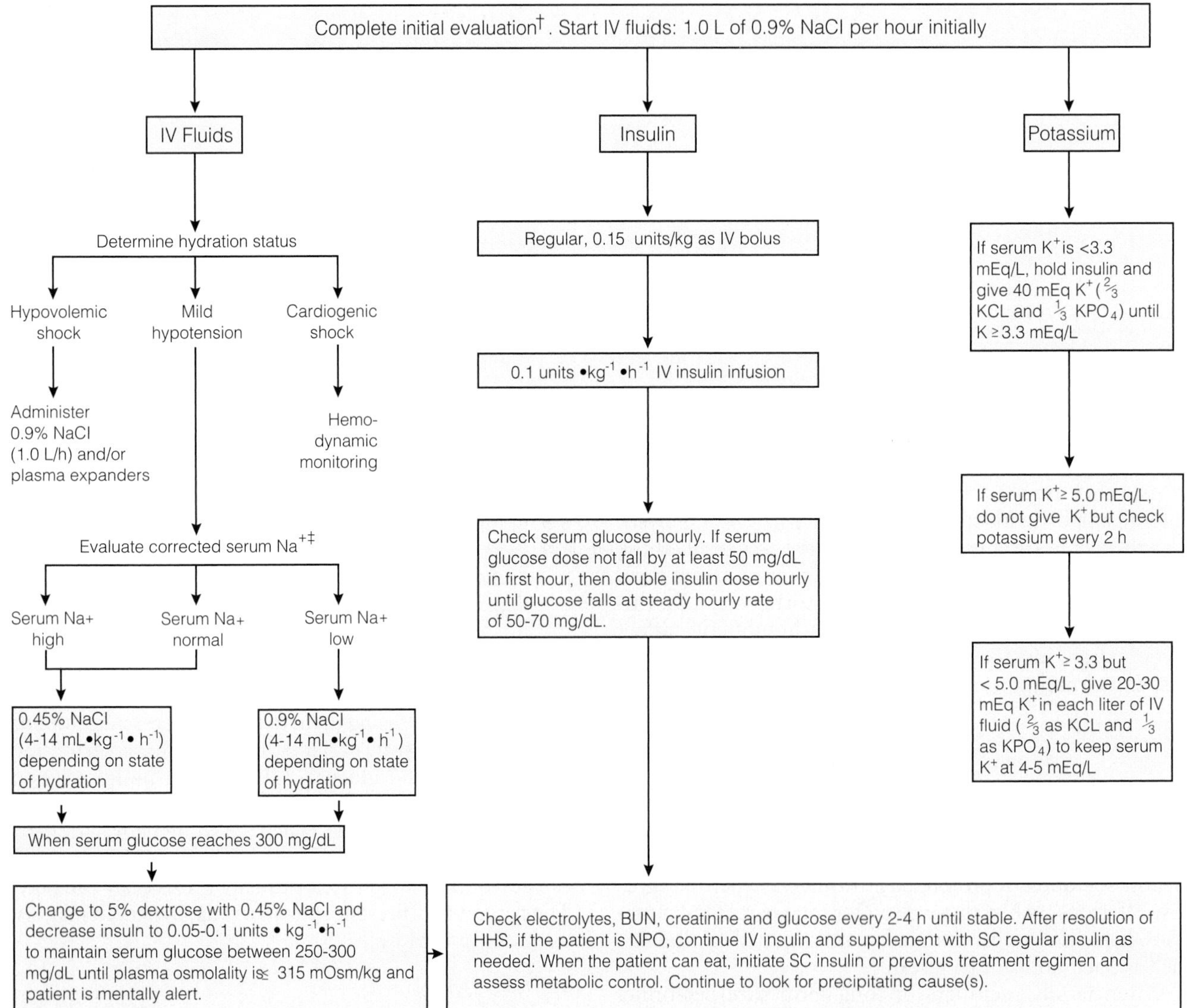

figure 44-8 Management of adults with hyperglycemic hyperosmolar state (HHS). *Diagnostic criteria: blood glucose >600 mg/dL, arterial pH >7.3, bicarbonate >15 mEq/L, mild ketonuria or ketonemia, and effective serum osmolality >320 mOsm/kg H_2O. This protocol is for patients admitted with mental status change or severe dehydration who require admission to an intensive care unit. Effective serum osmolality calculation: 2 [measured Na (mEq/L)] + glucose (mg/dL)/18. †After history and physical examination, obtain arterial blood gases, complete blood count with differential, urinalysis, plasma glucose, blood urea nitrogen (BUN), electrolytes, chemistry profile, and creatinine levels STAT as well as an electrocardiogram. Obtain chest X-ray and cultures as needed. ‡Serum Na should be corrected for hyperglycemia (for each 100 mg/dL glucose >100 mg/dL, add 1.6 mEq to sodium value for corrected serum value). IV, intravenous; SC, subcutaneous. Copyright © 2002 American Diabetes Association. (From Diabetes Care [Suppl 1]: S100–S108, 2002. Reprinted with permission from The American Diabetes Association.)

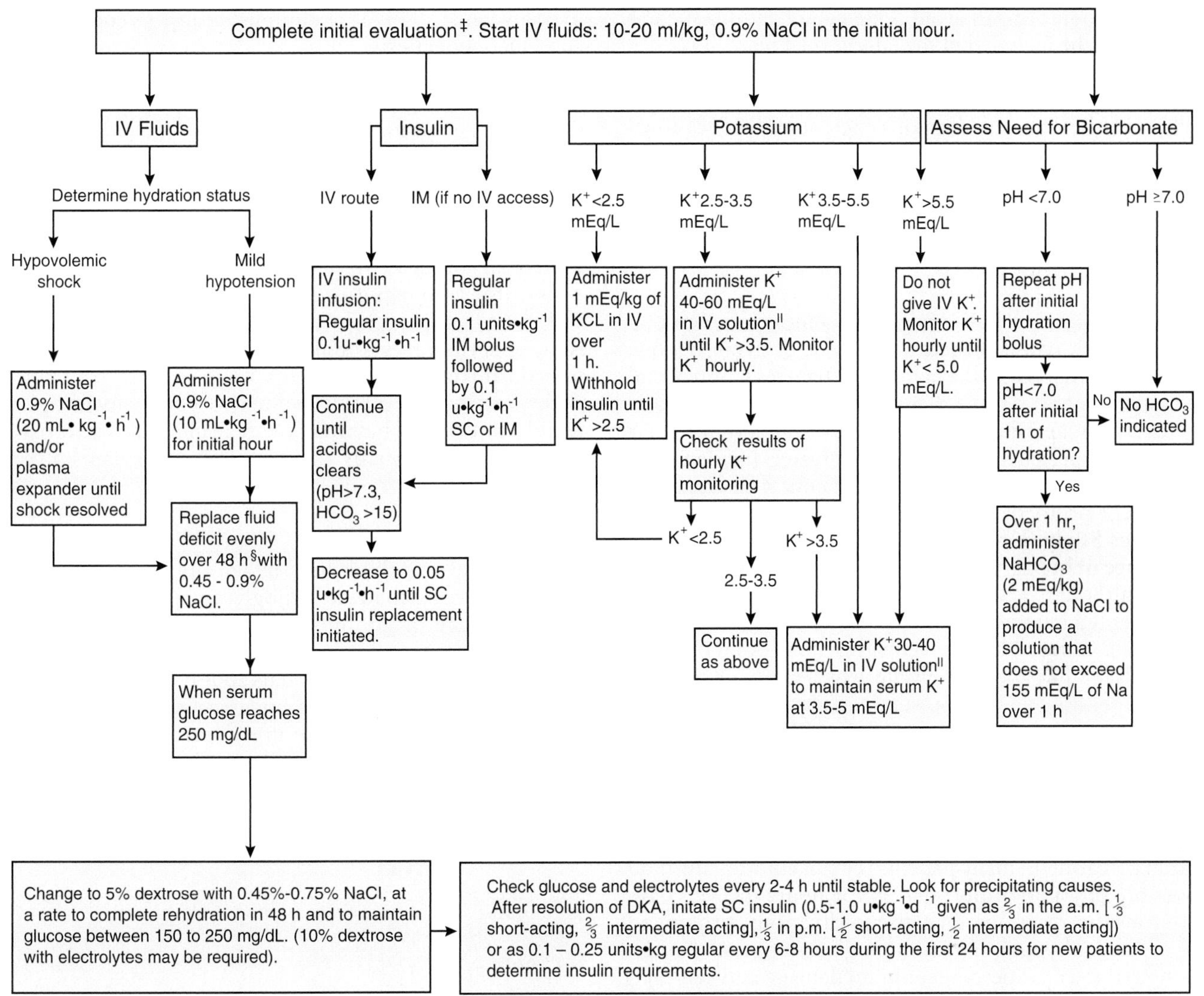

figure 44-9 Management of pediatric patients with diabetic ketoacidosis or hyperglycemic hyperosmolar state (HHS). *DKA diagnostic criteria: blood glucose >250 mg/dL, venous pH <7.3, bicarbonate <15 mEq/L, moderate ketonuria or ketonemia. †HHS diagnostic criteria: blood glucose >600 mg/dL, venous pH >7.3, bicarbonate >15 mEq/L, and altered mental status or severe dehydration. ‡After the initial history and physical examination, obtain blood glucose, venous blood gases, electrolytes, blood urea nitrogen (BUN), creatinine, calcium, phosphorous, and urine analysis STAT. §Usually 1.5 times the 24 h maintenance requirements (~5 ml · kg^{-1} · h^{-1}) will accomplish a smooth rehydration; do not exceed two times the maintenance requirement. ||The potassium in solution should be ⅓ KPO_4 and ⅔ KCl or Kacetate. IM, intramuscular; IV, intravenous; SC, subcutaneous. Copyright © 2002 American Diabetes Association. (From Diabetes Care [Suppl 1]: S100–S108, 2002. Reprinted with permission from The American Diabetes Association.)

toneal dialysis, medications) should be removed while treating the hyperglycemic state.

Older patients who develop HHS have frequent complications and high mortality rates. They often have difficulty handling the fluid volume shifts that occur during the development and treatment of this syndrome. Fluid should be given slowly to avoid complications associated with cerebral edema. These patients are also at risk for intravascular thrombosis and focal seizures because of the hemoconcentration of the blood and the hyperosmolar state. These patients should be placed on seizure precautions at all times. Because these patients usually have a pre-existing cardiac or renal history that predisposes them to complications, fluid resuscitation should proceed slowly and carefully.

PATIENT EDUCATION

As with patients with DKA, the patient and family experiencing HHS need education. Many cases of HHS and DKA can be prevented by better access to medical care, proper education, and effective communication with a health care provider during an intercurrent illness. Many uninsured or underinsured patients stop insulin for economic reasons. The nurse must assess for this possibility.

For the person with newly diagnosed diabetes, the nurse needs to provide information about the pathophysiology of the disease, the signs and symptoms of complications, and methods of treatment, including medications, diet, and exercise. Information about how to manage "sick days" and other tips to avoid acute complications such as HHS must be included in the educational plan.

The patient may need instruction on home management and glucose testing. Often the critical care staff consults with the diabetes educator as the patient's educational plan is being formulated. The main theme should focus on effective techniques to avoid emergency intervention in the future.

Hypoglycemia

Hypoglycemia is a well-recognized complication among patients with type 1 diabetes. The issue of hypoglycemia is well documented in the landmark Diabetes Control and Complications Trial (DCCT), in which people with diabetes who maintained strict, intensive therapy for their diabetes experienced a threefold greater incidence of severe hypoglycemia than those patients with less strict treatment protocols. The United Kingdom Prospective Diabetes Study (UKPDS) demonstrated some increased incidence of hypoglycemia among people with type 2 diabetes, although few severe, life-threatening cases were documented in the study.

Insulin-induced hypoglycemia reactions often occur in the midst of the patient's daily life, which can be, at the very least, embarrassing, and at worst, dangerous. Mild hypoglycemia causes unpleasant symptoms and discomfort; however, severe hypoglycemia can lead to life-threatening complications such as seizures, coma, and even death if not reversed. Even though measurable recovery from hypoglycemia is rapid and complete within minutes after proper treatment, many patients remain emotionally (and possibly physiologically) shaken for hours or even days after insulin reactions. In extreme situations, prolonged or recurrent hypoglycemia, although uncommon, has the potential to cause permanent brain damage and can even be fatal.

PATHOPHYSIOLOGY

Minute-to-minute dependence of the brain on glucose supplied by the circulation results from the inability of the brain to burn long-chain free fatty acids, the lack of glucose stored as glycogen in the adult brain, and the unavailability of ketones. The brain recognizes its energy deficiency when the serum glucose level falls abruptly to about 45 mg/dL. The term *neuroglycopenia* refers to the degree of hypoglycemia sufficient to cause brain dysfunction resulting in personality changes and intellectual deterioration. The exact level at which symptoms occur varies widely from person to person, however, and it is not uncommon for levels as low as 30 to 35 mg/dL to occur (e.g., during glucose tolerance tests) with no symptoms whatsoever among the long-term diabetic population.

Symptoms result from either the sympathetic nervous system response to hypoglycemia or from the neuroglycopenic response. The hypothalamus reacts to the lower glucose levels to mount the adrenergic response, including tachycardia, palpitations, tremors, and anxiety. The goal is to activate the counter-regulatory hormones (glucagon, catecholamines, cortisol, growth hormone) to raise the glucose level and protect vital organs from hypoglycemia. This is accomplished by glycogenolysis and gluconeogenesis.

ASSESSMENT

Occasional reactions happen in even the most stable insulin-dependent diabetic patient. As long as the reactions are mild, they can usually be tolerated without difficulty and are not cause for alarm or for changes in regimen. Frequently, the precipitating event is clear (e.g., a skipped meal or an unusually strenuous bout of exercise). Box 44-14 reviews the common causes of hypoglycemia.

When hypoglycemic reactions are frequent, recurrent, or severe, it is important to identify the cause and prevent further reactions. Otherwise patients may limit their functional activities and may become unwilling or unable to drive. They may overeat in an effort to prevent reactions. Usually the underlying mechanism can be discovered.

History and Physical Examination

The nurse asks about food intake and exercise because these often contribute to hypoglycemia. Problems with insulin dosage or administration may be noted. Every detail of insulin therapy should be investigated thoroughly, including insulin purchase and its appearance, species, and units; syringes, injection sites, and injection technique; and especially any recent change in any part of the regimen. The nurse explores for flaws and inconsistencies in reporting. Prescription errors, mismatched syringe and insulin units, use of new injection sites, and other errors may emerge.

box 44-14
Common Causes of Hypoglycemia

- Insulin shock
- Insulinoma
- Inborn errors of metabolism
- Stress
- Weight loss
- Postgastrectomy
- Alcohol-related
- Glucocorticoid deficiency
- Fasting hypoglycemia
- Profound malnutrition
- Prolonged exercise
- Severe liver disease
- Severe sepsis
- Drug effects
  - Ethanol
  - Salicylates
  - Quinine
  - Haloperidol
  - Insulin
  - Sulfonylureas
  - Sulfonamides
  - Allopurinol
  - Clofibrate
  - Beta-adrenergic agents

The administration or withdrawal of other drugs may be the precipitating event for recurrent insulin reactions. For example, salicylates in large doses can reduce blood sugar and, in combination with insulin, can produce hypoglycemia. Also, use of glucocorticoid medications should be determined. Because these medications cause insulin resistance, insulin doses are often raised to meet the increased insulin demand. If the steroids are then tapered without reducing the insulin dose, hypoglycemic reactions can occur. Alcohol often causes hypoglycemia. Not only do patients often eat less when they have a few drinks, but alcohol shuts off gluconeogenesis by interfering with intermediate biochemical steps in the liver. When combined with injected insulin, this frequently leads to hypoglycemia. Oral hypoglycemic agents can also produce severe and long-lasting hypoglycemia. Patients who experience such episodes tend to be older and undernourished with impaired renal or hepatic function. Nevertheless, any patient on oral agents can become hypoglycemic, especially when the oral agents are potentiated by other agents, such as salicylates and alcohol.

Another common mechanism that can cause hypoglycemia is an atypical (e.g., early or late) response to insulin therapy. Once the response pattern is defined, the insulin regimen can be adjusted and insulin reactions can be eliminated. Occasionally, when a stable, reaction-free patient begins to experience hypoglycemic episodes, the possibility of insulin sensitivity due to weight loss or the onset of azotemia should be explored.

As the blood sugar level falls below normal, the CNS responds in two distinct fashions: first, with impairment of higher cerebral functions, and soon thereafter with an "alarm" response in vegetative functions. Patients most commonly describe the symptoms of mild or early insulin reactions as fuzziness in the head, trouble thinking or concentrating, shakiness, light-headedness, or giddiness. These changes occur when the cerebral cortex is deprived of its main energy supply, usually when the blood glucose has fallen to 50 mg/dL or less or is rapidly declining. This part of the brain is apparently the most sensitive to the loss of glucose.

Changes in personality and behavior vary with the person and may not be apparent to them during an insulin reaction. Changes range from silly, manic, inappropriate behavior to withdrawn, sullen, grumpy, irritable, suspicious behavior. There may be difficulties in motor function, such as trouble walking and slurred speech, and patients who are well into insulin reactions may closely resemble people who have been drinking alcohol.

Some patients experience aphasia, vertigo, localized weakness, and even focal seizures with their insulin reactions. Such focal changes usually occur when there is prior damage to a specific area of the cortex, such as a head injury or CVA.

Closely following the cortical changes is a series of autonomic neurological responses. The primary response is discharge from the centers that control adrenergic autonomic impulses. This results in the release of norepinephrine throughout the body and epinephrine from the adrenals. Tachycardia, pallor, sweating, anxiety, and tremor are characteristic signs of hypoglycemia and are important early warning signs for patients who recognize a reaction. Headache can occur, and the stress response can occasionally trigger secondary sequences of symptoms, including angina or pulmonary edema in patients with fragile cardiovascular disease.

As hypoglycemia persists and worsens, consciousness is progressively impaired, leading to stupor, seizure, or coma. This is characteristic of severe hypoglycemia. The autonomic centers controlling fundamental systems, such as respiration and blood pressure, are the most resistant to hypoglycemia and continue to function even when most other cerebral functions are lost.

The more profound the hypoglycemia and the longer it lasts, the greater the chance of transient or even permanent cerebral damage after blood glucose is restored. There does not seem to be a clear duration threshold for such damage, but severe hypoglycemia lasting more than 15 to 30 minutes can result in some symptoms that persist for a time after glucose is given. Blood sugar measurement, before the administration of glucose if possible, verifies the diagnosis.

MANAGEMENT

Treatment of insulin reactions is always glucose. If the patient can swallow, the glucose is most conveniently given as a glucose- or sucrose-containing drink because in this form it probably gets through the stomach and into the absorbing intestine in the shortest possible time. If the patient is too groggy, stuporous, or uncooperative to drink, a bolus of 25 g of 50% dextrose is given intravenously over several minutes. If this route or dosage is unavailable, 1 mg of glucagon given subcutaneously or intramuscularly reverses the symptoms by inducing a rapid breakdown and release of glucose into the bloodstream from hepatic glycogen stores.

The amount of glucose needed to reverse an insulin reaction acutely is not large. The blood sugar can be raised from 20 to 120 mg/dL with less than 15 g (3 tsp) of glucose in an average-size adult. Glucose in almost any oral form will serve. Typical treatments for hypoglycemia include 3 glucose tablets, 6 ounces of regular cola, 6 ounces of orange juice, 4 ounces of 2% or skim milk, or 6 to 8 Lifesaver candies. Starch, found in crackers and cookies, is broken down to free glucose after passing through the stomach and is absorbed so rapidly that blood sugar rises virtually as fast as with free glucose or sucrose.

As an extension of their fears that they might "never wake up" from a nocturnal insulin reaction, patients are frequently concerned about what to do if they do not respond to the initial therapy. They must be reassured that if the first bolus of glucose consumed does not seem to work, the sensible thing to do is to take in more. Insulin reactions are always reversible with enough glucose. The response to oral glucose, of course, takes time, perhaps 5 to 15 minutes, whereas the response to intravenous glucose should occur within 1 or 2 minutes at most.

Failure to respond fully in the appropriate time indicates that not enough glucose has been given, that the diagnosis is incorrect, or that the hypoglycemia has been long and severe enough to produce persistent, although not necessarily permanent, cerebral dysfunction.

PATIENT EDUCATION

All people with diabetes should be taught to report hypoglycemic reactions to their health care provider for adjustments in their medical regimen. If they are on insulin, they should know when to expect peak effects of the drug so they can predict high-risk times for hypoglycemia. They should always carry a high-glucose snack with them for emergency use, and they should be encouraged to carry medical alert information with them at all times.

clinical applicability challenges

Self-Challenge: Critical Thinking

1. *Examine assessment findings for patients with thyroid crisis and myxedema coma. Compare the findings for fluid volume, metabolic state and body temperature, tissue perfusion, and cardiac output. Then construct collaborative interventions for these clinical issues.*
2. *Consider the additional needs for steroids in the patient with adrenal insufficiency. Relate the general signs and symptoms of the disorder to the underlying pathophysiology of adrenal insufficiency. List high-risk groups of patients who would require close monitoring.*
3. *Compare and contrast fluid volume findings and underlying pathophysiology for patients with syndrome of inappropriate antidiuretic hormone secretion (SIADH) and diabetes insipidus. Formulate interventions to monitor fluid volume excess or deficit for each. Distinguish differences in interventions for patients with these two endocrine disorders.*
4. *Compare and contrast the disorders of diabetic ketoacidosis (DKA) and hyperglycemic hyperosmolar state (HHS) in terms of types of diabetic patients affected, age of the patient, causes, mortality rates, and expected laboratory values. Predict the overall management for both.*
5. *Plan care for the patient experiencing severe hypoglycemia, outlining specific measures to ensure against future occurrences.*

Study Questions

1. *Which one of the following pharmacological agents is indicated for the treatment of hyperthyroidism?*
   a. *Aspirin*
   b. *Synthroid*
   c. *Demeclocycline*
   d. *Propylthiouracil*
2. *Which laboratory value is most consistent with diabetes insipidus?*
   a. *Blood glucose greater than 200 mg/dL*
   b. *Hematocrit greater than 30%*
   c. *Serum osmolality greater than 295 mOsm/L*
   d. *Urine osmolality greater than 150 mOsm/L*
3. *Myxedema coma is characterized by all but which one of the following symptoms?*
   a. *Hypotension, bradycardia, hypothermia*
   b. *Tachycardia, hypotension, hypothermia*
   c. *Hypothermia, tachycardia, hypertension*
   d. *Hypoventilation, bradycardia, hyperthermia*
4. *The most serious underlying problem for the patient with adrenal insufficiency is*
   a. *hyperkalemia.*
   b. *dehydration.*
   c. *hyperglycemia.*
   d. *hypothyroidism.*
5. *Diabetic ketoacidosis (DKA) is often precipitated by which one of the following conditions?*
   a. *Overinsulinization*
   b. *Growth spurt*
   c. *Compliance with oral medications*
   d. *Taking insulin when acutely ill*
6. *Traditional therapy for diabetic ketoacidosis (DKA) consists of all but which one of the following?*
   a. *Fluid replacement with isotonic saline, insulin, possible potassium replacement*
   b. *Fluid replacement with normal saline, insulin, bolus of sodium bicarbonate*
   c. *Fluid replacement with dextrose in 5% lactated Ringer's solution (D_5LR) initially, insulin, chloride bolus*
   d. *Hemodialysis to correct underlying fluid and electrolyte disturbances, insulin, oxygen*
7. *During hyperglycemic hyperosmolar state (HHS),*
   a. *the anion gap is usually 15 mEq/L or greater.*
   b. *ketonemia is present.*
   c. *serum glucose levels may be 600 to 2,400 mg/dL.*
   d. *serum bicarbonate level is less than 10 mEq/L.*
8. *One initial treatment goal of hyperglycemic hyperosmolar state (HHS) is to*
   a. *bring the blood glucose level to a normal range quickly.*
   b. *alleviate ketosis.*
   c. *diurese the patient aggressively.*
   d. *rehydrate the patient slowly.*
9. *Severe hypoglycemia is usually caused by which one of the following?*
   a. *Missed meals or too much exercise*
   b. *Counter-regulatory hormones such as cortisol or epinephrine*
   c. *Skipping oral hypoglycemic medications*
   d. *Severe, critical illness in a patient with diabetes*
10. *Hypoglycemia can be treated by all of the following except*
   a. *glucagon injection.*
   b. *glipizide orally.*
   c. *dextrose intravenous push.*
   d. *orange juice orally.*

OTHER SUGGESTED READING

Allen C, et al: Risk factors for frequent and severe hypoglycemia in type 1 diabetes. Diabetes Care 24(11):1878–1881, 2001

American Diabetes Association: Position statement: Hyperglycemic crises in patients with diabetes mellitus. Diabetes Care 25(Suppl): S100–S108, 2002

American Diabetes Association: Clinical practice recommendations 2002. Diabetes Care 25(Suppl 1):S1–S47, 2002

Becker KL (ed): Principles and Practice of Endocrinology and Metabolism (3rd Ed). Philadelphia, Lippincott Williams & Wilkins, 2001

Brook CGD, Marshall NJ: Essential Endocrinology (4th Ed). Oxford, Blackwell Science, 2001

Carson PP: Emergency: Adrenal crisis. Am J Nurs 100(7):49–50, 2000

Corbett JV: Diagnostic Procedures with Nursing Diagnosis (4th Ed). Stamford, CT, Appleton and Lange, 1996

Cooper DS, DeAngelis CD: Diabetes mellitus: A call for papers. JAMA 286(8):968–969, 2001

Cypress M: Acute complications [Diabetes update: CE articles]. RN 64(4):26–28, 30–32, 2001

Diabetes Control and Complications Trial (DCCT) Research Group: The effect of intensive treatment of diabetes on the development and progression of long-term complications in insulin-dependent diabetes mellitus. N Engl J Med 329:977–986, 1993

Felner EI, White PC: Improving management of diabetic ketoacidosis in children. Pediatrics 108(3):735–740, 2001

Fischbach F: Common Laboratory and Diagnostic Tests (3rd Ed). Philadelphia, Lippincott Williams & Wilkins, 2002

Heater DW: If ADH goes out of balance: Diabetes insipidus. RN 62(7):42–46, 1999

Heater DW: If ADH goes out of balance: SIADH. RN 62(7):47–50, 1999

Kacsoh B: Endocrine Physiology. New York, McGraw-Hill, 2000

Korenman SG (series ed): Atlas of Clinical Endocrinology, Vol I: Thyroid Diseases. Philadelphia, Current Medicine, 2000

Korenman SG (series ed): Atlas of Clinical Endocrinology, Vol IV: Neuroendocrinology and Pituitary Disease. Philadelphia, Current Medicine, 2000

Miller CD, et al: Hypoglycemia in patients with type 2 diabetes mellitus. Arch Intern Med 161(13):1653–1659, 2001

Miller J: Management of diabetic ketoacidosis. J Emerg Nurs 25(6): 514–519, 578–582, 1999

Mokdad AH, Bowman BA, Ford ES, et al: The continuing epidemics of obesity and diabetes in the United States. JAMA 286(10):1195–1200, 2001

Porth CM: Pathophysiology: Concepts of Altered Health States (6th Ed). Philadelphia, Lippincott Williams & Wilkins, 2002

Smeltzer SC, Bare BG: Brunner & Suddarth's Textbook of Medical–Surgical Nursing (10th Ed). Philadelphia, Lippincott Williams & Wilkins, 2004

Tkacs NC: Hypoglycemia unawareness: Your patient with diabetes won't always know when their blood sugar is low. Am J Nurs 102(2):34–41, 2002

Wilber JF: Contemporary Diagnosis and Management of Thyroid Disorders. Newtown, PA, Handbooks in Health Care, 2000

Wilson JD, et al: Williams Textbook of Endocrinology (9th Ed). Philadelphia, WB Saunders, 1998

PART

one
two
three
four
five
six
seven
eight
nine
ten
eleven
twelve

Hematological and Immune Systems

INTERNET RESOURCES

Topic	Web Page Address
AIDS.Org	www.immunet.org
American Cancer Society	www.cancer.org
American Organ Transplant Association	www.a-o-t-a.org
America Society of Clinical Oncology	www.oncology.com
American Society of Hematology	www.hematology.org
American Society of Pediatric Hematology	www.aspho.org
Association of Nurses in AIDS Care	www.anacnet.org
The Body: An AIDS and HIV Information Resource	www.thebody.com
Cancer Source Nursing	www.cancersourcern.com
Community AIDS Treatment Information Exchange	www.catie.ca
HIV InSite	http://hivinsite.ucsf.edu
HIV/AIDS Treatment Information Service	www.hivatis.org
International Transplant Nurses Society	www.itns.org
Johns Hopkins AIDS Service	www.hopkins-aids.edu
Leukemia and Lymphoma Society	www.leukemia.org
National AIDS Treatment Advocacy Project	www.natap.org
National Association on HIV Over Fifty	www.hivoverfifty.org
National Cancer Institute	www.cancer.gov
North American Transplant Coordinators Organization	www.Natco1.org
Oncolink: U of Penn Cancer Center Resource	www.oncolink.upenn.edu
Oncology Nursing Society	www.ons.org
Scientific Registry of Transplant Recipients	www.ustransplant.org
Tumor Cell and Tissue Banking	www.cryoma.com
United Network for Organ Sharing	www.unos.org
United States Website for Organ Donation	www.organdonor.gov

chapter

45

Anatomy and Physiology of the Hematological and Immune Systems

THOMASINE GUBERSKI ■ ANNE BELCHER

objectives

Based on the content in this chapter, the reader should be able to:

- Describe the blood and its components, and the function of each component.
- Delineate the clotting factors and the role each plays in coagulation.
- Describe the anatomy and physiology of the immune system.
- Differentiate between humoral and cell-mediated immunity.

The hematological and immune systems are complex; a change in one system can manifest itself in the other system. For example, a decrease in the number of white blood cells results in an immune system that is less able to resist infection. The systems are interrelated partly because cells for both originate in bone marrow. The anatomy and physiology of these two systems are discussed separately in this chapter, but the reader should keep in mind their close relationship.

HEMATOLOGICAL SYSTEM

Veins, venules, capillaries, arterioles, and arteries constitute an intricate network of conduits for the transportation of blood, which carries respiratory gases, nutrients, and waste products to and from body tissue. Patency of the conduits and containment of blood within the vasculature depend on the integrity of the transporting conduits. A delicate balance must be maintained in the vasculature to ensure both its patency and a liquid state of blood so that neither thrombosis nor hemorrhage occurs. This delicate balance is provided by the hemostatic and fibrinolytic systems working in concert.

Blood and Its Functions

Blood is an aqueous solution of colloid and electrolytes that serves as a medium of exchange between body cells (interior environment) and the exterior, or external, environment. It has distinct characteristics, including variable color (arterial blood is bright red; venous blood is dark red), viscosity (blood is three to four times thicker than water), a pH of 7.35 to 7.4, and a volume of approximately 70 to 75 mL/kg of body weight (5 to 6 L). Plasma constitutes approximately 55% of blood volume, whereas cellular elements suspended in the plasma constitute the remaining 45%.

The vital functions of blood are as follows:

- Transport of oxygen and absorbed nutrients to cells
- Transport of carbon dioxide and other waste products to the lungs, kidneys, gastrointestinal system, and skin
- Transport of hormones from endocrine glands to target organs and tissues
- Protection of the body from life-threatening microorganisms
- Regulation of acid–base balance
- Protection from blood loss through hemostasis
- Regulation of body temperature by heat transfer

See Chapter 16 for a more detailed discussion of circulation.

Components of Blood

PLASMA

Plasma is the liquid portion of the blood and contains a wide variety of organic and inorganic components (Table 45-1). The concentration of these components is a reflection of diet, metabolic demand, hormones, and vitamins. Plasma is approximately 90% water and 10% dissolved solutes. The most prevalent solutes by weight are the plasma proteins and clotting factors. Serum is plasma that has had clotting proteins removed.

Plasma proteins play a role in transport, volume regulation, immune function, and coagulation. Most plasma proteins, including albumin and fibrinogen, are synthesized by the liver; however, the immunoglobulins are synthesized by B lymphocytes. Albumin is essential for regulation of the colloidal osmotic pressure, which is critical for movement of water and solutes through the microcirculation. It also is a carrier molecule for normal blood components and exogenous agents, such as drugs. Immunoglobulins (antibodies) are essential for defense against infectious microorganisms (see the Immune System section in this chapter for a further description). Fibrinogen is the clotting factor that forms the fibrin clot, which is essential to stop bleeding.

Lipoproteins, which include the plasma lipids, triglycerides, phospholipids, cholesterol, and fatty acids, are carried through the blood as complexes with the plasma proteins. Also contained within the plasma, electrolytes (sodium, potassium, calcium, magnesium, chloride, bicarbonate, phosphate, and sulfate) maintain the pH and osmolality of the blood. Plasma nutrients, such as glucose, and gases, such as oxygen and carbon dioxide, are circulated to and from the tissues. Waste products, a final component of plasma, are carried to the appropriate organ for excretion.

table 45-1 Organic and Inorganic Components of Plasma

Constituent	Amount/Concentration	Major Functions
Water	93% of plasma weight	Medium for carrying all other constituents
Electrolytes	Total <1% of plasma weight	Maintain water in extracellular compartment; act as buffers; function in membrane excitability
Sodium (Na)	142 mEq/L (142 mM)	
Potassium (K)	4 mEq/L (4 mM)	
Calcium (Ca)	5 mEq/L (2.5 mM)	
Magnesium (Mg)	3 mEq/L (1.5 mM)	
Chloride (Cl)	103 mEq/L (103 mM)	
Bicarbonate (HCO_3)	27 mEq/L (27 mM)	
Phosphate (mostly HPO_4)	2 mEq/L (1 mM)	
Sulfate (SO_4)	1 mEq/L (0.5 mM)	
Proteins	7.3 g/dL (2.5 mM)	Provide colloid osmotic pressure of plasma; act as buffers; bind other plasma constituents (e.g., lipids, hormones, vitamins, metals); clotting factors; enzymes; enzyme precursors; antibodies (immune globulins); hormones
Albumins	4.5 g/dL	
Globulins	2.5 g/dL	
Fibrinogen	0.3 g/dL	
Gases		
Carbon dioxide (CO_2) content	22–29 mmol/L plasma	Byproduct of oxygenation, most carbon dioxide content from bicarbonate and acts as a buffer
Oxygen (O_2)	PaO_2 80 mm Hg or greater (arterial); PvO_2 30–40 mm Hg (venous)	Oxygenation
Nitrogen (N_2)	0.9 mL/dL	Byproduct of protein catabolism
		Provide nutrition and substances for tissue repair
Nutrients		
Glucose and other carbohydrates	100 mg/dL (5.6 mM)	
Total amino acids	40 mg/dL (2 mM)	
Total lipids	500 mg/dL (7.5 mM)	
Cholesterol	150–250 mg/dL (4–7 mM)	
Individual vitamins	0.0001–2.5 mg/dL	
Individual trace elements	0.001–0.3 mg/dL	
Waste products		
Urea (BUN)	7–18 mg/dL (5.7 mM)	End product of protein catabolism
Creatinine (from creatine)	1 mg/dL (0.09 mM)	End product from energy metabolism
Uric acid (from nucleic acids)	5 mg/dL (0.3 mM)	End product of protein metabolism
Bilirubin (from heme)	0.2–1.2 mg/dL (0.003–0.018 mM)	End product of red blood cell destruction
Individual hormones	0.000001–0.5 mg/dL	Functions specific to target tissue

From Vander AS, Sherman JH, Luciana DS: Human Physiology: The Mechanisms of Body Function (6th Ed.). New York, McGraw-Hill, 1994.

CELLULAR ELEMENTS

Summarized in Table 45-2 along with their functions, the cellular elements of the blood are erythrocytes (red blood cells), leukocytes (white blood cells), and platelets. All blood cell types are believed to be derived from a single stem cell, as shown in Figure 45-1. The production of blood cells (hematopoiesis) occurs in the bone marrow and is a two-stage process that involves mitotic division (proliferation) and maturation (differentiation). Each blood cell type results from pluripotential cells that become committed to a specific cell line when they receive specific biochemical signals. These signals occur when one or more populations of circulating cells have decreased to a certain level. Mitosis occurs, and proliferation continues until the needed number of mature daughter cells enters the circulation.

Erythrocytes

There are approximately 5 million erythrocytes per cubic millimeter of blood. They are produced in the red bone marrow found in the sternum, ribs, skull, vertebrae, and bones of the hands, feet, and pelvis. Normal cell formation requires nutrients such as iron, vitamin B_{12}, folic acid, and pyridoxine. Reticulocytes are released from the bone marrow and circulate for 1 to 2 days while maturing into adult cells. The average life span of an erythrocyte is 115 to 130 days. Dead red blood cells are eliminated mainly by phagocytosis in the liver and spleen.

The erythrocyte is a small, biconcave disk that is reversibly deformable. The flattened, biconcave shape has a surface area to volume ratio that is optimal for the diffusion of gases into and out of the cell. Reversible deformability allows the cell to alter its shape to squeeze through the microcirculation and then return to its normal shape.

Hemoglobin is the iron-containing substance of the erythrocyte. The normal amount of hemoglobin in the body is 12 to 18 g/dL of blood, with a lower level in women and a higher level in men. It is composed of a red compound called *heme* (which contains iron and porphyrin) and a simple protein called *globin*. Each red blood cell contains 200 to 300 million molecules of hemoglobin, which combines with oxygen to form oxyhemoglobin. It also combines with carbon dioxide. Thus, the blood can carry oxygen to the tissues and carbon dioxide to the alveoli of the lungs, where it is expelled into the atmosphere. One iron atom is present for each heme molecule. Total body iron ranges from 2 to 6 g. Two thirds of this is in hemoglobin, whereas the rest is stored in the bone marrow, spleen, and liver. When red blood cells break down, hemoglobin splits into heme and globin factors. The liver stores the iron portion of heme for production of new hemoglobin, and the remainder is converted into bilirubin, which is excreted in feces and urine after conjugation by the liver. This conjugation

table 45-2 **Cellular Components of the Blood**

Cell	Structural Characteristics	Normal Amounts in Circulating Blood	Function	Life Span
Erythrocyte (red blood cell)	Non-nucleated cytoplasmic disk containing hemoglobin	4.2–6.2 million/mm³	Gas transport to and from tissue cells and lungs	80–120 days
Leukocyte (white blood cell)	Nucleated cell	5,000–10,000/mm³	Bodily defense mechanisms	See below
Lymphocyte	Mononuclear immunocyte	25%–33% of leukocyte count (leukocyte differential)	Humoral and cell-mediated immunity	Days or years, depending on type
Monocyte and macrophage	Large mononuclear phagocyte	3%–7% of leukocyte differential	Phagocytosis; mononuclear phagocyte system	Months or years
Eosinophil	Segmented polymorphonuclear granulocyte	1%–4% of leukocyte differential	Phagocytosis; antibody-mediated defense against parasites, allergic reactions; associated with Hodgkin's disease, recovery phase of infection	Unknown
Neutrophil	Segmented polymorphonuclear granulocyte	57%–67% of leukocyte differential	Phagocytosis, particularly during early phase of inflammation	4 days
Basophil	Segmented polymorphonuclear granulocyte	0–0.75% of leukocyte differential	Unknown, but associated with allergic reactions and mechanical irritation	Unknown
Platelet	Irregularly shaped cytoplasmic fragment (not a cell)	140,000–340,000/mm³	Hemostasis following vascular injury; normal coagulation and clot formation/retraction	8–11 days

From McCance KL, Huether SE: Pathophysiology: The Biologic Basis for Disease in Adults and Children (4th Ed), pp 813–814. St. Louis, Mosby, 2002.

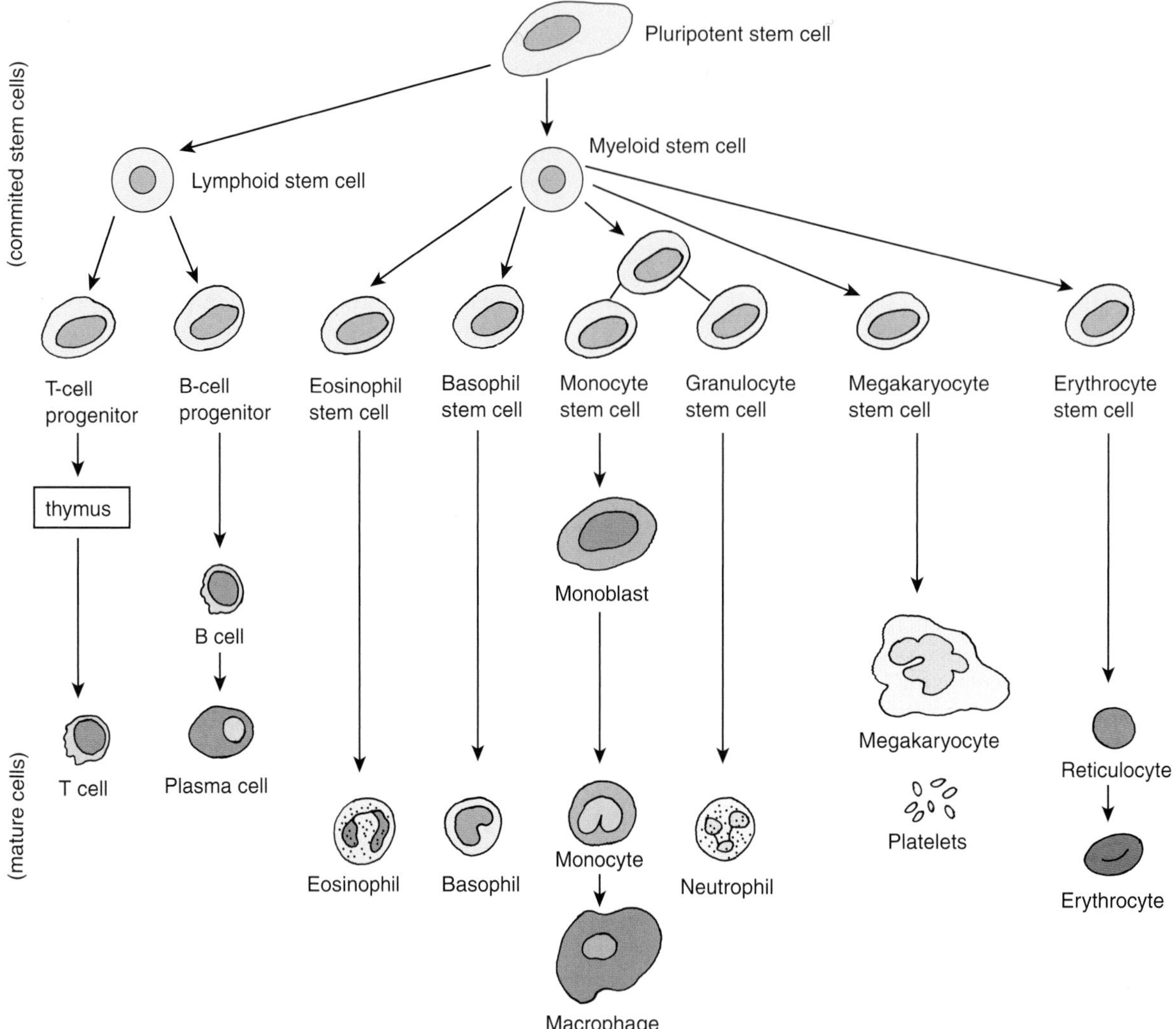

figure 45-1 Major maturational stages of blood cells. (From Porth CM: Pathophysiology: Concepts of Altered Health States [6th Ed], p 255. Philadelphia, Lippincott Williams & Wilkins, 2002.)

process is important to the excretion of bilirubin, which causes jaundice when it accumulates in the tissues (see Chapter 38).

Respiration is a major function of erythrocytes. Hemoglobin combines with oxygen in the lungs. The saturation of hemoglobin with oxygen is influenced by the partial pressure of oxygen available in the lungs, the temperature of the blood, the pH of the blood, and the amount of intracellular 2,3-biphosophyglycerate. For example, people who live at sea level and vacation in high altitudes, where the partial pressure of oxygen in the lungs is lower, may experience shortness of breath because less oxygen is available to combine with hemoglobin.

Leukocytes

Leukocytes, or white blood cells, are transported in the circulation but act primarily in the body tissues, defending the body against microorganisms and foreign antigens and removing debris such as dead or injured host cells. There are approximately 5,000 to 10,000 white blood cells per cubic millimeter of blood. The two major categories of leukocytes are granulocytes and agranulocytes.

Granulocytes comprise approximately 70% of all white blood cells and include neutrophils, eosinophils, and basophils. They are produced by the bone marrow, and their function depends on the type of enclosed granule. Polymorphonuclear leukocytes (PMNs), or neutrophils, fight bacterial infections and digest foreign particulate matter or break down products from cells through phagocytosis. Neutrophils are present during the early acute phase of an inflammatory reaction. After bacterial invasion or tissue injury, they migrate from the capillaries into the inflamed area, reaching their peak in 6 to 12 hours. In the inflamed area they destroy and ingest microorganisms and other debris. They die in 1 or 2 days, releasing digestive enzymes that dissolve cellular debris and prepare the inflamed site for healing.

Eosinophils are particularly important in detoxifying foreign protein. They ingest antigen–antibody complexes, attack parasites, and are elevated during allergic reactions.

Eosinophils have surface receptors for immunoglobulins and histamine.

Basophils contain cytoplasmic granules with vasoactive amines (histamine, bradykinin, and serotonin), which are thought to play a role in the symptoms of acute systemic allergic reactions. Basophils also contain the anticoagulant heparin, histamine, and other vasoactive substances.

Agranulocytes (monocytes, macrophages, and lymphocytes) are leukocytes that do not contain lysosomal granules in their cytoplasm. Monocytes (immature macrophages) and macrophages comprise the mononuclear phagocyte system (formerly called the reticuloendothelial system). They are responsible for the phagocytosis of dead leukocytes and erythrocytes in the blood and for the processing of antigenic material as the neutrophils start to decrease in number. Some of the circulating macrophages migrate out of the blood vessels in response to inflammation or infection, whereas others migrate to fixed sites in lymphoid tissues of the liver, spleen, lymph nodes, peritoneum, or gastrointestinal tract, where they may remain active for months or years. Lymphocytes are immunocompetent cells that are involved in producing antibodies and maintaining the immune response. The most important classifications are B and T lymphocytes, which are discussed later in the chapter.

Platelets

Platelets are disk-shaped cytoplasmic fragments formed from stem cells in the bone marrow, specifically, a giant cell called the *megakaryocyte.* Platelets maintain capillary integrity, accelerate coagulation, and retract clots. There are approximately 250,000 to 500,000 platelets per cubic millimeter of blood; one third of them reside in a reserve pool in the spleen. Platelets live about 10 days; when they die, they are removed from the circulation by macrophages, mostly in the spleen.

Blood Coagulation

Hemostatic homeostasis is maintained through three interdependent components: blood vessels, platelets, and blood coagulation factors. In the course of normal wear and tear, the endothelial lining of blood vessels is subject to damage that requires local repair to prevent blood leakage. The body repairs the vessels through a process called *coagulation.* In this process, damage to, or sloughing of, the endothelium exposes the underlying collagen. This exposed collagen attracts and activates platelets to adhere to it, which begins the formation of platelet plugging. With the attraction of platelets to the exposed collagen, an initial barrier of platelets is formed. These platelets release small amounts of adenosine diphosphate, which causes additional platelets to be attracted and stick to each other. Following this process, there is a release of platelet factor 3 from the platelet membrane, which interacts with various blood coagulation proteins and accelerates clotting.

Platelets play two major roles in the clotting process. First, the platelet plug temporarily plugs the leak in the blood vessel. This plug provides the architectural foundation for the building of the fibrin clot. Second, platelets initiate clotting by way of the intrinsic pathway through the release of platelet factor 3.

COAGULATION FACTORS

Coagulation factors are designated by Roman numerals and numbered according to the order in which they were first identified. When the factors are in active form, they are designated by a lowercase "a" (e.g., factor XIIa). Box 45-1 lists the factors by Roman numeral and common name.

COAGULATION PATHWAYS

Blood coagulation proteins, or coagulation factors, are found in the extrinsic and intrinsic pathways to coagulation. The trigger for coagulation activates either the extrinsic or intrinsic pathway. Recent information about the coagulation cascade indicates some interplay between the extrinsic and intrinsic pathways. Specifically, factor VII, found in the extrinsic pathway, can activate intrinsic pathway factor XI. Likewise, several factors in the intrinsic pathway activate factor VII.[1]

Extrinsic Pathway

The extrinsic pathway is a series of chemical reactions that originate outside the injured structure (Fig. 45-2). Injury to tissues and blood vessels triggers coagulation and results in the release of factor III (thromboplastin) into the circulation. Factor III, catalyzed by factor VII (proconvertin), activates factor X (Stuart-Prower factor). In the presence of calcium ions, factor V (proaccelerin), and platelet factor 3, factor Xa catalyzes the conversion of factor II (prothrombin) to IIa (thrombin) and factor I (fibrinogen) to the fibrin clot.

The result of the interaction among the blood vessels, platelets, and blood coagulation factors is the formation of factor Xa, which, as noted, converts prothrombin to thrombin and results in fibrin formation. The intrinsic and extrinsic pathways merge at factor Xa into a final common pathway to clot formation. See Figure 45-2 for a diagram of the sequence of clot formation. Note that the activation of factor VIII (antihemophiliac factor A) by thrombin causes the activation of factor X, resulting in a self-perpetuating effect.

Calcium plays an important role along the clotting cascade. Many coagulation factors carry two negative charges.

box 45-1
Coagulation Factors

I. Fibrinogen
II. Prothrombin (thrombin in active form–IIa)
III. Thromboplastin
IV. Calcium
V. Proaccelerin
VI. Unassigned
VII. Proconvertin; prothrombinogen; convertin
VIII. Antihemophiliac factor A (factor VIIIR–von Willebrand)
IX. Antihemophiliac factor B; Christmas factor; platelet cofactor II
X. Stuart-Prower factor; prothrombinase
XI. Plasma thromboplastin antecedent
XII. Hageman factor; glass factor
XIII. Fibrin-stabilizing factor; Laki-Lorand factor

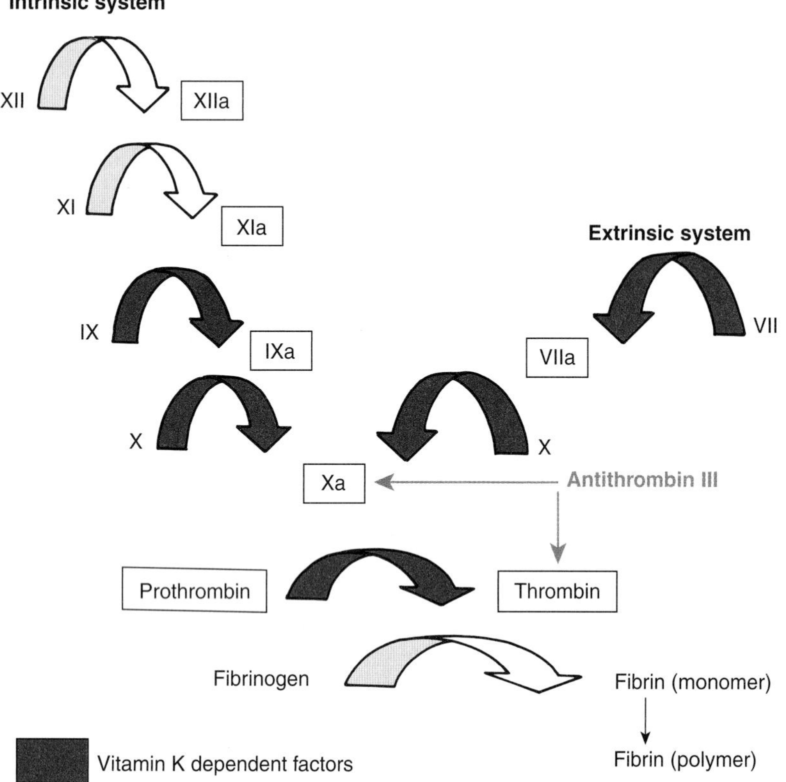

figure 45-2 The coagulation cascade. (From Porth CM: Pathophysiology: Concepts of Altered Health States [6th Ed], p 261. Philadelphia, Lippincott Williams & Wilkins, 2002.)

Calcium, with its two positive charges, creates a strong affinity for the factors to bind at the site of clotting.

Intrinsic Pathway

Normally, blood coagulation factors circulate in the blood in an inactive state. After an initiating stimulus, changes in the coagulation factors occur immediately. The stimulus causes molecular alteration in any inactive coagulation factor, known as a *proenzyme*, converting it to an active form. The product of this enzymatic reaction activates the next coagulation factor in a chainlike reaction, leading to final clot formation. This chain of chemical reactions is termed the *intrinsic pathway*, which indicates its origin from within the tissue.

The release of platelet factor 3 initiates the activation of the intrinsic pathway by activating factor XII (Hageman factor). It is also a necessary component for complex reactions at the levels of factors V and VIII. The exposed collagen, phospholipids from injured erythrocytes and granulocytes, antigen–antibody complexes, and endotoxins are thought to be other activators of factor XII. These activators convert factor XII to the active enzymatic form XIIa, which acts on the next clotting proenzyme, factor XI (plasma thromboplastin antecedent), converting it to XIa. Factor XIa is responsible for the activation of factor IX (antihemophiliac factor B), which requires calcium ions. The activation of the next factor, factor X, requires factor VIII and platelet factor 3. The conversion of factor II to factor IIa (thrombin) requires factor V, platelet factor 3, and calcium ions. Thrombin acts on fibrinogen, converting it to fibrin. This initial soluble fibrin clot is stabilized by factor XIII in the presence of calcium.

Again, the activation of factor VIII by thrombin creates the activation of factor X, resulting in a self-perpetuating effect. Thrombin enhances the activity of factor VIII so that it interacts more rapidly with factor IXa and thus catalyzes the activation of factor X. Thrombin also interacts with platelets, resulting in the release of platelet factor 3, which activates factor XII.

COAGULATION INHIBITORS

Unchecked activation of the blood clotting factors would cause clots to form on top of the platelet plug, releasing thrombin in the process of clotting, further attracting platelets to the clot site, and causing additional clots to form at the local site of the vessel leak (Fig. 45-3). There would be total vessel occlusion if there were no mechanisms operating to maintain the blood in a fluid state and prevent uncontrolled clotting.

There is, however, a well-controlled balance between clot formation and clot inhibition. Through the action of physiological coagulation inhibitors, the blood is maintained in its fluid state and vessels remain patent. These inhibitors—adequate blood flow, mast cells, antithrombin III, the mononuclear phagocyte system, and the fibrinolytic system—work by limiting reactions that promote clotting and by lysing any clots that do form, thereby preventing total occlusion of the vessels. Maintaining adequate blood flow facilitates the quick delivery of dilute-activated clotting factors to the liver, where they are cleared from circulation. Also, mast cells, which are located in most body tissues, produce heparin (which has a low anticoagulant activity compared with that of commercially produced heparin). Next, the liberation of

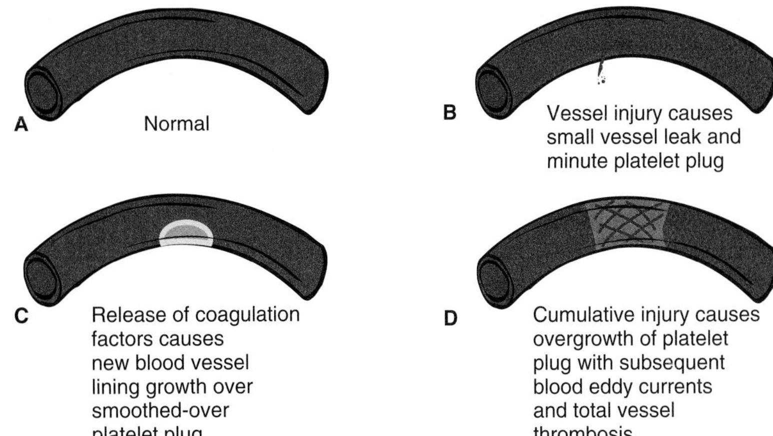

figure 45-3 Sequence of thrombus formation in blood vessels.

antithrombin III in response to thrombin inactivates the circulating thrombin and neutralizes activated factors XII, XI, and X. This retards the conversion of fibrinogen to fibrin, thereby stopping sequential activation of clotting factors. Also, the mononuclear phagocyte system, composed of tissue macrophages located throughout the body, inhibits coagulation by clearing activated factors from the blood. Finally, the fibrinolytic system interferes with thrombin at its site of action on fibrinogen. It also involves a chain reaction whereby activation of a series of proenzymes produces lytic enzymes capable of dissolving clots.

The proenzyme plasminogen circulates in the blood. It is believed that the endothelial cells that constitute the endothelial lining of blood vessels release plasminogen activator, converting plasminogen to plasmin. In addition, activated factor XII, thrombin, kallikrein, and substances in the tissues are thought to be involved in the conversion of plasminogen to plasmin. Plasminogen activator levels are transiently elevated in response to exercise, stress, anoxia, and pyrogen. Plasmin, then, is the dissolving, or lytic, enzyme that lyses fibrin and attacks factors V, VIII, IX, and fibrinogen.

Finally, the lysis of fibrinogen and fibrin results in the liberation of fibrin degradation products (FDPs). FDPs inhibit platelet aggregation, exhibit an antithrombotic effect, and interfere with formation of the fibrin clot.

FIBRINOLYTIC SYSTEM INHIBITORS

Similar to coagulation inhibitors, there are inhibitors of the fibrinolytic system. These inhibitors prevent inappropriate lysis of needed clot formation. The mononuclear phagocyte system clears FDPs from the circulation. Also, antiplasmin, a protein circulating in the blood, binds with plasmin and renders it inactive. The level of circulating antiplasmin far outweighs plasmin concentrations, and plasmin is neutralized rapidly.

It is evident that the systems of hemostasis and fibrinolysis in conjunction with their system inhibitors function within a narrow margin to ensure the liquidity of the blood and patency of the vasculature. An upset in these systems can result in clinical evidence of thrombosis, hemorrhage, or the catastrophic event of disseminated intravascular coagulation.

IMMUNE SYSTEM

The immune system is composed of the following organs and cells: spleen, lymph nodes, thymus, bone marrow, appendix, tonsils and adenoids, B and T lymphocytes, eosinophils, basophils, and phagocytes. The organs of the system are connected with one another and with other organs through a network of lymphatic vessels. Immune cells and foreign particles are conveyed through the vessels in lymph fluid.

As noted, the hematological and immune systems are closely related. In addition to both originating in the bone marrow, blood carries components of the immune system throughout the body. The following are functions of a healthy immune system:

- Protection of the body from destruction by foreign agents and microbial pathogens
- Degradation and removal of damaged and dead cells
- Surveillance and destruction of malignant cells

Immune Response

The immune system is the body's internal response to substances recognized as foreign. Individuals have two types of immunity: general, or innate, immunity and specific, or acquired, immunity. Innate immunity is the body's capacity to resist invasion by foreign agents, whereas acquired immunity is the specific capacity of an individual's immune system to identify a substance as foreign. Acquired immunity occurs when an individual develops his or her own antibodies in response to an antigen exposure. Acquired immunity also happens when another source supplies an individual with antibodies. The maternal-to-fetal transfer of antibodies is an example of one individual supplying antibodies to another.

Basically, the immune system protects the body, or "self," from invasion by "nonself" (also called *antigens*). Any foreign substance capable of eliciting a specific immune response is referred to as an antigen. Antigens are most often composed of proteins, but polysaccharides, complex lipids, and nucleic acids also can act as antigenic materials; bacteria, viruses, fungi, parasites, and foreign tissue are all antigens. For instance, transplant rejection occurs when the body recognizes transplanted tissues or organs as foreign. Markers on antigens enable the immune system to identify target cells, against which destructive forces are directed. The intensity of the system's response is affected by the route of invasion, the dosage of the antigen, and its degree of foreignness.

Immunological competence refers to the immune system's capacity to identify and reject foreign materials. The system's failure to recognize antigens and mobilize effective defenses results in infection or malignancy. Failure to recognize markers of self can result in autoimmune diseases, such as multiple sclerosis, rheumatoid arthritis, or systemic lupus erythematosus. The system's "battle against imaginary enemies," such as pollen or dust, may result in allergies.

The major histocompatibility complex (MHC) is a group of genes contained in a section of chromosome 6 that encode molecules that mark a cell as self. These genes vary widely in structure from one person to another. Their presence is a factor in transplant rejection because they determine to which antigens one responds and how strongly. They also allow immune cells to recognize and communicate with one another.

GENERAL IMMUNITY

General immunity is present in all healthy people and forms the first line of defense against illness. Previous exposure to an organism or toxin is not required. Also, mechanisms of general immunity do not distinguish among microorganisms of different species and do not alter in intensity on reexposure. General immunities include physical, chemical, and mechanical barriers; biological defenses; phagocytosis; inflammatory processes; and cytokines.

Physical, Chemical, and Mechanical Barriers

Physical barriers prevent harmful organisms and other substances from gaining entrance into the body or body cavities. These barriers include skin, mucous membranes, the epiglottis, respiratory tract cilia, and sphincters. Chemical barriers such as antibacterial agents, antibodies, and acid solutions create an environment hostile to many pathogens. Lysozymes in tears, lactic acid in vaginal secretions, and hydrochloric acid in gastric secretions all act as chemical barriers. Mechanical barriers help rid the body of potentially harmful substances through some action (e.g., lacrimation, intestinal peristalsis, urinary flow).

Biological Defenses

Under normal conditions, large areas of the human body are colonized with microorganisms. The skin and mucous membranes of the oropharynx, nasopharynx, intestinal tract, and parts of the genital tract each have their own microflora, referred to as normal flora. These microorganisms influence patterns of colonization by competing with more harmful organisms for essential nutrients and by producing substances that inhibit the growth of other microorganisms.

Phagocytes and Phagocytosis

Phagocytosis is a process by which injured cells and foreign invaders are ingested by leukocytes, specifically, neutrophils and mononuclear phagocytes (monocytes and macrophages). Both cell types originate from stem cells in the bone marrow and, although structurally different, approach phagocytosis in a similar manner.

Surface receptors on their cell membranes allow them to attach to foreign substances and then engulf, internalize, and destroy these substances using enzymes present in their cellular interior. Neutrophils provide the "first-wave" cellular attack on invading organisms during the acute inflammatory process. The number of neutrophils at the site peaks in 6 to 12 hours after inflammation begins. The second wave of cells is primarily monocytes. Monocytes spend only a short time in the bloodstream before escaping through the capillary membranes into the tissue. Once in the tissue, they swell to much larger sizes to become macrophages, which either attach to certain tissues and destroy bacteria, or wander through the tissue phagocytizing foreign matter. These cells are strategically placed throughout the body tissues, where they can exist for months and even years. Macrophages in different tissues differ in appearance because of environmental variations and are known by different names (i.e., Kupffer's cells in the liver, alveolar macrophages in the lungs, histiocytes in the skin and subcutaneous tissue, and microglia in the brain).

Inflammatory Responses

Inflammation is an acute physiological nonspecific response of the body to tissue injury caused by factors such as chemicals, heat, trauma, or microbial invasion. It is the primary process through which the body repairs tissue damage and defends itself against infection. The initial inflammatory response is localized, but may lead to systemic consequences such as fever, malaise, and neutrophilia. The inflammatory response contains three stages:

1. The vascular stage, which is an immediate but short-term vasoconstriction, followed by vasodilation of arterioles and venules and hyperemia and swelling resulting from the secretion of histamine, prostaglandins, and kinins.
2. The cellular exudate stage, characterized by neutrophilia, secretion of colony-stimulating factors into the interstitial fluid, and formation of exudate, a clear serous fluid with a high protein count. The functions of exudate are to transport leukocytes and antibodies to the inflammatory site, dilute toxins and irritating substances, and transport materials necessary for tissue repair. As the inflammatory process continues, the serous exudate changes to a creamy white fluid containing cellular debris.
3. The tissue repair and replacement stage, in which inflammatory material is removed and connective tissue cells proliferate. Collagen synthesis occurs, resulting in tissue replacement.

The most important result of these processes is accumulation at the site of injury of large numbers of neutrophils and macrophages, which inactivate or destroy invaders, remove debris, and begin the initial tissue repair.

Cytokines

Cytokines are chemical messengers functioning as immune system hormones. They enhance cell growth, promote cell activation, direct cellular traffic, stimulate macrophage function, and destroy antigens. They are also called *interleukins* (ILs) because they serve as messengers between leukocytes.

Interleukin-1 (IL-1) augments the synthesis of IL-2, IL-3, IL-4, gamma-interferon, and IL-2 receptors. It can also activate lymphokine-activated killer cells. IL-2 binds to specific receptors on activated T cells and markedly enhances the cytolytic activity of natural killer cells (NKCs), which are a specialized group of lymphoid cells that act directly, without prior sensitization, to lyse a variety of malignant and virus-infected cells. IL-3 and B-cell differentiation factor provide critical signals for the growth and maturation of antigen-primed B cells.

Cytokines can be classified as either lymphokines (secreted by lymphocytes) or monokines (secreted by monocytes or macrophages). Interferons (a type of lymphokine) provide some protection to the body against invasion by viruses until more slowly reacting specific immune responses take over. Interferons are produced when a virus infects a cell; they affect the transcription and translation of viral genes. In addition, interferons appear to be involved in protecting the body against some forms of cancer. Specifically, these substances have been demonstrated to interfere with cellular division and proliferation of abnormal cells. They also enhance the activity of NKCs.

SPECIFIC IMMUNITY

If a foreign agent persists in spite of general immune responses, the activation of specific immune responses occurs. To be most effective, these responses require previous exposure to a foreign agent or organism. The cellular components of these types of responses are capable of distinguishing among microorganisms and can alter their intensity and response time significantly on re-exposure.

Two types of specific immune responses have been identified: cell-mediated immunity and humoral immunity. Most foreign substances stimulate both cellular and humoral immune responses; this results in an overlapping of their reactions and maximum protection against damage from the invading substances.

B and T Lymphocytes

B and T lymphocytes originate from stem cells produced in the bone marrow. During fetal development and shortly after birth, primary lymphoid organs are the site where these cells differentiate and mature into the competent cells responsible for cell-mediated and humoral immune responses. For B lymphocytes, this preprocessing is believed to occur in the bone marrow and, possibly, the fetal liver; for T lymphocytes, it occurs in the thymus gland.

As they develop, both B and T lymphocytes acquire receptors for specific antigens that commit them to a single antigenic specificity for their lifetime. Subsequently, each of these "preprogrammed" B or T lymphocytes (on activation by its specific antigen) is capable of producing tremendous numbers of clones or duplicate lymphocytes. The different types of T cells produced are categorized according to their function, as shown in Table 45-3.

Lymphoid System

After preprocessing in the primary lymphoid organs, B and T lymphocytes migrate to secondary lymphoid tissues, where the interaction with antigens and immune responses actually occurs. Secondary lymphatic tissue is located extensively in the lymph nodes. It is also found in special lymphoid tissue, such as that of the spleen, tonsils, adenoids, appendix, bone marrow, and gastrointestinal tract. This lymphoid tissue is placed advantageously throughout the body to intercept invading organisms or toxins before they can enter the bloodstream and disseminate widely.

Cell-Mediated Immune Response

Cell-mediated immunity provides a response to fungi, parasites, and intracellular bacteria. It also plays a major role in the rejection or acceptance of certain tissue grafts, the stimulation and regulation of antibody production, and defense against various malignant changes. As noted, T lymphocytes contain an antigen receptor that allows for the binding of a specific type of antigen. Each of these

table 45-3 Types of T Cells and Their Functions

Cell Type	Function
Cytotoxic T cells (T8)	Direct-attack cells capable of killing many microorganisms; predominant effector cell Virus-infected cells, cancer cells, and transplanted cells especially susceptible
Helper-inducer T cells (T4)	Most numerous Play pivotal role in overall regulation of immune response Often called "master conductor" Secrete lymphokines
Suppressor T cells (T8)	Act as negative feedback controllers of T4 cells May also limit ability of immune system to attack body tissues
Memory T cells	Sensitized to antigens during specific immune responses Remain stored in body Capable of initiating far more rapid response by T cells on re-exposure to same antigen

T cells, on activation by its specific antigen, is capable of producing large numbers of clones. After preprocessing, T cells migrate to lymphoid tissue where they act as effector cells (directly attacking antigens and malignant cells) and regulators of both the cellular and humoral immune response.

Antigenic stimulation of T lymphocytes initiates the cell-mediated response. This step of the response may be mediated by macrophages that bind to the antigen, facilitating its recognition. The macrophages then produce cytokines, which stimulate T lymphocytes, increase B-lymphocyte proliferation, and activate phagocytes.

Humoral Immune Response

The humoral immune response is extracellular; that is, it occurs in blood and tissue fluid. It begins in response to most bacteria, bacterial toxins, and the extracellular phase of viral invasion. Humoral immunity involves two types of serum proteins, immunoglobulins (Igs) and complement.

Immunoglobulins are antibody molecules made by B lymphocytes that differentiate to plasma cells and memory cells. The plasma cells then secrete antibodies that bind to antigens; the resulting antigen–antibody complexes are ingested by phagocytes. After the complexes are eliminated, the memory cells remain in circulation and in lymphoid tissue to mature into plasma cells when the antigen is encountered again. Immunoglobulins are specific to antigens and are of several types:

- IgA (two types) concentrates in body fluids, such as tears, saliva, and secretions of respiratory and gastrointestinal tracts; it guards entrances to the body.
- IgM tends to remain in the bloodstream, where it is effective in killing bacteria.
- IgG (four types) is able to enter tissue spaces and works efficiently to coat microorganisms before phagocytosis occurs.
- IgD is found mostly in the membrane of B cells, where it is believed to regulate the cells' activation.
- IgE is normally present in only trace amounts; it is responsible for symptoms of allergy.

Complement is a nonspecific series of 15 proteins that circulate in inactive form in the bloodstream. These proteins activate one another in a cascading sequence when the first complement molecule C1 encounters an antigen–antibody complex. The end product of the cascade is a cylinder that lyses the cell membrane of the target cell, allowing fluids and molecules to flow in and out, which kills the target cell (Fig. 45-4).

Complement also facilitates the interaction of antigens and antibodies and enhances all aspects of the inflammatory process, especially increasing vascular permeability and phagocytosis.

Combined Immune Responses

The specific immune response is complex and involves the interaction of macrophages, complement proteins, and the cellular components of both the cellular and humoral systems (Fig. 45-5). Macrophages initially function to recognize, process, and present the antigen to antigen-specific T lymphocytes in the lymphoid tissues. Helper-inducer T4 cells are subsequently activated with the help of a chemical factor (IL-1) released by the presenting macrophage. The T4 cells proliferate and produce their own chemical substances, known as lymphokines, which in turn stimulate the activation and proliferation of antibody-producing B lymphocytes, cytotoxic T cells, suppressor T cells, and phagocytic macrophages. The production of antibodies leads to the activation of complement proteins. All of these components work together to destroy the antigen, either through complex processes involving direct attack or through modulation by chemical processes. Suppressor T cells provide feedback to the T4 helper cells to halt these defense reactions when they are no longer needed, and memory cells reactivate them on re-exposure to the antigen.

Impaired Host Resistance

The various components of the immune system provide a complex network of mechanisms that, when intact, defend the body against foreign microorganisms and malignant cells. In some situations, however, components of the system can fail, resulting in impaired host resistance. Often the state of immunosuppression is chemically induced by drugs or medications such as corticosteroids and cytotoxic chemotherapeutic agents. People who acquire an infection because of a deficiency in any of their host defenses are referred to as immunocompromised, or immunosuppressed.

The exact effects of, and symptoms related to, defects in host defense vary according to the part of the immune system affected (Table 45-4). General features associated with compromised host resistance include recurrent infections, infections caused by usually harmless agents (opportunistic organisms), chronic infections, skin rashes, diarrhea, growth impairment, and increased susceptibility to certain cancers.

clinical applicability challenges

Self-Challenge: Critical Thinking

1. *Hypothesize the impact of red blood cell lysis on the major functions of the hematological system.*
2. *Examine the role of T-cell immunodeficiencies on the immune response.*

Study Questions

1. *The humoral-mediated immune response has its effect primarily through the action of*
   a. *T cells.*
   b. *null cells.*
   c. *complement.*
   d. *B cells.*
2. *The major function of neutrophils is to*
   a. *mediate the immune response.*
   b. *initiate hypersensitivity reactions.*
   c. *phagocytize bacteria.*
   d. *stimulate nerve endings.*

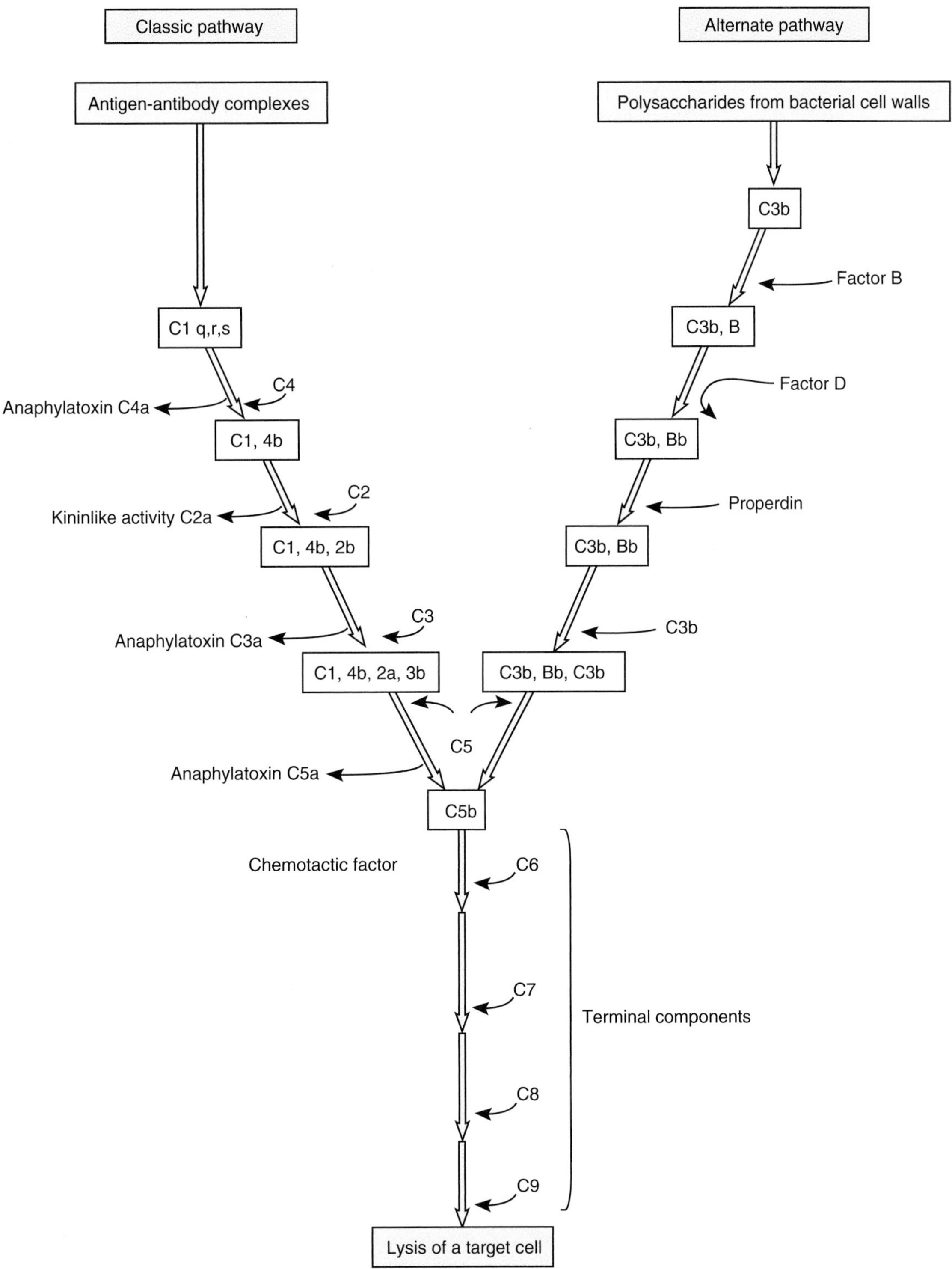

figure 45-4 The complement cascade. The classic pathway is activated by antigen–antibody complexes through component C1. The sequence of action of the initial components is based on their order of discovery (C1, C4, C2, C3, C5, C6, C7, C8, C9); the later-acting components are numbered according to their order of reaction. The alternative pathway is activated by numerous agents, such as bacterial polysaccharides. Although the complement system is basically a protective mechanism for the body, uncontrolled activation of this system produces inflammation and destruction of body tissues. (Bb is the activated form of factor B.)

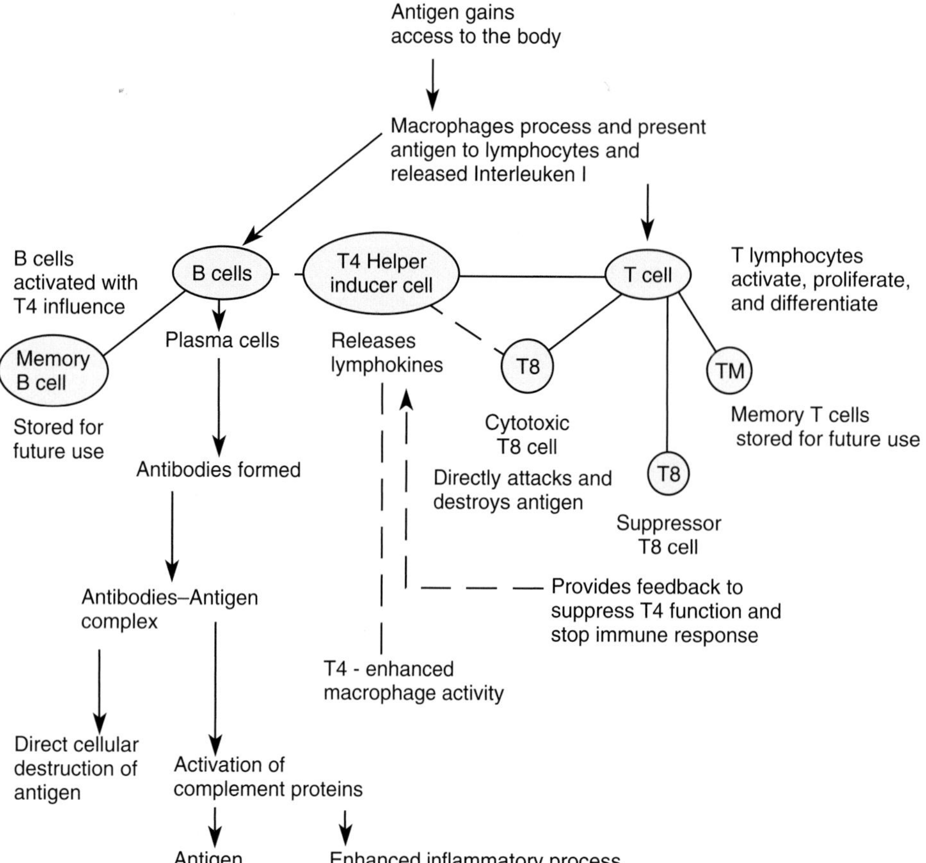

figure 45-5 A schematic representation of the combined immune responses.

table 45-4 Risk Factors for Compromised Host Defenses

Host Defect	Diseases, Therapies, and Other Conditions Associated With Host Defects
Impaired phagocyte functioning	Radiation therapy Nutritional deficiencies Diabetes mellitus Acute leukemias Corticosteroids Cytotoxic chemotherapeutic drugs Aplastic anemia Congenital hematological disorders Alcoholism
Complement system deficiencies	Liver disease Systemic lupus erythematosus Sickle cell anemia Splenectomy Congenital deficiencies
Impaired cell-mediated (T lymphocyte) immune response	Radiation therapy Nutritional deficiencies Aging Thymic aplasia AIDS Hodgkin's disease/lymphomas Corticosteroids Antilymphocyte globulin Congenital thymic dysfunctions

(continued)

table 45-4 Risk Factors for Compromised Host Defenses (Continued)

Host Defect	Diseases, Therapies, and Other Conditions Associated With Host Defects
Impaired humoral (antibody) immunity	Chronic lymphocytic leukemia Multiple myeloma Congenital hypogammaglobulinemia Protein-losing enteropathies (inflammatory bowel disease)
Interruption of physical/mechanical/chemical barriers	Traumatic injury Decubitus ulcers/skin defect Invasive medical procedures Vascular disease Skin diseases Nutritional impairments Burns Respiratory intubation Mechanical obstruction of body drainage systems, such as lacrimal and urinary systems Decreased level of consciousness
Impaired mononuclear phagocyte system	Liver disease Splenectomy

3. *The cells of the hematopoietic system that contribute to osmotic plasma pressure are*
   a. *coagulation factors.*
   b. *plasma proteins.*
   c. *red blood cells.*
   d. *thrombocytes.*
4. *The electrolyte that plays an important role in the coagulation cascade is*
   a. *calcium.*
   b. *potassium.*
   c. *sodium.*
   d. *vitamin K.*

REFERENCE

1. Harmening DM (ed): Clinical Hematology and Fundamentals of Hemostasis (3rd Ed). Philadelphia, FA Davis, 1997

OTHER SELECTED READING

Groer M: Advanced Pathophysiology: Application to Clinical Practice. Philadelphia, Lippincott Williams & Wilkins, 2001

Kinney M, Dunbar S, Brooks-Brunn J, et al: AACN Clinical Reference for Critical Care Nursing. St. Louis, Mosby, 1998

McCance KL, Heuther SE: Pathophysiology: The Biologic Basis for Disease in Adults and Children (4th Ed). St. Louis, Mosby-Year Book, 2002

Porth CM: Pathophysiology: Concepts of Altered Health States (6th Ed). Philadelphia, Lippincott Williams & Wilkins, 2002

chapter

46

Patient Assessment: Hematological and Immune Systems

PAULA TIMMERMAN

objectives

Based on the content in this chapter, the reader should be able to:

- Identify areas of a patient's history and physical assessment pertinent to assessing hematological and immune disorders.
- Differentiate diagnostic tests used to assess hematological and immune disorders.
- Synthesize the results of a patient's history, physical examination, and diagnostic tests to identify hematological and immune disorders.

Hematological and immune disorders encompass numerous ailments, many of which are life-threatening. In general, hematological disorders can be classified as overproduction or underproduction of hematological components or dysfunction of these components. Immune disorders usually are caused by underactivity or overactivity of immune system elements. The hematological and immune systems are complex and closely interrelated; therefore, disorders or dysfunctions of one system often alter the effectiveness of the other.

ASSESSMENT

History

A thorough patient history is essential when evaluating a patient for a potential hematological or immune disorder. When asked about his or her chief complaint, a patient may state symptoms that seem vague and unrelated. It is important to keep in mind the complex physiology of these systems when assessing a patient's health history (see Chapter 45). After obtaining information concerning the onset and duration of the chief complaint, the nurse inquires about the patient's medical history, previous therapies, and family medical history. Table 46-1 summarizes conditions and treatments that may predispose patients to hematological and immune disorders (see Chapter 49). Boxes 46-1 and 46-2 summarize special considerations for older patients and children, respectively.

The following are some specific questions to guide the interview process:

- What is the patient's chief complaint?
- Has the patient had a history of frequent infections (upper respiratory, lower respiratory, urinary tract, vaginal, oral cavity)?

table 46-1 Hematological and Immune Disorders Based on Patient History

Patient History	Potential Disorder
Chronic disease (inflammation, infection)	Anemia
Nutritional deficiencies (iron, folate, vitamin B_{12})	Anemia
Nutritional deficiencies (vitamin K, malabsorption)	Coagulopathy
Endocrine (thyroid, pituitary) dysfunction	Anemia
Hypersplenism	Anemia, thrombocytopenia
Acquired immunodeficiency syndrome	Anemia, neutropenia
Malignancy	Pancytopenia
Chemical exposure	Neutropenia, hemolytic anemia
Prosthetic heart valve or vascular graft	Hemolytic anemia
Collagen vascular disorder	TTP
Hypersensitivity reaction	TTP
Viral, bacterial, or fungal infection	TTP
Uremia	Coagulopathy
Chronic alcoholism	Coagulopathy
Liver disease	Coagulopathy, thrombosis
Vasculitis	Thrombosis
Atherosclerosis	Thrombosis
Chronic obstructive pulmonary disease	Polycythemia
Smoking	Polycythemia
Congenital cardiac disease	Polycythemia
Previous Therapies/Medications	
Heparin	Thrombocytopenia
Antibiotics	Agranulocytosis
Carbamazepine	Agranulocytosis
Alkylating agents	Leukemia, lymphoma, pancytopenia
Blood transfusion	Anemia
Aspirin, nonsteroidal anti-inflammatory drugs	Coagulopathy
Warfarin	Coagulopathy
Steroids	Leukocytosis
Various drugs, chemicals, and toxins (see Box 49-2)	Hemolytic anemia
Family History	
Sickle cell anemia	Anemia
Thalassemia	Anemia
Congenital hemolytic anemia	Anemia
Polycythemic disorders	Polycythemia vera
von Willebrand's disease	Bleeding disorder
Hemophilia	Bleeding disorder

TTP, thrombotic thrombocytopenic purpura.

- Has the patient had episodes of bruising or bleeding (unexplained bruises, epistaxis, bleeding gums, heavy menstruation, hemoptysis, blood in urine, gastrointestinal disturbances, tarry stools)?
- How does the patient describe his or her energy level and activity tolerance?
- Has the patient experienced frequent headaches, dizziness, visual disturbances, cerebral incidents (e.g., a transient ischemic attack [TIA], a cerebrovascular accident [CVA]), or lethargy?
- Has the patient noticed any enlarged lymph nodes or skin eruptions?
- Has the patient experienced fevers, night sweats, or unintentional weight loss?
- Has the patient been exposed to any foreign substances or chemicals?
- Is there a family history of bleeding disorders, anemia, hematological malignancy, or immune disorders?
- What medications has the patient been taking and for what duration?

Physical Examination

A thorough physical examination is necessary to identify physical signs that may indicate a hematological or immune system disorder. Table 46-2 summarizes physical findings that may suggest various disorders of these systems. (Many of these disorders are further described in Chapter 49.)

The nurse examines the patient's skin for pallor, jaundice, or facial plethora, as well as for signs of abnormal bleeding. He or she also evaluates the patient's joints for pain, swelling, and limited range of motion, which may suggest hemarthrosis from coagulopathy or sickle cell anemia. Superficial mucocutaneous bleeding and a dependent distribution of petechiae can indicate thrombocytopenia, whereas clusters of palpable, pruritic petechiae can suggest

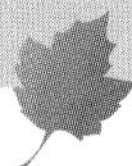

box 46-1

Factors That Place the Older Patient at Risk for Hematological Disorders

- Decreased iron intake, resulting from poor dentition (difficulty chewing meat) or a fixed income (making sources of iron such as meat or supplements unaffordable), can place the older adult at risk for iron deficiency anemia. Older adults may also experience low-grade gastrointestinal bleeding as a result of nonsteroidal anti-inflammatory drug use for the treatment of arthritis, from hemorrhoids and polyps, or from undiagnosed colon cancer. This blood loss may also place them at risk for iron deficiency anemia.
- Poor absorption of vitamin B_{12} (as a result of atrophic gastritis) places the older adult at risk for megaloblastic anemia.
- Declining immune function places the older adult at risk for leukemia, lymphoma, and multiple myeloma.
- Anticoagulation therapy (e.g., to treat atrial fibrillation) can result in platelet dysfunction and places the older adult at risk for hemorrhage. This is a particularly significant risk in older adults who are disoriented or have decreased mobility.

vasculitis. Extensive superficial purpura, deep hematomas, or hemarthroses may indicate a coagulation disorder.[1] The nurse also notes skin rashes, pruritus, and excoriations. Extremities are assessed for areas of redness, tenderness, warmth, or swelling, which can indicate thrombophlebitis. The lips and nail beds should be assessed for cyanosis; digital clubbing may also be present in patients with chronic hypoxemia. Leg and ankle ulcers may be present in patients with sickle cell anemia.

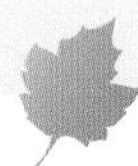

box 46-2

Hematological and Immune Disorders

- Iron deficiency anemia
- Macrocytic anemia
  - Folate deficiency
  - Vitamin B_{12} deficiency (rare)
- Anemia secondary to lead poisoning
- Sickle cell anemia
- Thalassemia
- Hemolytic anemia
  - Hemolytic disease of the newborn
  - Glucose-6-phosphate dehydrogenase deficiency
  - Pyruvate kinase deficiency
- Immune thrombocytopenia
- Hemophilia
- Thrombophilia
- Leukemia
- Hodgkin's disease
- Congenital immunodeficiencies

The nurse also examines the patient's eyes and mouth. Visual changes can indicate hyperviscosity from polycythemia or retinal infarcts from sickle cell anemia. The nares, gums, and the mucous membrane of the mouth should be assessed for signs of bleeding. Pallor of the oral mucosa can be a significant indicator of anemia. Tongue changes can occur in patients with an iron deficiency and megaloblastic anemias. Inspection of the throat and palpation of lymph nodes should be performed to assess for infection or malignancy.

Tachycardia and tachypnea may be present in patients with anemia or infection. An S_4 heart sound may be auscultated in a person with severe anemia. Dyspnea on exertion and orthostatic changes in blood pressure can be other symptoms of anemia. Thorough lung auscultation and inspection of sputum, if present, should be performed to rule out respiratory infection and hemoptysis. Symptoms of intermittent claudication (see Chapter 19) and angina pectoris (see Chapter 21) indicate problems with oxygen delivery in patients with polycythemia. These patients commonly experience hypertension as well.

Pertinent physical assessment findings of the abdominal and pelvic region include lymphadenopathy, splenomegaly, and hepatomegaly, which can indicate a number of hematological or immune conditions. The nurse should also thoroughly assess for infection of the urinary, vaginal, and perirectal areas. Body secretions or fluids (stool, urine, emesis, or gastric secretions) that may be present should be inspected for the presence of blood.

Neurological abnormalities may be present in patients with hematological conditions. For instance, headache and dizziness are symptoms of anemia. These symptoms, along with a sensation of fullness in the head, may indicate polycythemia. Confusion, headache, altered mental status, paresis, aphasia, dysphasia, coma, seizures, paresthesia, and visual problems may be caused by thrombotic thrombocytopenic purpura (TTP; see Chapter 49). An altered level of consciousness, headache, papilledema, vomiting, and bradycardia with widening pulse pressure are signs of increased intracranial pressure, which may be caused by intracranial bleeding in patients with coagulopathy.

DIAGNOSTIC STUDIES AND RESULTS INTERPRETATION

Laboratory tests determine whether components of the hematological and immune systems are being produced in adequate amounts. Further testing may be required to ascertain if the components are functioning properly. Because patients with severe presentations of hematological and immune conditions may be seen in the intensive care unit (ICU), tests to differentiate the conditions and their causes are presented here.

Tests to Evaluate Red Blood Cells

Red blood cells (RBCs) are essential for oxygenating tissues. An overproduction of RBCs results in polycythemia, which is indicated by a high hematocrit level and an increased RBC mass (see Chapter 48). Anemia is a condition marked by a decrease in the RBC mass caused by decreased production

table 46-2 **Findings Indicating Possible Hematological or Immune Disorders**

Physical Findings*	Related Information From Patient History	Possible Disorder
Pallor, dyspnea, dizziness, tachycardia, glossitis	Fatigue Headache Pica (compulsive craving for clay, laundry starch, earth, or ice)	Iron deficiency anemia
As above, also smooth tongue, stomatitis, icterus, paresthesias, gait ataxia, mental status changes	Fatigue Headache Premature graying of hair	Megaloblastic anemia
Bleeding (ecchymosis, petechiae, epistaxis, hemorrhage), pallor, dizziness, tachycardia	Fatigue Headache History of frequent infections (e.g., upper respiratory, cellulitis, perirectal) Previous viral infection (hepatitis, infectious mononucleosis, HIV, cytomegalovirus) Family history of aplastic anemia	Aplastic anemia
Pallor of conjunctiva, mucous membranes, palms and soles of feet; dyspnea; dizziness; tachycardia; bone pain; pain in chest or abdomen; splenomegaly; fever; leg and ankle ulcers; painless hematuria	African American descent Family history of sickle cell anemia Frequent infections Impaired vision Damage to joints Chronic renal failure History of stroke	Sickle cell anemia
Pallor, dyspnea, dizziness, jaundice, splenomegaly, cholelithiasis	Mediterranean descent, also Middle Eastern, South and Southeast Asian, and African	Thalassemia
Splenomegaly, hepatomegaly, facial and conjunctival plethora, hypertension, pruritus, dizziness, headache, thrombosis, thrombophlebitis	Visual disturbances Epigastric distress Cardiovascular insufficiency Bleeding tendency Numbness and burning of toes (from peripheral vascular insufficiency)	Polycythemia
Mouth sores, sore throat, lymphadenopathy, splenomegaly, hepatomegaly, infection (signs of infection may be minimal)	History of recurrent, severe infections Fatigue Recent radiation or chemotherapy treatment	Leukopenia
Infection, bleeding, bone pain, splenomegaly, skin and gum lesions, leukostasis if WBC count is extremely high (headache, confusion, CNS infarcts, acute respiratory insufficiency, pulmonary infarcts)	History of recurrent infections Fatigue Anorexia Weight loss	Acute or chronic leukemia
Bone pain, pallor, weakness, fatigue	History of recurrent infections Renal insufficiency Hypercalcemia (thirst, lethargy, confusion, polyuria, constipation)	Multiple myeloma
Weight loss, fever, night sweats, painless lymphadenopathy, splenomegaly, abdominal pain	Fatigue Anorexia History of infections	Hodgkin's disease or non-Hodgkin's lymphoma
Superficial mucocutaneous bleeding, petechiae on dependent areas of the body, epistaxis, hemoptysis, hematemesis, hematuria, rectal bleeding, vaginal bleeding, intra-abdominal hemorrhage (diffuse abdominal pain, restlessness, anxiety, pallor, rigidity, dusky coloration of abdominal skin, tachycardia, tachypnea, and hypotension), intracranial bleeding (headache, vomiting, decreasing level of consciousness, papilledema, bradycardia)	History of viral or bacterial infection Hypersplenism Malignancies affecting the bone marrow History of immune disorders Alcoholism Pregnancy	Thrombocytopenia

(continued)

table 46-2 Findings Indicating Possible Hematological or Immune Disorders (Continued)

Physical Findings*	Related Information From Patient History	Possible Disorder
Confusion, headache, altered mental status, paresis, aphasia, dysphagia, coma, seizures	Paresthesias Visual disturbances	TTP
Superficial purpura, mucocutaneous bleeding, hemorrhage, joint pain and swelling (from bleeding into joints), deep hematomas	History of excessive or recurrent bleeding in patient or family members Alcoholism Hepatitis Liver disease Malnutrition Malabsorption syndromes (affects absorption of vitamin K from gastrointestinal tract)	Coagulation disorder

CNS, central nervous system; TTP, thrombotic thrombocytopenic purpura; WBC, white blood cell.
*Findings listed may not always be present.

of RBCs, increased RBC destruction, a combination of these two conditions, or acute blood loss. All patients being evaluated for anemia should have a complete blood count (CBC) with RBC indices, a reticulocyte count, iron studies, and a peripheral smear analysis. Abnormalities in these test results indicate the need for subsequent testing.

COMPLETE BLOOD COUNT

The CBC provides an overall indication of bone marrow production of RBCs, white blood cells (WBCs), and platelets. It also indicates the patient's hemoglobin level, hematocrit level, RBC indices, and WBC differential.

RED BLOOD CELL INDICES

Red blood cell indices refer to laboratory values that indicate characteristics of RBC structure or function. Table 46-3 presents RBC indices and some of the conditions that can cause abnormal laboratory results.

PERIPHERAL SMEAR

The peripheral smear can indicate disorders of the structure of RBCs. Various abnormalities detected by examining the peripheral smear are listed in Table 46-4, along with further testing that may be appropriate.

Mature RBCs do not contain a nucleus. Nucleated RBCs mature in the bone marrow and are not normally present in peripheral blood. They appear in the peripheral smear after profound stimulation, such as that from acute hemorrhage, hypoxemia, hemolytic anemia, or megaloblastic anemia. If these causes are ruled out, the appearance of nucleated RBCs may be caused by infiltrative processes in the bone marrow from malignancy, myelofibrosis, or granuloma. Nucleated RBCs may also be seen in asplenic patients because the spleen normally recognizes and removes these abnormal cells.

Spherocytes and elliptocytes are abnormally shaped RBCs. They usually appear in patients with a hereditary disorder that causes RBC membrane defects. These irregular cells are trapped and destroyed in the spleen, causing hemolytic anemia. Testing for red blood cell osmotic fragility demonstrates that these cells are more likely to lyse than normal RBCs. Serum lactate dehydrogenase and serum bilirubin levels should be ordered if hemolysis is suspected.

The presence of Rouleaux formations (the RBCs on the peripheral smear resemble a stack of coins) can indicate multiple myeloma. If clinical findings support this suspicion, serum protein electrophoresis and urine analysis for Bence Jones protein are the next steps in determining a diagnosis.

Target cells, sickled cells, and red blood cell cytoplasmic inclusions on the peripheral smear suggest the need for hemoglobin electrophoresis and hemoglobin F and A_2 levels. The most common anemias diagnosed in this manner are beta-thalassemia and sickle cell anemia.

The presence of schistocytes in a patient with a prosthetic heart valve may indicate mechanical hemolysis. Schistocytes in a patient with fever, thrombocytopenia, renal dysfunction, and neurological abnormalities require immediate interventions for suspected TTP (see Chapter 49).

Tests to Evaluate White Blood Cells

Because white blood cells detect and destroy pathogens, an elevated WBC count usually indicates infection and tends to correlate with the severity of the infection.

WHITE BLOOD CELL COUNT

The WBC count measures circulating leukocytes and should always be assessed in conjunction with the WBC differential and the patient's clinical condition. The WBC differential describes the percentages of the WBC subtypes (neutrophils, eosinophils, basophils, monocytes, and lymphocytes). See Chapter 45 for a description of the different types of WBCs. Table 46-5 indicates normal values for the WBC count and the differential.

Conditions other than infection that may elevate the WBC count include use of steroids, trauma, stress, leukemia, hemorrhage, tissue necrosis, and dehydration. Table 46-6 summarizes abnormalities of WBC overproduction and potential physiological causes. In some cases, patients with leukemia have WBC counts greater than 100,000 cells/mm^3 because of excessive bone marrow production of blast cells (immature granulocytes). These patients are at risk for leukostasis, in which blasts aggregate in the capillaries of the brain and lungs. Clinical findings of leukostasis include headache, confusion,

table 46-3 Red Blood Cell Indices: Laboratory Abnormalities

Test	Normal Value	Significance	Possible Causes for Abnormal Results
Mean corpuscular volume	82–98 m^3	Indicates the average volume of an RBC in the blood sample. Low value indicates RBCs are smaller than normal (microcytic). High value indicates RBCs are larger than normal (macrocytic).	Decreased: Anemia (iron deficiency, sickle cell, hemolytic), alpha- or beta-thalassemia, chronic disease, radiation therapy, endocarditis, diverticulitis, warm autoantibodies Increased: Alcoholism, cirrhosis, folate deficiency, vitamin B_{12} deficiency, pancreatitis, chronic lymphocytic leukemia, aplastic anemia
Mean corpuscular hemoglobin	26–34 pg	Indicates the average weight of hemoglobin in each RBC.	Decreased: Anemia (iron deficiency, microcytic, normocytic) Increased: Anemia (macrocytic, pernicious), cold agglutinin conditions, presence of monoclonal blood proteins, heparin sodium, heparin calcium
Mean corpuscular hemoglobin concentration	31–38%	Indicates the amount of hemoglobin in the RBC compared with its size. Results expressed as hypochromic or normochromic, referring to the concentration of hemoglobin and color of RBCs.	Decreased: Anemia (iron deficiency, chronic, megaloblastic, microcytic, sideroblastic) Increased: Cold agglutinins, hereditary spherocytosis, intravascular hemolysis, heparin calcium, heparin sodium
Red cell distribution width	13.4–14.6%	Measures the amount of homogeneity in the RBC width in the blood sample. Much variation in RBC width indicates the red cell distribution width is elevated. RBCs of similar size indicates red cell distribution width is low.	Decreased: Defects in iron reutilization Increased: Iron deficiency
Reticulocyte count	1–2%	Indicates the amount of immature RBCs that have been recently released from the bone marrow, expressed as a percentage of the total RBCs. Low reticulocyte count in presence of decreased RBCs indicates possible bone marrow dysfunction.	Decreased: Alcoholism, anemia (aplastic, iron deficiency, megaloblastic, pernicious), chronic infection, myxedema, radiation therapy Increased: Hemolytic anemia, hemorrhage, leukemia, malaria, polycythemia, pregnancy, sickle cell anemia, thalassemia, thrombotic thrombocytopenic purpura
Serum iron	Adult men 50–160 μg/dL Adult women 40–150 μg/dL	Indicates the amount of iron in the serum. Low serum iron needs to be correlated with other testing (i.e., ferritin, transferrin, and total iron binding capacity) to determine if iron deficiency anemia is present.	Decreased: Acute blood loss, iron deficiency anemia, gastrectomy, malabsorption, malignancy, rheumatoid arthritis, uremia Increased: Acute hepatitis, aplastic anemia, blood transfusion, hemochromatosis, lead poisoning, pernicious anemia, thalassemia, vitamin B_6 deficiency
Serum ferritin	Adult men 15–200 ng/mL Adult women ≤40 y 11–122 ng/mL Adult women >40 y 12–263 ng/mL	Correlates well to the size of iron stores in the body. Ferritin is stored in the liver and reticuloendothelial system and released into the serum to meet the body's demand for iron.	Decreased: Hemodialysis, inflammatory bowel disease, iron deficiency anemia, gastrointestinal surgery, pregnancy Increased: Anemia (chronic, hemolytic, megaloblastic,

(continued)

table 46-3 Red Blood Cell Indices: Laboratory Abnormalities (Continued)

Test	Normal Value	Significance	Possible Causes for Abnormal Results
			pernicious, sideroblastic), chronic infection, chronic inflammation, chronic renal disease, excess ingestion of iron, hepatic disease, liver disease, malignancy, multiple blood transfusions, rheumatoid arthritis, thalassemia
Total iron binding capacity	250–400 mg/dL	Indicates the maximum amount of iron that can be bound to transferrin. Useful for differentiating anemia from chronic inflammatory disorders.	Normal: Chronic inflammatory disorders Increased: Iron deficiency anemia
Serum transferrin	200–400 mg/dL	Plasma protein that transports iron by binding iron to serum transferrin receptors. Emerging as more sensitive indicator of iron deficiency and may replace more conventional indices (serum iron and ferritin).	Decreased: Cirrhosis, hemochromatosis, inflammatory states, renal disease, hemorrhage, hepatitis, hypothyroidism, microcytic anemia, pernicious anemia, thalassemia Increased: Iron deficiency states

From Chernecky CC, Berger BJ: Laboratory Tests and Diagnostic Procedures (2nd Ed). Philadelphia, WB Saunders, 1997.

central nervous system infarcts, acute respiratory insufficiency, and pulmonary infiltrates.

A low WBC count usually indicates decreased production caused by immunosuppressive therapy or a disorder of bone marrow production due to infiltrative processes or bone marrow failure. Decreases in circulating neutrophils may be caused by decreased production from bone marrow injury, bone marrow infiltration, nutritional deficiencies, or congenital defects of the stem cells in the bone marrow. Other causes of neutropenia are splenic sequestration and destruction, immune-mediated granulocyte destruction, or overwhelming infection. Lymphocytopenia is most commonly caused by malignancy, followed by collagen vascular disease. Acquired immunodeficiency syndrome (AIDS) and AIDS-related complex are other notable causes of lymphocytopenia (see Chapter 48).

There are numerous potential abnormalities in the WBC differential. A *left shift* refers to an increase in the number of bands (neutrophil precursors), which usually indicates an infectious process. The presence of blasts in the peripheral blood is always an aberrant finding and suggests the presence of leukemia or a myeloproliferative disorder.

T AND B LYMPHOCYTE TESTS

As discussed in Chapter 45, lymphocytes are classified as T cells and B cells. T cells are important in the body's ability to distinguish between self and nonself. Monoclonal antibodies against specific lymphocyte surface proteins are used to identify types of circulating lymphocytes and their subset populations, which can be useful in characterizing hematological malignancies and identifying immunological and autoimmune diseases. A specific example of this is assessment of the $CD4^+$ subpopulation of T cells in patients with AIDS; a $CD4^+$ count of less than 400/mm^3 is associated with a poorer prognosis. Table 46-7 lists possible causes of lymphocytosis and lymphopenia.

When an antigen stimulates B cells, they differentiate into plasma cells and produce antibodies. Although plasma cells reside in lymphoid tissue, their antibody production can be evaluated through serum and urine protein electrophoresis. Autoimmune diseases occur when the body produces antibodies directed against its own tissues. These diseases can be organ specific (e.g., Graves' disease) or widely disseminated and involve multiple organs (e.g., systemic lupus erythematosus). Laboratory testing involves the detection of serum antibodies against various tissues. C-reactive protein, antinuclear antibody, rheumatoid factor, and erythrocyte sedimentation rate are additional tests used in diagnosing autoimmune disorders.

Tests to Evaluate Disorders of Primary Hemostasis

Any laboratory testing to evaluate for hematological dysfunction should be guided by the information gathered in the history and physical examination. Family history, underlying clinical conditions, and the duration and type of abnormal bleeding can indicate appropriate testing and diagnostic workup.

Disorders of primary hemostasis are caused by disorders of platelets and small blood vessels, resulting in mucocutaneous bleeding, petechiae, and superficial purpura. Decreased platelets or increased capillary fragility can cause the sudden appearance of petechiae, especially in dependent areas, such as the lower extremities.

PLATELET COUNT

The primary phase of hemostasis involves aggregation of platelets at the site of vessel injury. These platelets

table 46-4 ■ Peripheral Smear Red Blood Cell Abnormalities

Abnormality	Potential Diagnoses	Further Testing
Nucleated RBCs	Acute hemorrhage, hypoxia, megaloblastic anemia	Vitamin B_{12} and folate levels; assess for bleeding; O_2 saturation, arterial blood gases for hypoxia
Spherocytes, elliptocytes	Hemolytic anemia from hereditary spherocytosis, hereditary elliptocytosis	Reticulocyte count, serum bilirubin, serum lactate dehydrogenase, direct Coombs', osmotic fragility
Rouleaux formations	Multiple myeloma	Serum protein electrophoresis, urine for Bence Jones proteins
Target cells, sickle cells, red cell cytoplasmic inclusions	Sickle cell anemia, thalassemia	Hemoglobin studies (hemoglobin electrophoresis, hemoglobin F and A_2)
Schistocytes	Thrombotic thrombocytopenic purpura, mechanical hemolysis	Reticulocyte count, serum lactate dehydrogenase, serum bilirubin, coagulation studies, cardiac auscultation

table 46-5 ■ Normal Values for the White Blood Cell Count and Differential

Test	Normal Value
WBC count	4,500–11,000 cells/mm^3
Differential (expressed as a percentage of the total WBC count)	
Granulocytes	
Segmented neutrophils	54–62%
Band neutrophils	3–5%
Eosinophils	1–3%
Basophils	0–0.75%
Monocytes	3–7%
Lymphocytes	25–33%

From Chernecky CC, Berger BJ: Laboratory Tests and Diagnostic Procedures (2nd Ed). Philadelphia, WB Saunders, 1997.

initiate the coagulation cascade, which results in fibrin being deposited at the site of injury to stabilize the clot (secondary hemostasis). See Figure 45-2 for an illustration of the processes that occur during hemostasis.

When evaluating primary hemostasis, one first obtains a platelet count from the CBC. A platelet count of less than 150,000/mm^3 is abnormal, but bleeding from thrombocytopenia alone usually does not happen unless the platelet count falls below 20,000/mm^3. However, bleeding from surgery or trauma may be prolonged with platelet counts of 40,000 to 50,000/mm^3. Severe, spontaneous hemorrhage may occur when platelet counts reach 5,000 to 10,000/mm^3. Thrombocytopenia can be caused by decreased bone marrow production, splenic sequestration due to splenomegaly, or peripheral destruction of platelets by the body's own immune system. Disseminated intravascular coagulation (DIC) and TTP (see Chapter 49) are other serious disorders that involve low platelet counts. There are also

table 46-6 Potential Causes of Elevated White Blood Cell Count

Abnormality	Potential Causes
Neutrophilia	Infections, inflammatory disorders, tissue destruction, malignancies, drug induced hemolysis, diabetic ketoacidosis, myeloproliferative disorders, idiopathic
Eosinophilia	Allergies, hypersensitivity reaction, parasitic infections, immunological disorders, adrenal insufficiency
Basophilia	Myeloproliferative disorders, allergic conditions, myxedema, ulcerative colitis, basophilic leukemia
Monocytosis	Malignancies, infections, recovery from neutropenia, rheumatic disorders, monocytic leukemia, inflammatory bowel disease, cirrhosis, sarcoidosis, drug reactions
Lymphocytosis	Infection (especially viral), pertussis, acute infectious lymphocytosis, immunological disorders, lymphoproliferative disorders

people who produce adequate numbers of platelets, but ones that function abnormally.

An elevated platelet count greater than 400,000/mm^3 indicates increased platelet production or decreased platelet destruction. These platelets may function abnormally, causing aberrant bleeding and clotting. Primary thrombocytosis is caused by bone marrow disease. Reactive thrombocytosis may be caused by chronic inflammation, infection, malnutrition, acute stress, malignancy, splenectomy, or the postoperative state.

table 46-7 Possible Causes of Lymphocytosis and Lymphopenia

Finding	Possible Causes
Lymphocytosis	Cytomegalovirus infection, hepatitis, infectious mononucleosis, lymphocytic leukemia, syphilis, diverticulitis, endocarditis, pertussis, toxoplasmosis Drugs and chemicals include aspirin, haloperidol, lead intoxication, levodopa, phenytoin, carbon disulfate poisoning, tetrahydrochloride poisoning
Lymphopenia	Aplastic anemia, Cushing's syndrome, malignancy, chronic myelogenous leukemia, systemic lupus erythematosus, radiation therapy to the lymphatics, immunoglobulin deficiencies, uremia Drugs include chemotherapeutic agents, glucocorticoids, lithium, niacin, epinephrine

From Chernecky CC, Berger BJ: Laboratory Tests and Diagnostic Procedures (2nd Ed). Philadelphia, WB Saunders, 1997.

PERIPHERAL SMEAR

A peripheral blood smear may reveal megathrombocytes (large platelets), which may be present during premature platelet destruction. Also, note that some patients' platelets clump when exposed to EDTA (the anticoagulant used in the "purple top" CBC tube). Examination of the peripheral smear shows this clumping, and a repeat CBC in a heparinized "green top" blood collection tube reveals an accurate platelet count.

BLEEDING TIME

A bleeding time assesses the length of time required for a clot to form at the site of vessel injury. A prolonged bleeding time in a patient with a normal platelet count may indicate a disorder of platelet function that requires further testing. A deficiency in factor VIIIR (von Willebrand's disease) results in decreased ability of the platelets to adhere to the injured vessel wall. Uremia from renal failure, drugs (especially aspirin), foods, and spices can also cause abnormal platelet function. Box 46-3 lists some drugs known to decrease platelet production or function. Platelet aggregation studies are done to detect inherited or acquired disorders in platelet function.

PROTHROMBIN TIME AND ACTIVATED PARTIAL THROMBOPLASTIN TIME

Screening for coagulation abnormalities includes evaluating the prothrombin time (PT) and the activated partial thromboplastin time (aPTT). Prolongation of either of these tests indicates coagulation factor deficiencies or inhibition. PT screens for dysfunction in the extrinsic portion (tissue thromboplastin, factor VII) and the common pathway (factors X, V, II, fibrinogen) of the coagulation

box 46-3 ***Drugs That Decrease Platelet Production or Function***

- Aspirin
- Benzene and benzene derivatives
- Cimetidine
- Chemotherapeutic agents
- Chloramphenicol
- Chlorothiazides
- Digitalis
- Digoxin
- Estrogen
- Furosemide
- Gold
- Heparin
- Penicillin
- Phenytoin
- Quinidine
- Streptomycin
- Sulfonamides
- Tetracycline
- Vitamin E

From Doyle B, Porter DL: Thrombocytopenia. AACN Clin Issues 8:469–480, 1997.

system. Prolongation of PT can result from disorders such as liver disease, vitamin K deficiency, clotting factor deficiencies, or DIC. Numerous medications, including allopurinol, aspirin, beta-lactam antibiotics, chlorpropamide, digoxin, diphenhydramine, and phenytoin sodium, can also cause a prolonged PT. PT is also used to monitor patient response to anticoagulation therapy with warfarin.

In 1983, the World Health Organization introduced the international normalized ratio (INR) to provide a common standard for interpretation of PT. The INR value depends on the sensitivity ratio of the thromboplastin reagent used in the laboratory to the International Reference Preparation. It is now widely accepted practice to assess the level of anticoagulation and warfarin dosing based on the INR ratio.

The aPTT measures how well the coagulation sequences of the intrinsic pathway (factors XII, XI, IX, VIII) and the common pathway (factors X, V, II, and fibrinogen) are functioning. An elevated aPTT could indicate disorders of any coagulation factors except VII and XIII. Clinical conditions associated with an elevated aPTT include DIC, von Willebrand's disease, and liver disease. Drugs that may affect aPTT include chlorpromazine, codeine, phenothiazines, salicylates, and warfarin. aPTT is also used to monitor patient response to heparin therapy.

- Thrombin time: Thrombin time is a test that measures the clotting time of a sample of plasma to which thrombin has been added. Thrombin is important in converting fibrinogen to fibrin in the final phase of the coagulation cascade. Thrombin time is increased in conditions such as DIC, liver disease, clotting factor defeciencies, shock, and hematological malignancies. Decreased thrombin time occurs with thrombocytosis.
- Fibrinogen level: Fibrinogen is converted by thrombin to fibrin, which then combines with platelets to form a stable clot. Patients with DIC, severe liver disease, sepsis, TTP, or trauma have a low fibrinogen level. Elevated fibrinogen levels occur in conditions involving tissue damage and inflammation.
- Fibrin degradation product level: Fibrin degradation products (FDPs) accumulate when a large amount of clotting has occurred and then been broken down. Increased FDPs, along with an elevated PT/aPTT, decreasing platelets, and a low fibrinogen level, indicate possible DIC (see Chapter 49).
- D-dimer: D-dimer is a more specific test than FDP measurement for detecting an event in which fibrin is being broken down. Its indications include ruling out and monitoring DIC, deep venous thrombosis, pulmonary embolism, and venous and arterial thrombotic conditions, and the monitoring of thrombolytic therapy.

Tests to Evaluate Disorders of Secondary Hemostasis

Disorders of secondary hemostasis involve clotting factor deficiencies and are characterized by recurrent oozing of blood and hematoma formation. The onset of these symptoms may be delayed because of the initial plugging of the vessel injury; however, defective clotting mechanisms fail to provide a stable fibrin clot.

When assessing disorders of secondary hemostasis, one must determine whether the disorder is congenital or acquired. A history of excessive or recurrent bleeding in the individual or family members suggests a congenital disorder as the more likely cause. Potential complications experienced by people with congenital bleeding disorders are described in Table 46-8. The most common congenital bleeding disorders are von Willebrand's disease, hemophilia A, and hemophilia B. PT and aPTT are ordered for patients with suspected congenital disorders, along with factor VIIIR, factor VIII, and factor IX assays. A deficiency in von Willebrand's factor (VIIIR) results in the decreased ability of platelets to adhere to the injured vessel wall and a deficiency of factor VIII. A deficiency of factor VIII causes hemophilia A; a deficiency of factor IX causes hemophilia B. Table 46-9 summarizes laboratory abnormalities that indicate these congenital disorders.

An acute bleeding problem without a prior history of chronic bleeding suggests an acquired disorder. Acquired disorders of hemostasis occur with vitamin K deficiency, severe trauma, hemorrhage, massive transfusion, overwhelming infection, severe liver disease, and DIC.[1] A deficiency of vitamin K decreases synthesis of prothrombin, factor VII, factor IX, and factor X. Liver disease impairs the absorption of vitamin K by decreased production of bile salts necessary for vitamin K absorption from the gut or through obstruction of the biliary system. Dysfunctional hepatocytes in the liver are unable to produce the vitamin K–dependent factors, as well as fibrinogen; factors V, XI, XII, and XIII; and other clotting factors. Some patients with liver disease may demonstrate thrombotic tendencies caused by decreased liver synthesis of anticoagulants, such as protein C, protein S, plasminogen, and antithrombin III.[2]

Laboratory testing for an acquired disorder of hemostasis varies based on the suspected etiology of the disorder. In general, testing includes PT, aPTT, thrombin time, bleeding time, liver enzyme and liver function tests, fibrinogen levels, and FDPs. Table 46-10 summarizes laboratory abnormalities that indicate some of the acquired coagulation disorders.

table 46-8 Potential Complications in Congenital Bleeding Disorders

Site	Potential Complication
Abdomen (e.g., retroperitoneal)	Hypotension, hypovolemic shock
Muscle	Compartment syndrome
Joint	Hemarthrosis with destruction of bone and cartilage in joint capsule
Intracranial	Increased intracranial pressure
Retropharyngeal	Airway obstruction
Gastrointestinal	Anemia, melena
Urinary tract	Hematuria; clots in ureters may occur after factor administration

From Stabler SP: Hemophilia. In Wood ME (ed): Hematology/Oncology Secrets. Philadelphia, Hanley & Belfus, 1999.

table 46-9 Laboratory Abnormalities in Congenital Bleeding Disorders*

	PT	aPTT	vWF	vWF Antigen	VIII	IX	BT†
von Willebrand's	N	↑	↓	↓	↓	N	↑
Hemophilia A	N	↑	N	N	↓	N	↑
Hemophilia B	N	↑	N	N	N	↓	↑

*Other congenital bleeding abnormalities are rare and not mentioned in this text.

† Bleeding time (BT) depends on the severity of the condition; it may be normal in mild cases.

PT, prothrombin time; aPTT, activated partial thromboplastin time; vWF, von Willebrand's factor; VIII, factor VIII; IX, factor IX; BT, bleeding time; N, normal.

A hypercoagulable state causes an increased tendency for thrombosis. Box 46-4 summarizes some of the risk factors for hypercoagulability. Hereditary thrombotic disease is a group of genetic abnormalities causing defects of coagulation, fibrinolysis, or their regulatory systems. Laboratory abnormalities in hereditary hypercoagulability include deficiencies of antithrombin III, protein C, protein S, plasminogen, tissue plasminogen activator, and dysfibrinogen; however, 65% to 70% of the causes remain unknown. Lupus anticoagulant (LA) is an autoimmune disorder in which patients have an elevated aPTT, yet thrombosis develops in 30% of the patients. LA is confirmed by the presence of anticardiolipin antibodies, positive platelet neutralization procedure, or positive dilute Russell viper's venom test.[3]

Tests to Evaluate Hematological and Immune Disorders

Bone marrow aspiration and biopsy is the most important diagnostic test for determining bone marrow function. It is a means of examining the precursors of the peripheral blood components to determine if hematological abnormalities are due to disorders of blood cell production. Bone marrow examination is useful in detecting infiltrative processes, such as malignancy, which may be affecting blood cell production. This procedure is also performed to determine response to therapy in patients with hematological malignancies or solid tumor infiltration of the bone marrow.

Tissue biopsy may be performed on skin lesions in which malignancy (e.g., cutaneous T-cell lymphoma) or an autoimmune process (e.g., pemphigus) is suspected. *Lymph node biopsy* is required for lymphadenopathy that does not appear to be caused by an infectious process.

Internal lymph nodes of the chest, abdomen, and pelvis can be evaluated by *computed tomography (CT) scanning.* A CT scan may be used to determine the presence of masses in suspected malignancy, especially lymphoma. Positron emission tomography (PET) is used in lymphoma and non-Hodgkins lymphoma to diagnose and stage cancer, evaluate response to therapy, and assess for recurrence. Liver disease, an important factor in coagulopathy, and splenomegaly may also be evaluated through a CT scan. A *skeletal survey* (skull, vertebrae, ribs, pelvis, arms, forearms, thighs, and lower legs) is done in patients with suspected multiple myeloma to assess for the typical "punched-out" lytic lesions that occur in this condition.

Intradermal skin testing with various antigens for delayed-type hypersensitivity is used to evaluate cell-mediated immunity. Commonly used antigens include mumps, *Candida*, trichophytin, and tuberculin. Failure to respond to the injected antigens is called *cutaneous anergy* and implies a defect in the patient's cellular immunity. Causes of cutaneous anergy include AIDS; acute leukemia; chronic lymphocytic leukemia; carcinoma; Hodgkin's disease; non-Hodgkin's lymphoma; congenital immune conditions; bacterial, fungal, or viral infections; immunosuppressive medications; cirrhosis; and malnutrition.

table 46-10 Laboratory Abnormalities in Acquired Bleeding Disorders

	PT	aPTT	TT	FDP	Plt
Vitamin K deficiency	X	X			
Liver disease:					
Acute hepatitis, early liver disease	X				
Chronic liver disease	X	X	X	X	X
DIC	X	X	X	X	X
Massive transfusion	X	X	X		X

PT, prothrombin time; aPTT, activated partial thromboplastin time; TT, thrombin time; FDP, fibrin degradation products; Plt, platelets; DIC, disseminated intravascular coagulation; X, elevated laboratory result.

box 46-4 ***Risk Factors for Hypercoagulability***

Physiological
- Pregnancy
- Postpartum
- Venous stasis
- Age >40 y
- Immobilization
- Varicose veins
- Previous venous thromboembolism

Pathological
- Malignancy
- Liver disease
- Disseminated intravascular coagulation
- Polycythemia
- Lupus anticoagulant
- Vascular injury
- Sepsis
- Heart failure
- Myocardial infarction
- Inherited abnormalities

Environmental
- Smoking
- Stress
- Heat

Iatrogenic
- Surgery
- Postsurgical
- Oral contraceptives
- Estrogens

ASSESSMENT OF THE IMMUNOCOMPROMISED PATIENT

Immunocompetence refers to the body's ability to protect itself against disease (see Chapter 45). Figure 46-1 illustrates areas to be assessed for immunocompetence.

It is essential that critically ill patients' immunocompetence be assessed at frequent intervals. Physical and psychological stress from overwhelming illness or trauma in the critically ill patient can depress functioning of the immune system. Invasive procedures, indwelling catheters, intravenous lines, mechanical ventilation, nutritional compromise, and the intensive care environment itself can predispose patients to infections and sepsis. Protective measures, such as handwashing and aseptic technique, are essential to minimize exposure to infectious organisms. The nurse should closely monitor potential sites of infection, changes or fluctuations in body temperature, nutritional status, and laboratory findings for indications of compromised immune function or the onset of infection. Septic shock is a life-threatening complication that can develop rapidly in immunocompromised patients. Patient outcomes are greatly improved when septic shock is detected in its early stages and interventions are instituted promptly. Signs of early septic shock are given in Box 46-5 (also see Chapter 54).

History

Obtaining a thorough history to identify susceptibility to infection is of major importance when assessing a patient's immunocompetence. The type of infection often provides the first clue regarding the nature of the immune defect. For example, patients with defects in humoral immunity may have recurrent or chronic bacterial infections, such as meningitis or bacteremia. Repeated viral or fungal infections can indicate a defect in cell-mediated immunity. (See Chapter 45 for a review of humoral and cell-mediated immunity.)

Risk Factors for Immunocompromise

Certain factors, such as chronological age, place critically ill patients at a higher risk of immunocompromise. A patient who has a chronic disease or is already immunosuppressed may also be predisposed to further immune difficulties. Finally, certain medications and treatments can alter a patient's immunocompetence, as can his or her nutritional status and skin integrity. Nurses should be

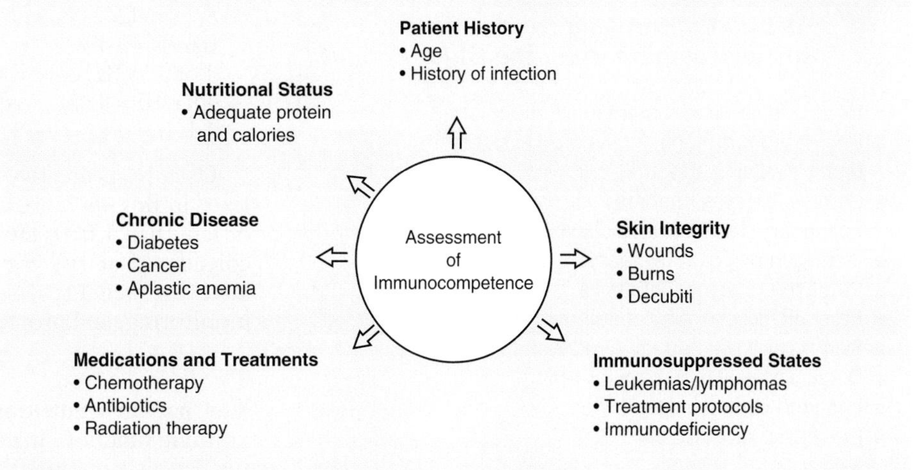

figure 46-1 In addition to obtaining his or her history, assessment of the immunocompromised patient should cover six major areas.

box 46-5 ***Signs of Early Septic Shock***

- Fever
- Chills
- Confusion
- Irritability
- Tachycardia
- Tachypnea
- Decreased peripheral pulses
- Hypotension
- Warm, dry skin

especially aware of these risk factors during their assessment of immunocompetence.

AGE

The patient's chronological age influences immunocompetence. Immune response may be depressed in the very young because of the underdevelopment of the thymus gland. Older patients experience a decline in immune system function, making them more susceptible to infections. Thus, they should be closely assessed for alterations in their immunocompetence. Box 46-6 describes factors that contribute to the overall decline of immunocompetence in older persons.

CHRONIC DISEASE

Many chronic diseases are associated with compromised immune functioning. Diabetes, cancer, and aplastic anemia are just a few examples of diseases in which immune deficiencies occur. Because many critically ill patients have an underlying chronic disease, the existence and severity of such diseases should be considered contributing factors to immunocompromise when these patients are assessed.

IMMUNOSUPPRESSED STATES

Patients with leukemia, lymphoma, multiple myeloma, and other hematological conditions can experience impaired immunity and recurrent infections. Immunodeficiency states can be congenital or acquired. People with congenital immunodeficiencies frequently do not survive childhood. Immunodeficiency syndromes in adults may occur through a spontaneous defect in the immune system or through infection with the human immunodeficiency virus (see Chapter 48).

Patients who are severely immunosuppressed have impaired responses to infectious agents and may not display the typical signs of infection. Fever and redness or pus at infection sites may be diminished because of the decreased numbers of WBCs required to promote these physical signs. Nurses should thus be extremely vigilant about monitoring for potential infection.

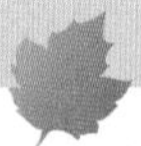

box 46-6

Factors Contributing to Diminished Immunocompetence in the Older Patient

- Decline in immune system functioning
- Decreased nutritional intake (decreased taste, poor teeth, declining appetite)
- Chronic illnesses (diabetes, chronic obstructive pulmonary disease, renal disease)
- Increased risk of malignancy
- Possible urinary incontinence
- Prostatic hypertrophy and urinary retention
- Skin breakdown and impaired wound healing
- Decreased ability to care for self
- Impaired communication
- Decreased mobility

MEDICATIONS AND TREATMENTS

Many medications affect immunocompetence. Antibiotics such as tetracycline and chloramphenicol impair bone marrow function. Steroids display many immunological effects, including decreased lymphocyte and antibody concentration. Patients who have received organ or bone marrow transplants (see Chapter 47) often must remain on medications (e.g., cyclosporine) that severely suppress the immune system. Patients placed on treatment regimens with any immunosuppressive medications should be monitored for early symptoms of infection that would indicate compromise in immune functioning.

Various treatments also impair immunocompetence. Treatment protocols for patients with cancer can lead to life-threatening complications, such as infection and sepsis. Biological therapy with interferon-alpha and interleukin-2 can cause leukopenia. Patients who receive multiple transfusions with RBCs can demonstrate suppressed immunity. Most chemotherapeutic agents and radiation to the pelvis, spine, ribs, sternum, skull, and metaphyses of the long bones can adversely affect the bone marrow's ability to produce WBCs. The lowest point in WBC levels, or the *nadir*, may not be seen until several days or weeks after the initiation of treatment. The absolute neutrophil count (ANC) is calculated in neutropenic patients to determine the degree of immunosuppression. The ANC is calculated as follows:

1. Add segmented neutrophils and band neutrophils (from the WBC differential).
2. Multiply the total WBC count by the total obtained in step 1.

Example:
Segs = 42%
Bands = 10%
Total WBC count = 4,100 cells/mm^3
42 + 10 = 52%
4,100 × 0.52 = 2,132 ANC

Usually, protective measures, such as those summarized in Box 46-7, are instituted for patients with an ANC of less than 1,000. However, all patients in the ICU are considered at risk for immunocompromise and should have the benefit of scrupulous handwashing, rigorous monitoring, and protective interventions.

NUTRITIONAL STATUS

The patient's nutritional status has a major impact on immune function. Inadequate intake of protein and calories can alter immune responses and resistance to infection

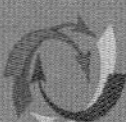

box 46-7 nursing interventions for the Immunocompromised Patient*

- Provide a private room or uninfected roommate.
- Use a laminar flow or positive pressure room.
- Maintain strict handwashing with antiseptic soap.
- Use no rectal thermometers, enemas, or suppositories.
- Restrict staff and visitors with infections (or require masks).
- Provide patient with a mask when he or she goes to other departments or crowded areas.
- Permit cooked foods only.
- Allow no fresh flowers or live plants.
- Avoid sources of stagnant water (vases, water pitchers, humidifiers, denture cups).

*Precautions taken may vary according to institutional policy and the severity of immunosuppression.

by decreasing lymphocyte and antibody production and impairing wound healing. A multidisciplinary approach using a nutritionist can assist the nurse in assessing dietary intake and nutritional requirements for the critically ill immunocompromised person. Supplemental intravenous or enteral feedings may be necessary to prevent further deterioration of the body's nutritional status and ability to fight infection.

SKIN INTEGRITY

The integumentary system, including the skin and mucous membranes, provides a physical barrier to infection. Surgical or traumatic wounds, burn injuries, or pressure sores breach these physical defenses and predispose the critically ill patient to infection. Also, in a critical care setting in which intravenous and intra-arterial catheters, urethral catheters, or endotracheal tubes are used, multiple portals of entry for pathogens can provide simultaneous sites for potential infection. Therefore, all wounds and portals of entry should be carefully monitored for signs and symptoms of infection.

clinical applicability challenges

Self-Challenges: Critical Thinking

1. *Patients in the ICU experience a higher rate of nosocomial (hospital-acquired) infections than patients in many other areas of the hospital. List the potential factors that place patients at risk for infections in the ICU and develop preventive nursing interventions for each factor.*
2. *A patient is admitted to the ICU from the emergency department. Her condition requires extensive abdominal surgery. During the health history interview she mentions frequent bruising, heavy menstrual periods, and a family history of "bleeding." Discuss further workup of this patient that needs to occur before surgery can proceed.*

Study Questions

1. *A low reticulocyte count in a patient with anemia most likely indicates*
   a. *sickle cell anemia.*
   b. *risk of thrombocytosis.*
   c. *possible bone marrow underproduction of RBCs.*
   d. *hemophilia.*
2. *When assessing the WBC differential, a "left shift" (increased number of bands) usually indicates*
   a. *acute leukemia.*
   b. *hypersensitivity reaction.*
   c. *immunosuppression.*
   d. *an infectious process.*
3. *A patient with chronic severe alcoholism should be assessed for a potential bleeding disorder related to*
   a. *vitamin K deficiency and insufficient production of coagulation factors.*
   b. *overproduction of platelets.*
   c. *congenital bleeding disorder.*
   d. *bone marrow dysfunction.*
4. *Which of the following is NOT related to the role of nutrition in preventing infection?*
   a. *Lymphocyte function and antibody production*
   b. *Hemostasis*
   c. *Wound healing*
   d. *Skin integrity maintenance*

REFERENCES

1. Baz R, Mekhail R: The evaluation of bleeding disorders. Cleveland Clinic Foundation, 2003. Available at: http://www.clevelandclinicmeded.com/diseasemanagement/hematology/bleeding
2. O'Hara J, Sanchez J, Allen M: Approach to the bleeding patient. Pathology Update, 4. Texas Tech University, 2002. Available at: http://www.elp.ttuhsc.edu/Pathology/images/PUNo4.pdf
3. Barger AP, Hurley R: Evaluation of the hypercoagulable state. Postgrad Med Online 108(4), 2000. Available at: http://www.postgradmed.com/issues/2000/09_00/barger.htm

OTHER SELECTED READING

Agaliotis DP: Hemophilia, overview. EMedicine, 2002. Available at: http://www.emedicine.com/topic3528.htm

Escolano S, Golmard JL, Korinek AM, et al: A multi-state model for evolution of intensive care unit patients: Prediction of nosocomial infection and deaths. Stat Med 19:3465–3482, 2000

Heyland DK, Novak F, Drover JW, et al: Should immunonutrition become routine in critically ill patient? JAMA 286:944–953, 2001

Holcomb SS: Anemia: Pointing the way to deeper problem. Nursing 2001 31:36–43, 2001

Thiagarajan P: Platelet disorders. EMedicine, 2002. Available at: http://www.emedicine.com/med/topic987.htms

chapter **47**

Organ and Hematopoietic Stem Cell Transplantation

SANDRA A. MITCHELL ■ JOANN SIKORA

objectives

Based on the content in this chapter, the reader should be able to:

- Analyze the criteria used to evaluate and prepare patients for transplantation.
- Evaluate the principles of organ and hematopoietic stem cell compatibility and immunosuppression.
- Describe the complications of organ and hematopoietic stem cell transplantation.
- Discuss nursing assessment and management for patients with organ transplants (kidney, liver, heart, pancreas, lung) and hematopoietic stem cell transplants.

Transplant research began in the early 1900s, but kidney transplantation did not become a realistic treatment for chronic renal failure in humans until the early 1950s. Heart and liver transplants followed in the 1960s and have steadily increased in frequency as a treatment for end-stage organ failure since the 1980s. Pancreas transplantation also began in the mid-1960s and achieved good graft survival rates in the 1980s. The number of lung transplants is small, primarily because of a lack of medically suitable donors. Survival rates for solid organ transplants are given in Table 47-1.

Over the past 20 years, hematopoietic stem cell transplantation (HSCT) has evolved from an experimental treatment for patients with advanced acute leukemia to a therapeutically effective modality that is now standard therapy for selected diseases. HSCT, which is known to be curative in several malignant and nonmalignant disorders, is a transplant using hematopoietic stem cells at various stages of differentiation and maturation. Decreased treatment-associated mortality and improved supportive care have helped make this possible.

table 47-1 Graft and Patient 1-Year Survival Rates for Adult Solid Organ Transplants Performed in 2001

Organ	Graft Survival Rate	Patient Survival Rate
Kidney	91%	95%
Heart	85%	85%
Lung	76%	77%
Liver	81%	86%
Pancreas	78%	96%
Kidney–pancreas	92%	95%

Data from the 2002 Annual Report of the U.S. Scientific Registry for Transplant Recipients and the Organ Procurement and Transplant Network–Transplant Data: 2000–2002 UNOS, Richmond, VA, and the Division of Transplantation, Bureau of Health Resources Development, Health Resources and Services Administration, U.S. Department of Health and Human Services, Rockville, MD, 2002.

Astute nursing care is essential to prevent treatment-related complications and death. Other factors that may affect the outcomes of HSCT include the type and stage of disease at the time of transplantation, the type of transplant (allogeneic versus autologous), the degree of human leukocyte antigen (HLA) matching in allogeneic transplants, the ages of both the donor and the recipient, and the experience of the transplantation center. In general, the transplant-related mortality risk in allogeneic HSCT is about 20% to 30% higher than in autologous HSCT. The transplant-related mortality rate in autologous HSCT is less than 5% at most centers.

Even when a patient is cured of the original disease, he or she may experience delayed and long-term complications that can shorten or negatively affect the quality of his or her remaining life. These complications include infections, chronic graft-versus-host disease (GVHD; seen in allogeneic HSCT), thyroid dysfunction, pulmonary complications, cataracts, and the development of second malignancies. In general, autologous transplantation has fewer long-term complications, largely because no GVHD is associated with autologous transplantation. Disease-free survival at 5 years after HSCT varies substantially (Table 47-2). Advances in histocompatibility matching, immunosuppression, stem cell collection, and cryopreservation techniques, and the development of more effective drugs to manage post-transplantation infections and stimulate hematopoiesis have helped to increase the success of HSCT.

This chapter includes the major aspects of care for patients receiving kidney, liver, heart, pancreas, and lung transplants, and HSCT. It covers principles that apply to all types of transplantation and discusses content unique to specific types of transplants.

INDICATIONS FOR TRANSPLANTATION

Many factors influence the indications and patient eligibility for transplantation. Currently, end-stage disease is the primary reason for most organ transplants. HSCT is now used when bone marrow is defective or destroyed by a disease process or as a result of treating an underlying disease.[1] New information concerning patient outcomes, complications, surgical techniques, immunosuppressive drugs, and availability of organs and hematopoietic stem cells is also considered. Table 47-3 presents indications for transplantation.

table 47-2 Disease-Free Survival at 5 Years After Hematopoietic Stem Cell Transplantation (HSCT)

Disease and Stage	Allogeneic (% Survival)	Autologous (% Survival)
Acute myeloid leukemia		
First complete remission	45–65	30–50
Second complete remission	20–45	20–40
Acute lymphoid leukemia		
First complete remission	40–70	30–50
Second complete remission	25–45	15–25
Chronic myelogenous leukemia		
Chronic phase	60–75	0–5
Accelerated phase	30–45	0–5
Blast crisis	10–20	0–5
Hodgkin's and non-Hodgkin's lymphoma		
First relapse, second remission	40–60	40–60
Advanced disease	10–25	10–25

Data from: Applebaum FR: The use of bone marrow and peripheral stem cell transplantation in the treatment of cancer. CA Cancer J Clin 46(3):142–164, 1996 and Armitage JO: Bone marrow transplantation. N Engl J Med 330(12): 827–838, 1994.

PATIENT EVALUATION AND CONTRAINDICATIONS TO TRANSPLANTATION

Selecting the ideal candidate for transplantation is an intricate process. To evaluate a patient's suitability for transplantation, a comprehensive multisystem analysis is performed. This includes both physiological and psychosocial factors that will affect the patient's chance for a successful transplant. During this evaluation phase, newly diagnosed conditions are treated, and plans are made to ensure adequate nutrition, mobility, and muscle strength. The goal is to have the patient in the best possible physical condition for transplantation. When transplantations are performed earlier rather than later in the disease process, there are fewer disabilities and a greater chance for survival.

Financial guidance is provided so that patients and families know what their insurance will cover and the nature and amount of their expected out-of-pocket expenses. Costs for transplants range from $80,000 to $250,000. Medications after transplantation can cost $10,000 to $16,000 a year.[2–4] Transplantation centers may require proof of the patient's ability to pay before accepting a patient for transplantation.

table 47-3 Indications for Transplantation

Organ	Indications for Transplantation	Common Causes
Kidney	End-stage renal disease	Hypertension, diabetes mellitus, glomerular nephritis, urological disorders, cancer, nephrotoxins, trauma, hemolytic disorders, congenital anomalies
Liver	Adults: irreversible liver disease, malignancy, and hepatic failure resulting in synthetic liver dysfunction Children: biliary atresia, α_1-antitrypsin deficiency	Acute or chronic hepatitis, primary sclerosing cholangitis, primary biliary cirrhosis, hepatocellular carcinoma, Budd-Chiari syndrome, alcoholic cirrhosis
Heart	End-stage heart failure	Ischemic cardiomyopathy, idiopathic cardiomyopathy, valvular heart disease, congenital anomalies
Pancreas	Type 1 diabetes mellitus with end-stage renal disease either alone or in combination with a kidney transplant	Diabetes mellitus
Lung	Chronic obstructive pulmonary disease (COPD)	Emphysema and bronchiectasis, idiopathic pulmonary fibrosis, emphysema due to α_1-antitrypsin deficiency, primary pulmonary hypertension
Heart-lung	Eisenmenger's syndrome	Pulmonary hypertension with irreversible right-sided heart failure not amenable to heart transplantation alone
Hematopoietic stem cell	Malignant disorders	Leukemias, myelodysplastic syndrome, Hodgkin's lymphoma, non-Hodgkin's lymphoma, multiple myeloma, and selected solid tumors (e.g., renal cell tumors, germ cell tumors, neuroblastoma, pinealoblastoma)[1]
	Nonmalignant disorders	Aplastic, sickle cell, and Fanconi's anemias; selected metabolic disorders; thalassemia; and immunodeficiency syndromes[1]

The following general criteria guide the selection for transplantation:

- Age is evaluated individually. Ages may range from newborn (patients who may have heart transplantation for hypoplastic left heart syndrome) to 70 years. People older than 55 years of age may be at increased risk for complications.
- Acute or chronic infection is absent or has been treated. Localized liver infection may be an exception. Inflammatory diseases, such as systemic lupus erythematosus, do not rule out transplantation but should be quiescent at the time of the procedure.
- For the patient undergoing HSCT for a malignancy, care is taken to distinguish patients who can be saved by transplantation from those who may relapse or succumb to the rigors and toxicities of treatment.

Organ-specific criteria for transplantation are listed in Table 47-4.

In general, evaluation common to all transplants includes the following:

- ABO typing
- Tissue typing, HLA matching, mixed lymphocyte culture (MLC) matching
- Transfusion history
- Infectious disease screening (tuberculin skin test, human immunodeficiency virus [HIV], hepatitis B surface antigen, hepatitis C virus, Epstein-Barr virus, cytomegalovirus [CMV], toxoplasmosis titers, herpes simplex, varicella virus, venereal disease)
- Liver function studies
- Renal function studies
- Complete blood count (CBC)
- Coagulation studies
- Gastrointestinal evaluation (depending on age and history)
- Gynecological examination
- Electrocardiogram (ECG)
- Chest radiograph
- Dental examination to rule out infection
- Social history, review of patient motivation, and ability to follow postoperative regimen; possible psychological evaluation

Contraindications are based on conditions and behaviors that decrease the chance of survival. For solid organ transplantation, these include serious active infection or sepsis, recent cancer (unless that is the reason for transplantation), current substance abuse, HIV infection, severe cachexia, active peptic ulcer disease, psychiatric disorders that impair the ability to give informed consent or adhere to the treatment regimen, and repeated noncompliance. Table 47-4 lists these contraindications.

DONOR SELECTION

After a person is determined to be a candidate for transplantation, a donor source must be selected.

table 47-4 Criteria, Contraindications, and Evaluations in Transplantation

Organ	Specific Criteria	Contraindications	Specific Evaluation
Kidney	• End-stage or near end-stage renal failure (defined as a glomerular filtration rate of <10 mL/min) • Pre–end stage preferable for some patients (i.e., children, patients with diabetes mellitus, and those for whom there is a living donor)	• Severe or uncorrectable coronary artery disease, peripheral vascular disease, or pulmonary disease • Severe cardiomyopathy	• Voiding cystourethrogram to evaluate for obstruction or reflux (medical history dependent) • Cardiac evaluation (age and medical history dependent)
Liver	• Malnutrition • Severe blood clotting abnormalities • Variceal bleeding • Hepatic encephalopathy • Severe, intractable ascites • Severe, intractable pruritus	• Multiple uncorrected congenital anomalies • Advanced cardiopulmonary disease • Severe pulmonary hypertension	• Abdominal computed tomography (CT) scan (to detect hepatoma) • Doppler ultrasound (to identify patency of portal vein) • Liver disease studies and autoimmune markers, such as ceruloplasmin, carcinoembryonic antigen (CEA), alpha-fetoprotein (AFP), antimitochondrial and antinuclear antibody • Endoscopic retrograde cholangiopancreatography (ERCP)/ cholangiogram (if indicated, usually for patients with cholestasis) • Liver biopsy (if indicated) • Upper and lower endoscopy (if indicated)
Pancreas	• End-stage renal failure (combine kidney and pancreas transplant) • Absence of (or corrected) coronary artery disease	• Severe or uncorrectable coronary artery disease, peripheral vascular disease, or pulmonary disease • Previous major amputation • Blindness (not absolute contraindication) • Severe cardiomyopathy	• Thallium stress test or coronary angiogram • Cardiology consult • Gastric emptying study • Ophthalmology evaluation • Endocrine studies: glycosylated hemoglobin, serum amylase and lipase, islet cell antibody, urine and serum peptide measurements
Heart	• Cardiac disease, New York Heart Association Class IV (or advanced III) • Condition not amenable to other forms of medical or surgical therapy • End-stage cardiac disease with less than a 25% likelihood of survival at 1 year without a transplant • Patients with potentially fatal arrhythmia not amenable to other therapies	• Fixed pulmonary hypertension with pulmonary vascular resistance: >6–8 Wood units (>480–640 dynse/sec/cm^{-5} or pulmonary arteriolar gradient >15 mm) • Recent unresolved pulmonary infarct (increased post-transplant risk of pulmonary infection) • Advanced or poorly controlled diabetes mellitus	• Right heart catheterization; full cardiac catheterization if indicated • Cardiopulmonary exercise testing (MVO_2) • Pulmonary function tests, including diffusion capacity (DLco) • Cardiac rehabilitation consultation • Multigated acquisition analysis (MUGA) or echocardiogram
Lung	• Untreatable end-stage pulmonary disease (parenchymal or vascular) • Medical therapy ineffective • Estimated survival (without lung transplant) less than probability of survival with lung transplant	• Significant coronary artery disease • Poor nutritional status (i.e., <10%–15% of ideal body weight) • Previous cardiothoracic surgery • Corticosteroid use >15 mg/d • Ventilation dependency	• Quantitative ventilation/perfusion scan • Cardiac evaluation • Full pulmonary function testing, including DLco, arterial blood gases, lung volume • 6-min walk test (rehabilitation assessment) • Nutritional assessment

(continued)

table 47-4 Criteria, Contraindications, and Evaluations in Transplantation (Continued)

Organ	Specific Criteria	Contraindications	Specific Evaluation
Hematopoietic stem cells	• **Malignant disorders:** replacement of hematopoietic and immune system destroyed by high-dose chemotherapy or radiation with new immune system that can recognize malignant cells as foreign and mount immunologic response against tumor • **Nonmalignant disorders:** replacement of an immune or hematopoietic system that is either defective or has failed	• Poor or no response to conventional-dose chemotherapy for malignant disorders (exception is acute leukemia that fails to respond to induction therapy [primary induction failure]; high-dose chemotherapy and allogeneic transplant is an accepted indication) • Poor performance status (using Karnofsky Performance Status scale to assess physical functioning) • Advanced cardiopulmonary or renal disease (left ventricular ejection fraction [LVEF] <50%; DLco <70; creatinine clearance, 60 mL/min [exception may be multiple myeloma patients]) • Brain metastasis • Age >70 years	• Disease restaging, including CT scans, nuclear medicine scans, bone marrow aspirate and biopsy, lumbar puncture, immunoglobulin levels, cytogenetics, molecular diagnostics, and measures of minimal residual disease • DNA procurement for future engraftment studies • ABO and Rh typing • HLA typing and HLA-matched platelet transfusion support (allogeneic transplant patients only) • Chest x-ray, ECG and MUGA scan, pulmonary function tests, including DLco, 24-hour urine for creatinine clearance • Baseline CT scans of chest and sinuses, particularly if there are symptoms or a history of repeated infections • Dental evaluation, including full mouth x-rays and cleaning • Sperm/fertilized embryo banking • Autologous stem cell backup if patient is undergoing unrelated or mismatched transplantation • Consultations with radiation therapy and infectious disease

Determining Compatibility

ORGAN TRANSPLANTATION

Two major antigen systems are evaluated in transplantation. The primary determinant for solid organ transplantation is ABO grouping. A mismatch in compatibility may cause an immediate reaction leading to organ loss. The rules of compatibility that apply to the administration of blood products also apply to organ transplantation: type A blood has the A antigen, type B blood has the B antigen, type AB blood has both A and B antigens, and type O blood has neither antigen.

Histocompatibility testing (tissue typing) is the evaluation of donor antigens against recipient antibodies. This determines the compatibility between donor and recipient, which predicts the chances of graft acceptance. In the HLA antigen system, antigens that compose a person's tissue type are coded by genes of the major histocompatibility complex. These genes contain information for cell surface antigens that differentiate self from nonself. These antigens (HLAs) are found on the surface of lymphocytes. The major histocompatibility complex involved in the immune response include class I antigens (A, B) and class II, the DR antigens. Each person has two A-, B-, and DR-locus antigens that are inherited as a haplotype (i.e., a single unit) from each parent. Many possible antigens may occur at each locus, resulting in a large number of HLA combinations. Therefore, it is rare for people who are unrelated to have identical antigens.

The higher the number of antigens that match, the higher the likelihood of compatibility, and the lower the risk of rejection. A six-antigen match is associated with the greatest potential for successful transplantation. HLA matching is performed for solid organ and bone marrow transplants. It is most important in kidney and bone marrow transplantation. Transplantation requires the suppression of the normal immune response with the postoperative administration of antirejection medications to prevent graft rejection. The greater the similarity of the donor and recipient tissue type, the less likely the occurrence of rejection.

In the case of living related donors, a direct white blood cell (WBC) cross-match may be performed. The sera of the donor and the recipient are tested and evaluated for cell death. For those patients not receiving living related donation, screening is routinely performed against a pool of lymphocyte samples from multiple random donors against the sera of the recipient. The percentage of samples to which the recipient reacts is referred to as the panel reactive antibody percentage (PRA). A high PRA is predictive of a high risk of rejection, and a prospective cross-match, such as is used in living donors, would be advised. PRA should be repeated monthly because the titer may change from time to time.

Blood transfusions are avoided if possible in patients awaiting organ transplantation because of the risk of antibody production and a resultant high PRA or positive cross-match between donor and recipient. If blood transfusions are necessary, leukocyte-filtered blood should be administered.

HEMATOPOIETIC STEM CELL TRANSPLANTATION

Selection of a donor for HSCT is based on the type and stage of the underlying disease, age, comorbidities, and the availability of an appropriate HLA- and MLC-matched donor. MLC is performed to observe for interaction between the potential donor's cells and recipient cells. Low reactivity indicates greater compatibility.

There are many sources of hematopoietic stem cells. The types of HSCT may be differentiated in terms of the hematopoietic stem cell donor, the method used to collect the cells, and the intensity of the conditioning regimen (Box 47-1).

For patients who receive hematopoietic stem cells from another person (i.e., allogeneic transplant), donor selection is based on the availability of HLA- and MLC-matched donors, who may or may not be related. A related donor is usually a sibling (siblings have the greatest chance of matching on both HLA and on other minor and as yet unrecognized antigens). If more than one donor is HLA-identical to the patient, donor selection is based on sex compatibility with the patient, ABO compatibility with the patient, negative viral titers, overall health, younger donor age, minimal exposure to blood products, and nulliparity, because all of these factors are associated with an improved outcome of HSCT.

If the patient does not have a suitable family donor, a search for an unrelated donor may be undertaken. The National Marrow Donor Program (NMDP), a donor registry developed in 1986, allows patients without a related donor to find an HLA-matched unrelated donor (Box 47-2). Umbilical cord blood is another potential stem cell source, particularly in pediatric allogeneic transplantation.

A difference in ABO blood groups between patient and donor does not interfere with donor selection; however, it does present unique clinical problems. The hematopoietic stem cell product may have to be depleted of red blood cells (RBCs) to prevent, during infusion, a hemolytic reaction caused by ABO antibodies still circulating in the patient's bloodstream. After engraftment and approximately 100 days after transplantation, the patient will seroconvert to the ABO type of the donor.

Living Donors

Living donors are increasingly being used in kidney, liver, pancreas, and lung transplantation. Living donors are used exclusively in bone marrow transplantation. There is an increase in the use of living organ donors, but there is a dire shortage of organs for transplantation. The number of transplant candidates is growing, and the number of cadaveric organ donors has remained relatively constant.

Once identified, a potential donor has a thorough medical evaluation to determine that the organ functions normally, there is no underlying disease, and donation would not jeopardize the donor's well-being in any obvious way. Once this evaluation is completed successfully, a living donor transplantation may be performed.

Ethical questions continue to be raised about the use of living donors. Long-term studies of living donors have

box 47-1
Types of Hematopoietic Stem Cell Transplantation

Differentiated based on *donor* source for stem cells

- *Auto*logous: self
- *Syn*geneic: identical twin
- *Allo*geneic: nonself
  - Related
  - Unrelated (National Marrow Donor Program)
- *Cord blood*
  - Related
  - Unrelated (cord blood bank)

Differentiated based on *method* of collecting stem cells

- Bone marrow harvest
- Peripheral blood stem cell collection by apheresis

Differentiated based on *intensity* of conditioning regimen

- *Myeloablative:* High doses of chemotherapy and sometimes radiation therapy given to destroy hematopoietic and immune systems of recipient. Transplantation of new stem cells allows hematopoietic and immune reconstitution. Higher morbidity and mortality rates restrict this treatment to younger patients and those in good medical condition.
- *Nonmyeloablative:* Lower chemotherapy doses (those that do not fully destroy patient's own hematopoietic and immune systems) are given along with immunosuppression to facilitate engraftment of donor hematopoietic cells. Significant long-term risks for infection and graft-versus-host disease (GVHD) persist.

box 47-2
Bone Marrow Registries

The National Marrow Donor Program (NMDP) is a federally funded registry established in 1986 to corrdinate the donor search and matching process. The program was initially formed by bone marrow transplant family members. The NMDP maintains the world's largest and most diverse registry of more than 5 million volunteer blood stem cell donors and more than 28,000 cord blood units. The NMDP works with the American Red Cross and with international registries. The office of patient advocacy is reached at 1-800-MARROW-2.

The American Bone Marrow Donor Registry is a private registry with more than 1/2 million donors. It also coordinates international searches.

Data from www.marrow.org.

shown that the risks and adverse effects of donation are rare, and, in fact, some donors report beneficial psychological effects from donating. However, some question the risk of coercion in living donors, especially when the donor is the parent of a child who will die without a transplant. To ensure freely given and informed consent, there may be an assessment by a psychiatrist, involvement of a non–transplant-related physician, and education of the donor.

KIDNEY DONOR

Living donors historically have been blood relatives because tissue matching was considered more likely. However, more recently, living kidney donors have been spouses and friends, and the results have been comparable with those obtained with living blood-related donors. Although either kidney may be used for transplantation, the left is preferred because the left renal vein is longer than the right.[5]

LIVER DONOR

Living related liver transplantation involves the removal of a portion of a liver in a living adult with transplantation into a child. The 1-year graft survival rate in the United States is 81%.[2]

PANCREAS DONOR

Transplanting part of the pancreas from a living person is rarely performed. The donor must not be at risk for diabetes mellitus.

LUNG DONOR

Recently, the use of living related donors in lung transplantation has been successful. Either the lobe of one lung from one parent is transplanted into the child, or one lobe from each parent is used for a bilateral lobar transplant. The major advantage of lobar transplantation is that it enables children to have the transplant either at a time when they are in the best condition or when they become critically ill and a cadaveric donor is unavailable.

Cadaveric Donors

If a cadaveric donor is needed, the recipient is placed on the national waiting list. The United States is divided into approximately 60 areas; an organ procurement organization (OPO) is responsible for recovering and transporting organs to transplantation hospitals in each area. The United Network for Organ Sharing (UNOS) is the private, nonprofit organization that administers organ waiting lists and allocates organs throughout the United States on behalf of the recipients.[3]

Patients are placed on the UNOS national list based on blood type and listing date. The size of hearts, lungs, and livers is important for donation. The waiting time varies by organ. Patients awaiting heart transplantation are risk stratified based on condition and classified according to status. A patient awaiting heart transplantation who requires the use of inotropic medications or a ventricular assist device may be placed at higher priority (status 1) than those waiting at home on stable oral heart failure medications (status 2). Patients awaiting liver transplants are also risk stratified. Status rankings 1, 2A, 2B, and 3 are used based on the severity of the disease process. A patient who is projected to live less than 7 days without transplantation is status 1, whereas a patient who is living at home with chronic liver disease is status 3.[3]

Despite the continued need for transplants, the supply of donor organs remains inadequate. According to the Scientific Registry of Transplant Recipients, in 2002, more than 80,000 patients awaited organ transplantation in the United States. The predicted annual number of brain-dead potential organ donors in the United States is between 10,500 and 13,800. The overall predicted consent rate is 42%. Lack of consent to a request for donation is the primary cause of the gap between the number of potential donors and the number of actual donors.[6]

A major factor in the discrepancy between potential and actual donors is lack of education for potential donor families. When a patient is determined to be brain dead, or support is withdrawn from a patient who is not brain dead, many hospitals alert the local organ procurement agency as a matter of policy. In some larger institutions, a nurse with advanced training in the area of organ donation and family support is trained as a donor advocate. The role of this nurse is to support the family in their grieving process while initiating the discussion of organ donation.

It is important that all potential organ donors be identified. Potential donors often are victims of trauma or cerebral aneurysm or a variety of other circumstances. Criteria for organ donation vary widely. Therefore, it is recommended that any patient for whom the possibility of donation is considered be referred to the local OPO.

DETERMINATION OF DEATH

With current technology, death can be determined in two ways. The absence of cardiopulmonary function is the better-known method; however, the absence of brain function (brain death) also is a common method of determining death (see Chapter 36 for neurological criteria for determining death). Most patients who are organ donors are pronounced dead based on the absence of brain function. The critical care nurse should be familiar with the laws in his or her state related to "brain death" and with the institutional policies for the determination of death.

ROLE OF THE NURSE

Critical care nurses are an integral part of the organ donation team. Almost all organ donors die in critical care units; therefore, the critical care nurse is a key person in identifying potential donors. Moreover, the nurse plays an important role as advocate by making certain that all efforts are made to determine and act on the patient's wishes regarding donation. Nurses also play a vital role in supporting the family psychologically, particularly when they are trying to accept the donor's death. When a decision is made for organ donation, the nurse also plays an important role in supporting the donor physiologically.

The care of the potential donor, once identified, becomes the responsibility of the OPO. A nurse, who is specially trained to maintain hemodynamic stability of the donor, works with the bedside nurse to care for the patient. It is essential to maintain hemodynamic stability so that the vital organs are perfused adequately. To accomplish this, hypotension is treated by administering fluids and plasma volume expanders. If vasopressors are necessary, dopamine, phenylephrine (Neo-Synephrine), or vasopressin is administered to maintain systolic blood pressure. Epinephrine or dobutamine may be administered to maintain the cardiac index. As the need for inotropes or vasopressors increases, the possibility for multiorgan recovery decreases.

It is also essential to assess urine output hourly to detect diabetes insipidus. This is common in organ donors and is caused by failure of the posterior pituitary to produce or release antidiuretic hormones. Aqueous vasopressin or desmopressin acetate may be ordered to reduce urine output and help maintain fluid balance.

Laboratory results, such as electrolytes, CBC, liver and renal function tests, and arterial blood gases (ABGs), are necessary to assess organ function and determine appropriate intervention. An ECG and echocardiogram are required for heart donation, and serial chest radiographs, sputum for Gram stain, bronchoscopy, and visual inspection at the time of organ procurement are required for lung donation.

ROLE OF THE DONOR COORDINATOR

The role of the donor coordinator has developed as a result of the need to make organs available for transplantation. Kidneys are the most commonly transplanted organ and hearts, lungs, livers, pancreata, corneas, skin, bone, and perhaps other organs or tissue may also be donated. The donor coordinator is involved in the coordination and procurement of all transplantable organs. In addition, the donor coordinator usually ensures that the family has the information necessary to give informed consent and provides them with access to bereavement support. The donor coordinator also serves as a resource for the health care team and as a liaison between the transplant program and the critical care area. Cooperation between the critical care staff and the transplant program helps ensure that the option of donation is offered to families of all potential donors.

PRESERVATION TIME

There is a broad range of acceptable preservation times for organs. However, the goal is to transplant organs as soon as possible. Kidneys can be stored for up to 48 hours using pulsatile perfusion preservation and for 24 to 36 hours using cold storage. Livers can be stored for up to 20 hours, pancreata up to 12 hours, and hearts and lungs for 4 to 6 hours. Organs are stored in a cold solution specifically designed to decrease cellular injury. Solutions are different for each organ and are based on the metabolic needs of the organ. The focus of preservation is to protect the organ from ischemic injury.[7]

ASSESSMENT AND MANAGEMENT IN ORGAN TRANSPLANTATION

The role of the transplant coordinator exists across the continuum of care. The role spans pre-evaluation of potential recipients through transplantation and follow-up. This individual is responsible for coordinating the evaluation and teaching the recipient and family about the evaluation testing process, the listing process, and organ allocation. A major contribution is reviewing preoperative through postoperative procedures, the immunosuppressive regimen, and follow-up care. In many institutions, a nurse practitioner, who also provides medical care and follow-up for the patients, fulfills this role.

Preoperative Phase

The immediate preoperative phase, which is usually only a matter of hours, includes comprehensive laboratory studies, chest radiograph, ECG, and, for kidney transplant recipients, dialysis within 24 hours of transplantation. Laboratory studies usually include CBC, prothrombin time (PT), partial thromboplastin time (PTT), electrolytes, blood sugar, blood urea nitrogen (BUN), creatinine, liver function tests, type and cross-match, and urinalysis.

Surgical Procedure

KIDNEY

Typically, the kidney is placed retroperitoneal in the iliac fossa. The hypogastric or internal artery and the external iliac vein are usually used for anastomosis. When it is mechanically difficult to access these vessels, as with children, it may be necessary to anastomose the renal vessels to the inferior vena cava and aorta.

Two common types of ureteral anastomoses can be performed. In the first procedure, the donor ureter is implanted into the recipient's bladder by a vertical cystotomy and a submucosal antireflux tunnel, because the ureter lacks innervation and normal peristalsis. In the second type, used less frequently, the donor kidney is anastomosed at the ureteropelvic junction to the recipient ureter. An indwelling catheter is used for both types of anastomoses, and occasionally a ureteral stent may be used. In either case, hematuria is present for several days. In the first, more common procedure, clots may be seen in the urine because of the vascular nature of the bladder. In the second, less common, procedure, the urine changes to pink within the first postoperative day because there are no sutures in the bladder.

LIVER

The liver is transplanted orthotopically, that is, in its normal position after the native liver is removed. Four vascular anastomoses must be performed: the suprahepatic vena cava, the infrahepatic vena cava, the portal vein, and the hepatic artery (Fig. 47-1). Then the liver is reperfused, and the bile duct is anastomosed, usually to the recipient bile duct.[8] A T tube is usually inserted. During liver transplantation, a rapid infusion system is used for administering blood and blood products, a cell saver is often used to limit the amount of banked blood required, and a pump for venovenous bypass is often used in adults to return blood to the heart. This is performed by inserting a catheter into the saphenous or femoral vein and another into the axillary vein (usually on the left side), which allows blood to circulate from the lower extremities back to the heart. Surgery usually takes between 8 and 16 hours.

HEART

Orthotopic Transplantation

Orthotopic heart transplantation (OHT) is the most common heart transplantation performed. The recipient's

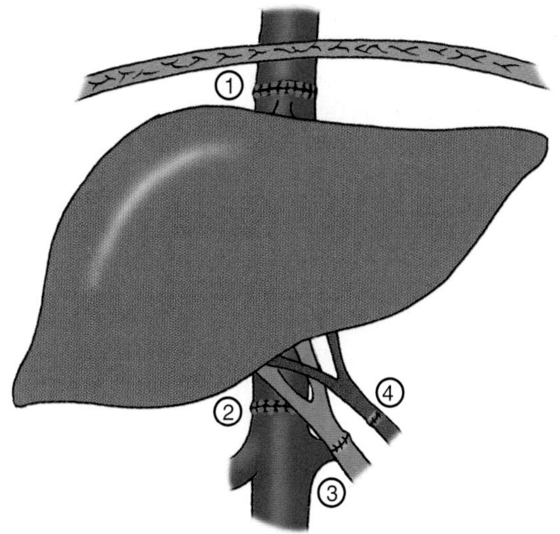

figure 47-1 Diagram of vascular anastomoses in liver transplantation. (1), Suprahepatic vena cava; (2), infrahepatic vena cava; (3), portal vein; and (4), hepatic artery.

heart is excised, and the donor heart is implanted in its place. A median sternotomy incision is made, cardiopulmonary bypass is initiated, and the recipient's heart is removed by incising the left and right atria, pulmonary artery, and aorta. The Lower and Shumway technique has been the gold standard for OHT. The atrial septum and posterior and lateral walls of the recipient's atria are left intact, including the areas of the sinoatrial node, inferior and superior venae cavae to the right atrium, and pulmonary veins to the left atrium. The remnant atria serve as anchors for the donor heart.

The donor atria are trimmed to preserve the anterior arterial walls, sinoatrial node, and internodal conduction pathways. Then anastomoses are made between the recipient and donor left and right atria, the pulmonary arteries, and the aortas. Atrial and ventricular pacing wires are placed at the time of surgery so that temporary pacing can easily be initiated. Cardiopulmonary bypass is weaned off, and the donor heart assumes the role of providing the cardiac output (Fig. 47-2A).

An alternative to the atrial-to-atrial cuff technique is the bicaval technique (Fig. 47-2B), which preserves atrial anatomy disrupted by the Lower and Shumway technique. The donor atria are intact, and the anastomoses are between the donor and recipient inferior and superior venae cavae rather than the atria. This avoids the loss of atrial anatomy, which has been demonstrated to be responsible for the development of post-transplantation complications such as mitral and tricuspid regurgitation, atrial thrombus formation, and tachydysrhythmia.[9]

Heterotopic Transplantation

Heterotopic transplantation, or piggyback procedure, is an infrequently used technique. The recipient's heart is left in place, and the donor heart is placed next to it in the right chest. The two hearts are connected in parallel by anastomoses made between the donor and recipient left and right atria, aortas, and pulmonary arteries using a synthetic tube graft. By allowing blood to flow through either or both hearts, two functional hearts work together to provide the cardiac output (Fig. 47-3).

Heterotopic transplantation may be used in patients with pulmonary hypertension in whom the donor heart alone would not have a strong enough right ventricle to pump against the increased pulmonary vascular resistance. It can also be used as a life-saving procedure in urgent cases if the only available donor heart is too small for the size of the recipient. Limitations of heterotopic transplantation include thromboembolism from the native heart with need for anticoagulation, limited space in the chest cavity, and, in ischemic heart disease, ongoing angina and the possibility of ischemia-induced dysrhythmias in the native heart. The survival rates are less favorable for heterotopic transplantation than for orthotopic transplantation.

PANCREAS

Transplantation of the entire pancreas is performed most commonly. A pancreas transplantation may be performed in combination with a kidney transplantation for recipients with end-stage renal disease secondary to diabetes mellitus. The pancreas and kidney may be transplanted at the same time or months apart. Segmental pancreas and islet cell transplantations are less frequent.

The pancreas is placed into a heterotopic position, usually the right iliac area. Techniques vary for vascular and exocrine anastomoses. The most controversial aspect of the surgical technique is the approach for draining exocrine secretions. The exocrine duct may be occluded, or exocrine secretions may drain either into the small bowel or bladder. There is no consensus about the best approach, and all have advantages and disadvantages.

LUNG

Both single and double lung transplantations are performed. In single lung transplants, the left lung mainstem bronchus is longer, which makes the procedure easier technically. The preferred lung is based on perfusion abnormalities (as determined by ventilation–perfusion scan) and functional abnormalities. Anastomoses are made at the mainstem bronchus, pulmonary artery, and at the cuff of atrium containing pulmonary veins. Cardiopulmonary bypass is not always necessary and depends on the patient's pulmonary artery pressure, blood pressure, and gas exchange. Incision is made at the fifth intracostal space using a posterior lateral thoracotomy for single lung transplants, whereas a median sternotomy incision or a clamshell incision is made for double lung transplants. Surgeons telescope the recipient's bronchus into the donor lung or vice versa, or perform an end-to-end anastomosis with omentopexy in which an omental flap is wrapped around the tracheal anastomosis to increase blood supply to the area.

Postoperative Phase

Immediately after surgery, transplant recipients are cared for in a closely monitored area until stable. Kidney transplant recipients often go to a postanesthesia care unit and

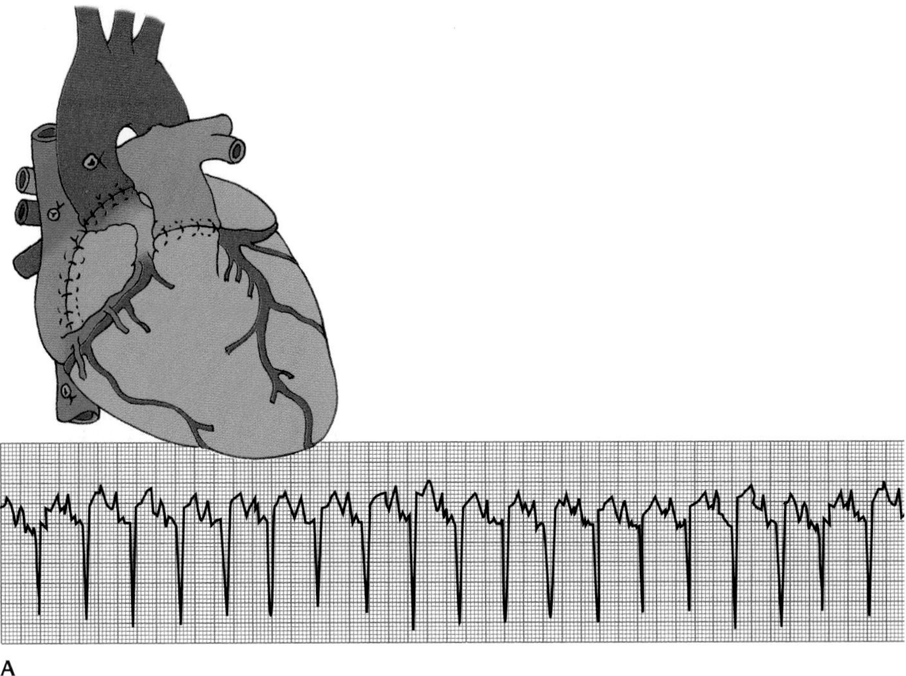

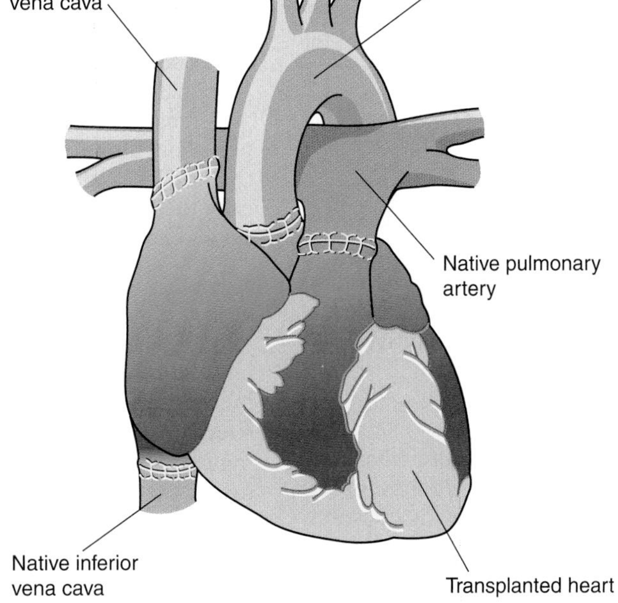

figure 47-2 Orthotopic method of transplantation. (**A**) Lower and Shumway technique. Both the donor and the recipient sinoatrial nodes are intact (**X**), resulting in this ECG tracing. Note the double P wave at independent rates. (**B**) Bicaval technique. The anastomoses are made between the inferior and superior venae cavae rather than the atria. (**B** from Smeltzer SC, Bare BG: Brunner & Suddarth's Textbook of Medical–Surgical Nursing [10th Ed], p 775. Philadelphia, Lippincott Williams & Wilkins, 2004.)

then directly to a transplant unit. Other organ recipients go to an intensive care unit (ICU) from the operating room. When a patient arrives in the postanesthesia or intensive care area, the following assessments are made:

- Blood pressure, heart rate, respirations, oxygenation and ventilator settings, temperature, central venous pressure, and cardiopulmonary hemodynamics. In renal transplant recipients, blood pressure should be taken on an extremity that does not have a functioning vascular access site because even momentary interference with arterial blood flow may lead to access malfunction.
- Patient's level of consciousness and degree of pain
- Number of intravenous and arterial lines, noting the site, type of solution, and flow rate
- Abdominal or chest dressing for drainage, noting the presence of drains and amount and type of drainage
- Presence of bladder and possible ureteral catheters and patency and urinary drainage

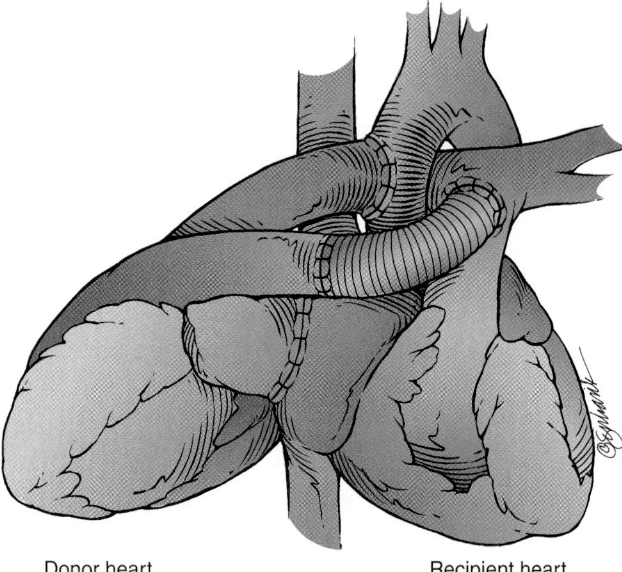

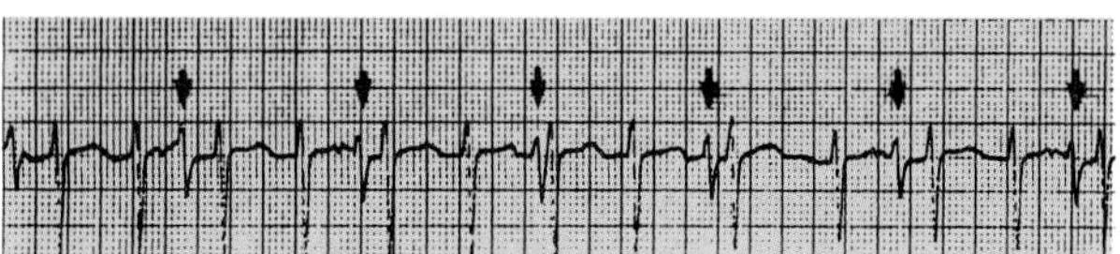

figure 47-3 Heterotopic method of heart transplantation. The donor heart is anastomosed with a Dacron graft to the recipient's heart, resulting in this ECG tracing. Note the "extra" QRS at an independent rate. (From Smeltzer SC, Bare BG: Brunner & Suddarth's Textbook of Medical–Surgical Nursing [10th Ed], p 775. Philadelphia, Lippincott Williams & Wilkins, 2004.)

- Attachment of nasogastric tube to appropriate drainage system and amount and character of drainage
- Most recent hemodynamic and intraoperative laboratory results

KIDNEY

Care of the kidney transplant recipient is centered around assessing renal function and administering immunosuppressive therapy. Therefore, answers to the following questions help guide care:

- Are the patient's own kidneys present in addition to the graft, and if so, how much urine do they produce daily? This information helps determine how much urine is from the transplanted kidney.
- What are the preoperative results of laboratory tests (BUN, creatinine, hematocrit)?
- How much and what kind of intravenous fluid has the patient received?
- What immunosuppressive drugs were given before or during surgery? What immunosuppressive therapy should be given after surgery?

In addition, the vascular access is located, and its patency determined by placing either fingers or a stethoscope directly over the access site and feeling or listening for a characteristically loud, pulsating noise called a *bruit*. If the patient has been maintained on peritoneal dialysis and the catheter is in place, the catheter system must be sterile and capped.

Nursing responsibilities involve the following:

- Observing the function of the transplanted kidney
- Monitoring fluid and electrolyte balance
- Helping avoid sources of infection
- Detecting early signs of complications
- Supporting the patient and family through the recovery phase

Renal Graft Function

The amount of urine produced by the transplanted kidney varies from a large amount (200 to 1,000 mL/hour) to small amounts (less than 20 mL/hour). The degree of renal function is related to ischemic injury in the donor kidney, usually from either hypotensive periods in a cadaveric donor or from the time the kidney is stored outside the body (preservation time). Renal function is better when kidney preservation time is less than 24 hours. Most post-transplantation dysfunction is reversible but may take up to 4 weeks to return to normal.

Renal function is assessed by periodic serum urea nitrogen and creatinine levels and in some centers by a beta-microglobulin test. This low–molecular-weight globulin is filtered readily by the glomerular basement membrane and is reabsorbed and metabolized almost completely by the proximal renal tubules.

A renal scan is a radionuclide test used to determine renal perfusion, filtration, and excretion. It is usually performed in the first 24 hours to obtain baseline data and then periodically thereafter when laboratory values or clinical changes suggest an alteration in renal function.

Urinary Drainage Problems

When a change in urinary output occurs, such as a large volume one hour and a diminished amount the next, mechanical factors that interfere with urinary drainage should be suspected. Clotted, kinked, or compressed tubing in the urinary drainage system may be the cause of the decreased output. When the catheter is occluded by a clot, the patient may complain of pain, feel an urgency to void, or have bloody leakage around the catheter. Milking is the preferred way to dislodge clots because irrigation, even under aseptic conditions, increases the risk of infection. However, gentle irrigation with strict aseptic technique may be necessary. Small amounts of irrigant (no more than 30 mL) are recommended because patients commonly have small bladders. Vigorous irrigation also could cause extravasation at the ureteral anastomosis site.

Urinary Leakage

Urinary leakage on the abdominal dressing and severe abdominal discomfort or distension may indicate retroperitoneal leakage from the ureteral anastomosis site. Decreased urinary output or severe abdominal pain in the presence of good renal function and adequate pain medication should be reported because technical and surgical complications can result in loss of graft function.

Hyperkalemia

The most frequent electrolyte disturbance in the acute postoperative phase is hyperkalemia. If the graft functions and excretes a high volume of urine, it is usually also able to excrete the excessive serum potassium created by surgical tissue damage. If the patient is oliguric or anuric after surgery, the serum potassium may increase to unacceptable levels. Interventions include administration of glucose and insulin to transport potassium into the cell and administration of oral polystyrene sulfonate.

LIVER

Immediate postoperative care is focused on hemodynamic stability, adequate oxygenation, fluid and electrolyte balance, adequate hemostasis, and graft function. An arterial line and pulmonary artery catheter are in place. The pulmonary artery catheter readings help monitor cardiac function and fluid status because high cardiac output and low systemic vascular resistance related to the effects of end-stage liver disease continue immediately after surgery.

Vasopressors and additional fluid boluses may be required in the first 24 to 36 hours. Central venous pressure should be maintained at greater than 10 cm H_2O to balance the importance of good cardiac function against the risk of passive congestion of the liver. Hypotension is most often caused by intra-abdominal bleeding. An increase in abdominal girth or excess bloody drainage from Jackson-Pratt drains is indicative of a severe problem.

Oxygenation

Adequate ventilation is crucial for graft perfusion and helps reduce the risk of pulmonary complications. Ventilator settings are determined by the critical care team, and the arterial (SaO_2) and mixed venous ($S\bar{v}O_2$) oxygen saturations are monitored. Pulse oximetry may be used, but severe jaundice may interfere with saturation measurements. Postoperative pleural effusion is common due to the presence of ascites and risk of injury to the diaphragm during surgery. A chest tube may be required for drainage.

Ventilator support is usually withdrawn when the patient is fully awake. However, if the patient is going to receive a monoclonal antibody, such as muromonab-CD3, the first dose should be given before extubation because there is a risk of pulmonary edema as a reaction to the medication.

Coagulation

Abnormal clotting factors, anastomosis site bleeding, and decreased graft function may all contribute to problems with hemostasis. Therefore, PT, PTT, fibrinogen, and factor V level are monitored along with the amount, color, and consistency of bleeding from the incision and drainage tubes.

The patient may need infusions of platelets, RBCs, or cryoprecipitate. Blood products should be filtered to avoid introduction of CMV, especially if the patient is negative for CMV. Care is taken to avoid overcorrecting coagulation deficiencies, which could lead to vascular thrombosis of the extremities or the graft. As a result of the venovenous bypass system, there is also a risk of phlebitis or thrombosis in the femoral and axillary access site. This may be indicated by ipsilateral swelling in these extremities. Anticoagulation or an inferior vena cava filter may be necessary if deep venous thrombosis develops.

Electrolyte Balance

Hyperglycemia; hyperkalemia; metabolic alkalosis; and calcium, phosphorus, and magnesium disorders may occur. Hyperglycemia is an indication that the liver is able to store glycogen and convert it to glucose. Hyperkalemia can indicate nonfunctional hepatocytes and in turn, a nonfunctional graft. Metabolic alkalosis is related to the citrate in stored blood (metabolized to bicarbonate), hypokalemia, diuretic therapy, and the administration of large volumes of fresh frozen plasma. This usually resolves spontaneously, but hypoventilation in response to the alkalosis may slow weaning from mechanical ventilation. Calcium, phosphorus, and magnesium disturbances are primarily due to the administration of fluid and blood products.

Some degree of postoperative renal dysfunction is also common due either to hepatorenal syndrome or hypotension during surgery. In addition, some immunosuppressive medications are nephrotoxic. This can affect fluid and electrolyte balance. On occasion, when dialysis is needed, continuous arteriovenous or venovenous hemofiltration is used because it interferes least with hemodynamic stability.

Liver Function

Function of the transplanted liver can range from excellent to primary nonfunction. Although the cause of primary nonfunction is not known, it is believed to be related to preservation injury, and retransplantation is necessary. Liver function is initially assessed by bile production, coagulation factors, and later by liver function tests. Measuring bile production from the biliary drainage tube helps assess the excretory function of the liver and is a good early indicator of graft function. PT and the international normalized ratio (INR) provide a measure of the synthetic function of the liver. Aminotransferases (alanine aminotransferase and aspartate aminotransferase) provide information about the degree of hepatic injury related to preservation. Liver function is also assessed by improvement in the clearance of lactate, encephalopathy, and glucose metabolism. All liver function test results are elevated initially and gradually decrease.

HEART

Postoperative care of the heart transplant recipient is similar to that for any person undergoing cardiac surgery. However, there are several major differences, including changes in cardiac rhythm and function caused by denervation of the donor heart and the potential for right ventricular failure. Only the more common orthotopic transplant is discussed here.

Remnant P Waves

In the standard atrial cuff technique, the recipient sinoatrial node and portions of the recipient atria are left intact at the time of surgery. Therefore, two P waves are usually seen on the ECG. The recipient sinoatrial node initiates an impulse that depolarizes the remnant recipient atria; however, this depolarization wave usually does not cross the atrial suture line. The donor sinoatrial node initiates the impulse that causes depolarization of the entire donor heart and elicits the QRS complex. Because the two sets of atria beat independently of each other, two different P waves may appear on the ECG. Remnant P waves may be identified by their dissociation or lack of relationship to the QRS complexes. They usually occur at a slower rate than the donor P waves, and their rate may speed up or slow down because the remnant P waves are still under autonomic nervous system influence, whereas the donor P waves are denervated. The two sets of atria may also be in different rhythms. For example, the recipient atrial remnants may be in atrial fibrillation while the donor heart is in normal sinus rhythm.

Effects of Denervation

During removal of the donor heart, the nerve supply is severed, resulting in a lack of autonomic nervous system innervation of the transplanted heart. Because of the loss of vagal influence, the resting sinus rate is higher than normal—usually between 90 and 110 beats/minute—and heart rate variations due to respiration do not occur.

Decreased donor sinoatrial node automaticity can also occur after transplantation as a result of injury to the node during procurement, transport, surgical procedure, or postoperative edema of the atrial suture line. Usually, these problems resolve within 1 to 2 weeks after transplantation, but temporary pacing may be needed to maintain an adequate heart rate. Atropine, which blocks vagal stimulation, is ineffective in treating bradydysrhythmias in the transplanted heart because there is no parasympathetic innervation. If the sinus rate is reduced, junctional rhythms can occur earlier than normal because of the loss of vagal tone.

Normal cardiovascular reflexes are also removed by denervation. In the normal heart, increased body metabolic demands cause direct compensatory stimulation of the heart by the sympathetic nervous system, which immediately increases heart rate, contractility, and cardiac output. Because direct sympathetic nervous system stimulation of the transplanted heart is absent, this response is mediated through release of circulating catecholamines from the adrenal medulla. Therefore, increases in heart rate, contractility, and cardiac output occur much more slowly than normal. With exercise, heart rate and cardiac output increase gradually over 3 to 5 minutes and remain elevated longer after exercise. Prolonged warm-up before and cool-down after exercise help compensate for these changes.

Orthostatic hypotension can occur because the normal, immediate reflex tachycardia, which compensates for venous pooling with position change, does not occur. When patients begin ambulating, they should be cautioned to change position gradually to prevent orthostatic hypotension.

Because of denervation, the cardiac effects of medications normally mediated by the autonomic nervous system are abnormal. Atropine, which increases heart rate by blocking parasympathetic influence, is ineffective. Isoproterenol, a positive chronotropic agent, has been widely used, because it stimulates myocardial receptors directly for pharmacological management of symptomatic bradydysrhythmias. However, isoproterenol is not widely available. Instead, dobutamine and epinephrine, along with temporary epicardial pacing, are frequently used.

Digitalis preparations are ineffective in decreasing the heart rate or increasing the atrioventricular nodal refractory period because these effects are mediated primarily by the parasympathetic nervous system. Digitalis does increase myocardial contractility by its direct action on myocardial cells. Beta-blocking drugs or calcium channel blockers (e.g., verapamil) can be used to control supraventricular tachydysrhythmias in the transplanted heart; carotid sinus pressure, the Valsalva maneuver, and digitalis are ineffective.

Finally, denervation prevents transmission of pain impulses from ischemic myocardium to the brain, so the patient does not experience angina. Severe myocardial ischemia or infarction may go unnoticed. For this reason, ECG stress testing and annual coronary angiography or coronary vascular ultrasonography are usually performed.

Potential for Ventricular Failure

Post-transplantation ventricular failure, causing decreased cardiac output, occurs for the same reasons as in other cardiac surgical procedures. In addition, a prolonged ischemia time, inotropic support of the donor, or rejection can cause myocardial depression in a transplant recipient.

Right ventricular failure is the most common cause of primary graft failure after transplantation. Reasons for right-sided heart dysfunction are not entirely clear but are related to acute changes in pulmonary vascular resistance. The newly transplanted heart is required to work against elevated pulmonary pressures secondary to long-standing heart failure in the recipient.[10] Postoperative changes in pH or ABGs can cause pulmonary vascular spasm. Both pulmonary hypertension and spasm increase the pulmonary vascular resistance or resistance to ejection of blood by the right ventricle. The normal right ventricle of the donor heart may be unable to increase its output acutely to overcome a high preexisting pulmonary vascular resistance. Signs of acute right ventricular failure include elevated central venous pressure and jugular venous distension. Left ventricular cardiac output decreases because the right ventricle is unable to pump enough blood through the lungs.

Treatment of post-transplantation right-sided heart failure involves the use of drugs to decrease right heart afterload (dobutamine, milrinone, inhaled nitric oxide). Inhaled nitric oxide, a direct pulmonary vasodilator, may be administered through the ventilator circuit, thereby avoiding the systemic affects of the drugs that are administered intravenously. Conditions that increase right heart afterload (e.g., hypoxia, acidosis, excessive blood transfusions) should be avoided.

PANCREAS

Pancreas transplant recipients may be cared for briefly in the critical care setting. Their care is somewhat similar to patients who have had abdominal surgery. The differences relate to pancreatic function, the type of surgical procedure, and secondary effects of diabetes mellitus.

Blood glucose response usually returns within the first few postoperative hours; however, an insulin drip may be required until blood glucose is normal. Pancreatic function is monitored by glucose levels before and after meals, by the results of glycosylated hemoglobin, and sometimes glucose tolerance testing. Even minor abnormalities may indicate rejection or vascular thrombosis of the graft.

When a section of duodenum is used for exocrine drainage, the prevention of infection is particularly challenging. Antibiotics are usually administered until the intraoperative culture of the duodenum is reported. When the bladder is used for exocrine drainage, bicarbonate wasting in the urine may occur. Intravenous and oral sodium bicarbonate are given to help maintain normal bicarbonate levels. With this surgical approach, an indwelling catheter is placed to prevent bladder distension, which can result in stress on suture lines and pancreatitis. Depending on the patient's ability to void, the catheter may be needed for several days or possibly weeks if there is long-standing neurogenic bladder dysfunction secondary to diabetes mellitus.

A nasogastric tube is kept in place until bowel activity returns. This may take 3 to 5 days if there is diabetic gastroparesis. If the nasogastric tube remains in place, enteral or parenteral feedings may be necessary.

LUNG

The lung transplant recipient is anesthetized, intubated, and mechanically ventilated on arrival to the ICU. Usually, extubation occurs 24 to 36 hours after surgery. Patients with emphysema and a single lung transplant are usually extubated more quickly than patients with pulmonary hypertension, who may need a longer intubation period.

The lung transplant recipient does not have a cough reflex because of denervation. Therefore, when suctioning, avoid inserting the catheter where it can cause damage. Frequent bronchoscopy is performed by the surgical team to ensure intact anastomoses and for pulmonary toileting. A common problem in the immediate post-transplantation period is pulmonary edema due to a phenomenon known as "reperfusion" injury. As a result, the patient is maintained in a relatively hypovolemic state for the first few days. Diuresis is started when the patient is hemodynamically stable.

The lungs are constantly exposed to the outside world, and therefore prevention of infection is especially important after lung transplantation. Antibiotics are given prophylactically and are determined by donor cultures, preoperative serology results, and sputum samples. Patient care measures to prevent infection include giving oral care, encouraging physical activity early in the postoperative course, and performing daily respiratory and chest physiotherapy. Continuous pulse oximetry is used to monitor oxygen saturation, and daily chest radiographs help monitor progress. Infection control measures by staff include washing hands, and using aseptic suctioning technique. Staff and visitors with active infections should avoid caring for or visiting the patients.

ASSESSMENT AND MANAGEMENT IN HEMATOPOIETIC STEM CELL TRANSPLANTATION

HSCT involves replacing diseased, destroyed, or nonfunctioning hematopoietic cells with healthy progenitor cells, also called *stem cells*. Stem cells are primitive hematopoietic cells capable of self-renewal, and they are pluripotent, meaning that they are capable of maturation into an RBC, WBC, or platelet. These stem cells may be collected directly from the bone marrow spaces by a bone marrow harvest procedure, or from the peripheral blood, by apheresis. HSCT is an important advance in restoring hematopoietic function in patients whose bone marrow has been destroyed by high-dose chemotherapy and radiation therapy (see Table 47-1).

In both autologous and allogeneic HSCT, peripheral blood stem cells have become the preferred source of hematopoietic stem cells for grafting. Collection of cells through apheresis is easier and less costly and may also result in a more rapid recovery of neutrophil and platelet counts. In unrelated allogeneic transplantation, the source of stem cells may be either a bone marrow harvest procedure or a peripheral blood stem cell collection. Box 47-3 outlines the benefits and limitations of the various sources of stem cells for transplantation. Special considerations for the pediatric patient are shown in Box 47-4. A detailed comparison of autologous and allogeneic stem cell transplantation is presented in Table 47-5.

Stem Cell Harvesting, Mobilization, and Collection

Stem cells are most numerous in the bone marrow spaces, and some circulate in the peripheral blood. The process of harvesting and collecting hematopoietic stem cells differs depending on the type of transplant. Progenitor cells may be obtained through a bone marrow harvest or collected through the peripheral blood.

box 47-3
Sources of Stem Cells: Benefits and Limitations

Peripheral Blood Stem Cell Collection/Apheresis

- Easier collection for autologous patients and potentially easier for allogeneic donors
- Shorter duration of myelosuppression
- In theory, there is thought to be less tumor contamination from peripherally derived stem cells
- Incidence of graft-versus-host disease (GVHD) may be same or higher

Bone Marrow Harvest

- Harvest-related pain
- General anesthesia required
- May be more cost-effective or more convenient for donors

Cord Blood

- Plentiful and relatively easy to harvest if obstetricians are trained
- Inexpensive
- Excellent source to increase pool of unrelated donors
- May be associated with less GVHD
- Currently limited to individuals who weigh less than 50–70 kg; with ex vivo expansion, techniques may become more widespread

box 47-4

Organ and Hematopoietic Stem Cell Transplantation in the Pediatric Patient

- Growth and development
- Education, play, and socialization
- Response to illness, hospitalization, treatment, and sequelae
- Body image and self-esteem
- Family role and relationships
- Effect of child's illness on parents (i.e., fear of child's death, separation, sick role issues, financial concerns)

When stem cells are obtained from the bone marrow, the harvesting procedure is performed in the operating room with the patient anesthetized. Multiple aspirations are obtained from each posterior iliac crest using large-bore needles until a total of 2 to 3 × 10^8 nucleated cells per kilogram of recipient body weight is obtained. The total volume of aspirate is 1 to 2 L. The marrow is placed in a heparinized tissue culture medium and filtered for the removal of fat and bone particles, and the cells are taken directly to the recipient's room for infusion. The bone marrow harvest procedure usually takes 1 to 2 hours. Pressure dressings are applied to the aspirate sites, and the donor is usually admitted for overnight observation. The harvest sites may be mildly uncomfortable for 2 to 7 days after the procedure.

Hematopoietic stem cells may also be collected from the peripheral blood. However, because stem cells are not abundant in the peripheral blood, chemotherapy or colony-stimulating factors (granulocyte colony-stimulating factor [G-CSF] or granulocyte–macrophage colony-stimulating factor [GM-CSF]) must be given before collection to drive progenitor cells into the peripheral circulation. This process is termed *mobilization* or *priming*. The chemotherapy that patients receive for stem cell mobilization is also useful for tumor reduction. For related and unrelated donors, colony-stimulating factors alone are used to increase the number of stem cells in the peripheral blood. Protocols vary, but G-CSF or GM-CSF is given by a subcutaneous injection daily. Stem cell collections begin after 4 or 5 days of cytokine injections.

Hematopoietic progenitor cells are collected from the peripheral blood by a method called *leukapheresis*. A commercial cell separator machine collects the progenitor cells and returns the remainder of the plasma and cellular components to the bloodstream. This is performed either through wide-bore double-lumen central catheters or large-bore antecubital Angiocaths. The procedure takes approximately 3 to 4 hours, and the number of leukapheresis procedures required is determined by the number of stem cells harvested at each session. The goal is to collect 5 × 10^6 CD34-positive cells per kilogram of recipient body weight. The CD34-positive antigen is an antigen

table 47-5 Comparison of Autologous and Allogeneic Stem Cell Transplantation

	Autologous	Allogeneic
Indications	Hematological malignancies and solid tumors Possible role in treatment of autoimmune disorders Future role in combination with gene therapy to treat genetic disorders and HIV infection	Hematological malignancies, aplastic anemia, congenital bone marrow disorders, immune deficiency states, some inborn errors of metabolism
Source of stem cells	Stem cells collected from bone marrow or peripheral blood of the patient and then reinfused after high-dose conditioning regimen Stem cells given to rescue the patient from hematological toxicity of conditioning regimen	Marrow, peripheral blood, cord blood, family donors, unrelated donors, HLA-matched or partially matched
Preparative regimen	High-dose chemotherapy to eradicate malignant disease	High-dose chemotherapy and sometimes total-body radiation as intensive therapy for malignant disease and to provide immunosuppression to allow engraftment (makes "space" for incoming stem cells)
Post-transplantation treatment	Supportive care, transfusions, growth factors, immune manipulation	Supportive care, transfusions, growth factors, immune manipulation, prophylaxis and treatment of GVHD
Risk of infectious complications	Lower risk; infections occur mainly in early post-transplantation period	Higher risk; sustained risk of infection for months or years
Major complications	Preparative regimen toxicity, disease recurrence or progression Treatment-related mortality rate usually <5%	Preparative regimen toxicity, disease recurrence or progression, GVHD, immunodeficiency
Treatment-related mortality rate	Usually <5%	5%–30% depending on many patient-, donor-, and disease-related factors

Adapted from Barrett J, Warwick R: In Barrett J, Treleaven J (eds): The Clinical Practice of Stem Cell Transplantation. Oxford: Isis Medical Media, 1998.

expressed on the surface of early progenitor cells. With autologous hematopoietic progenitor cells, the cells are immediately cryopreserved and stored in liquid nitrogen until the recipient is ready for reinfusion. The donor may experience a transient hypocalcemia reaction with chills, fatigue, tingling in the lips and extremities, and vertigo resulting from the citrate infusion, which is used to prevent clotting of the blood during the procedure. The symptoms can be prevented or treated by taking a calcium supplement, such as Tums.

Conditioning Regimen

After the progenitor cells have been obtained, the patient begins the conditioning regimen designed to prepare him or her to receive transplanted stem cells. The goal of the conditioning regimen depends in part on whether the transplant is autologous or allogeneic and on the nature of the patient's underlying disease. In allogeneic transplantation, the purpose of conditioning is to eradicate any malignant disease, eliminate the bone marrow to create a space for the new donor stem cells, and provide sufficient immunosuppression to allow engraftment of the transplanted stem cells. In autologous transplantation, immunosuppression is not required, because the patient is the source of the hematopoietic stem cells. However, the high-dose therapy is still needed to eradicate malignant disease.

High-dose chemotherapy treatment is based on the hypothesis that increasing the total dose or dose rate will kill more tumor cells, resulting in improved response and survival rates. Drugs with different (i.e., nonoverlapping) nonhematologic dose-limiting toxicities are combined in maximal doses.[11,12] Alkylating agents (cyclophosphamide, carboplatin, busulfan, thiotepa, cisplatin, melphalan, carmustine), etoposide, cytarabine, and sometimes total-body irradiation are used to destroy the bone marrow and eradicate disease. The regimen is administered over 2 to 8 days. The individual drugs that may be used in combination as part of the transplant conditioning regimen may have several adverse effects (Table 47-6).

The patient is then allowed 1 to 2 rest days to clear the chemotherapy from the system before the infusion of stem

table 47-6 ■ Nonhematological Adverse Effects of High-Dose Therapy Regimens

Drug or Therapy	Adverse Effects
Busulfan	Interstitial pulmonary fibrosis, hepatic dysfunction (including veno-occlusive disease of the liver), acute cholecystitis, generalized seizures, mucositis, skin adverse effects (hyperpigmentation, desquamation, acral erythema), nausea and vomiting
Carmustine (BCNU)	Hepatic, pulmonary, and central nervous system adverse effects, cardiac adverse effects (dysrhythmias and hypotension), nausea and vomiting
Cytosine arabinoside (Ara-C)	Cerebellar toxicity, encephalopathy, seizures, conjunctivitis, skin adverse effects (rash, acral erythema), nausea and vomiting, diarrhea, renal insufficiency, liver function abnormalities, pancreatitis, noncardiogenic pulmonary edema, fever, arthralgias
Cyclophosphamide	Cardiac adverse effects (cardiomyopathy, congestive heart failure, hemorrhagic cardiac necrosis, pericardial effusion, ECG abnormalities), interstitial pulmonary fibrosis, hemorrhagic cystitis, elevation in liver enzymes, nausea and vomiting, metabolic adverse effects (syndrome of inappropriate antidiuretic hormone secretion [SIADH])
Carboplatinum	Nausea and vomiting, nephrotoxicity, liver function abnormalities (including veno-occlusive disease of the liver), ototoxicity
Cisplatinum	Nausea and vomiting, neurotoxicity (peripheral neuropathy, ataxia, visual disturbances), ototoxicity, renal adverse effects
Etoposide	Hypersensitivity reactions, hypotension, liver function abnormalities and chemical hepatitis, renal dysfunction, nausea and vomiting, metabolic adverse effects (metabolic acidosis), mucositis, stomatitis, painful skin rash (on the palms, soles, and periorbital area)
Ifosfamide	Hemorrhagic cystitis, nausea, vomiting
Melphalan	Acute hypersensitivity reaction, renal adverse effects, mucositis, nausea and vomiting, hepatic toxicity (including veno-occlusive disease of the liver)
Thiotepa	Hyperpigmentation, acute erythroderma, dry desquamation, liver function abnormalities (including veno-occlusive disease of the liver), mucositis, esophagitis, dysuria, hypersensitivity reactions
Total-body irradiation	Nausea and vomiting, diarrhea, parotitis, xerostomia, stomatitis, erythema, pneumonitis, veno-occlusive disease of the liver

cells. Bone marrow aplasia occurs within days after the conditioning regimen is completed. The acute toxicity from the regimen can last for a few weeks or until engraftment occurs.

Research is underway to study whether a nonmyeloablative conditioning regimen followed by allogeneic HSCT is improved treatment for malignancies. Nonmyeloablative transplantation may provide a treatment option for patients who, because of advanced age or preexisting lung, kidney, or liver damage, cannot tolerate the toxicities of a traditional allogeneic transplant.[13] The theory behind a nonmyeloablative transplantation is that the immune-mediated graft-versus-tumor effect provided by the new immune system, rather than the conditioning regimen itself, cures the disease. Specific regimens under investigation include fludarabine, single-dose total-body irradiation, and a combination of potent immunosuppressive medications. These regimens are not without risk, and patients undergoing nonmyeloablative transplantation still experience many of the expected complications of myeloablative allogeneic transplantation. The problems encountered in the early post-transplantation period, such as infection, bleeding, and regimen-related toxicities, may be reduced after nonmyeloablative transplantation, but the risk of GVHD and the long-term risks of infection continue to be important.

Transplantation/Hematopoietic Stem Cell Infusion

In allogeneic HSCT, the stem cells are usually infused immediately after they are collected. Autologous stem cells are cryopreserved with dimethylsulfoxide (DMSO) and must be thawed in a warm normal saline bath at the bedside immediately before reinfusion.

The actual infusion of stem cells is a relatively simple procedure, much like a blood transfusion. The cells are infused into a central venous catheter over 30 to 60 minutes, depending on the total volume of the product. Patients usually are premedicated with acetaminophen, hydrocortisone, and diphenhydramine, and prehydrated to maintain renal perfusion. Diuretics, mannitol, and antihypertensives may be required to prevent volume overload and manage hemodynamic changes during infusion. Vital signs are monitored, and oxygen and cardiac monitoring are readily available.

Complications of allogeneic HSCT may include pulmonary edema, hemolysis, infection, and anaphylaxis; however, these are rare. A garlicky odor or taste may occur; this is caused by excretion of DMSO. DMSO-associated RBC hemolysis may also occur, and patients require vigorous hydration to prevent renal toxicity. An infusion reaction that may include bradycardia (rarely heart block), hypertension, and an acute hypersensitivity reaction is another potential adverse effect of DMSO during the administration of cryopreserved autologous HSCT. During HSCT, patients are also monitored for volume overload and for complaints suggestive of embolism such as chest pain, dyspnea, and cough. Patients may also experience an acute hemolytic transfusion reaction if they are receiving hematopoietic stem cells from an ABO-mismatched donor.

Engraftment

After intravenous infusion, the hematopoietic stem cells migrate to the bone marrow spaces, where they are attracted by chemotactic factors. Engraftment occurs when the transplanted progenitor cells begin to grow and manufacture new hematopoietic cells in the bone marrow. Engraftment is generally defined as an absolute neutrophil count greater than 0.5×10^9/L for 3 consecutive days, and a platelet count greater than $20{,}000 \times 10^9$/L achieved without transfusion support. The rate of engraftment depends on the source of the progenitor cells, the total progenitor cell dose, the use of colony-stimulating factors, the complications the patient experiences in the pre-engraftment period, and the choice of prophylaxis against GVHD. Time to engraftment in HSCT varies according to the origin of the hematopoietic stem cells: for bone marrow–derived stem cells, 2 to 3 weeks; for peripheral blood stem cells, 11 to 16 days; and for cord blood–derived stem cells, 26 days (average; as long as 42 days).

Patients usually receive their conditioning treatment and immediate post-transplantation care in an inpatient unit. However, improved symptom management and technological advances, including the use of hematopoietic growth factors, have allowed earlier discharge from hospital. The criteria for hospital discharge after HSCT are presented in Box 47-5. Many institutions now have outpatient care facilities available for transplant recipients that permit outpatient treatment and evaluation 7 days per week.[14]

After the transplantation but before complete hematopoietic cell engraftment, patients experience severe pan-

box 47-5
Criteria for Hospital Discharge After Hematopoietic Stem Cell Transplantation

Discharge from hospital is usually permitted when:

- The patient has been afebrile for at least 24 hours
- A 24-hour outpatient medical facility is available
- Family caregiver support is available
- The patient is independent in basic activities of daily living
- Acute post-transplantation complications have been resolved or controlled
- The patient is achieving oral intake of at least 1,500 mL per day, or a plan to meet the patient's fluid needs through self-administration of intravenous fluids or daily intravenous fluid administration in clinic is in place
- Nausea and vomiting are controlled
- The patient is able to tolerate oral medications
- Availability of appropriate transfusion support in a clinic environment and access to irradiated blood products have been determined
- The patient's platelet count is supportable with no more frequent than daily platelet product
- The patient's white blood cell count is greater than 1,000/µL
- A hematocrit of 25% is supportable with no more than daily transfusion of one unit of packed red blood cells

cytopenia and immunosuppression, and the resulting complications may include infection and bleeding. Hematopoietic growth factors (e.g., G-CSF, GM-CSF) are given to accelerate neutrophil recovery, thereby reducing the period of pancytopenia and the highest risk of infection. While patients have pancytopenia, until their blood counts begin to recover, they typically receive broad-spectrum antimicrobial drugs directed at bacteria, viruses, and fungi, as well as blood components such as platelets and packed red blood cells.

All blood products given to HSCT recipients should be filtered to remove WBCs that may transmit CMV, and irradiated to prevent transfusion-associated GVHD. Studies have determined that leukodepletion by either bedside filtration during transfusion or by prestorage leukocyte depletion of blood products is an effective method of preventing transfusion-associated CMV infection in HSCT, because CMV is transmitted by leukocytes.[14,15] In addition, filtered blood products may also prevent febrile transfusion reactions and delay alloimmunization.[15–17] However, use of a leukocyte depletion filter does not affect the risk of transmission of viral hepatitis.

Transfusion-associated GVHD is a rare but almost uniformly fatal complication of transfusion, resulting from the infusion of immunocompetent lymphocytes capable of proliferation into an immunocompromised recipient who is unable to destroy them.[14] The infused lymphocytes recognize host tissues as foreign, and mount a reaction.

To prevent transfusion-associated GVHD, all cellular blood products, except for stem cell grafts and donor lymphocytes given for graft-versus-tumor effect, should be irradiated to 2,500 cGy.[15] The blood component should be labeled as irradiated. It is not radioactive, and no additional precautions for handling the blood product are required. Blood products that have been irradiated can be used by other patients; the irradiating process does not alter the efficacy or cellular content of the product and does not harm the recipient in any way. Patients who have undergone allogeneic or autologous HSCT should receive irradiated cellular components, both before and after stem cell transplantation.[14] Most centers recommend that allogeneic stem cell recipients receive irradiated blood products for the rest of their lives. Box 47-6 shows a Collaborative Care Guide for the patient with allogeneic HSCT.

IMMUNOSUPPRESSIVE THERAPY

In solid organ transplantation, the transplanted organ is foreign to the recipient, whose immune system eventually will recognize this and mobilize to reject the transplanted organ. Therefore, immunosuppressive therapy is necessary to suppress the immune response so the transplanted organ will be accepted. In allogeneic HSCT, because the immune system is generated from donor cells, immunosuppressive therapy is used to prevent GVHD, a response in which donor T lymphocytes attack the recipient's cells. The challenge of immunosuppressive therapy is to provide the recipient with adequate immunosuppression without undue toxicity, unfavorable reactions, and excess susceptibility to opportunistic infections. Therapeutic regimens may be individualized based on the needs of a particular patient.

Several drugs may be given to solid organ transplant recipients to suppress the immune response (Table 47-7). A single medication usually cannot do this effectively. Therefore, immunosuppressive regimens include medications that complement each other and increase the effectiveness of the immunosuppression. The foundation of most immunosuppressant regimens for solid organ transplantation is triple, or three-drug, therapy. The combination of drugs used for organ transplantation and HSCT may differ.

Triple therapy is a combination of low-dose prednisone, azathioprine, and cyclosporine A or tacrolimus. The dose of each drug is lower so that patients experience fewer adverse effects than they would from one drug alone. For example, the risk of aseptic necrosis, diabetes mellitus, cataracts, and gastrointestinal complications attributed to chronic steroid therapy is greatly reduced with the combination therapy. Because the dosage of azathioprine is low, the potential for hepatotoxicity and leukopenia is decreased. Problems associated with higher doses of cyclosporine A, including lymphoma, hirsutism, hepatotoxicity, gingival hyperplasia, seizures, and gastrointestinal disturbances, rarely occur.

Quadruple, or sequential, therapy uses the same three drugs that are used in triple therapy (prednisone, azathioprine, and cyclosporine A or tacrolimus) plus antithymocyte antibody preparations or monoclonal antibody, monomurab-CD3. Cyclosporine A is not included until renal function is present. All four drugs are given for several days, after which the polyclonal or monoclonal antibody preparation is discontinued. A triple-drug regimen is used for maintenance therapy.

The primary advantage of quadruple therapy is that cyclosporine can be withheld in the absence of renal function. Because of the nephrotoxicity of cyclosporine and its cumulative effect in the absence of renal function, both broad and specific immunosuppression can be accomplished without it. The disadvantage of quadruple therapy is the potential inability to use the polyclonal or monoclonal antibody preparation for treatment of rejection or as "rescue" therapy.

COMPLICATIONS OF TRANSPLANTATION

Complications after solid organ transplantation and HSCT are usually due to graft function, problems with immunosuppression, or the adverse effects of the transplantation preconditioning regimen. GVHD and infection are other common complications after HSCT.

Organ Transplantation

ORGAN REJECTION

Because the transplanted organ is not immunologically identical to the recipient, it acts as an antigen or foreign substance and triggers the immune system to reject it. Rejection can vary in degree from mild to severe and may

(text continues on page 1110)

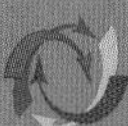

box 47-6 collaborative care guide
allogeneic hematopoietic stem cell transplantation

OUTCOMES | **INTERVENTIONS**

Oxygenation/Ventilation

Outcomes

The patient will demonstrate pulmonary hygiene techniques, including coughing, deep breathing, incentive spirometry, and daily exercise as tolerated.

Patient will demonstrate improvement in respiratory pattern and lung sounds, with subjective reduction in complaints of dyspnea, weakness, or pain.

Patient's risk of aspiration will be eliminated or minimized.

Interventions

- Auscultate lung sounds and vital signs and pulse oximetry q4h and PRN.
- Note skin color capillary refill and presence of central or peripheral cyanosis.
- Assess the quality of respirations including use of accessory muscle, nasal flaring, and grunting.
- Note cough and complaints of shortness of breath, orthopnea, or pleuritic pain.
- Determine effects of medications that may affect respiratory status, including narcotics and sedatives.
- Suction oropharynx or nasotrachea to remove secretions.
- Encourage deep-breathing and coughing exercises, and teach patient proper use of incentive spirometry.
- Encourage patient to maintain optimal level of activity, including walking, exercise bicycle, and working daily with physical therapist.
- Instruct patient on methods of preventing respiratory complications related to mucositis or aspiration, such as avoiding drinking liquids after using topical local anesthetics, keeping head of bed elevated and having oral suction in a convenient location.
- Implement measures to control bleeding, if present.
- Administer supplemental oxygen as indicated.
- Administer diuretics as ordered.

Circulation/Perfusion

Outcomes

The patient will exhibit the absence of or control of signs and symptoms of potential physiological problems:

Bleeding/hemorrhage
Hypotension secondary to sepsis, hemorrhage, medication side effects, or dehydration
Hypertension secondary to medication side effects
Dehydration secondary to decreased oral fluid intake as a result of nausea, vomiting, or mucositis, or increased fluid losses through fever, diarrhea, or insensible fluid losses through the skin

Interventions

- Develop a nursing plan to manage individual cardiovascular problems. Cardiovascular problems may include hypertension, orthostatic hypotension, sepsis-induced hypotension, dysrhythmias, pericarditis, superior vena cava syndrome, thrombus formation, and myocardial infarction.
- Replace fluid losses with packed red blood cells or hydration.
- Use appropriate measures to decrease fluid losses secondary to fever, diarrhea, vomiting, or hemorrhage.
- Administer antihypertensives, diuretics, antidysrhythmics, or vasoactive drugs as ordered and monitor their effectiveness.
- Provide information to patient and family regarding cardiac status, and rationale for specific nursing interventions.
- Monitor platelet count carefully, especially in patients experiencing hypertension.
- Instruct patient about appropriate safety measures during period of altered cardiac status. Patients who are orthostatic may become dizzy when standing. Provide assistance as needed.
- Although hypotension and hypertension may occur without symptoms, alert patient to these signs and symptoms, and encourage prompt reporting to the health care team. Common signs of hypertension include headache and visual disturbance. Hypotension may be associated with dizziness, visual disturbances, tachycardia, and cool or diaphoretic skin.
- Emphasize the importance of taking oral antihypertensive medications when scheduled.

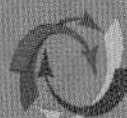

box 47-6 collaborative care guide
allogeneic hematopoietic stem cell transplantation (Continued)

OUTCOMES	INTERVENTIONS
Fluids/Electrolytes The patient will exhibit the absence of or control of signs and symptoms of potential physiological problems: **Veno-occlusive disease of the liver,** as manifested by sudden weight gain, increase in bilirubin, aspartate aminotransferase, and alkaline phosphatase levels, hepatomegaly, ascites, and encephalopathy **Renal insufficiency/failure,** as manifested by a decreased urine output or rising serum creatinine **Dehydration** secondary to decreased oral fluid intake as a result of nausea, vomiting, or mucositis, or increased fluid losses through fever, diarrhea, or insensible fluid losses through the skin. **Electrolyte disorders** secondary to steroid-induced hyperglycemia, syndrome of inappropriate antidiuretic hormone secretion (SIADH), tumor lysis syndrome, or medication-induced electrolyte shifts	▪ Strictly monitor intake, output and fluid balance q4–8h. ▪ Check weight twice daily. ▪ Measure abdominal girth daily in patients with veno-occlusive disease. ▪ Perform pulmonary assessment, including pulse oximetry, respiratory rate, quality, and presence of adventitious breath sounds. ▪ Perform cardiac assessment, noting presence of orthostatic hypotension, extra heart sounds, or neck vein distension. ▪ Assess for peripheral and sacral edema. ▪ Monitor serum electrolytes, liver function tests, and urine specific gravity qd or bid as ordered. ▪ Monitor for and treat steroid-induced hyperglycemia. ▪ Adjust dose or eliminate nephrotoxic drugs in patients with renal insufficiency or renal failure. ▪ Administer fluids as ordered to replace gastrointestinal losses and to supplement inability to consume sufficient oral fluids. ▪ Administer electrolyte replacements as ordered. ▪ Administer antiemetics and antidiarrheal agents as ordered. ▪ Monitor stools for volume, consistency, color, and odor. ▪ Monitor for fluid losses through sloughing of the skin.
Mobility/Safety The patient will: Maintain baseline strength and endurance, and minimize focal muscle weakness, fatigue, and dyspnea Participate in measures to prevent a decrease in strength and endurance Experience minimal complications from decreased mobility Use safety measures to prevent injury	▪ Encourage patient to continue daily activities throughout the transplantation course. Provide rationale and explain the complications of inactivity to both patient and family. ▪ Develop an individualized plan to address factors contributing to limited mobility, including pain, nonadherence, depression, medication side effects, nausea, generalized weakness and malaise, and altered level of consciousness. ▪ Refer to physical and occupational therapy for assessment and treatment. ▪ Encourage focused exercises that provide proximal muscle strengthening in patients on corticosteroids. ▪ Encourage patient to maintain maximal independence in ADLs and self-care. ▪ Develop a schedule that allows adequate rest by coordinating all activity and treatments (ADLs, medications, health team rounds, patient's habits). ▪ Identify signs of impaired activity tolerance and set specific goals for improving tolerance/endurance in activities.
Skin Integrity The patient will: Maintain skin integrity Demonstrate techniques of skin care Demonstrate basic understanding of skin GVHD Exhibit control of symptoms associated with skin GVHD	▪ Assess skin daily for maculopapular rash, erythema, sloughing, or open lesions. ▪ Monitor skin for the development of infection in areas of skin involved with GVHD. ▪ Apply skin emollients and other topical agents, including topical antimicrobial agents, as ordered. ▪ Consider use of antipruritic or steroid topical agents to manage symptoms of itching and inflammation.

(continued)

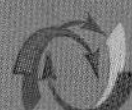

box 47-6 collaborative care guide *allogeneic hematopoietic stem cell transplantation (Continued)*

OUTCOMES	INTERVENTIONS
	■ If skin breakdown occurs, consult enterostomal therapist or wound management specialist concerning nonadherent, absorptive dressings and the role of special beds/mattresses. ■ Monitor patient for dehydration if there are increased insensible losses of fluid through the skin. ■ Teach patient and family the importance of avoiding direct sun exposure, and the importance of using sun block and protective clothing when outdoors, because sun exposure can initiate a flare of GVHD of skin.
Nutrition The patient will: Have nutritional balance maintained through diet and parenteral nutrition Demonstrate understanding of dietary restrictions related to a specific gastrointestinal problem Demonstrate methods for maintaining nutritional requirements as an outpatient	■ Evaluate oral mucosal integrity and note presence of oral problems. ■ Note subjective data, including complaints of nausea, loss of appetite, taste changes, early satiety, pain or abdominal cramping, and any precipitating factors. ■ Monitor calorie counts, intake and output totals, and weights to determine adequacy of nutritional intake. ■ Develop a multidisciplinary plan for nutritional management. Discuss approaches to use when experiencing taste changes, thick, viscous saliva and mucus, xerostomia, early satiety, nausea/vomiting, mucositis or esophagitis, and other troubling symptoms. ■ If patient is receiving high-dose steroids, ensure increased protein intake and calcium and vitamin D supplementation. Consider restricted concentrated carbohydrate intake if hyperglycemia is present. Consider restricted sodium intake if fluid retention is especially problematic. ■ Increase protein intake in patients with extensive skin or gastrointestinal GVHD. ■ Consider multiple vitamin without iron (to prevent iron overload), and folic acid supplementation 1 mg orally qd. ■ Maintain nutritional requirements through use of hyperalimentation as required. ■ Encourage patient to try different foods as tolerated. ■ Advance diet as tolerated and note response to advancement. ■ Encourage small, frequent meals, and a bedtime snack. ■ Medicate for nausea or pain as needed. ■ Encourage family members to be supportive and patient. Pressure from family, staff, and peers can produce anxiety that will have a negative effect on eating habits.
Comfort/Pain Control Patient will be able to: Identify activities that increase or decrease pain Relate location and characteristics of pain as well as degree of pain relief to the health care team Participate in daily care without interference from pain or side effects of pain control measures Achieve acceptable level of pain control	■ Monitor for the potential sources of pain/discomfort in the hematopoietic stem cell transplant recipient, including: Procedural pain Pain associated with diagnostic procedures Neuropathic pain secondary to immunosuppressive medications Mucositis/esophagitis Rectal pain/hemorrhoids Painful urination from hemorrhagic cystitis Abdominal pain secondary to infections, severe diarrhea/enteritis, or liver distension Cutaneous discomfort secondary to GVHD of skin

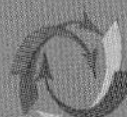

box 47-6 collaborative care guide
allogeneic hematopoietic stem cell transplantation (Continued)

OUTCOMES	INTERVENTIONS
	■ Teach patient importance of reporting pain and the effectiveness of pain relief measures to health care team. ■ Assess location, onset, frequency, intensity, and quality of pain. Use a 0–10 pain scale to assess patient's perception of pain and to assist in evaluating effectiveness of treatment. For patients unable to communicate, monitor changes in vital signs, and observe for increased restlessness, which could indicate inadequate pain control. ■ Premedicate patient before potentially painful procedures. ■ Teach proper and safe use of patient-controlled analgesia if ordered. ■ For patients receiving continuous infusion, consider the need for a bolus of analgesic before disconnecting patient from continuous infusion, while disconnected, and after resuming continuous infusion. ■ Suggest consultation with pain management team if indicated. ■ Monitor narcotic dosages and patient response carefully in patients with hepatic dysfunction secondary to veno-occlusive disease or GVHD. ■ In the nonventilated patient, adjust analgesic dosages in the presence of markedly deceased respiratory rate or markedly altered level of consciousness.
Psychosocial—Individual and Family Patient and family will be able to: Identify effective and ineffective coping patterns Identify personal strengths Verbalize their needs Actively participate in problem solving Use resources and support systems to strengthen their coping skills	■ Provide opportunities for patient and family to communicate with each other, as well as with psychosocial support professionals and other health care team members. ■ Reinforce successful coping skills (i.e., clearly verbalizing needs, using activities that reduce stress, and effective patient/family/team communication). ■ Provide reassurance and review support systems, options, and resources available to support effective coping. ■ Establish trust and congruence in goals and objectives. ■ Provide information in a timely and specific manner. ■ Allow patient as much choice and control as appropriate and feasible. ■ Avoid the use of approaches that foster dependency (coercion, persuasion, manipulation). ■ Demonstrate caring, respect, and concern for patient and family. ■ Use positive reinforcement.
Teaching/Discharge Planning The patient and family will demonstrate knowledge of: The overall process of hematopoietic stem cell transplantation, and the expected complications and self-care requirements, including preparative regimen and side effects, infusion of peripheral stem cells and side effects, engraftment, complications, discharge criteria, follow-up care, symptoms to report, protective precautions (neutropenic and thrombocytopenic precautions), dietary restrictions, and specific psychomotor skills, including central venous catheter care, medication administration, and vital sign monitoring	■ Introduce staff and approach patient with respectful caring attitude. ■ Orient patient to unit, room environment, ancillary services, and general routines. The patient and family may be initially overwhelmed by the amount of new information and may require reinforcement of information. ■ Allow patient and family to share concerns and request additional information about the transplantation process. ■ Encourage questions throughout the transplantation process, and provide clarification on all aspects of treatment.

(continued)

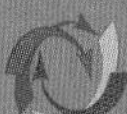

box 47-6 collaborative care guide
allogeneic hematopoietic stem cell transplantation (Continued)

OUTCOMES	INTERVENTIONS
The structure of the inpatient unit, unit routines, and the programs and resources available to make their inpatient stay more comfortable and facilitate their self-care The importance of the active involvement of patient and family in the daily care and decision making throughout the hematopoietic stem cell transplantation process On discharge, patient and family will demonstrate knowledge of: Signs and symptoms that should be reported immediately to the health care team, including fever, chills, skin rash, bleeding, nausea, vomiting, diarrhea or abdominal pain, shortness of breath, cough, dyspnea, and an inability to take oral medication or consume sufficient fluids Names of medication, rationale for each medication, the required schedule for administration, and potential side effects Contact telephone numbers for day and after-hours care Psychomotor skills necessary for administration of oral and intravenous (IV) medications, self-care of central venous catheter, and any other self-care skills such as administration of total parenteral nutrition and home IV hydration	■ Explain the need for active patient and family involvement in daily care and decision making throughout the hematopoietic stem cell transplantation process. ■ Teach the importance of daily hygiene, diligent oral care, daily exercise, nutrition, and other routines. ■ Encourage patient to maintain open communication with health care team. ■ Integrate discharge teaching while fostering patient family participation in daily care. ■ Provide patient with written instructions on outpatient self-care guidelines, medication schedule, and other self-care activities. ■ Refer to home health agency for continued education and support of patient at home, as indicated. ■ Provide teaching/instruction using methods adapted to patient's learning style. Discuss with patient how he or she learns best: by doing, by listening, or by watching. ■ Document teaching provided, areas requiring continued reinforcement and follow-up, and learning outcomes achieved in the patient's record.

be irreversible. Rejection may occur at any time, but the risk is highest in the first 3 months after transplantation. The earlier and more severe the rejection, the worse the prognosis for graft survival. Biopsy of the transplanted organ is usually needed to diagnose rejection definitively. Four types of rejection are defined: hyperacute, accelerated, acute, and chronic, although all types do not occur in all transplanted organs.

Hyperacute Rejection

Hyperacute rejection occurs in the operating room immediately after transplantation. It is a humoral immune response in which the recipient has preformed antibodies that immediately react against antigens of the donor organ. Vascular damage occurs, resulting in severe thrombosis and graft necrosis. In kidney and heart transplantation, hyperacute rejection always results in graft failure and the need for retransplantation. Fortunately, hyperacute rejection is uncommon and can usually be prevented by pretransplantation cross-matching.

Accelerated Rejection

Accelerated rejection is defined only in kidney transplantation, and it occurs within 1 week after transplantation. Clinically, the patient may have anuria, increased BUN and creatinine, and pain at the graft site. Accelerated rejection is due to either preformed antibodies against the donor antigens in the recipient's blood or to lymphocytes in the recipient that are already sensitized to some of the donor antigens. Like hyperacute rejection, accelerated rejection is seen infrequently because of improved tissue typing and cross-matching. It is treated aggressively with immunosuppressants and usually results in loss of the transplanted kidney.

Acute Rejection

Acute rejection occurs within the first 3 months after transplantation. This is the most common type of rejection, and most patients experience at least one episode. Acute rejection occurs when antigens on the donor organ trigger lymphocytes to mature into helper T cells. The helper T cells increase the production of cytotoxic killer T cells, which bind to the transplanted organ and damage it by secreting lysosomal enzymes and lymphokines. Acute rejection is also the type of rejection that responds best to immunosuppressive therapy.

Chronic Rejection

Chronic rejection is not completely understood. Most likely it is a combination of a cell-mediated response and a response to circulating antibodies. Second in frequency to acute rejection, chronic rejection usually occurs from 3 months to years after transplantation and is accompanied by deteriorating organ function.

Kidney. Acute rejection occurs after the first postoperative week. It is the most frequently seen form of rejection and the type that responds best to therapy. Changes in laboratory values are the earliest and most reliable indicators that graft function is deteriorating. Clinical manifestations of rejection are more subtle and may not be seen.

(text continues on page 1113)

table 47-7 ■ Selected Immunosuppressive Drugs Used in Solid Organ Transplantation

Drug	Adverse Reactions	Dosing/Administration	Comments
Methylprednisolone (Solu-Medrol) (IV) Prednisone (PO)	Increased susceptibility to infection	Initial: 0.5–3 mg/kg of body weight, tapered to an adequate oral maintenance dose	
	Masks symptoms of infection Peptic ulcer, GI bleeding		An antacid and H_2 blockers are given while patient is on steroids to reduce the risk of gastric irritation and ulceration; cimetidine may also be used to decrease ulcerogenic tendencies.
	Increased appetite, weight gain Increased sodium and water retention, which exaggerate hypertension Delayed healing Negative nitrogen balance Adrenal gland suppression Behavior and personality changes Diabetogenic effect Muscle weakness Osteoporosis with long-term therapy Skin atrophy, striae Easy bruising Glaucoma, cataracts Hirsutism Acne Avascular/aseptic necrosis	During rejection: methylprednisolone may be given in IV boluses up to 1 g/dose	Cardiac arrest can occur if IV bolus of 1 g is given rapidly. Sodium restriction may be necessary when steroid dosage is high or when fluid retention increases.
Azathioprine (Imuran) (IV or PO)	Bone marrow suppression: leukopenia, thrombocytopenia, anemia, pancytopenia Rash Alopecia Liver damage, jaundice Increased susceptibility to infection	Regulated to keep WBC 5,000–10,000; drug usually stopped when WBC 3,000 or less Initial 2–5 mg/kg of body weight Maintenance: 2–3 mg/kg of body weight During rejection: maximum of 3 mg/kg of body weight, dose not usually increased with rejection	The dose is lowered when allopurinol is added to medication regimen because allopurinol delays metabolism of azathioprine (allopurinol and azathioprine are synergistic).
Cyclosporine (Sandimmune) (IV or PO) Neoral (PO, microemulsion)	Nephrotoxicity Hepatotoxicity	Initial: 4 mg/kg/day (IV) Maintenance: 5–15 mg/kg/day PO may be used as part of triple-therapy regimen (prednisone, azathioprine, cyclosporine), or quadruple-therapy regimen (same as triple therapy plus ALG or OKT3)	Initially, nephrotoxicity and hepatotoxicity seem to be dose related and respond to dose reduction.
	Hypertension Hirsutism Gum hyperplasia Malignancy Nausea, vomiting, diarrhea Tremors/seizures Diabetogenic effects Anaphylactic reactions have been seen with IV administration	The dose for Sandimmune and Neoral are not interchangeable due to differences in bioavailability. When preparations are changed, dose adjustments are based on blood levels. Dosage altered by monitoring drug levels at least during initial period	Long-term nephrotoxicity is a major concern. Nephrotoxicity is sometimes difficult to differentiate from rejection or acute tubular necrosis in renal patients. Metabolized by cytochrome P-450 enzymes. Drugs that are inducers or inhibitors for P-450 enzymes may increase or decrease cyclosporine concentrations. Trough levels done to monitor and titrate dosage. Drug interactions can raise or lower blood levels.

(continued)

table 47-7 ■ Immunosuppressive Drugs Used in Solid Organ Transplantation (Continued)

Drug	Adverse Reactions	Dosing/Administration	Comments
			Risk of anaphylaxis is reduced if slow continuous infusion is given.
Tacrolimus (Prograf)	Infection Nephrotoxicity Neurotoxicity Hypertension Diabetogenesis Tremors	Dosage varies 0.10 mg/kg/day IV 0.05–0.2 mg/kg/day PO (given in divided doses)	Dose based on trough levels. May be able to discontinue steroids. Monitor renal and liver function. Drug interactions and liver function can affect blood levels. P-450 enzyme system is affected.
Muromonab-CD3 (Orthoclone OKT3)	Febrile reactions; fever, chills, tremor Respiratory: dyspnea, chest pain, wheezing, pulmonary edema GI: nausea, vomiting, diarrhea Anemia, thrombocytopenia	2.5–5 mg/day IV bolus over 30–60 s, for 10–14 days	Reactions are greatest with first dose and occur within 30–60 min. To minimize first dose reaction, pretreat with methylprednisolone, acetaminophen, and diphenhydramine hydrochloride. Monitor vital signs q15min for 2 h, then q30min first two doses. Have emergency equipment and cooling blanket available. Repeat administrations may cause serious reactions if antibodies develop.
Antilymphocyte globulin (ALG)	Anaphylactic shock due to hypersensitivity to animal serum	Skin test for hypersensitivity to animal serum performed before initial dose	
Antithymocyte globulin (ATG) Antilymphocyte serum (ALS) Antithymocyte serum (ATS) (usually IV, IM, or deep SC)	Fever (up to 105°F or 40.6°C) and chills Increased susceptibility to infections due to decreased lymphocytes IM or deep SC injection site swollen, red, and painful, with abscess formation Difficulty walking if IM or SC injection given in thigh	Dosage may vary	Lymphocytes or platelets decrease sharply with drug administration; therefore, blood work for lymphocyte and platelet counts should be drawn before infusion is started. Usually given only for short period of time either to prevent or treat rejection; not a long-term immunosuppressant.
Cyclophosphamide (Cytoxan)	Leukopenia, thrombocytopenia Increased susceptibility to infections Metabolites direct irritants to bladder mucosa and may cause hemorrhagic cystitis	1–2 mg/kg (or 1/2 to 2/3 of azathioprine dosage)	Given in place of azathioprine when it causes hepatotoxicity. Administer on awakening to avoid accumulation of metabolites in bladder while sleeping. Observe for hematuria. Fluid intake should be encouraged to dilute metabolites.
Mycophenolate mofetil (Cellcept)	Alopecia Nausea Vomiting Diarrhea Dyspepsia	Usual dosage 1 g bid (250-mg capsules)	GI symptoms may be dose related and may improve with decrease. Preferable to take on an empty stomach unless GI symptoms are intolerable.
Methotrexate (MTX)	Myelosuppression Mucositis Hepatotoxicity	15 mg/m^2 day 1, then 10 mg/m^2 day 3, 6, 11	No other regimen has proven superior to a methotrexate/cyclosporine combination for prevention of GVHD in allogeneic bone marrow transplant recipients. The consequences of MTX exposure can be reversed by leukovorin if it is administered before irreversible changes lead to cell death (usually when plasma levels are greater than 4×10^{-8})

table 47-7 ■ Immunosuppressive Drugs Used in Solid Organ Transplantation (Continued)

Drug	Adverse Reactions	Dosing/Administration	Comments
			Most of the drug is excreted through the kidney, with a small fraction excreted through the bile. Standard doses in patients with good renal function, bilirubin less than 10 mg/dL and without effusions or ascites are not likely to produce serious toxicity
Sirolimus (Rapamune)	Hypercholesterolemia Elevated triglycerides Thrombocytopenia (dose related) Leukopenia	Loading dose 6–15 mg Maintenance dose 2–5 mg/day	Monitoring by trough levels Therapeutic levels: 5–20 ng/mL
Daclizumab	Common Cough Dizziness, fatigue, headache, tremor Dysuria GI effects, vomiting Insomnia Pain Serious Anaphylaxis Bleeding, thrombosis Dyspnea Edema, hypertension, hypotension, tachycardia Fever Infection Lymphoproliferative disorders	1 mg/kg IV beginning within 24 hours before transplantation, then 1 mg/kg IV every 14 days for a total of five doses	Used for induction therapy to prevent acute rejection early in transplant. **Not** used for treatment of acute rejection.
Basiliximab	Common Abdominal pain Vomiting Asthenia Dizziness Insomnia Serious Acute hypersensitivity reaction Anemia Candidiasis (frequent) Cytomegalovirus infection	20 mg IV within 2 h before transplantation surgery; then another 20-mg IV dose day 4 after surgery	Used for induction therapy to prevent acute rejection early in transplant. **Not** used for treatment of acute rejection.

GI, gastrointestinal; IM, intramuscular; IV, intravenous; PO, oral; SC, subcutaneous.

The patient may experience any, all, or none of the following during an acute rejection episode.

Laboratory Findings

- Increased serum creatinine, BUN, serum β_2-microglobulin
- Decreased creatinine clearance
- Decreased urine creatinine
- Possibly decreased urine sodium
- Decreased blood flow on renal scan

Clinical Manifestations

- Decreased urine output
- Weight gain
- Edema
- Temperature at least 100°F (37.8°C)
- Tenderness over the graft site, with possible swelling of the kidney
- General malaise
- Increased blood pressure

Chronic rejection is the result of repeated episodes of acute rejection in which the vessels become infarcted due to the vasculitis, and the renal tissue becomes scarred. This gradually leads to deteriorating kidney function. The symptoms are similar to acute rejection except for fever and graft enlargement. Laboratory findings are similar to those of acute rejection but also include signs of chronic renal failure, such as a declining hematocrit and calcium–phosphorus imbalance. The rate of deterioration can vary from months to years. A transplant nephrectomy is not usually required unless the kidney becomes necrotic and life-threatening.

Liver. Acute rejection in liver transplantation is suspected when liver function tests, specifically PT/INR (most sensitive), aminotransferases, alkaline phosphatase, and total bilirubin, are increased. Clinical signs, such as decreased bile production and perigraft tenderness, may or may not occur.[8] Chronic rejection is not completely understood but is believed to be due to multiple acute rejection episodes or a positive cross-match. A definitive diagnosis is made when a biopsy shows portal and bile duct inflammation and the presence of inflammatory cells, such as T lymphocytes.[8]

Heart. Although acute rejection is often asymptomatic, subtle signs and symptoms may include decreased cardiac output, atrial flutter or fibrillation, elevated WBC count, and low-grade fever. Endomyocardial biopsy is performed weekly for the first month and then less frequently to diagnose rejection. Acute rejection is a major cause of death in the first year after transplantation.

Chronic rejection is the leading cause of death after the first year of cardiac transplantation. The prevalence within 5 years of transplantation is at least 60%. This cell-mediated rejection causes progressive myocardial fibrosis, leading to heart dysfunction. The lesions in allographic vasculopathy are concentric, not focal, unlike in typical atherosclerosis, and allographic vasculopathy can often be missed on standard cardiac catheterization. Angina cannot be used as a warning sign for coronary artery disease because the heart is denervated. Instead, decreased exercise tolerance during stress testing or intravascular ultrasonography are used for diagnosis.[18]

Pancreas. Rejection is a major cause of graft loss in pancreas transplantation. This may be attributed to the difficulty in diagnosing rejection. Elevated blood glucose is a late sign of rejection and may occur too late to initiate successful treatment. When the bladder is used for exocrine drainage, urinary amylase levels reflect rejection before hyperglycemia becomes obvious. In combined kidney–pancreas transplantation, an elevated serum creatinine may indicate rejection, although rejection can occur in one organ and not the other. Some experts state that chronic pancreas rejection may not occur in combined kidney–pancreas transplantation. The best pancreas transplant survival rate occurs when the procedure is performed simultaneously with kidney transplantation[2] (see Table 47-1). Needle biopsy during cystoscopy is used for definitive diagnosis.

Lung. The signs and symptoms of lung transplant rejection are difficult to distinguish from pulmonary infection. Decreased lung function (i.e., forced expiratory volume), dyspnea, cough, decreased breath sounds, fever, and tachypnea may occur in both rejection and infection. Immediately after surgery, rejection may also be confused with volume overload, reperfusion injury, or ischemic injury secondary to preservation. Chest radiographs showing interstitial and perihilar edema may be signs of rejection and signal the need for biopsy. Even so, biopsies must be carefully interpreted to rule out infectious complications, such as infection with CMV or *Pneumocystis carinii*, which can have histological findings similar to those of acute rejection.

Chronic rejection is known as *obliterative bronchiolitis* and occurs in approximately 15% to 25% of lung transplant recipients. Acute rejection and infection are believed to play a role in obliterative bronchiolitis.[18]

INFECTION

Infection is the most common post-transplantation complication. Alterations in the integrity of mucosal barriers and severe neutropenia from the pretransplantation conditioning regimen produce an environment conducive to serious bacterial and fungal infection.

The causative agents are often from the patient's own flora, particularly from the gastrointestinal tract and integumentary system. Pathogens may be bacteria, fungi, viruses, and even protozoa. The latter three groups of organisms are referred to as *opportunistic* pathogens. Normally harmless and found in humans and in the environment, they pose serious threats to patients with compromised immune systems. They take advantage of the decreased host defenses—hence the term "opportunistic." Examples of opportunistic infections include herpes simplex and herpes zoster viruses, CMV, *Candida albicans*, *P. carinii*, *Aspergillus fumigatus*, and *Cryptococcus neoformans*.

All transplant recipients are at risk for bacterial infections due to intravascular lines and urinary drainage catheters, but organ transplant recipients can also acquire postoperative wound and lung infections. Usually broad-spectrum antibiotics are given prophylactically for 48 hours after organ transplantation or until invasive lines and drains are removed. HSCT recipients receive antibiotics prophylactically for months after transplantation. Infections caused by bacteria and other organisms that commonly occur after allogeneic HSCT are listed in Table 47-8.

Recipients of organ transplants are at high risk for infection during the first 3 months post-transplantation because they receive high dosages of immunosuppres-

table 47-8 Infections After Allogeneic Hematopoietic Stem Cell Transplantation

Period of Neutropenia (Days 0–30)	Period of Acute GVHD (Days 30–100)	Period of Chronic GVHD (Days 100+)
Gram-negative bacteria	Gram-negative bacteria	Encapsulated bacteria
Gram-positive bacteria	Gram-positive bacteria	Varicella-zoster virus
Herpes simplex	Cytomegalovirus	Cytomegalovirus
Candida species	Polyomavirus (BK virus)	*P. carinii*
Aspergillus species	Adenovirus	*Aspergillus* species
	Varicella-zoster virus	
	Candida species	
	Aspergillus species	
	Pneumocystis carinii	
	Toxoplasma gondii	

Adapted from Burt RK, Walsh T: Infection prophylaxis in bone marrow transplant recipients: Myths, legends and microbes. In Burt RK, Deeg HJ, Lothian S, et al (eds): Bone Marrow Transplantation, pp 438–451. Austin, TX, Landes Bioscience, 1998.

sants. Infections in the post–stem cell transplantation period usually follow a predictable pattern based on the recovery of the immune system. Therefore, recipients of HSCT are at high risk of infection during the first month, which is the pre-engraftment phase, because of neutropenia. HSCT recipients may receive colony-stimulating factors to reduce their risk of infection by accelerating WBC recovery. They remain at high risk for infection if they are receiving immunosuppressive medications to prevent or treat GVHD.

During the first month, the predominant fungal infections in recipients of HSCT are *Aspergillus* species and *Candida* species, for which amphotericin B or fluconazole may be used prophylactically. The most frequent viral infection is herpes simplex, and 80% of the patients who were seropositive before transplantation experience a reactivation of herpes simplex unless they receive acyclovir prophylactically.[19]

After the first month, the most common infection in all transplant recipients is CMV. To prevent CMV infection, patients who are CMV seronegative should receive only CMV-negative blood products. Many centers require that all blood transfusions be filtered. Patients who are CMV seropositive and symptomatic and those receiving increased immunosuppression for an episode of acute organ rejection may be treated with ganciclovir. HSCT recipients are closely monitored for CMV reactivation, and early preemptive treatment is initiated. Prevention is important in heart transplant recipients because there is a connection between CMV and coronary artery disease.[20,21] CMV may affect many organ systems; therefore, signs and symptoms of hepatitis, retinitis, enteritis, pneumonitis, fever, chills, and malaise may occur.

A small number of HSCT recipients contract severe and potentially fatal infections 3 months or more posttransplantation, during the late recovery phase, due to cellular immune deficiencies. The most frequent causes of these infections are *Pneumococcus, Staphylococcus aureus, Candida* species, and varicella-zoster virus.

If infection develops in immunosuppressed patients, the usual signs and symptoms may be absent. For these patients, even a small increase in temperature (99°F [37.2°C]) may be significant. The WBC count is monitored daily. After organ transplantation, the leukocyte count is usually slightly elevated because of surgery and steroid treatment. However, infection may be present if the elevation persists, a rapid elevation occurs after a decline, or there is an increase in immature WBCs (bands).

It is essential to prevent infection in transplant recipients, who are immunosuppressed and may be neutropenic. Important nursing responsibilities include maintaining protective environments, practicing consistent and thorough provider handwashing and good oral and skin hygiene, monitoring vital signs frequently, and performing head-to-toe assessments. In some centers, additional protective measures include protective isolation systems, air filtration, gut and skin decontamination, and low-microbial diets. The benefit of these interventions has been debated, and their application is institution or protocol specific.[22]

In combined kidney–pancreas transplantation, immunosuppressive drugs may be discontinued in the presence of a severe infection to mobilize the patient's immune system. Consequently, the graft may be lost to save the patient. In heart, lung, and liver transplantation, immunosuppression may be decreased but must be continued.

BLEEDING

Bleeding, oozing from the surface of the transplanted organ, or the presence of hematoma or lymphocele may occur postsurgery. The heart transplant recipient is at risk of bleeding because the pericardial sac has stretched to accommodate an enlarged heart. When a smaller, healthy heart is implanted, the larger pericardial sac becomes a reservoir that can conceal postoperative bleeding. This may result in cardiac tamponade. Long-term coagulation therapy and liver congestion from pretransplantation heart failure also increase the risk for bleeding.

After liver transplantation, bleeding may occur as a result of coagulopathy because of liver dysfunction or from small vessels that continue to bleed after surgery. When the bladder drainage technique is used for exocrine drainage in pancreas transplantation, patients may have postoperative hematuria if the transplanted duodenal segment becomes ulcerated or if cystitis develops. Electrocautery using cystoscopy may be required for severe bleeding.

GASTROINTESTINAL COMPLICATIONS RELATED TO STEROID THERAPY

Chronic steroid therapy increases the risk of peptic ulceration and erosive gastritis because it increases the secretion of hydrochloric acid and pepsinogen. Massive gastrointestinal bleeding may occur not only from steroid therapy but from stress and decreased tissue viability caused by long-term protein restriction. For these reasons, patients usually are given histamine type 2 receptor (H_2) antagonists, such as nizatidine or ranitidine. The degree of renal function dictates which antacid is selected. Liquid preparations are considered more effective.

Other serious gastrointestinal complications include acute pancreatitis, diverticulitis, *Candida* infection, esophagitis, obstruction from bowel adhesions, and ulcerative colitis. Infection becomes an added risk if the patient has an intestinal perforation. Ischemic bowel disease has been observed in the early posttransplantation period as a result of dehydration or ischemia due to low cardiac output.

More than one complication may occur simultaneously. In addition, signs and symptoms of gastrointestinal bleeding or perforation may be obscured by the anti-inflammatory effects of steroids. Therefore, complaints and changes in the patient's progress require thorough and prompt assessment.

The gastrointestinal tract of the patients who have had HSCT may also be affected by the total-body irradiation and chemotherapy used in the preparatory regimen. Symptoms may include mucositis, nausea, vomiting, diarrhea, cramping, dyspepsia, anorexia, taste changes, and xerostomia.

Hematopoietic Stem Cell Transplantation

GRAFT FAILURE

Graft failure is usually defined precisely by institutional protocols. However, all definitions include a complete absence of engraftment or a seemingly initial hematopoiesis post-transplantation, with later decreasing blood cell counts and an absence of hematopoiesis.[23] The clinical features of graft failure include neutropenia, anemia, and thrombocytopenia occurring beyond the initial period expected as a result of high-dose chemotherapy or chemoradiation therapy.

The overall incidence of graft failure is less than 5%, and it occurs most often in patients with aplastic anemia or those receiving unrelated donor transplants. The etiology is multifactorial. An important component in the evaluation is differentiating graft failure from disease recurrence or drug-induced myelosuppression. Table 47-9 describes graft failure in terms of its risk factors, possible causes, and treatment and preventive measures.

The HSCT recipient may be more susceptible to the myelosuppressive effects of various drugs after the transplantation. Drugs with a potential to cause myelosuppres-

table 47-9 Graft Failure After Hematopoietic Stem Cell Transplantation: Risk Factors, Causes, and Preventive Measures

	Risk Factors	Causes	Preventive/Supportive Measures
Autologous stem cell transplants	• Patients with acute myelocytic leukemia, patients extensively pretreated • Low cell dose • Purged marrow • Marrow-suppressive drugs • Viral infection	• Defective marrow microenvironment with stromal cell damage • Collection of damaged stem cells due to extensive previous treatment • Drug-induced myelosuppression • Viral effects on stroma of bone marrow	• Harvest autologous stem cells early, before multiple cycles of potentially stem cell–toxic regimens have been given • Maximize number of infused cells (minimum number of autologous peripheral blood stem cells that results in consistent engraftment is at least 1×10^6 CD34+ cells/kg of body weight, below which engraftment may be incomplete or there may be failure of engraftment) • Avoid all myelosuppressive drugs after transplantation • Adjust doses of medications for renal dysfunction • Treat/prevent viral infections • Keep unmanipulated cells as backup in case or purged or manipulated grafts • Ensure that there is no folate or vitamin B_{12} deficiency • Administer G-CSF and rEPO as needed
Allogeneic stem cell transplants	• Diseases associated with a defective marrow microenvironment, including aplastic anemia and myelofibrosis • Stem cell source from HLA-mismatched, unrelated, or cord blood donor • Pre-transplant transfusions, especially from a related donor • T-cell depletion, low cell dose, purging • Patients whose clinical condition precludes a sufficiently intensive conditioning regimen • Inadequate post-transplantation immunosuppression • Marrow-suppressive drugs • Viral infection, including infection with CMV	• Defective marrow microenvironment with stromal cell damage • Histocompatibility barriers • Allosensitization by transfusions • Damaged or inadequate number of stem cells infused • Persistence of host hematopoiesis • Persistence of immunocompetent host lymphocytes • GYHD-associated damage to bone marrow microenvironment • Drug-induced myelosuppression • Viral effects on stroma of bone marrow	• Avoid pretransplantation transfusions, especially from relatives • Select histocompatible donors • Ensure that the conditioning regimen is adequately immunosuppressive • Provide sufficient stem cell dose (minimum number of allogeneic peripheral blood stem cells that results in consistent engraftment is at least 2×10^6 CD34+ cells/kg of body weight, below which engraftment may be incomplete or there may be failure of engraftment) • Use post-transplantation immunosuppression with cyclosporine, tacrolimus, or methotrexate • Avoid all myelosuppressive drugs after transplantation • Adjust doses of medications for renal dysfunction • Treat/prevent viral infections • Ensure that there is no folate or vitamin B_{12} deficiency • Administer G-CSF, rEPO as needed • Consider cryopreserving autologous peripheral blood stem cells pre-allograft for possible use in the event of graft failure and overwhelming clinical problems such as hemorrhage or life-threatening infection

rEPO, recombinant erythropoietin.
Based on information from references 23, 77, and 83.

sion should be used very cautiously, if at all, to minimize the risk of drug-induced graft failure. In patients with delayed engraftment, it is prudent to review all medications and consider eliminating those that are not absolutely essential.

VENO-OCCLUSIVE DISEASE OF THE LIVER

Veno-occlusive disease of the liver is a potentially fatal liver disease that occurs in 15% to 20% of recipients of HSCT. Veno-occlusive disease is a complication of the conditioning regimen and usually develops within 2 weeks of transplantation. The risk of veno-occlusive disease is increased in patients who have received total-body irradiation. Veno-occlusive disease may be severe; some studies report an incidence of 25% and a mortality rate close to 50%.[24–27]

Veno-occlusive disease occurs when fibrous material accumulates, resulting in obstruction of small venules in the liver. Subsequently, portal hypertension, acute liver congestion, and destruction of liver cells develop. Liver disease ranges from mild to severe, and severe liver failure may occur. In addition, veno-occlusive disease affects the kidneys; there is a decrease in renal blood flow, causing further water and sodium retention. Mild veno-occlusive disease persists until liver tissue heals and resumes normal function, usually 10 to 14 days after onset. Severe disease may result in multisystem failure.

Clinical manifestations of veno-occlusive disease usually begin during the first 3 weeks after transplantation and are characterized by hyperbilirubinemia, rapid weight gain, ascites, right upper quadrant pain, hepatomegaly, splenomegaly, and jaundice.[25] Treatment is supportive and focuses on maintaining intravascular volume and renal perfusion while minimizing fluid accumulation. This may require central venous pressure monitoring and mechanical ventilation, and pulmonary artery pressure monitoring if excess fluids accumulate in the lungs. Sodium is restricted, and spironolactone is given to decrease extravascular accumulation. Other supportive strategies may include renal-dose dopamine infusion, avoidance of diuretics that deplete intravascular volume, and chest physiotherapy to avoid pulmonary atelectasis.[25]

Strategies for prevention of veno-occlusive disease of the liver are currently undergoing investigation. These include anticoagulation with heparin, fibrinolytics such as tissue plasminogen activator or antithrombin III concentrates, prostaglandin E, and ursodeoxycholic acid (Actigall).[24,26,28]

PULMONARY COMPLICATIONS

Pulmonary complications develop in 30% to 60% of patients after HSCT.[29] Pulmonary complications may result from (1) infection, pulmonary edema, aspiration pneumonia, acute respiratory distress syndrome (ARDS), and septic shock; and (2) from lung damage from total-body irradiation or pulmonary toxic chemotherapy agents.[29–33] The pulmonary complications of HSCT are listed in Table 47-10.

table 47-10 Pulmonary Complications of Hematopoietic Stem Cell Transplantation

Time Line	Complication
Acute (before day +30)	Pulmonary edema (secondary to fluid overload, cardiac dysfunction, or allergic reaction to medications/therapy) Oropharyngeal mucositis Aspiration pneumonia Pulmonary hemorrhage/diffuse alveolar hemorrhage Bacterial or fungal pneumonia Atelectasis Pleural effusion Recall radiation pneumonitis Allergic bronchospasm Transfusion-associated lung injury ARDS and septic shock
Early (before day +100)	Idiopathic interstitial pneumonitis Pulmonary embolism Viral pneumonia (CMV, herpes simplex virus, varicella-zoster virus, respiratory syncytial virus, adenovirus, parainfluenza, influenza) Protozoal pneumonia (*Pneumocystis carinii* pneumonia) Fungal pneumonia Bacterial pneumonia Transfusion-associated lung injury ARDS and septic shock
Late (after day 100)	Idiopathic interstitial pneumonitis Bacterial, fungal, or viral pneumonia Bronchiolitis obliterans/GVHD of lung

ARDS, acute respiratory distress syndrome.

GRAFT-VERSUS-HOST DISEASE

GVHD, which is unique to allogeneic HSCT, results when the infused donor stem cells (graft) recognize the recipient (host) as foreign tissue. The graft then mounts an immunologic response attacking the host tissues, resulting in a T-cell–mediated reaction in the skin (rash), gastrointestinal tract (enteritis), and liver (elevated liver function test results). Figure 47-4 shows examples of the skin and gastrointestinal tract manifestations that may occur in acute GVHD.

The incidence of GVHD is 30% to 60% in cases involving histocompatible, sibling-matched allografts, with more GVHD occurring when there is greater HLA mismatch between the donor and recipient.[34] The mortality rate due directly or indirectly to GVHD may reach 50%.[34] Risk factors other than histoincompatibility include sex mismatching; donor parity; older age; post-transplantation infectious complications, especially viral infections; the use of donor lymphocyte infusions post-transplantation; and the type of GVHD prophylaxis used.[35]

GVHD is a serious complication, but it also has a beneficial effect in controlling the patient's malignancy in that immunocompetent donor cells are able to recognize the patient's malignant cells as foreign and eliminate them. This effect was originally identified in leukemia patients and was termed "graft-versus-leukemia" effect. Leukemia relapse was seen less often in patients with GVHD than in those without GVHD. The absence of GVHD in autologous transplant recipients is suspected to play a role in the higher disease relapse rates these patients experience. Recently, researchers are applying the graft-versus-tumor effect to prevent disease recurrence after stem cell

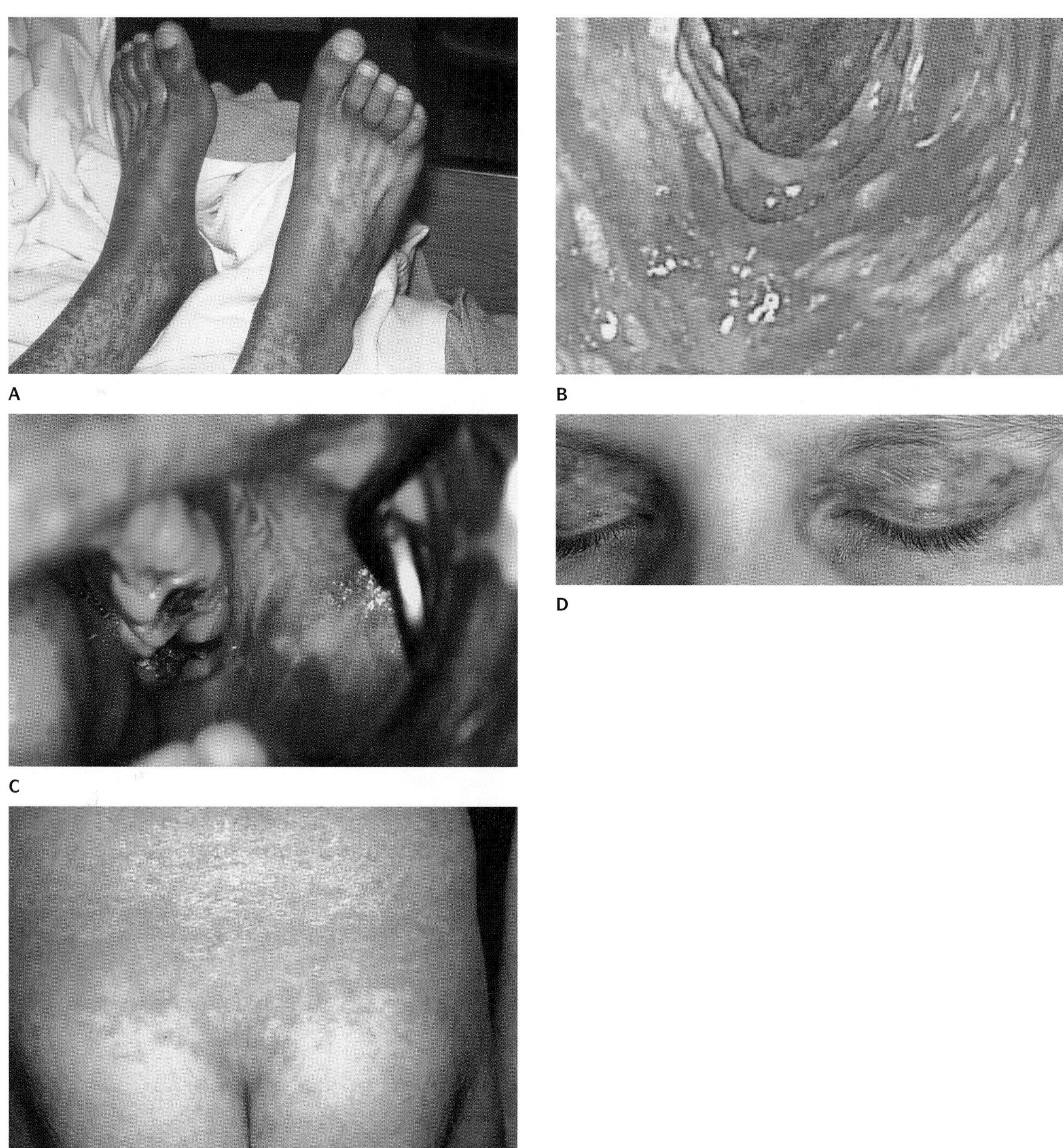

figure 47-4 Acute graft-versus-host disease (GVHD) (**A**) GVHD of the skin is characterized by fine, discrete, or confluent, erythematous macules and papules. Lesions may be pruritic or slightly tender with palpation. Earliest skin findings are usually seen on the face, palms and soles, and upper trunk. (**B**) GVHD of the gastrointestinal tract. Images obtained during endoscopy demonstrate tissue edema, extensive erythema, and mucosal ulcerations. (Photo courtesy of Bruce Greenwald, MD, University of Maryland Medical System, Baltimore, Maryland.) (**C**) Oral lichen planus changes in a patient with GVHD more than 130 days after allogeneic peripheral blood stem cell transplantation. Note the confluent, smooth, white papules that create a lacy pattern on the buccal mucosa. (Photo courtesy of Jane Fall-Dickson, RN, PhD, AOCN, National Institutes of Health, Bethesda, Maryland.) (**D**) Chronic GVHD of the skin with irregularly shaped, deeply hyperpigmented macular lesions. Note the atrophy of the dermal and subcutaneous tissues, with paper-thin skin giving an easily wrinkled or shiny appearance. The term *poikiloderma* is used to describe the classic features of patchy hypopigmentation and hyperpigmentation, dermal atrophy, and telangiectasies (small-diameter linear blood vessels seen on the skin's surface). (Photo courtesy of T.L. Diepgen and G. Yihune, Dermatology Online Atlas [www.dermis.net/doia], used with permission.) (**E**) Lichenoid chronic GvHD of the skin of the lumbar region, with flat-topped, violaceous papules; the surface is shiny and has a lacy white pattern. The eruption is confluent in some areas and hypertrophic plaques have developed. Postinflammatory hyperpigmentation may develop. (Photo courtesy of T.L. Diepgen and G. Yihune, Dermatology Online Atlas [www.dermis.net/doia], used with permission.)

transplantation by the infusion of donor lymphocytes. This approach is called *donor lymphocyte infusion* (DLI). Research is also underway to devise strategies to induce GVHD in autologous recipients of HSCT.

Acute Graft-Versus-Host Disease

Acute GVHD may occur as early as 7 to 21 days post-transplantation but peaks at 30 to 40 days post-transplantation. Acute GVHD targets the skin, liver, and gastrointestinal system. Skin reactions, which often occur first, include an itchy maculopapular, erythematous rash on the palms, soles, ears, face, and trunk. This may resolve or progress to generalized erythroderma and desquamation. Gastrointestinal symptoms include nausea, vomiting, anorexia, abdominal cramping, and large-volume diarrhea that is green and watery. Stool may be guaiac-positive as a result of intestinal mucosa sloughing. An enlarged liver, right upper quadrant pain, jaundice, and elevated bilirubin and alkaline phosphatase levels may occur. The severity and extent of acute GVHD are evaluated using a grading system (Table 47-11).

Chronic Graft-Versus-Host Disease

Chronic GVHD usually occurs in patients who have had acute GVHD, although it can occur in the absence of acute GVHD. Among patients who survived 150 days after allogeneic stem cell transplantation, chronic GVHD was observed in 33% to 49% of HLA-identical related transplants, and in 64% of matched unrelated donor transplants.[36,37]

Risk factors for chronic GVHD include previous acute GVHD, older recipient age, and sex mismatching (female donor and male recipient).[38] The incidence of chronic GVHD may also be higher in recipients of peripheral blood stem cells than in recipients of bone marrow–derived stem cells.[39] Another significant risk factor for the development of chronic GVHD is a continuing need for corticosteroids for control of GVHD by day +100.[40]

Clinical manifestations of chronic GVHD, which may be limited or extensive, are present in the skin, liver, eyes, oral cavity, lungs, gastrointestinal system, neuromuscular system, and a variety of other body systems. Chronic GVHD typically occurs 100 to 400 days after transplantation. Table 47-12 summarizes the clinical features, screening and evaluation, and interventions recommended for patients with chronic GVHD.[41–56]

Treatment and Prophylaxis of Graft-Versus-Host Disease

The first and most important way to limit GVHD is to find an HLA-matched donor. Despite such optimal matching of donor and recipient, further strategies to limit GVHD must be taken. The two major approaches to the prophylaxis of GVHD after HSCT are T-cell depletion of the graft and pharmacological therapy to prevent and treat GVHD.

T cells play a major role in the recognition of self from nonself proteins, and decreasing the number of T cells in the graft before transplantation may decrease the incidence and severity of GVHD. Methods of T-cell depletion involve physical, immunological, and pharmacological techniques. The desired outcome is a reduction or elimination of T cells capable of initiating life-threatening GVHD. However, T cells also play a role in engraftment, and T-cell depletion carries greater risks for infection, graft failure, and disease relapse.

table 47-11 Staging and Grading System for Acute Graft-Versus-Host Disease

Clinical Staging of Individual Organ Systems

Organ	Stage	Description
Skin*	+1	Maculopapular eruption over <25% of body area
	+2	Maculopapular eruption over 25%–50% of body area
	+3	Generalized erythroderma
	+4	Generalized erythroderma with bullous formation and often with desquamation
Liver	+1	Bilirubin 2.0–3.0 mg/dL
	+2	Bilirubin 3.1–6.0 mg/dL
	+3	Bilirubin 6.1–15 mg/dL
	+4	Bilirubin >15 mg/dL
Gut	+1	Diarrhea >500 mL/day
	+2	Diarrhea >1,000 mL/day
	+3	Diarrhea >1,500 mL/day
	+4	Diarrhea >2,000 mL/day, or severe abdominal pain, or ileus

Overall Grade

Grade	Skin	Liver		Gut
I	+1 to +2	0		0
II	+1 to +3	+1	and/or	+1
III	+2 to +3	+2 to +3	and/or	+2 to +3
IV	+2 to +4	+2 to +4	and/or	+2 to +4

*If no skin disease is present, the overall grade is the higher single-organ stage.

table 47-12 Chronic Graft-Versus-Host Disease: Clinical Manifestations, Screening/Evaluation, and Interventions

Organ/System	Clinical Manifestations	Screening Studies/ Evaluation	Interventions
Dermal	Dyspigmentation, xerosis (dryness), erythema, hyper-keratosis, pruritus, sclero-derma, lichenification, onychodystrophy (nail ridging/nail loss), alopecia, second malignancies	Clinical examination Skin biopsy—3-mm punch biopsy from forearm and posterior iliac crest areas	• Immunosuppressive therapy • PUVA; extracorporeal photopheresis • Topical tacrolimus ointment (Prograf) • Topical with steroid creams, moisturizers/ emollient, antibacterial ointments to prevent suprainfection; aggressive lubrication of the skin • If the sweat glands are affected, avoid over-heating because heat prostration and heat stroke can occur • Avoid sunlight exposure, use sun block lotion with a large hat that shades the face when outdoors
Oral	Lichen planus, xerostomia, ulceration, second malignancies	Oral biopsy from inner lower lip	• Steroid mouth rinses, oral PUVA, pilocarpine and anetholetrithione for xerostomia, fluoride gels/rinses to decrease caries • Careful attention to oral hygiene; regular dental evaluations
Ocular	Keratitis, sicca syndrome, increased risk for cataracts secondary to protracted use of post-transplantation steroids	Schirmer's test, ophthalmic evaluation	• Regular ophthalmological follow-up • Preservative-free tears and moisturizing ophthalmic ointments • Temporary or permanent lacrimal duct occlusion • Consider therapy with retinoic acid • Consider trial of cyclosporine ophthalmic emulsion
Hepatic	Jaundice, abdominal pain	Liver function tests (alanine and aspartate amino-transferases, alkaline phosphatase, bilirubin)	• Consider bile acid displacement therapy with ursodeoxycholic acid (Actigall) 300 mg PO tid
Pulmonary	Obstructive/restrictive pul-monary disease, shortness of breath, cough, dyspnea, wheezing, fatigue, hypoxia, pleural effusion	Pulmonary function studies, peak flow, arterial blood gas, chest CT	• Prevent and treat pulmonary infections, including *Pneumocystis carinii* and *Streptococcus pneumoniae* • Aggressively investigate changes in pulmonary function because these may represent GVHD of lung/bronchiolitis obliterans • Encourage smoking cessation
Gastrointestinal	Nausea, odynophagia, dys-phagia, anorexia, early satiety, malabsorption, diarrhea, weight loss	Stool cultures, esophago-gastroduodenoscopy, colonoscopy, nutritional assessment, fecal fat excretion studies, serum amylase, D-xylose absorption test, CT of the abdomen	• Referral to gastroenterologist; consultation with nutritionist and nutrition support • Consider empirical trial of pancreatic enzyme supplementation • Aggressive management of gastrointestinal symptoms such as nausea and vomiting • Consider the use of cholestyramine (Questran) in the management of diarrhea • Consider a trial of oral beclomethasone
Nutritional	Protein and calorie deficiency, malabsorption, dehydration, weight loss, muscle wasting	Weight, fat store measure-ment, prealbumin	• Nutritional monitoring, supplementation, symptom specific interventions • Trial of megestrol (Megace) or other approaches to appetite stimulation (e.g., mirtazapine [Remeron] or similar antidepressants, dronabinol [Marinol])
Genitourinary	Vaginal sicca, vaginal atrophy, stenosis or inflammation	Pelvic examination	• Consider trial of mucosal application of cortico-steroid ointment, cyclosporine ointment, or tacrolimus ointment • Vaginal lubricants • Sexual counseling

table 47-12 Chronic Graft-Versus-Host Disease: Clinical Manifestations, Screening/Evaluation, and Interventions (Continued)

Organ/System	Clinical Manifestations	Screening Studies/ Evaluation	Interventions
Immunological	Hypogammaglobulinemia, autoimmune syndromes, recurrent infections including CMV, herpes simplex virus, varicella-zoster virus, fungus, PCP and encapsulated bacteria	Quantitative immunoglobulin levels, CD4/CD8 lymphocyte subsets	• Intravenous immunoglobulin supplementation as indicated, and prophylactic antimicrobials (rotating antibiotics for recurrent sinopulmonary infections, PCP prophylaxis, topical antifungals) • Screening for CMV and other opportunistic infections with frequent surveillance cultures and antigen detection • Consider vaccination against influenza and pneumococcus
Musculoskeletal	Contractures, debility, muscle cramps/aches, carpal spasm	Performance status, formal quality-of-life evaluation (e.g., FAHCT-BMT), formal evaluation of rehabilitation needs (CARES)	• Physical therapy • Correct electrolyte imbalances • Consider clonazepam treatment for muscle cramping or myalgias

CT, computed tomography; PCP, *Pneumocystis carinii* pneumonia; PUVA, psoralen and ultraviolet A.

A variety of immunosuppressive agents, alone or in combination, have been used prophylactically for acute GVHD.[57] Immunosuppressive medications minimize the newly developing donor immune system's ability to recognize the host or patient as foreign, and limit the immune response. Immunosuppressive drugs may need to be taken for months or years after an allogeneic HSCT. Immunosuppression may be achieved with a single drug (often tacrolimus or cyclosporine A) or with a combination of drugs (methotrexate, tacrolimus, cyclosporine A, steroids, antithymocyte globulin), sometimes in combination with T-cell depletion.[56,58] The immunosuppressive agents commonly used in patients undergoing HSCT and the associated nursing implications are presented in Table 47-13.[34,57–71]

For patients at higher risk for GVHD, especially those undergoing matched unrelated HSCT, more intensive strategies for GVHD prevention are necessary. Many drug–drug interactions are associated with cyclosporine A and tacrolimus. Table 47-14 lists drugs that may interact with cyclosporine A and tacrolimus. Patients should be instructed to take their immunosuppressive medication exactly as instructed by the health care team and to contact their physician before starting any new medication.

Prospective, randomized trials have demonstrated that combination therapy is superior to single-drug therapy in the prevention of acute GVHD. However, to date, research has not shown that any one prophylactic regimen is superior in preventing acute GVHD or improving overall outcome.[56,57,72–74] The most widely used pharmacological regimen for the prophylaxis of acute GVHD is a combination of methotrexate and either cyclosporine A or tacrolimus.[75] Other drugs included in some GVHD prophylaxis regimens are corticosteroids, antithymocyte globulin, daclizumab, and mycophenolate mofetil.[75] Several sample regimens for GVHD prophylaxis are presented in Table 47-15.

If grade II to IV acute GVHD develops, treatment is usually required.[56] Corticosteroids are the main component of therapy, along with continuing treatment with the immunosuppressive agent used for prophylaxis (tacrolimus or cyclosporine A). High doses of methylprednisolone may be used (1 to 50 mg/kg/day). However, these high-dose regimens are associated with fatal infections and cannot be administered for more than a few days, and the dose of methylprednisolone is rapidly tapered to 2 mg/kg/day in divided doses. Once maximal improvement is achieved, the steroids are tapered over 8 to 20 weeks, based on patient response.

For patients with GVHD in whom initial therapy has failed, a variety of salvage or secondary regimens, including mycophenolate mofetil, infliximab, and daclizumab, are available. Once chronic GVHD develops, it is usually treated with steroids, cyclosporine A, tacrolimus, and a variety of other immunosuppressive agents.[54] Gut rest, pain control, and antimicrobial prophylaxis coupled with hyperalimentation, if needed, are important aspects of the supportive care of patients with acute GVHD.[76] The outcome of treatment of acute GVHD is predicted by the overall grade of acute GVHD; higher overall grades are associated with poorer outcomes.[35] Response to treatment is another key determinant of outcome, and mortality is greatest in patients who do not achieve a complete response to the initial treatment strategy for acute GVHD.[56]

LONG-TERM CONSIDERATIONS

Organ transplantation can lead to long-term survival. Increasing numbers of recipients lead healthier and longer lives. However, complications may occur long after transplantation.

Long-term care focuses on monitoring the patient's progress and adherence to the health care regimen. A major cause of graft loss in the long term is failure of patients to adhere to the medication regimen. Patients must also be

(text continues on page 1130)

table 47-13 ■ Selected Immunosuppressive Drugs Used in Allogeneic [Hematopoietic] Stem Cell Transplantation

Agent/Drug	Mechanism of Action	Dosing/Administration	Adverse Reactions	Comments
Cyclosporine A (Sandimmune, Neoral)	Prevents IL-2 gene expression, and thus impairs IL-2 synthesis, and activation of T lymphocytes	Total daily dose: usually 1.5 mg/kg IV q12h, 0.75 mg/kg q6h or 3 mg/kg/day as a continuous infusion, with dosage adjusted to achieve therapeutic levels IV to PO conversion: approximately 1:3 Dosage dependent on achieving and sustaining therapeutic blood levels based on laboratory evaluation Therapeutic monitoring not required once drug is being tapered	Metabolic: hyperkalemia and hyperglycemia, hypomagnesemia, hyperlipidemia, hyperuricemia, diabetes mellitus Neurotoxicity: headache, tremor, insomnia, paresthesia, dizziness, seizures GI: diarrhea, nausea, constipation, anorexia, vomiting, abdominal pain, ascites, elevated liver function tests Renal: elevated creatinine, nephrotoxicity Cardiovascular: hypertension, chest pain Hematological: anemia Cutaneous: acneiform rash, striae Other: peripheral edema, infection, impaired wound healing, osteoporosis, gingival hyperplasia, flushing, sweating, hirsutism	• Bioavailability differs between oral solution and capsule formulation. Once regimen is established, patients should be instructed not to change formulation or brand. • Take with food. • Instruct patient on importance of strict adherence to administration schedule and to notify health care team immediately if unable to take due to GI side effects. • Monitor serum creatinine, BUN, potassium, magnesium, glucose, and triglyceride levels. • Avoid potassium-sparing diuretics. • Replete electrolytes as indicated. • Coadministration with grapefruit juice may increase cyclosporine levels and should be avoided. • Drug–drug interactions can lead to subtherapeutic or toxic cyclosporine levels. Drugs that inhibit or induce cytochrome P-450 are most responsible (see Table 47-14). • Cyclosporine trough levels to be drawn before administration of morning dose. Therefore, doses are usually timed for 10 AM and 10 PM to allow trough blood draw at morning clinic visit. Instruct patient to bring dose to clinic, and to administer once trough level drawn. • Should not be used simultaneously with tacrolimus. • Tacrolimus should be discontinued 24 hours before starting cyclosporine. In the presence of increased tacrolimus levels, initiation of cyclosporine should usually be further delayed. • Doses should be adjusted for renal dysfunction. • Monitor levels carefully in patients with renal or hepatic dysfunction.
Tacrolimus (Prograf)	Impaired synthesis of IL-2 prevents T-lymphocyte proliferation; interferes with the gene transcription for a variety of cytokines including IFN-γ, TNF-α	Total daily dose: usually 1–2 mg PO q12h; 0.05–0.1 mg/kg/day as a continuous infusion, with dosage adjusted to achieve therapeutic levels	Metabolic: hyperkalemia and hypokalemia, hyperglycemia, hypomagnesemia, hyperlipidemia, hypophosphatemia, diabetes mellitus	• Take on empty stomach. • Instruct patient on importance of strict adherence to administration schedule and to notify the health care team immediately if unable to take due to GI side effects.

		IV to PO conversion: approximately 1:4 Dosage dependent on achieving and sustaining therapeutic blood levels based on laboratory evaluation Therapeutic monitoring not required once drug is being tapered	Neurotoxicity: headache, tremor, insomnia, paresthesia, dizziness, seizures GI: diarrhea, nausea, constipation, anorexia, vomiting, abdominal pain, ascites, elevated liver function tests Renal: elevated creatinine, nephrotoxicity Cardiovascular: hypertension, chest pain Hematological: anemia, leukocytosis, thrombocytopenia Cutaneous: pruritus, acneiform rash Pulmonary: pleural effusion, atelectasis, dyspnea Other: peripheral edema, infection, impaired wound healing, osteoporosis	• Monitor serum creatinine, BUN, potassium, magnesium, phosphorus, glucose, and triglyceride levels. • Avoid potassium-sparing diuretics. • Replete electrolytes as indicated • Coadministration with grapefruit juice may increase tacrolimus levels and should be avoided. • Drug–drug interactions can lead to subtherapeutic or toxic tacrolimus levels. Drugs that inhibit or induce cytochrome P-450 are most responsible (see Table 47-14). • Tacrolimus trough levels to be drawn before administration of morning dose. Therefore doses are usually timed for 10 AM and 10 PM to allow trough blood draw at morning clinic visit. Instruct patient to bring dose to clinic, and to administer once trough level drawn. • Should not be used simultaneously with cyclosporine. • Cyclosporine should be discontinued 24 hours before starting tacrolimus. In the presence of elevated cyclosporine levels, initiation of tacrolimus is delayed. • Doses should be adjusted for renal dysfunction. • Monitor levels carefully in patients with renal or hepatic dysfunction.
Steroids	Decreases cytotoxic T-cell proliferation, inhibits production of IL-1 and IFN-γ, prevents production of IL-2, inhibits neutrophils function by stabilizing leukocyte lysosomal membrane and inhibiting chemotaxis	Dosage varies according to institutional protocols Dosage: 0.5–2 mg/kg/day q12h, with tapering schedule determined based on starting dose and patient response	Metabolic: fluid and electrolyte imbalance, diabetes mellitus, hyperlipidemia Neurotoxicity: tremors, seizures, headache, difficulty concentrating, insomnia GI: GI irritation Cardiovascular: hypertension, dysrhythmias Cutaneous: bruising, fragile skin Neurotoxicity: tremors, seizures, headache	• Usually used in combination with cyclosporine or tacrolimus. • Consult physical therapy for proximal muscle strengthening exercise program. • Instruct patient in strategies to prevent or treat hyperglycemia, and in diabetic self-management. • Administer oral corticosteroids with food/milk to minimize GI upset. • Administer H_2 blockers as ordered. • May increase tacrolimus or cyclosporine levels. • Report complaints of visual changes and consult ophthalmology.

(continued)

table 47-13 Selected Immunosuppressive Drugs Used in Allogeneic [Hematopoietic] Stem Cell Transplantation (Continued)

Agent/Drug	Mechanism of Action	Dosing/Administration	Adverse Reactions	Comments
			Other: hunger, peripheral edema, infection, impaired wound healing, hirsutism, osteoporosis, weight gain, steroid myopathy, cataracts/glaucoma, cushingoid changes, psychiatric disturbances (steroid psychosis, mood changes, confusion)	• For patients on long-term steroids or otherwise at risk for or experiencing osteopenia (e.g., patients with acute lymphocytic leukemia, postmenopausal) ensure regular dual-energy x-ray absorptiometry scans, calcium and vitamin D supplementation and specific treatment for osteopenia with antiresorptive agents such as pamidronate, aledronate. • Tapering calendar specifying the dosage to be taken each day can help facilitate adherence in patients who are on tapering doses of steroids, or an alternate-day steroid regimen.
Mycophenolate mofetil (MMF) (Cellcept)	Antimetabolite that selectively inhibits the proliferation of T and B lymphocytes by interfering with purine nucleotide synthesis	Dosage: 1–1.5 g IV or PO q12h depending on institutional guidelines	Metabolic: hyperkalemia and hypokalemia, hyperlipidemia, hypophosphatemia, hyperglycemia Neurotoxicity: headache, insomnia, tremors, seizures GI: diarrhea, nausea, constipation, anorexia, vomiting, abdominal pain, hepatotoxicity Renal: elevated creatinine, nephrotoxicity Cardiovascular: hypertension, hypotension, dysrhythmias Hematological: anemia, leukocytosis, thrombocytopenia Cutaneous: acneiform rash Pulmonary: cough, dyspnea Other: fever, edema, pain, infection, muscle weakness, anxiety, depression	• MMF should be taken on an empty stomach. • Monitor complete blood count at regular intervals and adjust dosage for pancytopenia, as ordered. • Monitor liver function tests (bilirubin and serum aminotransferases) at regular intervals, adjust dosage for liver function abnormalities, as ordered. • Monitor serum levels of the MMF metabolic to guide treatment in patients with renal dysfunction. • In the setting of renal impairment, or when coadministered with probenicid, acyclovir, or ganciclovir, the drug concentrations of MMF and of these drugs may increase. • There may be decreased MMF absorption when coadministered with magnesium oxide, aluminum- or magnesium-containing antacids, or cholestyramine.
Azathioprine (Imuran)	Antimetabolite that selectively inhibits the proliferation of T and B lymphocytes by interfering with purine nucleotide synthesis	Usual dose: 2–2.5 mg/kg/day. Oral dose same as IV dose	Alopecia, myelosuppression, hepatotoxicity, infection, nausea, vomiting, diarrhea, mucosal ulceration, esophagitis, second malignancies	• Dose decrement is required when given with allopurinol. • May lead to anemia and leukopenia when given with angiotensin-converting enzyme inhibitors; synergistic with other bone marrow suppressants. • Use with caution in patients with hepatic or renal impairment. • Teratogenic; advise patient and partner about need for contraception.

Methotrexate	Antimetabolite that inhibits dihydrofolate reductase, thereby hindering DNA synthesis and cell reproduction, and thus inhibiting lymphocyte proliferation	Institutional protocols vary Usual dose: 5–15 mg/m^2 given IV on days 1, 3, 6, and 11 after transplantation	Myelosuppression, mucositis, photosensitivity, interstitial pneumonitis, hepatotoxicity, nephrotoxicity	• Dose and schedule for methotrexate prophylaxis for GVHD varies by institution. Common regimen is 5–15 mg/m^2 on days 1, 3, 6 and 11 post-transplantation. • Doses may be adjusted or held for severe mucositis and renal or liver insufficiency. Doses may need to be adjusted for hypoalbuminemia. • Wait until at least 24 hours after stem cell infusion to give day +1 dose.
Daclizumab (Zenapax)	Monoclonal antibody against the IL-2 receptor expressed on activated T cells. Binds to the IL-2 receptor in a non-activating fashion, competing with IL-2 and thereby inhibiting IL-2 driven proliferation of the activated T lymphocyte IL-2–induced proliferation of activated (antigen stimulated) T lymphocytes is a critical step in proliferation and ultimately tissue destruction	Institutional protocols vary Usual dose: 1 mg/kg by IV administration	Constipation, nausea, vomiting, diarrhea, abdominal pain, abdominal distension, edema, tremor, headache, dizziness, nephrotoxicity, chest pain, tachycardia, fever, pain, fatigue, hypertension, hypotension, dyspnea, pulmonary edema, coughing, musculoskeletal pain, back pain	• Anaphylactoid reactions after the administration of daclizumab have not been observed but can occur after the administration of proteins. Medications for the treatment of severe hypersensitivity reactions should be available for immediate use. • The calculated volume of daclizumab should be mixed with 50 mL of sterile 0.9% sodium chloride solution and administered through a peripheral or central vein over a 15-min period. Once the infusion is prepared, it should be administered intravenously within 4 h. If it must be held longer, it should be refrigerated between 2°–8°C (36°–46°F) for up to 24 h. After 24 h, the prepared solution should be discarded. • No incompatibility between daclizumab and PVC or polyethylene bags or infusion sets has been observed. • No dosage adjustment is necessary for patients with severe renal impairment.
Infliximab (Remicade)	Monoclonal antibody against TNF-α Binds to soluble and membrane-bound TNF-α, producing reduction in serum IL-1 and reduced levels of nitric oxide synthase	Institutional protocols vary Usual dose: 10 mg/kg by IV administration Administer over at least 2 h Must be given with a low protein-binding filter of 1.2 μm or less	Headache, nausea, abdominal pain, fatigue, fever and coughing Infusion reactions, including fever, chills, chest pain, hypotension, headache, and urticaria can occur during the infusion and for up to 2 h after the infusion is complete. There is no increase in the incidence of reactions after the initial infusion.	• Monitor patient for development of infusional toxicities. • Consider premedication with acetaminophen and dyphenhydramine (Benadryl). • Initiate therapy at 10 mL/h × 15 min, increase to 20 mL/h × 15 min, and then increase to 40 mL/h × 15 min, then 80 mL/hr × 15 min, then 150 mL/h × 30 min, and then 250 mL/h × 30 min to complete infusion in 2 h. • Stop or slow infusion and give Benadryl, acetaminophen, or Solu-Cortef to treat mild to moderate infusion reaction. Resume infusion at 10 mL/h once reaction controlled or abated.

(continued)

table 47-13 Selected Immunosuppressive Drugs Used in Allogeneic [Hematopoietic] Stem Cell Transplantation (Continued)

Agent/Drug	Mechanism of Action	Dosing/Administration	Adverse Reactions	Comments
			Delayed, serum sickness–like reactions including myalgias, arthralgias, fever, rash, sore throat, dysphagia, and hand and facial edema can be seen 3–12 days after infusion. Patients may develop human antichimeric antibody.	• Medications for treating hypersensitivity reactions (e.g., acetaminophen, antihistamines, corticosteroids, or epinephrine) and supplemental oxygen should be available for immediate use in the event of a reaction. • Incompatible with PVC equipment or devices. Use glass infusion bottles and polyethylene-lined administration sets.
Antithymocyte globulin (Atgam, equine) (Thymoglobulin, rabbit)	Polyclonal immunoglobulin composed of horse or rabbit antibodies capable of destroying human leukocytes	Institutional protocols vary Usual dose: 10–40 mg/kg/day for equine ATG, and 2.5 mg/kg/day for rabbit ATG	Seizures, laryngospasm, anaphylaxis, pulmonary edema, leukopenia, and thrombocytopenia. ATG is a foreign xenogeneic protein and an antibody, which may cause serum sickness, including myalgias, arthralgias, fever, rash, sore throat, dysphagia and hand and facial edema.	• Monitor patient closely both during infusion and after infusion for signs of serum sickness and anaphylaxis. Consider premedication with corticosteroids, acetaminophen, and H_1 and H_2 blockers. • Medications for treating hypersensitivity reactions (e.g., acetaminophen, antihistamines, corticosteroids, or epinephrine) and supplemental oxygen should be available for immediate use in the event of a reaction. • Because transient and at times severe thrombocytopenia may occur after ATG administration, in patients with platelet counts less than 100,000, monitor platelet count 1 h after ATG administration, and transfuse platelets as indicated.
Alemtuzumab (Campath)	Monoclonal antibody directed against the cell surface antigen CD52, which is expressed on B and T lymphocytes	Institutional protocols vary Usual dose: 20 mg/day IV given over several hours for 5 days, beginning before transplantation	Infusional toxicities may be severe, and include fever and rigors in more than 80% of patients. Other adverse effects include neutropenia, anemia, thrombocytopenia, nausea, vomiting, rash, fatigue, and hypotension.	• Premedicate patient with acetaminophen and Benadryl. • Medications for treating hypersensitivity reactions (e.g., acetaminophen, antihistamines, corticosteroids, or epinephrine) and supplemental oxygen should be available for immediate use in the event of a reaction. • Consider treatment with mepedridine to control infusional rigors. • Administer fluid bolus as ordered to treat hypotension. • Produces profound and rapid lymphopenia; therefore, patients require broad antifungal, antibacterial, antiviral, and antiprotozoal prophylaxis for at least 4 mo after treatment.

Sirolimus (Rapamune)	Structurally similar to tacrolimus and cyclosporine; however, it has a distinct immunosuppressant activity Inhibits response of B and T lymphocytes to cytokine stimulation by IL-2 and inhibits antibody production by B cells	Long half-life permits once-daily dosing Monitor trough blood levels	Hyperlipidemia, thrombocytopenia, leukopenia, headache, nausea, anorexia, dizziness	• May suppress hematopoietic recovery if used in patients who have recently undergone high-dose therapy. • Oral bioavailability is variable and is improved with high-fat meals. • Like tacrolimus and cyclosporine, [sirolimus] is metabolized through the cytochrome P-450 3A system.
N-Acetylcysteine	Inhibits B7-1/CD28 expression in vitro Thought to interfere with T-cell/antigen-presenting cell costimulator pathways May also counterbalance tissue damage from free radicals and oxidative stress	Bolus of 150 mg/kg IV followed by continuous IV infusion of 50 mg/kg/day over at least 7–21 days.		• Monitor vital signs every 15 min during initial bolus infusion. • Compatibilities with other therapies such as total parenteral nutrition are unknown; separate intravenous access should be used for drug infusion.
Thalidomide (Thalomid)	Immunosuppressive and anti-inflammatory properties, including impaired neutrophil phagocytosis and chemotaxis; reduced antibody production in response to antigenic stimulation; increased T-suppressor cells and reduced T-helper cells; inhibition of TNF-α production by monocytes	100 mg PO qhs, increasing gradually to 400–600 mg PO qhs	Neutropenia, skin rash, skin ulceration, peripheral neuropathy, somnolence, lightheadedness, constipation, bradycardia, hypothyroidism, hypotension	• Thalidomide is a potent teratogen and is contraindicated in patients who are, or are likely to become pregnant. Systematic counseling and education program, written informed consent, and participation in a confidential survey program at the start of treatment and throughout treatment are required for all patients receiving thalidomide. Both men and women who are of childbearing potential must practice protected sex while on this drug. • Perform pregnancy test before initiating treatment with thalidomide. • The combination of thalidomide with certain antibiotics, HIV protease inhibitors, rifampin, griseofulvin, phenytoin, or carbamazepine may decrease the effectiveness of oral contraceptives. • Obtain baseline ECG before treatment. • Thalidomide should not be started if the ANC is less than 750/mm^3, and therapy should be reevaluated if the ANC drops below this level.

(continued)

table 47-13 ■ Selected Immunosuppressive Drugs Used in Allogeneic [Hematopoietic] Stem Cell Transplantation (Continued)

Agent/Drug	Mechanism of Action	Dosing/Administration	Adverse Reactions	Comments
				• Always administer doses in the evening to minimize impact of drowsiness on lifestyle and safety. • Teach patient to use caution when taking thalidomide with other drugs that can cause drowsiness or neuropathy. • Teach patient to rise slowly from a supine position to avoid lightheadedness. • Teach patient to report immediately signs or symptoms suggestive of peripheral neuropathy, including numbness or tingling in the hands or feet or the development of skin rash or skin lesion. These may require immediate cessation of the drug until the patient can be evaluated for the neuropathy or skin rash. • Teach patient to use protective measures (e.g., sunscreens and protective clothing) against exposure to ultraviolet light or sunlight. • Control or manage constipation with a stool softener or mild laxative.
Methoxsoralen (Oxsoralen)	When photoactivated by ultraviolet light, drug inhibits mitosis by binding covalently to pyrimidine bases in DNA	400 μg/kg PO 1.5–2 h before exposure to ultraviolet light		• Patients who have received cytotoxic chemotherapy or radiation and who are taking methoxsoralen are at increased risk for skin cancers, and long-term use may increase the risk of skin cancer. • Toxicity increases with concurrent use of phenothiazines, thiazides, and sulfanilamides. • Severe burns may occur from sunlight or ultraviolet A exposure if dose or treatment frequency is exceeded. • Pretreatment eye examinations are indicated to evaluate for the presence of cataracts. Repeat eye examinations should be performed every 6 mo while patients are undergoing psoralen and ultraviolet A therapy.

ANC, absolute neutrophil count; GI, gastrointestinal; IFN, interferon; IL, interleukin; IV, intravenous; PO, oral; PVC, polyvinyl chloride; TNF, tumor necrosis factor.

table 47-14 Drugs That May Alter Levels of Cyclosporine and Tacrolimus

Effects	Known Interactions	Suspected Interactions
Increase serum levels	Erythromycin Clarithromycin Itraconazole Fluconazole Ketoconazole Corticosteroids	H_2 antagonists Cephalosporins Thiazide diuretics Furosemide Acyclovir Warfarin Calcium channel blockers (i.e., diltiazem, verapamil, nicardipine) Oral contraceptives Doxycycline Metoclopramide Coadministration with grapefruit juice
Decrease serum levels	Phenytoin or phenobarbital Rifampin or isoniazid Sulfadiazine + trimethoprim (intravenous)	Sulfinpyrazone Carbamazepine Anticonvulsants
Cause additive nephrotoxicity	Amphotericin B Aminoglycosides Melphalan Trimethoprim-sulfamethoxazole	Nonsteroidal anti-inflammatory drugs
Alter immunosuppressive effects		Propranolol Verapamil Etoposide

Based on information from Melocco T, Kerr S, McKenzie C: Drug toxicity and interactions posttransplant. In Atkinson K (ed): Clinical Bone Marrow Transplantation: A Clinical Textbook, pp 396–409. Cambridge, United Kingdom, Cambridge University Press, 1994.

table 47-15 Examples of Commonly Used Drug Regimens for Prophylaxis of Acute GVHD

Regimen	Dosing Schedule
Cyclosporine/steroids	Cyclosporine 3 mg/kg/day IV infusion from day –2, taper 10% weekly starting day +180* Methylprednisolone 0.25 mg/kg bid days +7 to +14, 0.5 mg/kg bid days +15 to +28, 0.4 mg/kg bid days +29 to +42, 0.3 mg/kg bid days +43 to +58, 0.25 mg/kg bid days +59 to +119, and 0.1 mg/kg daily days +120–180.
Cyclosporine/methotrexate/steroids	Cyclosporine 5 mg/kg/day IV infusion from day –2, taper 20% every 2 wk starting day +84* Methotrexate 15 mg/m² on day +1, 10 mg/m² on days +3 and +6 Methylprednisolone 0.25 mg/kg bid days +7 to +14, 0.5 mg/kg bid days +15 to +28, 0.4 mg/kg bid days +29 to +42, 0.3 mg/kg bid days +43 to +58, 0.25 mg/kg bid days +59 to +119, and 0.1 mg/kg daily days +120–180
Tacrolimus/minimethotrexate	Tacrolimus 0.03 mg/kg/day infusion from day –2, taper 20% every 2 wk starting day +180* Methotrexate 5 mg/m² on days +1, +3, +6, and +11
Antithymocyte globulin (ATG)/cyclosporine/methotrexate	ATG 20 mg/kg IV days –3, –2, and –1 Cyclosporine 5 mg/kg/day IV infusion from day –1, taper 10% weekly starting day +180* Methotrexate 10 mg/m² on days +1, +3, +6, and +11

*Either tacrolimus or cyclosporine has been used with this methotrexate or steroid dose schedule.

monitored for the development of late complications, including hypertension and cardiovascular disease, chronic rejection, and recurrence of the original disease, such as hepatitis in liver transplantation and recurrent glomerulonephritis in kidney transplantation. There is also increased incidence of post-transplantation lymphoproliferative disease (PTLD) in solid organ transplant recipients who are receiving long-term immunosuppression.

Weight gain can be a significant complication post-transplantation as a result of steroid use or because of general improved well-being related to the organ transplantation. Osteoporosis secondary to high steroid use is also a long-term issue for organ transplant recipients, more often for heart and liver than kidney transplant recipients.

The refinement and success of HSCT has resulted in a large population of patients who have achieved control of their underlying disease. However, these patients must often deal with long-term sequelae and late effects of HSCT. In addition to chronic GVHD and infectious risks, they may experience a wide range of complications, as summarized in Box 47-7.[37,44,45,53,77–80] Most transplantation centers have unique requirements for continued follow-up care that depends on protocols. The frequency of clinic visits is determined by the nature of the complications the patient is experiencing. Table 47-16 presents guidelines for screening and management of late effects in HSCT recipients.[28,45,57,77–87]

box 47-7
Early and Late Complications of Autologous and Allogeneic Hematopoietic Stem Cell Transplantation

Early (Occurring Before Day +100)

Regimen-related toxicity
- Hemorrhagic cystitis
- Veno-occlusive disease of the liver
- Pulmonary complications
- Renal complications
- Neurological complications

Nutritional complications
Idiopathic pneumonitis
Graft failure
Infection
- Viral
- Bacterial
- Fungal

Graft-versus-host disease
Relapse

Late (Occurring After Day +100)

Regimen-related toxicity
- Cataracts
- Neurological conditions (peripheral and autonomic neuropathies)
- Gonadal dysfunction
- Endocrine dysfunction

Immunodeficiency
Infection
Musculoskeletal
- Osteoporosis
- Avascular necrosis

Chronic graft-versus-host disease
Relapse of malignancy
Secondary malignancy

case study ■ CARDIAC TRANSPLANT

H.W. is a 59-year-old man who has carditis and aortic regurgitation as a result of rheumatic fever at age 16 years. Congestive heart failure symptoms began in 1991, and the patient's ejection fraction at that time was noted to be 23%. In November 1993, the patient underwent an aortic valve replacement with a St. Jude prosthesis. An automatic implantable cardioverter–defibrillator (AICD) was placed in 1998 due to the presence of ventricular dysrhythmias. In the spring of 1999, the patient noted worsening dyspnea with minimal exertion and increased fluid retention in his abdomen with exacerbations of his congestive heart failure.

The patient's heart transplant evaluation revealed an O+ blood type panel reactive antibody percentage (PRA) of 4%. His blood urea nitrogen (BUN) level was 23 mg/dL with a creatinine level of 1.0 mg/dL. Serologies were negative for cytomegalovirus (CMV) and hepatitis B and C antibodies. Serologies were positive for toxoplasmosis, Epstein-Barr virus (EBV), and herpes simplex virus type 1 (HSV-1). Echocardiography revealed an ejection fraction of 15% with moderate mitral regurgitation and mild aortic regurgitation. Right heart catheterization revealed elevated pulmonary artery pressures of 60/23 mm Hg with a mean pulmonary artery pressure of 5 mm Hg, cardiac output of 4.05 L/min, transpulmonary gradient of 30 mm Hg, and pulmonary vascular resistance (PVR) of 7.4 Woods units, indicating the presence of pulmonary hypertension secondary to long-standing heart failure. Reversibility of pulmonary hypertension was demonstrated after 0.4 mg of sublingual nitroglycerin was administered, with a decrease in the patient's PVR to 2.6 Woods units. The patient was deemed a suitable candidate for cardiac transplantation and was listed in the summer of 1999.

An appropriate donor for the cardiac transplant was identified in July 2002. Operative bleeding was problematic due to significant chest wall adhesions from the patient's prior sternotomy. The operative procedure took approximately 4 hours. The patient was transported to the cardiothoracic ICU on dopamine and dobutamine. The patient's prior history of pulmonary hypertension led to some right-sided heart failure because the donor heart was not used to pumping against this type of resistance. Nitroglycerin was added secondary to rising central venous pressures of 18 to 20 mm Hg to provide vasodilation of the pulmonary bed. Dopamine, dobutamine, and nitroglycerin were gradually weaned over the first 6 postoperative days.

Immunosuppression was started immediately after surgery with steroids, mycophenolate mofetil (MMF), and sirolimus (Rapamune). Tacrolimus, a known renal toxin, was initiated in a delayed fashion on postoperative day 5 to preserve renal function as the patient's BUN and creatinine levels rose to 67 mg/dL and 1.5 mg/dL, respectively. MMF was discontinued 8 days post-transplantation when

table 47-16 Evaluation and Screening of Late Effects of Hematopoietic Stem Cell Transplantation

System/Dimension	Possible Late Effects	Evaluation and Screening
Disease status	Relapse/recurrence	Determined based on site of original disease, but may include CT scans, bone marrow aspirate and biopsy, lumbar puncture, cytogenetics, and engraftment studies Evaluation for minimal residual disease (if available)
Engraftment	Graft failure/marrow dysfunction with cytopenia	CBC with differential Bone marrow aspirate and biopsy Engraftment studies: to detect differences between DNA of donor and recipient and thus establish engraftment: variable nucleotide tandem repeats or restriction fragment length polymorphisms; cytogenetic studies may also be used to establish engraftment if the donor and recipient are of opposite sexes
Immunological function/recovery	Disorders of B- and T-lymphocyte quantity and function Hypogammaglobulinemia	CD4/CD8 lymphocyte subsets Quantitative immunoglobulin levels Vaccination titers
Cardiopulmonary effects	Interstitial pneumonitis Bronchiolitis obliterans Hypertension, cardiomyopathy, pericardial damage, peripheral vascular disease	Chest x-ray Pulmonary function tests with diffusing capacity of lungs for carbon monoxide Electrocardiogram Echocardiogram History and physical examination
Neurological effects	Peripheral and autonomic neuropathies Cognitive changes, shortened attention span, difficulty with concentration Leukoencephalopathy Ototoxicity	Health history Neurological examination Neuropsychological testing Rehabilitation medicine Audiological testing
Gastrointestinal effects	Liver dysfunction Malabsorption syndromes	Liver function tests Hepatitis B serologies, hepatitis C polymerase chain reaction qualitative
Genitourinary effects	Renal dysfunction Radiation nephritis Hematuria, proteinuria Cancer of the bladder	BUN, creatinine Urinalysis with microscopy 24-Hour urine for creatinine clearance, total protein, if indicated
Endocrine		
Thyroid function	Hypothyroidism	TSH, T_3, T_4, free T_4
Gonadal function	Decreased production of gonadal hormones	LH, FSH, estradiol (women) Pelvic examination LH, FSH, testosterone (men)
Hypothalamic–pituitary	Abnormal pituitary gland function	Prolactin levels, FSH, LH, TSH
Ophthalmic	Cataracts	Ophthalmological examination to include slit-lamp examination and Schirmer's test
Dental/oral cavity	Sicca syndrome Caries Periodontal disease Xerostomia Oral malignancy	Regular dental evaluations Careful attention to oral hygiene Fluoride gels/rinses
Musculoskeletal	Osteoporosis Avascular necrosis Myopathy	Dual-energy x-ray absorptiometry scan MRI if pain in a joint, limited range of motion, or a limp MRI, neurological examination, electromyogram
Second malignancy	Nonmelanoma skin cancer	Complete physical examination with biopsy of suspect lesions; skin photographs may also help to monitor status
	Breast cancer	Mammogram, self-examination

(continued)

table 47-16 Evaluation and Screening of Late Effects of Hematopoietic Stem Cell Transplantation (Continued)

System/Dimension	Possible Late Effects	Evaluation and Screening
	Thyroid cancer	History and physical examination, ultrasound, I^{131} scan
	Acute leukemia	CBC with differential
	Myelodysplastic syndrome	Bone marrow aspirate and biopsy (if CBC abnormal)
	PTLD	CT scans if PTLD suspected
	Cancer of the uterine cervix	Gynecological examination with Papanicolaou smear
	Cancer of the bladder	Urinalysis with micro to detect microhematuria, urine cytology, follow-up cystoscopy
Integumentary	Increased incidence of benign and malignant nevi	Complete physical examination Skin biopsy of suspect lesions
Psychological/ rehabilitation, quality of life	Changes in body image, roles, family relationships, lifestyle, occupation, discrimination, overcoming stigma, living with compromises, coping with symptoms	Assessment of individual adjustment, achievement of normal developmental tasks, marital stress, sexual function, body image, rehabilitation needs, symptom distress through systematic and structured evaluation

CBC, complete blood count; CT, computed tomography; FSH, follicle-stimulating hormone; LH, luteinizing hormone; MRI, magnetic resonance imaging; PTLD, post-transplantation lymphoproliferative disorder; T_3, triiodothyronine; T_4, thyroxine; TSH, thyroid-stimulating hormone.

tacrolimus trough levels were approximately 5 to 7 ng/mL. An endomyocardial biopsy was performed on postoperative day 8 and the patient was found to have acute grade 3A rejection. Solumedrol (1 g intravenously) was administered every day for 3 days. The patient remained hemodynamically stable and was asymptomatic. Repeat biopsy 10 days post-treatment indicated resolving rejection.

After surgery, the patient also experienced transient episodes of sinus bradycardia with heart rates in the 40s. Theophylline was administered orally in an attempt to prevent further bradycardia. This therapy proved to be unsuccessful and due to persistent intermittent bradycardia a permanent pacemaker was inserted.

Due to CMV mismatch (recipient negative/donor positive), the patient was started on prophylactic valganciclovir (900 mg twice daily). CMV antigenemias were checked weekly to evaluate for early CMV disease. The patient was discharged to home after teaching was complete and he could verbalize his medication regimen and self-care needs. ■

clinical applicability challenges

Self-Challenge: Critical Thinking

1. *Analyze the similarities and differences in the care of transplant recipients and that of other postoperative patients.*
2. *Based on the case study in this chapter, determine H.W.'s preoperative and postoperative risks. Develop a care plan for him based on your analysis.*
3. *Based on the case study in this chapter, what is H.W.'s greatest risk for transplant coronary artery disease?*

Study Questions

1. *Mr. Jones is receiving high-dose conditioning therapy for 2 days consisting of total-body irradiation 1,125 cGy and cyclophosphamide (Cytoxan) 60 mg/kg. His antiemetic regimen consists of dexamethasone 40 mg orally (PO) each day, granisetron (Kytril), 1 mg intravenously (IV) each day, prochlorperazine (Compazine) 10 mg PO/IV every 4 hours prn for nausea, and lorazepam (Ativan). Which of the following adverse effects would you least expect with this regimen?*
   a. *Parotitis*
   b. *Abnormalities on electrocardiogram (ECG)*
   c. *Fever*
   d. *Hypoglycemia*
2. *Mr. Jones is day 2 post–allogeneic transplantation after conditioning with total-body irradiation and cyclophosphamide (Cytoxan). Laboratory studies show white blood cells 0.1 × 10^9/L, hemoglobin 8.2 g/dL, hematocrit 24.6%, platelets 17,000/mm^3, sodium 126 mEq/L, potassium 3.0 mEq/L, chloride 98 mEq/L, carbon dioxide 18 mEq/L, BUN 11 mg/dL, creatinine 0.6 mg/dL. Vital signs are temperature 98.1°F (36.7°C); pulse 100 beats/minute; respirations 22 breaths/minute; blood pressure 108/55 mm Hg. The patient's 24-hour fluid balance shows intake = 5,600 mL, output = 2,105 mL. He complains of nausea, vomiting, diarrhea, and abdominal pain. Based on these data, which of the following findings would be most likely on physical examination?*
   a. *Rales, peripheral edema, jugular venous distension*
   b. *Firm abdomen with absent bowel sounds and rebound tenderness, cardiac gallop (S_3), skin rash*
   c. *Skin pallor, rales, peripheral edema, tenderness of the right upper quadrant*
   d. *Erythema or shallow ulcerations of the oral cavity, weakness, erythema of the skin, conjunctival pallor, petechial skin rash*
3. *In addition to pancytopenia and gastrointestinal toxicity, Mr. Jones demonstrates which of the following acute complications of high-dose therapy?*
   a. *Syndrome of inappropriate antidiuretic hormone secretion (SIADH)*
   b. *Veno-occlusive disease of the liver*
   c. *Renal insufficiency*
   d. *Sepsis*

4. *Which of the following statements concerning irradiation of blood products in patients undergoing hematopoietic stem cell transplantation (HSCT) is correct?*
   A. *Irradiation inactivates immunologically competent T lymphocytes contained in the blood product.*
   B. *Transfusion-associated graft-versus-host disease (GVHD) develops when immunocompetent allogeneic lymphocytes are transfused into a severely immune compromised host.*
   C. *Gamma irradiation to 2,500 cGy is currently the most efficient and effective mode of irradiation.*
   D. *Blood products that have been irradiated cannot be used by other patients because the irradiating process alters the efficacy of the blood product.*
      a. *A, B, C*
      b. *A, C*
      c. *A, C, D*
      d. *All of the above*
5. *Which of the following would place a patient at a higher risk for the development of acute graft-versus-host disease (GVHD)?*
   a. *T-cell depletion*
   b. *Related, sex-matched donor as source of hematopoietic stem cells*
   c. *Younger patient or donor*
   d. *Post-transplantation cytomegalovirus (CMV) or other viral infections*
6. *Mr. Jones is taking cyclosporine A to prevent acute graft-versus-host disease (GVHD). Which of the following statements would be an expected outcome of the teaching provided to Mr. Jones regarding cyclosporine A?*
   A. *Mr. Jones states that headache, tremor, or confusion may occur intermittently while taking cyclosporine A and these symptoms do not reflect a serious problem.*
   B. *To make up for a missed dose of cyclosporine A, Mr. Jones takes 1.5 times the usual dose at the next regularly scheduled time.*
   C. *Mr. Jones takes his usual cyclosporine A dose immediately before the clinic visit when drug levels are drawn.*
   D. *Mr. Jones substitutes cyclosporine A capsules for cyclosporin elixir because the elixir has an oily, aversive taste and the capsules are easier to swallow.*
      a. *A, B, D*
      b. *B, C, D*
      c. *None of the above*
      d. *A, B, C, D*
7. *Which of the following immunosuppressive drugs must be monitored by drug levels?*
   a. *Prednisone*
   b. *Mycophenolate mofetil*
   c. *Tacrolimus*
   d. *Imuran*
8. *Mr. Smith is 4 hours post–orthotopic heart transplantation. You note that his central venous pressure (CVP) has increased from 10 to 22 cm H_2O. His pulmonary artery pressures have gradually increased to 47/24 from 30/15 mm Hg. His systolic blood pressure is averaging 110 mm Hg. The physician suspects that Mr. Jones is experiencing right-sided heart dysfunction secondary to the acute change in pulmonary vascular resistance during transplantation of a healthy heart into the pulmonary bed of the previously failing heart. Which of the following medications is the physician most likely to prescribe?*
   a. *Epinephrine*
   b. *Dopamine*
   c. *Vasopressin*
   d. *Inhaled nitric oxide*
9. *Which of the following is an absolute contraindication to solid organ transplantation?*
   a. *Recent infection*
   b. *Recipient age >65 years*
   c. *Current substance abuse*
   d. *Diabetes mellitus*

REFERENCES

1. Williams LA, McCarthy PL: Diseases treated with peripheral stem cell transplantation. In Buchsel PC, Kapustay PM (eds): Stem Cell Transplantation: A Clinical Textbook, pp 3.3–3.21. Pittsburgh, Oncology Nursing Press, 2000
2. Scientific Registry of Transplant Recipients. 2002. Available at: www.ustransplant.org. Accessed August 2003
3. United Network for Organ Sharing. Available at: www.unos.org. Accessed August 2003
4. Medicare. Available at: wwww.medicare.org. Accessed August 2003
5. Danovitch GM (ed): Handbook of Kidney Transplantation. Philadelphia, Lippincott Williams & Wilkins, 2001
6. Sheehy E, Conrad SL, Brigham LE, et al: Estimating the number of potential organ donors in the United States. N Engl J Med 349: 667–674, 2003
7. Dubernard JM, Dawahra M, McMaster P (eds): Organ Preservation and Transplant Surgery. New York, Taylor & Francis, 2003
8. Penko ME: An overview of liver transplantation. AACN Clin Issues 10:176–184, 1999
9. Aziz TM, Burgess MI, El-Gamel A, et al: Orthotopic cardiac transplantation technique: A survey of current practice. Ann Thorac Surg 68:1242–1246, 1999
10. Poston RS, Griffith BP: Heart transplantation. J Intensive Care Med 19(1):3–12, 2004
11. Petros WP, Gilbert CJ: High-dose alkylating agent pharmacology/toxicity. In Burt RK, Deeg HJ, Lothian S, et al (eds): Bone Marrow Transplantation, pp 123–130. Austin, TX, Landes Bioscience, 1998
12. Rees C, Beale P, Judson I: Theoretical aspects of dose intensity and dose scheduling. In Barrett J, Treleaven J (eds): The Clinical Practice of Stem Cell Transplantation, pp 17–29. Oxford, Isis Medical Media, 1998
13. Wong R, Giralt SA, Martin T, et al: Reduced-intensity conditioning for unrelated donor hematopoietic stem cell transplantation as treatment for myeloid malignancies in patients older than 55 years. Blood 102(8):3052–3059, 2003
14. Schmit-Pokorny K, Franco T, Frappier B, et al: The cooperative care model: An innovative approach to deliver blood and marrow stem cell transplant care. Clin J Oncol Nurs 7(5):509–514, 556, 2003
15. Fox MC: Transfusions. In Burt RK, Deeg HJ, Lothian S, et al (eds): Bone Marrow Transplantation, pp 54–68. Austin, TX, Landes Bioscience, 1998
16. Johnston E, Crawford J: The hematologic support of the cancer patient. In Berger AM, Portenoy RK, Weissman DE (eds): Principles and Practice of Supportive Oncology, pp 549–569. Philadelphia, Lippincott Williams & Wilkins, 1998
17. Morgan M, Dodds A: ABO incompatibility and blood product support. In Atkinson K (ed): Clinical Bone Marrow Transplantation: A Clinical Textbook, pp 291–296. Cambridge, United Kingdom, Cambridge University Press, 1994
18. Westall GP, Michaelides A, Williams TJ, et al: Bronchiolitis obliterans syndrome and early human CMV DNAemia dynamics after lung transplantation. Transplantation 75(12):2064–2068, 2003
19. Burt RK, Walsh T: Infection prophylaxis in bone marrow transplant recipients: Myths, legends and microbes. In Burt RK, Deeg HJ, Lothian S, et al (eds): Bone Marrow Transplantation, pp 438–451. Austin, TX, Landes Bioscience, 1998
20. Hosenspud JD: Coronary artery disease after heart transplant and its relation to cytomegalovirus. Am Heart J 138:S469–S472, 1999

21. Fateh-Moghadam S, Bocksch W, Wessely R, et al: Cytomegalovirus infection status predicts progression of heart transplant vasculopathy. Transplantation 76:1470–1474, 2003
22. Shelton BK: Evidence-based care for the neutropenic patient with leukemia. Semin Oncol Nurs 19(2):133–141, 2003
23. Shapiro T, Davison D, Rust D: A Clinical Guide to Stem Cell and Bone Marrow Transplantation. Boston, Jones and Bartlett, 1997
24. Bearman SI: The syndrome of hepatic veno-occlusive disease after marrow transplantation. Blood 85:3005–3020, 1995
25. Gluckman E: Veno-occlusive disease. In Atkinson K (ed): Clinical Bone Marrow Transplantation: A Clinical Textbook, pp 356–359. Cambridge, United Kingdom, Cambridge University Press, 1994
26. McDonald BG: Venoocclusive disease of the liver following marrow transplantation. Marrow Transpl Rev 3(4):129–134, 1994
27. Philpott NJ, Kanfer EJ: Complications in the early post-transplant period. In Barrett J, Treleaven J (eds): The Clinical Practice of Stem Cell Transplantation, pp 768–785. Oxford, Isis Medical Media, 1998
28. Ruutu T, Eriksson B, Remes K, et al: Ursodeoxycholic acid for the prevention of hepatic complications of allogeneic stem cell transplantation. Blood 100:1977–1983, 2002
29. Afessa B, Litzow MR, Tefferi A: Bronchiolitis obliterans and other late onset non-infectious pulmonary complications in hematopoietic stem cell transplant. Bone Marrow Transplant 28:425–434, 2001
30. Bryant D: Pulmonary complications. In Atkinson K (ed): Clinical Bone Marrow Transplantation: A Clinical Textbook, pp 467–474. Cambridge, United Kingdom, Cambridge University Press, 1994
31. Height S, Shields M: Problems following bone marrow transplantation: Pulmonary complications. In Treleaven J, Wiernik P (eds): Color Atlas and Text of Bone Marrow Transplantation, pp 169–180. London, Mosby-Wolfe, 1995
32. Crawford S: Supportive care in bone marrow transplantation: Pulmonary complications. In Winter J (ed): Blood Stem Cell Transplantation, pp 231–254. Boston, Kluwer Academic, 1997
33. Atkinson K: Interstitial pneumonitis. In Atkinson K (ed): Clinical Bone Marrow Transplantation: A Clinical Textbook, pp 360–371. Cambridge, United Kingdom, Cambridge University Press, 1994
34. Lazarus HM, Vogelsang GB, Rowe JM: Prevention and treatment of acute graft-versus-host disease: The old and the new. A report from the Eastern Cooperative Oncology Group (ECOG). Bone Marrow Transplant 19:577–600, 1997
35. Socie G, Cahn JY: Acute graft-versus-host disease. In Barrett J, Treleaven J (eds): The Clinical Practice of Stem Cell Transplantation, pp 596–618. Oxford, Isis Medical Media, 1998
36. Przepiorka D, Anderlini P, Saliba R, et al: Chronic graft versus host disease after allogeneic blood stem cell transplantation. Blood 96: 1695–1700, 2001
37. Sullivan KM, Angura E, Anasetti C, et al: Chronic graft versus host disease and other late complications of bone marrow transplantation. Semin Hematol 28:250–259, 1991
38. Carlens S, Ringden O, Remberger M, et al: Risk factors for chronic graft versus host disease after bone marrow transplantation: A retrospective single center analysis. Bone Marrow Transplant 22:755–761, 1998
39. Cutler C, Giri S, Jeyapalan S, et al: Acute and chronic graft-versus-host disease after allogeneic peripheral-blood stem cell and bone marrow transplantation: A meta-analysis. J Clin Oncol 19:3685–3691, 2001
40. Wagner JL, Flowers MED, Longton G, et al: The development of chronic graft versus host disease: An analysis of screening studies and the impact of corticosteroid use at 100 days after transplant. Bone Marrow Transplant 22:139–146, 1998
41. Abdelsayed RA, Sumner T, Allen C, et al: Oral precancerous and malignant lesions associated with graft-versus-host disease: Report of 2 cases. Oral Surg Oral Med Oral Pathol 93:75–80, 2002
42. Akpek G, Valladares JL, Lee L, et al: Pancreatic insufficiency in patients with chronic graft versus host disease. Bone Marrow Transplant 27:163–166, 2001
43. Aristei C, Allessandro M, Santucci A, et al: Cataracts in patients receiving stem cell transplantation after conditioning with total body irradiation. Bone Marrow Transplant 29:503–507, 2002
44. Baker KS, DeFor TE, Burns LJ, et al: New malignancies after blood or marrow stem-cell transplantation in children and adults: Incidence and risk factors. J Clin Oncol 21:1352–1358, 2003
45. Buchsel PC, Leum EW, Randolph SR: Delayed complications of bone marrow transplantation: An update. Oncol Nurs Forum 23:1267–1291, 1996
46. Chao NJ: Graft-versus-host disease. In Burt RK, Deeg HJ, Lothian S, et al (eds): Bone Marrow Transplantation, pp 478–497. Austin, TX, Landes Bioscience, 1998
47. Gold P, Flowers M, Sullivan K: Outpatient management of marrow and blood stem cell transplant patients. In Burt RK, Deeg HJ, Lothian S, et al (eds): Bone Marrow Transplantation, pp 524–531. Austin, TX, Landes Bioscience, 1998
48. Grigg AP, Angus PW, Hoyt R, et al: The incidence, pathogenesis, and natural history of steatorrhea after bone marrow transplantation. Bone Marrow Transplant 31:701–703, 2003
49. Lash AA: Sjögren's syndrome: Pathogenesis, diagnosis and treatment. Nurse Practitioner 26(8):50–58, 2001
50. Lee SJ, Vogelsang G, Flowers ME: Chronic graft versus host disease. Biol Blood Marrow Transplant 9(4):215–233, 2003
51. Loughran TP, Sullivan KM, Morton T, et al: Value of day 100 screening studies for predicting the development of chronic graft versus host disease after allogeneic bone marrow transplantation. Blood 76:228–234, 1990
52. Seber A, Vogelsang G: Chronic graft-versus-host disease. In Barrett J, Treleaven J (eds): The Clinical Practice of Stem Cell Transplantation, pp 620–634. Oxford, Isis Medical Media, 1998
53. Treleaven J: Late effects of bone marrow transplantation. In Treleaven J, Wiernik P (eds): Color Atlas and Text of Bone Marrow Transplantation, pp 193–200. London, Mosby-Wolfe, 1995
54. Vogelsang G: How I treat chronic graft-versus-host disease. Blood 97:1196–1201, 2001
55. Wagner JL, Flowers MED, Longton G, et al: Use of screening studies to predict survival among patients who do not have chronic graft-versus-host disease at day 100 after bone marrow transplantation. Biol Blood Marrow Transplant 7:239–240, 2001
56. Sullivan KM: Graft-versus-host disease. In Thomas ED, Blume KG, Forman SJ (eds): Hematopoietic Cell Transplantation (2nd Ed), pp 515–536. Oxford, Blackwell Science, 1999
57. Chao N: Graft-Versus-Host Disease. Austin, TX, RG Landes, 1999
58. Chao N: Pharmacology and use of immunosuppressive agents after hematopoietic cell transplantation. In Thomas ED, Blume KG, Forman SJ (eds): Hematopoietic Cell Transplantation (2nd Ed), pp 176–185. Oxford, Blackwell Science, 1999
59. Bush WW: Overview of transplantation immunology and the pharmacotherapy of adult solid organ transplant recipients: Focus on immunosuppression. AACN Clin Issues 10(2):253–269, 1999
60. Cather JC: Cyclosporine A and tacrolimus in dermatology. Dermatol Clin North Am 19(1):119–137, 2001
61. Chan B: The pharmacology of peripheral blood stem cell transplantation. In Buchsel PC, Kapustay PM (eds): Stem Cell Transplantation: A Clinical Textbook, pp 8.3–8.24. Pittsburgh, Oncology Nursing Press, 2000
62. Charuhas PM: Medical nutrition therapy in bone marrow transplantation. In McCallum PD, Polisena CG (eds): The Clinical Guide to Oncology Nutrition, pp 90–98. Chicago, American Dietetic Association, 2000
63. Cronin DC, Faust TW, Brady L, et al: Modern immunosuppression. Clin Liver Dis 4:619–655, 2000
64. Gaziev D, Galimberti M, Lucarelli G, et al: Chronic graft-versus-host disease: Is there an alternative to conventional treatment? Bone Marrow Transplant 25:689–696, 2000
65. Goldman DA: Thalidomide use: Past history and current implications for practice. Oncol Nurs Forum 28:471–477, 2001
66. Lanuza DM, McCabe MA: Care before and after lung transplant and quality of life research. AACN Clin Issues 12(2):186–201, 2001
67. National Home Infusion Association Monograph: Infliximab therapy in patients with rheumatoid arthritis and Crohn's disease. Infusion 7(6):1–13, 2001
68. Nunes F, Lucey M: Gastrointestinal complications of immunosuppression. Gastroenterol Clin 28(1):233–246, 1999
69. Perlman SE, Rudy SJ, Pinto C, Townsend-Akpan C: Caring for women with childbearing potential taking teratogenic dermatologic drugs. J Reprod Med 46(2 Suppl):153–161, 2001
70. Seeley K, DeMeyer E: Nursing care of patients receiving Campath. Clin J Oncol Nurs 6(3):138–143, 2002
71. Solimando D: Medications. In Burt RK, Deeg HJ, Lothian S, et al (eds): Bone Marrow Transplantation, pp 544–566. Austin, TX, Landes Bioscience, 1998
72. Locatelli F, Bruno B, Zecca M, et al: Cyclosporin A and short-term methotrexate versus cyclosporin A as graft versus host disease pro-

phylaxis in patients with severe aplastic anemia given allogeneic bone marrow transplantation from an HLA identical sibling: Results of a GITMO/EBMT randomized trial. Blood 96:1690–1697, 2000

73. Ogawa H, Soma T, Hosen N, et al: Combination of tacrolimus, methotrexate, and methylprednisolone prevents acute but not chronic graft versus host disease in unrelated bone marrow transplantation. Transplantation 74:236–243, 2002
74. Chao N, Snyder D, Jain M, et al: Equivalence of 2 effective graft versus host disease prophylaxis regimens: Results of a prospective double blind randomized trial. Biol Blood Marrow Transplant 6:254–261, 2000
75. Przepiorka D: Prevention of acute graft-versus-host disease. In Ball ED, Lister J, Law P (eds): Hematopoietic Stem Cell Therapy, pp 452–469. New York, Churchill Livingstone, 2000
76. Wagner ND, Quinones VW: Allogeneic peripheral blood stem cell transplantation: Clinical overview and nursing implications. Oncol Nurs Forum 25:1049–1055, 1998
77. Deeg HJ: Delayed complications. In Burt RK, Deeg HJ, Lothian S, et al (eds): Bone Marrow Transplantation, pp 512–522. Austin, TX, Landes Bioscience, 1998
78. Deeg HJ, Socie G: Malignancies after hematopoietic stem cell transplantation: Many questions, some answers. Blood 91:1833–1844, 1998
79. Sanders J: Late effects after bone marrow transplantation. In Schwartz CL, Hobbie W, Constine LS, et al (eds): Survivors of Childhood Cancer: Assessment and Management, pp 293–318. St. Louis, Mosby, 1994
80. Shalet S: Endocrine and reproductive dysfunction in adults. In Barrett J, Treleaven J (eds): The Clinical Practice of Stem Cell Transplantation, pp 850–854. Oxford, Isis Medical Media, 1998
81. Deeg HJ: Graft failure. In Burt RK, Deeg HJ, Lothian S, et al (eds): Bone Marrow Transplantation, pp 309–316. Austin, TX, Landes Bioscience, 1998
82. Meadows AT, Fenton JG: Follow-up care of patients at risk for the development of second malignant neoplasms. In Schwartz CL, Hobbie W, Constine LS, et al (eds): Survivors of Childhood Cancer: Assessment and Management, pp 319–328. St. Louis, Mosby, 1994
83. Mehta J, Singhal S: Graft failure: Diagnosis and management. In Barrett J, Treleaven J (eds): The Clinical Practice of Stem Cell Transplantation, pp 646–658. Oxford, Isis Medical Media, 1998
84. Schwartz C, Hobbie W, Constine L: Algorithms of late effects by disease. In Schwartz CL, Hobbie W, Constine LS, et al (eds): Survivors of Childhood Cancer: Assessment and Management, pp 7–19. St. Louis, Mosby, 1994
85. Ruccione KS: Issues in survivorship. In Schwartz CL, Hobbie W, Constine LS, et al (eds): Survivors of Childhood Cancer: Assessment and Management, pp 329–337. St. Louis, Mosby, 1994
86. Constine L, Hobbie L, Schwartz C: Facilitated assessment of chronic treatment by symptom and organ systems. In Schwartz CL, Hobbie W, Constine LS, et al (eds): Survivors of Childhood Cancer: Assessment and Management, pp 21–79. St. Louis, Mosby, 1994
87. Harpham WS: Long-term survivorship: Late effects. In Berger A, et al (eds): Principles and Practice of Supportive Oncology, pp 889–907. Philadelphia, Lippincott Williams & Wilkins, 1998

OTHER SELECTED READING

Banner NR, Polak JM, Yacoub MH (ed): Lung Transplantation. Cambridge, Cambridge University Press, 2003

Baumgartner WA, Reitz B, Kasper E, et al (eds): Heart and Lung Transplantation (2nd Ed). Philadelphia, WB Saunders, 2002

Burns JM, Tierney DK, Long GD, et al: Critical pathway for administering high-dose chemotherapy followed by peripheral blood stem cell rescue in the outpatient setting. Oncol Nurs Forum 22:1219–1224, 1995

Bush WW: Overview of transplantation immunology and the pharmacotherapy of adult solid organ transplant recipients: Focus on immunosuppression. AACN Clin Issues 10:253–269, 1999

Couples SA, Ohler L (eds): Transplantation Nursing Secrets. Philadelphia, Hanley & Belfus, 2003

Hakim N, Stratta R, Gray D (eds): Pancreas and Islet Transplantation. Oxford, Oxford University Press, 2002

Kapustay PM, Buchsel PC: Process, complications, and management of peripheral stem cell transplantation. In Buchsel PC, Kapustay PM (eds): Stem Cell Transplantation: A Clinical Textbook, pp 5.3–5.28. Pittsburgh, Oncology Nursing Press, 2000

Kaufman DB, Shapiro R, Lucey MR, et al: 2003 SRTR report on the state of transplantation: Immuno Suppression: Practice and Trends. Am J Transplantation 4 (Suppl 9):38–53, 2004

Kirkland JK, Young JB, McGiffin DC (eds): Heart Transplantation. Philadelphia, Churchill Livingstone, 2002

Maddrey WC, Shiff ER, Sorrell MF (eds): Transplantation of the Liver. Philadelphia, Lippincott Williams & Wilkins, 2001

Maurer JR, Frost AE, Estenne M, et al: International guidelines for the selection of lung transplant candidates. J Heart Lung Transplant 17:703–709, 1998

Mitchell SA: Hematopoietic stem cell transplantation. In Lin EM (ed): Advanced Practice in Oncology Nursing, pp 151–212. Philadelphia, WB Saunders, 2001

Philpott NJ, Kanfer EJ: (1998). Complications in the early post-transplant period. In Barrett J, Treleaven J (eds): The Clinical Practice of Stem Cell Transplantation, pp 768–785. Oxford, Isis Medical Media, 1998

Taylor DO: Cardiac transplantation: Drug regimens for the 21st century. Ann Thorac Surg 75:S72–S78, 2003

Barrett J, Treleaven J (eds): The Clinical Practice of Stem Cell Transplantation. Oxford, Isis Medical Media, 1998

Rubin RH: Medical progress: Infection in organ-transplant recipients. N Engl J Med 328:1741–1751, 1998

Ruccione KS: Issues in survivorship. In Schwartz CL, Hobbie W, Constine LS, et al (eds): Survivors of Childhood Cancer: Assessment and Management, pp 329–337. St. Louis, Mosby, 1994

Socie G, Cahn JY: Acute graft-versus-host disease. In Barrett J, Treleaven J (eds): The Clinical Practice of Stem Cell Transplantation, pp 596–618. Oxford, Isis Medical Media, 1998

Wagner ND, Quinones VW: Allogeneic peripheral blood stem cell transplantation: Clinical overview and nursing implications. Oncol Nurs Forum 25:1049–1055, 1998

Walker F, Roethke S, Martin G: An overview of the rationale, process, and nursing implications of peripheral blood stem cell transplantation. Cancer Nurs 17(2):141–148, 1994

chapter 48

Common Immunological Disorders

KIMMITH JONES ■ BRENDA SHELTON

objectives

Based on the content in this chapter, the reader should be able to:

- Describe the etiology and immunopathology associated with human immunodeficiency virus (HIV) infection and acquired immunodeficiency syndrome (AIDS).
- Discuss the use of nucleoside reverse transcriptase inhibitors and protease inhibitors in the treatment of HIV infection and AIDS.
- Explain standard precautions and transmission-based precautions and their implementation in the intensive care unit.
- Describe the pathophysiological processes of the oncological emergencies.
- Identify appropriate assessment data for each oncological emergency derived from patient history and physical examination, clinical manifestations, and diagnostic studies.
- Explain the anticipated medical management and rationale for the treatment of selected oncological emergencies.
- Describe relevant aspects of nursing management for each of the oncological emergencies.

Normally, an intact immune system provides protection from disease. When one or more components of this system is weakened or adversely altered, a person becomes susceptible to disease. An immunodeficiency that is congenital or inherited is classified as primary. Examples of primary immunodeficiencies include hypogammaglobulinemia, Bruton's disease, and Wiskott-Aldrich syndrome. If acquired later in life, the immunodeficiency is known as secondary. Examples of secondary immunodeficiency are human immunodeficiency virus (HIV) infection; acquired immunodeficiency syndrome (AIDS); any form of neoplastic disease; or immunosuppression as a result of drug therapy, such as cortisone or cyclophosphamide.

This chapter deals with two areas of secondary immunodeficiency, HIV infection and AIDS, and emergent situations precipitated by commonly occurring neoplastic disorders. The reader is encouraged to review Chapter 45, Anatomy and Physiology of the Hematological and Immune Systems. Especially important is the material relating to the immune mechanisms (humoral and cell-mediated immunity, complement system, and phagocytosis). This review will help the reader appreciate the pathophysiological changes occurring in the conditions discussed in this chapter.

HUMAN IMMUNODEFICIENCY VIRUS INFECTION

The hallmark of AIDS, which is caused by HIV, is impaired cellular immunity. In 1981, AIDS was first recognized. In 1982, AIDS was defined by the Centers for Disease Control (CDC), and in 1993, the case definition for AIDS was expanded and updated to include the latest research. To be diagnosed with AIDS, a person with HIV infection must have one of the indicator conditions (Box 48-1).

HIV infection is a chronic illness. Currently, it is not curable. Initially, it was believed that people were exposed to HIV, became HIV positive, contracted AIDS, and died within a very short period. The long-term survival for patients infected with HIV has improved considerably because of advances in antiretroviral therapy and in the prophylaxis and treatment of opportunistic infections. Survival for patients receiving antiretroviral agents and therapy for opportunistic infections is now about 20 years. The rate of progression to AIDS is significantly higher in people who are HIV positive and not receiving therapy. The higher the CD4 count and lower the viral load, the lower the risk of progression to AIDS (Table 48-1).

Many people with HIV infection require sophisticated medical and nursing care during the course of their illness. People may be admitted to the intensive care unit (ICU) for one of the common opportunistic infections; for a completely unrelated problem, such as trauma; or for a surgical procedure. Their admission to the ICU may be the first indication of their HIV-positive status. To achieve a positive patient outcome, it is essential to understand how HIV infection contributes to the reason for ICU admission. Critical care nurses must be knowledgeable about the disease process and the multisystem complications that may occur.

Epidemiology

An estimated 40 million people worldwide are living with HIV/AIDS. Of these, 37.2 million are adults and 2.7 million are children (in this case, children are defined as people younger than 15 years of age). Women represent 17.6 million of the adults and account for 47% of all adults with HIV. Most cases of AIDS in the United States are in urban areas. The 10 metropolitan areas with the highest cumulative totals of reported AIDS cases are, in descending order, New York City, Los Angeles, San Francisco, Miami, Washington, DC, Chicago, Philadelphia, Houston, Newark, and Atlanta.[1]

About 46% of the total number of reported AIDS cases in the United States occur among men who have had sex with men. The rate of new HIV infection in these men has decreased considerably in the past decade because of changes in sexual behavior resulting from the use of safer sexual practices. Heterosexual women now represent the fastest-growing group of HIV-affected people.[2] HIV is now the fourth leading cause of death in women between 25 and 44 years of age, and it is the leading cause of death in African-American women.[3]

Figure 48-1 depicts the change in the number of deaths related to AIDS from 1985 to 1999. The decrease in the number of deaths can be attributed to the improvement in treatment and the implementation of safer sexual practices.

Pathophysiology

Immune defects seen in HIV infection are caused by a viral agent (HIV) from the group of viruses known as retroviruses. Retroviruses are transmitted from person to person by blood and intimate (sexual) contact and have a strong affinity for T lymphocytes.

VIRAL REPLICATION

HIV is considered a retrovirus. A retrovirus is composed of a small outer envelope, an inner core of genetic material (RNA), and three enzymes necessary for reproduction: reverse transcriptase, integrase, and protease. Like all viruses, HIV cannot reproduce on its own. It must attach to and invade other cells, in this case, helper T4 lymphocytes, to reproduce. The process of viral replication is illustrated in Figure 48-2.

box 48-1
Case Definition of AIDS for Surveillance Purposes: Indicator Conditions

- Candidiasis of bronchi, trachea, or lungs
- Candidiasis, esophageal
- Cervical cancer, invasive*
- Coccidioidomycosis, disseminated or extrapulmonary
- Cryptococcosis, extrapulmonary
- Cryptosporidiosis, chronic intestinal (>1 month duration)
- Cytomegalovirus disease (other than liver, spleen, or nodes)
- Cytomegalovirus retinitis (with loss of vision)
- Encephalopathy, HIV-related
- Herpes simplex: chronic ulcer(s) (>1 month duration); or bronchitis, pneumonitis, or esophagitis
- Histoplasmosis, disseminated or extrapulmonary
- Isosporiasis, chronic intestinal (>1 month duration)
- Kaposi's sarcoma
- Lymphoma, Burkitt's (or equivalent)
- Lymphoma, immunoblastic (or equivalent)
- Lymphoma, of brain, primary
- *Mycobacterium avium* complex or *Mycobacterium kansasii,* disseminated or extrapulmonary
- *Mycobacterium tuberculosis,* any site (pulmonary* or extrapulmonary)
- *Mycobacterium,* other species or unidentified species, disseminated or extrapulmonary
- *Pneumocystis jiroveci* pneumonia
- Pneumonia, recurrent bacterial*
- Progressive multifocal leukoencephalopathy
- *Salmonella* septicemia, recurrent
- Toxoplasmosis of brain
- Wasting syndrome due to HIV
- $CD4^+$ count ≤200 cells/mL*

*Added in the 1993 expansion of the AIDS surveillance case definition.
From Centers for Disease Control and Prevention: 1993 Revised classification system for HIV infection and expanded surveillance case definition for AIDS among adolescents and adults. Morb Mortal Wkly Rep 41(RR-17), 1992.

table 48-1 Probability of Developing an AIDS-Defining Opportunistic Infection Within 3 Years in the Absence of Antiretroviral Therapy, Based on Baseline CD4 Count and Viral Load

		% AIDS-Defining Complication		
Viral Load (RT-PCR)*	*N*	*3 y*	*6 y*	*9 y*
CD4 <350 cells/mm³				
1,500–7,000*	30	0	18.8	30.6
7,000–20,000	51	8.0	42.2	65.6
20,000–55,000	73	40.1	72.9	86.2
>55,000	174	72.9	92.7	95.6
CD4 350–500 cells/mm³				
1,500–7,000	47	4.4	22.1	46.9
7,000–20,000	105	5.9	39.8	60.7
20,000–55,000	121	15.1	57.2	78.6
>55,000	121	47.9	77.7	94.4
CD4 >500 cells/mm³				
<1,500	110	1.0	5.0	10.7
1,500–7,000	180	2.3	14.9	33.2
7,000–20,000	237	7.2	25.9	50.3
20,000–55,000	202	14.6	47.7	70.6
>55,000	141	32.6	66.8	76.3

Data from Multicenter AIDS Cohort Study.
*Plasma HIV RNA levels in cells per milliliter using reverse transcriptase–polymerase chain reaction.
From Bartlett JG: The 2002 Abbreviated Guide to Medical Management of HIV Infection, p 23. Baltimore, Johns Hopkins University, Division of Infectious Diseases, 2002.

HIV enters the bloodstream, attaches to a T lymphocyte, and then sheds its outer envelope. Viral RNA is then transcribed into DNA by way of the enzyme reverse transcriptase. The viral DNA is incorporated into the DNA of the T lymphocyte, in essence, tricking the T lymphocyte into making components for more virus. The components are assembled into units called *virions*, which are structurally intact and infectious virus particles.

The T lymphocytes reproduce the viral components at varying rates depending on the person. It is unclear why the cells of some patients reproduce slowly and others reproduce more rapidly.[4,5] Although new virions are being produced, there is a period of clinical latency in which the patient is asymptomatic. This latency may last for many years.[6]

Eventually, the new virions undergo a process of coating and are then expelled from the host cell by budding. During budding, the parent cell releases a daughter cell with its cytoplasmic material, which begins existence as a separate cell. These daughter cells disseminate through the bloodstream and infect other cells. About 10 billion new virions are produced each day in the HIV-infected person who is not receiving treatment. Each virion has a half-life of less than 6 hours.[7]

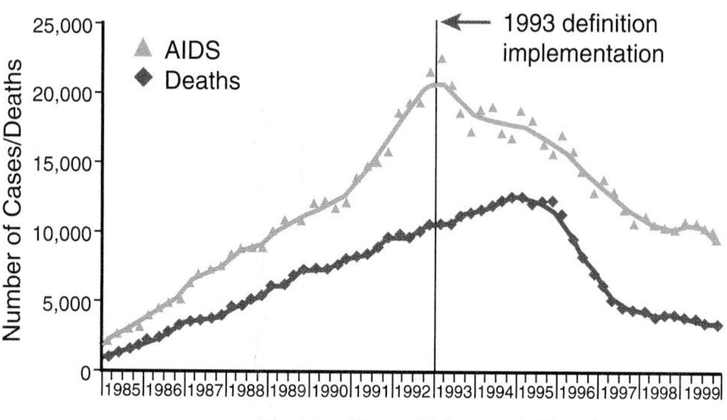

figure 48-1 Estimated incidence of AIDS and deaths of adults and adolescents with AIDS, 1985–1999, in the United States (adjusted for reporting delays). (From Centers for Disease Control and Prevention: AIDS Surveillance Trends 1985–1999. Available at www.cdc.gov/hiv/graphics/trends.htm.)

IMMUNE DEFECTS

Patients with HIV infection exhibit impaired activation of both cellular and humoral immunity. HIV primarily infects the helper T4 cell of the immune system. As discussed in Chapter 45, the helper T4 cell plays a major role in the overall immune response. Infection of the helper T4 cell with HIV results in profound lymphopenia with decreased functional abilities, including decreased response to antigens and loss of stimulus for T- and B-cell activation. In addition, the cytotoxic activity of the T8 killer cell is impaired. Functional abilities of macrophages also are affected, with decreased phagocytosis and diminished chemotaxis. In humoral immunity, there is diminished antibody response to antigens, along with deregulation of antibody production. In essence, serum antibodies are increased, but their functional abilities are decreased. The total effect of these immune defects is increased susceptibility to opportunistic

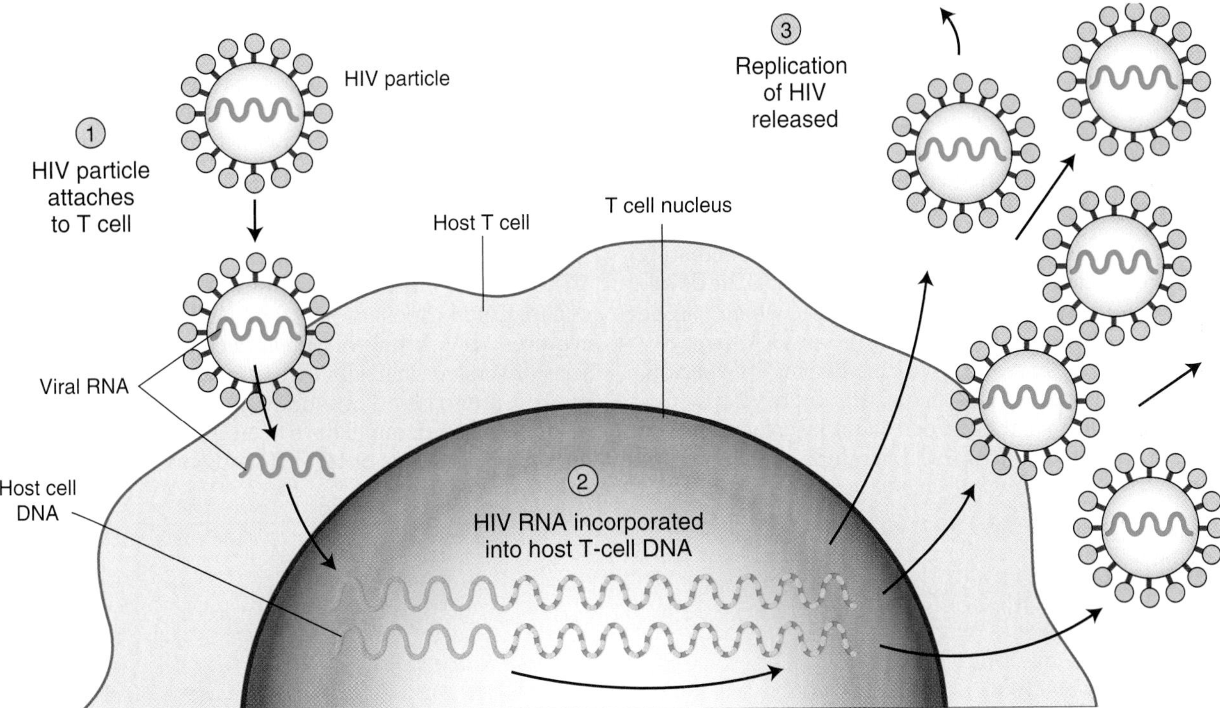

figure 48-2 Process of viral replication. (**1**) Human immunodeficiency virus (HIV) attaching itself to a host cell, most often a T cell, and injecting its genetic material (RNA). (**2**) The genetic material for HIV becomes part of the cell's genetic material. This changes the host cell into an HIV-producing machine. (**3**) Many new copies of HIV are produced from the host T cell. These new copies infect even more T cells. (Redrawn from Glaxo Wellcome: HIV: Understanding the Disease. Research Triangle Park, NC, Author, 1995, with permission.)

infections and neoplasms. A summary of the immune defects associated with AIDS is presented in Figure 48-3.

HIV TRANSMISSION

HIV is a fragile virus and cannot survive long outside the body. Survival time depends on the size of the liquid droplet in which it exists; the larger the droplet, the longer HIV can remain alive. As the droplet dries, HIV dies.

HIV has been isolated from all types of body fluids and tissues. However, not all body fluids have been implicated in the transmission of HIV. The four fluids from which large amounts of virus have been isolated and that have been implicated in transmission include blood, semen, vaginal fluid, and breast milk.

The infectiousness of a fluid depends on the amount of virus present in the fluid and the ability of that fluid to reach the target cell, in this case the T lymphocyte. Although HIV has been isolated in all types of body fluids, the amount of virus present is very low (except in the four fluids associated with HIV transmission). In addition, for HIV to cause infection, it must leave the body of the infected person, travel to the body of another person, penetrate the skin barrier, enter the bloodstream, and attach itself to a T lymphocyte. The likelihood this series of events will occur is low, especially because a certain amount of virus is required to cause an infection. Small tears in the anus or vagina provide a portal of entry for virus present in blood, semen, and vaginal fluid. The virus in breast milk can

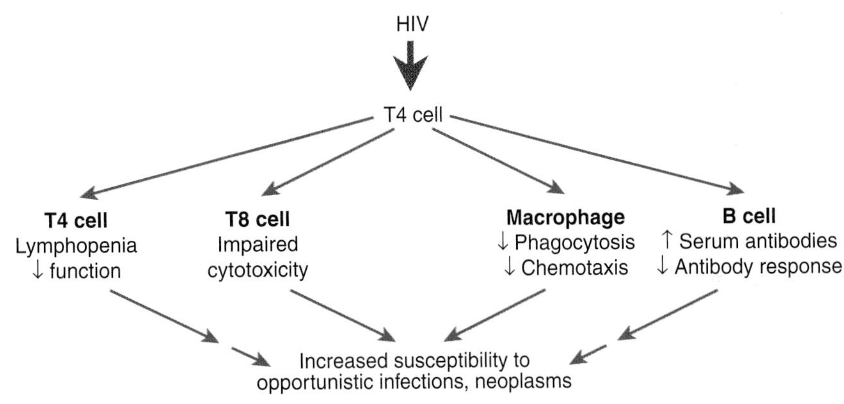

figure 48-3 Summary of immune defects in AIDS.

enter through cuts or irritation in the gastrointestinal tract of the infant.

There are three known modes of transmission of HIV:

- Unprotected vaginal or anal sexual contact with an infected person
- Inoculation with infected blood or blood products
- Pregnancy, delivery, or breastfeeding

A person does not become HIV positive immediately after the virus enters the body. Seroconversion is the development of antibodies from HIV exposure, which can be detected in the blood. In other words, an HIV-negative result becomes an HIV-positive one. During this period, the body recognizes HIV as an invader and develops antibodies to it, which will then be detectable by enzyme-linked immunosorbent assay (ELISA). Therefore, there is a 2- to 12-week period when a person can unknowingly transmit the virus because his or her ELISA may not be positive. In most people, seroconversion occurs 10 to 14 days after exposure to HIV.[8,9] In others, the process takes 3 to 4 weeks, and the process occurs within 6 months in almost all people.[9]

The risk of HIV transmission to health care workers is low if Standard Precautions and Transmission-Based Precautions are followed[10] (Box 48-2). As of June 2000, 56 health care workers had acquired HIV infection through occupational exposure, and 132 health care workers had acquired HIV through a *possible* occupational exposure. All seroconversions in health care workers have been the result of exposure to blood or bloody fluids. All seroconversions in laboratory personnel have been the result of exposure to high concentrations of HIV. The reported seroconversion

box 48-2

Summary of Recommended Practices for Standard and Transmission-Based Precautions

Standard Precautions

- Wash hands after touching blood, body fluids, secretions, excretions, and contaminated items, regardless of whether gloves are worn. Wash hands immediately after gloves are removed, between patient contacts, and whenever indicated to prevent transfer of microorganisms to other patients or environments. Use plain soap for routine handwashing and an antimicrobial or waterless antiseptic agent for specific circumstances.
- Wear clean, nonsterile gloves when touching blood, body fluids, excretions or secretions, contaminated items, mucous membranes, and nonintact skin. Change gloves between tasks on the same patient as necessary, and remove gloves promptly after use.
- Wear mask, eye protection, or face shield during procedures and care activities that are likely to generate splashes or sprays of blood or body fluids. Use gown to protect skin and prevent soiling of clothing.
- Ensure that used patient care equipment that is soiled with blood or identified body fluids, secretions, and excretions is handled carefully to prevent transfer of microorganisms, or cleaned and appropriately reprocessed if used for another patient.
- Use adequate environmental controls to ensure that routine care, cleaning, and disinfection procedures are followed.
- Handle, transport, and process linen soiled with blood and body fluids, excretions, and secretions in a manner that prevents skin and mucous membrane exposures, contamination of clothing, and transfer of microorganisms.
- Use previously identified techniques and equipment to prevent injuries when using needles, sharps, and scalpels, and place these items in appropriate puncture-resistant containers after use.

Transmission-Based Precautions

The following precautions are recommended in addition to Standard Precautions:

Airborne Precautions

- Place the patient in private room that has monitored negative air pressure in relation to surrounding areas, 6 to 12 air changes per hour, and appropriate discharge of air outside or monitored filtration if air is recirculated. Keep the door closed and the patient in the room.
- Use respiratory protection when entering room of patient with known or suspected tuberculosis. If patient has known or suspected rubeola (measles) or varicella (chickenpox), respiratory protection should be worn unless person entering room is immune to these diseases.
- Transport the patient out of the room only when necessary, and place a surgical mask on the patient if possible.
- Consult Centers for Disease Control and Prevention Guidelines for additional prevention strategies for tuberculosis.

Droplet Precautions

- Use a private room, if available. Door may remain open.
- Wear a mask when working within 3 feet of the patient.
- Transport the patient out of the room only when necessary, and place a surgical mask on the patient if possible.

Contact Precautions

- Place the patient in a private room if available.
- Change gloves after having contact with infective material. Remove gloves before leaving the patient environment, and wash hands with an antimicrobial or waterless antiseptic agent.
- Wear a gown if contact with infectious agent is likely or patient has diarrhea, an ileostomy, colostomy, or wound drainage not contained by a dressing.
- Limit movement of the patient out of the room.
- When possible, dedicate the use of noncritical patient care equipment to a single patient to avoid sharing equipment.

From Centers for Disease Control and Prevention: Guideline for isolation precautions in hospitals: Part II. Recommendations for isolation precautions in hospitals. Am J Infect Control 24(1):32–52, 1996.

rate with percutaneous exposure (needlestick) is 0.25% to 0.30%.[11] Of the 56 health care workers who acquired HIV infection through occupational exposure, symptoms developed in most within 2 to 6 weeks, but a few did not show symptoms or seroconvert until 6 months postexposure.[11]

Postexposure prophylaxis (PEP) should be started as soon as possible after exposure to HIV. The decision about when to initiate PEP should be based on the type of exposure, risk assessment of the incident, and the risk assessment for HIV. The median time between exposure and treatment for 432 health care workers exposed to HIV between October 1996 and September 1998 was 1.8 hours.[6] Combination therapy using two or three drugs is recommended in PEP; the number of drugs depends on the type of exposure and the risk status of the source individual. Health care workers exposed to HIV should have serological testing at the time of exposure and 6 weeks, 3 months, and 6 months afterward.

Assessment

HISTORY AND PHYSICAL EXAMINATION

The spectrum of clinical findings ranges from asymptomatic infection with HIV, to a variety of infections and symptoms of decreasing immunocompetence, to unquestionable AIDS. Patients with HIV infection may become seriously ill, requiring frequent hospitalizations and care in the ICU. The critical care nurse more often encounters patients with AIDS when they have life-threatening opportunistic infections. Patients are often admitted to the ICU for an opportunistic illness and are diagnosed with AIDS at the same time.

The most common opportunistic infection requiring admission to the ICU is *Pneumocystis* pneumonia (PCP), which is caused by *Pneumocystis jiroveci*, formerly known as *Pneumocystis carinii*. The organism is considered a fungus based on its genetic makeup. Even though the name has changed, the abbreviation PCP is still used to describe the pathogen. PCP is the AIDS indicator condition in 38% of patients; PCP is the most common AIDS-defining condition.[12] The classic triad of symptoms in PCP is fever, exertional dyspnea, and nonproductive cough, but only 50% of patients present with these symptoms. They may have dyspnea, tachypnea, cyanosis, and initial uncompensated respiratory alkalosis.[12]

The major indication for critical care of patients with PCP is impending or actual respiratory failure. Symptoms of respiratory compromise often are more severe than diagnostic studies, such as chest radiographs and blood gas values, indicate. Therefore, early aggressive therapy for PCP using intravenous (IV) trimethoprim and sulfamethoxazole (Bactrim, Septra), and corticosteroids is the treatment of choice. Corticosteroids are given to reduce the inflammation caused by the death of *P. jiroveci* in the lungs. Even with urgent, aggressive treatment, many patients require mechanical ventilation for progressive alveolar hypoventilation. Adverse reactions to trimethoprim and sulfamethoxazole, including nausea and vomiting, maculopapular rash, bone marrow suppression, hepatitis, and drug fever, reportedly occur in more than 50% of patients.[12]

The research related to HIV was originally conducted in men. This body of knowledge could not be generalized to women because women did not participate in the studies. Many recent studies, which have included women, suggest that men and women do not differ in terms of the general characteristics of HIV disease.[2] The clinical course of infection, including time from HIV infection to AIDS, risk factors for HIV seroconversion, number and type of opportunistic illnesses, protection against infections, and the effectiveness of potent antiretroviral agents all appear similar[3] in both men and women.

No organ system escapes involvement in HIV infection. Single infections may develop in critically ill patients with AIDS, but patients often have multiple infections occurring simultaneously and requiring a variety of treatment strategies. The multisystem manifestations that develop are caused by the decrease in immune system functioning, resulting in an increase in opportunistic infections. Figure 48-4 presents manifestations of HIV infection and AIDS. Box 48-3 lists examples of nursing diagnoses for patients with HIV infection.

In 1992, the CDC revised the classification system for AIDS in which clinical categories and CD4 counts are used to determine where on the disease continuum a person fits. There are three clinical categories and three CD4 cell categories (Table 48-2). When a person has either one of the clinical conditions in category C or a CD4 lymphocyte count less than 200 cells/mm^3, the diagnosis of AIDS is made. However, if the person falls within category A1, A2, B1, or B2, he or she is considered HIV positive.

The AIDS indicator conditions in category C are disorders caused by viruses, fungi, parasites, and bacteria, as well as cancers (see Box 48-1 for a detailed list of these conditions). All of these agents are always present in the environment. In the immunocompetent person, the immune system keeps these opportunists under control, but in the immunosuppressed person, such as one who is HIV positive, the immune system loses this ability. Table 48-3 illustrates the correlation between CD4 counts and various infections and noninfectious complications seen in HIV infection.

LABORATORY AND DIAGNOSTIC STUDIES

Tests Used to Detect HIV

Several serological tests are used to determine if a person has been exposed to HIV. Table 48-4 describes the U.S. Food and Drug Administration (FDA)–approved diagnostic tests for HIV. The most widely used test is the ELISA, which determines the presence of antibodies for HIV. The results of this rapid and inexpensive test are available in a few hours. ELISA is reported as reactive (positive) or nonreactive (negative) and has a sensitivity and specificity of greater than 99%.[9] Unfortunately, the presence of other antibodies may lead to a false-positive result, which means that the test result was HIV positive, but the person is actually HIV negative. With ELISA, the false-positive rate is 0.0004%, or 1 per 251,000.[13] A positive ELISA is always repeated, and if the second ELISA is positive, another confirmatory test is performed. Low production of antibodies at the time the test is performed may lead to a false-negative result in 0.3% of cases.[9] A false-negative result means that

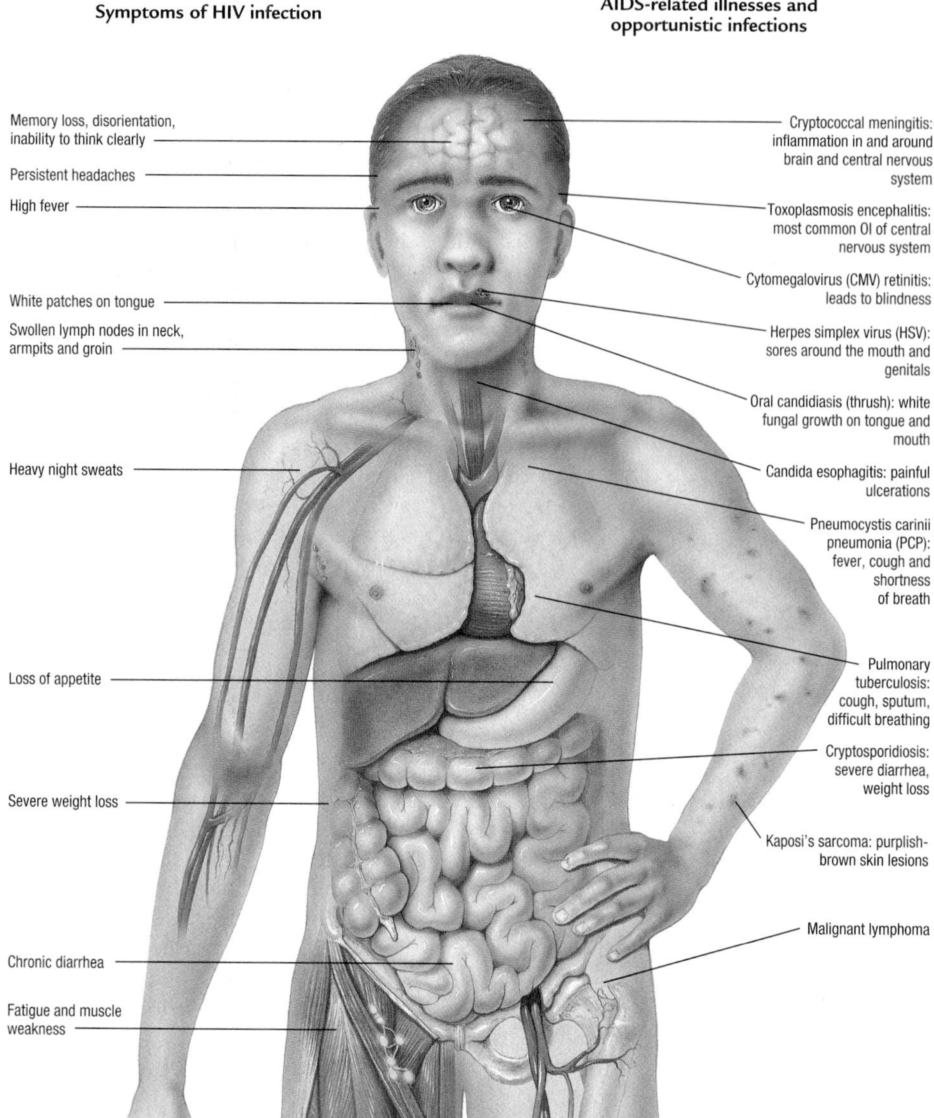

figure 48-4 Manifestations of HIV infection and AIDS. (From Anatomical Chart Company: Atlas of Pathophysiology, p 251. Springhouse, PA, Springhouse, 2002.)

box 48-3 ***Examples of Nursing Diagnoses and Collaborative Problems for the Patient With HIV Infection***

- Risk for Infection related to HIV immunodeficiency
- Risk for Impaired Gas Exchange related to alveolar–capillary membrane changes with *Pneumocystis jiroveci* pneumonia infection
- Risk for Deficient Fluid Volume related to diarrhea, dysphagia
- Risk for Infection Transmission related to HIV
- Anxiety related to critical illness, fear of death
- Deficient Knowledge related to illness and impact on patient's future
- Risk for Disturbed Thought Processes related to HIV or opportunistic infection of central nervous system

the test result was HIV negative, but the person is actually HIV positive.

The Western blot analysis is the most widely used confirmatory test and is as specific as the ELISA. The Western blot identifies the presence of antibodies to individual viral components. It should always be used in combination with the ELISA because it has a 2% false-positive rate.[11] The Western blot is more expensive and requires more skill in interpretation than the ELISA.

Several alternative FDA-approved HIV detection methods are available, but usually they are not used as screening tests for adults. Most of them require traditional serological testing to confirm the presence of HIV.

Two home kits were approved by the FDA in 1994. Results can be obtained in about 7 days by calling and listening to a prerecorded message. The test requires the person to use a lancet and filter strip with blotted blood, which is mailed to a laboratory using an anonymous code. People

table 48-2 Assessment Parameters in Classification of HIV Disease

CD4 Cell Categories	Clinical Categories: A Asymptomatic, or PGL or Acute HIV Infection	B Symptomatic* (not A or C)	C† AIDS Indicator Condition (1987)
1. >500/mm³ (≥29%)	A1	B1	C1
2. 200–499/mm³ (14%–28%)	A2	B2	C2
3. <200/mm³ (<14%)	A3	B3	C3

*Symptomatic conditions not included in Category C that are (1) attributed to HIV infection or indicative of a defect in cell-mediated immunity, or (2) considered to have a clinical course or management that is complicated by HIV infection. Examples of B conditions include but are not limited to bacillary angiomatosis; thrush; vulvovaginal candidiasis that is persistent, frequent, or poorly responsive to therapy; cervical dysplasia (moderate or severe); cervical carcinoma in situ; constitutional symptoms such as fever (38.5°C) or diarrhea >1 mo; oral hairy leukoplakia; herpes zoster involving two episodes or >1 dermatome; idiopathic thrombocytopenic purpura; listeriosis; pelvic inflammatory disease (especially if complicated by a tubo-ovarian abscess); and peripheral neuropathy.

†All patients in categories A3, B3 and C1–3 (shown in gray) are reported as AIDS, based on the AIDS indicator conditions and/or a CD4 cell count <200/mm³.

PGL, persistent generalized lymphadenopathy

From Centers for Disease Control and Prevention: 1993 Revised classification system for HIV infection and expanded surveillance case definition for AIDS among adolescents and adults. MMWR Morb Mortal Wkly Rep 41(RR-17), 1992.

table 48-3 Correlation Between CD4 Count and HIV Complications

CD4 Count* (as cells/mm³)	Infectious Complications	Non-infectious† Complications
>500	Acute retroviral syndrome Candidal vaginitis	Persistent generalized lymphadenopathy Guillain-Barré syndrome Myopathy Aseptic meningitis
200–500	Pneumococcal and other bacterial pneumonia Pulmonary tuberculosis (TB) Herpes zoster Oropharyngeal candidiasis (thrush) Cryptosporidiosis, self-limited Kaposi's sarcoma Oral hairy leukoplakia	Cervical intraepithelial neoplasia Cervical cancer B-cell lymphoma Anemia Mononeuronal multiplex Idiopathic thrombocytopenic purpura Hodgkin's lymphoma Lymphocytic interstitial pneumonitis
<200	*Pneumocystis jiroveci* pneumonia Disseminated histoplasmosis and coccidioidomycosis Miliary/extrapulmonary TB Progressive multifocal leukoencephalopathy	Wasting Peripheral neuropathy HIV-associated dementia Cardiomyopathy Vacuolar myelopathy Progressive polyradiculopathy
<100	Disseminated herpes simplex Toxoplasmosis Cryptococcosis Cryptosporidiosis, chronic Microsporidiosis Candidal esophagitis	
<50	Disseminated cytomegalovirus Disseminated *Mycobacterium avium* complex	Central nervous system lymphoma

*Most complications occur with increasing frequency at lower CD4 counts.

†Some conditions categorized as noninfectious are often microbially mediated, such as lymphoma (Epstein-Barr virus), cervical carcinoma (human papillomavirus).

From Bartlett JG: The 2002 Abbreviated Guide to Medical Management of HIV Infection, p 6. Baltimore, Johns Hopkins University, Department of Infectious Diseases, 2002.

table 48-4 Diagnostic Tests for HIV Approved by the US Food and Drug Administration

Test Category/Test	Clinical Use	Comments
Antibody-based tests		
Enzyme-linked immunosorbent assay (ELISA)	Primary screening test	Sensitivity and specificity >99%. Patients recently infected with HIV have a "window period" between infection and reactivity.
Western blot	Most commonly used supplemental test to confirm the presence of HIV antibodies	Specificity of 97.8%. About 4% to 20% of sera that are repeatedly reactive by HIV-1 ELISA are interpreted as indeterminate by Western blot.
Indirect immunofluorescence assay	Confirms the presence of HIV antibodies	Sensitivity and specificity similar to Western blot.
Detection of viral antigens p24 antigen	Diagnostic aid	Used to evaluate acute symptomatic HIV disease and as a screening test in blood donors to reduce the "window period."
Viral nucleic acid detection PCR and branched-chain DNA assays	Monitor HIV progression and effectiveness of antiretroviral therapy	Useful in diagnosis of acute HIV infection in a high-risk patient with a negative or indeterminate Western blot test. A low-level positive viral load may be a false positive.
Viral culture HIV culture	Diagnostic aid	Highly specific but relatively insensitive, due to varying degrees of viremia and technical difficulties.
Alternative diagnostic modalities Single-Use Diagnostic System	Rapid test; notify patient in one visit	Sensitivity and specificity >99%. Positive results must be confirmed with a Western blot or indirect immunofluorescence assay.
OraSure oral test	Alternative to blood drawing	The patient places collection pad between cheek and gum. A health care professional then places pad in preservative solution and mails to a central laboratory. Initial studies reported a sensitivity and specificity >99%.
Calypte urine test	Alternative to blood drawing	Lower sensitivity and specificity than oral mucosal transudate testing.
Home Access Health Corporation	Home kit; patient reluctant to visit a health care facility	The blood-spot specimen is sent to a central laboratory. Results are available by phone within 3 to 7 days. Patients with positive results are referred to a physician.

Laboratory testing for infection with the human immunodeficiency virus: Established and novel approaches. Am J Med 109:571, 2000.

whose results are positive receive counseling and a referral to a health care provider.

One rapid test, the Single Use Diagnostic System (SUDS) test, was approved by the FDA in 1992. The SUDS test requires a trained laboratory technician to obtain the sample and perform the test. Results can be obtained in 10 to 15 minutes. The test has a sensitivity of 99.9% and a specificity of 99.6%.[9] Negative results can be reported as definitive because of the high sensitivity and specificity; however, positive results require confirmation by standard serology. SUDS is used when rapid confirmation regarding a person's HIV status is required, such as after exposure to a pregnant woman in labor or after possible exposure in a health care worker; PEP is attempted as soon as possible.

An oral HIV test was approved by the FDA in 1994. The test involves collecting saliva and testing it for the presence of antibodies to HIV. The person places a specially treated pad between his or her lower cheek and gum for 2 minutes. Results are available by phone or fax within 3 days.

A urine HIV test was approved by the FDA in 1996. The test uses the ELISA technology and is administered by a physician. Positive results must be confirmed by standard serology testing. The test has a sensitivity of 99% and a specificity of 94%.[9]

The p24 antigen test is used as a diagnostic tool. One of the core proteins of HIV is p24. Initially, p24 can be detected in the blood; however, during the latent phase of HIV, the protein drops to very low levels. As the virus becomes more active, p24 again becomes detectable in the blood. Some clinicians monitor p24 antigen to determine how rapidly the virus is multiplying.

Viral culture is used to grow HIV. It is mainly used in infants to detect HIV and in research. It is expensive and very labor intensive.

Periodic testing for HIV is recommended in people who practice high-risk behaviors, such as IV drug use and unprotected vaginal or anal sexual contact. Most authorities recommend 6- to 12-month intervals; the time interval is arbitrary.[14]

Tests Used to Evaluate Progression of HIV Infection

HIV nucleic acid testing, also called *viral load testing*, in combination with the CD4 count is currently the best method available to determine progression on the HIV disease continuum. The viral load measures the amount of viral particles in 1 mL (mm^3) of blood. The higher the viral load, the more rapid the progression to AIDS.[4] Three methods can be used to determine the viral load: polymerase chain reaction (PCR), branched-chain DNA, and nucleic acid sequence–based amplification.[15] PCR is the most common method. The test results are used to determine the best time to begin antiretroviral therapy and when a change in therapy may be indicated.[4]

The CD4 count is another important evaluation tool used to stage the HIV disease and to make decisions concerning the initiation of antiretroviral therapy and prophylactic treatment for opportunistic organisms. The normal CD4 count is about 1,000 cells/mm^3, and the count declines over time in the person with AIDS (Fig. 48-5). There is an inverse relationship between the viral load and CD4 count (Fig. 48-6). As HIV/AIDS progresses, the number of CD4 cells declines, and the amount of HIV in the blood increases.

Other tests used to evaluate HIV infection include complete blood count (CBC), rapid plasma reagin, chest radiograph, serum chemistries, Papanicolaou (Pap) smears in women, purified protein derivative skin test, hepatitis serology, toxoplasmosis serology, and cytomegalovirus antibody serology.

Management

Management of patients with HIV disease involves a complex, multisystem assessment, including diagnostic tests that establish a baseline, to determine the appropriateness of therapy. Prognosis is based on the type and number of opportunistic infections that occur and the degree of immunocompromise. Patients with multiple opportunistic infections tend to be more seriously immunosuppressed and have a poorer prognosis.

CONTROL OF OPPORTUNISTIC INFECTION

The primary goal of management in critically ill HIV-infected patients is the prevention or resolution of opportunistic infections and nosocomial infections. Opportunistic infections are the leading cause of death in patients with HIV infection; therefore, prevention is the cornerstone of treatment. Treatment of opportunistic infections is aimed at support of the involved system or systems. Standards of care have been developed for prophylaxis against several organisms associated with opportunistic infections. The current organisms for which prophylaxis is strongly recommended include *P. jiroveci*, *Mycobacterium tuberculosis*, and *Toxoplasma gondii*. Organisms that should be considered for prophylaxis include *Streptococcus pneumoniae*, *Mycobacterium avium* complex, and varicella-zoster. Organisms and the preferred choice for prophylaxis are listed in Table 48-5. Organisms that usually receive prophylaxis include *S. pneu-*

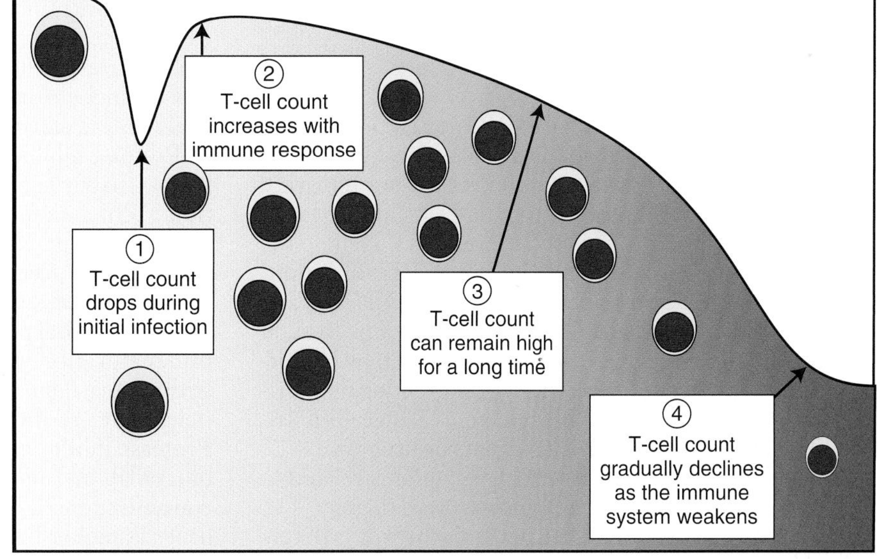

①
T-cell count
drops during
initial infection
②
T-cell count
increases with
immune response
③
T-cell count
can remain high
for a long time
④
T-cell count
gradually declines
as the immune
system weakens
Early stage
(briefly symptomatic)
Intermediate stage
(asymptomatic)
Advanced stage
(symptomatic)

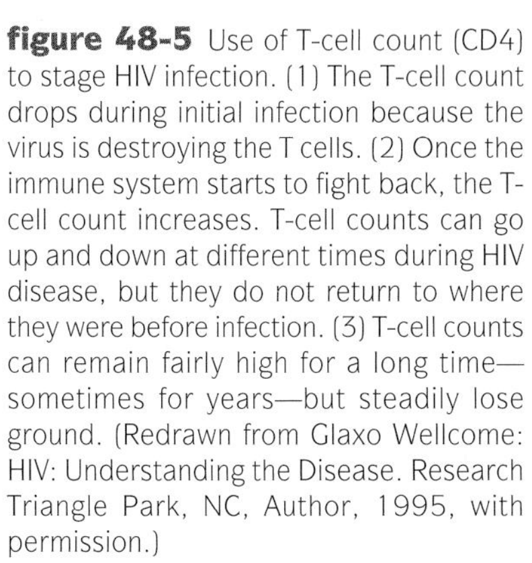
figure 48-5 Use of T-cell count (CD4) to stage HIV infection. (1) The T-cell count drops during initial infection because the virus is destroying the T cells. (2) Once the immune system starts to fight back, the T-cell count increases. T-cell counts can go up and down at different times during HIV disease, but they do not return to where they were before infection. (3) T-cell counts can remain fairly high for a long time—sometimes for years—but steadily lose ground. (Redrawn from Glaxo Wellcome: HIV: Understanding the Disease. Research Triangle Park, NC, Author, 1995, with permission.)

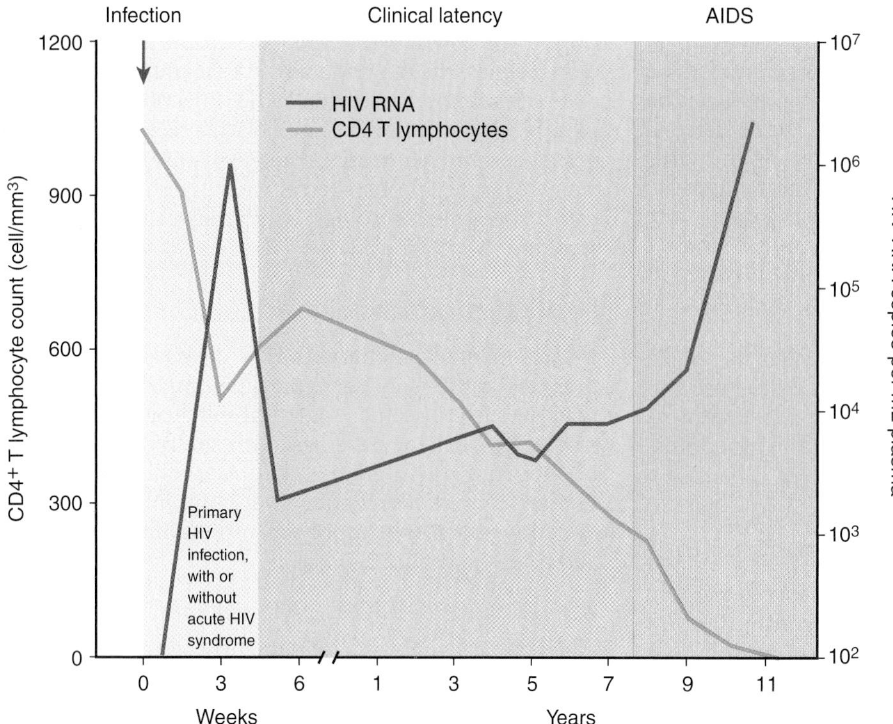

figure 48-6 Typical course of HIV infection (From Understanding Disease and Management, available at www.Roche-hiv.com. Modified from Fauci AS, et al., Ann Intern Med 124(7):654–663, 1996.)

moniae, hepatitis B, influenza, and hepatitis A. Safe infection control measures to prevent bacterial contamination and complications in the ICU must be maintained when working with patients with AIDS.

The use of highly active antiretroviral therapy (HAART) has had a significant impact on the treatment of opportunistic infections. The number of opportunistic infections has significantly decreased because of advances in antiretroviral therapy[16] (Fig. 48-7). Prophylactic or suppressive treatment for PCP, toxoplasmosis, cytomegalovirus infection, *Mycobacterium avium* complex infection, leishmaniasis, cryptococcosis, and candidal thrush may be discontinued if the patient's CD4 count increases sufficiently.[7] Administration of HAART also can rapidly reduce viral load, thereby decreasing the incidence of complications.

ANTIRETROVIRAL THERAPY

Originally, it was believed that HIV-infected people progressed to AIDS and died within a short time, but we now know that HIV-positive people who receive antiretroviral therapy can survive for many years after being infected with the virus. The drug groups used to treat HIV include the nucleoside reverse transcriptase inhibitors (NRTIs), nonnucleoside reverse transcriptase inhibitors (NNRTIs), and protease inhibitors (Fig. 48-8). The drug groups work at different points along the replication cycle, thereby inhibiting the development of new virions or preventing new virions from becoming mature and infectious. Table 48-6 lists the FDA-approved antiretroviral agents by drug type.

All patients who are experiencing symptoms related to HIV infection should be offered antiretroviral therapy. The decision to initiate or change a person's therapy is determined by the presence or absence of symptoms along with the degree of immunosuppression that the patient is experiencing. The guidelines are based on the virological, immunological, and clinical status of the patient, not the sex of the person.[2] The approach becomes more complicated when the patient is asymptomatic and requires an analysis of the risks and benefits of initiating therapy. All antiretroviral drugs, regardless of type, have adverse effects. Table 48-7 outlines the most common adverse effects of the antiretroviral drugs.

Specific Antiretroviral Drugs

Both NRTIs and NNRTIs block the conversion of viral RNA to viral DNA through inhibition of the enzyme reverse transcriptase (see Fig. 48-8). Even though both groups of drugs inhibit reverse transcriptase, the mechanism used to accomplish the inhibition is different. NNRTIs include drugs such as nevirapine, delavirdine, and efavirenz. NRTIs include drugs such as zidovudine, didanosine, zalcitabine, and stavudine.

Protease inhibitors, which began to be used in 1996, are proving to be of great benefit in the treatment of HIV infection.[10] Protease inhibitors add to the arsenal against HIV and when used in combination with NRTIs and NNRTIs, provide even greater antiretroviral coverage. Protease is an enzyme necessary for breaking down large polyproteins into smaller viral proteins that are necessary for viral assembly, maturation, and budding. Protease inhibitors bind with protease and block this process, resulting in viral particles that are immature and noninfectious (Fig. 48-9). Protease inhibitors have limitations, including a low oral bioavailability and short half-life, that produce low trough concentrations. This may require the administration of the drugs at higher frequency and dose to achieve the desired effect.[17] Other adverse effects include neurological, gastrointestinal, and urological complications; insulin intolerance;

table 48-5 Prophylaxis to Prevent First Episode of Opportunistic Disease Among Adults and Adolescents Infected With Human Immunodeficiency Virus

	Preventive Regimen	
Pathogen	***Indication***	***First Choice***
Strongly Recommended as Standard of Care		
Pneumocystis jiroveci	CD4+ counts of <200/µL or oropharyngeal candidiasis	Trimethoprim-sulfamethoxazole (TMP-SMZ), 1 double-strength tablet (DS) by mouth, daily (AI) or TMP-SMZ 1 single-strength tablet (SS) by mouth daily (AI)
Mycobacterium tuberculosis		
Isoniazid-sensitive	Tuberculin skin test (TST) reaction ≥5 mm or prior positive TST result without treatment or contact with person with active tuberculosis, regardless of TST result (BIII)	Isoniazid, 300 mg by mouth plus pyridoxine, 50 mg by mouth daily for 9 mo (AII) or isoniazid, 900 mg by mouth plus pyridoxine, 100 mg by mouth, twice weekly for 9 mo (BII)
Isoniazid-resistant	Same as previous pathogen; increased probability of exposure to isoniazid-resistant tuberculosis	Rifampin, 600 mg by mouth daily (AIII) or rifabutin, 300 mg by mouth (BIII) daily for 4 mo
Multidrug-resistant (isoniazid and rifampin)	Same as previous pathogen; increased probability of exposure to multidrug-resistant tuberculosis	Choice of drugs requires consultation with public health authorities; depends on susceptibility of isolate from source patient
Toxoplasma gondii	Immunoglobulin G antibody to *Toxoplasma* and CD4+ count of <100/µL	TMP-SMZ, 1 DS by mouth daily (AII)
Mycobacterium avium complex	CD4+ count of <50/µL	Azithromycin, 1,200 mg by mouth weekly (AI) or clarithromycin, 500 mg by mouth twice daily (AI)
Varicella-zoster virus (VZV)	Substantial exposure to chickenpox or shingles for patients who have no history of either condition or, if available, negative antibody to VZV	Varicella-zoster immune globulin (VZIG), 5 vials (1.25 mL each) intramuscularly, administered ≤96 h after exposure, ideally in ≤48 h (AIII)
Usually Recommended		
Streptococcus pneumoniae	CD4+ count of ≥200/µL	23-valent polysaccharide vaccine, 0.5 mL intramuscularly (BII)
Hepatitis B virus	All susceptible patients (i.e., antihepatitis B core antigen–negative)	Hepatitis B vaccine: 3 doses (BII)
Influenza virus	All patients (annually, before influenza season)	Inactivated trivalent influenza virus vaccine: one annual dose (0.5 mL) intramuscularly (BII)
Hepatitis A virus	All susceptible patients at increased risk for hepatitis A infection (i.e., antihepatitis A virus–negative) (e.g., illegal drug users, men who have sex with men, hemophiliacs) or patients with chronic liver disease, including chronic hepatitis B or C	Hepatitis A vaccine: two doses (BIII)

System used to rate the strength of recommendations and quality of supporting evidence: A, Both strong evidence for efficacy and substantial clinical benefit support recommendation for use; should always be offered; B, Moderate evidence for efficacy or strong evidence for efficacy, but only limited clinical benefit, supports recommendation for use; should usually be offered; I, Evidence from at least one correctly randomized, controlled trial; II, Evidence from at least one well-designed clinical trial without randomization, from cohort or case-controlled analytic studies (preferably from more than one center), or from multiple time-series studies, or dramatic results from uncontrolled experiments; III, Evidence from opinions of respected authorities based on clinical experience, descriptive studies, or reports of consulting committees.

From Centers for Disease Control and Prevention: Guidelines for preventing opportunistic infections among HIV-infected persons: 2002 recommendations of the U.S. Public Health Service and the Infectious Diseases Society of America. MMWR Morb Mortal Wkly Rep 51(RR-8): 1–51, 2002.

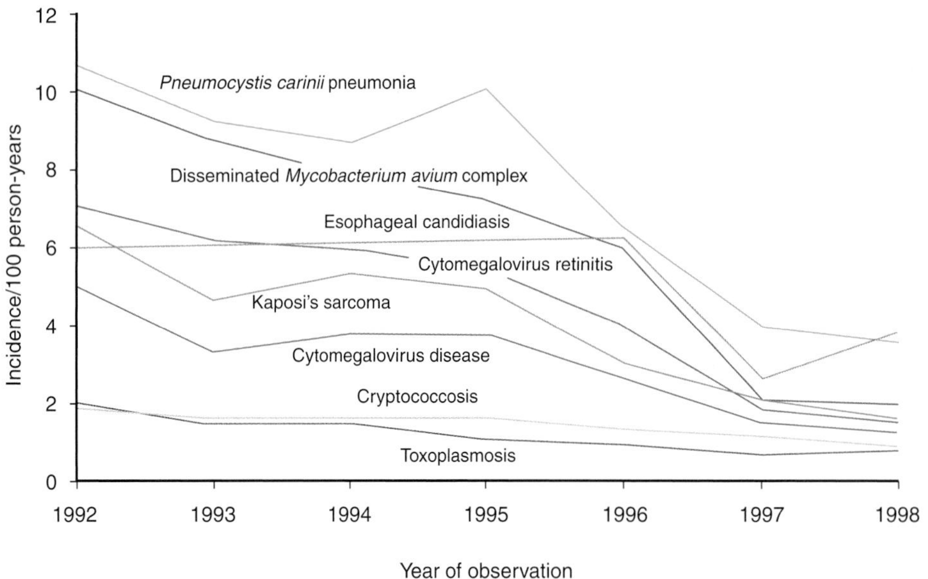

figure 48-7 Trends for opportunistic infections in HIV-infected adults and adolescents, ASD (Adult and Adolescent Spectrum of Disease) Project, 1992–1998. Data are standardized to the population of AIDS cases reported nationally in the same years by age, sex, race, HIV-exposure mode, country of origin, and CD4+ count. The median CD4+ count of reported patients with AIDS is 100 to 110/μL; therefore, rates indicate the incidence of opportunistic infections among persons with CD4+ counts in this range. The number of subjects included in the analysis are 10,441, 11,589, 11,276, 10,048, 9,250, 8,897, and 8,074, respectively, for the years 1992–1998. (From Kaplan JE, Hanson D, Dworkin MS, et al: Epidemiology of human immunodeficiency virus–associated opportunistic infections in the United States in the era of highly active antiretroviral therapy. Clin Infect Dis 30 [Suppl 1]: S6, 2000.)

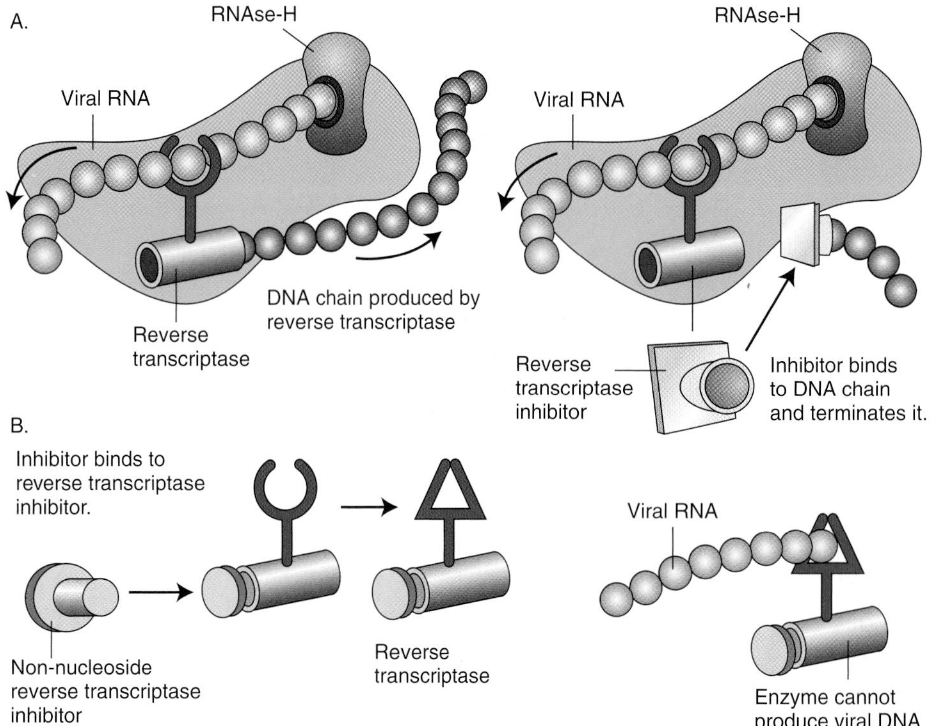

figure 48-8 Mechanism of action of nucleoside and non-nucleoside reverse transcriptase inhibitors. To enable HIV to be integrated into the host DNA, the single-strand viral RNA must be converted to double-stranded DNA by the viral enzyme reverse transcriptase while the enzyme RNAse-H hydrolyses the RNA after it has been copied. Nucleoside and non-nucleoside reverse-transcriptase inhibitors are two classes of antiretroviral drugs that suppress HIV replication by attacking reverse transcriptase. (**A**) Nucleoside reverse transcriptase inhibitors are similar in structure to the building blocks that make up DNA. By incorporating themselves into the DNA nucleoside chain being produced by reverse transcriptase, they stop attachment of further nucleosides and prevent ongoing viral DNA synthesis. (**B**) Non-nucleoside reserve transcriptase inhibitors attach to the reverse transcriptase and affect the activity of the enzyme by restricting its mobility and making it unable to function. (From Richman DD: HIV chemotherapy. Nature 410:998, 2001.)

table 48-6 FDA-Approved Antiretroviral Agents

Agent	Brand Name	Manufacturer	FDA Approval
Nucleoside Reverse Transcriptase Inhibitors			
Abacavir (ABC)	Ziagen	GlaxoSmithKline	12/98
AZT/3TC	Combivir	GlaxoSmithKline	10/97
AZT/3TC/ABC	Trizivir (TZV)	GlaxoSmithKline	11/00
Didanosine (ddl)	Videx, Videx EC	Bristol-Myers Squibb	10/91
Lamivudine (3TC)	Epivir	GlaxoSmithKline	11/95
Stavudine (d4T)	Zerit	Bristol-Myers Squibb	06/94
Zalcitabine (ddC)	HIVID	Roche	06/92
Zidovudine (AZT, ZDV)	Retrovir	GlaxoSmithKline	03/87
Nucleotide Reverse Transcriptase Inhibitor			
Tenofovir (TDF)	Viread	Gilead	10/01
Protease Inhibitors			
Amprenavir (APV)	Agenerase	GlaxoSmithKline	04/99
Indinavir (IDV)	Crixivan	Merck	03/96
Lopinavir/Ritonavir (LPV/RTV)	Kaletra	Abbott	09/00
Nelfinavir (NFV)	Viracept	Agouron	03/97
Ritonavir (RTV)	Norvir	Abbott	03/96
Saquinavir (SQV, FTV)	Fortovase	Roche	11/97
Saquinavir mesylate (INV)	Invirase	Roche	12/95
Non-Nucleoside Reverse Transcriptase Inhibitors			
Delavirdine (DLV)	Rescriptor	Agouron	04/97
Efavirenz (EFV)	Sustiva	Bristol-Myers Squibb	09/98
Nevirapine (NVP)	Viramune	Boehringer Ingelheim	06/96
Other Drugs			
Hydroxyurea (HU)	Droxia, Hydrea	Bristol-Myers Squibb	—

From Bartlett JG: The 2002 Abbreviated Guide to Medical Management of HIV Infection, p 29. Baltimore, Johns Hopkins University, Department of Infectious Diseases, 2002.

elevated cholesterol and triglycerides; and redistribution of body fat, with loss of fat from the face and limbs, along with central adiposity.[7,17] This latter side effect is known as lipodystrophy. Currently, three protease inhibitors have been approved by the FDA: saquinavir, indinavir, and ritonavir. Indinavir is more potent than saquinavir and seems to have fewer short-term side effects and fewer drug interactions than ritonavir.

Highly Active Antiretroviral Therapy

HAART is the coadministration of two NRTIs plus one NNRTI or one protease inhibitor.[7,16,18] HAART, which became the standard of practice in 1996, has four goals:[4,17,19]

- To suppress and maintain the viral load at nondetectable levels for as long as possible
- To restore and preserve immunological function
- To improve quality of life
- To reduce HIV-associated morbidity and mortality

The most recent guidelines recommend that HAART be offered to patients with a CD4 count of less than 350 cells/mm^3 or a plasma HIV-RNA (viral load) level greater than 55,000 copies/mL (Table 48-8). The use of HAART commonly results in an increase in CD4 count of 100 to 250 cells/mm^3.[16] This increase may return the patient's number of cells to the normal range; this is known as *immune reconstruction*.[18]

The effectiveness of HAART is evaluated using HIV-RNA levels. Once therapy has begun, a decrease in HIV-RNA should occur within 2 to 8 weeks. Within 4 to 6 months after starting HAART, the patient's HIV-RNA level should be nondetectable (i.e., not measurable by current technology). The current threshold for detectability of HIV-RNA is 50 copies/ml.[10] Viral load assessment should be repeated every 3 to 4 months to monitor effectiveness.[19]

Failure of therapy is defined as the presence of a measurable viral load at the 4- to 6-month mark. Reasons for antiretroviral failure may include nonadherence to the prescribed medications, inadequate potency of drugs or suboptimal levels of drugs, or viral resistance to the drugs.[7] Nonadherence to therapy, which is a significant contributor to drug resistance, is the most common reason.[18]

VACCINES

Research concerning vaccine development has been active ever since the causative agent in HIV infection and AIDS was isolated. Unfortunately, to develop a vaccine that

(text continues on page 1152)

table 48-7 Antiretroviral and Other Medications Used in HIV/AIDS and Their Common or Clinically Significant Side Effects

Medication	Common Side Effects or Clinically Significant Side Effects
Protease Inhibitors	
Saquinavir (Invirase; Fortovase)	Headache Nausea Diarrhea
Indinavir sulfate (Crixivan)	Nephrolithiasis Hyperbilirubinemia Fatigue Headache Nausea Abdominal pain
Nelfinavir (Viracept)	Mild diarrhea Elevated liver enzymes
Ritonavir (Norvir)	Nausea and vomiting Anorexia; abdominal discomfort Diarrhea Taste alterations; dry mouth Paresthesia—hands, feet, lips
Amprenavir (Agenerase*)	Stevens-Johnson syndrome (1%) Nausea and vomiting Diarrhea Taste disorders Paresthesia—oral/perioral, peripheral Depression or mood disorders Rash
Non-nucleoside Reverse Transcriptase Inhibitors (NNRTIs)	
Nevirapine (Viramune)	Rash Fever Nausea Elevated liver enzymes
Delavirdine (Rescriptor)	Rash Fever Elevated liver enzymes Nausea and vomiting
Efavirenz (Sustiva)	Central nervous system symptoms (50%)—dizziness, impaired concentration, somnolence, abnormal dreams, insomnia Psychiatric symptoms Rash
Nucleoside Reverse Transcriptase Inhibitors (NRTIs)	
Zidovudine (ZDV; AZT; Retrovir)	Neutropenia Anemia Nausea Malaise Headache Insomnia Myalgia Asthenia
Didanosine (ddI; Videx)	Peripheral neuropathy Abdominal pain Dry mouth Diarrhea Pancreatitis Rash

table 48-7 Antiretroviral and Other Medications Used in HIV/AIDS and Their Common or Clinically Significant Side Effects (Continued)

Medication	Common Side Effects or Clinically Significant Side Effects
Zalcitabine (ddc; Hivid)	Peripheral neuropathy Pancreatitis Rash Fever Aphthous ulcers Anemia Liver enzyme elevation
Stavudine (d4T; Zerit)	Peripheral neuropathy Liver enzyme elevation Nausea Diarrhea Myalgia
Lamivudine (3TC; Epivir)	Rash Headache Diarrhea
Abacavir (Ziagen)	Hypersensitivity reaction (5%) Anorexia Nausea and vomiting Malaise and fatigue Diarrhea
Other Drugs	
Azithromycin dihydrate (Zithromax)	Headache, dizziness, fatigue Nausea, diarrhea, abdominal pain Hypoglycemia, hyperkalemia
Trimethoprim-sulfamethoxazole (Bactrim)	Nausea, vomiting Rash Aplastic anemia Headache, insomnia, fatigue
Dapsone	Hemolytic anemia, blood dyscrasias Peripheral motor weakness Liver damage
Atovaquone (Mepron)	Headache, insomnia Cough Nausea, diarrhea Rash Fever
Fluconazole (Diflucan)	Headache Nausea, vomiting, diarrhea Abdominal pain Rash
Clarithromycin (Biaxin)	Abnormal taste Nausea, diarrhea Abdominal pain Hepatotoxicity Headache
Isoniazid (INH)	Peripheral neuropathy Toxic encephalopathy, convulsions Agranulocytosis, hemolytic aplastic anemia, thrombocytopenia Eosinophilia Methemoglobinemia Jaundice, fatal hepatitis
Ethambutal (Myambutol)	Optic neuritis, blurred vision Nausea, vomiting, anorexia Peripheral neuritis

(continued)

table 48-7 Antiretroviral and Other Medications Used in HIV/AIDS and Their Common or Clinically Significant Side Effects (Continued)

Medication	Common Side Effects or Clinically Significant Side Effects
Ciprofloxacin (Cipro)	Nausea, vomiting Abdominal pain Diarrhea
Sulfadiazine	Anaphylaxis Nausea, vomiting Hepatitis Leukopenia, thrombocytopenia, agranulocytosis, hemolytic anemia, aplastic anemia Stevens-Johnson syndrome Renal failure, toxic nephrosis
Pyrimethamine (Daraprim)	Nausea, vomiting, anorexia Thrombocytopenia, leukopenia, pancytopenia, megaloblastic anemia, agranulocytosis
Hydroxyurea (Hydrea)	Leukopenia, anemia, thrombocytopenia Rash

*Agenerase capsules and oral solution contain large amounts of vitamin E, which exceed the Recommended Dietary Allowance. Warn patients not to take supplemental vitamin E.
From Burns J: HIV/AIDS: Impact on healing. Ostomy Wound Manage 46(3):32–33, 2000.

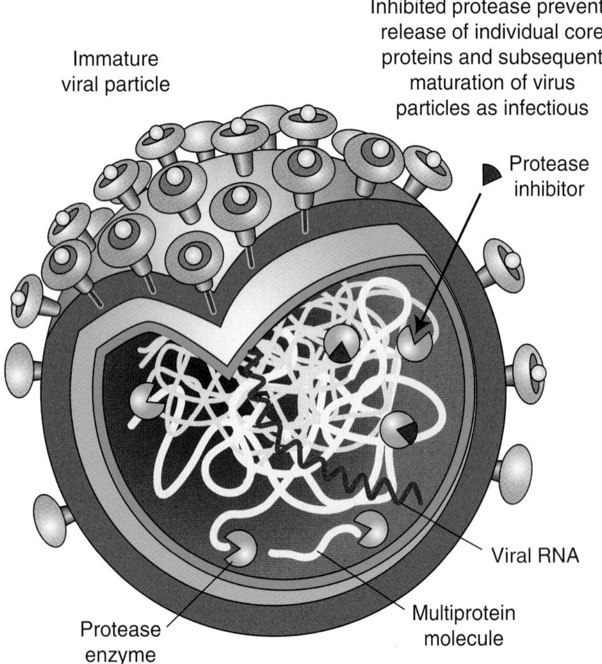

figure 48-9 Mechanism of action of protease inhibitors. After transcription in the nucleus, viral mRNA enters the cytoplasm and uses the host's cellular machinery to manufacture virus proteins. The viral components then gather at the cell membrane and immature viruses bud off the cell. Core proteins are produced as part of long polypeptides, which must be cut into smaller fragments by the enzyme protease in order to form mature, fuctional proteins. Protease inhibitors bind to the site where protein cutting occurs and prevent the enzyme from releasing the individual core proteins. As a result of this, the new viral particles are unable to mature or become infectious. (From Richman DD: HIV chemotherapy. Nature 410:998, 2001.)

protects against HIV infection, a large population of people with a well-defined resistance to HIV infection is needed to identify the immune parameter. To date, no such populations have been identified.[7] Vaccine research is progressing, and many phase 1 (dose-escalation safety and toxicity), phase 2 (expanded safety and dose optimization), and phase 3 (efficacy) clinical trials have taken place.[20] The lack of knowledge about the immune parameter and the genetic diversity of the virus are the most challenging obstacles to developing an effective vaccine.

case study ■ HIV/AIDS

Ms. Lewis is a 41-year-old African-American woman with hypertension who has been HIV positive for 15 years. She was exposed to the virus through unprotected sex. The man did not tell her he was HIV positive; he became sick, was diagnosed with AIDS, and died within 2 years. When the patient learned that the man was HIV positive, she went to her physician to have an HIV test. ELISA was used initially, and Western blot analysis confirmed the positive result. The patient's viral load at the time of testing was 2,000 cells/mL. The patient was diligent about her follow-up visits and had a relatively low viral load for 8 years. However, 7 years ago her viral load increased to 26,000 copies/mL, and her CD4 count decreased to 250 cells/mm^3. At that time, she was started on an antiretroviral regimen consisting of lamivudine/zidovudine (Combivir) and indinavir.

The patient has remained healthy for the past 7 years on this regimen until recently, when she began to experience shortness of breath. She has been unable to walk 25 feet without dyspnea. She has had a fever of 100.4°F (38°C) for

table 48-8 Recommended Antiretroviral Agents for Initial Treatment of Established HIV Infection

Recommendation	Column A	Column B
Strongly recommended	Efavirenz Indinavir Nelfinavir Ritonavir plus indinavir*† Ritonavir plus lopinavir*§ Ritonavir plus saquinavir* (soft-gel capsule¶ or hard-gel capsule¶)	Didanosine plus lamivudine Stavudine plus didanosine** Stavudine plus lamivudine Zidovudine plus didanosine Zidovudine plus lamivudine
Recommended as alternatives	Abacavir Amprenavir Delavirdine Nelfinavir plus saquinavir (soft-gel capsule) Nevirapine Ritonavir Saquinavir (soft-gel capsule)	Zidovudine plus zalcitabine
No recommendation because of insufficient data††	Hydroxyurea in combination with antiretroviral drugs Ritonavir plus amprenavir* Ritonavir plus nelfinavir* Tenofovir§§	
Not recommended and should not be offered (All monotherapies whether from column A or B¶¶)	Saquinavir (hard-gel capsule)***	Stavudine plus zidovudine Zalcitabine plus didanosine Zalcitabine plus lamivudine Zalcitabine plus stavudine

This table is a guide to using available treatment regimens for patients with no previous or limited experience with HIV therapy. In accordance with established therapy goals, priority is assigned to regimens in which clinical trial data demonstrate (1) sustained suppression of HIV plasma ribonucleic acid (including among patients with high baseline viral load); (2) sustained increase in CD4+ T cell count (for the majority of patients, during 48 weeks); and (3) favorable clinical outcome (i.e., delayed progression to acquired immunodeficiency syndrome and death). Regimens that have been compared directly with other regimens that perform sufficiently well with regard to these parameters are included in the strongly recommended category. Other factors considered included the regimen's pill burden, dosing frequency, food requirements, convenience, toxicity, and drug-interaction profile compared with other regimens. All antiretroviral agents, including those in the strongly recommended category, have potentially serious toxic and adverse events associated with their use. Clinicians should consult CDC Guidelines[19] before formulating an antiretroviral regimen for their patients. Antiretroviral drug regimens include one choice each from columns A and B of this table. Drugs are listed in alphabetical, not priority order.

*See CDC Guidelines[19] for additional information regarding optimizing protease inhibitor exposure with ritonavir.

†Recommendation is based on the opinions of specialists in HIV treatment.

§Coformulated as Kaletra (Abbott Laboratories).

¶Saquinavir (soft-gel capsule) refers to Fortovase (Roche Laboratories, Inc.); Saquinavir (hard-gel capsule) refers to Invirase (Roche Laboratories, Inc.).

**Pregnant women might be at increased risk for lactic acidosis and liver damage when treated with stavudine plus didanosine. This combination should be used for pregnant women only when the potential benefit outweighs the potential risk.

††This category includes drugs or combinations for which information is too limited to allow a recommendation for or against use.

§§Data from clinical trials are limited to use in salvage. Data from trials of tenofovir as initial therapy should be available in the future.

¶¶Zidovudine monotherapy can be considered for prophylactic use among pregnant women with low viral load and high CD4+ T cell counts to prevent perinatal transmission.

***Use of saquinavir (hard-gel capsule) (i.e., Invirase) is recommended only in combination with ritonavir.

From Centers for Disease Control and Prevention: Guidelines for using antiretroviral agents among HIV-infected adults and adolescents: Recommendations of the Panel on Clinical Practices for Treatment of HIV. MMWR Morb Mortal Wkly Rep 51(RR-7):40, 2002.

the past 3 days as well as a nonproductive cough. During the night, the patient's shortness of breath became worse, and she decided to go to the hospital. On arrival at the emergency department, the patient's vital signs are as follows: temperature 101.2°F (38.4°C); respirations 32 breaths/minute; heart rate 126 beats/minute; and blood pressure 118/60 mm Hg. A chest radiograph shows pulmonary infiltrates throughout both lung fields. A sputum sample is sent to the laboratory for gram stain and silver stain. Arterial blood gases (ABGs) reveal an uncompensated respiratory alkalosis (pH 7.53; $Paco_2$ 27 mm Hg; Pao_2 86 mm Hg; HCO_3 24 mm Hg; and Sao_2 93%).

These signs and symptoms lead the health care team to believe that the patient has *Pneumocystis* pneumonia (PCP). It is the patient's first experience with this opportunistic infection. She receives her first dose of trimethoprim-sulfamethoxazole (TMP-SMZ) by IV infusion. Within 30 minutes, a significant skin rash with urticaria develops in the patient. The TMP-SMZ is discontinued, and she is given clindamycin 600 mg IV every 8 hours instead.

The patient's respiratory status becomes worse during her stay in the emergency department. Her respiratory rate increases to 44 breaths/minute and respiratory acidosis develops, indicating that she is getting tired. ABGs are pH

7.26; $PaCO_2$ 50 mm Hg; PaO_2 80 mm Hg; HCO_3 25 mm Hg; and SaO_2 90%. The patient agrees to be intubated; this is successfully accomplished. She is then transferred to the ICU for continued evaluation and monitoring.

In the ICU, clindamycin is continued, and prednisone 40 mg IV twice daily is started. The patient is placed on bed rest. Deep venous thrombosis prophylaxis, with bilateral compression devices on her lower extremities, and gastrointestinal prophylaxis are both started. The head of the bed is maintained at 30 degrees or more.

Over the next 2 days, the patient's oxygenation worsens. On day 3 in the ICU, her oxygenation begins to improve. On day 5, she is breathing independently on continuous positive airway pressure with a fraction of inspired oxygen (FIO_2) of 0.5, 5 cm H_2O of positive end-expiratory pressure, and 10 cm H_2O pressure support. The decision is to made to extubate the patient, and she receives 40% oxygen by face mask. Her FIO_2 is continually weaned down, and she is no longer receiving oxygen by day 7.

On day 8, the patient is discharged home in the care of her brother. The patient is instructed to follow up with her primary care physician in 2 to 3 days and to continue taking the oral clindamycin and prednisone. The patient is educated about the need to continue with medication until her immune system is capable of keeping the PCP under control (i.e., her CD4 count is greater than 350 cells/mm^3), at which time her physician may decide to discontinue the drug.

Currently, the patient's CD4 count is 275 cells/mm^3, so she remains on PCP prophylaxis at home. She has not experienced any additional opportunistic infections and understands the importance of healthy eating, exercising, safe sexual practices, and stress reduction. ■

ONCOLOGICAL COMPLICATIONS AND EMERGENCIES

As much as 20% of people diagnosed with cancer have at least one oncological emergency during the course of their disease.[21] The incidence of these emergencies increases as patients with cancer live longer. The nurse must recognize patient-specific risk factors for the development of critical illness and plan appropriate assessment and intervention strategies for the most common oncological emergencies. These emergencies are classified by pathophysiological mechanism: hematological, anatomical–structural, and metabolic. Hematological complications involving bone marrow dysfunction, such as engraftment syndrome and leukostasis, commonly occur in neoplastic disorders. Anatomical–structural disorders such as cardiac tamponade, carotid artery rupture, hepatic veno-occlusive disease, obstruction of the superior vena cava, pleural effusion, spinal cord compression, and tracheobronchial obstruction are the result of tumor invasion or treatment-related destruction of normal anatomical structures. Metabolic disruptions from cancer or its treatment such as hypercalcemia, syndrome of inappropriate antidiuretic hormone secretion (SIADH), and tumor lysis syndrome may involve hormone stimulation, procoagulant activity, and electrolyte imbalances.

General Principles in the Critical Care of Patients With Cancer

Patients with cancer present unique concerns for the critical care nurse. A knowledge of preexisting illness, nature of the malignancy, treatment-related considerations, and prognostic implications must be incorporated into patient care. In addition, it is necessary to appreciate the psychosocial factors related to caring for patients with a chronic disease. Box 48-4 lists management factors in the evaluation and treatment of an oncological emergency. Ideally, before any acute event, the oncologist or primary care physician has discussed end-of-life care and the oncological crises that should be treated and those that should not be treated with the patient and family members. However, this is not often the case, and the critical care nurse is an important liaison between the primary care physician and the intensivist. Each time a patient with cancer presents with critical illness, prognostic variables and information regarding treatment of the presenting condition should be used to

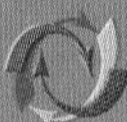

box 48-4 nursing interventions for *Evaluation and Treatment of an Oncological Emergency*

Symptoms and Signs

1. Are the symptoms and signs due to the tumor or to complications of treatment?
2. How quickly are the symptoms of the oncological emergency progressing?

Natural History of the Primary Tumor

1. Is there a previous diagnosis of malignancy?
2. What is the disease-free interval between the diagnosis of the primary tumor and onset of the emergency?
3. Has the emergency developed in the setting of terminal disease?

Efficacy of Available Treatment

1. Has there been no prior therapy or extensive pretreatment?
2. Should treatment be directed at the underlying malignancy or the urgent complications?
3. Will the patient's general medical condition influence the ability to administer effective treatment?

Treatment and Goals

1. What is the potential for cure?
2. Is prompt palliation required to prevent further debilitation?
3. What is the risk versus benefit ratio of treatment?
4. Should treatment be withheld if there is a minimal chance of response to available antitumor therapies?

Used with permission from Murphy GP, Lawrence W, Lenhard RE: Clinical Oncology, p 597. Atlanta, GA, American Cancer Society, 1995.

advise the patient of the best course of action. Clearly there are times when the risk–benefit ratio of a lifesaving measure does not warrant its use; yet there are also many other situations in which a lifesaving intervention in a hopelessly ill patient may also enhance the quality of life. For example, a patient with advanced cancer may present with a potentially life-threatening pericardial effusion that can be effectively treated with insertion of a pericardial catheter. This patient may require a limited amount of intensive care after catheter insertion and fluid drainage, but the symptom relief may be advantageous in enhancing the quality of the last few weeks of the patient's life. Aggressive management of most oncological emergencies is indicated if a histological diagnosis of cancer has not been established, if the patient has a good prognosis or can achieve prolonged palliation with treatment, or if there is the possibility of restoring functional status. The nursing intervention guidelines in Box 48-4 are presented as a list of clinical questions that should be considered when making a decision about whether to provide critical care interventions to the patient with cancer.

To provide high-quality, individualized care to patients with oncological emergencies, the critical care nurse should know a few facts regarding critical illness and the patient with cancer. Box 48-5 presents important conclusions drawn from multiple studies of critical illness in patients with cancer. Box 48-6 lists nursing diagnoses and collaborative problems for patients with oncological emergencies.

box 48-5
Critical Care of Cancer Patients: Conclusions From the Literature

Incidence of Critical Illness

- Affects about 20% of patients
- More common in patients with hematological malignancy
- Most common critical illnesses:
  Respiratory distress
  Refractory hypotension
  Oncological emergencies

Prognostics of Critical Illness

- Survival is better in the newly diagnosed who have not yet received antineoplastic therapy.
- Survival from specific interventions:

Cardiac arrest:	<2% alive to discharge
Mechanical ventilation:	12%–45% alive to discharge (worst prognosis in patients receiving blood and marrow transplant, best prognosis in patients with a newly diagnosed solid tumor)
Dialysis:	21%–40% alive to discharge (prognosis has been improving with use of continuous renal replacement therapies)

- Most important predictor of survival: status of the underlying malignant disease
- Other poor prognostic variables:
  Age extremes
  Concomitant health problems
  Severity of cancer
  Aggressiveness/potency of treatment
  Reversibility of the specific crisis

Hematological Complications

BONE MARROW SUPPRESSION

Cancer and its treatment often cause suppression of hematopoietic cell production or differentiation. Causes of bone marrow suppression are commonly associated with cancer invasion of the bone, chemotherapy and some radiation treatments, or blood and marrow transplantation. The clinical consequences are symptoms related to decreased red blood cell production (anemia), decreased platelet production (thrombocytopenia), and decreased white blood cell production (leukopenia). Table 48-9 is a summary of the key clinical features and nursing implications of these three types of bone marrow suppression. These disorders are not uniquely oncological, but they are common in patients with cancer and influence the patient's response to other critical illnesses.

Other causes of bone marrow suppression must be considered if cancer-related etiological factors are not present. When serum tests are unclear in elucidating the etiology of bone marrow suppression, a bone marrow aspirate or biopsy may be performed to confirm the pathophysiological process. This test usually requires sedation and a local anesthetic before a large coring needle is used to remove the liquid red bone marrow from either the hip or sternum. Bone marrow biopsy determines whether the bone marrow defect is present during the cellular production phase, and it may be a basis for clinical management.

Management of bone marrow suppression as a cluster involves determining whether the cause is time-limited and ascertaining the amount of supportive therapy required. Treatment may include administration of bone marrow growth factors specific to the deficient cellular component,[22] infusion of blood components, or prophylactic clotting enhancement and antimicrobial therapy to prevent life-threatening bleeding or infectious complications.

ENGRAFTMENT SYNDROME

Engraftment syndrome, also known as *cytokine release syndrome* or *cytokine storm*, is a recently identified disorder that occurs infrequently in association with the return of bone marrow growth after treatment of hematological malignancies and blood and marrow transplantation. Patients most at risk for engraftment syndrome are women, those with acute leukemia (especially lymphocytic subtype), those who have just had allogeneic blood or marrow transplantation (especially with human leukocyte antigen–mismatched donors), and those who have had transplantation for autoimmune disorders or solid tumors.[23,24] Patients who have had early engraftment after high-dose marrow-ablative treatment are also at risk for engraftment syndrome.

box 48-6 *Example of Nursing Diagnoses and Collaborative Problems for Patients With Oncological Emergencies*

- Risk for Infection related to impaired or deficient leukocytes
- Risk for Injury related to thrombocytopenia and bleeding.
- Risk for Ineffective Tissue Perfusion due to reduced erythrocytes, or vascular disruption by tumor
- Potential for Impaired Gas Exchange due to cancer involvement of the lungs or alterations in fluid status
- Potential for Impaired Sensorimotor Function due to spinal cord compression
- Potential for Imbalanced Fluid Volume due to disease or treatment
- Potential for Fatigue due to malignant illness or its treatment
- Potential for Impaired Mobility due to disease complications
- Anxiety related to fear of disease or treatment
- Deficient Knowledge related to disease, or anticancer therapies
- Potential for Ineffective Coping related to severity of illness or prognosis
- Potential for Role Conflict due to chronic serious illness

Pathophysiology

Regrowth of bone marrow cells, particularly myelocytes, results in release of inflammatory cytokines that produce vasodilation and capillary leaking similar to sepsis. Lymphocytes and myelocytic precursors engraft the bone marrow earliest, and patients often still appear leukopenic at the onset of symptoms. Patients with engraftment syndrome often present with signs and symptoms similar to infection at a time when their blood counts are still low and they are equally at risk for engraftment syndrome and severe infection. Therefore, it is extremely difficult to distinguish the two disorders.

Assessment

History. Engraftment syndrome often begins with fever, total body erythema, and symptoms of respiratory distress[24] and these symptoms may be the only manifestations. However, many patients exhibit additional signs or symptoms of cytokine effects such as oliguria or hematuria with elevated creatinine, abdominal discomfort with elevated aminotransferases, and gastrointestinal bleeding. The onset of symptoms is rapid, usually occurring over 24 to 48 hours, and they dissipate after the neutrophils engraft and the white blood cell count reaches about 2,500 to 3,000/mm^3. Box 48-7 outlines key clinical manifestations that distinguish sepsis and engraftment syndrome.

Diagnostic Studies. There is no clearly definitive diagnostic test that can differentiate engraftment syndrome from sepsis, which it closely resembles. The cornerstones of diagnosis are the constellation of clinical symptoms, subsequent increase in white blood cell count in patients with previous leukopenia, and absence of a positive microbial culture.[25]

Management

Engraftment syndrome is managed supportively and conservatively. Patients are presumed septic and treated with broad-spectrum antimicrobial agents. Acetaminophen and diphenhydramine are administered as needed for erythema and pruritus. Hepatic dysfunction requires cautious monitoring and adjustment of fluids and medication doses as appropriate. IV fluids are used to prevent vasodilatory hypotension but, occasionally, potent constricting agents such as phenylephrine are required. Rapid-acting IV corticosteroids have been used effectively when clinical symptoms are strongly suggestive of this disorder.[24,26] Mechanical ventilation and renal replacement therapy are initiated as indicated, with the understanding and presumption that the syndrome is usually very short-lived.

Complications

The long-term outcome for most patients with engraftment syndrome is excellent, and there are no significant clinical sequelae.[23] Rarely do patients die or have long-term ischemic organ damage. In situations where negative sequelae have occurred, it has been difficult to determine whether engraftment syndrome or sepsis was the primary pathophysiological process. For example, patients with a rapid onset and progression of respiratory distress syndrome may die of refractory hypoxemia, yet whether this has been caused by undiagnosed and untreated infection or engraftment syndrome cannot be determined.

LEUKOSTASIS

Leukostasis is a disorder of excess circulating white blood cells, resulting in hyperviscosity and microvascular occlusions.[27] Cancers such as acute leukemias are the primary cause of leukostasis.

Pathophysiology

Excess numbers of circulating white blood cells, such as commonly occur in patients with acute leukemia, can cause a hyperviscosity syndrome that may lead to microcirculatory occlusion with ischemia and vessel rupture. Several types of leukemia can cause elevated white blood cell counts. The immature myelocytes (blasts) found in acute nonlymphocytic leukemia have the greatest propensity for "stickiness" due to adhesion molecules and their interaction with endothelial vessel linings and are most likely to cause leukostasis.[28] Risk of leukostasis is considered greatest when the white blood cell count is greater than 100,000/mm^3, although significant clinical symptoms may be present even when counts are in the 50,000/mm^3 range, especially if the white blood cell count is increasing rapidly or the cells are immature.[28] Vascular occlusion of the lungs and brain are most common, although coronary artery occlusion, renal failure, and splenic or bowel infarctions have been reported.[29]

Assessment

History. Patients with leukostasis usually first present with respiratory or neurological symptoms.[27,30] Onset of symptoms is acute (several hours to 1 day). Severe respiratory distress with hypoxemia and inflammatory alveolar

table 48-9 Key Clinical Features of Bone Marrow Suppression

Feature	Anemia	Thrombocytopenia	Leukopenia
Definition	General criteria • Hemoglobin <12 mg% • RBC count <3.0 × 10^6/mm^3 • Hematocrit <32% Specific to types of anemia • Aplastic anemia • Nutritional anemia • Hemolytic anemia	Classified according to severity of thrombocytopenia and risk of bleeding: • Mild <100,000/mm^3 • Moderate <50,000/mm^3 • Severe <20,000/mm^3	Classified according to severity of leukopenia and risk of infection Decreased granulocytes (granulocytopenia) classified by severity of ANC • Mild <1000/mm^3 • Moderate <500/mm^3 • Severe <100/mm^3 Decreased lymphocytes (lymphocytopenia) classified by severity of absolute lymphocyte count • Mild <250 cells/mm^3 • Moderate <100 cells/mm^3 • Severe <50 cells/mm^3
Pathophysiology			
Etiology/ contributing factors	General • Bone marrow suppression (e.g., chemotherapy, radiation to axial skeleton) • Nutritional deficits—iron, protein, B vitamins • Medications (estrogens, allopurinal [Zyloprim]) Aplastic anemia • Congenital disorders (e.g., Fanconi's syndrome, maternal ingestion of thiazides) • Viral infection • Medications Nutritional anemia • Iron deficiency • B vitamin deficiency Hemolytic anemia • Immune hemolysis (viral illness, autoimmune disease) • Sickle cell anemia • PNH	• Bone marrow suppression (e.g., chemotherapy, radiation to axial skeleton) • Medications (nonsteroidal anti-inflammatory drugs)	• Bone marrow suppression (e.g., chemotherapy, radiation to axial skeleton) • Nutritional deficits • Medications
Clinical manifestations	• Due to decreased oxygen carrying and tissue delivery: fatigue, oliguria, chest pain, decreased bowel sounds and constipation • Due to decreased body insulation and vascular volume: hypothermia, hypotension, orthostasis • Due to compensation for inadequate oxygen delivery to the tissue: tachycardia, tachypnea, cool extremities	• Due to decreased platelet plugging for normal vascular wear and tear: gum oozing, petechiae, occult blood in urine and stool • Related to inadequate platelet response to injury: ecchymoses, hematomas, bleeding around procedure sites, frank hematuria, or gastrointestinal bleeding	Granulocytopenia • Due to decreased phagocytic properties and recognition of invading microbes: fever, pain at site of potential infection, bacterial and fungal infecting organisms (after 7–10 days of granulocytopenia) • Related to diminished inflammatory response: lack of localized erythema, swelling or exudates Lymphocytopenia • Due to decreased cellular immune responses and recognition of foreign tissue or proteins: tissue anergy to pathogens, (opportunistic and viral infections more common)

(continued)

table 48-9 Key Clinical Features of Bone Marrow Suppression (Continued)

Feature	Anemia	Thrombocytopenia	Leukopenia
Diagnostic tests	General • RBC count • Hematocrit and hemoglobin • RBC morphology Aplastic anemia • Bone marrow aspirate and biopsy Nutritional anemia • Ferritin level • Transferrin level • Total iron-binding capacity (TIBC) • Folate level • Vitamin B_{12} level Hemolytic anemia • Total and direct bilirubin • Erythrocyte sedimentation rate (ESR) • RBC morphology • Hemoglobin electrophoresis (sickle cell, PNH) • Indium-tagged RBC survival studies	• Platelet count • Bleeding time tests platelet quality to identify whether symptoms may be partly related to platelet function rather than number	• White blood cell count is initial screening tool, but analysis of actual cell count may be helpful • ANC demonstrates the true number of granulocytes available for phagocytic activity • Absolute lymphocyte count demonstrates the true number of lymphocytes available for recognition of foreign tissue and proteins
Common nursing problems	• Fatigue • Activity intolerance • Hypoxemia • Digestion disorders	• Bleeding • Altered body image	• Infection • Risk of hemodynamic instability
Medical management	• Erythropoietin injections • RBC transfusions • Energy conservation	• Interleukin-1 (Oprelvekin) injections • Platelet transfusions • Bleeding precautions	• Granulocyte colony-stimulating factor (G-CSF) or granulocyte–macrophage colony-stimulating factor (GM-CSF) injections • Broad-spectrum antimicrobial therapy

ANC, absolute neutrophil count; PNH, paroxysmal nocturnal hemoglobinuria; RBC, red blood cell.

infiltrates are the hallmarks of pulmonary involvement. It is difficult to determine the severity of hypoxemia because the immature white blood cell blasts consume the oxygen in the arterial blood gas (ABG) specimen, making the arterial blood oxygen level appear even lower than suspected based on clinical evidence. Oxygen saturation may be low (e.g., 82% to 90%), but ABG oxygen levels may be only 30 mm Hg. It is believed that immediate icing and rapid transit may reduce but not eliminate this testing problem. Neurological leukostasis presents as mental status changes with clear focal deficits; vascular occlusions cause thrombotic or embolic strokes.[31]

box 48-7
Distinguishing Between Engraftment Syndrome and Sepsis

SEPSIS	ENGRAFTMENT SYNDROME
▪ Fever, variable clinical features ▪ Variable symptom onset ▪ Variable skin manifestations ▪ Dyspnea, often with distinct infiltrates on chest radiography ▪ Thrombocytopenia; occasional mucous membrane bleeding ▪ Hypotension-related oliguria and elevated creatinine ▪ Hypotension-related hepatomegaly, elevated aminotransferases	▪ Fever, sudden onset, often high and continuous ▪ Sudden symptom onset over 24–48 h near engraftment period ▪ Erythema with or without pruritic total body rash ▪ Dyspnea; bilateral diffuse alveolar infiltrates on chest radiography ▪ Gastrointestinal bleeding ▪ Unprecipitated oliguria, elevated creatinine, hematuria ▪ Unprecipitated hepatomegaly, elevated aminotransferases

Diagnostic Studies. Leukostasis may be suspected in high-risk groups but the diagnosis is primarily made on the basis of clinical manifestations. In many instances, the existence of pathophysiological complications such as infarction or stroke may validate the presumed diagnosis. Patients have specific diagnostic tests performed to assess their presenting symptoms. Chest radiography is often sufficient to diagnosis pulmonary leukostasis. A head computed tomography (CT) scan may reveal neurological leukostasis. Ultrasonography and magnetic resonance imaging (MRI) may also be performed. In pulmonary leukostasis, ABG results are used with a clear understanding of their diagnostic limitations.

Management

In leukostasis, the preferred management is to identify high-risk or early symptomatic patients and perform leukapheresis before the cells cause organ damage. Therapeutic leukapheresis removes 20,000 to 40,000 white blood cells per treatment, and once- or twice-daily treatments are often required until the white blood cell count is less than 30,000 to 40,000/mm^3.[28] If leukapheresis cannot be performed immediately, large amounts of IV fluids should be administered to dilute the blood and enhance renal excretion of metabolic toxins. If leukapheresis is still not possible within a 12- to 24-hour period, and the patient's symptoms continue to worsen, exchange transfusions may be used.[29]

Many patients also receive immediate concomitant chemotherapy to prevent rapid cell regrowth or spontaneous tumor lysis syndrome with renal failure.[30] If possible, it is preferred to complete the necessary leukapheresis cycles before starting chemotherapy; however, many patients are too sick for such treatment. When this occurs, the critical care nurse must administer antimicrobial agents or chemotherapy between leukapheresis or continuous renal replacement therapy (CRRT). Low-dose cranial radiation (100 to 300 Gy) was once believed to stabilize cell membranes and destroy malignant cells, but this practice is now not recommended.[27,28] Patients with leukostasis receive supportive drug therapy with agents such as antimicrobials, diuretics, bronchodilators, and allopurinol, which are aimed at stabilizing their symptoms.

It is important to recognize interventions that worsen the hyperviscosity of leukostasis and avoid these actions. Patients with acute leukemia are often anemic, but blood products should be administered with extreme caution and in combination with crystalloid fluids to avoid increased blood viscosity. Diuretics may be given to enhance renal excretion of uric acid associated with tumor cells lysis, but also only in combination with crystalloid fluids to maintain normal vascular osmolarity. Supportive interventions to reduce intracranial hemorrhage may include elevating the head of the bed and administering corticosteroids. Box 48-8 lists nursing interventions aimed at reducing the risk of leukostasis-related complications.

Complications

Even in the face of appropriate, definitive treatment, patients with leukostasis may experience stroke, respiratory failure, bowel infarction, renal failure, or myocardial infarction. In many, some degree of reversible organ ischemia develops, requiring supportive treatment.[27]

Anatomical–Structural Complications

CARDIAC TAMPONADE

Cardiac tamponade is the result of accumulation of excess pericardial fluid or the presence of a tumor that compresses the heart. At autopsy, as much as 20% of people with cancer are found to have cardiac or pericardial metastases.

Pathophysiology

The pericardium is a double-walled sac that surrounds the heart and great vessels. A visceral layer lines the surface of the heart and the parietal layer (or outer layer) moves freely. The pericardium supports the heart in a stable position and provides a frictionless sac for cardiac contractions. The pericardial cavity lies between the two layers and contains 10 to 50 mL of serous fluid.

Neoplastic cardiac tamponade results from the formation and accumulation of excessive amounts of fluid in the pericardial sac. This emergent condition may also be caused by encasement of the heart by tumor or postradiation pericarditis. The severity of the tamponade is in direct proportion to the rate of fluid formation and the volume of fluid accumulated. Slow accumulation may stretch the pericardium so that cardiac contractility is not adversely affected for months. Normal diastolic filling is impaired by elevated pericardial pressures, and stroke volume is reduced. As stroke volume continues to fall, hypotension, compensatory tachycardia, and equalization and elevation of the mean left atrial, pulmonary arterial and venous, right atrial, and vena caval pressures occur. In an attempt to

box 48-8 nursing interventions for *Leukostasis*

- Recognize patients at risk for leukostasis—acute myelocytic leukemia (with circulating blasts), white blood cell count >100,000/mm^3, renal dysfunction, dehydration.
- Administer large volumes of intravenous fluids to dilute cells and aid excretion of lysis components.
- Perform leukapheresis as soon as possible.
- Treat organ system–specific leukostatic symptoms (e.g., elevation of head of bed, bronchodilators).
- Administer corticosteroids to reduce inflammatory cytokine symptoms.
- Administer blood components cautiously early in the disease when hyperviscosity is problematic.
- Plan assessment interventions aimed at monitoring for ischemia or infarction of the body organs.

maintain arterial pressure, increase blood volume, and improve venous return, tachycardia and peripheral vasoconstriction develop. If the tamponade goes undiagnosed or untreated, circulatory collapse ensues.

Cancers of the esophagus or lung grow by direct extension into the pericardium, whereas distant primary cancers (e.g., renal cell) metastasize to the pericardium through the bloodstream. Large chest tumors may also cause pericardial effusion due to lymphatic obstruction of pericardial fluid recirculation. The primary tumors most commonly associated with pericardial effusion are tumors of the breast, lung, or esophagus, lymphoma, gastrointestinal carcinomas, melanoma, sarcoma, and leukemia. Radiation pericarditis may be a causative factor, especially if the patient's heart was in the treatment field and if the total dose of radiation to this field exceeded 4,000 rad (40 Gy). Biotherapeutic agents such as interleukin-2 (Aldesleukin) and interferon alfa cause increased capillary permeability and clinically significant pericardial effusions.

Assessment

History. Signs and symptoms reflect the rapidity with which the fluid accumulates in the pericardial sac, and in the patient with cancer, are mainly those of right-sided heart failure due to slow accumulation. Signs of tamponade include rapid, weak pulse; distant heart sounds; distended neck veins during inspiration (Kussmaul's sign); pulsus paradoxus (inspiratory decrease in arterial blood pressure of more than 10 mm Hg from baseline); ankle or sacral edema; edema; ascites; hepatosplenomegaly; hepatojugular reflex; lethargy; and altered level of consciousness. The patient may complain of dyspnea, cough, and retrosternal pain that is relieved by leaning forward. On occasion, a patient with a large effusion experiences epigastric pain, hiccups, hoarseness, nausea, and vomiting.

Diagnostic Studies. A variety of studies are used to determine the presence and severity of cardiac tamponade. A chest film is used to determine the presence of cardiac enlargement, mediastinal widening, or hilar adenopathy. The electrocardiogram (ECG) may show nonspecific abnormalities, including low QRS complex voltage in limb leads, sinus tachycardia, precordial ST segment elevations, and T-wave changes. Echocardiography is the most sensitive and most specific noninvasive test for the presence of tamponade and is used routinely in most settings. Two distinct echoes may be identified, one from effusion and the other from the posterior heart border. Spaces between these echoes indicate the size of the effusion or the thickness of the pericardium. Catheterization of the right side of the heart reveals pericardial tamponade or constriction but is performed infrequently because echocardiograms are routinely available. Pericardiocentesis gives a positive cytological result in the patient with metastatic cancer.

Management

First, volume expansion is necessary because it increases venous pressure so that it is greater than pericardial pressure, allowing increased venous return and improved cardiac output. Oxygen should be administered, although assisted or mechanical ventilation may increase thoracic pressures, further impeding venous return and worsening the tamponade.

The definitive treatment for pericardial effusion is fluid drainage. Acute or life-threatening symptoms are indications for emergent pericardial drainage by needle or catheter *pericardiocentesis* (Box 48-9). Without definitive treatment to alleviate the fluid in the pericardium, cardiac arrest will occur. Tamponade is likely to recur in 24 to 48 hours if treatment to prevent pericardial fluid reaccumulation is not initiated quickly.

Factors to be considered when selecting a therapeutic option include the sensitivity of the primary tumor to specific treatment modalities, previous treatment, and the patient's life expectancy. If effective drugs are available (e.g., as in lymphoma and small cell lung cancer), systemic chemotherapy may be initiated after the patient is clinically stable. This treatment may also be effective in patients with leukemia, lymphoma, and breast cancer who have pericardial effusion. In radiosensitive tumors such as lymphoma and breast cancer, radiation therapy may be the treatment of choice. Radiation therapy has been reported to control more than 50% of malignant pericardial effusions.[32] Insertion of a pericardial catheter guided by fluoroscopy or echocardiography to permit rapid fluid drainage is often the preferred immediate treatment. The catheter may be left in place while anticancer therapy is initiated. Pericardial sclerosis through the pericardial catheter, which is rarely used, can control tamponade by causing adherence of the two pericardial layers and inhibiting fluid accumulation.

In patients with a longer life expectancy and adequate performance status, an inferior pericardiotomy may be performed thoracoscopically. In this procedure, a pleural–pericardial window is created, which provides immediate relief of cardiac compression and tissue specimens for histological diagnosis. Fewer than 5% of patients have recurrence of symptoms after this procedure. Pericardectomy is performed if radiation-induced pericardial disease is not responsive to conservative medical management. This procedure should not be performed if an extensive pericardial tumor is present because surgical morbidity and mortality rates are high.

CAROTID ARTERY RUPTURE

Carotid artery rupture (or "blowout") is caused by tumor erosion or rupture of the carotid artery. Such rupture results in the loss of large amounts of blood that, without rapid intervention, becomes life-threatening hemorrhage. Patients at risk for this oncological emergency are primarily those with cancer of the head and neck, especially after surgery or radiation, or with a wound infection. Affected

box 48-9 ***Signs and Symptoms of Neoplastic Cardiac Tamponade***

The life-threatening symptoms listed indicate the need for emergent pericardial drainage.

- Cyanosis, dyspnea with hypoxemia, impaired consciousness, or shock
- Pulsus paradoxus >50% of the pulse pressure
- Decrease >20 mm Hg in pulse pressure
- Peripheral venous pressure >13 mm Hg

patients occasionally have thyroid cancer, lymphoma, or melanoma. Patients with a palpable pulse on top of a tumor, or in close proximity to it, have a greater risk of carotid vessel erosion.

Pathophysiology

Rupture of a carotid artery is likely to occur when that vessel is weakened by invasion of tumor or by surgical manipulation. Other causes of vessel weakness include simultaneous infection or skin flap necrosis.

Assessment

The rupture of the artery may occur suddenly with forceful expulsion of large volumes of blood from the damaged vessel; however, the first sign of erosion or rupture usually is a small trickle of blood from the neck area or unexplained oral bleeding. If the skin over the artery is intact, the patient may have darkened or ecchymotic skin changes, swelling, difficulty swallowing or breathing, retrosternal or high epigastric chest pain, and mental status changes. A unilateral headache or visual disturbance may also signal carotid artery bleeding. Box 48-10 lists the cardinal signs and symptoms of carotid artery rupture.

Management

Patients identified as high risk for carotid artery rupture may have vascular stents placed during surgery as a preventive measure. In addition, IV access should be in place, and blood should be typed and available for immediate transfusion.[29]

Gauze, irrigation saline, and vascular clamps should be readily available at all times. Constant digital pressure with saline-soaked cotton dressing wrapped around the two middle fingers and applied directly to the area over the artery is the first emergency intervention in suspected carotid artery rupture. The nurse must not lessen pressure to see whether the bleeding has stopped or attempt to apply a hemostat. Either of these steps increases the likelihood of further blood loss. Maintenance of the airway is essential. Only after the patient is in the operative suite and the operative area has been prepared should the pressure be released. The surgical treatment of choice is ligation of the damaged artery. Embolization or stent placement may be alternatives. Chapter 22 contains a detailed discussion of carotid artery surgery with assessment and nursing care.

Complications

The overall mortality rate of carotid artery rupture is 40% to 60%.[33] About 60% of patients who survive this complication have long-term neurological deficits, the most common of which is hemiparesis. The risk of hemiparesis is reduced by the prevention of shock and replacement of fluid for adequate perfusion of the brain through the opposite internal carotid artery.

box 48-10 ***Cardinal Signs and Symptoms of Carotid Artery Rupture***

- Oozing blood from neck wound
- Unexplained oral bleeding
- Ecchymoses over neck region
- Sudden neck edema
- Retrosternal or epigastric chest pain
- Sense of impending doom, anxiety, or restlessness

HEPATIC VENO-OCCLUSIVE DISEASE

Hepatic veno-occlusive disease, occlusion of the venous vessels of the liver, is a recently identified complication of high-dose radiation therapy and chemotherapy. Its incidence is as low as 5% to 10% in some chemotherapy and monoclonal antibody regimens but as high as 60% in some patients receiving blood and marrow transplants.[34] Hepatic veno-occlusive disease is most likely to develop in patients receiving high-dose alkylating agents (e.g., cyclophosphamide, busulfan) or abdominal radiation, although the disease also occurs in patients receiving the leukemic monoclonal antibody gemtuzumab (Mylotarg).[35] Other risk factors are extensive pretreatment in patients with cancer, older age, and previous history of hepatitis.[36]

Pathophysiology

Through uncertain mechanisms, etiological agents cause fibrotic changes in the endothelial layer that lines the walls of the veins and sinusoids in the liver, resulting in narrowed and stiff-walled venules that have a tendency for thrombosis. Venous flow through the liver is reduced, and there is congestion and eventual pressure-related hepatic damage.

Assessment

History. The earliest manifestations of hepatic veno-occlusive disease are fluid retention, elevated serum bilirubin, and nonspecific abdominal pain. The onset of these symptoms occurs an average of 8 to 20 days after therapy; the time varies with the causative agent.[36] The clinical course begins primarily as one of portal hypertension with ascites, painful hepatomegaly, and right-sided heart failure; it progresses over 1 to 3 weeks to include hepatic destruction with coagulopathies, thrombocytopenia, hyperammonemia, metabolic alkalosis, increased vagal tone, and hepatorenal failure.[34] Box 48-11 lists early and late

box 48-11 ***Signs and Symptoms of Hepatic Veno-occlusive Disease***

Early Findings

- Weight gain
- Fluid retention, edema
- Painful hepatomegaly
- Increased total and direct bilirubin
- Increased aspartate aminotransferase and alkaline phosphatase

Late Findings

- Coagulopathies, thrombocytopenia
- Hyperammonemia
- Metabolic alkalosis
- Hepatorenal syndrome
- Right-sided heart failure
- Elevated aminotransferases
- Increased vagal tone

clinical findings in hepatic veno-occlusive disease. Most patients with hepatic veno-occlusive disease have mild, reversible disease, and only 10% to 20% have severe, life-threatening manifestations.[37]

Diagnostic Studies. The first and most specific diagnostic test is the elevation of total and indirect bilirubin.[36] Aspartate transaminase (AST; previously known as serum glutamic oxaloacetic transaminase [SGOT]) and alkaline phosphatase also increase early, and when progressive liver failure develops, hepatic aminotransferases also increase. Abdominal ultrasonography confirms hepatic enlargement and is used to rule out causal conditions such as cholestasis and hepatic abscess.[38,39] Once a cholestatic process has been ruled out, diagnosis is made based on clinical findings and development of progressive hepatic and renal dysfunction.

In late or severe disease, the platelet count decreases, and coagulation studies such as prothrombin time (PT) or partial thromboplastin time (PTT) are prolonged. A definitive diagnosis may be made only on the basis of liver biopsy. When it is necessary to differentiate hepatic veno-occlusive disease from other clinically similar processes, such as graft-versus-host disease (GVHD), a liver biopsy may be performed; it shows venule fibrosis.[40]

Management

Because the pathological mechanisms of hepatic veno-occlusive disease are uncertain, therapy is still presumptive and not clearly effective. Once hepatic veno-occlusive disease is suspected, supportive therapies such as balancing fluid administration and diuresis are implemented. Transjugular intrahepatic portosystemic shunt (TIPS) procedures have been used in an attempt to enhance portal blood outflow.[41,42] Patients may require platelet transfusions, vasopressors, and ammonia-lowering therapies, such as lactulose. Modest reports of successful symptom resolution have been noted with high-dose methylprednisolone,[43] glutamine with high-dose vitamin E,[44] ursodiol,[44,45] and tissue plasminogen activator.[37,45] Renal replacement therapy is often required; continuous venovenous hemofiltration is often the preferred method of therapy because of increased vagal tone and a tendency for vasodilatory hypotension. Some experts advocate early implementation to preserve renal function and reduce the need for respiratory support. Before the advent of CRRT, patients often required mechanical ventilation to control fluid imbalance–induced respiratory distress.

No methods to prevent hepatic veno-occlusive disease have yet proved successful. Use of low-dose heparin subcutaneously or intravenously is being studied as a potential preventive agent to prevent hepatic veno-occlusive disease.[44,46] Defibrotide is also a subject of research.[43,47,48]

Complications

Patients with mild to moderate hepatic veno-occlusive disease experience complete reversal of the pathological process. It is uncertain whether supportive therapies have any influence on this outcome. Well-controlled studies clearly show that patients with total bilirubin levels greater than 15 to 18 mg/dL have a high mortality rate.

SUPERIOR VENA CAVA SYNDROME

Superior vena cava syndrome (SVCS)—obstruction of the superior vena cava—results in venous blockage that produces pleural effusion and facial, arm, and tracheal edema. Severe obstruction may result in impaired cardiac filling and cerebral edema.

Pathophysiology

The superior vena cava is a thin-walled, low-pressure blood vessel in the mediastinal cavity that collects blood from the venous vessels that drain the head and neck and the upper thoracic cavity. The mediastinum is a rigid anatomical structure that contains the trachea, the vertebral column, the sternum and ribs, and the lymph nodes.

Most cases of SVCS result from mediastinal malignancies or involved lymph nodes that cause extrinsic compression or invade the vessel.[49] More than 75% of cases are secondary to small cell or squamous cell lung cancers, and 10% to 15% are secondary to mediastinal lymphomas. Obstruction of the vessel lumen by a thrombus may also occur; it is most commonly caused by a central venous catheter or a hypercoagulability syndrome due to cancer. Causes of SVCS are summarized in Box 48-12.

Assessment

History. Signs and symptoms of SVCS depend on the rapidity of compression of the superior vena cava. If it is compressed gradually and collateral circulation develops, indications of SVCS may be more subtle. Initial symptoms are most prominent in the early morning and include periorbital and conjunctival edema, facial swelling, and Stokes' sign (tightness of the shirt collar). These signs may disappear after the patient has been upright for a few hours. The patient may also complain of visual disturbances and headache. Altered consciousness and focal neurological signs may result from brain edema and impaired cardiac filling. Late signs and symptoms include distension of the veins of the thorax and upper extremities, dysphagia, dyspnea, cough, hoarseness, and tachypnea. All patients, including children, most commonly visit health care providers because of dyspnea. Box 48-13 describes special considerations in the pediatric population.

box 48-12
Risk Factors for Superior Vena Cava Syndrome

- Chest, neck, or epigastric tumors (e.g., lung cancer, breast cancer, lymphoma, head and neck cancer, thyroid cancer, gastric cancer, esophageal cancer, pancreatic cancer, metastatic renal cell cancer, metastatic colorectal cancer, melanoma)
- Devices in the superior vena cava (e.g., large-bore, multilumen central lines, especially if placed in the subclavian site)
- Hypercoagulability syndromes (disseminated intravascular coagulation, hypercoagulability of malignancy [e.g., mucin-producing adenocarcinomas, brain tumors, Trousseau's syndrome])

box 48-13

Oncological Emergencies: Considerations for the Pediatric Patient

Children presenting with large mediastinal tumors (usually lymphoma) and respiratory distress are often presumed to have a disorder known as *superior mediastinal syndrome* (SMS), which involves obstruction of both the superior vena cava and the major airways. Children's relative size, the flexibility of their airways, and a propensity for airway edema result in an increased risk for this syndrome. SMS in children signifies a heightened sense of emergency compared with the same disease does in adults. Because of the tumor and the respiratory distress, compression of the superior vena cava and large airways produces profound dyspnea. Symptoms of SMS in children are similar to those in adults and include cough, hoarseness, orthopnea, and chest pain. Neurological symptoms such as anxiety, confusion, headache, visual disturbances, and syncope are considered serious signs of altered brain perfusion and warrant emergent management.

From National Institutes of Health, National Cancer Institute. Available at www.thecancerweb.com/lung/svc.htm, revised February, 1999.

Diagnostic Studies. Until recently, diagnostic evaluation required multiple tests to validate the location, size, and vena cava involvement of tumors or thrombus. Conventional chest CT with IV contrast, venography, angiography, and radionuclide scans were used. Currently, the spiral CT scan with contrast, which provides accurate information about tumor location and involvement of the vena cava, may be the only diagnostic test performed.[49] However, biopsy or cytological tests may be required to establish a diagnosis in many patients because this syndrome is the presenting symptom at the time of diagnosis of cancer.

Management

The primary treatment of choice for SVCS caused by a tumor is radiation therapy. Dosage depends on the size of the tumor and its radiosensitivity. Radiation therapy is initially given in high daily fractions (total dose of 30 to 50 rads), and symptom relief occurs in 7 to 14 days. Radiation therapy is palliative for SVCS in 70% of patients with lung cancer and for more than 95% of patients with lymphoma. Radiation of the mediastinal, hilar, and supraclavicular lymph nodes and any adjacent parenchymal lesions is appropriate in patients with locally advanced non–small cell lung cancer.

Patients who receive radiation therapy experience increased cough within 3 days of the start of therapy. During the initial 7 to 10 days, secretions are increased because of inflammation, but a dry irritation then develops, resulting in a dry, hacking cough with few secretions but possible bleeding.

Chemotherapy may be the treatment of choice for SVCS in patients with disseminated disease, such as small cell anaplastic carcinoma or lymphoma. The agents used most often include high-dose regimens containing cyclophosphamide, cisplatin, bleomycin, and doxorubicin. The adverse effects of these agents include bone marrow suppression, cardiac toxicity, and renal dysfunction.

Treatment of SVCS caused by a thrombus around a central venous catheter may include antifibrinolytics or anticoagulants and possibly surgical removal of the catheter. In any case, chest and neck central venous catheter placements should be avoided until effective treatment has been delivered.

In some circumstances, the placement of stents or vascular grafts in the superior vena cava provides immediate symptomatic relief while patients receive definitive therapy.[49] It is unclear whether long-term anticoagulation is required.

Supportive care of the patient is essential. Maintenance of a patent airway is of the highest priority. Because many patients have severe dyspnea, they are unable to lie flat for their radiation therapy, and short-term airway intubation may be required. Oxygen therapy, diuretics, steroids, and heparin may be prescribed and must be administered with careful observation of patient response. If necessary, corticosteroids are administered for 3 to 7 days to decrease the edema associated with the disease and treatment. The patient should be taught not to bend over and to avoid Valsalva maneuvers. When the patient is in bed, the head should be at least in a semi-Fowler's position. Elevation of the patient's arms on pillows helps alleviate swelling; however, the legs should not be elevated because this increases fluid volume in the torso.

Complications

Several complications may occur in patients with SVCS. Right-sided heart failure is the most common complication. Such heart failure is usually self-limiting and is treated symptomatically with fluid restrictions, diuretics, and digoxin. Vessel rupture in SVCS when a tumor invades the vena cava is a great risk because the tumor shrinks with treatment. The incidence of vessel rupture is highest in patients with esophageal and lung cancer; peak incidence is 3 to 4 weeks after initiation of therapy. Warning signs of vessel rupture are acute and sudden dyspnea, hypoxia, cough, and vascular collapse. Radiation pneumonitis, an inflammatory response in the radiation field that correlates with breath sound and radiographic changes reflective of alveolar capillary permeability, may occur in patients who receive chest radiation for SVCS. Treatment of radiation pneumonitis involves corticosteroids and supportive therapy. SVCS recurs in 10% to 30% of patients.[49]

PLEURAL EFFUSION

Pathophysiology

There is normally 30 to 150 mL of fluid between the visceral and parietal pleura that helps maintain a negative pleural pressure to facilitate lung expansion with minimum work of breathing. A pleural effusion is excess accumulation of fluid in the pleural space with subsequent impaired lung expansion and hypoxemia. When lymphatic obstruction (particularly of the thoracic duct), venous congestion, pleural inflammation, or excess capillary permeability occurs, the amount of fluid increases or does not drain properly. Although many nonmalignant conditions (e.g., congestive heart failure, hypothyroidism) may cause pleural effusion, malignant conditions involving lymphatic obstruction or infiltration with malignant cells may also have the same result. Pleural effusions that occur due to volume overload, capillary permeability, or lymphatic obstruction produce a transudate characterized by the presence of albumin and the absence of cell fragments or enzymes in the pleural fluid. Malignant cell infiltration causes pleural inflammation and exudates characterized by the release of red blood cells, white blood cells, and lactate dehydrogenase into the pleural fluid. As much as 15% of patients with cancer experience pleural effusions during the course of their disease.[50]

Accumulation of pleural fluid leads to increased (more positive) pleural pressure. Higher pleural pressures increase the work of breathing, and collapsed alveoli cause decreased gas exchange and hypoxemia.

Assessment

History. The clinical findings in pleural effusion are related to the two major physiological mechanisms: increased work of breathing and alveolar collapse. Excess pleural pressures decrease lung compliance ("stiff lungs"). Patients feel short of breath and must use their accessory muscles to breathe, and chest excursion on the affected side is reduced. When patients are in an upright position, fluids are pulled down by the force of gravity, and breath sounds are diminished to the level of fluid. The pleural fluid takes up space in the chest, impeding lung expansion with consequent alveolar collapse. Symptoms that relate to this pathological process are diminished breath sounds, tracheal shift away from the effusion, and signs of hypoxemia (e.g., dyspnea, anxiety, confusion, oliguria, decreased bowel sounds).

Diagnostic Studies. The first diagnostic test performed to confirm the presence of pleural effusion is an upright chest radiograph. The fluid accumulates in the lower lung, causing a blunted diaphragmatic dome and decreased radiolucence in the lower lung. Fluid accumulation often produces a meniscus of decreased radiolucence and a thickened lateral pleural lining, indicating fluid tracking up the side. After a pleural effusion is confirmed, a cytological evaluation is performed by extracting a sample of fluid and sending it for fluid chemistry and cytology. Pleural fluid is categorized as transudative or exudative, which provides clues to the cause of the effusion. Cytological studies confirm the presence or absence of malignant cells, which influences treatment decisions.

Management

The treatment of pleural effusion depends on the etiological mechanism, rapidity of symptom onset, and degree of respiratory compromise. When pleural effusions are small or have a nonmalignant cause, observation without definitive treatment may be indicated. Aggressive antineoplastic therapy may be indicated when a large tumor causes lymphatic obstruction, heart failure, or pneumonitis that in turn causes pleural effusion.

When malignant cells are present in the pleural fluid, management may be determined by overall treatment goals. Repeated therapeutic thoracenteses are often the preferred choice; this assumes that the ultimate cause of the pleural effusion is being treated or that the patient's life expectancy does not warrant more interventional measures.

When the patient's life expectancy is longer, and the pleural effusions do not resolve with anticancer therapy and intermittent thoracenteses, the preferred treatment is pleurodesis through a chest catheter. Pleurodesis, also called *pleural sclerosing,* involves intrapleural administration of a chemical (e.g., doxycycline, bleomycin) or a mechanical agent (e.g., talc slurry) to alter the pH of the pleural fluid and cause inflammatory adherence of the visceral and parietal pleura to each other. Sclerosed pleura do not have the normal lubricating pleural fluid, and restrictive lung disease is the long-term consequence. Pleurodesis is successful only about 67% of the time, necessitating the availability of additional treatment options. Box 48-14 presents nursing interventions related to the management of pleurodesis.

Pleurectomy is a thoracic surgical procedure that removes the entire pleura. Pleurectomy is effective but can be difficult to perform when long-term inflammation and pleurodesis attempts cause a friable pleura that is not easily separated. Chronic, long-term pleuroperitoneal shunts or implanted access devices have been used, but development of fibrin sheaths on the catheters often causes occlusion. Newer, small-bore chest catheters that permit home

box 48-14 nursing interventions for *Pleurodesis*

- Be certain pleural drainage from chest tube in previous 24 h is <150 mL.
- Obtain sclerosing agent (bleomycin, doxycycline, or talc slurry) and postsclerosing flush solution (preservative-free sterile water or normal saline or lidocaine [Xylocaine] 1% or 2%).
- Plan to inject sclerosing agent into the chest drainage tube.
- Set up an extra Pleur-Evac with tubing to connect if tubing leaks after injecting sclerosing agent.
- Clamp tubing for 4–6 h after instillation of sclerosing agent.
- Have patient be as mobile as possible, but scheduled body rotation is not necessary to ensure distribution of the agent throughout the pleura.
- Unclamp chest tube and observe drainage (effective 67%–70% of time). If effective, drainage is minimal to absent.
- Assist with removal of chest tube and monitor patient for air tracking and pneumothorax, or reaccumulation of fluid.

drainage of the pleural fluid have recently become available. Box 48-15 summarizes home care considerations for patients with malignant pleural effusions.

Complications

Untreated pleural effusions that continue to accumulate lead to clinically significant alveolar collapse and respiratory failure, which may be caused by loss of gas-exchanging airways or mediastinal shifting with major airway obstruction. Progressive hypoxemia leads to profound respiratory acidosis and ischemic organ failure.

SPINAL CORD COMPRESSION

Spinal cord compression occurs when tumor cells or collapsed vertebrae in the epidural space exert pressure on the spinal cord, which may result in permanent dysfunction (including paralysis) if not diagnosed and treated promptly. Epidural tumors have been found in more than 5% of patients with metastatic disease at autopsy.

Pathophysiology

Two major pathophysiological mechanisms are likely to result in spinal cord compression: (1) tumors arising within the epidural space through vertebral or lymphatic spread, and (2) bony metastasis causing vertebral collapse with spinal cord and nerve root compression. Permanent neurological damage from proximal tumors may also occur if spinal circulation is compromised such as in prolonged ischemia or hemorrhage. Other disorders producing signs and symptoms of cord compression are paraneoplastic syndromes, radiation myelopathy, herpes zoster, pain from a pelvic or long bone metastasis, or cytotoxic drug effects. Tumors most likely to cause cord compression and the location of compression are noted in Table 48-10.

box 48-15
Oncological Emergencies: Pleural Effusions

Malignant pleural effusions are a common cause of severe debilitating disease and impaired quality of life in patients with end-stage cancer. Effectiveness of pleurodesis is only 65% to 70%; many patients do not achieve resolution of their pleural effusions with standard therapy. Multiple devices such as pleuroperitoneal shunts or access ports inserted into the pleural space have been used to permit home drainage of pleural effusions, with limited success. Newer, small-bore thoracostomy catheters have now been developed that permit these patients to return to their homes with a comfortable chest catheter drainage system. Small-bore thoracostomy tubes are connected to a one-way valve similar to the flutter valve, and a drainage bag that resembles a Foley catheter drainage bag.

From Sahin U, Unlu M, Akkaya A, et al: The value of small-bore catheter thoracostomy in the treatment of malignant pleural effusions. Respiration 68(5):501–505, 2001.

Assessment

History. When a primary tumor presses on the spinal cord, signs and symptoms usually develop slowly. Problems develop more rapidly with metastatic disease. Most patients with spinal cord compression complain of progressive central or radicular back pain that often is aggravated by weight bearing, lying down, coughing, sneezing, or performing the Valsalva maneuver. The pain is relieved by sitting.

The earliest neurological symptoms are sensory changes, such as numbness, paresthesia, and coldness. Compression occurs most often in the thoracic section of the spinal cord, causing neurogenic bladder with urinary retention and incontinence. Patients may also lose the urge to defecate and be unable to bear down. Men on occasion lose the ability to have or maintain an erection. Metastases to the cauda equina frequently produce impaired urethral, vaginal, and rectal sensations; bladder dysfunction; decreased sensation in the lumbosacral dermatomes; and saddle anesthesia. Box 48-16 describes spinal cord considerations in the older adult.

The level of cord compression can be determined by the patient's report of pain during straight leg raising, neck flexion, or vertebral percussion. The upper limit of the sensory level is usually one or two vertebral bodies below the site of compression. Lessened rectal tone and perineal sensation are observed with autonomic dysfunction. Deep tendon reflexes can be brisk with cord compression and diminished with nerve root compression.

Once patients experience pain, motor weakness and ataxia often follow. They may complain that the arms or legs feel heavy. Some patients lose the ability to sense light touch, pain, and temperature. Over time, weakness may progress to spasm, paralysis, and muscle atrophy; sensations of deep pressure and position may disappear.

Diagnostic Studies. MRI is highly sensitive for neurological tissues and can clearly demonstrate all epidural deposits as well as complete or partial block of the spinal cord. Therefore, it is the diagnostic test of choice. A myelogram or CT scan may reveal spinal tumors, but these studies are less sensitive for diagnosing the presence and extent of cord compression. Lumbar puncture is used to obtain cerebrospinal fluid, which reveals malignant cells in the presence of epidural disease.

Management

Factors considered in the selection of the best therapeutic option are the level of cord compression, the rate of neurological deterioration, and previous use of radiation therapy. Corticosteroids are used to decrease peritumoral edema and neurological dysfunction. Dexamethasone 10 mg is administered to patients with neurological symptoms before emergency diagnostic procedures are performed and is continued during radiation therapy (4 to 20 mg every 6 hours) and then tapered. It is not clear whether such steroid therapy affects final patient outcome.

Radiation therapy is used when the tumor is determined to be radiosensitive and should be initiated as soon as the diagnosis of cord compression has been confirmed. Radiation portals include the entire area of blockage and two vertebral bodies above and below this area. More than 50%

table 48-10 Spinal Cord Compression: Etiology and Clinical Presentation

Location of Lesion	Common Malignant Etiologies	Physical Symptoms	Autonomic Symptoms
Cervical spine	• Head and neck cancers • Melanoma	• Radicular pain in the neck, occipital region, and shoulders (pain is often provoked by neck movement) • Quadriplegia • Upper extremity weakness (may be spastic or atrophic) • Sensory loss in area of weakness • Weakness or paralysis of the diaphragm may occur with lesion at or above C4 (may be unilateral or bilateral)	• Hypotension • Bradycardia • Loss of temperature autoregulation • Autonomic hyperreflexia • Gastric hypersecretion and paralytic ileus • Reflex bowel, bladder, and erection • Hoffman's sign (flicking of the middle finger induces flexion of the ipsilateral thumb or index finger)
Thoracic spine	• Breast cancer • Gastric cancer • Lung cancer • Lymphoma • Pancreatic cancer	• Pain (may be local, radicular, or both) • Paraplegia • Sensory loss below the level of the lesion • Reflex abnormalities distal to the lesion	• Venous stasis and associated complications • Reflex bowel, bladder, and penile erection
Lumbar spine	• Ovarian cancer • Renal cell cancer • Prostate cancer	• Bowel and bladder dysfunction • Extensor plantar response	• Venous stasis and associated complications • Reflex bowel, bladder, and penile erection
Cauda equina	• Bladder cancer • Prostate cancer	• Pain (may be local, referred, or radicular) • Sphincter disturbances • Loss of buttock and leg sensation • Lower extremity weakness/paralysis	• Areflexic bowel, bladder, and penile erection

of patients with rapid neurological deterioration improve with radiation therapy; however, patients with autonomic dysfunction or paraplegia have a poor prognosis with any therapy.

Laminectomy, with or without placement of stabilization rods in the nearby vertebral bodies, may result in immediate decompression of the spinal cord and nerve roots. The posterior approach is preferred but is often difficult because most metastases arise in the vertebral bodies anterior to the spinal cord. Anterior laminectomy is used for people in cases in which the tumor is believed to be resectable, making the clinical risks worth the aggressive surgical intervention. Postoperative radiation therapy is used to shrink residual tumor, relieve pain, and improve the patient's functional status. Surgery is usually contraindicated if there is a collapsed vertebral body or if there are several areas of cord compression. If there is no previous histological diagnosis of cancer or if infection or epidural hematoma must be ruled out, then laminectomy can be used for both diagnosis and treatment. If high cervical cord compression precludes surgery, the patient's neck should be stabilized in halo traction to prevent respiratory paralysis. If the patient continues to deteriorate neurologically despite high doses of steroids and radiation therapy, then emergency decompression should be attempted.

If the tumor is chemosensitive, chemotherapy may be administered concurrently with or soon after completion of radiation therapy or surgery. Chemotherapy may also be effective in patients with multiple myeloma who have had previous radiation therapy. Systemic chemotherapy or hormonal therapy may be used with certain types of tumors, such as lymphoma or prostatic cancer.

Pain management should include administration of appropriate analgesics, bed rest, and patient support during

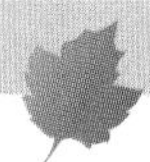

box 48-16

Spinal Cord Compression in the Older Patient

Signs and symptoms of spinal cord compression often begin as subtle and nonspecific back pain and sensory changes. The older patient may have concomitant diabetes mellitus or osteoarthritis that produces overlapping symptoms, delaying diagnosis of the oncological complication. In addition, older persons often have bowel and bladder changes causing constipation or urinary incontinence, mimicking the more serious autonomic changes that occur in later spinal cord compression. People at high risk for spinal cord compression, such as those with known bone metastases, should be taught the importance of reporting and having evaluated all back pain and sensory changes, especially in the lower extremities. In spinal cord compression, palpable vertebral tenderness is more often present than with other nononcologic disorders.

position changes and transfer. Range-of-motion exercises are useful in patients with motor and sensory deficits. Bowel retraining and intermittent urinary catheterization may be needed by the patient. Frequent skin care is essential. Surgical wounds are particularly susceptible to skin breakdown (with possible wound dehiscence) due to limited mobility and the effects of concomitant corticosteroid therapy.

TRACHEOBRONCHIAL OBSTRUCTION

Pathophysiology

Obstruction of the trachea or major branches of the bronchi with tumor results in respiratory distress and hypoxemia. The severity of symptoms depends on the rapidity of obstruction and degree of closure. Tumors most likely to cause airway obstruction are lung cancer and lymphoma, although other metastatic tumors (e.g., head and neck cancer, melanoma, breast cancer) and nonmalignant disorders such as amyloidosis or bronchomalacia may also cause airway obstruction.

Assessment

History. Patients with tracheobronchial obstruction present with varying degrees of dyspnea depending on the amount and location of the obstruction and the rapidity of onset. Some patients with slowly developing tumors have compensated respiratory acidosis and minimal symptoms even with near-complete obstruction. Other patients, especially those with lymphoma or small cell lung carcinoma, have rapidly growing tumors and severe symptoms even when the airway is less than 75% obstructed. Stridor is present in tracheal obstruction, and wheezing with unequal chest excursion is seen with bronchial obstruction.

Diagnostic Studies. Bronchoscopy makes it easy to detect tracheal or bronchial obstruction and grade its severity. However, bronchoscopy does not always reveal whether the airways are compressed extrinsically or invaded with tumor. Bronchoscopy is used in conjunction with spiral CT scans to provide a comprehensive description of the obstructive process that is used to guide therapy.

Management

Clinically significant obstruction of the major airways always requires immediate treatment, although the treatment plan varies according to tumor-specific factors and therapeutic goals. Laser therapy for tumors invading the major airways is highly effective in prolonging life as well as improving quality of life. Laser therapy is performed with a rigid bronchoscope under anesthesia, and patients usually experience a rapid recovery with little more than a sore throat and annoying cough for a few days afterward. Endobronchial brachytherapy involves endotracheal intubation with precisely directed radiation therapy through an endobronchial catheter. In both laser therapy and endobronchial brachytherapy, patients are observed closely for airway bleeding, and cough suppressants or low-dose corticosteroids may be prescribed to reduce the incidence of bleeding.

Airway opening with tracheal or bronchial stents may provide temporary symptomatic relief while definitive anticancer treatment is implemented for palliative relief of symptoms near the end of life. Airway stents are inserted using a rigid bronchoscope and light anesthesia, and multiple bronchoscopic procedures to assess or adjust placement are required. The most common problem with stents, especially if placed before shrinking the tumor, is displacement because the airway naturally opens with the reduction of tumor. Displaced stents usually cause severe and sudden respiratory distress and require immediate interventional adjustment. In rare circumstances, or when stenting is not possible, patient positioning to shift the chest tumor off the major airway (e.g., prone positioning) may provide temporary symptomatic relief while cancer therapy is used to shrink the tumor.

Complications

Two severe complications that may occur are total airway occlusion and hemorrhage caused by tumor erosion into the nearby pulmonary vessels. Total obstruction is treated the same way as partial obstruction when an improvement in symptoms can be reasonably expected as a result of therapy. Hemorrhage may be treated with embolization when recognized before massive bleeding occurs. If severe hemorrhage occurs, a dual-lumen endotracheal tube should be inserted and the bleeding lung occluded while ventilating the good lung until surgical repair can be performed. Airway obstruction may also lead to erosion through the airway and accompanying pneumothorax. In these circumstances, supportive therapy such as chest tube insertion may be used but is rarely helpful.

Metabolic Complications

HYPERCALCEMIA

Hypercalcemia exists when the corrected serum calcium level is above 11 mg/dL (normal range, 8.5 to 10.5 mg/dL). This oncological emergency develops when the bones release more calcium into the extracellular fluid than can be filtered by the kidneys and excreted in the urine.

Pathophysiology

Ninety-nine percent of the calcium in the body is in an insoluble form in the bones. The remaining 1% is freely exchangeable calcium. The calcium of importance is the ionized calcium, which must be maintained within a precise range. Serum calcium levels are regulated by parathyroid hormone and calcitonin. The release of parathyroid hormone from the parathyroid glands stimulates an increase in serum calcium levels, whereas the release of calcitonin produces a decrease in serum calcium levels.

Destruction of the bone by metastatic invasion is believed to be the most common cause of malignant hypercalcemia; however, 20% of patients with solid tumors usually associated with hypercalcemia do not show evidence of bony involvement. Certain humoral substances, such as parathyroid hormone–like substances or osteolytic prostaglandins, are secreted by tumor cells. In patients with multiple myeloma, osteoclast-activating factor (OAF) is produced by the abnormal plasma cells; however, hypercalcemia does not develop in these patients unless they have inadequate renal function. Patients with adult T-cell lymphoma have severe hypercalcemia related to the ectopic production of OAF, colony-stimulating factor, interferon gamma, and an active vitamin D metabolite. Additional causes of hypercalcemia in the presence of malignancy include immobilization, renal insufficiency, high dietary calcium or vitamin D intake, and low phosphate levels. Box 48-17 lists causes of hypercalcemia in malignancy.

Hypercalcemia develops in as much as 40% to 50% of women with metastatic breast cancer. There is a risk of bone metastasis, and estrogen and antiestrogens stimulate breast cancer cells to produce osteolytic prostaglandins and to increase bone resorption.

Assessment

History. The severity of signs and symptoms of hypercalcemia often correlates with the serum calcium level. Common presenting symptoms include nausea, constipation, polyuria, and mental status changes. Most patients present with somnolence, combativeness, or confusion.

Diagnostic Studies. Elevated serum calcium and elevated ionized calcium are the hallmark diagnostic findings in hypercalcemia. The serum calcium measurement is often reported as an absolute number without considering that only the calcium bound to albumin is counted. The serum calcium may be corrected for a low albumin by subtracting the patient's albumin from low normal, multiplying this number by a correction factor of 0.8, and adding this number to the reported calcium. Serum ionized calcium levels are accurate, but because the normal value is 1.0 mEq/L (± 0.02), it is a less sensitive indicator of clinically significant hypocalcemia.

In addition to increased calcium levels, there are also elevations in alkaline phosphatase and immunoreactive parathyroid hormone. Serum phosphate and serum potassium are decreased. Symptomatic patients usually have ECGs that show a bradycardia and prolonged PR, QRS, and QT intervals.

Management

Medical management of hypercalcemia involves the use of IV fluids and drug therapy to enhance renal excretion of calcium and to decrease bone resorption. Acute hypercalcemia is initially treated with IV 0.9% normal saline to dilute calcium levels and increase urinary calcium excretion. When hypercalcemia is life-threatening, aggressive hydration (250 to 300 mL/hour) and IV loop diuretics such as furosemide are prescribed.

Most patients are effectively treated with hydration, diuretics, appropriate antitumor therapy, and mobilization. Patients who are not responsive to these therapies must be maintained on hypocalcemic therapy indefinitely. Bisphosphonates are most frequently used to treat hypercalcemia. Currently, the most potent bisphosphonate available is zoledronic acid. It is administered as an 8-mg 15-minute IV infusion daily for 3 days unless serum calcium levels decrease before that time. Until recently, pamidronate has been the mainstay of bisphosphonate therapy, and it may still be preferred by some clinicians. It is usually given as a 90-mg, 24-hour infusion with continued hydration, possibly diuretics, and careful monitoring of calcium levels. However, because of clinical safety and efficacy studies, many clinicians give this dose over 90 to 120 minutes.

If possible, patients should ambulate to prevent osteolysis. Constipation, usually caused by an increased level of calcium in the blood, should be eliminated. Reduced oral intake of calcium or increased salt intake may be of some help. Medications such as thiazide diuretics and vitamins A and D should not be prescribed because they elevate the calcium level. Fluid status must be closely monitored. Patients may receive up to 10 L of IV fluids daily, and intake and output should be carefully measured. The patient should be carefully observed for signs of overhydration. Potassium supplements may be prescribed. Hypercalcemia is a common oncological emergency that can be prevented or diminished in a large number of patients with the appropriate education and precautions. A teaching guide for patients with hypercalcemia is presented in Box 48-18.

Complications

Permanent renal tubular abnormalities may develop in patients with prolonged hypercalcemia. Sudden death from cardiac dysrhythmias may result from an acute increase in serum calcium.

box 48-17
Causes of Hypercalcemia in Malignancy

- Bone demineralization due to bone metastases (most common in breast cancer, colorectal cancer, renal cell cancer)
- Tumor production of a parathormone-like substance (thyroid cancer, multiple myeloma, leukemia, lymphoma, gastric cancer, pancreatic cancer, lung cancer)
- Renal insufficiency
- Immobilization
- Dehydration

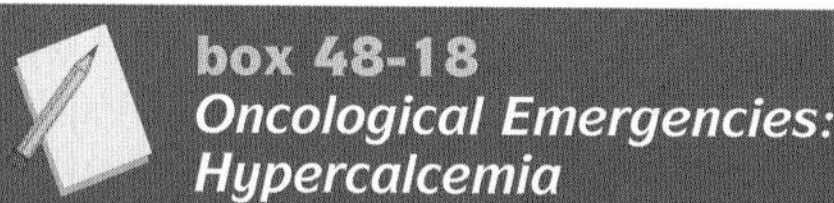

box 48-18
Oncological Emergencies: Hypercalcemia

Patients at high risk for malignancy-associated hypercalcemia include those with:
- Bone metastases (most common in breast, lung, and colon cancer)
- Lung cancer
- Gastrointestinal cancers (gastric, pancreatic, colon)
- Hematological cancers (leukemia, lymphoma, multiple myeloma)
- Renal (kidney) cancer
- Thyroid cancer

Other factors that increase the risk of developing hypercalcemia include:
- Lack of physical activity
- Low fluid status
- Poor kidney function

Suggestions for prevention of hypercalcemia include:
- Drink at least six to eight glasses of water every day
- Eat salty foods
- Remain physically active
- Limit dairy products and vitamin D–enriched foods such as milk, cheese, and yogurt

SYNDROME OF INAPPROPRIATE ANTIDIURETIC HORMONE SECRETION

The syndrome of inappropriate antidiuretic hormone secretion (SIADH) is a clinical disorder characterized by excess stimulation of pituitary excretion of antidiuretic hormone (ADH). Under normal circumstances, the posterior pituitary gland releases ADH in response to changes in plasma osmolality (concentration of solutes) and circulating blood volume. ADH release causes decreased urine production and volume and increased water resorption. SIADH has several specific causes related to cancer and its treatment. The clinical consequences of SIADH and its management strategies are discussed in Chapter 44.

Pathophysiology

When thoracic or mediastinal tumors press on major cardiac vessels, the obstruction may impede cardiac output. The posterior pituitary gland perceives this to be a fall in circulatory volume and compensates by inappropriately secreting ADH, which in turn suppresses urinary output. The resulting volume expansion improves cardiac output but leaves the patient with a relative sodium deficit (dilutional hyponatremia).

In addition to the pressure of thoracic or mediastinal tumors on cardiac vessels, SIADH can also be precipitated by the cancers and treatment-related factors. Small cell lung cancers release an ADH-like substance. Certain chemotherapeutic agents, such as cyclophosphamide and vincristine, as well as morphine, may stimulate ADH release or potentiate its effects on the kidneys.

Management

Treatment of the underlying malignancy is of primary importance in cancer-related SIADH. Clinical evidence of excess ADH is present until the primary tumor stops compressing the major cardiac vessels, or producing ADH-like substances. Antineoplastic therapy may include chemotherapy, radiation therapy, or corticosteroids. Fluid intake is limited to 500 to 1,000 mL/day, which should result in a corrected fluid balance in 7 to 10 days. Demeclocycline, an antibiotic that inhibits ADH secretion, may be prescribed; patients with chronic SIADH may receive demeclocycline 900 to 1,200 mg/day. Adverse effects include diarrhea, nausea, dysphagia, and photosensitivity.

Diuretics are not ordered except in severe circumstances because they may produce additional electrolyte imbalances. However, the patient who is comatose or convulsing is given 3% IV hypertonic saline and a potent loop diuretic, such as furosemide.

TUMOR LYSIS SYNDROME

Tumor lysis syndrome is a metabolic imbalance caused by rapid cancer cell death. Most patients experience this complication 1 to 5 days after initiation of therapy in patients with chemosensitive or radiosensitive tumors. However, there are documented instances of tumor lysis syndrome in rapidly proliferating disease even before treatment initiation.

Patients at greatest risk for tumor lysis syndrome are those with bulky tumors having a high growth rate (e.g., acute leukemia or Burkitt's lymphoma), and those with highly radiosensitive or chemosensitive tumors such as small cell lung cancer and most malignant lymphomas. Patients with preexisting renal dysfunction may be at greatest risk for tumor lysis syndrome due to their difficulty in clearing the metabolic waste products fast enough to prevent clinical complications. Other patients at high risk for tumor lysis syndrome are those with Merkel's tumor, hepatoblastoma, and medulloblastoma.[49]

Pathophysiology

Rapid cell death causes the release of intracellular contents (potassium, phosphorus, and nucleic acids) into the circulating serum. The normal filtration mechanisms in the kidneys should immediately detect the levels of metabolic waste products and attempt to excrete them. If production is more rapid than excretion or renal insufficiency is present, accumulation of electrolytes and uric acid occurs in the serum. The most common abnormalities include hyperkalemia, hyperphosphatemia, and hyperuricemia. High phosphorus causes the kidneys to excrete calcium, causing hypocalcemia. Hyperuricemia causes deposition of uric acid crystals in the urinary tract and may lead to renal failure.

Assessment

History. Signs and symptoms of tumor lysis syndrome are related to the specific electrolyte imbalances involved and renal dysfunction. Hyperkalemia, hyperphosphatemia, hypocalcemia, hyperuricemia, and acidosis may occur. Box 48-19 lists the typical clinical signs and symptoms associated with the metabolic abnormalities of tumor lysis syndrome.

Diagnostic Studies. The electrolyte panel is used to identify key abnormalities in patients at risk for tumor lysis syndrome. Elevated serum potassium, phosphate, uric acid, blood urea nitrogen (BUN), and creatinine, with a low calcium are reported. Acidosis may be present in patients with severely compromised renal function. The urinary uric acid-to-creatinine ratio is greater than one. Renal ultrasonography is used to exclude ureteral obstruction.

Management

Treatment involves recognition of high-risk patients and promoting prevention through aggressive hydration, urinary alkalinization, and administration of phosphate-binding agents and allopurinol for at least 48 hours before beginning chemotherapy. Agents that block tubular reabsorption of uric acid should be avoided (e.g., aspirin, radiographic contrast, probenecid, thiazide diuretics). The goal is to keep the serum uric acid level within normal limits and the urine pH above 7.0. Electrolyte disturbances are specifically treated as needed.

IV fluids are given to ensure a urine volume of more than 3 L/day. IV sodium bicarbonate (4 g initially, then 1 to 2 g every 4 hours) is administered to alkalinize the urine and reduce uric acid crystallization in the kidney tubules. A Foley catheter is usually inserted into the bladder to measure urine output more accurately. If oliguria or anuria develops, ureteral obstruction must be excluded. Phosphate-binding agents such as aluminum hydroxide are given every 2 to 4 hours in an effort to keep phosphate levels below 4 mg/dL. Elevated serum potassium levels not prevented with hydration may be managed with concomitant

box 48-19 ***Signs and Symptoms of Tumor Lysis Syndrome***

Hyperkalemia
- Peaked T waves on ECG
- Dysrhythmias (tachycardia, ventricular ectopy/torsade de pointes [especially when potassium >6.8 mEq/L])
- Muscle flaccidity, weakness
- Hyperactive bowel sounds, abdominal cramping, diarrhea

Hyperphosphatemia
- Muscle weakness
- Bone marrow suppression (thrombocytopenia, leukopenia)
- Bone demineralization with tendency for pathological fractures
- Renal dysfunction

Hypocalcemia
- Muscle tetany
- Seizures
- Short PR and QT intervals on ECG
- Dysrhythmias (tachycardia, ventricular ectopy/torsade de pointes)
- Hyperactive bowel sounds, abdominal cramping, diarrhea

Hyperuricemia
- Uric acid crystals in urine
- Hematuria
- Oliguria, anuria
- Flank pain
- Renal failure

Acidosis
- Tachypnea
- Hypotension

diuresis or medications such as Kayexalate that enhance gastrointestinal excretion of potassium. Allopurinol is a xanthine oxidase inhibitor that blocks uric acid production and is administered in doses ranging from 300 to 900 mg/day. Because it is now available in an IV form given as 200 to 400 mg/m^2/day, rapid normalization of uric acid levels is an achievable objective. A new agent, rasburicase (Elitek), acts like the natural enzyme urate oxidase to oxidize uric acid to allantoin for excretion.[51]

If diuresis does not occur within a few hours after the initiation of treatment, renal replacement therapy is needed. An initial hemodialysis treatment usually reduces the patient's uric acid levels by 50%, but most patients then receive several additional days of CRRT until electrolyte abnormalities and hyperuricemia resolve. A low-calcium dialysate is used to prevent calcium phosphate precipitation. If peritoneal dialysis is used, albumin is added to the dialysate to increase uric acid protein binding and removal.

The focus of nursing care is on careful monitoring of fluid therapy, intake and output, and electrolyte balance. The incidence and severity of tumor lysis syndrome have been reduced by the use of prophylactic allopurinol, aggressive hydration, and early intervention with CRRT.

case study ■ SQUAMOUS CELL CANCER OF THE LUNG

Daryl Lopez is a 60-year-old man with squamous cell cancer of the lung being treated with radiation. He is brought to the emergency department by his family because of his increasing lethargy. Over the past 10 days, he has lost his appetite, and 2 days ago became drowsy and difficult to arouse and was vomiting after consuming food or fluids. When examined by a nurse, he appears to be cachectic and chronically ill. His blood pressure is 130/90 mm Hg, and his pulse is 90 beats/minute. His mucous membranes are dry. Bronchial breath sounds and dullness are noted in the left lung base. He falls asleep several times during the examination. His laboratory values are serum calcium 14.4 mg/dL; serum phosphorus 3.5 mg/dL; potassium 3.6 mEq/L; urea nitrogen 45.0 mg/dL; and creatinine 2.2 mg/dL.

Treatment includes IV fluids (0.9% sodium chloride 100 to 250 mL/hour) to correct volume depletion. Administration is continued at a slower rate as needed to promote renal calcium excretion and hydration. Pamidronate disodium 60 mg IV over 24 hours is ordered. A Foley catheter is inserted, and an accurate intake and output record is maintained. Safety precautions include side rails in the upright position at all times and frequent assessment of the patient's level of consciousness.

Mr. Lopez's serum calcium level is 10.5 mg/dL within 24 hours. He is eating well, drinking adequate amounts of fluid, and has no further vomiting. He is alert and oriented, has sufficient urinary output and clear breath sounds, and has begun to ambulate. Plans are made for resumption of radiation therapy treatments. Mr. Lopez is encouraged to maintain a program of moderate exercise, avoid bed rest, and eat a diet adequate in sodium. Family members are taught early signs and symptoms of hypercalcemia to report to Mr. Lopez's physician. ■

clinical applicability challenges

Self-Challenge: Critical Thinking

For questions 1 to 3, refer to the Case Study: HIV/AIDS.

1. *What combination of antiretroviral medications is appropriate for a person who is starting treatment?*
2. *Why is Ms. Lewis, the patient in the case study, started on prednisone when she arrives in the ICU?*
3. *What are alternative medications that may be given to a patient with an allergy to trimethoprim-sulfamethoxazole?*

For questions 4 to 7, refer to Case Study: Squamous Cell Cancer of the Lung.

4. *In a patient with a known large mediastinal tumor, several oncological emergencies may occur. Describe the emergent conditions Mr. Lopez experienced in the case study. Include the physiological basis of these emergencies in your answer.*

5. *Patients and families often are surprised by an oncological emergency. Develop a teaching plan for Mr. Lopez and his family.*
6. *Explore the ethical dimensions of treating patients with advanced cancer who present to the emergency department with an oncological emergency.*
7. *A patient at risk for tumor lysis syndrome may have several electrolyte and metabolic disorders. Develop a comparative list of symptoms for each of the different metabolic disorders that shows the overlapping and widely different symptoms.*

Study Questions

1. *The test(s) most widely used to evaluate HIV disease progression is*
   a. *enzyme-linked immunoassay (ELISA).*
   b. *viral load.*
   c. *p24 antigen.*
   d. *single-use diagnostic system (SUDS).*
2. *The average time from exposure to HIV and conversion to seropositivity in most people is*
   a. *10 to 14 days.*
   b. *2 to 6 weeks.*
   c. *6 weeks to 3 months.*
   d. *6 to 12 months.*
3. *The four body fluids that have been implicated in the transmission of HIV are*
   a. *blood, saliva, semen, vaginal fluid.*
   b. *tears, saliva, urine, sweat.*
   c. *blood, semen, vaginal fluid, breast milk.*
   d. *urine, semen, vaginal fluid, breast milk.*
4. *A male patient is diagnosed with Pneumocystis jiroveci pneumonia. When teaching the patient about his treatment, you explain that*
   a. *he will be receiving therapy for the rest of his life.*
   b. *his CD4 count is too low to start therapy.*
   c. *he must be isolated from others during his acute illness to prevent exposing others.*
   d. *his therapy will be stopped if his CD4 count rises above 200 cells/mm³ for more than 3 months.*
5. *A 65-year-old man with head and neck cancer calls the nurse to his room complaining of indigestion and a taste of blood in his mouth. He has a dry, nonproductive cough. He is most likely experiencing*
   a. *tracheal obstruction.*
   b. *carotid artery rupture.*
   c. *cardiac tamponade.*
   d. *superior vena cava syndrome.*
6. *Hypercalcemia can be prevented or lessened by which intervention?*
   a. *Allopurinol*
   b. *Urinary alkalinization*
   c. *Increasing fluid intake*
   d. *Limiting activity*
7. *A 59-year-old patient with small cell lung cancer is admitted with severe dyspnea and upper body edema. The first diagnostic test performed probably is*
   a. *chest CT scan.*
   b. *echocardiogram.*
   c. *electrocardiogram.*
   d. *multigated acquisition (MUGA) scan.*
8. *Patients with acute leukemia are at greatest risk for which of the following complications?*
   a. *Cardiac tamponade, syndrome of inappropriate antidiuretic hormone secretion (SIADH)*
   b. *Hypercalcemia, carotid artery rupture*
   c. *Pleural effusions, superior vena cava syndrome (SVCS)*
   d. *Cytokine release syndrome, tumor lysis syndrome*

REFERENCES

1. Centers for Disease Control and Prevention: HIV/AIDS Surveillance Report 13(2): 2001
2. Hader SL, Smith DK, Moore JS, et al: HIV infection in women in the United States: Status at the millennium. JAMA 285(9):1186–1192, 2001
3. Ahdieh L: Pregnancy and infection with human immunodeficiency virus. Clin Obstet Gynecol 44(2):154–166, 2001
4. Burns J, Pieper B: HIV/AIDS: Impact on healing. Ostomy Wound Manage 46(3):30–47, 2000
5. Mindel A, Tenant-Flowers M: Natural history and management of early HIV infection. BMJ 322:1290–1293, 2001
6. Pantaleo G, Cohen O, Graziosi C, et al: Immunopathogenesis of human immunodeficiency virus infection. In DeVita VT, Hellman S, Rosenberg SA (eds): AIDS: Etiology, Diagnosis, Treatment and Prevention (4th Ed). Philadelphia, Lippincott-Raven, 1997
7. Richman DD: HIV chemotherapy. Nature 410:995–1001, 2001
8. Centers for Disease Control and Prevention: Guidelines for preventing opportunistic infections among HIV-infected persons: 2002 recommendations of the U.S. Public Health Service and the Infectious Diseases Society of America. MMWR Morb Mortal Wkly Rep 51(RR-8):1–51, 2002
9. Mylonakis E, Paliou M, Lally M, et al: Laboratory testing for infection with the human immunodeficiency virus: Established and novel approaches. Am J Med 109:568–576, 2000
10. Trzcianowska H, Mortensen E: HIV and AIDS: Separating fact from fiction. Am J Nurs 101(6):53–59, 2001
11. Centers for Disease Control and Prevention: Updated U.S. Public Health Services guidelines for the management of occupational exposures to HBV, HCV, and HIV and recommendations for postexposure prophylaxis. MMWR Morb Mortal Wkly Rep 50(RR-11):1–53, 2001
12. Wilkin A, Feinberg J: *Pneumocystis carinii* pneumonia: A clinical review. Am Fam Physician 60:1699–1714, 1999
13. Kleinman S, Busch MP, Hall L, et al: False-positive HIV-1 test results in a low-risk screening setting of voluntary blood donation. JAMA 280(12):1080–1085, 1998
14. Barlett J: The 2002 Abbreviated Guide to Medical Management of HIV Infection. Baltimore, Johns Hopkins University, Division of Infectious Diseases, 2002
15. Weiser JK: Diagnostic testing in HIV disease. In Ungvarski PJ, Flaskerud JH (eds): HIV/AIDS: A Guide to Primary Care Management. Philadelphia, WB Saunders, 1999
16. Kaplan JE, Hanson D, Dworkin MS, et al: Epidemiology of human immunodeficiency virus-associated opportunistic infections in the United States in the era of highly active antiretroviral therapy. Clin Infect Dis 30(Suppl 1):S5–S14, 2000
17. John L, Marra F, Enson M: Role of therapeutic drug monitoring for protease inhibitors. Ann Pharmacother 35:745–754, 2001
18. Madge S, Singh S: The GP's role in HIV and AIDS care. Practitioner 244:772–777, 2000
19. Centers for Disease Control and Prevention: Guidelines for using antiretroviral agents among HIV-infected adults and adolescents: Recommendations of the Panel on Clinical Practices for Treatment of HIV. MMWR Morb Mortal Wkly Rep 51(RR-7):1–55, 2002
20. Nabel GJ: Challenges and opportunities for development of an AIDS vaccine. Nature 410:1002–1007, 2001
21. Shelton BK: Preventing crises in the patient with cancer. Oncol Nurs Forum 27(6):905–913, 2000
22. Oncology Nursing Society: Chemotherapy and Biotherapy Guidelines and Recommendations for Practice. Pittsburgh, Oncology Nursing Press, 2001

23. Marin D, Baerrade J, Ferra C, et al: Engraftment syndrome and survival after respiratory failure post-bone marrow transplantation. Intensive Care Med 24(7):732–735, 1998
24. Spitzer TR: Engraftment syndrome following hematopoietic stem cell transplantation. Bone Marrow Transplant 27(9):893–898, 2001
25. Ravenel JG, Scalzetti EM, Zamkoff KW: Chest radiographic features of engraftment syndrome. J Thorac Imaging 15(1):56–60, 2000
26. Capizzi SA, Kumar S, Huneke NE, et al: Peri-engraftment respiratory distress syndrome during autologous stem cell transplantation. Bone Marrow Transplant 27(12):1299–1303, 2001
27. Porcu P, Cripe LD, Ng EW, et al: Hyperleukocytic leukemias and leukostasis: A review of pathophysiology, clinical presentation and management. Leuk Lymphoma 39(1):1–18, 2000
28. Porcu P, Farag S, Marucci G, et al: Leukocytoreduction for acute leukemia. Ther Apher 6(1):15–23, 2002
29. Shelton BK: Oncologic emergencies. In Varricchio C (ed): A Cancer Source Book for Nurses (7th Ed), pp 214–230. Boston, Jones and Bartlett, 1998
30. Wurthner JU, Kohler G, Behringer D, et al: Leukostasis followed by hemorrhage complicating the initiation of chemotherapy in patients with acute myeloid leukemia and hyperleukocytosis: A clinicopathologic report of four cases. Cancer 85(2):368–374, 1999
31. Chim CS, Ooi CG: Cerebral leukostasis manifesting as multifocal intracerebral hemorrhage. Haematologica 86(11):1231, 2001
32. Chernecky C, Shelton B: Pulmonary complications in patients with cancer. Am J Nurs 101(5):24A–24H, 2001
33. Macdonald S, Gan J, McKay AJ, et al: Endovascular treatment of acute carotid blow-out syndrome. J Vasc Interv Radiol 11:1184–1188, 2000
34. Richardson P, Guinan E: Hepatic veno-occlusive disease following hematopoietic stem cell transplantation. Acta Haematol 106:57–68, 2001
35. Tack DK, Letendre L, Kamath PS, et al: Development of hepatic veno-occlusive disease after Mylotarg infusion for relapsed acute myeloid leukemia. Bone Marrow Transplant 28(9):895–897, 2001
36. Bearman SI: Avoiding hepatic veno-occlusive disease: What do we know and where are we going. Bone Marrow Transplant 27(11): 1113–1120, 2001
37. Carreras E: Veno-occlusive disease of the liver after hematopoietic cell transplantation. Eur J Haematol 64(5):281–291, 2000
38. Yoshimoto K, Yakushiji K, Ijuin H, et al: Colour Doppler ultrasonography of a segmental branch of the portal vein is useful for early diagnosis and monitoring of the therapeutic course of veno-occlusive disease after allogeneic haematopoietic stem cell transplantation. Br J Haematol 115(4):945–948, 2001
39. McCarville MB, Hoffer FA, Howard SC, et al: Hepatic veno-occlusive disease in children undergoing bone-marrow transplantation: Usefulness of sonographic findings. Pediatr Radiol 31(2): 102–105, 2001
40. Arai S, Lee LA, Vogelsang GB: A systematic approach to hepatic complications in hematopoietic stem cell transplantation. J Hematother Stem Cell Res 11(2):215–229, 2002
41. Zenz T, Rossle M, Bertz H, et al: Severe veno-occlusive disease after allogeneic bone marrow or peripheral stem cell transplantation: Role of transjugular intrahepatic portosystemic shunt (TIPS). Liver 21(1):31–36, 2001
42. Azoulay D, Castaing D, Lemoine A, et al: Transjugular intrahepatic portosystemic shunt (TIPS) for severe veno-occlusive disease of the liver following bone marrow transplantation. Bone Marrow Transplant 25(9):987–992, 2000
43. Sayer HG, Will U, Schilling K, et al: Hepatic veno-occlusive disease (VOD) with complete occlusion of liver venules after tandem autologous stem cell transplantation: Successful treatment with high-dose methylprednisolone and defibrotide. J Cancer Res Clin Oncol 128(3):148–152, 2002
44. Pegram AA, Kennedy LD: Prevention and treatment of veno-occlusive disease. Ann Pharmacother 35(7–8):935–942, 2001
45. Bearman SI: Veno-occlusive disease of the liver. Curr Opin Oncol 12(2):103–109, 2000
46. Simon M, Hahn T, Ford LA, et al: Retrospective multivariate analysis of hepatic veno-occlusive disease after blood or marrow transplantation: possible beneficial use of low molecular weight heparin. Bone Marrow Transplant 27(6):627–633, 2001
47. Mor E, Pappo O, Bar-Nathan N, et al: Defibrotide for the treatment of veno-occlusive disease after liver transplantation. Transplantation 72(7):1237–1240, 2001
48. Chopra R, Eaton JD, Grassi A, et al: Defibrotide for the treatment of hepatic veno-occlusive disease: Results of the European compassionate-use study. Br J Haematol 111(4):1122–1129, 2000
49. Gucalp R, Dutcher J: Oncologic emergencies. 2002. Available at www.merck.praxis.md
50. American Thoracic Society: Management of malignant pleural effusions. Am J Respir Crit Care Med 162:1987–2001, 2000
51. Brandt JM: Rasburicase: An innovative new treatment for hyperuricemia associated with tumor lysis syndrome. Clin J Oncol 2002 (*in press*)

OTHER SELECTED READING

Chiles C, Woodward PK, Gutierrez FR, et al: Metastatic involvement of the heart and pericardium: CT and MR imaging, Radiographics 21(2):439–449, 2001

Donato V, Bonfili P, Bulzonetti N, et al: Radiation therapy for oncological emergencies. Anticancer Res 21(3C):19–24, 2001

Esch JF, Frank SV: HIV drug resistance and nursing practice. Am J Nurs 101(6):30–36, 2001

Finley JP: Hypercalcemia. In Ziegfeld CR, Lubejko BG, Shelton BK (eds): Oncology Fact Finder: Manual of Oncology Care, pp 425–430. Philadelphia, Lippincott Williams & Wilkins, 1998

Finley JP: Tumor lysis syndrome. In Ziegfeld CR, Lubejko BG, Shelton BK (eds): Oncology Fact Finder: Manual of Oncology Care, pp 420–424. Philadelphia, Lippincott Williams & Wilkins, 1998

Fristoe B: Long-term cardiac and pulmonary complications in cancer care. Nurse Practitioner Forum 9(3):177–184, 1998

Garcia-Riego A, Cuinas C, Vilanova JJ: Malignant pericardial effusion. Acta Cytol 45(4):561–566, 2001

Hemann R: Superior vena cava syndrome. Clin Excel Nurse Pract 5(2):85–87, 2001

Jones LM, Mair EA, Fitzpatrick TM, et al: Multidisciplinary airway stent team: A comprehensive approach and protocol for tracheobronchial stent treatment. Ann Otol Rhinol Laryngol 109(10 Pt 1):889–898, 2000

Jones SG: Taking HAART: How to support patients with HIV/AIDS. Nursing 31(12):36–41, 2001

Lamy O, Jenzer-Closuit A, Burckhardt P: Hypercalcemia of malignancy: An undiagnosed and undertreated disease. J Intern Med 250(1):73–79, 2001

Lanciego C, Chacon JL, Julian A, et al: Stenting as first option for endovascular treatment of malignant superior vena cava syndrome. AJR Am J Roentgenol 177(3):585–593, 2001

Little K, Surjadi M: A scientific overview of the development of AIDS vaccines. J Assoc Nurses AIDS Care 11(6):19–28, 2000

Makimoto T, et al: Risk factors for severe radiation pneumonitis in lung cancer. Jpn J Clin Oncol 29(4):192–197, 1999

Marasso A, Bernardi V, Gai R, et al: Radiofrequency resection of bronchial tumors in combination with cryotherapy: Evaluation of a new technique. Thorax 53(2):106–109, 1998

Migueles SA, Tuazon CU: Endocrine disorders in human immunodeficiency virus infection. In Becker KL (ed): Principles and Practice of Endocrinology and Metabolism (3rd Ed). Philadelphia, Lippincott Williams & Wilkins, 2001

Moren D: Editorial response: Serological screening tests for antibody to human immunodeficiency virus—the search for perfection in an imperfect world. Clin Infect Dis 25:101–103, 1997

Mundy GR: The evolving role of bisphosphonate: Cancer treatment-induced bone loss. Oncol 18(5 Suppl 3):9–10, 2004

Oderich GS, Treiman GS, Schneider P, et al: Stent placement for treatment of central and peripheral venous obstruction: A long-term multi-institutional experience. J Vasc Surg 32(4):760–769, 2000

Polverosi R, Vigo M, Baron S, et al: Evaluation of tracheobronchial lesions with spiral CT: Comparison between virtual endoscopy and bronchoscopy. Radiol Med 102(5–6):313–319, 2001

Prevost A, Costa B, Elamarti R, et al: Long-term effect and tolerance of talc slurry for control of malignant pleural effusions. Oncol Rep 8(6):1327–1331, 2001

Ribaud P, Gluckman E: Hepatic veno-occlusive disease. Pediatr Transplant 3(Suppl 1):41–44, 1999

Shannon M: Antiretroviral therapy in HIV-infected pregnant women and their infants: Current interventions and challenges. J Perinat Neonat Nurs 16(2):1–25, 2002

Shelton BK: Superior vena cava syndrome. In Ziegfeld CR, Lubejko BG, Shelton BK (eds): Oncology Fact Finder: Manual of Oncology Care, pp 401–409. Philadelphia, Lippincott Williams & Wilkins, 1998

Shelton BK: Spinal cord compression. In Shelton BK, Ziegfeld CR, Olsen M (eds): Johns Hopkins Manual of Cancer Nursing, pp 548–559, Philadelphia, Lippincott Williams & Wilkins, 2004

Shepherd FA: Malignant pericardial effusion. Curr Opin Oncol 9(2):70–74, 1997

Smith U: Professional development. HIV and AIDS 1: Epidemiology, virology and immunology. Part 1 of 3. Nurs Times 98(5):43–46, 2002

Stephens KE Jr, Wood DE: Bronchoscopic management of central airway obstruction. J Thorac Cardiovasc Surg 119(2):289–296, 2000

Swanepoel E, Apffelstaedt JP: Malignant pericardial effusion in breast cancer: Terminal event or treatable condition? J Surg Oncol 64(4): 308–311, 1997

Taubert J: Management of malignant pleural effusion. Nurs Clin North Am 36(4):665–683, 2001

Tomkowski W, Szturmowicz M, Fijakowska A, et al: New approaches to the management and treatment of malignant pericardial effusions. Support Care Oncol 5(1):64–66, 1997

Ungvarski PJ: The past 20 years of AIDS through the eyes of one nurse. Am J Nurs 101(6):26–29, 2001

Vonk-Noordegraaf A, Postmus PE, Sutedja TG: Tracheobronchial stenting in the terminal care of cancer patients with central airways obstruction. Chest 120(6):1811–1814, 2001

Wang SA, Panlilio AL, Doi PA, et al: Experience of healthcare workers taking postexposure prophylaxis after occupational HIV exposures: Findings of the HIV postexposure prophylaxis registry. Infect Control Hosp Epidemiol 21(12):780–785, 2000

Weller IVD, Williams IG: Treatment of infections. BMJ 322:1350–1354, 2001

Witt C, Dinges S, Schmidt B, et al: Temporary tracheobronchial stenting in malignant stenoses. Eur J Cancer 33(2):204–208, 1997

Wood DE: Airway stenting. Chest Surg Clin North Am 11(4):841–860, 2001

chapter 49

Common Hematological Disorders

PAULA TIMMERMAN ■ MARTHA KENNEDY ■ BRENDA SHELTON

objectives

Based on the content in this chapter, the reader should be able to:

- Describe pathophysiological principles for hematological disorders.
- Discuss assessment findings and diagnostic studies for the patient with disseminated intravascular coagulation (DIC).
- Describe the clinical syndrome of thrombosis and hemorrhage related to DIC.
- Explain the anticipated management and rationale for the treatment of DIC.

DISORDERS OF RED BLOOD CELLS

Red blood cell disorders may be seen in the intensive care unit (ICU) as an incidental condition in a patient admitted to the unit for another acute illness or as an acute condition requiring intensive monitoring and intervention. Laboratory assessment to evaluate anemia is discussed in Chapter 46. Nursing interventions primarily are supportive of treatment protocols and of measures to identify the underlying cause. Other important actions include assessing for adverse effects of replacement therapy and for signs and symptoms indicative of decreased perfusion secondary to anemia, such as tachycardia, chest pain, dyspnea, and dizziness. All patients with red blood cell disorders must receive appropriate instructions in fatigue management and ways to effectively manage their chronic conditions to promote optimal quality of life and prevent or minimize complications.

Deficiency Anemias

Deficiency anemias include iron-deficiency anemia, megaloblastic anemia, and anemia of chronic disease (Table 49-1).

IRON-DEFICIENCY ANEMIA

Iron deficiency is the most common cause of anemia. It occurs when there is excessive loss of iron through chronic

table 49-1 Common Anemias and Primary Interventions

Type of Anemia	Primary Interventions
Iron-deficiency anemia	Iron supplements; correction of underlying stressor
Megaloblastic anemia	Vitamin B_{12} replacement; folic acid supplement
Anemia of chronic disease	Transfusion; recombinant erythropoietin (rEPO); correction of underlying disorder

bleeding, or when there is inadequate iron intake or absorption. When the cause is chronic bleeding, treatment is to correct the underlying bleeding, if possible, and replace iron using oral supplements. An increase in the patient's hemoglobin will be noticed over a period of weeks. If an increase does not occur, the patient may be noncompliant with therapy or have malabsorption of iron from the gastrointestinal system. When the cause is malabsorption, or when the patient has poor tolerance for oral iron, parenteral iron may be given. Intramuscular iron injection may be painful and stain the patient's skin. Instead, intravenous injection is recommended. Close patient observation is necessary because severe anaphylactic reactions may occur with this treatment. Transfusion of packed red blood cells is reserved for managing severe, active bleeding and when the patient is experiencing serious symptoms from anemia.

MEGALOBLASTIC ANEMIA

Megaloblastic anemias are a group of anemias, most of which are caused by a deficiency of vitamin B_{12} (cobalamin), folate, or both. Treatment entails correcting the deficiency, once the patient's particular vitamin deficiency is ascertained.

Vitamin B_{12} is poorly absorbed from the gut, and intramuscular or subcutaneous injection is required. Most patients require maintenance injections monthly for the remainder of their lives. The hematocrit may improve within a matter of days with vitamin B_{12} therapy. However, if neurological symptoms are present, these symptoms may take up to 6 months to improve.

Body stores of folate can be restored with an oral folate supplement given daily for approximately 4 weeks. Once the deficiency is corrected, maintenance therapy is rarely necessary unless underlying factors, such as chronic alcoholism, are present. In patients who are receiving an oral folate supplement, an increase in the hematocrit is expected by the second week, with a normal hematocrit being achieved by 8 weeks. Drugs that interfere with folate metabolism are listed in Box 49-1.

ANEMIA OF CHRONIC DISEASE

Finally, anemia is seen with a number of chronic disorders, such as renal failure, infections, malignancies, and connective tissue diseases (such as rheumatoid arthritis). Several mechanisms cause anemia of chronic disease. One defect is the apparent inability of the mononuclear phagocyte system to recycle iron from phagocytosed, senescent red blood cells. This causes a decrease in the iron stores available for erythropoiesis. A significant increase in macrophage production also occurs. These cells release cytokines (interleukin-1 alpha, tumor necrosis factor, and interferon) that directly suppress red blood cell production. Other factors are a decreased red blood cell survival time and low serum erythropoietin levels.

Treatment involves correcting the underlying cause, if possible. Transfusion may be of temporary benefit, although the survival of the transfused red blood cells is reduced. Recombinant erythropoietin (rEPO) may be the treatment of choice for many individuals. The patient's or caregiver's ability to administer injections or come for clinic visits, the cost of rEPO, and adequate iron stores are important considerations before beginning therapy. Complications of rEPO are infrequent and seen mostly in patients on renal dialysis. Side effects of rEPO include hypertension, seizures, arteriovenous shunt thromboses, and increased blood viscosity.

box 49-1
Drugs That Interfere With Folate Metabolism

- Alcohol
- Methotrexate
- Carbamazepine
- Diphenylhydantoin
- Triamterene
- Trimethoprim
- Pyrimethamine

Hemolytic Anemias

Hemolytic anemias are those resulting from destruction of red blood cells. They may be congenital or acquired and can vary greatly in the degree to which the anemia is experienced.

CONGENITAL HEMOLYTIC ANEMIA

The most common types of congenital hemolytic anemias are caused by enzyme defects or red blood cell membrane defects (Table 49-2). Approximately 90% of congenital red blood cell enzymatic deficiencies are glucose-6-phosphate dehydrogenase (G-6-PD) and pyruvate kinase deficiencies.[1] Enzyme defects cause the red blood cells to lyse when exposed to certain stressful conditions, such as drugs, chemicals, infections, surgery, or pregnancy. Substances to which individuals with G-6-PD deficiency may be susceptible are listed in Box 49-2. Hydration and avoiding causative agents (especially oxidative drugs) is standard treatment for patients with hemolytic anemia resulting from G-6-PD deficiency. Patients with pyruvate kinase deficiency may require transfusion and splenectomy.

Hemolytic anemia from hereditary spherocytosis or elliptocytosis is caused by a red blood cell membrane defect that gives the red blood cell an abnormal shape. These red blood cells are sequestered in the spleen and destroyed.

table 49-2 Congenital Hemolytic Anemias and Primary Interventions

Type of Defect	Primary Interventions
Enzyme defects	
Glucose-6-phosphate dehydrogenase	Avoidance of agents that trigger hemolysis; hydration
Pyruvate kinase deficiency	Transfusion; splenectomy
Red blood cell membrane defects	
Hereditary spherocytosis	Splenectomy; folic acid supplements
Hereditary elliptocytosis	Usually no treatment required; folic acid supplements
Paroxysmal nocturnal hemoglobinuria	Corticosteroids, androgens, recombinant erythropoietin, iron therapy; transfusion as needed; anticoagulation therapy if thrombotic events; possible bone marrow transplantation

Patients with hereditary spherocytosis usually require splenectomy and folic acid supplements. Most anemias from hereditary elliptocytosis are not as severe; usually no treatment is required other than folic acid supplements. Paroxysmal nocturnal hemoglobinuria (PNH) is caused by aberrant stem cells that produce red blood cells, white blood cells, and platelets with abnormal surface membranes. These cells are destroyed by the immune system, causing intravascular hemolysis. Exacerbations of hemolysis occur at night. Because of defective white blood cell production, these patients are susceptible to severe infections, and ineffective platelet production predisposes them to thromboses. Treatment of PNH includes corticosteroids, androgens, iron replacement, and transfusion. Bone marrow transplantation may be considered to replace the defective stem cells with healthy marrow.

ACQUIRED HEMOLYTIC ANEMIA

Acquired hemolytic anemias can be caused by several different factors (Table 49-3). In microangiopathic hemolytic anemia, red blood cells are fragmented by vasculitis, abnormal microvasculature, collagen vascular disease, abnormal cardiac valves, arteriovenous malformations, thrombotic thrombocytopenic purpura (TTP), or disseminated intravascular coagulation (DIC). These red blood cell fragments are called *schistocytes* and are seen on the peripheral smear. Treatment focuses on removing the causative factor, such as replacing the abnormal heart valve or repairing the arteriovenous shunt. If this is not possible, the patient may be maintained on iron and folate supplements and periodic transfusions of red blood cells.

Infectious agents may cause hemolytic anemia indirectly by causing splenomegaly or directly by invading the red blood cell and destroying its membrane. Malaria is an example of the latter. These patients are treated with transfusion support and anti-infective agents to address the underlying cause.

Abnormally shaped red blood cells are frequently noticed in patients with liver disease. These patients may also have congestive splenomegaly, which causes sequestration and destruction of red blood cells. In severe hemolysis, splenec-

box 49-2
Substances That May Cause Hemolytic Anemia in Susceptible Individuals

Congenital Hemolytic Anemia (G-6-PD Deficiency)

- Acetanilid
- Nalidixic acid
- Ciprofloxacin niridazole
- Norfloxacin
- Methylene blue
- Chloramphenicol
- Phenazopyridine
- Vitamin K analogs
- Doxorubicin
- Isobutyl nitrite
- Naphthalene
- Phenylhydrazine
- Pyridium
- Mothballs
- Fava beans (Mediterranean variant of G-6-PD deficiency)

Acquired Hemolytic Anemia

- Chloramines
- Nitrobenzene
- Isobutyl nitrates
- Aniline dyes
- Arsine gas
- Sodium chlorate
- Potassium chlorate
- Wasp and bee stings
- Spider bites
- Snake bites
- Copper
- Lead
- Paraquat
- Quinine
- Quinidine
- Acetanilid
- Furazolidone
- Isobutyl nitrite
- Nalidixic acid
- Naphthalene
- Niridazole
- Methyldopa
- Levodopa
- Procainamide
- Nonsteroidal anti-inflammatory drugs (NSAIDs)
- Penicillins
- Cephalosporins

table 49-3 Acquired Hemolytic Anemias and Potential Interventions

Acquired Hemolytic Anemia	Interventions
Microangiopathic	Removal of causative factor; iron and folate supplements; transfusion
Infectious agents	Treatment of underlying infection; transfusion
Liver disease	Splenectomy; transfusion
Autoimmune	
Warm antibody	Glucocorticoids; splenectomy; immunosuppressive agents; transfusion
Cold-reactive	Avoidance of exposure to cold; transfusion; plasma exchange
Drug-induced	Discontinuation of drug; transfusion

tomy and supportive red blood cell transfusions may be required.

Some patients can experience autoimmune hemolytic anemias. Warm autoimmune hemolytic anemia is the most common of these types. Approximately one half of all cases are idiopathic; known causative factors include collagen diseases, lymphoproliferative disorders, and drug reactions (see Box 49-2). Immunoglobulin G (IgG) is the autoantibody that attaches to the red blood cell membrane, causing its destruction by macrophages in the peripheral circulation and the spleen. The peripheral smear reveals microschistocytes due to incomplete red blood cell destruction. The Coombs' test is positive for autoantibody on the red blood cell surface. The reticulocyte count and the indirect bilirubin level are elevated. Primary therapy is oral glucocorticoids to suppress the immune system. Patients who do not respond to glucocorticoids or require high doses are candidates for splenectomy. Patients who undergo splenectomy usually still require low maintenance doses of glucocorticoids. If no response is noted after these interventions, immunosuppressive agents, such as azathioprine, cyclophosphamide, or vinca alkaloids, may be used. Intravenous immunoglobulin and cyclosporine are also potential interventions.[2]

Cold-reactive autoimmune hemolytic anemia is a disorder in which exposure to cold triggers complement-fixing IgM antibodies to attach to red blood cells in susceptible individuals, causing agglutination and hemolysis. Agglutination in the blood vessels is thought to produce the characteristic acrocyanosis of fingers, toes, earlobes, and nose. Often these patients have an underlying lymphoproliferative disorder; others may have *Mycoplasma pneumoniae* infection, infectious mononucleosis, or hepatitis. The peripheral smear shows spherocytes, and the reticulocyte count, serum lactate dehydrogenase (LDH), and indirect bilirubin are elevated. Susceptibility to cold varies among individuals and correlates with the severity of hemolysis. The anemia from this condition is usually not as severe as that from warm autoimmune hemolytic anemia. If these patients require transfusion, a blood warmer and measures to keep the patient warm are recommended. Steroids and splenectomy are ineffective in this disorder; intervention focuses on avoiding exposure to cold.

Hemolytic anemia can be induced by exposure to various drugs, chemicals, or toxins (see Box 49-2). Some drugs, such as penicillin, bind to the red blood cell membrane and cause antibodies to react against the drug itself. The red blood cell is destroyed during this reaction. Other drugs (sulfonamides, phenothiazines, quinine) may bind to antibodies in the patient's plasma, then attach to the red blood cell, causing its complement-mediated destruction. Finally, a drug such as methyldopa may induce the formation of autoantibodies against the red blood cells. All of these mechanisms cause a positive direct Coombs' test. Treatment is discontinuation of the suspected drug and red blood cell transfusions, if required.

Sickle Cell Anemia

Sickle cell anemia is caused by a structural abnormality in hemoglobin that causes the formation of abnormally shaped red blood cells. Cells are elongated, sickle shaped, and rigid. Sickled red blood cells are unable to pass through the microvasculature, causing decreased delivery of oxygen, obstruction of vessels, and inflammation.

Increased sickling of red blood cells occurs under the conditions of low oxygen levels, low pH, increased serum osmolarity, or sluggish blood flow. Destruction of the abnormal red blood cells causes varying degrees of hemolytic anemia, as well as jaundice and decreased cardiac output.[3] Rapid hemolysis of red blood cells can cause increased levels of bilirubin, which can lead to the formation of gallstones. The microvasculature of the spleen, lungs, brain, retina, kidneys, penis, and skeletal system can be occluded by the sickled red blood cells. Splenic obstruction predisposes the patient to overwhelming infection, especially pneumococcal sepsis. Acute chest syndrome is caused by pulmonary infarction. Strokes can occur in children, and repeated occlusion and revascularization in the retinal periphery can lead to retinal detachment and blindness. Damage to the vasculature in the kidneys causes impaired renal tubular function and eventual chronic renal failure. Priapism is painful engorgement of the penis by sickled red blood cells. Bone pain is one of the most severe symptoms experienced by persons with sickle cell disease. It is caused by avascular necrosis of active bone marrow. Pediatric patients may experience dactylitis, which is painful swelling of the hands and feet. Leg and ankle ulcers may also develop due to poor tissue perfusion.

Initial treatment of sickle cell crisis includes hydration to decrease blood viscosity and maintain renal perfusion. Oxygen administration and red blood cell transfusion are usually required. The patient is evaluated for infection because this is often the underlying cause of the crisis. Exchange transfusion, in which blood is removed from the patient while red blood cells are transfused, may be required for more acute situations. A recent study has shown an 85% disease-free survival rate in patients with severe sickle cell disease who underwent ablation of their own marrow and received stem cells from a sibling donor.[4] Although not without risks, this is a promising intervention that, when performed early in a patient's life, may help to prevent a great deal of future physical debilitation as a result of sickle cell disease.

The pain experienced by patients in sickle cell crisis is intense. Patients require around-the-clock dosing with a strong narcotic, such as morphine. Frequent, lower doses of narcotics avoid the erratic levels of analgesia caused by infrequent doses of stronger narcotics. Timed-release narcotics and patient-controlled analgesia (PCA) are two methods of delivering steady doses of pain medication. Patients with sickle cell crisis may not display overt signs of pain, as is typical for patients who experience chronic pain. The patient's report of pain should be used in assessing pain, as well as clinical indicators. Although there are rare instances of physical dependency for narcotics developing in patients, most narcotic-seeking behavior is due to undermedication.

The patient with sickle cell crisis must be closely monitored for response to interventions to promote tissue perfusion, treat infection, and effectively manage pain.

Polycythemia

Polycythemia is a disorder of increased red blood cell production, as indicated by a high hematocrit and an increased red blood cell mass. Increased red blood cell production results in increased blood viscosity, vascular insufficiency, decreased tissue oxygenation, and risk of thrombosis.

Polycythemia vera is a myeloproliferative disorder of uncontrolled red blood cell production that is independent of erythropoietin. These patients may also have leukocytosis, thrombocytosis, splenomegaly, and hypercellular bone marrow. Normal blood stem cells are also present but appear to be suppressed. Table 49-4 lists additional clinical findings in polycythemia vera. As the disease progresses, the patient may enter the "spent" phase, characterized by bone marrow fibrosis, increasing splenomegaly, anemia, and increasing numbers of abnormal white blood cells. Acute leukemia may develop in a small percentage of patients.

table 49-4 Clinical Findings and Related Causes in Polycythemia Vera

Clinical Finding	Cause
Dizziness, headache	Increased blood viscosity
Thrombosis	Increased blood viscosity, thrombocytosis, platelet defects
Pruritus	Elevated blood levels of histamine and/or increased skin mast cells
Bleeding tendency	Increased RBC-to-fibrin ratio; engorged capillaries and venules due to increased blood volume
Epigastric distress	Engorgement of gastric mucosa; increased blood histamine levels
Numbness and burning of toes	Peripheral vascular insufficiency
Cardiovascular insufficiency	Impaired tissue oxygenation due to increased blood viscosity

Thrombosis and bleeding complications are the major concerns for these patients. The patient with polycythemia vera is at increased risk for thromboembolic events due to hyperviscosity, especially myocardial and cerebral infarction, deep venous thrombosis, and pulmonary embolism. Measures to prevent thromboembolic complications, such as lower extremity compression devices or facilitating ambulation if the patient's condition permits, should be instituted.

Patients 40 years of age or younger who do not have vascular disease may be maintained by phlebotomy alone. The disadvantage of phlebotomy is that it stimulates bone marrow production, which leads to increased numbers of defective, sticky platelets. Antiplatelet aggregating agents, such as aspirin or dipyridamole, do not reduce thrombotic events and may increase the risk of bleeding. Older patients with vascular disease are at high risk for thrombosis and require bone marrow suppression in addition to phlebotomy. Long-term therapy with bone marrow suppressing agents has been associated with an increased risk of acute leukemia, so the potential benefits must be weighed against the anticipated duration of therapy. Hydroxyurea is the agent of choice because it has not been shown to increase the incidence of acute leukemia, as has been the case with some other alkylating agents. The use of aspirin and dipyridamole to decrease thrombotic events has been associated with an increased risk of hemorrhage in older patients. Therapy with a lower aspirin dose has been suggested, but its effectiveness has not yet been demonstrated.[5]

Secondary polycythemia is an increase in the red blood cell mass caused by increased red blood cell production. This may be a result of chronic hypoxia or autonomous erythropoietin production. Conditions causing chronic hypoxia include living at high altitudes, chronic obstructive pulmonary disease (COPD), sleep apnea, morbid obesity, arteriovenous malformation, and exposure to carbon monoxide. Causes for autonomous erythropoietin production include renal lesions, such as renal cysts, renal artery narrowing, or hydronephrosis, and exogenous production by malignant or benign tumors. Although the number of red blood cells is increased to help compensate for hypoxic conditions, the patient is also at risk for thrombosis. Treatment is to correct the underlying cause with long-term oxygen therapy, smoking cessation, weight loss, or surgical intervention as indicated. If these measures are ineffective, repeated phlebotomy to maintain a hematocrit of 45% or less is required.

DISORDERS OF WHITE BLOOD CELLS

Disorders of white blood cells include neutropenia, lymphoproliferative disorders, and myeloproliferative disorders. The major goals of nursing care for the patient with a white blood cell disorder include preventing infection and preventing and managing bleeding related to

■■■ **insights into clinical research**

Androne AS, Katz SD, Lund L, et al: Hemodilution is common in patients with advanced heart failure. Circulation 107(2):226–229, 2003.

In patients with congestive heart failure (CHF), anemia may be present due to increased plasma volume (hemodilution) or reduced blood cell volume (true anemia). A total of 137 patients with CHF were assessed for the presence of anemia. Sixty-one percent of the patients evaluated were anemic. In patients with New York Heart Association class II heart failure, the prevalence of anemia was 33%. In patients with class IV heart failure, the prevalence increased to 68%. The number of patients with true anemia versus anemia from hemodilution was approximately equal (54% versus 46%).

Patients with CHF and anemia have a poor prognosis. Patients with anemia due to hemodilution fare worse than patients with true anemia, suggesting that volume overload contributes to the poor outcome in anemic patients with CHF.

associated disorders of disseminated intravascular coagulation (DIC), thrombocytopenia, or leukostasis. Nursing interventions are guided by the treatment modality (e.g., chemotherapy, radiation, bone marrow transplantation). Meticulous attention to infection control procedures and vigilant surveillance of invasive lines and equipment are mainstays of care. Assessment for early indications of infection (e.g., fever, chills, tachycardia, tachypnea) may allow for prompt and aggressive initiation of pharmacological therapies to reduce morbidity and mortality associated with infection in patients with white blood cell disorders.

Patients with leukocyte counts greater than 100,000 cells/mm^3 are at risk for leukostasis, in which blasts aggregate in the capillaries. Manifestations include headache, confusion, central nervous system infarcts, acute respiratory insufficiency, and pulmonary infiltrates. Leukophoresis (removal of white blood cells from the circulation) may be performed to treat leukostasis. Central nervous system radiation may also be indicated. Leukostasis in patients with chronic myelogenous leukemia (CML) responds well to hydroxyurea.

Some of the leukemias and Hodgkin's disease can affect adolescents and young adults. Special considerations for this population with a white blood cell disorder are given in Box 49-3.

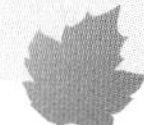

box 49-3

Considerations for the Adolescent/Young Adult Patient With a White Blood Cell Disorder

Hodgkin's disease and some leukemias may occur in late adolescence and young adulthood. People at this stage in life are developing increasing independence. Serious, life-threatening illness and severe treatment sequelae can profoundly affect the patient's perception of personal control and autonomy, resulting in anger, frustration, anxiety, withdrawal, and depression. Adolescents in particular may have concerns regarding their body image and appearing different from their peers. Hair loss, central venous catheters, and surgical scars are visible signs of treatment that may be areas of deep concern. Treatment schedules and physician appointments may disrupt normal activities and become a source of resentment or noncompliance.

Nurses assist the patient with sorting through conflicting feelings of independence and dependence. Support groups with people of similar ages may be extremely beneficial in addressing psychosocial issues. Attending school or working may be advisable for the peer contacts and the normality of such activities, but limitations during treatment should be discussed with the treating physician. Emotional support, information, and encouragement regarding the temporary nature of the physical changes and the anticipated time span for treatment should be provided to the patient and his or her family.

Neutropenia

Neutropenia refers to an abnormally low number of neutrophils in the blood. Neutropenia can be caused by infection, autoimmune disorders, splenomegaly, or bone marrow suppression. These patients are susceptible to overwhelming infection and sepsis. Treatment involves managing the underlying cause, and the use of anti-infectives and recombinant granulocyte colony-stimulating factor (rG-CSF). rG-CSF stimulates bone marrow production of neutrophils and enhances the activity of circulating neutrophils. Intravenous immunoglobulin and steroids may be used to treat immune-related neutropenia.

Lymphoproliferative Disorders

Lymphoproliferative disorders (disorders in which lymphoid tissue increases by reproducing itself) may originate in the bone marrow or the lymph nodes and thymus. Lymphoproliferative disorders of the bone marrow are leukemias and multiple myeloma; lymphoproliferative disorders of the lymph nodes and thymus are lymphomas.

NON-HODGKIN'S LYMPHOMA

Non-Hodgkin's lymphoma (NHL) is a diverse group of malignancies that originate in the lymphoid cells. NHL can occur as a discreet mass, such as a single lymph node, or as a widespread disease that affects multiple organ systems. Lymphomas are classified according to stage, or the extent of spread in the body, and by growth patterns, cellular subsets, and disease aggressiveness. Symptoms seen are related to the body area affected by the disease. People with extensive chest disease experience increasingly severe dyspnea. Bulky chest disease can cause compression of the superior vena cava, causing pressure and congestion of the face, neck, and upper thorax. Abdominal disease can cause obstruction of bowel or ureters. Bone marrow involvement can lead to decreased production of red blood cells, white blood cells, and platelets. Lymphoma of the central nervous system can cause headaches, visual disturbances, motor dysfunction, and increased intracranial pressure (ICP). Extensive involvement of the lymphatic system can lead to impaired immune function and frequent, severe infections.

The treatment of NHL varies according to the subclassification, the clinical stage, and the grade or aggressiveness of the disease. Low-grade, early-stage NHL may be treated with radiation therapy alone or with watchful waiting. Combination chemotherapy and radiation may be used to treat the more aggressive phases of this condition. Combination chemotherapy is the standard treatment for intermediate and high-grade lymphomas. Radiation therapy may also be used to reduce the mass of bulky tumors. Lymphoma that involves the central nervous system is treated with intrathecal chemotherapy, cranial irradiation, or intravenous chemotherapy. Patients with relapsed NHL may receive high-dose chemotherapy followed by peripheral blood stem cell infusion. Rituximab, a monoclonal antibody directed against the CD20 antigen, has been an effective agent for managing NHL.

HODGKIN'S DISEASE

Hodgkin's disease is a cancer of the lymphatic system. A diagnosis of Hodgkin's disease is confirmed by the presence of Reed-Sternberg cells in tissue that is biopsied. These cells are not present in NHL. There are subtypes of Hodgkin's disease that are based on molecular and immunological analysis of the malignant tissue. The patient's prognosis may vary depending on the subtype classification. The subtype classification may also be used to determine if more or less aggressive treatment is indicated.

As stated previously, clinical manifestations depend on the body site(s) affected. Early-stage disease may be treated with radiation alone. More advanced Hodgkin's disease is treated with chemotherapy followed by radiation therapy to sites considered high risk for relapse. Relapsed Hodgkin's disease is treated with further chemotherapy if the relapse occurs more than 12 months after initial treatment. Relapse less than 12 months after chemotherapy is treated with high-dose chemotherapy followed by peripheral blood stem cell infusion.

MULTIPLE MYELOMA

Multiple myeloma is a disorder of malignant plasma cells. Plasma cells differentiate from B lymphocytes and produce immunoglobulins, which are necessary for humoral immunity. Malignant plasma cells accumulate in the bone marrow and produce excessive amounts of an immunoglobulin, usually IgG or IgA; these excess immunoglobulins are collectively referred to as M proteins.

Malignant plasma cells can crowd bone marrow, causing decreased production of red blood cells, white blood cells, and platelets. M proteins can increase plasma volume, causing hyperviscosity and electrolyte imbalances. Perfusion of the kidneys is affected, causing renal dysfunction. Cytokines produced by the M proteins can cause bone destruction, which results in pain, fractures, and hypercalcemia. M proteins can suppress the production of normal immunoglobulins, causing impaired immunity and the potential for sepsis. Spinal cord compression and paralysis can result from disease affecting the spine.

Chemotherapy, often combined with glucocorticoids, is the optimal treatment for multiple myeloma. Alpha interferon has shown benefit in some studies and no benefit in others. Thalidomide is a newer treatment for multiple myeloma that is showing promising results. High-dose chemotherapy with peripheral blood stem cell infusion may be used for patients with resistant or relapsed disease, but because multiple myeloma usually occurs in older patients with comorbid conditions, there are limitations to the usefulness of high-dose chemotherapy. Radiation therapy is used for painful bony lesions, usually with very satisfactory results in relieving pain and associated morbidity. Impending fractures may require surgical fixation and stabilization before radiation therapy can be initiated. Spinal cord compression requires immediate intervention with radiation therapy and glucocorticoids to prevent permanent neurological damage and paralysis. Bisphosphonates are a class of drugs that inhibit bone resorption. Pamidronate and zoledronic acid are two drugs that are highly effective in treating hypercalcemia, relieving bone pain, and reducing skeletal fractures.

CHRONIC LYMPHOCYTIC LEUKEMIA

Chronic lymphocytic leukemia (CLL) is a disorder in which there is an increase in functionally incompetent lymphocytes in the bone marrow and peripheral blood. In most cases the lymphocytes are B cells derived from a single clone. These B cells function poorly, resulting in progressive humoral immunodeficiency. The T-cell pool in the peripheral blood expands, but most of these cells are helper/suppressor T cells, causing further immunosuppression. The onset of CLL may be gradual, with few symptoms. As the disease progresses, the patient may experience recurrent infections such as pneumonia, herpes simplex, and herpes zoster. Other clinical findings include bulky lymphadenopathy, anemia, thrombocytopenia, weight loss, and hepatosplenomegaly.

CLL is incurable, so therapy focuses on controlling the disease and managing recurrent infections. Early-stage CLL does not require treatment; progressive disease requires treatment with a chemotherapeutic agent, such as fludarabine. Monoclonal antibody therapy with Campath-1H and rituximab appears to be promising for these patients. Patients experiencing recurrent bacterial infections may respond to treatment with intravenous immunoglobulin. Death most commonly occurs from infectious complications caused by the disease itself or immunosuppressive therapy. CLL can transform into acute leukemia or immunoblastic sarcoma.

ACUTE LYMPHOBLASTIC LEUKEMIA

Acute lymphoblastic leukemia (ALL) is a disorder in which a clone of immature lymphocytes proliferates and replaces the normal cells of the bone marrow. The leukemic clones proliferate and infiltrate other normal tissues, such as the liver, spleen, and lymph nodes. A diagnosis of ALL depends on the presence of 30% or more lymphoblasts in the patient's bone marrow. Anemia, thrombocytopenia, and granulocytopenia are common. Patients experience weakness, fatigue, easy bruising, weight loss, and frequent infections. The spleen, liver, thymus, and lymph nodes are usually enlarged. A small percentage of patients have meningeal involvement at the time of diagnosis.[6]

Treatment involves induction chemotherapy for weeks to months to eradicate the leukemic cells and achieve remission. If this is successful, the next step is to prolong the remission through cyclical administration of chemotherapy in the consolidation phase. Lower doses of drugs may be given over many months in the maintenance phase. The central nervous system is prophylactically treated after remission with intrathecal methotrexate. Relapsed ALL has a poor response to secondary chemotherapy and requires bone marrow transplantation. Bone marrow transplantation should be offered to young, high-risk patients in first remission. Young patients who are not high-risk should reserve bone marrow transplantation for relapse if it occurs. Older patients with adverse features (e.g., comorbidities) and relapsed ALL should consider investigational therapies.

Myeloproliferative Disorders

Myeloproliferative disorders encompass numerous defects in bone marrow production. Some of these disorders are discussed later in this chapter. Chronic and acute myelogenous leukemias are discussed here.

CHRONIC MYELOGENOUS LEUKEMIA

Chronic myelogenous leukemia (CML) is caused by a chromosomal abnormality that results in the proliferation of mature and immature granulocytes, along with splenomegaly. The chronic phase of CML lasts for several years. In addition to leukocytosis and splenomegaly, many patients experience fatigue and weakness. Less common symptoms are bleeding, bone and joint pain, fevers, sweating, and weight loss. The acute phase of CML is called a *blast crisis*, and in most instances is similar to acute myelogenous leukemia (AML). One third of the cases, however, may resemble ALL. The transformation may be gradual or abrupt. It is characterized by worsening of the aforementioned symptoms, as well as increasing numbers of blasts in peripheral blood and bone marrow, and increasing myelofibrosis.

Previously, CML was treated with oral chemotherapy, such as hydroxyurea or busulfan. Alpha interferon also produced a response in some patients. Bone marrow transplantation was performed on low-risk patients in the chronic phase. However, a new agent, STI571 or imatinib, was recently approved for first-line therapy for CML. This novel agent has produced remarkable responses, with progression-free survival rates exceeding 90%. The long-term survival data are still being monitored, but this agent appears very promising.[7]

ACUTE MYELOGENOUS LEUKEMIA

A malignant disorder of hematopoietic stem cells, AML causes abnormal production of the myeloid cell lines (erythrocyte, neutrophil, megakaryocyte, macrophage). The malignant clones proliferate but do not differentiate into mature, functional cells. The blood, bone marrow, or both contains more than 30% blast cells. The proliferation of immature cells and bone marrow infiltration results in anemia, neutropenia, and thrombocytopenia; patient symptomatology is related to these conditions. The leukemic cells infiltrate the bone marrow and other body tissues. Splenomegaly is present in approximately one third of patients. Patients may require immediate interventions at the time of diagnosis for infections or anemia, or to achieve hemostasis.

The goal of treatment is to eradicate the leukemic clone and restore normal bone marrow function. Induction therapy with one to two cycles of chemotherapy results in a complete remission rate of approximately 60% to 65%.[8] Consolidation therapy is given to prolong the remission. Some patients undergo bone marrow transplantation after first remission; others undergo bone marrow transplantation when relapse occurs. Gemtuzumab ozogamicin is a monoclonal antibody for AML in first relapse that is mainly used in elderly patients who are not candidates for more aggressive therapy.

DISORDERS OF BONE MARROW FAILURE

Bone marrow failure describes numerous conditions in which the marrow fails to produce precursor cells for the peripheral components, resulting in cytopenias. This section discusses aplastic anemia, myelodysplastic syndrome (MDS), and myelofibrosis. Nursing interventions for the patient with a disorder of the bone marrow depends on the choice of treatment and the seriousness of the illness. Prevention of infection, assessment for signs and symptoms of bleeding, and institution of bleeding precautions are paramount. Most patients in the ICU setting are seen as a result of bone marrow transplantation, which is the curative treatment for most of these disorders.

Aplastic Anemia

Aplastic anemia is a condition of pancytopenia of the peripheral blood and bone marrow. Bone marrow is hypocellular and mostly replaced by fat. In many cases, the cause of aplastic anemia is unknown. Possible factors include drugs, chemicals, viruses, and immunological and congenital disorders (Box 49-4). In some patients, aplastic anemia is thought to result from replacement of normal cells by clones of cells that are incapable of normal hematopoiesis. Aplastic anemia causes anemia, neutropenia, and thrombocytopenia; clinical features are related to these conditions and include anemia, infections, and bleeding.

Mild aplastic anemia is treated by removing any known causative agents and administering supportive care (i.e., transfusions) as indicated. Oral androgens and glucocorticoids may be of some benefit. Hematopoietic growth factors may be of temporary benefit in patients who still have some residual bone marrow function. Most patients with mild aplastic anemia spontaneously recover; however, others may experience mild aplasia for years, which may progress to severe aplastic anemia in some cases. Transfusions should be used cautiously in patients who may require bone marrow transplantation.

Severe aplastic anemia is treated with transfusion support, immunosuppressive agents, and bone marrow transplantation. Drugs to stimulate marrow function are of no benefit in this condition. Bone marrow transplantation, preferably from a human leukocyte antigen (HLA)–matched

box 49-4
Causative Factors in Aplastic Anemia

Congenital (20% of Cases)
- Fanconi's anemia
- Congenital dyskeratosis
- Shwachman-Diamond syndrome
- Dubowitz's syndrome
- Diamond-Blackfan syndrome
- Familial aplastic anemia

Acquired (80% of Cases)
- Idiopathic
- Irradiation
- Drugs
  - Chloramphenicol
  - Phenylbutazone
  - Quinine derivatives
  - Sulfonamides
  - Cimetidine
  - Gold salts
  - Hydantoins
- Chemicals
  - Benzene and benzene derivatives
  - Insecticides
  - Cleaning solvents
- Infections
  - Non-A, non-B hepatitis
  - Epstein-Barr virus
  - Human immunodeficiency virus
  - Parovirus
  - Mycobacteria
- Immunological
  - Graft-versus-host disease
  - Systemic lupus erythematosus
  - Thymoma
- Pregnancy

sibling donor, should be considered for patients younger than 60 years of age. These patients should be considered for immediate transplantation and should not receive any transfusions or drug therapy before transplantation, if possible. Immunosuppressive therapy with antithymocyte globulin, cyclosporine, or methylprednisolone may be of benefit for older patients or those without a compatible donor for bone marrow transplantation. Bone marrow transplantation may be used for patients who fail immunosuppressive therapy, although the results are not as successful.

Myelodysplastic Syndrome

In a group of clonal hematopoietic diseases called *myelodysplastic syndrome* (MDS), the precursor cells do not mature, resulting in peripheral cytopenias. Unlike acute leukemia, the abnormal clone expands slowly and retains the ability to differentiate. Over time, however, the abnormal clone suppresses normal bone marrow function, causing severe and fatal pancytopenia or acute leukemia. In most cases, the cause of MDS is unknown. Known causative agents include alkylating agents, irradiation, and benzene. Symptoms are related to bone marrow failure and include pallor, fatigue, infection, bruising, and bleeding. The peripheral blood shows pancytopenia, often with monocytosis and abnormal cells from all three cell lines.

Treatment for MDS focuses on treating symptoms and improving quality of life. Hematopoietic growth factors are indicated to attempt to stimulate production of blood cells. Transfusions of red blood cells and platelets are required on an ongoing basis. Anti-infective agents and possible transfusion of granulocytes are needed to treat life-threatening infections. Bone marrow transplantation with a matched donor is used in patients 55 years and younger who are in late stages of MDS. However, most patients with MDS are elderly and are not candidates for bone marrow transplantation.

Myelofibrosis

Myelofibrosis is fibrosis of the bone marrow that occurs as a result of hematological disease or as a response to other disorders, such as malignant infiltration of bone marrow, infectious agents, or granulomatous disorders. Primary myelofibrosis, also known as *idiopathic myelofibrosis* (IMF), is caused by clonal proliferation of an abnormal hematopoietic progenitor and is considered a myeloproliferative disorder. The abnormal hematopoietic clone may produce a substance that results in the proliferation of fibroblasts in the bone marrow. Patients experience a slowly progressive anemia due to ineffective red blood cell production and low-grade hemolysis. Thrombocytopenia occurs as IMF worsens, and immature myeloid precursors are noted in the peripheral blood smear. Other clinical findings are pallor, fever, night sweats, anorexia, fatigue, and hepatosplenomegaly. No aspirate is usually obtained from the bone marrow, and biopsy shows fibrosis and osteosclerosis.

Asymptomatic IMF requires no treatment. Symptomatic anemia is treated with transfusion; some patients also respond to androgens. Corticosteroids are used if hemolysis is present. Thrombocytopenia is treated with platelet transfusions, but long-term management is difficult because of hypersplenism and alloimmunization. Hypersplenism may be treated with irradiation, splenectomy, busulfan, or alpha interferon. Few patients have received bone marrow transplantation. Survival averages approximately 5 years. Refractory thrombocytopenia and neutropenia develop in most patients with IMF, and death results from bleeding or infection.

DISORDERS OF HEMOSTASIS

Hemostasis may be impaired by disruption of numerous interactions in the coagulation pathway or deficiencies or dysfunction in the required components for coagulation. Disorders of hemostasis include bleeding disorders, immune thrombocytopenic purpura (ITP), and thrombotic thrombocytopenic purpura (TTP).

Patients with disorders of hemostasis may be critically ill. Assessment of the extent of bleeding or the risk for bleeding is a primary nursing intervention. The risk of bleeding increases exponentially when the platelet count drops below 20,000/mm^3. Platelet counts below 10,000/mm^3 are associated with gastrointestinal bleeding and the possibility of spontaneous intracranial hemorrhage. Avoidance of trauma is essential and may even preclude the placement of central venous catheters in some situations.

If platelet transfusions are indicated, the patient must be monitored for allergic reactions, anaphylaxis, and volume overload. Evaluation of continued blood loss and assessment of laboratory data for adequacy of the platelet count and other parameters of hemostasis are important measures. Further nursing interventions are dictated by other treatment protocols, such as the use of immunosuppressive drugs and plasmapheresis.

Bleeding Disorders

Disorders of hemostasis may be congenital or acquired. The most common congenital bleeding disorders are von Willebrand's disease, hemophilia A, and hemophilia B. Of these three disorders, von Willebrand's disease is the most common. A deficiency in von Willebrand's factor results in the decreased ability of platelets to adhere to the injured vessel wall and a deficiency of factor VIII. Hemophilia A is caused by a deficiency of factor VIII, and hemophilia B is caused by a deficiency of factor IX.

Management of bleeding disorders involves correcting the coagulation factor deficiency and treating sequelae that occur as a result of abnormal bleeding. Bleeding disorders vary greatly in their severity; not all patients with a bleeding disorder require intervention. Treatment of most bleeding disorders is administered by the patient at home at the start of the bleeding episode. However, more recent evidence suggests that complications in hemophilia, such as hemarthroses, may be minimized with regular, prophylactic administration of factor. This intervention may be instituted in patients as young as 1 to 2 years of age and has greatly helped to prevent the painful sequelae of hemarthroses and joint deterioration. Patients with mild hemophilia A and mild von Willebrand's factor deficiency may respond to intravenous or nasal spray administration of desmopressin acetate, a hormone that temporarily stimulates the release of factor VIII to control bleeding.[9]

More severe cases of hemophilia A or active bleeding require intravenous infusion of factor VIII concentrate. Bleeding in hemophilia B is controlled with intravenous infusions of factor IX concentrate. Patients with more severe presentations of von Willebrand's disease require factor VIII concentrate that contains von Willebrand's factor. Von Willebrand's factor is also found in cryoprecipitate, and factors VIII and IX are in fresh frozen plasma. Aminocaproic acid is an antifibrinolytic agent used in bleeding disorders to control mucous membrane bleeding in the mouth and nose.

Numerous complications can occur as a result of bleeding disorders (Table 49-5). Additional difficulties experienced by patients with bleeding disorders include the high cost of factor replacement therapy; the need for intravenous access; increased risk of acquiring viral illnesses, including hepatitis and acquired immunodeficiency syndrome (AIDS); and chronic pain from joint destruction.

table 49-5 Complications in Bleeding Disorders

Bleeding Site	Complication
Abdomen	Hypotension, hypovolemic shock
Muscle	Compartment syndrome
Joint	Hemarthrosis with destruction of bone and cartilage in joint capsule
Intracranial	Increased intracranial pressure
Retropharyngeal	Airway obstruction
Gastrointestinal	Anemia, melena
Urinary tract	Clots in ureters (especially after factor administration)

Immune Thrombocytopenic Purpura

Immune thrombocytopenic purpura (ITP) is an immune-mediated disorder of platelet destruction. There are two distinct forms of ITP. The acute form typically occurs in childhood and may resolve spontaneously in several weeks. Autoimmune platelet destruction appears to be stimulated after a viral illness. Chronic ITP usually occurs in adults. The platelet membrane is coated with an autoantibody (usually IgG), and the sensitized platelets are destroyed in the reticuloendothelial system of the spleen and liver. In at least 50% of patients with ITP, no known causative agent is identified; other patients may have underlying autoimmune, rheumatic, or lymphoproliferative diseases or human immunodeficiency virus (HIV) infection. The main clinical feature of ITP is bleeding that may have a gradual or abrupt onset. ITP is diagnosed by ruling out other disorders of platelet destruction, including DIC, TTP, and drug-induced thrombocytopenia.

Patients with mild to moderate thrombocytopenia without bleeding require no treatment. The severity of thrombocytopenia in these patients can be exacerbated, however, by even mild viral infections. Initial therapy for ITP may be immunosuppression with corticosteroids. A short course of prednisone may be sufficient to induce a remission, but only 10% to 30% of patients obtain long-term remission with steroids alone. Patients refractory to steroids or unable to tolerate steroid tapering may require splenectomy, which has a sustained remission rate of approximately 60%.[10] Intravenous immunoglobulin (IV IgG) is a highly successful treatment in patients at high risk for bleeding who require intervention. IV IgG is also used in thrombocytopenic patients who have undergone splenectomy. Platelets are given only if the patient is actively bleeding or the risk of intracranial hemorrhage is high. Patients refractory to the previous interventions may receive treatment with plasmapheresis or drugs such as azathioprine, vincristine, cyclophosphamide, colchicine, and danazol.

Thrombotic Thrombocytopenic Purpura

In thrombotic thrombocytopenic purpura (TTP), a rare, acute, often fatal disorder, platelets become sensitized and clump in blood vessels, causing occlusion. This process causes

- Thrombocytopenia and bleeding due to increased consumption of platelets
- Microangiopathic hemolytic anemia due to rupture of red blood cells as they try to pass through partially occluded blood vessels

- Fluctuating and often bizarre neurological abnormalities, transient ischemic attacks, and strokes due to interrupted blood flow to the brain
- Renal dysfunction due to obstruction of intraglomerular capillaries and infarction of the renal cortex
- Fever, which is possibly due to hemolysis or vascular infarction of the hypothalamus[11]

Not all five characteristics must necessarily be present. Clinical features are described further in Table 49-6. Initiation of the disease process may be related to immune-mediated endothelial damage, causing platelet aggregation. Autoimmune disorders, viral and bacterial infections, toxic agents, and genetic predisposition may also be involved in the development of TTP.

Primary treatment of TTP is based on the knowledge that patients with TTP have absent or decreased levels of platelet-aggregating factor inhibitor, which is normally present in plasma.[11] Simple plasma transfusion may be adequate to replace whatever factors are missing in the patient's plasma. Acutely ill patients may require plasma exchange, in which plasmapheresis is used to remove 2 to 3 L of the patient's plasma and an equal amount of fresh plasma is given as replacement. Plasmapheresis is initiated as quickly as possible and repeated daily for 5 to 10 days. To protect the endothelium from further damage, prednisone is also initiated immediately. Antiplatelet agents, such as aspirin and dipyridamole, may be used to inhibit platelet aggregation, although the effectiveness of this is in question. IV IgG and splenectomy may be used if the patient relapses after the initial response; vincristine may also be given as an immunosuppressive agent. Platelet transfusion is contraindicated even in severe thrombocytopenia because it may exacerbate the thrombotic process, causing myocardial infarction and stroke. Despite the aforementioned interventions, acute, severe TTP has a mortality rate of 30% to 40%.[11] Early recognition and prompt initiation of treatment may improve patient survival. Long-term follow-up of patients with TTP is required; 13% to 36% relapse after the initial remission.[12]

table 49-6 ■ Clinical Manifestations of Thrombotic Thrombocytopenic Purpura (TTP)

Abnormality	Findings
Thrombocytopenia	Bleeding, ecchymosis, purpura at various sites
Hemolytic anemia	Schistocytes, reticulocytosis, elevated serum lactate dehydrogenase and bilirubin, jaundice, pallor, weakness
Neurological abnormalities	Headache, mental changes, confusion, visual problems, seizures, coma, aphasia, dysphasia, paresthesias
Renal dysfunction	Proteinuria, microscopic hematuria, elevated blood urea nitrogen and creatinine, renal failure
Fever	Persistent elevation of temperature during acute phase
Other	Abdominal pain, malaise, nausea, vomiting, weakness, ECG changes

case study ■ THROMBOTIC THROMBOCYTOPENIC PURPURA

Mrs. Venable is a 41-year-old African-American woman with a recent history of diarrheal illness. She presented to the emergency department complaining of worsening fatigue, bruising, and persistent vaginal bleeding. Her responses during the history and physical examination were vague and disorganized, and she complained of blurred vision and a persistent headache. Vital signs were as follows: pulse 112 beats/minute; respirations 26 breaths/minute; blood pressure 100/64 mm Hg; temperature 37.1°C (98.8°F). Examination of the skin and mucous membranes revealed multiple ecchymoses, gingival oozing, bright red vaginal bleeding, and jaundiced sclera. Neurological examination revealed an alert patient with intact cranial nerve reflexes and pupils that were equal and reactive to light, but blurred vision and altered mental processes. Examination of the chest revealed lungs that were clear to auscultation and a tachycardic but regular heart rhythm with no S_3 or S_4. Abdominal examination revealed soft, slight epigastric discomfort and active bowel sounds. Hemoccult-positive stool was found on digital rectal examination.

Laboratory tests were ordered and the results came back as follows: hemoglobin 6.2 g/dL; hematocrit 18.1%; platelets 8,000/mm^3; reticulocytes, 5.9%; peripheral blood smear—schistocytes; serum lactate dehydrogenase (LDH) 997 U/L; serum bilirubin 4.3 mg/dL; blood urea nitrogen (BUN) 32 mg/dL; serum creatinine 1.4 mg/dL; urine red blood cells—many; urine white blood cells—few; urine protein 11 mg/dL.

Based on the evidence of thrombocytopenia, microangiopathic hemolytic anemia, neurological changes, and renal dysfunction, a diagnosis of TTP was made, and the patient was admitted to the ICU.

The patient's mental status quickly deteriorated in the ICU; she became agitated and confused and required restraints to prevent injury to herself. Because a computed tomography scan of the brain was negative, the mental status changes were thought to be due to transient ischemia from microvascular thrombi in the intracranial arterioles. Oxygen therapy was begun at 5 L/minute and titrated according to oxygen saturation levels. Prednisone 2 mg/kg daily was initiated, along with ranitidine to prevent gastrointestinal bleeding. Two units of packed red blood cells were transfused. Repeat transfusions of packed red cells were required on days 2, 4, 6, and 10. Arrangements were made for plasmapheresis and plasma exchange. Because this treatment was not immediately available at the hospital, fresh frozen plasma was administered. Several hours later, the necessary equipment and personnel had arrived, and plasmapheresis and exchange of 2 L of plasma daily was begun and ordered to continue for the next 10 days.

The patient continued to demonstrate a mild proteinuria over the next 10 days, but her BUN and creatinine levels remained stable during this time. The patient's blood sugar ranged between 280 and 320 mg/dL. This was thought to be due in part to the prednisone, but thrombotic lesions of the pancreatic islet cells could not be ruled out. The hyperglycemia was covered with sliding-scale insulin and returned to normal as the steroids were tapered. The patient's platelet count initially rose to 32,000/mm^3. Vincristine was administered for further immune suppression. This resulted in a platelet count of 62,000/mm^3 by day 12. Plasmapheresis and exchange were extended through day 14, then decreased to every other day for the next week, then twice weekly for a month.

The patient experienced noticeable improvement in her neurological status by day 7. Her serum LDH and bilirubin levels had returned to near normal by day 14, although schistocytes remained on her peripheral blood smear for a month. This was thought to be due to ineffective clearing of the ruptured red blood cells by the reticuloendothelial system, because her hematocrit remained stable. Two months after her discharge, the patient returned to the hospital with relapsed TTP after a viral illness that was detected on routine complete blood count. This relapse was treated promptly with prednisone, fresh frozen plasma, and plasmapheresis and exchange and was resolved without incident by day 11. ■

DISSEMINATED INTRAVASCULAR COAGULATION

Pathophysiology

Disseminated intravascular coagulation (DIC) is defined by the inappropriate triggering of the coagulation cascade and a breakdown in the normal feedback mechanisms in the body that allow for the dissolution of clots. Instead of a localized response to tissue damage or vascular injury, there is a release of prothrombotic mediators into the circulation with widespread intravascular clotting. Eventually coagulation factors become depleted as the body attempts to dissolve the newly formed clots. In essence, there is an imbalance between the natural procoagulant and anticoagulant systems in the body. The result is disproportionate creation of thrombi in the vascular system, consumption of coagulation factors necessary for clot formation, and increased fibrinolytic activity. Clinical consequences include systemic ischemia from the thrombi formation, as well as minor or major hemorrhage from ongoing fibrinolysis and depletion of clotting factors.

Inherent to the development of DIC is an underlying condition that serves as the initial triggering event for the inappropriate intravascular coagulation. There are a number of etiologies leading to the development of DIC. Common to them all is the inappropriate stimulation of clotting. This involves the activation of any of the coagulation pathways. The extrinsic pathway is activated with damage to the endothelial lining of blood vessels and subsequent release of tissue thromboplastin from the endothelial cells. When thromboplastin and factor VII connect, the extrinsic pathway is activated. Common causes include surgery, burns, heat stroke, bacterial endotoxin, and malignant tumors. The intrinsic pathway is activated when subendothelial tissue is exposed to the bloodstream and circulating factor XII comes in contact with the exposed tissue. The exposure may follow vascular injury or damage from immune complexes or bacterial endotoxins. The result is clot formation and activation of the coagulation cascade.

In all of these states, the presence of injured or lysed cells causes the release of tissue phospholipid into the bloodstream, which can then trigger activity of the intrinsic pathway. Endotoxins released by Gram-negative bacteria and the resulting sepsis are significant triggers of DIC, accounting for approximately 20% of cases.[13] Shock or low flow states can result in metabolic acidosis, tissue ischemia, and necrosis, which may also lead to clot formation. In cancer, a common etiology of DIC, the condition is caused by tumors eroding tissue with subsequent release of thromboplastin or stimulation of factor XII from vascular injury, as well as by the autolysis of tumor cells in rapidly proliferating tumors. In cancers that are able to autolyse (e.g., acute leukemia, Burkitt's lymphoma, small cell lung cancer), the cell fragments that result from the lysis are seen as "foreign bodies" and stimulate clotting. Still other cancers release procoagulants that enhance clotting (e.g., mucin-producing adenocarcinomas, prostate and renal cancer, promyelocytic leukemias, and brain tumors).[14] Box 49-5 outlines some malignant and nonmalignant states of physiological disequilibrium that can be precipitating factors for DIC.

Regardless of the precipitating event in DIC, the triggering stimulus initiates systemic coagulation activity, resulting in diffuse intravascular fibrin formation and deposition of fibrin in the microcirculation. The result is the accumulation of clot in the body's capillaries, the total length of which exceeds 100,000 miles in the average adult. Because of the rapidity of intravascular thrombin formation, clotting factors are used up in the capillary clotting process at a rate exceeding factor replenishment. The normal clotting/clot dissolution balance is also disturbed because the availability of thrombin neutralizers such as antithrombin III, heparin cofactor II, protein C, and protein S is greatly decreased compared with thrombin activity. The result is unregulated thrombin activity, microvasculature thrombi, platelet consumption, and microangiopathic hemolytic anemia.

Activation of coagulation mechanisms also activates the fibrinolytic system. (Activated factor XII, thrombin, endothelial cells, and tissue substances stimulate the release of plasminogen activators.) As thrombin is activated, plasmin is generated. Plasmin cleaves fibrin and factors I, V, and VII. The breakdown of fibrin and fibrinogen results in fibrin degradation products (FDPs) and D-dimers. These products interfere with platelet function and the formation of the fibrin clot. In addition, the plasmin can activate the complement and kinin systems, leading to increased vascular permeability, hypotension, and shock. Thus, the patient has a simultaneous, self-perpetuating combination of thrombotic and bleeding activity occurring in response

box 49-5
Selected Disease States Associated With Disseminated Intravascular Coagulation (DIC)

Nonmalignant
- Bacterial infections (gram-negative, gram-positive)
- Viremias (human immunodeficiency virus, cytomegalovirus, hepatitis)
- Burns
- Heat stroke
- Brain injury
- Crush injuries and necrotic tissue
- Obstetrical complications (amniotic fluid embolism, missed abortion, eclampsia, retained dead fetus, abruptio placentae)
- Intravascular hemolysis (hemolytic transfusion reactions, massive blood replacement therapy)
- Acute liver disease
- Intravascular prosthetic devices
- Prolonged low cardiac output states (cardiac failure, prolonged cardiopulmonary bypass, hemorrhagic shock, cardiopulmonary arrest)
- Vasculitis
- Immunological disorders (immune complex disorders, allograft reaction, incompatible blood transfusion)
- Surgery
- Other (snake venom, vascular malformations, fat embolism)

Malignant
- Leukemias (acute promyelocytic, acute myelomonocytic, others)
- Solid tumors (adenocarcinoma, lung cancer, breast cancer, hepatic cancer, colon cancer, prostate cancer, brain cancer)
- Chemoradiation therapy

to the precipitating event, as well as the potential for hemodynamic instability (Fig. 49-1).

A patient with DIC is vulnerable to a wide variety of complications resulting from the thrombotic or hemorrhagic disease processes. Thrombosis may result in ischemia or infarction in any organ, with concomitant loss of function. With depletion of clotting factors and platelets, bleeding into subcutaneous tissues, skin, and mucous membranes, or more serious hemorrhage, may result.

Assessment

All critically ill patients are at risk for development of DIC because many are in the state of physiological disequilibrium characterized by hypovolemia, hypotension, hypoxia, and acidosis, all of which have procoagulant effects. In addition, the patient's critical illness may have been triggered by an injury that in itself could result in the development of DIC. Increased awareness of DIC as a potentially catastrophic complication in the critically ill patient has resulted in earlier recognition and intervention. The critical care nurse who is armed with a knowledge of physiological norms and who uses a systemic approach to assessment may be the first person to identify the early signs of coagulation dysfunction and its probable trigger.

HISTORY AND PHYSICAL EXAMINATION

DIC may be acute in presentation, evidenced by severe clinical deterioration, or chronic in presentation, evidenced by mildly abnormal laboratory values and minimal, varied clinical symptomatology. In the patient with chronic DIC, thrombosis is the prevalent disorder and the degree of symptomatology is related to the ability of the liver and bone marrow to compensate for the disorder. These patients may have low-grade bleeding if factors become depleted, unexpected thrombotic events (including large vessel thrombi), or both. Chronic DIC must be ruled out in patients with multiple thrombotic sites developing simultaneously, serial thromboses, superficial venous thromboses, or arterial thromboses, especially in the presence of malignancy.[15]

However, most critical care nurses care for patients with acute DIC. It is important to realize that the assessment varies as the disease state evolves. Clinical assessment is organized according to the basic pathological process of DIC: clot formation with resulting emboli and perfusion defects, or unchecked clot dissolution with resultant bleeding. The nurse evaluates the patient for signs and symptoms of inappropriate clotting: cyanosis, gangrene, mental status changes, altered level of consciousness, cerebrovascular accident, pulmonary embolus, bowel ischemia and infarction, and renal insufficiency or failure. Thrombosis may involve both arteries and veins, and clinical examination may reveal demarcation cyanosis (total occlusion of microvessels, most common in digits but may be evident in earlobes). The nurse also evaluates the patient for signs of bleeding: bleeding from the nose, gums, lungs, gastrointestinal tract, surgical sites, injection sites, and intravascular access sites; hematuria; acral cyanosis; petechial rashes; and purpura fulminans. Bleeding is a manifestation of later disease because it is evidence of depletion of clotting factors, bleeding diathesis, or both.

Assessment of the patient with possible DIC requires constant reassessment and interpretation of findings. For example, the patient with a dull headache is likely to have a thrombotic defect, whereas a sudden and acute headache is more likely to be hemorrhagic. Dyspnea can be from a thrombotic disorder (pulmonary embolism) or from a hemorrhagic disorder (bleeding in the lungs). Either condition my present with hemoptysis and blood with suctioning. Hypotension may result from myocardial infarction (a thrombotic disorder) or cardiac tamponade (a hemorrhagic disorder). Ischemic bowel is characterized by decreased bowel sounds and a crampy and painful abdomen, with potential gastrointestinal bleeding when the mucosal layer sloughs, whereas gastrointestinal bleeding always presents with heme-positive to melanotic stool and hyperactive bowel sounds. Patients with DIC must be monitored closely for signs and symptoms of onset of shock, either hypovolemic or ischemic in origin. Constant assessment of all body systems and critical thinking are required when caring for a patient at risk for DIC.

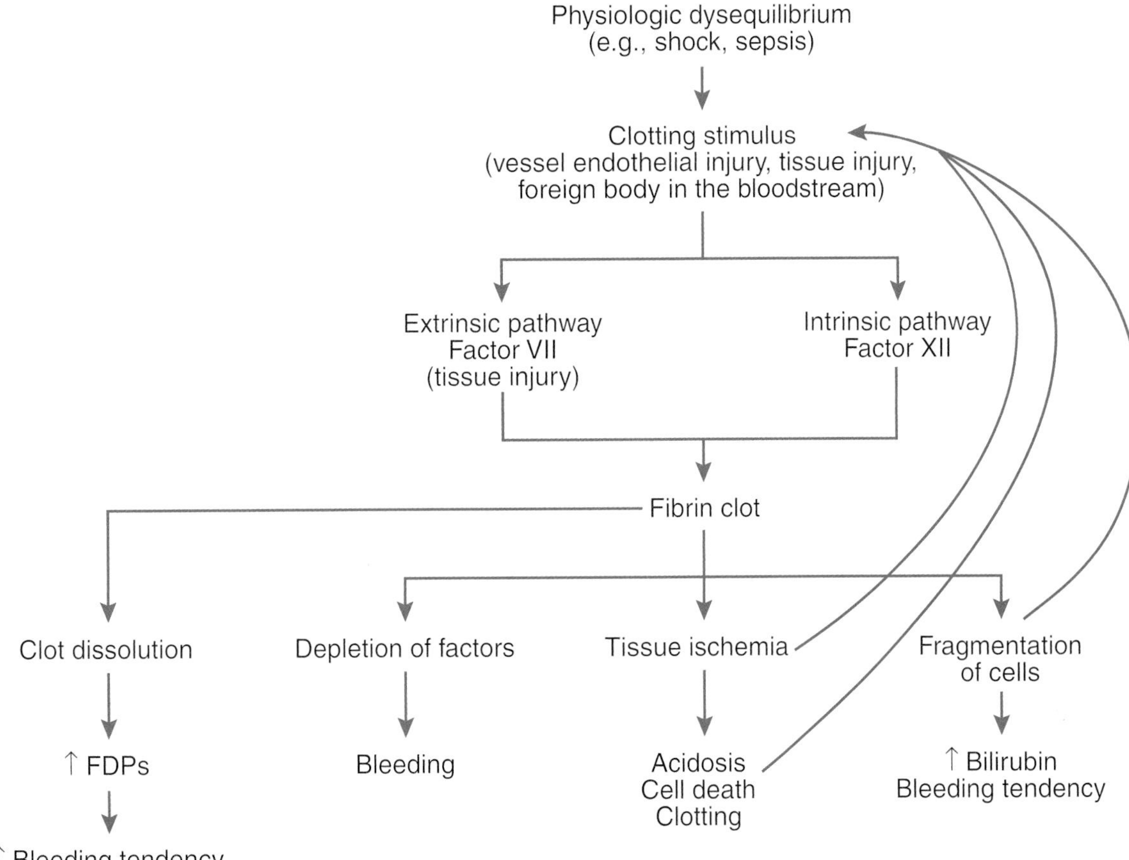

figure 49-1 Self-perpetuating cycle of thrombosis and bleeding in disseminated intravascular coagulation (DIC).

LABORATORY STUDIES

Regardless of the inciting event, four basic diagnostic components of DIC can be appreciated: excessive rate of clot formation; increased rate of clot dissolution; consumption of essential clotting factors; and end-organ damage resulting from the excessive clotting process.[16]

Table 49-7 outlines studies that are commonly used to assess DIC. These studies, unfortunately, are neither specific nor sensitive, and results vary throughout the course of the disease. For the average patient, thrombocytopenia occurs as platelets are consumed during the unchecked clotting, followed by hypofibrinogenemia. Normal fibrinogen levels do not preclude DIC because it is an acute-phase reactant. Serial measurements of platelet count, prothrombin time (PT), partial thromboplastin time (PTT), and fibrinogen level help gauge disease progression. Peripheral smears may reveal the presence of schistocytes reflecting fragmentation of red blood cells moving through clots or partially occluded vessels.

Management

The backbone of therapy for DIC is elimination of the causative agent. The factor that activates the clotting factors must be "turned off," be it through antibiotic/antifungal therapy for sepsis, antineoplastic therapy, rehydration, increasing oxygenation, or resolution of low flow states (Box 49-6). Unfortunately, some causes (e.g., burns, crush injury, brain injury) cannot be easily "turned off." General treatment principles include avoiding vasoconstriction that may worsen perfusion defects, maintaining adequate fluid volume status, and screening for and eliminating all medications that may enhance bleeding. In addition, for patients who are at risk for development of DIC as a result of sepsis, the recently approved agent activated protein C (drotrecogin alfa [activated], marketed as Xigris), may be used to slow the development of uncontrolled clotting that may result from the septic process.[17] There are stringent criteria for the use of activated protein C. The argument for use of activated protein C is that with aggressive treatment of the causative agent (sepsis), it may be possible to decrease the rate of clot formation, slow the clotting cascade, and reclaim the balance between clotting and fibrinolysis. This agent has not been investigated for its potential benefit in patients with confirmed DIC.

MANAGEMENT OF THROMBOTIC DISEASE

Attention is directed to correction of hypovolemia, hypotension, hypoxia, and acidosis, all of which have procoagulant effects. Primary to the management of the underlying

(text continues on page 1190)

table 49-7 ■ Laboratory Findings in Acute Disseminated Intravascular Coagulation (DIC)

Test	Normal Value	Value in DIC
Massive Intravascular Clotting		
Platelet count	150,000–400,000/mm³	Decreased
Fibrinogen level	200–400 mg/100 mL	Decreased
Thrombin time	7.0–12.0 sec	Prolonged
Protein C level	4 μg/mL	Decreased
Protein S level	23 μg/mL	Decreased
Secondary Depletion of Essential Clotting Factors		
Prothrombin time (PT)	11–15 sec	Prolonged
Activated partial thromboplastin time (aPTT)	30–40 sec	Prolonged
International normalized ratio (INR)	1.0–1.2 times normal	Prolonged
Excessive/Accelerated Fibrinolysis		
Fibrin degradation products (FDPs)	<10 mg/mL	Increased
D-dimer assay	<50 μg/dL	Increased
Antithrombin III level	89%–120%	Decreased
Clinical Effects of Microvascular Clotting/Cell Destruction		
Schistocytes on peripheral smear		Present
Bilirubin level	0.1–1.2 mg/dL	Increased
Blood urea nitrogen (BUN)	8–20 mg/dL	Increased

box 49-6 collaborative care guide
for the Patient With Disseminated Intravascular Coagulation (DIC)

OUTCOMES	INTERVENTIONS
Oxygenation/Ventilation	
Arterial blood gases are within normal limits.	■ Monitor pulse oximetry and arterial blood gases. ■ Validate significant changes in pulse oximetry with co-oximetry arterial saturation measurement. ■ Transfuse as necessary to increase oxygen carrying capacity. ■ Turn, cough, deep breathe, and use incentive spirometer q2h.
Breath sounds are clear bilaterally.	■ Suction oropharynx and trachea carefully when necessary (see Chapter 25, Box 25-7) ■ Turn, cough, deep breathe, and use incentive spirometer q2h.
Circulation/Perfusion	
Patient will achieve/maintain tissue perfusion.	■ Monitor tissue perfusion: color, temperature, pulses, capillary refill, level of consciousness, urinary output, and PaO_2. ■ Monitor vital signs qh–4h based on clinical condition. ■ Monitor cardiac output, stroke volume, systemic vascular resistance, and pulmonary artery pressures q4h hours if pulmonary artery catheter in place.
Serum lactate will be within normal limits.	■ Monitor lactate qd or more frequently until it is within normal limits. ■ Administer red blood cells, positive inotropic agents, IV infusions as ordered to increase oxygen delivery. ■ Assess patient for potential sources of lactate (e.g., ischemic bowel, ischemic distal digits) or decreased ability to clear lactate (liver dysfunction).

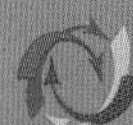

box 49-6 collaborative care guide
for the Patient With Disseminated Intravascular Coagulation (DIC) (Continued)

OUTCOMES	INTERVENTIONS
Hematological Patient will not experience bleeding related to coagulopathies.	■ Monitor PT, PTT, complete blood count (CBC), fibrin split products, and fibrinogen levels daily; more frequently if monitoring for acute changes or response to therapy. ■ Assess q4h for signs of bleeding, including thrombotic and hemorrhagic manifestations. ■ Quantify degree of bleeding (weigh dressings, count pads, measure bodily drainage; test stool, urine, drains, and emesis for heme). ■ Assess individual organs for signs and symptoms of bleeding: crackles, decreased Sao_2 with pulmonary bleeding; visual changes (diplopia, blurred vision, visual field deficit) with retinal thrombosis/hemorrhage; back pain, flank pain, abdominal pain consistent with visceral organ bleeding. ■ Administer blood and coagulation factors as indicated. ■ Maintain strict adherence to bleeding precautions. ■ Avoid invasive procedures and treatments. ■ Avoid medications that inhibit coagulation or promote thrombosis. ■ Apply pressure to puncture sites for 3–5 min, then use pressure dressing.
Fluids/Electrolytes Patient is euvolemic.	■ Take daily weights. ■ Monitor intake and output; replace/diurese as required. ■ Maintain IV access and fluid replacement therapy.
Mineral and electrolyte levels are within normal limits.	■ Monitor and replace electrolytes Mg and PO_4 qd and PRN.
Mobility/Safety There is no evidence of bruising due to preventable injury.	■ Institute bleeding precautions, including padded side rails, no sharp objects at or around bedside, assistance out of bed, and padded self-protective devices (if necessary). ■ Assess for bleeding/bruising q2h or more frequently.
Skin Integrity Skin will remain intact.	■ Assess skin q8h and each time patient is repositioned for pressure areas, petechiae, and ecchymosis. ■ Turn q2–4h. ■ Consider pressure relief/reduction mattress, avoid shearing forces. ■ Perform range-of-motion exercises every shift. ■ Use Braden Scale to assess risk of skin breakdown.
Nutrition Caloric and nutrient intake meets metabolic requirements per calculation (e.g., basal energy expenditure).	■ Provide parenteral feeding if NPO. ■ Assess for gastrointestinal bleeding and report. ■ Consult dietitian or nutritional support service.
Comfort/Pain Control Patient will be as comfortable as possible as evidenced by stable vital signs or cooperation with treatments or procedures.	■ Objectively assess comfort/pain using a pain scale. ■ Correlate pain ratings with sites of potential ischemia/infarction/hemorrhage. Notify house officer for correlation. ■ Provide warm compresses to promote vasodilation and decrease ischemic pain as indicated (with MD/NP/PA approval). ■ Provide analgesia and sedation as indicated by assessment. ■ Monitor patient response to medication.

(continued)

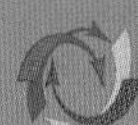

box 49-6 collaborative care guide for the Patient With Disseminated Intravascular Coagulation (DIC) (Continued)

OUTCOMES	INTERVENTIONS
Psychosocial	
Patient demonstrates decreased anxiety.	■ Educate patient and family regarding disease process, actions taken to correct disorder. ■ Provide areas of control to patient and family as possible (e.g., performance of ADLs, visitors) ■ Provide explanations and reassurance before procedures. ■ Consult social services, clergy as appropriate. ■ Provide for adequate rest and sleep.
Teaching/Discharge Planning	
Patient/significant others understand procedures and tests needed for treatment.	■ Prepare the patient and family for procedures, such as blood transfusions and laboratory studies. ■ Educate the patient and family regarding clinical parameters and patient presentation required for safe discharge from unit/hospital.

thrombotic process is removal of the cause of the DIC, if possible. Previously, heparin therapy was initiated to minimize further clotting. However, the risk of increased bleeding is always a major concern. In acute DIC, there have been few clinical studies showing heparin's effectiveness in slowing the coagulation cascade. Occasionally, nurses may see low-dose heparin therapy used in patients with DIC resulting from obstetrical accidents, severe arterial occlusion, or acute promyelocytic leukemia.[16]

MANAGEMENT OF BLEEDING OR POTENTIAL BLEEDING AND REPLACEMENT OF DEPLETED FACTORS

Correction of the imbalances between clotting and repletion clotting factors is the focus of the treatment for bleeding patients with DIC. Platelet transfusions are usually used only for patients with active bleeding and a platelet count of less than 50,000/mm^3, or for patients with inactive bleeding and a platelet count below 20,000 mm^3. Fresh frozen plasma contains components of both the coagulation and fibrinolytic systems. The recommended dose is 15 to 20 mL/kg. Cryoprecipitate may be used for patients with plasma fibrinogen levels below 100 mg/dL. A single unit provides 200 mg of fibrinogen, as well as factor VIII, factor XII, and von Willebrand's factor. The usual adult dose is 5 to 10 units, with each unit raising the fibrinogen level by 5 to 10 mg/dL. Depleted antithrombin III (necessary to balance clot production) can be replaced using heat-treated pooled plasma concentrates, and has been shown to shorten the duration of DIC.[18] Red blood cell transfusions, although not useful for repleting coagulation factors, are given to increase hemoglobin and oxygen-carrying capacity.

Localized bleeding can be minimized when possible. With venipuncture or removal of vascular access from compressible sites, pressure is applied for a minimum of 15 to 30 minutes or until bleeding has stopped. Sites are reassessed frequently for rebleeding because the initial clot may dissolve if the patient is deficient of the factors required to maintain hemostasis. Topical hemostatics may be used to provide topical hemostasis.

clinical applicability challenges

Self-Challenge: Critical Thinking

1. *Genetic testing and selection of embryos without a genetic defect are options available to couples who may have a genetic predisposition to a hematological disorder (e.g., Fanconi's anemia, hemophilia). Consider the ethical and financial implications of such interventions.*
2. *Immunosuppressive drugs and splenectomy are interventions used to manage a number of hematological disorders. Develop nursing interventions and a patient teaching plan for someone who is receiving this type of immunosuppressive therapy.*
3. *A variety of malignant factors can cause disseminated intravascular coagulation (DIC). Distinguish between factors that initiate the intrinsic and extrinsic pathways of coagulation.*
4. *Biochemical mediators are implicated in the activation and acceleration of the innate inflammatory response (IIR), which can precipitate DIC. Develop a plan of care directed to reducing the inflammatory response in a multiple trauma patient.*

Study Questions

1. *Iron-deficiency anemia may be caused by*
   a. *inadequate intake of iron in the diet.*
   b. *malabsorption of oral iron.*
   c. *chronic blood loss.*
   d. *all of the above.*
2. *The most effective treatment for chronic myelogenous leukemia (CML) is*
   a. *alpha interferon.*
   b. *bone marrow transplantation.*
   c. *STI571.*
   d. *glucocorticoids.*

3. *An acute episode of bleeding in a patient with hemophilia A would be managed with administration of*
   a. *von Willebrand's factor.*
   b. *factor VIII.*
   c. *factor IX.*
   d. *platelet transfusion.*
4. *Normal inhibitors of coagulation include all but which of the following?*
   a. *Adequate cardiac output, which dilutes activated factors*
   b. *Antithrombin III, which inactivates thrombin*
   c. *Tissue thromboplastin, which interferes with fibrin formation*
   d. *Plasminogen converting to plasmin*
5. *An early indication of a disseminated intravascular coagulation (DIC) process is bleeding associated with*
   a. *a decreased platelet count.*
   b. *a decreased prothrombin time (PT).*
   c. *decreased levels of fibrin degradation products (FDPs).*
   d. *increased fibrinogen.*
6. *Patients with disseminated intravascular coagulation (DIC), a hypercoagulable syndrome, bleed because of all of the following except:*
   a. *depleted clotting factors.*
   b. *increased levels of fibrin degradation products (FDPs).*
   c. *diffuse microthrombosis.*
   d. *decreased plasminogen levels.*

REFERENCES

1. Conrad ME: Anemia. Emedicine. Available at http://www.emedicine.com/med/topic123.htm. Accessed February 15, 2002
2. Branda RF, Kolhouse JF: Hemolytic anemias. In Wood ME (ed): Hematology/Oncology Secrets. Philadelphia, Hanley & Belfus, 1999
3. Godwin PF: Hematologic disorders. In Swearigen PL, Ross DG (eds): Manual of Medical-Surgical Nursing Care. St. Louis, Mosby, 1999
4. Dotts T: Are allogeneic stem cell transplants a "cure" for sickle cell disease? Hematol Oncol Today 4(1):2, 2003
5. Besa EC, Woerman U: Polycythemia vera. Emedicine. Available at http://www.emedicine.com/med/topic1864.htm. Accessed April 8, 2002
6. Seiter K: Acute lymphoblastic leukemia. Emedicine. Available at http://www.emedicine.com/med/topic3146.htm. Accessed February 7, 2002
7. Dotts T: STI571 should be standard for first-line CML. Hematol Oncol Today 4(1):11, 2003
8. Seiter K: Acute myelogenous leukemia. Emedicine. Available at http://www.emedicine.com/med/topic34.htm. Accessed December 31, 2001
9. Agaliotis DP: Hemophilia, overview. Emedicine. Available at http://www.emedicine.com/topic 3528.htm. Accessed May 31, 2002
10. Kovachy RJ, Schrier DM: Idiopathic thrombocytopenic purpura. In Wood ME (ed): Hematology/Oncology Secrets. Philadelphia, Hanley & Belfus, 1999
11. Hassell KL: Thrombotic thrombocytopenic purpura and hemolytic uremic syndrome. In Wood ME (ed): Hematology/Oncology Secrets. Philadelphia, Hanley & Belfus, 1999
12. Wun T, Bahou WF: Thrombotic thrombocytopenic purpura. Emedicine. Available at http://www.emedicine.com/topic2265.htm. Accessed February 20, 2002
13. Levi M, ten Cate H: Disseminated intravascular coagulation. N Engl J Med 341:586, 1999
14. Ziegfeld C, Shelton BK, Olsen M: Manual of Oncology Nursing. Philadelphia, Lippincott Williams & Wilkins, 2005
15. Messmore HL, Wehrmacher WH: Disseminated intravascular coagulation: A primer for primary care physicians. Postgrad Med 111(3), 2002
16. Geiter H: Disseminated intravascular coagulopathy. Dimens Crit Care Nurs 22(3):108–114, 2003
17. Bernard G, Vincent JL, Laterre PF, et al: Efficacy and safety of recombinant human activated protein C for severe sepsis. N Engl J Med 344:699–709, 2001
18. Riewald M, Reiss H: Treatment options for clinically recognized disseminated intravascular coagulation. Semin Thromb Hemost 24:53–59, 1998

OTHER SELECTED READING

Barbui T, Falana A: Disseminated intravascular coagulation in acute leukemia. Semin Thromb Hemost 27(6):593–604, 2001

Bick RL: Disseminated intravascular coagulation. A review of etiology, pathophysiology, diagnosis, and management: guidelines for care. Clin Appl Thromb Hemost 8(1):1–31, 2002

Cleveland K: Argatroban: A new treatment option for heparin-induced thrombocytopenia. Crit Care Nurse 23(6):61–69, 2003

DeSancho MT, Rand JH: Bleeding and thrombotic complications in critically ill patients with cancer. Crit Care Clin 17:599–622, 2001

Gilcreast D, Avella P, Camarillo E, et al: Treating severe anemia in a trauma patient who is a Jehovah's Witness. Crit Care Nurse 21(2): 69–82, 2001

Levi MM, Vink R, deJonge E: Management of bleeding disorders by prohemostatic therapy. Int J Hematol 76(Suppl 2):139–144, 2002

Maxson JH: Management of disseminated intravascular coagulation. Crit Care Clin North Am 12(3):341–352, 2000

Montoya V, Wink D, Sole ML: Adult anemia: Determination of clinical significance. Nurse Practitioner 27(3):38–53, 2002

Pearl RG, Pohlman A: Understanding and managing anemia in critically ill patients. Crit Care Nurse 22(12 Suppl):1–14, 2002

ten Cate H: Pathophysiology of disseminated intravascular coagulation in sepsis. Crit Care Med 28(9 Suppl):S9–S11, 2000

Williams E: Disseminated intravascular coagulation. In Loscalzo J, Schafer AI (eds): Thrombosis and Hemorrhage. Philadelphia, Lippincott Williams & Wilkins, 2003

Yu M, Nargella BS, Pechet L: Screening tests of disseminated intravascular coagulation: Guidelines for rapid and specific laboratory diagnosis. Crit Care Med 28:1777–1780, 2000

PART

one two three four five six seven eight nine ten

eleven

twelve

Integumentary System

INTERNET RESOURCES

Topic	Web Page Address
Alberta Burn Rehabilitation Society	www.burnrehab.com
The Alisa Ann Ruch Burn Foundation	www.aarbf.org
American Academy of Wound Management	www.aawm.org
American Burn Association	www.ameriburn.org
Burn Prevention Foundation	www.burnprevention.org
Dr. Koop's Online	www.drkoop.com
Medline Plus: Skin Cancer	www.nlm.nih.gov/medlineplus/skincancer.html
National Center for Injury Prevention & Control	www.cdc.gov/ncipc/default.htm
National Pressure Ulcer Advisory Panel	www.npuap.org
Ostomy Wound Management	www.o-wm.com
The Phoenix Society	www.phoenix-society.org
Regranex Gel Information	www.regranex.com
Shriners Hospitals for Children	www.shrinershq.org
Skin Care Physicians Homepage	www.skincarephysicians.com
U.S. Fire Administration	www.usfa.fema.gov
University of Michigan Trauma Burn Center	www.traumaburn.org
Wound Care Education Institute	www.wcei.net
Wound Care Information Network	www.medicaledu.com
Wound Care Resource	www.wounds1.com
Wound Care Strategies Homepage	www.woundcarestrategies.com
Wound Management Information	www.woundvac.com
Wound Management Practice Resource Center	www.smtl.co.uk/wmprc/index.html
Wound Ostomy & Continence Nurses Society	www.wocn.org
Woundcare Network	www.woundcarenet.com
Wounds: Clinical Research and Practice	www.woundsresearch.com

chapter

50

Anatomy and Physiology of the Integumentary System

JOAN DAVENPORT

objectives

Based on the content in this chapter, the reader should be able to:

- Describe the features of the epidermis, dermis and hypodermis.
- Identify the homeostatic functions of the skin.
- Explain the mechanism of infection resistance afforded by the integumentary system.
- Describe the appendages of the skin and state the purpose of each.
- Contrast features of the skin of the older adult and the child with the adult client.

The skin is described as protective, sensitive, reparative, and capable of maintaining an individual's homeostasis. These physiological features are explored in this chapter as functions of the anatomy of the skin and its appendages. The skin covers 1.2 to 2.3 m^2 of area and is the heaviest organ of the body.[1] The three layers of the skin are the outer epidermis, middle dermis, and the underlying hypodermis or subcutaneous tissue. The appendages include the hair, nail, eccrine and apocrine sweat glands, and the sebaceous glands. Figure 50-1 pictures the structures and layers of the skin. The functions of the skin include protection, sensation, water balance, temperature regulation, and vitamin production.

EPIDERMIS

This outer layer of the skin serves to protect underlying structures from invasion by microbes and other foreign substances. The cornified, external layer of the epidermis helps in the body's regulation of water loss. The innermost sublayer bends into the dermis and serves as the basis for the glands, nails, and hair roots. The epidermis does not have vascular supply; it depends on the dermal level for its nourishment.

Melanin and keratin are formed in the inner cellular layer of the epidermis. Melanocytes provide melanin, a pigment for both the skin and hair. This pigment provides the color for the skin and, more important, provides protection for the underlying structures from ultraviolet light exposure by absorbing and scattering the radiation.[2]

Keratin is a tough protein that makes up hair, nails, and the tough, outer epidermal surface. These flattened scales of the skin slough continually and are replaced every 2 to 4 weeks.[3] The epidermis is actually made up of five distinct layers; the keratinocytes move from inner to outer sublayers as they mature. At the top, outermost layer the keratinocytes are dead and are arranged in various thicknesses depending on the area of the body. In areas of the face there is a thin stratum made up of a layer 15 cells deep. This is contrasted to the thicker soles of the feet and palms of the hands, with at least 100 layers of keratinized cells.[2] It is these tough protein cells that serve to protect the underlying structures of the body.

DERMIS

The middle layer of the skin, the dermis, provides support for the outer epidermal layer. It is a very vascular connective tissue and the blood vessels are integral to regulation of body temperature and blood pressure. The arteriovenous anastomoses, under control of the sympathetic nervous system and found in the dermal layer, are able to

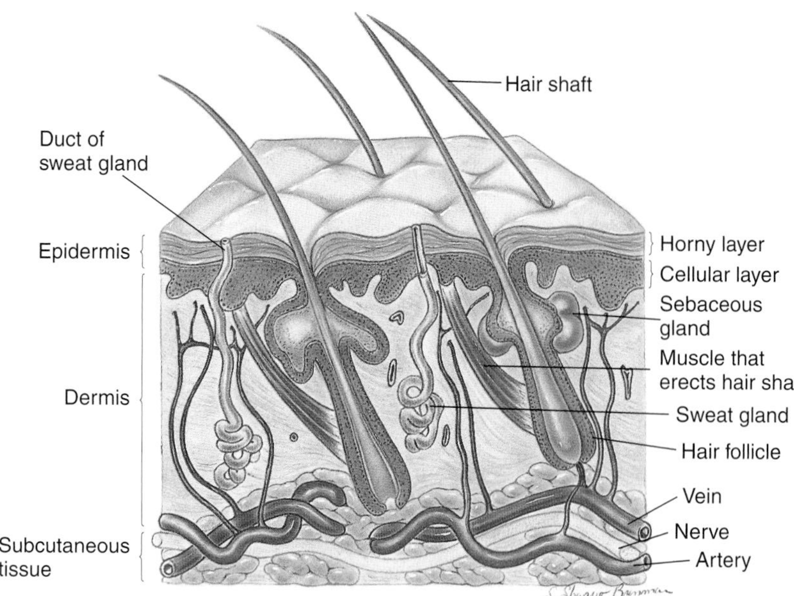

figure 50-1 Layers of the skin. (From Bickley LS, Szilagyi PG: Bates' Guide to Physical Examination and History Taking [8th Ed], p 95. Philadelphia, Lippincott Williams & Wilkins, 2003.)

dilate or constrict in response to environmental conditions of heat and cold and to internal stimulation from anxiety or blood volume loss.

The sensory function of the skin includes receptors for heat, cold, touch, pressure, and pain; these are located in the dermal layer. There is a great variety in the function of the nerve endings; multiple stimuli are mediated centrally and result in patterned responses.[2]

The dermis is composed of two distinct layers. The papillary dermis is the more superficial of the two layers, lying just beneath the epidermis. This layer provides the attachment for the epidermis as the epidermal basal cells project into the papillary dermis.[4]

The thicker underlayer of the dermis is the reticular dermis. Collagen is organized in a three-dimensional mesh pattern in this portion of the dermis. It is this mesh arrangement that allows the dermis to stretch with movement. Immune system components of the skin are found in the dermal layer and include macrophages, mast cells, T cells, and fibroblasts.[2]

HYPODERMIS

The hypodermis or subcutaneous skin layer consists of connective tissue interspersed with fat. The fat of the hypodermis has the protective functions of heat retention and cushioning the underlying structures. In addition, the fat of the subcutaneous skin layer serves as storage for calories.[5]

SKIN APPENDAGES

The hair, nails, and sebaceous and sweat glands are considered a part of the skin. These structures arise from or extrude through the epidermal or dermal skin layers.

Sweat Glands

Eccrine sweat glands are distributed throughout the surface of the skin. These glands arise from the dermis and open at the skin surface. These specialized glands secrete sweat for the purpose of internal body temperature regulation.

Apocrine sweat glands are not as widespread as the eccrine glands, are larger than eccrine glands, and open through a hair follicle of the axillae, nipples, areolae, groin, eyelids, and external ears.[5] Another difference between the two types of sweat glands is that the larger, less abundant apocrine glands secrete an oily substance with a particular odor. This odor is used by animals to recognize the presence of other animals. In humans, the odor, known as *body odor*, is produced when the secretions come in contact with bacteria and when the fluid begins to decompose.[2,5]

Sebaceous Glands

The sebaceous glands secrete sebum, a combination of triglycerides, cholesterol, and wax, through the hair follicle. These glands are situated over the entire surface of the skin except for the palms and soles of the feet. Sebaceous glands are inactive until puberty. At this time, they enlarge and are stimulated to secrete sebum by a rise in sex hormones. The sebum serves to keep the skin and hair from drying out.[5] By protecting the outer layer of the epidermis from undue drying, the sebum helps to conserve body heat. Table 50-1 summarizes the location and function of the eccrine, apocrine, and sebaceous glands.[6]

Hair

Epidermal cells in the dermis form the hair. Together with the sebaceous gland, the hair follicle forms the pilosebaceous unit. Vellus hair is unobtrusive, soft, and less pigmented than terminal hair. Terminal hair is darker, coarser, and more obvious. The follicular bulb is the site of vascular papilla, which nourishes and maintains the hair follicle. Hair color is determined by the melanocytes also found at the bulb. Under the sebaceous gland, adjacent to the hair follicle, are the arrector pili muscles. Contraction of the arrector pili causes gooseflesh, a reduction of skin surface area, and reduced surface area for heat loss (Fig. 50-2).

table 50-1 Sweat and Sebaceous Glands

Type of Gland	Location	Function
Eccrine sweat glands	All over body Numerous in thick skin Extended from dermis to epidermis	Regulate body temperature Respond to emotional distress Respond to physiological stimuli
Apocrine sweat glands	Axillae Nipples, breasts Anogenital region External ear canal Eyelids	Respond to hormonal influences Respond to emotional distress
Sebaceous glands	All over body except palms of hands, dorsum, and soles of feet	Produce sebum to lubricate hair and skin

From Allwood J, Curry K: Normal and altered functions of the skin. In Bullock BA, Henze RL (eds): Focus on Pathophysiology, p 842. Philadelphia, Lippincott Williams & Wilkins, 2000.

Nails

Hardened plates of epidermal keratin cells grow from a curved groove over the distal dorsal fingertips. These nails serve to protect the fingers and toes and increase physical dexterity. Approximately one fourth of the nail is covered by the proximal nail fold; the cuticle extends from the fold and serves to waterproof the space between the plate and the fold. The lunula is the white, "half-moon"–shaped edge distal to the cuticle. The angle between the proximal nail fold and the nail plate is expected to be less than 180 degrees (Fig. 50-3).

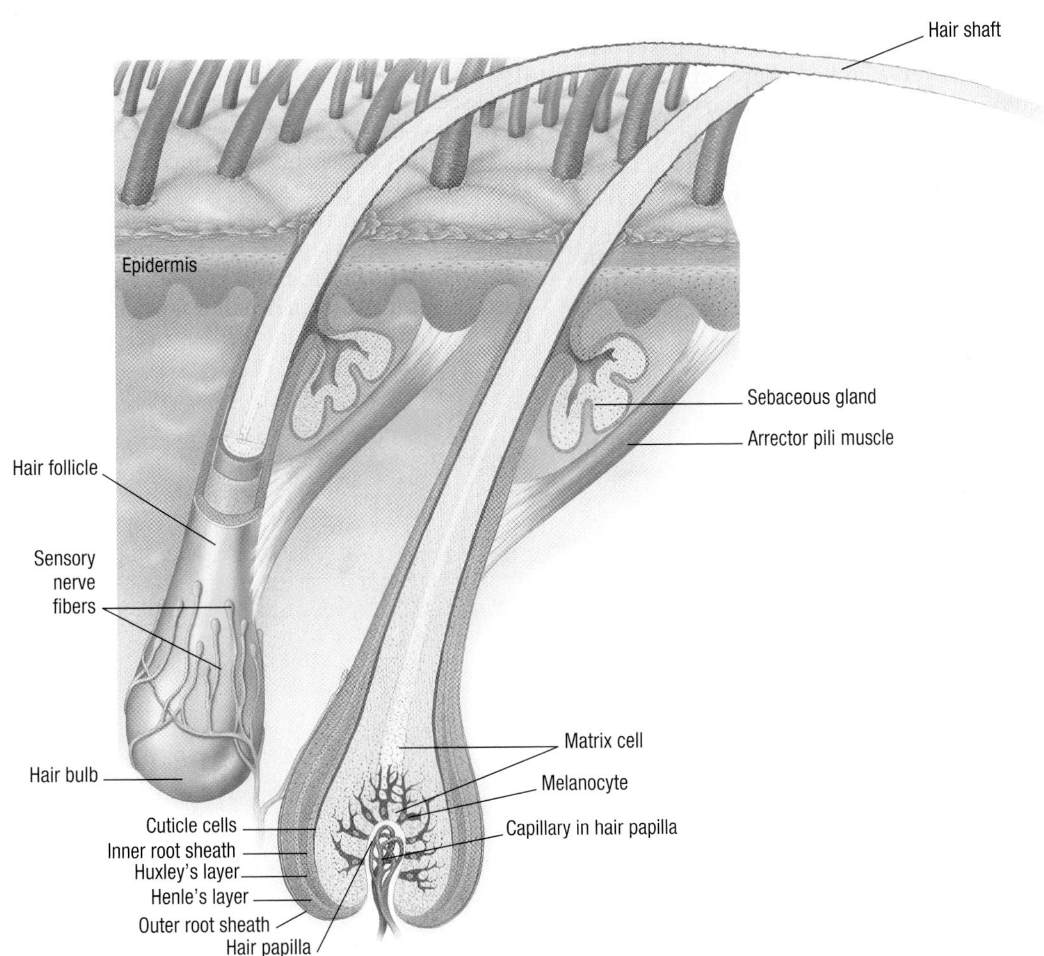

figure 50-2 Anatomical structures of hair. (From Anatomical Chart Company: Atlas of Human Anatomy, p 329. Springhouse, PA, Springhouse, 2001.)

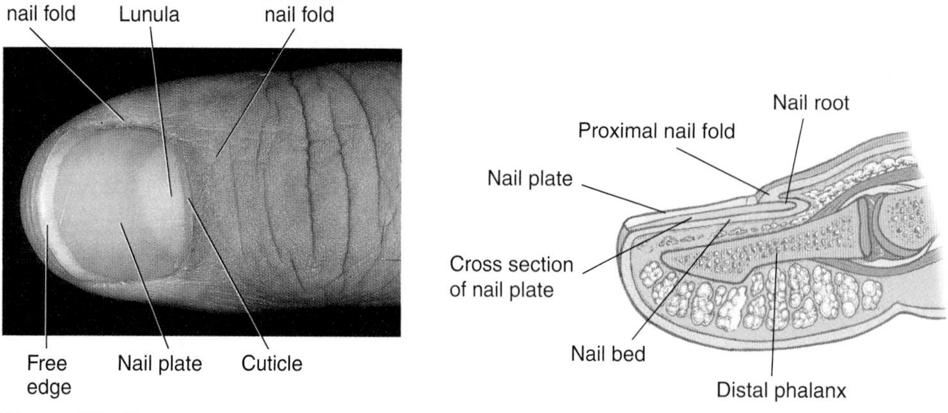

figure 50-3 The normal nail. (From Bickley LS, Szilagyi PG: Bates' Guide to Physical Examination and History Taking [8th Ed], p 96. Philadelphia, Lippincott Williams & Wilkins, 2003.)

FUNCTIONS OF THE SKIN

The epidermal layer of the integument provides protection against microbes, ultraviolet light exposure, and countless other threats. This tough, hardened outer layer also restricts water loss and thus helps to maintain organism homeostasis. The vascular dermis, with its rich supply of blood vessels, provides blood pressure and temperature regulatory features. Immune functions performed by macrophages, mast cells, T cells, and fibroblasts are also housed in the dermis. Nerve endings here supply receptors for heat, cold, touch, pressure, and pain. The skin's ability to stretch with movement is also provided by the dermal collagen's mesh formation. The underlying hypodermal layer of connective tissue and fat serve to retain heat and as a cushion for underlying structures. The appendages of the skin, the hair, nails, and glands, contribute to the homeostatic function primarily by controlling heat loss with the hair's arrector pili muscles and secretions by the sebaceous and sweat glands. The integument is vital to an individual's survival.

During critical care hospitalizations, there are many insults to the skin. Surgical wounds, vascular catheter insertions, opportunistic infections of the skin, nutritional compromise, and persistent pressure that leads to reduced blood flow are only a few of the challenges faced by the patient's integument. Attention to the skin and appendages by the nurse maximizes this organ's functioning and results in protection of the patient.

SKIN OF THE OLDER ADULT

In the older adult, it is expected that the skin may become thinner and drier, with less perspiration and increased itching; have increased wrinkles; bruise more easily; and have dark patches or old-age spots (solar lentigo). In addition, the older adult's hair may become gray and thinner, and terminal hair transitions to softer, vellus hair.[5,7] Each of these changes is attributed to physiological changes occurring over time, and they are summarized in Table 50-2.

SKIN OF THE CHILD

Expected differences in the skin, hair, nails, and glands depend on the age of the child. Infants and children, without exposure to the sun or wind, are expected to have very smooth-textured skin without coarse adult terminal hair. Infants, up to about 14 days of age, may be covered with lanugo, a fine, silky-textured hair.[5] Infants also have less developed hypodermal fat and, as a result, are at risk for hypothermia. The sweat glands do not begin to function until 1 month of age and are not fully functional until adolescence.

In the young child, the most noticeable variation may be that of bruising as the child increases activity and play becomes more aggressive. It is important to note the location and color changes of bruising indicating the stage of healing. Bruising is more common and not unexpected on the lower legs and the face. Bruising on the upper arms, buttocks, and abdomen occurs less often and may be indicative of abuse and warrant further investigation.[5]

table 50-2 **Skin Changes in the Older Adult**

Changes Seen in the Older Adult	Physiological Cause
Dryness, itching, and decreased perspiration	Decreased sebaceous and sweat gland activity
Thinning of skin	Decreased vascularity of the dermis
Increased bruising	Thinning of the hypodermal layer with less fat protection
Solar lentingo	Chronic sun exposure
Increased wrinkles	Loss of dermal elasticity, collagen, and mass
Thinning hair	Hormonal changes
Graying hair	Decreased melanin

table 50-3 Expected Skin of the Child

Age Group	Expected Variant
Infant	Smooth skin Lack of terminal hair Lanugo Less hypodermal fat Decreased sweat gland activity
Child	Some bruising*
Adolescent	Sweat and sebaceous gland activity begins Terminal axillary and pubic hair development

*NOTE: It is very important to attend to bruising seen in the child; it may be associated with abusive situations.

In the adolescent, the sweat glands and sebaceous glands become fully functional. The adolescent may be expected to experience body odor, increasing axillary perspiration, and acne.[8] The development of axillary and pubic hair is expected related to the increasing levels of circulating androgen levels in both male and female adolescents.[5] Each of these expected variants for the integument of the child is included in Table 50-3.

clinical applicability challenges

Self-Challenge: Critical Thinking

1. *In what ways does the skin help to maintain homeostasis?*
2. *In what ways is protection against ultraviolet light afforded by the skin and appendages?*

Study Questions

1. *Which layer of the skin does not have its own blood supply?*
   a. *Dermis*
   b. *Epidermis*
   c. *Hypodermis*
   d. *Sebaceous glands*
2. *Eccrine sweat glands help to maintain*
   a. *blood flow to the subdermal layer.*
   b. *epidermal skin integrity.*
   c. *internal body temperature.*
   d. *skin color.*
3. *What is the function of melanin?*
   a. *It provides a tough outer layer to protect underlying structures.*
   b. *It promotes skin sloughing and replacement by the epidermal layer.*
   c. *It is necessary for sebaceous gland activity.*
   d. *It provides the skin with color and protection from light exposure.*
4. *What accounts for the thinning of skin seen in the older adult?*
   a. *Decreased vascularity of the dermis*
   b. *Decreased sweat gland function*
   c. *Increased fat deposits in the subdermal layer*
   d. *Increased hormone production*
5. *The ability to sense touch, pain, and temperature is provided by*
   a. *the epidermis.*
   b. *the dermis.*
   c. *the hypodermis.*
   d. *the outer surface of the nails.*

REFERENCES

1. Bickley LS, Szilagyi PG: The skin. In Bickley LS, Szilagyi PG (eds): Guide to Physical Examination and History Taking (8th Ed), pp 95–113. Philadelphia, Lippincott Williams & Wilkins, 2003
2. Simandl G: Control of integumentary function. In Porth CM (ed): Pathophysiology: Concepts of Altered Health States (6th Ed), pp 1393–1400. Philadelphia, Lippincott Williams & Wilkins, 2002
3. Lewis SM, Heitkemper MM, Dirksen SR: Medical-Surgical Nursing: Assessment and Management of Clinical Problems (5th Ed). St. Louis, Mosby, 2000
4. Wysocki AB: Skin anatomy, physiology, and pathophysiology. Nurs Clin North Am 34:777–798, 2000
5. Wilson SF, Giddons JF: Skin, hair, and nails. In Wilson SF, Giddons JF (eds): Health Assessment for Nursing Practice (2nd Ed), pp 257–287. St. Louis, Mosby, 2002
6. Allwood J, Curry K: Normal and altered functions of the skin. In Bullock BA, Henze RL (eds): Focus on Pathophysiology, pp 837–873. Philadelphia, Lippincott Williams & Wilkins, 2000.
7. American Academy of Dermatology: Agingskinnet. Skincare physicans.com, 2000. Available at http://www.skincarephysicians.com/agingskinnet/Q&A. Accessed July 1, 2003
8. Hockenberry MJ, Wilson D, Winkelstein ML, et al (eds): Wong's Nursing Care of Infants and Children (7th Ed). St. Louis, Mosby, 2003

OTHER SELECTED READING

Hayes KVD: Skin wellness and illness. In Condon MC (ed): Women's Health. Upper Saddle River, NJ, Prentice-Hall, 2004

Tortora GJ, Grabowski S: Principles of Anatomy and Physiology (9th Ed), pp 140–159. New York, John Wiley & Sons, 2000

chapter

51

Patient Assessment: Integumentary System

JOAN DAVENPORT

objectives

Based on the content in this chapter, the reader should be able to:

- Identify the assessment skill necessary for the critical care nurse to use when evaluating the health of a patient's skin.
- Identify expected differences in skin color related to racial or skin tone characteristics.
- Describe and recognize abnormal changes in skin color.
- Recognize and describe skin lesions resulting from increased vascularity.
- Describe the significance of rashes related to infection or to allergic reaction.
- Identify the pitting and nonpitting edema.
- Explain the cause of pressure ulcers and at least one scale used to assess a patient for pressure ulcer development.
- Describe the features of malignant skin diseases.

The skin of a critically ill person is exposed to insults ranging from diminished blood flow and the resultant risk of pressure ulceration to rashes from hypersensitivity drug reactions and opportunistic infections. There is often ample opportunity for the critical care nurse to assess the skin—the intimacy involved in providing care to someone who is critically ill, the relative level of undress of the patient, and the attention to detail implicit in critical care nursing make integument assessment an ongoing and vital process.

HISTORY

When caring for patients with skin disorders, it is important to obtain information from the health history (Box 51-1). The information is useful in guiding the physical examination and in determining appropriate interventions.

PHYSICAL EXAMINATION

The assessment techniques necessary for an evaluation of the integument involve inspection and palpation.

Inspection

Inspection of the general appearance of the skin includes assessment of color; determination of the presence of lesions, rashes, or increased vascularity; and assessment of the condition of the nails and hair.

COLOR

Skin color is expected to be uniform over the body, except for the areas with greater degrees of vascularity. The genitalia, upper chest, and cheeks may appear pink or have a reddish tone in people with light skin. These same areas may appear darker in people with dark skin. Additional normal variations in skin color include those listed in Table 51-1.

box 51-1
Patient History—Skin Disorders

Patient history relevant to skin disorders may be obtained by asking the following questions:

When did you first notice this skin problem? (Also investigate duration and intensity.)
Has it occurred previously?
Are there any other symptoms?
What site was first affected?
What did the rash or lesion look like when it first appeared?
Where and how fast did it spread?
Do you have any itching, burning, tingling, or crawling sensations?
Is there any loss of sensation?
Is the problem worse at a particular time or season?
How do you think it started?
Do you have a history of hay fever, asthma, hives, eczema, or allergies?
Who in your family has skin problems or rashes?
Did the eruptions appear after certain foods were eaten? Which foods?
When the problem occurred, had you recently consumed alcohol?
What relation do you think there may be between a specific event and the outbreak of the rash or lesion?
What medications are you taking?
What topical medication (ointment, cream, salve) have you put on the lesion (including over-the-counter medications)?
What skin products or cosmetics do you use?
What is your occupation?
What in your immediate environment (plants, animals, chemicals, infections) might be precipitating this disorder? Is there anything new, or are there any changes in the environment?
Does anything touching your skin cause a rash?
How has this affected you (or your life)?
Is there anything else you wish to talk about in regard to this disorder?

From Smeltzer SC, Bare BG: Brunner & Suddarth's Textbook of Medical-Surgical Nursing (10th Ed), p 1645. Philadelphia, Lippincott Williams & Wilkins, 2004.

Skin color is determined by the presence of four pigments: melanin, carotene, hemoglobin, and deoxyhemoglobin. The amount of melanin is genetically determined and produces varying degrees of dark skin tone. Carotene, a yellow pigment, is in subcutaneous fat and is most evident in those areas with the most keratin, the palms and soles of the feet. Skin color abnormalities, such as pallor, cyanosis, jaundice, and erythema, manifest differently depending on the person's normal skin tone (Table 51-2).

The degree of oxygenation affects skin color. Hemoglobin, attached to red blood cells, transports oxygen to the tissues. A diminished flow of oxyhemoglobin through the cutaneous circulation results in pallor. In people with light skin, the skin appears very pale, without the usual pink undertones. In people with darker skin, pallor manifests as a yellowish-brown or ashen appearance (again, because the usual pink undertones are lost).

table 51-1 Normal Variations in Skin Color

Normal Variation	Description
Moles (pigmented nevi)	Tan to dark brown; may be flat or raised
Stretch mark (striae)	Silver or pink; may be caused by weight gain or pregnancy
Freckles	Flat macules anywhere on the body
Vitiligo	Unpigmented skin area; more prevalent in people with dark skin
Birthmarks	Generally flat marks anywhere on the body; may be tan, red, or brown

As hemoglobin gives up its oxygen to the tissues, the hemoglobin changes to deoxyhemoglobin. When deoxyhemoglobin is present in the cutaneous circulation, the skin takes on a blue cast and the individual is said to be cyanotic.[1] In light-skinned people, cyanosis may be seen as a grayish-blue color, especially in the palms and soles of the feet, the nail beds, the earlobes, the lips, and the mucous membranes. In those with darker skin, cyanosis evidences itself as an ashen-gray color seen easiest in the conjunctiva, oral mucous membranes, and nail beds.[2]

The yellowish hue of jaundice is indicative of liver disease or of hemolysis of red blood cells. In dark-skinned people, jaundice is seen as a yellowish-green color in the sclera, palms of the hands, and soles of the feet. In light-skinned people, jaundice is seen as a yellow coloration of the skin, sclera, lips, hard palate, and underside of the tongue. Bickley and Szilagyi recommend using a transparent slide pressed against the lips to "blanch out the red color," making the yellow of jaundice more easily seen.[1]

Another skin color abnormality is erythema. Erythema manifests as a reddish tone in light-skinned people and a deeper brown or purple tone in dark-skinned people. It is indicative of increased skin temperature caused by inflammation. The process of inflammation increases vascularity of the tissues and this, in turn, produces the color alteration seen with erythema. Erythema may be expected when associated with a surgical wound, due to the inflammatory process inherent in any tissue trauma. It is also seen in disease processes affecting the skin, such as cellulitis. In either case, the erythema is indicative of inflammation.

LESIONS

Skin lesions are variously described by their color, shape, cause, or general appearance (Table 51-3). They are considered abnormal conditions and arise from many factors. In general, it is important to note the anatomical location, distribution, color, size, and pattern of any abnormal skin lesion. In addition, details about the lesion's borders or edges, as well as whether the lesion is flat, raised, or sunken, should be noted. Finally, the length of time the lesion has

table 51-2 Skin Color Abnormalities

Skin Color Abnormality	Underlying Cause	Manifestation in Light-Skinned People	Manifestation in Dark-Skinned People
Pallor	Decreased blood flow (decreased oxyhemoglobin flow to tissues)	Excessively pale skin	Yellowish-brown or ashen color to the skin
Cyanosis	Increased deoxyhemoglobin in the cutaneous circulation	Grayish-blue color of the palms and soles of the feet, the nail beds, the lips, the earlobes, and the mucous membranes	Ashen-gray color of the conjunctiva, oral mucous membranes, and nail beds
Jaundice	Increased red blood cell hemolysis, liver disease	Yellow color of the sclera, lips, and hard palate	Yellow-green color of the sclera and palms and soles of the feet
Erythema	Inflammation	Reddish tone	Deeper brown or purple tone

table 51-3 Types of Skin Lesions

Lesion	Description
Blister	Fluid-filled vesicle or bulla
Bulla	Blister larger than 1 cm
Comedo	Plugged and dilated pore, called blackhead or whitehead
Crust	Dried exudate over a damaged epithelium; may be associated with vesicle, bullae, or pustules
Cyst	Semisolid or fluid-filled mass, encapsulated in deeper layers of skin
Desquamation	Shedding or loss of debris on skin surface
Erosion	Loss of epidermis; may be associated with vesicles, bullae, or pustules
Excoriation	Epidermal erosion usually caused by scratching
Fissure	Crack in the epidermis usually extending into the dermis
Macule	Flat area of skin with discoloration, less than 5 mm in diameter
Nodule	Solid, elevated lesion or mass, 5 mm to 5 cm in diameter
Papule	Solid, elevated lesion less than 5 mm in diameter
Plaque	Raised, flattened lesion greater than 5 mm in diameter
Pustule	Papule containing purulent exudate
Scale	Skin debris on the surface of the epidermis
Tumor	Solid mass, larger than 5 cm in diameter; usually extends to dermis
Ulceration	Loss of epidermis, extending into dermis or deeper
Urticaria	Raised wheal-like lesion
Vesicle	Small fluid-filled lesion, less than 1 cm in diameter
Wheal	Transient, irregular pink elevation with surrounding edema

From Allwood J, Curry K: Normal and altered functions of the skin. In Bullock BA, Henze RL (eds): Focus on Pathophysiology, pp 837–873, Philadelphia, Lippincott Williams & Wilkins, 2000

been present, and any environmental or medication exposure that may be considered contributory, are also noted.[3]

Vascular lesions can be either a normal variation or an abnormal finding. Vascular changes considered to be normal variants include nevus flammeus (port-wine stain), immature hemangioma (strawberry mark), telangiectasis, cherry angioma, and capillary hemangioma (Table 51-4). Abnormal vascular findings include petechiae, purpura, ecchymoses, spider angiomas, and urticaria (hives). These findings may indicate disease or injury and warrant further investigation by the critical care nurse.

Petechiae are purple or red, small (1- to 3-mm) lesions easily seen on light-skinned individuals and more difficult to see in those with dark skin (Fig. 51-1A). They may be seen on the oral mucosa and in the conjunctiva. They do not disappear when pressure is applied to them.[2] Petechiae result from tiny hemorrhages in the dermal or submucosal layers. Purpura are very similar to petechiae, only larger. Purpura may appear brownish-red.

Ecchymoses are bruises. They may appear as purple to yellowish-green rounded or irregular lesions, and are more easily seen in people with light skin (see Fig. 51-1B). Ecchymoses occur as a result of trauma, when blood leaks from damaged blood vessels into the surrounding tissue.

Spider angiomas are fiery red lesions that are most often located on the face, neck, arms, or upper trunk (see Fig. 51-1C). Spider angiomas are seldom seen below the waist. They have a central body that is sometimes "raised and surrounded by erythema and radiating legs."[1] These lesions are most often associated with liver disease and vitamin B deficiency.[2]

Urticaria is a reddened or white, raised, nonpitting plaque that often occurs as a result of an allergic reaction. The lesion often changes shape and size during the course of the reaction. The edema associated with urticaria is a result of local vasodilation and inflammation, which is followed by transudation of serous vascular fluid into the surrounding tissue.

RASHES

Rashes identified during inspection may indicate infection or a reaction to drug therapy. Some of these rashes are identified by the names listed in Table 51-3. Identifying the type of lesion may help in identifying the cause of the rash. Attention to the development of a rash in association with a change in pharmacotherapy is essential to help identify the occurrence of an allergic hypersensitivity reaction.[4] The development of urticaria is often associated with food or drug reactions. Urticaria usually resolves completely over days to several weeks as the excess local fluid is reabsorbed. These lesions are often pruritic, and patient scratching may precipitate secondary skin abrasions, which can place the patient at risk for localized skin infections.

Skin infections are most often caused by fungi or yeasts, and may range from superficial tinea pedis (athlete's foot) to intermediate yeast infections (e.g., moniliasis resulting from *Candida albicans* infection) to deep fungal infections (e.g., aspergillosis) that invade the underlying tissues. Most often in the critical care setting, fungal and yeast infections are of the intermediate type and are the result of an opportunistic infection by normal flora. Antibiotics and corticosteroids place the patient at risk for these infections. Candidiasis presents in the groin and under the breasts of female patients with "erythema, a whitish pseudomembrane, and peripheral papules and pustules."[5] Oral candidiasis, also known as *thrush*, manifests as a whitish coating of the oral mucosa, especially the tongue. This painful condition may produce fissures on the tongue and often restricts a patient's oral intake, further compromising the patient from a nutritional perspective.

CONDITION OF THE HAIR

The patient's terminal hair is inspected daily, noting the hair's quantity, distribution, and texture. Scalp hair should be resilient and evenly distributed.

Alopecia refers to hair loss and can be diffuse, patchy, or complete. Hair loss in the critical care setting can be associated with pharmacotherapy. Chemotherapy used in oncology treatment produces alopecia. Other drugs, such as heparin, used for a prolonged time may also be responsible for hair loss.[6] Hirsutism or increased facial, body, or pubic hair growth is an abnormal finding in the examination of women and children. Hirsutism has a familial pattern and is associated with menopause, endocrine disorders, and certain pharmacotherapies (e.g., corticosteroids and androgenic medications).[2]

A change in the hair's texture may indicate ongoing health concerns. Hair that is thin and brittle occurs in

table 51-4 Vascular Lesions: Normal Variations

Normal Variation	Description
Nevus flammeus (port-wine stain), immature hemangioma (strawberry mark)	Range from dark red to pale pink in color and are considered birthmarks
Cherry angioma	Small, slightly raised, bright red lesions on the face, neck, and trunk; increase in size and number with advancing age
Capillary hemangioma	Red, irregular patch caused by capillary dilation in the dermis of the skin
Telangiectasis	Irregular, fine red lines caused by permanent dilation of a group of superficial vessels

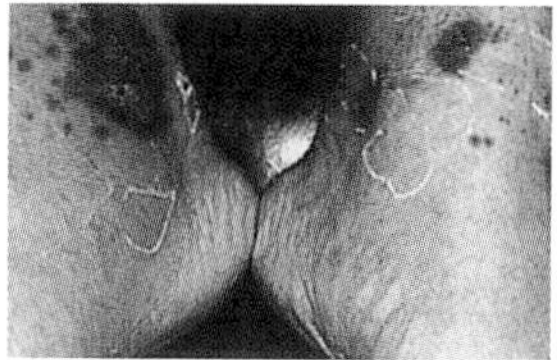

A. Petechiae/purpura

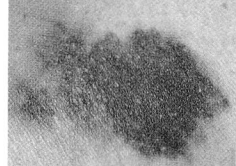

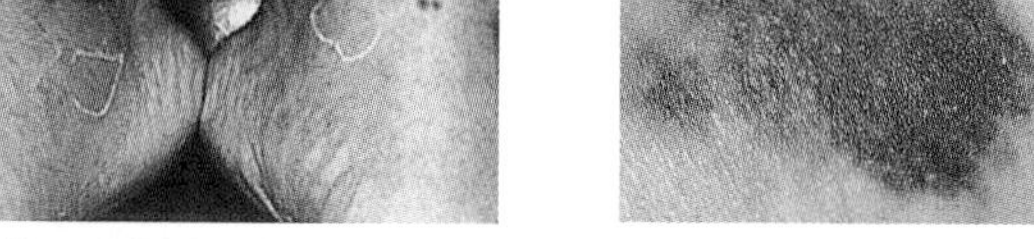

B. Ecchymosis

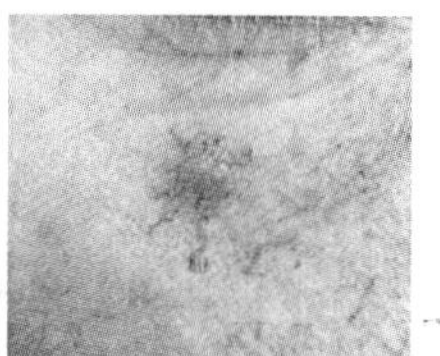

C. Spider angioma

figure 51-1 Abnormal vascular lesions. (**A,** used with permission from Kelley WN: Textbook of Internal Medicine. Philadelphia, JB Lippincott, 1989. **B,** used with permission from Bickley L: Bates' Guide to Physical Examination and History Taking [8th Ed], p 106. Philadelphia, Lippincott Williams & Wilkins, 2003. **C,** used with permission from Marks R: Skin Disease in Old Age. Philadelphia, JB Lippincott, 1987.)

hypothyroidism. In those with severe protein malnutrition, the hair color may appear reddish or bleached and the hair texture is described as coarse and dry.[7]

Also not to be overlooked is the presence of infection or infestation of the scalp and hair. The patient's scalp and body hair is inspected regularly for evidence of flaking, sores, lice, louse eggs, and ringworm.[7] During the inspection, the hair is parted in several areas to reveal the underlying scalp.

CONDITION OF THE NAILS

Nails, like hair, can be overlooked in the rush of critical care nursing; however, a careful inspection as part of the "routine" assessment can reveal information about the patient's general state of health. The nail bed is very vascular and is an excellent location for assessing the adequacy of the patient's peripheral circulation. The capillary refill test, done by blanching the nail beds and then releasing the pressure, should indicate a return of the pink tones in less than 3 seconds. Nail beds that are bluish or purplish in tint may be indicative of cyanosis; nail beds that are pale may indicate reduced arterial blood flow.

When the angle of the nail is 180 degrees or greater, clubbing is said to be present (see Chapter 24, Fig. 24-2). Clubbing is attributed to chronic hypoxemia. Other shapes that the nail takes on may provide clues to deficient nutritional states of the patient. Chronic disease states such as cirrhosis, heart failure, and type 2 diabetes mellitus may affect the nails by producing Terry's nails.[1] These nails are whitish with a distal band of dark reddish-brown color, and the lunulae may not be visible (Fig. 51-2). A spoon-shaped nail, called *koilonychias,* is associated with iron-deficiency anemia. Bands across the nails, especially in the older adult, may indicate protein deficiency. White spots on the nails are associated with zinc deficiency.[7]

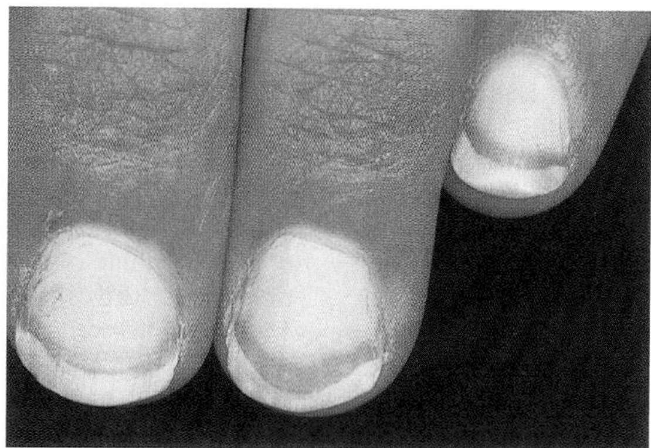

figure 51-2 Terry's nails, seen in people with chronic diseases such as cirrhosis, congestive heart failure, and type 2 diabetes mellitus. (Used with permission from Bickley L: Bates' Guide to Physical Examination and History Taking [8th Ed], p 110. Philadelphia, Lippincott Williams & Wilkins, 2003.)

Palpation

The skin is palpated for texture, moisture, temperature, mobility and turgor, and edema. In addition, during palpation any evidence of discomfort arising from the areas palpated is noteworthy.

TEXTURE

Texture refers to the smoothness of the skin surface. It requires gentle palpation to assess. Rough skin occurs in patients with hypothyroidism.

MOISTURE

The skin may be described as dry, oily, diaphoretic, or clammy. Dry skin may be seen in the patient with hypothyroidism. Skin is oily with acne and with increased activity of the sebaceous glands, as in Parkinson's disease. Diaphoresis may be a response to increased temperature or increased metabolic rate. *Hyperhidrosis* is the term given to excessive perspiration. *Bromhidrosis* refers to foul-smelling perspiration. Low cardiac output states may produce skin that is referred to as *clammy.*

TEMPERATURE

Temperature is usually assessed with the dorsal surface of the hand to identify the general skin temperature as warm or cool. The skin's temperature can also be used to assess the possibility of reduced blood flow from an arterial insufficiency. In this case, the skin may be noticeably cooler distal to an occluding lesion.

MOBILITY AND TURGOR

Mobility and turgor provide information about the health of the skin and may yield information about the patient's fluid volume balance. When assessed centrally, over the clavicles, the skin is expected to lift up easily and quickly return into place. Skin mobility may be decreased in scleroderma or in a patient with increased edema. Skin turgor is decreased in the patient with dehydration.[1]

EDEMA

Edema is classified as either nonpitting or pitting. Nonpitting edema is that which does not depress with palpation. Nonpitting edema is seen in patients with a local inflammatory response and is caused by capillary endothelial damage. In addition to the edema, the skin is usually red, tender, and warm. Pitting edema is usually in the skin of the extremities and in dependent body parts. Pitting edema is identified as edema that retains the depression made when palpated. This type of edema can be further classified by the depth of the depression and, occasionally, by the amount of time it takes the pit to rebound (Table 51-5).

ASSESSMENT OF PRESSURE ULCERS

The development of pressure ulcers in the critically ill patient is a preventable complication. The difficulty arises in the patient with multiple-system dysfunction with concomitant fluid, electrolyte, and nutritional deficiencies. Common pressure ulcer points include the occiput, scapula, sacrum, buttocks, ischium, heels, and toes. It is the pressure applied by the weight of the body that causes a reduction in arterial and capillary blood flow, leading to these ischemic events. Therefore, frequent position changes are required to prevent the development of pressure ulcers. Pressure ulceration on the toes occurs as a result of the pressure of the bed linen on the feet. Dressing devices and wound appliances can place pressure on underlying skin, resulting in reduced blood flow. The back of the neck of the patient with a tracheostomy tube must be assessed because the tube holder may be applied too tightly. The tape securing a nasogastric tube must be regularly removed and the condition of the tip of the nose and nares assessed for changes resulting from pressure from the tube.

Assisting the patient with frequent position changes is crucial in preventing pressure ulcers from developing. In addition, keeping the skin clean and dry is requisite in the prevention of pressure ulceration. Moisture increases the risk for maceration of the skin and promotes its breakdown. Infectious matter in wound drainage or feces increases the risk that an ulcer will progress and become a major source of sepsis.

Patients with decreased sensation (e.g., from brain or spinal cord injury or from a peripheral neuropathy such as that caused by diabetes) are at greater risk for ulceration because they do not recognize the discomfort from being in one position for extended periods. Similarly, patients with sedation or frequent analgesic dosing are at increased risk for problems related to their immobility. Patients with poor circulation, such as that caused by hypotension, heart failure, or peripheral vascular insufficiency, are also at higher risk because of the underlying possibility of tissue hypoxia. Lack of movement then serves only to accelerate the process of pressure ulcer development.

Identifying those individuals most at risk for pressure ulcer development is a focus of assessment. Recognizing that there are certain features that increase a patient's risk for development of pressure ulcers allows the critical care nurse to increase surveillance and implement preventative treatment modalities. Problems with sensory perception, moisture, activity, mobility, nutrition, and friction and shearing forces increase the patient's risk for development of pressure ulcers, which are debilitating and expensive to treat. Critically ill patients are among those with the most significant limitations of these parameters, and therefore are at very high risk for the development of pressure ulcers.

Many tools for assessing pressure ulcer risk use a point system.[8,9] The Braden Scale for Predicting Pressure Sore Risk, recommended in the guidelines set forth by the U.S. Agency for Health Care Policy and Research and widely used in hospital settings, requires the daily assessment of six parameters and provides a numerical score ranging from a very high risk score of 6 to a very limited risk or minimal risk score of 23[10] (Fig. 51-3). Adults with a score below 16 (18 for older adults) are considered at risk and specific interventions to prevent the development of ulceration are recommended. There has been some work done to establish the relative risk among those with darker-pigmented skin using a higher cut-off score of 18.[11] A 2002 study by Bergstrom and Braden compared cut-off scores for black and white populations and found no difference between scores, but a score of 18 best predicts pressure ulcer risk for both groups.[12]

During assessment of the skin, the nurse must be vigilant for signs of skin breakdown (Fig. 51-4).

ASSESSMENT OF SKIN TUMORS

Benign nevus and seborrheic keratosis are common, benign skin lesions. The benign nevus or mole appears in the first two to three decades and its appearance remains unchanged

table 51-5 Pitting Edema Scale

Scale (1+ to 4+)	Measurement	Description	Time to Rebound
1+/4	2 mm	Barely detectable	Immediate
2+/4	4 mm	Deeper pit	Few seconds
3+/4	6 mm	Deep pit	10–20 sec
4+/4	10 mm	Very deep pit	> 20 sec

Braden Scale
FOR PREDICTING PRESSURE SORE RISK

Patient's Name__________ Evaluator's Name__________ Date of Assessment

SENSORY PERCEPTION Ability to respond meaningfully to pressure-related discomfort	**1. Completely Limited:** Unresponsive (does not moan, flinch, or grasp) to painful stimuli, due to diminished level of consciousness or sedation. OR limited ability to feel pain over most of body surface.	**2. Very Limited:** Responds only to painful stimuli. Cannot communicate discomfort except by moaning or restlessness. OR has a sensory impairment which limits the ability to feel pain or discomfort over 1/2 of body	**3. Slightly Limited:** Responds to verbal commands, but cannot always communicate discomfort or need to be turned. OR has some sensory impairment which limits ability to feel pain or discomfort in 1 or 2 extremities.	**4. No Impairment:** Responds to verbal commands. Has no sensory deficit which would limit ability to feel or voice pain or discomfort.	
MOISTURE Degree to which skin is exposed to moisture	**1. Constantly Moist:** Skin is kept moist almost constantly by perspiration, urine, etc. Dampness is detected every time patient is moved or turned.	**2. Very Moist:** Skin is often, but not always, moist. Linen must be changed at least once a shift.	**3. Occasionally Moist:** Skin is occasionally moist, requiring an extra linen change approximately once a day.	**4. Rarely Moist:** Skin is usually dry, linen only requires changing at routine intervals.	
ACTIVITY Degree of physical activity	**1. Bedfast:** Confined to bed	**2. Chairfast:** Ability to walk severely limited or nonexistent. Cannot bear own weight and/or must be assisted into chair or wheelchair.	**3. Walks Occasionally:** Walks occasionally during day, but for very short distances, with or without assistance. Spends majority of each shift in bed or chair.	**4. Walks Frequently:** Walks outside the room at least twice a day and inside room at least once every 2 hours during waking hours.	
MOBILITY Ability to change and control body position	**1. Completely Immobile:** Does not make even slight changes in body or extremity position without assistance.	**2. Very Limited:** Makes occasional slight changes in body or extremity position but unable to make frequent or significant changes independently.	**3. Slightly Limited:** Makes frequent though slight changes in body or extremity position independently.	**4. No Limitations:** Makes major and frequent changes in position without assistance.	
NUTRITION Usual food intake pattern	**1. Very Poor:** Never eats a complete meal. Rarely eats more than 1/3 of any food offered. Eats 2 servings or less of protein (meat or dairy products) per day. Takes fluids poorly. Does not take a liquid dietary supplement. OR is NPO and/or maintained on clear liquids or IVs for more than 5 days.	**2. Probably Inadequate:** Rarely eats a complete meal and generally eats only about 1/2 of any food offered. Protein intake includes only 3 servings of meat or dairy products per day. Occasionally will take a dietary supplement. OR receives less than optimum amount of liquid diet or tube feeding.	**3. Adequate:** Eats over half of most meals. Eats a total of 4 servings of protein (meat, dairy products) each day. Occasionally will refuse a meal, but will usually take a supplement if offered. OR is on a tube feeding or TPN regimen which probably meets most of nutritional needs.	**4. Excellent:** Eats most of every meal. Never refuses a meal. Usually eats a total of 4 or more servings of meat and dairy products. Occasionally eats between meals. Does not require supplementation.	
FRICTION AND SHEAR	**1. Problem:** Requires moderate to maximum assistance in moving. Complete lifting without sliding against sheets is impossible. Frequently slides down in bed or chair, requiring frequent repositioning with maximum assistance. Spasticity, contractures or agitation leads to almost constant friction.	**2. Potential Problem:** Moves feebly or requires minimum assistance. During a move skin probably slides to some extent against sheets, chair, restraints, or other devices. Maintains relatively good position in chair or bed most of the time but occasionally slides down.	**3. No Apparent Problem:** Moves in bed and in chair independently and has sufficient muscle strength to lift up completely during move. Maintains good position in bed or chair at all times.		

Braden Scale Scores
1 = Highly Impaired
3 or 4 = Moderate to Low Impairment
Total Points Possible: 23
Risk Predicting Score: 16 or Less

NPO: Nothing by Mouth
IV: Intravenously
TPN: Total parenteral nutrition

Total Score

figure 51-3 The Braden Scale is a widely used screening tool to identify people at risk for pressure ulcers. (Courtesy of Barbara Braden and Nancy Bergstrom. Copyright, 1988. Reprinted with permission.)

over time. These lesions have clearly defined borders, are uniform in color, and round or oval in shape. The nevus is periodically assessed for changes because a change may indicate dysplasia of the tissue and the risk of melanoma. Seborrheic keratoses are common, yellow to brown lesions that are described as velvety when touched[1] (Fig. 51-5A). These lesions are often multiple and often symmetrically distributed on the trunk and face. Precancerous lesions (actinic keratoses) are thick, rough patches that develop on sun-exposed areas of the skin, especially in fair-skinned people (see Fig. 51-5B). They are described as "white, scaly keratotic (horny) lesions on the exposed areas of the body." These lesions require attention because there is a risk for development of squamous cell carcinoma.[4]

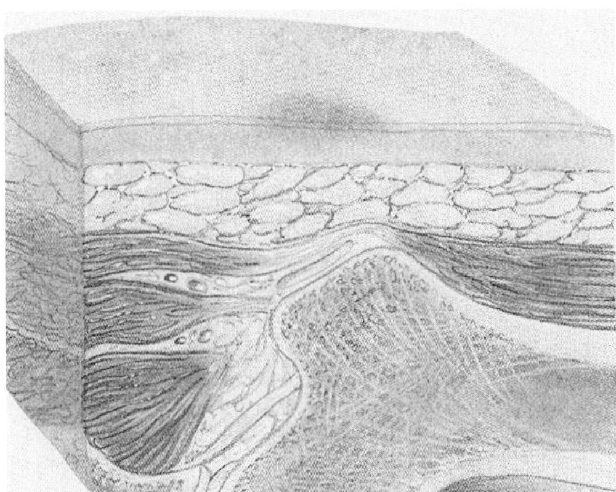

Stage I. Skin is unbroken but appears red; no blanching when pressed.

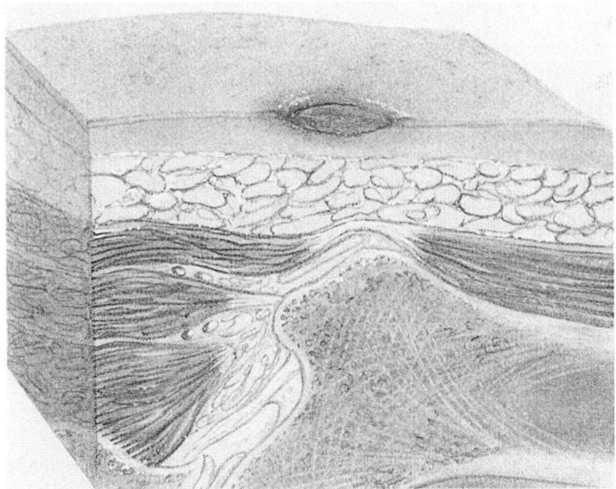

Stage II. Skin *is* broken, and there is superficial skin loss involving the epidermis alone or also the dermis. The lesion resembles a vesicle, erosion, or blister.

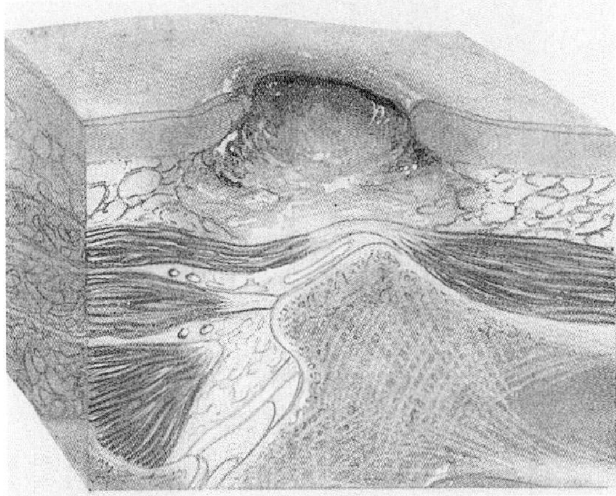

Stage III. Pressure area involves epidermis, dermis, and subcutaneous tissue. The ulcer resembles a crater. Hidden areas of damage may extend through the subcutaneous tissue beyond the borders of the external lesion but not through underlying fascia.

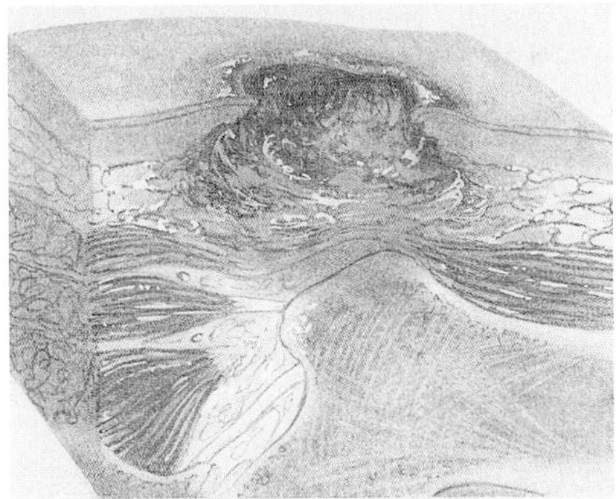

Stage IV. Pressure area involves epidermis, dermis, subcutaneous tissue, bone, and other support tissue. The ulcer resembles a massive crater with hidden areas of damage in adjacent tissue.

figure 51-4 Stages of pressure ulcers. (Used with permission from Weber J, Kelley J: Health Assessment in Nursing [2nd Ed], p 133. Philadelphia, Lippincott Williams & Wilkins, 2003. Illustrations used with permission from Makelbust J, Sieggreen MY: Pressure Ulcers: Guidelines for Prevention and Management. Springhouse, PA, Springhouse, 2001.)

Skin cancer is the most common type of cancer in the United States. It is estimated that 40% to 50% of those who live to age 65 years will be diagnosed with skin cancer at least once.[13] Basal cell and squamous cell cancers are often grouped as nonmelanoma skin cancers. Basal cell carcinomas are found exclusively in light-skinned people, and arise from the hair follicles on the head and neck. Prolonged and cumulative exposure to the sun is recognized as the cause of basal cell carcinoma. These tumors are slow growing and rarely metastasize but do cause local skin destruction and disfigurement. Basal cell carcinomas appear with pearly borders, depressed centers, and rolled edges[3,14] (see Fig. 51-5C).

Squamous cell carcinomas affect the skin and the mucous membranes. Like basal cell cancers, the primary cause is exposure to ultraviolet light. Radiation and tissue damage from scars, ulcers, and fistulas may give rise to squamous cell carcinomas. These cancers can be invasive and are more malignant than basal cell cancers if not treated promptly. As it develops, the carcinoma takes on a hyperkeratotic appearance and may ulcerate and bleed[3] (see Fig. 51-5D).

Malignant melanomas are highly metastatic lesions that come from the melanin-producing cells of the body. The worldwide frequency of malignant melanomas is growing more rapidly than any other cancer except lung cancer. Those at highest risk include those with fair complexions, those prone to sunburn, and those with a family history of melanoma.[14] The most common location for the development of these lesions is on the trunk in men and on the legs in women. The tumors have irregular borders, are dark brown or black, and are usually larger than 6 mm. The American Cancer Society (ACS) recommends a monthly self-assessment for melanoma using the "ABCDs."[15] *A* is for asymmetry; *B* is for borders (are they irregular, ragged, notched, or blurred?); *C* is for color (dark brown or black, red, white, or blue?); and *D* is for diameter.

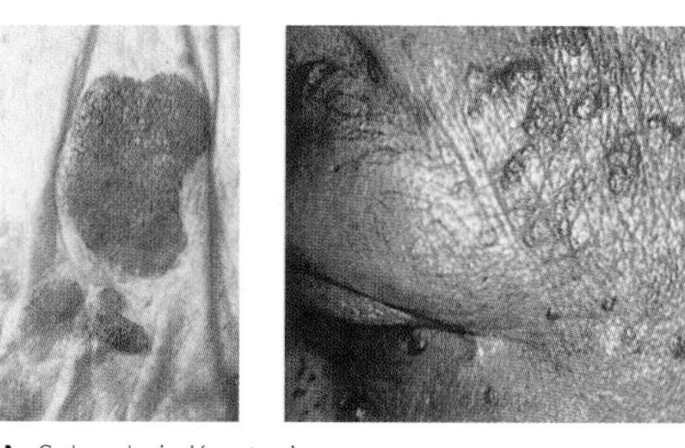

A. Seborrheic Keratosis

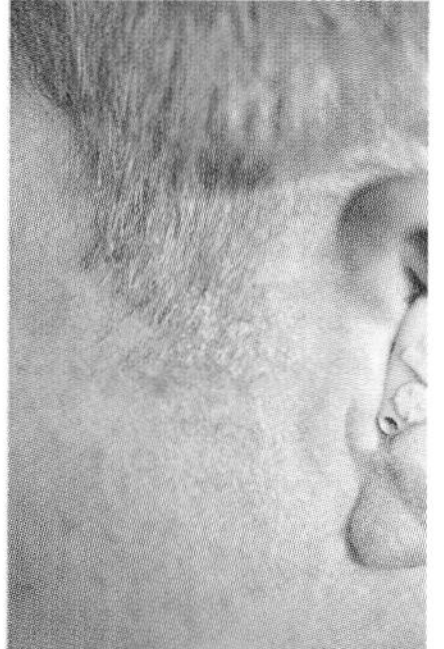

B. Actinic Keratosis

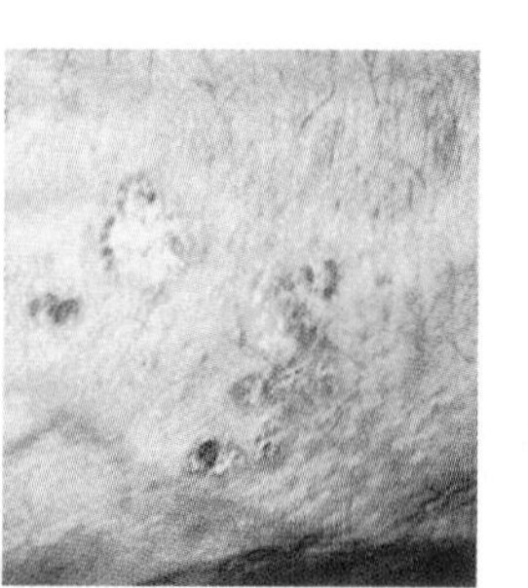

C. Basal Cell Carcinoma

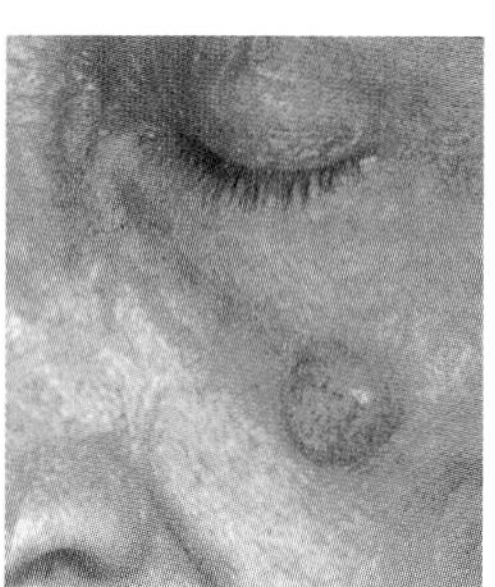

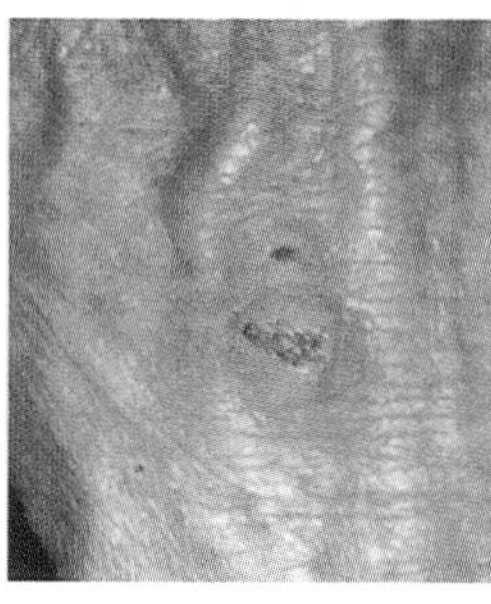

D. Squamous Cell Carcinoma

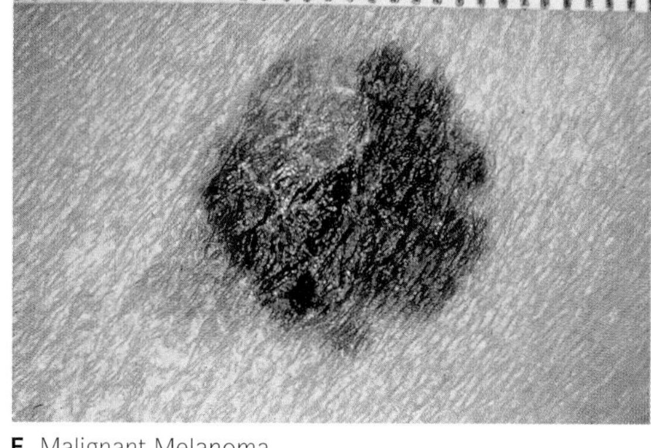

E. Malignant Melanoma

figure 51-5 Benign, premalignant, and malignant skin lesions. (**A, B,** and **D** courtesy of Sauer GC: Manual of Skin Diseases [5th Ed]. Philadelphia, JB Lippincott, 1985. **C,** Bickley L: Bates' Guide to Physical Examination and History Taking [8th Ed], p 107. Philadelphia, Lippincott Williams & Wilkins, 2003. **E,** American Cancer Society.)

Figure 51-5 provides pictures and descriptions of these benign, premalignant, and malignant lesions. While in a critical care setting, it is possible to do a thorough assessment for suspect skin lesions that may be cancerous, refer the patient to a dermatologist or oncologist, and have treatment initiated much sooner than would otherwise be the case.

ASSESSMENT OF THE SKIN IN OLDER ADULTS

With aging there are some expected changes to the integument (Box 52-2). With loss of underlying fat tissue and decreased vascularity of the dermal layer, the skin thins, wrinkles, and loses turgor. Prolonged or repeated sun exposure results in a yellowed or thickened appearance. Purple patches or macules from blood leaking into the tissues after minimal injury may appear. These lesions are called *actinic purpura* and occur because the underlying capillaries lose the protection from hypodermal fat. Dry and flaking skin results from decreased sebaceous and sweat gland activity and is not unexpected in the older adult patient.[1,2] Solar lentigo, sometimes called "liver spots," appear as light to dark brown, flat macules and may be seen in isolation or in clusters on sun-exposed areas of the face or hands.[4]

In the older adult, hair color often transitions to gray because of diminished melanin. Reduced hormone levels result in a change in the size of the hair follicle and produce the change from coarse terminal hair to softer vellus hair and the thinning of hair seen in both sexes. However, the opposite change, from vellus to terminal, occurs in the hair of the nares and on the tragus of men's ears.[2]

Decreased peripheral circulation produces changes in the nails. They grow more slowly but are often thicker and more brittle, and have a tendency to split into layers. Mobility restrictions over time may result in an unkempt appearance of nails in the older patient and may require attention and care by a podiatrist.

box 51-2

Expected Changes in the Integument of Older Patients

- Loss of underlying fat tissue and decreased vascularity of the dermal layer lead to thinning of the skin, increased wrinkling, loss of skin turgor, and actinic purpura.
- Sun exposure over a long period of time leads to yellowing and thickening of the skin and the development of solar lentigo.
- Decreased sebaceous and sweat gland activity leads to dry and flaking skin.
- Decreased melanin leads to graying of the hair.
- Reduced hormone levels lead to thinning of the hair and transition from terminal to vellus hair.
- Decreased peripheral circulation leads to slowed nail growth and brittle nails that split easily.

The risk of pressure ulcer formation in the older adult is increased because of greater mobility limitations and impaired peripheral circulation from cardiovascular, neurological, and metabolic disorders. Once developed, pressure ulcers in this population heal more slowly and are often complicated by the older patient's diminished immune response.

ASSESSMENT OF THE SKIN IN CHILDREN

The assessment of a child's skin is much the same as that of an adult's, but it is important to recognize that some findings take on a different significance because of the nature of the child's skin. Normally, the skin of a child is soft, smooth, and slightly dry. Skin that is locally very dry may indicate eczema, cradle cap, or diaper rash. Skin that is excessively dry throughout the body may indicate a vitamin A deficiency or may be related to frequent bathing.[16]

Because of reduced total sun exposure, dark lesions, considered an expected finding in an older adult, may indicate a malignant change in a child. Bruises in a child may indicate nonaccidental trauma and attention is paid to the location of the bruises and to the color. As a bruise ages, it changes color from purplish to greenish. The critical care nurse must be sure that special attention is paid to the skin of children in critical care settings related to lesions from infectious disease; the skin is assessed for any rashes that may indicate bacterial or viral infection.

clinical applicability challenges

Self-Challenge: Critical Thinking

Mrs. Louise Hooper, a 62-year-old widow, has been in the medical-surgical intensive care unit (ICU) for the past 2 weeks after a diagnosis of respiratory failure and pneumonia. This patient's medical history includes obesity, type 2 diabetes mellitus, and chronic obstructive pulmonary disease (COPD). She has been intubated and on mechanical ventilation. She has received continuous enteral feedings through a nasogastric tube, numerous antibiotics, and dopamine for blood pressure support during her first 3 days in the ICU. She has a triple-lumen central venous access catheter.

Mrs. Hooper is scheduled for a tracheostomy tomorrow and, at that time, will also have a percutaneous gastric feeding tube inserted. She has a continuous bladder catheter and an incontinence fecal bag in place draining liquid stool. Over the past 5 days, Mrs. Hooper has received a benzodiazepine for sedation at least once per day. Physical therapy consultation was made on day 3, and she is assisted by two caregivers with a pivot to a chair twice each day. Mrs. Hooper's family visits daily and helps her to communicate with a pencil and paper tablet.

1. *What is the role of the critical care nurse in the prevention of pressure ulcers for Mrs. Hooper?*
2. *What are Mrs. Hooper's risk factors for development of pressure ulcers?*
3. *How might the medications indicated (dopamine, numerous antibiotics, and benzodiazepine sedation) affect Mrs. Hooper's integument status?*

Study Questions

1. *The color change of erythema is related to*
   a. *increased oxyhemoglobin content.*
   b. *increased tissue vascularity.*
   c. *decreased hemoglobin levels.*
   d. *decreased interstitial pressures.*
2. *Urticaria is best described as a*
   a. *purple, irregular lesion caused by tissue trauma.*
   b. *fiery red, raised lesion with a central body and radiating legs.*
   c. *reddened or white, raised inflamed lesion with transudate vascular fluid in the surrounding tissue.*
   d. *small, pinpoint, nonblanching lesion.*
3. *Which one of the following statements about oral candidiasis is true?*
   a. *It is a painless manifestation of an opportunistic infection.*
   b. *It manifests itself as a white, crusty lesion of the patient's lips and hard palate.*
   c. *It is a painful white coating of the oral mucosa and tongue.*
   d. *It is the result of systemic Staphylococcus infection.*
4. *Skin turgor is best assessed*
   a. *peripherally over the patient's forearms and shins.*
   b. *peripherally at the nail beds.*
   c. *centrally over the trunk.*
   d. *centrally over the patient's clavicles.*
5. *Which of the following phrases describes basal cell carcinoma?*
   a. *Depressed center, rolled edge, pearly border*
   b. *Scaly white lesion*
   c. *Large, dark black lesion with irregular border*
   d. *Light brown lesion that feels velvety when touched*
6. *Cyanosis in an African-American patient can best be identified by assessment of the*
   a. *palms of the hands and soles of the feet.*
   b. *earlobes.*
   c. *conjunctiva and oral mucous membranes.*
   d. *dorsal surface of the forearm.*

REFERENCES

1. Bickley LS, Szilagyi PG: The skin. In Bickley LS (ed): Guide to Physical Examination and History Taking (8th Ed), pp 95–113. Philadelphia, Lippincott Williams & Wilkins, 2003
2. Wilson SF, Giddons JF: Skin, hair, and nails. In Wilson SF, Giddons JF (eds): Health Assessment for Nursing Practice (2nd Ed), pp 257–287. St. Louis, Mosby, 2002
3. Allwood J, Curry K: Normal and altered functions of the skin. In Bullock BA, Henze RL (eds): Focus on Pathophysiology, pp 837–873, Philadelphia, Lippincott Williams & Wilkins, 2000
4. American Academy of Dermatology: Agingskinnet. In Skincare physicans.com. 2000. Available at http://www.skincarephysicians.com/agingskinnet/Q&A. Accessed July 1, 2003
5. Stawiski MA, Price SA: Cutaneous infections. In Price SA, Wilson LM (eds): Pathophysiology (6th Ed), pp 1087–1096. St. Louis, Mosby, 2003

6. Buttry TS: Anticoagulant and antiplatelet drugs. In Gutierrez K (ed): Pharmacotherapeutics: Clinical Decision-Making in Nursing, pp 774–789. Philadelphia, WB Saunders, 1999
7. Kozier B, Erb G, Berman AJ, et al: Health assessment. In Kozier B, Erb G, Berman AJ, et al. (eds): Fundamentals of Nursing (6th Ed), pp 531–629. Upper Saddle River, NJ, Prentice-Hall, 2000
8. Bergstrom N, Braden BJ, Laguzza A, et al: The Braden Scale for predicting pressure sore risk. Nurs Res 36:205–210, 1987
9. Gosnell DJ: An assessment tool to identify pressure sores. Nurs Res 22(1):55, 1973
10. Agency for Health Care Policy and Research, Panel for the Prediction and Prevention of Pressure Ulcers in Adults: Pressure Ulcers in Adults: Prediction and Prevention. Clinical Practice Guideline no. 15, AHCPR publication no. 92-0047. Rockville, MD: Agency for Health Care Policy and Research, Public Health Service, U.S. Department of Heath and Human Services, 1992
11. Lyder CH, Yu C, Emerling J, et al: The Braden Scale for pressure ulcer risk: Evaluating the predictive validity in black and Latino/Hispanic elders. Appl Nurs Res 12(2):60–68, 1999
12. Bergstrom N, Braden BJ: Predictive validity of the Braden Scale among black and white subjects. Nurs Res 51:398–403, 2002
13. National Cancer Institute: What you need to know about skin cancer? 2002. Available at http://www.cancer.gov/cancerinfor/wyntk/skin. Accessed July 1, 2003
14. Huether SE: Structure, function, and disorders of the integument. In McCance KL, Huether SE (eds): The Biological Basis for Disease in Adults and Children (4th Ed), pp 1434–1468. St. Louis, Mosby, 2002
15. American Cancer Society: Detecting skin cancer. 2003. Available at http://www.cancer.org. Accessed July 1, 2003
16. Hockenberry MJ, Wilson D, Winkelstein ML, et al. (eds): Wong's Nursing Care of Infants and Children (7th Ed). St. Louis, Mosby, 2003

OTHER SELECTED READING

Byers PH, Carta SG, Mayrovitz HN: Pressure ulcer research issues in surgical patients. Adv Skin Wound Care 13:115, 2000

Cuzzell JZ: Wound assessment and evaluation. Dermatol Nurs 13(4):289, 2001

Hayes KVD: Skin wellness and illness. In Condon MC (ed): Women's Health. Upper Saddle River, NJ, Prentice-Hall, 2004

Finch A: Assessment of skin in older people: As the largest organ in the body, the skin can offer valuable information about the general health of an older person. Nurs Older People 15(2):29, 2003

Strayer SM, Reynolds P: Diagnosing skin malignancy: Assessment of predictive clinical criteria and risk factors. J Fam Pract 53:210, 2003

chapter

52

Patient Management: Integumentary System

SUSAN LUCHKA

objectives

Based on the content in this chapter, the reader should be able to:

- Define specific terms related to wounds: *acute wound, chronic wound, partial thickness, full thickness, stages of wound healing, primary intention, secondary intention, tertiary intention.*
- Explain the normal healing process.
- Describe the components of wound assessment.
- Discuss basic wound care for a variety of scenarios.
- Discuss the aspects of nutrition and pharmacotherapeutics and how they affect wound healing.

TYPES OF WOUNDS

A wound is simply a break in the skin integrity. Wounds may be acute or chronic. An acute wound is a wound that follows an orderly, sequential healing process, resulting in an area that has anatomical and functional integrity.[1,2] Acute wounds are caused by surgery or trauma. Conversely, a chronic wound fails to yield an area that has anatomical and functional integrity. Chronic wounds fail to follow an orderly, sequential process due to precipitating factors such as diabetes, pressure, malnutrition, peripheral vascular disease, immune deficiencies, and infection.[1,2] An acute wound may become a chronic wound at any time.

Acute and chronic wounds may be defined as partial- or full-thickness wounds. Partial-thickness wounds involve the epidermis and may involve the dermis. A partial-thickness wound is a shallow wound that is usually moist and painful (because the loss of the epidermis exposes the nerve endings). Full-thickness wounds involve the loss of the epidermis, dermis, and subcutaneous tissue, and they may involve muscle, tendons, ligaments, and bone. A full-thickness wound involves a large amount of tissue loss and appears as a crater or crevice.

Pressure ulcers and leg ulcers are two specific types of wounds that may be seen in the critical care setting. Critically ill patients are at risk for pressure ulcers. Leg ulcers are due to specific disease processes that may complicate the critically ill patient's overall recovery.

Pressure Ulcers

Pressure ulcers are wounds caused by pressure, shear, and friction. Pressure ulcers start as acute wounds but become chronic in patients with other risk factors. Risk factors for the development of pressure ulcers include prolonged and impaired mobility, incontinence, malnutrition, diabetes, spinal cord injuries, metastatic cancers, decreased level of consciousness, impaired mental status, and peripheral vascular disease.[1,2] A patient teaching guide for pressure ulcers is given in Box 52-1.

Pressure ulcers are the only type of wound that is staged. Staging of pressure ulcers is done when assessing and documenting the wound. Stage I is defined as nonblanchable erythema of intact skin. In patients with darker skin, the stage I pressure ulcer may be red, blue, or purple. Stage II involves partial-thickness tissue loss and presents as a blistered or denuded area, a shallow open wound. Stage III is a full-thickness wound involving the subcutaneous tissue and presents as a crater. Stage IV is also a full-thickness wound involving a large amount of tissue loss. The stage IV pressure ulcer extends through the subcutaneous tissue and deep into the fascia, involving muscle, bone, ligament, or tendon. It should be noted that reverse staging is inappropriate. The tissue that fills in the wound bed is not the same as the tissue lost. Lost muscle or subcutaneous tissue cannot be replaced. Therefore, it is appropriate to document, "healing stage IV wound," but it is not appropriate to document, "stage IV wound now stage III."

The standards of care for pressure ulcers are established by the Agency for Healthcare Research and Quality (AHRQ), formerly known as the Agency for Health Care Policy and Research (AHCPR) committee. The AHRQ is a component of the U.S. Department of Health and Human Services. The AHRQ publishes Clinical Practice Guidelines and a patient reference booklet on pressure ulcers. These guidelines are the basis for individual institutions' policies and procedures. The AHRQ guidelines address the economic impact of pressure ulcers and establish the basic standards for assessment, turning, dressings, wound cleansers, treatment of infections, operative repair, quality improvement, and education. In addition, the AHRQ guidelines include a glossary, an extensive reference list, clinical algorithms, and research methodology. The AHRQ guidelines are the gold standard for individual institution guidelines, journal articles, and other publications.

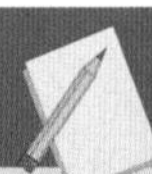

box 52-1
Pressure Ulcers

- Pressure ulcers are also known as *pressure sores* or *bed sores.*
- Pressure ulcers occur in people who have trouble moving around easily.
- At first, a pressure ulcer is just a reddened, tender area. If pressure is not relieved, the skin in this area may break down (open up or pull off, forming a blistered area). Pressure ulcers can destroy the underlying muscles, bone, ligaments, and tendons if they are not treated.
- Risk factors for pressure ulcers include difficulty moving around, medical problems (such as diabetes), spinal cord injury, incontinence of urine and stool, surgeries that limit mobility for an extended period (such as hip or knee replacement surgery), poor nutrition, and poor hydration (decreased fluid intake).
- Pressure ulcers occur most frequently over bony prominences (e.g., heels, sacral area, hips, and shoulder blades), but they can occur anywhere on the body where there is constant pressure that is unrelieved.
- Many times, pressure ulcers can be prevented by turning the person in bed at least every 2 hours and by placing a pillow under the person's ankles to keep the heels off the bed, thus relieving pressure. A specialty bed may also be used to decrease pressure.
- *Not all pressure ulcers can be prevented.* The person's medical condition, nutrition and hydration status, immune status, and overall health status are all factors that affect the person's risk for developing pressure ulcers.
- Treatment depends on the type of pressure ulcer and the person's health status.

Leg Ulcers

Leg ulcers are chronic wounds seen frequently in critically ill patients with underlying health problems, such as venous stasis ulcers, arterial ulcers, and diabetic foot ulcers. Although patients with leg ulcers may have a high risk for pressure ulcers, leg ulcers are not pressure ulcers and are not staged.

VENOUS STASIS ULCERS

Venous stasis ulcers are usually found on the medial aspect of the lower leg, superior to the medial malleolus.[1,2] The wound margins are irregular, and present as shallow craters.[1,2] The wound margins and lower leg may have a ruddy appearance or hemosiderin staining.[1,2] The drainage from venous stasis ulcers may vary from mild to heavy. The primary treatment for venous stasis ulcers is compression therapy.[2,3] Compression therapy may be administered using Unna boots or a multiple-wrap dressing. The affected leg is elevated above heart level to decrease edema (edema impedes the healing process).

ARTERIAL ULCERS

Arterial ulcers (ischemic ulcers) are usually found on the distal leg, medial malleoli, and the dorsal aspect of the foot and toes.[1,2] The wound margins of arterial ulcers are round, smooth (*not* irregular), and frequently described as having a "punched-out" appearance.[1,2] Arterial ulcers have pale wound beds and may be shallow or deep. The affected leg may be cool to touch, cyanotic, and pale with minimal hair distribution. The patient experiences increased pain to the affected area if the leg is elevated.[1,2] The primary dressing for arterial leg ulcers is an occlusive dressing.[3] Healing will not occur unless the vascular deficit is addressed surgically.

DIABETIC FOOT ULCERS

Diabetic foot ulcers are found in patients with diabetes and are frequently not recognized early, due to the patient's accompanying neuropathy. The primary location for diabetic foot ulcers is the plantar aspect of the foot, heels, and metatarsals.[1,2] To promote wound healing, a dressing that provides a moist environment is used most often. The ulcer area usually needs debridement and must be assessed carefully for infection. Other treatment modalities include off-loading the patient's weight using special shoes. Osteomyelitis is always a concern in patients with diabetic foot ulcers. Healing is a prolonged process due to the diabetes.

WOUND HEALING

Phases of Wound Healing

Optimal wound healing occurs in a moist (not extremely wet or dry) environment. The wound healing process is composed of three phases (Fig. 52-1). The first phase is the *inflammatory phase*, which occurs immediately after the wound occurs. At the time of injury, there is immediate vasoconstriction; this is the body's way of controlling bleeding. Once vasoconstriction occurs, platelets collect at the site and deposit fibrin to form a clot. The vasoconstriction is holding the wound together and the platelets with their fibrin clot formation essentially "plug the hole." Phagocytosis also occurs during the inflammatory phase. Phagocytosis is the release of macrophages at the site of injury to destroy any bacteria that may be present and to remove the wound's cellular debris. This is the body's way of providing the optimal environment for wound healing (i.e., a clean wound bed). It is at this time that growth factors are also present at the site of the injury. Overall, the inflammatory phase is estimated to last between 4 and 6 days. Visual assessment of the wound during the inflammatory phase reveals a wound with erythema, edema, and pain.

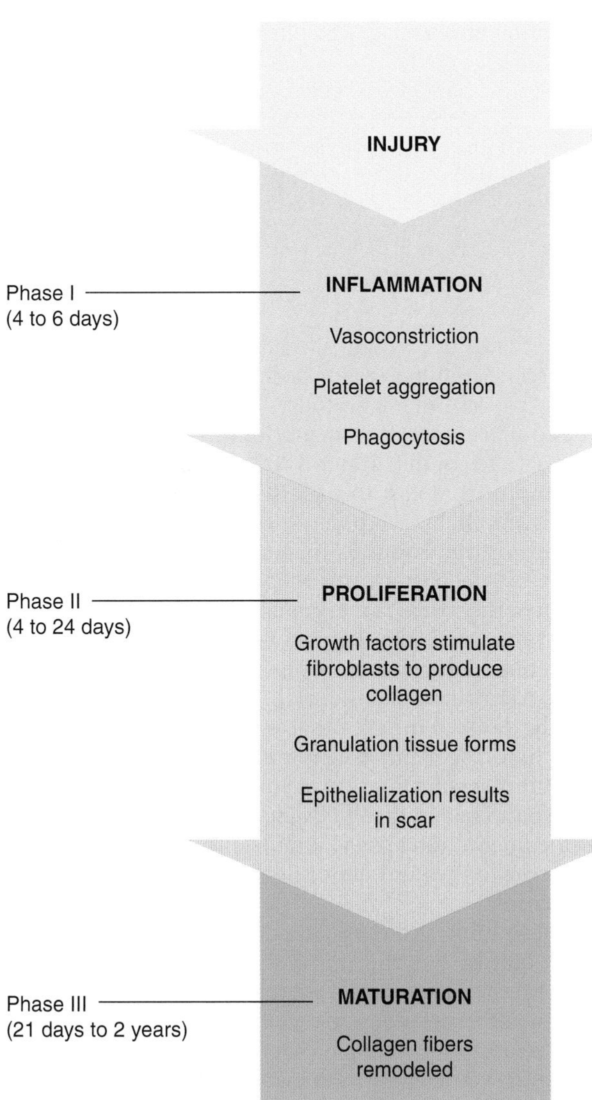

figure 52-1 The stages of wound healing.

The second phase of wound healing is the *proliferation phase*. Growth factors stimulate the fibroblast to produce collagen. Collagen, along with new blood vessels and connective tissue, creates granulation tissue. Visual assessment of the wound at this point reveals a wound that is beefy red and shiny with a grainy or bumpy appearance. The appearance of granulation tissue prompts the wound margins to contract. Pulling together of the wound edges decreases the overall size of the wound. The last step of the proliferation phase is *epithelialization* or *reepithelialization*. Epithelialization results in a scar. The estimated overall duration of the proliferation phase is anywhere from 4 to 24 days.

The final and third phase of wound healing is the *maturation phase*. During the maturation phase, the collagen fibers are remodeled. The goal is to increase the tensile strength of the scar tissue. It has been estimated that only 70% to 80% of the skin's original strength is attained when the wound is healed.[1] The maturation phase can extend from 21 days to 2 years. The outcome is always an area of tissue that is at greater risk for breakdown and more fragile than undamaged tissue.

If the wound becomes extremely wet or dry, the phases of wound healing occur, but at a slower rate. This may affect the final quality of the scar tissue with respect to anatomical and functional integrity, as well as tensile strength. The patient's age and physical status also have an impact on how well the healing process functions (Boxes 52-2 and 52-3).

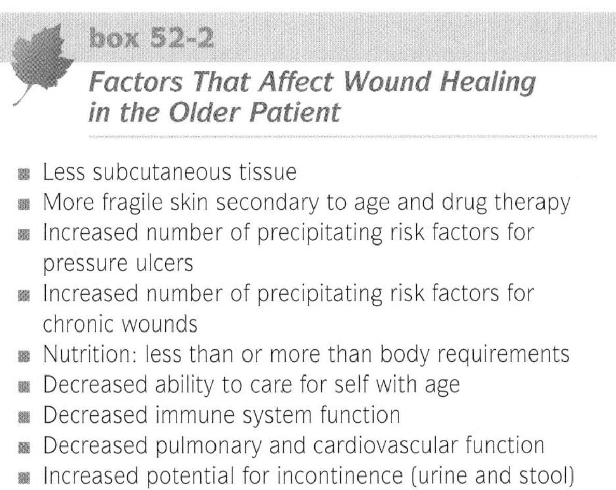

box 52-2

Factors That Affect Wound Healing in the Older Patient

- Less subcutaneous tissue
- More fragile skin secondary to age and drug therapy
- Increased number of precipitating risk factors for pressure ulcers
- Increased number of precipitating risk factors for chronic wounds
- Nutrition: less than or more than body requirements
- Decreased ability to care for self with age
- Decreased immune system function
- Decreased pulmonary and cardiovascular function
- Increased potential for incontinence (urine and stool)

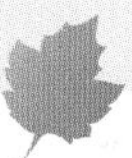

box 52-3

Factors That Affect Wound Healing in the Pediatric Patient

- Preterm status (preterm infants have extremely fragile skin and therefore are at very high risk for skin breakdown)
- Less subcutaneous tissue
- Inability to care for self (based on age)
- Incontinence until child is toilet trained
- Ambulatory deficit, decreases with age
- Diet concerns due to lack of dentition, decreases with age

Methods of Wound Healing

Wounds can heal through primary intention, secondary intention, or tertiary intention. *Primary intention* is used for acute or surgical wounds. The edges of the wound are drawn together (approximated), shortening the time required for the wound to heal to about 4 to 14 days overall. Primary intention is associated with a decreased risk of infection and minimal scarring. With primary intention, not only is scarring minimal and the risk of infection decreased, but the amount of tissue loss is decreased.

Secondary intention is seen most frequently in chronic wounds, but can occur in acute wounds, when the wound edges cannot be approximated to each other due to a significant tissue loss. An example of secondary intention would be a pressure ulcer or a venous stasis ulcer. The potential for infection is increased because of the inability to approximate the edges, thus leaving the area open to bacteria. Scarring may also be significant, depending on the amount of tissue loss.

The last form of wound repair is *tertiary intention*, which may also be called *delayed primary intention*. Tertiary (delayed primary) intention should not be confused with primary intention. With this type of wound healing, the wound is not closed for a period (usually 3 to 5 days) to allow infection, edema, or both to resolve. During this time, the wound is packed or irrigated to remove exudate and cellular debris. When the edema and risk of infection have decreased, the wound edges are approximated and the wound is closed as it is in primary intention. Scarring is usually greater than that seen with primary intention but less than that seen with secondary intention.

WOUND ASSESSMENT

Wound assessment is done in an orderly, sequential manner (Box 52-4).

The location of the wound is defined as precisely as possibly using anatomical terminology (e.g., "medial aspect of the left lower leg, 10 cm distal to the knee"). Using correct anatomical terminology allows other health care professionals to visualize the location of the wound. Correct location is especially important if the patient has more than one wound.[2,4,5] Photography may be used and is more frequently used in chronic wounds than acute wounds.

box 52-4

Wound Assessment

Location: Document the location, using anatomical positions.

Size: Document the size, in centimeters or millimeters. Measure the length from 1200 to 1800 position. Measure the width from the 0900 to 0300 position.

Depth: Use a sterile swab to determine the depth (see Fig. 52-2).

Undermining or tunneling: Document the presence or absence of undermining or tunneling (see Fig. 52-3).

Tissue type: Describe the wound bed. If the wound bed is not visible, document the presence and condition of the eschar (scab), sutures, staples, or other wound closure.

Drainage: Note the presence or absence of drainage. If drainage is present, describe its odor, color, amount, and consistency.

Wound margins: Describe the wound margins (approximation, condition of surrounding tissue).

Drains and tubes: Note the type of drain or tubing, and its location (using anatomical or clock positions).

Condition of dressing: Describe the amount and type of drainage on the dressing, as well as the ease with which the dressing was removed.

Pain: Evaluate on a 0 to 10 scale (or other institution-approved assessment scale). Provide pain relief as needed before, during, and after wound assessment or dressing.

The size of the wound should always be measured in centimeters, millimeters, or both.[2,4,5] Avoid terminology such as "the size of a half dollar." This leads to inconsistent and inaccurate documentation. Length is measured from north to south (1200 to 1800 clock position). Width is measured from east to west (0900 to 0300 clock position; Fig. 52-2).

Depth of the wound is measured by placing a sterile swab in the deepest area of the wound and marking the location of the wound's margin on the swab.[2] Dip the sterile swab in normal saline before inserting it into the wound; this decreases the chance of leaving cotton fibers in the wound. After removing the swab, measure from the distal tip of the swab to the area that was marked. Documentation includes the depth in centimeters and also the location where the assessment was made (e.g., "depth 5.8 cm in the distal wound bed in the 0900 clock position"). Clear, concise documentation allows other health care professionals to reassess the wound depth in the same area with each reevaluation.

Undermining and tunneling do not usually occur with acute wounds, but the nurse should always assess the wound for their presence. Undermining occurs when there is the loss of tissue along the wound margins, similar to a "lip of tissue."[2] Tunneling is exactly what it implies, a tunnel opening somewhere in the wound bed. Tunneling can begin in acute wounds in which there are drains. (Note that if tunneling occurs, the wound is not an acute wound but

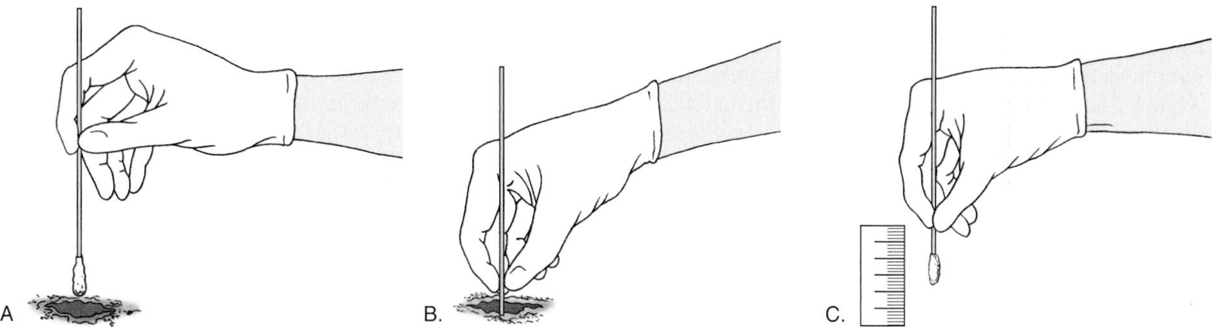

figure 52-2 Procedure for measuring wound depth. (**A**) Put on gloves. Gently insert the swab into the deepest portion of the wound that you can see. (**B**) Grasp the swab with your thumb and forefinger at the point corresponding to the wound margin. (**C**) Carefully withdraw the swab while maintaining the position of your thumb and forefinger. Measure from the tip of the swab to that position. (From Thomas Hess C: Clinical Guide: Wound Care [4th Ed], p 98. Philadelphia, Lippincott Williams & Wilkins, 2001.)

has become a chronic wound.) The process for assessing the direction and depth of tunneling is shown in Figure 52-3.[2]

Determining the tissue type entails visual assessment of the wound bed. The tissue in the wound bed should be beefy red (as opposed to pale). Note the presence or absence of granulation tissue (shiny red, grainy, or bumpy tissue). Assess for necrotic tissue, which presents as black or brown tissue. Slough may also be present in the wound bed. Slough is yellow and stringy in appearance. Describe what you see even if you are unsure of the correct terminology. If the wound bed is not visible, document the presence or absence of eschar (scab), sutures, staples, Steri-Strips, or wound adhesives.

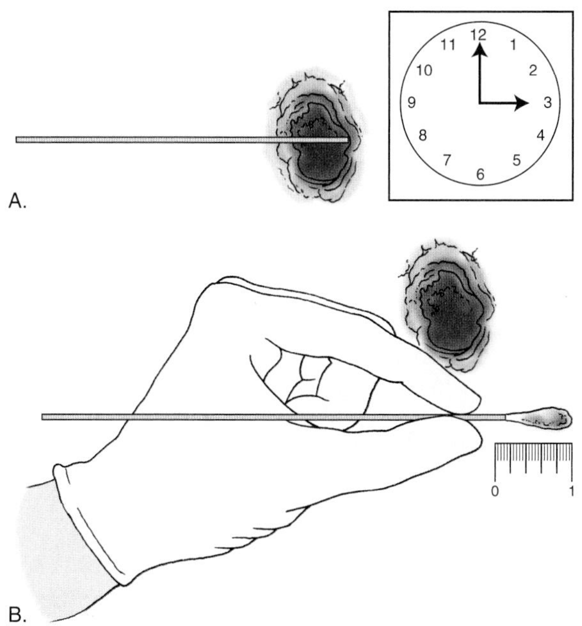

figure 52-3 Procedure for determining the direction and depth of tunneling. (**A**) To assess the direction of tunneling, put on gloves and insert the swab into the sites where tunneling occurs. Progressing in a clockwise direction, document the deepest sites where the wound tunnels. (12 o'clock points in the direction of the patient's head, so in this example, tunneling occurs at 3 o'clock.) (**B**) To assess the depth of tunneling, insert the swab into the tunneling areas and grasp the swab where it meets the wound margin. Remove the swab, place it next to a measuring guide, and document the measurement in centimeters. (From Thomas Hess C: Clinical Guide: Wound Care [4th Ed], p 100. Philadelphia, Lippincott Williams & Wilkins, 2001.)

The presence or absence of drainage is also important to note, along with the location of the drainage or exudate (e.g., "drainage/exudate noted at the proximal end of the wound").[6] The drainage or exudate needs to be assessed for odor, color, consistency, and amount (e.g., "abdominal dressing of multiple 4 × 4s is saturated with serosanguineous drainage every 2 hours").

The wound margins are also assessed when performing a wound assessment. Are the edges well approximated? Is the surrounding tissue clean, dry, reddened, edematous, pale, intact, or blistered? Again, describe your findings and be as exact as possible to paint an accurate picture of the wound margins for the next health care professional.

Drains or tubes may be present in or near the wound bed. Drains or tubes must also be assessed for location, the appearance of the surrounding tissue, and the characteristics of the drainage. Consider the insertion site of a drain or tube as an acute wound in itself!

The dressing is assessed after it is removed. Clearly describe the soiled dressing's condition (e.g., "saturated"), the ease with which the dressing was removed (e.g., "sticking"), and the location and type of drainage on the dressing. If the dressing came off without being removed by the nurse, note this as well (e.g., "dressing found lying in bed—wound uncovered").

One last area, but of the utmost importance in wound assessment, is that of pain. Pain is assessed using an institution-approved standardized scale, such as the 0 to 10 scale. Pain medication is always administered before dressing changes, if needed. The patient should never be in pain while a wound is assessed or dressed. If the patient experiences pain during the dressing change procedure, stop and medicate the patient before completing the procedure. The choice of pain medication and delivery method depend on the patient's status. Delivery methods may include continuous drips, epidurals, patient-controlled analgesia (PCA) pumps, or local anesthesia.

Wound documentation includes all descriptions and measurements, the presence and absence of pain during the procedure, and the type of dressing applied.[1,2,4,5] Many institutions use special wound measurement tools, wound assessment tools, and documentation tools (e.g., flow sheets) for wound documentation. The flow sheet format allows the health care provider to track the wound healing process and to identify, early on, those wounds that may not be following an orderly, sequential healing process.

WOUND CARE

Nursing diagnosis for patients with wounds revolves around a few basic themes[7] (Box 52-5). Wound care seeks to address these problems.

Wound Closure

The goal of all wound care is ultimately the closure of the wound and restoration of skin integrity. Wound closure is usually promoted by various types of treatments and dressings.

VACUUM-ASSISTED WOUND CLOSURE

Vacuum-assisted wound closure (VAC) is a system that assists wound closure by providing localized negative pressure to the wound bed and wound margins. The occlusive dressing promotes a moist environment for healing and the negative pressure removes excessive wound drainage, assisting in pulling the wound margins together.[8]

Tubing, similar to that of suction tubing, is placed into a special foam dressing. The foam dressing is shaped in wedges that are cut to fit the wound. The sponge wedge and tubing are then covered with an occlusive transparent dressing. The tube is then connected to the vacuum unit, at low suction levels (as directed by the manufacturer). The negative pressure acts to draw the wound edges together by collapsing the foam dressing and removing wound fluids while maintaining a moist wound environment that promotes healing. If the dressing is not collapsed, there is a leak in the VAC system and the dressing must be replaced with attention given to the transparent occlusive dressing application. The transparent occlusive dressing must be securely in place to maintain negative pressure in the wound. Dressings have the appearance of being "vacuum packed" when the dressing is secure and occlusive.

With the VAC system, granulation tissue is stimulated, infection and bacterial colonization are decreased, and wound closure occurs in a moist "vacuum" environment.

box 52-5 *Examples of Nursing Diagnoses and Collaborative Problems for the Patient With an Acute or Chronic Wound*

- Acute Pain related to debridement and wound care
- Ineffective Tissue Perfusion
- Impaired Tissue Integrity related to wound
- Imbalanced Nutrition: Less than body requirements
- Risk for Infection related to wound and presence of bacteria
- Disturbed Body Image related to dysfunctional open wound or scarring
- Risk for Deficient Fluid Volume related to increased metabolism

In addition, the VAC system decreases the frequency of dressing changes, thus decreasing patient discomfort and nursing time.[8]

The VAC system can be used in both acute and chronic wounds.[8] The VAC system may be indicated for chronic wounds (including diabetic and nonhealing stage III and IV pressure ulcers); flaps and grafts (both acute surgical wounds); dehisced incisions; acute and traumatic wounds; and burns. The VAC system should be used with extreme caution in patients with active bleeding, those who are on anticoagulant therapy, or patients with a history of uncontrolled bleeding.[8] The VAC system is contraindicated for any patient with untreated osteomyelitis, necrotic tissue with eschar, malignancies of the wound, fistulas, exposed blood vessels or organs, or wounds close to major organs.[8] VAC sponges must be positioned on viable tissue; therefore, if necrotic tissue or devitalized tissue is present, the wound needs to be debrided before the VAC sponges can be placed.[8] The VAC system may be used in an infected wound, but only with appropriate antibiotic therapy.[8]

It is the nurse's responsibility to be familiar with the operation and maintenance of the VAC system. Nursing responsibilities include wound assessment and documentation, along with placing the patient on the vacuum system, changing the canister, and maintaining the system. The wound should demonstrate progressive healing. If documentation fails to demonstrate progressive wound healing within 30 days, then alternative therapies must be evaluated.

SUTURES, STAPLES, AND WOUND ADHESIVES

Sutures or staples must be cleaned with sterile normal saline or a wound cleanser. Immediately after surgery, the wound needs to be covered with a dry sterile dressing. Frequently after the initial postoperative period, the staples or sutures are left open to air.

Wound adhesives may be used on surgical or traumatic wounds to approximate the wound margins, in which case sutures are used to close the underlying tissue and the wound adhesive is applied topically to the wound margins as they are drawn together. The wound adhesive has the appearance of a shiny, clear coating over the incision. Caution is needed when applying wound adhesives due to their liquid status. Wound adhesives may inadvertently spread to other areas. Incisions in which wound adhesives are used are not cleansed or soaked with any wound cleaner, although they may be gently rinsed. Wounds in which a wound adhesive has been used are left uncovered.

Wound Drainage

Often, a drain is inserted in the wound to prevent the pooling of exudate in the wound bed. Pooling of exudate in the wound bed decreases healing and increases the potential for infection. The most common types of drains are Hemovac drains, Penrose drains, and Jackson-Pratt drains, and chest tubes. Basic care of all drains and chest tubes includes cleansing with sterile normal saline and applying a dry sterile dressing. The dressing stabilizes the drain and prevents the drain insertion site from coming in contact with drainage and other potentially infectious surfaces. Drain and tube insertion sites are never left open to air due to the risk of infection. If drainage from another source may potentially saturate the dressing (over the drain site), then the dressing also needs to be occlusive. Drain tubing is stabilized with tape to decrease the potential for inadvertent dislodgement and removal. Inadvertent removal of a drain potentiates pain and infection and puts the person at risk for an acute wound becoming a chronic one.

Bacitracin or Neosporin may be applied, although hydrogen peroxide and povidone-iodine (Betadine) ointment are always avoided because they destroy granulation tissue and prolong the healing process. Normal saline causes no damage to the wound bed and is physiologically normal and cost-effective. Some institutions may use prepared wound cleansers. Most wound cleansers have some potential to destroy granulating tissue (compared with normal saline), but are less toxic to granulating tissue than hydrogen peroxide or Betadine. Prepared wound cleansers are improving rapidly, becoming less cytotoxic and more time-efficient and cost-effective.

Impregnated gauzes for packing and various solutions (e.g., Betadine and Dakin's solution) may be used in the event that the wound is infected, but should not be used as a routine wound treatment for a prolonged time because they destroy granulating tissue and inhibit the normal healing process. Remember that the use of these products signals that the wound itself is not an acute wound, but has become a chronic wound.

Wound Dressings

The goal of wound dressings is to protect the wound from infection and promote a moist environment. There are hundreds of dressing products available. The dressing of choice depends on the wound. Skin tears (partial-thickness wounds) are acute wounds secondary to tape or transparent occlusive dressings and should be cared for using an Adaptic-type dressing (without iodine/Betadine additives) that is then covered with a Kling- or Kerlix-type dressing to avoid further tearing of the skin. It is important to minimize the use of adhesives in all forms for patients prone to skin tears.

WET-TO-DRY DRESSINGS

A wound healing by secondary or tertiary intention is frequently packed with wet-to-dry dressings. The use of wet-to-dry dressings is controversial.[9] Wounds need a moist environment to heal without impediment. Changing a wet-to-dry dressing every 8 or 12 hours leads to the dressing becoming exceptionally dry. Thus, when it is removed, indiscriminate debridement of both necrotic and granulating tissue occurs. This constant debriding of the wound increases the patient's discomfort, promotes infection (due to frequent dressing changes), and slows the healing process. Although wet-to-dry dressings are frequently used in clinical practice, research has shown they are actually detrimental to the wound.[9] If a wet-to-dry dressing must be used, the optimal method would be wet-to-moist, changing the dressing every 4 hours and covering the wet-to-dry dressing with a transparent dressing to promote and maintain a moist wound environment.

CALCIUM ALGINATES AND FOAM DRESSINGS

Wound healing by secondary or tertiary intention may also be promoted with calcium alginates or foam dressings (as opposed to wet-to-dry dressings). Calcium alginates are made from brown seaweed. They come in ropelike or flat pieces that must be "fluffed" and packed into the wound bed. Calcium alginates have an absorptive quality and can hold up to 20 times or more their weight in wound drainage. As the calcium alginate absorbs the wound drainage, its appearance changes from dry, fluffed strands to that of a gel that is easily removed from the wound. Calcium alginates may be covered with a hydrocolloid or a transparent dressing.

Foam dressings have the advantage of being highly absorptive. They are available in various shapes and sizes and are placed over the wounds. When it is time to remove the foam dressing, it is simply lifted off the wound. Minimal trauma occurs to the wound bed and surrounding tissue. Foam dressings, like calcium alginates, provide a moist wound environment.

Contraindications to calcium alginates and foam dressings vary according to the manufacturer. Caution should always be used if the wound is infected.

HYDROCOLLOIDS

A hydrocolloid is most frequently used in the care and treatment of stage I and II pressure ulcers. Hydrocolloids are occlusive, self-adhesive, and absorptive, although their absorptive capacity is not as great as that of calcium alginates or foam dressings. The advantage of a hydrocolloid is that it is changed only every 3 to 5 days, or if it is inadvertently removed. Contraindications to hydrocolloids depend on the manufacturer's recommendations and, again, caution is always used if the wound is infected.

Wound Debridement

At times, both acute and chronic wounds need to be debrided. Debridement is defined as the removal of necrotic (dead) or devitalized tissue. Necrotic or devitalized tissue presents as dark brown, black, yellow, pale, cyanotic, or crusty eschar. To promote optimal wound healing, this tissue needs to be removed from the wound. Debridement may be done in several ways: autolytic, chemical, mechanical, or laser. Occasionally, a combination of debridement methods may be used throughout the healing process. Combination therapy depends on the type of wound and its location, the patient's status, and physician preference.

AUTOLYTIC DEBRIDEMENT

In autolytic debridement, the body breaks down necrotic or devitalized tissue. Hydrocolloid dressings are frequently used to promote autolytic debridement. Autolytic debridement is not the optimal choice in wounds that have large amounts of necrotic tissue. Autolytic debridement takes time for the body to use its own ability to lyse and dissolve necrotic tissue.

CHEMICAL DEBRIDEMENT

Chemical debridement is done using proteolytic enzymes or collagen-based drugs applied topically to the wound. Examples of chemical debridement medications include Collagenase Santyl, Accuzyme, and Panafil. Chemical debridement agents dissolve nonviable tissue. Chemical debridement requires caution because some enzyme agents may destroy healthy tissue while debriding the wound of necrotic and devitalized tissue. Product instructions must be reviewed before use.

MECHANICAL DEBRIDEMENT

Mechanical debridement can be accomplished by wet-to-dry dressings, whirlpools, or the use of sharps. Although wet-to-dry dressings are an effective method of debridement, care must be taken to change to another method of wound care when the wound bed is debrided. Use of the whirlpool is controversial because although it does debride (but not effectively), the potential for infection is increased with multiple patients using a static number of whirlpools (even though they are cleaned between patients). Use of whirlpools also leaves the wound margins macerated, which increases tissue loss, impeding wound closure. In sharps debridement, using a scalpel or scissors, the wound bed is cleared of all necrotic and devitalized tissue surgically. This is a surgical procedure that may require anesthesia, intravenous conscious sedation, a local anesthetic, or a combination of the three.

LASER DEBRIDEMENT

Laser debridement may also be used to provide a clean wound bed. Currently laser debridement is not done as frequently as autolytic, chemical, and mechanical debridement. As technology advances, the use of laser debridement will become more common.

Wound Cultures

Routine wound cultures are not recommended unless there are signs and symptoms of infection such as fever, erythema, edema, induration, purulent exudates, and an elevated white blood cell count. All wounds are considered contaminated and have the potential to become infected. Several methods may be used to culture a wound, including fluid biopsy, wound (tissue) biopsy, and surface culture (culture swab).

A surface culture is usually done first. The wound is cleansed or irrigated with sterile normal saline before swabbing the wound. Exudate and necrotic tissue are not cultured—doing so provides invalid results. After the wound is cleansed, the swab is gently rolled or rotated, starting at the 12 o'clock position and moving in a zig-zag pattern from side to side down the wound to the 6 o'clock position.[2] Optimally, there should be 10 points of contact[2] (Fig. 52-4). A colony count of 100,000 organisms/mL indicates an infection that needs to be treated with the appropriate antibiotic.[10] At colony counts of greater than 100,000 organisms/mL, normal wound healing is inhibited and the wound becomes a chronic wound.[1,2] Wounds that do not respond to antibiotic treatment need to be recultured. The most appropriate form of culture in this scenario is a wound biopsy. Wounds that contain necrotic tissue or tunneling need both aerobic and anaerobic cultures.

Use of Pressure-Relieving Devices

Pressure relief is a major component of wound care. A variety of methods may be used, ranging from low- to high-technology.[2,3,4,11] The easiest and most effective treatment for pressure ulcers on the heels is to keep the heels off the bed by placing a pillow under the lower legs (a low-technology, cost-effective treatment). Turning schedules are effective, easy to implement, and cost-effective. A critically ill patient may require a specialty bed that is designed to reduce pressure. Many specialty beds inflate, deflate, alternate pressures, and laterally rotate. In many institutions, patients must meet specific criteria to qualify for a specialty bed. Another pressure-relieving device is the Vollman-Turner device, which places the patient in the prone position (thus relieving all pressure on the patient's back). The Vollman-Turner device is not a specialty bed. Rather, it is a device that is attached to the bed frame. The advantage of the Vollman-Turner device is that only a minimal number of people are needed to turn the patient when this device is used. Programs that use both high- and low-technology solutions and adapt to meet the patient's needs at various stages in the recovery process tend to be the most successful.

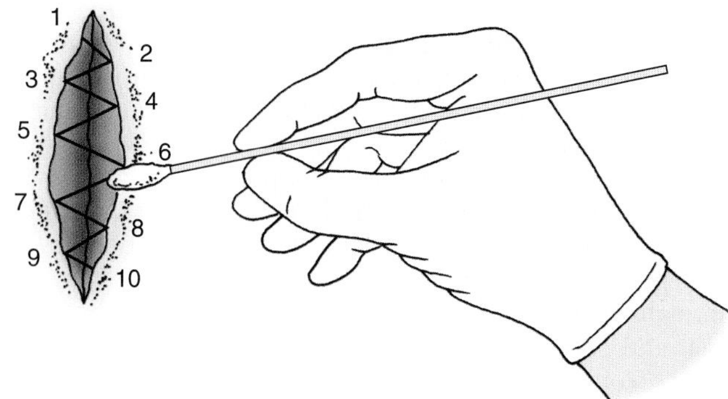

figure 52-4 Procedure for collecting a wound culture. The wound edges are swabbed using 10-point coverage. (From Thomas Hess C: Clinical Guide: Wound Care [4th Ed], p 18. Philadelphia, Lippincott Williams & Wilkins, 2001.)

Pain Management

In all areas of wound care (assessment, cleansing, and dressing changes), the nurse needs to focus on pain assessment and control. No procedure should occur without assessing for pain and then medicating the patient as needed. Wound assessment and wound care should be stopped if needed to ensure that the patient's pain is controlled. Once pain is controlled, the nurse may proceed with the wound care. The choice of pain medication and the delivery method used (e.g., continuous drip, epidural, PCA pump, local anesthesia) depends on the patient's status.

Pharmacotherapy

Pharmacotherapy in wound care entails the use of pain medications and, in some cases, growth hormones and steroids. Pain medications are used to control pain during wound assessment, cleansing, and dressing changes. Growth hormones (e.g., becaplermin [Regranex Gel 0.01%]) may be used to stimulate wound healing. Regranex is applied topically to the wound in measured doses that are recalculated weekly or biweekly. The gel is spread evenly over the wound and covered with gauze moistened with saline. Topical steroid creams, such as clocortolone pivalate (Cloderm) and doxepin hydrochloride (Prudoxin), may be prescribed for wound care to relieve surface inflammation and pruritus of the wound margins.

CARE OF SPECIFIC WOUNDS

Pressure Ulcers

Pressure ulcer treatment depends on the stage of the wound. Stage I and II pressure ulcers are usually treated with hydrocolloid dressings. Stage III and IV pressure ulcers may be dressed using wet-to-dry dressings packed into the wound bed or with calcium alginates "fluffed" and placed into the wound bed and then covered with a hydrocolloid or occlusive transparent dressing. Although they are used, wet-to-dry dressings are not optimal, as discussed earlier. Other options for stage III and IV pressure ulcers are foam dressings and the VAC system.

Burns

Burns are acute wounds, graded as first, second, or third degree, and described as partial or full thickness.[12] Wound care goals in burns are a clean wound free from infection. Burns are cleaned with sterile normal saline or a mild soap and water. Topical ointments such as bacitracin, polymyxin, or silver sulfadiazine may be applied.[12] After cleaning the wound, a dressing is applied. The type of dressing depends on the type of burn, the amount of tissue involved, institutional policy, and physician preference. Another choice is a dressing that releases silver into the wound bed when dampened, such as Acticort or Aquacel. Hydrocolloids, calcium alginates, and foam dressings may also be used, depending on the type and location of burn.

Broad-spectrum antibiotic therapy is not used routinely due to the potential for antibiotic resistance. Infection is treated only if it occurs and is documented with positive cultures. The antibiotic chosen is based on sensitivity results. A more thorough discussion of care of the patient with burns is given in Chapter 53.

High-Volume Draining Wounds

Some wounds may have high volumes of exudate (drainage). Exudate is the response of the body to the inflammatory phase. Wound drainage is composed of neutrophils, macrophages, cellular debris, proteins, and toxins.[6] High-volume draining wounds generate more drainage than traditional gauze pad dressings can manage, in which case hydrocolloids, calcium alginates, hydrogels, or foam dressings may be used. A composite dressing may also be used. These dressings combine the physical attributes of two or more dressings to enhance the absorptive capability.

If the exudate cannot be controlled with these measures, alternatives must be considered. The goal of wound care in this instance is to contain the drainage and protect the surrounding tissue from breakdown. Frequently, the wound may be "pouched" or "bagged." The same supplies used for ostomy pouching are used for pouching a wound[2] (Fig. 52-5), or a product designed specifically for pouching high-volume draining wounds may be used. Pouching the high-volume draining wound allows for accurate measurement of output from the wound and protects the surrounding wound margins.

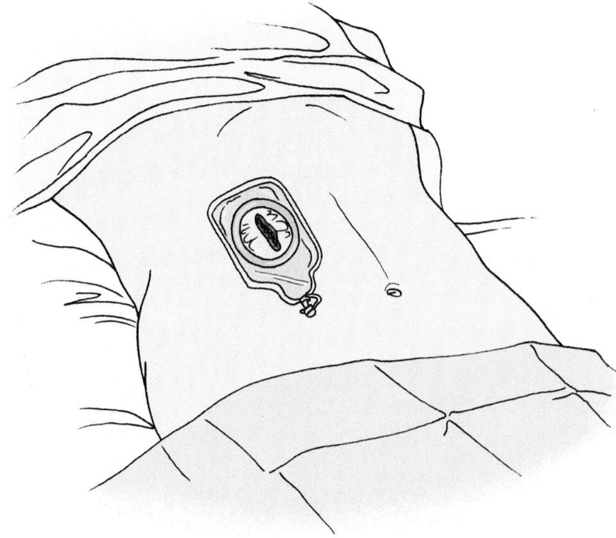

figure 52-5 Procedure for "pouching" or "bagging" a high-volume draining wound. (From Thomas Hess C: Clinical Guide: Wound Care [4th Ed], p 27. Philadelphia, Lippincott Williams & Wilkins, 2001.)

To pouch a wound, the skin is first cleaned with saline or an antibacterial soap and water, then dried. The skin may then be prepared with a protective skin barrier wipe, which protects the skin and enhances the adherence of the wafer. The wound is measured or traced, and a wafer is cut to fit. Stoma paste is applied around the cut-out area to prevent leakage of the drainage onto the skin. A one- or two-piece pouching system may be used. With a one-piece pouching system, the wafer/pouch is applied to the wound. With a two-piece system, the wafer is applied first, and then the pouch is attached. Both systems need a clamp closure device at the end of the pouch. A benefit of a two-piece system is that it allows for pouch removal so that the wound can be assessed without disturbing the wafer.

NUTRITION AND WOUND HEALING

One of the most overlooked aspects of wound care is nutrition. Nutrition is paramount in the critically ill patient or the patient with wounds, whether the wounds are acute or chronic. To heal properly, the body needs adequate carbohydrates, fats, proteins, minerals, calories, vitamins, and hydration[2] (Table 52-1).

Protein is a basic and key component of all cellular activity. Without proteins, the inflammatory process is impaired and the risk of infection increases. Proteins also affect oncotic pressure, which predisposes the patient to edema. Edema in the wound decreases the diffusion of oxygen and nutrients, impeding the healing process even more.[13]

table 52-1 Necessary Nutrients for Wound Healing

Nutrient	Function	Results of Deficiency
Proteins	• Wound repair • Clotting factor production • White blood cell production and migration • Cell-mediated phagocytosis • Fibroblast proliferation • Neovascularization • Collagen synthesis • Epithelial cell proliferation • Wound remodeling	• Poor wound healing • Hypoalbuminemia and generalized edema, which slows oxygen diffusion and metabolic transport mechanisms from the capillaries and cell membranes • Lymphopenia • Impaired cellular immunity
Carbohydrates	• Supply cellular energy • Spare protein	• Body uses visceral and muscle proteins for energy
Fats	• Supply cellular energy • Supply essential fatty acids • Cell membrane structure • Prostaglandin production	• Inhibited tissue repair • Use of visceral and muscle proteins for energy
Vitamin A	• Collagen synthesis • Epithelialization	• Poor wound healing • Impaired immunity
Vitamin C	• Membrane integrity • Antioxidant	• Impaired immunity • Poor wound healing • Capillary fragility
Vitamin K	• Normal blood clotting	• Increased risk of hemorrhage and hematoma formation
Iron	• Collagen synthesis • Enhances leukocytic bacterial activity • Hemoglobin synthesis	• Anemia, leading to increased risk of local tissue ischemia • Impaired tensile strength
Zinc	• Cell proliferation • Cofactor for enzymes • Vitamin A utilization	• Impaired collagen cross-linkage • Slow healing • Alteration in taste • Anorexia • Impaired immunity
Copper	• Collagen cross-linkage • Red blood cell synthesis	• Decreased collagen synthesis • Anemia
Pyridoxine, riboflavin, and thiamine	• Energy production • Cellular immunity • Red blood cell synthesis	• Decreased resistance to infection • Impaired wound healing
Arginine	• Increases local wound immune system • Nitrogen-rich (32% nitrogen, whereas the average amino acid is 16% nitrogen) • Precursor to proline, which is converted to hydroxyproline and then to collagen	• Decreased local wound immune system
Glutamine	• Primary fuel for fibroblasts • Preservation of lean body mass	• Less fuel for fibroblasts

From Hess CT: Clinical Guide: Wound Care (4th Ed), p 46. Springhouse, PA, Springhouse, 2002.

Although protein is a key component in the healing process, other nutrients play major roles. Carbohydrates are the body's fuel source and spare the proteins so they can be used in cellular construction. Fats maintain cell membrane function and assist with the movement of minerals and fat-soluble vitamins in and out of the cell. Vitamins act as catalysts in the body's chemical reactions and are also needed for protein synthesis and cellular replication. Minerals are needed in the body's biochemical reactions and control the movement of fluids into and out of the cell, through the process of osmosis.

table 52-2 **Nutrient Needs Based on Body Weight**

Nutrient	Requirements
Calories	
Normal	25 to 30 kcal/kg/day
Protein-calorie malnutrition (PCM)*	30 to 35 kcal/kg/day
Critically ill or injured*	35 to 40 kcal/kg/day
Protein	
Recommended daily allowance (RDA)	0.8 g/kg/day
PCM	1.5 g/kg/day
Critically ill or injured*	1.5 to 2.0 g/kg/day
Fat	<30% kcal
Water	30 mL/kg body weight or 1 L/1,000 kcal

*Nutrient supplementation required
From Hess CT: Clinical Guide: Wound Care (4th Ed), p 42. Springhouse, PA, Springhouse, 2002.

An adequate caloric intake is required for a wound to heal. Normal adult caloric intake is 25 to 30 kcal/kg/day, and the normal adult protein intake is 0.8 g/kg/day.[2] In a critically ill or critically injured patient, caloric and protein intakes must be dramatically increased. Caloric intake requirements increase to 35 to 40 kcal/kg/day and protein requirements increase to 1.5 to 2 g/kg/day[2] (Table 52-2). Optimal nutritional care for the patient with wounds can be achieved by consulting a dietitian and monitoring laboratory test results along with the patient's basic intake, output, and daily weights.

Serum albumin is of particular interest in that it is a key indicator of protein available for cellular construction and replication. Table 52-3 demonstrates the various albumin requirements at specific ages.[10] In each case, if the albumin level is less than the minimal parameter, replacement therapy is needed to provide the optimal wound healing environment. Normal serum albumin is defined as 3.8 to 5 g/dL. In an adult, a serum albumin level of less than 3.5 g/dL necessitates replacement therapy.

Serum total protein levels are also monitored. Normal levels for serum total protein are 6 to 8 g/dL[10] (see Table 52-3). As stated earlier, protein also affects the oncotic pressure, and levels less than 6 g/dL lead to edema. Note that the serum total protein level, like the albumin level, varies according to age.

Along with electrolytes, complete blood count (CBC), serum albumin, and serum total protein, two other laboratory tests that may be assessed are serum transferrin and the total lymphocyte count (TLC). The serum transferrin level is an indicator of the body's ability to transfer iron through the plasma. The normal serum transferrin level is 180 to 260 mg/dL.[10] Decreased serum transferrin levels lead to anemia, as demonstrated by the CBC. TLC normal parameters are 1,500 to 3,000 cells/μL.[10,13] A TLC assists in the assessment of the patient's immune status and may be decreased in states of malnutrition.

Patients who are NPO for longer than 24 to 48 hours are at risk for slowed healing due to the lack of an adequate supply of protein, carbohydrates, and other nutrients. Nutritional management includes monitoring laboratory test results; documenting intake and output and daily weights; a nutritional assessment by a dietitian; total parental or peripheral parental nutrition or enteral feedings; and calorie counts. Nutrition needs to be addressed early in the patient's admission to promote the optimal opportunity and environment for healing.[13] In critical care, monitoring nutritional status is as important as monitoring hemodynamics.

Adequate hydration is paramount to ensure oxygen delivery to the tissues. If the patient is hypovolemic, then oxygen transport to the peripheral tissues will be impaired. The optimal goal is to maintain hemodynamic stability (Table 52-4). In the critically ill patient, tissue perfusion must be addressed based on the symptom and cause. For example, if the cardiac output is decreased, systolic blood pressure is decreased, the heart rate is tachycardic, and the pulmonary artery wedge pressure is decreased, the patient is hypovolemic. To improve tissue perfusion for this critically ill patient, fluids are given. The hemoglobin and hematocrit must also be assessed and, if low, the patient should be transfused. By improving hydration and correcting the anemia, the circulating volume and the oxygen-carrying capacity of the blood are increased, thus improving tissue perfusion. Improved tissue perfusion enhances the environment for wound healing.

table 52-3 **Normal Values for Serum Total Protein and Serum Albumin**

Age of Patient	Total Protein	Albumin
Adult	6.0–8.0 g/dL or 60–80 g/L	3.5–5.0 g/dL or 38–50 g/L
10–19 y	6.3–8.6 g/dL or 68–86 g/L	3.7–5.6 g/dL or 37–56 g/L
7–9 y	6.2–8.1 g/dL or 62–81 g/L	3.7–5.6 g/dL or 37–56 g/L
4–6 y	5.9–7.8 g/dL or 59–78 g/L	3.5–5.2 g/dL or 35–52 g/L
1–3 y	5.9–7.0 g/dL or 59–70 g/L	3.4–4.2 g/dL or 34–42 g/L
<5 days	5.4–7.0 g/dL or 54–70 g/L	2.6–3.6 g/dL or 26–36 g/L

From Fischbach FT: Nurse's Quick Reference to Common Laboratory and Diagnostic Tests (3rd Ed), p 564, Philadelphia, Lippincott Williams & Wilkins, 2002.

table 52-4 Hemodynamic Stability

Parameter	Normal Value
Cardiac index	2.5–4 L/min/m²
Cardiac output	4–8 L/min
Pulmonary artery systolic pressure	15–30 mm Hg
Pulmonary artery diastolic pressure	8–15 mm Hg
Pulmonary artery wedge pressure	8–15 mm Hg
Central venous pressure	2–8 mm Hg
Heart rate	Sinus 60–100 beats/min
Urinary output	>30 mL/h
Oxygen saturation	>92%
Capillary refill	<3 sec
Systolic blood pressure	≥90 mm Hg; ≤140 mm Hg
Diastolic blood pressure	≤80 mm Hg

PATIENT TEACHING AND DISCHARGE PLANNING

Patient teaching and discharge planning are ongoing processes that occur throughout the patient's hospital stay. Discharge planning for patients with wounds is a multidisciplinary challenge. Multiple factors must be considered if discharge is to be successful (Box 52-6). An important part of discharge planning is ensuring that the patient or a family member knows how to care for the wound once he or she leaves the hospital. Examples of patient teaching guides for wound care are given in Boxes 52-7 through 52-10.

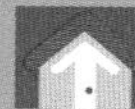

box 52-6 *Wounds*

- Determine whether the patient can be discharged home, or whether skilled nursing will be necessary.
- Evaluate the home environment for safety.
- Determine the availability of financial resources for expenses such as dressing supplies and home support.
- Determine the patient's or family member's readiness to learn wound care.
- Determine the type of treatment or wound care. This will be dictated by the type of wound (e.g., stage, acute, chronic, burn).
- Determine the patient's access to transportation to and from the health care provider's office for follow-up.
- Before discharge, a nutritional assessment must be completed and dietary concerns need to be addressed by the nurse and dietitian.
- Self-care deficits must be addressed. A home health nurse or a home health aide may need to follow at discharge if the patient is unable to perform activities of daily living (ADLs). Family members may need instruction in assisting the patient at home.
- Document the location of the wound and instruct the patient and family members on how to perform wound care.
- Assess the patient's psychosocial support system. Referrals to various community programs may be needed.
- Supply the patient and family members with readily available resources to troubleshoot problems (for example, specific instructions about when to call 911, versus the primary care provider's office).

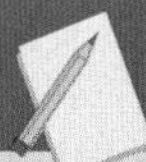

box 52-7
Wound Care (Sutures, Staples, and Wound Adhesives)

Wound Closure

- Sutures are threadlike. They are placed using a needle to pull the skin together. You may see "knots."
- Staples are special surgical staples. They are placed using a special staple gun to pull the skin together.
- Wound adhesives are a type of glue that holds the edges of the skin together.

Patient Activity

- Keep your sutures/staples/wound adhesive clean and dry.
- Wash your hands before you start.
- Do not rub or pull the area.
- Clean the wound gently with mild soap and water and rinse, or use a wound cleanser as directed by your physician. Do not "soak" the sutures/staples/wound adhesive. Gently pat the area dry.
- A dry gauze dressing may be applied to keep your wound clean or pad the area if your clothes rub.
- Wash your hands when you are done.

When To Call Your Physician

- Call if you find any redness, tenderness, pus-type drainage, swelling, missing sutures or staples, or increased pain, or if the area is warm or hot to the touch.
- Call if you have a fever of more than 101°F.
- Call immediately and go to the emergency department if your incision "pulls open."

Medications

- Take your medications as prescribed.
- If you are taking an antibiotic, take all pills prescribed. Do not stop taking them when you feel better!

Safety

- You may drive, climb stairs, work, begin sexual activity, and lift when instructed by the physician.

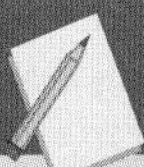

box 52-8
Wound Care (Dry Dressing)

Patient Activity

- Change your dressing every day.
- Wash your hands before you start.
- Clean the wound with normal saline, mild soap and water, or a wound cleanser as directed.
- Cover the wound with a dry gauze dressing.
- Wash your hands when you are done.

When to Call Your Physician

- Call if you find any redness, tenderness, pus-type drainage, swelling, missing sutures or staples, or increased pain, or if the area is warm or hot to the touch.
- Call if you have a fever of more than 101°F.
- Call immediately and go to the emergency department if your incision "pulls open."

Medications

- Take your medications as prescribed.
- If you are taking an antibiotic, take all pills prescribed. Do not stop taking them when you feel better!

Safety

- You may drive, climb stairs, work, begin sexual activity, and lift when instructed by the physician.

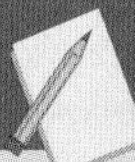

box 52-9
Wound Care (Calcium Alginate)

Calcium alginate is a dressing that can be packed (lightly) into your wound. It is made of a special type of seaweed that has healing properties. Calcium alginates look similar to "angel hair" when "fluffed."

Patient Activity

- Change your dressing every 3 days unless otherwise directed by your physician.
- Wash your hands before you start.
- Remove the old dressing (it will appear to be a gelatinous mass, not the fibrous "angel hair" that you put in).
- Clean your wound with normal saline or with a wound cleanser as directed.
- Take the calcium alginate out of the package and gently "fluff" it (pull it apart slightly so that it has a light, fluffy look).
- Place the "fluffed" calcium alginate into the wound.
- Cover the wound and (calcium alginate) with the type of covering you were directed to use.
- Wash your hands when you are done.

When to Call Your Physician

- Call if you find any redness, tenderness, pus-type drainage, swelling, missing sutures or staples, or increased pain, or if the area is warm or hot to the touch.
- Call if you have a fever of more than 101°F.

Medications

- Take your medications as prescribed.
- If you are taking an antibiotic, take all pills prescribed. Do not stop taking them when you feel better!

Safety

- You may drive, climb stairs, work, begin sexual activity, and lift when instructed by the physician.

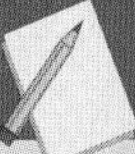

box 52-10
Wound Care (Hydrocolloid)

A hydrocolloid is a thicker type of wound covering that can be placed over open wounds such as bed sores (pressure sores). A hydrocolloid may also be placed over a wound in which calcium alginate has been packed. A hydrocolloid comes in various shapes and sizes. It has an adhesive (sticky) side. The adhesive side goes over the wound.

Patient Activity

- Change your dressing every 3 to 5 days unless otherwise directed by your physician, or when it comes off.
- Wash your hands before you start.
- Gently peel the old hydrocolloid off, being careful not to peel too quickly or roughly.
- Clean your wound with normal saline or with a wound cleanser as directed.
- If you are packing the wound with calcium alginate, do it at this time.
- Peel the paper off the adhesive of the hydrocolloid.
- Place the "adhesive side down" over the wound.
- Press gently and smooth the hydrocolloid over the wound.
- Place your hand on top of the hydrocolloid for about 1 minute. This helps the adhesive to stick better.

When to Call Your Physician

- Call if you find any redness, tenderness, pus-type drainage, swelling, missing sutures or staples, or increased pain, or if the area is warm or hot to the touch.
- Call if you have a fever of more than 101°F.

Medications

- Take your medications as prescribed.
- If you are taking an antibiotic, take all pills prescribed. Do not stop taking them when you feel better!

Safety

- You may drive, climb stairs, work, begin sexual activity, and lift when instructed by the physician.

clinical applicability challenges

Self-Challenge: Critical Thinking

William Bowman is a 46-year-old African-American man with a history of hypertension and sickle cell disease. His last sickle cell crisis was 9 months ago. He is admitted to the intensive care unit (ICU) with an acute inferior wall myocardial infarction. Three days after myocardial infarction, he has a cardiac arrest. After arrest, he remains ventilated with a fraction of inspired oxygen (FIO_2) of 50%, tidal volume of 750, synchronized intermittent mandatory ventilation (SIMV) of 14, and pressure support of 5 cm H_2O. Mr. Bowman has dopamine infusing at a rate of 15 µg/kg/minute and dobutamine at a rate of 9 µg/kg/minute through the proximal port of a triple-lumen catheter. Through the medial port of the triple-lumen catheter, a nitroglycerin drip is infusing at a rate of 40 µg/minute. Infusing through the distal port of the triple-lumen catheter is a lidocaine drip at a rate of 2 mg/minute and a maintenance intravenous infusion of 5% dextrose in water (D_5W) at a rate of 40 mL/hour. Mr. Bowman's vital signs are as follows: blood pressure, 90/48 mm Hg; heart rate, 110 beats/minute; respirations, 14 breaths/minute. His cardiac output is 2.8 L/minute; pulmonary artery wedge pressure 4 mm Hg; central venous pressure, 0 mm Hg; urinary output, 10 mL/hour; and oxygen saturation, 94%.

1. *Discuss Mr. Bowman's potential for skin breakdown. What are the risk factors? Of these risk factors, which can be modified?*
2. *Describe your plan of care for Mr. Bowman. Prioritize this plan of care.*
3. *Of the following treatment modalities, explain why each is of importance and which would be most effective considering the patient's present status: nutrition, oxygenation, hydration.*

Study Questions

1. *On assessment of a patient, you find pale, punched-out wounds on her distal leg. These are*
   a. *venous stasis ulcers.*
   b. *arterial ulcers.*
   c. *healing by secondary intention.*
   d. *healing by delayed primary intention.*
2. *The inflammatory phase can best be described as*
   a. *an initial phase, lasting 4 to 6 days, in which phagocytosis and vasoconstriction occur.*
   b. *an initial phase in which growth factors stimulate fibroblast to produce collagen.*
   c. *a secondary phase, lasting 4 to 24 days, with the focus on collagen production and granulation tissue.*
   d. *the third and final phase, where the goal is to increase tensile strength of the scar tissue.*
3. *Identify which of the following nursing notes best describes a wound.*
   a. *Half-dollar-size stage II on buttock, cleansed with normal saline, hydrocolloid dressing applied.*
   b. *Two inch by two inch stage I–II on sacral area cleansed, dressing applied.*
   c. *Stage II length 3.4 cm, width 1.8 cm, depth N/A, on sacrum, cleansed with NS, hydrocolloid dressing applied.*
   d. *Pressure ulcer stage II sacrum, cleansed with normal saline, hydrocolloid dressing applied.*
4. *The vacuum-assisted wound closure (VAC) system can be used in which of the following situations?*
   a. *Flaps, grafts, dehisced incisions, heels with eschar*
   b. *Flaps, grafts, acute and traumatic wounds*
   c. *Acute and traumatic wounds with necrotic tissue*
   d. *Acute and traumatic wounds with untreated osteomyelitis*
5. *An example of autolytic debridement would be*
   a. *proteolytic enzymes.*
   b. *whirlpool.*
   c. *application of a wet-to-dry dressing.*
   d. *application of a hydrocolloid dressing.*
6. *What is happening when a wound is left open for 3 to 5 days due to infection and edema?*
   a. *The wound is being allowed to heal by primary intention.*
   b. *The wound is being allowed to heal by secondary intention.*
   c. *The wound is being allowed to heal by delayed primary (tertiary) intention.*
   d. *The wound is in the proliferation phase.*

REFERENCES

1. Bryant RA: Acute and Chronic Wounds: Nursing Management (2nd Ed). St. Louis, Mosby, 2000
2. Thomas Hess C: Clinical Guide: Wound Care (4th Ed). Springhouse, PA, Springhouse, 2002
3. Cullum N: Pressure ulcer prevention and treatment. Crit Care Nurs Clin North Am 13:547–554, 2001
4. Hahn JF, Olsen CL, Tomaselli N, et al: Wounds: Nursing care and product selection—Part I. Nursing Spectrum, 2003. Available at http://nsweb.nursingspectrum.com/ce/ce80.htm. Accessed August 4, 2003
5. McCarty R, Tarboton S: Developing an assessment tool for acute wounds. Nurse Prescriber/Commun Nurse (April): 55–56, 1999
6. Staiano-Coico L, Higgins PJ, Schwartz SB, et al: Wound fluids: A reflection of the state of healing. Ostomy Wound Manage 46(1A): 85s–93s, 2000
7. Ackley BJ, Ladwig GB: Nursing Diagnosis Handbook (5th Ed.). St. Louis, Mosby, 2002
8. Kinetic Concepts, Inc. The V.A.C. Available http://www.kci1.com/products/vac/vac/index.asp. Accessed January 29, 2003
9. Ovington LG: Hanging wet to dry dressings out to dry. Adv Skin Wound Care 15(2):79–84, 2002
10. Fischbach FT: Nurse's Quick Reference to Common Laboratory and Diagnostic Tests (3rd Ed). Philadelphia, Lippincott Williams & Wilkins, 2002
11. Junkin J: Failure to thrive in wounds: Prevention and early intervention. Infect Control 1(2):1–8, 2002
12. Wiebelhaus P, Hansen SL: How to manage burn emergencies. Dimens Crit Care Nurs 20(4):2–9, 2001
13. Whitney JD, Heitkemper M: Modifying perfusion, nutrition and stress to promote wound healing in patients with acute wounds. Heart Lung 28(2):128–133, 1999

OTHER SELECTED READING

Biala K: Case conferencing for wound care patients. Home Healthcare Nurse 20(2):120–126, 2002

Bergstrom N, Allman R, Alvarez O, et al: Treatment of Pressure Ulcers. Clinical Practice Guideline no. 15. AHCPR publication no. 95-0652. Rockville, MD: U.S. Department of Health and Human Services, Public Health Service, 1994

Clever K, Smith G, Bower C, et al: Evaluating the efficacy of a uniquely delivered skin protectant and its effect on the formation of sacral/buttock pressure ulcers. Ostomy Wound Manage 48(12):60–67, 2002

Convatec, Inc. Available at www.woundcarehelpline.com/conva.edu.htm. Accessed July 24, 2003

Flynn MB, Fink R: Committing to evidence-based skin care practices. Crit Care Nurs Clin North Am 13:555–568, 2001

Frantz RA: Chronic wound healing. University of Iowa, Nursing Education, 2003. Available at: http://coninfo.nursing.uiowa.edu/sites/chronicwounds. Accessed July 24, 2003

Franz MG, Kuhn MA, Wright TE, et al: Use of the wound healing trajectory as an outcome determinant for acute wound healing. Wound Repair Regen 8(6):511–516, 2000

Hahn JF, Olsen CL, Tomaselli N, et al: Wound: Nursing care and product selection—Part II. Nursing Spectrum, 2003. Available at http://nsweb.nursingspectrum.com/ce/ce81.htm. Accessed July 24, 2003

Krasner D: Chronic Wound Care: A Clinical Source Book for Healthcare Professionals (3rd Ed). King of Prussia, PA, Health Management Publications, 2001

Kuznar W: Adjunctive approaches aid in acute wound healing. Dermatol Surg (May):58, 2002

Mendez-Eastman S: New advances in wound therapy. 2003. Available at http://www.wounds1.com/hero/hero.cfm. Accessed April, 2003

Nayduch DA: Trauma wound management. Nurs Clin North Am 34(4):895–907, 1999

Ovington LG: Wound care products: How to choose. Home Healthcare Nurse 19(4):224–232, 2001

Ovington LG: Dealing with drainage: The what, why and how of wound exudate. Home Healthcare Nurse 20(6):368–374, 2002

Thomas DW, Hill CM, Lewis MA, et al: Randomized clinical trial of the effect of semi-occlusive dressings on the microflora and clinical outcome of acute facial wounds. Wound Repair Regen 8(4):258–263, 2000

Trengrove NJ, Stacey MC, Macauley S, et al: Analysis of the acute and chronic wound environments: The role of proteases and their inhibitors. Wound Repair Regen 7(6):442–452, 1999

chapter **53**

Burns

TONYA APPLEBY

objectives

Based on the content in this chapter, the reader should be able to:

- Describe the pathophysiology of a burn injury.
- Explore the mechanism of a burn injury.
- Review the physiological changes associated with each organ system in relation to a burn injury.
- Discuss the initial priorities of a patient with a burn injury.
- Formulate a plan of care for a patient who has sustained a burn injury.
- Select appropriate wound care coverings for a patient with a burn injury.
- Evaluate the collaborative efforts of the burn team in relation to desired outcomes in a patient with a burn injury.

Great strides have been made in the technological and pharmacological care of the burned patient. The past two decades have witnessed a significant decline in the number of burn injuries and hospitalizations. Total burn injuries have decreased from 2.5 million to approximately 1 million per year. Burn injuries account for 700,000 emergency department visits per year. The average size of a burn is about 14% of the total body surface area (TBSA). The trend toward outpatient management has contributed to the decreased number of hospitalized patients.[1]

Acute hospitalization resulting from a burn injury has declined 50% since the 1970s. Before the 1970s, a patient with a 50% TBSA burn had a 40% chance of survival. Today, a patient with a 75% TBSA burn has a 50% chance of survival.[1]

Despite the dramatic decreases in incidence, an acute burn injury is the third leading cause of death in children between the ages of 1 and 9 years and is the fifth leading cause of death in the remainder of the population. There are an estimated 4500 fire and burn deaths per year.[1,2] Safety measures for preventing burns are given in Box 53-1.

Each year, about 45,000 patients who sustain a burn injury are hospitalized. Of these 45,000, about half are treated at specialized burn centers. Burn treatment centers are comprised of nurses, physicians, physical therapists, occupational therapists, recreational therapists, nutritionists, psychologists, social workers, and spiritual support staff. The American Burn Association has established guidelines for transfer and referral of these patients. Despite specialized management, about 6% of all patients admitted to burn centers do not survive.[1]

CLASSIFICATION OF BURN INJURIES

Burn injuries are described by causative agent, depth, and severity.

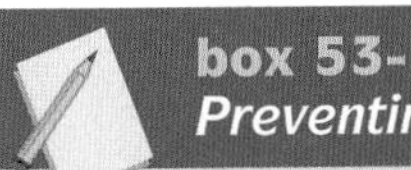

box 53-1
Preventing Burns

Prevent Accidents in the Home

- Never leave children unattended in a bathtub.
- Set your hot water heater no higher than 120°F.
- Never leave candles unattended, and always be sure candles are fully extinguished.
- Exercise caution with foods that are cooked in a microwave.
- Have your furnace serviced once a year.
- Install a carbon monoxide detector.
- Install a smoke detector on each floor of your house; change the batteries twice a year.
- Plan an exit route in your house in the event of a fire and have routine fire drills once a month.
- Exercise caution with cooking. Avoid wearing clothes with sleeves that may dangle and accidentally ignite clothing.
- Keep pot and skillet handles turned in toward the stove.
- Never use the oven as a heating source.
- Never allow children to stand on an open oven door, as this may cause the entire stove to collapse.

Prevent Accidents Outside the Home

- Only a responsible adult should handle fireworks. Never leave fireworks out where children can have access.
- Exercise caution with campfires.
- If an electrical wire is found in a tree, do not touch! Call the local electric company as soon as possible.
- Use sunscreens! Choose a sunscreen with ultraviolet A (UVA) and ultraviolet B (UVB) protection and a sun protection factor (SPF) of 30. Apply every 2 to 3 hours.

Should a Burn Occur

- Stop the burning process by removing the source!

Causative Agent

A burn injury usually results from energy transfer from a heat source to the body. The heat source may be thermal, chemical, or electrical.

THERMAL BURNS

Thermal burns may be caused by a flame source such as a house fire, a cooking accident, or a fiery explosion. Scald burns from steam or contact from a hot object, such as a cooking pan or hot steel, may also cause thermal injury.

CHEMICAL BURNS

Chemical injuries are commonly encountered after exposure to acids and alkali, including hydrofluoric acid, formic acid, anhydrous ammonia, cement, and phenol. Other specific chemical agents that cause chemical burns include white phosphorus, certain elemental metals, nitrates, hydrocarbons, and tar.

Contact time is a critical element in determining the severity of injury. Initiation of hydrotherapy is crucial to limit the effects of the chemical. Regardless of the causative agent, the irrigation must continue once the patient arrives at the emergency department. Time should not be wasted attempting to neutralize the acid or alkali. For all chemical burns, hydrotherapy treatment should continue for 2 to 3 hours.

ELECTRICAL BURNS

The effects of electricity on the body are determined by seven factors: the type of current, the amount of current, the pathway of the current, the duration of contact, the area of contact, the resistance of the body, and the voltage. Humans are sensitive to very small electric currents because of their highly developed nervous system. Electricity travels the path of least resistance; therefore, tissue, nerves, and muscle are easily damaged, whereas bone is not.

Low-voltage injuries are considered to be caused by 380 volts or less. Low-voltage injuries tend to occur at home and involve the hands and oral cavities. The most common cause of low-voltage electric burns of the hand is contact with an extension cord in which the insulating material has worn off, either from wear or misuse. A low-voltage burn of the hand usually consists of a small, deep burn that may involve vessels, tendons, and nerves. These burns involve a small area of the hand, yet they may be severe enough to require amputation of a finger. Low-voltage electricity can also damage the oral cavity, leaving a permanent scar. These injuries occur most frequently in children between the ages of 1 and 2 years. Most are caused by sucking on, or biting, an extension cord socket. Low-voltage current usually follows the path of least resistance (nerves, blood vessels), whereas high-voltage current takes a direct path between entrance and ground. Current is concentrated at its entrance to the body, then diverges centrally, and finally converges before exiting. Unfortunately, the most severe damage to tissue occurs at the sites of contact, which are commonly referred to as the entrance and exit wounds. High-voltage electric entry wounds are charred, centrally depressed, and leathery in appearance, whereas exit wounds are more likely to "explode" as the charge exits.

Depth

Many factors alter the response of body tissues to heat. The degree or depth of burn depends on (1) the temperature of the injuring agent, (2) the duration of exposure to the injuring agent, and (3) the areas of the body that are exposed to the injuring agent. Damage to the skin is frequently described according to the depth of injury and is defined in terms of superficial, partial-thickness, and full-thickness injuries, which correspond to the various layers of the skin (Table 53-1; Fig. 53-1).

SUPERFICIAL BURNS

Superficial burn injuries are commonly known as *first-degree burns.* Superficial burns affect the epidermal layer and heal with minimal intervention. Sunburn is a familiar example of a first-degree superficial burn injury. The burned skin is painful at first, and later itches because of the stimulation of sensory receptors. Because of the continuous replacement of epidermal epithelial cells, this type of injury heals spontaneously without scarring. Care of superficial burns is summarized in Box 53-2.

table 53-1 Characteristics of Burns of Various Depths

Depth	Tissues Involved	Usual Cause	Characteristics	Pain	Healing
Superficial (first-degree)	Minimal epithelial damage	Sun	Dry Blisters after 24 h Pinkish red Blanches with pressure	Painful	About 5 days No scarring
Superficial partial-thickness (second-degree)	Epidermis, minimal dermis	Flash Hot liquids	Moist Pinkish or mottled red Blisters Some blanching	Pain Hyperesthetic	21–28 days Minimal scarring
Deep partial-thickness (second-degree)	Entire epidermis, part of dermis: epidermal-lined hair and sweat glands intact	Above plus hot solids, flame, and intense radiant injury	Dry, pale, waxy No blanching	Sensitive to pressure	30 days to months Late hypertrophic scarring; marked contracture formation
Full-thickness (third-degree)	All of above, and portion of subcutaneous fat; may involve connective tissue, muscle, bone	Sustained flame, electrical, chemical, and steam	Leathery, cracked avascular, white, cherry red, or black	Little pain	Cannot self-regenerate; needs grafting

PARTIAL-THICKNESS BURNS

Partial-thickness burns are differentiated into superficial and deep partial-thickness burns. Superficial partial-thickness burns affect the epidermal and superficial dermal layers and heal with minimal intervention (see Box 53-2). Deep partial-thickness burns affect the epidermal and deep dermal layers. Fluid resuscitation, nutritional status, and the presence of premorbid conditions may affect the healing potential of a deep partial-thickness burn injury. Deep partial-thickness burn injuries may take as long as 3 weeks to heal spontaneously. Delayed healing may result in scarring and loss of function.

FULL-THICKNESS BURNS

Full-thickness burns (third-degree burns) expose the fat layer, which is composed of poorly vascularized adipose

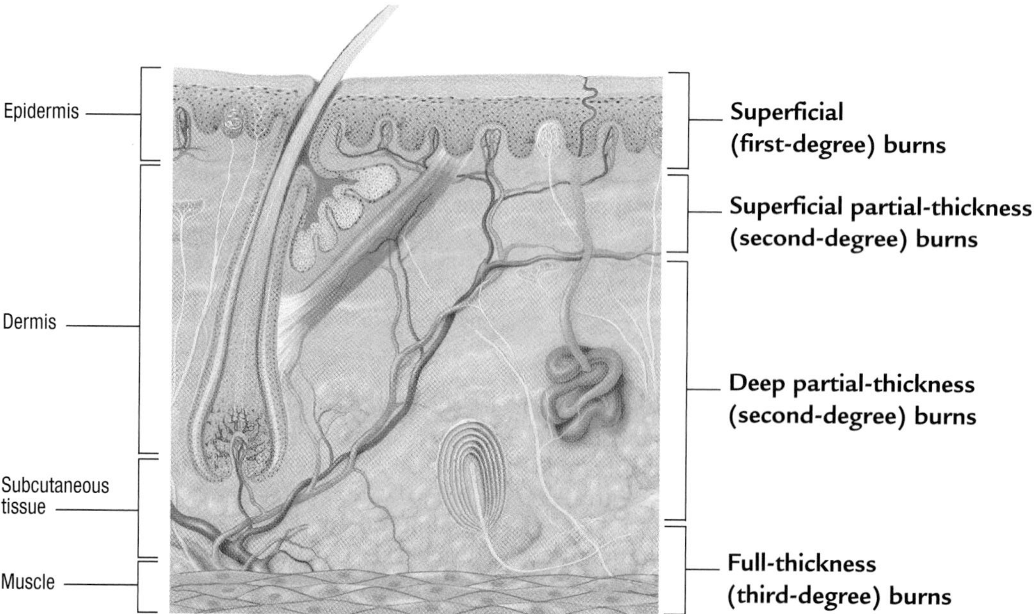

figure 53-1 Classification of burns by depth of injury. (Source: Anatomical Chart Company: Atlas of Pathophysiology, p 361. Springhouse, PA, Springhouse, 2001.)

box 53-2
Care of Superficial (First-Degree) Burns and Superficial Partial-Thickness (Second-Degree) Burns

Superficial (First-Degree) Burns

- Apply ice packs or cold compresses.
- No dressing is required.
- Aloe gel with lidocaine can be applied topically as necessary for localized relief.
- Acetaminophen, aspirin, or ibuprofen can be taken as necessary for generalized discomfort.

Superficial Partial-Thickness (Second-Degree) Burns

- If the skin or blister is broken, wash the area with water and mild antiseptic soap.
- Apply a layer of silver sulfadiazine or bacitracin.
- Apply a layer of nonadherent gauze and secure with a gauze roll.
- Dressings should be changed twice a day.
- Wrap fingers and toes individually to prevent "webbing" of healing granulation tissue.
- The patient may continue his or her usual activity depending on the burned site.
- Dependent extremities should be elevated above the level of the heart to prevent excessive edema and promote venous return.
- The patient should be aware of signs and symptoms of infection, including fever, marked tenderness and erythema surrounding the burn wound, purulent drainage of pus, red streaks radiating from the wound, or pain that cannot be controlled with analgesics.
- The patient should follow up in 2 days with a primary care provider.

tissue. This layer contains the roots of the sweat glands and hair follicles. All epidermal and dermal elements are destroyed. These burns may appear white, red, brown, or black. Reddened areas do not blanch in response to pressure because the underlying blood supply has been interrupted. Thrombosed blood vessels and capillaries may be visualized. These burns are completely anesthetic because the sensory receptors have been completely destroyed. In addition, they may appear sunken because of the loss of underlying fat and muscle.

A small wound (<4 cm) may be allowed to heal by granulation and migration of healthy epithelium from the wound margins. Extensive, open full-thickness wounds, however, leave the patient highly susceptible to overwhelming infection and malnutrition. Wound closure by skin grafting restores the integrity of the skin.

Severity

Burn severity is determined by the extent and depth of the burn and the causative agent, time, and circumstances surrounding the burn injury. To assess the severity of the burn, several factors must be considered:

- The percentage of body surface area burned
- The depth of the burn
- The anatomical location of the burn
- The age of the person (Boxes 53-3 and 53-4)
- The person's medical history
- The presence of concomitant injury
- The presence of inhalation injury

Several methods using percentages of TBSA may be used to estimate the extent of a burn (Fig. 53-2). The "rule of nines" divides the body parts into multiples of 9%. The head is considered to account for 9% of TBSA; each arm, 9%; each leg, 18%; the anterior trunk, 18%; the posterior trunk, 18%; and the perineum, 1%, making a total of 100%. Burns may involve only one surface of a body part, or they may be circumferential. For example, if only the anterior surface of the arm is burned, then the TBSA is estimated to be 4.5%. However, if the burn circles the entire arm, then the value is 9%.

The Lund and Browder chart is another method of measuring burn size. This method is highly recommended because it corrects for the large head-to-body ratio of infants and children. Surface measurements are assigned to each body part in terms of the age of the patient. For estimating small scattered burns (e.g., scald and grease burns), the "rule of palms" allows for quick assessment until a Lund and Browder assessment can be done. The patient's palm equals 1% TBSA.

A burn injury may range from a small blister to a massive full-thickness burn. Recognizing the need for a clear description of terms, the American Burn Association developed the Injury Severity Grading System, which is used to determine the magnitude of the burn injury and to provide

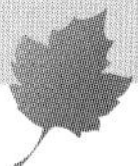

box 53-3
Considerations for the Older Patient With Burns

Older patients respond differently to burn injuries because of age-related changes and diminished physiological reserve. Pre-existing medical conditions and complications as a result of injury are significant factors leading to mortality of the older burn patient. The adverse effects of trauma, including burns, can persist for an extended period after injury. Once injured, elderly patients may never regain their preinjury level of health. Postdischarge destination and care are challenging obstacles in discharge planning. Family interest in assuming caregiver responsibility, ability of the patient to render self-care, insurance, and financial limitations must be considered in planning for discharge. Many independent elderly patients will no longer be able to return home alone after a burn injury. Rehabilitation and long-term care facilities can create an emotional and financial burden on the family. In addition, acute rehabilitation requires the patient to participate in 3 hours of therapy each day. Many elderly patients are unable to meet this requirement, and thus may not be eligible for acute rehabilitation.

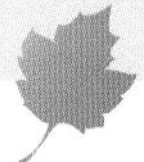

box 53-4

Considerations for the Pediatric Patient With Burns

The National Burn Information Exchange is a voluntary burn patient registry that was established in 1964. As of 1991, metadata revealed that children from birth through 4 years of age have a disproportionately high number of burn accidents. This age group accounts for nearly 52% of all burns in children. After 4 years of age, the incidence of burn injury tapers off, but rises again as adolescents enter the workforce.

In those younger than 4 years of age, the most common burns are scald injuries. The kitchen area presents numerous hazards for a toddler. Hot beverages, foods, and stovetops can cause significant injury to an unattended toddler in a matter of seconds. If a nonaccidental burn is suspected, the family members should be interviewed separately. The histories are then compared for consistency. Scalding burns of lower extremities in which the entire foot is burned, with a well-demarcated line of injury around the leg and absence of splash marks, suggest forced immersion into hot water. Accidental scalding usually results in partial-thickness burns; deep full-thickness burns caused by scalding are suspect and suggest sustained contact with hot water. Evidence of other trauma, such as bruising or numerous healed wounds, should be noted. A child who has a depressed affect may be chronically abused. A call to the local child protective services in these cases is mandatory.

optimal criteria for hospital resources for patient care. The severity of burn injury has been categorized into minor, moderate, and major burns, as outlined in Box 53-5. Minor burn injuries can be treated in the emergency department with outpatient follow-up every 48 hours, until the risk of infection is reduced and wound healing is underway. Patients with moderate, uncomplicated burn injuries or major burn injuries should be referred to a regional burn center and, if appropriate, transferred for specialized care.

PATHOPHYSIOLOGY

Localized Tissue Response

Cellular injury is started when tissues are exposed to an energy source (thermal, chemical, electrical, or radiation). The depth of the thermal injury is demonstrated by the extent of injury down through the layers of skin. Figure 53-3 represents the concentric zones of a burn injury. The zone of hyperemia heals rapidly and has no cell death. In the zone of stasis, the cells can recover or become necrotic in the initial 24 hours. In the zone of coagulation, temperatures have reached 113°F (45°C). The tissues are black, gray, khaki, or white and have undergone protein coagulation and cell death.

Systemic Response

Major changes at the cellular level are responsible for the tremendous systemic response noted in a patient with burns. The localized response causes a coagulation of cellular proteins, leading to irreversible cell injury with local production of complement, histamine, and oxygen free radicals (i.e., byproducts of oxidative processes). Oxygen free radicals alter cell lipids and proteins, affecting the integrity of the cell membrane. This is particularly problematic in the endothelium of the microvascular circulation because disruption of the cell membrane leads to increased vascular permeability.[3] Increased vascular permeability leads to loss of plasma proteins and results in a marked decrease in circulating volume. Complement (particularly C5a) activation and histamine release contribute to the increased vascular permeability by increasing production of oxygen free radicals.[3] Increased vascular permeability leads to the formation of interstitial edema, which usually peaks within 24 to 48 hours of injury. It is postulated that the microvasculature takes weeks to restore itself completely to its premorbid state. The pulmonary vasculature is not spared and pulmonary interstitial edema forms, with intra-alveolar hemorrhages.[3] This initial pulmonary insult is thought to be a precursor to the development of acute respiratory distress syndrome (ARDS).

Systemically, a burn injury causes a release of vasoactive substances such as histamine, prostaglandins, interleukins, and arachidonic acid metabolites. These substances initiate the systemic inflammatory response syndrome (SIRS). The potent mediators and cytokines (nitric oxide, platelet-activating factor [PAF], serotonin, thromboxane A_2, and tumor necrosis factor [TNF]) deplete the intravascular volume, decreasing blood flow to the kidneys and the gastrointestinal tract. If left uncorrected, hypovolemic shock, metabolic acidosis, and hyperkalemia may occur. A review of the literature suggests that translocation of bacteria occurs at this time, as seen in septic shock states.[3]

Nitric oxide relaxes smooth muscle and produces vasodilation and hypotension. It may also depress myocardial function and block platelet aggregation and adhesion. PAF initiates neutrophil and white blood cell activation and produces tissue inflammation. PAF increases permeability of vessels, thereby decreasing myocardial contractility, causing vasodilation and hypotension. Some prostaglandins cause vasoconstriction and increased blood flow. A fever may also accompany prostaglandin activation. Serotonin causes vasodilation, hypotension, and increased vessel permeability. Thromboxane A_2 is responsible for inflammation, platelet aggregation, and polymorphonuclear cell adherence. TNF is responsible for numerous cellular responses, including increased formation of oxygen free radicals, which leads to injury of the lungs, gastrointestinal tract, and kidneys; increased cytokine production; initial hyperglycemia followed by hypoglycemia; hypotension; metabolic acidosis; coagulopathy; and activation of the coagulation cascade.

The end results of the local and systemic responses are dramatic, if the burn covers more than 20% of the TBSA. The person with a major burn injury experiences a form

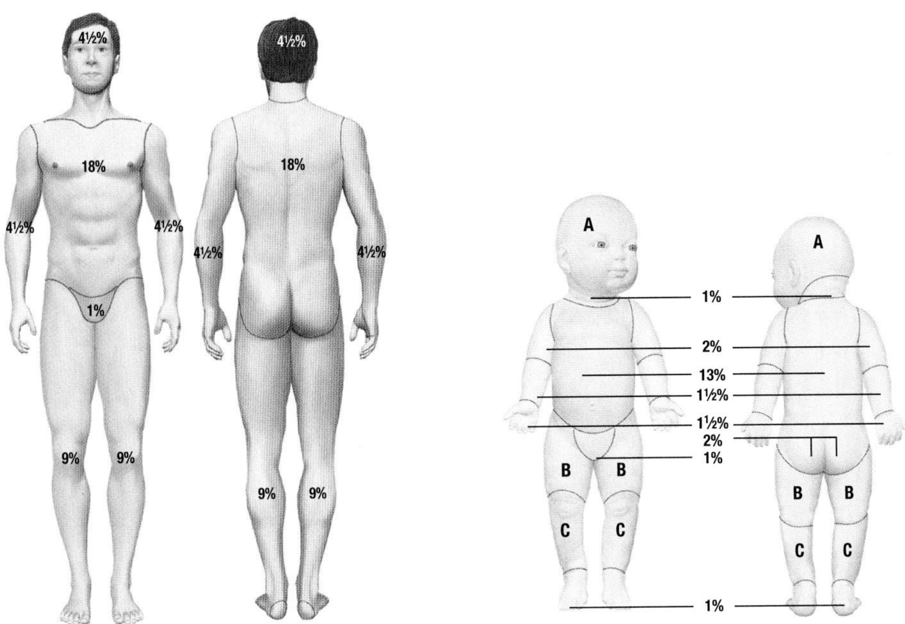

A. Rule of Nines

AREA	PERCENT OF BURN					SEVERITY OF BURN		TOTAL PERCENT
	0-1 Year	1-4 Years	5-9 Years	10-15 Years	Adult	2°	3°	
Head	19	17	13	10	7			
Neck	2	2	2	2	2			
Ant. Trunk	13	13	13	13	13			
Post. Trunk	13	13	13	13	13			
R. Buttock	2½	2½	2½	2½	2½			
L. Buttock	2½	2½	2½	2½	2½			
Genitalia	1	1	1	1	1			
R. U. Arm	4	4	4	4	4			
L. U. Arm	4	4	4	4	4			
R. L. Arm	3	3	3	3	3			
L. L. Arm	3	3	3	3	3			
R. Hand	2½	2½	2½	2½	2½			
L. Hand	2½	2½	2½	2½	2½			
R. Thigh	5½	6½	8½	8½	9½			
L. Thigh	5½	6½	8½	8½	9½			
R. Leg	5	5	5½	6	7			
L. Leg	5	5	5½	6	7			
R. Foot	3½	3½	3½	3½	3½			
L. Foot	3½	3½	3½	3½	3½			
Total	**Blue areas indicate 2°** **Red areas indicate 3°**			**Total**				

B. Lund and Browder chart

figure 53-2 (**A**) The "rule of nines" method for determining percentage of body area with burn injury. (**B**) Lund and Browder method for determining percentage of body area with burn injury. (Source for part *A:* Anatomical Chart Company: Atlas of Pathophysiology, p 361. Springhouse, PA, Springhouse, 2001.)

box 53-5
Classification of Extent of Burn Injury

Minor burn injury
- Second-degree burn of <15% total body surface area (TBSA) burn in adults or <10% TBSA in children
- Third-degree burn of <2% TBSA not involving special care areas (eyes, ears, face, hands, feet, perineum, joints)
- Excludes all patients with electrical injury, inhalation injury, or concurrent trauma; all poor-risk patients (i.e., extremes of age, intercurrent disease)

Moderate, uncomplicated burn injury
- Second-degree burns of 15%–25% TBSA in adults or 10%–20% in children
- Third-degree burns of <10% TBSA not involving special care areas
- Excludes all patients with electrical injury, inhalation injury, or concurrent trauma; all poor-risk patients (i.e., extremes of age, intercurrent disease)

Major burn injury
- Second-degree burns of >25% TBSA in adults or 20% in children
- All third-degree burns of ≥10% TBSA
- All burns involving eyes, ears, face, hands, feet, perineum, joints
- All patients with inhalation injury, electrical injury, or concurrent trauma; all poor-risk patients

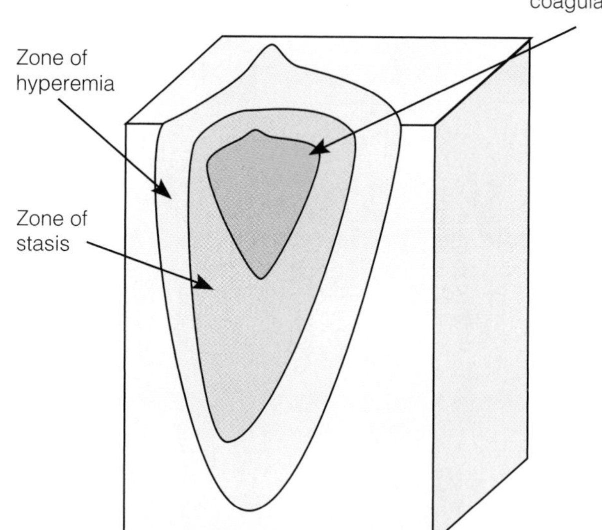

figure 53-3 The concentric zones of a burn injury.

of hypovolemic shock known as *burn shock* (Fig. 53-4). Within minutes of thermal injury, a marked increase in capillary hydrostatic pressure occurs in the injured tissue, accompanied by an increase in capillary permeability. This results in a rapid shift of plasma fluid from the intravascular compartment across heat-damaged capillaries, into interstitial areas (resulting in edema), and to the burn wound itself. The loss of plasma fluid and proteins results in a decreased colloid osmotic pressure in the vascular compartment. As a result, fluid and electrolytes continue to leak from the vascular compartment, resulting in additional edema formation in the burned tissue and throughout the body.

This "leak," which consists of sodium, water, and plasma proteins, is followed by a decrease in cardiac output, hemoconcentration of red blood cells, diminished perfusion to major organs, and generalized body edema. The pathophysiological response after burn injury is biphasic. In the early postinjury (ebb) phase, generalized organ hypofunction develops as a consequence of decreased cardiac output. Peripheral vascular resistance increases as a result of the neurohumoral stress response after trauma. This increases cardiac afterload, resulting in a further decrease in cardiac output. The increase in peripheral vascular resistance (selective vasoconstriction) and the hemoconcentration resulting from plasma fluid loss may cause the blood pressure to appear normal at first. If fluid replacement is inadequate, however, and plasma protein loss continues, hypovolemic shock soon occurs.

In patients receiving adequate fluid resuscitation, the cardiac output usually returns to normal in the latter part of the first 24 hours after burn injury. As plasma volume is replenished during the second 24 hours, the cardiac output increases to hypermetabolic levels (hyperfunction phase) and slowly returns to more normal levels as the burn wounds are closed.[4,5]

In some instances, with burns exceeding 60% of the TBSA, depressed cardiac output does not respond to aggressive volume resuscitation. A myocardial depressant factor capable of depressing ventricular contractility by 60% has been identified. Myocardial depression in the early postburn period may also be the result of reduced coronary blood flow.[5]

The response of the pulmonary vasculature is similar to that of the peripheral circulation. Pulmonary vascular resistance, however, is greater and lasts longer. Immediately after burn injury, the patient may experience a mild, transient pulmonary hypertension. A decrease in oxygen tension and lung compliance may also be evident.

The loss of fluid throughout the body's intravascular space results in a thickened, sluggish flow of the remaining circulatory blood volume. The effects reach all body systems. This slowing of circulation permits bacteria and cellular material to settle in the lower portions of blood vessels, especially in the capillaries, which results in sludging.

The antigen–antibody reaction to burned tissue adds to circulatory congestion by the clumping or agglutination of cells. Coagulation problems occur as a result of the release of thromboplastin by the injury itself and the release of fibrinogen from injured platelets. If thrombi occur, they may cause ischemia of the affected part and lead to necrosis. The increased coagulation process may develop into disseminated intravascular coagulation (DIC).

CONCOMITANT PROBLEMS

Pulmonary Injury

Pulmonary damage usually appears within 24 to 48 hours of the injury and is secondary to the inhalation of combustible products, or it may be the result of inhaled superheated

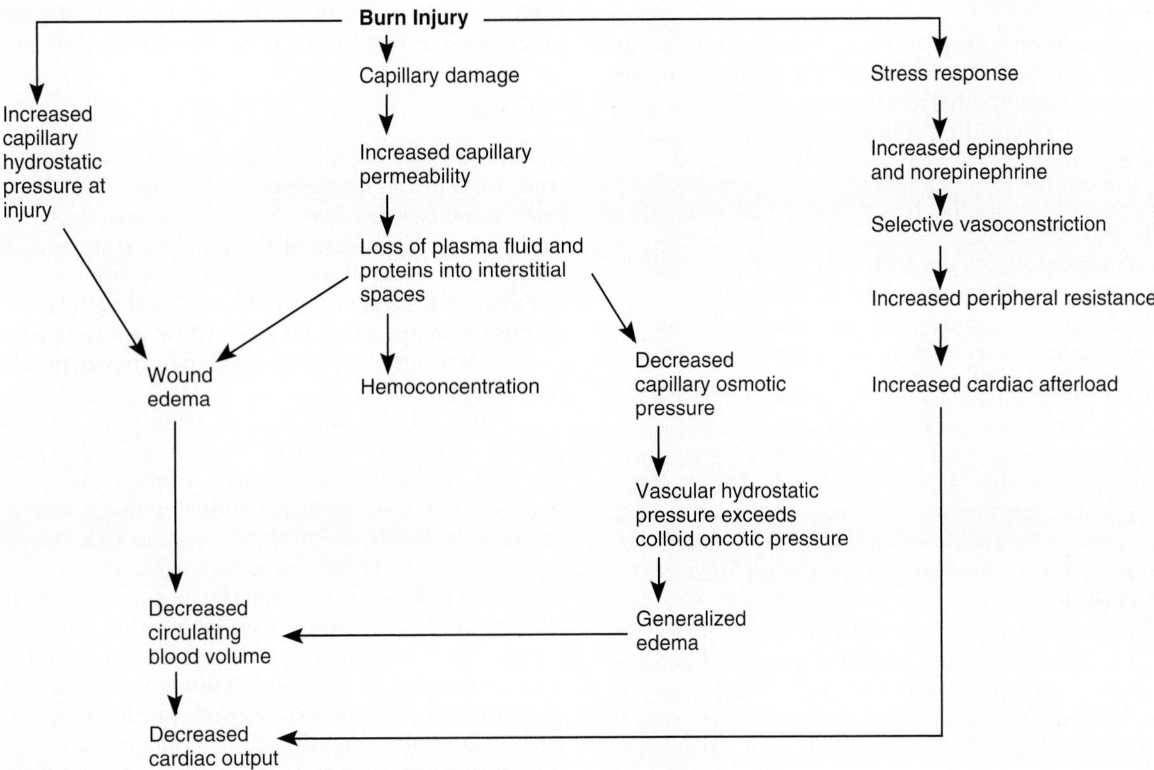

figure 53-4 Fluid shifts in burn shock.

air. Pulmonary injury may also be the result of a systemic process related to SIRS.

CARBON MONOXIDE TOXICITY

Carbon monoxide is a nonirritating, odorless, colorless gas that is formed as a result of incomplete combustion of any carbon fuel. Carbon monoxide is found in a variety of sources, including exhaust from hot water heaters and furnaces, vehicular exhaust fumes, and tobacco smoke. Carbon monoxide poisoning produces its effect on the body by competing with oxygen for uptake by hemoglobin, thereby acting as an asphyxiant. Because hemoglobin has 200 times the affinity for carbon monoxide that it has for oxygen, carbon monoxide readily displaces the oxygen, leading to the formation of carboxyhemoglobin and a reduction in systemic arterial oxygen content. Carboxyhemoglobin shifts the oxyhemoglobin dissociation curve to the left, further decreasing the ability of the red blood cells to release oxygen to body tissues.[6] This may lead to severe anoxia and related brain injury.

The patient with a clear history of exposure to carbon monoxide is usually found in a closed environment in the presence of combusted gases, such as smoke, automobile exhaust, or fumes from a faulty furnace. The signs of carbon monoxide poisoning depend on the amount of carboxyhemoglobin that is present in the patient's blood (Table 53-2).

When carbon monoxide poisoning is suspected, 100% high-flow oxygen is administered. Carbon monoxide has a half-life of 4 hours if the patient breathes room air and 1 hour if the patient is breathing 100% oxygen. Serial arterial blood gas (ABG) measurements are the most accurate way to assess responsiveness to oxygen therapy. It is important to know that pulse oximetry is an inaccurate tool in the presence of an elevated carboxyhemoglobin level.

table 53-2 Signs and Symptoms of Carbon Monoxide Poisoning

Carboxyhemoglobin Saturation (%)	Clinical Presentation
10	No symptoms
20	Headache, vomiting, dyspnea on exertion
30	Confusion, lethargy, changes on electrocardiogram (ECG)
40–60	Coma
More than 60	Death

INHALATION INJURY

Besides carbon monoxide poisoning, smoke inhalation can result in thermal injury to the airway. Pulmonary damage, primarily as a result of inhalation injury, accounts for 20% to 84% of burn mortality. Three stages of injury have been described:

1. Acute pulmonary insufficiency may occur during the first 36 hours.
2. Pulmonary edema occurs in 5% to 30% of burn patients between 6 and 72 hours after injury.
3. Bronchopneumonia appears in 15% to 60% of burn patients 3 to 10 days after injury.

Upper airway injury is the result of inhalation of superheated air, which may cause blisters and edema in the supraglottic area around the vocal cords. This situation may cause airway obstruction and edema. Hoarseness, stridor, dyspnea, carbonaceous sputum, and tachypnea indicate airway compromise, which must be addressed immediately. Early intubation may thwart such disastrous occurrences.

Tracheobronchial and parenchymal lung injuries are usually a result of incomplete combustion of chemicals (e.g., aldehyde, acrolein) and result in a chemical pneumonitis. Inflammatory changes in the trachea and alveoli occur within 24 hours of injury. The pulmonary tree becomes irritated and edematous. The alveoli may collapse, causing a decreased compliance, which leads to atelectasis. ARDS may develop rapidly. Changes may not become apparent, however, until the second 24 hours. Pulmonary edema is a possibility any time from the first few hours to 7 days after the injury. Subtle changes in the patient's sensorium may indicate hypoxia.

History and physical assessment findings that should alert the nurse to the potential for inhalation injury are given in Box 53-6. Serial ABGs show a falling arterial oxygen tension (PaO_2). Usually, the admission chest film appears normal because changes are not reflected until 24 to 48 hours postburn. A sputum specimen is obtained for culture and sensitivity studies. Laryngoscopy and bronchoscopy may be of value in determining the presence of extramucosal carbonaceous material (the most reliable sign of inhalation injury) and the state of the mucosa (blistering, edema, erythema). More specific confirmation of inhalation injury is achieved with the use of fiberoptic bronchoscopy, which permits direct examination of the proximal airway, and xenon-133 scintigraphy (ventilation–perfusion scanning). Xenon-133 scintigraphy is helpful in establishing a diagnosis of injury to small airways and lung parenchyma.

box 53-6 ***History and Physical Examination Findings Suggestive of Inhalation Injury***

- History of incident occurring in a confined area
- Singed nasal hairs
- Burns of the oral or pharyngeal mucous membranes
- Burns in the perioral area or neck
- Carbonaceous sputum
- Change in voice

Infection

There is no greater problem for the burn patient than infection. Loss of the mechanical barrier between the human body and the environment is the first step in the weakening of defenses. All aspects of the immune system, including phagocytosis, soluble mediators of innate immunity such as complement, antibody production, and cellular (T-cell) defense systems, are compromised by severe burn injury. The most common cause of death in burn patients after the first 7 days is infection.

Actions of the health care team can compromise patient survival. All catheters invading the body, including endotracheal tubes, central venous catheters, and bladder catheters, must be handled with as clean a technique as possible. Although the skin and gut are the source of endogenous bacteria, a greater threat to the patient is colonization with antibiotic-resistant pathogens carried by the burn team from other patients. The hands must be washed without fail after handling the patient, the patient's bed, or equipment. When dressings are removed and wounds exposed, sterile gloves must be worn. Compulsive handwashing alone probably prevents infection more than any other single action. Infection control policies vary from burn center to burn center, but the philosophy remains the same: Make every effort to minimize the transmission of bacteria from patient to patient.

Diagnosis of invasive infection in the burn patient is unusually difficult. Most burn patients have elevated core temperatures and white blood cell counts. The significance of these signs becomes blunted in the burn patient. In a patient with burns, a more useful sign of infection is the appearance of sugar in the urine, particularly if this appears paradoxically when the blood sugar level is within normal limits. Hyperglycemia and increased difficulty in controlling the blood sugar in a person with diabetes are signs of threatening sepsis. A drop in the platelet count, particularly in children, is an early warning sign of sepsis. Manifestations of multisystem organ dysfunction (MODS), such as hypotension, hypoxia, decreased pulmonary compliance, renal failure, or hepatic dysfunction, are almost certain signs of septic shock.

Qualitative wound cultures done by swabbing the wound yield no new information other than the nature of the bacterial species colonizing the surface of the wound. On the other hand, a biopsy of the burn wound permits a quantitative assay of the number of colony-forming units (CFU) of bacteria per gram of tissue. Burn wound sepsis is likely if the colony count is greater than 10^5 CFU/g, and the quantitative culture also allows isolation and identification of the invading organism.

Trauma

Concomitant injuries such as fractures and head trauma pose significant risk for the burn patient. Ensuring adequate airway, breathing, and circulation takes precedence over caring for specific injuries. Cervical spine injuries should be stabilized and cleared. If head trauma is suspected, a CT scan is obtained.

MANAGEMENT

The initial assessment of the burn patient is like that of any trauma patient. The American Burn Association has identified criteria for referral to a burn center (Box 53-7). Patients with these burns should be treated in a specialized burn facility after initial assessment and treatment at an emergency department. Whether the patient stays at the initial hospital or is transferred to a burn center facility, the resuscitation phase begins immediately after the burn insult has occurred. The primary and secondary surveys are completed before transfer. Proper stabilization of the patient is crucial for successful transfer. As with any major trauma, the first hour is crucial and the next 24 to 36 hours are also important. The management of fluid balance, nutrition, and the respiratory system are vital and all systems have a major impact on the patient's survival.

Resuscitative Phase

PRIMARY SURVEY

The following parameters are assessed in the primary survey:

- Airway maintenance with cervical spine protection
- Breathing and ventilation
- Circulation with hemorrhage control
- Disability (assess neurological deficit)
- Exposure (completely undress the patient, but maintain temperature)

box 53-7
Criteria for Referral to a Burn Center

- Partial-thickness burns >10% of total body surface area (TBSA)
- Burns that involve the face, hands, feet, genitalia, perineum, or major joints
- Third-degree burns in any age group
- Electrical burns, including lightning injury
- Chemical burns
- Inhalation injury
- Burn injury in patients with pre-existing medical disorders that could complicate management, prolong recovery, or affect mortality
- Concomitant trauma, in which the burn injury poses the greatest risk of morbidity or mortality*
- Children with burns in hospitals without qualified personnel or equipment for the care of children
- Patients with burns who will require special social, emotional, or long-term rehabilitative intervention

*In such cases, if the trauma poses the greater immediate risk, the patient may be initially stabilized in a trauma center before being transferred to a burn unit. Physician judgment is necessary in such situations and should be in concert with the regional medical control plan and triage protocols.

Airway

On initial assessment of the burned patient, the airway must be assessed immediately. The compromised airway may be controlled by a chin lift, jaw thrust, insertion of an oropharyngeal airway in an unconscious patient, or endotracheal intubation. It is crucial not to hyperextend the neck in any suspected cervical spine injuries.

Breathing and Ventilation

Ventilation requires adequate functioning of the lungs, chest wall, and diaphragm. To assess for breathing and ventilation, the nurse must listen to the chest and verify breath sounds in each lung, assess adequacy of rate and depth of respiration, administer high-flow oxygen at 15 L/minute using a nonrebreathing mask, and assess for circumferential full-thickness burns of the chest that may impair ventilation.

Circulation

Assessment of the circulation includes a measurement of blood pressure and heart rate. Intravenous cannulation is performed by inserting two large-bore catheters into the skin that is unburned, if possible. Doppler ultrasonography can be used to assess for pulses. Box 53-8 lists risk factors for impaired circulation.

Disability

Typically, the patient is alert and oriented. If not, associated injuries such as inhalation, head trauma, substance abuse, or pre-existing medical conditions should be considered. The assessment is initiated by determining the patient's level of consciousness using the AVPU (Alert, responds to Verbal stimuli, responds to Painful stimuli, Unresponsive) method.

Exposure

All the patient's clothing and jewelry is removed to complete the primary and secondary survey. After examination, the patient is covered with a dry sheet and warm blankets to prevent evaporative cooling. If possible, intravenous fluids are warmed to 98.6°F (37°C) to 104°F (40°C).

SECONDARY SURVEY

The secondary survey consists of a detailed history and physical examination of the patient as well as a complete history of the accident. Every attempt is made to determine exactly what happened (Box 53-9). A detailed neurological examination is completed and initial radiographic and laboratory studies are done. Resuscitative measures are ongoing and constantly evaluated.

box 53-8 ***Risk Factors for Impaired Circulation***

- Decreased sensation
- Progressive worsening of pain
- Paresthesias
- Decreased capillary refill
- Pallor of extremity

box 53-9
Information Obtained During a Secondary Survey

Thermal Burns

- How did the burn occur?
- Did the burn occur inside or outside?
- Did the clothes catch fire?
- How long did it take to extinguish the fire?
- Were there any explosions?
- Was the patient found in a smoke-filled room?
- How did the patient escape?
- Did the patient jump out of a window?
- Were there other people injured or killed at the scene?
- Was the patient unconscious at the scene?
- Was there a motor vehicle crash?
- Was the car severely damaged?
- Was there a car fire?
- Are the purported circumstances of the injury consistent with the burn characteristics (is there possibility of abuse)?

For Scald Injuries

- How did the burn occur?
- What was the temperature of the liquid?
- What was the liquid; how much liquid was involved?
- What was the burn cooled with?
- Who was present when the burn took place?
- Where did the burn take place? Is there possibility of abuse?

Chemical Burns

- What was the agent?
- How did the exposure occur?
- What was the duration of contact?
- Did contamination take place?

Electrical Burns

- What kind of electricity was involved?
- Did the patient lose consciousness?
- Did the patient fall?
- What was the estimated voltage?
- Was cardiopulmonary resuscitation (CPR) administered at the scene?

A complete history and physical examination is the hallmark of the secondary survey. It is not uncommon for patients to have comorbid diseases. Pre-existing diseases such as diabetes, hypertension, asthma, cancer, and stroke should be documented. A medication list should be obtained from the patient if possible, or a family member should be asked to provide the information. In addition, any allergies, the person's tetanus immunization history, and the time of the person's last meal should be documented. Burn depth and burn size are assessed.

Burn injuries require a global assessment. The following laboratory and diagnostic studies are indicated for burn patients:

- Complete blood count (CBC)
- Comprehensive chemistry panel, including blood urea nitrogen (BUN)
- Creatinine level
- Urinalysis
- ABGs with a carboxyhemoglobin
- Electrocardiogram (ECG)
- Chest radiograph

After the primary and secondary surveys are complete, the burned area is usually covered with a dry sheet. This prevents infection and keeps the patient warm. Ice can be applied to small superficial burns. If the patient has an electrical burn, continuous cardiac monitoring is provided. If the patient has a chemical burn, the area is immediately flushed with large amounts of water to remove the chemical, and all contaminated clothing is removed and bagged. If the patient is going to be transferred to a burn center, initiation of fluid resuscitation, insertion of a nasogastric tube, and insertion of a Foley catheter may be carried out during the secondary assessment.

Reparative Phase

Once the patient is stabilized, measures are taken to promote healing and prevent infection. As noted earlier, burn wounds can have profound effects on nearly every organ system. Box 53-10 lists nursing diagnoses for burn patients,

box 53-10 ***Examples of Nursing Diagnoses and Collaborative Problems for the Burn Patient***

- Ineffective Airway Clearance related to impaired cough, oropharyngeal and tracheal swelling, or artificial airway
- Impaired Gas Exchange related to inhalation injury, atelectasis, acute respiratory distress syndrome, or carbon monoxide poisoning
- Ineffective Breathing Pattern related to circumferential chest burn, upper airway obstruction, or acute respiratory distress syndrome
- Impaired Peripheral Tissue Perfusion related to edema or circumferential burn
- Deficient Fluid Volume related to altered capillary permeability, insensible and third spacing losses
- Risk for Fluid Volume Excess related to fluid resuscitation and subsequent fluid mobilization 3 to 5 days postburn
- Impaired Skin Integrity related to burn injury or surgical interventions
- Hypothermia related to impaired integument
- Imbalanced Nutrition: Less than Body Requirements related to hypermetabolic response to burn injury, paralytic ileus
- Impaired Urinary Elimination related to indwelling urinary catheter
- Risk for Infection related to loss of integument, invasive procedures, and immunocompromise
- Pain related to exposure of nerve endings, invasive procedures, surgical procedures, and dressing changes
- Ineffective Individual and Family Coping related to altered body image and fear
- Anxiety related to traumatic injury, fear of dying, fear of disfigurement, change in body image, and change in role relationships

and Box 53-11 contains a collaborative care guide for the patient with burns.

PROVIDING HEMODYNAMIC SUPPORT

Therapy for burn shock is aimed at supporting the patient through the period of hypovolemic shock until capillary integrity is restored. Fluid resuscitation is the primary intervention in the resuscitative phase in the intensive care unit (ICU). Goals in fluid resuscitation are as follows:

- Correct fluid, electrolyte, and protein deficits.
- Replace continuing losses, and maintain fluid balance.
- Prevent excessive edema formation.
- Maintain a urine output in adults of 30 to 70 mL/hour.

Formulas for Fluid Administration

Numerous formulas have been developed for fluid resuscitation (Box 53-12). Each has advantages and disadvantages. They differ primarily in terms of recommended volume administration and salt content. In general, lost crystalloid and colloid solutions must be replaced rigorously. Free water, given as 5% dextrose in water (D_5W) with or without added electrolytes, is regulated so that insensible fluid loss is covered. Lactated Ringer's solution is used as the crystalloid solution because it is a balanced salt solution, which closely approximates the composition of extracellular fluid (ECF).

The Baxter (Parkland) formula is the most commonly used resuscitation regimen in the United States. This formula requires 4 mL of lactated Ringer's solution per kilogram of body weight per percentage TBSA burn. This amount is administered in the first 24 hours postinjury. One-half is given in the first 8 hours postinjury, and the remainder is administered over the subsequent 16 hours postinjury. The Baxter formula and other fluid resuscitation formulas are guidelines, and individual patients may require more or less than 4 mL/kg per percentage TBSA during the first 24 hours.

Other formulas contain various amounts of hypertonic saline or colloid. Hypertonic saline resuscitation lowers the amount of fluid that needs to be given to selected patients; however, it can cause severe hypernatremia and must be used cautiously. The argument against colloid administration within 12 hours of injury is that during this time, the diffuse postburn capillary leak allows colloids to extravasate through endothelial junctions. Therefore, colloid administration does not produce any demonstrable oncotic benefit over administration of a crystalloid while the capillary leak is present. The time postinjury at which capillary integrity is restored varies among individuals, but usually is between 12 and 14 hours. Many physicians administer colloids at this point to restore albumin levels to 2.0 to 3.0 mg/dL. Controversy exists over the type of colloid to be administered, with some centers using salt-poor albumin and others using fresh frozen plasma.

Nonprotein collagens may be used in burn shock resuscitation. Dextran and hetastarch are high–molecular-weight solutions that generate colloid osmotic pressure when given intravascularly. Allergic responses have been reported with dextran, but the risk virtually is eliminated by pretreatment with Promit, a very low–molecular-weight dextran.

Care must be taken to avoid fluid overload and pulmonary edema. This is often difficult because large amounts of fluids are given over a short period during fluid resuscitation immediately after the burn. For example, according to the Baxter formula, a patient weighing 75 kg who received burns over 50% of his body would require 15,000 mL of fluid (4 mL × 75 kg × 50% = 15,000 mL). Of this, 7500 mL is to be administered during the first 8 hours, and 3750 mL is to be administered in the second and third 8-hour periods. It is extremely difficult to avoid fluid overload and pulmonary edema when it is necessary to infuse large amounts of fluids so rapidly.

After the first 24 hours postinjury, replacing the massive evaporative water loss is a major consideration in fluid management. The primary solution given at this time is D_5W, with the goal of keeping the patient's sodium concentration at 140 mEq/L. The fluid volume depends on the severity of injury, the age of the patient, the physiological status of the patient, and any associated injuries. Consequently, the volume recommended by a resuscitation formula must be modified according to the individual's response to therapy (Fig. 53-5).

Urine output is the single best indicator of fluid resuscitation in patients with previously normal renal function. The onset of spontaneous diuresis is a hallmark indicating the end of the resuscitative phase. Infusion rates can be decreased by 25% for 1 hour if the urine output is satisfactory and can be maintained for 2 hours; the reduction may then be repeated. It is essential that urinary outputs be maintained within normal limits (30 to 50 mL/hour). Other indications of adequate fluid replacement are listed in Box 53-13.

Patients are usually weighed daily. A gain of 15% of admission weight may be expected. Intake and output must be monitored meticulously. Patients who sustain deep muscle injury (i.e., second- or third-degree burns) are at risk for development of acute renal insufficiency. This renal dysfunction may be the result of inadequate fluid resuscitation or it may be the consequence of the liberation of the myoglobin and hemoglobin from damaged cells. These compounds, sometimes called *hemochromogens*, may precipitate in renal tubules, resulting in acute tubular necrosis (ATN). Hemochromogens produce a clear reddish-brown color in the urine. Should hemochromogens appear in the urine, acidosis should be corrected promptly and intravenous fluids increased to maintain a brisk urine output until the urine returns to its normal clear yellow and there is no urinary myoglobin.

PROVIDING PULMONARY SUPPORT

Inhalation injury is the leading cause of death in the first 24 hours after burn injury, and increases the mortality rate by 20% to 60% when combined with pneumonia.[7] Goals for the successful treatment of inhalation injury include improving oxygenation and decreasing interstitial edema and airway occlusion.

The conventional treatment for inhalation injury is largely supportive. Humidified oxygen is administered to prevent drying and sloughing of the mucosa. Upper airway edema peaks at 24 to 48 hours after injury. If the

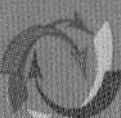

box 53-11 collaborative care guide *for the Patient With a Burn*

OUTCOMES	INTERVENTIONS
Oxygenation/Ventilation	
Patent airway is maintained. Lung is clear on auscultation.	■ Auscultate breath sounds q2–4h and PRN. ■ Assess for inhalation injury, and anticipate intubation. ■ Assess quantity and color of tracheal secretions. ■ Suction endotracheal airway when appropriate (see Collaborative Care Guide for Patient on Ventilator). ■ Hyperoxygenate and hyperventilate before and after each suction pass.
Peak, mean, and plateau pressures are within normal limits for a patient on a ventilator.	■ Monitor airway pressures q1–2 h. ■ Monitor lung compliance q8h (see Chapter 24). ■ Administer bronchodilators and mucolytics. ■ Perform chest physiotherapy q4h. ■ Monitor airway pressures and lung compliance for improvement after interventions.
There is no evidence of atelectasis or infiltrates.	■ Turn side to side q2h. ■ Consider kinetic therapy or prone positioning. ■ Take daily chest x-ray.
Arterial blood gases are within normal limits.	■ Monitor carboxyhemoglobin and carbon monoxide levels. ■ Monitor arterial blood gases using cooximeter analysis of arterial saturation. (Pulse oximeter and calculated Sa_{O_2} are inaccurate measures in the presence of carbon monoxide.) ■ Provide humidified oxygen. ■ Consider hyperbaric therapy.
Circulation/Perfusion	
Blood pressure, heart rate, central venous pressure (CVP), and pulmonary artery pressures are within normal limits.	■ Assess vital signs q1h. ■ Assess hemodynamic pressures q1h if patient has pulmonary artery (PA) catheter. ■ Administer intravascular volume as ordered to maintain preload (see below).
Temperature is within normal limits.	■ Monitor temperature q1h. ■ Maintain a warm environment, and use warming lights or blankets to prevent hypothermia. ■ Treat fever with antipyretics and cooling blankets.
Perfusion to extremities is maintained; pulses are intact.	■ Monitor perfusion using pulse oximetry, Doppler, palpation q1h. ■ Elevate burned extremities. ■ Prepare for escharotomy or fasciotomy.
Fluids/Electrolytes	
Restore and maintain fluid balance: Urine output 30–70 mL/h or 0.5 mL/kg. CVP, 8–12 mm Hg; pulmonary artery wedge pressure (PAWP), 12–18 mm Hg; blood pressure, within normal limits; heart rate, <120 bpm.	■ Assess intake and output q1h. ■ Give lactated Ringer's 4 mL/kg/% burn, divided into first 24 h postburn. ■ Monitor for spontaneous diuresis, and reduce IV infusion rate as indicated. ■ Take daily weight.
Electrolytes, mineral, and renal function values are within normal limits.	■ Monitor and replace minerals and electrolytes. ■ Monitor BUN, creatinine, myoglobin, and urine electrolytes and glucose. ■ Monitor neurological status. ■ Monitor and treat dysrhythmias.

(continued)

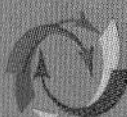

box 53-11 collaborative care guide *for the Patient With a Burn (Continued)*

OUTCOMES	INTERVENTIONS
Mobility/Safety	
Patient is free of joint contractures.	■ Provide passive and active range-of-motion exercises q1–2h. ■ Apply positioning splints as needed.
There is no evidence of complications related to immobility.	■ Turn and reposition q2h. ■ Consider kinetic therapy.
There is no evidence of infection.	■ Consider deep venous thrombosis (DVT) prophylaxis. ■ Maintain strict sterile technique, and monitor technique of others. ■ Maintain sterility of invasive catheters and tubes. ■ Per hospital protocol, change dressings and invasive catheters. Culture wounds, blood, urine, as necessary. ■ Monitor systemic inflammatory response syndrome criteria: increased white blood cell (WBC) count, increased temperature, tachypnea, tachycardia.
Skin Integrity	
Unburned skin will remain intact.	■ Assess skin q4h and each time patient is repositioned. ■ Turn q2h. ■ Consider pressure relief/reduction mattress.
Burns begin healing without complications.	■ Treat burns per hospital protocol; apply topical medications and debride as indicated. ■ Monitor skin graft viability. ■ Protect grafted areas (e.g., bed cradle, dressings). ■ Consider air fluidized bed to enhance healing and relieve pressure from burned surface.
Nutrition	
Caloric and nutrient intake meets metabolic requirements per calculation (e.g., Basal Energy Expenditure).	■ Provide parenteral or enteral nutrition within 24 h of injury. ■ Consult dietitian or nutritional support service to assess nutritional requirements with team. ■ Monitor protein and calorie intake. ■ Monitor albumin, prealbumin, transferrin, cholesterol, triglycerides, glucose.
Comfort/Pain Control	
Patient will have minimal pain, <5 on pain scale, and discomfort.	■ Assess pain and discomfort using objective pain scale q4h, PRN, and following administration of pain medication. ■ Administer analgesics prior to procedures, and monitor patient response. ■ Use nonpharmacological pain management techniques (e.g., music, distraction, touch).
Psychosocial	
Patient demonstrates decreased anxiety.	■ Assess vital signs during treatments, discussions, and so forth. ■ Administer sedatives before treatments/procedures. ■ Consult social services, clergy, and so forth as appropriate. ■ Provide for adequate rest and sleep. ■ Encourage discussion regarding long-term effects of burns, available resources, and coping strategies.

(continued)

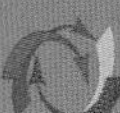

box 53-11 collaborative care guide *for the Patient With a Burn (Continued)*

OUTCOMES	INTERVENTIONS
Teaching/Discharge Planning	
Patient/significant others understand procedures and tests needed for treatment.	■ Prepare patient/significant others for procedures, such as debridement, escharotomy, fasciotomy, intubation, and mechanical ventilation.
Significant others understand the severity of the illness, ask appropriate questions, anticipate potential complications.	■ Explain the potential effects of burns and the potential for complications, such as infection, respiratory or renal failure. ■ Encourage significant others to ask questions related to the management of burns, disfigurement, coping, and so forth.

injury is mild or moderately severe, placing the patient in a high Fowler's position and administering aerosolized racemic epinephrine may be sufficient to limit further edema formation. Severe upper airway obstruction may require endotracheal intubation to protect the airway until the edema subsides.

In patients with mild tracheobronchial injury, atelectasis may be prevented by frequent pulmonary toilet, including a high Fowler's position, coughing and deep breathing, chest physiotherapy, repositioning, frequent tracheal suctioning, and incentive spirometry. Patients with more severe inhalation injury require more frequent suctioning and, possibly, bronchoscopic removal of debris. These patients usually require endotracheal intubation and mechanical ventilatory support. The objective of ventilatory support is to provide adequate gas exchange at the lowest possible inspired oxygen concentration and airway pressure, in an attempt to reduce the incidence of oxygen toxicity and pulmonary barotrauma. Recent studies[7,8] support the use of volumetric diffusive respiration (VDR), which appears to offer advantages over conventional mechanical ventilation. In VDR, subtidal volume breaths accumulate and build to a set airway pressure, which is then followed by passive exhalation. During inspiration, high-frequency pulsations of air are continuously administered to the patient. This method of inspiration seems to aid in ventilation and recruitment of partially obstructed alveoli.

Patients with bronchospasm are treated with aerosolized or intravenously administered bronchodilators. Respiratory parameters are monitored closely and constant attention is

box 53-12
Fluid Resuscitation Formulas

Baxter (Parkland) Formula

- **First 24 hours:** Lactated Ringer's solution (4 mL/kg/%TBSA); half given over first 8 hours, remaining half given over next 16 hours
- **Second 24 hours:** Dextrose in water, plus potassium- and colloid-containing fluid (0.3–0.5 mL/kg/%TBSA)

Brooke Formula

- **First 24 hours:** Lactated Ringer's solution (1.5 mL/kg/%TBSA) plus colloid solution (0.5 mL/kg/%TBSA); half given over first 8 hours, remaining half given over next 16 hours
- **Second 24 hours:** Lactated Ringer's solution (0.5–0.75 mL/kg/%TBSA), plus 5% dextrose in water (2 L)

Modified Brooke Formula

- **First 24 hours:** Lactated Ringer's solution (2 mL/kg/%TBSA); half given over first 8 hours, remaining half given over next 16 hours
- **Second 24 hours:** Colloid solution (0.3–0.5 mL/kg/%TBSA), plus 5% dextrose in water to maintain adequate urine output

Consensus Formula

- **First 24 hours:** Lactated Ringer's solution (2–4 mL/kg/%TBSA in adults; 3–4 mL/kg/%TBSA in children); half given over first 8 hours, remaining half given over next 16 hours
- **Second 24 hours:** Colloid-containing fluid (0.3–0.5 mL/kg/%TBSA), plus electrolyte-free fluid (in adults) or half-normal saline (in children) to maintain adequate urine output

Dextran Formula

- **First 8 hours:** Dextran 40 in saline (2 mL/kg/h), plus lactated Ringer's solution infused to maintain urine output at 30 mL/h
- **Second 8 hours:** Fresh frozen plasma (0.5 mL/kg/h) for 18 hours, plus additional crystalloid to maintain adequate urine output

Evans Formula

- **First 24 hours:** 0.9% normal saline (1 mL/kg/%TBSA), plus colloid solution (1 mL/kg/%TBSA); half given over first 8 hours, remaining half given over next 16 hours
- **Second 24 hours:** 0.9% normal saline (0.5 mL/kg/%TBSA), plus 5% dextrose in water (2 L)

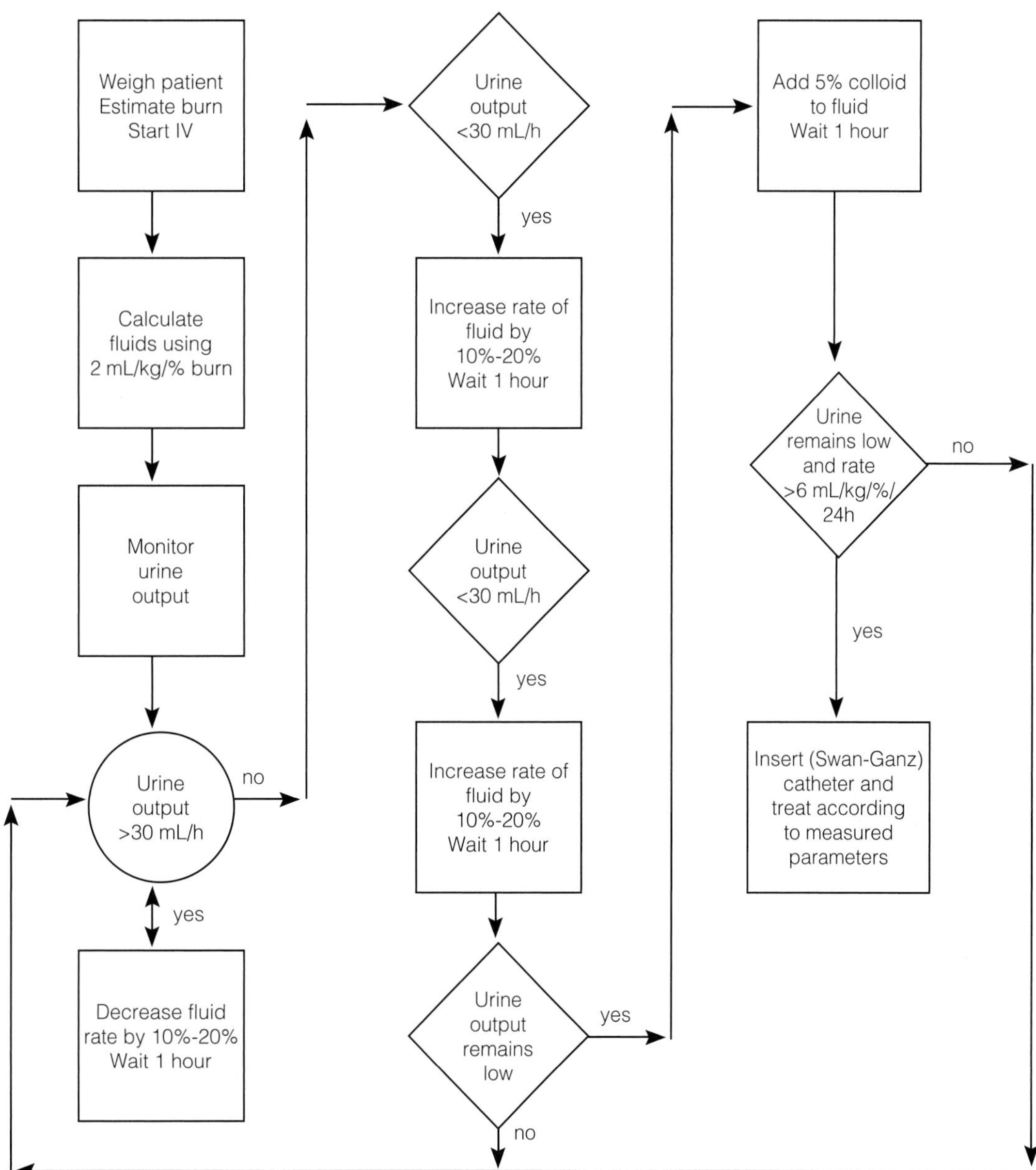

figure 53-5 Initial 24-hour fluid management. (From Rue LW, Cioffi WG: Resuscitation of thermally injured patients. Crit Care Nurs Clin North Am 3[2]:186, 1991.)

box 53-13
Indications of Adequate Fluid Replacement*

Blood pressure	Normal to high ranges
Pulse rate	<120
Central venous pressure (CVP)	<12 cm H_2O
Pulmonary artery wedge pressure (PAWP)	<18 mmHg
Urinary output	30–70 mL/h
Lungs	Clear
Sensorium	Clear
GI tract	Absence of nausea and adynamic ileus

*Central lines and Swan-Ganz catheters are not inserted routinely because of the danger of sepsis; however, they are used in selected instances.

paid to breath sounds and vital signs to detect fluid overload as early as possible.

Bronchopneumonia may be superimposed on other respiratory problems at any time and may be hematogenous or airborne. Airborne bronchopneumonia is most common, with an onset occurring soon after injury. It is often associated with a lower airway injury or aspiration. Hematogenous, or miliary, pneumonia begins as a bacterial abscess secondary to another septic source, usually the burn wound. The time of onset usually is 2 weeks after injury.

Prophylactic antibiotics and steroids have not been demonstrated to prevent the common complications of infection encountered in patients with inhalation injury. New methods to decrease the incidence of nosocomial pneumonia in critically ill patients that are currently under investigation include selective decontamination of the orodigestive tract.

ENSURING OPTIMAL NUTRITION

Before the unique nutritional needs of burn patients were fully recognized in the late 1970s, those with severe burn injuries who survived languished in a hospital ward with minimal oral intake until they became severely cachectic. It is currently clear that appropriate nutrition plays a significant role in improving outcome for people with severe burn injuries.

Although early parenteral feeding has been associated with increased mortality because of an increase in the risk of infections, early enteral feeding has been proposed because it may reduce the translocation of bacteria from the intestinal lumen. Passage of bacteria from the gut into the intestinal lymphatics or portal venous system probably occurs in all healthy individuals. However, the intestinal edema that accompanies the burn resuscitation period and the immunosuppression that follows makes it difficult for the body to clear these microorganisms effectively. Microbial products—either live organisms or cell wall fragments—disseminate through the body, prompting the release of cytokines such as TNF, interleukin-1 (IL-1), and IL-6. These cytokines exacerbate the hypermetabolic response and may initiate SIRS.

The rationale for enteral feeding within the first 24 hours of injury is that the presence of food in the gut lumen reduces the rate of microbial translocation. Although not proven definitively in the clinical setting of burn patients, safety and simplicity of early feeding have been demonstrated. One approach is to slowly infuse tube feedings through the nasogastric tube at a rate of 10 to 20 mL/hour. Although this clearly does not meet the nutritional needs of adult patients, it is enough to protect the gut mucosa. Long feeding tubes can be placed into the small bowel using endoscopy or fluoroscopy. The advantages of such tubes are higher and earlier rates of infusion, and continuous feeding of patients during surgical procedures requiring general anesthesia.

Despite the theoretical advantages of enteral feeding, difficulties exist. Patients receive, on average, only 80% of the goal rate for enteral feedings because of frequent interruptions for patient care, including radiological procedures and surgery. This deficit increases when patients develop intestinal ileus, as typically occurs with major infection. Osmotic diarrhea is troublesome, particularly when the patient's feces soil the burn dressings. A variety of techniques combat diarrhea, including replacement of intestinal flora with lactobacillus granules and nonpasteurized yogurt, and retardation of small bowel motility with diphenoxylate hydrochloride. Despite the theoretical advantages and need for the calories provided by enteral feeding, difficulties exist, and the technique cannot be used in all patients.

The estimated caloric and protein needs of a patient may be met more reliably with parenteral than enteral feeding. The central venous catheter, which predisposes the patient to invasive infections (particularly *Candida* species infections), is a disadvantage. Reports suggest the rate of bacterial translocation is increased with the use of parenteral nutrition compared with enteral nutrition, and that infection rates are higher. Long-term use of parenteral nutrition alone is associated with hepatobiliary dysfunction, including cholestatic hepatitis and acalculous cholecystitis. Nevertheless, parenteral nutrition can be used for patients who do not tolerate enteral feedings because of paralytic ileus of the intestine or diarrhea, and for patients returned to the operating room frequently for serial escharotomies.

Burn injury results in an increase in the metabolic expenditure. Initial investigative work performed in the 1970s demonstrated that some burn patients needed as many as 7000 or 8000 kcal/day to maintain weight. Although burn patients still become hypercatabolic after injury, they do not become so to the same degree because of changes in management. Because of the effect of earlier enteral feeding and the introduction of procedures that promote early wound closure, the increase in metabolic rate has diminished. Recently, indirect calorimetry has shown that the most severe injuries require no more calories than twice the resting energy expenditure as described in the Harrison-Benedict formula. The resting energy expenditure calculated by the Harrison-Benedict formula is multiplied by a stress factor in direct proportion to the size of the burn (Box 53-14). The stress factor is judged conservatively to avoid overfeeding, which is associated with increased susceptibility to infection. Studies suggest that although indirect calorimetry prevents gross underestimation or overestimation of the patient's caloric needs, in most patients it is probably not superior to estimating their needs from a formula (such as the Harrison-Benedict formula) alone.

Wound repair depends on amino acids, which are the building blocks of proteins. The type of amino acids used in enteral feedings varies. The amino acids arginine and glutamine have immune-enhancing properties, improve nitrogen retention, and maintain lean body mass. Formulas containing arginine supplements have been reported to reduce infections in trauma patients and to reduce length of stay of critically ill patients.

box 53-14
Stress Factors for Energy Expenditure Related to Burn Size (Harrison-Benedict Equations)

Women: REE = 655 + [4.3 × Wt (lb)] + [4.3 × Ht (in)] – [4.7 × age]

Men: REE = 65 + [6.2 × Wt (lb)] + [12.7 × Ht (in)] – [6.8 × age]

TBSA	STRESS FACTOR
0–10%	1.4
11–20%	1.5
21–30%	1.6
31–40%	1.7
41–50%	1.8
51–60%	1.9
>60%	2.0

REE, resting energy expenditure.

Judging the amount of protein necessary for recovery from burn injuries is difficult. Massive and unquantified loss of protein from the burn wound exudates precludes nitrogen balance studies based on urine excretion alone. Sequential measurements of serum proteins such as transferrin and prealbumin are a better index of the body's response to the amount and type of dietary protein given; however, few clinical studies show a correlation between an increase in serum proteins and improved clinical outcome. It is important to avoid overfeeding of protein because it predisposes patients to sepsis. Amounts of protein greater than 3 g/kg/day in adults are usually not tolerated because of azotemia. Dietary protein should be started at an administration rate of 1.2 g/kg/day and should be increased if there is not a subsequent increase in serum protein markers. A patient's diet can also be supplemented with vitamins A and C, and with the trace element zinc, all of which improve wound healing.

Successful weaning of patients from nutritional supplements sometimes occurs earlier than expected. A regular diet with liquid supplements is offered within 24 hours of extubation. The increased thirst of burn patients is used to encourage the intake of protein-containing solutions, either soy- or milk-based supplements, or protein-containing fruit drinks. Using supplements, patients can take up to 2000 kcal each day. It is preferable to feed patients or allow them to feed themselves because of the inherent risks of feeding tubes and central lines.

PROVIDING MUSCULOSKELETAL SUPPORT

Physical and occupational therapy begins on day one of a burn injury. Independent of the patient's general condition, injured upper and lower extremities can be elevated to allow adequate venous drainage and reduce edema. Passive exercises are initiated and, if alert and cooperative, the patient should participate in these exercises. Active and passive exercises to maintain joint range of motion are continued throughout hospitalization and the outpatient rehabilitation period.

Two important axioms influence rehabilitation. First, the burn wound will shorten by contraction until it meets an opposing force. Across a flexor surface, this results in a contracture. Second, the position of comfort is the position of contracture. Range-of-motion exercises prevent tendon shortening and restriction of joint motion by burn scar contractures. As patients begin to recover and participate actively in therapy, exercises are designed to increase muscle strength and endurance. A return to activities of daily living frequently takes months.

An unfortunate consequence of contractures and immobility is heterotopic ossification. Heterotopic ossification develops when there is an abnormal deposition of calcium phosphate crystals in joint spaces or along tendons. Heterotopic ossification restricts the motion of joints, particularly in elbows and knees. Unlike the heterotopic ossification seen in patients with spinal cord injuries, the heterotopic ossification seen in patients with burns does not respond to treatment with etidronate disodium, and early surgical removal is not indicated. Resolution occurs with time in most patients, and few need surgical removal of the ossified crystals in the joints.

MANAGING PAIN

The pain associated with burns is managed aggressively. All narcotics are given intravenously because malabsorption of the drug may occur if given intramuscularly. Patients are given anxiolytics for anxiety related to appearance, procedures, and fear. Patient-controlled analgesia (PCA) is ideal for patients who are awake and sufficiently oriented to use the pump. PCA pumps can provide a continuous pain medication, with a "dose" available every 6 to 8 minutes for intermittent pain. The nurse can give the patient a "bolus" dose for procedures such as dressing changes and physical therapy. Recommended narcotics include morphine, fentanyl, and hydromorphone.

CARE OF THE WOUND

Cleansing

All burn center and hospital wound protocols vary, but the most common wound cleansing involves water and chlorhexidine or saline and povidone-iodine (Betadine). Wounds are cleansed at each dressing change and are observed for signs of infection and rate of healing.

Some centers immerse patients in a Hubbard tank to loosen exudates, clean and assess the wound, and provide range-of-motion exercises. Bath solutions vary, and may contain salt, povidone-iodine solutions, and bleaches. Because baths are usually painful, patients should receive an analgesic 20 to 30 minutes before the bath. In addition, the patient should receive a complete explanation of, and assistance with, pain-controlling techniques (e.g., imagery). Additional support should be offered by providing ongoing explanations of what is to be done and why, and by permitting the patient to participate in care as much as possible. Limiting the time the procedure takes is important to the patient's pain tolerance and temperature control. Hydrotherapy should be limited to 20 minutes to prevent extreme chilling, which increases metabolic demand.

Care must be taken to avoid cross-contamination of wounds during bathing procedures. For this reason, many centers no longer immerse patients in Hubbard tanks. Portable shower trolleys can provide hydrotherapy without the risk of contamination. Clean or healing wounds should be cleaned separately from contaminated ones.

Application of Topical Antimicrobial Agents

The choice of topical antimicrobial agents depends on the wound depth, location, and condition, and on the presence of specific organisms. Common antimicrobial agents used from time of admission to a burn unit include 0.5% silver nitrate, mafenide acetate (Sulfamylon), nitrofurazone, povidone-iodine, silver sulfadiazine, gentamycin, and nystatin (Table 53-3). No single agent is totally effective against all burn wound infections. Treatment is guided by in vitro testing or in vivo results. Eschar and granulating wound surfaces may be biopsied three times weekly to identify contaminating organisms and determine antibiotic sensitivity.

Silver sulfadiazine is the primary topical agent of choice on admission. The most common adverse reaction is leukopenia; therefore, serial CBCs must be monitored. If the white blood count falls below 3000 cells/mm^3, the physician will probably change to another topical agent. When

table 53-3 Agents for Burn Wound Management

Agent	Advantages	Disadvantages	Nursing Considerations
Mafenide acetate	Broad-spectrum, penetrates eschar	Painful application, acid–base imbalances	Apply twice a day, leave open to air
Silver nitrate	Painless application, broad-spectrum, rare sensitivity	No eschar penetration, discolors wound and environmental surfaces, must be kept moist	Wet-to-wet dressing with non-adhering layer, followed by a gauze layer every 24 h
Silver sulfadiazene	Painless application, broad-spectrum, easy application	May cause transient leukopenia, minimal eschar penetration	Apply a moderate layer and wrap in a gauze dressing every 12 h
Bacitracin	Painless application, nonirritating	No eschar penetration, antimicrobial spectrum not as wide as above agents	Apply a thin layer and nonadhering dressing; if used on face, leave open to air
Mupirocin	Antimicrobial spectrum broader than bacitracin	Expensive	Apply a thin layer and nonadhering dressing; if used on face, leave open to air
Neomycin	Painless application	Antimicrobial spectrum not as wide as above agents	Apply a thin layer and nonadhering dressing; if used on face, leave open to air

the leukocyte count returns to normal (4000 to 5000 cells/mm^3), silver sulfadiazine therapy may be reinstituted.

If the colony counts increase, the topical agent of choice is usually mafenide acetate cream, an effective broad-spectrum bacteriostatic agent. Mafenide acetate diffuses through third-degree eschar to the burn wound margin within 3 hours of application. It inhibits carbonic anhydrase, resulting in metabolic acidosis. This acidosis initially is compensated for by hyperventilation. Oral administration of sodium citrate dihydrate (Bicitra) or intravenous sodium bicarbonate usually corrects this acid–base imbalance.

The application of topical antimicrobial agents inhibits the rate of wound epithelialization and may increase the metabolic rate. Electrolyte imbalances (e.g., sodium leaching by silver nitrate) and acid–base abnormalities may occur. The best topical agents are water soluble because they do not hold in heat and macerate the wound. With the application of any topical agent, it is important to use sterile technique.

Debridement

Eschar covers the burn wound until it is excised or has separated spontaneously. In theory, burn wound management is simple. It calls for debridement of the eschar and skin graft closure before the eschar becomes infected. However, the sometimes serious systemic complications of burn injury, such as hypovolemia and sepsis, may delay this course of action significantly.

Mechanical Debridement. Mechanical debridement may be accomplished using forceps and scissors to gently lift and trim loose necrotic tissue. Another form of mechanical debridement is dressing the wound with coarse gauze in the form of wet-to-dry or wet-to-wet dressings. Wet-to-dry dressings consist of layers of moistened coarse mesh gauze. As the inner layer dries, it adheres to the wound, entrapping exudate and wound debris. The dressing should be removed at a 90-degree angle, and every effort should be made to avoid damaging fragile, newly granulating tissue. As the wound forms increasing amounts of granulation tissue, wet-to-wet dressings may be used to prevent desiccation and trauma. These dressings remain moist until the next dressing change. The dressing should be removed by first gently lifting from the edges toward the center of the wound, and then removing the dressing at a 180-degree angle. This procedure prevents detachment of newly formed epithelial tissue.

Enzymatic Debridement. Enzymatic debridement involves the application of a proteolytic substance to burn wounds to shorten the time of eschar separation. Travase and Elase are the most commonly used agents. The wound is first cleaned and debrided of any loose necrotic material. The agent is then applied directly to the wound bed and covered with a layer of fine-mesh gauze. A topical antimicrobial agent is applied next, and the entire area is covered with saline-soaked gauze. The dressing is changed two to four times per day.

Enzymatic debridement has the advantage of eliminating the need for surgical excision; however, certain complications must be considered. Hypovolemia may occur as a result of excessive fluid loss through the wound. Hence, no more than 20% TBSA should be treated in this manner. Cellulitis and maceration of normal skin may occur around the wound periphery, and patients often complain of a burning sensation lasting 30 to 60 minutes after enzyme application.

Surgical Debridement. In surgical excision, the wound is excised to viable bleeding points while minimizing the loss of viable tissue. Early excision has contributed significantly to the survival of people with major burns. The open burn causes hypermetabolism and a stress response that is not corrected until wound closure occurs. Surgical excision should be done as soon as the patient is hemodynamically stable, usually within 72 hours.

After excision is complete, hemostasis must be achieved. This may be accomplished by topical thrombin sprayed on the wound or application sponges soaked in a 1:10,000 epinephrine solution. After removal of necrotic tissue, the exposed underlying structures must be dressed with a temporary or permanent covering to provide protection and prevent infection.

Grafts

The ideal substitute for lost skin is an autograft of similar color, texture, and thickness from a close location on the body. Sheets of the patient's epidermis and a partial layer of the dermis are harvested from unburned locations using a dermatome. These grafts, referred to as *split-thickness grafts*, can be applied to the wound as a sheet grafts or mesh grafts. In a sheet graft, the harvested skin is applied to the surgically excised area. It is usually covered with a petroleum-based gauze dressing. The graft must be inspected frequently for collections of fluid under the graft. Fluid accumulation is prevented by rolling a cotton-tipped applicator over the graft to express any trapped fluid. Over exposed areas, such as the face and hands, sheet grafts give a more natural appearance than do mesh grafts.

In a mesh graft, the harvested skin is slit and then the graft is placed on the burn site. The slits (or interstices) allow the skin to expand, providing for greater coverage and drainage and facilitating draping over uneven surfaces. Mesh grafts frequently have to be expanded to get maximum coverage from each piece of autograft. An expansion ratio of 1:3 or 1:4 is often practical. Sometimes ratios such as 1:6 or 1:7 are used to cover large burns. With these larger ratios, the expanded autograft is covered with either cadaver skin allografts or synthetic skin (Biobrane; Winthrop Pharmaceuticals). In addition to physically stabilizing the fragile mesh, the cover decreases evaporation, heat loss, and bacterial contamination.

Dressings are used after surgery to immobilize the grafted area and prevent shearing and dislodging of the graft. Postoperative dressings also provide a degree of compression to minimize hematoma and seroma formation, but may be a source of vascular compression in the extremities. Pulse checks distal to the dressings are documented every 4 hours for 24 hours after surgery. The dressings are usually left in place until the third postoperative day. Until that time, the dressings are moistened every 6 hours with a solution containing normal saline and polymyxin. The antibiotic solution keeps the fragile meshed grafts moist and protects against infection. On postoperative day 3, the dressings are removed and evaluated by the physician, who determines the success of the grafting. This is expressed in terms of percentages. The grafted area is then covered with a nonadherent dressing and a gauze layer, which are secured with a gauze roll. All components of the dressing are moistened with the antibiotic solution.

The donor site is covered during surgery with a single layer of fine-mesh gauze (Scarlet Red or Biobrane). Usually the Scarlet Red is kept in place until it begins to separate itself from the donor site. Positioning to prevent pressure on the site is important. Daily inspection of the donor site is essential to detect early signs of infection or cellulitis.

A new technique that involves the growth and subsequent graft placement of cultured epithelial autografts has become an important adjunct to permanent coverage of extensive burn wounds. Biopsies are taken from unburned skin and cells are cultured in the laboratory. Sheets of cultured epithelial cells are attached to petroleum jelly gauze and applied to the wound. After 7 to 10 days, the petroleum jelly gauze is removed, and a nonadherent dressing is applied to prevent mechanical trauma.

Escharotomy

Any circumferential burn to an arm or leg may mimic compartment syndrome. Edema formation in the tissues under the tight, unyielding eschar of a circumferential burn of a deep partial-thickness or full-thickness injury produces significant vascular compromise in the affected limb.

To minimize the risk of circulatory compromise, the patient's rings, watch, or other jewelry are removed during the initial examination. Elevation and active motion of the injured extremity may alleviate minimal degrees of circulatory distress. Skin color, sensation, capillary refill, and peripheral pulses are assessed and documented hourly in an extremity with a circumferential burn. Doppler ultrasonography is the most reliable means of assessing arterial blood flow and the need for an escharotomy. In the upper extremity, the radial, ulnar, and palmar arch pulses are checked hourly. In the lower extremity, the posterior tibial and dorsalis pedis pulses are checked hourly. Loss—or a progressive diminution (decrease)—of the ultrasonic signal is an indication for escharotomy.

The escharotomy is carried out as a bedside procedure, using a sterile field and scalpel, an electrocautery device, or both. Taking the patient to the operating room is not necessary and causes unacceptable delay. Local anesthesia is rarely needed because full-thickness injuries are insensate. However, small doses of narcotics and benzodiazepines assist in patient comfort. The incision should be placed along either the mid-medial or mid-lateral aspect of the extremity and should extend through the eschar down to the subcutaneous fat to permit adequate separation of the cut edges for decompression (Fig. 53-6).

PROVIDING PSYCHOLOGICAL AND FAMILIAL SUPPORT

Providing psychological support for the newly admitted burn patient and family is not the least of the many tasks facing the critical care nurse. The patient most often is awake and alert, although anxious and overwhelmed by the suddenness and magnitude of injuries. With high anxiety levels and lack of knowledge pertaining to burns, the family approaches the burn unit with fear, hesitancy, and sometimes hysteria. The physical appearance of the patient and the high-technology atmosphere of the burn unit are frightening. Preparing the family for the initial visit by explaining what to expect and escorting them to the bedside is extremely important. Visitors often are overwhelmed on the first visit and stand silently with feelings of anxiety and hopelessness growing. Burn injuries are dramatic and are psychologically traumatic for the patient and for those witnessing the accident. Counseling for the

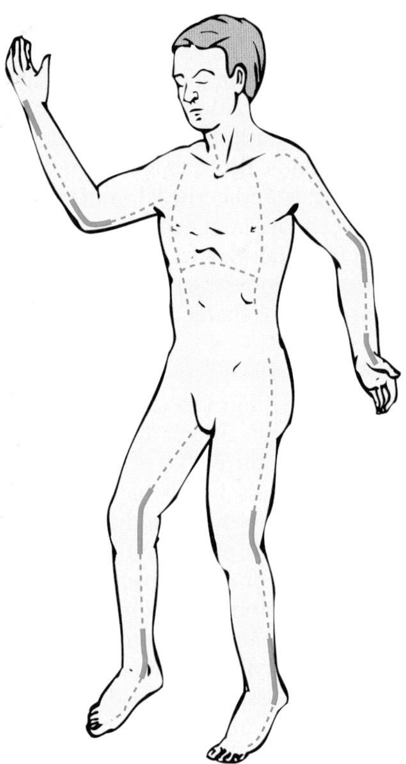

figure 53-6 Preferred sites of escharotomy incisions.

patient and the family begins on the day of admission. Families require constant support and the burn team should plan weekly family meetings to discuss the patient's care plan and progress. This is often the all-important basis for establishing a trusting relationship for the long months of rehabilitation ahead. The trusting relationship that is established initially provides a strong base for patient and family teaching and rehabilitation in the months to follow. Critically ill burn patients are on a roller coaster ride between life and death that does not stop until the burn wounds are closed, which can be 2 to 3 months after injury. The family needs to be informed and provided with the means to care for their own physical and psychological needs. It is particularly stressful for families of patients who were transferred from a great distance and who lack nearby support systems. The need to provide support for families cannot be overemphasized.

Burn patients often become depressed and withdrawn, asking to be left alone and not to be made uncomfortable. The nurse should respond by making certain expectations of the patient clear. That is, the nurse should make it clear to the patient that he or she is to feed himself or herself, go to the bathroom, or do as much as his or her physical condition permits, while communicating to the patient that the situation is not hopeless and that recovery is expected.

The best way to handle regression in a burn patient is to acknowledge it. First, the nurse must accept the fact that the patient may be unable to cope on an adult level and that the patient may be unstable emotionally and physically. Second, the nurse must devise ways to help the patient cope on an appropriate level. Interventions that usually help include following a regular schedule so that the patient knows what is expected, rewarding the patient for adult behavior, and permitting the patient as much control and choice as possible.

It is not uncommon for severely burned patients to transfer their fears to a specific caregiver (physician, nurse, therapist) and to complain that they are being treated unjustly or unkindly. Working with a psychiatric liaison nurse may help the burn survivor recognize and deal with his or her fears more effectively and help the caregiver support the patient by responding therapeutically.

Hallucinations, confusion, and combativeness are common in severely burned patients for physical and mental reasons. Exhaustion, pain, and medications may distort reality and produce schizophrenic behavior.

Although the patient tends to concentrate on the present, the family members look to the future and want to know what to expect. Information about the patient's condition and treatments should be shared with them using an honest and open approach.

Rehabilitative Phase

Patients with extensive burns require many months for recovery and rehabilitation. Physical and psychological rehabilitation measures are begun in the ICU and continued throughout the recovery period.

PHYSICAL REHABILITATION

The diet of the burn patient should remain high in protein until all wounds have healed. As healing takes place, the diet should be tapered to meet normal caloric requirements. Burn patients may become accustomed to eating frequently and in large amounts. After healing is complete, metabolism returns to normal, and weight will be gained if eating habits are not controlled properly.

PREVENTION OF SCARRING AND CONTRACTURES

Once regarded as inevitable, hypertrophic scarring and joint contractures are now largely preventable. Preventive measures start when the person is admitted to the hospital and continue for at least 12 months or until the scar is fully mature.

These preventive measures (i.e., positioning the body and helping the patient perform range-of-motion exercises) are not new to the nurse. Positioning the body with the extremities extended is extremely important. Although tightly flexed positions are preferred by patients for comfort, they will result in severe contractures. The range-of-motion exercises should be carried out with each dressing change or more often if indicated. Special splints are used to maintain arm, legs, and hands in extended, yet functional, positions. Later, when the wounds have healed sufficiently, the person is custom-fitted for a special pressure garment. By applying continuous uniform pressure over the entire area of the burn, the garment prevents hypertrophic scarring. The garment must be worn 24 hours a day for approximately 1 year. The smooth elastic garment forms a shield that permits the person to wear normal clothing and resume ordinary activities much sooner.

Healed and grafted skin will be dry and tight. Itching is a major patient complaint as healing occurs. Massaging a mild, nonirritating lotion into the healed skin provides lubrication and aids in range of motion.

PSYCHOLOGICAL REHABILITATION

The burn survivor may have many psychological issues once discharge is nearing. The patient may have post-traumatic stress disorder, anxiety, depression, or a combination of these. To ensure that these issues are effectively managed, the multidisciplinary team caring for the burn patient must include mental health professionals.

case study ■ A 58% TOTAL BODY SURFACE AREA (TBSA) BURN

Mr. Bowman is a 32-year-old white man who has sustained a 58% TBSA burn as the result of an indoor explosion in a sawmill where he is employed. Mr. Bowman is a well-nourished, slender man who has been healthy until this event. He does not smoke, but reports drinking one case of beer a week for the last 5 years. He has never been seriously ill or had any operations. Mr. Bowman is married and the father of two healthy children. His family history indicates no hypertension; diabetes; or heart, lung, or kidney disease.

Mr. Bowman was airlifted to the regional burn trauma center about 4 hours after the explosion. The referring local hospital had initially stabilized Mr. Bowman by intubating him, starting intravenous therapy, placing a Foley catheter, inserting a nasogastric tube, and performing bilateral upper extremity escharotomies.

On admission to the burn unit, initial assessment revealed that Mr. Bowman had received a 58% TBSA burn. He was observed to have full-thickness burns on his face, both arms (circumferential), the dorsal surfaces of both hands, and the posterior surfaces of both thighs. These full-thickness burns account for 40% of the TBSA that is burned. The burned areas are dry, hard, and leathery in appearance. He stated that these areas were not painful when touched or exposed to the air, before intubation. The remaining 18% of the TBSA that is burned demonstrates partial-thickness burns. The areas include the posterior head and neck, the buttocks, and the palms, and the anterior areas of his thighs. The wounds are red in appearance with serous fluid seeping from many open areas. Thin-walled blisters have formed in the areas, causing significant pain.

Mr. Bowman received 6000 mL of lactated Ringer's solution before admission to the burn center. His urine output is maintaining 30 mL/hour since catheterization. Further examination reveals that he is developing periorbital edema. Examination of Mr. Bowman's pharynx reveals carbonaceous soot on his vocal cords and chest auscultation reveals coarse rhonchi. His respirations are 30 breaths/minute, shallow and labored. Cardiac status reveals a regular heart rate with no ectopic beats or sounds. There is marked swelling and tightness of the skin on both arms and hands. Mr. Bowman is medicated with a continuous drip of morphine and lorazepam for comfort and sedation.

Initial laboratory values are as follows: white blood count 20,000 cells/mm^3; hematocrit 55.5%; sodium 120 mEq/L; potassium 3.4 mEq/L; chloride 101 mEq/L; bicarbonate 24 mEq/L; blood urea nitrogen (BUN) 17 mg/dL; and creatinine 0.7 mg/dL. Initial vitals signs are as follows: blood pressure (supine) 124/78 mm Hg; heart rate 128 beats/minute; respirations 30 breaths/minute; and rectal temperature 101.3°F (38.5°C).

Fluid resuscitation is accomplished within the first 24 hours by using the Baxter (Parkland) fluid resuscitation formula (4 mL/75 kg/58%). On the basis of body weight and burn area, it is calculated that Mr. Bowman requires 17.4 L of fluid in the first 24 hours. Half of the 17.4 L will be infused in the first 8 hours and the second half will be infused in the next 16 hours. A colloid-containing fluid (25 mL of 25% albumin in 1 L of 0.9% normal saline) will be used for fluid resuscitation over the next 24 hours. (The colloid is calculated using 0.5 mL colloid/75 kg/58%.)

Burn treatment consists of cleaning the burned areas twice a day with chlorhexidine solution. This is followed by application of Bacitracin ointment to the face, mafenide acetate to the ears, and silver sulfadiazine to the trunk and extremities. A gauze dressing is applied to the trunk and extremities.

On postburn day 5, Mr. Bowman's urine output is decreased to 15 to 20 mL/hour. It subsequently falls to less than 10 mL/hour. The urine is dark yellow. Urinalysis reveals the following: urine specific gravity 1.021 and urine sodium 10 mEq/L. The BUN level is 43 mg/dL and the serum creatinine level is 1.3 mg/dL. Mr. Bowman's Foley catheter irrigates easily.

Mr. Bowman progresses clinically from the prerenal failure caused by shock to intrarenal failure from renal tubular damage. His urine sodium level falls to 7 mEq/L and his urine specific gravity is 1.020. He appears to be normovolemic, even though his kidneys are not functioning well. It is determined that Mr. Bowman has acute renal failure caused by acute tubular necrosis (ATN). Cellular casts and epithelial debris sloughed off by the dying tubular wall appear in his urine, as well as moderate to heavy protein. He continues to be oliguric despite a cautious attempt to increase his renal blood flow and to flush out the debris with drugs that dilate renal arteries and prevent sodium resorption in the tubules (dopamine and diuretics). Unfortunately, he has no response to the treatments and they are discontinued.

The following day Mr. Bowman is asynchronous with the ventilator and is agitated, despite continued sedation and analgesia therapies. His vital signs are as follows: heart rate 98 beats/minute; blood pressure 168/92 mm Hg; respirations 24 breaths/minute, deep and asynchronous with the ventilator; and pulses normal. A third heart sound (S_3) is present. Mr. Bowman has gained 15 kg over 36 hours and gross edema remains to his face, hands, and feet. His lungs have crackles bilaterally one-third up from the bases. An electrocardiogram reveals tall, peaked T waves and widening intervals. Laboratory studies reveal the following: BUN 94 mg/dL; creatinine 4.1 mg/dL; potassium 7.5 mEq/L; and bicarbonate 10 mEq/L. Arterial blood gases (ABGs) are as follows: pH 7.29; arterial carbon dioxide tension ($Paco_2$) 20 mm Hg, and arterial oxygen tension (Pao_2) 69 mm Hg. Hemodialysis is initiated immediately. The treatment goal is to correct Mr. Bowman's electrolyte imbalance, metabolic acidosis, and fluid overload.

On postburn day 21, Mr. Bowman's laboratory values are trending down to baseline after receiving hemodialysis 3 days per week. He is now extubated and receiving vigorous pulmonary toileting to prevent atelectasis and pneumonia. The BUN level is 33 mg/dL and the creatinine level is 2.0

mg/dL. Mr. Bowman's metabolic acidosis is corrected and his urine output is 35 to 75 mL/hour. By postburn day 45, hemodialysis is no longer necessary. Because Mr. Bowman had nearly 40% TBSA full-thickness injuries, excision and grafting of burned skin began on postburn day 9 and his wounds are healing without difficulty. Mr. Bowman undergoes numerous grafting surgeries during his admission. On postburn day 58, nearly 2 months after his accident, he is discharged to an inpatient rehabilitation facility for a concentrated exercise and strengthening program. ■

clinical applicability challenges

Self-Challenge: Critical Thinking

1. *Refer to the case study at the end of this chapter. Discuss the clinical rationale for intubating Mr. Bowman within 1 hour of his injury, versus waiting to see if he develops respiratory compromise.*
2. *How do you perform a neurovascular assessment in a patient who is intubated?*
3. *Relate the pathophysiology of burn shock to the development of acute tubular necrosis (ATN).*

Study Questions

1. *What is the best fluid to use for fluid resuscitation of a burn patient during the first 24 hours?*
   a. *Packed red blood cells*
   b. *5% dextrose in normal saline solution (D_5NSS)*
   c. *Albumin*
   d. *Lactated Ringer's solution*
2. *A patient has been burned in a house fire. She sustained burns that damaged the epidermis, dermis, and subcutaneous tissue. Which one of the following classifications of burns best describes this patient's injuries?*
   a. *First-degree*
   b. *Full-thickness*
   c. *Superficial*
   d. *Partial-thickness*
3. *Which of the following statements best describes the development of burn shock?*
   a. *Increased capillary permeability causes an increase in vascular colloid osmotic pressure and a decrease in hydrostatic pressure.*
   b. *Release of epinephrine produces increased heart rate, but it is ineffective, and cardiogenic shock occurs.*
   c. *Increased capillary permeability results in decreased capillary colloid osmotic pressure.*
   d. *The stress response (epinephrine and norepinephrine) causes selective vasoconstriction, resulting in shock.*
4. *A patient complains of headache, nausea, and vertigo. What might these symptoms indicate?*
   a. *Smoke inhalation*
   b. *Carbon monoxide poisoning*
   c. *Cerebral edema*
   d. *Overhydration*
5. *A patient has sustained burns to his entire right arm and his anterior trunk. Using the "rule of nines" method, what is the percentage of his burn injury?*
   a. *48%*
   b. *27%*
   c. *18%*
   d. *9%*
6. *During the resuscitative phase, an elevated serum potassium level may occur. This is primarily the result of*
   a. *cellular injury.*
   b. *fluid volume loss.*
   c. *increased capillary permeability.*
   d. *interstitial edema.*
7. *Intramuscular injection of analgesics during the resuscitative phase is not recommended because*
   a. *narcotics can severely depress the respiratory system.*
   b. *narcotics can further decrease the blood pressure.*
   c. *inadequate peripheral perfusion results in uneven absorption of the medication.*
   d. *tolerance to pain medication develops easily.*
8. *Which of the following nursing actions is appropriate when using silver sulfadiazine?*
   a. *Premedicate the patient for pain before application.*
   b. *Monitor acid–base balance.*
   c. *Monitor white blood cell count.*
   d. *Observe for signs of hepatotoxicity.*

REFERENCES

1. American Burn Association: Available at: http://www.ameriburn.org
2. National Center for Injury Prevention and Control: Available at: http://www.cdc.gov/ncipc/default.htm
3. Sommers M: Multisystem. In Alspach JG (ed): Core Curriculum for Critical Care Nursing, pp 715–798. Philadelphia, WB Saunders, 1998
4. Shaw A, Anderson J, Hayward A, et al: Pathophysiological basis of pain management. Br J Hosp Med 52(11):583–587, 1994–1995
5. Carleton SC, Tomassoni AJ, Alexander J: Cardiac problems associated with burns. Cardiol Clin 3(2):257–262, 1995
6. Mackey D: Pulmonary emergencies. In Kitt S, Selfridge-Thomas J, Proehl J, et al (eds): Emergency Nursing: A Physiologic and Nursing Perspective, pp 207–211. Philadelphia, WB Saunders, 1995
7. Rue LW, Cioffi WG, Mason AD, et al: The risk of pneumonia in thermally injured patients requiring ventilatory support. J Burn Care Rehabil 16(3 Pt 1):262–268, 1995
8. Rodeberg DA, Housinger TA, Greenhalgh DG, et al: Improved ventilatory function in burn patients using volumetric diffusive respiration. J Am Coll Surg 179(5):518–522, 1994

OTHER SELECTED READING

Ahrns K: Trends in burn resuscitation: Shifting the focus from fluids to adequate endpoint monitoring, edema control, and adjuvant therapies. Crit Care Nurs Clin North Am 16(1):75–98, 2004

Bishop JF: Burn wound assessment and surgical management. Crit Care Nurs Clin North Am 16(1):145–178, 2004

Flynn MB: Nutritional support of the burn-injured patient. Crit Care Nurs Clin North Am 16(1):139–144, 2004

Honari S: Topical therapies and antimicrobials in the management of burn wounds. Crit Care Nurs Clin North Am 16(1):1–12, 2004

LaBorde P: Burn epidemiology: The patient, the nation, the statistics, and the data resources. Crit Care Nurs Clin North Am 16(1): 13–26, 2004

Merrel P, Mayo D: Inhalation injury in the burn patient. Crit Care Nurs Clin North Am 16(1):27–38, 2004

Merz J, Schrand C, Mertens D, et al: Wound care of the pediatric burn patient. AACN Clin Issues 14(4):429–441, 2003

Montgomery RK: Pain management in burn injury. Crit Care Nurs Clin North Am 16(1):39–50, 2004

Santucci S, Gobara S, Santos C, et al: Infections in a burn intensive care unit: Experience of seven years. J Hosp Infection 53(1):6–13, 2003

Smith M, Doctor M, Boulter T: Unique considerations in caring for a pediatric burn patient: A developmental approach. Crit Care Nurs Clin North Am 16(1):99–108, 2004

Supple K: Physiologic response to burn injury. Crit Care Nurs Clin North Am 16(1):109–118, 2004

PART
one
two
three
four
five
six
seven
eight
nine
ten
eleven
twelve

Multisystem Dysfunction

INTERNET RESOURCES

Topic	Web Page Address
The Agency For Toxic Substances and Disease Registry	www.atsdr.cdc.gov
Alcoholics Anonymous	www.alcoholics-anonymous.org
The American Academy of Clinical Toxicology	www.clintox.org
American Association of Poison Control Centers	www.aapcc.org
American Association for the Surgery of Trauma	www.aast.org
The American College of Medical Toxicology	www.acmt.net
American Society for Microbiology	www.asm.org
American Society of Surgical Technologists	www.ast.org
American Trauma Society	www.amtrauma.org
Association for Professionals in Infection Control and Epidemiology	www.apic.org
Association of Rehabilitation Nurses	www.rehabnurse.org
British Trauma Society	www.trauma.org
Community Anti-Drug Coalitions of America	www.cadca.org
The Eastern Association for the Surgery of Trauma	www.east.org
Emergency Nurses Association	www.ena.org
Infectious Disease Society of America	www.idsociety.org
International Council on Alcohol, Drugs and Traffic Safety	www.icadts.org
International Society for Biomedical Research on Alcoholism	www.isbra.com
Johns Hopkins Division of Infectious Diseases Antibiotic Guide	www.hopkins-abxguide.org
National Association of Orthopaedic Nurses	www.orthonurse.org
Orthopaedic Trauma Association	www.ota.org
Society of Critical Care Medicine	www.sccm.org
Society of Trauma Nurses	www.traumanursesoc.org
Toxicology Data Network	www.toxnet.nlm.nih.gov
The U.S. Department of Education's Higher Education Center for Alcohol and Other Drug Abuse and Violence Prevention	www.edc.org/hec

chapter **54**

Shock, Systemic Inflammatory Response Syndrome, and Multiple Organ Dysfunction Syndrome

MARY BETH FLYNN ■ SANDRA MCLESKEY

objectives

Based on the content in this chapter, the reader should be able to:

- Describe common pathophysiological processes involved in the generalized shock response.
- Compare and contrast the etiology and clinical manifestations of the major categories of shock.
- Explain the anticipated medical management and rationale for treatment of the various shock states.
- Describe patients at risk for development of shock and complications associated with the various shock states.
- Discuss nursing management principles for patients with shock, systemic inflammatory response syndrome, and multiple organ dysfunction syndrome.

PATHOPHYSIOLOGY OF SHOCK

Under normal conditions, the body provides sufficient oxygen to the cells to meet metabolic needs. Under stress, the body consumes its oxygen more rapidly, and compensatory mechanisms are initiated to meet the increased demands of the body and restore oxygen and perfusion to cells. These compensatory mechanisms are the same, regardless of the clinical condition causing the cellular hypoperfusion. Clinical conditions that result in cellular hypoperfusion are often referred to as *shock states.*

This chapter discusses various clinical conditions that create states of cellular hypoperfusion, or shock. These states include hypovolemia, cardiogenic shock, anaphylaxis, neurogenic shock, and septic shock. In addition, this chapter describes systemic inflammatory response syndrome (SIRS) and multiple organ dysfunction syndrome (MODS), which both represent progression of shock states. Patients in critical care are at significant risk for development of any one of these clinical conditions. Early recognition of shock and appropriate intervention are necessary to prevent or limit SIRS or MODS.

Tissue Oxygenation and Perfusion

Oxygenation of all organs and tissues is directly related to the ability of the body to provide oxygen to the blood and transport the oxygenated blood to cells. The pulmonary system provides for the diffusion of oxygen into the blood through the process of respiration (ventilation [partial pressure of arterial carbon dioxide, or $PaCO_2$] and oxygenation [partial pressure of arterial oxygen, or PaO_2]). The cardiovascular system assists in the transport of the oxygenated blood to the cells for metabolism; hemoglobin in the blood acts as the carrier for the oxygen (arterial oxygen saturation [SaO_2]). Typically, cells consume about 25% of the oxygen delivered; this utilization of oxygen is referred to as *oxygen consumption* ($\dot{V}O_2$). The body's ability to provide oxygen to the cells is called *oxygen delivery* (DaO_2). Box 54-1 shows how oxygen parameters are calculated.

Under normal conditions, $\dot{V}O_2$ is independent of DaO_2. This means that when cells need to consume additional oxygen to produce energy, they can extract the necessary amount required to produce energy in the form of adenosine triphosphate (ATP). However, during times of physiological stress, $\dot{V}O_2$ becomes dependent on DaO_2. Initial respiratory, endocrine, and circulatory compensatory mech-

box 54-1
Procedure for Calculating Oxygen Parameters

CALCULATED OXYGEN PARAMETERS	NORMAL PARAMETERS
Assessment of Pulmonary Function	
Ventilation $Paco_2$	35–45 mm Hg
Oxygenation Pao_2	80–100 mm Hg
Arterial oxygen saturation (Sao_2)	>95%
Venous oxygen saturation ($S\bar{v}o_2$)	>65%–75%
Oxygen Carrying Capacity	
Hemoglobin	12–18g/dL
Tissue Perfusion	
CO	4–8L/min
Heart rate	80–100 bpm
Stroke volume	55–100 mL/beat/m^2
Oxygen Delivery	
$Dao_2 = CO \times Hbg \times Sao_2 \times 1.39 \times 10$	Normal, 800–1,200 L/min
$Dao_2I = \frac{Dao_2}{BSA}$	Normal range depends on patient's body surface area
Oxygen consumption	
$\dot{V}o_2 = CO \times (Ca - v)O_2 \times 10$	Normal, 180–250 L/min
$\dot{V}o_2 = \frac{\dot{V}o_2}{BSA}$	Normal range depends on patient's body surface area

Technique

1. Calculate the $\dot{V}o_2$ to determine the cellular energy requirements of the patient with an oxygenation/perfusion problem.
2. Calculate the Dao_2.
3. Increase the Dao_2 by manipulating elements of the equation (↑CO, ↑Hgb, ↑oxygenation) through titration of vasoactive and inotropic agents or fluids, administration of blood, maximized oxygenation, and ventilatory support. As Dao_2 is increased, $\dot{V}o_2$ of the cellular energy needs will be met, maintaining aerobic metabolism.

CO, cardiac output; Ca − v, content of arterial oxygen (obtained from arterial blood gas) − content of venous oxygen (obtained from mixed venous blood gas); BSA, body surface area; I, indexed

anisms respond to the cells' need for oxygen by increasing elements of DaO_2. If additional oxygen is required, and the cells cannot extract the oxygen, they must use anaerobic metabolism to produce ATP. Anaerobic metabolism is not an efficient method of energy production, and the ATP produced is insufficient to meet cellular demands. Moreover, anaerobic metabolism produces lactic acid as a byproduct, increasing the amount of acid that must be eliminated. If oxygen continues to be insufficient to meet cellular demands for energy, cell death ensues. As more cells die, tissues and organs eventually become progressively dysfunctional.

During shock states or poor perfusion, oxygen is consumed at a much greater rate than it is delivered, but it is difficult to predetermine the amount of oxygen the cells will require. To meet the increased need for cellular $\dot{V}O_2$, the DaO_2 must be increased. Although it is not possible to manipulate cellular $\dot{V}O_2$ directly, many nursing interventions can be implemented to manipulate and increase DaO_2. In shock states, the primary goal is to maximize DaO_2 to meet cellular oxygen requirements in an ongoing effort to prevent tissue and cell death and maintain end-organ perfusion.

Compensatory Mechanisms

Cellular perfusion depends on the synergy of multiple physiological processes. The pulmonary, endocrine, and circulatory systems maintain an intricate balance of oxygen exchange and delivery to the cells by generation of an adequate oxygenated blood supply and cardiac output (Fig. 54-1). The autonomic nervous system assists in the orchestration of this delicate balance.

During states of hypoxia, activated compensatory mechanisms increase the depth and rate of respiration. The

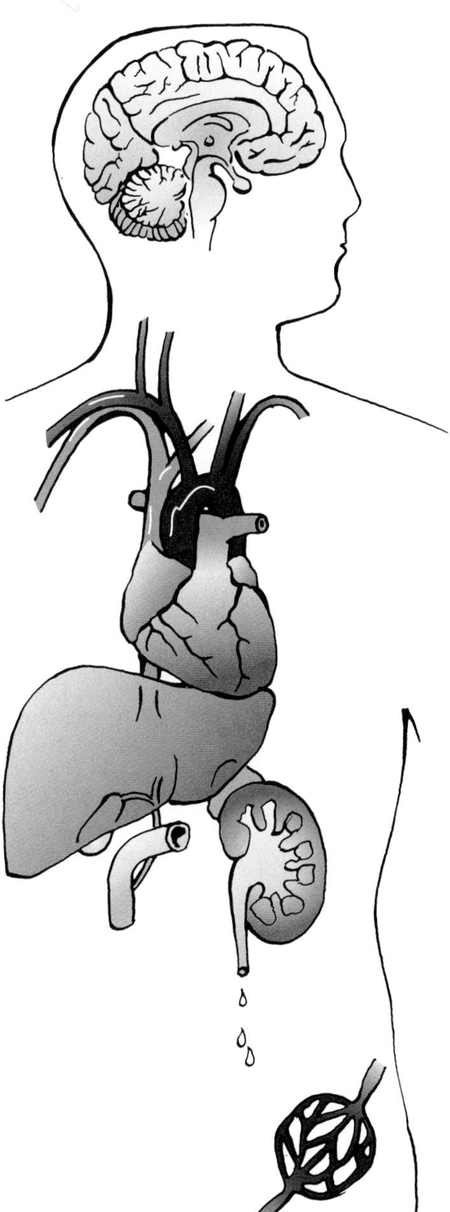
Brain
• Thirst
• Increased production and release of ADH
Cardiovascular system
• Increased heart rate
• Increased force of cardiac contraction
• Increased systemic vascular resistance
• Decreased blood flow to the
kidney
gastrointestinal tract
skin
skeletal muscles
• Constriction of the veins
Adrenal gland
• Increased production and release of aldosterone by the adrenal cortex
• Increased production and release of the catecholamines (epinephrine and norepinephrine) by the adrenal medulla
Liver
• Constriction of veins and sinusoids with mobilization of blood stored in the liver
Kidney
• Increased retention of sodium and water
• Decreased urine output
Capillary bed
• Increased reabsorption of water into the capillary from the interstitial spaces due to constriction of the arterioles with a resultant decrease in capillary pressure

figure 54-1 Compensatory mechanisms in hypovolemic shock. *ADH*, antidiuretic hormone. (From Porth CM: Pathophysiology: Concepts of Altered Health States [6th Ed], p 562. Philadelphia, Lippincott Williams & Wilkins, 2002.)

cardiovascular system increases cardiac output to increase oxygen delivery to the cells. During states of low perfusion (low blood pressure), compensatory mechanisms are initiated and result in increases in heart rate, systemic vascular resistance (SVR), preload, and cardiac contractility in an effort to restore appropriate circulatory volume. (Review Chapter 16 for a discussion of these terms.) The fall in systemic blood pressure activates a series of neurohormonal responses aimed at reestablishing sufficient cardiac output and perfusion to vital organs. The fall in blood pressure results in decreased stimulation of baroreceptors and eventually an increase in sympathetic response.

Continued sympathetic stimulation causes an increased heart rate and contractile force, increasing the cardiac output. Arteriolar vasoconstriction (increased SVR) increases blood pressure and also shunts blood from less vital organs such as the stomach and intestines to vital organs such as the heart, lungs, and brain. The preload and subsequently the cardiac output are increased by venoconstriction. The kidneys respond to sympathetic stimulation and local hypoperfusion by activating the renin–angiotensin system, which also increases vasoconstriction of the arterioles and veins, increasing cardiac output and SVR. Activation of the renin–angiotensin system also stimulates the adrenal cortex to release aldosterone, which acts on the kidney to conserve sodium and water, increasing circulating volume. A drop in blood pressure also causes the pituitary gland to release antidiuretic hormone, which also increases vascular tone and stimulates water and sodium retention by the kidney, further increasing preload. An increase of preload (from multiple sources) increases cardiac output, thereby increasing blood pressure. Collective compensatory responses act together to increase the body's circulating volume, blood pressure, and cardiac output to provide perfusion and oxygen to the cells (Fig. 54-2).

The goal in treating patients in shock states is to reestablish perfusion and oxygenation adequate to the needs to the cells as quickly as possible. Early recognition of signs of shock and ongoing assessments guide therapeutic interventions. The nurse plays a key role in the ongoing assessment of shock. The patient's clinical presentation depends on the cause of the shock state and degree of compensation. Clinical assessment parameters should be evaluated frequently to establish effectiveness of interventions and progression of shock state. Traditional assessment parameters include altered level of consciousness, tachypnea (PaO_2, $PaCO_2$, SaO_2), tachycardia, hypotension, decreased urine output, and metabolic acidosis (base deficit and serum lactate levels), which are commonly found in all states of hypoperfusion. Recent advances in technology provide

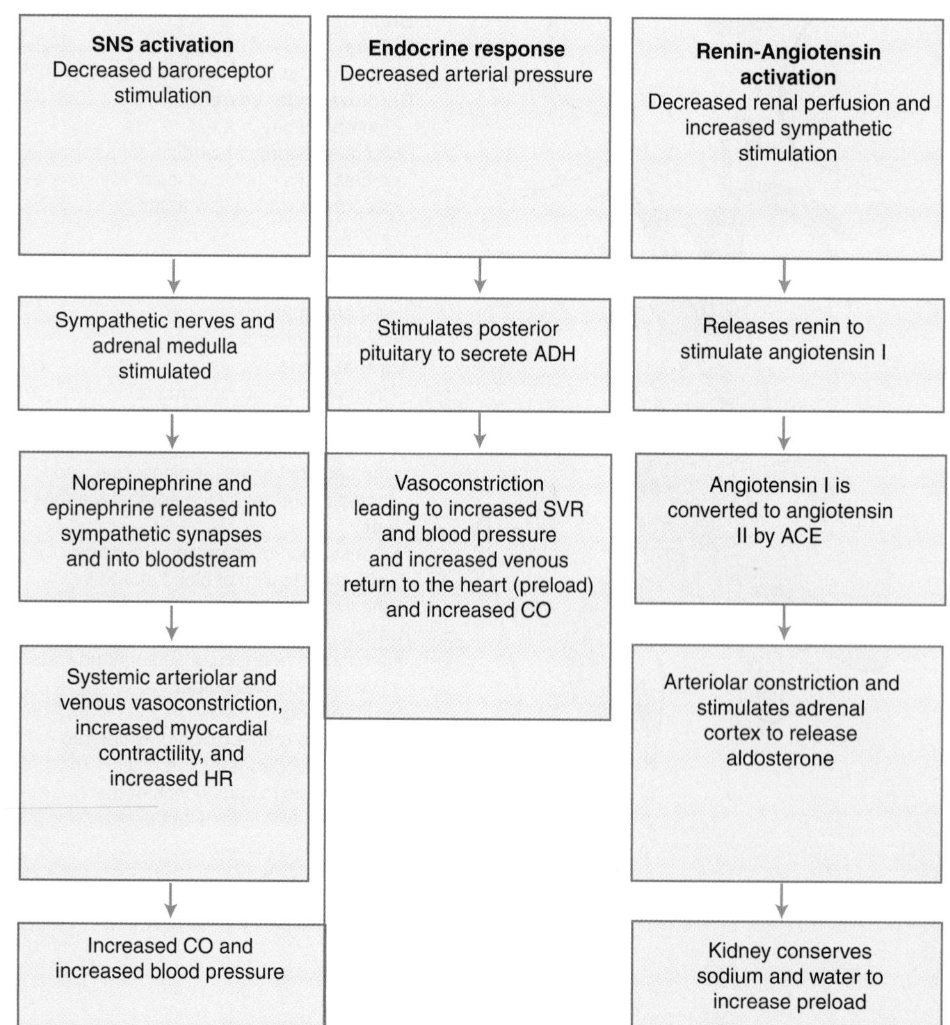

figure 54-2 Compensatory mechanisms in shock. *ACE,* angiotensin-converting enzyme; *ADH,* antidiuretic hormone; *CO,* cardiac output; *HR,* heart rate; *SNS,* sympathetic nervous system.

methods for earlier assessment of the patient's tissue oxygenation and perfusion using measures of gastric pH, sublingual end-tidal carbon dioxide ($ETCO_2$), and central mixed venous oxygen saturation ($cS\bar{v}O_2$).[1] The newer technologies also allow for earlier assessment of metabolic acidosis.

CLASSIFICATION OF SHOCK

Shock states have historically been classified according to the causal failing organ or system. *Hypovolemic shock* results in a state of hypoperfusion because of a loss of circulation volume. *Cardiogenic shock* is caused by a significant insult to the myocardium, resulting in the loss of the structural and mechanical function of the heart. *Anaphylactic shock* is the body's overwhelming allergic response to an antigen. *Neurogenic shock* is caused by the disruption of sympathetic tone. Last, *septic shock* is a state of overwhelming infection and inflammatory response causing a maldistribution of the circulating blood volume, resulting in organ hypoperfusion.

HYPOVOLEMIC SHOCK

Etiology

Hypovolemic shock is a result of inadequate circulating volume. Most commonly, hypovolemic shock is caused by sudden blood loss or severe dehydration. Some injuries, such as burns, cause significant fluid shifts from the intravascular space to the interstitial space, resulting in hypovolemia (see Chapter 53). Volume disorders in critically ill patients may be classified as either depletion or expansion disorders and involve both intracellular and extracellular compartments. Acute fluid volume loss does not allow the normal compensatory mechanisms to restore an appropriate circulating volume rapidly enough. If left untreated, hypovolemia may lead to a variety of secondary complications, such as hypotension, electrolyte and acid–base disturbances, and organ dysfunction due to hypoperfusion (Fig. 54-3).

Pathophysiology

A sudden loss of intravascular volume decreases venous return to the heart and results in a reduction in cardiac output. Compensatory mechanisms are initiated to increase the circulating volume through the activation of the sympathetic nervous system and neurohormonal responses. If the condition persists, existing blood volume is shunted to the vital organs (heart, lungs, and brain), causing hypoperfusion to such organs as the liver, stomach, and kidneys. If volume is not replaced, compensatory mechanisms eventually become ineffective. The failure of the compensatory mechanisms to restore adequate circulating volume causes cellular hypoperfusion and inability to meet cellular oxygen requirements for metabolism. The cells must use anaerobic metabolism in an effort to meet their ATP requirements, resulting in lactic acidosis.

Failed compensatory mechanisms, which were initiated to restore cardiac output, eventually cause the myocardium to fatigue. Sympathetic stimulation to increase heart rate, contractility, and SVR escalates the workload of the heart. Ejection of a higher volume of blood against a higher SVR requires production of more oxygen and energy. Such stress on the heart causes an increase in myocardial metabolism and myocardial oxygen consumption ($M\dot{V}O_2$). The continued lack of circulating volume prevents appropriate oxygen delivery to the heart, creating a vicious cycle. Inability of the circulatory system to provide end-organ perfusion with enough oxygen forces conversion to anaerobic metabolism to meet cellular energy needs. Anaerobic metabolism cannot provide enough ATP to meet energy demands; thus, ischemic damage may ensue. If the situation continues, end-organ failure may occur (see Fig. 54-3).

Assessment

Clinical findings are directly related to the severity and acuity of volume loss (Table 54-1). Some patients, especially older patients or those who have chronic diseases, have more subtle compensatory responses, which may be overlooked. Box 54-2 lists considerations in older patients. Serial assessments of physical and laboratory findings may uncover trends that guide treatment and prevent vascular collapse.

HISTORY

A thorough history of the patient's presenting problem may reveal risk factors for hypovolemic shock. Patients experiencing significant blood loss because of gastric hemorrhage or liver or splenic rupture from trauma require a rapid replacement of circulating blood volume to prevent the consequences of hypovolemia. Both very young and older patients are at greater risk of hypovolemia that may be caused by severe dehydration or other medical illness, rather than trauma.

PHYSICAL FINDINGS

Patients with hypovolemic shock have the following signs and symptoms caused by poor organ perfusion:

- Altered mentation, ranging from lethargy to unresponsiveness
- Rapid and deep respirations, which gradually become labored and shallower as the patient's condition deteriorates
- Cool and clammy skin, with weak and thready pulses
- Tachycardia due to activation of the sympathetic nervous system
- Decreased urine output; urine is dark and concentrated because the kidneys are conserving fluid

LABORATORY STUDIES

Useful laboratory studies include determinations of serum lactate, arterial pH, and base deficit to assess the presence of anaerobic metabolism. Test results can be used to measure the effectiveness of fluid replacement therapy. Metabolic laboratory studies and electrolyte determinations assist with adjustment of fluid and electrolytes. Serial hemoglobin and hematocrit determinations and coagulation panels may be drawn to assess the need for blood product replacement. However, the hemoglobin and hematocrit may not directly reflect the severity of blood loss due to either hemoconcentration caused by dehydration or hemodilution caused by intravenous (IV) fluid therapy.

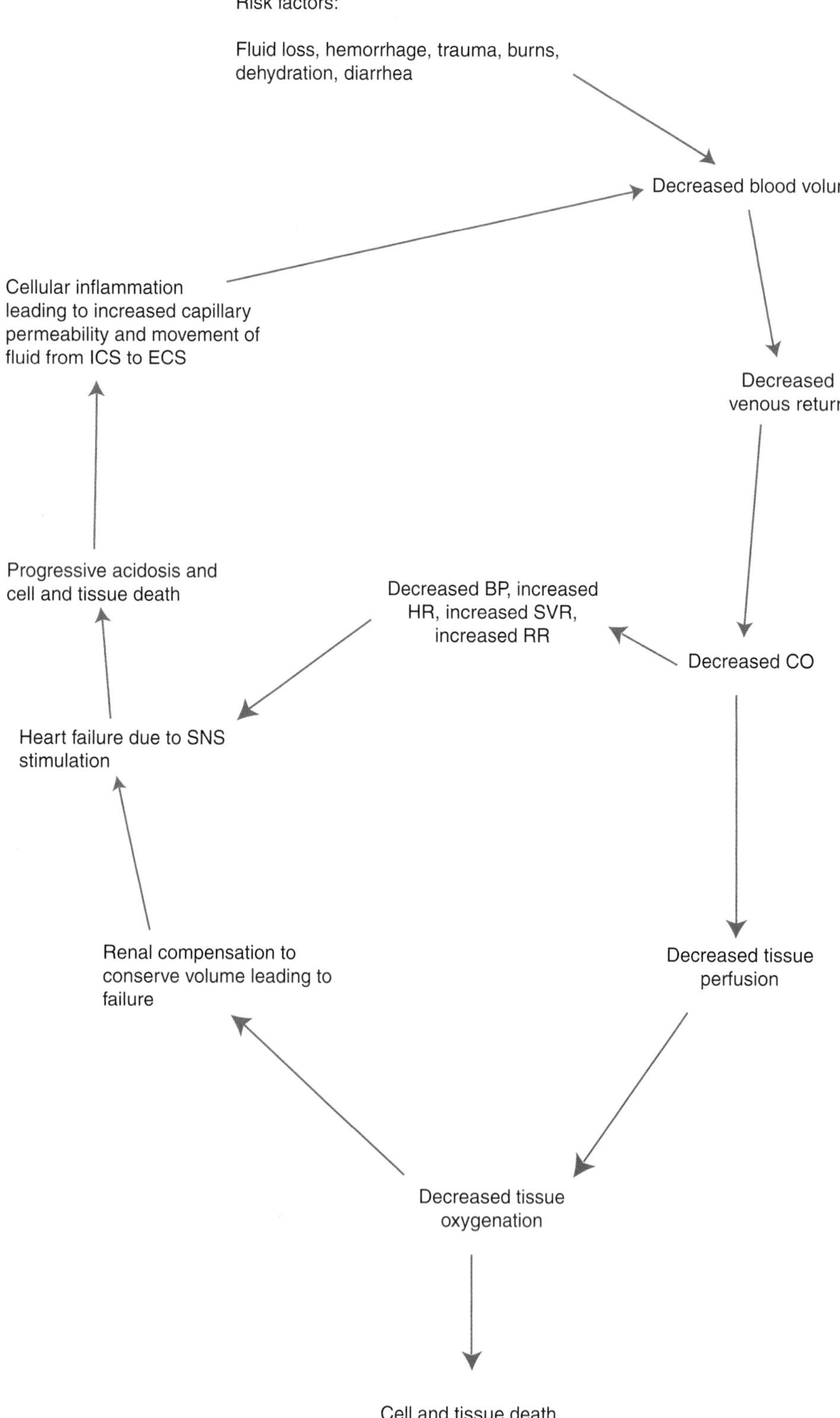

figure 54-3 Hypovolemic shock. *BP*, blood pressure; *CO*, cardiac output; *ECS*, extracellular space; *HR*, heart rate; *ICS*, intracellular space; *RR*, respiratory rate; *SNS*, sympathetic nervous system; *SVR*, systemic vascular resistance.

Management

Management focuses on restoring circulating volume and resolving the cause of volume loss. Composition of volume replacement therapy depends on what was lost. Crystalloid solutions are used primarily as first-line therapy. Isotonic solutions, such as lactated Ringer's solution or 0.9% normal saline solution, are preferred over hypotonic solutions (5% dextrose solution). Blood products and other colloid solutions (albumin and synthetic volume expanders) may be used to assist in the resuscitation process, especially if blood loss is the primary cause. The

table 54-1 Correlation of Clinical Findings Associated With Volume Loss in Hemorrhagic Shock

Estimated Blood Loss	Clinical Findings
<500 mL	None
500–1,000 mL	• Tachycardia (↑HR >20% of patient's baseline) • Hypotension (↓SBP >10% of patient's baseline) • ↓Urine output • Pulses weaker • Skin and extremities cool to touch • Hemodynamics: within normal limits CO, ↑SVR • Mild acidosis (↑base deficit, ↑lactic acid, ↓gastric pH)
1,000–2,000 mL	• Tachycardia (↑HR >20%–30% of patient's baseline) • Hypotension (↓SBP >10%–20% of patient's baseline) • Tachypnea (↑RR >10% of patient's baseline) • Oxygen saturation may not be altered dependent on the percentage of exogenous oxygen the patient is receiving • $S\bar{v}O_2$ <60% • ↓Urine output (<30 mL/h) • Altered level of consciousness: restlessness, agitation, confusion, or obtunded • Cool, diaphoretic skin • Poor peripheral pulses • Hemodynamics: ↓CO, ↑SVR • Progressive acidosis (↑base deficit, ↑lactic acid, ↓gastric pH)
2,000–3,000 mL	• Tachycardia (↑HR >20%–30% of patient's baseline) • Hypotension (↓SBP >10%–20% of patient's baseline) • Tachypnea (↑RR >10%–20% of patient's baseline) • ↓Oxygen saturation • $S\bar{v}O_2$ <55%–60% • Oliguria → anuria • Mental stupor • Marked peripheral vasoconstriction: cold extremities, poor peripheral pulses, pallor • Hemodynamics: ↓CO, ↑SVR • Severe acidosis (↑base deficit, ↑lactic acid, ↓gastric pH)

SBP, systolic blood pressure; SVR, systemic vascular resistance; CO, cardiac output; RR, respirations; HR, heart rate.

use of packed red blood cells is of utmost importance if hypotension is due to hemorrhage, and may be useful in other hypovolemic states.

Nursing management of hypovolemic shock focuses on the restoration of circulating volume through volume administration. Obtaining and maintaining adequate IV access is essential. Ideally, large IV catheters are inserted in the antecubital space or central venous system to assist with the rapid infusion of fluids. Care must be taken to administer fluids as rapidly as possible without compromising the pulmonary system. Fluids given too rapidly may cause pulmonary congestion and inhibit adequate oxygenation, further compromising oxygen delivery to the tissues. Fluids should also be warmed during infusion to limit the negative effects of hypothermia. Lower extremities may be elevated to prevent distal venous pooling and enhance blood return to the heart. Frequent documentation of vital signs, heart rate, respiratory rate and depth, oxygen saturation, urine output, and mentation, as well as laboratory results and interventions, is essential.

The use of colloids in the early phase of fluid replacement is controversial. During shock, a state of increased capillary membrane permeability causes a shift of intravascular volume into the extravascular space. However, in some cases, colloids may enter the extravascular space, further shifting fluids from the intravascular space to the extravascular space and thereby worsening the hypovolemia. A recent review of the literature by Vincent[2] suggests that although a consensus on whether to use colloids has yet to be achieved, if only crystalloids are used for resuscitation, more fluid is needed to achieve adequate intravascular fluid volume.

Complications

Complications associated with hypovolemic shock depend on the length of time and severity of the hypotensive crisis. Complications may range from renal damage to cerebral anoxia and death.

CARDIOGENIC SHOCK

Etiology

Cardiogenic shock is actually extreme congestive heart failure and therefore results from loss of critical contractile function of the heart. Usually, cardiogenic shock is

box 54-2

Response to Shock States in the Older Patient

As an individual ages, normal physiological changes may limit the ability of the body to respond efficiently to shock states. The nurse should be aware of physiological changes of aging and monitor closely for changes in the older patient's baseline assessment(s). The patient's medical history indicates other chronic disease states that further compromise normal physiological changes seen with aging.

Cardiovascular system: Increased dysrhythmias, increased atrial size and irritability, left ventricular myocardial thickening leading to decreased compliance and lower ejection fraction; thickened heart valves that interfere with forward flow; decreased response to sympathetic nervous system; decreased sensitivity of baroreceptors; generalized stiffening of arterial vessels, including aorta

Pulmonary system: Decreased tidal volume and respiratory muscle strength, decreased alveolar surface area, increased dead space at end-expiration, decreased elastic recoil of lungs, increased resting respiratory rate, increased risk of infection as a result of decreased number of cilia, blunted response to hypoxemia, decreased gag and cough reflex leading to increased risk for infection, aspiration

Hematologic system: Decreased ability of bone marrow to produce cells (red blood cells, white blood cells, platelets), increased anemia, decreased immune function (decreased production of T and B lymphocytes) leading to increased infections, lower baseline temperature, gradual changes in temperature in the elderly versus spikes (101.3°F [38.5°C]), increased risk of adverse drug reactions

diagnosed by the presence of systemic and pulmonary hemodynamic alterations, which result from inadequate cardiac output and tissue perfusion. Typically, this occurs when greater than 40% of ventricular mass is damaged. The most common cause of cardiogenic shock is an extensive left ventricular myocardial infarction. The reported incidence of cardiogenic shock due to myocardial infarction ranges from 15% to 20% and carries a mortality rate of 75% of 85%.[3] It is believed that this rate has decreased since the introduction of rapid invasive monitoring and revascularization procedures.[4] Although cardiogenic shock may develop within a few hours after the onset of myocardial infarction symptoms, it often occurs after hospitalization. Other causes of cardiogenic shock include papillary muscle rupture, ventricular septal rupture, cardiomyopathy, acute myocarditis, valvular disease, and dysrhythmias.

Box 54-3 shows independent predictors for development of cardiogenic shock. Patients with all five risk factors have a greater than 50% chance for developing cardiogenic shock. Research indicates that mortality rates for patients who present with cardiogenic shock compared with those in whom it develops in the hospital are similarly high. Identifying patients at risk for development of cardiogenic shock and formulating strategies for prevention are extremely important.

box 54-3 ***Risk Factors for Inpatient Development of Cardiogenic Shock***

- Increased age (elderly)
- Left ventricular ejection fraction <35% on hospital admission
- Large myocardial infarction
- History of diabetes mellitus
- Previous myocardial infarction

Pathophysiology

Cardiogenic shock is caused by loss of ventricular contractile force, which results in decreased stroke volume and decreased cardiac output. Neuroendocrine compensatory mechanisms, which are discussed in detail in the section on hypovolemic shock, are activated to increase preload through retention of sodium and water. Vasoconstriction also increases afterload (SVR). Ventricular filling pressures increase because of the increased preload, but lack of contractility prevents complete ejection. The ventricle becomes distended, further impairing effective contraction, and cardiac output continues to decrease. Compensatory mechanisms continue the vicious cycle of elevated ventricular filling pressures and SVR in combination with an inability of the heart to eject an adequate volume of blood into circulation. Blood pools in the pulmonary circulation, resulting in pulmonary congestion. Pulmonary capillaries are under increased pressure and leak fluid into the interstitium and alveoli, preventing pulmonary diffusion of oxygen and reducing oxygen tension in the blood (PaO_2; Fig. 54-4).

The body's cells become ischemic because of the decreased cardiac output, adding to an already tenuous state of myocardial functioning by further stimulating compensatory mechanisms to increase perfusion to the cells. Increased sympathetic stimulation increases the heart rate even more, further escalating myocardial oxygen demands and compounding the crisis. Associated hypotension prevents adequate oxygenation of myocardial tissue, exacerbating the anaerobic metabolism of the myocardial tissue and further decreasing the contractile state of the heart. These stressors placed on the failing heart may result in extension of a myocardial infarction.

Assessment

Patients admitted with the diagnosis of myocardial infarction require close monitoring. Assessment parameters are similar to the signs and symptoms of congestive heart failure but are more extreme. Assessment findings should be followed over time to allow the nurse to perceive the subtle changes that signal the beginning of cardiogenic shock.

HISTORY

A thorough history provides the information necessary to predict patients at risk for development of cardiogenic

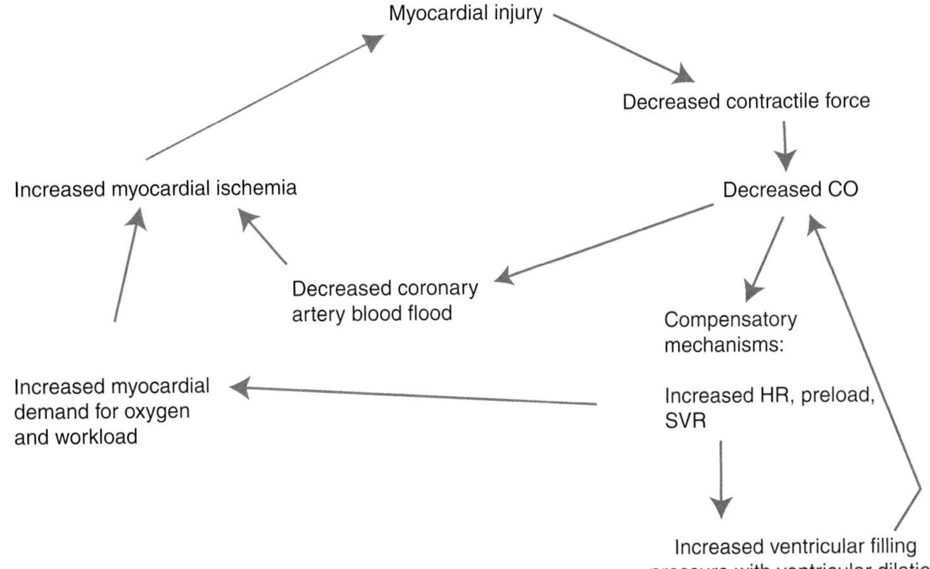

figure 54-4 Cardiogenic shock. *CO*, cardiac output; *HR*, heart rate; *SVR*, systemic vascular resistance.

shock. Cardiogenic shock frequently occurs in individuals who have suffered an extensive myocardial infarction, have an admission ejection fraction of less than 35%, have diabetes mellitus, or are elderly (see Box 54-3). These patients in particular should be closely monitored; the existence of these predisposing factors should alert the clinician to assess for the initial phases of shock, allowing for rapid, lifesaving intervention. It is important to rule out other causes of decreased cardiac output before initiating therapy. Some complications associated with myocardial infarction may require further intervention, including surgery.

PHYSICAL FINDINGS

Clinical manifestations associated with cardiogenic shock are outlined in Box 54-4. In addition to the signs and symptoms listed in the box, patients with cardiogenic shock often experience recurrent chest pain, which is suggestive of infarct extension. Other clinical findings are directly related to the decrease in cardiac output.

LABORATORY STUDIES

Presence of elevated myocardial tissue markers accompanied by progressive hemodynamic compromise and clinical deterioration are often hallmarks of extensive myocardial necrosis, which may precipitate cardiogenic shock. Laboratory studies suggestive of myocardial tissue death reveal a continuous release of myocardial bands of creatine phosphokinase (MB-CPK) and cardiac troponin I into the circulation. These cardiac markers are released from dying cardiac cells into the bloodstream. Each marker has a time course for its peak level indicative of myocardial injury. Brain natriuretic peptide (BNP), another cardiac marker that may be assessed by laboratory analysis, is produced and released by the ventricle in response to pressure overload.[5] An elevated BNP does not correlate with myocardial ischemia; however, it may provide information about the patient's ventricular compliance, providing additional data that may place the patient at higher risk for cardiogenic shock after a myocardial infarction.

Management

Management is aimed at increasing myocardial oxygen delivery, maximizing cardiac output, and decreasing left ventricular workload. The first goal of treatment is to correct reversible problems, protect the ischemic myocardium, and improve tissue perfusion. Early treatment is imperative to preserve myocardial muscle. Reversing the hypoxemia and acidosis can improve the response to other therapies. Fluids should be managed to provide adequate filling pressure without overdistension of the ventricle. Left ventricular filling pressures are often elevated; therefore, diuresis

box 54-4
Clinical Manifestations of Cardiogenic Shock

Hemodynamic findings
Systolic blood pressure <90 mm Hg
Mean arterial pressure <70 mm Hg
Cardiac index <2.2 L/min/m^2
Pulmonary artery wedge pressure >18 mm Hg

Noninvasive findings
Thready, rapid pulse
Narrow pulse pressure
Distended neck veins
Arrhythmias
Chest pain
Cool, pale, moist skin
Oliguria
Decreased mentation

Pulmonary findings
Dyspnea
↑Respiratory rate
Inspiratory crackles, possible wheezing
Arterial blood gases show ↓ in Pao_2
Respiratory alkalosis

Radiographic findings
Enlarged heart
Pulmonary congestion

may be indicated to achieve optimal preload. Electrolytes, specifically potassium, calcium, and magnesium, may need to be replaced to provide optimal conditions for the damaged myocardial muscle.

Nursing management for the patient with cardiogenic shock is centered on conserving myocardial energy and decreasing the workload of the heart. Use of narcotic analgesics and sedatives to minimize the sympathetic nervous system response can increase venous capacitance and decrease resistance to ejection. Narcotics also relieve ischemic pain. Increasing the oxygen concentration of inspired air is a simple but important step, but may require initiation of mechanical ventilation. Nurses need to provide physical care and periods of rest to minimize myocardial energy expenditure.

Dysrhythmias often occur with acute myocardial infarction, ischemia or acid–base imbalances and can further decrease cardiac output. Correcting these problems with antidysrhythmic agents, cardioversion, or pacing can help restore a stable heart rhythm and enhance cardiac output. The critical care nurse must obtain, follow, and carefully interpret the patient's hemodynamic parameters to achieve the goal of optimizing cardiac output without causing poor outcomes. If the goal is overshot, symptoms of pulmonary edema occur, and diuretics may be necessary.

Optimal filling pressures assist in restoring cardiac output but must be attained cautiously. As mentioned, left ventricular filling pressures may be elevated, and diuresis should be used to reduce these pressures. If the left ventricular filling pressure is too low, fluids may be used, but they must be stopped when filling pressures increase without a subsequent increase in cardiac output. In general, a preload (left ventricular end-diastolic pressure [LVEDP]) of 14 to 18 mm Hg should be maintained (see Chapter 18). Achieving an "optimal filling pressure" through the administration of fluids and diuretics is not always an easy task. Frequently, use of a pulmonary artery catheter is necessary. Slow fluid administration or diuresis requires a diligent assessment of the effectiveness of the interventions.

Pharmacological agents can be used to augment cardiac output, but they too must be used cautiously. Many agents can increase $M\dot{V}O_2$ without having an appreciable effect on cardiac output. Decisions to use some pharmacological agents are based on overall risk–benefit considerations. The sympathomimetic drugs norepinephrine and epinephrine hydrochloride may enhance cardiac output by increasing contractility, heart rate, or SVR but increase cardiac work. In addition, stimulation of $beta_2$ receptors by epinephrine may produce dilation in peripheral vascular beds that robs vital organs of blood. Therefore, this agent is used with caution. Agents with positive inotropic effects that have little activity on vascular tone, such as low-dose dopamine hydrochloride, dobutamine hydrochloride, amrinone lactate, and milrinone, are used more frequently with favorable results. Table 54-2 lists pharmacological agents used in the treatment of patients in shock states.

table 54-2 Pharmacologic Agents Used in the Treatment of Shock*

Drug Category	Heart Rate	Effects on Contractility	Systemic Venous Resistance	Nursing Considerations
Vasoconstrictors				
Dopamine (Intropin)	↑	↑↑	↑	Hemodynamic effects are dose dependent
Epinephrine (Adrenaline)	↑↑	↑↑	↑	May induce ventricular dysrhythmias May exacerbate $M\dot{V}O_2$ demands $Beta_2$ activity may dilate peripheral beds
Norepinephrine (also known as levarterenol [Levophed])	↑	↑	↑↑↑	Monitor peripheral circulation closely; may increase $M\dot{V}O_2$
Phenylephrine (Neo-synephrine)			↑↑	May induce dysrhythmias
Vasopressin (Pitressin)		↑	↑↑	Monitor peripheral circulation closely; may increase $M\dot{V}O_2$
Vasodilators				
Sodium nitroprusside (Nipride)	↑		↓↓	Hemodynamic effects are dose dependent; adjust dosage slowly
Nitroglycerine (Tridil)	↑		↓	Hemodynamic effects are dose dependent; adjust dosage slowly; tolerance may develop
Angiotensin-converting enzyme (ACE) inhibitors	↑		↓	
Inotropic Agents				
Amrinone (Inocor)	↑	↑	↓	May exacerbate $M\dot{V}O_2$ demands
Milrinone (Primacor)	↑	↑↑	↓	May exacerbate $M\dot{V}O_2$ demands Monitor for tachyarrhythmias
Dobutamine (Dobutrex)	↑	↑↑	↓	May exacerbate $M\dot{V}O_2$ demands Monitor for tachyarrhythmias

$M\dot{V}O_2$, myocardial oxygen consumption.
*All agents should be administered through a great vein (central access) and using a volumetric pump.

Decreasing the workload of the left ventricle can be accomplished through pharmacological afterload reduction or mechanical support devices. Vasodilators, such as sodium nitroprusside, nitroglycerin, or angiotensin-converting enzyme inhibitors, reduce SVR and, consequently, LVEDP. This produces an increase in the cardiac output and improved left ventricular function. Mechanical support for the failing ventricle includes the intra-aortic balloon pump and left ventricular assist device. Both devices reduce the workload of the left ventricle by supplementing pumping ability.

New therapies that involve invasive cardiac procedures, such as percutaneous transluminal coronary angioplasty, thrombolytic therapy, stent placement, and rotoblade therapy, are designed to expedite revascularization. The earlier these procedures are performed, the greater the survival rate. (See Chapter 18 for discussion of these management modalities.)

ANAPHYLACTIC SHOCK

Anaphylaxis results from an allergic reaction to a specific allergen that evokes a life-threatening hypersensitivity response. If left untreated, vascular collapse occurs, resulting in greatly decreased tissue perfusion. Prompt intervention is critical. Predisposing factors, such as age, sex, race, occupation, allergic tendencies, or geographical location, do not seem to play a role in development of anaphylaxis.

Etiology

Antigens, the substances that elicit the response, can be introduced through injection or ingestion, or through the skin or respiratory tract. Substances capable of evoking anaphylaxis in humans include a multitude of factors (Box 54-5).

Anaphylaxis may be either immunoglobulin E (IgE) or non-IgE mediated. Non-IgE responses occur without the presence of IgE antibodies and are called *anaphylactoid reactions*. It is thought that direct activation of mediators causes this response. Anaphylactoid reactions are commonly associated with nonsteroidal anti-inflammatory drugs (NSAIDs), including aspirin. If there has been an anaphylactoid reaction to one agent, restrictions should include all NSAIDs because any of them could elicit a second reaction.

IgE-mediated anaphylaxis occurs as a result of the immune response to a specific antigen. The first time the immune system is exposed to the antigen, a very specific IgE antibody is formed and circulates in the blood. When a second exposure to this antigen occurs, the antigen binds to this circulating IgE, which then activates mast cells and basophils, triggering release of histamine, prostaglandins, leukotrienes, and other biochemical mediators that initiate anaphylaxis.

Pathophysiology

The antibody–antigen reaction causes antibody-specific mast cells and basophils to secrete substances such as histamine, leukotrienes, eosinophil chemotactic substance, heparin, prostaglandins, neutrophil chemotactic substance, and platelet-activating factor[2] (Fig. 54-5). These substances, particularly histamine, prostaglandins, and leukotrienes, cause systemic vasodilation, increased capillary permeability, bronchoconstriction, coronary vasoconstriction, and urticaria (hives). Some of the other substances precipitate a continued downward spiral by causing myocardial depression, inflammation, excessive mucus secretion, and peripheral vasodilation. The diffuse arterial vasodilation creates a maldistribution of blood volume to tissues, and venous dilation decreases preload, decreasing cardiac output. Increased capillary permeability leads to loss of vascular volume, further decreasing cardiac output and subsequently impairing tissue perfusion. Initial symptoms include itching, urticaria, and some difficulty breathing due to bronchoconstriction. Death due to circulatory collapse or extreme bronchoconstriction may occur within minutes or hours.

box 54-5 ***Agents Commonly Implicated in Anaphylactic and Anaphylactoid Reactions***

Antibiotics	Penicillin and its synthetics, cephalosporins, erythromycin, streptomycin, tetracyclines
Anti-inflammatory agents	Salicylates, aminopyrine, ibuprofen, naproxen, and others
Narcotic analgesics	Morphine, codeine
Other medications	Protamine, chlorpropamide, parenteral iron, iodides, thiazide diuretics
Anesthetics	Procaine, lidocaine, cocaine, thiopental
Anesthetic adjuncts	Succinylcholine, tubocurarine
Blood products	Red blood cell, white blood cell, and platelet transfusions; gamma globulin
Immune sera	Rabies, tetanus, diphtheria antitoxin, snake and spider antivenom
Diagnostic agents	Iodinated radiocontrast agents
Venoms	Bees, wasps, hornets, spiders, snakes, jellyfish
Hormones	Insulin, corticotropin, pituitary extract
Enzymes and other biologicals	Acetylcysteine, pancreatic enzyme supplements
Extracts used in desensitization	Food, pollen, venoms
Foods	Eggs, fish, shellfish, milk, nuts, legumes
Textiles	Latex

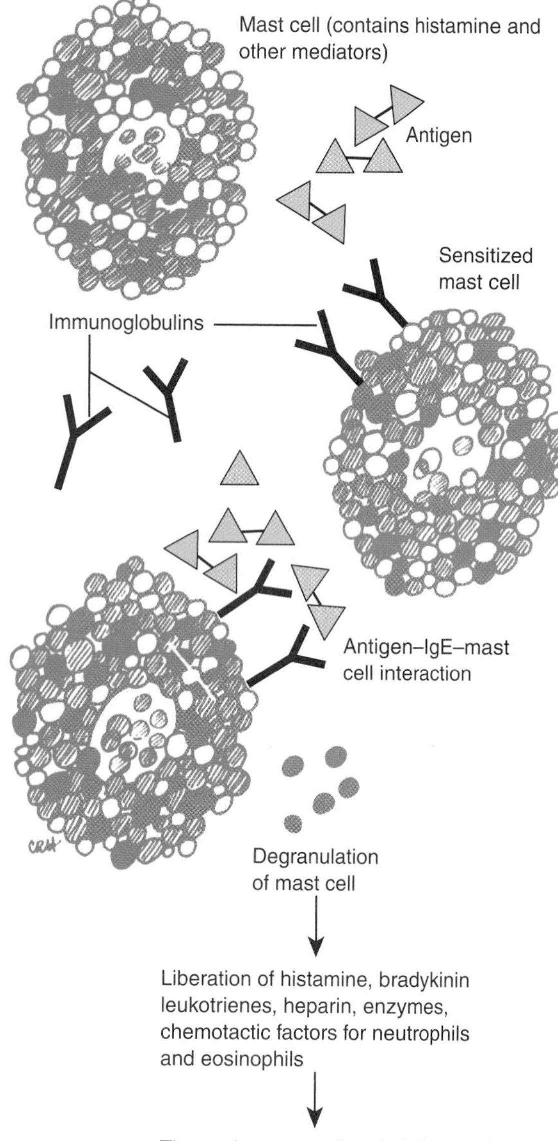

figure 54-5 Inflammatory/immune response: type 1 IgE-mediated hypersensitivity reaction. (From Porth CM: Pathophysiology: Concepts of Altered Health States [6th Ed], p 367. Philadelphia, Lippincott Williams & Wilkins, 2002.)

Assessment

HISTORY

Avoiding known allergens is usually the best way to prevent anaphylactic shock. It is necessary to obtain a thorough history of allergies and responses to drugs, foods, blood products, or anesthetic agents. Anaphylactic shock may have no predisposing factors. Thus, it is important to recognize the various clinical presentations.

PHYSICAL FINDINGS

Generalized erythema, urticaria, pruritus, and subsequent angioedema may occur. The earlier the symptoms appear after exposure to the antigen, the more severe the response. Later symptoms may include anxiety and restlessness, dyspnea, wheezing, a warm feeling, and even pain. As the episode progresses, severe respiratory manifestations, such as laryngeal edema or severe bronchoconstriction with stridor, may develop. Hypotension from vasodilation soon occurs and leads to circulatory collapse. As circulatory collapse or hypoxia due to severe bronchoconstriction progresses, the level of consciousness deteriorates to unresponsiveness.

Management

Early recognition and treatment of anaphylaxis is essential. Therapeutic goals include removal of the offending antigen, reversal of effects of the biochemical mediators, and restoration of adequate tissue perfusion. Regardless of the cause of the anaphylactic reaction, treatment depends on clinical symptoms. If the symptoms are mild, immediate therapy includes oxygen and subcutaneous or IV administration of an antihistamine, such as diphenhydramine, to block the effects of histamine, and possibly an epinephrine injection to reverse the vasodilation and bronchoconstriction (Box 54-6). Other pharmacotherapy includes corticosteroids, bronchodilators, and, if necessary, vasoconstrictors and positive inotropic agents to combat circulatory collapse.

Nursing care involves maintaining an adequate airway and monitoring patient response to the antigen. The nurse also monitors respirations, heart rate, blood pressure, and level of anxiety, and institutes comfort measures related to the dermatological manifestations. Patient education regarding prevention and treatment is critical for any person who experiences a significant anaphylactic or anaphylactoid reaction.

NEUROGENIC SHOCK

Neurogenic shock results from loss or disruption of sympathetic tone, which causes peripheral vasodilation and subsequent decreased tissue perfusion. The disturbance of sympathetic tone may be caused by any event that disrupts the sympathetic nervous system. The most common cause of neurogenic shock is a spinal cord injury above the level of T6. Other causes include spinal analgesia, emotional stress, pain, drugs, or other central nervous system problems. (Refer to Chapter 37 for a thorough discussion of spinal cord injury and neurogenic shock.)

box 54-6
Epinephrine Dosage in Anaphylaxis

- Adults—0.5 mL of a 1:1,000 solution intramuscularly or 3–5 mL of a 1:10,000 solution intramuscularly or slowly intravenously
- Children—0.01 mL of a 1:1,000 solution per kg intramuscularly or 0.1 mL of a 1:10,000 solution per kg intravenously

The dosage is not one ampoule

Fisher M: Treatment of acute anaphylaxis. Br Med J 311:731–734, 1995 (used with permission)

SEPTIC SHOCK

Septic shock is a complex and generalized process that involves all organ systems. Sepsis, severe sepsis, and septic shock represent progressive stages of the same illness. In 1991, the Society of Critical Care Medicine and the American College of Chest Physicians established universal definitions for the term *sepsis* and other associated clinical conditions.[6] These organizations wished to promote earlier detection of and intervention for these states, improve outcomes, and standardize the terminology used in research protocols to make the information derived easier to disseminate and apply to practice. In 2002, a second consensus conference was held to modify the existing definitions for accuracy, reliability, and clinical utility of the diagnosis of sepsis[7,8] (Box 54-7).

Etiology

In the United States, there are approximately 750,000 new episodes of sepsis each year and an associated 200,000 deaths.[9] Estimated annual costs of treatment exceed $16 billion.[9] In patients in the intensive care unit (ICU), sepsis has the highest incidence of any other major disease, including congestive heart failure, breast and colon cancer, trauma, and acquired immunodeficiency syndrome (AIDS).[10] The same factors that increase the risk of hypoperfusion may increase the risk of septic shock, and certain invasive therapies and medical devices also increase this risk (Box 54-8). The high incidence of sepsis may reflect an increased number of resistant microorganisms; a heightened awareness and rate of diagnosis; an increased number of aging individuals; and a growing number of chronically ill or immunocompromised patients,[11] who live longer because of improved medical therapy but have greater risk for sepsis.

Septic shock is initiated by an infection. Infections may be due to invading gram-negative or gram-positive bacteria, fungi, and viruses. In many patients, multiple causative organisms are identified. Bacteria may be introduced either through the pulmonary system, urinary tract, or gastrointestinal system; through wounds; or through invasive devices. Both gram-negative and gram-positive organisms may directly stimulate the inflammatory response and other aspects of the immune system that activate cytokines, complement, and coagulation systems.

Pathophysiology

In sepsis, cytokines are released from white blood cells (WBCs) and other cells in response to an infection to protect from additional injury and to begin the healing process. Cytokines are proteins that regulate numerous functions

box 54-7
Clinical Terminology: Sepsis and Organ Failure

Definitions developed by the Consensus Conferences of the Society of Critical Care Medicine and American College of Chest Physicians.

Bacteremia: The presence of viable bacteria in the blood.

Hypotension: A systolic blood pressure of <90 mm Hg or a reduction of >40 mm Hg from baseline in the absence of other causes for hypotension.

Infection: Microbial phenomenon characterized by an inflammatory response to the presence of microorganisms or the invasion of normally sterile host tissue by those organisms.

Multiple organ dysfunction syndrome: Presence of altered organ function in an acutely ill patient such that homeostasis cannot be maintained without intervention.

Sepsis: The systemic response to infection. This systemic response is manifested by two or more of the following conditions as a result of infection:

- Temperature >38°C or <36°C (100.4°F or 96.8°F)
- Heart rate >90 beats/minute
- Respiratory rate >20 breaths/minute or $Paco_2$ <32 mm Hg (<4.3 kPa)
- WBC count >12,000 cells/mm³, <4,000 cells/mm³, or >10% immature (band) forms

The **PIRO mnemonic** may be used to diagnose and track the progression of sepsis:

- **P**atient predisposition and response to infection based on genetics
- **I**nfection
- **R**esponse to inflammation
- **O**rgan dysfunction

Severe sepsis: Sepsis associated with organ dysfunction, hypoperfusion, or hypotension. Hypoperfusion and perfusion abnormalities may include, but are not limited to, lactic acidosis, oliguria, or an acute alteration in mental status.

Septic shock: Sepsis with hypotension, despite adequate fluid resuscitation, along with the presence of perfusion abnormalities that may include, but are not limited to, lactic acidosis, oliguria, or an acute alteration in mental status. Patients who are on inotropic or vasopressor agents may not be hypotensive at the time that perfusion abnormalities are measured.

Systemic inflammatory response syndrome: The systemic inflammatory response to a variety of severe clinical insults. The response is manifested by two or more of the following conditions:

- Temperature >38°C or <36°C (>100.4°F or <96.8°F)
- Heart rate >90 beats/minute
- Respiratory rate >20 breaths/minute or $Paco_2$ <32 mm Hg (<4.3 kPa)
- WBC count >12,000 cell/mm³, <4,000 cells/mm³, or >10% immature (band) forms

Adapted from Levy MM: Definitions of sepsis revisited: Results of the SSSM/ESICM/ACCP/ATS consensus conference. In Levy MM, Vincent JL (eds): Sepsis: Pathophysiologic Insights and Current Management, pp 39–42. Chicago, Society of Critical Care Medicine, 2003.

box 54-8 ***Risk Factors for Hypoperfused States***

Host Factors

- Extremes of age
- Malnutrition
- General debilitation
- Chronic debilitation
- Chronic illness
- Drug or alcohol abuse
- Neutropenia
- Splenectomy
- Multiple organ failure

Treatment-Related Factors

- Use of invasive catheters
- Surgical procedures
- Traumatic or thermal wounds
- Invasive diagnostic procedures
- Drugs (antibiotics, cytotoxic agents, steroids)

of the inflammatory response.[10] Cytokines account for the signs and symptoms seen early in the infective process; they promote vasodilation and hypotension, increased capillary permeability, fever, and decreased myocardial contractility.

Neutrophils are released from the bone marrow as part of the inflammatory response, adhere to vessel walls in the area of the infection, exit the circulation by diapedesis, and travel through tissues to the site of infection. They release cytokines that increase the inflammatory response and enzymes that destroy invading organisms. Unfortunately, these enzymes can also damage vascular endothelial linings.[9–11] This in turn increases the inflammatory response due to vessel damage, and the damaged endothelial cells release more cytokines.

Bacteria and neutrophils continue to stimulate the release of inflammatory mediators such as endotoxin, interleukin-1 (IL-1) and IL-6, tumor necrosis factor (TNF), and tissue factor. Tissue factor stimulates a procoagulant state and formation of fibrin clots. Normally, this procoagulant state is counter-regulated by mediators of anticoagulation and/or fibrinolysis such as thrombin-activated fibrinolysis inhibitor, plasminogen activator inhibitor, and activated protein C (APC).[9–12] Studies have shown that APC is deficient in sepsis, and therefore the procoagulant state is not balanced by sufficient fibrinolysis. The end result is the formation of microcirculatory clots that inhibit perfusion to cells and tissues. This process is believed to be pivotal to the progression from sepsis to SIRS, MODS, and death. In sepsis, the intravascular coagulation and thrombolytic responses are out of balance (Fig. 54-6).

PERFUSION IMBALANCE

In septic shock, there is hypoperfusion of vital organs and tissue ischemia. Inflammatory mediators such as cytokines and bacterial endotoxins produce profound vasodilation and increase capillary permeability. This results in low SVR and inadequate volume in the arterial tree. In response to the decreased SVR and circulating volume, the cardiac output may be high but inadequate to maintain tissue and end-organ perfusion. Preload is not optimal because of venous dilation, further limiting the ability of the heart to produce a cardiac output adequate to maintain the blood pressure.

Activation of the sympathetic nervous system causes preferential vasoconstriction of the splanchnic circulation and vessels of the skin with dilation of skeletal muscle beds and preservation of blood flow to the heart, lungs, and brain. Increased capillary permeability causes tissue edema. Activation of the coagulation cascade by inflammatory mediators may cause microthrombi to form in multiple small vessels, which obstruct blood flow to structures distal to the thrombi. Net effects are unequal perfusion of various capillary beds with inadequate or poor blood flow in many tissues, resulting in regions of tissue hypoxia and concomitant organ damage. Inability of the circulatory system to meet cellular oxygen demands causes cells to resort to anaerobic metabolism for energy production. Lactic acid, the end product of anaerobic metabolism, is measured clinically to evaluate the effectiveness of end-organ tissue perfusion.

MYOCARDIAL ALTERATIONS

In septic shock, there is evidence of depressed myocardial performance in the form of decreased ventricular ejection fraction and impaired contractility,[13] which may be caused by circulating myocardial depressants. A proposed causative agent, myocardial depressant factor, is thought to originate from ischemic pancreatic tissue.[13] Other studies suggest that impaired coronary perfusion is at fault or that other mediators, including TNF and IL-1, may also depress cardiac contractility.[9,10,14] Lactic acidosis, which decreases myocardial responsiveness to catecholamines, may also be partly responsible. Whatever the mechanism, the heart demonstrates impaired contractility and ventricular performance.

Early in septic shock, it is believed that the heart is hyperdynamic, with high cardiac output and low SVR. However, evidence indicates that even at this stage, the heart is performing less than optimally. Later, as circulating cardiac depressants increase, the heart becomes hypodynamic, with low cardiac output and increased SVR. Hemodynamic parameters, including $cS\bar{v}O_2/S\bar{v}O_2$ and measures of metabolic acidosis, should be followed over time to recognize early and progressive cardiac failure.

PULMONARY ALTERATIONS

Events initiated by activation of the inflammatory response and its mediators affect the lungs both directly and indirectly. Activation of the sympathetic nervous system and release of epinephrine from the adrenal medulla produce bronchodilation. However, this may be overridden by activity of cytokines, and the net result is bronchoconstriction. More important, inflammatory mediators and activated neutrophils cause capillary leak into the pulmonary interstitium, resulting in interstitial edema, areas of poor pulmonary perfusion (shunting), pulmonary hypertension, and increased respiratory work. As fluid collects in the interstitium, pulmonary compliance is reduced, gas exchange is impaired, and hypoxemia occurs.

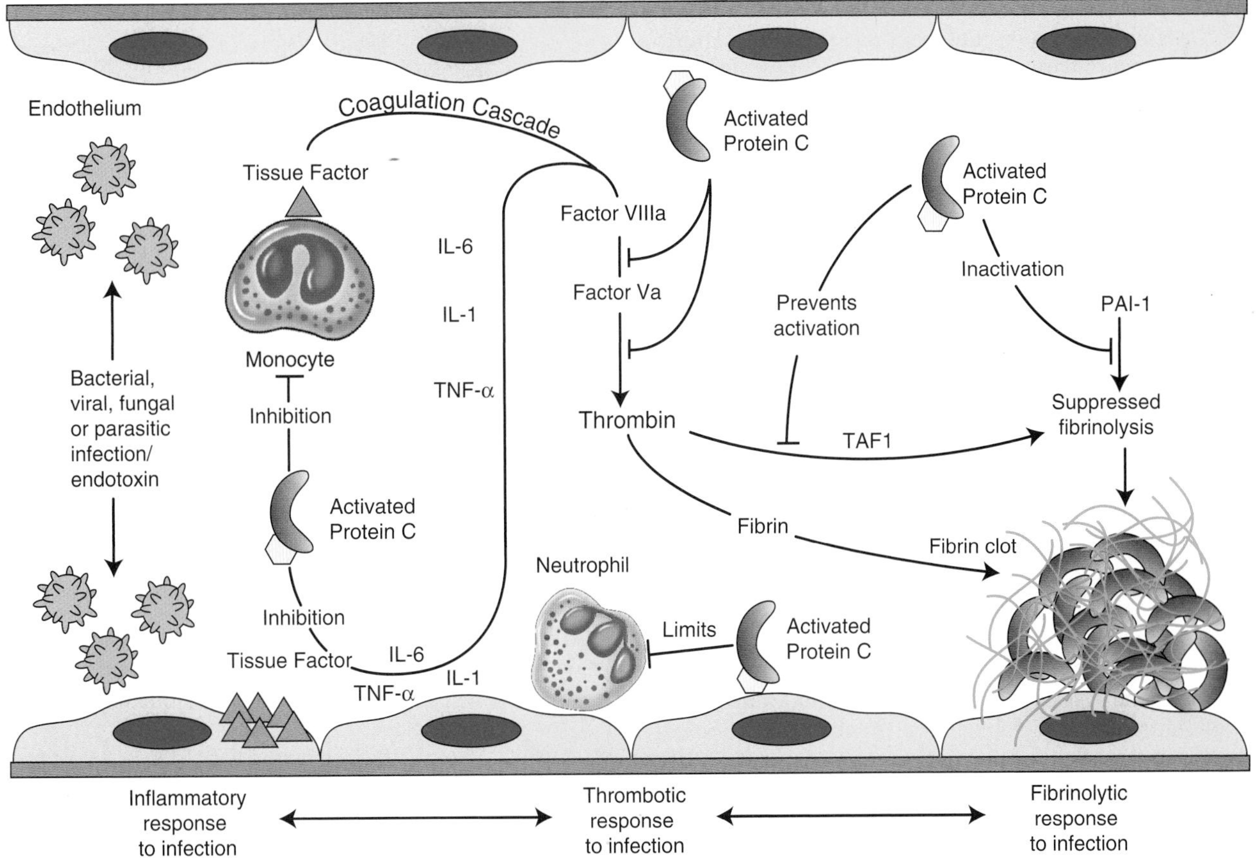

figure 54-6 Inflammatory/immune response in septic shock. *IL-1,* interleukin 1; *IL-6,* interleukin-6; *TNF-α,* tumor necrosis factor-α; *TAFI,* thrombin-activated fibrinolysis inhibitor; *PAI-1,* plasminogen activator inhibitor-1.

The pulmonary alterations described previously may culminate in acute respiratory distress syndrome (ARDS), which is frequently associated with septic shock. Forty to 60% of all patients with septic shock are at risk for ARDS. Moreover, continued fluid accumulation in the pulmonary interstitium may finally spill over into the alveoli, producing alveolar infiltrates that provide fertile areas for bacterial growth. Mechanical ventilation, which is common in patients with ARDS, may provide an avenue of entry for lung infections. Therefore, a secondary pneumonia may develop, possibly caused by a different organism than that which produced the sepsis.

HEMATOLOGICAL ALTERATIONS

Bacteria or their toxins cause activation of the complement cascade. Sepsis involves a global inflammatory response; therefore, over-reactive complement activation may contribute to responses that eventually become detrimental rather than protective. Complement causes mast cells to release histamine, which further stimulates vasodilation and increased capillary permeability. These actions further contribute to the circulatory alterations in volume distribution and the development of interstitial edema.

Platelet abnormalities also occur in septic shock because endotoxin indirectly causes platelet aggregation and subsequent release of more vasoactive substances (serotonin and thromboxane A_2). Circulating platelet aggregates have been identified in the microvasculature of septic patients. These cause obstruction to blood flow and compromised cellular metabolism. Overactivation of the coagulation cascade without the counterbalance of adequate fibrinolysis compromises tissue perfusion both regionally and globally. Over time, clotting factors are depleted and a coagulopathy results, with the potential of progressing to disseminated intravascular coagulation.

METABOLIC ALTERATIONS

Widespread metabolic disturbances are associated with septic shock. Excessive catecholamine release stimulates gluconeogenesis and insulin resistance. Cells are progressively unable to use glucose, protein, and fat as energy sources. Hyperglycemia that is resistant to insulin therapy is a frequent finding in early shock. Eventually, all glycogen energy stores are depleted, cells lack ATP, and cellular pumps fail, progressing to tissue and organ death.

In response to lack of effect of insulin, proteins break down, as shown by high blood urea nitrogen and urinary nitrogen excretion. Muscle protein is broken down to amino acids, some of which are used as energy sources for the Krebs cycle or as substrates for gluconeogenesis. In later stages of shock, the liver is unable to use the amino acids because of its own metabolic dysfunction. Amino acids then accumulate in the bloodstream.

As shock progresses, adipose tissue is broken down (lipolysis) to furnish the liver with lipids for energy production. Hepatic triglyceride metabolism produces ketones, which circulate to peripheral cells that can use them in the Krebs cycle for ATP production. However, as liver function decreases, triglycerides are not broken down and collect in the mitochondria, inhibiting the Krebs cycle and resulting in increased anaerobic metabolism and lactate production.

The net effect of these metabolic derangements is that cells become energy starved. This energy deficit is implicated in the emergence of multiple organ failure that frequently develops regardless of interventions designed to support the circulatory and organ systems.

Assessment

A thorough understanding of the mediator responses that occur during sepsis aids in the assessment and evaluation of response to treatment.

PHYSICAL FINDINGS

Some of the earliest signs of septic shock include changes in mental status (confusion or agitation), increased respiratory rate as compensation for the metabolic acidosis, and either fever or hypothermia. Because of the exaggerated inflammatory response with release of vasoactive mediators, the clinical presentation of the patient is complex. The patient is edematous yet intravascularly depleted, and areas of microthrombi and vasoconstriction obstruct perfusion. As fluid replacement occurs, the leaking capillary beds shift the fluid interstitially, requiring more fluid resuscitation, which may further exacerbate interstitial edema. Because of the inappropriate systemic activation of the coagulation system, clotting factors are depleted, and spontaneous bleeding may occur. Perfusion imbalances cause ischemia in some vascular beds, such as the splanchnic circulation, skin, and extremities, which may lead to necrosis. Cardiac output may be unusually high, but it is insufficient to maintain adequate perfusion due to circulating myocardial depressant factors. Compensatory mechanisms, such as activation of the sympathetic nervous system, continue to increase cardiac output. However, inflammatory mediators prevent necessary vasoconstriction, and the SVR remains inappropriately low, thereby perpetuating the hypoperfusion crisis.

As sepsis progresses and organ hypoperfusion persists, cells in hypoperfused organs begin to die, and the organs begin to fail. This may lead to MODS.

LABORATORY STUDIES

Laboratory and diagnostic studies that may be helpful in the identification of sepsis are summarized in Box 54-9. Despite the use of such testing, the early diagnosis of sepsis and septic shock is usually made on the basis of patient risk factors and clinical findings (see Box 54-7).

box 54-9
Physiological Data Helpful in Diagnosing Sepsis

- Cultures: blood, sputum, urine, surgical or nonsurgical wounds, sinuses, and invasive lines; positive results are not necessary for diagnosis.
- CBC: WBCs usually will be elevated and may decrease with progression of shock.
- Sequential multiple analysis-7 (SMA-7): hyperglycemia may be evident, followed by hypoglycemia in later stages.
- Arterial blood gases: metabolic acidosis with possibly compensating respiratory alkalosis ($Paco_2$ <35 mm Hg) is present in sepsis, with mild hypoxemia (Pao_2 <80 mm Hg)
- CT scan may be needed to identify sites of potential abscesses.
- Chest and abdominal radiographs may reveal infectious processes.
- $S\bar{v}o_2$ pulmonary artery catheter will assist in the assessment of oxygen delivery and consumption needs of the tissues and cells.
- Lactate level: decreasing levels of lactate in the serum indicates aerobic metabolism is able to meet cellular energy requirements. Elevated levels indicate inadequate perfusion and anaerobic metabolism to meet cellular energy requirements.
- Base deficit: elevated levels indicate inadequate perfusion and anaerobic metabolism.
- $ETco_2$: may detect early indications of inadequate regional and global tissue perfusion

Management

Septic shock requires a prompt, aggressive, multidisciplinary team approach with monitoring and treatment facilities found in an ICU. The primary goals of treatment are to maximize oxygen delivery above cellular oxygen consumption requirements and to halt the exaggerated inflammatory response. The collaborative care guide in Box 54-10 outlines some of the care given in septic shock.

PREVENTION

Because diagnosis of sepsis is so complex and mortality from septic shock so high, it is imperative that preventive infection control measures be in place. Defense mechanisms may be impaired, and protection from hospital-acquired (nosocomial) infections is essential. The estimated cost of treating nosocomial infections is nearly $5 billion dollars per year.[15] Therefore, a critical aspect of nursing care involves adherence to aseptic techniques, thorough handwashing, and a continuing awareness of multiple sites and causes of infection. Sources of equipment-related infections are listed in Box 54-11.

IDENTIFICATION AND TREATMENT OF INFECTION

Identification of the infecting organism and use of appropriate antibiotic treatment are of utmost importance. Before the causal organism has been identified, empiric broad-spectrum antibiotic therapy is initiated, usually with multiple antibiotics with coverage against gram-negative and gram-positive bacteria and anaerobes. However, once the infectious organism has been isolated,

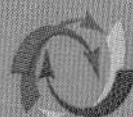

box 54-10 collaborative care guide *for the Patient in Septic Shock*

OUTCOMES	INTERVENTIONS
Oxygenation/Ventilation	
Patent airway is maintained. Lungs are clear on auscultation.	■ Auscultate breath sounds q2–4h and PRN. ■ Suction endotracheal airway when appropriate (see Collaborative Care Guide for Patient on Mechanical Ventilation, Chapter 25, Box 25-7). ■ Hyperoxygenate and hyperventilate before and after each suction pass.
Arterial blood gases are within normal limits.	■ Monitor pulse oximetry and end tidal CO_2 ($ETCO_2$). ■ Monitor arterial blood gases as indicated by changes in noninvasive parameters. ■ Monitor intrapulmonary shunt ($\dot{Q}s/\dot{Q}t$ and Pao_2/Fio_2)
Peak, mean, and plateau pressures are within normal limits.	■ Monitor airway pressures q1–2h.
There is no evidence of atelectasis or infiltrates.	■ Turn side to side q2h. ■ Consider kinetic therapy.
There is no evidence of acute respiratory distress syndrome (ARDS).	■ Do daily chest x-ray (see Collaborative Care Guide for Patient with ARDS, Chapter 27).
Circulation/Perfusion	
Blood pressure, heart rate, central venous pressure (CVP), and pulmonary artery pressures are within normal limits.	■ Assess vital signs q1h. ■ Assess hemodynamic pressures q1h if patient has pulmonary artery catheter. ■ Administer intravascular volume as ordered to maintain preload.
Vascular resistance is within normal limits.	■ Assess SVR and peripheral venous resistance (PVR) q6–12h. ■ Administer intravascular volume and vasopressors as ordered.
Oxygen delivery is >600 mL O_2/m^2 and oxygen consumption is >150 mL O_2/m^2.	■ Monitor cardiac output, Dao_2, and $\dot{V}o_2$ q6–12h. ■ Administer red blood cells, positive inotropic agents, colloid infusion as ordered to increase oxygen delivery. ■ Consider monitoring gastric mucosal pH as a guide to systemic perfusion.
Serum lactate will be within normal limits.	■ Monitor serum lactate qd until it is within normal limits.
Fluids/Electrolytes	
Urine output is >30 mL/h (or >0.5 mL/kg/h).	■ Monitor intake and output q1h. ■ Administer fluids and diuretics to maintain intravascular volume and renal function, per order.
There is no evidence of electrolyte imbalance or renal dysfunction.	■ Monitor electrolytes daily and PRN. ■ Replace electrolytes as ordered. ■ Monitor blood urea nitrogen (BUN), creatinine, serum osmolality, and urine electrolytes daily.
Mobility/Safety	
There is no evidence of complications related to bed rest and immobility.	■ Initiate deep vein thrombosis prophylaxis. ■ Reposition frequently. ■ Mobilize to chair when acute phase is past, and hemodynamic stability and hemostasis are achieved. ■ Consult physical therapist. ■ Conduct range-of-motion and strengthening exercises.

(continued)

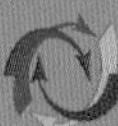

box 54-10 collaborative care guide for the Patient in Septic Shock (Continued)

OUTCOMES	INTERVENTIONS
Normalization of temperature and WBC and negative blood cultures as evidence that source and microorganisms causing sepsis are obliterated.	■ Identify source of infection: obtain urine, sputum, and blood cultures; central vascular line tip cultures; wound cultures. ■ Administer antibiotics as directed by culture results. ■ Monitor serum antibiotic levels. ■ Obtain infectious disease consult. ■ Monitor systemic inflammatory response syndrome criteria: increased WBCs, increased temperature, tachypnea, tachycardia.
There is no evidence of new infection.	■ Use strict aseptic technique during procedures, and monitor technique of others. ■ Maintain sterility of invasive catheters and tubes. ■ Per hospital protocol, change chest tube and other dressings and invasive catheters.
Skin Integrity	
Skin will remain intact.	■ Assess skin q4h and each time patient is repositioned. ■ Turn q2h. ■ Consider pressure relief/reduction mattress. ■ Use Braden Scale to assess risk of skin breakdown.
Nutrition	
Caloric and nutrient intake meet metabolic requirements per calculation (e.g., basal energy expenditure).	■ Provide parenteral or enteral nutrition within 24 h of onset. ■ Consult dietitian or nutritional support service. ■ Monitor lipid intake. ■ Monitor albumin, prealbumin, transferrin, cholesterol, triglycerides, glucose.
Comfort/Pain Control	
Patient will be as comfortable as possible as evidenced by stable vital signs or cooperation with treatments or procedures.	■ Objectively assess comfort/pain using a pain scale. ■ Provide analgesia and sedation as indicated by assessment. ■ Monitor patient's cardiopulmonary and pain response to medication.
Psychosocial	
Patient demonstrates decreased anxiety.	■ Assess vital signs during treatments, discussions, and so forth. ■ Cautiously administer sedatives. ■ Consult social services, clergy, and so forth as appropriate. ■ Provide for adequate rest and sleep.
Teaching/Discharge Planning	
Patient/significant others understand procedures and tests needed for treatment.	■ Prepare patient/significant others for procedures, such as pulmonary artery catheter insertion, blood cultures, intubation, and mechanical ventilation.
Significant others understand the severity of the illness, ask appropriate questions, anticipate potential complications.	■ Explain the causes and effects of sepsis and the potential for complications, such as ARDS or renal failure and MODS. ■ Encourage significant others to ask questions related to the ventilator, pathophysiology, monitoring, treatments, and so forth.

box 54-11 ***Equipment-Related Sources of Infections***

Intravascular catheters
Endotracheal/tracheostomy tubes
Indwelling urinary catheters
Surgical wound drains
Intracranial monitoring devices and catheters
Orthopedic hardware
Nasogastric tubes
Gastrointestinal tubes

antibiotic therapy should be changed so specific antibiotics that are effective against that organism are used to try to minimize development of antibiotic resistance.[15] Other definitive measures to alleviate the cause of sepsis might include resection or drainage of purulent tissues or secretions.

However, antimicrobial treatment of sepsis is not sufficient to treat the generalized inflammatory reactions seen with septic shock. Supportive measures establish and maintain adequate tissue perfusion, and other therapies aim to block or interfere with the action of the various mediators implicated in shock. Aspects of supportive care include the following:

- Restoring intravascular volume
- Maintaining an adequate cardiac output
- Ensuring adequate ventilation and oxygenation
- Restoring balance between coagulation and anticoagulation
- Providing an appropriate metabolic environment

RESTORATION OF INTRAVASCULAR VOLUME

Adequate volume replacement is important for reversing hypotension. Patients may require several liters or more of fluid because of mediator-induced vasodilation and capillary leak. Fluid replacement should be guided by hemodynamic parameters, urine output, and indicators of metabolic acidosis ($ETCO_2$, base deficit, lactic acid levels). Patients usually require pulmonary artery and arterial catheterization for close monitoring. Invasive catheters that also monitor venous oxygen saturation ($cS\bar{v}O_2$ or $S\bar{v}O_2$) are helpful in guiding fluid resuscitation.[16] A downward trend in the markers of metabolic acidosis is a good indicator of improvement in tissue perfusion.

The use of crystalloid or colloid fluids for fluid replacement is controversial in clinical practice (see Management, Hypovolemic Shock). The underlying condition and response to fluid administration help determine which fluids should be used. Blood products may be administered even in the absence of bleeding to enhance the delivery of oxygen to cells. Administering the fluid and closely monitoring the response to fluid therapy are important nursing responsibilities (see Box 54-10).

MAINTENANCE OF ADEQUATE CARDIAC OUTPUT

In the early phase of septic shock, cardiac output may be normal or elevated. However, the cardiac output is not adequate to maintain tissue oxygenation and perfusion because of decreased SVR and peripheral vasodilation. As septic shock progresses, cardiac output begins to decrease because of cardiac dysfunction. Therefore, maintenance of cardiac output is an essential therapeutic goal.

If adequate volume replacement does not improve tissue perfusion, vasoactive drugs are administered to support circulation. Low-dose dopamine, which increases SVR and improves renal and mesenteric blood flow, may be used. Dobutamine or milrinone may be added for its inotropic effects on the heart. Vasoconstricting drugs frequently used include levarterenol (norepinephrine [Levophed]), epinephrine, vasopressin, and phenylephrine (Neo-Synephrine). Some patients with low cardiac output and high SVR may benefit from the use of vasodilators such as nitroprusside (Nipride) to redistribute blood flow and improve perfusion. Often, no single drug can achieve the desired hemodynamic effects. In these situations, various combinations of drugs are individualized to the patient's response. The nurse's role is to administer the drugs, usually titrating the dosage to a desired response or effect, and closely monitor the patient for response and potentially harmful side effects (see Box 54-10).

MAINTENANCE OF ADEQUATE VENTILATION AND OXYGENATION

Maintaining a patent airway, augmenting ventilation, and ensuring adequate oxygenation in the patient with septic shock usually require endotracheal intubation and mechanical ventilation. Because of the ARDS-like picture, positive end-expiratory pressure frequently is necessary to aid oxygenation (for nursing management issues on ventilation, see Chapter 25).

Assessment of circulatory support, ventilation, and oxygenation is essential. The patient's DaO_2 and $\dot{V}O_2$ needs should be evaluated frequently. The goal is to maximize DaO_2 to ensure that $\dot{V}O_2$ remains independent of DaO_2. Aerobic metabolism is maintained, and tissue energy needs are satisfied through the delivery of adequate oxygen to the cells.

RESTORATION OF BALANCE BETWEEN COAGULATION AND ANTICOAGULATION

There has been intense investigation of drugs aimed directly at the bacterial toxins and mediators implicated in the inflammatory response seen in sepsis and SIRS. Recently, the U.S. Food and Drug Administration approved drotrecogin alfa (activated) (Xigris). This agent reestablishes homeostasis of coagulation and fibrinolysis that is lost in septic shock states (see Fig. 54-6), and research has shown that it reduces morbidity and mortality in patients with severe sepsis.[12] Further studies will evaluate the best use of this agent.

MAINTENANCE OF APPROPRIATE METABOLIC ENVIRONMENT

The many and varied metabolic derangements associated with septic shock necessitate frequent monitoring of hematological, renal, and hepatic function. Nutritional stores are depleted, and the patient requires supplemental nutrition to prevent malnutrition and to optimize cellular function. Enteral nutrition is the preferred route of nutritional support because it maintains the integrity of the gastrointestinal tract, decreases infection, and decreases length of stay and days of mechanical ventilation.[17] Intolerance of enteral feeding may necessitate the use of total parenteral nutrition (TPN), but, ideally, a small amount of enteral nutrition can still be delivered. Recent research suggests that specific nutrients typically found in enteral nutrition and some in TPN may help support the immune system during states of stress. Essential nutrients for immune support include glutamine and arginine.[18] (See Chapter 40 for a discussion of nutritional support.)

FEATURES COMMON TO ALL SHOCK STATES

Although shock states have different causes and different presentations, researchers have gradually concluded that some features, such as hypoperfusion, hypercoagulability, and activation of the inflammatory response, are common to all shock states. Moreover, it has become clear that once a shock state develops, the subsequent course may have more to do with the physiological response to shock, including activation of the sympathetic nervous system, the inflammatory response, and the immune system, rather than with the initial cause of the shock. These findings have led to a unified theory of shock as a derangement of compensatory mechanisms that results in further circulatory and respiratory hypofunction with subsequent multiple organ damage.

STAGES OF SHOCK

Shock is believed to progress through three increasingly severe stages, the last of which cannot be reversed by known means. It is difficult to determine the stage of shock in a particular individual at a particular time for three reasons: (1) shock has diverse causes, (2) the exact time of onset is unknown in many cases, and (3) there is a lack of diagnostic tests that give a clear-cut measurement of the extent of shock at a given time. Nevertheless, the stages are useful because they allow shock to be viewed as a progressive, rather than a static, process.

In the initial, nonprogressive stage (stage 1), the previously described compensatory mechanisms are effective in maintaining relatively normal vital signs and cerebral perfusion. During stage 1, shock is poorly diagnosed and frequently goes unrecognized. However, if the cause of the shock is successfully treated at this time, the patient may make a full recovery.

In the intermediate, progressive phase (stage 2), compensatory mechanisms that maintain normal perfusion begin to fail, metabolic and circulatory derangements become more pronounced, and activation of the inflammatory and immune responses may become fully developed. At this point, interventions that target both the cause of the shock and the resultant metabolic, circulatory, and inflammatory responses may result in salvage of the patient. At this time, signs of failure in one or more organs may become apparent.

In the final, irreversible stage (stage 3), cellular and tissue injury is so severe that even if metabolic, circulatory, and inflammatory derangements are corrected, life is not sustainable. At this point, full-blown MODS may become evident.

SYSTEMIC INFLAMMATORY RESPONSE SYNDROME

Assessment of the severity of shock is often difficult (see Stages of Shock). It has become clear that progressive shock states involve systemic activation of the inflammatory response, with resultant damage to tissues and organs. Efforts have been made to identify patients in whom this systemic reaction is occurring, with the thought that prompt, effective intervention might prevent progression of the shock to the irreversible stage. The term *systemic inflammatory response syndrome* (SIRS) has been developed to describe patients in whom the inflammatory response is fully and systemically activated, no matter what the underlying cause of shock.

Etiology

SIRS is defined by inclusion and exclusion criteria because there are many causes of shock and no definitive diagnostic tests (see Box 54-7). Patients who meet these criteria do not have a new disease. Rather, they have reached a particular point in the continuum of shock. SIRS may frequently occur in patients with septic shock, but it may be caused by any type of shock. Moreover, in cases of SIRS that occur as the result of progression of septic shock, the infecting organism may be undetectable by the time SIRS is identified because of previous antibiotic therapy. Therefore, blood cultures are negative in many patients. SIRS should be suspected in any patient with shock or any condition that might lead to shock (Fig. 54-7).

Pathophysiology

Normally, the inflammatory response is an essential, tightly regulated, and controlled protective mechanism of *local* response to invasion by microorganisms or to *local* tissue damage. In response to mediators released by injured tissue, such as TNF-α or IL-1, blood vessels dilate and become leaky, discharging coagulation factors and fibrinogen into the immediate area and resulting in local activation of the coagulation cascade. Fibrin, the end product of the coagulation cascade, walls off the area and isolates it from the rest of the body. Mediators also attract phagocytic WBCs to the area and activate the complement cascade. The combination of activity of WBCs and complement proteins may result in elimination of the invading microorganism.

The endothelial cells that line blood vessels are central players in the development of a local inflammatory response. Important functions of endothelial cells include providing an anticoagulant surface and controlling permeability of vessels.[10] In a local inflammatory response, endothelial cells near the site of inflammation become activated as a result of mediators released by injured tissue cells. The activated endothelial cells express cell surface proteins that attract platelets and neutrophils. A procoagulant endothelial surface is formed in the area. WBCs, platelets, and

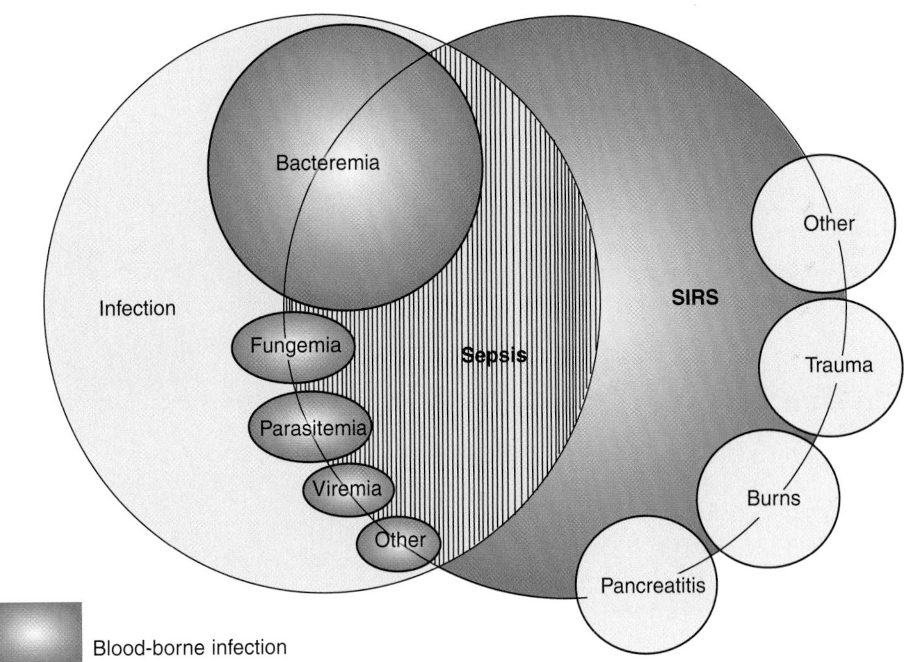

figure 54-7 The interrelationship between systemic inflammatory response syndrome (SIRS), sepsis, and infection.

activated endothelial cells themselves release vasodilating compounds such as nitric oxide, histamine, and bradykinin. These compounds and other substances also promote leakiness of local vessels, resulting in local extravasation of plasma with coagulation factors.

In SIRS, the inflammatory response is *systemic;* it occurs throughout the body. The result is overwhelming, unregulated inflammation with uncontrolled coagulation, widespread leakiness of vessels with maldistribution of circulating volume, and unbalanced oxygen supply and demand. Endothelial cells become activated in many vessels throughout the body, resulting in widespread extravasation of fluid into the interstitial compartment and systemic activation of the immune system and coagulation cascade. There is substantial extravascular fluid accumulation and widespread microthrombi in vessels and in the interstitium. The combination of intravascular coagulation and low circulating volume results in decreased perfusion of vital organs, increasing the likelihood of MODS and death.

Events surrounding the complex interactions of the mediators of SIRS remain an active area of clinical research. Several mediators are believed to play a key role in the maldistribution of blood flow and oxygen delivery and consumption imbalance associated with SIRS and sepsis. Table 54-3 lists these key mediators and summarizes their activity.

Management of SIRS is similar to that of septic shock. Therapies are aimed at tissue perfusion and adequate oxygenation.

MULTIPLE ORGAN DYSFUNCTION SYNDROME

MODS represents another point in the continuum of shock. MODS is a consequence of the inability to maintain end-organ perfusion and oxygenation, resulting in injury and organ failure (inability of an organ to maintain function). For example, the inability of the pulmonary system to oxygenate the blood adequately through ventilation and gas exchange is considered pulmonary failure.

Etiology

Overall, MODS has an associated mortality rate up to 75%[10] and may be responsible for up to 80% of ICU deaths. Table 54-4 gives the mortality rate from MODS according to the number of organ systems involved.

The etiology of MODS is unknown. Systemic inflammatory mediators found in SIRS (see Table 54-3) may play a role in the etiology of MODS. In addition, a loss of integrity of mucosal barrier function may liberate bacterial toxins from the gut. These toxins circulate systemically, damaging multiple organs. Finally, tissue hypoxia caused by microvascular thromboses probably also contributes to MODS.

Pathophysiology

Damage to organs may be primary or secondary and cause organ failure. A primary insult refers to a direct injury to an organ that results in organ dysfunction. For example, severe blunt chest trauma injures the lungs and may cause ARDS. Secondary insult is due to mechanisms operable in shock states. For example, a wound infection may cause sepsis, but the resultant septic shock or SIRS may cause ARDS. (ARDS is discussed in Chapter 27.) Typically, the first organs to manifest signs of dysfunction are the lungs, heart, and kidneys. Liver failure tends to occur later because the liver has a considerable compensatory capacity. If the shock state persists, eventually all vital organs fail, and death occurs. It is paramount that interventions increase end-organ perfusion and oxygenation and lessen the inflammatory response during the clinical management of shock states.

table 54-3 Mediators of the Inflammatory/Immune Responses (IIR)

Mediator	Description of Activity	Clinical Response
Endotoxin	• Activates complement system and coagulation cascades • Activates macrophages, which release TNF and IL-1	• Increased microvascular permeability, vasodilation, third-spacing, microthrombi formation • Inflammatory response
Tumor necrosis factor (TNF)	• Released by monocyte–macrophages • Multiple effects locally and systemically • Stimulates other mediator activity	• Hypotension, tachycardia, myocardial depression, tachypnea, hyperglycemia, metabolic acidosis, third spacing, fever, microvascular vasoconstriction
Interleukin-1 (IL-1)	• Released by monocyte–macrophages • Stimulates leukocytosis • Triggers production of acute phase proteins and release of amino acids from skeletal muscle • Activates procoagulant activity • Decreases vascular responsiveness to catecholamines	• Increased white blood cells • High urinary nitrogen excretion and muscle wasting • Elevated coagulation laboratory values • Decreased SVR, which is not as responsive to low dosages of vasopressor or synthetic catecholamine agents
Interleukin-6 (IL-6)	• Released by monocytes, T helper cells and macrophages • Increases inflammatory response • B cell stimulation and differentiation • Synergistic with IL-1	• Fever • Antibody secretion
Complement cascade	• Inflammatory process • Opsonization and lysis of foreign particles and cells • Stimulates neutrophils (and oxygen radicals) and IL-1 • Degranulation of mast cells and basophils	• Edema formation, vasodilation, vascular permeability, third spacing • All effects of IL-1
Platelet aggregating factor (PAF)	• Released by mast cells, basophils, macrophages, neutrophils, platelets, and damaged endothelium • Increases platelet aggregation • Increases neutrophil adhesion • Increases vascular permeability and bronchoconstriction • Negative inotropic effects on the heart	• Microthrombi formation interfering with perfusion • Third spacing • Bronchoconstriction, rhonchi and wheezes, increased pulmonary airway pressures • Decreased heart contractility and force, which is not as responsive to low dosages of vasopressor and inotropic agents
Arachidonic acid metabolites (AA)	• Stimulation of AA causes the release of metabolites prostaglandins (PG), thromboxanes (TX), and leukotrienes (LT) • PGF and TXA_2 cause pulmonary hypertension, vasoconstriction, and platelet activation and aggregation • PGE, PGD, and prostacyclin cause vasodilation and decreased platelet aggregation • Leukotrienes increase neutrophil chemotaxis, vascular constriction, and vascular permeability • Increase gastric permeability to gram-negative bacteria • Inhibits leukocyte adhesion and platelets	• Oxygenation and ventilation difficulties, increased airway resistance, wheezing • Third spacing and edema formation • Vasolidation, increased capillary permeability, and hypotension
Oxygen radicals	• Generate metabolites (O_2^-, H_2O_2, OH^-) during the respiratory burst of the neutrophils • Damage cell structure and interfere with cell activities • Damage endothelial cells, which stimulate the coagulation system • Increase permeability	• Inflammatory response, edema formation, fever • Microthrombi formation • Third spacing

table 54-4 Survival Rates in the Intensive Care Unit as a Function of the Number of Failing Organ Systems

Number of Failing Systems	Mortality (%)
0	0.8
1	6.8
2	26.2
3	48.5
4	68.8
5	83.3

From Irwin RS, Rippe JM: Irwin and Rippe's Intensive Care Medicine (5th Ed), p 1837. Philadelphia, Lippincott Williams & Wilkins, 2003.

box 54-12 *Examples of Nursing Diagnoses and Collaborative Problems for the Patient With Shock States, SIRS, or MODS*

- Ineffective Tissue Perfusion
- Altered Cardiac Output
- Deficient Fluid Volume and Electrolytes
- Ineffective Breathing Pattern
- Impaired Gas Exchange
- Prolonged Immobility
- Altered Pain Management
- Fear and Anxiety

The concept of MODS reflects that no organ is independent of any other. Therefore, failure of a particular organ makes the failure of a second or third organ more likely. Moreover, restoration of function to the organ system that failed first may not save the patient because organ systems that subsequently failed may be damaged beyond repair.

Assessment: Monitoring Organ Function

Like SIRS, MODS is a concept developed to help define the extent of the shock state, follow a patient's deterioration or improvement, and enable appropriate treatment of a particular patient. Nursing diagnoses for shock states, SIRS, and MODS are shown in Box 54-12.

MODS is presumed to exist if failure exists in two or more organ systems. Multiple scoring systems exist to determine the extent of MODS. The Sepsis-Related Organ Failure Assessment (SOFA) system[19] is presented in Table 54-5. Other scoring systems include the Acute Physiology and Chronic Health Evaluation (APACHE)[20] and the Mortality Probability Models (MPM) systems.[21] Each of these has been validated in critically ill populations as a predictor of mortality. Moreover, these scoring systems may also be used to determine staffing levels and third-party reimbursement and to determine inclusion or exclusion criteria in research settings.

Management

Unfortunately, there is no specific treatment for MODS other than supportive care. Treatment directed at specific organ systems has not been shown to result in improved survival in patients with MODS. This may reflect the interdependence of organ systems and the systemic character of MODS. However, there is evidence that early identification (7 to 72 hours after admission) of patients with a high likelihood of developing MODS and early normalization of $S\bar{v}O_2$, arterial lactate concentration, base deficit, and pH lead to a more benign hospital course with decreased inpatient mortality.[16] These data, which require confirmation, point out the systemic nature of MODS. Other treatments that target the inflammatory nature of SIRS or MODS include drotrecogin alfa (Xigris). Corticosteroids may be used but are controversial.

case study ■ CARDIOGENIC AND SEPTIC SHOCK CAUSED BY MYOCARDIAL INFARCTION

Mrs. Cox, a 52-year-old woman, presents to the emergency department with new-onset chest pain that is not relieved by rest. She had been grocery shopping and began to experience diaphoresis and chest heaviness while bringing the grocery bags into the house. The chest heaviness progressed to pain and she called 911. Medical history includes hypertension and type 2 diabetes mellitus. After the diagnosis of hypertension 1 month ago, Mrs. Cox began taking metoprolol (Lopressor) 100 mg/day. She was also started on glyburide (DiaBeta) 5 mg twice daily. Mrs. Cox does not exercise regularly, is a social drinker (one to two alcoholic beverages per week), and has smoked approximately one-half pack of cigarettes per day for the past 20 years.

On physical examination, Mrs. Cox is obese and diaphoretic, and her chest pain is 8 on a scale from 1 to 10. Two 18-gauge IV lines are started in the bilateral antecubital spaces. $D_{5 1/2}$ normal saline (NS) is infusing at 75 mL/hour. Vital signs on admission are temperature 99.7°F (37.6°C); respiration rate 32 breaths/minute; heart rate 116 beats/minute; blood pressure 136/96 mm Hg. A Foley catheter is inserted, and 7 mL of concentrated urine is obtained. Laboratory values are hemoglobin 12.2 g/dL; hematocrit 35%; WBC count 9.9 mm^3; glucose 167 mg/dL; sodium 141 mEq/L; potassium 3.7 mEq/L; blood urea nitrogen 26 mg/dL; creatinine 1.2 mg/dL; magnesium 1.8 mg/dL; calcium 8.7 mg/dL; and total creatine phosphokinase (8 hours after onset of chest pain) 154.4 IU/dL (normal, 0 to 20 IU/dL). Cardiac markers are MB-CPK 5.42 IU/dL (normal less than 0.7 IU/dL); and cardiac troponin 124 ng/mL.

Mrs. Cox is admitted to the hospital with a diagnosis of acute myocardial infarction, and she is transported to the cardiac catheterization laboratory for evaluation of the

table 54-5 Sepsis-Related Organ Failure Assessment (SOFA) Scoring System

	SOFA Score			
Organ System	**1**	**2**	**3**	**4**
Respiration				
Partial pressure of oxygen/fraction of inspired oxygen (mm Hg)	<400	<300	<200 with respiratory support	<100
Coagulation				
Platelets × 10^3 mm^3	<150	<100	<50	<20
Liver				
Bilirubin (mg/dL)	1.2–1.9	2.0–5.9	6.0–11.9	>12
Cardiovascular				
Hypotension	MAP <70 mm Hg	Dopamine ≤5 or dobutamine any dose	Dopamine >5 or epinephrine ≤0.1 or norepinephrine ≤0.1	Dopamine >15 or epinephrine >0.1 or norepinephrine >0.1
Central nervous system				
Glasgow Coma Scale score	13–14	10–12	6–9	<6
Renal				
Creatinine (mg/dL) or urine output	1.2–1.9	2.0–3.4	3.5–4.9 or <500 mL/day	>5.0 or <200 mL/day

MAP, mean arterial pressure.
From Irwin RS, Rippe JM: Irwin and Rippe's Intensive Care Medicine (5th Ed), p 1836. Philadelphia, Lippincott Williams & Wilkins, 2003.

coronary arteries and possible stent placement. Her left anterior descending coronary artery is 90% occluded, and her right coronary artery is 75% occluded. Two stents are successfully inserted. Mrs. Cox experiences increased chest pain during the procedure, requiring placement of a central venous catheter to administer the following: IV fluids, dopamine 5 μg/kg/minute, dobutamine 2.5 μg/kg/minute, and nitroglycerin 100 μg/minute. Blood pressure (72/46 mm Hg) during the procedure is low, and she is now diagnosed with cardiogenic shock. An intra-aortic balloon (IAB) catheter is placed to reduce the workload of the heart, and she is transferred to the ICU.

On arrival in the ICU, Mrs. Cox experiences respiratory arrest. She is emergently intubated and placed on mechanical ventilation. An arterial line and pulmonary artery catheter (PAC) are inserted. Initial parameters are cardiac output (CO) 2.1 L/minute; pulmonary artery wedge pressure (PAWP) 24 mm Hg; SVR 1,567 dynes/second/cm^{-5}; blood pressure 72/54 mm Hg; mean arterial pressure (MAP) 66 mm Hg; and heart rate 132 beats/minute. Arterial blood gases (ABGs) reveal respiratory acidosis: pH 7.30; Pco_2 62 mm Hg; Po_2 62 mm Hg; HCO_3 24 mEq/L. Mrs. Cox receives 80 mg of furosemide, and the dobutamine is increased to 5 μg/kg/minute. She is also started on heparin at 900 units/hour. The IAB is set to a 1:1 ratio for maximal cardiac support.

Mrs. Cox continues to be treated with IAB, dobutamine, dopamine, nitroglycerin, and heparin. Morphine and midazolam are given for pain and sedation. IV fluids are administered at 50 mL/hour, and a 200-mL bolus is ordered if the PAWP falls below 18 mm Hg. The diuretic furosemide 20 mg IV is ordered PRN every 4 hours if the PAWP rises above 22 mm Hg. Potassium chloride 20 mEq IV PRN is ordered if the serum potassium falls to less than 4.0 mEq/L.

On ICU day 2, Mrs. Cox is more stable hemodynamically. Her vital signs are improving: temperature 99.7°F (37.6°C); heart rate 110 to 116 beats/minute; and blood pressure 92/56 mm Hg on 5 μg/kg/minute dobutamine and 5 μg/kg/minute dopamine. The IAB catheter remains at a 1:1 ratio. Pulmonary artery readings are cardiac output 5.7 L/minute; PAWP 18 mm Hg; and SVR 879 dynes/second/cm^{-5}. Trials to wean her from ventilator support begin, and she requires fewer medications for pain and sedation.

On ICU day 3, Mrs. Cox is extubated and placed on 40% oxygen by mask. The IAB ratio slowly begins to increase. She has suffered a larger anterior wall myocardial infarction but is recovering from the cardiogenic shock without other serious organ involvement.

On ICU day 4, the IAB is removed from Mrs. Cox, and the PAC is changed to a multilumen central line. Orders to wean the dobutamine and dopamine are obtained, and a liquid diet is ordered. Ten hours later, Mrs. Cox becomes more irritable and begins pulling at her IV lines and Foley catheter. Her vital signs are temperature 102.0°F (38.9°C); respiration rate 32 breaths/minute; heart rate 124 breaths/minute; and blood pressure 82/44 mm Hg. Blood and urine are sent for culture. Mrs. Cox is electively reintubated, and a PAC is reinserted. Initial hemodynamic readings are cardiac output 8.2 L/minute; PAWP 22 mm Hg; and SVR 660 dynes/second/cm^{-5}. Mrs. Cox is diagnosed with septic shock, and broad-spectrum antibiotics are ordered. Large amounts of fluids are necessary to support her blood pressure; however, her myocardial injury requires diuresis to optimize preload. Acute pulmonary edema develops, and furosemide 100 mg IV is administered. Phenylephrine is initiated at 0.05 μg/kg/minute, with orders to titrate to a MAP greater than 70 mm Hg.

ABGs reveal a metabolic acidosis and a serum lactate of 5.8 mmol/L. The WBC count increases to 12.4 mm^3, and preliminary blood cultures are positive for gram-negative rods. Mrs. Cox is not responsive to pain and is unable to follow commands. She is receiving intermittent doses of midazolam and morphine.

Four hours later, sustained ventricular tachycardia develops in Mrs. Cox and progresses to ventricular fibrillation. Resuscitation is unsuccessful. ■

clinical applicability challenges

Self-Challenge: Critical Thinking

1. *Compare and contrast medical and nursing management interventions directed at the inflammatory response system SIRS, sepsis, and MODS.*
2. *Compare and contrast hemodynamic assessment parameters (blood pressure, heart rate, central venous pressure, cardiac output, systemic vascular resistance) for each shock state.*
3. *Explain the pathophysiology of compensatory mechanism in early shock.*
4. *Discuss nursing priorities for the care of the patient in shock states.*

Study Questions

1. *Which intervention(s) might the nurse consider when caring for a patient in shock to improve delivery of oxygen to the cells?*
   a. *Administering packed red blood cell products*
   b. *Maximizing oxygenation*
   c. *Maximizing cardiac output*
   d. *All of the above*
2. *What parameters other than vital signs might the nurse assess to determine whether adequate amounts of oxygen are being delivered to the tissues?*
   a. *Serum lactate levels or base deficit*
   b. *Peripheral pulses*
   c. *Bowel sounds*
   d. *Electrolytes*
3. *M.J. is a 82-year-old man who is admitted with severe dehydration and hypovolemic shock. The physician has ordered intravenous crystalloid fluids to be administered at a rate of 750 mL/hour. In carrying out this order, the nurse understands that rapid administration of fluids to this patient may result in*
   a. *acute renal failure.*
   b. *hyperthermic response.*
   c. *pulmonary edema.*
   d. *hepatic failure.*
4. *A female patient tells you that when taking some antibiotics, she develops an itchy rash. This information should alert the nurse that the patient may be more likely to experience what form of shock?*
   a. *Hypovolemic*
   b. *Cardiogenic*
   c. *Anaphylactic*
   d. *Septic*
5. *Medications that may be ordered in the treatment of cardiogenic shock to optimize preload are*
   a. *diuretics.*
   b. *intravenous fluids.*
   c. *antibiotics.*
   d. *both intravenous fluids and diuretics.*
6. *The complex physiology of sepsis and SIRS involves an activation in the inflammatory/immune response. Which of the following are mediators of this activation?*
   a. *Cytokines of inflammation*
   b. *Endothelial cells*
   c. *Coagulation system*
   d. *All of the above*
7. *The primary etiology of MODS is believed to be related to*
   a. *inadequate tissue perfusion causing cell death.*
   b. *inflammatory/immune response mechanisms that activate the coagulation cascade.*
   c. *history of chronic disease.*
   d. *a and b.*

REFERENCES

1. Falk JL, Anderson PN, Meyer KC: Emergency department monitoring of trauma patients. In Ferrera PC, Colucciello SA, Marx JA, et al (eds): Trauma Management: An Emergency Medicine Approach, pp 103–111. St. Louis, Mosby, 2001
2. Vincent JL: Correcting the deficits: Fluids, pressors, and RBCs in resuscitation. In Levy MM, Vincent JL (eds): Sepsis: Pathophysiologic Insights and Current Management, pp 103–111. Chicago, Society of Critical Care Medicine, 2003
3. Pahor M, Elam MB, Garrison RJ, et al: Emerging noninvasive biochemical measures to predict cardiovascular risk. Arch Intern Med 159:237–245, 1999
4. Urban N, Porth CM: Heart failure and circulatory shock. In Porth CM (ed): Pathophysiology: Concepts of Altered Health States (5th Ed), pp 427–456. Philadelphia, Lippincott Williams & Wilkins, 1998
5. Hachey DM, Smith T: Use of nesiritide to treat acute decompensated heart failure. Crit Care Nurse 23(1):53–58, 2003
6. American College of Chest Physicians/Society of Critical Care Medicine: Consensus conference: Definitions for sepsis and multiple organ failure and guidelines for use of innovative therapies in sepsis. Crit Care Med 20:864–874, 1992
7. Levy MM: Definitions of sepsis revisited: Results of the SSSM/ESICM/ACCP/ATS consensus conference. In Levy MM, Vincent JL (eds): Sepsis: Pathophysiologic Insights and Current Management, pp 39–42. Chicago, Society of Critical Care Medicine, 2003
8. Sommers MS: The cellular basis of septic shock. Crit Care Nurs Clin North Am 15:13–25, 2003
9. Angus DC, Linde-Zwirble WT, Lidicker J, et al: Epidemiology of severe sepsis in the United States: Analysis of incidence, outcome, and associated costs of care. Crit Care Med 29(7):1303–1310, 2001
10. Schulman CS: New thoughts on sepsis. Dimens Crit Care Nurs 22(1):20–30, 2003
11. Kleinpell RM: The role of the critical care nurse in the assessment and management of the patient with severe sepsis. Crit Care Nurs Clin North Am 15:27–34, 2003
12. Bernard GR: Drotrecogin alfa (activated) for the treatment of severe sepsis. Crit Care Med 31(1 Suppl):S85–S93, 2003
13. Kellum J, Pinsky M: Use of vasopressor agents in critically ill patients. Curr Opin Crit Care 8(3):236–241, 2002
14. Ward N: Anti-inflammatory mediators. In Levy MM, Vincent JL (eds): Sepsis: Pathophysiologic Insights and Current Management, pp 31–38. Chicago, Society of Critical Care Medicine, 2003
15. Houghton D: Antimicrobial resistance in the intensive care unit: Understanding the problem. AACN Clin Issues 13(3):410–420, 2002
16. Rivers E, Nguyen B, Havstad S, et al: Early goal directed therapy in the treatment of severe sepsis and septic shock. N Engl J Med 345(19):1368–1377, 2001
17. Braunschweig C, Levy P, Sheean P, et al: Enteral compared with parenteral nutrition: A meta analysis. Am J Clin Nutr 74:534–542, 2001

18. DeLegge M: Enteral access: The foundation of feeding. JPEN J Parenter Enteral Nutr 25(2):S8–S13, 2001
19. Vincent JL, et al: The SOFA (Sepsis-Related Organ Failure Assessment) score to describe organ dysfunction/failure. On behalf of the Working Group on Sepsis-Related Problems of the European Society of Intensive Care Medicine. Intensive Care Med 22: 707–710, 1996
20. Knaus WA, et al: APACHE II: A severity of disease classification system. Crit Care Med 13:818–828, 1985
21. Lemeshow SD, et al: Mortality Probability Models (MPM II) based on an international cohort of intensive care unit patients. JAMA 270:2478–2486, 1993

OTHER SUGGESTED READING

Ahrens T, Sona C: Capnography application in acute and critical care. AACN Clin Issues 14(2):123–132, 2003

Bernard GR, Vincent JL, Laterre PF, et al: Efficacy and safety of recombinant human activated protein C for severe sepsis. N Engl J Med 344(10):699–709, 2001

Bone RC: Definitions for sepsis and organ failure and guidelines for the use of innovative therapies in sepsis. Chest 101:1644–1653, 1992

Chavez JA, Brewer C: Stopping the shock. RN 65(9):30–35, 2002

Ely EW, Kleinpell RM, Goyette RE: Advances in the understanding of clinical manifestations and therapy of severe sepsis: An update for critical care nurses. Am J Crit Care 12(2):120–135, 2003

Leeper B: Monitoring right ventricular volumes: A paradigm shift. AACN Clin Issues 14(2):208–219, 2003

Mitchel RN, Cotran RS: Hemodynamic disorders, thrombosis and shock. In Cotran RS, Kumar VK, Collins T (eds): Robbins Pathologic Basis of Disease (6th Ed), pp 113–138. Philadelphia, WB Saunders, 1999

Reigle B, Dienger M: Sepsis and treatment-induced immunosuppression in the patient with cancer. Crit Care Nurs Clin North Am 15(1): 109–118, 2003

Rote NS: Inflammation. In McCance KL, Huether SE (eds): Pathophysiology: The Biologic Basis for Disease in Adults and Children (4th Ed), pp 197–226. St. Louis, Mosby, 2002

Sommers M: The cellular basis of septic shock. Crit Care Nurs Clin North Am 15(1):13–26, 2003

Truog R, Cist A, Brackett S, et al: Recommendations for end-of-life care in the intensive care unit: The Ethics Committee of the Society of Critical Care Medicine. Crit Care Med 29(12):2332–2348, 2001

Vary T, McLean B, VonRueden K: Shock and multiple organ dysfunction syndrome. In McQuillan K, VonRueden KI, Hartsock R, et al (eds): Trauma Nursing From Resuscitation Through Rehabilitation (3rd Ed), pp 173–200. Philadelphia, WB Saunders, 2002

Waikar S, Chertow G: Crystalloids versus colloids for resuscitation in shock. Curr Opin Nephrol Hypertens 9(5):501–504, 2000

Wheeler AP, Bernard GR: Treating patients with severe sepsis. N Engl J Med 340(3):207–214, 1999

Workman ML: The cellular basis of bacterial infection. Crit Care Nurs Clin North Am 15(1):1–12, 2003

chapter 55

Trauma

CARLA A. ARESCO

objectives

Based on the content in this chapter, the reader should be able to:

- Describe phases of initial assessment and related care of the trauma patient.
- Discuss the assessment of patients with thoracic, abdominal, musculoskeletal, and maxillofacial trauma.
- Contrast the response of solid and hollow abdominal organs to trauma.
- Explain the management and nursing care of patients with thoracic, abdominal, musculoskeletal, and maxillofacial trauma.
- Describe immediate, early, and late complications of trauma and the impact of these complications on mortality.

Trauma is defined by the *American Heritage Dictionary* as "a wound, especially one produced by sudden physical injury."[1] *Injury* is defined by the National Committee for Injury Prevention and Control as "unintentional or intentional damage to the body resulting from acute exposure to thermal, mechanical, electrical, or chemical energy or from the absence of such essentials as heat or oxygen."[2] This chapter specifically discusses mechanical injury.

Unintentional injury includes motor vehicle crashes (MVCs), poisonings, falls, drownings, fires, and burns. In 2000, unintentional injuries accounted for 97,300 deaths and 20,500,000 disabling injuries. The total cost of fatal and nonfatal unintentional injuries to employers and insurers was 512.4 billion dollars in the year 2000. To put this in perspective, the total cost is equivalent to 51 cents of every dollar paid in federal personal income taxes or 54 cents of every dollar spent on food in the United States.[2]

Of these numbers, MVCs accounted for 43,000 deaths and 2,300,000 disabling injuries. The total cost of MVCs to consumers was 201.5 billion dollars. This figure is equivalent to

- What it would cost to purchase 610 gallons of gas for each registered motor vehicle in the United States, or
- Approximately 1,100 dollars per licensed driver, or
- Greater than 25 times the combined profits reported by Ford and General Motors.[2]

Unintentional injuries are the leading causes of death in people between the ages of 1 and 34 years. In the 35- to 44-year age bracket, unintentional injury is second only to cancer as a leading cause of death. Unintentional injuries are the fifth leading cause of death among people of all ages. In 2000, unintentional injuries accounted for 15,127 deaths (11,078 male and 4,049 female victims).[2]

Intentional injuries (e.g., suicide attempts, assaults, and homicides) include injuries from poisoning, hanging, drowning, firearms, cutting, and jumping. In 1998, these injuries accounted for 30,575 deaths. Of these, 17,424 were caused by firearms.[2]

MECHANISM OF INJURY

Knowing the mechanism of injury is important. The mechanism of injury can help explain the type of injury, predict the eventual outcome, and identify common injury combinations.[3] In addition, an injury may exist in a trauma patient without the classic signs. The mechanism of injury may indicate the need for additional diagnostic workup and reassessment.

The mechanism of injury is related to the type of injuring force and the subsequent tissue response. Injury occurs when the force deforms tissues beyond their failure limits. Wounds vary depending on the injuring agent. The effect of injury also depends on personal and environmental factors, such as the person's age and sex, the presence or absence of underlying disease process, and the geographic region.

Force may or may not be penetrating. The injury delivered from force depends on the energy delivered and the area of contact. In penetrating injury, the concentration of force is to a small area. In blunt or nonpenetrating injury, the energy is distributed over a large area. The predominant feature affecting the impact is speed, or acceleration:

$$\text{Force} = \text{mass} \times \text{acceleration}$$

Blunt Injury

Mechanisms of blunt injury include MVCs, falls, assaults, and contact sports. Multiple injuries are common with blunt trauma, and these injuries are often more life-threatening than penetrating injuries because the extent of the injury is less obvious and the diagnosis can be more difficult.

Blunt injury is caused by a combination of forces. These forces include acceleration, deceleration, shearing, crushing, and compressive resistance:

- *Acceleration* is an increase in the velocity (or speed) of a moving object.
- *Deceleration*, on the other hand, is a decrease in the velocity of a moving object.
- *Shearing* occurs across a plane when structures slip relative to each other.
- *Crushing* occurs when continuous pressure is applied to a body part.
- *Compressive resistance* is the ability of an object or structure to resist squeezing forces or inward pressure.

In blunt trauma it is the direct impact that causes the greatest injury. Injury occurs when there is direct contact between the body surface and the injuring agent. Indirect forces are transmitted internally with dissipation of energy to the internal structure. The extent of injury from an indirect force depends on transference of energy from an object to the body. Injury occurs as a result of energy released and the tendency for the tissues to be displaced on impact.[3] Acceleration–deceleration injuries are the most common causes of blunt trauma.

In an MVC, the vehicle size and design change injury patterns. Small cars are involved in more crashes per mile and cause more deaths than larger vehicles. Before the crash, the occupant and the car are traveling at the same speed. During the crash, both the occupant and the car decelerate to zero, but not necessarily at the same rate. There are actually three collisions involved in one crash. The first is the car into another object; the second is the occupant's body with the interior of the car; and the third is the internal tissues impacting against the rigid body surface structure. For example, rapid deceleration in an MVC can cause direct injury to tissue. Subsequently, injury occurs as internal organs impinge on bony internal structures and cause major vessels to undergo stretching and bowing.

Wearing shoulder and lap restraints reduces the incidence and severity of injury by reducing the force with which a person strikes a surface, thereby preventing the occupant from striking multiple surfaces and being ejected from the vehicle[3] (Fig. 55-1). The occupant's position in the vehicle also makes a difference in the blunt injury received. When a vehicle strikes a pedestrian it is important to visualize the size of the vehicle and the size of the pedestrian. The area of impact can vary depending on these factors (Fig. 55-2).

Penetrating Injury

Penetrating trauma refers to an injury produced by foreign objects penetrating the tissue. The severity of the injury is related to the structures damaged. The mechanism of injury is caused by the energy created and dissipated by the penetrating object into the surrounding areas.[3] The amount of tissue damaged by a bullet is determined by the amount of energy that transfers into the tissue along with the amount of time it takes for the transfer to occur. The surface area over which the transfer is distributed also contributes to tissue damage.[4]

Velocity determines the extent of cavitation and tissue damage (Fig. 55-3). Low-velocity missiles localize the injury to a small radius from the center of the tract and have little disruptive effect. They cause little cavitation and blast effect, essentially only pushing the tissue aside.

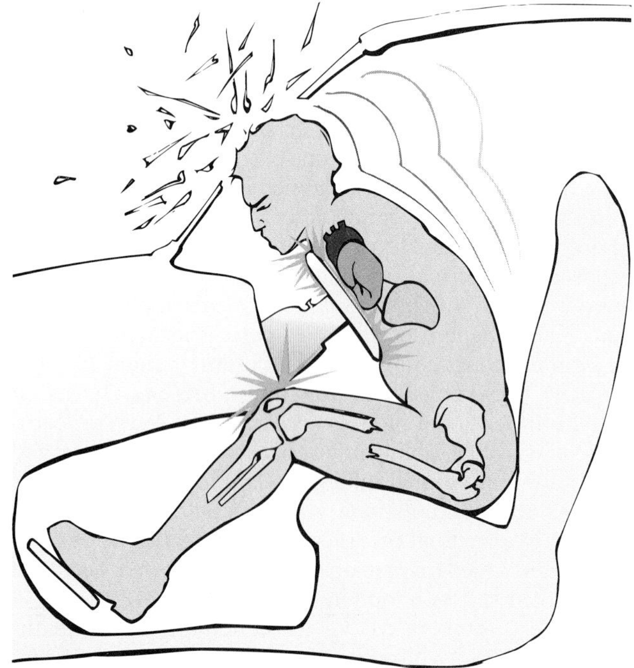

figure 55-1 In a motor vehicle accident, if the driver is not wearing a seat belt, damage may occur in various sections of the body. Common injuries occur to the skull, scalp, face, sternum, ribs, heart, liver, or spleen. Bones of the pelvis and lower extremities also may be damaged.

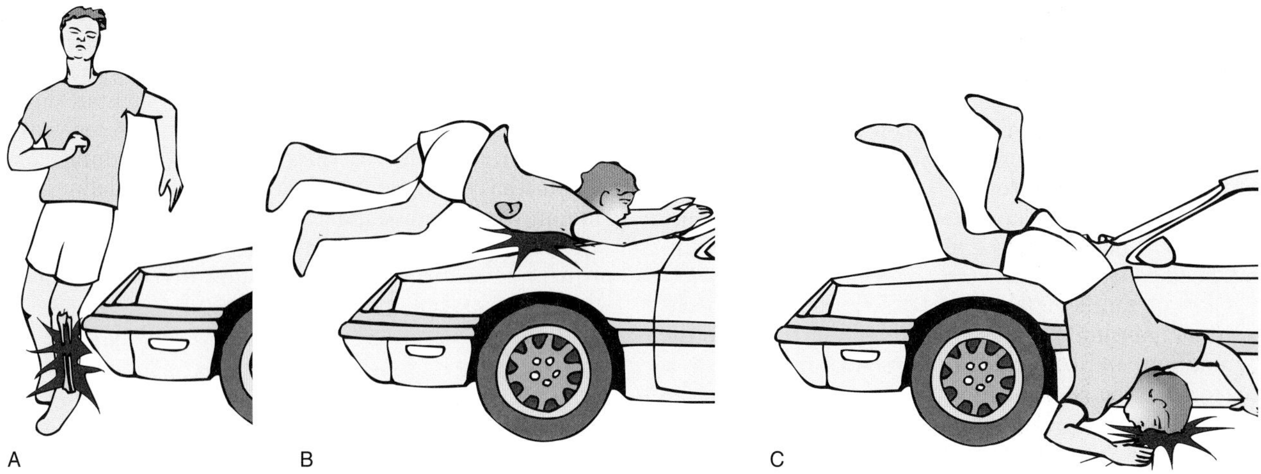

figure 55-2 Pedestrians may be hurt critically when hit by a moving vehicle. (**A**) A common injury is the fracture of the tibia and fibula at the time of impact. (**B**) Impact when the pedestrian strikes the hood of the car may cause fractured ribs and a ruptured spleen. (**C**) Injuries to the head and additional fractures of the extremities may occur as the pedestrian rolls off the braking car or is thrown by the impact.

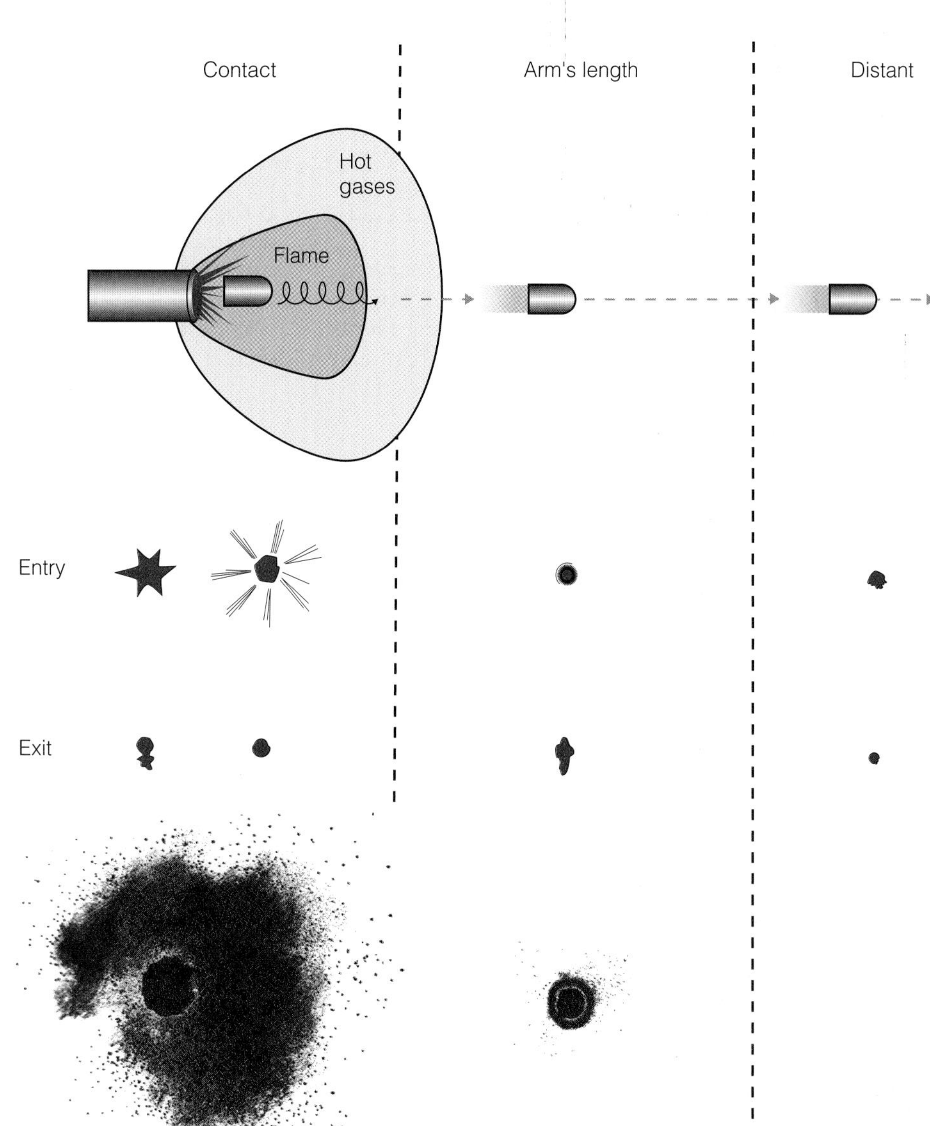

figure 55-3 Diagrammatic views of the effects of gunshot wounds on the body surface. Kinetic energy is dependent on the distance from which the weapon is fired and the tissue involved. Entry and exit wounds are shown when in direct contact, at arm's reach, and at a distance. The bottom illustrations show entry wounds of .22 rifle at 5-cm range (*left*) and at 20-cm range (*right*). The drilled-in entry wound and faint power markings are indicated.

High-velocity missiles can cause more serious injury because of the amount of energy and cavitation produced. The damage depends on three factors: the density and compressibility of the tissue injured, the missile's velocity, and the fragmentation of the primary missile. High-velocity bullets compress and accelerate tissue away from the bullet, causing a cavity to form around the bullet and its entire tract.

Shotguns are short-range, low-velocity weapons that use multiple lead pellets encased in a larger shell for ammunition. Each pellet is a missile (Fig. 55-4).

It is important to obtain a brief description of the mechanism of gunshot injuries, including the weapon, the ammunition, and ballistics. This essential information is used to guide the assessment of patients who sustain injuries from these weapons. All trauma patients must be undressed and inspected for entrance and exit wounds during the assessment process.

Stab Wounds and Impalements

A stab wound or impalement is a low-velocity injury. The main injury determinants are length, width, and trajectory of the penetrating object and the presence of vital organs in the area of the wound. Although the injuries tend to be localized, deep organs and multiple body cavities can be penetrated.

INITIAL ASSESSMENT AND MANAGEMENT

When a trauma patient is brought to the emergency department or the trauma resuscitation unit, it is imperative to obtain a thorough history of the preceding events. This initial evaluation aids in assessment and treatment, and can decrease morbidity and mortality. During this initial assessment, it is important to obtain as much detail as possible about the circumstances surrounding the injury, including the mechanism of injury. To facilitate initial assessment, intervention, and triage of the trauma victim, the American College of Surgeons (ACS) Committee on Trauma has developed guidelines. These guidelines provide an organized, standardized approach to the initial assessment of trauma patients, increasing the speed of the primary assessment and minimizing the risk that injuries will be overlooked.

Prehospital Management

The trauma patient has a greater chance of a positive outcome if definitive care is initiated within 1 hour of injury. Care begins in the prehospital arena and is continued throughout the hospital stay. There are currently two theories about prehospital management of patients, the "stay and play" theory and the "scoop and run" theory.[5] Proponents of the "stay and play" theory believe that "time in the field can be well spent stabilizing the patient's physiologic status,"[5] whereas proponents of the "scoop and run" theory believe that "only life-threatening issues should be addressed in the field."[6] Several studies demonstrated that the time taken to establish intravenous access was longer than the transport time to definitive care.[5] This prolongation of transport was associated with an increase in patient mortality. Therefore, it was suggested that each emergency medical system (EMS) evaluate its approach to prehospital management, taking into account the transport time to definitive care. For example, in an urban area, the "scoop and run" theory may be appropriate because transport time to a definitive care setting is very short. In a rural area, however, the extra minutes that it may take to stabi-

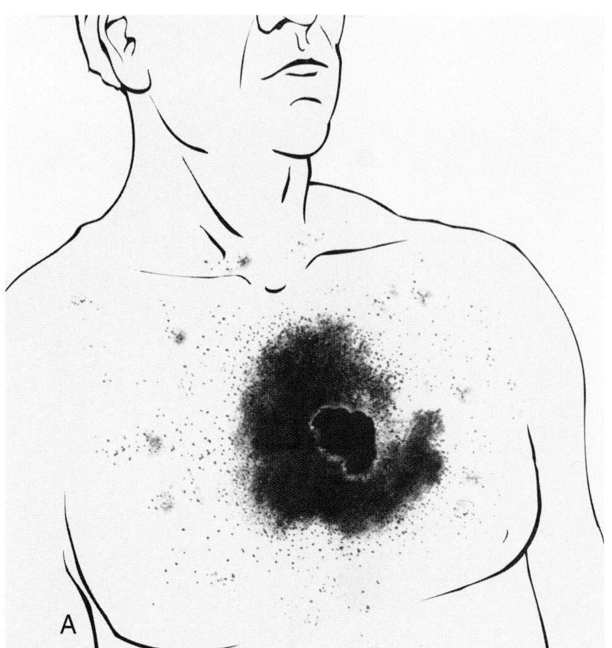

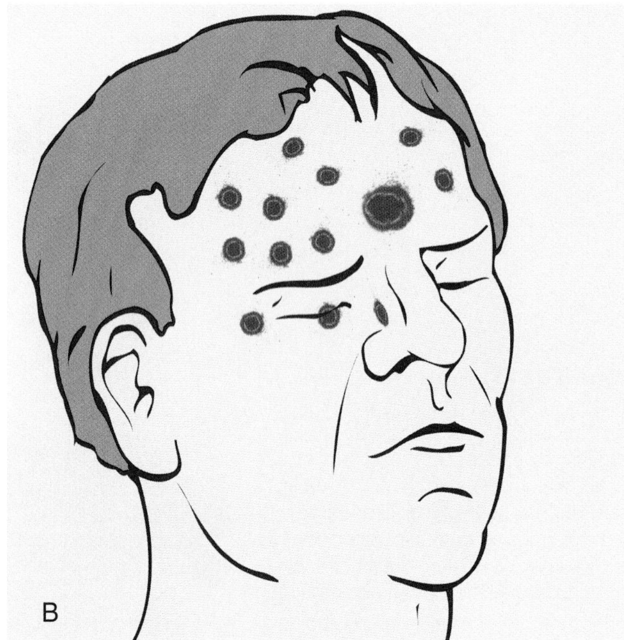

figure 55-4 Damage is caused by shotguns at two different distances. (**A**) At close range, opening is extensive and is surrounded by blood splatters and powder burns. (**B**) At medium range (8–10 feet), the larger entry wound is surrounded by individual pellet wounds.

lize the patient may have a positive impact on the overall outcome because of the long transport time.

The advanced trauma life support (ATLS) guidelines state that the emphasis for assessment and management in the prehospital phase should be placed on maintaining the airway, ensuring adequate ventilation, controlling external bleeding and preventing shock, maintaining spine immobilization, and transporting the patient immediately to the closest appropriate facility.[7]

The prehospital priority of maintaining adequate airway, breathing, and circulation (ABCs) may be difficult to attain owing to the mechanism of injury. It is imperative that cervical spine immobilization be maintained at all times during airway management and transport to definitive care. After assessing and managing the ABCs, the trauma patient's neurological status is assessed, including level of consciousness and pupil size and reaction. Once this primary assessment is complete, a secondary assessment is done to determine any other injuries.

The prehospital providers must consider the facility that will receive the patient (Table 55-1). Transporting the patient to a level I facility allows definitive care to be initiated earlier in the process, thereby reducing patient mortality. Transport of the patient to a lesser facility for "stabilization," followed by transport to the definitive care setting later on, is associated with higher patient mortality rates.

In-Hospital Management

In-hospital patient management entails a rapid primary evaluation and resuscitation of vital functions, a more detailed secondary survey, and initiation of definitive care. Table 55-2 shows the process, commonly referred to as the "ABCDEs" of trauma care. According to the ACS, adhering to this sequence allows for the efficient identification of life-threatening conditions.[7]

PRIMARY SURVEY

During the primary survey, each priority of care is dealt with in order. The patient's assessment does not continue to the next phase until each preceding priority is effectively managed. For example, if a patient does not have a patent airway, breathing and ventilation cannot be established. Therefore, it is during this initial phase that life-threatening injuries are identified and managed. So, if the patient does not have a patent airway, endotracheal intubation, chest tube insertion, and central line access may be initiated and intravenous fluid and blood products may be administered to maintain life-sustaining vital signs before moving on to the next phase of the evaluation.

Assessing the patient for evidence of hypovolemia is essential. Blood loss can result from an external injury, associated with obvious bleeding, or from an internal injury, where bleeding may not be obvious. Any of these injuries can lead to inadequate tissue perfusion, which equals traumatic shock. It is necessary to first stop the bleeding with compression or surgery and then replace the lost intravascular volume. Some signs of hypovolemia include pallor, poor skin integrity, diaphoresis, tachycardia, and hypotension. Usually, trauma patients arrive at the trauma center with a large-bore intravenous line already in place, with intravenous fluid running in rapidly.

During the resuscitation period, an electrocardiogram (ECG) is done. The patient is placed on a monitor with pulse oximetry and end-tidal carbon dioxide monitoring. A Foley catheter and a nasogastric or orogastric tube are placed, and bloodwork is sent to the laboratory for evaluation. Bloodwork analysis includes evaluation of electrolytes, hemoglobin and hematocrit, blood type and crossmatch, and arterial blood gases (ABGs), if the patient is expected to have a high level of injury.

The patient is also assessed for hypothermia. The trauma patient is often subjected to environmental factors, which, along with his or her altered physiological state and possible wet clothing, predispose the patient to hypothermia. Measures taken by health care professionals, such as the infusion of room-temperature intravenous fluids or exposure of the patient's body to inspect for injuries, can exacerbate hypothermia. Warm fluids and blankets are used whenever possible to increase body temperature or maintain normothermia.

table 55-1 Trauma Center Designation

	Level I	Level II	Level III	Level IV
Admission requirements	1200 patients per year; 20% with an Injury Severity Score (ISS) ≥15 or 35 patients per surgeon with an ISS ≥15	Varies depending on geographical area, population, resources available, and system maturity	No requirement	No requirement
Surgeon availability	24-hour in-house attending surgeon	Rapidly available	Promptly available	24-Hour emergency coverage
Research center	Required	Not required	Not required	Not required
Education, prevention, and outreach	Required	Required	Required	Required

Source: Scalea TM, Boswell SA: Initial management of traumatic shock. In McQuillan KA, Von Rueden KT, Hartsock RL, et al. (eds): Trauma Nursing (3rd Ed). Philadelphia, WB Saunders, 2002.

table 55-2 Initial Assessment and Management of the Patient With Trauma

Parameter	Assessment	Interventions
Airway	Air exchange Airway patency	Jaw thrust, chin lift Removal of foreign bodies Suctioning Oropharyngeal or nasopharyngeal airway Endotracheal intubation (orally or nasally) Cricothyrotomy
Breathing	Respirations (rate, depth, effort) Color Breath sounds Chest wall movement and integrity Position of trachea	Supplemental oxygen Ventilation with bag–valve device Treatment of life-threatening conditions (e.g., tension pneumothorax)
Circulation	Pulse, blood pressure Capillary refill Obvious external bleeding Electrocardiogram	Hemorrhage control: direct pressure, elevate extremity, pneumatic antishock garment Intravenous therapy: crystalloids, blood transfusion Treatment of life-threatening conditions (e.g., cardiac tamponade) Cardiopulmonary resuscitation
Disability	Level of consciousness Pupils	—
Exposure	Inspection of body for injuries	—

SECONDARY SURVEY

Once the primary survey is completed, a more detailed secondary survey is initiated. This survey begins at the head and works down to the patient's feet. Non–life-threatening injuries are revealed during this survey. During this time, a plan is developed and the appropriate diagnostic tests (e.g., x-rays, ultrasound studies, computed tomography [CT] scans, angiographic studies) are ordered for the patient. This is also the time when a more detailed patient history can be obtained, as well as important information regarding the mechanism of injury. The nurse asks the field providers for information regarding the incident because the patient may not be able to speak or may not remember the event. Family and friends might be helpful in providing additional information about the patient.

Questions the nurse asks before or during the trauma patient's arrival to the hospital include the following:

- Was the person involved in an MVC? Was the person wearing a restraining device? If the person was hit by a vehicle, was the person on foot or on a bike? What kind of vehicle was involved? Where was the person at the time of impact? What was the speed, point of impact, type of impact? Was there a fatality at the scene?
- Are we concerned with blunt or penetrating trauma?
- Did the patient fall? How far? Was the fall off a ladder, or down a flight of stairs?

Based on the information obtained from field providers or family members of the patient, other injuries may be suspected and further investigation may be warranted. This is especially true in intubated, comatose, or paralyzed patients who are unable to verbalize their complaints. The nurse continuously reassesses the trauma patient because injuries often go undetected.

FLUID RESUSCITATION

Most trauma patients have a fluid volume deficit that must be corrected. The goals of fluid resuscitation are to maintain physiological support of circulation and oxygen transport while avoiding physiological and hemostatic deficiencies.[8] It is essential to have adequate intravascular volume and oxygen-carrying capacity to transport needed nutrients to the tissues. To guide fluid resuscitation, the nurse uses the patient's physical assessment and hemodynamic parameters.

Crystalloids

Typically, crystalloids are used in the trauma patient. Crystalloids contain water and other electrolytes that are premixed into the fluid. These electrolytes may include sodium, potassium, and chloride. Crystalloids can be further broken down by their tonicity. The tonicity is based on the amount of sodium in the solution. Crystalloids can be classified as isotonic, hypotonic, and hypertonic (Table 55-3).

Hypertonic saline has been shown to enable a more rapid restoration of cardiac function with a smaller volume of fluid. It is supplied either in a 3%, 7.5%, or 23.4% sodium chloride (NaCl) solution. As little as 4 mL/kg, if given rapidly, may have the same hemodynamic effect as several liters of isotonic crystalloid.[9] Hypertonic saline has the effect of shifting water into the plasma. This water comes from the red blood cells, interstitial space, and tissue. The result is a rapid increase in blood volume, which supports and improves hemodynamics.[10] Hypertonic saline increases the mean arterial pressure and cardiac output,

table 55-3 Intravenous Fluid

Isotonic	• Example: 0.9 normal saline • Equivalent to the tonicity of the human body • Causes minimal shifts between intracellular and extracellular fluid
Hypotonic	• Example: 5% dextrose in water (D_5W) • Tonicity is less than that of human body • May cause swelling, pulls into extra-cellular space
Hypertonic	• Example: 3% saline • Tonicity is more than that of human body • Pulls fluid into the intravascular space

Modified from American Association of Critical-Care Nurses: Clinical Reference for Critical-Care Nursing (4th Ed). Aliso Viejo, CA, American Association of Critical-Care Nurses, 1998.

which then leads to peripheral vasodilation. The peripheral vasodilation allows for an increase in total splanchnic, renal, coronary, and mesenteric blood flow.[11]

The initial management of trauma patients often requires the rapid infusion of 2 L of isotonic crystalloid as rapidly as possible, while trying to obtain a normal heart rate and blood pressure. However, research has shown that the infusion of crystalloids in patients with hypotension can cause more harm by displacing a hemostatic clot, only to cause more bleeding.[8,10–12] The infusion of crystalloid also further dilutes the patient's hemoglobin and can increase intraperitoneal blood loss.

Colloids

Colloids can also be given to resuscitate a trauma patient. Colloids, such as albumin, dextran, and hetastarch, create oncotic pressure, which encourages fluid retention and movement of fluid into the intravascular space. Proponents for colloid use have argued that less volume of fluid is necessary to achieve hemodynamic stability and the fluid is retained in the intravascular space longer. Despite possible advantages, there is no clear evidence that colloids are superior to crystalloids for resuscitation of the trauma patient. Potential complications, such as anaphylaxis and coagulopathy, have been reported with certain colloids. These potential adverse affects, together with higher costs, make colloid use less desirable than crystalloid use for resuscitation of trauma patients.

Blood Products

Blood products are considered an excellent resuscitation fluid.[12] Red blood cells increase oxygen-carrying capacity and allow for volume expansion. Blood also stays in the intravascular space for longer periods of time compared with the other resuscitation fluids.[12] Although there is some concern about bloodborne pathogens and transfusion reactions, it is essential to understand the advantages offered by blood transfusion.

Blood should be transfused when patients are hemodynamically unstable or are showing signs of tissue hypoxia despite crystalloid infusion.[13] Crossmatched blood is preferred but is not always possible if emergent transfusion prohibits type and crossmatching of the patient's blood. O-negative blood is the preferred type of uncrossmatched blood, especially in women of childbearing age. O-positive blood may be used in male and postmenopausal female patients. If the patient requires large amounts of blood, transfusion of fresh frozen plasma and platelets is initiated.[13] It is important to replace coagulation factors and platelets not contained in blood. In the event of massive blood transfusions, the risk of acute respiratory distress syndrome (ARDS) and disseminated intravascular coagulation (DIC) is heightened. An extended period of hypotension increases the possibility of renal failure.

Autotransfusion is another common modality used in the hemorrhaging trauma patient. Obviously, the nature of trauma prevents patients from donating their own blood, as they could in an elective surgery. However, sometimes blood is salvaged from wounds, drains, and body cavities.[8] Most often blood is saved from a chest tube underwater seal device. A cell saver is connected into the system and the blood from the wound collects there. Once full, the cell saver is disconnected from the underwater seal device and this blood is then transfused into the patient using a macroaggregate filter.[8]

Blood Substitutes

Blood substitutes have been developed but have not been approved for use in all countries. These agents do not require crossmatching and do not carry the risk of bloodborne pathogen transmission. Blood substitutes have a long shelf life and are not immunosuppressive. They also have a lower viscosity then blood, which promotes flow and peripheral oxygen delivery.[12]

DEFINITIVE CARE

Increasingly, trauma care consists of nonoperative management of stable patients. Traditionally, solid organ injuries, both blunt and penetrating, were treated with surgery. Today, many trauma surgeons are choosing nonoperative management for their patients whenever possible. Ever more sophisticated techniques for visualization of internal structures, such as CT, ultrasonography, and angiography, have reduced the need for immediate surgical exploration in many cases. In addition to being used for diagnosing a person's injury, many of these techniques can be used to manage the person's condition as well. For example, angiographic interventions may be used to embolize a hemorrhaging internal vessel, obviating the need for invasive surgical intervention. Nonoperative diagnosis and management reduces the need for blood transfusion, minimizes the number of missed injuries, and places the patient at lower risk for delayed bleeding.[14] Patients who are treated nonoperatively require frequent assessment and are admitted to the intensive care unit to facilitate this.

To observe the patient effectively, the nurse must be aware of potential injuries and associated signs and symptoms. Examples of nursing diagnoses and collaborative problems are given in Box 55-1. Attention is also given to the management of pre-existing medical conditions and the identification of injuries missed during treatment of life-threatening problems. Once again, knowledge regarding the mechanism of injury is necessary. Finally, the patient is monitored for the development of complications. The

box 55-1 *Examples of Nursing Diagnoses and Collaborative Problems for the Person With Trauma*

- Deficient Fluid Volume related to hemorrhage, "third spacing"
- Impaired Gas Exchange related to pulmonary trauma, respiratory complications (e.g., acute respiratory distress syndrome [ARDS], pain)
- Impaired Tissue Integrity related to trauma, surgery, invasive procedures, immobility
- Anxiety related to critical illness, fear of death or disfigurement, role changes within social setting, or permanent disability
- Risk for Ineffective Tissue Perfusion: Multiple Organs related to decreased cardiac output, decreased oxygenation, decreased gas exchange
- Risk for Infection related to trauma, invasive procedures
- Pain related to trauma
- Impaired bowel elimination related to intraabdominal trauma, ileus, or both
- Increased Risk for Ineffective Family and Individual Coping related to trauma

critical care nurse must be aware of potential complications and related risk factors associated with various injuries. Certain situations, such as prolonged extrication, prolonged hypothermia, respiratory or cardiac arrest, massive fluid resuscitation, or massive blood transfusions, suggest an increased likelihood of severe injuries and a greater chance of complications and death after trauma. A Collaborative Care Guide for the patient with multisystem trauma is given in Box 55-2.

ASSESSMENT AND MANAGEMENT OF SPECIFIC INJURIES

Although this section discusses traumatic injuries related to specific areas of the body, the nurse must keep in mind that head-to-toe assessment is required for each trauma patient. Physical assessment of each organ system is indicated, as described in previous chapters throughout this text.

Thoracic Trauma

Thoracic injuries are responsible for 25% of all trauma-related deaths and are second only to central nervous system (CNS) injuries as the leading cause of all trauma deaths.[15–17] MVCs are responsible for approximately 70% of thoracic injuries.[15] One seventh of all deaths by injury now involve violence. A significant number of these deaths are from penetrating gunshot or stab wounds to the chest.[18]

TRACHEOBRONCHIAL TRAUMA

Injuries to the trachea or bronchi can be caused by blunt or penetrating trauma and frequently are accompanied by esophageal and vascular damage. Ruptured bronchi often are present in association with upper rib fractures and pneumothorax. Severe tracheobronchial injury has a high mortality rate; however, with continued improvements in prehospital care and transport, more of these patients are surviving.

Airway injuries often are subtle. Presenting signs include dyspnea (occasionally the only sign), hemoptysis, cough, and subcutaneous emphysema. A chest x-ray can alert the physician to a possible injury; however, diagnosis usually is made with bronchoscopy or during surgery. Tracheobronchial injury is considered whenever a persistent air leak accompanies a pneumothorax.

Small lung lacerations or pleural tears can be managed conservatively with mechanical ventilation delivered through an endotracheal tube or tracheostomy. Larger injuries may require surgical repair. Simultaneous independent lung ventilation, where each lung is ventilated separately (each with a dedicated ventilator), may also be used.

Nursing care involves the assessment of oxygenation and gas exchange, along with appropriate pulmonary care. During the first few days, the physician may perform a bronchoscopy to visualize the repair site and provide more effective secretion removal. Pneumonia is a potential short-term complication, whereas tracheal stenosis may occur later.

BONY THORAX FRACTURES

Rib fractures, sternal fractures, and flail chest are thoracic fractures commonly seen in trauma patients. The greatest concerns for nurses caring for patients with such injuries are pain, ineffective ventilation, and secretion control. Ribs 1 and 2 are usually protected by the clavicle, scapula, humerus, and surrounding muscles. If these ribs are fractured, it often signifies high-impact trauma and other injuries, such as to the aorta, the thorax, and the spine, are very likely and should be investigated. Ribs 3 through 9 are most commonly fractured in blunt trauma. These fractures are often associated with underlying lung injuries. Fractures of the lower ribs can also be associated with injury to the liver or other abdominal structures. Sternal fractures are associated with blunt trauma.

Flail chest is an injury that involves multiple rib fractures. These fractures can be anterior, posterior, or lateral, and usually a sternal fracture is present as well. The stability of the thorax is disrupted and the rib cage no longer moves in unison. The injured area does not respond to the action of the respiratory muscles; rather, it moves in accordance with the changes in intrapleural pressure. The flail segment movement is paradoxical, hence the term *paradoxical breathing*. The flail segment causes a decrease in the normal negative pressure of the chest, thereby decreasing ventilation and causing some degree of hypoxia.

Initial management of patients with bony thorax fractures includes airway management, pain management, and oxygen therapy to maintain adequate saturation. The nurse must consider the underlying structures and the possible injury to them. Treatment of flail chest includes turning the patient with the injured side down to improve oxygenation. This is often difficult to perform because of the need to maintain cervical spine immobilization. Other treatment modalities include internal splinting, accomplished by placing the intubated patient on positive-

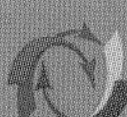

box 55-2 collaborative care guide *for the Patient With Multisystem Trauma*

OUTCOMES	INTERVENTIONS
Oxygenation/Ventilation	
The patient will maintain a patent airway.	■ Auscultate breath sounds. ■ Perform frequent assessments. ■ Intubate if needed. ■ Provide supplemental oxygen PRN.
The patient will maintain an Sao_2 ≥95% and have adequate ABGs.	■ Provide pulmonary toilet (chest physiotherapy and incentive spirometry). ■ Intubate. ■ Monitor ABGs.
The patient will be able to take deep breaths and will be free of anxiety.	■ Use mechanical ventilation if necessary to support adequate ventilation. ■ Provide adequate pain medication to promote deep breathing (patient-controlled analgesia [PCA], epidural, around-the-clock medications) ■ Medicate before pain increases. ■ Use antianxiety drugs as necessary.
Circulation/Perfusion	
The patient will maintain an adequate blood pressure, heart rate, and respiratory rate.	■ Monitor respiratory rate and depth. ■ Use ECG monitor. ■ Administer intravenous (IV) fluids and packed red blood cells to ensure adequate intravascular volume and oxygen-carrying capacity. ■ Administer medications, such as vasoactive and inotropic agents, after intravascular volume is restored. ■ Install pulmonary artery catheter/A-line. ■ Assess skin color and capillary refill time.
The patient will not experience deep venous thrombosis.	■ Use prophylactic anticoagulants unless contraindicated. ■ Apply TED stockings. ■ Use pneumatic compression devices.
Fluids/Electrolytes	
The patient will maintain an adequate intake and output.	■ Monitor blood pressure, heart rate, central venous pressure, pulmonary capillary wedge pressure, IV fluid ■ Use Foley catheter to monitor urine output. ■ Consider insensible fluid loss in output. ■ Monitor laboratory values.
The patient will maintain electrolyte balance.	■ Replace electrolytes PRN. ■ Monitor ECG.
Mobility/Safety	
The patient's range of motion will be maintained.	■ Consult Physical/Occupational Therapy. ■ Use splints PRN. ■ Do range-of-motion exercises every 8 hours. ■ Out of bed as tolerated.
Skin Integrity	
The patient will not experience skin breakdown.	■ Monitor skin every 4 hours. ■ Turn patient every 2 hours and PRN. ■ Use pressure-relieving devices. ■ Remove splints to monitor skin. ■ Provide prescribed wound care. ■ Monitor wound for evidence of infection.

(continued)

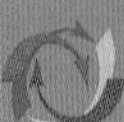

box 55-2 collaborative care guide *for the Patient with Multisystem Trauma (Continued)*

OUTCOMES	INTERVENTIONS
Nutrition	
The patient will maintain an adequate calorie intake to meet metabolic needs.	▪ Arrange dietary/nutrition consult. ▪ Use total parenteral nutrition (TPN)/lipids if enteral nutrition contraindicated. ▪ Tube feeds: encourage enteral nutrition when possible. ▪ Check prealbumin and electrolytes. ▪ Monitor for weight loss.
Comfort/Pain Control	
The patient will maintain a pain score of less than 5.	▪ Administer adequate pain medication. ▪ Use PCA/epidural PRN. ▪ Arrange pain consult if needed. ▪ Use sedation as needed. ▪ Monitor vital signs.
Psychosocial	
The patient will maintain as much control as possible.	▪ Inform patient of procedures. ▪ Establish a schedule with the patient if possible. ▪ Provide an alternate means of communication if necessary, such as lip reading, writing, and a communication board.
The patient and family will cope effectively with the traumatic event.	▪ Provide repeated information. ▪ Encourage use of appropriate coping. ▪ Encourage use of support systems. ▪ Arrange social work consult.
Teaching/Discharge Planning	
Patient will be involved in discharge planning.	▪ Discuss discharge with patient. ▪ Allow patient to make decisions if possible. ▪ Provide patient with list of injuries.
Patient will understand injuries and complications of injuries.	▪ Provide discharge instructions accordingly with injury.

pressure ventilation. Sometimes surgical repair is done, especially if a thoracotomy is necessary for other reasons. Surgical repair may help decrease the need for prolonged mechanical ventilation.

PLEURAL SPACE INJURIES

For the purpose of this chapter, the term *pleural space injuries* is used in reference to pneumothorax (intrapleural air collection), hemothorax (intrapleural blood collection), and hemopneumothorax (interpleural air and blood collections). Pleural space injuries are caused by disruption of an intrathoracic structure that allows air or blood to build up in the pleural layers, thereby leading to a decrease in negative intrathoracic pressure. Sometimes air and blood continue to build up in the pleural cavity, causing increased tension, which leads to a tension pneumothorax or a tension hemothorax. Either blunt or penetrating trauma may result in a pleural space injury.

The mechanism of injury may lead the nurse to suspect a pleural space injury. For example, an unrestrained driver whose chest hits the steering wheel has a great potential for this injury. When assessing the patient, respiratory distress may be evident along with altered ventilation, which leads to impaired gas exchange. Impaired gas exchange may be evidenced by restlessness, anxiety, tachypnea, decreased oxygenation, poor color, and diaphoresis. The nurse continuously reassesses the patient because even if the original injury is small, it can expand, causing a life-threatening emergency.

Chest radiography is usually used to diagnose pleural space injuries. Sometimes if the pneumothorax is less than 20% of the chest cavity, it may not be seen initially on chest film. A chest CT scan often shows the smaller pleural space injuries.

Treatment of pleural space injuries includes appropriate management of the patient's airway, ventilation, and oxygenation. A large-bore chest tube, such as a 40-French tube, is often inserted to re-expand the lung and drain the air or blood. This tube is inserted in the fourth or fifth intercostal space at the mid-axillary line. For trauma patients with a simple pneumothorax, a chest tube may be placed in the second intercostal space at the mid-clavicular line. Once the tube is inserted, it is attached to an underwater seal system and then attached to suction. The effects of treatment are assessed by chest x-ray, physical examination, and noting of improved oxygenation. Often there is an air leak in the underwater seal system of the chest tube drainage device that ceases within a few days.

The nurse monitors the amount of blood that drains into the chest tube drainage device. Drainage of more than 200 mL/hour for 2 consecutive hours may indicate a missed injury or the need for further exploration, and should be reported.[7]

A massive hemothorax is defined as 1.5 to 4 L of intrathoracic blood loss and truly constitutes a life-threatening injury. A massive hemothorax is often caused by severe thoracic injuries, and the source of bleeding is a large systemic blood vessel or mediastinal structure. Patients with massive hemothorax often arrive at the emergency department or trauma resuscitation unit in cardiopulmonary arrest. These patients require immediate thoracotomy to control bleeding. The patients who are not in cardiopulmonary arrest present with signs of hypovolemic shock (see Chapter 50), dyspnea, tachypnea, and cyanosis. Initial management of these patients includes treatment of the shock state. Two large-bore intravenous lines should be established and resuscitation fluid administered. The amount of fluid administered depends on the patient's response.[19]

A left massive hemothorax is more common than a right one, and is often associated with aortic rupture.[7] The chest cavity is large enough to hold most of the patient's circulating blood volume. Because of this, the bleeding stops only when the pressure in the pleural cavity is equal to or greater than the pressure in the damaged vessel. Placement of a chest tube in a patient with massive hemothorax could lead to exsanguination by eliminating the tamponade caused by a closed chest injury. If a chest tube is inadvertently placed, it should be clamped until exploratory thoracotomy can be performed.

Tension pneumothorax is a life-threatening condition that requires immediate recognition. It may be the result of a primary injury to the thorax or a delayed complication related to tracheobronchial injury or mechanical ventilation. Tension pneumothorax is caused by air entering the pleural space and becoming trapped without an exit. A one-way valve closed system is formed. This causes a compression of one or more of the intrathoracic structures (trachea, heart, lungs, and great vessels) and prohibits them from functioning adequately. The outcome is ventilation failure, compromised venous return, and insufficient cardiac output.

Tension pneumothorax is often difficult to diagnose in the trauma patient because of other injuries the patient may have, as well as the presence of a shock state. It may not be diagnosed until the patient has decompensated. The nurse may notice that it is difficult to ventilate the patient, despite an open airway. There is often a drop in the patient's oxygenation. Other signs of tension pneumothorax include chest asymmetry, tracheal shift, neck vein distension (unless the patient is hypovolemic), decreased breath sounds on the affected side, and evidence of decreased cardiac output (e.g., decreased blood pressure and poor tissue perfusion).

Treatment of tension pneumothorax requires immediate decompression of the trapped air. This is done initially by placing a 14- or 16-gauge needle into the pleural space, usually between the second to fourth anterior intercostal space. An immediate rush of air should escape and the patient's ventilation should improve. Supplemental oxygen is provided to the patient before decompression. After emergent decompression, the needles are changed to chest tubes. This is done to allow the lungs to expand as well as to prevent a reoccurrence. Last, additional assessment is necessary to determine the cause of tension pneumothorax. The nurse must continue to assess and reassess the patient.

PULMONARY CONTUSION

A pulmonary contusion is a bruising of the lung parenchyma, often caused by blunt trauma. This disorder may not be diagnosed on the initial chest x-ray; however, the presence of a scapular fracture, rib fractures, or a flail chest should lead to the suspicion of a possible underlying pulmonary contusion.

Pulmonary contusion occurs when rapid deceleration ruptures capillary cell walls, causing hemorrhage and extravasation of plasma and protein into alveolar and interstitial spaces. This results in atelectasis and consolidation, leading to intrapulmonary shunting and hypoxemia. Presenting signs and symptoms include dyspnea, rales, hemoptysis, and tachypnea. Severe contusions also result in increasing peak airway pressures, hypoxemia, and respiratory acidosis. Pulmonary contusion may mimic acute respiratory distress syndrome (ARDS); both are poorly responsive to high fractions of inspired oxygen (FIO_2). ARDS is discussed in detail in Chapter 27.

Treatment of pulmonary contusion is supportive. Patients with a mild contusion require close observation with frequent ABG measurements or pulse oximetry monitoring. Additional nursing interventions include frequent respiratory assessment, pulmonary care, and pain control. Chest physiotherapy and continuous epidural analgesia also may be beneficial. An oximetric pulmonary artery catheter and arterial line usually are placed to facilitate monitoring of ABGs, hemodynamics, and respiratory parameters (oxygen delivery, oxygen consumption, intrapulmonary shunt).

Severe pulmonary contusion may require ventilatory support with positive end-expiratory pressure (PEEP). Although alveolar ventilation improves as PEEP is added, blood flow to alveoli may diminish, leading to an increased intrapulmonary shunt. To optimize tissue perfusion and oxygenation, each change in PEEP requires assessment of the status of the shunt, oxygen delivery, and other indicators of tissue perfusion (cardiac output, blood pressure, and urine output). Adequate pain control is necessary and may require epidural or intrapleural infusions of analgesics or an intracostal nerve block. In severe cases of respiratory compromise, increased sedation or paralysis may be indicated to decrease energy expenditure and oxygen requirements. A rotation bed also may be considered to promote pulmonary toilet and respiratory gas exchange. Positioning the patient with the injured side up is beneficial in the case of a severe unilateral contusion. In rare instances, when the patient is not responding to traditional mechanical ventilation, prone positioning and high-frequency jet ventilation may be used.[20,21] Another mode of ventilation commonly used is airway pressure-release ventilation (APRV).

Fluid management also is important. Intake and output, daily weights, central venous pressure, and pulmonary artery and capillary wedge pressures are monitored to guide fluid administration. Medications may need to be more concentrated to compensate for excess fluid intake, and diuretics may be required periodically. Severe fluid restriction is not indicated. Instead, fluid balance should be maintained at a normal level (euvolemia) to support optimal cardiac output and oxygen delivery. The contused lung should show radiographic signs of improvement within 72 hours. The presence of persistent infiltrates may indicate complications, such as pneumonia or superimposed ARDS. Long-term sequelae include prolonged reduced functional residual capacity, dyspnea, and fibrosis.

BLUNT CARDIAC INJURIES

Blunt cardiac injuries include cardiac wall rupture, valvular disruption, coronary artery dissection, and cardiac contusions. Cardiac contusions, the most common form of blunt cardiac injuries, are usually caused by blunt trauma as the heart hits the sternum during rapid deceleration. A contusion can also develop if the heart is compressed between the sternum and the spine.

Symptoms of cardiac contusion vary from none (common) to severe congestive heart failure and cardiogenic shock. Complaints of chest pain must be evaluated carefully after trauma. Nonspecific ECG changes are frequently seen, and can include any type of dysrhythmia. Atrial dysrhythmias and conduction disturbances may be seen with injuries to the right side of the heart; ventricular disturbances are more likely after a left-sided cardiac injury.

A cardiac contusion is suspected when there is a history of severe anterior blunt trauma and the patient has chest wall bruising and fractures of the ribs or sternum. Twelve-lead ECG is done to detect any electrical abnormalities. Most patients with cardiac contusions have ECG abnormalities on admission. These patients are placed on continuous cardiac monitoring and blood is drawn for cardiac isoenzyme and troponin studies. In particular, an elevation in troponin I or the myocardial band of the creatine kinase (CK-MB) is clinically significant with this injury.[22,23]

Controversy exists over the standard of care for patients with cardiac contusion.[22] Because there is no standard in diagnosing this injury, there is also no standard in treatment. Continuous monitoring must be done to evaluate for symptomatic arrhythmias, especially ventricular irritability and conduction defects. Echocardiography or multigated angiography (MUGA) may be helpful in determining any muscle defect or damage. In general, patients are treated to relieve their symptoms.

PENETRATING CARDIAC INJURY

In most cases, a penetrating injury to the heart results in prehospital death. In the remainder of patients, hemorrhage and shock are common presenting signs. The right ventricle is injured most often because of its anterior location. Occasionally, small stab wounds to the ventricles seal themselves owing to the thick ventricular musculature. Treatment of hemodynamically stable patients remains controversial. In some instances, monitoring the patient with serial CT scanning or with pericardial and pleural ultrasound is acceptable.[24] In other cases, surgery to create a thoracoscopic pericardial window may be necessary to aid in the diagnosis of ongoing hemorrhage and to drain pericardial fluid collections.[25] In the presence of ongoing hemorrhage and shock, lost blood volume is replaced, and the patient is immediately transported to the operating room for a median sternotomy and exploration. In severe cases, a thoracotomy in the emergency department may be required as a life-saving measure.

After surgical repair, a pulmonary artery catheter and arterial line are placed to facilitate careful hemodynamic monitoring. Vasopressors or inotropic agents may be necessary to maintain adequate blood pressure and cardiac output. Fluid and electrolyte balance, along with cardiac rhythm, must be monitored closely. Heart sounds are assessed to detect murmurs, indicating valvular or septal defects, and for signs of congestive heart failure. Chest and mediastinal tube drainage are recorded frequently. Fresh frozen plasma and platelets are administered, as indicated, to correct coagulopathies. Complications include continued hemorrhage and postcardiotomy syndrome.

CARDIAC TAMPONADE

Cardiac tamponade, known as both a symptom and injury, can result from both penetrating and blunt trauma. It is a life-threatening injury that needs to be immediately assessed and treated. It is caused by blood filling the pericardium and compressing the heart, causing decreased cardiac filling, which leads to reduced cardiac output and eventually shock. Bleeding into the pericardial sac (hemopericardium) or a small pericardial rupture may or may not cause cardiac tamponade, depending on the amount of pressure in the pericardium.[17]

The pericardial sac normally holds about 25 mL of fluid, which serves to cushion and protect the heart. Only a small amount of pericardial blood (50 to 100 mL) is necessary to increase intrapericardial pressure. Continued bleeding increases the pressure rapidly and the patient presents with signs and symptoms of cardiac tamponade.

Classic symptoms include decreased blood pressure, muffled heart sounds, and increased central venous pressure manifested by distended neck veins (Beck's triad). Because these signs may be obscured in the hypovolemic trauma victim, patients with a history of precordial trauma must be treated with a high index of suspicion. A pericardiocentesis may be diagnostic and therapeutic; however, thoracotomy often is necessary to identify and repair the source of bleeding. Postoperative nursing care is similar to that for a penetrating cardiac injury.

AORTIC INJURIES

Thoracic aortic disruption from blunt trauma is the leading cause of death in people who fall, people who are struck by motor vehicles, and people who are passengers in vehicles involved in MVCs.[16] A recent study stated that 22% of patients who sustained a ruptured aorta died before reaching the hospital, another 37% died during initial resuscitation or in the operating room, and another 14% died after surgery. Of those who survived, 19% had paraplegia or paresis.[26] These statistics alone indicate the severe nature of these injuries.

There are three common locations of vessel rupture. Because the thoracic aorta is very mobile, the tears occur at points of fixation. The most common is at the aortic isthmus, just distal to the left subclavian artery, where the vessel is attached to the chest wall by the ligamentum arteriosum. The two other sites of rupture are in the ascending aorta, where the aorta leaves the pericardial sac, and at the entry to the diaphragm. The inner layers of the vessel tear on impact from deceleration. The outer layers remain intact and balloon out into a pseudoaneurysm. A partial circumferential hematoma may also be tamponaded by surrounding tissues. Both of these mechanisms may prolong survival, but only for a limited time.

An understanding of the injury history can raise the suspicion of aortic injury. Penetrating mediastinal injuries or thoracic injuries caused by blunt trauma should raise suspicion. Other injuries that may raise suspicion include first or second rib fractures, high sternal fractures, clavicular fractures at the sternal margin, and massive left-sided hemothorax.

Loss of effective blood transport because of major vessel rupture is the main physiological problem associated with aortic rupture. The goal of assessment is to identify evidence of poor perfusion beyond the aortic lesion. Many patients are asymptomatic on presentation. Findings associated with aortic injuries are given in Box 55-3.

A supine chest x-ray is obtained to aid in diagnosis of an aortic injury. After spinal injury has been ruled out, an upright chest x-ray may be obtained as well. If a widened mediastinum is detected on chest x-ray, additional evaluation is necessary for definitive management. Although an aortic tear is sometimes seen on CT scan, aortography is the study used for definitive diagnosis.[26]

A positive aortogram indicates the need for surgical repair. The torn aorta may require end-to-end anastomosis or, more commonly, the placement of a synthetic graft. Cardiopulmonary bypass may be necessary for repair of the ascending aorta or the aortic arch. However, repair of the descending thoracic aorta is usually accomplished during aortic cross-clamping. Because this maneuver occludes distal blood flow, it is imperative that the cross-clamp time be as short as possible (preferably less than 30 minutes). To prevent leakage from the repair site, vasodilators may be administered after surgery to reduce afterload. After replacement of intravascular volume, a vasopressor may be added to support adequate blood pressure. Nursing care focuses on hemodynamic monitoring with a pulmonary artery catheter and titrating medications to maintain optimal blood pressure. Autotransfusion may also be necessary.

Complications are related to the level of the tear and the extent of altered perfusion. Hypoperfusion and resulting damage to organs below the level of the laceration can result from the injury itself or from prolonged cross-clamping during repair. Serious complications resulting from prolonged cross-clamp time include renal failure, bowel ischemia, lower extremity weakness, or permanent paralysis of the lower extremities. Other sequelae, such as ARDS or DIC, can be a consequence of hemorrhagic shock and multiple blood transfusions.

box 55-3 ***Signs and Symptoms of Aortic Injuries***

- Pulse deficit in any area, particularly lower extremities or left arm
- Hypotension unexplained by other injuries
- Upper extremity hypertension relative to lower extremities
- Interscapular pain or sternal pain
- Precordial or interscapular systolic murmur caused by turbulence across the disrupted area
- Hoarseness caused by hematoma pressure around the aortic arch
- Respiratory distress or dyspnea
- Lower extremity neuromuscular or sensory deficit

Adapted from Sherwood SF, Hartsock RL: Thoracic injuries. In McQuillan KA, Von Rueden KT, Hartsock RL, et al (eds): Trauma Nursing (3rd Ed), pp 543–590. Philadelphia, WB Saunders, 2002.

Abdominal Trauma

Abdominal injuries rank third in the causes of trauma deaths.[27] They account for 13% to 15% of trauma deaths, primarily as a result of hemorrhage. Deaths that occur more than 48 hours after abdominal injury are due to sepsis and its complications.[28] In intra-abdominal trauma, rarely does single-organ injury or single-system injury occur.

Abdominal trauma can be caused by both blunt and penetrating injuries. MVCs are the most common cause of blunt abdominal trauma. Diagnosing blunt abdominal trauma can be difficult, especially if there are multisystem injuries. If the patient has abdominal tenderness or guarding, hemodynamic instability, lumbar spine injury, pelvic fracture, retroperitoneal or intraperitoneal air, or unilateral loss of the psoas shadow on x-ray, visceral damage should be suspected.

The abdominal cavity contains solid and hollow organs. Blunt trauma is likely to cause serious damage to solid organs, and penetrating trauma most often injures the hollow organs. The compression and deceleration of blunt trauma lead to fractures of solid organ capsules and parenchyma, whereas the hollow organ can collapse and absorb the force. The bowel, however, which occupies most of the abdominal cavity, is prone to injury by penetrating trauma. In general, solid organs respond to trauma with bleeding. Hollow organs rupture and release their contents into the peritoneal cavity, causing inflammation and infection.

Stab wounds, impalements, and gunshot wounds can cause penetrating trauma. If the mechanism of penetrating trauma is from a stab wound, knowledge of the size, shape and length of the instrument used is helpful in determining the extent of intra-abdominal damage. Impalement is considered a "dirty" wound. "Dirty" wounds can result in high mortality secondary to the infection that is caused by bacterial contamination and subsequent multisystem organ failure. Gunshot wounds (missile injuries) are difficult to evaluate. The amount of major vessel disruption and multiple organ involvement are predictors of mortality. The velocity and amount of energy dispersed by the bullet often determines the extent of injury. A bullet can rebound off organs or bones, changing its trajectory and causing massive internal damage to organs and vessels. The blast effect from bullets can also cause significant intra-abdominal injury.

Abdominal trauma requires continual assessment. Unrecognized abdominal trauma is a frequent cause of preventable death.[7,29] The nurse must be organized and methodical in the approach to patient assessment. The nurse needs to understand the mechanism of injury as well as the patient's complaints to perform an adequate assessment and identify potentially life-threatening abdominal injuries.

Usually, a primary survey is completed and the patient is resuscitated before the abdomen is assessed. During the secondary survey, the abdomen is assessed and reassessed and laboratory and diagnostic tests are performed. An orogastric or nasogastric tube and a Foley catheter are placed during the secondary survey phase.

Diagnostic testing may include focused abdominal sonography for trauma, (FAST), diagnostic peritoneal lavage (DPL), a chest x-ray (to determine gross abnormalities as well as any organ displacement), and an abdominal CT scan. Many trauma centers are performing FAST on all trauma patients. This is a relatively quick examination that provides valuable information.[30] It is performed by placing an ultrasound probe over various areas on the abdomen to determine if free fluid is located in those areas. The areas evaluated are the Morison's pouch in the right upper quadrant, the pericardial sac, the splenorenal region in the left upper quadrant, and the pelvis (Douglas' pouch). If the results of FAST are positive and the patient is hemodynamically unstable, an exploratory laparotomy is performed.

A DPL is a quick diagnostic procedure that is used during the resuscitation phase of care in hemodynamically unstable trauma patients to diagnose intra-abdominal bleeding (Box 55-4). Other indications for use may include:

1. Unexplained hypotension, decreased hematocrit, or shock
2. Equivocal results of abdominal examination
3. Altered mental status caused by brain injury or alcohol or drug intoxication
4. Spinal cord injury
5. Distracting injuries, such as major orthopedic fractures or chest trauma[28]

If the results of DPL are positive and the patient is hemodynamically unstable, an exploratory laparotomy is performed.

There are several contraindications to performing a DPL. These include morbid obesity, third-trimester pregnancy, advanced cirrhosis, a history of coagulopathy, and a history of multiple abdominal surgeries.[28] There is an increased risk of omental laceration and visceral or vascular perforation if DPL is performed in patients with these findings.

When performing DPL, it is important to first ensure that the patient has a Foley catheter and an orogastric or nasogastric tube in place to decompress the stomach and the bladder. Decompression of the stomach and bladder guards against accidental perforation when the lavage catheter is placed. Once the Foley catheter and an orogastric or nasogastric tube are placed, the lavage catheter is inserted into the peritoneal space. If less than 10 mL of frank blood is returned, a liter bag of warm crystalloid (lactated Ringer's solution or 0.9% normal saline) is infused into the peritoneum. After the infusion is complete, the intravenous bag is placed in a dependent position to allow the fluid to exit the abdomen by gravity. A sample of the fluid is then sent to the laboratory for evaluation.

box 55-4
Diagnostic Peritoneal Lavage (DPL)

Indications

- Blunt abdominal injury with:
  - Altered mental status
  - Unexplained hypotension, decreased hematocrit, shock
  - Equivocal results of abdominal examination
  - Spinal cord injury
  - Distracting injuries (e.g., orthopedic fractures, chest trauma)
- Penetrating abdominal trauma (if exploration is not indicated)

Possible Contraindications

- History of multiple abdominal operations
- Third trimester pregnancy
- Advanced cirrhosis of the liver
- Morbid obesity
- Known history of coagulopathy

Technique

1. Insert lavage catheter into peritoneal cavity through 1- to 2-cm incision.
2. Attempt to aspirate peritoneal fluid.
3. Infuse normal saline or Ringer's lactate by gravity.
4. Turn patient from side to side (unless contraindicated).
5. Allow fluid to run back into bag by gravity.
6. Send specimens to laboratory.

Positive Results

- 10–20 mL gross blood on initial aspirate
- Greater than 100,000 red blood cells/mm^3
- Greater than 500 white blood cells/mm^3
- Elevated amylase level
- Presence of bile, bacteria, or fecal matter

CT scans are now being used more often in hemodynamically stable patients. Often, the CT scan is done with both intravenous and oral contrast to visualize the organs and note any disruption. The CT scan allows visualization of the peritoneal, retroperitoneal, and pelvic areas and permits estimation of the amount of fluid in these areas. CT scans are also used to grade solid organ injuries. Limitations to the use of CT include the amount of time required to perform the study, the need to transport the patient out of the resuscitation area, and the requirement that the patient must be hemodynamically stable and have limited movement during the study.

TRAUMA TO THE STOMACH AND SMALL BOWEL

Significant gastric injury is rare. Small bowel injuries are much more common. Although frequently damaged by penetrating trauma, the small bowel can also burst when subjected to blunt trauma. The multiple convolutions occasionally form a closed loop, which, when subjected to increased pressure caused by impact with a steering wheel or seatbelt, can rupture. The bowel's mobility around fixed points (such as the ligament of Treitz) predisposes it to shearing injuries with deceleration.

Blunt small bowel or gastric injury can present with blood in the nasogastric aspirate or hematemesis. Physical signs often are absent, and CT findings may be subtle and nonspecific. Close observation is required; often diagnosis is not made until peritonitis develops. Penetrating injuries usually cause positive results on DPL. Although a mild bowel contusion can be managed conservatively (gastric decompression and withholding oral intake), surgery usually is necessary to repair penetrating wounds or bowel rupture.

Postoperative decompression with a gastric tube is maintained until bowel function returns. In most cases, a feeding jejunostomy tube is placed distal to the repair site, and tube feedings can be initiated early in the postoperative course. As the concentration and rate of feedings are advanced slowly, frequent assessment for signs of intolerance (distension, vomiting) is essential.

Because the stomach and small bowel contain an insignificant amount of bacteria, the risk of sepsis is small after rupture of these organs. On the other hand, the acidic gastric juice is irritating to the peritoneum and may cause peritonitis. Potential complications related to stomach and small bowel trauma are listed in Box 55-5. Some of these conditions may necessitate additional surgical procedures.

TRAUMA TO THE DUODENUM AND PANCREAS

The pancreas and duodenum are discussed together because these retroperitoneal organs are closely related anatomically and physiologically. A great deal of force is necessary to injure these organs because they are well protected deep in the abdomen. Injuries to adjacent organs almost always are present. The retroperitoneal location makes these injuries difficult to diagnose with DPL. An abdominal CT scan is very useful in this instance. Signs and symptoms may include an acute abdomen, increased serum amylase levels, epigastric pain radiating to the back, nausea, and vomiting.

Small lacerations or contusions may require only the placement of drains, whereas larger wounds need surgical repair. Most pancreatic injuries require postoperative closed suction drainage to prevent fistula formation. Distal pancreatectomy and Roux-en-Y anastomosis are two procedures commonly performed for injuries to the body and tail of the pancreas. Occasionally, the spleen also must be removed owing to the multiple vascular attachments it has to the pancreas. Damage to the head of the pancreas is associated with duodenal injury and severe hemorrhage because of the close proximity of vascular structures. Surgical procedures used in these cases include pancreaticoduodenectomy, Roux-en-Y anastomosis, and, on rare occasions, total pancreatectomy.

Postoperative nursing assessment and care are similar for the various procedures. Patency of drains must be maintained and the patient must be monitored for the development of fistulas, the most common complication. Skin protection is important if a cutaneous fistula does develop because of the high enzyme content of pancreatic fluid. Assessment of fluid and electrolyte balance is also important because a pancreatic fistula results in fluid loss, along with loss of potassium and bicarbonate. Pancreatic stimulation can be decreased by administering parenteral hyperalimentation or jejunal feedings instead of an oral diet. The onset of diabetes mellitus is rare unless a total pancreatectomy is performed.

Primary repair or resection with reanastomosis is sufficient to manage most penetrating duodenal injuries. A duodenostomy tube may be placed for decompression and a jejunostomy tube for feeding. Blunt trauma to the duodenum can cause an intramural hematoma, which may lead to duodenal obstruction. The diagnosis is made with a diatrizoate (Gastrografin) upper gastrointestinal study. A complete obstruction usually requires surgical drainage of the hematoma.

box 55-5 ***Complications Related to Stomach and Small Bowel Trauma***

- Intolerance to tube feedings
- Peritonitis
- Postoperative bleeding
- Hypovolemia caused by "third-spacing"
- Development of a fistula or obstruction

TRAUMA TO THE COLON

Usually, colon injury results from penetrating trauma. The nature of the injury most often dictates surgical exploration (exploratory laparotomy). Primary repair is the treatment of choice for lacerations of the colon.[31] In some situations, such as injury to the left colon or when there is massive blood loss, an exteriorized repair or colostomy is required. A cecostomy tube may be placed for colon decompression. Subcutaneous tissue and skin of the incision site are often left open to decrease the chance of wound infection. The colon has a high bacteria count; spillage of the contents predisposes the patient to intra-abdominal sepsis and abscess formation.

Postoperative nursing care focuses on prevention of infection. Dressing changes are necessary for open incisions, and prophylactic antibiotics may be used. In the case of an exteriorized colon repair, resection and end-to-end anastomosis is performed, and the repair site is exteriorized to facilitate identification of a leak. The exteriorized colon must be kept moist and covered with a nonadherent dressing or bag to protect the integrity of the sutures. Because sepsis is a major complication of colon injuries, a series of radiographic and surgical procedures may be required to locate and drain abscesses.

A Teaching Guide for patients who have undergone a laparotomy can be found in Box 55-6.

TRAUMA TO THE LIVER

After the spleen, the liver is the most commonly injured abdominal organ. Both blunt and penetrating trauma can cause hepatic injuries. Fractures of the right lower ribs increase suspicion for a liver injury. Presenting signs and symptoms may include right upper quadrant pain, rebound

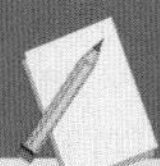

box 55-6
After a Laparotomy

Patient Activity

- No tub baths or showers while the staples/stitches are in place.
- If you are tired, rest.
- Only lift what you can easily lift with one hand.
- You may eat your normal diet.
- Take your temperature once a day at the same time and write it down.
- Maintain a normal schedule with your bowel movements.
- If you become constipated, drink more fruit juices.
- Do not drive until you have your doctor's permission.

Wound Care

- It is important to keep the staple/stitch line clean.
- Monitor your wound closely.
- Cleanse the area once a day. To do this, you will need 4″ × 4″ gauze pads and a solution of half peroxide/half saline.
- Wash your hands.
- Open the gauze pad and leave it on the paper.
- Pour a small amount of the peroxide/saline solution on the center of the pad while it is laying on the paper.
- Pick up the pad, pulling all four corners together without touching the center.
- Wipe over the stitches/staples from top to bottom, covering them well with the solution. It is normal to see bubbles when cleaning with this solution. Wipe the area only once with a single gauze pad.
- Repeat.
- Allow the area to dry.
- Tape a gauze pad over the stitch/staple line to prevent rubbing or irritation caused by a belt or waistband.

Signs of Infection

- Swelling around the site
- Increased redness
- Increased tenderness
- Warmth around the site
- Wound edges separating
- Increased drainage
- Foul-smelling drainage
- Change in color of drainage
- Temperature of 101°F or higher
- Vomiting, diarrhea, or constipation

tenderness, hypoactive or absent bowel sounds, or signs of hypovolemic shock.

Hemodynamically stable patients may be managed nonoperatively. In this case, serial CT scans are done to verify bleeding cessation. In many cases, however, the patient's unstable clinical condition dictates the need for surgery. Hepatic trauma can cause a large blood loss into the peritoneum, but bleeding may stop spontaneously. In some instances, bleeding vessels may be ligated or embolized. Small lacerations are repaired, whereas larger injuries may require segmental resection or debridement. In the case of uncontrollable hemorrhage, the liver is packed. After packing, the abdomen may be closed or simply covered and left open. An additional surgical procedure is required within the next few days to remove the packing and repair the laceration. Large liver injuries also need postoperative drainage of bile and blood with closed suction drains.

After surgery, coagulopathies may be present. Incomplete hemostasis also is a possibility and must be differentiated from coagulopathy-induced bleeding. Severe bleeding resulting from incomplete hemostasis requires clot removal, packing, and additional repair. With a coagulopathy, bleeding arises from numerous sites, whereas with incomplete hemostasis, the bleeding is mainly from the surgical site. Nursing care includes the replacement of blood products while monitoring the hematocrit and coagulation studies. Assessment of the character and amount of tube drainage, along with fluid balance, also is essential. Potential complications of liver injury include hepatic or perihepatic abscess, biliary obstruction or leak, sepsis, ARDS, and DIC.

TRAUMA TO THE SPLEEN

The spleen is the most commonly injured abdominal organ, usually as a result of blunt trauma. Presence of left lower rib fractures increases suspicion for a splenic injury. Presenting signs and symptoms include left upper quadrant pain radiating to the left shoulder (Kehr's sign), hypovolemic shock, and the nonspecific finding of an increased white blood cell count. DPL or abdominal CT is usually necessary for diagnosis.

Adults with minor injuries and most children are treated nonoperatively with observation (serial abdominal examinations, serial hematocrits) and gastric decompression. Because the spleen and stomach are both in the left upper quadrant, decompression of the stomach reduces pressure on the injured spleen. Preferred surgical treatment is splenorrhaphy, although in some cases splenectomy is necessary. Splenic autotransplantation, a fairly new procedure, consists of implanting splenic fragments into pockets of omentum after splenectomy. Splenic autotransplantation may be performed after severe injuries to retain the normal splenic immune functions.[32,33]

Early complications include recurrent bleeding, subphrenic abscess, and pancreatitis resulting from surgical trauma. Late complications consist of thrombocytosis and overwhelming postsplenectomy sepsis (OPSS). Because the spleen plays an important role in the body's response to infection, a splenectomy predisposes the patient to an increased risk for infection. This risk is especially high among children and highest in those younger than 2 years. *Pneumococcus*, an encapsulated microorganism resistant to phagocytosis, is the organism that most often infects patients after splenectomy. OPSS frequently begins with the onset of pneumococcal pneumonia, which progresses to a fulminant sepsis. Postsplenectomy patients can increase their immunity toward pneumococcal infections by receiving a polyvalent pneumococcal vaccine (Pneumovax). Complications of OPSS include adrenal insufficiency and DIC. OPSS has a high incidence and mortality rate, especially within 1 year of surgery. Patient and family teaching should focus on information about signs and symptoms of infection. Splenic autotransplantation may prove beneficial in decreasing the incidence of OPSS.

TRAUMA TO THE KIDNEYS

Injury to the kidney may lead to a "free" hemorrhage, contained hematoma, or the development of an intravascular thrombus. Sudden deceleration injury can cause the kidney to move, avulsing smaller renal vessels or tearing the renal artery intima, which also may lead to vessel thrombosis. Blunt and penetrating trauma can also cause a laceration or contusion of the renal parenchyma or rupture of the collecting system. Lower rib or lumbar vertebral fractures, along with liver and spleen injuries, should raise suspicion of an associated renal injury.[34] Signs and symptoms, when present, consist of hematuria, pain, a flank hematoma, or ecchymosis over the flank.[34] Because the bleeding is retroperitoneal, it can be difficult to detect. A helical CT scan, ultrasound, or an intravenous pyelogram (less commonly used) usually provides the diagnosis.

Renal injuries are classified based on their severity. Many renal injuries can be managed conservatively with observation and bed rest until gross hematuria resolves. However, in some instances (mainly for vascular injury), surgical repair or nephrectomy is necessary.

Postoperative assessment and support of renal function are imperative. Optimal fluid balance must be maintained. Low-dose dopamine may be ordered to promote renal perfusion. Major complications consist of arterial or venous thrombosis and acute renal failure. Other complications include bleeding, perinephric abscess, the development of a urinary fistula, and late onset of hypertension.

TRAUMA TO THE BLADDER

The bladder can be lacerated, ruptured, or contused, most often as the consequence of blunt trauma (usually because of a full bladder at the time of injury).[34] Bladder injuries frequently are associated with pelvic fractures. Gross hematuria is typically noted with bladder rupture. Presence of blood at the urethral meatus, a scrotal hematoma, or a displaced prostate gland requires examination for urethral injuries with a CT scan or conventional cystography before the insertion of a urinary catheter.[34]

A bladder injury can cause intraperitoneal or extraperitoneal urine extravasation. Extraperitoneal extravasation, usually associated with pelvic fractures, can often be managed with urinary catheter drainage. Intraperitoneal extravasation (associated with a high-force injury), however, requires surgery. This injury has a high mortality rate because of associated injuries that occur secondary to the force involved.[34] A suprapubic cystostomy tube may be placed. Complications are infrequent, but infection due to the urinary catheter or sepsis from extravasation of infected urine can occur. Patients may complain of an inability to void or of shoulder pain (caused by urine extravasation into the peritoneal space).

Musculoskeletal Injuries

Although musculoskeletal injuries take a long time to heal and can often result in lifelong disability, they are usually not considered life-threatening injuries unless there is a traumatic amputation or pelvic fracture. Routinely, the musculoskeletal assessment is done in the secondary survey after hemodynamic stabilization. These injuries do require prompt recognition and stabilization to promote optimal recovery and function.

There are approximately 33 million musculoskeletal injuries per year. This includes 20 million fractures, dislocations, and sprains, with approximately 8,000 deaths.[35] Although there are a variety of causes of trauma-related musculoskeletal injuries, the major ones include MVCs; falls; industrial, farming, and home accidents; and assaults. Musculoskeletal injuries are often associated with other injuries to the body.

It is important to understand the circumstances surrounding, and the mechanism involved in, musculoskeletal trauma. Force might be applied to one area but the transferred energy and distribution of force may cause injury somewhere else. For example, in a person who falls off a two-story building and lands on his or her feet, one would expect to find calcaneus or ankle fractures, but the transference of energy may also cause a pelvic or lumbar spine fracture. Obviously, if the patient is conscious, he or she can verbalize his or her pain. However, many times, fractures and sprains go unrecognized because the patient is not able to verbalize and communicate the location of his or her pain.

As in all trauma patients, initial assessment begins with the primary survey. Once this is complete and the patient is hemodynamically stable, the secondary assessment is conducted. When trauma patients are admitted to the resuscitation unit, cervical spine, chest, and pelvis films are obtained first. Sometimes thoracic and lumbar spine films are obtained, depending on the mechanism of injury. The initial pelvic film tells the nurse if the patient has a life-threatening pelvic fracture. If this is the case, immobilization of the pelvis should be maintained to prevent exsanguination. Immobilization of the pelvis is achieved with a C-clamp, external fixator, pelvic binder, or sheets wrapped tightly around the patient to attempt to stop the bleeding.

During the secondary survey, if limb swelling, ecchymosis, or deformity is noted, that extremity should be immobilized. Proper films are ordered to determine the extent of the injury. The nurse tests the extremities for capillary refill (less than 2 seconds is normal), pulses, crepitus, muscle spasm, movement, sensation, and pain.

The most common studies used to diagnose musculoskeletal injuries are plain x-rays, CT, and magnetic resonance imaging (MRI). When obtaining x-rays on a patient it is important to get two views of the affected area. It is also important to assess the joint above and below the injured area. If the affected area is in a place that is difficult to visualize on plain films, a CT scan usually gives a better picture. An MRI also gives more specific detail about the area surrounding the injury and about the injury itself.

There are many types of musculoskeletal injuries, including fractures, fracture–dislocations, amputations, and trauma to the soft tissue (i.e., skin, muscle, tendons, ligaments, and cartilage). Fracture classification is based on type, cause, and anatomical location.[36] Several fracture types are shown in Figure 55-5. If the skin is broken at the fracture site, the injury is considered to be an "open" fracture. If the skin is intact, the injury is said to be a "closed" fracture. An open fracture is further classified as grade I, II, or III, depending on the tissue damage involved.

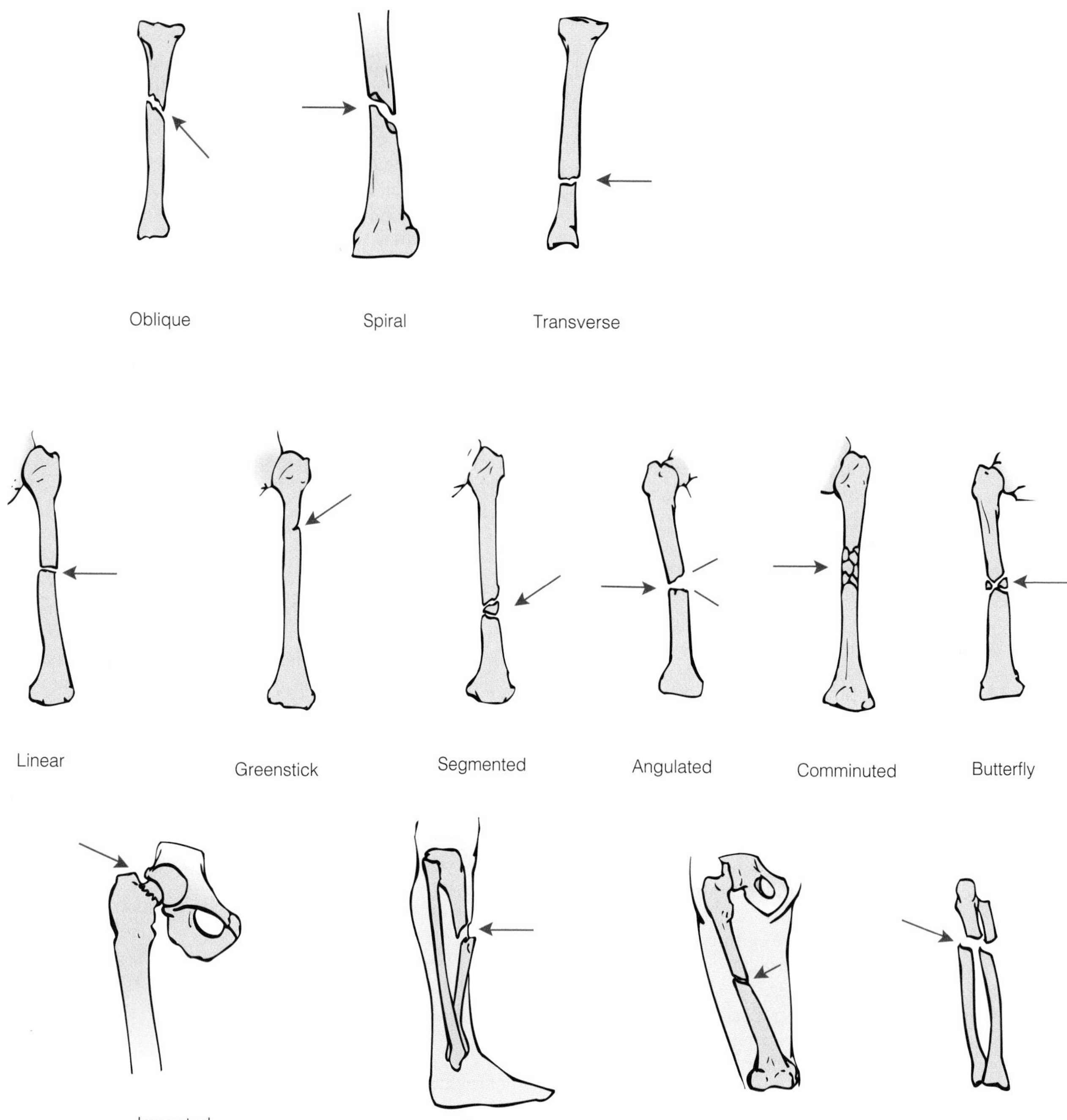

figure 55-5 There are many different types of fractures.

Dislocation occurs when the articulating surfaces of a joint are no longer in contact because of joint disruption. Joint mobility may be restricted. There may also be associated vascular or nerve injury with dislocations. Ligamentous injury usually accompanies dislocations because ligaments stretch or tear at the time of dislocation.

Amputations are classified according to the amount of tissue, nerve, and vascular damage. A cut or guillotine amputation has clean lines and well-defined edges, whereas a crush amputation has more soft tissue damage and the edges are not as well defined. An avulsion amputation occurs when a force stretches and tears away tissues, causing nerves and vessels to be torn in different areas than the bone.

As with any injury, musculoskeletal trauma requires continuous assessment. It is not uncommon for vascular or neurological compromise, or both, to develop in patients with musculoskeletal injury. Any musculoskeletal injury involving bone or soft tissue can cause neurological or vascular compromise because nerves and blood vessels are located in such close proximity to the bones and muscles. The nerves and muscles are very sensitive to impaired circulation and compression.

It is also important to continually assess the patient for hypovolemia. As stated earlier, traumatic amputation and major pelvic ring fractures are known for their extensive blood loss. Other orthopedic injuries can also cause substantial blood loss. Very rarely do patients sustain severe musculoskeletal injuries without other systemic injuries; therefore, other sources of blood loss should also be investigated.

Infection is common in open injuries. Ideally, patients with musculoskeletal trauma are brought to the operating room within 6 hours of injury for a washout of the affected area. Sometimes antibiotic prophylaxis is started; however, this practice is controversial. A tetanus booster is given if indicated to all patients with open injuries.

Other serious complications of musculoskeletal injuries include compartment syndrome, deep venous thrombosis (DVT), pulmonary embolus, and fat embolus syndrome.

COMPARTMENT SYNDROME

Compartment syndrome occurs when the pressure within the fascia-enclosed muscle compartment is increased, causing blood flow to the muscles and nerves in the compartment to become compromised, thereby resulting in tissue ischemia.[37] This ischemia then leads to tissue damage, which compromises nerve and muscle function. A prolonged elevation of compartmental pressure leads to death of the muscles and nerves involved.[38] Intracompartmental pressures that exceed 30 to 40 mm Hg can cause muscle ischemia, and pressures greater than 55 to 65 mm Hg cause irreversible muscle death.[37,38]

Patients with compartment syndrome complain of increased pain in the affected area. The pain is described as being "out of proportion" to the injury.[37,38] The most reliable early sign of compartment syndrome is decreased sensation.[37] The compartment involved is firm and the patient eventually has paresthesia. Pallor and pulselessness are late signs of compartment syndrome. When the compartment syndrome has progressed to the point that the patient is showing late signs, loss of the affected extremity is threatened. The nurse must constantly monitor the affected extremity and compare it with the nonaffected extremity. If any of the signs or symptoms of compartment syndrome are present, the orthopedic or general surgeon should be notified immediately so compartment pressures can be measured. If it is deemed that the compartment pressures are high, a fasciotomy is performed to release the pressure and save the extremity.

DEEP VENOUS THROMBOSIS

DVT is a significant risk for all trauma patients, especially those with musculoskeletal injuries. It is known as a "common, life threatening complication" of major trauma.[39] The danger of DVT is that it may progress to pulmonary embolus. The administration of low-dose heparin or low–molecular-weight heparin and the use of intermittent pneumatic compression devices are recommended to prevent DVT.[39]

The pathophysiology of DVT, and later pulmonary embolus, is related to Virchow's triad:

1. Venous stasis from decreased blood flow, decreased muscular activity, and external pressure on the deep veins
2. Vascular damage or concomitant pathological state
3. Hypercoagulability[35]

The nurse assesses for signs and symptoms of DVT on a regular basis. These include the presence of Homans' sign (calf pain on dorsiflexion of the foot), swelling of the affected area, tachycardia, fever, and distal skin color and temperature changes. If these signs or symptoms are found, they should be reported immediately. Sometimes an acute pulmonary embolus is the first indication of DVT.

PULMONARY EMBOLUS

A pulmonary embolus occurs when a blood clot dislodges from the vein, travels through the heart, and lodges in the pulmonary artery, obstructing blood flow. Sudden onset of dyspnea is the classic sign of a pulmonary embolus, but signs and symptoms vary, depending on the size of the clot and the number of vessels occluded. Signs and symptoms may include a decline in oxygenation, substernal chest pain, hypovolemic relative shock, tachypnea, shortness of breath, anxiety, a feeling of impending doom, a low-grade fever, an altered level of consciousness, and a pale, dusky, or cyanotic skin color.

FAT EMBOLISM SYNDROME

Fat emboli are fat globules in the lung tissue and peripheral circulation after a long bone fracture or major trauma.[40] Fat emboli may or may not cause systemic symptoms. Fat embolism syndrome is a serious (but rare) manifestation of fat emboli that involves progressive respiratory insufficiency, thrombocytopenia, and a decrease in mental status. It usually occurs within 72 hours of injury.[40] Clinical indications of this syndrome include tachypnea, dyspnea, cyanosis, tachycardia, and fever.[35,40] Nurses should be aware of the potential for fat embolism syndrome to develop and monitor the patient for hypoxemia with pulse oximetry. The patient's neurological status is also monitored for signs of a decreasing mental status.

Maxillofacial Trauma

Despite laws that mandate lower speed limits and the use of air bags and seat belts, the incidence of maxillofacial trauma remains high because the face is unprotected during rapid deceleration.[41,42] The degree of maxillofacial injury is directly related to the force at impact when the face makes contact with a stationary object. As the force increases, the amount of energy that is dispersed increases, causing an increase in injury. Penetrating injury is less common than blunt injury in patients with maxillofacial trauma.

As with any trauma patient, initial management priorities remain airway, breathing, and circulation. The trauma team cannot be distracted from these priorities by obvious deformities that may be associated with maxillofacial injuries. Maxillofacial trauma can cause airway obstruction and death if airway and breathing are not adequately and urgently established. When the primary survey is completed, an adequate assessment of the maxillofacial injuries is performed.

When assessing for maxillofacial injuries, soft tissues are assessed as well as bony structures. The face is inspected for symmetry and then palpated systematically to observe for any movement of bony structures. Cranial nerves are assessed. Often, maxillofacial injuries coincide with head injuries, reinforcing the importance of a thorough neurological examination (see Chapter 33). Any midface fractures that communicate through the orbit require a thorough ocular assessment and frequent reassessment.

Most maxillofacial injuries involve the soft tissue. In any soft tissue injury there is potential for contamination. Therefore, each patient's immunization to tetanus is assessed. If needed, a tetanus booster is given. All wounds are assessed for dirt, grease, particles, and other contaminants. Many wounds require an operation for washout to debride the tissue and clean the area. These injuries are usually not life-threatening and are treated in the appropriate order. However, even a small abrasion to a person's face can lead to a lifetime of disfigurement; therefore, all injuries must be attended to appropriately.

As stated earlier, in any type of trauma, but especially in maxillofacial trauma where the patient's airway may be compromised, it is imperative continuously to assess and maintain an adequate airway for the patient. Loss of an artificial airway (e.g., inadvertent removal of the endotracheal tube) can be life-threatening because of soft tissue swelling. It is also essential to assess for and treat hypovolemia secondary to hemorrhage from facial arteries. Epistaxis may also occur with any fracture that communicates with the nose. The nurse also continuously assesses the patient's neurological status and reports any abnormalities. The patient's pain and anxiety must be assessed and treated. Many patients with maxillofacial injuries are robbed of their senses. They may be unable to see, smell, taste, or speak secondary to their injury. This is an anxiety-provoking situation; patients require continuous reassurance and medication as necessary. Many maxillofacial injuries require multiple surgeries before the patient is definitively treated.

box 55-7 ***Delayed Complications of Multiple Trauma***

Hematologic
- Hemorrhage, coagulopathy, disseminated intravascular coagulation (DIC)

Cardiac
- Dysrhythmia, heart failure, ventricular aneurysm

Pulmonary
- Atelectasis, pneumonia, emboli (fat or thrombotic), acute respiratory distress syndrome (ARDS)

Gastrointestinal
- Peritonitis, adynamic ileus, mechanical bowel obstruction, acalculous cholecystitis, anastomotic leak, fistula, bleeding

Hepatic
- Liver abscess, liver failure

Renal
- Hypertension, myoglobinuria, renal failure

Orthopedic
- Compartment syndrome

Skin
- Wound infection, dehiscence, skin breakdown

Systemic
- Sepsis

COMPLICATIONS OF MULTIPLE TRAUMA

Complications associated with multiple trauma are numerous (Box 55-7). Because most trauma patients are in the intensive care unit when these complications develop, the nurse plays an essential role in detecting, preventing, and treating these sequelae.

The unexpected nature of trauma tends to amplify fear and anxiety. Therefore, nursing care must also provide psychosocial support for the seriously injured patient and his or her family. A multidisciplinary approach that recognizes concerns and offers frequent explanations is recommended. Special considerations for pediatric and older trauma patients can be found in Boxes 55-8 and 55-9, respectively.

Death after multiple traumatic injuries, when it occurs, may occur immediately, or it may occur as a result of early or late complications. Immediate deaths occur at the scene and within minutes of the injury. Most common causes of immediate deaths are brainstem or high spinal cord injury, cardiac rupture, transection of the great vessels, and airway obstruction.

Early Complications

Severe head injuries and hemorrhage are the early complications of multiple trauma most often responsible for causing death within hours of the injury, usually in the emergency department or operating room. Often, death at this stage can be prevented with quick assessment, resuscitation, and management of injuries.

Management of head injuries is discussed in Chapter 35. To prevent exsanguination, hemorrhage must be controlled and volume resuscitation begun with the infusion of crystalloids and blood. Patients may require emergent surgical ligation or packing, or embolization by angiography. Massive hemorrhage complicated by hypothermia, metabolic acidosis, and coagulopathy is highly lethal.

Late Complications

Late complications of multiple trauma include hypovolemic shock, infection and septic shock, ARDS, and multiple organ dysfunction syndrome (MODS).

HYPOVOLEMIC SHOCK

Massive hemorrhage or continued bleeding because of incomplete hemostasis or an undiagnosed injury can lead to hypovolemic shock and eventually decreased organ perfusion. The various organs respond differently to the decrease in perfusion caused by hypovolemia. Multiple blood transfusions are often necessary, further increasing the likelihood of ARDS and MODS.

INFECTION AND SEPTIC SHOCK

Another frequent and potentially serious complication of multiple trauma is infection. The risk of infection is increased after close-range shotgun blasts, high-velocity

box 55-8

Considerations for the Pediatric Patient With Trauma

General Principles

- Trauma is the leading cause of death in people between the ages of 1 and 19 years, with motor vehicle crashes being the leading cause.
- Blunt injury is more common then penetrating injury and should raise a high level of suspicion.
- The anatomy of a child is more vulnerable to traumatic injury:
  - *Head:* A child's head is proportionately larger in relation to body mass. Head injury is the most common cause of death in children.
  - *Chest:* A child's chest is more compliant than an adult's. Therefore, bony injuries are less common in children than in adults.
  - *Abdomen:* Liver and spleen injuries are most common in children, followed by bowel and pancreatic injuries. The kidney is less protected in children and often sustains more damage than the bladder and urethra, as seen in adults.
- When treating a child, it is extremely important to consider the entire family in the plan of care.
- When caring for a child, it is important to develop a trusting relationship. Involve the parents, offer a toy, speak to the child on his or her level, and protect the child.
- Children have a decreased reserve, compared with adults.
  - A child has a greater insensible water loss per unit of body weight (due to a larger surface area and an increased metabolic rate). Therefore, the child's fluid requirement is increased. A child's urine output should average 0.5 to 1 mL/kg/h.
  - A child experiences a rapid loss of body temperature secondary to increased surface area.
  - Shock is caused by hypoxia and blood loss. There is a small margin of error in treating shock in a child.
  - Hypovolemia occurs more rapidly in children. A child can compensate up to 25% of blood loss.

Primary Survey

- Airway: Use an uncuffed tube until the child is 7 years of age.
- Breathing: Watch for chest rise and fall.
- Circulation: Central and peripheral pulses are used to determine adequate circulation and capillary refill.
  - *Intraosseous infusion:* A bone marrow needle is inserted into the medial flat surface of the anterior tibia, approximately two fingerbreadths below the tibial tuberosity.
  - *Volume resuscitation:* 20 mL/kg × 1; if no response, give a second bolus. Volume resuscitation is guided by vital signs before and after infusion.

Adapted from Moloney-Harmon PA: Pediatric trauma. In McQuillan KA, Von Rueden KT, Hartsock RL, et al (eds): Trauma Nursing (3rd Ed), pp 747–771. Philadelphia, WB Saunders, 2002.

penetrating injuries, penetrating wounds to the colon, prolonged surgery, multiple blood transfusions, and injury to multiple organs. Other risk factors include advanced age, underlying immunosuppression, and a history of diabetes mellitus.

Infections can range from a minor wound infection to fulminant sepsis syndrome and septic shock. In septic shock, the release of toxins causes dilation of vessels, leading to venous pooling that results in a decreased venous return. Initially, cardiac output increases to compensate for decreased systemic vascular resistance. Eventually, the compensatory mechanisms fail, and cardiac output falls along with blood pressure and organ perfusion (i.e., septic shock).

The source of infection must be found and eradicated to treat sepsis effectively. The nurse must watch for the sometimes subtle indicators of sepsis. Hyperthermia or hypothermia and altered mental status are often present early in the septic process, as well as tachycardia, tachypnea, and an increase in the white blood cell count. These findings should prompt further assessment to detect a possible infectious source.

When sepsis is suspected, cultures are obtained, antibiotics are prescribed, radiological studies are done, and exploratory surgery frequently is performed. Intra-abdominal abscess is a frequent cause of sepsis. Some abscesses can be drained percutaneously, whereas others require surgery. After the surgical drainage of an abdominal abscess, the incision is left open with drains in place to allow healing and prevent recurrence. Other sources of infection are invasive lines, the urinary tract, and the lungs. Pneumonia is a common cause of sepsis in trauma patients. Risk factors for pneumonia include advanced age, aspiration, underlying pulmonary disease, thoracic or abdominal surgery, and prolonged intubation.

Hemodynamics are altered and metabolic demands are increased during sepsis. The typical patient exhibits elevated cardiac output, decreased systemic vascular resistance, and increased oxygen consumption. Hemodynamics must be supported and a balance between oxygen delivery and oxygen consumption maintained. Research suggests that early nutritional support decreases the development of sepsis and MODS. Enteral feeding should be used whenever possible because it is associated with a lower incidence of sepsis than total parenteral nutrition.

ACUTE RESPIRATORY DISTRESS SYNDROME

Sepsis may predispose the patient to ARDS (see Chapter 27). In addition to sepsis, specific injuries (e.g., head trauma, pulmonary contusion, multiple major fractures), massive blood transfusions, aspiration, and pneumonia can also increase the likelihood of ARDS. With a mortality rate of about 50% to 70%, ARDS is characterized by hypoxemia with shunting, decreased lung compliance, tachypnea, dyspnea, and the appearance of diffuse bilateral pulmonary infiltrates. The syndrome requires intensive ventilatory support with PEEP.[43,44] Oxygen delivery is assessed and supported.

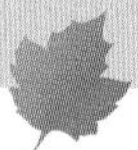

box 55-9

Considerations for the Older Patient With Trauma

- By 2030, 20% of the United States population will be older than 65 years of age. This is the fastest-growing segment of our population.
- Trauma is the seventh most frequent cause of death in this population.
- The older person is injured less frequently than the younger person; however, when an older person does sustain injuries, the injuries are more likely to be life-threatening.
- The injuries occurring in this population tend to be less severe but are associated with a greater risk of death.
- Falls are the most prominent cause of trauma in the older person.
- Constant monitoring is essential with the older trauma patient.
- Providers should have a decreased threshold for invasive monitoring with this population, secondary to predisposing conditions and past medical history.
- Management considerations are as follows:
  - Consider cervical osteoarthritis when intubation is necessary.
  - Pain management should be more local if possible (e.g., epidural catheter, nerve block).
  - Fluid management should be done cautiously. This population requires adequate rapid fluid replacement without excess. Consider a pulmonary artery or central venous pressure line for guidance in fluid replacement.
  - This population tends to become hypothermic more quickly than the younger population.
  - Use warm fluid and warming devices as indicated.

Adapted from Atwell SL: Trauma in the elderly. In McQuillan KA, Von Rueden KT, Hartsock RL, et al (eds): Trauma Nursing (3rd Ed), pp 772–787. Philadelphia, WB Saunders, 2002.

MULTIPLE ORGAN DYSFUNCTION SYNDROME

More than 10% of critically injured patients experience MODS.[45] Many factors have been associated with the development of MODS, including hemorrhage, massive blood transfusion, hypovolemic shock, and sepsis. Characterized by the failure of two or more organs, MODS accounts for more than 50% of late deaths in trauma patients.[45] Usually the lungs are the first organs to fail (heralded by the onset of ARDS), followed by the liver, gastrointestinal tract, and kidneys.[46,47]

Liver failure can result from initial damage, vascular compromise, shock, or sepsis. Jaundice is a common indicator of deteriorating liver function, although other causes, such as post-traumatic biliary obstruction, must be ruled out. Liver function tests are diagnostic. Liver failure can lead to a decreased level of consciousness, abnormal clotting study results, and hypoglycemia (see Chapter 41).

Gastrointestinal failure manifests with hemorrhage from stress ulcers requiring blood transfusion. Prophylactic neutralization of gastric acid can minimize the risk of bleeding (see Chapter 41).

Renal failure can be precipitated by a renal injury, ischemia, radiographic contrast material, rhabdomyolysis, hypovolemia (due to hemorrhage, third spacing), or sepsis. Initial signs include increasing blood urea nitrogen (BUN) and serum creatinine levels. Renal failure may be polyuric or oliguric. Dialysis may be necessary (see Chapter 30).

Cardiovascular failure, DIC, metabolic changes (e.g., hyperglycemia, metabolic acidosis), and CNS changes, ranging from confusion to obtundation, also may be evident in MODS (see Chapter 49 for a discussion of DIC).

case study ■ MOTOR VEHICLE TRAUMA

A 35-year-old woman was admitted to the resuscitation unit after being struck by a motor vehicle. She arrived unresponsive, but the paramedics stated that eyewitnesses reported that the woman had landed on the windshield of the car after being thrown into the air by the impact. It was reported that she broke the windshield on impact. Her initial vital signs were as follows: blood pressure 70/50 mm Hg; pulse rate 120 beats/minute; respiratory rate 4 to 6 breaths/minute with assisted ventilation by Ambu bag. Her arterial oxygen saturation (SaO_2) was 85%.

The patient was urgently intubated and multiple x-rays and CT scans were obtained. These studies revealed a subarachnoid hemorrhage, pulmonary contusions, a ruptured bladder, a right acetabular fracture, bilateral upper extremity fractures, a right open humerus fracture, and possibly aortic injury. Despite multiple transfusions and fluid resuscitation, the patient was unable to sustain a systolic blood pressure greater than 90 mm Hg. She was then taken to angiography for further diagnosis and treatment of her injuries. It was determined that she did not have an aortic injury; however, her bladder rupture could not be repaired and the patient was transferred to the operating room for an emergent exploratory laparotomy and repair of her fractures.

After the operation, the patient was transferred to the multitrauma intensive care unit, where she was monitored continuously and maintained on mechanical ventilation. Her abdomen and right upper extremity were left open. Despite continuous monitoring and frequent transfusions, the patient remained hemodynamically unstable. A pulmonary artery catheter and arterial line were inserted for more invasive monitoring. Laboratory values were assessed every 6 hours and indicated a rising lactate level and decreasing hematocrit and hemoglobin.

During an assessment, the nurse noted an increased amount of drainage from the patient's right upper extremity wound. The dressing was removed and an arterial bleed was noted. After the application of direct pressure, the artery was cauterized and the wound redressed. The next set of laboratory values indicated a stable hematocrit and hemoglobin, but the lactate was unchanged and the patient remained unresponsive. It was also noted that the patient had an increased temperature and worsening lung sounds. The results of blood, sputum, urine, and wound cultures suggested that the patient was septic and antibiotics were initiated. A repeat head CT indicated a swollen brain with a new contusion.

After several days without improvement, the patient was removed from life support according to the wishes of her family, who felt that she would not want to be kept alive indefinitely by machines. ■

clinical applicability challenges

Self-Challenge: Critical Thinking

1. *Refer to the case study at the end of this chapter. What other information would have been helpful from the prehospital providers to ensure that this patient received the appropriate care on arrival to the resuscitation unit?*
2. *What complications should the nurse be aware of after a patient sustains the amount of force this patient received and requires this much fluid/blood resuscitation?*
3. *What are the concerns regarding end-of-life decisions, and what services should be provided to the family and the patient?*

Study Questions

1. *A 50-year-old man is admitted to the trauma resuscitation unit. He is intubated on arrival. What is the next step in the primary survey?*
   a. *Obtain a chest x-ray to determine tube placement.*
   b. *Listen to lung sounds to assess for ventilation.*
   c. *Assess the patient's blood pressure and peripheral pulses.*
   d. *Initiate large-bore intravenous catheter placement and replace fluid.*
2. *A patient is admitted to the emergency department after being involved in a motor vehicle crash (MVC). The patient was wearing a seat belt but the air bag did not deploy. What injuries should the nurse be looking for, given the circumstances of the accident?*
   a. *Head injuries*
   b. *Pleural space injuries*
   c. *Abdominal injuries*
   d. *All of the above*
3. *In what phase of care would the health care provider listen for bowel sounds?*
   a. *Primary survey*
   b. *Secondary survey*
   c. *Definitive care*
   d. *Resuscitation*
4. *A patient presents to the intensive care unit after an exploratory laparotomy related to trauma. The patient is hypotensive and tachycardic. This is most likely due to which of the following?*
   a. *Hypovolemia*
   b. *Pain*
   c. *Hypothermia*
   d. *All of the above*
5. *A 40-year-old woman is involved in an equestrian accident. She presents with chest pain, shortness of breath, and difficulty breathing. Her arterial oxygen saturation (Sao_2) is 85% and her respiratory rate is 40 breaths/minute. A 40-French chest tube is placed and the nurse observes a return of 300 mL blood into the system. What is the nurse's next step?*
   a. *Clamp the chest tube and notify the surgeon immediately.*
   b. *Call for a chest x-ray.*
   c. *Place the patient on oxygen.*
   d. *Explain to the patient what is happening to decrease her anxiety.*
6. *A 16-year-old is admitted to the floor after a football injury. The patient has a femur fracture. An external fixation device was applied in the operating room. This patient is at an increased risk for developing which of the following?*
   a. *Deep venous thrombosis (DVT)*
   b. *Post-traumatic stress disorder*
   c. *Pulmonary embolism*
   d. *None of the above*

REFERENCES

1. The American Heritage Dictionary (2nd Ed). Boston, Houghton Mifflin, 1991
2. National Safety Council: Accident Facts, 2000. Chicago, National Safety Council, 2000
3. Weigelt JA, Klein JD: Mechanism of injury. In McQuillan KA, Von Rueden KT, Hartsock RL, et al (eds): Trauma Nursing (3rd Ed), pp 149–172. Philadelphia, WB Saunders, 2002
4. Yee DA, Devitt JH: Mechanisms of injury: Causes of trauma. Anesthesiol Clin North Am 17(1):1–16, 1999
5. Reines HD, Bartlett RL, Chudy NE, et al: Is advanced life support appropriate for victims of motor vehicle accidents? The South Carolina Highway Trauma Project. J Trauma 28:563–570, 1988
6. Sampalis JS, Lavoie A, Williams JI, et al: Impact of on-site care, prehospital time, and level of in-hospital care on survival in severely injured patients. J Trauma 34:252–261, 1993
7. American College of Surgeons' Committee on Trauma: Advanced Trauma Life Support: Program for Physicians. Chicago, American College of Surgeons, 1997
8. Landers DF, Dullye KK: Vascular access and fluid resuscitation in trauma. Anesthesiol Clin North Am 17(1):125–139, 1999
9. Younes RN, Aun F, Accioly CQ, et al: Hypertonic solutions in the treatment of hypovolemic shock: A prospective, randomized study in patients admitted to the emergency room. Surgery 111(4):380–385, 1992
10. Orlinsky M, Shoemaker W, Reis ED, et al: Current controversies in shock and resuscitation. Surg Clin North Am 81(6)1217–1262, 2001
11. McCunn M, Karlin A: Nonblood fluid administration: More questions than answers. Anesthesiol Clin North Am 17(1):107–123, 1999
12. Henry S, Scalea TM: Trauma care in the new millennium: Resuscitation in the new millennium. Surg Clin North Am 79(6):1259–1267, 1999
13. Drummond JC, Petrovich CT: The massively bleeding patient. Anesthesiol Clin North Am 19(4):633–649, 2001
14. Knudson MM, Maull KI: Trauma care in the new millennium: Nonoperative management of solid organ injuries, past, present and future. Surg Clin North Am 79(6):1357–1371, 1999
15. Fulda G, Brathwaite CEM, Rodriguez A, et al: Blunt traumatic rupture of the heart and pericardium: A ten-year experience (1979–1989). J Trauma 31(2):167–173, 1991
16. Flynn MB: Blunt chest trauma: Case report. Crit Care Nurse 19(5):68–77, 1999
17. Sherwood SF, Hartsock RL: Thoracic injuries. In McQuillan KA, Von Rueden KT, Hartsock RL, et al (eds): Trauma Nursing (3rd Ed), pp 543–590. Philadelphia, WB Saunders, 2002
18. Moschella JM, Wilson D: The cycle of violence: Important considerations for the EMS providers. J Emerg Med Serv 24(6):46–56, 1999
19. Velmahos GC, Chan L, Cornwall EE: Is there a limit to massive blood transfusion after severe trauma? Arch Surg 133(9):947–952, 1998
20. Voggenreiter G, Neudeck F, Aufmkolk M, et al: Clinical investigations, intermittent prone positioning in the treatment of severe

and moderate posttraumatic lung injury. Crit Care Med 27(11): 2375–2382, 1999

21. Riou B, Zaier K, Kalfon P, et al: Case reports: High-frequency heat ventilation in life-threatening bilateral pulmonary contusion. Anesthesiology 94(5):927–930, 2001
22. Adams JE, Davila-Roman VG, Bessey PQ, et al: Improved detection of cardiac contusion with cardiac troponin I. Am Heart J 131(2):308–312, 1996
23. Orliaguet G, Ferjani M, Riou B: The heart in blunt trauma. Anesthesiology 95(2):544–548, 2001
24. Feliciano DV: Advances in the diagnosis and treatment of thoracic trauma. Surg Clin North Am 79(6):1417–1429, 1999
25. Morales CH, Salinas CM, Henao CA, et al: Thoracoscopic pericardial window and penetrating cardiac trauma. J Trauma 42(2):273–275, 1997
26. Morgan PB, Buechter KJ: Blunt thoracic aortic injuries: Initial evaluation and management. South Med J 93(2):173–175, 2000
27. Tumbarello C: Ultrasound evaluation of abdominal trauma in the emergency department. J Trauma Nurs 5(3):67–72, 1998
28. Montonye JM: Abdominal injuries. In McQuillan KA, Von Rueden KT, Hartsock RL, et al (eds): Trauma Nursing (3rd Ed), pp 591–619. Philadelphia, WB Saunders, 2002
29. Amoroso TA: Evidence based emergency medicine: Evaluation and diagnostic testing, evaluation of the patient with blunt abdominal trauma. An evidence based approach. Emerg Med Clin North Am 17(1):63–75, 1999
30. Boulanger BR, Rozycki GS, Rodriguez A: Trauma care in the new millennium: Sonographic assessment of traumatic injury—future developments. Surg Clin North Am 79(6):1297–1316, 1999
31. Miller PR, Fabian TC, Croce MA, et al: Improving outcomes following penetrating colon wounds: Application of a clinical pathway. Ann Surg 235(6):775–781, 2002
32. Zhang H, Chen J, Kaiser G, et al: The value of partial splenic autotransplantation in patients with portal hypertension: A prospective randomized study. Arch Surg 137(1):89–93, 2002
33. Power RE, Kaye E, Kelly CJ, et al: Factors that may influence splenic autotransplantation and regeneration. Br J Surg 88(5):751, 2001
34. Dreitlein DA, Sriner S, Basler J: Genitourinary emergencies: Genitourinary trauma. Emerg Med Clin North Am 19(5), 2001
35. Walsh C: Musculoskeletal injuries. In McQuillan KA, Von Rueden KT, Hartsock RL, et al (eds): Trauma Nursing (3rd Ed), pp 646–689. Philadelphia, WB Saunders, 2002
36. Snyder P: Fractures. In Maher AB, Salmond SW, Pellino TA, (eds): Orthopedic Nursing (2nd Ed). Philadelphia, WB Saunders, 1998
37. Hoover TJ, Siefert JA: Orthopedic emergencies: Soft tissue complications of orthopedic emergencies. Emerg Med Clin North Am 18(1):115–139, 2000
38. Rosenberg AD, Bernstein RL: Trauma: Perioperative anesthetic management of orthopedic injuries. Anesthesiol Clin North Am 17(1):171–182, 1999
39. Geerts WH, Heit JA, Clagett GP, et al: Prevention of venous thromboembolism. Chest 119(1):132s–175s, 2001
40. Bulger EM, Smith DG, Maier RV, et al: Fat embolism syndrome: A 10 year review. Arch Surg 132:435–439, 1997
41. Hogg NJV, Stewart TC, Armstrong JEA, et al: Epidemiology of maxillofacial injuries at trauma hospitals in Ontario, Canada, between 1992 and 1997. J Trauma 49(3):425–431, 2000
42. Robertson BC, McQuillan KA: Maxillofacial injuries. In McQuillan KA, Von Rueden KT, Hartsock RL, et al (eds): Trauma Nursing (3rd Ed), pp 462–483. Philadelphia, WB Saunders, 2002
43. McIntyre RC, Pulido EJ, Bensard DD, et al: Reviews: Thirty years of clinical trials in acute respiratory distress syndrome. Crit Care Med 28(9):3314–3331, 2000
44. Brower RG, Ware LB, Berthiaume Y, et al: Reviews: Treatment of ARDS. Chest 120(4):1347–1367, 2001
45. Nast-Kolb D, Aufmkolk M, Rucholtz S, et al: Multiple organ failure still a major cause of morbidity but not mortality in blunt multiple trauma. J Trauma 51(5):835–842, 2001
46. Lee CC, Marill KA, Carter WA, et al: Review: A current concept of trauma-induced multiorgan failure. Ann Emerg Med 38(2):170–176, 2001
47. Khadaroo RG, Marshall JC: ARDS and the multiple organ dysfunction syndrome: Common mechanisms of a common systemic process. Crit Care Clin 18(1):127–141, 2002

OTHER SELECTED READING

DePalma JA, Fedorka P, Simko LC: Quality of life experienced by severely injured trauma survivors. AACN Clin Issues 14(1):54–63, 2003

Epstein CD, Peerless J, Martin J, Malangoni M: Oxygen transport and organ dysfunction in the older trauma patient. Heart Lung 31(5): 315–326, 2002

Fort CW: How to combat three deadly trauma complications. Nurs 2003 33(5):58–64, 2003

Frawley PM, Cowan J: Airway pressure release ventilation: The future of trauma ventilatory support? J Trauma Nurs 9(3):75–82, 2002

Morse JM, Pooler C: Patient-family-nurse interactions in the trauma-resuscitation room. Am J Crit Care 11(3):240–249, 2002

Pudelek B: Geriatric trauma: Special needs for a special population. AACN Clin Issues 13(1):61–72, 2002

Richmond TS, Kauder D, Hinkle J, Shults J: Early predictors of long-term disability after injury: Am J Crit Care 12(3):197–205, 2003

Wetzel RC, Burns RC: Multiple trauma in children: Critical care overview. Crit Care Med 30(11):Supplement S486–S477, 2002

chapter 56

Drug Overdose and Poisoning

ERIC R. SCHUETZ ■ JULIE SCHUETZ

objectives

Based on the content in this chapter, the reader should be able to:

- Explain the initial assessment and management of acutely poisoned or overdosed patients.
- Compare and contrast methods used to prevent absorption and enhance elimination of a drug or toxin.
- Describe the groups of symptoms that may help identify the drug(s) or toxin(s) to which a patient may have been exposed.
- Formulate a plan of care for the poisoned patient.

In 2001, more than 2 million exposures to various drugs and toxins were reported to the American Association of Poison Control Centers. Of these exposures, 1,074 resulted in death. The largest age group of human exposures was children younger than 6 years (42.4%); however, the largest age group for fatalities was adults (95%).[1] The types of toxic exposure reported to poison control centers are diverse: herbal remedies purchased at health food stores, snake and arthropod envenomations, alcohol or drugs, fumes emitted by faulty furnaces, poisonous plants, and industrial hazardous material spills or releases.

Because of clinical experience and new research information, therapy for toxic exposure changes rapidly. Health care professionals may find it challenging to keep abreast of the most advanced therapy. Fortunately, phone consultation with poison control centers offers rapid access to this information. A local poison control center can be reached nationwide by calling 1-800-222-1222. The services of a local poison control center are a useful resource for both health care professionals and the public. Nurses, pharmacists, and physicians with specialized training in clinical toxicology staff such centers.

This chapter presents general guidelines for the assessment and management of the acutely poisoned or overdosed patient. It lists commonly observed poisonings and contains a collaborative care guide for the patient with cocaine toxicity. The chapter ends with a section discussing prevention through patient teaching.

THE POISONED OR OVERDOSED PATIENT

Poisonings and drug overdoses can cause quick physical and mental changes in a person. Bystanders usually are the ones who must initiate care and call a poison control center or emergency number. Commonly observed poisonings or drug overdoses are caused by (but certainly not limited to) acetaminophen, amphetamines, benzodiazepines, carbon monoxide, cocaine, fluorinated hydrocarbons, lysergic acid diethylamide (LSD), methanol, opiates, salicylates, and tricyclic antidepressants. These particular substances and care of the toxic patient exposed to them are described later in the chapter.

Poisoning

The most common routes of exposure in poisoning are inhalation, ingestion, and injection. Toxic chemical reactions compromise cardiovascular, respiratory, central nervous, hepatic, gastrointestinal (GI), and renal systems.

Most exposures to toxic fumes occur in the home. Poisoning may result from the improper mixing of household cleaning products or malfunctioning household appliances that release carbon monoxide. Burning wood, gas, oil, coal, or kerosene also produces carbon monoxide. Carbon monoxide gas is colorless, odorless, tasteless, and nonirritating, which makes it especially dangerous. Prevention and patient teaching are discussed at the end of this chapter.

The ingestion of poisons and toxins occurs in various settings and in different age groups. Poisoning in the home usually occurs when children ingest household cleaners or medicines. Improper storage of these items contributes to such accidents. Plants, pesticides, and paint products are also potential household poisons. Because of mental or visual impairment, illiteracy, or a language barrier, older adults may ingest incorrect amounts of medications. In addition, poisoning may occur in the health care environment when medications are administered improperly.

Similarly, poisoning can also occur in the health care environment when a medication normally given only by the subcutaneous or intramuscular route is given intravenously, or when the incorrect medication is injected. Poisoning by injection can also occur in the setting of substance abuse, as when a heroin addict inadvertently injects bleach or too much heroin.

Substance Abuse and Overdose

Admission of most poisoned patients to a critical care unit is for an intentional or suspected suicidal overdose. As part of their histories, these patients frequently have mental illness, substance abuse problems, or both. Often, withdrawal symptoms and syndromes complicate the assessment of potential toxidromes. A toxidrome is a group of signs and symptoms (syndrome) associated with overdose or exposure to a particular category of drugs and toxins.

Commonly abused substances are nicotine, alcohol, heroin, marijuana, narcotic analgesics, amphetamines, benzodiazepines, and cocaine. Some children and adolescents turn to common household substances because they are readily available. People who attempt to manage stress through substance abuse require a comprehensive treatment program to address their coping and adaptation problems.

■■■ insights into clinical research

Bond GR. Home syrup of ipecac use does not reduce emergency department use of improve outcome. Pediatrics 112(5):1061-1064, 2003.

Since the early 1980s, the American Academy of Pediatrics has recommended that parents keep syrup of ipecac at home to treat poisonings. It was believed that having syrup of ipecac readily available would allow the safe management of poison in the home.

The use of syrup of ipecac as a home remedy for poisoning has been challenged in recent years by physicians in the United States and in Europe. Many poison centers no longer recommend the use of syrup of ipecac. The purpose of this study was to determine if the use of syrup of ipecac in children at home is associated with reduced utilization of emergency department (ED) resources or improved outcome after unintended exposure to a pharmaceutical.

Retrospective data were collected from the American Association of Poison Control Centers' Toxic Exposure Surveillance System Database. Data were obtained for the years 2000 and 2001 involving children under 6 years of age (754,602 telephone calls to poison centers) who unintentionally ingested a pharmaceutical agent and in which the call to the poison control center came from the home. Data included ED referral rate, actual rate of ED use, actual home use of syrup of ipecac, and outcome.

The mean rate of ED referral was 9% (range 3%–18%). The mean home use of syrup of ipecac was 1.8% (range 0.2%–14%). Increased use of home syrup of ipecac was not associated with referral to the ED. Adverse outcome was rare at 0.6% (range 0.2%–2.1%).

Based on their findings, the researcher concluded that there is no reduction in resource utilization or improvement in patient outcome from use of syrup of ipecac in the home. However, the conclusions are limited because the study only investigated calls to the poison center related to pharmaceutical ingestion. Poisoning from other ingested substances was not examined in this study.

ASSESSMENT

A health care facility's systematic approach to the assessment of the poisoned or overdosed patient includes performing triage, obtaining the patient's history, performing a physical examination, and conducting laboratory studies.

Triage

Although some type of triage usually is performed at the scene or by an emergency response team, triage is always the first step performed in the emergency department. Two essential questions to be considered in the triage evaluation are:

1. Is the patient's life in immediate danger?
2. Is the patient's life in potential danger?

If the patient's life is in immediate danger, the goals of immediate treatment are patient stabilization and evaluation and management of airway, breathing, and circulation (ABCs).

History

A history of the patient's exposure provides a framework for managing the poisoning or overdose. Key points include identifying the drug(s) or toxin(s), the time and duration of the exposure, first aid treatment given before arrival at the hospital, allergies, and any underlying disease processes or related injuries. This information may be obtained from the patient, family members, friends, rescuers, or bystanders. In some cases, family or police may need to search the patient's home for clues. Clothing and personal effects may supply additional information.

Physical Examination

A quick but thorough physical examination is essential. Preliminary examination results lead to the in-depth evaluation and serial assessment of affected systems (actual or anticipated). As noted previously, a toxidrome is a group of signs and symptoms associated with overdose or exposure to a particular category of drugs and toxins. Recognizing the presence of a toxidrome may help identify the toxin(s) or drug(s) to which the patent was exposed, and the crucial body systems that may be involved. Table 56-1 lists four common toxidromes with their signs and symptoms and common causes.

Laboratory Studies

Relevant clinical laboratory data are vital to the assessment of the poisoned or overdosed patient. Tests that provide clues to the agent(s) taken by the patient include electrolytes, hepatic function, urinalysis, electrocardiography, and serum osmolality tests. A serum level measurement of acetaminophen is obtained in all patients who have overdosed because acetaminophen is a component of many prescription and over-the-counter preparations. In the event of an acetaminophen overdose, the result of the level is plotted against the time since ingestion on the Rumack-Matthew nomogram (Fig. 56-1). Serum level measurements are also available for carbamazepine, iron, ethanol, lithium, aspirin, and valproic acid and may be obtained if these agents are suspected in an overdose.

MANAGEMENT

Management of the poisoned or overdosed patient seeks to prevent absorption of and further exposure to the agent. After triage to determine the status of the patient's airway, breathing, and circulation, the patient must be stabilized. Treatment begins with first aid at the scene and continues in the emergency department and often the intensive care unit (ICU). Advanced general management involves further steps to prevent absorption and enhance elimination of the agent. For instance, antidotes, antivenins, or antitoxins may be administered. The health care team must further support vital functions and monitor and treat multisystem effects. Patient and family teaching to prevent future exposures is another part of the nurse's management strategy. Nursing diagnoses for the poisoned or overdosed patient are listed in Box 56-1.

Stabilization

Stabilization of patients includes performing the steps summarized in Box 56-2, which are also discussed in the following list:

- *Airway:* Nasotracheal or endotracheal intubation may be necessary to adequately maintain and protect the patient's airway.
- *Breathing:* Mechanical ventilation may be necessary to support the patient. Many drugs and toxins, such as heroin, depress the respiratory drive. Patients therefore may require ventilator assistance until the drugs or toxins are eliminated from the body.
- *Circulation:* Complications range from shock caused by fluid loss to fluid overload, and are often related to the patient's hydration status and the ability of the cardiovascular system to adjust to drug- or toxin-induced changes. For example, rattlesnake envenomations often cause third-spacing of fluid into the area of the bite, leading to intravascular hypovolemia. As a consequence, the patient develops hypotension, which

table 56-1 Toxidromes

Toxidrome	Signs/Symptoms	Common Causes
Anticholinergic	Delirium; dry, flushed skin; dilated pupils; elevated temperature; decreased bowel sounds; urinary retention; tachycardia	Antihistamines, atropine, Jimson weed
Cholinergic	Excessive salivation, lacrimation, urination, diarrhea, and emesis; diaphoresis, bronchorrhea, bradycardia, fasciculations, central nervous system depression, constricted pupils	Organophosphate insecticides (e.g., Malathion, Diazinon); carbamate insecticide (e.g., carbaryl, propoxur)
Opioid	Central nervous system depression, respiratory depression, constricted pupils, hypotension, hypothermia	Opiates (e.g., codeine, morphine, propoxyphene, heroin), diphenoxylate (e.g., diphenoxylate/atropine sulfate [Lomotil])
Sympathomimetic	Agitation, tachycardia, hypertension, seizures, metabolic acidosis	Amphetamines, cocaine, theophylline, caffeine

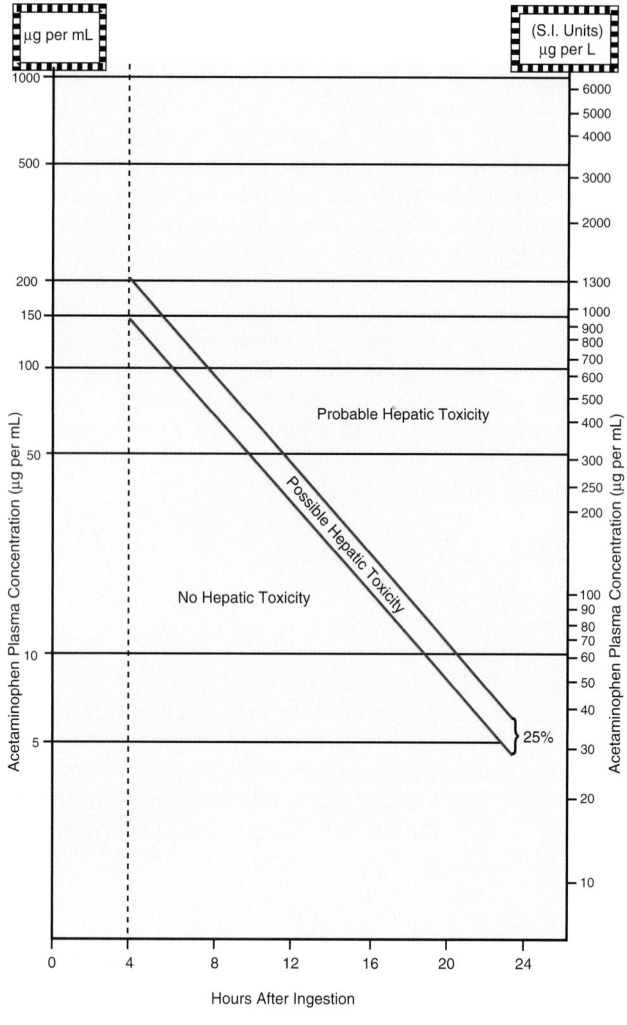

RUMACK – MATTHEW NOMOGRAM FOR ACETAMINOPHEN POISONING

CAUTION FOR USE OF THIS CHART
1) The time coordinates refer to time of ingestion.
2) Serum levels drawn before 4 hours may not represent peak levels.
3) The graph should be used only in relation to a single acute ingestion.
4) The lower solid line is 25% below the standard nomogram is included to allow for possible errors in acetaminophen plasma assays and estimated time from ingestion of an overdose.

figure 56-1 Semilogarithmic plot of plasma acetaminophen levels versus time. (With permission from Rumack BH, Matthew HJ: Acetaminophen poisoning and toxicity. Pediatrics 55:871–876, 1975.)

usually responds to aggressive intravenous (IV) fluid therapy. Some toxic drug ingestions impair myocardial contractility, and fluid overload may result because of the heart's inability to pump effectively. In these cases, fluid balance needs to be carefully controlled. Invasive monitoring (e.g., central venous pressure, pulmonary artery catheter, Foley catheter with urometer) and drug therapy may be necessary to prevent or minimize complications such as pulmonary edema.

- *Cardiac function:* Many drugs and toxins cause cardiac conduction delays and arrhythmias. The history of the drug(s) or toxin(s) involved may not be reliable or even known, especially when patients are found unconscious or have attempted suicide. In these cases, continuous cardiac monitoring and 12-lead electrocardiograms help detect cardiotoxic effects.
- *Acid–base balance and electrolyte homeostasis:* Electrolyte abnormalities and metabolic acidosis frequently occur and may require serial measurements of electrolytes and arterial blood gases (ABGs), and other specific laboratory tests. For example, serial measurements of electrolytes, ABGs, and salicylate levels are the means of evaluating aspirin toxicity. Aspirin, in large ingestions, may form a solid mass in the gastrointestinal (GI) tract, called a *concretion*, instead of breaking apart and dissolving. As a result, absorption is delayed, and the development of toxic effects, such as hypokalemia, metabolic acidosis, and respiratory alkalosis, may not be observed for several hours.
- *Mentation:* Many factors can affect the patient's mental status. Hypoglycemia and hypoxemia are two that can be life-threatening but easily addressed by administering oxygen and IV dextrose until laboratory results are available. Patients with chronic alcoholism also have a special risk called Wernicke-Korsakoff syndrome, which is characterized by ataxia and altered mentation. Early IV or intramuscular administration of thiamine (vitamin B_1) may prevent exacerbation of the syndrome. Naloxone (Narcan) is a narcotic antagonist that reverses narcotic-induced central nervous system (CNS) and respiratory depression. It is often initially given to comatose patients. It must be given cautiously, however, because it can precipitate withdrawal in narcotic-dependent individuals, which may present as violent, agitated behavior, thus placing nurses and other health care providers in danger. In the critical care unit it may be necessary to continue to administer boluses of naloxone to a patient because of its short duration of action compared with the duration of action of most opioids. In such circumstances it may be necessary to give naloxone by con-

box 56-1 *Examples of Nursing Diagnoses and Collaborative Problems for the Poisoned or Overdosed Patient*

- Poisoning
- Ineffective Breathing Pattern
- Impaired Gas Exchange
- Ineffective Tissue Perfusion
- Fluid Volume Imbalance, Risk for
- Impaired Thought Processes
- Violence, Risk for (to self or others)
- Self-Esteem Disturbance
- Ineffective Individual/Family Coping
- Injury, Risk for
- Ineffective Role Performance
- Acidosis/Alkalosis, Risk for
- Atelectasis
- Hypoxemia
- Dysrhythmias
- Hypovolemia
- Electrolyte Imbalances

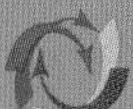

box 56-2 nursing interventions for *Stabilization of the Poisoned or Overdosed Patient*

- Assess, establish, and maintain the airway.
- Evaluate respiratory effort.
- Maintain adequate circulation.
- Monitor cardiac function.
- Maintain or correct acid–base balance and electrolyte homeostasis.
- Assess mentation.
- Identify injuries and disease processes that increase risk.
- Measure vital signs and temperature frequently to track changes.

tinuous infusion.[2] Because it is often unclear why a patient is comatose, emergency response personnel may administer what is commonly referred to as a "coma cocktail," consisting of D50, vitamin B_1, and naloxone, at the scene. These agents are well tolerated and have minimal toxicities. Proceeding with this therapy at the scene addresses all three easily correctable possibilities (hypoglycemic, alcoholic, or narcotic coma) without wasting time waiting for laboratory results to become available.

- *Injuries associated with toxic exposure and underlying disease processes:* Any injuries associated with toxic exposure and other underlying disease processes identified during the initial physical examination are treated or monitored, or both. For example, the street drug phencyclidine (PCP) may provoke violent, agitated, bizarre behavior, leading to trauma during the acute toxic phase. Also, for instance, the patient with pre-existing ischemic heart disease may not be able to tolerate the hypoxemia associated with carbon monoxide poisoning as well as a young, healthy patient.
- *Vital signs and temperature:* The critical or potentially critical patient's vital signs and temperature are measured frequently to track changes indicating additional problems.

Initial Decontamination

First aid may be given by a bystander, health care provider, or emergency response team, or in the emergency department. The physicochemical properties of the agent and the amount, route, and exposure time help determine the type and extent of management required. Decontamination methods for ocular, dermal, inhalation, and ingestion exposures follow.

OCULAR EXPOSURE

Many substances can accidentally splash into the eyes. When this happens, the eyes must be flushed to remove the agent. Immediate irrigation with lukewarm water or normal saline is recommended. Continuous flooding of the eyes with a large glass of water or low-pressure shower should be done for 15 minutes. The patient should blink the eyes open and closed during the irrigation. If necessary, the pH of the eyes can be tested. If the pH is abnormal, irrigation should continue until the pH normalizes. An ophthalmologic examination is needed when ocular irritation or visual disturbance persists after irrigation.

DERMAL EXPOSURE

When dermal exposure occurs, the patient should flood the skin with lukewarm water for 15 to 30 minutes. Most companies that produce or use chemical agents have showers for this purpose. The patient should remove any clothing that may have been contaminated. After standing under running water for the allotted time, the patient should then wash the area gently with soap and water and rinse thoroughly.

Some toxins may require further decontamination. For example, three separate soap and water washings or showers are recommended to decontaminate organophosphate pesticides (e.g., Malathion or Diazinon). Protective clothing should be worn to reduce the risk for toxicity while handling contaminated clothing or assisting with skin decontamination.

Although it may seem logical to apply an acid to neutralize a base exposure and a base to neutralize an acid exposure, this can be quite dangerous. Neutralization is the reaction between an acid and a base, in which the H^+ of the acid and the OH^- of the base react to produce H_2O (water) and heat. The heat produced by this reaction is significant enough to cause burns. Therefore, neutralizing the skin after a dermal exposure is not recommended.

INHALATION EXPOSURE

A victim of an inhalation exposure should be moved to fresh air as quickly as possible. The responder must also protect himself or herself from the airborne toxin. Further evaluation is needed if the patient experiences respiratory irritation or shortness of breath. Large-scale exposures or those that occur at the workplace may require consultation with a HAZMAT team, a group of individuals specially trained to manage exposures to hazardous materials.

INGESTION EXPOSURE

Milk or water dilutes ingested irritants such as bleach or caustics such as drain cleaner. After such an ingestion, adults should drink 8 oz of milk or water and children should drink 2 to 8 oz (based on their size). Further evaluation is necessary after dilution if there is mucosal irritation or burns. Because of the risk of aspiration, ingestions should not be diluted when they are accompanied by seizures, depressed mental status, or loss of the gag reflex. Again, neutralization is not used because of the risk of thermal burn.

Gastrointestinal Decontamination

Gastric lavage, adsorbents, cathartics, and whole-bowel irrigation are used to prevent absorption of, and forestall toxicity from, almost all drugs and a variety of toxins.

The American Academy of Pediatrics no longer recommends the use of emetics (such as syrup of ipecac) for GI decontamination.

GASTRIC LAVAGE

Gastric lavage is a method of GI decontamination. Fluid (usually normal saline) is introduced into the stomach through a large-bore orogastric tube and then drained in an attempt to reclaim part of the ingested agent before it is absorbed. A small-bore nasogastric tube is ineffective for lavage because particulate matter such as tablets or capsules are too large to pass through the tube. If airway protection is necessary, the patient should be intubated before lavage begins.

As noted, a large-bore orogastric tube (a 36 to 40 French in adults and a 16 to 28 French in children) is used to evacuate particulate matter, including whole tablets and capsules. For the lavage, the patient is positioned in the left lateral decubitus position, with the head lower than the feet. Before beginning, the tube should be coated with a jelly lubricant such as hydroxyethylcellulose. The position of the tube must be confirmed after passing, either by aspirating and checking the pH of the aspirate, or by insufflation of air, while listening over the stomach. The lavage is accomplished by attaching a funnel or syringe to the end of the tube and instilling aliquots of 150 to 200 mL (50 to 100 mL in children) of 100°F (38°C) saline into the stomach. Placing the funnel and tube below the patient allows the fluid to return by gravity. This procedure is repeated until clear fluid returns or 2 L of fluid has been used. The contents of the stomach can then be collected for drug or toxin identification.

Complications of gastric lavage include esophageal perforation, pulmonary aspiration, electrolyte imbalance, tension pneumothorax, and hypothermia (when cold lavage solutions are used). Lavage is contraindicated in cases of ingestion of caustics or hydrocarbons with a high aspiration potential. Because of the associated risks and the lack of clear evidence supporting its use, gastric lavage should be used only if the patient has ingested a life-threatening amount of a substance and the procedure is undertaken within an hour of the ingestion.[3]

ADSORBENTS

An adsorbent is a solid substance that has the ability to attract and hold another substance to its surface ("to adsorb"). Activated charcoal is an effective nonspecific adsorbent of many drugs and toxins. Activated charcoal adsorbs, or traps, the drug or toxin to its large surface area and prevents absorption from the GI tract. Box 56-3 identifies both drugs and toxins that are adsorbed effectively by activated charcoal and those not adsorbed effectively.

Activated charcoal is a fine, black powder that is given as a slurry with water, either orally or by nasogastric or orogastric tube, as soon as possible after the ingestion. Commercially available activated charcoal products may be mixed with 70% sorbitol to decrease grittiness, increase palatability, and serve as a cathartic. The usual dose that is given is one 50-g bottle. Administration of more than one dose is controversial, and usually limited to overdoses of large quantities of aspirin, valproic acid, and theophylline. Activated charcoal is used cautiously in patients with diminished bowel sounds and is contraindicated in patients with bowel obstruction.[3]

box 56-3
Adsorption of Drugs and Toxins by Activated Charcoal

Drugs and Toxins Well Adsorbed by Activated Charcoal
- Acetaminophen
- Amphetamines
- Antihistamines
- Aspirin
- Barbiturates
- Benzodiazepines
- Beta blockers
- Calcium channel blockers
- Cocaine
- Opioids
- Phenytoin
- Theophylline
- Valproic acid

Drugs and Toxins Not Well Adsorbed by Activated Charcoal
- Acids
- Alkalis
- Alcohols
- Iron
- Lithium
- Metals

CATHARTICS

A cathartic is a substance that causes or promotes bowel movements. The use of cathartics alone in the management of poisoning is not an acceptable means of GI decontamination. In theory, cathartics decrease the absorption of drugs and toxins by speeding their passage through the GI tract, thereby limiting their contact with mucosal surfaces. Magnesium citrate or 70% sorbitol often is used. Currently, however, there is no clinical evidence that shows that a cathartic can reduce the bioavailability of drugs or improve the outcome of poisoned patients.[3] Data regarding the effectiveness of mixing cathartics with activated charcoal are not yet available. Clearly, more research needs to be done in this area of clinical practice.[3]

WHOLE-BOWEL IRRIGATION

The goal of whole-bowel irrigation is to give large volumes of a balanced electrolyte solution rapidly (1 to 2 L/hour) to flush the patient's bowel mechanically without creating electrolyte disturbances. Used as a bowel preparation for colonoscopy, it is also used as a GI decontamination procedure for patients who have ingested bags or vials of narcotics to avoid arrest, for drug smugglers who pack their GI tracts with narcotics (either orally or rectally), and for patients who have overdosed on modified-release pharmaceuticals.

Commercial products used in whole-bowel irrigation include GoLYTELY and Colyte. Both products are dispensed as powders and are given after adding water. Whole-bowel irrigation is contraindicated in the patient with bowel obstruction or perforation.[3]

Enhanced Elimination of the Drug or Toxin

The pharmacological and kinetic characteristics of a drug or toxin greatly influence the severity and length of the clinical course in the acutely poisoned or overdosed patient. The absorption rate, body distribution, metabolism, and elimination must be considered when choosing methods to eliminate the drug or toxin from the body. There are six methods of enhanced elimination:

1. Multiple-dose activated charcoal
2. Alteration of urine pH
3. Hemodialysis
4. Hemoperfusion
5. Chelation
6. Hyperbaric oxygenation (HBO) therapy

MULTIPLE-DOSE ACTIVATED CHARCOAL

Administering multiple doses of activated charcoal can result in greater adsorption of certain drugs such as aspirin, valproic acid, and theophylline. Multiple-dose activated charcoal is given orally, by nasogastric tube, or by orogastric tube every 2 to 6 hours. Complications of multiple-dose activated charcoal include aspiration and bowel obstruction.[3]

ALTERATION OF URINE pH

Alkalinizing the patient's urine enhances excretion of drugs that are weak acids by increasing the amount of ionized drug in the urine. This form of enhanced elimination is also termed *ion trapping*. The urine is alkalinized by administering a continuous IV infusion of one to three ampules of sodium bicarbonate per liter of fluid. Urine alkalinization is frequently used in patients experiencing a salicylate overdose. Complications of alkalinization include cerebral or pulmonary edema and electrolyte imbalances.

Urine acidification is no longer recommended because of low drug clearance and the risk of complications such as rhabdomyolysis.

HEMODIALYSIS

Hemodialysis is the process of altering the solute composition of blood by removing it from an artery, diffusing it across a semipermeable membrane (between the blood and a salt solution), then returning it into a vein. It is used in moderate to severe intoxications to remove a drug or toxin rapidly when more conservative methods (e.g., gastric lavage, activated charcoal, antidotes) have failed or in patients with decreased renal function. Hemodialysis requires consultation with a nephrologist and specially trained nurses to perform the procedure and monitor the patient. Low molecular weight, low protein binding, and water solubility are factors that make a drug or toxin suitable for hemodialysis. Drugs and toxins that may be removed by hemodialysis include ethylene glycol (commonly found in antifreeze), methanol, lithium, salicylates, and theophylline.[4]

HEMOPERFUSION

Hemoperfusion removes drugs and toxins from the patient's blood by pumping the blood through a cartridge of adsorbent material, such as activated charcoal. An advantage of hemoperfusion over hemodialysis is that the total surface area of the dialyzing membrane is much greater with the hemoperfusion cartridges. As in hemodialysis, drugs that have high tissue-binding characteristics and a large volume distributed outside the circulation are not good candidates for hemoperfusion because little drug is found in the blood. Although rarely used in the poisoned and overdosed population, hemoperfusion has been used successfully in patients experiencing a theophylline overdose.[4]

CHELATION

Chelation involves the use of binding agents to remove toxic levels of metals from the body, such as mercury, lead, iron, and arsenic. Examples of chelating agents are dimercaprol (BAL in oil), calcium disodium edetate (EDTA), succimer (DMSA), and deferoxamine. Concerns about the toxicity of the chelators; their tissue distribution characteristics; and the stability, distribution, and elimination of the chelator–metal complex make chelation a complicated procedure.

HYPERBARIC OXYGENATION THERAPY

In HBO therapy, oxygen is administered to a patient in an enclosed chamber at a pressure greater than the pressure at sea level (e.g., 1 atmosphere absolute). This therapy has been used in carbon monoxide and methylene chloride poisonings (methylene chloride is metabolized to carbon monoxide in the body). The result is enhanced elimination of carbon monoxide: The half-life of carbon monoxide in room air is 5 to 6 hours, in 100% oxygen it is 90 minutes, and in an HBO chamber it is 20 minutes. Another use of HBO therapy is the treatment of diving sickness (the "bends"). However, the small number of HBO chambers and lack of around-the-clock staffing limits the wide use of this therapy.

Complications of HBO therapy include pressure-related otalgia, sinus pain, tooth pain, and tympanic membrane rupture. Confinement anxiety, convulsions, and tension pneumothorax also have been observed in patients receiving HBO therapy.[5]

Antagonists, Antitoxins, and Antivenins

In pharmacology, an antagonist is a substance that counteracts the action of another drug. Although the general public often believes there is an antidote for every drug or toxin, the opposite is closer to the truth. There are, in fact, very few antidotes. Antidotes for specific intoxications are listed in Table 56-2.

Antitoxins neutralize a toxin. For instance, botulism antitoxin trivalent (equine) is available through the Centers for Disease Control and Prevention to counteract the effects of botulism.

Antivenins are antitoxins that neutralize the venom of the offending snake or spider. There are several antitoxins; each is active against a specific venom. For example, antivenin Crotalidae polyvalent (equine) is active against

table 56-2 ■ Antidotes for Specific Drugs and Toxins

Drug/Toxin	Antidote
Acetaminophen	*N*-acetylcysteine (Mucomyst)
Anticholinergics	Physostigmine (Antilirium)
Benzodiazepines	Flumazenil (Romazicon)
Beta-blocking agents	Glucagon
Calcium channel blockers	Glucagon, calcium chloride
Carbon monoxide	Oxygen
Cyanide	Lilly Cyanide Antidote Kit: amyl nitrite, sodium nitrite, and sodium thiosulfate
Digoxin	Digoxin-specific fab fragments (Digibind)
Ethylene glycol	Fomepizole (Antizol)[6], ethanol
Methanol	Fomepizole (Antizol)[7], ethanol
Nitrites	Methylene blue
Opioids	Naloxone (Narcan)
Organophosphate insecticides	Atropine, pralidoxime

venoms of the family Crotalidae, which are pit viper snakes native to North, Central, and South America. Because this agent is derived from horse serum (and therefore recognized as "foreign" by the human immune system), significant side effects such as anaphylactic or anaphylactoid reactions are common. Recently approved by the U.S. Food and Drug Administration (FDA) is Crotalidae polyvalent immune Fab (CroFab), a product that is produced using a purification process that removes the Fc fragment and leaves only the Fab fragments of the immunoglobulins. Typically, this process results in a product that causes fewer reactions in humans. Antivenin (*Lactrodectus mactans;* equine) is available for black widow spider bites as well as for envenomations by the eastern and Texas coral snake (*Micrurus fulvius;* equine). However, there are many venomous snakes and spiders for which no antivenin exists. Envenomation from one of these species is treated with symptomatic and supportive care.[8]

Continuous Patient Monitoring

Seriously poisoned or overdosed patients may require continued monitoring for hours or days after exposure. Physical examination, the use of diagnostic tools, and careful assessment of clinical signs and symptoms provide information about the patient's progress and direct medical and nursing management. Diagnostic tools include the following:

- *Electrocardiography:* Electrocardiography can provide evidence of drugs causing arrhythmias or conduction delays (e.g., tricyclic antidepressants).
- *Radiology:* Many substances are radiopaque, or can be visualized using a contrast-enhanced computed tomography (CT) scan (e.g., heavy metals, button batteries, some modified-release tablets or capsules, aspirin concretions, cocaine or heroin containers). Chest radiographs provide evidence of aspiration and pulmonary edema.
- *Electrolytes, ABGs, and other laboratory tests:* Acute poisoning can cause an imbalance in a patient's electrolyte levels, including sodium, potassium, chloride, carbon dioxide content, magnesium, and calcium. Signs of inadequate ventilation or oxygenation include cyanosis, tachycardia, hypoventilation, intercostal muscle retractions, and altered mental status. Such signs should be evaluated by pulse oximetry and ABG measurements. Seriously poisoned patients require routine screening of electrolytes, ABGs, creatinine, and glucose; complete blood count; and urinalysis.
- *Anion gap:* The anion gap is a simple, cost-effective tool that uses common serum measurements, such as sodium, chloride, and bicarbonate, to help evaluate the poisoned patient for certain drugs or toxins. The anion gap represents the difference between unmeasured anions and cations in the blood. Using measured anions and a cation, the anion gap is calculated using the following formula:

$$[Na] - ([Cl] + [HCO_3]) = \text{anion gap}$$

The normal value for the anion gap is approximately 8 to 16 mEq/L. An anion gap that exceeds the upper normal value can indicate metabolic acidosis caused by an accumulation of acids in the blood. Drugs, toxins, or medical conditions that can produce an elevated anion gap include iron, isoniazid (INH), lithium, lactate, carbon monoxide, cyanide, toluene, methanol, metformin, ethanol, ethylene glycol, salicylates, hydrogen sulfide, strychnine, diabetic ketoacidosis, uremia, seizures, and starvation. Although these substances and processes can cause an elevated anion gap, a normal anion gap alone does not preclude a toxic exposure.

- *Osmolal gap:* The osmolal gap is the difference between the measured osmolality (using the freezing point depression method) and the calculated osmolality. The calculated osmolality is derived using laboratory values for the major osmotically active substances in the serum, such as sodium, glucose, and blood urea nitrogen (BUN). Like the anion gap, it is a simple, cost-effective tool for evaluating the poisoned patient for certain drugs or toxins. The calculated osmolality (using serum electrolyte values) is defined as follows:

$$2(\text{Na}^+) + \frac{\text{glucose}}{18} + \frac{\text{BUN}}{2.8} = \text{calculated osmolality}$$

The osmolal gap is then calculated as follows:

$$\text{Measured osmolality} - \text{calculated osmolality} = \text{osmolal gap}$$

An osmolal gap that exceeds 10 mOsm is abnormal. Toxins that can cause an elevated osmolal gap include ethanol, ethylene glycol, and methanol. If an ethanol level is known, it can be factored into the following equation:

$$2(\text{Na}^+) + \frac{\text{glucose}}{18} + \frac{\text{BUN}}{2.8} + \frac{\text{BAL}}{4.6} = \text{calculated osmolality}$$

where BAL is the blood alcohol level measured in milligrams per deciliter.

- *Toxicology screens:* A toxicology screen is a laboratory analysis of a body fluid or tissue to identify drugs or toxins. Although saliva, spinal fluid, and hair may be analyzed, blood or urine samples are used more frequently. The number and type of drugs assessed by toxicology screens vary. Each screen tests for specific drugs or agents. For example, drug abuse screens usually identify several common street or prescription drugs, whereas a coma panel detects common drugs that cause CNS depression. Comprehensive screens include many drugs (ranging from antidepressants to cardiac drugs to alcohols) and are more expensive. A number of factors limit the role of toxicology screens in managing poisonings or overdoses. The test sample must be collected while the drug or toxin is in the body fluid or tissue used for testing. For example, cocaine is a rapidly metabolized drug; however, its metabolite, benzoylecgonine, can be detected in the urine for several hours after cocaine use. Also, a toxicology screen with a negative result does not necessarily mean that no drug or toxin is present, but rather that none of the drugs or toxins for which a patient has been screened is present. For example, gamma-hydroxybutyrate (GHB) is not included in toxicology screens because it is rapidly metabolized to small, unmeasurable molecules. The sample must also be properly collected, and there must be a laboratory near enough to obtain results quickly. For many smaller, rural laboratories, these tests are taken by a courier service or mailed to a larger laboratory, and the results are not available for several days. In these situations, the value of the test for managing the immediate overdose or poisoning needs to be considered.

Patient care in some of the more common poisonings and overdoses is summarized in Table 56-3. Clinical manifestations are included in the table. Management of the patient who is toxic with cocaine is summarized in Box 56-4.[12]

Patient Teaching

One of the interventions the nurse can perform in the emergency department or intensive care unit is preventive teaching. All patients (and parents of pediatric patients) who have survived a toxic encounter should be taught how to prevent such an incident from recurring. Parents of young children need information on child-proofing their home. Teaching information related to the prevention of childhood poisoning is given in Box 56-5. Family teaching guidelines for lead poisoning are included in Box 56-6. Finally, a summary of poison prevention for the older patient can be found in Box 56-7.

In addition, carbon monoxide detectors alert families to problems in their homes. Utility companies and local health and fire authorities can help identify and remove sources of fumes.

case study ■ SUICIDAL OVERDOSE

Mr. S., a 48-year-old, 176-lb (80-kg) man, was brought to the emergency department by emergency medical services (EMS). The patient's family had called EMS to the scene after a suspected suicidal overdose. Mr. S. was uncooperative, refusing to answer questions, but seemingly alert. His initial vital signs were blood pressure 140/90 mm Hg, pulse 120 beats/minute, and respirations 30 breaths/minute and nonlabored. His pupils were equal and reactive to light. His skin was warm and dry. EMS started an IV with lactated Ringer's solution at a keep vein open (KVO) rate, and initial blood draws were performed. The family reported that the patient had recently stopped taking his medications for bipolar disorder, and had taken approximately 200 aspirin tablets within the last hour.

On initial examination in the emergency department, his vital signs were blood pressure 142/92 mm Hg, pulse 132 beats/minute, respirations 30 breaths/minute, and temperature 99°F (37.2°C). He complained of feeling tired and nauseous. His pupils remained normal, and all reflexes were intact. A nasogastric tube was placed, some stomach contents were withdrawn, and 50 g of activated charcoal was instilled. Within minutes he vomited.

The nurse in the emergency department called the poison control center, which initially recommended an antiemetic to control the nausea and vomiting, instillation of a second 50-g dose of activated charcoal, cardiac monitoring, seizure precautions, measurement of ABGs, and serial (every 2 hours) measurements of the patient's blood salicylate and electrolyte levels. IV hydration with fluids containing two to three ampules of sodium bicarbonate and 40 mEq of potassium chloride was also recommended. In addition, a blood acetaminophen level was recommended to rule out the possibility of coingestion.

The initial salicylate level drawn by EMS approximately 1 hour after ingestion was 30 mg/dL. The patient's acetaminophen level was less than 10 µg/mL. His initial basic metabolic panel levels were sodium 142 mEq/L,

(text continues on page 1314)

table 56-3 Common Patient Care in Poisonings and Overdoses

Drug/Substance	Clinical Presentation and Assessment	Intervention

Acetaminophen (APAP):
Common OTC antipyretic and analgesic
Often sold as a component of combination drugs for pain, cough, cold, and sleep
Examples: OTC remedies such as Tylenol, Tylenol Extended Relief, Tempra, Liquiprin, Panadol, Excedrin PM (diphenhydramine-APAP) and in controlled-substance combination drugs such as oxycodone-APAP (Percocet), codeine-APAP (Tylenol #3), hydrocodone-APAP (Vicodin)
Acetaminophen toxicity: Hepatotoxicity and occasionally renal dysfunction, 1–3 days postingestion
	• Phase 1 (up to 24 h postingestion): anorexia, nausea, malaise
	• Phase 2 (24–48 h postingestion): clinical picture improves, increase in AST, ALT, and total bilirubin, prolongation of prothrombin time
	• Phase 3 (72–96 h postingestion): peak hepatotoxicity usually observed
	• Coagulopathies
	• Jaundice
	• AST and ALT may rise into the 10,000–20,000 IU/L range and return to normal without the patient experiencing long-term sequelae
	• Chronic toxicity well described in the medical literature
		Prevention of absorption:
		• Activated charcoal
		Laboratory:
		• Draw acetaminophen level at 4 h (or later if patient presents late to the health care facility), plot level on the Rumack-Matthew nomogram (see Fig. 56-1) to determine if antidote is indicated.
		• Monitor daily AST, ALT, total bilirubin, BUN, creatinine, and prothrombin time in patients with a toxic acetaminophen level.
		Treatment:
		• Antidote: *N*-acetylcysteine (NAC, Mucomyst)
		  • Loading dose: 140 mg/kg orally
		  • Maintenance doses: 79 mg/kg orally every 4 h for a total of 17 maintenance doses
		  • Dilute NAC (20% solution) 3:1 with a soft drink or juice
		  • Repeat any dose not retained 1 h, may need large doses of antiemetics to control vomiting[9]
		• Supportive care

Amphetamines Group of drugs used therapeutically for narcolepsy, short-term treatment of obesity, and attention-deficit disorder As drugs of abuse, used for ability to stimulate central nervous system to combat fatigue or produce a "high" Prescription amphetamines and related agents: methylphenidate (Ritalin), dextroamphetamine (Dexedrine), mixed salts of amphetamine (Adderall) Street names: speed, uppers, crank, E, X, ecstasy, ice, crystal	• Flushing • Diaphoresis • Restlessness • Talkativeness • Irritability • Confusion • Panic • Seizures • Intracranial hemorrhage • Hypertension • Tachycardia • Chest pain • Myocardial infarction • Cardiac arrhythmias • Palpitations • Peripheral vasoconstriction • Nausea • Vomiting • Chronic amphetamine toxicity may lead to the development of paranoia or hallucinations • IV abusers may also have complications such as hepatitis, sepsis, abscesses, and HIV infection	Prevention of absorption: • Activated charcoal Laboratory: • Monitor electrolytes and acid–base status • Urine drug screen may detect amphetamines Treatment: • External cooling measures for hyperthermia • Benzodiazepines to control agitation • Severe hypertension controlled with IV nitroprusside (Nipride), other drugs suggested • Supportive care
Benzodiazepines Antianxiety agents, anticonvulsants, muscle relaxants, and sedatives Examples: alprazolam (Xanax), clonazepam (Klonopin), diazepam (Valium), Lorazepam (Ativan), midazolam (Versed) Primarily cause CNS and respiratory depression. Due to their low order of toxicity, fatalities unlikely unless ingested with other CNS depressants	• Respiratory depression • Airway protection/gag reflex • Lethargy • Coma • Confusion • Slurred speech • Ataxia	Prevention of absorption: • Activated charcoal Laboratory: • Urine drug screen may detect benzodiazepines. Treatment: • Flumazenil reverses CNS and respiratory depression; due to risk in unmasking controlled seizures, flumazenil is contraindicated in the face of simultaneous potential seizure causing overdose.[10] • Supportive care

table 56-3 Common Patient Care in Poisonings and Overdoses (Continued)

Drug/Substance	Clinical Presentation and Assessment	Intervention
Carbon Monoxide Colorless, odorless gas that is a component of automobile exhaust, natural gas or propane furnace emissions, cigarette smoke, wood stove emissions, and pollution Methylene chloride, a component found in some paint strippers, is metabolized in the body to carbon monoxide after inhaled or ingested It displaces oxygen from the hemoglobin, leading to hypoxia It is absorbed rapidly by inhalation and combines readily with hemoglobin due to a greater affinity than oxygen Fetal carboxyhemoglobin levels are possibly 10–15% greater than the maternal carboxyhemoglobin level	• Flulike symptoms • Headache • Nausea • Vomiting • Syncope • Fatigue • Weakness • Lack of concentration • Irritability • Chest pain, especially in people with underlying cardiovascular disease • Occasionally, irreversible changes in memory and personality • Fetotoxicity • People usually report feeling better when not in the area of the carbon monoxide; for example, if the exposure is occurring in the home because of a faulty furnace, the person will often report a decrease or resolution of symptoms when away from the home	Prevention of absorption: • Fresh air Laboratory: • Carboxyhemoglobin levels Treatment: • 100% oxygen until all signs and symptoms resolve • Thorough neurological examination • Hyperbaric oxygen therapy (HBO) to decrease half-life; however, due to lack of available HBO chambers, use is limited and efficacy not well documented by research • Supportive care
Cocaine Common street drug that produces a temporary feeling of well-being for the user Routes of exposure: IV, snorting, smoking Street names: crack, rock, coke, snow, blow Toxic effects related to the rapid onset of CNS and cardiac stimulation	• Tachycardia • Hypertension • Cardiac arrhythmias • Chest pain • Myocardial infarction • Aortic dissection • Bowel infarction • Hyperthermia • Anxiety • Seizures • Tactile hallucinations ("cocaine bugs") • Cerebral hemorrhage • Cerebral infarction • Rhabdomyolysis • Rapid onset of toxic effects • In pregnant women, abruptio placentae or abortion possible • Chronic snorting, nasal septal perforation If clinical presentation is inconsistent with cocaine alone, possibly adulterants, substitutes, co-ingestants, or withdrawal	Prevention of absorption (for ingested packets): • Activated charcoal • Whole-bowel irrigation Laboratory: • Urine drug screen to detect metabolite of cocaine: benzoylecgonine • Cardiac enzymes as indicated to rule out myocardial infarction Treatment: • Benzodiazepines such as diazepam (Valium) usually control hyperactivity, hypertension, tachycardia, anxiety, hyperthermia, and seizures • Phenobarbital may be necessary if seizures not controlled with benzodiazepines • Life-threatening hyperthermia may be reduced by external cooling measures • Cardiac monitoring and serial 12-lead electrocardiogram are used to evaluate arrhythmias and myocardial ischemia[11] • Monitor for other organ ischemia or infarction • Provide supportive care

(continued)

table 56-3 Common Patient Care in Poisonings and Overdoses (Continued)

Drug/Substance	Clinical Presentation and Assessment	Intervention
Halogenated Hydrocarbons Agents used as propellants and refrigerants Freon, dichlorodifluoromethane (freon 12), and trichloromonofluoromethane (freon 11) included in this category Exposures to leaking household air conditioners are usually minor, causing transient eye, nose, and throat irritation; dizziness; and palpitations More concentrated exposures such as in industrial spills or deliberate abuse ("huffing") associated with possible fatal ventricular arrhythmias (due to myocardial sensitization to catecholamines) and pulmonary edema	• Eye, nose, and throat irritation • Cough • Dizziness • Disorientation • Palpitations • Bronchial constriction • Pulmonary edema • Ventricular arrhythmias • Frostbite possible with dermal exposures	Prevention of absorption: • Fresh air Laboratory: • No specific laboratory tests Treatment: • Quiet environment • Cardiac monitoring • Frostbite: complete rewarming • Supportive care
Heroin Common street drug that produces a temporary euphoria in the user Routes of exposure: IV, snorting Street names: dope, smack, junk	• Miosis • Decreased respiratory drive • Decreased level of consciousness • "Nodding"	Prevention of absorption: • Not applicable Laboratory: • As clinically indicated • Serum toxicology screen Treatment: • Careful administration of naloxone • Referral to substance abuse counselor
LSD Common name for psychedelic drug lysergic acid diethylamide Common drug of abuse since its rise in popularity in the 1960s Street drug: available in tablet, capsule, sugar cubes, or as a substance on blotting paper known as "blotter acid" One source of LSD is ingestion of morning glory seeds In addition to the psychedelic experience, may result in physical effects and behavior-related trauma during the acute toxic phase	• Anxiety • Impaired color perception • Impaired judgment • Paranoia or ideas of persecution • Time distortions • Blood pressure normal • Tachycardia • Tachypnea • Slight temperature elevation • Flashbacks (transient recurrences of a psychedelic experience) possible after a period of abstinence, may recur for years • Trauma due to behavioral changes associated with LSD use	Prevention of absorption: • Activated charcoal • Cathartic Laboratory: • Urine drug screen Treatment: • Acute anxiety may be managed with IV or oral diazepam (Valium) • A quiet, nonstimulating environment may be useful while trying to help the patient who is experiencing a bad reaction • Evaluate for evidence of trauma • Provide supportive care

(continued)

table 56-3 Common Patient Care in Poisonings and Overdoses (Continued)

Drug/Substance	Clinical Presentation and Assessment	Intervention
Methanol Highly toxic antifreeze and solvent Available forms: most windshield washer fluids, Sterno canned heat, and components of some paints, gasoline additives, and shellacs Toxic effects: life-threatening acidosis and irreversible blindness, caused by the toxic metabolite, not the methanol itself	• Blurred vision • Decreased visual acuity • Subjective description of vision as if walking in a snowstorm • Retinal edema • Hyperemia of the optic disk • Headache • Vertigo • Lethargy • Confusion • Coma • Nausea • Vomiting • Abdominal pain • Metabolic acidosis	Prevention of absorption: • Syrup of ipecac • Gastric lavage • Activated charcoal and cathartic are of little value Laboratory: • Methanol level drawn 1 h postingestion • Serial electrolytes • If using ethanol therapy, serial glucose and blood ethanol level monitored every hour initially Treatment: • Treatment is aimed at preventing the formation of toxic metabolites with either Antizol (4-methylpyrazole: 4-MP) or ethanol • Hemodialysis usually indicated for methanol levels >50 mg/dL, visual changes, renal failure, or refractory acidosis • Folic acid administration to assist with oxidation of the toxic metabolite formic acid to carbon dioxide • Supportive care
Salicylates Group of drugs used primarily for anti-inflammatory, antipyretic, and analgesic properties Common sources: aspirin, some formulations of Alka-Seltzer, Aspergum, PeptoBismol, sunscreens, liniments such as Icy Hot, and oil of wintergreen (methylsalicylate) Life-threatening metabolic acidosis, cerebral edema, and pulmonary edema from salicylism Aspirin ingestions difficult to manage due to the formation of a mass of aspirin in the gastrointestinal tract called a *concretion* Concretion formation leads to delayed absorption and therefore delayed toxicity Chronic salicylism more common in older adults and easily missed due to lack of careful history taking Higher salicylate levels tolerated with acute overdose as opposed to chronic toxicity	• Tinnitus • Tachypnea • Pulmonary edema • Confusion • Lethargy • Seizures • Cerebral edema • Respiratory alkalosis coupled with metabolic acidosis (initially) • Hypokalemia • Platelet dysfunction • Hypothrombinemia • Gastrointestinal hemorrhage • Nausea • Vomiting • Hyperthermia • Dehydration	Prevention of absorption: • Syrup of ipecac • Gastric lavage • Multiple-dose activated charcoal • Single-dose cathartic Laboratory: • Serial salicylate levels • Serial electrolytes • Arterial blood gas as indicated • Hematological and coagulation studies Treatment: • IV hydration • Urinary excretion is enhanced by urine alkalinization (urine pH = 7.5–8.0); IV fluid is usually D_5W with 20–40 mEq KCl and two to three ampules of sodium bicarbonate per liter to infuse at a rate of 2–3 mL/kg/h to achieve equal urine output (Note: It is difficult to alkalinize the urine without a normal serum potassium level) • Potassium is replaced intravenously as needed • Monitor onset of cerebral or pulmonary edema; chest radiograph is taken as needed • Hemodialysis is indicated for renal failure, cerebral edema, pulmonary edema, refractory acidosis, chronic salicylate level >50 mg/dL, or acute salicylate level >100 mg/dL postingestion • Provide supportive care Note: Treatment is based on serial salicylate levels and clinical presentation; each case is individually assessed and managed

(continued)

table 56-3 Common Patient Care in Poisonings and Overdoses (Continued)

Drug/Substance	Clinical Presentation and Assessment	Intervention
Tricyclic Antidepressants (TCA) Class of drugs prescribed for depression and chronic pain Examples: amitriptyline (Elavil), clomipramine (Anafranil), desipramine (Norpramin), doxepin (Adapin, Sinequan), imipramine (Tofranil), nortriptyline (Pamelor, Aventyl), protriptyline (Vivactil), and trimipramine (Surmontil)	• Tachycardia • Ventricular arrhythmias (including ventricular tachycardia and ventricular fibrillation) • Cardiac conduction delays (e.g., QRS >100 msec) • Hypotension • Agitation • Sedation • Seizures • Coma • Dry, flushed skin • Decreased gastrointestinal motility • Urinary retention • Metabolic acidosis	Prevention of absorption: • Syrup of ipecac contraindicated because of the rapid onset of sedation or seizures • Gastric lavage • Activated charcoal • Cathartic Laboratory: • Serum TCA levels not clinically useful in managing overdoses • Urine drug screen for TCAs • Serial electrolytes and arterial blood gases as indicated Treatment: • Prepare for rapid onset of cardiovascular collapse • Seizures may be treated initially with intravenous benzodiazepines (diazepam, lorazepam), and, if necessary, phenytoin (Dilantin) and phenobarbital • Ventricular arrhythmias may initially be controlled with systemic alkalinization (keeping blood pH +7.45–7.55 using intravenous boluses of sodium bicarbonate or intubation and hyperventilation); ventricular arrhythmias not controlled with systemic alkalinization may be controlled with lidocaine or bretylium (Bretylol); do not use procainamide (Pronestyl) or quinidine due to effects on cardiac conduction similar to those of TCAs • Cardiac conduction delays (e.g., QRS >100 msec) also are treated with systemic alkalinization as outlined in previous point; conduction delays not responsive to systemic alkalinization may be treated with phenytoin • Hypotension may be addressed initially with Trendelenburg position and IV fluids; if necessary, follow with dopamine infusion; norepinephrine (Levophed) may be necessary • Provide supportive care

ALT, alanine aminotransferase; AST, aspartate aminotransferase; OTC, over the counter.

potassium 4.0 mEq/L, chloride 100 mEq/L, carbon dioxide 14 mEq/L, BUN 10 mg/dL, creatinine 0.9 mg/dL, and glucose 140 mg/dL. His ABGs were pH 7.48, $P{CO_2}$ 20 mm Hg, $P{O_2}$ 85 mm Hg, and bicarbonate 12 mEq/L. The patient had received 10 mg of IV metoclopramide (Reglan) and was able to tolerate a second 50-g dose of activated charcoal by nasogastric tube, without vomiting. IV fluids had been changed to 5% dextrose in water (D_5W) with two ampules of sodium bicarbonate and 40 mEq of potassium chloride at 15 mL/hour. Mr. S. was admitted to the ICU for continued treatment and monitoring.

While Mr. S. was in the ICU, the second salicylate level came back at 88 mg/dL (drawn approximately 3.5 hours after ingestion). The nurse in the ICU called the poison control center with this information and asked for further recommendations. The poison control center recommended another 50-g dose of activated charcoal and a renal consultation to consider hemodialysis. An abdominal CT scan to look for a possible concretion was also recommended.

Repeated laboratory studies obtained on arrival in the ICU included measurements of the patient's salicylate level, basic metabolic panel levels, and ABGs. The third salicylate level drawn approximately 7 hours after ingestion was 122 mg/dL. Basic metabolic panel levels were sodium 144 mEq/L, potassium 3.6 mEq/L, chloride 110 mEq/L, carbon dioxide 20 mEq/L, BUN 10 mg/dL, creatinine 1.0 mg/dL, and glucose 152 mg/dL. His ABGs were pH 7.50, $P{CO_2}$ 34 mm Hg, $P{O_2}$ 88 mm Hg, and bicarbonate 16 mEq/L. The patient remained lethargic and tachycardic at 120 beats/minute with a respiratory rate of 16 breaths/minute. A nephrology consultation

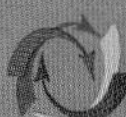

box 56-4 collaborative care guide *for the Patient With Cocaine Toxicity*

OUTCOMES	INTERVENTIONS
Oxygenation/Ventilation	
Arterial blood gases are within normal limits.	■ Monitor pulse oximetry and arterial blood gases. ■ Validate significant changes in pulse oximetry with co-oximetry arterial saturation measurement.
Respiratory rate and depth are within normal limits.	■ Monitor q15min, then q1h. ■ Prepare for intubation and mechanical ventilation (see Collaborative Care Guide for the Patient on a Ventilator).
Circulation/Perfusion	
Blood pressure, heart rate are within normal limits. Patient is free of dysrhythmias. There is no evidence of myocardial dysfunction, such as altered electrocardiogram (ECG) or cardiac enzymes.	■ Monitor vital signs q15min then q1h. ■ Provide continuous ECG monitoring. ■ Monitor 12-lead ECG qd and PRN. ■ Monitor cardiac enzymes, magnesium, phosphorus, calcium, and potassium as ordered. ■ Assess for chest pain. ■ Monitor ECG for dysrhythmias and changes consistent with evolving myocardial infarction.
Patient is euthermic.	■ Assess temperature q15–30min, then q1h. ■ Provide a cool environment, and institute cooling strategies (e.g., hypothermia blanket, tepid sponge bath), as indicated.
Fluids/Electrolytes	
Patient's urine output >30 mL/h (or >0.5 mL/kg/h).	■ Take intake and output q1h. ■ Administer fluids and diuretics to maintain intravascular volume and renal function per order.
There is no evidence of electrolyte imbalance or renal dysfunction.	■ Monitor electrolytes daily and PRN. ■ Replace electrolytes as ordered. ■ Monitor BUN, creatinine, serum osmolality, and urine electrolytes daily.
Mobility/Safety	
There is no evidence of seizure activity.	■ Monitor for seizure activity. ■ Administer anticonvulsants. ■ Assess anticonvulsant levels qd if indicated. ■ Maintain calm, quiet environment.
Patient does not harm self.	■ Institute seizure precautions. ■ Institute fall precautions. ■ Assess need for physical or chemical restraint to protect from self-injury. ■ Monitor agitation and administer sedation when appropriate. ■ Evaluate risk for suicide and take measures to protect patient.
Skin Integrity	
There is no evidence of skin breakdown.	■ Document skin integrity q8h. ■ Turn and reposition q2h. ■ Use Braden Scale to assess risk of skin breakdown.
Nutrition	
Caloric and nutrient intake meet metabolic requirements per calculation (e.g., Basal Energy Expenditure).	■ Provide parenteral or enteral nutrition if patient is NPO. ■ Consult dietitian or nutritional support service. ■ Monitor protein and calorie intake. ■ Monitor albumin, prealbumin, transferrin, cholesterol, triglycerides, glucose.

(continued)

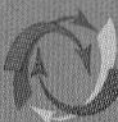

box 56-4 collaborative care guide
for the Patient With Cocaine Toxicity (Continued)

OUTCOMES	INTERVENTIONS
Comfort/Pain Control	
Patient will have minimal discomfort related to withdrawal from cocaine and other substances.	■ Obtain toxicology screen to identify other substances used by the patient. ■ Treat drug withdrawal and overdose symptoms promptly and with appropriate intervention (e.g., remove from circulation, administer antidote, administer methadone).
Psychosocial	
Patient and family acknowledge substance abuse.	■ Assess patient and family response to overdose. ■ Support healthy coping behaviors. ■ Consult substance abuse counselor and social worker. ■ Encourage patient discussion regarding use of illegal drugs, support system, financial concerns, and readiness for substance abuse treatment.
Teaching/Discharge Planning	
Patient and family have information about treatment and self-help resources.	■ Assess patient and family knowledge and understanding of substance abuse. ■ Provide literature and explanations to patient and family regarding substance abuse, treatment, relapse, legal issues, and self-help groups.
Patient and family each have a plan for follow-up care.	■ Refer family to self-help resources. ■ If patient agrees, initiate referral for substance abuse rehabilitation. ■ Coordinate referral with patient, family, and social worker to address other possible issues (e.g., housing, financial issues, long-term care planning).

box 56-5
Prevention of Childhood Poisoning

- Keep all medications and toxic products in original containers in a locked cabinet out of the reach of children.
- Read labels carefully before using drugs or toxic products.
- Use toxic chemical products in a well-ventilated area.
- Do not mix common household cleaning products.
- Identify any poisonous house plants, and keep seeds, bulbs, leaves, and fruits of such plants away from children.
- Do not treat medicines as candy.
- Measure and give medicine in well-lit areas to avoid error.
- Use child-resistant containers when available.
- Recap containers immediately after measuring dose.
- Destroy all old medications in a safe way, such as flushing them down the toilet.
- Keep Poison Control Center telephone numbers posted by the phone.
- Do not take medications in front of children.
- Keep all household products and drugs in original containers. Never put chemicals in empty food or drink containers.

box 56-6
Lead Poisoning

- Lead is commonly found in old homes, in paint, plumbing, and dinnerware.
- Lead is excreted more slowly than it is absorbed, leading to a buildup of lead in the body.
- Accumulation of lead in high levels is frequently missed through lack of blood lead level screening, and not detected until effects such as learning disabilities are diagnosed.
- Children can be tested for lead by their health care providers.
- The local health department can provide lead poisoning treatment and information about lead abatement programs.

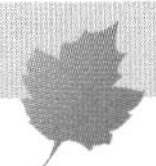

box 56-7

Accidental Poisoning in the Older Patient

- Poison Control Centers receive many calls from or related to older adults regarding accidental poisonings.
- Telephone numbers for the health care provider and the Poison Control Center should be in a readily accessible place.
- The older population uses more medicine than any other age group.
- Older people may be more susceptible to the effects of drugs.
- When questions arise concerning drugs, a responsible adult should not hesitate to call a health care provider.
- The patient should not change the dose or discontinue taking prescription drugs without first consulting the physician or nurse.
- It is not wise to double medication when a pill is forgotten. The patient should seek the advice of his or her physician, nurse, or pharmacist.
- Medications and alcohol should not be mixed without first checking with the pharmacist for possible interactions.
- The pharmacist can provide large-print labels.
- A medication calendar or diary will help the older person keep track of the dosing schedule.
- Pill dispensers are helpful for the patient who has to take a variety of pills or who has trouble remembering the prescribed schedule.
- When a drug is discontinued, the remaining medication should be thrown away.

resulted in the placement of an intravascular catheter for hemodialysis to allow better management of the high salicylate level and more rapid correction of the electrolyte and ABG abnormalities. The abdominal CT scan failed to show a concretion. In the ICU, Mr. S. continued to receive 50-g doses of activated charcoal every 4 hours for a total of three doses. He began passing activated charcoal rectally in combination with stool. The fourth salicylate level drawn approximately 10 hours after ingestion was 120 mg/dL, and hemodialysis was initiated. The patient received one 4-hour run of hemodialysis and experienced a significant improvement in symptoms. His salicylate level after hemodialysis was 20 mg/dL, with normal measurements of electrolytes and ABGs. Supportive care continued, and he was discharged on the third hospital day. ■

clinical applicability challenges

Self-Challenge: Critical Thinking

1. *Formulate a nursing plan of care for the patient who arrives at the emergency department with a sustained-release salicylate overdose. The plan should include initial stabilization, assessment, and follow-up care provided in the ICU.*
2. *Debate the risks and benefits of the different methods of GI decontamination, and discuss why certain methods are preferable or contraindicated in the management of different poisonings or overdoses.*

Study Questions

1. *The first step in the approach to the poisoned patient is*
   a. *identification of the toxidrome.*
   b. *correction of any electrolyte abnormalities.*
   c. *evaluation and maintenance of airway, breathing, and circulation.*
   d. *administration of an antidote.*
2. *Administration of activated charcoal is indicated in preventing absorption from a recent overdose of*
   a. *acetaminophen.*
   b. *aspirin.*
   c. *amitriptyline.*
   d. *all of the above.*
3. *All of the following symptoms are part of the anticholinergic toxidrome except*
   a. *tachycardia.*
   b. *miosis.*
   c. *flushed skin.*
   d. *decreased bowel sounds.*
4. *Management of an intravenous heroin overdose includes*
   a. *administration of activated charcoal.*
   b. *administration of a cathartic.*
   c. *whole-bowel irrigation.*
   d. *naloxone.*

REFERENCES

1. American Association of Poison Control Centers: 2001 Toxic exposure surveillance system poisoning data. Retrieved on January 11, 2003. Available at: www.aapcc.org
2. Sporer KA: Acute heroin overdose. Ann Intern Med 130:584–590, 1999
3. American Academy of Clinical Toxicology, European Association of Poison Centers and Clinical Toxicologists: Position statements. J Toxicol Clin Toxicol 35:699–762, 1997
4. Goldfrank L, Flomenbaum N, Lewin N, et al: Toxicologic Emergencies (6th Ed), pp 56–58. Stamford, CT, Appleton & Lange, 1998
5. Ford M, Delaney K, Ling L, et al: Clinical Toxicology, pp 661–665. Philadelphia, WB Saunders, 2001
6. Brent J, McMartin K, Phillips S, et al: Fomepizole for the treatment of methanol poisoning. N Eng J Med 344:424–429, 2001
7. Brent J, McMartin K, Phillips S, et al: Fomepizole for the treatment of ethylene glycol poisoning. N Engl J Med 340:832–838, 1999
8. Haddad L, Shannon M, Winchester J: Clinical Management of Poisoning and Drug Overdose (3rd Ed), pp 343–347. Philadelphia, WB Saunders, 1998
9. Wright RO, Anderson AC, Lesko SL, et al: Effect of metoclopramide dose on preventing emesis after oral administration of N-acetylcysteine for acetaminophen overdose. J Toxicol Clin Toxicol 37:35–42, 1999
10. Barnett R, Grace M, Boothe P, et al: Flumazenil in drug overdose: Randomized, placebo-controlled study to assess cost effectiveness. Crit Care Med 27:78–81, 1999
11. Tanen DA, Graeme KA, Curry SC: Crack cocaine ingestion with prolonged toxicity requiring electrical pacing. J Toxicol Clin Toxicol 38:653–657, 2000
12. Hoffman RS: Cocaine overdose: Clinical manifestations and treatment. J Toxicol Clin Toxicol 38:181–182, 2000

OTHER SELECTED READING

Bara V: Antihypertensive drug overdose. Emerg Nurse 7(4):13–18, 1999

Bates N: Acute poisoning: Bleaches, disinfectants and detergents. Emerg Nurse 8(10):14–19, 2001

Clark J: Acetaminophen poisoning and the use of intravenous N-acetylcysteine. Air Med J 20(4):16–17, 2001

Cohen SM: Lead poisoning: A summary of treatment and prevention. Pediatr Nurs 27(2):125–126, 129–130, 147–148, 2001

Dines A, Cullen G: Lead poisoning. Emerg Nurse 9(4):16–21, 2001

Goldfrank L, Flomenbaum N, Lewin N, et al: Toxicologic Emergencies (6th Ed). Stamford, CT, Appleton & Lange, 1998

James LP, Wells E, Beard RH, et al: Predictors of outcome after acetaminophen poisoning in children and adolescents. J Pediatr 140:522–526, 2002

Kearns GL: Acetaminophen poisoning in children: Treat early and long enough. J Pediatr 140:495–498, 2002

Koschel MJ: Emergency. Where there's smoke, there may be cyanide: Cyanide poisoning—a common but often overlooked consequence of smoke inhalation. Am J Nurs 102(8):39–42, 2002

McDrea S: Antiepileptic drug overdose. Emerg Nurse 9(9):13–18, 2002

Olson K, Anderson I, Benowitz N, et al: Poisoning and Drug Overdose (3rd Ed). Stamford, CT, Appleton & Lange, 1999

Pickford M: Antipsychotic drug overdose. Emerg Nurse 7(9):17–22, 2000

Schwab M, Oetzel C, Morike K, et al: Using trade names: A risk factor for accidental drug overdose. Arch Intern Med 162:1065–1066, 2002

APPENDIX one two

ACLS Guidelines

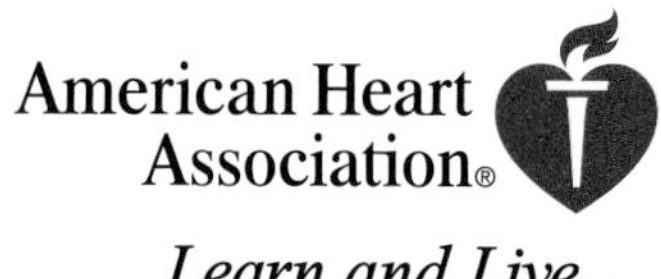

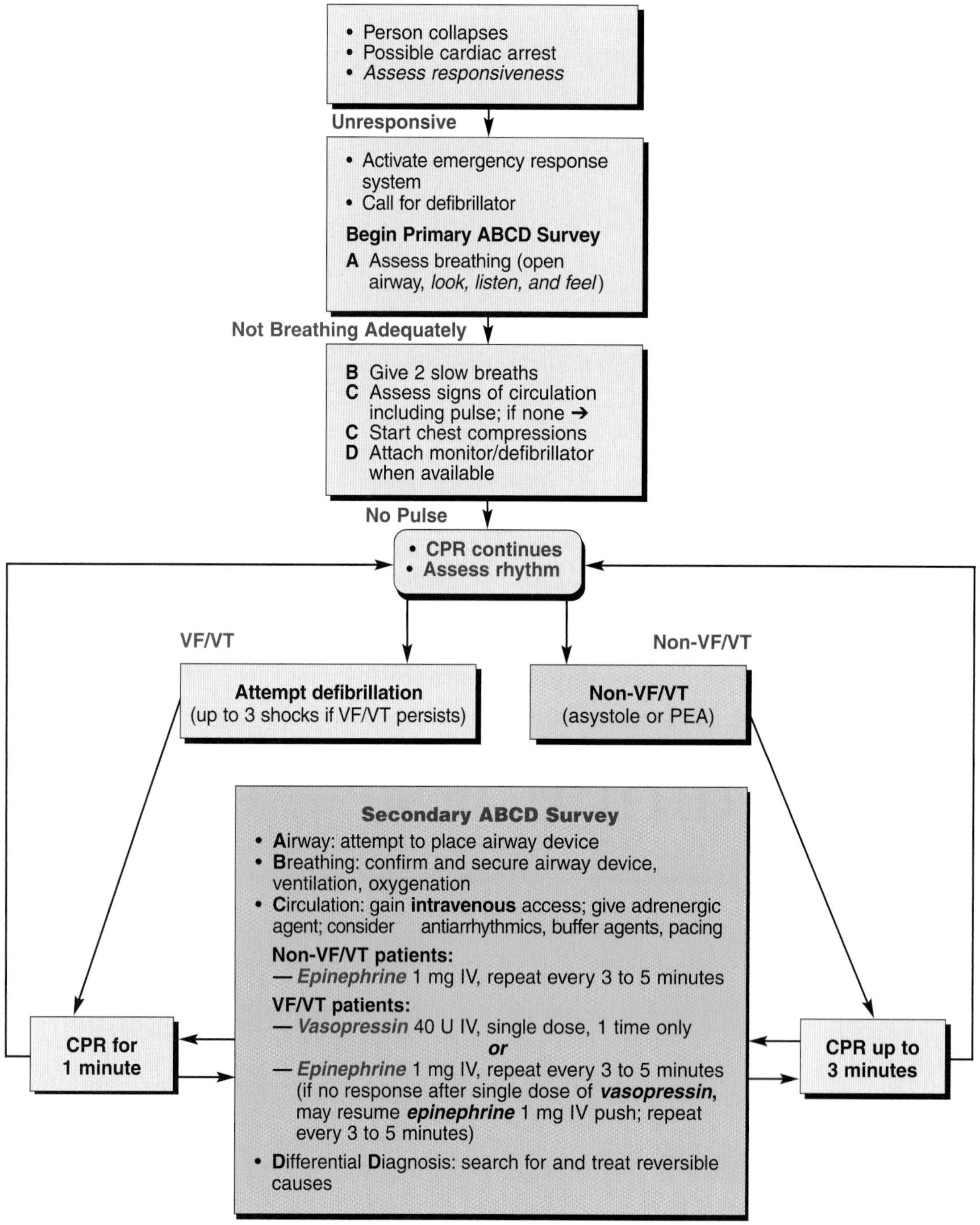

- Person collapses
- Possible cardiac arrest
- *Assess responsiveness*

Unresponsive ↓

- Activate emergency response system
- Call for defibrillator

Begin Primary ABCD Survey

A Assess breathing (open airway, *look, listen, and feel*)

Not Breathing Adequately ↓

B Give 2 slow breaths
C Assess signs of circulation including pulse; if none →
C Start chest compressions
D Attach monitor/defibrillator when available

No Pulse ↓

- **CPR continues**
- **Assess rhythm**

VF/VT

Attempt defibrillation
(up to 3 shocks if VF/VT persists)

Non-VF/VT

Non-VF/VT
(asystole or PEA)

Secondary ABCD Survey

- **A**irway: attempt to place airway device
- **B**reathing: confirm and secure airway device, ventilation, oxygenation
- **C**irculation: gain **intravenous** access; give adrenergic agent; consider antiarrhythmics, buffer agents, pacing

Non-VF/VT patients:
— ***Epinephrine*** 1 mg IV, repeat every 3 to 5 minutes

VF/VT patients:
— ***Vasopressin*** 40 U IV, single dose, 1 time only
or
— ***Epinephrine*** 1 mg IV, repeat every 3 to 5 minutes (if no response after single dose of ***vasopressin,*** may resume ***epinephrine*** 1 mg IV push; repeat every 3 to 5 minutes)

- **D**ifferential **D**iagnosis: search for and treat reversible causes

CPR for 1 minute

CPR up to 3 minutes

figure 1 Universal algorithm for adult emergency cardiac care.

American Heart Association®

Learn and Live℠

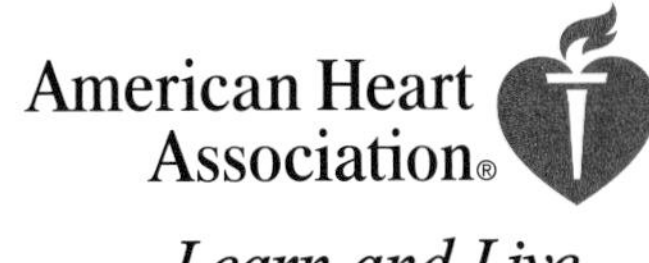

Primary ABCD Survey

Focus: *basic CPR and defibrillation*

- **Check** responsiveness
- **Activate** emergency response system
- **Call** for defibrillator

A **Airway:** open the airway

B **Breathing:** provide positive-pressure ventilations

C **Circulation:** give chest compressions

D **Defibrillation:** assess for and shock VF/pulseless VT, up to 3 times (200 J, 200 to 300 J, 360 J, or equivalent *biphasic*) if necessary

↓

Rhythm after first 3 shocks?

↓

Persistent or recurrent VF/VT

↓

Secondary ABCD Survey

Focus: *more advanced assessments and treatments*

A **Airway:** place airway device as soon as possible

B **Breathing:** confirm airway device placement by exam plus confirmation device

B **Breathing:** secure airway device; purpose-made tube holders preferred

B **Breathing:** confirm effective oxygenation and ventilation

C **Circulation:** establish IV access

C **Circulation:** identify rhythm → monitor

C **Circulation:** continue CPR, administer drugs appropriate for rhythm and condition

D **Differential Diagnosis:** search for and treat identified reversible causes

→

- ***Epinephrine*** 1 mg IV push, repeat every 3 to 5 minutes

or

- ***Vasopressin*** 40 U IV, **single dose**, 1 time only

↓

Resume attempts to defibrillate

1 · 360 J (or equivalent *biphasic*) within 30 to 60 seconds

↓

Consider antiarrhythmics:

- ***Amiodarone*** (IIb for persistent or recurrent VF/pulseless VT)
- ***Lidocaine*** (Indeterminate for persistent or recurrent VF/pulseless VT)
- ***Magnesium*** (IIb if known hypomagnesemic state)
- ***Procainamide*** (Indeterminate for persistent VF/pulseless VT; IIb for recurrent VF/pulseless VT)

↓

Resume attempts to defibrillate

Give shock(s) after each drug or each minute of CPR.

figure 2 Ventricular fibrillation/pulseless ventricular tachycardia (VF/VT) algorithm.

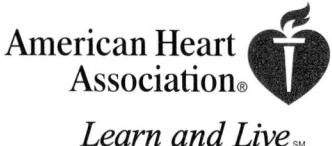

Pulseless Electrical Activity
(**PEA** = rhythm on monitor, without detectable pulse)

↓

Primary ABCD Survey
Focus: *basic CPR and defibrillation*

- **Check** responsiveness
- **Activate** emergency response system
- **Call** for defibrillator

A **Airway:** open the airway
B **Breathing:** provide positive-pressure ventilations
C **Circulation:** give chest compressions
D **Defibrillation:** assess for and shock VF/pulseless VT

↓

Secondary ABCD Survey
Focus: *more advanced assessments and treatments*

A **Airway:** place airway device as soon as possible
B **Breathing:** confirm airway device placement by exam plus confirmation device
B **Breathing:** secure airway device; purpose-made tube holders preferred
B **Breathing:** confirm effective oxygenation and ventilation
C **Circulation:** establish IV access
C **Circulation:** identify rhythm → monitor
C **Circulation:** administer drugs appropriate for rhythm and condition
C **Circulation:** assess for occult blood flow ("pseudo-EMD")
D **Differential Diagnosis:** search for and treat identified reversible causes

↓

Review for most frequent causes*

- **H**ypovolemia
- **H**ypoxia
- **H**ydrogen ion — acidosis
- **H**yper-/hypokalemia
- **H**ypothermia
- "**T**ablets" (drug OD, accidents)
- **T**amponade, cardiac
- **T**ension pneumothorax
- **T**hrombosis, coronary (ACS)
- **T**hrombosis, pulmonary (embolism)

*Advanced providers may use 6 H's by adding hypo-/hyperglycemia and 6 T's by adding trauma.

↓

Epinephrine 1 mg IV push, repeat every 3 to 5 minutes

→

Atropine 1 mg IV (if PEA rate is ***slow***), repeat every 3 to 5 minutes as needed, to a total dose of 0.04 mg/kg

figure 3 Pulseless electrical activity (PEA) algorithm (electromechanical dissociation [EMD]).

American Heart Association®
Learn and Live℠

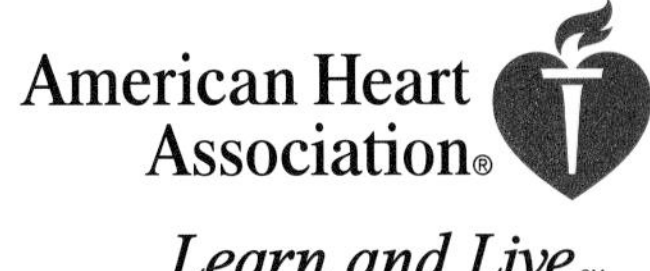

Asystole

↓

Primary ABCD Survey
Focus: *basic CPR and defibrillation*

Rapid scene survey: is there any evidence that personnel should ***not*** attempt resuscitation (eg, DNAR order, signs of death)?

- **Check** responsiveness
- **Activate** emergency response system
- **Call** for defibrillator

A **Airway:** open the airway
B **Breathing:** provide positive-pressure ventilations
C **Circulation:** give chest compressions
C **Confirm** true asystole
D **Defibrillation:** assess for VF/pulseless VT; shock if indicated

↓

Secondary ABCD Survey
Focus: *more advanced assessments and treatments*

A **Airway:** place airway device as soon as possible
B **Breathing:** confirm airway device placement by exam plus confirmation device
B **Breathing:** secure airway device; purpose-made tube holders preferred
B **Breathing:** confirm effective oxygenation and ventilation
C **Circulation:** confirm true asystole
C **Circulation:** establish IV access
C **Circulation:** identify rhythm → monitor
C **Circulation:** give medications appropriate for rhythm and condition
C **Circulation:** assess for occult blood flow ("pseudo-EMD")
D **Differential Diagnosis:** search for and treat identified reversible causes

↓

Transcutaneous pacing:
If considered, perform immediately

↓

Epinephrine 1 mg IV push,
repeat every 3 to 5 minutes

↓

Atropine 1 mg IV,
repeat every 3 to 5 minutes
up to a total of 0.04 mg/kg

→

Asystole persists
Withhold or cease resuscitative efforts?
- Consider quality of resuscitation?
- Atypical clinical features present?
- Support for cease-efforts protocols in place?

figure 4 Asystole treatment algorithm.

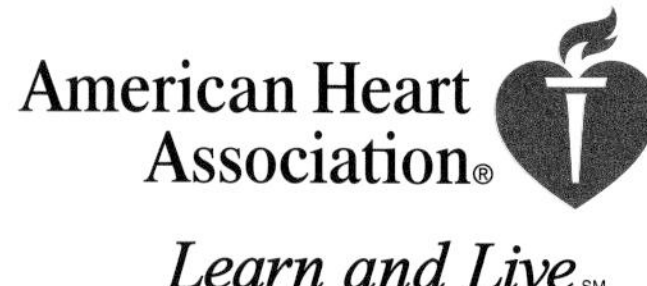

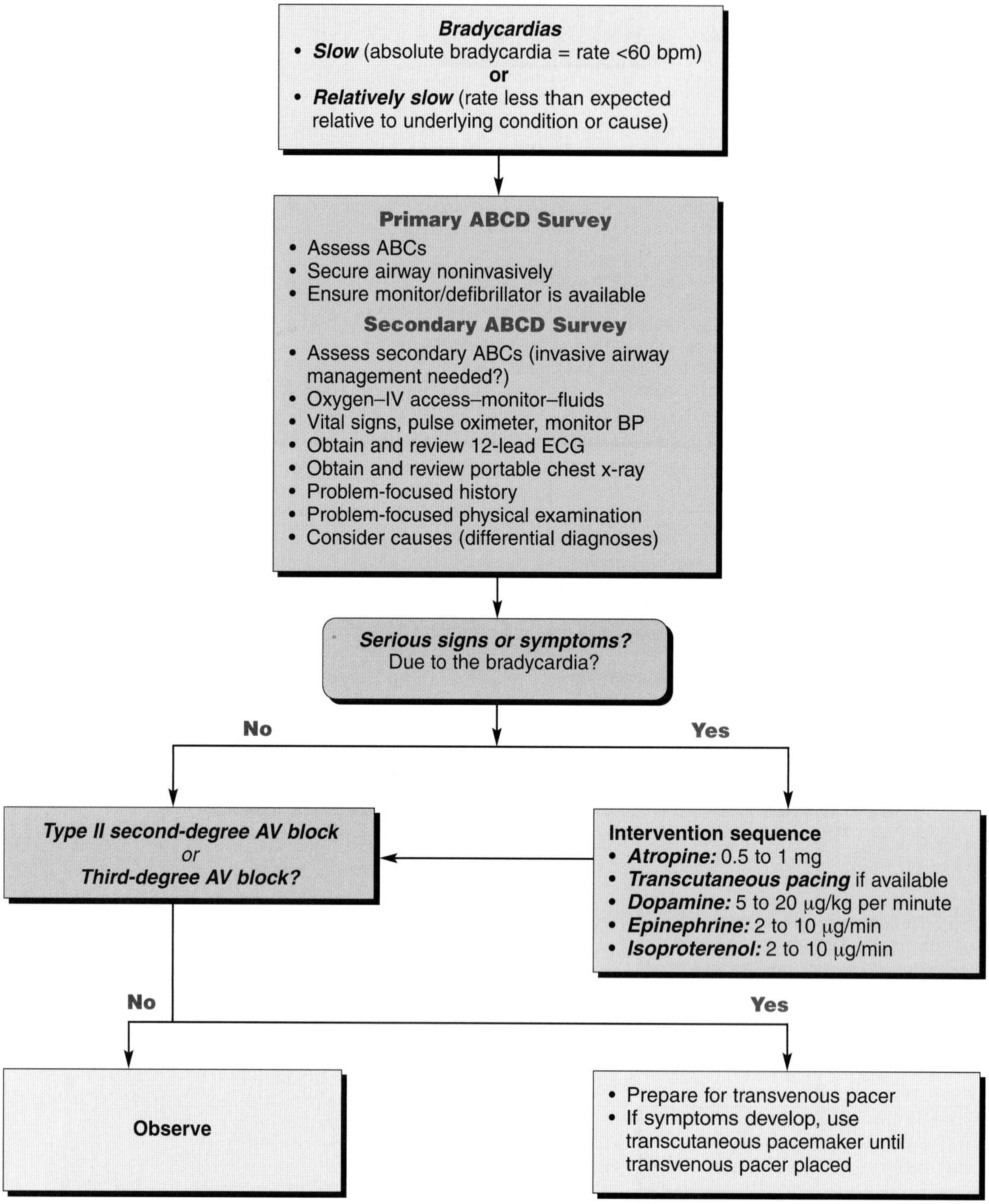

Bradycardias
- ***Slow*** (absolute bradycardia = rate <60 bpm)

or
- ***Relatively slow*** (rate less than expected relative to underlying condition or cause)

↓

Primary ABCD Survey
- Assess ABCs
- Secure airway noninvasively
- Ensure monitor/defibrillator is available

Secondary ABCD Survey
- Assess secondary ABCs (invasive airway management needed?)
- Oxygen–IV access–monitor–fluids
- Vital signs, pulse oximeter, monitor BP
- Obtain and review 12-lead ECG
- Obtain and review portable chest x-ray
- Problem-focused history
- Problem-focused physical examination
- Consider causes (differential diagnoses)

↓

Serious signs or symptoms?
Due to the bradycardia?

No → ***Type II second-degree AV block*** *or* ***Third-degree AV block?***

Yes → **Intervention sequence**
- ***Atropine:*** 0.5 to 1 mg
- ***Transcutaneous pacing*** if available
- ***Dopamine:*** 5 to 20 μg/kg per minute
- ***Epinephrine:*** 2 to 10 μg/min
- ***Isoproterenol:*** 2 to 10 μg/min

(Intervention sequence → *Type II second-degree AV block or Third-degree AV block?*)

Type II second-degree AV block or Third-degree AV block?

No → **Observe**

Yes →
- Prepare for transvenous pacer
- If symptoms develop, use transcutaneous pacemaker until transvenous pacer placed

figure 5 Bradycardia algorithm (patient is not in cardiac arrest).

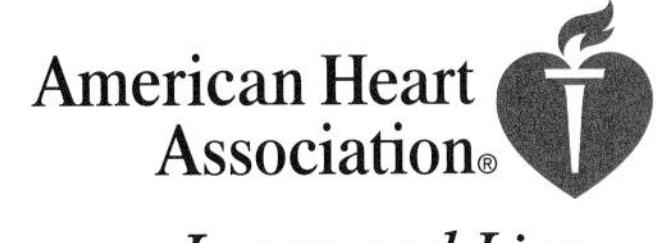

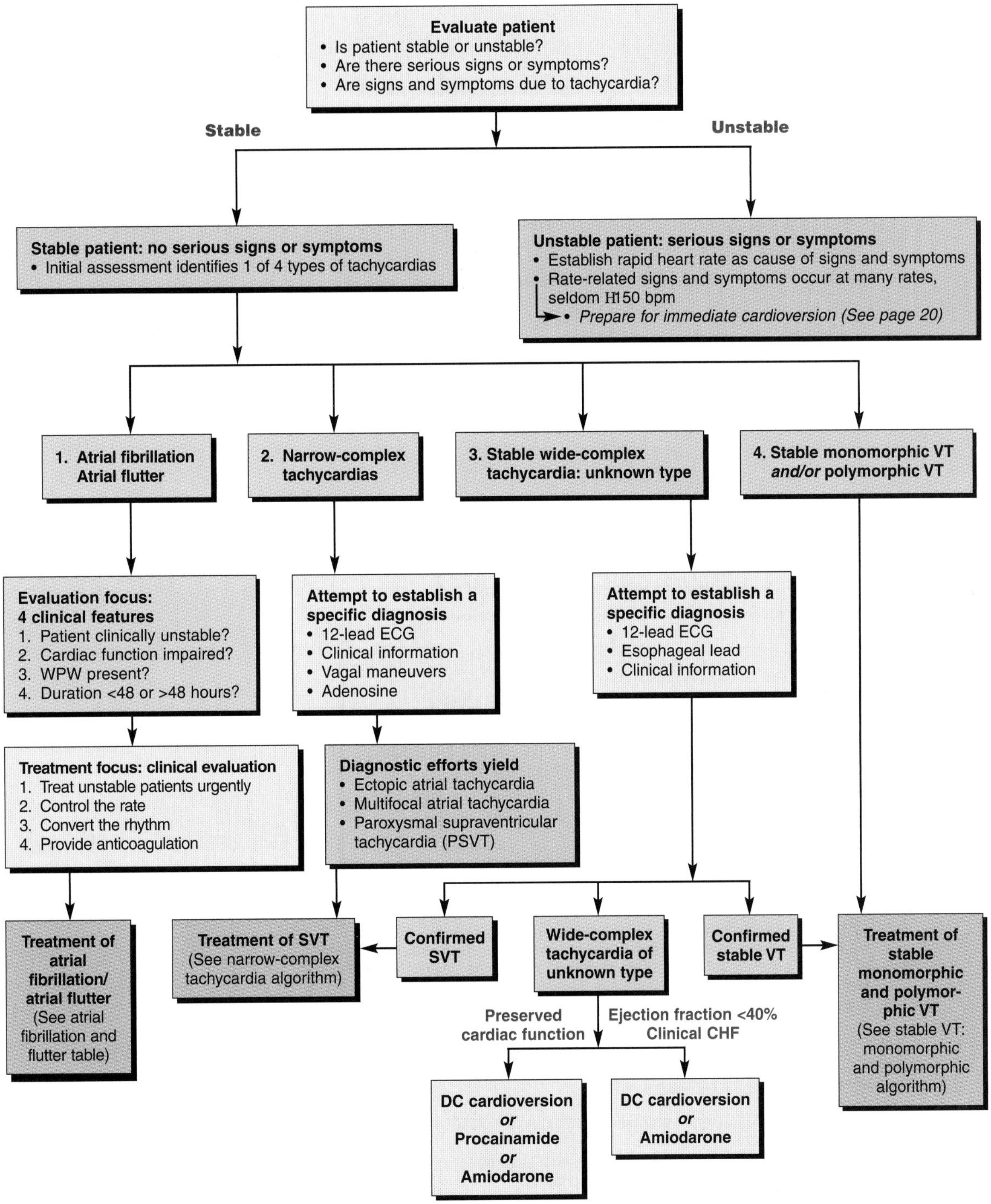

Evaluate patient
- Is patient stable or unstable?
- Are there serious signs or symptoms?
- Are signs and symptoms due to tachycardia?

Stable

Stable patient: no serious signs or symptoms
- Initial assessment identifies 1 of 4 types of tachycardias

Unstable

Unstable patient: serious signs or symptoms
- Establish rapid heart rate as cause of signs and symptoms
- Rate-related signs and symptoms occur at many rates, seldom H150 bpm
  - *Prepare for immediate cardioversion (See page 20)*

1. Atrial fibrillation Atrial flutter

Evaluation focus: 4 clinical features
1. Patient clinically unstable?
2. Cardiac function impaired?
3. WPW present?
4. Duration <48 or >48 hours?

Treatment focus: clinical evaluation
1. Treat unstable patients urgently
2. Control the rate
3. Convert the rhythm
4. Provide anticoagulation

Treatment of atrial fibrillation/ atrial flutter
(See atrial fibrillation and flutter table)

2. Narrow-complex tachycardias

Attempt to establish a specific diagnosis
- 12-lead ECG
- Clinical information
- Vagal maneuvers
- Adenosine

Diagnostic efforts yield
- Ectopic atrial tachycardia
- Multifocal atrial tachycardia
- Paroxysmal supraventricular tachycardia (PSVT)

Treatment of SVT
(See narrow-complex tachycardia algorithm)

3. Stable wide-complex tachycardia: unknown type

Attempt to establish a specific diagnosis
- 12-lead ECG
- Esophageal lead
- Clinical information

Confirmed SVT → **Treatment of SVT**

Wide-complex tachycardia of unknown type
- Preserved cardiac function → **DC cardioversion** *or* **Procainamide** *or* **Amiodarone**
- Ejection fraction <40% Clinical CHF → **DC cardioversion** *or* **Amiodarone**

Confirmed stable VT → **Treatment of stable monomorphic and polymorphic VT**

4. Stable monomorphic VT *and/or* polymorphic VT

Treatment of stable monomorphic and polymorphic VT
(See stable VT: monomorphic and polymorphic algorithm)

figure 6 Tachycardia algorithm.

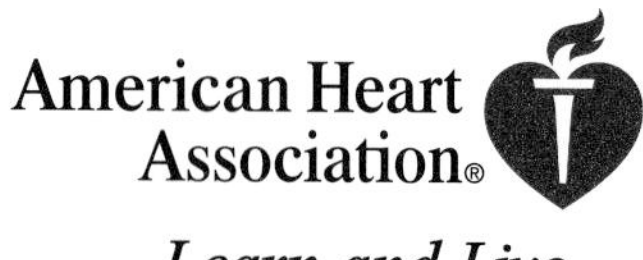

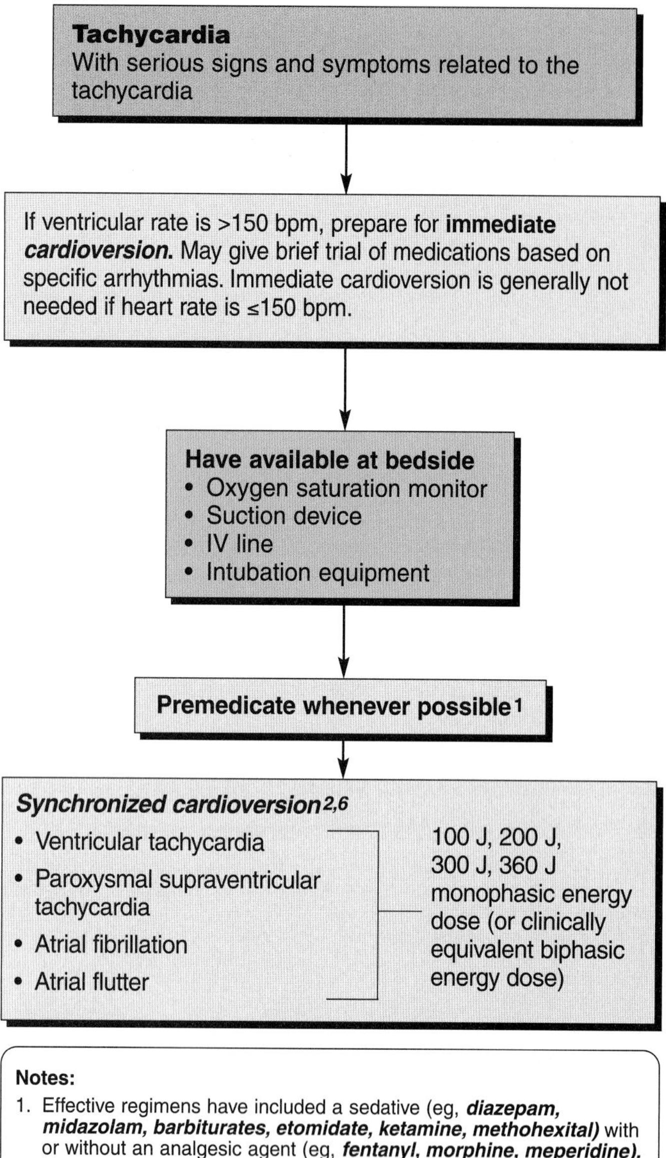

Tachycardia
With serious signs and symptoms related to the tachycardia
If ventricular rate is >150 bpm, prepare for immediate cardioversion. May give brief trial of medications based on specific arrhythmias. Immediate cardioversion is generally not needed if heart rate is ≤150 bpm.
Have available at bedside
• Oxygen saturation monitor
• Suction device
• IV line
• Intubation equipment
Premedicate whenever possible 1
Synchronized cardioversion 2,6
• Ventricular tachycardia
• Paroxysmal supraventricular tachycardia
• Atrial fibrillation
• Atrial flutter
100 J, 200 J, 300 J, 360 J monophasic energy dose (or clinically equivalent biphasic energy dose)

Notes:

1. Effective regimens have included a sedative (eg, ***diazepam, midazolam, barbiturates, etomidate, ketamine, methohexital)*** with or without an analgesic agent (eg, ***fentanyl, morphine, meperidine).*** Many experts recommend anesthesia if service is readily available.
2. Both monophasic and biphasic waveforms are acceptable if documented as clinically equivalent to reports of monophasic shock success.
3. Note possible need to resynchronize after each cardioversion.
4. If delays in synchronization occur and clinical condition is critical, go immediately to unsynchronized shocks.
5. Treat polymorphic ventricular tachycardia (irregular form and rate) like ventricular fibrillation: see ventricular fibrillation/pulseless ventricular tachycardia algorithm (Figure 3).
6. Paroxysmal supraventricular tachycardia and atrial flutter often respond to lower energy levels (start with 50 J).

figure 7 Electrical cardioversion algorithm (patient is not in cardiac arrest).

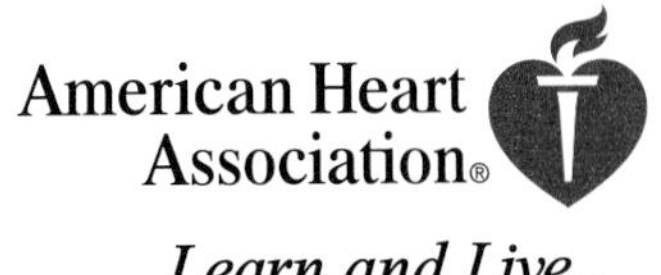

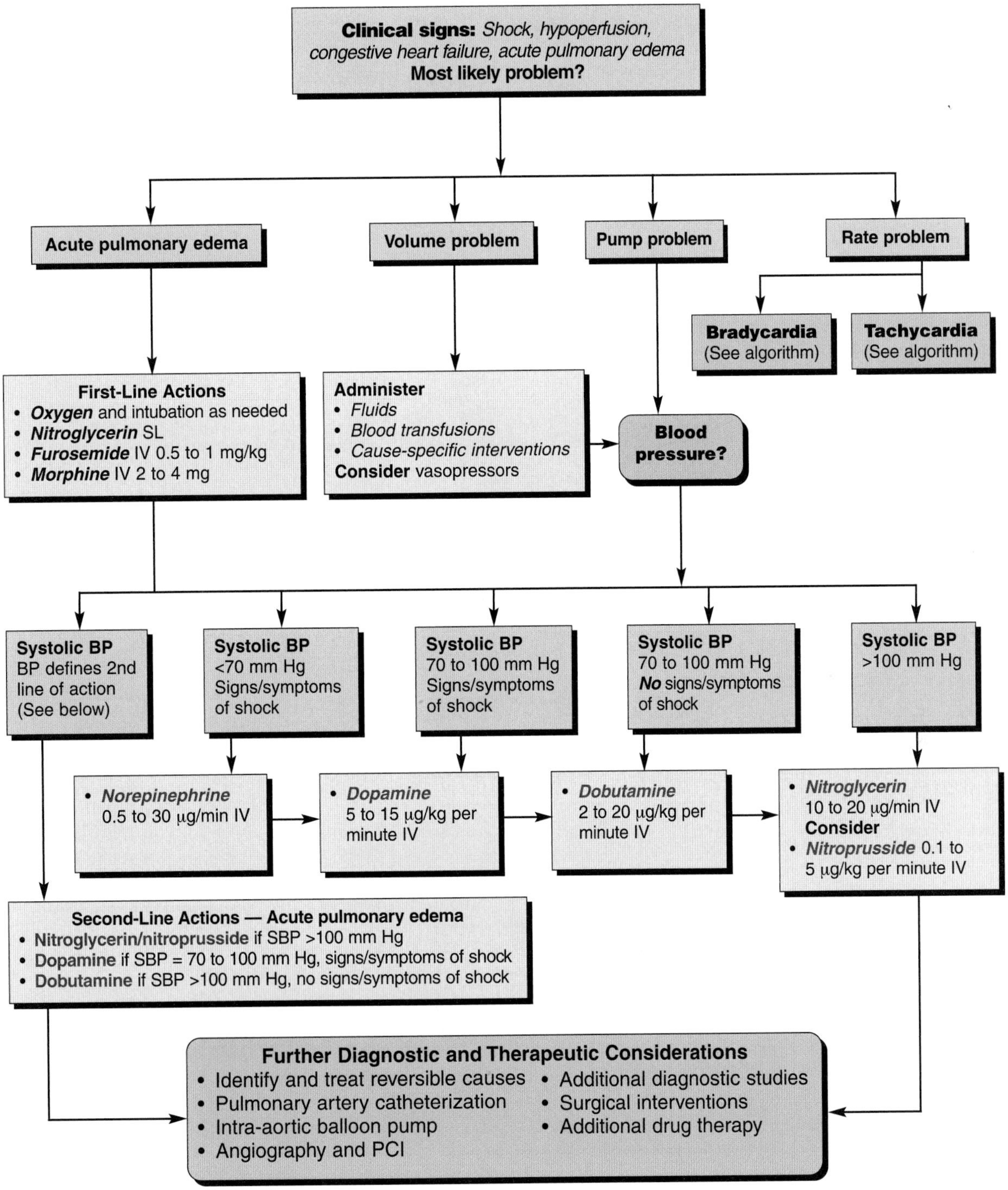

Clinical signs: *Shock, hypoperfusion, congestive heart failure, acute pulmonary edema*
Most likely problem?

- **Acute pulmonary edema**
  - **First-Line Actions**
    - ***Oxygen*** and intubation as needed
    - ***Nitroglycerin*** SL
    - ***Furosemide*** IV 0.5 to 1 mg/kg
    - ***Morphine*** IV 2 to 4 mg
- **Volume problem**
  - **Administer**
    - *Fluids*
    - *Blood transfusions*
    - *Cause-specific interventions*
  - **Consider** vasopressors
  - → **Blood pressure?**
- **Pump problem** → **Blood pressure?**
- **Rate problem**
  - **Bradycardia** (See algorithm)
  - **Tachycardia** (See algorithm)

Systolic BP
BP defines 2nd line of action
(See below)

Systolic BP
<70 mm Hg
Signs/symptoms of shock
→ • ***Norepinephrine*** 0.5 to 30 μg/min IV

Systolic BP
70 to 100 mm Hg
Signs/symptoms of shock
→ • ***Dopamine*** 5 to 15 μg/kg per minute IV

Systolic BP
70 to 100 mm Hg
No signs/symptoms of shock
→ • ***Dobutamine*** 2 to 20 μg/kg per minute IV

Systolic BP
>100 mm Hg
→ • ***Nitroglycerin*** 10 to 20 μg/min IV
Consider
• ***Nitroprusside*** 0.1 to 5 μg/kg per minute IV

Second-Line Actions — Acute pulmonary edema
- **Nitroglycerin/nitroprusside** if SBP >100 mm Hg
- **Dopamine** if SBP = 70 to 100 mm Hg, signs/symptoms of shock
- **Dobutamine** if SBP >100 mm Hg, no signs/symptoms of shock

Further Diagnostic and Therapeutic Considerations
- Identify and treat reversible causes
- Pulmonary artery catheterization
- Intra-aortic balloon pump
- Angiography and PCI
- Additional diagnostic studies
- Surgical interventions
- Additional drug therapy

figure 8 Acute pulmonary edema/hypotension/shock algorithm.

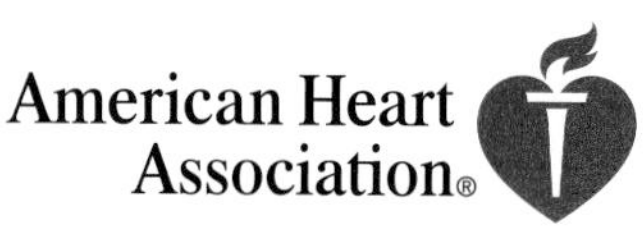

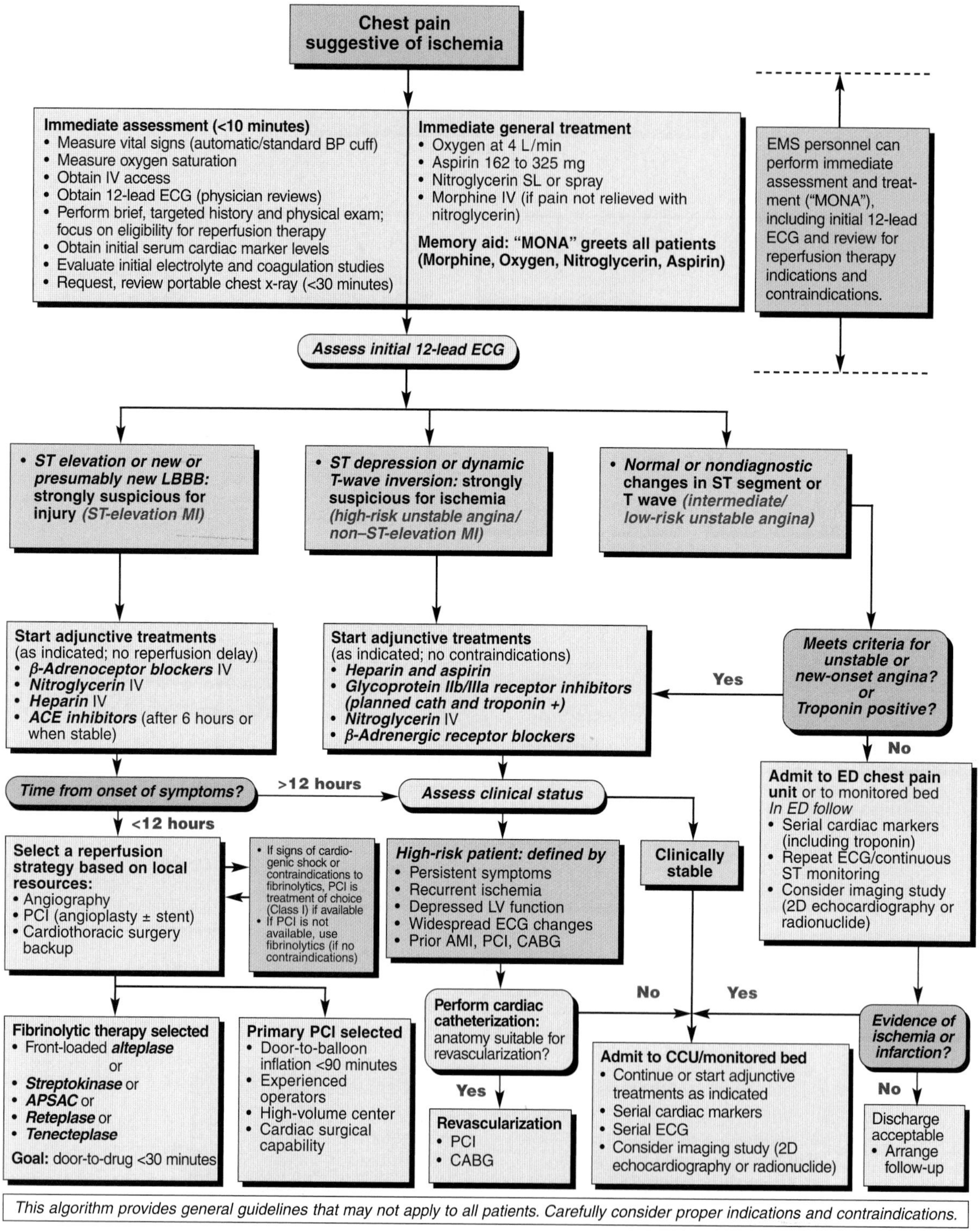

Chest pain suggestive of ischemia

Immediate assessment (<10 minutes)
- Measure vital signs (automatic/standard BP cuff)
- Measure oxygen saturation
- Obtain IV access
- Obtain 12-lead ECG (physician reviews)
- Perform brief, targeted history and physical exam; focus on eligibility for reperfusion therapy
- Obtain initial serum cardiac marker levels
- Evaluate initial electrolyte and coagulation studies
- Request, review portable chest x-ray (<30 minutes)

Immediate general treatment
- Oxygen at 4 L/min
- Aspirin 162 to 325 mg
- Nitroglycerin SL or spray
- Morphine IV (if pain not relieved with nitroglycerin)

Memory aid: "MONA" greets all patients (Morphine, Oxygen, Nitroglycerin, Aspirin)

EMS personnel can perform immediate assessment and treatment ("MONA"), including initial 12-lead ECG and review for reperfusion therapy indications and contraindications.

Assess initial 12-lead ECG

- ***ST elevation or new or presumably new LBBB:* strongly suspicious for injury *(ST-elevation MI)***

- ***ST depression or dynamic T-wave inversion:* strongly suspicious for ischemia *(high-risk unstable angina/ non–ST-elevation MI)***

- ***Normal or nondiagnostic* changes in ST segment or T wave *(intermediate/ low-risk unstable angina)***

Start adjunctive treatments
(as indicated; no reperfusion delay)
- ***β-Adrenoceptor blockers*** IV
- ***Nitroglycerin*** IV
- ***Heparin*** IV
- ***ACE inhibitors*** (after 6 hours or when stable)

Start adjunctive treatments
(as indicated; no contraindications)
- ***Heparin and aspirin***
- ***Glycoprotein IIb/IIIa receptor inhibitors (planned cath and troponin +)***
- ***Nitroglycerin*** IV
- ***β-Adrenergic receptor blockers***

Meets criteria for unstable or new-onset angina? or Troponin positive?

Yes → Start adjunctive treatments (as indicated; no contraindications)

No →

Admit to ED chest pain unit or to monitored bed
In ED follow
- Serial cardiac markers (including troponin)
- Repeat ECG/continuous ST monitoring
- Consider imaging study (2D echocardiography or radionuclide)

Time from onset of symptoms?

>12 hours → *Assess clinical status*

<12 hours →

Select a reperfusion strategy based on local resources:
- Angiography
- PCI (angioplasty ± stent)
- Cardiothoracic surgery backup

- If signs of cardiogenic shock or contraindications to fibrinolytics, PCI is treatment of choice (Class I) if available
- If PCI is not available, use fibrinolytics (if no contraindications)

Assess clinical status

High-risk patient: defined by
- Persistent symptoms
- Recurrent ischemia
- Depressed LV function
- Widespread ECG changes
- Prior AMI, PCI, CABG

Clinically stable

Fibrinolytic therapy selected
- Front-loaded ***alteplase***

  or
- ***Streptokinase*** or
- ***APSAC*** or
- ***Reteplase*** or
- ***Tenecteplase***

Goal: door-to-drug <30 minutes

Primary PCI selected
- Door-to-balloon inflation <90 minutes
- Experienced operators
- High-volume center
- Cardiac surgical capability

Perform cardiac catheterization: anatomy suitable for revascularization?

Yes →

Revascularization
- PCI
- CABG

No → Admit to CCU/monitored bed

Admit to CCU/monitored bed
- Continue or start adjunctive treatments as indicated
- Serial cardiac markers
- Serial ECG
- Consider imaging study (2D echocardiography or radionuclide)

Evidence of ischemia or infarction?

Yes → Admit to CCU/monitored bed

No →

Discharge acceptable
- Arrange follow-up

This algorithm provides general guidelines that may not apply to all patients. Carefully consider proper indications and contraindications.

figure 9 Acute myocardial infarction algorithm. Recommendations for early management of patients with chest pain and possible AMI.

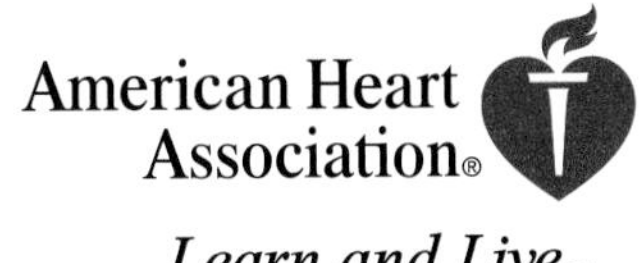

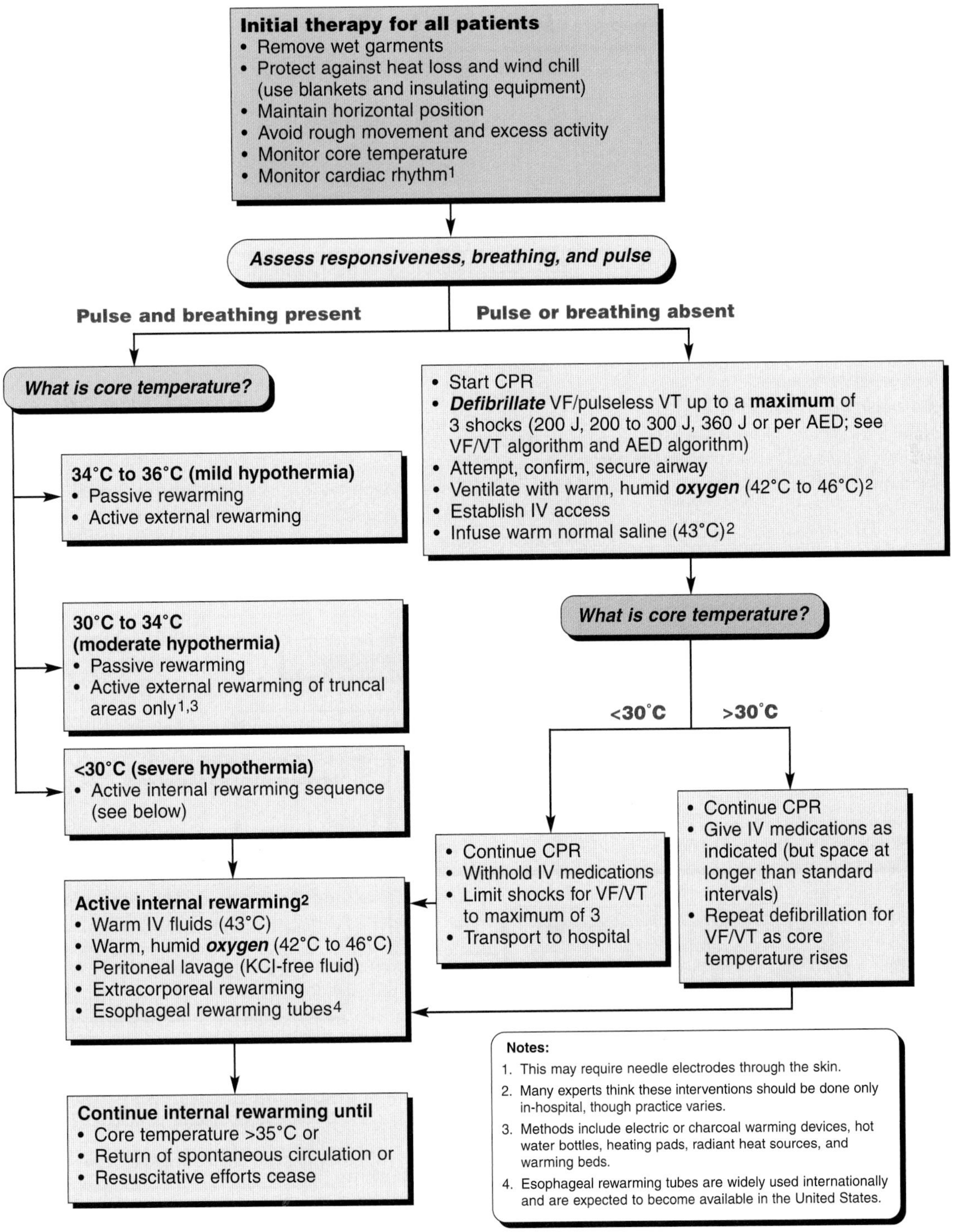

Initial therapy for all patients
- Remove wet garments
- Protect against heat loss and wind chill (use blankets and insulating equipment)
- Maintain horizontal position
- Avoid rough movement and excess activity
- Monitor core temperature
- Monitor cardiac rhythm[1]

Assess responsiveness, breathing, and pulse

Pulse and breathing present

What is core temperature?

34°C to 36°C (mild hypothermia)
- Passive rewarming
- Active external rewarming

30°C to 34°C (moderate hypothermia)
- Passive rewarming
- Active external rewarming of truncal areas only[1,3]

<30°C (severe hypothermia)
- Active internal rewarming sequence (see below)

Pulse or breathing absent

- Start CPR
- ***Defibrillate*** VF/pulseless VT up to a **maximum** of 3 shocks (200 J, 200 to 300 J, 360 J or per AED; see VF/VT algorithm and AED algorithm)
- Attempt, confirm, secure airway
- Ventilate with warm, humid ***oxygen*** (42°C to 46°C)[2]
- Establish IV access
- Infuse warm normal saline (43°C)[2]

What is core temperature?

<30°C
- Continue CPR
- Withhold IV medications
- Limit shocks for VF/VT to maximum of 3
- Transport to hospital

>30°C
- Continue CPR
- Give IV medications as indicated (but space at longer than standard intervals)
- Repeat defibrillation for VF/VT as core temperature rises

Active internal rewarming[2]
- Warm IV fluids (43°C)
- Warm, humid ***oxygen*** (42°C to 46°C)
- Peritoneal lavage (KCl-free fluid)
- Extracorporeal rewarming
- Esophageal rewarming tubes[4]

Continue internal rewarming until
- Core temperature >35°C or
- Return of spontaneous circulation or
- Resuscitative efforts cease

Notes:
1. This may require needle electrodes through the skin.
2. Many experts think these interventions should be done only in-hospital, though practice varies.
3. Methods include electric or charcoal warming devices, hot water bottles, heating pads, radiant heat sources, and warming beds.
4. Esophageal rewarming tubes are widely used internationally and are expected to become available in the United States.

figure 10 Hypothermia algorithm (adult advanced cardiac life support).

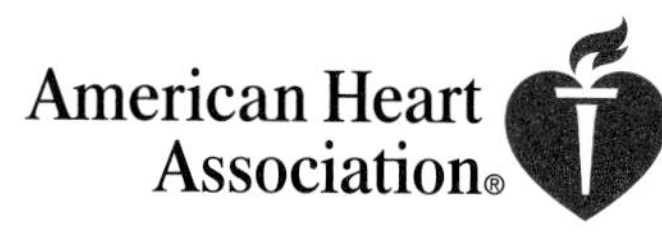

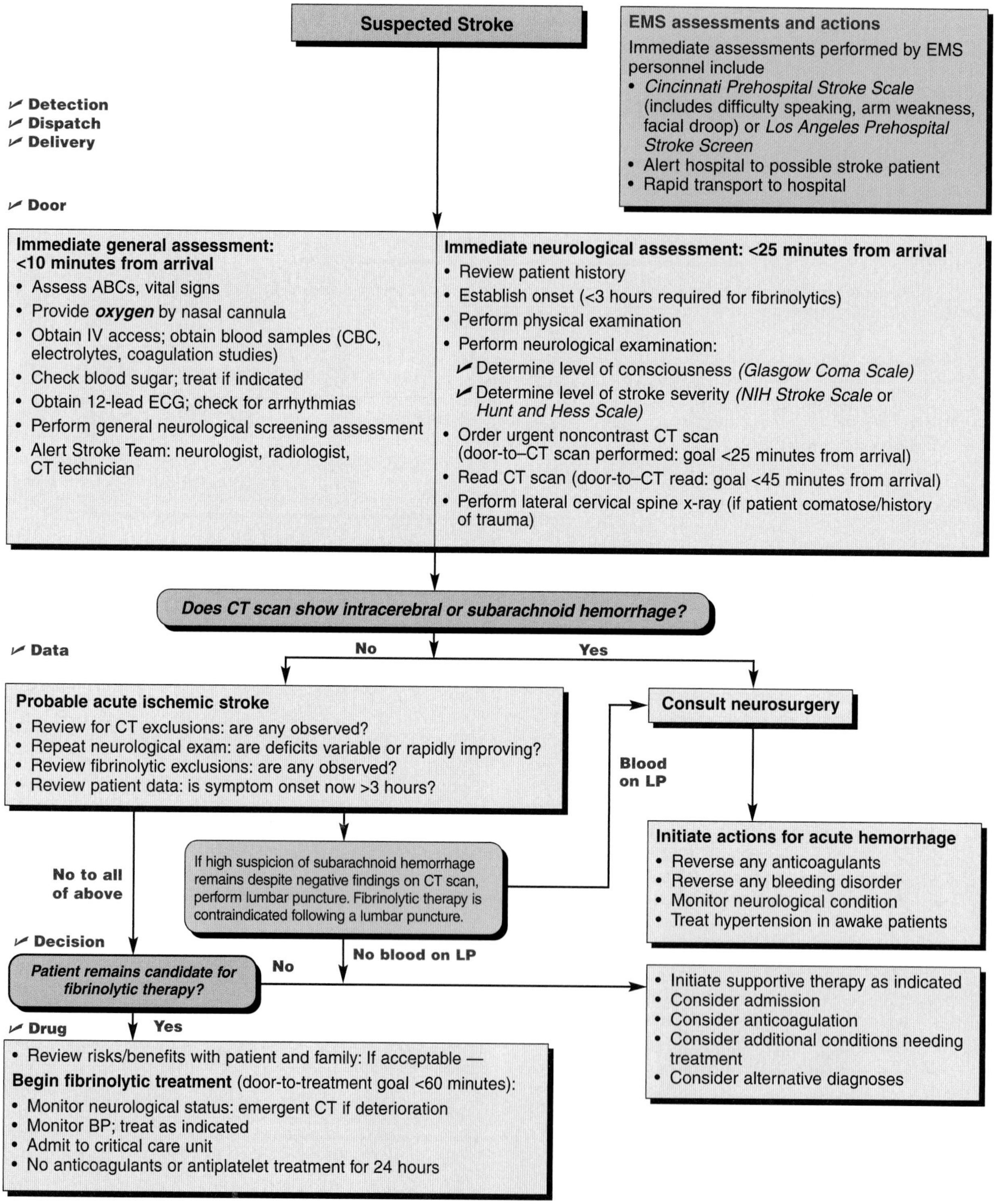

Suspected Stroke

EMS assessments and actions
Immediate assessments performed by EMS personnel include
- *Cincinnati Prehospital Stroke Scale* (includes difficulty speaking, arm weakness, facial droop) or *Los Angeles Prehospital Stroke Screen*
- Alert hospital to possible stroke patient
- Rapid transport to hospital

✓ **Detection**
✓ **Dispatch**
✓ **Delivery**

✓ **Door**

Immediate general assessment: <10 minutes from arrival
- Assess ABCs, vital signs
- Provide ***oxygen*** by nasal cannula
- Obtain IV access; obtain blood samples (CBC, electrolytes, coagulation studies)
- Check blood sugar; treat if indicated
- Obtain 12-lead ECG; check for arrhythmias
- Perform general neurological screening assessment
- Alert Stroke Team: neurologist, radiologist, CT technician

Immediate neurological assessment: <25 minutes from arrival
- Review patient history
- Establish onset (<3 hours required for fibrinolytics)
- Perform physical examination
- Perform neurological examination:
  - ✓ Determine level of consciousness *(Glasgow Coma Scale)*
  - ✓ Determine level of stroke severity *(NIH Stroke Scale* or *Hunt and Hess Scale)*
- Order urgent noncontrast CT scan (door-to–CT scan performed: goal <25 minutes from arrival)
- Read CT scan (door-to–CT read: goal <45 minutes from arrival)
- Perform lateral cervical spine x-ray (if patient comatose/history of trauma)

Does CT scan show intracerebral or subarachnoid hemorrhage?

✓ **Data**

No →

Probable acute ischemic stroke
- Review for CT exclusions: are any observed?
- Repeat neurological exam: are deficits variable or rapidly improving?
- Review fibrinolytic exclusions: are any observed?
- Review patient data: is symptom onset now >3 hours?

If high suspicion of subarachnoid hemorrhage remains despite negative findings on CT scan, perform lumbar puncture. Fibrinolytic therapy is contraindicated following a lumbar puncture.

Blood on LP → Consult neurosurgery

No blood on LP → supportive therapy (below)

No to all of above →

✓ **Decision**

Patient remains candidate for fibrinolytic therapy?

No →
- Initiate supportive therapy as indicated
- Consider admission
- Consider anticoagulation
- Consider additional conditions needing treatment
- Consider alternative diagnoses

✓ **Drug**

Yes →
- Review risks/benefits with patient and family: If acceptable —

Begin fibrinolytic treatment (door-to-treatment goal <60 minutes):
- Monitor neurological status: emergent CT if deterioration
- Monitor BP; treat as indicated
- Admit to critical care unit
- No anticoagulants or antiplatelet treatment for 24 hours

Yes →

Consult neurosurgery

Initiate actions for acute hemorrhage
- Reverse any anticoagulants
- Reverse any bleeding disorder
- Monitor neurological condition
- Treat hypertension in awake patients

figure 11 Algorithm for initial evaluation of acute stroke patients (adult advanced cardiac life support).

APPENDIX

one

two

Answer Key to Study Questions With Rationales

Chapter 1: CRITICAL CARE NURSING PRACTICE: AN INTEGRATION OF CARING, COMPETENCE, AND COMMITMENT TO EXCELLENCE

1. **d** As health care changes continue at monumental rates, tradition and previous education are inadequate to provide state-of-the-science critical care nursing care. The first step to evidence-based nursing practice is to recognize that health care is continually evolving. After accepting this fact, a nurse can then identify a need for change of practice, frame a clinical question, search the literature, synthesize and evaluate the evidence, and change practice if warranted.
2. **c** In today's health care system, quality outcomes require nurses to appreciate the care environment from a perspective that recognizes holistic interrelationships, hence systems thinking. The ongoing process of questioning and evaluating practice is called *clinical inquiry*. Response to diversity recognizes, appreciates, and incorporates differences in the provision of care. Facilitating the learning of others and fostering the work of others blends collaboration with facilitating of learning.
3. **b** In this situation, the domestic partner desires to learn skin care, which illustrates the patient characteristic of participation in care. In response, the nurse is sensitive to recognize, appreciate, and incorporate differences of family configuration, exemplifying a response to diversity.
4. **c** Following the introduction of a new pharmacologic agent to treat coronary ischemia, the critical care nurse facilitates learning through formal in-service education.
5. **a** The cognitive skills associated with critical thinking require analyzing, information seeking, applying standards, logical reasoning, and transforming knowledge. Through case study analysis and reading clinical journals, the certified critical care nurse uses a variety of learning methods to enhance critical thinking skills, resulting in clinical excellence.

Chapter 2: THE PATIENT'S EXPERIENCE WITH CRITICAL ILLNESS

1. **d** Anxiety occurs whenever there is a threat to well-being. This includes anything that threatens the patient's sense of wholeness, security, and control.
2. **b** Encouraging patients to discuss their fears and concerns and listening will let patients know that these fears and concerns are important to, and accepted by, the nurse.
3. **d** Order and predictability in routine and staff follow-through, offering choices, and having patients make as many decisions as possible about their own care are actions that foster a sense of control.
4. **a** In cognitive reappraisal, the patient clearly identifies the sources of stress and identifies his or her usual responses to the stimuli, then attempts to change these responses through the use of positive thinking.
5. **d** Laughter produces all of the listed effects: a psychological sense of well-being, muscle relaxation, and reduced tension.
6. **b** Reassurance is useful for responding to exaggerated fears, calming a patient, and reducing an increased respiratory rate associated with anxiety. It should not stifle expression of feelings or emotions.
7. **d** Denial occurs in the first stage of loss. This time helps the patient temporarily block out the loss and provides time to regroup energy. Stripping away the denial will increase the sense of helplessness.

Chapter 3: THE FAMILY'S EXPERIENCE WITH CRITICAL ILLNESS

1. **c** Providing opportunities and choices for the family whenever possible helps them to develop a sense of control over the situation.
2. **b** Definition of a problem associated with a crisis assists the family in identifying the parameters of the problem, as well as increasing their sense of understanding.
3. **d** Events with lasting consequences, such as an inability to problem solve and a disturbed equilibrium, all increase the probability that the family will enter a crisis.

Chapter 4: IMPACT OF THE CRITICAL CARE ENVIRONMENT ON THE PATIENT

1. **a** When patients feel safe, this indicates that their other needs are being met. Sleep periods should be longer than 2 hours, and family members should be allowed more liberal access than only twice per day. Opioids are an important intervention in pain relief, but if a patient feels safe, this is an indication that he or she is receiving adequate analgesia.
2. **b** Music entrains body rhythms, including breathing. Music lowers, not raises, sympathetic tone. There is no evidence that the body relaxes first in music therapy. While music may provide distraction, pain medication is typically still indicated.
3. **b** Untreated pain and anxiety is the number one reason patients complain of poor sleep. Bed baths on the night shift interrupt sleep. Family visiting does not interfere with sleep and may actually enhance it. Altered melatonin levels may be a problem, but the scientific evidence is just emerging.
4. **d** Soothing, calm colors are most important to consider in intensive care unit (ICU) design. Carpets are not appropriate in most ICUs and may make moving beds and equipment a hazard for back injuries. Patient rooms, not waiting rooms, should be redesigned to accommodate families. Overhead lighting is an irritant to patients who are critically ill.

Chapter 5: RELIEVING PAIN AND PROVIDING COMFORT

1. **b** Unrelieved pain can result in hypertension, not hypotension. In addition, unrelieved pain can cause myocardial ischemia, atelectasis, and musculoskeletal contractions or spasms.
2. **c** The patient's self-report is the most reliable source of information about pain, because pain is a subjective experience. Even though critical care nurses are frequently more attuned to objective indicators of pain, if the patient can communicate, the critical care nurse must accept the patient's description of pain as valid.
3. **c** The best way to manage an opioid-related side effect is to reduce the dose of the opioid. This strategy is directed at the cause of the side effect. Side effects are usually seen with excessively high serum levels of the drug. Decreasing the opioid dose can alleviate the side effect while still providing pain relief.
4. **c** Naloxone is a pure opioid antagonist that reverses opioid effects.
5. **d** Propofol is a rapid-acting sedative with an ultra-short half-life. It can be reversed simply by stopping the infusion. Patients awaken within minutes.

Chapter 6: PATIENT AND FAMILY EDUCATION IN CRITICAL CARE

1. **d** All of the factors listed negatively affect the patient's attention span and ability to concentrate. Background noise, such as bedside alarms, may decrease the patient's learning because it dis-

rupts the patient's ability to focus on information that the nurse is attempting to teach. Interrupted sleep patterns reduce concentration and attention span. Lack of privacy can make patients feel self-conscious about asking questions that might be overheard by others.

2. **d** The critical care nurse must assess the following principles of learning: the need to know, readiness to learn, and motivation to learn. Adults need to understand why they need to learn something before they are willing to engage in learning. Adults are ready to learn when the information applies to them specifically. Adults are motivated more by internal forces, such as quality of life, improved self-esteem, and personal satisfaction.

Chapter 7: ETHICAL ISSUES IN CRITICAL CARE NURSING

1. **b** An ethic of care is primarily based on recognition of the uniqueness of individuals, the value of relationships, and the importance of emotions in moral judgments.
2. **d** Ethics helps people to reach answers to moral dilemmas by clarifying the moral issues and principles involved in a situation, helping the person to examine his or her responsibilities and obligations, and providing an ethically adequate rationale for a decision.
3. **b** A nurse who refuses to give a patient care and leaves the workplace is violating the principles of beneficence and fidelity.
4. **a** The statement, "Withholding life-sustaining treatment is ethically acceptable, but withdrawing such treatment is not" is false.

Chapter 8: LEGAL ISSUES IN CRITICAL CARE NURSING

1. **c** The doctrine of respondeat superior is the legal theory under which an employer is vicariously liable for the negligent acts of its employees, as long as they act within the scope of employment.
2. **c** The Patient Self-Determination Act requires hospitals, nursing homes, and certain other health care providers to provide patients with information about all types of advance directives applicable in the state in which they live.
3. **a** A living will is applicable when a patient is incapacitated and terminally ill.

Chapter 9: GENETIC ISSUES IN CRITICAL CARE NURSING

1. **c** The ability to diagnose a genetic disease is not a core competency as defined by the *National Coalition for Health Professional Education in Genetics* (NCHPEG).
2. **b** Amino acids assembled into proteins are the final product of translation.
3. **b** Most mutations are "silent" and cause no disease.
4. **a** Multifactorial disorders are the most common types of genetically influenced disorders in the adult population.

Chapter 10: BUILDING A PROFESSIONAL PRACTICE MODEL FOR EXCELLENCE IN CRITICAL CARE NURSING

1. **c** Bernice Buresh and Suzanne Gordon are non-nurses who authored *From Silence to Voice: What Nurses Know and Must Communicate to the Public.* Ottawa, Canada: Canadian Nurses Association, 2000. Abraham Flexner (a non-nurse) and Lucie Young Kelly (a nurse) do not specifically address "voice;" their work identifies overall characteristics of professionalism. Barbara DeAngelis (a clinical psychologist) does not address "specific nursing issues." Her work identifies overall components on how to "put balance" in life.
2. **c** The survey conducted in 2000 by the American Association of Critical-Care Nurses (AACN) revealed that approximately 65,000 nurses were members.
3. **d** Six attributes are identified as components of "A Professional Practice Model for Critical Care Nursing Excellence": values, vision, mastery, passion, action, and balance.
4. **a** We can no longer remain "silent." It is our professional responsibility to advance critical care nursing through as many forums as possible. In our critical care units, we can advocate "evidenced-based practice" and eliminate "we've always done it this way" practice. In our grade schools to our high schools, we can educate counselors about the exciting field of "high-tech and high-touch" critical care nursing. In our communities, we can be visible and passionate about public health issues so that "our voice is heard."
5. **d** Excellence comes from an inner core deep inside all of us. The attributes for a professional practice model of critical care nursing excellence (values, vision, mastery, action, passion, and balance) provide a framework for ongoing self-reflection. The direction for individual professional and personal goals can then be determined on how best to bring critical care nursing excellence to patients, families, and the profession.

Chapter 11: THE CRITICALLY ILL PEDIATRIC PATIENT

1. **a** Decreased systemic perfusion is an early sign of shock in the pediatric patient. This is manifested by diminished pulses, delayed capillary refill time, cool extremities, color changes, decreased level of consciousness, and decreased urine output. These are considered red flags of cardiovascular collapse. Hypotension, decreased pulse pressure, and bradycardia are all late signs of shock.
2. **c** The formula for determining the correct size endotracheal tube is 16 plus age (in years) divided by 4. This child is 8 years old; therefore, he requires a 6.0-mm endotracheal tube ($[16 + 8]/4 = 6$). There should always be a tube that is one half size smaller and one half size larger immediately available.
3. **a** Oxygen is administered immediately to all patients with signs of respiratory insufficiency. Oxygen exchange is often inadequate in these patients because of limited pulmonary gas exchange.

Chapter 12: THE CRITICALLY ILL PREGNANT WOMAN

1. **b** Indications for hemodynamic monitoring in obstetrics are much the same as in any area of medicine/surgery. Patients with severe preeclampsia further complicated by oliguria, pulmonary edema, or both will need close and accurate hemodynamic monitoring.
2. **c** Immediate resuscitation of the pregnant woman must occur first in order for the fetus to survive.
3. **a** Amniotic fluid embolism (AFE) resembles anaphylactic shock. Signs and symptoms may include hemorrhage, pulmonary edema, and vascular collapse that leads to cardiac arrest.
4. **b** Signs and symptoms of magnesium toxicity include hyporeflexia, respiratory suppression, and decreased level of consciousness.

Chapter 13: THE CRITICALLY ILL OLDER PATIENT

1. **d** Anemia is not a normal age-related change. If a decline in hemoglobin and hematocrit is noted, further work-up is necessary

to determine the underlying cause. Reduced sensory and perceptual activity, reduced glomerular filtration rate (GFR), and decreased amounts of connective and collagen tissue are all normal age-related changes.

2. **a** Drug absorption in older adults is influenced by changes in albumin levels, changes in the gastrointestinal villi, and altered gastrointestinal motility. The gastrointestinal pH does not increase with age; therefore, this is not a factor that influences drug absorption in the older adult.
3. **b** Bone loss in an older adult who is hospitalized may be exacerbated by bed rest, which results in increased burn turnover. Neither dehydration, infection, nor delirium affect bone loss in hospitalized older adults.
4. **d** In older adults, depression does not present with classic signs and symptoms, such as sadness and melancholy, an acute physical problem, or an acute change in cognition. A more likely presentation is pseudohypochondriasis, such as an obsession with a common problem (e.g., constipation).
5. **d** Blurred vision and blunted visual acuity are the most common symptoms of cataracts. A person with cataracts would be unlikely to complain of pain, drainage from the eye, or decreased peripheral vision.
6. **a** In an older adult, the presentation of an acute illness, such as an infection, is generally atypical. For example, rather than presenting with fever and chills or leukocytosis, an older adult with an infection may present with a change in cognition, function, or behavior.

Chapter 14: THE POSTANESTHESIA PATIENT

1. **a** Dantrolene sodium is the specific drug therapy used for treating malignant hyperthermia. An initial dose of 2.5 mg/kg IV should be followed by repeated doses of 1–2 mg/kg to a total of 10 mg/kg, depending on the patient's response.
2. **d** Propofol has the lowest incidence of associated nausea and vomiting and in small bolus doses may treat nausea.
3. **d** Atelectasis may cause intrapulmonary right-to-left shunting, leading to hypoxemia.
4. **a** The pulse oximeter is the fastest noninvasive method used to assess the postoperative patient. The pulse oximeter provides oxygen saturation level, heart rate, and, depending on the available technology, waveform analysis to assist in correlating the accuracy of the data.
5. **a** A negative inspiratory force greater than –20 cm H_2O is associated with the ability to generate appropriate muscle movement to support spontaneous ventilation.
6. **d** A nasal cannula is usually all that is required to correct mild-to-moderate hypoxemia in a postanesthesia patient.

Chapter 15: INTERFACILITY TRANSPORT OF THE CRITICALLY ILL PATIENT

1. **a** If a patient requires stabilization and the facility is capable of providing that level of care, stabilization should be done at the sending facility, prior to the arrival of the transport team and the departure of the receiving facility.

Chapter 16: ANATOMY AND PHYSIOLOGY OF THE CARDIOVASCULAR SYSTEM

1. **a** The mitral valve sits between the left atria and the left ventricle.
2. **c** The sinoatrial node (SA) node is the pacemaker site for the heart because it discharges faster than other cells of the heart.
3. **c** The coronary arteries are the only arteries of the body to fill during diastole. The coronary arteries derive from the aorta and lie between myocardial fibers. Blood flows to the coronary arteries during diastole.
4. **a** The left anterior descending artery provides blood to the anterior wall of the left ventricle, the anterior ventricular septum, and the bundle branches.
5. **d** Cardiac output is the product of heart rate times stroke volume. Stroke volume is determined by preload, afterload, and contractility. Cardiac output for the normal heart is 4 to 8 liters per minute.
6. **c** The workload of the right side of the heart is less than the workload of the left. The right side pumps blood to the lungs whereas the left side pumps blood to the aorta (systemic circulation). Therefore, the walls of the right ventricle are not as thick as the left ventricle.
7. **d** The atrioventricular valves are the tricuspid and the mitral valves. These valves sit between the atria and the ventricles and prevent the backward flow of blood during ventricular systole.
8. **b** The endocardium consists of endothelial tissue and is the layer of the heart that lines the inner surface of the chambers and the valves.
9. **c** The tricuspid valve is located between the right atria and the right ventricle. When the pressure in the right atria exceeds the pressure in the right ventricle, the tricuspid valve opens.

Chapter 17: PATIENT MANAGEMENT: CARDIOVASCULAR SYSTEM

Cardiac History and Physical Examination

1. **d** Mrs. J has the risk factors of advanced age (74 years) and a history of hypertension and hyperlipidemia. Age is a risk factor that cannot be modified. Hypertension and hyperlipidemia are modifiable risk factors.
2. **b** The normal location of the apical pulse, also known as the point of maximal impulse, is the left midclavicular line, at the fourth or fifth intercostals space.
3. **c** S_2 represents the start of diastole. The sound is produced by the vibrations from the closure of the pulmonic and aortic valves.

Cardiac Laboratory Studies

1. **b** Troponin is not affected by skeletal muscle damage and is highly specific for cardiac muscle. LDH isoforms are found in several organ systems in addition to the heart. CK is released from several muscle groups in the presence of injury and can be found in other tissues besides the heart. Myoglobin is released on skeletal muscle damage and is not specific to the heart.
2. **c** With myocardial damage, CK-MB isoforms are released. The ratio of CK-MB_2 to CK-MB_1 is usually greater than the normal ratio of 1:1 and therefore indicative of myocardial damage.
3. **c** Serum troponin levels peak later than CK and remain elevated for several days after myocardial insult, thereby allowing for a definitive diagnosis of injury past the time when other markers have returned to normal. Troponin is not affected by noncardiac muscle damage.

Cardiac Diagnostic Studies

1. **b** Use of an implantable loop monitor is the best mechanism to evaluate syncopy because it can continually monitor the patient over time. A Holter monitor, a signal-averaged electrocardiogram, and a standard 12-lead electrocardiogram only view the patient episodically, or at one moment in time.
2. **a** Transesophageal echocardiography is a superior means to evaluate cardiac and vascular structures. Other diagnostic procedures do not provide the scope of information that can be obtained with transesophageal echocardiography. M-mode echocardiography can view cardiac structures, but transesophageal

echocardiography provides better access to view the aorta, atria, and valves. Phonocardiography and Doppler echocardiography are more specific for assessing blood flow rather than cardiac or vascular structures.

3. **b** Presence of a cardiac pacemaker is an absolute contraindication to MRI. A tissue valve replacement does not contain metal and is therefore not a contraindication. Artificial limbs can be removed if they contain metal. The presence of surgical staples is not usually a problem.
4. **a** Patients who have had a cardiac catheterization must keep their leg straight for at least 6 hours after the procedure to ensure hemostasis. Monitoring vital signs, checking the catheterization puncture site for bleeding, and checking the coagulation status are all standards of care in the postcatheterization period.

Electrocardiographic Monitoring

1. **a** The positive electrode is placed in the desired monitoring lead position. The negative electrode for a modified chest lead is always placed under the left clavicle.
2. **b** According to Einthoven's triangle, in lead II the positive electrode is on the left side of the body below the level of the heart and the negative electrode is placed under the right clavicle.
3. **c** Wide QRS complex rhythms such as bundle branch blocks are best seen in chest leads V_1 and V_6.

Arrhythmias and the 12-Lead Electrocardiogram

1. **c** Electrocardiographic waves always represent electrical activity, not contraction of the muscle. The QRS complex represents the electrical excitation of the ventricles, which is known as ventricular depolarization.
2. **d** These changes from sinus bradycardia to sinus tachycardia are often seen based on the low metabolic demands of sleep and the higher metabolic demands of exercise.
3. **a** Patients who have atrial fibrillation are at increased risk of formation of clots in the atria and the movement of these clots out of the atria, causing problems such as pulmonary embolus.
4. **c** In atrial flutter, the atrioventricular node serves as the "gatekeeper" and only allows some of the atrial excitation to pass into the ventricles.
5. **d** The absence of a P wave indicates that the extra beat did not originate in the atria. The wide QRS complex indicates that the ventricles were depolarized at a slower than normal rate. These are both indicators of premature ventricular contractions.
6. **c** In junctional rhythm, the AV junction serves as the pacemaker site. The atria may be depolarized before (inverted P wave before QRS), with (absent P wave), or after (inverted P wave after QRS) ventricular depolarization.
7. **b** In third-degree heart block (complete heart block), the SA node fires, but the impulses do not reach the ventricles. A focus in the ventricle takes control, but that focus is often slow and unreliable.
8. **a** Tall, peaked T waves may be an indication of hyperkalemia, whereas the presence of U waves is associated with hypokalemia.
9. **a** A prolonged QT interval is seen with hypocalcemia, whereas a shortened QT interval is associated with hypercalcemia.

Hemodynamic Monitoring

1. **b** The normal systolic pulmonary artery pressure is 20–30 mm Hg and the normal diastolic pulmonary artery pressure is 8–15 mm Hg. The normal pulmonary artery systolic pressure is equivalent to the normal right ventricular systolic pressure. The normal pulmonary artery diastolic pressure is equivalent to the normal pulmonary artery wedge pressure.
2. **a** The most common complication during PA catheter insertion is arrhythmias due to the irritation of the ventricle by the catheter.
3. **b** Arterial and wedge pressures of the PA provide an indication of left heart function. When the PA pressures increase, it often means the left ventricle is failing; in this case, the failure is due to myocardial infarction.
4. **d** When the cardiac output decreases, the heart attempts to compensate by increasing the heart rate (cardiac output = heart rate × stroke volume).
5. **c** The steady CVP readings indicate that the right heart is adequately handling the venous return. If the value is low, it indicates low preload perhaps due to dehydration.

Chapter 18: PATIENT MANAGEMENT: CARDIOVASCULAR SYSTEM

1. **c** Tenecteplase is given as a single bolus over 5 seconds; alteplase and streptokinase are given as an intravenous infusion; lidocaine is an antiarrhythmic drug.
2. **d** The Advanced Cardiac Life Support guidelines recommend amiodarone for both atrial and ventricular arrhythmias.
3. **a** Inotropic drugs increase the force of myocardial contraction and increase cardiac output. These drugs increase myocardial oxygen requirements and may actually increase the risk of myocardial ischemia or infarction. Epinephrine is the only inotropic drug that can be given through an endotracheal tube.
4. **d** Angiotensin-converting enzyme inhibitors are used to treat congestive heart failure, hypertension, acute myocardial infarction, and asymptomatic left ventricular dysfunction.
5. **b** The addition of coronary stenting to the PTCA procedure helps promote the successful opening of the artery, and because of the presence of the stent, helps prevent restenosis. Intracoronary stenting may result in a lower stenosis rate in native and vein graft lesions of approximately 10%.
6. **c** Primary angioplasty is a dilation of an infarct-related coronary artery during the acute phase of a myocardial infarction without prior administration of a thrombolytic agent.
7. **a** Restenosis is a term used to describe a blockage of a coronary artery. About 20% to 30% of patient who have had a PTCA will have a restenosis within the first 6 months.
8. **a** When a patient experiences an acute closure of a coronary artery after an interventional procedure, the blood supply to the heart muscle is interrupted. ST segment elevations are a classic sign of lack of adequate oxygen to the heart. When the heart lacks adequate oxygen, the patient experiences chest pain. The lack of adequate perfusion to the heart also causes cardiac dysrhythmias.
9. **c** A patient who undergoes an interventional procedure may experience bleeding at the insertion site of the catheter; a myocardial infarction due to the inability to open the vessel, or the restenosis of the vessel. Hyperlipidemia is a chronic condition not caused by an interventional procedure.
10. **b** Gene therapy has not been approved by the Food and Drug Administration. A magnetic resonance angiography is not a treatment; it is a diagnostic procedure.
11. **a** Coronary artery perfusion occurs during the diastolic phase of the cardiac cycle.
12. **b** The closure of the aortic valve occurs when the pressure in the aorta exceeds the pressure in the left ventricle. This activity is represented by the dicrotic notch on arterial waveforms regardless of where the arterial line originates.
13. **a** Inflation occurs at the onset of diastole, which is represented by the dicrotic notch.
14. **c** The presence of family members may encourage nutritional intake for patients.
15. **b** AAIRO alone allows intrinsic AV conduction when pacing. In this mode, the pacemaker paces and senses in the atrium and provides rate response with activity. The AV node then receives the impulse and normal conduction through AV node follows, in the absence of AV block. This mode is usually used in patients with sinus node dysfunction with chronotropic incompetence with intact AV node conduction.

16. **c** Mr. Wood had epicardial patches and myocardial sensing leads. A transvenous lead usually requires an insertion site in the subclavicular region, even if the lead is tunneled to the abdomen.
17. **b** The symptoms accompanied by the monitored rhythm reveal PACs, which can persist after AV node modification. Ablation failure can only be proven by breakthrough, sustained dysrhythmia.
18. **a** Hypokalemia and digitalis toxicity are relative contraindications to cardioversion. In view of renal insufficiency and the fact that amiodarone can potentiate digitalis levels, digitalis toxicity should be ruled out even in the absence of symptoms.
19. **a** Amiodarone can increase defibrillation threshold levels, and ICD testing through PES should be done to confirm adequate safety margins. Testing when appropriately functioning (shocks for sustained VT, no shocks for NSVT) is unnecessary. PES has no role at present for new onset atrial fibrillation.
20. **b** The sensitivity setting should be adjusted to a less sensitive setting to avoid oversensing of T waves. Since the patient does not appear to be pacemaker dependent, it would be not appropriate to make the setting asynchronous since this could cause competition and possibly R on T phenomenon.
21. **d** Any patient must be assessed when a change in their condition is suspected. When a patient is on a cardiac monitor, the rhythm may not be indicative of the patient's actual status.
22. **b** Elderly women are predisposed to have osteoporosis. This includes a weakening of the sternum. Compressions are continued, but adequate depth of compression must be assessed to ensure that circulation is restored.
23. **a** Many victims of sudden cardiac arrest can be resuscitated if interventions are begun promptly.
24. **c** Family members may witness resuscitative efforts by the health care team, but the ability to conduct the resuscitation is of paramount concern.

Chapter 19: COMMON CARDIOVASCULAR DISORDERS

1. **c** Fever, heart murmurs, and petechiae are signs and symptoms of endocarditis. Peripheral edema and urinary frequency are not associated with endocarditis.
2. **b** Pain on inspiration associated with pericarditis is due to contact between the inflamed pericardium, which is adjacent to the diaphragm, and the trachea.
3. **d** Key clinical findings in the assessment of the patient with suspected acute arterial occlusion include pain, absent distal pulses, pallor, and paresthesia. Polydipsia and polyphagia are not associated with acute dissection.
4. **c** Risk factors for the development of acute aneurysms include diabetes, hypertension, and a family history of aneurysm. Pericarditis is not a risk factor for the development of aortic aneurysms.
5. **d** Factors that contribute to a high rate of re-hospitalization among the elderly include lack of family support, confusion, and the presence of comorbidities. There is usually no additional difficulty in establishing the diagnosis or determining therapy because the patient is elderly.

Chapter 20: HEART FAILURE

1. **b** Heart failure is a collection of symptoms, such as shortness of breath and dyspnea on exertion, associated with impaired filling (diastolic dysfunction) or emptying (systolic dysfunction) of the left ventricle. Right-sided heart failure causes liver congestion because pulmonary artery pressures are high. They may be elevated because of left-sided heart failure, but there are other causes as well. Decreased ejection fraction may exist without symptoms of heart failure, as does dilated cardiomyopathy.
2. **d** Heart failure cannot currently be cured with standard treatment. The goal is to minimize symptoms and help the patient to maintain as normal a life as possible.
3. **b** Dobutamine is an inodilator that increases cardiac output by decreasing afterload and increasing contractility. As cardiac output increases and the heart empties more completely, the left ventricular end-diastolic pressure (and therefore, the pulmonary capillary wedge pressure) decrease as well.
4. **a** Nitrates such as nitroglycerin decrease preload by dilating the venous bed and decreasing venous return. This is felt to lower pulmonary artery pressures and decrease orthopnea.
5. **a** Angiotensin-converting enzyme (ACE) inhibitors inhibit renin in the kidney, which leads to increased reabsorption of potassium. If the patient depends on renin to maintain renal perfusion (as in bilateral renal artery stenosis or dehydration), blood urea nitrogen (BUN) and creatinine levels will rise. Careful monitoring of these parameters is required, especially as the ACE inhibitor is initiated and titrated, decreases the risk of life-threatening side effects.

Chapter 21: ACUTE MYOCARDIAL INFARCTION

1. **d** Pleuritic pain, unlike anginal pain, is made worse by a deep breath, swallowing, and coughing. The patient often has a fever of less than 38.6 degrees centigrade.
2. **c** An elevated ST segment is the hallmark indicator of an acute injury process. Q waves indicate myocardial infarction. Inverted T waves and ST segment depressions usually indicated myocardial ischemia.
3. **a** Pain management for patients with an acute myocardial infarction is a priority. The drug of choice is intravenous morphine sulfate.
4. **d** The inferior wall is seen in leads II, III, and aVF. The anterior wall is viewed in leads V_1, through V_4. The lateral wall is seen in leads I, aVL, V_5, and V_6. The posterior wall is viewed in leads V_7 through V_9.
5. **b** Obesity is a major risk factor for heart disease that the patient can control. Age is an uncontrollable risk factor. Stress and excessive alcohol intake are contributing risk factors.

Chapter 22: CARDIAC SURGERY

1. **a** The internal mammary artery (IMA) graft is preferred over the saphenous vein graft (SVG) because it remains patent longer. Using the IMA graft may take more time for the dissection from the chest wall, so it is technically a more difficult procedure to perform. Fibrointimal hyperplasia *does* occur with the SVG. There is no difference in postoperative pain with either procedure.
2. **b** Acute mitral insufficiency can occur because of myocardial infarction, an acute condition. Rheumatic heart disease, myxoma, and left ventricular dilatation can lead to chronic mitral insufficiency (i.e., mitral insufficiency that occurs over a long period of time).
3. **d** Syncope occurs in the later stages of aortic stenosis because the stenotic ("stiff") aortic valve decreases forward flow, especially when it is needed with increased tissue oxygen demand. Aortic stenosis leads to left ventricular hypertrophy, but that is not what causes syncope. Myocardial ischemia and stroke can cause syncope, but as a result of other pathology, not aortic stenosis.
4. **c** The mechanical valve is a good choice for a younger patient because it will last for a longer period of time, compared with a tissue valve. However, the disadvantage is that anticoagulation is required for life.
5. **d** The bypass machine will damage the endothelium because major vessels are accessed with the large-bore intravenous (IV)

access. This activates the endothelium, which activates the platelets and the other proteins of the coagulation cascade.

6. **a** The subtle cognitive changes that occur in patients who have cardiac surgery using the bypass machine were a major reason for the development of the off-pump coronary artery bypass graft (OPCABG) procedure. The OPCABG procedure does produce an inflammatory response, leading to vasodilation and an increase in activation of antidiuretic hormone (ADH) that may lead to hemodilution.
7. **c** The principles to follow when volume resuscitating a patient are: (1) to infuse volume quickly, using a pressure bag if needed; and (2) to infuse the volume through a large-bore intravenous (IV) access, which is shorter in length. A 16-gauge peripheral IV that is inserted into a large peripheral vein will not meet the above-mentioned criteria.
8. **d** Recognizing cardiac tamponade early is very important. Equalization of pulmonary artery and central venous pressures occurs very late in the process. Sudden increases in vasoactive drugs may be the result of a decrease in cardiac output leading to a decrease in blood pressure as the right side of the heart has a significant decreases in preload.
9. **c** The facial nerve traverses the surgical area involved in carotid endarterectomy. It is the nerve that innervates the muscles that are used when smiling.
10. **d** Fever in combination with an increase in bands (immature white blood cells) indicates that the body is attempting to respond to a foreign body in the system. This foreign body is usually a microorganism, found in either the blood, urine, or sputum.

Chapter 23: ANATOMY AND PHYSIOLOGY OF THE RESPIRATORY SYSTEM

1. **a** Intrapleural pressure, a slightly negative pressure, creates a suction that holds the lungs open to their resting level. Without this negative pressure to hold the lungs against the chest wall, elastic recoil properties of the lung would cause them to collapse.
2. **d** The conducting airways include the nasopharynx, oropharynx, trachea, bronchi, bronchioles, and terminal bronchioles (Figure 23-4). The conducting airways contain no alveoli and do not participate in gas exchange.
3. **b** The extent to which the lungs expand is called compliance. Compliance is a measurement of distensibility, or how easily a tissue is stretched. If compliance is reduced, it is more difficult to expand the lungs for inspiration. Conversely, if compliance is increased, it is easier to expand lung tissue.
4. **c** Diffusion, or movement of molecules, occurs from an area of high concentration to low concentration. Fick's law describes the diffusion of gases through the alveolar-capillary membrane (Figure 23-14). Fick's law states that the rate of transfer of gas through a semipermeable membrane is proportional to the surface area and the difference in gas pressures between the two sides and inversely proportional to tissue thickness.
5. **a** When perfusion exceeds ventilation, the ratio is low and a shunt is present. Blood passes by the alveoli without gas exchange occurring. A low ventilation–perfusion ratio is seen with pneumonia, atelectasis, tumor, or mucus plug (Figure 23-16B).

Chapter 24: PATIENT ASSESSMENT: RESPIRATORY SYSTEM

1. **c** Vesicular breath sounds are heard over the periphery of the lung. Bronchial breath sounds are heard over the trachea, and bronchovesicular breath sounds are heard over the major airways.
2. **a** Normally mixed venous saturation of oxygen is 60% to 80%. The arterial oxygen saturation is normally 93% to 99%.
3. **d** The pH is less than 7.40, representing acidosis. The $PaCO_2$ is elevated above 35 to 45 mm Hg, indicating a respiratory acidosis. The bicarbonate is within normal limits. The oxygen level is normal for sea level. This represents uncompensated respiratory acidosis.
4. **a** By definition, *respiratory* alkalosis will be a dysfunction in the $PaCO_2$, the respiratory parameter. By definition, *alkalosis* in the respiratory parameter occurs from low levels of $PaCO_2$.
5. **c** Hypothermia decreases oxygen demand, thus allowing more oxygen to return to the venous side. Pain, anxiety, and hyperthermia increase oxygen demand, thus less oxygen is returned to the venous side. Anemia results in a decreased supply of oxygen and therefore causes a lowered $S\bar{v}O_2$.
6. **a** End-tidal CO_2 should be measured at the end of the alveolar plateau, just before the inspiratory downstroke. It is this point right before inspiration that best measures the very end of expiration.
7. **b** Patient education is always required prior to any procedure. The chest x-ray helps to identify the region or lung to be tapped, and the coagulation studies are essential to ensure that the patient does not have a coagulopathy that might cause profuse bleeding from trauma of the needle stick.
8. **a** As long as the organ system will NOT be affected by manipulation during the exam, it is always acceptable to start with the least invasive element and move toward auscultation. However, in the case of the abdomen, where the system would be affected by manipulation, auscultation occurs prior to palpation and percussion.
9. **a** Three cultures are necessary to ascertain whether or not the patient harbors mycobacterium. The specimens should be collected first thing in the morning each day for 3 days.
10. **b** The $PaCO_2$ is usually 2 to 5 mm Hg higher than the $ETCO_2$. This is typically attributed to pulmonary blood flow.
11. **c** A kink in the ventilator tubing will cause the carbon dioxide to remain near the sensor for an extended period of time, thereby influencing the censor and creating an elevated $ETCO_2$ reading.

Chapter 25: PATIENT MANAGEMENT: RESPIRATORY SYSTEM

1. **d** The correct answer is over the ribs in the areas designated for bronchial drainage. Percussion and vibration are never performed over the clavicles, breast tissue, sternum, shoulder blades, spine, waist, abdomen, surgical or chest tube sites, or below the thoracic cage. This can cause pain, trauma, or both to those sites.
2. **b** The patient should be positioned with the healthy lung down. Positioning the patient with the diseased lung down is likely to cause hypoxemia with ventilation–perfusion mismatching and shunting. Positioning is different, however, if the patient has a lung abscess. In this case, the preferred position is with the diseased lung down, because if the abscessed lung is placed in a gravity-dependent position, purulent material will drain into the opposite, healthy lung.
3. **d** If the oxygen concentration must be constant, the system used is the Venturi mask. It is a high-flow device that delivers an exact percentage of oxygen, regardless of the patient's tidal volume. Patients with chronic obstructive pulmonary disease (COPD) may require oxygen delivery by the Venturi system. The CO_2 level can be detected through serial arterial blood gas (ABG) monitoring, which reveals large increases in $PaCO_2$ with small increases in oxygen flow.
4. **d** Patients who are ventilated benefit from having the head of the bed elevated 30 degrees at all times. This promotes lung expansion and prevents aspiration that can occur in intubated patients in the recumbent position.
5. **a** The criteria that may terminate weaning from mechanical ventilation include a respiratory rate greater than 30 breaths/

min, increased use of accessory muscles, an SaO_2 of less than 90%, or changes on the electrocardiogram (ECG).

6. **c,d** Pressure support ventilation (PSV) or synchronized intermittent mandatory ventilation (SIMV) may be used for weaning.
7. **b** The normal amount of pleural fluid found within the pleural space is 5 to 15 mL.
8. **d** In order to decrease bronchospasm, albuterol works on the $beta_2$ receptors.
9. **b** DNase assists in improving airflow in patients with cystic fibrosis by breaking down large molecules in thick secretions.
10. **c** Management and weaning of the patient on mechanical ventilation are best accomplished with a collaborative approach to planning and delivering care. The patient requiring mechanical ventilation often has a complex illness and pre-existing health problems. Successful outcomes require the input and interventions of representatives from all appropriate disciplines—nurses; doctors; respiratory, physical, and occupational therapists; dietitians; pharmacists; and others as needed.
11. **d** In any ventilated patient, but especially in a frail, elderly patient, successful weaning depends on taking care of *all* basic needs. Lack of nutrition or adequate rest can leave the patient without the strength or endurance to regain independent spontaneous ventilation. Alterations in bowel elimination can cause abdominal distension (limiting lung expansion), metabolic abnormalities, or both. The agitated patient may waste energy fighting the ventilator and the anxious patient can easily develop psychological as well as physical dependence on mechanical support.

Chapter 26: COMMON RESPIRATORY DISORDERS

1. **a** There is a proportionate loss of ventilation and perfusion in the lung in severe chronic obstructive pulmonary disease (COPD). Air is trapped in the lungs during forced expiration, leading to abnormally high residual volume, decreased forced expiratory volume, and increased total lung capacity.
2. **c** Passively breathing cigarette smoke and smoking are the most important causes of emphysema. Smoking plays a role in the increased inflammatory cells in the alveoli, enhanced release of elastase from neutrophils, increased elastase activity in macrophages, and activated mast cells, which stimulate release of mast cell elastases.
3. **a** Treatment of chronic bronchitis with airflow obstruction primarily includes inhaled bronchodilators ($beta_2$-adrenergic agents, anticholinergic agents, corticosteroids) and theophylline.
4. **d** The presence of a productive cough with sputum greater than 250 mL per day for at least 3 months per year over 2 consecutive years is consistent with the diagnosis of chronic bronchitis.
5. **b** According to the Centers for Disease Control and Prevention (CDC) theoretical framework for pneumonia, aspiration is the primary route for organisms to enter the lower respiratory tract. Organisms colonize the oropharynx and are then aspirated into the lower respiratory tract.
6. **c** Congestive heart failure is the most common cause of pleural effusions in critically ill patients.
7. **a** Transudative pleural effusions are an ultrafiltrate of plasma, indicating the pleural membranes are not diseased. A pleural effusion is caused by at least one of five mechanisms: (1) increased pressure in the subpleural capillaries, (2) increased capillary permeability, (3) decreased colloid osmotic pressure of the blood, (4) increased intrapleural negative pressure, and (5) impaired lymphatic drainage of the pleural space.
8. **c** Invasive procedures and barotrauma are the most common cause of pneumothorax in critically ill patients.
9. **b** Pulmonary embolism produces an increase in pulmonary artery pressure and central venous pressure. When compensatory mechanisms (increased heart rate, increased right ventricular stroke volume, and recruitment and distention of pulmonary vessels) are activated, a decrease in cardiac output and a dramatic increase in right atrial pressure occur, producing increased pulmonary artery and central venous pressureS.

Chapter 27: ACUTE RESPIRATORY DISTRESS SYNDROME

1. **b** In late-stage ARDS, it is the fibrotic lung changes that are associated with increasing risk of barotrauma, development of increased airway pressures, and poor compliance, resulting in inadequate oxygenation and ventilation and development of barotrauma. The scarring and remodeling that occurs in late-stage ARDS contribute directly to mechanical ventilation difficulties after several weeks for patients with ARDS. Interstitial pulmonary edema and neutrophil infiltration of the vascular system relate to the pathological changes in the lung in early ARDS.
2. **a** One of the major research findings for supportive care in ARDS has been low-volume ventilation. In patients with ARDS, regional lung changes result in normal lung tissue co-existing with injured lung tissue. Traditional ventilation strategies result in stimulation of inflammatory mediators and further lung damage. The combination of low tidal volumes with plateau pressures set at safe maximal peak alveolar pressure limits airway pressures, thus preventing over-distension of compliant lung regions.
3. **b** Positive end-expiratory pressure (PEEP) can be altered to help reduce the fraction of inspired oxygen (FIO_2) required to maintain an adequate arterial oxygen tension (PaO_2). The high FIO_2 levels seen to adequately oxygenate patients with ARDS have traditionally been accepted recognizing that the risk of oxygen toxicity is a possible consequence in the face of limited other options. Changes in PEEP and use of PEEP studies help to reduce FIO_2 and maximize oxygen delivery at optimal levels.
4. **d** The risk of intracranial hemorrhage is associated with interventions such as extracoporeal membrane oxygenation (ECMO) and therefore is not considered a complication of ARDS. Immobility may result in deep venous thrombosis (DVT). Multiorgan failure is a consequence of systemic inflammatory response syndrome (SIRS). Pneumothorax occurs in approximately 15% of patients with ARDS.
5. **c** To date, the only effective treatment for ARDS is early removal of the cause, thus preventing further stimulation of mediators. Lung protective ventilation and prone positioning prevent further damage, but have not demonstrated improvements in mortality. Multiple ventilation strategies are needed to optimize oxygenation and ventilation, and these are considered supportive.

Chapter 28: ANATOMY AND PHYSIOLOGY OF THE RENAL SYSTEM

1. **b** In the glomerulus, filtration promotes the movement of fluid and substances from the blood to the tubular lumen. Secretion and reabsorption occur as the tubular fluid moves through the nephron.
2. **b** Aldosterone increases the reabsorption of sodium to promote water reabsorption. A secondary effect is the loss of potassium in the urine, which is due to the cation exchange system of sodium and potassium. Therefore, one possible consequence of elevated plasma aldosterone levels is hypokalemia.
3. **b** Osmolarity is determined by the concentrations of sodium, glucose, and urea/nitrogen. Under normal circumstances, glucose and urea/nitrogen do not greatly affect the osmolarity. With hyperglycemia, however, the osmolarity increases, triggering the loss of sodium with water to follow.

4. **d** Parathyroid hormone (PTH) causes the absorption of calcium from the bone, which in turn causes the plasma levels of calcium to increase. Calcium and phosphorus are inversely related; therefore measures that will increase one will decrease the other.

Chapter 29: PATIENT ASSESSMENT: RENAL SYSTEM

1. **c** Creatinine is produced at a constant rate and excreted in the urine primarily during filtration, although some creatine may be secreted as well. Thus, creatinine is an estimate of glomerular function or dysfunction. Blood urea nitrogen (BUN) is influenced by several factors, such as nutrition and liver function, and is not as reliable in estimating renal function.
2. **d** Both renal angiography and ultrasonography can assess blood flow to the kidneys. Renal angiography is a more sensitive test, particularly when specific measurements are required. Computed tomography will only assess kidney size and shape.
3. **d** Under the influence of aldosterone during volume depletion, the kidneys will reabsorb sodium to promote water reabsorption, resulting in a decreased level in the urine. The fractional excretion of sodium (FE_{Na}) measures urinary sodium while removing the confounding effect of water.
4. **c** Acidosis will result in hyperkalemia due to intracellular shifts of potassium. Potassium can be lost anywhere along the gastrointestinal tract.
5. **d** Calcium is required for muscular depolarization and contraction. Lack of calcium can result in muscular excitability, as evidenced by positive Chvostek's and Trousseau's signs, cramping, and tetany.

Chapter 30: PATIENT MANAGEMENT: RENAL SYSTEM

1. **b** Heparin is *not* always needed to keep blood from clotting in the system. Critically ill patients may already be anticoagulated due to the underlying disease. As with any medication regimen, it is necessary to review all costs and benefits prior to initiation of therapy.
2. **c** The nurse administers a saline bolus to inspect the circuit for clotting. Assessment always precedes intervention to avoid unnecessary administration of medications. In the event a clot does exist, changing of the circuit may indeed be necessary.
3. **a** If the drained fluid is cloudy during a peritoneal fluid exchange, the nurse first obtains a sample of the drained fluid, sends it to the laboratory for culture and sensitivity and cell count, and obtains an order for an antibiotic. Peritonitis is a serious but manageable complication of peritoneal dialysis. Early assessment and therefore early treatment will ensure positive outcome.
4. **a** The formula required to calculate hourly fluid balance for patients on continuous renal replacement therapies (CRRT) is fluid balance = total negative balance + total positive balance + replacement fluid. Assessment of hourly balance is the sum of all output and input during that hour. Some settings on CRRT may mean that there is an output (removal of fluid), an infusion of fluid (fluid bolus), or a replacement fluid (CVVH).
5. **c** D_5 NS would be the best choice for restoration of fluid balance for a patient with pancreatitis. Pancreatitis is a disease where a capillary leak may be present and induce hypotension. In these cases, infusing a fluid that will stay predominately in the vascular space will assist in restoration of adequate vascular volume.
6. **b** Starch compounds may cause coagulopathies. The mechanism for this is not completely understood. As a hypertonic solution, hetastarch will pull volume from the interstitium into the vascular space, expanding the volume beyond the milliliter of fluid infused, placing the patient at risk for volume overload. Because hetastarch is a starch, a rise in amylase may occur. Dextran, not hetastarch, may cause difficulty with cross-matching.
7. **b** Intravenous calcium will immediately help to restore cell membrane stability. Administration of sodium polystyrene will help to remove potassium from the body but has a longer onset of action, and therefore will not immediately reverse the hyperkalemic effects. Intravenous fluids will help to remove potassium from the body to some degree, but will not immediately restore cell membrane stability. A 12-lead electrocardiogram (ECG), while it may be included in the plan of care, is a diagnostic test and not a management strategy.
8. **b** Magnesium is required to maintain plasma potassium levels.

Chapter 31: RENAL FAILURE

1. **c** Both aminoglycosides and radiocontrast dye are nephrotoxic and are major causes of hospital-acquired acute tubular necrosis (ATN), a type of intrarenal acute renal failure (ARF). Calculi in the ureters and hypovolemic shock (choice b) and Foley catheter obstruction and benign prostatic hypertrophy (choice d) are causes of postrenal ARF, not intrarenal ARF. Dehydration and *decreased* cardiac output are prerenal causes of ARF.
2. **b** The oliguric phase of acute tubular necrosis (ATN) is marked by fluid overload, electrolyte abnormalities of renal failure (i.e., hyperkalemia), gastrointestinal bleeding, and infection. The onset phase starts with the initial insult to the kidney and ends when actual renal injury occurs. Electrolyte abnormalities and complications of fluid overload from renal failure are not yet manifested. Fluid volume *deficits* and *hypokalemia* are major risks of the diuretic phase of ATN. During the recovery phase of ATN, kidney function is returning to normal and thus electrolyte or fluid complications are less frequent.
3. **d** In prerenal acute renal failure (ARF), the kidneys are able to respond to a hypoperfused state by avid sodium and water reabsorption, resulting in a low fractional excretion of sodium (FE_{Na}). The blood urea nitrogen to serum creatinine ratio (BUN:Cr) in prerenal ARF is high (greater than 20:1) because as the tubules reabsorb water, urea is also reabsorbed. Creatine is not reabsorbed, and although it rises because of a fall in the glomerular filtration rate (GFR), it does not rise in proportion to the urea. As there is no renal tubular damage in prerenal ARF, urinary sediment is normal.
4. **c** Chronic renal failure (CRF) is *irreversible* and is characterized by a *slow, progressive deterioration* in renal function that ultimately leads to end-stage renal disease (ESRD). Diabetes is the most common cause of CRF.
5. **b** Metabolic acidosis from renal failure is caused by decreased reabsorption of bicarbonate and decreased (rather than increased) secretion and excretion of hydrogen ions. Renal failure, especially acute renal failure (ARF), results in an increase in catabolism, which can contribute to metabolic acidosis. The increased exhalation of carbon dioxide is a response to metabolic acidosis, not a cause of it.
6. **c** Insulin causes potassium to go into the intracellular fluid; dextrose is given to avoid hypoglycemia. Calcium antagonizes the effects of excess potassium on the electrical conduction of the heart. Sodium polystyrene is an exchange resin that exchanges sodium for potassium in the intestine.
7. **c** Erythropoietin is a hormone, 90% of which is produced in the kidneys, that stimulates red blood cell production in response to hypoxia. When kidneys fail, this hormone is inadequately produced, resulting in decreased red blood cell production.

Chapter 32: ANATOMY AND PHYSIOLOGY OF THE NERVOUS SYSTEM

1. **c** The inside of the cell is negative.
2. **a** Basal ganglia: cerebral hemispheres; midbrain: brainstem; conus medullaris: spinal cord.
3. **b** Sleep: RAS, Emotion: Limbic system, CSF: Ventricles.
4. **c** Sight is not a function of cranial nerve III where the rest of the answers are.
5. **d** It is the right lower abdominal quadrant.

Chapter 33: PATIENT ASSESSMENT: NERVOUS SYSTEM

1. **a** The patient's Glasgow Coma Scale (GCS) score is 7T. Eye opening to pain receives a score of 2 points. Withdrawal from the stimulus receives 4 points. Because he is intubated, he has no verbal response and receives a point of 1 with the T to indicate intubation.
2. **d** Slow, writhing movements are called *athetosis*. Fasciculations are twitching of resting muscles secondary to peripheral nerve or cord injury. Myoclonus is a nonrhythmic movement consisting of single jerk-like responses. Chorea is an irregular movement involving limbs and facial muscles.
3. **b** The central cranial nerve VII (the facial nerve) is most likely to be affected by a stroke. Peripheral facial nerve paralysis is associated with Bell's palsy and other lower motor neuron lesions. It differs from central facial nerve paralysis in that the upper portions of the face (i.e., the forehead and eyes) are predominantly affected. Cranial nerve I (the olfactory nerve) is not usually affected in stroke, but most likely is associated with frontal lobe damage or sinus dysfunction. Cranial nerve VIII (the acoustic nerve) controls hearing and equilibrium and is not commonly affected in stroke.
4. **c** Rhinorrhea is drainage of cerebrospinal fluid (CSF) from the nose and is suggestive of cribriform plate fracture. Otorrhea is drainage of CSF from the ear and is usually associated with fracture of the petrous portion of the temporal bone. Battle's sign is bruising over the mastoid area suggestive of basal skull fracture. Kernig's sign is pain in the neck when the thigh is flexed and the leg extended, and is a manifestation of meningeal irritation.
5. **b** Evoked potentials evaluate the brain's response to an external stimulus and is of particular interest in multiple sclerosis and Guillain-Barré syndrome. An electroencephalogram (EEG) measures the electrical activity of the brain and is useful in the diagnosis of seizures. Myelography is a contrast study of the spinal cord and is helpful when evaluation of the nerve roots is needed. Digital subtraction angiography is a study for the evaluation of cerebrovascular problems.

Chapter 34: PATIENT MANAGEMENT: NERVOUS SYSTEM

1. **d** Monitoring of intracranial pressure (ICP) may be indicated when the brain computed tomography (CT) scan is abnormal, when the patient is unable to obey commands or utter recognizable words despite cardiopulmonary stabilization, and when the patient scores less than 8 on the Glasgow Coma Scale.
2. **b** Interventions to decrease increased intracranial pressure (ICP) include the administration of mannitol, the administration of morphine as needed, and maintaining the patient's head in a neutral neck position. Hypoventilation is not an appropriate intervention for the patient with increased ICP.
3. **c** The patient *should* receive sedation with neuromuscular blockading (NMB) agents. The patient receiving NMB agents must be mechanically ventilated, and he or she will require adjunctive analgesia therapy. Depth of neuromuscular blockade is measured using a peripheral nerve stimulator.
4. **a** Opiate analgesics *can* be administered to a patient with a head injury. When opiates are administered to a patient with a head injury, a visual or verbal pain score is used to assess pain. As-needed dosing of an opiate analgesic provides more effective pain relief than a continuous infusion of an analgesic agent. The lowest dose possible of an opiate analgesic should be administered to provide adequate pain relief.

Chapter 35: COMMON NEUROSURGICAL AND NEUROLOGICAL DISORDERS

1. **c** The most common primary brain tumor is glioblastoma multiforme.
2. **d** A definitive diagnosis of brain tumor is obtained through pathological examination of tumor tissue.
3. **b** Epilepsy is the condition of recurrent abnormal or excessive discharges of cerebral neurons.
4. **b** The most common type of stroke is ischemic stroke.
5. **a** A recent history of surgery is a contraindication for receiving tissue plasminogen activator (t-PA).
6. **b** Intravenous colloid solutions are administered to prevent vasospasm.
7. **a** Guillain-Barré syndrome typically presents as a rapid ascending paralysis.
8. **a** The defect at the neuromuscular junction in myasthenia gravis is caused by antibody attack on acetylcholine receptor sites.

Chapter 36: HEAD INJURY

1. **c** Elevating the head of bed will promote drainage of venous blood from the head, reducing intracranial contents; therefore, this is the action that should be taken during the acute phase of caring for a head-injured patient. Cervical immobilization devices should not be removed until a physical examination can be made and the patient can be questioned about neck pain, which may indicate ligamentous injury. The cerebral perfusion pressure should be maintained at levels greater than 60 mm Hg, not less than 60 mm Hg. Critically ill patients should be turned, albeit carefully, in order to prevent skin breakdown and assist with pulmonary toilet. Sedation can be used to blunt spikes in the intracranial pressure (ICP) when turning.
2. **d** When evaluating the oculovestibular response, cranial nerves III (the oculomotor nerve), VI (the abducens nerve), and the vestibular portion of cranial nerve VIII (the acoustic nerve) are tested.
3. **d** Syndrome of inappropriate antidiuretic hormone secretion (SIADH) is a state in which an excessive amount of antidiuretic hormone (ADH) is released, causing an increased intravascular volume due to reabsorption of water in the kidneys. Therefore, SIADH is characterized by decreased sodium levels, decreased urinary output, and a high urine specific gravity.
4. **c** Ecchymosis behind the ear (also called *Battle's sign*) indicates a fracture in the base of the middle fossa. Basilar skull fractures in the anterior fossa are often accompanied by ecchymosis around the eyes or "raccoon eyes." Both Battle's sign and raccoon eyes are late signs of basilar skull fractures.

Chapter 37: SPINAL CORD INJURY

1. **d** The patient with a suspected cervical spinal cord injury is at high risk for respiratory failure because of an ineffective breathing pattern due to inadequate innervation of the respiratory muscles. Therefore, respiratory assessment is an assessment priority.

2. **b** Hypotension and bradycardia are findings associated with spinal shock. Spinal shock is caused by the sudden cessation of impulses from the higher brain centers, resulting in loss of motor, sensory, reflex, and autonomic function below the level of injury.
3. **d** Osteoporosis is an adverse effect of methylprednisolone that is more often seen in long-term use. Euphoria, hyperglycemia, and heart failure are potential adverse effects of methylprednisolone when administered in the emergency setting.
4. **c** As long as the weights are on the floor, no traction is applied and cervical alignment is not maintained. Therefore, the patient must be repositioned in bed until the weights are off the floor. This should only be done by staff who have been educated in the proper procedure. If the nurse does not know how to correctly move the patient, then the physician or nurse practitioner should be notified.
5. **a** On discovering a stage I pressure ulcer, the nurse should assess the area for blanching. If the area does not blanch, the patient is at risk for further breakdown and progression to a stage II pressure ulcer.
6. **d** A heating pad or hot water bottle may present a danger to body parts with no sensation. Therefore, using a heating pad for a patient with a spinal cord injury and ineffective thermoregulation is contraindicated.
7. **a** Spasticity is the return of spinal reflex activity. It does not indicate returning voluntary control of motor activity.
8. **d** A patient with paraplegia is at risk for autonomic dysreflexia, a condition characterized by extreme hypertension, a throbbing headache, flushing, blurred vision, and nasal congestion. When autonomic dysreflexia is recognized, the head of the bed should be raised immediately. The physician or nurse practitioner should also be notified, but this is secondary to raising the head of the bed.

Chapter 38: ANATOMY AND PHYSIOLOGY OF THE GASTROINTESTINAL SYSTEM

1. **d** Pancreatic juice is capable of nearly completing digestion of food in the absence of all other digestive enzymes; these enzymes require a pH close to neutrality for optimal activity.
2. **d** Excitation and inhibition of gastric hydrochloric acid secretion occurs in three phases and are identified by the region in which a stimulus acts to modify the rate of secretion (cephalic, gastric, and intestinal).
3. **a** Of all the gastrointestinal peptides, cholecystokinin (CCK) is the most potent regulator of gallbladder contraction. CCK is also responsible for pancreatic and biliary secretion and gastric emptying.
4. **b** The lower esophageal sphincter (LES) is the major barrier between the acid-filled stomach and the predominately alkaline esophageal lumen.
5. **c** Propulsive mass movements occur in the colon, usually after a meal, and are often followed by the desire to defecate.

Chapter 39: PATIENT ASSESSMENT: GASTROINTESTINAL SYSTEM

1. **d** The triceps skinfold thickness provides an estimate of body fat based on the amount of fat in subcutaneous tissue.
2. **c** A tympanic sound is heard over air, as in the gastric bubble or air-filled intestine.
3. **b** Loud, high-pitched, tinkling bowel sounds are most likely to be heard in a patient with early intestinal obstruction. Intestinal obstruction occurs when blockage prevents the normal flow of contents through the intestinal tract. An accumulation of intestinal contents, fluid, and gas develops above the intestinal obstruction. High-pitched, tinkling sounds indicate that fluid and air are under tension in the intestine, which may signal an early intestinal obstruction.
4. **a** Ammonia is produced in the liver, intestine, and kidneys as the end product of protein metabolism. When the liver is functioning properly, it converts ammonia into urea, which is then excreted by the kidneys. Ammonia levels rise when the liver is unable to convert ammonia to urea.
5. **c** Endoscopic retrograde cholangiopancreatography (ERCP) provides visualization of the common bile duct, hepatic bile ducts, and pancreatic ducts with a flexible fiberoptic endoscope. Therapeutic biliary or pancreatic procedures can be accomplished during ERCP, such as tissue biopsy or brushings, fluid cytology, placement of biliary or pancreatic stents, or retrieval of retained gallstones.

Chapter 40: PATIENT MANAGEMENT: GASTROINTESTINAL SYSTEM

1. **c** Although checking air over the gastric region and aspirating secretions are helpful, an abdominal x-ray is the gold standard for feeding tube placement.
2. **c** Enteral nutrition may be initiated immediately after surgery, with or without the presence of bowel sounds; however, the rate should be started and advanced at a slower rate (which is often significantly less volume than goal rates.) Parenteral nutrition is inappropriate at this point as there is no contraindication to enteral nutrition and that is the preferred physiological route. Maintenance IV fluids provide no nutritional value to the patient, other than minimal calories. *Clostridium difficile* cultures may be an appropriate intervention if the patient is concurrently receiving antibiotics and the initial intervention of slowing the enteral infusion rate does not correct the diarrhea.
3. **b** Postpyloric residuals are inaccurate often due to the fact that the intestinal lumen is not a reservoir and the narrow feeding tubes tend to collapse upon themselves during aspiration. It is best to monitor the patient for nausea and vomiting as a sign of intolerance. Small intestinal infusion rates should be no faster than 150 cc/hour. Holding tube feedings and diluting them with water will place the patient at risk for inadequate nutrition, especially if this is done frequently and adjustments are not made to supplement the patient. Parenteral nutrition is not indicated.
4. **d** Protein, or amino acids, is the building blocks for tissue maintenance and repair, and hence wound healing. All the other nutrients are important for metabolic functioning, but protein would be increased in order to promote wound healing.

Chapter 41: COMMON GASTROINTESTINAL DISORDERS

1. **c** Myocardial ischemia is the most likely etiology of the chest pain since coronary and systemic vasospasm is one of the major side effects of vasopressin therapy.
2. **c** In this situation, the critical care nurse's first responsibility is to cut and remove the Sengstaken-Blakemore tube. If the Sengstaken-Blakemore gastric balloon ruptures, the tension on the tubing will dislodge it into the upper airway and block respirations. The number one safety rule with this tube is to have scissors available to cut and remove the tube if sudden respiratory distress occurs.
3. **a** In acute pancreatitis, both serum amylase and lipase are elevated. Additionally, decreased serum albumin and, subsequently, decreased serum calcium levels are noted.
4. **c** Hypocalcemia from acute pancreatitis causes increased muscle spasm and tetany, and may result in positive Chvostek's and Trousseau's signs. Low albumin levels contribute to decreased

serum calcium levels (as a result of decreased protein available for calcium to bind to), but hypoalbuminemia does not directly affect these physical findings. Serum amylase and lipase are not involved in these physical findings.

5. **c** Administration of intravenous fluids is the top priority for a patient with acute pancreatitis due to the potential of these patients to develop hemodynamic instability and renal failure from decreased renal perfusion. Insertion of a nasogastric tube and Foley catheter are a part of the supportive care needs of this patient, but not a priority over intravenous fluid administration. Oral intake is discouraged, to decrease pancreatic stimulation for secretion of digestive enzymes.
6. **d** Hypoactive bowel sounds are associated with an ileus. Diarrhea is associated with hyperactive bowel sounds, and early intestinal obstruction is associated with high-pitched tinkling bowel sounds. Portal hypertension does not have a direct influence on bowel sounds.
7. **c** Small bowel obstruction is the most likely diagnosis due to the patient's recent surgical history (and potential for surgical adhesions). Colicky pain is a result of the intestine contracting in an attempt to overcome the obstruction. Failure to bypass the obstruction leads to vomiting of fecal material.
8. **d** Biliary disease is a common cause of extrahepatic-induced noninfectious hepatitis and acute pancreatitis. Cholestasis is not associated with small or large bowel obstruction.
9. **b** Based on this patient's history, physical examination, and laboratory results, he most likely has acute hepatitis B virus (HBV) infection. Acute hepatitis B infection is marked by a positive hepatitis B surface antigen (HBsAg), positive hepatitis B core antibody (anti-HBc IgM), and positive anti-hepatitis B core antigen (HBeAg). Serial markers for hepatitis A virus (HAV) and hepatitis C virus (HCV) were negative.

Chapter 42: ANATOMY AND PHYSIOLOGY OF THE ENDOCRINE SYSTEM

1. **a** Gluconeogenesis and glycogenolysis are the two main mechanisms for glucose elevation via glucocorticoids. Glucocorticoids also stimulate the anti-inflammatory response and suppress histamine responses. Glucocorticoids promote water reabsorption in the kidney.
2. **c** Glucagon is the hormone responsible for regulation of serum glucose along with insulin. Calcitonin, aldosterone, and antidiuretic hormone (ADH) affect other hormonal systems.
3. **a** Stimulation of the renin–angiotensin–aldosterone system is accomplished to restore extracellular fluid compartments. Events such as hemorrhage, hypovolemia, and hypoxia stimulate the system.
4. **c** Antidiuretic hormone (ADH) stimulants include hypovolemia, hypoxia, pain, positive pressure ventilation, and several drugs. Inhibition of ADH results from alcohol, low serum osmolality, hypervolemia, and exposure to cold.
5. **c** Lower levels of triiodothyronine (T_3) and thyroxine (T_4) are associated with hypothyroidism. Thyroid-stimulating hormone (TSH) levels would be elevated in an attempt to stimulate thyroid gland production of T_3 and T_4.

Chapter 43: PATIENT ASSESSMENT: ENDOCRINE SYSTEM

1. **b** Increased serum osmolality results from the ensuing dehydration in the absence of adequate antidiuretic hormone (ADH). The serum osmolality will decrease in the presence of too much or ectopic ADH, as is seen with syndrome of inappropriate antidiuretic hormone secretion (SIADH).
2. **a** The healthy thyroid is nonpalpable, without visible nodules or masses. The best way to assess the thyroid is to approach the patient from behind while palpating the gland. The best way to visualize the gland is to observe the thyroid while the patient swallows water.
3. **c** Tetany results in a positive Trousseau's sign (carpedal spasm) when pressure is applied to the patient's arm with a blood pressure cuff for several minutes. Tetany also can result in facial nerve irritation and spasm (Chvostek's sign).
4. **c** The American Diabetes Association guidelines include two separate fasting glucose levels greater than 126 mg/dL as diagnostic for type 2 diabetes. The guidelines do not include glycosylated hemoglobin (HbA_{1c}) in the diagnostic criteria. Although the patient with gestational diabetes is at higher risk for future development of type 2 diabetes, the presence of gestational diabetes is still not considered a criterion for diagnosis.
5. **b** The patient with diabetic ketoacidosis (DKA) sustains major fluid and electrolyte loss, shifts, or both secondary to the hyperglycemia and resultant dehydration. Not all patients with DKA have sepsis or fever, and hypokalemia usually does not lead to profound neurological symptoms initially.

Chapter 44: COMMON ENDOCRINE DISORDERS

1. **d** Propylthiouracil is the only medication that is appropriate for a patient with hyperthyroidism. Aspirin is contraindicated because it can exacerbate circulating triiodothyronine (T_3) and thyroxine (T_4) levels. Synthroid is exogenous T_4 and should not be given. Demeclocycline is given to block antidiuretic hormone (ADH) effects on the kidney in patients with syndrome of inappropriate antidiuretic hormone secretion (SIADH).
2. **c** Patients with diabetes insipidus become quite dehydrated and will display unusually high serum osmolality. Hematocrit and blood sugar levels may become slightly elevated as a result of hemoconcentration, but they will not be this abnormal. Urine osmolality will be quite low, reflective of the copious, dilute urine that accompanies diabetes insipidus.
3. **a** Patients with extreme hypothyroidism disorder will be bradycardic, hypotensive, and hypothermic, and will hypoventilate. All of these symptoms result from inadequate thyroid hormone.
4. **b** The patient with adrenal insufficiency will quickly dehydrate in the absence of cortisol and aldosterone.
5. **b** Diabetic ketoacidosis (DKA) is often precipitated by counter-regulatory hormone activation: growth hormone, cortisol, and epinephrine. Using insulin when ill will protect the patient from DKA.
6. **a** Initial treatment for diabetic ketoacidosis (DKA) includes rapid fluid replacement with isotonic or hypotonic saline, insulin, and supportive care. Typically, the patient will not require sodium bicarbonate, chloride, or other electrolytes since fluid will usually correct the problem.
7. **c** In hyperglycemic hyperosmolar state (HHS), the patient still produces sufficient insulin to avoid ketosis and will not display ketoacidosis or abnormally low bicarbonate. The patient will develop extremely high glucose levels and may also display lactic acidosis.
8. **d** In hyperglycemic hyperosmolar state (HHS), the patient is usually frail and elderly with a multitude of other medical complications. Fluid resuscitation must proceed slowly in order to avoid cerebral edema and pulmonary edema.
9. **a** Missed meals and excessive exercise will lower glucose levels. Counter-regulatory hormones (such as cortisol and epinephrine), skipping oral hypoglycemic medications, and severe illness in a person with diabetes elevate the glucose level.

10. **b** Glipizide is a potent oral sulfonylurea drug that will aggravate hypoglycemia. Glucagon injection, dextrose IV push, and orange juice orally will all correct hypoglycemia.

Chapter 45: ANATOMY AND PHYSIOLOGY OF THE HEMATOLOGICAL AND IMMUNE SYSTEMS

1. **d** B cells manufacture immunoglobulins, which are the major factors in the humoral-mediated immune response.
2. **c** The cell structure of neutrophils promotes their attachment to bacteria and facilitates the bacteria being engulfed.
3. **b** Plasma proteins, because of their size and structure, regulate the movement of water and solute, thereby contributing to osmotic plasma pressure.
4. **a** Calcium is negatively charged, binds with coagulation factors, and creates an affinity for clotting factors to bind at the site of clotting.

Chapter 46: PATIENT ASSESSMENT: HEMATOLOGICAL AND IMMUNE SYSTEMS

1. **c** Underproduction of RBCs is reflected by a low reticulocyte count. A person with sickle cell anemia may have an elevated reticulocyte count, especially in sickle cell crisis. Platelet overproduction and coagulopathy are not reflected by the reticulocyte count.
2. **d** Increased numbers of bands in the WBC differential can indicate an infectious process. In acute leukemia, the WBC differential may show the presence of blasts. An allergic reaction may be shown by increased numbers of eosinophils.
3. **a** Liver dysfunction from chronic alcoholism causes decreased production of coagulation factors. Overproduction of platelets is related to bone marrow dysfunction. A congenital bleeding disorder is an inherited coagulopathy that is not acquired through alcohol abuse. Bone marrow dysfunction is not caused by alcohol abuse.
4. **b** Hemostasis could be affected by a decreased intake of vitamin K, but this is not related to prevention of infection. Nutrition is an important factor in lymphocyte function, antibody production, wound healing, and skin integrity maintenance.

Chapter 47: ORGAN AND HEMATOPOIETIC STEM CELL TRANSPLANT

1. **d** Hypoglycemia is unlikely to occur in a patient with a history of diabetes mellitus who is receiving steroids. Parotitis and fever may occur as a result of the total body irradiation, although usually the steroids administered as antiemetics also assist with the management of these symptoms. Electrocardiogram (ECG) abnormalities, including sinus tachycardia and arrhythmias, can occur in association with the administration of high-dose cyclophosphamide (Cytoxan).
2. **d** Physical findings consistent with pancytopenia, including petechiae and pallor of the skin and mucous membranes, would be expected. Erythema or shallow ulcerations of the oral cavity may occur.
3. **a** Total body irradiation causes a generalized erythema of the skin. Although the patient has an intake greater than output for a 24-hour period, the sodium is extremely low. The decreased urine output and hyponatremia suggest SIADH, probably as a result of high-dose cyclophosphamide (Cytoxan). Additional studies would include a high urine osmolality and decreased serum osmolality. Right upper quadrant tenderness would suggest veno-occlusive disease of the liver. The patient is at risk for veno-occlusive disease of the liver at this stage, and his positive 24-hour fluid balance suggests weight gain. However, without liver function tests; an assessment of the abdomen, which demonstrates hepatomegaly or ascites; and an abdominal ultrasound, not right upper quadrant tenderness alone; it is unclear whether this patient is developing veno-occlusive disease. Congestive heart failure and renal failure are therefore unlikely causes of the decreased urine output; thus, signs of congestive heart failure such as rales, peripheral edema, jugular venous distension, and a third heart sound (S_3) would not be expected. Although the urine output is reduced, there is no evidence of renal insufficiency as the blood urea nitrogen (BUN) and creatinine levels are within normal limits. There is no evidence of sepsis such as fever or mental status changes.
4. **a** Transfusion-associated graft-versus-host disease (GVHD) is a rare but almost uniformly fatal complication of transfusion resulting from the infusion of immunocompetent lymphocytes capable of proliferation that the recipient is unable to destroy. The infused lymphocytes recognize host tissues as foreign and mount a reaction. All cellular blood products, except for stem cell grafts and lymphocytes given for graft-versus-tumor effect, must be irradiated to 2500 cGy to prevent transfusion-associated GVHD. Blood products that have been irradiated can be used by other patients; irradiation does not alter the efficacy or cellular content of the product and does not harm the recipient in any way. Patients who have undergone allogeneic or autologous hematopoietic stem cell transplantation should receive irradiated cellular components, both in the period before stem cell transplantation and in the post-transplant period. Most centers recommend that allogeneic stem cell recipients receive irradiated blood products for the rest of their life.
5. **d** T-cell depletion reduces the risk of developing graft-versus-host disease (GVHD). However, T-cell depleted transplants have a higher risk of infectious complications and poor engraftment. An unrelated donor or a sex-mismatched donor as the source of hematopoietic stem cells, increased patient/donor age, and the occurrence of cytomegalovirus or other viral infections post-transplant are all associated with a higher risk for the development of GVHD.
6. **c** Patients taking cyclosporine should be instructed to report any neurologic side effects such as headache, tremor, or confusion, because these symptoms may reflect cyclosporine A–induced neurotoxicity. Missed doses of cyclosporine A cannot be corrected by increasing the next dose of cyclosporine A. Patients must be instructed on the importance of adherence to the medication schedule, and asked to notify the health care team immediately if they are unable to take their medications due to gastrointestinal side effects. Cyclosporine trough levels are to be drawn prior to administration of the morning dose of cyclosporine A. Doses are usually timed for 10 AM and 10 PM to allow trough blood draw at morning clinic visit. The patient should be instructed to bring the dose to the clinic and to administer it once the trough level is drawn. Bioavailability differs between oral solution and capsule formulation. Patients should be instructed that once a regimen is established, changes should not be made to the formulation or brand of cyclosporine A.
7. **c** Tacrolimus must be monitored by level. Insufficient levels may lead to rejection. Elevations in levels may be nephrotoxic or neurotoxic.
8. **d** Inhaled nitric oxide is a selective pulmonary vasodilator that can be administered via the ventilatory circuit without effect on the systemic system. Given that the patient's systolic blood pressure is averaging 110 mm Hg, nitric oxide would be the preferred agent. Epinephrine, dopamine, and vasopressin are vasoconstrictors and would be contraindicated in this case.
9. **c** Current substance abuse is an absolute contraindication to solid organ transplantation. Recent infection, age, and diabetes mellitus are relative contraindications. The patient's age must be evaluated on a case-by-case basis, although older patients gener-

ally have more complications. Recent infection, if treated and not active, would not preclude a patient from receiving a solid organ transplant. Diabetes mellitus is an indication for pancreas transplant. In other solid organ transplants, the presence of diabetes mellitus must be evaluated on a case-by-case basis as further diabetic complications can occur with steroid use for immunosuppression.

Chapter 48: COMMON IMMUNOLOGICAL DISORDERS

1. **b** Viral load is the measure of HIV RNA in the person's body and is currently the standard test used to determine and monitor an individual's disease progression. Patients with higher viral loads have more advanced disease. The enzyme-linked immunosorbent assay (ELISA), Single Use Diagnostic System (SUDS), and p24 antigen tests are used to detect the presence of HIV.
2. **a** For most people, seroconversion occurs within 10 to 14 days after exposure to HIV. Some people may take longer to convert.
3. **c** The four body fluids that have been implicated in the transmission of HIV are blood, semen, vaginal fluid, and breast milk. HIV has been isolated in a variety of other fluids, but none have been implicated in the transmission of the virus.
4. **d** The current standard for treating opportunistic infections is to stop therapy when the individual's immune system has become competent and can fight off potential infections. *Pneumocystis jiroveci* can produce an infection when the CD4 count drops below 200 cells/mm^3. This level is used as the "goalpost" for discontinuing treatment.
5. **b** Indigestion, a taste of blood in the mouth, and a dry, nonproductive cough are signs and symptoms of carotid artery rupture.
6. **c** Hypercalcemia can be prevented or lessened by increasing fluid intake.
7. **a** A chest computed tomography (CT) scan would most likely be the first diagnostic test performed for a patient with small cell lung cancer who is admitted with severe dyspnea and upper body edema, to evaluate for superior vena cava syndrome (SCVS).
8. **d** Patients with acute leukemia are at greatest risk for cytokine release syndrome and tumor lysis syndrome.

Chapter 49: COMMON HEMATOLOGICAL DISORDERS

1. **d** Iron deficiency anemia may be caused by inadequate intake of iron in the diet, malabsorption of oral iron, or chronic blood loss.
2. **c** STI571 is a new and extremely successful treatment for chronic myelogenous leukemia (CML) with very few side effects.
3. **b** An acute episode of bleeding in a patient with hemophilia A would be managed by administering factor VIII, which is deficient in these patients.
4. **c** Normal inhibitors of coagulation include adequate cardiac output, the presence of antithrombin III, and plasminogen converting to plasmin. Tissue thromboplastin in the circulation causes activation of the extrinsic pathway through activation of factor VII.
5. **a** An early indication of a disseminated intravascular coagulation (DIC) process is a decreased platelet count. Platelets are consumed in the initial hypercoagulable state to form platelet plugs and to initiate clotting via the intrinsic pathway through the release of platelet factor 3.
6. **d** Patients with disseminated intravascular coagulation (DIC) bleed because of depleted clotting factors, increased levels of fibrin degradation products (FDPs), and diffuse microthrombosis. Decreased plasminogen levels result in decreased levels of plasmin. Plasmin is the lytic enzyme that acts to break down fibrin. Hence, decreased plasmin levels result in decreased clot breakdown, lessening the chance of bleeding and consumption of clotting factors.

Chapter 50: ANATOMY AND PHYSIOLOGY OF THE INTEGUMENTARY SYSTEM

1. **b** The epidermal layer is nourished by the blood vessels from the dermal layer; it does not have its own blood supply.
2. **c** The eccrine sweat glands help to maintain the internal body temperature. The loss of sweat provides for heat loss from the body by evaporation of the fluid from the skin surface.
3. **d** Melanin, produced by melanocytes at the epidermal layer, determines the skin color and protects underlying structures from light exposure.
4. **a** As blood flow to the dermal layer is reduced, the skin becomes thinner. This explains why an older adult's skin may be shiny and "parchment-like" in appearance, and why the older adult's skin is more at risk for tearing.
5. **b** The sensory afferent fibers, which transmit stimuli for touch, pain, and temperature from the surface of the skin to the spinal cord and the brain for interpretation and response, are located in the dermis.

Chapter 51: PATIENT ASSESSMENT: INTEGUMENTARY SYSTEM

1. **b** Erythema is the result of inflammation, which produces increased blood flow to the tissue. This increased vascularity produces a red tone in light-skinned people and a deeper brown or purple tone in dark-skinned people.
2. **c** Urticaria is best described as a reddened or white raised inflamed lesion with transudate vascular fluid in the surrounding tissue. A purple irregular lesion caused by tissue trauma is a bruise. A fiery red, raised lesion with a central body and radiating legs is a spider angioma. Small, pinpoint nonblanching lesions are petechiae.
3. **c** Oral candidiasis (also called *thrush*) is a painful white coating of the oral mucosa and tongue. The discomfort caused by oral candidiasis or thrush may restrict the patient's oral intake and compromise nutritional status.
4. **d** Turgor provides information about the patient's fluid volume status. Turgor is assessed centrally over the patient's clavicles. Peripheral assessment sites may be influenced by peripheral blood vessel disease, whereas the clavicles are easily accessed and reflect central fluid status.
5. **b** A basal cell carcinoma presents as a scaly white lesion. Squamous cell carcinoma presents with a depressed center, rolled edge, and pearly border. Melanomas are typically large, dark black or brown lesions with irregular borders. Seborrheic keratosis is a light brown lesion that feels velvety when touched.
6. **c** In people with darker skin tones, cyanosis is best identified by assessing the conjunctiva and oral mucous membranes.

Chapter 52: PATIENT MANAGEMENT: INTEGUMENTARY SYSTEM

1. **b** This patient has arterial ulcers. These are typically described as wounds with pale wound beds; a "punched-out" appearance; and round, smooth margins that are usually found on the distal leg, medial malleoli, and the dorsal aspects of the feet and toes.
2. **a** The inflammatory phase is the first phase of wound healing, which begins immediately after a wound occurs. There is immediate vasoconstriction to control bleeding and allow a fibrin clot to form. Phagocytosis occurs with the release of macrophages, which remove bacteria and cellular debris from the wound bed.

3. **c** This choice provides the most accurate documentation—the wound is staged (stage II); the location is stated precisely, using anatomic terms ("sacrum"); the length and width are stated in centimeters ("3.4 by 1.8 cm"); the depth is noted ("nonapplicable"); and the wound care is documented ("cleansed with normal saline and hydrocolloid dressing applied").
4. **b** The vacuum-assisted wound closure (VAC) system may be used with flaps, grafts, and acute or chronic wounds. VAC is contraindicated in wounds with uncontrolled bleeding, eschar, necrotic tissue, malignancies, exposed organs and blood vessels, and untreated osteomyelitis.
5. **d** Hydrocolloids and calcium alginates are used in autolytic debridement. A proteolytic enzyme is an example of chemical debridement. Whirlpool and wet-to-dry dressings are examples of mechanical debridement.
6. **c** The wound is being allowed to heal by delayed primary intention. Delayed primary (tertiary) intention is used when a wound is infected or edematous. Primary intention requires the wound to be closed at the time of surgery or injury. In secondary intention, due to the amount of tissue loss, the wound cannot be closed. The proliferation phase is the second phase of wound healing.

Chapter 53: BURNS

1. **d** Lactated Ringer's solution is the best fluid to use for fluid resuscitation of a burn patient during the first 24 hours.
2. **b** Burns damaging the epidermis, dermis, and subcutaneous tissue are classified as full-thickness burn injuries.
3. **c** In burn shock, increased capillary permeability causes a loss of plasma fluid and proteins into the interstitial spaces, which results in decreased capillary colloid osmotic pressure.
4. **b** Headache, nausea, and vertigo are experienced with a carbon monoxide saturation of 20%. Prompt recognition of carbon monoxide injuries is essential for patient survival.
5. **b** A patient who has sustained burns to his entire right arm and his anterior trunk has sustained injury to 27% of his body. The entire right arm counts for 9% and the anterior trunk counts for 18%, adding up to 27% total body surface area (TBSA).
6. **a** During the resuscitative phase, the patient may have an elevated serum potassium level. Burn injuries result in tissue and cellular destruction. Cellular injuries result in a release of potassium into the intravascular space.
7. **c** Intramuscular injection of analgesics during the resuscitative phase is not recommended because inadequate peripheral perfusion results in uneven absorption of the medication.
8. **c** When administering silver sulfadiazine, the nurse must monitor the patient's white blood cell count because an adverse effect of silver sulfadiazine is a transient leukopenia. After discontinuing the medication, the leukopenia resolves without sequela. Silver sulfadiazine has a painless application and does not alter acid–base balance. In addition, it is not associated with hepatotoxicity.

Chapter 54: SHOCK, SYSTEMIC INFLAMMATORY RESPONSE SYNDROME, AND MULTIPLE ORGAN DYSFUNCTION SYNDROME

1. **d** Oxygen delivery involves interventions that aid in optimal pulmonary and cardiovascular function. In addition, adequate hemoglobin levels are necessary to transport oxygen to the cells.
2. **a** Vital signs may not be abnormal in early stages of shock. If tissues are underperfused, lactic acid, a byproduct of anaerobic metabolism, is present in the blood and can be measured to assess the adequacy of tissue perfusion.
3. **c** The heart and lungs become less compliant with increasing age and cannot readily adapt to rapid changes in intravascular volume; this age-related physiological change is normal. Rapid administration of large volumes of intravenous fluid may result in acute pulmonary congestion in the elderly patient.
4. **c** A history of a previous, possibly allergic reaction increases the likelihood of occurrence of allergic reactions that may progress to anaphylactic shock.
5. **d** In cardiogenic shock, failure of the heart to eject the blood volume causes excessively high preload in the heart. A combination of intravenous fluids and diuretics is used to facilitate an appropriate preload.
6. **d** Research has shown that the loss of homeostasis of the cytokines, endothelial cells, and coagulation systems during insults increases the risk of septic shock, SIRS, and MODS.
7. **d** MODS is initiated by underperfused states of organs, which in turn activate a systemic inflammatory response. Activation of the inflammatory response results in the development of microthrombi that further decrease perfusion to the organs, creating a cycle of lack of perfusion, eventual organ dysfunction, and possible death.

Chapter 55: TRAUMA

1. **b** Listening to lung sounds to assess for ventilation is the next step in the ABCs. Once an airway is established, breathing is the next priority to be assessed. This is done while waiting for the chest x-ray.
2. **d** All of the stated injuries (head, pleural space, and abdominal) can occur in a motor vehicle crash (MVC) when the vehicle is not equipped with an air bag or the air bag does not deploy.
3. **b** Bowel sounds are part of the secondary survey.
4. **a** The patient is most likely hypovolemic upon arrival in the intensive care unit. Many trauma patients are not adequately resuscitated prior to going to the operating room. These patients need continuous monitoring and fluid replacement until they are hemodynamically stable.
5. **a** The chest tube should be clamped and the surgeon notified immediately. When a chest tube puts out more than 200 mL an hour, the patient may need a thoracotomy. The patient should already be on oxygen. A chest x-ray is important but most likely will not alter the plan of care. It is important to explain to the patient what is happening, but this explanation should not take precedence over managing a life-threatening emergency.
6. **a** The teenage patient with the leg injury is at risk for developing deep venous thrombosis (DVT), the most common complication associated with long bone injury.

Chapter 56: DRUG OVERDOSE AND POISONING

1. **c** Evaluation and maintenance of the ABCs (airway, breathing, and circulation) is the first step in managing any patient, regardless of diagnosis.
2. **d** Activated charcoal may be indicated in exposure to acetaminophen, aspirin, or amitriptyline.
3. **b** Mydriasis (pupil dilation), not miosis (pupil contraction), is part of the anticholinergic toxidrome. Remember: blind as a bat, mad as a hatter, hot as a hare, red as a beet, dry as a bone.
4. **d** Management of an intravenous heroin overdose includes the administration of naloxone, an opioid receptor antagonist. Administration of activated charcoal or a cathartic and whole-bowel irrigation would be suitable if gastrointestinal decontamination were necessary, but this patient has sustained an intravenous heroin overdose.

Index

Note: Page numbers followed by b indicate boxed material; those followed by f indicate figures; those followed by t indicate tables.

B

D

E

F

J

K

L

M

N

S

T

W

X

Z